Andrews'

DISEASES OF THE SKIN

Clinical Dermatology

Eighth Edition

HARRY L. ARNOLD, Jr., A.B., M.S., M.D., F.A.C.P.

Clinical Professor of Dermatology
University of California, San Francisco
San Francisco, California

Clinical Professor of Medicine
John A. Burns School of Medicine
University of Hawaii

RICHARD B. ODOM, M.D.

Clinical Professor of Dermatology
University of California, San Francisco
San Francisco, California

WILLIAM D. JAMES, M.D.

Chief, Dermatology Service
Walter Reed Army Medical Center
Washington, D.C.

W.B. SAUNDERS COMPANY   **1990**
Harcourt Brace Jovanovich, Inc.
Philadelphia   London   Toronto   Montreal   Sydney   Tokyo

W. B. SAUNDERS COMPANY
Harcourt Brace Jovanovich, Inc.

The Curtis Center
Independence Square West
Philadelphia, PA 19106

Library of Congress Cataloging-in-Publication Data

Arnold, Harry Loren, 1912–

Andrews' diseases of the skin : clinical dermatology.—8th ed. /
Harry L. Arnold, Jr., Richard B. Odom, William D. James.

p. cm.

Previous ed. cataloged under: Andrews, George Clinton, 1891–.
Includes bibliographical references.

1. Skin—Diseases.   I. Andrews, George Clinton, 1891–
Diseases of the skin.   II. Odom, Richard B., 1937–
III. James, William, 1950–   .   IV. Title.   V. Title:
Diseases of the skin.   [DNLM: 1. Skin Diseases. WR 140
A755a]

RL71.A76 1990   616.5—dc20   89–10820

ISBN 0–7216–2424–3   DNLM   DLC   CIP

The opinion or assertions contained herein are the private views of the author(s) and
are not to be construed as official or as reflecting the views of the Department of the
Army or the Department of Defense.

Editor: William Lamsback
Designer: Dorothy Chattin
Production Manager: Carolyn Naylor
Manuscript Editor: Phyllis Skomorowsky
Illustration Coordinator: Walt Verbitski
Indexer: Roger Wall
Cover Designer: Maureen Sweeney

Andrews' Diseases of the Skin: Clinical Dermatology, 8/e   ISBN 0–7216–2424–3

Printed in the United States of America.

Last digit is the print number: 9   8   7   6   5   4   3   2

Contributors

Herbert Goldschmidt, M.D.
Clinical Professor of Dermatology,
University of Pennsylvania Medical School;
Attending Physician,
Department of Dermatology,
University of Pennsylvania Hospital,
Philadelphia, Pennsylvania
X-Ray Therapy

Roy C. Grekin, M.D.
Assistant Clinical Professor of Dermatology and
Chief of Dermatologic Surgery,
University of California,
San Francisco, School of Medicine,
San Francisco, California
Physical Modalities of Dermatologic Therapy

Preface

In June, 1986, I was invited by the two senior authors, Harry Arnold and Richard Odom, to collaborate in the revision and updating of the seventh edition of *Andrews' Diseases of the Skin,* published in 1981. During the past three years I have been privileged to interact with two giants of dermatology on a regular basis in bringing the eighth edition to fruition. It has taken hours upon hours of reading, collecting references, reading or rereading published papers, listening to and learning from colleagues across the country or across the sea, and writing or rewriting about half the text.

Together, the three coauthors of this text have participated in the revision of all the chapters except the two that have been rewritten by invited experts: x-ray therapy, by Herbert Goldschmidt, and fundamentals of surgery, by Roy Grekin. We feel this is a major strength of such an uncommon effort. It brings a coherent, unified approach to the book as well as to the philosophy of one's approach to skin disease in general. In addition, this cooperation allows the book to be more concise and compact, because each disease is discussed, in general, in only one chapter of the text, avoiding repetitive discussions.

As with all previous editions of *Andrews',* a primary goal was to maintain it as a single volume, with strong clinical orientation, for desk-top rather than library use. It is intended to be useful to students, interns and residents, internists and other medical specialists, family practitioners, and indeed all physicians, dermatologists included.

Many major changes have been made in this edition. About half the text has been rewritten. This was necessary to reflect the new information gained over the past decade and to delete a great deal of obsolete material. The clinical descriptions, always a strength of past editions, were changed the least. Discussions of etiopathogenesis and treatments were changed the most, reflecting the extensive advances made in these areas.

Molecular biology, advances in immunology and the understanding of the skin as an immunologically active organ, the development of new dermatologic subspecialties (dermatologic surgery and immunodermatology, for example), continued advances in dermatopathology with immunohistochemical analysis leading the way, and the identification of microorganisms that have been newly found to cause known skin diseases, as well as new cutaneous infections, are among the new knowledge that had to be incorporated into the current edition's discussions of etiopathogenesis.

Many new therapeutic advances have been made in the past decade. Retinoids, antiviral agents, new laser technology, new generations of antibiotics, minoxidil, interferons, extracorporeal photochemotherapy, and cyclosporine necessitated complete revision of several sections because of their impact on dermatologic therapeutics. Old drugs have been rediscovered and found useful in a wider range of diseases. We have included in the discussion of therapy not only the best-accepted drugs of choice but also many suggested modalities that have been mentioned only in isolated case reports, in order to expand the available options in difficult, resistant cases.

The advances in technology, basic science, and therapeutics required extensive revisions and additions, and the recognition of numerous new disorders also required many additions to several chapters. Major new diseases such as AIDS—the acquired immunodeficiency syndrome—and other retroviral infections have been included. Over 100 other entities have been added in this edition, including oxalosis, calciphylaxis, histiocytic cytophagic panniculitis, Olmstead's syndrome, Haber's syndrome, focal acral hyperkeratosis, porokeratotic eccrine ostial and dermal duct nevus, *Vibrio vulnificus* infection, pneumococcal cellulitis, DF2 septicemia, oral hairy leukoplakia, neutrophilic dermatosis of malignancy, annular erythema of infancy, rheumatoid neutrophilic dermatitis, episodic angioedema with eosinophilia, sialidosis, Proteus syndrome, neutral lipid storage disease, peeling skin syndrome, Kindler's syndrome, atrichia with papular lesions, loose anagen syndrome, tufted angioma, restrictive dermopathy, epithelioid hemangioendothelioma, POEMS syndrome, clear-cell papulosis, papillary eccrine adenoma, aggressive digital papillary adenoma and adenocarcinoma, vulvar and penile melanosis, acquired dyskeratotic leukoplakia, inherited patterned lentiginosis in blacks, syringoacanthoma, Birt-Hogg-Dubé syndrome, and Schnitzler's syndrome.

Discovering or understanding better the etiology of several disease states has required some reorganization of the chapters. Many diseases could have been discussed in any of several chapters; in deference to conciseness, we have discussed each entity in one section only. Examples are the realization that granulomatous slack skin, lymphomatoid granulomatosis, and angioendotheliomatosis are actually lymphomas; that cat-scratch disease is a bacterial infection; that deep fungal classification systems have been reorganized and renamed in many areas; that xanthomatoses have been reclassified to reflect advances in the recognition of genetic defects that lead to different phenotypes; that serologic/genetic/immunologic findings have led to a reclassification of lupus erythematosus; and that identification of molecular antigens involved in the blistering diseases has unified (or split) syndromes among both the primary bullous diseases and the mechanobullous disorders. We have at times discussed diseases under their old chapters: for example, lymphomatoid granulomatosis, since it is still included among the vasculitides in most classification systems. At times old concepts have been left in place to provide historical perspective and because such placement retains a certain utility. An example is the histiocytosis X ("L-cell") syndromes, which are first discussed as one, and then separately as Letterer-Siwe disease, Hand-Schüller-Christian disease, and eosinophilic granuloma.

The emphasis on recent references is easily seen on scanning the text. Most older references from the seventh edition have been deleted to achieve conciseness, even though some are still referred to in the text. Such references can easily be found in the seventh edition or in the bibliographies of current articles. We feel that a 1988 or 1989 reference to the *Archives of Dermatology*, the *British Journal of Dermatology*, or the *Journal of the American Academy of Dermatology* is more useful to a practicing physician than a 20-year-old classic source; it is likely to be more quickly available and will summarize earlier data.

I include thanks to my wife Ann and my children Dan and Becky for their patience and support; to the staff and residents at Walter Reed Army Medical Center, especially Dr. O. G. Rodman, for their support and their input into my continued education; to Bill Lamsback, our editor at Saunders; to Cheryl A. Currie for all the extra typing; and finally to the senior authors, for asking me to participate and for their continued patience, support, teaching, and dedication to this project.

WILLIAM D. JAMES
Washington, D. C.

It is fitting that Dr. James should have been asked to write the preface to this edition, because he has since mid-1986 borne the burden of updating and reorganizing the text of the seventh edition, almost singlehanded. Dr. Odom, with the assistance and the use of the photographic collection of Dr. Axel W. Hoke, has replaced scores of illustrations and added many new ones. Dr. Arnold has edited the text and the legends.

During the course of typesetting this book, we were permitted to supplement and edit galley proofs until mid-1989 (a privilege once reserved to authors of the eminence of Winston Churchill), with the result that references as recent as mid-1989 could be added. Electronic typesetting has made this possible.

The chapter on x-ray therapy was rewritten by Dr. Herbert Goldschmidt of Bala-Cynwyd, Pennsylvania, dean of American dermatologic radiologists, and the chapter on dermatologic surgery by Dr. Roy C. Grekin of San Francisco, a graduate of my (H.L.A.) old department at the University of Michigan. These chapters reflect the newest practices in these fields without any attempt at an encyclopedic coverage of them, since both topics are covered in separate textbooks.

The references have been moved from the ends of the chapters into the body of the text, where they are far more readily accessible, and (as pointed out by Dr. James) they have been pruned of most older citations.

We believe this is the best edition of *Andrews'* ever. The traditional usefulness and practicality of the book have been preserved intact, and to these has been added an almost encyclopedic review of the most recent developments in etiopathogenesis and therapy. Despite its increased size (28 fewer, but larger, pages), it is still the eminently practical "what is it?" and "how to" book it has always been. Enjoy!

HARRY L. ARNOLD, JR.
RICHARD B. ODOM
San Francisco, California

Contents

1

The Skin: Basic Structure and Function

The skin is composed of two layers: **epidermis** and **dermis**. Beneath these is the subcutaneous tissue, referred to as the subcutis or the fatty **panniculus** (Fig. 1–1).

The **epidermis,** the outermost layer, is directly contiguous with the environment. It is formed by an ordered arrangement of cells called keratinocytes, whose basic function is to synthesize keratin, a filamentous protein which serves a protective function.

The **dermis** is the inner layer. Its principal constit-

uent is the fibrillar structural protein, collagen. The dermis lies upon the **panniculus** or subcutis, which is composed principally of lobules of lipocytes or fat cells.

Inflammatory conditions generally begin in either the dermis or panniculus, but are quickly reflected in the other, and in the epidermis as well. Thus in psoriasis, erythema (beginning as vasodilatation in the dermis) is soon reflected in the epidermis as accelerated proliferation of keratinocytes, which results in rapid cornification, and the cornified cells

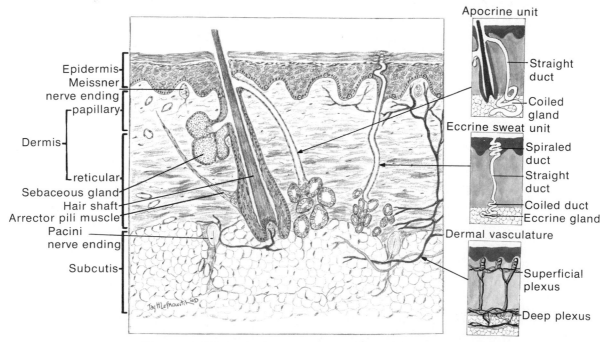

Figure 1–1. Diagrammatic cross section of the skin and panniculus.

1

accumulate on the surface as scale. Allergic reactions to ingested substances—food, for example, or drugs—may lead to inflammation in the dermis, by ectasia of blood vessels and the appearance of a variety of white blood cells, which percolate through the collagen bundles. A specific type of inflammation of the subcutaneous fat can result from the release of enzymes into the general circulation secondary to pancreatitis or pancreatic carcinoma. These enzymes lyse fat cells, resulting in the formation of a granulomatous reaction primarily involving the fat lobules.

Benign and malignant neoplasms of the skin, like their inflammatory counterparts, principally involve one of the three anatomic layers. They reflect autonomous proliferation of a specific cell type and are best illustrated when the specific cells of the skin are examined in detail.

All skin sites are composed of these three anatomically distinct layers, although there is considerable regional variation in their relative thickness. The epidermis is thickest on the palms and soles, measuring approximately 1.5 mm. It is very thin on the eyelids, where it measures less than 0.1 mm. The dermis is thickest on the back, where it is 30 to 40 times as thick as the overlying epidermis. The amount of subcutaneous fat is generous on the abdomen and buttocks compared to the nose and sternum, where it is meager.

Ebling FJG: The normal skin, in Rook A, Wilkinson DS, Ebling FJG (eds): Textbook of Dermatology, 4th Ed. Oxford, England, Blackwell Scientific Publications, 1986, pp 5–38.

Fitzpatrick TB, Eisen AZ, Wolff K, et al: Dermatology in General Medicine. New York, McGraw-Hill Inc, 1987.

Jakubovic HR, et al: Development, morphology, and physiology, in Moschella SL, Hurley HT (eds): Dermatology. Philadelphia, WB Saunders Co, 1985, pp 1–70.

Lever WF, Schaumburg-Lever G: Histopathology of the Skin, 6th ed. Philadelphia, JB Lippincott Co, 1983, pp 8–41.

Mehregan AH: Pinkus' Guide to Dermatohistopathology, 4th ed. Norwalk, CT, Appleton-Century-Crofts, 1986, pp 5–40.

Pinkus H: Anatomy and histology of skin, in Graham JH, Johnson WC, Helwig EB (eds): Dermal Pathology. Hagerstown, MD, Harper & Row, 1972, pp 1–24.

Zelickson AS: Ultrastructure of human epidermis, in Graham JH, Johnson WC, Helwig EB (eds): Dermal Pathology. Hagerstown, MD, Harper & Row, 1972, pp 24–45.

EPIDERMIS

During the first weeks of fetal life, the epidermis consists of a single sheet of contiguous, undifferentiated cells, which subsequently assume the characteristics of keratinocytes. Adnexal structures, particularly follicles and eccrine sweat units, originate during the third month of fetal life as downgrowths from the developing epidermis. Later, apocrine sweat units develop from the upper portion of the follicular epithelium, and sebaceous glands and ducts from the midregion of the follicle. The development of adnexal structures at specific skin sites, like the

regional variation in thickness of the three skin layers, is genetically modulated.

The adult epidermis is composed of three basic cell types: **keratinocytes, melanocytes**, and **Langerhans cells** (Fig. 1–2). Two additional types of cells, the **indeterminate dendritic cell** and the **Merkel cell**, can occasionally be found within the epidermis and at the undersurface of the epidermis and oral mucosa, respectively. The indeterminate dendritic cell is identifiable by electron microscopy and is characterized by the absence of both melanosomes and Langerhans granules. It is related to Langerhans cells, reacts with the monoclonal antibody OKT6, and is Ia antigen positive. The Merkel cell, located directly above the basement membrane, contains intracytoplasmic neurosecretorylike granules, and, through its association with neurites, is thought to mediate the sensation of touch. Despite its direct connection to adjacent keratinocytes by desmosomes, specialized attachment plates characteristic of ectodermal-derived cells, Breathnach believes the Merkel cell to be of neural crest origin rather than of either ectodermal or mesenchymal origin. Merkel cells probably belong to the amino precursor uptake and decarboxylation (APUD) cell system.

The Keratinocyte

The keratinocyte,* or squamous cell, is the principal cell of the epidermis. It is a cell of ectodermal origin which has the specialized function of producing keratin, a complex filamentous protein that not only forms the surface coat (stratum corneum) of the epidermis but also is the structural protein of hair and nails.

The epidermis may be divided into the following zones beginning with the innermost layer: **basal layer, malpighian** or **prickle layer, granular layer,** and **horny layer,** or **stratum corneum** (Fig. 1–3). These names reflect the changing appearance of the keratinocyte as it differentiates into a cornified cell.

A proportion of the basal cells proliferate, differentiate, and move in a stepwise fashion through the full thickness of the epidermis. As many as 50 per cent of basal cells are noncycling. As the proliferative cell moves upward through the epidermis, it changes morphologically. It flattens out, eventually the nucleus disappears, and the keratinocyte is then called a horn cell.

Just as there is regional variation in the thickness of the anatomic layers of the skin (epidermis, the dermis), and the subcutis, so also is there variation in the thickness of the different zones of the epidermis according to skin site. The horny layer and granular layer are thickest on the palms and soles, and virtually absent on the more delicate skin of the flexor aspect of the forearms and the abdomen. The

---

*So named in 1957 by Dr. Walter B. Shelley.

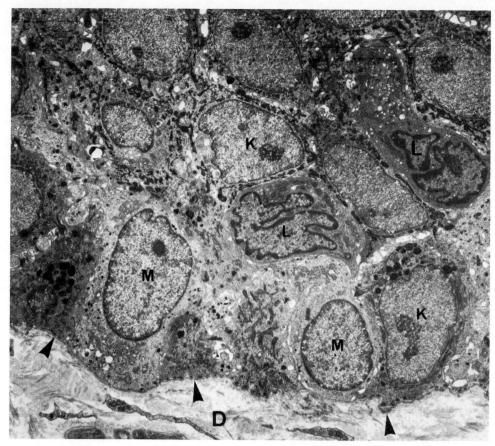

Figure 1–2. *Electron micrograph illustrating the three basic cell types in the epidermis and their relationships. Most of the cells are keratinocytes (prickle cells and basal cells), some labeled (K). Langerhans cells (L) with their characteristic cribriform nuclei are distributed among the keratinocytes in the Malpighian layer. Melanocytes (M) are located in the basal layer of the epidermis, which is separated from (and attached to) the dermis by the basement membrane zone (arrows).*

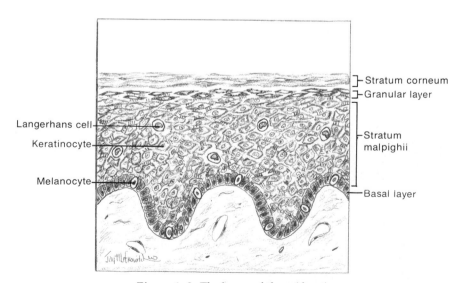

Figure 1–3. *The layers of the epidermis.*

basal layer, however, is generally one cell thick regardless of the skin site examined.

The process of keratinization remains incompletely understood. Matoltsy has suggested that the keratinocyte passes through first a synthetic and then a degradative phase on its way to becoming a horn cell. In the synthetic phase, the keratinocyte accumulates within its cytoplasm intermediate filaments composed of a fibrous protein arranged in an alpha-helical pattern. These **tonofilaments** are fashioned into bundles, which converge upon and terminate at the plasma membrane, where they end in specialized attachment plates called **desmosomes** (Fig. 1–4).

The plasma membranes of adjacent cells are separated by an intercellular space. Electron microscopic histochemical studies have shown that this interspace contains glycoproteins and lipids which are thought to contribute to cellular cohesion. Lamellar granules function in this space, primarily at the interface between the granular and cornified cell layers.

Keratinocytes of the granular zone contain, in addition to the keratin filament system, **keratohyaline granules,** composed of amorphous particulate material of high sulfur-protein content. This material is a precursor to filaggrin, so named because it is thought to be responsible for keratin filament aggregation. Conversion to filaggrin takes place in the granular layer, and this forms the electron-dense interfilamentous protein matrix of mature epidermal keratin. Lamellated organelles called **Odland bodies,** also referred to as membrane-coating granules or **keratinosomes,** are found intracellularly in upper-level keratinocytes and extracellularly at the junction of the granular and horny layers. Their appearance extracellularly coincides with the degradative phase of keratinization, which is characterized by the disappearance of cell organelles and the consolidation

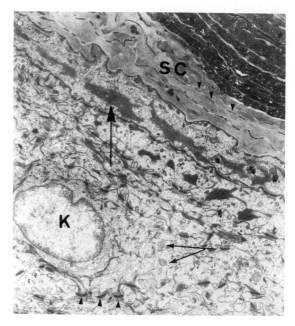

Figure 1–5. The upper portion of the epidermis. Keratinocytes (K) are flatter than those of the lower portion (see Fig. 1–2), and contain keratinosomes (thin arrows). Desmosomes (short arrows) become more obvious as the ratio of nucleus to cytoplasm increases. Keratinocytes of the granular layer have developed keratohyalin granules (broad, long arrow). The stratum corneum (SC) is composed of horny plates which retain only filaments and amorphous material enveloped in a thickened cell membrane. Horny cells, like other keratinocytes, are joined by desmosomes (short arrowheads).

of all contents into a mixture of filaments and amorphous materials enveloped by a thickened cell membrane (horn cell of the stratum corneum) (Fig. 1–5). They establish a barrier to water loss and, with filaggrin, mediate stratum corneum cell cohesion.

Keratinocytes play a role in the immune functioning of the skin. In certain diseases such as lichen planus, allergic contact dermatitis, mycosis fungoides, and graft-versus-host disease, keratinocytes may express the Ia antigen. This may enable them to participate in communication, interaction, and regulation of cell systems collaborating in the induction of the immune response. Also, keratinocytes release interleukin-1 or epidermal-cell–derived thymocyte activating factor (ETAF), which provides the second signal (the first having been antigen) necessary for T cell activation.

Fibronectin, recognized in 1985 as a fibroblast-binding protein, has lately been found to be important in causing keratinocytes to attach to one another and spread; they produce it, and move across it. It is present in abundance before the basement membrane is assembled.

A variety of skin diseases are manifestations of abnormal keratinization. Psoriasis is characterized by an abnormally rapid transformation of basal cells into horn cells. Instead of the normal transit time of 26 to 42 days, it may take only three or four days for a basal cell to become a horn cell. Loss of cohesion of

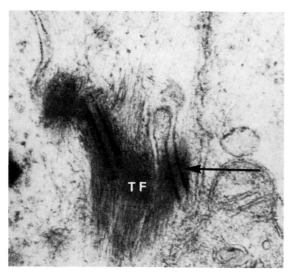

Figure 1–4. Ultrastructural appearance of the desmosome (arrow), the specialized attachment plate between adjacent keratinocytes. Tonofilaments (TF) within the cytoplasm of adjacent keratinocytes converge on the plasma membrane of each cell, where they condense to form an electron-dense zone.

keratinocytes results in the bullous lesions of pemphigus. Desmosomal attachments between keratinocytes are disrupted (acantholysis) and the cells become rounded and separate from one another. This pathologic process is associated with the presence of circulating antibodies directed at these attachments. In pemphigus foliaceus, they bind specifically to desmoglein I, a desmosomal core glycoprotein. Sybert et al have identified a defect in filaggrin synthesis correlating with the absence of keratohyalin granules in ichthyosis vulgaris.

The Melanocyte

The melanocyte is the pigment-producing cell of the epidermis. It is derived from the neural crest, and by the eighth week of development can be found within the fetal epidermis. In normal adult epidermis, melanocytes reside in the basal layer at a frequency of approximately one for every 10 basal keratinocytes. The number of melanocytes in the epidermis is the same regardless of race or color; rather, it is the number and size of the **melanosomes** or pigment granules, continuously synthesized by these melanocytes, which determine racial differences in skin color (Fig. 1–6).

In histologic sections of skin routinely stained by hematoxylin and eosin the melanocyte appears as a "clear" cell in the basal layer of the epidermis. The apparent "halo" is an artefact caused by separation of the melanocyte from adjacent keratinocytes during fixation of the specimen. This occurs because the melanocyte, lacking tonofilaments, cannot form desmosomal attachments with keratinocytes.

The melanocyte is actually a dendritic cell, a feature rarely appreciated at the light-microscope level. Ultrastructural and tissue culture studies demonstrate the octopuslike appearance of the melanocyte. Its dendrites extend for long distances within the epidermis, and any one melanocyte is therefore in contact with a great number of keratinocytes; together they form the so-called **epidermal melanin unit.**

Although the melanocyte is the pigment factory for the skin, **melanosomes** synthesized there are continuously transferred to adjacent keratinocytes, which serve as reservoirs for pigment in the skin. Melanosomes are synthesized in the Golgi zone of the cell and pass through a series of stages in which the enzyme tyrosinase acts upon melanin precursors to produce the densely pigmented granules. While this is occurring, the melanosome migrates to the tip of a dendrite, where it is transferred to an adjacent keratinocyte by apocopation, a phenomenon in which the keratinocyte phagocytoses the dendrite of the melanocyte. Other possible mechanisms of melanosome transfer are direct injection of melanosomes into keratinocytes and release of melanosomes into the extracellular space, followed by their uptake by keratinocytes.

Melanocytes of dark skin synthesize melanosomes larger than those produced in light skin. The size of the melanosome is the principal factor in determining how the melanosomes will be distributed within the keratinocytes. The larger melanosomes of dark skin are individually dispersed within the cytoplasm of keratinocytes; smaller melanosomes of light skin are packaged in membrane-bound complexes within the keratinocyte (Figs. 1–7, 1–8). Chronic sun exposure can stimulate the melanocyte to produce larger melanosomes, thereby making the distribution of melanosomes within keratinocytes resemble the pattern seen in dark-skinned individuals.

Areas of leukoderma or "whitening" of skin can be caused by very different phenomena. In **vitiligo,** the affected skin becomes white because of destruction of melanocytes, leading to decrease in their number. In **albinism,** the number of melanocytes is normal. However, they are unable to synthesize fully pigmented melanosomes. In the former case, the pigment factory has disappeared; in the latter, the tools for pigment synthesis are faulty.

Local areas of increased pigmentation can be due

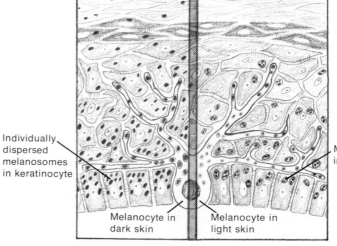

Figure 1–6. The epidermal melanin unit in dark (left) and light (right) skin.

Individually dispersed melanosomes in keratinocyte

Melanosome complex in keratinocyte

Melanocyte in dark skin

Melanocyte in light skin

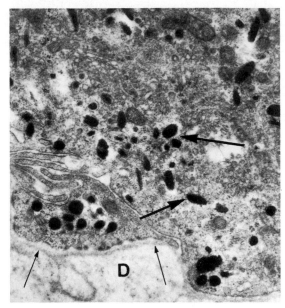

Figure 1–7. Portion of a melanocyte from dark skin, illustrating melanosomes (broad arrows) at various stages of development. Basement membrane zone (thin arrows) and dermis (D) are also seen.

to a variety of causes. The typical freckle is due to a localized increased production of pigment by a normal number of melanocytes. Nevi are benign proliferations of melanocytes. Melanomas are their malig-

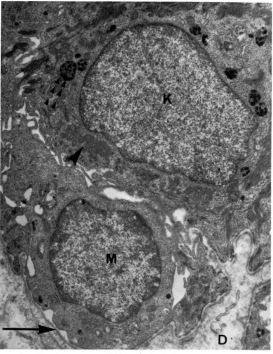

Figure 1–8. The relationship between melanocytes (M) and basal keratinocytes (K) in light skin. Melanocytes synthesize pigment granules (keratinosomes), which are transferred to keratinocytes, where they are contained within membrane-bound "melanosome complexes" (small arrowheads). Bundles of tonofilaments (broad arrowhead) identify the cell as a keratinocyte. The basement membrane zone (arrow) separates epidermis from dermis (D).

nant counterpart. Frequently, though, skin lesions are not pigmented because of hyperplasia or hyperactivity of melanocytes. Rather, they are colored by pigment within the keratinocyte. The seborrheic keratosis is a common example of such a benign pigmented epithelial neoplasm. An example of a malignant epithelial neoplasm which is pigmented—but not by an increase in the relative number of melanocytes—is the pigmented basal cell carcinoma.

The Langerhans Cell

Langerhans cells are normally found scattered among keratinocytes of the stratum spinosum, or prickle cell layer of the epidermis. They constitute 3 to 5 per cent of the cells in this layer. Like the melanocyte, they are not connected to adjacent keratinocytes by desmosomes. At the light-microscopic level, Langerhans cells are difficult to detect in routinely stained sections; however, they appear as dendritic cells in sections impregnated with gold chloride, a stain specific for Langerhans cells. They can, however, be stained with peroxidase-labeled monoclonal antibody OKT6, which stains them and also a small population of indeterminate cells that do not contain Birbeck granules. Ultrastructurally they are characterized by a folded nucleus and distinct intracytoplasmic organelles called Langerhans or **Birbeck granules** (Fig. 1–9). These organelles in their fully developed form are rod-shaped with a vacuole at one end, and resemble a tennis racquet.

Functionally, Langerhans cells are of the monocyte-macrophage lineage and are of bone marrow origin. They play a role in induction of graft rejection, primary contact sensitization, and immunosurveillance. If skin is depleted of them by exposure to ultraviolet radiation, it loses the ability to be sensitized until its population of Langerhans cells is replenished. Langerhans cells also produce some interleukin-1, which acts like that produced by keratinocytes, to aid in T-cell activation.

Silberberg and colleagues have shown that the Langerhans cell serves a primary role in immune reactions of the delayed hypersensitivity type, specifically, allergic contact dermatitis.

Breathnach AS: Aspects of epidermal ultrastructure. J Invest Dermatol 1975, 65:2.

Christophers E, et al: The formation of epidermal cell columns. J Invest Dermatol 1974, 62:555.

Choi KL: The role of the Langerhans cell and keratinocyte in epidermal immunity. J Leukocyte Biol 1986, 39:343.

Chu A, et al: Immunoelectron microscopic identification of Langerhans cells using a new antigenic marker. J Invest Dermatol 1980, 78:177.

Dinarello CA, et al: Lymphokines. N Engl J Med 1987, 317:940.

Ford MJ: Filaggrin. Int J Dermatol 1986, 25:547.

Hanau D: Langerhans cell in allergic contact dermatitis. Dermatologica 1986, 172–182.

Jimbow K, et al: Some aspects of melanin biology: 1950–1975. J Invest Dermatol 1976, 67:72.

Katz SI: The skin as an immunologic organ. JAAD 1985, 13:530.

Kolara G: Wound healing and the role of fibronectin. J Invest Dermatol 1987, 88:527.

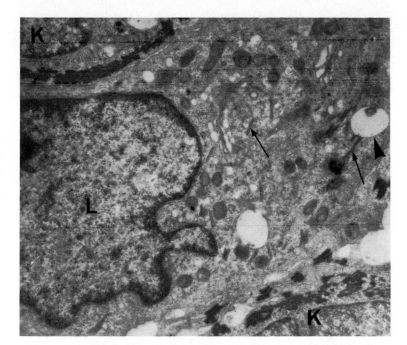

Figure 1–9. Ultrastructural appearance of the Langerhans cell (L). The characteristic intracytoplasmic Langerhans ("Birbeck") granules have a rod-shaped "handle" (thin arrow) and a wide "head" (broad arrowhead). The Langerhans cell is not connected to adjacent keratinocytes (K) by desmosomes.

Lazarus GS, et al: Lysosomes and the skin. J Invest Dermatol 1975, 65:259.

Matoltsy AG: Keratinization. J Invest Dermatol 1976, 67:20.

Niedecken H, et al: Differential expression of major histocompatibility complex class II antigens on human keratinocytes. JAAD 1988, 19:1030.

Osborn M: Components of the cellular cytoskeleton. J Invest Dermatol 1984, 82:443.

Shelley WB, Juhlin L: The Langerhans cell: Its origin, nature, and function. Acta Dermatovener (Stockh). 1978, Suppl. 79.

Silberberg I, et al: The role of Langerhans cells in allergic contact hypersensitivity. A review of findings in man and guinea pigs. J Invest Dermatol 1976, 66:210.

Stanley JR, et al: A monoclonal antibody to desmosomal glycoprotein desmoglein I binds the same polypeptide as human autoantibodies in pemphigus foliaceus. J Immunol 1986, 136:1227.

Sybert VP, et al: Ichthyosis vulgaris. J Invest Dermatol 1985, 84:191.

Toews GB, et al: Epidermal Langerhans cell density determines whether contact hypersensitivity or unresponsiveness follows skin painting with DNFB. J Immunol 1980, 124:445.

Voorhees JJ, et al: Regulation of cell cycles. J Invest Dermatol, 1976, 67:15.

The Epidermal-Dermal Junction

The junction of epidermis and dermis is formed by the basement membrane zone (Fig. 1–2). Ultrastructurally, this zone is composed of four components: the **plasma membranes** of the basal cells with their specialized attachment plates (hemidesmosomes); an electron-lucent zone called the **lamina lucida**; the **basal lamina**; and the **fibrous components** associated with the basal lamina, including anchoring fibrils, dermal microfibrils, and collagen fibers (Fig. 1–10). At the light-microscope level, the so-called PAS-positive basement membrane is composed solely of the fibrous components, which are of dermal origin. The basal lamina is synthesized by the basal cells of the epidermis.

Katz has reviewed in detail the many component layers of the basement membrane zone. Included is a discussion of the ultrastructural localization of the various immunoreactants in the chronic bullous dermatoses.

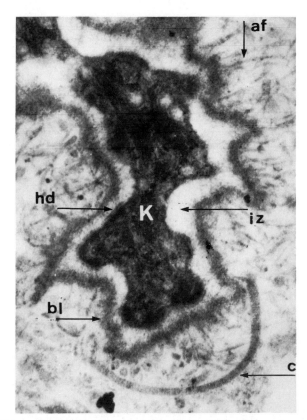

Figure 1–10. Ultrastructural appearance of the basement membrane zone at the junction of epidermis and dermis. The zone comprises four layers: the plasma membrane of basal keratinocytes (K) with their specialized attachment plates, the hemidesmosomes (hd); the clear lamina lucida or intermembranous space (iz); the basal lamina (bl); and the dermal fibrous components, including anchoring fibrils (af) and collagen fibers (c).

The basement membrane zone is considered to be a "porous" semipermeable filter, which permits exchange of cells and fluid between the epidermis and dermis. It further serves as a structural support for the epidermis and holds the epidermis and dermis together. The basement membrane zone serves the same functions for the skin appendages.

Briggaman RA, Wheeler CE Jr: The epidermal-dermal junction. J Invest Dermatol 1975, 65:71.
Katz SI: The epidermal basement membrane zone—structure, ontogeny, and role in disease. JAAD 1984, 11:1025.

EPIDERMAL APPENDAGES (The Adnexa)

Eccrine and apocrine glands and ducts and pilosebaceous units constitute the skin adnexa. Embryologically, they originate as downgrowths from the epidermis and are therefore ectodermal in origin. Melanocytes and other cells which are seen in the adult epidermis can be found within the adnexa. While the various adnexal structures serve specific functions, they all can function as "reserve" epidermis.

Re-epithelialization after injury to the surface epidermis occurs principally by virtue of the migration of keratinocytes from the adnexal epithelium along the skin surface. It is not surprising, therefore, that skin sites such as the face or scalp, which contain pilosebaceous units in abundance, re-epithelialize more rapidly than do skin sites such as the back, where adnexa of all types are comparatively scarce. Since those sites which contain numerous adnexa are also abundantly endowed with a rich network of nerves and blood vessels within the surrounding dermis, wound healing in general is more rapid there.

The Eccrine Sweat Unit

The eccrine sweat unit is composed of three sections which are modified from the basic tubular structure that formed during embryogenesis as a downgrowth of surface epidermis (Fig. 1–1). The *intraepidermal component* of the unit, the acrosyringium, which opens directly onto the skin surface, is called the **spiral duct.** It is derived from dermal duct cells through mitosis and upward migration. The duct consists of a single layer of inner or luminal cells and two or three outer rows of cells. Cornification takes place within the duct, and the horn cells become part of the stratum corneum of the epidermis. The straight dermal portion of the duct is composed of a double layer of cuboidal epithelial cells and is lined by an eosinophilic cuticle on its luminal side.

The secretory acinar portion of the unit, or **coil gland,** is found within the panniculus near the junc-

tion of dermis and subcutis. An inner layer of epithelial cells, the secretory portion of the gland, is surrounded by a layer of flattened myoepithelial cells. The secretory cells are of two types: glycogen-rich, large pale cells and smaller, darker-staining cells. The pale glycogen-rich cells are thought to initiate the formation of sweat. The darker cells may function in a manner similar to that of cells of the dermal duct, which actively reabsorb sodium, thereby modifying sweat from a basically isotonic solution to a hypotonic one by the time it reaches the skin surface. Sweat is similar in composition to plasma, containing the same electrolytes, though in a more dilute concentration.

Eccrine sweat units are found at virtually all skin sites. They are most abundant on the palms, soles, forehead, and axillae. Secretion of sweat is dependent upon many factors and is mediated by cholinergic innervation. Heat is a prime stimulus to increased sweating, but other physiologic stimuli, including emotional stress, are important as well. Increased sweat production in response to heat is part of the thermoregulatory system of the body: together with increased cutaneous blood flow, it can effectively dissipate excessive body heat. At friction surfaces, such as the palms and soles, eccrine secretion is thought to assist tactile sensibility and improve adhesion.

The Apocrine Unit

Adult apocrine units develop as outgrowths, not of the surface epidermis, but of the infundibular or upper portion of the hair follicle (Fig. 1–1). They are therefore intimately related, at least anatomically, if not functionally, to pilar units. Although immature apocrine units are found covering the entire skin surface of the human fetus, these regress and are absent by term.

The straight excretory portion of the duct, which opens into the infundibular portion of the hair follicle, is composed of a double layer of cuboidal epithelial cells. The coiled secretory gland is located at the junction of the dermis and subcutaneous fat. It is lined by a single layer of cells, which vary in appearance from columnar to cuboidal. This layer of cells is surrounded by a layer of myoepithelial cells.

The apexes of the columnar cells project into the lumen of the gland and in histologic cross section appear as if they are being extruded (so-called decapitation secretion). Controversy exists about the mode of secretion in apocrine secretory cells, whether merocrine, apocrine, holocrine, or all three.

The composition of the product of secretion is only partially understood. Protein, carbohydrate, ammonia, lipid, and iron are all found in apocrine secretion. It appears milky and is odorless until it reaches the skin surface, where it is altered by bacteria in such a way as to make it odoriferous.

Apocrine secretion is mediated by adrenergic innervation and by circulating catecholamines of adrenomedullary origin. Excretion, or the propulsion of the secretion through the duct, is episodic, though the actual secretion of the gland is continuous.

Apocrine gland secretion in man serves no known function; in animals it has a protective as well as a sexual function. In some species, it is important in thermoregulation as well.

Although occasionally found in an ectopic location, apocrine units of the human body are generally confined to the following sites: axillae, areolae, the anogenital region, the external auditory canal (ceruminous glands), and the eyelids (glands of Moll). Conditions such as Fox-Fordyce disease and hidradenitis suppurativa, traditionally thought to be apocrine gland dysfunctions, appear to be related etiologically to the excretory components of the apocrine unit, i.e., the apocrine ducts and their associated pilar units, rather than to any abnormality in apocrine secretion per se.

The Hair Follicle

During embryogenesis, mesenchymal cells in the fetal dermis collect immediately below the basal layer of the epidermis. Epidermal buds grow down into the dermis at these sites. The developing follicle forms at an angle to the skin surface and continues its downward growth. At its base, the column of cells widens and surrounds the small collections of mesenchymal cells forming the bulb. The hair is formed from cells just above the bulb, which also give rise to concentric zones of differentiated epithelial cells destined to form the inner and outer root sheaths. Along one side of the follicle, two buds are formed: an upper, which develops into the sebaceous gland, and a lower, which becomes the attachment for the arrector pili muscle. At skin sites destined to have apocrine units, a third epithelial bud develops from the opposite side of the follicle above the level of the sebaceous gland anlage. The uppermost portion of the follicle, which extends from its surface opening to the entrance of the sebaceous duct, is called the **infundibular segment.** The portion of the follicle between the sebaceous duct and the insertion of the arrector pili muscle is the **isthmus.** The **matrix,** or inferior portion, includes the lowermost part of the follicle and the hair bulb.

Hair follicles develop sequentially in rows of three. *Primary* follicles are surrounded by the appearance of two *secondary* follicles; other secondary follicles subsequently develop around the principal units. The density of pilosebaceous units decreases throughout life, mainly because of the poor development of the secondary follicles.

The actual hair shaft, as well as an inner and outer root sheath, develops from the mitotically active undifferentiated cells of the matrix portion of the hair bulb (Fig. 1–11). The sheaths and contained hair are derived from different regions of the bulb, and

they form concentric cylindrical layers. The hair shaft and inner root sheath move together as the hair grows toward the surface; the outer root sheath remains fixed in position. The epidermis of the upper part of the follicular canal is contiguous with the outer root sheath and includes the infundibular and isthmus zones of the follicle. This portion of the follicle is permanent; the portion of the follicle between the bulb and the upper limit of the inner root sheath is completely replaced at each new cycle of hair growth.

The rate of hair growth is dependent upon mitotic activity of the cells of the bulb matrix. Hair "form," or cross-sectional shape of the hair, depends upon the arrangement of cells in the bulb. Scalp hair of Caucasians is round; pubic hair, beard hair, and eyelashes are oval. The scalp hair of blacks is also oval. Curliness of black hair is due to this, and to a curvature of the follicle just above the bulb.

Basic hair color is due to the distribution of melanosomes within hair bulb cells, which become the cells of the hair shaft. Melanocytes of the hair bulb synthesize melanosomes and transfer them to the cells of the bulb matrix in a fashion similar to the transfer of melanosomes from melanocytes to keratinocytes in the surface epidermis. Larger melanosomes are found in the hair of blacks; smaller melanosomes, which are aggregated within membrane-bound complexes, are found in Caucasian hair. Red hair is characterized by spherical melanosomes. The intensity of color is most likely a reflection of the number of fully melanized melanosomes produced by the melanocytes. Graying of hair is a result of a decreased number of melanocytes, which produce fewer melanosomes. Lerner has likened the pathogenesis of graying of the hair to that of vitiligo. Both conditions show a decreased number of melanocytes in affected sites.

Human hair growth is cyclical but each follicle functions as an independent unit. Therefore, humans do not shed hairs synchronously as most animals do. Each hair follicle undergoes intermittent stages of activity and quiescence (Fig. 1–12). During the **growing phase** or **anagen,** the cells of the hair bulb actively divide and produce the growing hair. As this phase ceases, and the follicle goes into the **catagen,** or transitional phase of activity, the matrix cells stop dividing and the hair develops a brushlike zone (**club hair**) owing to incomplete keratinization of the cells. During catagen, the lower portion of the follicle disappears, leaving behind a thin strand of epithelial cells surrounded by a thick basement membrane zone. During the **telogen** or **resting phase** of the hair cycle, the epithelial strand subsequently shortens to the level of the arrector pili muscle and leaves in its wake a small aggregate of epithelial cells exposed to surrounding dermis. The club hair remains within the foreshortened follicle until a new anagen follicle develops in a fashion recapitulating its formation during embryogenesis, and the newly formed hair shaft dislodges the club hair.

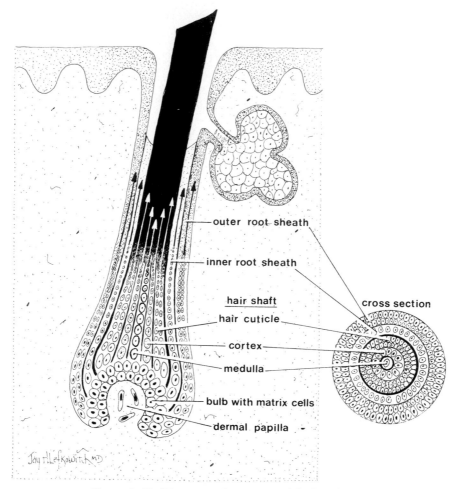

Figure 1–11. *Diagrammatic anatomy of the hair follicle.*

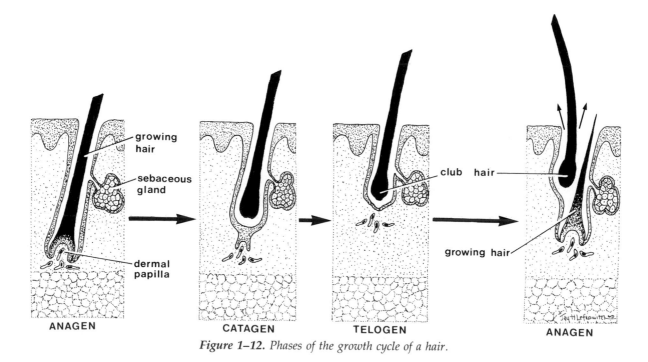

Figure 1–12. *Phases of the growth cycle of a hair.*

The temporal profile of the hair cycle is variable for hairs in different regions of the body. In man, the average period of growth of a scalp hair is three to four years, and the involutional and resting phases last for approximately three months. Normally, approximately 85 to 90 per cent of all scalp hairs are in the anagen phase, a figure which decreases with age and decreases faster in male pattern baldness.

Various exogenous and endogenous physiologic factors can modulate the hair cycle. An example is pregnancy, which is often accompanied by retention of an increased number of scalp hairs in the anagen phase. Three or four months after pregnancy ends, the normal complement of resting hairs plus those which had been temporarily retained in the anagen phase are lost, producing a transient alopecia. Patients on chemotherapy often have hair loss as the drugs interfere with the mitotic activity of the hair matrix, leading to the formation of a thin shaft, which breaks within the follicle.

The donor dominance of hair transplant plugs taken from the lower portions of the scalp attests to regional differences in the viability of hair follicles.

The Sebaceous Gland

The sebaceous gland is formed embryologically as an outgrowth from the upper portion of the hair follicle. It is composed of lobules of pale-staining cells with abundant lipid in their cytoplasm. At the periphery of the lobules are several layers of cells that resemble basal cells of the epidermis and are called **germinative cells.** These germinative cells give rise to the lipid-filled pale cells, which are continuously being extruded through the short sebaceous duct into the infundibular portion of the hair follicle (Fig. 1–1).

Sebaceous glands are found in greatest abundance on the face and scalp, although they are distributed throughout all skin sites except the palms and soles. They are always associated with hair follicles except at the following sites: the eyelids (Meibomian glands), the buccal mucosa and vermilion border of the lip (Fordyce's spots), the prepuce (Tyson's glands), and the female areolas (Montgomery's tubercles).

Although sebaceous glands are independent mini-organs in their own right, they are anatomically and functionally related to the hair follicle. Cutaneous disorders attributed to sebaceous glands, such as acne vulgaris, are really disorders of the entire pilosebaceous unit. The clinical manifestations of acne, namely the comedo, papule, pustule, and cyst, would not form, regardless of increased sebaceous gland activity, as long as the sebaceous duct and infundibular portion of the hair follicle remained patent and lipid and cell debris (sebum) were able to reach the skin surface.

Bell M: The ultrastructure of human axillary apocrine glands after epinephrine injection. J Invest Dermatol 1974, 63:147.

Ebling FJ: Hair. J Invest Dermatol 1976, 67:98.
Jarrett A (ed): The Physiology and Pathophysiology of the Skin: Vol 4, The Hair Follicle. London, Academic Press, 1977.
Knutson DD: Ultrastructural observations in acne vulgaris: The normal sebaceous follicle and acne lesions. J Invest Dermatol 1974, 62:228.
Lerner AB: On the etiology of vitiligo and gray hair. Am J Med 1971, 51:141.
Montagna W: An introduction to sebaceous glands. J Invest Dermatol 1974, 62:120.
Robertshaw D: Neural and humoral control of apocrine glands. J Invest Dermatol 1974, 63:160.
Strauss JS, et al: The sebaceous glands: Twenty-five years of progress. J Invest Dermatol 1976, 67:90.

THE DERMIS

The constituents of the dermis are mesodermal in origin except for nerves, which, like melanocytes, derive from the neural crest. Until the sixth week, fetal dermis is merely a pool of acid-mucopolysaccharide–containing, scattered, dendritic-shaped cells, which are the precursors of fibroblasts. By the twelfth week, fibroblasts are actively synthesizing **reticulum fibers, elastic fibers,** and **collagen.** A vascular network develops, and by the twenty-fourth week, fat cells have appeared beneath the dermis.

The principal component of the dermis is **collagen,** a fibrous protein that serves as the major structural protein for the entire body. It is found in tendons, ligaments, and the lining of bones as well as in the dermis. It represents 70 per cent of the dry weight of skin.

The fibroblast synthesizes the procollagen molecule, a helical arrangement of specific polypeptide chains that are subsequently secreted by the cell and assembled into collagen fibrils. Collagen is rich in the amino acids hydroxyproline, hydroxylysine, and glycine. Collagen is uniform in width and each fiber displays characteristic cross striations with a periodicity of 68 nm. Collagen fibers are loosely arranged in the upper (papillary) portion of the dermis. They are tightly bundled in a fasciclelike pattern within the lower, or reticular, portion of the dermis. Collagen fibers are continuously being degraded by proteolytic enzymes called collagenases, and replaced by newly synthesized fibers.

The fibroblast also synthesizes reticulum and elastic fibers, as well as the ground substance of the dermis, which is composed of glycosaminoglycans or acid mucopolysaccharides. **Reticulum fibers** are similar to collagen in their perodicity, although smaller in diameter. Large numbers are found within the upper part of the papillary dermis where they serve as the anchoring fibrils for the basal lamina (Fig. 1–10). **Elastic fibers** differ both structurally and chemically from collagen. They consist of aggregates of two components: protein filaments and elastin, an amorphous protein. The amino acids desmosine and isodesmosine are unique to elastic fibers. Elastic fibers in the papillary dermis are fine, whereas those in the reticular dermis are coarse. The extracellular matrix or ground substance of the dermis is composed of acid mucopolysaccharide, principally hyaluronic acid, chondroitin sulfate and dermatan sulfate, neutral mucopolysaccharides, and electrolytes.

Collagen is the major stress-resistant material of the skin. Elastic fibers contribute very little to resisting deformation and tearing of skin, although they appear to have a role in maintaining its elasticity. Although "connective tissue disease" is a term generally used to refer to a clinically heterogeneous group of autoimmune diseases, including lupus erythematosus, scleroderma, and dermatomyositis, only scleroderma involves a detectable abnormality in the metabolism of collagen. Like scleroderma, keloid and hypertrophic scar formation reflect abnormalities in the rates of collagen synthesis and degradation.

Defects in collagen synthesis have recently been described in a number of inheritable diseases, including Ehlers-Danlos syndrome, X-linked cutis laxa, and osteogenesis imperfecta. Increased degradation of collagen by increased collagenase activity has been demonstrated, in vitro, in a variety of diseases, including recessive epidermolysis bullosa dystrophica.

Vasculature

The **dermal vasculature** consists principally of three important intercommunicating **plexuses**: the *subpapillary plexus* courses within the papillary portion of the dermis parallel to the epidermis and furnishes a rich supply of capillaries, end arterioles, and venules to the dermal papillae. The *deeper plexuses* around the hair follicles and eccrine glands are composed of larger blood vessels than those of the superficial plexus (Fig. 1–1). The vasculature of the dermis is particularly well developed at sites of adnexal structures.

Associated with the vascular plexus are the **dermal lymphatics.**

Muscles

Smooth muscle occurs in the skin as **arrectores pilorum** (erectors of the hairs), as the tunica dartos (or **dartos**) of the scrotum, and in the areolas around the nipples. The arrectores pilorum are attached to the hair follicles below the sebaceous glands and, in contracting, pull the hair follicle upward, producing gooseflesh.

Striated (voluntary) muscle occurs in the skin of the neck as the platysma muscle and in the skin of the face as the muscles of expression.

Specialized aggregates of smooth muscle cells found between arterioles and venules are called **glomus bodies.** These serve to shunt blood from the arterial to the venous side of the vascular system, thereby avoiding the capillaries where exchange of oxygen and heat takes place. These arteriovenous anastomoses are best developed on the digits.

Nerves

The dermis is rich in **nerves.** *Touch* and *pressure* are mediated by Meissner corpuscles in the dermal papillae, particularly on the palms and soles, and by Vater-Pacini corpuscles located in the deeper portion of the dermis of weight-bearing surfaces. Mucocutaneous end-organs are found in the papillary dermis of modified hairless skin at the mucocutaneous junctions, namely, the glans, the prepuce, the clitoris, the labia minora, the perianal region, and the vermilion border of the lips. *Temperature, pain,* and *itch* sensation are transmitted by unmyelinated nerve fibers which terminate in the papillary dermis and around hair follicles. Impulses pass to the central nervous system by way of the dorsal root ganglia.

Postganglionic adrenergic fibers of the autonomic nervous system regulate vasoconstriction, apocrine gland secretions, and contraction of arrector pili muscles of hair follicles. Cholinergic fibers mediate eccrine sweat secretion.

Mast Cells

An important cellular constituent of the dermis is the **mast cell.** Some 6–12 microns in diameter, it is distinguished by containing up to 1000 granules, each measuring 0.6–0.7 microns in diameter. On the cell's surface are 100,000 to 500,000 glycoprotein receptor sites for immunoglobulin E (IgE).

The granules stain metachromatically because of their high content of heparin. They also contain histamine, neutrophil chemotactic factor, eosinophil chemotactic factor of anaphylaxis, tryptase, kininogenase, and beta-glucosaminidase. Slow reacting substance of anaphylaxis (leukotrienes C4 and D4), leukotriene B4, platelet activating factor, and prostaglandin D2 are formed only after IgE-mediated release of granules.

The mast cell is an active participant in several neoplastic or proliferative disorders: urticaria pigmentosa, cutaneous mastocytosis, and systemic mastocytosis, which are discussed under those headings in Chapter 28 (Dermal Tumors).

THE SUBCUTIS

Beneath the dermis lies the **subcutis** or **panniculus,** lobules of fat cells or lipocytes separated by fibrous septa composed of collagen and large blood vessels. The collagen in the septa is continuous with the collagen in the dermis. Just as the epidermis and the dermis vary in thickness according to skin site, so does the subcutis. Certain inflammatory dermatoses, known as the **panniculitides,** principally affect the subcutis, producing subcutaneous nodules. The pattern of the inflammation, specifically whether it primarily affects the septa or the fat lobules themselves, serves to distinguish various conditions which clinically may resemble one another.

Clark RAF: Cutaneous tissue repair. JAAD 1985, 13:701.

Cotta-Pereira G, et al: Oxytalan, eulanin, and elastic fibers in the human skin. J Invest Dermatol 1976, 66:143.

Kühn K: Structure and biochemistry of collagen. Aesth Plast Surg 1988, 9:141.

Melman SA: Mast cells and their mediators. Int J Dermatol 1987, 26:335.

Nagata H, et al: Fibronectin. Arch Dermatol 1985, 121:995.

Pierard GE: Skin in dermatosparaxis. Dermal microarchitecture and biochemical properties. J Invest Dermatol 1976, 66:2.

Prunieras M: Melanocytes, melanogenesis, and inflammation. Int J Dermatol 1986, 25:629.

Ryan TJ: The blood vessels of the skin. J Invest Dermatol 1976, 67:110.

Idem: Lymphatics of the skin. Int J Dermatol 1986, 25:411.

Serafin WE, et al: Mediators of immediate hypersensitivity. N Engl J Med 1987, 317:30.

Vitto J, et al: Defects in the biochemistry of collagen in diseases of connective tissue. J Invest Dermatol 1976, 66:59.

Yen A, et al: Ultrastructure of the human dermal microcirculation: The horizontal plexus of the papillary dermis. J Invest Dermatol 1976, 66:131.

2

Cutaneous Symptoms, Signs, and Diagnosis

The various diseases that affect the human skin may present similar symptoms and signs. Such identical features create problems in making a diagnosis; however, in most instances the appearance of many skin lesions may be so typical and so distinctive that a glance at the patient's skin will reveal the diagnosis. At times subjective symptoms and clinical signs in themselves are inadequate, and a complete history and laboratory examinations, including a biopsy, are essential to arrive at a diagnosis.

The same disease may show variations under different conditions and in different individuals. The appearance of the lesions may be modified by previous treatment or obscured by extraneous influences. Subjective symptoms may be the only evidence of a disease, as in pruritus. In most instances, however, the diagnosis is made by relying on the objective physical characteristics and location or distribution of one or more lesions that can be seen or felt.

Barr RJ: Cutaneous cytology. JAAD 1984, 10:163.
Goodman H: Nikolsky sign. Arch Dermatol Syph 1953, 68:334.

CUTANEOUS SYMPTOMS

The subjective symptoms consist of pruritus (itching), sensations of heat (burning), cold (tingling), prickling, biting, formication, pain, and numbness.

PRURITUS (Itching)

Itching, or pruritus, is defined by Dorland's Medical Dictionary as "an unpleasant cutaneous sensation which provokes the desire to scratch or rub the skin." It occurs when there is a weak stimulation of cutaneous nerves. Pruritus is by far the most common cutaneous symptom.

It may be a mere prickling, tingling, or formication, or its severity may be so intense as to be intolerable. There are regional differences in the severity of the body's reaction to the itch, and different persons react differently to the itch stimulus. The anogenital area is especially susceptible: common problems are pruritus ani and pruritus vulvae or scroti. Pruritus is commonly associated with eczematous dermatitis, urticaria, food allergy, dermatitis venenata, dermatitis herpetiformis, scabies, lichen planus, mycosis fungoides, and pediculosis; it is also encountered more or less in all inflammatory dermatoses, in malignant lymphoma, and in xerosis. Senile pruritus is due mainly to dryness of the skin (xerosis).

Pruritus may result from or be associated with systemic diseases. Among these are diabetes mellitus, biliary obstructive disease, iron deficiency anemia, internal cancer, and severe renal insufficiency. Endocrine imbalances resulting from thyroid dysfunction, menstruation, and menopause may cause pruritus.

In diabetes, the pruritus is generally assumed to be due to dryness of the skin (xerosis), which is a product of decreased surface lipid and a decreased hydrating capacity of the horny layer, producing

14

scaling and fissuring. Pruritus of the anogenital area, especially in diabetic women, may be associated with *Candida albicans* infection.

In biliary obstructive disease, icterus may be severe and still not cause pruritus. The increased bile salts in the system are probably the etiologic factor for pruritus.

In Hodgkin's disease, mycosis fungoides, non-Hodgkin's lymphoma, and leukemia, pruritus may be severe. Erythroderma may be a manifestation of the specific lymphoma that causes the severe pruritus.

Uremic pruritus is generalized and occurs in severe cases in which the skin has a yellowish brown discoloration. Gilchrist has been able to relieve uremic pruritus with ultraviolet phototherapy (UVB type). This has also been effective in patients on hemodialysis with severe pruritus.

Intractable pruritus may be the most frequent complaint in patients receiving hemodialysis. Tapia et al showed that intravenous lidocaine (200 mg in 100 ml physiologic saline) was remarkably effective in relieving this form of pruritus.

Itching due to urticaria, dermatitis, tinea, scabies, or other external cause rarely wakens a patient from sleep, and seldom raises the pain threshold so that scratching regularly produces bleeding, or scars, or causes lichenification. In circumscribed neurodermatitis (lichen simplex), nummular eczema, prurigo nodularis, atopic dermatitis, dermatitis herpetiformis, and neurotic excoriations, however, it is characteristically (though not exclusively) so timed, and

so severe. This feature is of great value in diagnosis. Itching is discussed in more detail in Chapter 4.

Arnold HL Jr: Paroxysmal pruritus. JAAD 1985, 11:322.
Denman ST: A review of pruritus. JAAD 1986, 14:375.
Edwards AE, et al: Pruritic skin diseases, psychological stress, and itch sensation. Arch Dermatol 1976, 112:339.
Hazelrigg DE: Paroxysmal pruritus (letter). JAAD 1985, 13:839.
Herndon JH Jr: Itching: The pathophysiology of pruritus. Int J Dermatol 1975, 14:465.
Lewiecki EW, et al: Pruritus. A manifestation of iron deficiency. JAMA 1976, 236:2319.
Martin J: Pruritus. Int J Dermatol 1985, 24:634.
Vickers CFH: Iron deficiency pruritus (letter). JAMA 1977, 238:129.

OTHER SYMPTOMS

Pain may be deep-boring and burning as in herpes zoster, shooting as in tabes dorsalis, or throbbing as in furuncles, carbuncles, and cellulitis. **Anesthesia** may be present in patches and if dissociated (i.e., only to cold or touch or pain), is considered pathognomonic of leprosy. Dissociation also occurs, however, in syringomyelia, in which the fingers may have loss of pain and temperature sensation but preservation of tactile sensations. Hypesthesia and hyperesthesia may also be seen. Sensory dissociation is also a feature, though an inconstant one, of follicular mucinosis. Anesthesia to pinprick was observed by Aeling in the pale halo surrounding the central red papules that may follow multiple mosquito bites.

CUTANEOUS SIGNS

According to the nature of the pathologic process, lesions assume more or less distinct characteristics. They may be uniform or diverse in size, shape, and color, and may be in different stages of evolution or of involution. The original lesions are known as the primary lesions. They may continue to full development or be modified by regression, trauma, or other extraneous factors.

PRIMARY LESIONS

Primary lesions are of the following forms—macules (or patches), papules (or plaques), nodules, tumors, wheals, vesicles, bullae, and pustules.

Macules (Maculae, Spots). Macules are variously sized, circumscribed changes in skin color, without elevation or depression. They may be circular, oval or irregular, and may be distinct in outline or fade into the surrounding area.

Macules may constitute the whole or part of the eruption, or may be merely an early phase. Occasionally the spots tend to become slightly raised; they are then designated papules, or sometimes, as in morbilliform eruptions, *edematous macules*.

Patches. A patch is a very large macule, perhaps 15 or 20 cm in diameter, as may be seen in nevus flammeus, or widespread vitiligo.

Papules (Papulae). Papules are circumscribed, solid elevations with no visible fluid, varying in size from a pinhead to a pea. They may be acuminate, rounded, conical, flat-topped, or umbilicated, and may appear white (as in milium), red (as in eczema), yellowish (as in xanthoma), reddish brown (as in lupus vulgaris), or black (as in melanoma).

Papules may be seated in the dermis, around sebaceous glands, at the orifices of the sweat ducts, or at the hair follicles. They may be of soft or firm consistency. The surface may be smooth or rough. If capped by scales, they are known as *squamous papules*, and the eruption is called papulosquamous.

Some papules are discrete and irregularly distributed, as in papular urticaria, while others are grouped, as in lichen nitidus. Some persist as papules, whereas those of the inflammatory type may progress to vesicles and even to pustules, or may form ulcers before regression takes place.

It should be noted that a **maculopapular** eruption is relatively rare, and that it is composed, not of "maculopapules," but of macules *and* papules. There may be "edematous macules" (see above), but there is no such thing as a "maculopapule."

Plaques. A plaque is a broad papule (or confluence of papules), 1 or more cm in diameter. It is generally flat, and may be centrally depressed or even clear.

Nodules. Nodules are a form of papules, but larger and deeper. They are generally persistent. Unlike papules, they arise in the dermis or even the panniculus.

Tumors. Tumors are soft or firm and freely movable or fixed masses of various sizes and shapes. General usage dictates the use of the word tumor to mean a neoplasm. They may be elevated or deep seated, and in some instances are pedunculated (fibromas). Tumors have a tendency to be rounded. Their consistency depends upon the constituents of the lesion. Some tumors remain stationary indefinitely, whereas others increase in size, or break down as a result of infection and necrosis.

Wheals (Hives). Wheals are evanescent, edematous, flat elevations of various sizes. They are usually oval or of bizarre contours, whitish or pinkish, and are surrounded by a pink areola. They may be discrete or may coalesce to form solid plaques. These lesions develop in a few seconds, but disappear slowly. Itching is almost always present. Dermographism may be evident.

Vesicles (Blisters). Vesicles are circumscribed epidermal elevations 1 to 10 mm in size, and usually contain a clear fluid. They may be pale or yellowish from serous fluid matter, or reddish from serum mixed with blood, and occasionally have deep reddish areolae. The apex may be rounded, acuminate, or umbilicated as in eczema vaccinatum. Vesicles may be discrete, irregularly scattered, grouped as in herpes zoster, or linear as in poison ivy dermatitis. They may arise directly or from a macule or papule, and generally lose their identity in a short time, breaking spontaneously or developing into bullae through coalescence or enlargement, or developing into pustules. When the contents are of a seropurulent character, the lesions are known as *vesicopustules.* Vesicles consist of either a single cavity (*unilocular*) or of several compartments (*multilocular*), containing fluid.

Bullae. Bullae are rounded or irregularly shaped blisters containing serous or seropurulent fluid. They differ from vesicles only in size, being larger than 1 cm. They are usually single-chambered but may be multilocular. Bullae may be located superficially in the epidermis, so that their walls are flaccid and thin and subject to rupture spontaneously or from slight injury. After rupture, remnants of the thin walls may persist and, together with the exudate, may dry to form a thin crust; or the broken bleb may leave a raw and moist base, which may be covered with seropurulent or purulent slough. More rarely, irregular vegetations may appear on the base (as in pemphigus vegetans). When the bullae are subepidermal, they are tense, and ulceration and scarring often result.

In pemphigus there is a lack of cohesion between the epidermal cells so that the overlayers can be easily rubbed off, leaving a raw moist erosion (**Nikolsky's sign**). Hemorrhagic bullae are common in pemphigus, herpes zoster, toxic epidermal necrolysis, and, infrequently, lichen sclerosus et atrophicus. The cellular contents of bullae may be diagnostic in pemphigus, herpes zoster, and herpes simplex.

Pustules (Pimples). Pustules are small elevations of the skin containing pus. They are similar to vesicles in shape, and usually have an inflammatory areola. They are usually whitish or yellowish, but may be reddish if they contain blood with the pus. They may originate as pustules or may develop from papules or vesicles, passing through transitory early stages during which they are known as *papulopustules* or *vesicopustules.*

SECONDARY LESIONS

Secondary lesions are of many kinds, of which the most important are scales, excoriations, fissures, crusts, erosions, ulcers, and scars.

Scales (Exfoliations, Squames, Squamae). Scales are dry or greasy laminated masses of keratin. The body ordinarily is constantly undergoing a scarcely perceptible desquamation in the form of tiny, thin epidermal particles. When the formation of keratin cells is rapid or the process of normal keratinization is interfered with, pathologic exfoliation results, producing scales. These vary in size, some being fine, delicate, and branny, as in tinea versicolor, others being coarser, as in eczema and ichthyosis, while still others are stratified, as in psoriasis. Large sheets of desquamated epidermis are seen in exfoliative dermatitis, toxic epidermal necrolysis, staphylococcal scalded skin syndrome, and scarlet fever. Generally, the exfoliations are thin, dry, brittle, shiny flakes, but sometimes they are greasy and dull from the sebum and sweat. They vary in color from whitishgrayish to yellowish or brown from the admixture of dirt or melanin. Occasionally they have a silvery sheen from trapping of air between their layers: these are *micaceous scales,* characteristic of psoriasis.

Scaling is common in a large number of inflammatory diseases of the skin, being associated with parakeratosis.

Excoriations (Abrasions, Scratch Marks). An excoriation is a punctate or linear abrasion produced by mechanical means, usually involving only the epidermis and rarely reaching the papillary layer of the dermis. Excoriations are caused by scratching with the fingernails in an effort to relieve itching in a variety of diseases (eczema, neurodermatitis, scabies), by other mechanical trauma, and even from constant friction. Although of various sizes and shapes, excoriations are generally small, linear lesions, the bright red or dark color resulting from dried blood. Frequently there is an inflammatory areola about the excoriation or a covering of yellowish dried serum over it.

Excoriations may be accompanied by inoculation

of pyogenic microorganisms and the formation of pustules, occasionally associated with enlargement of the neighboring lymphatic glands. The longer and deeper excoriations are, the more severe was the pruritus that provoked them.

Fissures (Cracks, Clefts). A fissure is a linear cleft through the epidermis, or rarely into the dermis, caused by disease or injury. These lesions may be single or multiple and vary from tiny cracks to clefts several centimeters in length with sharply defined margins. They may be dry or moist, reddish, straight, curved, irregular, or branching. They occur most commonly when the skin is thickened and inelastic from inflammation and dryness, especially in regions subjected to frequent movement. Such areas are the tips and flexural creases of the thumbs, fingers, and palms; the edges of the heels; the clefts between the fingers and toes; at the angles of the mouth; and about the nares, auricles, and anus. When the skin is dry and sensitive, exposure to cold and wind or the action of soap and water may produce a stinging, burning sensation and fissures—"**chapping**." Pain often accompanies movement of the parts by opening or deepening the cracks or forming new ones.

Crusts (Scabs). Crusts are dried serum, pus, or blood, usually mixed with epithelial and bacterial debris. They vary greatly in size, thickness, shape, and color, according to their origin, composition, and the amount of discharge. They may be dry, golden yellow, soft, friable, and superficial, as in impetigo contagiosa; yellowish, as in favus; thick, hard, and tough as in third-degree burns; or lamellated, elevated, brown, black, or green masses, as in late syphilis. The latter have been described as oyster-shell (ostraceous) crusts and are known as **rupia**. When thin crusts become detached, the base may be dry, or red and moist; it will usually heal leaving a smooth, normal skin surface.

Erosions (Erosio). Loss of all or portions of the epidermis alone, as in impetigo or herpes zoster or simplex after vesicles rupture, produces an erosion. It may or may not become crusted, but it heals without a scar.

Ulcers (Ulcera). Ulcers are rounded or irregularly shaped excavations that result from loss of dermis as well as epidermis. They vary in diameter from a few millimeters to several centimeters. They may be shallow, involving little beyond the epidermis, as in

dystrophic epidermolysis bullosa, the base being formed by the papillary layer, or they may extend deep into the dermis or even reach into the subcutaneous structures, as in basal cell cancer or decubitus. They heal with scarring.

Scars (Cicatrices). Scars are new formations of connective tissue that replace loss of substance in the dermis or deeper parts as a result of injury or disease, as part of the normal reparative and healing process. Their size and shape are determined by the form of the previous destruction. In certain dermatoses the process of absorption of cellular infiltration leads to scar formation, as in lupus and syphilis. In others, pressure leads to thin, atrophic scars or the fibrous elements develop into neoplastic overgrowths, as in keloid. Cicatrices may be smooth or rough, pliable or firm, and tend at first to be pink or violaceous, later becoming white, glistening, or rarely pigmented.

Scars with certain characteristics are typical of particular diseases of the skin, so that they have a diagnostic value. Those of lupus erythematosus are shiny, thin, telangiectatic, and minutely pitted, corresponding to glandular orifices; those from lupus vulgaris, tough and fibrous, occasionally cordlike or with scaling at the edges; those that follow burns are a mixture of thin, depressed, atrophic and hypertrophic, raised or fibrous lesions with keloidal tendency; those of scrofuloderma are linear and cordlike; those that follow the involution of syphilids are thin, crinkled, and papery. Some individuals and some areas of the body, such as the anterior chest, are especially prone to scarring.

Scars are persistent but are inclined to become less noticeable in the course of time. On the other hand, sometimes they grow thick, tough, and corded, forming a hypertrophic scar or keloid, and may cause severe pruritus.

Histologically, a useful diagnostic feature is the absence of interpapillary pegs overlying the scar. After destruction of the epidermis, the interpapillary pegs do not regenerate with the rest of the epidermis. The connective tissue in the dermis appears in broad bundles that interlace and blend with the neighboring normal fibrous tissue. In young scars the nuclei are larger and more closely placed, whereas in old scars the nuclei are sparse and small, and the bundles are smooth and hyalinized.

GENERAL DIAGNOSIS

Interpretation of the clinical picture is difficult, for identical manifestations may result from widely different causes. Moreover, the same etiologic factor may give rise to a great diversity of eruptions. However, there is one great advantage in dermatology, namely, that of dealing with an organ that can be seen and felt. Smears and cultures may be readily made for bacteria and fungi. By excision and microscopic examination of the lesion, its histopathology

can be studied in relation to the clinical appearance more directly in the skin than elsewhere.

HISTORY

Knowledge of the patient's age, health, occupation, hobbies, living conditions, and the onset, duration, and course of the disease, and its response to previous treatment, may be pertinent.

It may be useful to inquire about family tendencies to diabetes, allergies, hereditary diseases, psoriasis, and acne.

A complete drug history is perhaps the most important aspect of a thorough history. Drug reactions are frequently seen and may simulate many different diseases. Sedatives such as the barbiturates; laxatives such as phenolphthalein; anti-inflammatory agents, steroidal or nonsteroidal; and antibacterial agents such as the sulfas and penicillin may all produce distressing cutaneous changes. All these may simulate entities not usually attributed to drugs. It is equally important to inquire about topical agents that have been applied to the skin and mucous membranes for medicinal or cosmetic purposes, for these agents may cause cutaneous or systemic reactions.

Other illnesses; travel abroad, even for a few days; the patient's environment at home and at work; seasonal occurrences and recurrences of the disease; the temperature, humidity, and weather of the patient's environment are all important items in a dermatologic history. Habitation in certain parts of the world predisposes one to distinctive diseases for a particular geographic locale. Some such diseases are San Joaquin Valley fever (coccidioidomycosis); leprosy, endemic only in certain areas of the world; bejel and pinta in tropical climates; South American blastomycosis and keloidal blastomycosis in South America; and histoplasmosis in the Mississippi River valley.

Sexual orientation and practices may be relevant, as in suspected AIDS (acquired immune deficiency syndrome), AIDS-related disorders, and ulcerating (or other) genital lesions.

EXAMINATION

Examination should be conducted in a well-lighted room. Daylight is the ideal illumination. Some eruptions are more clearly visible in ultraviolet light, as in the case of faint macular eruptions that become prominent under it. In tinea capitis the use of ultraviolet light passed through Wood's filter, which is permeable to a wavelength of 365 nanometers (nm), is of assistance in diagnosis, for some species of fungi become fluorescent in these rays. This light is also valuable in the diagnosis of tinea versicolor, erythrasma, and vitiligo.

A magnifying lens is of inestimable value in examining minute lesions. It may be necessary to palpate the lesion for firmness and fluctuation; rubbing will elucidate the nature of scales; scraping will reveal the nature of the lesion's base. Pigmented lesions, especially in infants, should be rubbed in an attempt to elicit **Darier's sign** (whealing) in urticaria pigmentosa.

The manner of display of the diseased areas is important. The entire eruption must be seen in order to evaluate distribution and configuration. Laboratory tests may be necessary to complete the study.

DIAGNOSTIC DETAILS OF LESIONS

Distribution of Lesions. Lesions may be few or numerous, and in arrangement they may be discrete or may coalesce to form patches of peculiar configuration. They may appear over the entire body, sometimes following the lines of cleavage, or they may follow the course of nerves, as in herpes zoster and leprosy, or they may form groups, rings, crescents, or grotesque patterns. A remarkable degree of bilateral symmetry is characteristic of dermatitis herpetiformis, vitiligo, and pemphigoid (herpes) gestationis.

Evolution. Some lesions quickly attain complete formation without any intermediate stage (macules). Certain others remain the same (warts) during their entire existence. When lesions succeed one another in a series of crops, as they do in varicella and dermatitis herpetiformis, a *polymorphous* eruption results, with lesions in various stages of development or involution all present at the same time.

Involution. Certain lesions disappear completely, whereas others (lichen planus) leave pigment or scars, and still others do not involute.

Grouping. Certain lesions tend to be grouped in clusters, as in herpes zoster; or in a concentric manner, as in "iris" lesions of erythema multiforme. Grouping is a characteristic of dermatitis herpetiformis, herpes simplex, herpes zoster, and late syphilitic eruptions. Small lesions arranged around a large one are said to be in a *corymbose* arrangement. Rings within concentric rings, as in borderline leprosy or erythema multiforme, are said to be in a *cockade* pattern, like the tricolor cockades worn by French revolutionists. Flea and other arthropod bites are usually grouped and tend to be paired.

Configuration. Some lesions assume characteristic figures, either by enlargement or by coalescence. Circinate and annular lesions are encountered in dermatophytosis, erythema annulare centrifugum, granuloma annulare, syphilis, erythema multiforme, lichen planus, psoriasis, seborrheic dermatitis, and pityriasis rosea. Gyrate patterns are formed in erythema gyratum repens, psoriasis, mycosis fungoides, and sometimes syphilis. A serpiginous border is a characteristic of late syphilis and occasionally of dermatophytosis. In some syphiloderms and in the configurate type of seborrheic dermatitis there are crescentic formations. Some grotesque and bizarre patterns are found in mycosis fungoides, the other malignant lymphomas, and in dermatitis artefacta.

Color. The color of the skin is due to melanin, oxyhemoglobin, reduced hemoglobin, and carotene. Not only do the proportions of these components affect the color, but their depth within the skin and the thickness of the epidermis and hydration also play a role. The Tyndal effect modifies the color of skin and the color of lesions by the selective scattering of light waves of different wavelengths. The blue nevus and mongolian spots are examples of this light dispersion effect.

It is not advisable to place too much reliance on

the color of lesions as a diagnostic factor, for it is difficult to describe colors, and they appear differently to different individuals; but they may at least serve as a corroborative aid. In mycosis fungoides, scarlet fever, juvenile xanthogranuloma, erysipelas, erythema multiforme, erythroderma, xanthoma, steatocystoma multiplex, secondary syphilis, lupus vulgaris, and many other diseases, the characteristic color is of diagnostic aid.

Patches lighter in color than the normal skin—hypopigmented—suggest tinea versicolor, nevus anemicus, leprosy, hypomelanotic macules of tuberous sclerosis, hypomelanosis of Ito, idiopathic guttate hypomelanosis, and, when mottled about the neck, syphilis. Patches of seborrheic dermatitis and pityriasis alba may be light. Actual depigmentation should be distinguished from this; it suggests vitiligo, nevus depigmentosus, halo nevus, scleroderma, morphea, or lichen sclerosus et atrophicus. Leprosy never causes depigmentation, except in scars.

Darkening may be due to inflammation, nevi, lentigines, melasma; the result of pressure or rubbing; arsenical dermatitis; or due to deposits of metals such as silver, mercury, gold, or, in the gingiva, bismuth or lead deposits. When generalized or profuse, darker lesions may be a sequel of lichen planus, dermatitis herpetiformis, or photosensitivity reactions.

Hyperpigmented patches or lesions may be seen in Kaposi's sarcoma (typically violaceous papules or nodules), neurofibromatosis, acanthosis nigricans, urticaria pigmentosa, melanoma, xeroderma pigmentosum, incontinentia pigmenti, vagabond's disease (maculae caeruleae), tar melanosis, ochronosis, poikiloderma, lichen aureus, and many other diseases.

Consistency. *Palpation* is an essential part of the physical examination of lesions. Does the lesion blanch on pressure? If not, it may be purpuric. Is it fluctuant? If so, it may have free fluid in it. Is it cold? hot? If there is a nodule or tumor, does it sink through a ring into the panniculus, like a neurofibroma? Is it hard enough to make one suspect calcification, or merely very firm, like a fibroma or dermatofibroma? Or brawny, like scleredema? Or doughy, like the proximal muscles in dermatomyositis? Does the skin dimple when the lesion is picked up and compressed laterally? This is Fitzpatrick's "dimple sign," suggestive of a histiocytoma. Witkowski and Parish have considered this in a commentary.

Witkowski JA, et al: The touching question. Int J Dermatol 1981, 20:426.

DERMATOSES OF THE NEWBORN

Some of the more frequently encountered dermatoses of the newborn are prickly heat or miliaria, perianal dermatitis, impetigo contagiosa, intertrigo, diaper rash, candidiasis, scabies, seborrheic dermatitis (cradle cap), erythema toxicum neonatorum, transient neonatal pustular melanosis, contact dermatitis, dermatitis medicamentosa, icterus neonatorum, and insect bites. Less frequently seen dermatoses are congenital syphilis, congenital candidiasis, Letterer-Siwe disease, subcutaneous fat necrosis (adiponecrosis subcutanea neonatorum), sclerema neonatorum (sclerema adiposum), Leiner's disease, Ritter's disease, and congenital dysplasias.

DERMATOSES OF THE AGED

Among the dermatoses of the aged are actinic elastosis, purpura senilis, pruritus senilis, xerotic eczema, arteriosclerotic leg ulcer, varicose leg ulcer, thrombotic leg ulcer, corns, plantar callosities, alopecia senilis, seborrheic keratoses, comedones, keratoacanthomas, lentigines, actinic keratoses, cutaneous horns, senile telangiectasia, cherry angiomas, and skin carcinoma.

CUTANEOUS FINDINGS IN SYSTEMIC DISEASE

The human skin may mirror the presence of benign or malignant systemic disease in many different ways. Many times an unusual skin eruption may be a clue to some internal disorder that may not be obvious, and only by the presence of a dermatosis may it become evident that a systemic disease may be present.

Nodules. Subcutaneous or dermal metastatic nodules are the most frequent and most obvious manifestations of metastatic carcinoma. Although these nodules may arise anywhere on the skin, the most favored site is the trunk or scalp. They may be present for long periods with no lesions elsewhere. These nodules most frequently are metastases from carcinoma of the breast, gastrointestinal tract, lung, melanoma, ovary, or uterus. *Sister Mary Joseph's nodule* is a deep subcutaneous nodule that occurs periumbilically. It most commonly arises from a metastasizing gastric adenocarcinoma.

Multicentric reticulohistiocytosis may show numerous firm, red, brown, or yellow nodules 2 to 10 mm in width, occurring most frequently on the fingers and hands and less often over joints and bony prominences. Carcinoma may be present in up to 25 percent of cases.

Vascular Lesions. Petechiae, ecchymoses, "pinch purpura," and *caput medusae* are some of the vascular lesions associated with malignancies. "Pinch purpura," produced by pinching the skin, is seen most frequently on the forearms of the elderly, where it is known as senile (or better, actinic) purpura and is due to solar elastosis, or associated with systemic steroid therapy, with oral prednisone or, even more so, IM triamcinolone (steroid purpura). It may also be a characteristic presentation of amyloidosis of the skin. Purpura is a common sign of acute leukemia. Splinter hemorrhages may be present under the nails.

Flushing. Episodic flushing, especially of the face, lasting some 10 to 30 minutes, is a consistent sign of carcinoid syndrome. Bronchial carcinoid tumors may be manifested by severe and prolonged flushing episodes, facial and periorbital edema, excessive lacrimation, salivation, tachycardia, and hypotension.

Pruritus. Generalized pruritus may be seen in metastatic carcinoma, leukemia, myeloma, polycythemia vera, iron deficiency anemia, and especially Hodgkin's disease. The pruritus may be the sole cutaneous reaction, and may persist for years before the underlying cause can be identified. Hodgkin's disease is an example. Primary biliary cirrhosis, as already mentioned, is accompanied by intolerable pruritus and hyperpigmentation. Cholestatic jaundice usually itches severely. Diabetes mellitus may cause severe pruritus, although the dry skin that may accompany this malady certainly contributes to this pruritus. Anemia and thyroid disease may show pruritus. Carcinoid syndrome frequently is accompanied by pruritus, specifically of the palms and soles.

Eczema. A unilateral eczematous eruption on one nipple, though usually neurodermatitis, may be the first sign of Paget's disease of the breast with underlying intraductal carcinoma metastatic to the skin of the nipple. The early stages of mycosis fungoides may start with severe eczema over the various parts of the body, with intense pruritus. An eczematous eruption involving the hands, feet, nose, and ears is characteristic of Bazex's syndrome. This is associated with malignant neoplasms of the aerodigestive tract.

Vesicles and Bullae. Vesicles and eczematization are the signs of dermatitis herpetiformis, which may be associated with lymphoma of the small intestine. Abnormalities in the jejunal mucosa, indistinguish-

able from celiac disease, are associated with Duhring's disease (dermatitis herpetiformis). This is almost never of any clinical significance, however.

Grouped vesicles on an erythematous base occurring unilaterally are indicative of herpes zoster, which is only very rarely a sign of internal malignancy, especially of leukemia and lymphoma, or may presage the development of AIDS in a member of a predisposed patient population.

Erythema multiforme bullosum has a multiform morphology, ranging from single or multiple lesions of simple erythema to generalized exanthems with iris, polycyclic, or gyrate configuration. Vesicles and bullae may also be present. This type of eruption may occur in leukemia, drug reactions, or systemic infections.

Bullous pemphigoid in the elderly may occur with diabetes or with carcinoma, especially of the gastrointestinal tract. The lymphomas are less frequently associated with bullous pemphigoid. The association with cancer is no greater than in an age-matched population.

Ecthyma gangrenosum is manifested by rapidly enlarging hemorrhagic vesicles with surrounding erythema. It is caused by *Pseudomonas aeruginosa* as a secondary invader in patients with acute leukemia or other diseases causing immunosuppression.

Erythroderma (Exfoliative Dermatitis). Universal erythroderma, generally accompanied by scaling, may be associated with malignancy, usually lymphoma. This is characteristic of Sézary's syndrome. Severe drug reaction may also be the cause.

Erythema and Edema. Muscular weakness, especially with erythema and swelling and a purplish (heliotrope) discoloration of the eyelids, is indicative of dermatomyositis. Urticarial patches and erythema may appear, especially on the upper extremities and trunk. The incidence of neoplasia in patients over 40 years of age with dermatomyositis appears increased over that in the general population.

Tender, erythematous, edematous plaques on the upper part of the body associated with fever and leukocytosis characterize Sweet's syndrome. This may be the presenting sign of leukemia.

Erythematous Nodules. Erythema nodosum may occur in Hodgkin's and metastatic carcinoma. It may also be seen in leprosy, tuberculosis, sarcoidosis, histoplasmosis, coccidioidomycosis, blastomycosis, ulcerative colitis, and after drug use. The most common occurrence is following streptococcal pharyngitis.

Hyperkeratosis. Sézary's erythroderma, Hodgkin's disease, and lymphocytic leukemia may be accompanied by hyperkeratosis of the palms and soles, as may Bazex's syndrome. Howell-Evans has described a unique familial syndrome in which the hyperkeratosis of the palms and soles was followed by esophageal carcinoma. Of 48 members of a family with hyperkeratosis, 18 developed cancer. Of the 87 members of this family without hyperkeratosis, none developed cancer. Keratosis punctata palmaris et

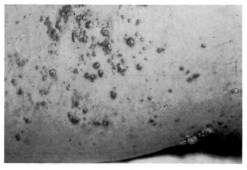

Figure 2–1. Metastases to the skin of the upper thigh from endometrial carcinoma, removed 4 years before.

plantaris has recently been linked to adenocarcinoma of the colon in one family by Bennion et al.

Hyperpigmentation. In metastatic melanoma a generalized darkening of the skin may occur. This is known as diffuse melanosis cutis. Usually melanuria is a prominent feature. Pituitary tumors may also cause this type of pigmentation as a result of increased secretion of melanocyte stimulating hormone (MSH) from the intermediate lobe. Bronze hyperpigmentation is seen in hemochromatosis and arsenic intoxication. Addisonian hyperpigmentation occurs in Addison's disease, which may be a manifestation of carcinoma metastatic to the adrenal glands.

Alopecia. When follicular mucinosis (alopecia mucinosa) occurs on the scalp or the bearded area, a sharply circumscribed area of alopecia occurs. This may be due to malignant lymphoma, specifically mycosis fungoides.

Hirsutism and Hypertrichosis. Adrenal or ovarian carcinomas may be the cause of excessive hair growth. Malignant down is an excessive growth of lanugo-like hair which is associated with malignant disease of the lung, colon, gallbladder, and uterus.

Urticaria. The chronic type may occur with necrotizing vasculitis, collagen vascular disease, penicillin or other drug sensitivity, serum sickness, and rarely in systemic mastocytosis. Hodgkin's disease may frequently be accompanied by urticaria. Cold urticaria with cryoglobulinemia is seen in multiple myeloma.

Sulfur Yellow Plaques on the Shins. Usually bilateral, these lesions have well-defined borders with a smooth glistening (glazed) surface. This is typical of necrobiosis lipoidica, with or without diabetes mellitus.

Dermatoses Associated with Systemic Disease. There are dermatoses that have various lesions connected with the entity and may be harbingers of systemic disease.

Gardner's Syndrome. Intestinal polyposis with dermal lipomas, fibromas, leiomyoma, epidermal cysts, and osteomas are typical of Gardner's syndrome. Intestinal malignant disease is believed to be inevitable with this syndrome.

Poikiloderma Vasculare Atrophicans. Lymphoma, Hodgkin's disease, mycosis fungoides, and rarely carcinoma may be associated with this rare disease.

Acanthosis Nigricans. The very rare juvenile or nevoid type of acanthosis nigricans is never associated with malignant disease. The vast majority of cases of the disorder are the result of obesity, sometimes associated with some endocrine disorder. Malignant acanthosis nigricans by definition is associated with internal malignancy, most frequently in the gastrointestinal tract, but carcinomas of the ovaries, lungs, and breasts may also cause it.

Other Skin Reactions. Numerous other cutaneous manifestations may be associated with systemic disease: for example, ichthyosis (lymphoma, AIDS, cancer), superficial migratory thrombophlebitis (cancer, especially pancreatic) telangiectasia (Bloom's syndrome, ataxia-telangiectasia), elastosis perforans serpiginosa (Down's syndrome), and erythema gyratum repens (cancer).

Bennion SD, et al: Keratosis punctata palmaris et plantaris and adenocarcinoma of the colon. JAAD 1984, 10:587.

Brownstein MH, et al: Metastatic tumors of the skin. Cancer 1972, 29:1298.

Catterall MD, et al: Multicentric reticulohistiocytosis and malignancy. Br J Dermatol 1978, 98:211.

Chanda JJ: Extramammary Paget's disease. JAAD 1985, 13:1009.

Chobanian SJ: Skin tags and colonic polyps. JAAD 1987, 16:407.

Dobson RL, et al: Palmar keratoses and cancer. Arch Dermatol 1965, 92:553.

Friedman-Kien AE, et al: Herpes zoster. JAAD 1986, 14:1023.

Hasan T, et al: Erythroderma: A follow-up of fifty cases. JAAD 1983, 8:836.

Holdiness MR: The sign of Leser-Trélat. Int J Dermatol 1986, 25:564.

Jemec GBE: Hypertrichosis lanuginosa acquisita. Arch Dermatol 1986, 122:805.

Jenkins D, et al: Histiocytic lymphoma occurring in a patient with dermatitis herpetiformis. JAAD 1983, 9:252.

Langlois JC, et al: Erythema gyratum repens unassociated with internal malignancy. JAAD 1985, 12:911.

Pecora AL, et al: Acrokeratosis paraneoplastica (Bazex's syndrome). Arch Dermatol 1983, 119:820.

Perry HO: Less common skin markers of visceral neoplasms. Int J Dermatol 1976, 15:19.

Powell FC, et al: Sister Mary Joseph's nodule: A clinical and histopathologic study. JAAD 1984, 10:610.

Wilkin JK: Flushing. Ann Intern Med 1981, 95:468.

3

Dermatoses Due to Physical Factors

The body requires a certain amount of heat, but beyond definite limits, insufficient or excessive amounts are injurious. The local action of excessive heat causes burns or scalds; on the other hand, undue cold causes chilblains, frostbite, and congelation. Thresholds of tolerance exist in all body structures sensitive to electromagnetic wave radiation of varying frequencies, such as x-rays and ultraviolet rays. The eye, which is sensitive to vibrations within the visible light range, is an example of a special sense organ that has similar limits. The skin, which is exposed to so many external physical forces, is more subject to injuries caused by them than is any other organ.

Page EH, et al: Temperature-dependent skin disorders. JAAD 1988, 18:1003.

HEAT INJURIES

THERMAL BURNS

A dermatitis of varying intensity may be caused by the action of excessive heat on the skin. If this heat is extreme, the skin and underlying tissue may even be destroyed. The changes in the skin due to dry heat or scalding are classified in four degrees. A **first-degree** burn of the skin results merely in an active congestion of the superficial blood vessels, causing an erythema that may be followed by epidermal desquamation (peeling). Ordinary sunburn is the most common example of a first-degree burn. The pain and increased surface heat may be severe, and it is not rare to have some constitutional reaction if the involved area is large.

When the burn is of **second degree** there is a transudation of serum from the capillaries, which causes edema of the superficial tissues. Vesicles and blebs are formed by the serum gathering beneath the outer layers of the epidermis. Complete recovery, without scar formation or other blemish, is usual in burns of these two degrees.

Third-degree burns are serious, as there is actual loss of tissue of the full thickness of the skin and even some of the subcutaneous tissues. The skin appendages are also destroyed, so that there is no epithelium available for regeneration of the skin. An ulcerating wound is produced, which in healing leaves a scar.

Fourth-degree burn is the destruction of the entire skin and subcutaneous fat with any underlying tendons. Both third- and fourth-degree burns require grafting for closure. All third- and fourth-degree burns are followed by constitutional symptoms of varied gravity, their severity depending upon the size of the involved surface, the depth of the burn, and particularly the location of the burned surface. It appears that the more vascular the involved area, the more severe the symptoms.

Symptoms of shock may appear within 24 hours after the burn. These are followed by symptoms of toxemia from absorption of destroyed tissue on the surface of the wound. Lastly, there may be symptoms from wound infection, the result of contamination with pyogenic organisms. The symptoms of these three conditions may merge so that differentiation is difficult.

The prognosis is poor in any patient in whom a large area of skin surface is involved. It is particularly serious if more than two thirds of the body surface has been burned. In addition to the infection of the wound and surrounding cutaneous tissue with cellulitis or erysipelas, sepsis, with seeding of internal organs, such as the meninges, lungs, or kidneys, may occur. Irregularities in electrolytes and fluid balance and loss of serum proteins are other complications.

Excessive scarring, with either keloidlike scars or flat scars with contractures, may produce deformities and dysfunctions of the joints as well as chronic ulcerations due to impairment of the local circulation. Later changes of a malignant nature in the scar may result in carcinoma or sarcoma. With modern reconstructive surgery these unfortunate end results can be minimized.

TREATMENT. Immediate first aid for minor thermal burns consists of prompt cold applications (ice water, or cold tap water if no ice is at hand) continued until pain does not return on stopping them.

The vesicles or blebs of second-degree burns should not be opened but should be protected from injury, since they form a natural barrier against contamination with microorganisms. If they become tense and unduly painful, the fluid may be evacuated under strictly aseptic conditions by puncturing the wall with a sterile needle, allowing the blister to collapse upon the underlying wound, and then applying a topical antibiotic. In severe deep burns silver sulfadiazine (Silvadene) ointment has been found effective in the control of burn wound infections. Recently developed skin substitutes, which employ collagen-synthetic bilaminate membranes, are enjoying increasing use in coverage of these wounds. In many centers, cultured epidermal grafts, both autologous and allogeneic, are being used, with promising results.

Morbidity and mortality following severe burns are often due to bacterial and fungal infection; therefore, treatment should be directed against this complication. After the usual first-aid treatment, definitive therapy consists of antishock measures, debridement of loose skin and dirt, and the application of 0.5 per cent silver nitrate solution wet dressings that are then encased in dry sheets and blankets. Antibiotics and fluid and electrolyte support are given, and good nutrition is maintained, with supplemental vitamins.

In severe deep second- and third-degree burns, large doses of heparin intravenously have relieved pain without the development of edema, toxic reactions, or shock.

Split-thickness grafts are applied after the eschar has been removed by tangential excision. Grafting should be done as soon as possible. Severe second- and third-degree burns require specialized teams of physicians working together to give the most effective treatment, because many problems are involved.

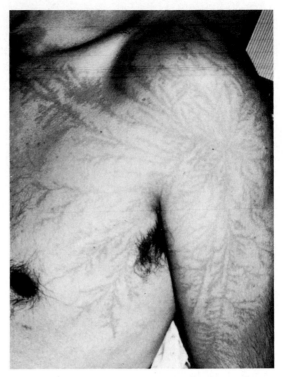

Figure 3–1. "Christmas tree" pattern in the skin, a characteristic marker of being struck by lightning. (Courtesy of Dr. C. W. Bartholome.)

Electrical Burns. These are of two varieties, contact and flash. A contact burn is small but deep, causing some necrosis of the underlying tissues, which later separate and are thrown off. Flash burns usually cover a large area and, being similar to any surface burn, are treated as such.

Hot Tar Burns. Demling has reported that the polyoxyethylene sorbitan in Neosporin ointment is an excellent dispersing agent that facilitates the removal of hot tar from burns.

Artz CP, et al: Management of burns. Military Med 1976, 141:673.
Demling R, et al: Management of hot tar burns. J Trauma 1980, 20:242.
Falanga VL: Occlusive wound dressings. Arch Dermatol 1988, 124:872.
Monafo WW: The treatment of burns with compresses wet with 0.5 per cent silver nitrate solution. Med Clin N Am 1967, 47:1029.
Pruitt BA, et al: Characteristics and uses of biologic dressings and skin substitutes. Arch Surg 1984, 119:312.
Saliba MJ Jr, et al: Large burns in humans—treatment with heparin. JAMA 1973, 225:261.
Spicer TE: Burns. Select Read Plastic Surg 1985, 3:1.

MILIARIA

The retention of sweat as a result of occlusion of eccrine sweat ducts and pores produces an eruption which is common in hot humid climates such as the tropics and during the hot summer months in the temperate climates. The occlusion prevents normal secretion from the sweat glands and eventually the

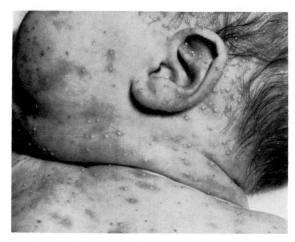

Figure 3–2. Miliaria crystallina: uniform minute crystal-clear vesicles. (Courtesy of Dr. Axel W. Hoke.)

back-up pressure causes rupture of the sweat gland or duct at different levels. The escape of sweat into the adjacent tissue produces anatomic changes to produce miliaria. Depending upon the level of the sweat gland or duct injury, several different forms of "prickly heat" are recognized.

TYPES

Miliaria Crystallina (Sudamina). This is characterized by small clear and very superficial vesicles without an inflammatory reaction; it appears in bedridden patients whose fevers produce increased perspiration. The lesions are asymptomatic and their duration is short-lived because of the tendency to rupture upon the slightest trauma.

The lesions are self-limited, and no treatment is required.

Miliaria Rubra (Prickly Heat, Heat Rash). These lesions appear as discrete, extremely pruritic, erythematous papulovesicles. They later may become confluent in a bed of erythema. The sites most frequently affected are the antecubital and popliteal fossae, the trunk, the inframammary areas (especially under pendulous breasts), the abdomen (especially at the waistline), and the inguinal regions; these sites frequently become macerated because evaporation of moisture has been impeded. The site of injury and sweat escape is in the prickle cell layer, where spongiosis is produced.

Miliaria Pustulosa. This type of miliaria is always preceded by some other dermatitis that has produced injury, destruction, or blocking of the sweat duct. The pustules are distinct, superficial, and independent of the hair follicle. The pruritic pustules occur most frequently on the intertriginous areas, on the flexure surfaces of the extremities, and on the scrotum. Contact dermatitis, lichen simplex chronicus, and intertrigo are some of the associated diseases, although pustular miliaria may occur several weeks after the diseases have subsided. Usually the contents of the pustules are sterile, but they may contain nonpathogenic cocci.

Miliaria Profunda. Nonpruritic flesh-colored vesi-

cles that appear to be uninflamed papules characterize this form of miliaria. With the exception of the face, axillae, hands, and feet, all the sweat glands are nonfunctional. The occlusion is in the upper dermis. This form is observed only in the tropics and usually follows a severe bout of miliaria rubra.

Postmiliarial Hypohidrosis. This results from occlusion of sweat ducts and pores and may be severe enough to impair one's ability to perform sustained work in heat. Affected persons may show decreasing efficiency, irritability, anorexia, drowsiness, vertigo, and headache; they may wander in a daze.

It has been shown that hypohidrosis invariably follows miliaria, and that the duration and severity of the hypohidrosis are related to the severity of the miliarial involvement. Further, sweating may be depressed to half the normal amount for as much as three weeks following miliaria.

Tropical Anhidrotic Asthenia. This is a rare form of miliaria with long-lasting poral occlusion, which produces anhidrosis and heat retention.

Occlusion Miliaria. A similar picture occurs with the application of extensive polyethylene film occlusion for 48 or more hours. Miliaria may be produced with accompanying anhidrosis and increased heat stress susceptibility.

TREATMENT. The most effective treatment for miliaria is to place the patient in a cool environment. Even one night in an air-conditioned room helps to alleviate the discomfort. Next best is the use of circulating air fans to aid in cooling the skin.

Anhydrous lanolin resolves poral occlusion and may help to restore normal sweat secretion. Hydrophilic ointment also helps to dissolve keratinous plugs and facilitates the normal flow of sweat.

Soothing, cooling baths containing Aveeno colloidal oatmeal or cornstarch are beneficial if used in moderation.

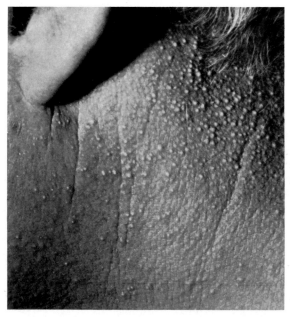

Figure 3–3. Miliaria pustulosa: red papules and pustules.

Mild cases may respond to dusting powders such as cornstarch or baby talcum powder. A lotion containing 1 per cent menthol and glycerin and 4 per cent salicylic acid in 95 per cent alcohol is also effective. This should be dabbed on the affected areas several times daily until desquamation sets in.

An oily shake lotion such as calamine liniment, with 1 or 2 per cent phenol, or a corticosteroid ointment (not cream) may be even more effective.

Ascorbic acid, 1 gm daily by mouth, is also purportedly helpful, though we cannot confirm it.

Griffin TB, et al: Miliaria and anhidrosis. J Invest Dermatol 1967, 49:379.
Rochmis PG, et al: Iatrogenic miliaria crystallina due to betanechol. Arch Dermatol 1967, 95:499.
Sulzberger MB, et al: Miliaria and anhidrosis. Arch Dermatol 1972, 105:845.

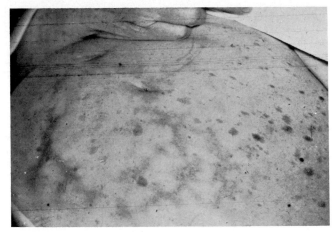

Figure 3–4. *Pigmentatio ab igne from years of application of a hot water bottle to the abdomen.*

ERYTHEMA (PIGMENTATIO) AB IGNE

Erythema ab igne, "toasted skin" syndrome, is a persistent erythema—or the coarsely reticulated residual pigmentation resulting from it—that is usually produced by long-continued exposure to excessive heat without the production of a burn. It begins as a mottling due to local hemostasis and becomes a reticulated erythema, leaving pigmentation. All the various phases usually are simultaneously present in a patch, the color varying from pale pink to old rose or dark purplish brown. After the cause is removed, the affection tends to disappear gradually, but sometimes the pigmentation is permanent.

Histologically, an increased amount of elastic tissue in the dermis is noted. The changes in erythema ab igne are similar to those of actinic elastosis, and it has been suggested these changes be termed "thermal elastosis."

Erythema ab igne is most common on the legs of women as a result of habitually warming them in front of open fireplaces, radiators, or heaters. Similar changes may be produced with a hot water bag or electric heating pad. The disease occurs also in cooks, stokers, invalids, and others exposed over long periods to the direct action of moderate heat. Epithelial atypia, including one instance of Bowen's disease, has rarely been reported to occur overlying erythema ab igne.

The use of bland emollients is helpful. There is no effective treatment, though Kligman's combination of 5 per cent hydroquinone in hydrophilic ointment containing 0.1 per cent retinoic acid and 0.1 per cent dexamethasone may help reduce unsightly pigmentation.

Arrington JH, et al: Thermal keratosis and squamous cell carcinoma in situ associated with erythema ab igne. Arch Dermatol 1979, 115:1226.
Finlayson GR, et al: Erythema ab igne. J Invest Dermatol 1966, 46:104.

COLD INJURIES

Local cold injuries are divided into chilblain, frostbite, and immersion foot. Whereas chilblain and frostbite occur sporadically in civil life, immersion foot is encountered almost entirely in the armed forces.

Intense vasoconstriction due to the local action of cold and reflex vasoconstrictor stimulation is reinforced by the passage of cold blood through the vasomotor center. Vasoconstriction provokes tissue anoxia. Decreased muscular activity further diminishes the blood supply. Ice crystal formation in the blood vessels does not usually occur, but when it does, necrosis ensues.

CHILBLAIN (Pernio)

CLINICAL SIGNS AND SYMPTOMS. Chilblain is a recurrent localized erythema and swelling caused by exposure to cold. Blistering and ulcerations may develop in severe cases. In people predisposed by poor peripheral circulation, even moderate exposure to cold may produce chilblain. Acute chilblain is the mildest form of cold injury. This occurs chiefly on the hands, feet, ears, and face, especially in children, the onset being favored by dampness. Patients are usually unaware of the injury at first, but later burning, itching, and redness call it to their attention.

The areas are bluish red, the color disappearing on pressure, and are decidedly cool to the touch. Sometimes the extremities are clammy because of excessive sweating.

Chronic chilblains occur repeatedly during cold weather and disappear during warm weather. The affected extremities are cold, cyanotic, and often hyperhidrotic. Cryoglobulinemia may be present and chilblain-like lesions may occur in discoid and systemic lupus erythematosus.

A condition was described by Toback et al in which painful plaques and vesicles developed on the hands of a group of campers who lived on a boat where there was exposure to cold and moisture. They called this "pulling boat" (the name of their open rowing/sailing craft) hands.

TREATMENT. The circulation should be improved by regular exercise. Vasodilators such as nicotinamide 100 mg three times a day or dipyridamole 25 mg three times a day are used for improvement of circulation. Systemic corticoid therapy is useful in chilblain lupus erythematosus, and Rustin et al showed that the calcium channel blocker nifedipine was effective. Trental should be effective.

The parts should be cleansed with water and massaged gently with warm oil each day and should be protected against further injury and exposure to cold or dampness. If the feet are affected, woolen socks should be worn at night during the cold months. Electric pads should be used to warm the parts. Smoking is prohibited.

Herman EW, et al: A distinctive variant of pernio. Arch Dermatol 1981, 117:26.

Millard LG, et al: Chilblain lupus erythematosus (Hutchinson). Br J Dermatol 1978, 98:497.

Rustin MHA, et al: Treatment of chilblains with nifedipine. Br J Dermatol 1989, 120:267.

Toback AC, et al: Pulling boat hands. JAAD 1985, 12:649.

FROSTBITE (Congelatio)

CLINICAL SIGNS. When the soft parts are frozen and locally deprived of blood supply, the affection is termed frostbite. The ears, nose, cheeks, fingers, and toes are most often affected. The frozen part becomes pale and waxy but there is scarcely any pain or discomfort. Various degrees of tissue destruction similar to those caused by burns are encountered. These are erythema and edema, vesicles and bullae, superficial gangrene, deep gangrene, and injury to muscles, tendons, periosteum, and nerves.

TREATMENT. Early treatment of frostbite before swelling develops should consist of covering the part with clothing or with the warm hand or other body surface to maintain a slightly warm temperature so that adequate blood circulation can be maintained. Rapid rewarming in a water bath between 100 and 110°F is the treatment of choice for all forms of frostbite. Slow thawing results in more extensive tissue damage. Analgesics, unless contraindicated, should be administered, owing to the considerable pain experienced with rapid thawing. When the skin flushes and is pliable, thawing is complete. Supportive measures such as bed rest, a high-protein–high-caloric diet, wound care, and avoidance of trauma are imperative. Any rubbing of the affected part should be avoided, but gentle massage of proximal portions of the extremity that are not numb may be helpful.

After swelling and hyperemia have developed, the patient should be kept in bed with the affected limb slightly flexed, elevated, and at rest. Exposing the affected limb to air at room temperature relieves pain and helps prevent tissue damage. Protection by a heat cradle may be desirable.

The use of anticoagulants to prevent thrombosis and gangrene has been advocated. Papaverine or

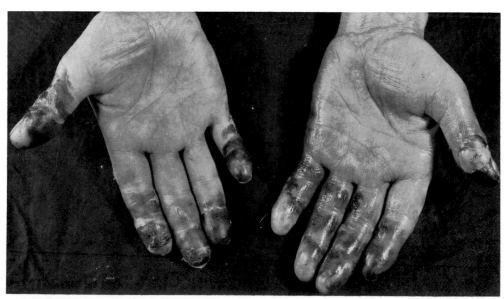

Figure 3–5. Frostbite. Note highlights, caused by hyperhidrosis. (Courtesy of Dr. H. Shatin.)

nicotinic acid may be given to reduce vasospasm. Antibiotics should be given as a prophylactic measure against infection, and tetanus immunization should be updated. Recovery may take many months.

Corbett DW: Cold injuries. J Assoc Milit Dermatol 1982, 8:34.
Lapp NL, et al: Frostbite. Mayo Clin Proc 1965, 49:932.

IMMERSION FOOT SYNDROMES

Trench Foot

Trench foot results from prolonged exposure to cold without actual freezing. The term is derived from "trench warfare" in World War I, when soldiers stood, sometimes for hours, in trenches with a few inches of cold water in them. The lack of circulation produces edema, paresthesias, and damage to the blood vessels. Gangrene may occur in severe cases.

Treatment consists of removal from the causal environment, bed rest, and restoration of the circulation. Other measures, such as those used in the treatment of frostbite, should be employed.

Tropical Immersion Foot

Immersion of the feet in warm water for 48 hours or more may produce a syndrome similar to trench foot, known as tropical immersion foot or **warm-water immersion foot.** It was common in Vietnam, where troops were exposed to prolonged or repeated wading in paddy fields or streams. It has been reported more recently in personnel wearing insulated boots for long periods—the "moon boot" syndrome.

The clinical manifestations are maceration, blanching, and wrinkling of the soles and sides of the feet. Itching and burning with erythema and swelling may persist a few days after removal of the cause, but disability is temporary.

Warm-water immersion foot can be prevented by allowing the feet to dry for a few hours out of every 24, or by greasing the soles with a silicone grease once a day. Recovery from it is usually rapid if the feet are thoroughly dried for a few hours.

Adnot J, et al: Immersion foot syndromes. J Assoc Milit Dermatol 1985, 11:87.

DERMATOSES WITH COLD HYPERSENSITIVITY

Exposure to cold may produce abnormal reactions in several dermatoses. The reactions are mediated most frequently through abnormal globulins such as cryoglobulin and cryofibrinogen. In addition, histamine, serotonin, leukotrienes, prostaglandins, kinins, and cold hemolysins may be involved.

Some of these reactions are those of Raynaud's phenomenon, ulcerations, necrotic plaques, urticaria, purpura, cyanosis, and hemorrhagic bullae.

ERYTHROCYANOSIS CRURUM

Various names have been given to this and similar diseases in which the chief characteristics are a slight swelling and a bluish pink tint of the skin of the legs and thighs of young girls and women. The disease may be unilateral. Atypical varieties are common, some presenting cinnabar red spots, bullae, indurations, and lichenoid papules. There may be a history of cramps in the legs at night. Upon palpation small tender nodules may be found as a result of fat necrosis in the deep dermis. These nodules may break down and form small, often multiple ulcers, as in erythema induratum. As a rule, the affected limbs are cold to the touch. The disease is seen mostly in northern countries and is considered to be an abnormal reaction of the blood vessels to prolonged exposure to cold.

ACROCYANOSIS

Acrocyanosis is a persistent cyanosis with coldness and hyperhidrosis of the fingers and hands and sometimes also of the toes and feet. It occurs chiefly in girls and young women, but is not rare in young men. At times, upon exposure to cold, a digit becomes stark white and insensitive (acroasphyxia). The etiology is unknown. In severe cases sympathectomy is the only treatment. Smoking, coffee, and tea should be avoided.

Remittent necrotizing acrocyanosis is a term applied to functional vascular spasm or organic occlusion that produces pain in the hands and feet, with areas of coldness and cyanosis and necrosis of the tips of the fingers and toes. This has occurred without prodromal or constitutional symptoms. It must be differentiated from acrosclerosis and Raynaud's syndrome.

Trental should be very helpful.

Bigby M, et al: Reddish-blue hands and feet. Arch Dermatol 1988, 124:263.

COLD PANNICULITIS

Following exposure to severe cold, well-demarcated erythematous warm plaques may develop, particularly on the cheeks of young children. The lesions usually develop within two days after exposure. The induration resolves spontaneously in about two weeks.

The lesions are readily reproducible in these patients by placing an ice cube on the volar aspect of the forearm for two minutes.

Laboratory findings are characteristically within normal limits. These include serum protein electrophoresis, cold agglutinins, cryoglobulins, cryofibrinogens, and immunoelectrophoresis.

This type of panniculitis is seen mostly in young children, who are believed to have excessive amounts of saturated fatty acids in the immature subcutaneous fat. There is also a higher solidification point of the saturated fatty acid.

Patients outgrow this susceptibility. No treatment is indicated.

Popsicle dermatitis is a temporary redness and induration of the cheek in children resulting from sucking popsicles. No connection has been found with true cold panniculitis.

Beacham et al described indurated, red, tender plaques which appeared on the upper outer thighs of young women who were horseback riding outdoors in winter. These were lesions of cold panniculitis.

Beacham BE, et al: Equestrian cold panniculitis in women. Arch Dermatol 1980, 116:1025.

Duncan WC, et al: Cold panniculitis. Arch Dermatol 1966, 94:722.

Rotman H: Cold panniculitis in children. Arch Dermatol 1968, 94:720.

ACTINIC INJURY

SUNBURN

Light from the sun consists of three types of radiation, one of which is visible radiation, in the spectral range of 400 to 760 nm (violet through red), which has little biological activity except for its ability to stimulate the retina. Beyond 760 nm is infrared radiation, experienced as radiant heat. Below 400 nm is the ultraviolet spectrum, divided into three bands, as shown in Table 3–1.

The usual ultraviolet light source, the mercury-vapor lamp or sunlamp bulb, produces mostly UVB, which is the strongest inducer of erythema (sunburn). "PUVA" light therapy uses bulbs that produce only UVA, so that burning may be avoided at therapeutic dose levels. Immediate pigment-darkening (IPD) is produced and maintained by UVA.

The sun, whose rays contain 100 times more UVA than UVB during the mid-day hours, still burns us with just UVB, which induces little IPD. A good UVB sunscreen puts UVB and UVA on an almost equal footing as a source of sunburn, and the fact that UVA is reflected from sand, snow, or ice much better than UVB puts it a little ahead again in the race to cause sunburn, but only with a screen and only late (or early) in the day. Mostly, we are burned by UVB.

CLINICAL SIGNS AND SYMPTOMS. Sunburn is a normal human reaction to sunlight in excess of an erythema dose: i.e., the amount that will induce reddening (after a latent period of four to eight hours) in an individual's skin. The initial evidence is reddening, then soreness, and finally, in severe cases, blistering, which may become confluent. Discomfort may be severe; edema commonly occurs in the extremities and face; chills, fever, nausea, shock, and a sense of impending dissolution may be present. In severe cases such symptoms may last for as long as a week. As the redness subsides and the blisters collapse, desquamation begins.

In the meantime, skin pigment undergoes two changes: immediate pigment-darkening (IPD, Meirowsky phenomenon); and delayed melanogenesis, beginning in two to three days and lasting 10 to 14 days. With large doses of UVA, the initial darkening is prolonged and may blend into the delayed melanogenesis, though the exfoliation after a burn will shed much of the new pigment that is formed.

ETIOLOGY. The burn is caused, when its source is sunlight, wholly by UVB, even though there is only 1/100 as much UVB as UVA in sunlight. Delayed melanogenesis is also induced very largely by UVB, though UVA also contributes to it and will produce it even when UVB is blocked by a sunscreen, or by the atmosphere before 9 AM or after 3 PM.

Reflection of the sun's rays exaggerates the effect of UVA more than that of UVB, and is significant off sand, snow, or ice at any time of day, but reflection off water is significant only before 9 AM or after 3 PM, since between those hours the sun's rays are almost completely absorbed by the water.

The intensity of sunlight and its reflection off water

Table 3–1. ULTRAVIOLET SPECTRUM

	UVA 340–390 NM	UVB 290–340 NM	UVC 200–290 NM
Abundance in mid-day sun	100	1	0
Immediate pigment darkening potency	10	0	0
Melanogenic stimulation	1	1000	?
Sunburn potency	1	1000	?
Penetration	Through dermis	Into dermis	To dermis

are affected not only by the time of day but also by season and latitude. Cloudiness, unless very heavy, absorbs mainly visible light and transmits most of the ultraviolet.

COMPLICATIONS OF SUNBURN. Acute sunburn, even if very slight, may trigger the recurrence or exacerbation of herpes simplex, lupus erythematosus, porphyria cutanea tarda, solar urticaria, polymorphous light eruption, erythema multiforme, and other photoaggravated disorders.

PATHOGENESIS. The vasodilatation that occurs in UVB-induced erythema appears to be mediated by prostaglandins PGE_2 and PGF_2. These increase in skin after exposure to UVB, whereas there is no associated increase in histamine or kinins. Prostaglandin inhibitors such as aspirin and indomethacin inhibit both the increase in prostaglandins and much of the associated erythema. Systemic symptoms, such as fever, appear to be mediated by interleukin-1. The mechanism of UVA- and PUVA-induced erythema is unknown and is apparently not mediated by prostaglandins.

TREATMENT. Though some slight relief can be obtained by ice-cold milk or water compresses, and by taking 10 grains of aspirin every two hours, a sunburn victim generally has to suffer through at least a day or two of discomfort and even pain before much relief occurs. An effective topical remedy for treatment of severe sunburn due to UVB is the following:

Indomethacin	100 mg
Absolute ethanol	57 ml
Propylene glycol	57 ml

Sig.: Spread widely over burned area with palms and let dry.

Indomethacin or aspirin taken orally is also helpful, probably by suppressing prostaglandin formation in the skin. A 2.5% solution of indomethacin appears to be an effective sunscreen, according to Gschnait et al. Richard Gange warns against topical use until percutaneous absorption and systemic toxicity have been evaluated; however, a 2-ml application would—even if completely absorbed—provide a dose of only 50 mg.

PROPHYLAXIS. Within a few hours after radiation exposure has occurred, sunburn due to UVB can still be prevented almost completely by a large dose of steroids, 60 to 80 mg of prednisone daily, or a comparable dose of any other steroid, either orally or parenterally. Very large accidental overdoses of UVB have been rendered harmless in this way. Such treatment is also highly effective, as one would expect, if given before the exposure occurs.

The opportunity to do this, however, is rare, and protection for the most part should consist of prudence in timing one's exposure to sunlight or artificial UV. Persons who know that they burn easily and tan poorly should in general expose themselves for only 10 minutes on each side the first day, and increase the time gradually. The various factors of weather, hour of day, season, latitude, clarity of atmosphere, paleness of skin, type of complexion, and type of sunscreen, make for a very complex determination of how long an exposure one can tolerate. One can only say that it is best to err on the side of conservatism.

For immediate protection of the easily burned person who wishes to spend some time in the sun for recreational or occupational reasons, hundreds of proprietary sunscreen preparations are available, all of which are reasonably effective, and some of which are very effective.

The sunscreening agent's efficacy in absorbing the UVB (sunburn-inducing) radiation is expressed by a Sun Protection Factor (SPV), which is the number of MEDs of radiation required to induce a burn through a thin film of the protecting cream or lotion.

The most efficient sunscreen is 5 per cent para-aminobenzoic acid (PABA) in ethanol lotion. This permits tanning by passing UVA and blocking UVB. The disadvantages of this otherwise efficient lotion are that it is drying and it stains. Such preparations include Pabanol, PreSun, Supershade, and Solar cream. Some of these (PreSun) now are also prepared in an emollient base.

The more cosmetically elegant preparations are those containing PABA esters. These contain emollients and also permit tanning. Some of these preparations are Eclipse, Total Eclipse, Pabafilm, Block Out, Sundown, and Coppertone Super Shade. All of these preparations are pleasant to use. Rarely, PABA may sensitize, and "PABA-free" sunscreens are now being marketed.

A new class of UVA-blocking sunscreens, the dibenzoylmethanes, has been introduced into the U.S., not for protection against sunburn, but for prevention of the photoallergic UVA-mediated reactions. Photoplex is such a screen.

Those sunscreens containing cinnamates and benzophenones are also efficient and cosmetically elegant; however, sensitization may occur rarely. Preparations of this type are Sundare lotion, Maxafil, Solbar, Uval, and Piz Buin.

The opaque sunscreens, zinc oxide, titanium dioxide, kaolin, talc, and iron oxide, which reflect and scatter ultraviolet, are the most effective sunscreens, but cosmetically less desirable. These are A-Fil, RVPaque, Shadow, Reflecta, and Covermark.

Patients who sunburn with only a few minutes' exposure can be helped to tolerate longer exposures by the use of psoralens, but it is unwise to achieve this, as it will permit increased sun exposure, and the danger of promoting the production of skin cancer is considerable. The advice given in our seventh edition is regretted, and withdrawn.

TANNING. There are two components of sun tan, the familiar darkening of the skin in sunlight that is experienced by most people. First to happen is immediate pigment-darkening (IPD, Meirowsky phenomenon), induced entirely by UVA. Its duration is proportional to the amount of irradiation received, within broad limits. All of the melanin already present, pathologic as well as normal, undergoes this oxidative darkening. IPD provides little protection against subsequent sunburn.

The second and more important component is melanogenesis: formation of new, additional melanin. It is stimulated far more by UVB than by UVA. The melanogenic response to a single exposure continues for about two weeks. It does provide significant protection against subsequent sunburn. A few individuals can get this response without prior sunburn, but most require a mild burn, and some individuals, notably red or sandy-haired individuals of Celtic ancestry, cannot acquire any new pigmentation without a prior severe sunburn. Therefore tanning may be impossible for them, and is inadvisable considering the adverse long-term effects of UVB in this patient population.

Gschnait F, et al: Topical indomethacin protects from UVB and UVA radiation. Arch Derm Res 1984, 276:131.
Pathak MA: Sunscreens, topical and systemic. JAAD 1982, 7:285.
Po-Fitzpatrick MB: The biologic action of solar radiation on skin with a note on sunscreens. J Dermatol Surg Oncol 1977, 3:199.
Willis I: Sunlight and the skin. JAMA 1971, 217:1088.

CHRONIC ACTINIC DAMAGE
(Chronic Solar Dermatitis)

This type of skin inflammation is precancerous and can lead to basal cell or squamous cell carcinoma. In addition, chronic sun exposure may lead to the development of vitiligo, telangiectasia, photoaging, immune suppression, actinic keratoses, solar elastosis, and various papillomas. It aggravates lupus erythematosus, porphyria cutanea tarda, xeroderma pigmentosum, and skin lesions of pellagra.

The most susceptible to the deleterious effects of sunlight are those blue-eyed fair-complexioned persons who do not tan readily; they are frequently of Irish, other Celtic, or Anglo-Saxon descent. Susceptibility to actinic degeneration of the skin and the development of carcinoma is diminished by the amount of pigment in the skin.

Sailor's Skin, Farmer's Skin. These are but two of the many terms used to describe the type of skin that develops in white people, especially the fair-skinned, after many years of almost constant exposure to sunlight. Many of the changes now known to be due to chronic sunlight exposure were formerly ascribed to aging. The skin becomes dry, thin, and inelastic; pigmented and white atrophic macules are observed.

The V area of the neck and chest, the face, and the backs of the hands are the usual sites of involvement. Changes in the elastic fibers and collagen degeneration occur as a result of sunlight exposure.

Prevention consists of the use of sunscreens while exposed and the regular use of emollients or moisturizing creams. Removal of the damaged skin by dermabrasion is the only effective treatment, and it is only possible to do it on the face or scalp; in other areas the results are poor.

Weiss et al published a small study in 1988 stating that the use of 0.1 per cent tretinoin cream would reverse the changes of photoaging, just as Kligman predicted a decade ago. The evidence is extremely persuasive.

Actinic Elastosis. *Solar elastosis* and *senile elastosis* are other terms frequently used for the type of skin that develops after prolonged exposure to the sun's rays. Small yellowish papules and plaques develop on the face and backs of the hands in fair-skinned persons who are overexposed to the sun over a period of years. The skin assumes a dull yellowish color with deep furrows and wrinkles. It becomes leathery and subject to the development of actinic keratoses and carcinomata.

Graham Smith has shown that there is increased elastic-tissue–staining in the dermis. This elastotic material, which is newly formed and differs from normal elastic tissue, is found in the upper part of the dermis. The fibroblast produces this elastotic material instead of collagen in actinic elastosis.

In addition to the elastic fiber changes, the collagen is also altered; there is reduction in proline and hydroxyproline; there is an increase in hexosamine, total acid mucopolysaccharides (acid glycosaminoglycans), and hyaluronic acid in the skin exposed to sunlight.

Poikiloderma of Civatte. This common sun-induced disorder consists of telangiectasia, hyperpigmentation, and slight atrophy of the sides of the neck, lower anterior neck, and V of the chest. The submental area, shaded by the chin, is spared.

Cutis Rhomboidalis Nuchae. The skin on the back of the neck becomes thickened, tough, and leathery so that the normal skin markings are exaggerated. This, together with tanning, produces a distinctive picture.

Farmers, sailors, and sportsmen who are exposed

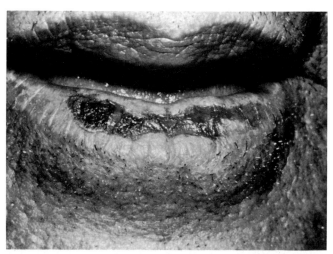

Figure 3–6. Severe actinic cheilitis. (Courtesy of Dr. Axel W. Hoke.)

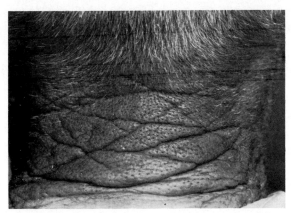

Figure 3–7. Cutis rhomboidalis nuchae, seen in men after years of exposure to sunlight. (Courtesy of Dr. A. Kaminsky.)

to a great amount of sunlight are especially prone to this.

Nodular Elastoidosis. Also known as **Favre-Racouchot syndrome,** this is seen mostly around the eyes and extends onto the cheeks in the elderly, especially in men. The lesions consist of giant comedones, follicular cysts, and large folds of furrowed and yellowed skin.

The elastoidosis may be accompanied by other solar degenerative changes such as cutis rhomboidalis nuchae, actinic keratoses, and carcinoma.

The Favre-Racouchot syndrome is seen in people who have spent much time outdoors. Sun, wind, and perhaps cold are some of the causative factors, but sun is paramount.

Treatment is the removal of the large comedones and cystic lesions. Retinoic acid cream 0.05 per cent applied nightly is effective in clearing the comedones.

Actinic Cheilitis. This occurs mostly on the lower lip, on which excessive sunlight exposure produces dryness, scaling, atrophy, and telangiectasia. Fissures, keratoses, leukoplakia, and carcinomas may also occur on the lips as a result of the chronic cheilitis. This type of cheilitis responds well to cryosurgery or to 5 per cent fluorouracil solution or cream, which should always be tried before resorting to cheiloplasty. Sunscreen lipsticks, Sun Stik, RVP Stik, PreSun, and Eclipse are available, and susceptible persons should use them.

Actinic Keratosis. This is also known as solar keratosis or senile keratosis. On the sun-exposed areas, especially on the face, ears, and backs of the hands, numerous 1- to 10-mm, erythematous, slightly scaling, ill-defined patches develop, especially in light-skinned middle-aged people who have a long history of frequent sunlight exposure. These are precancerous lesions. Microscopically they merge into intraepidermal, noninvasive carcinoma. They are discussed in more detail in Chapter 28.

Skin Cancer. Basal and squamous cell carcinomas and melanoma are enhanced by total hours of exposure to UVB and perhaps UVA as well. The risk of melanoma appears to be increased by intermittent severe sunburn, especially when these exposures take place in childhood.

PREVENTION. A sunscreen of SPF 15 or 20, used daily year round, is recommended. The only serious adverse effect is vitamin D deficiency, as reviewed by Prystowsky.

Goette DK, et al: Post-irradiation angiosarcoma. JAAD 1985, 12:922.
Idem: Post-irradiation malignant fibrous histiocytoma. Arch Dermatol 1985, 121:535.
Kligman LH, et al: Prevention of ultraviolet damage to the skin of hairless mice by sunscreens. J Invest Dermatol 1982, 78:181.
Prystowsky JH: Photoprotection and the vitamin D status of the elderly. Arch Dermatol 1988, 124:1844.

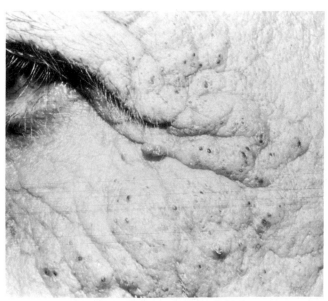

Figure 3–8. Periorbital elastosis and comedones of Favre-Racouchot syndrome. (Courtesy of Dr. Axel W. Hoke.)

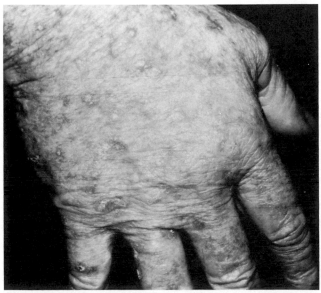

Figure 3–9. Actinic keratoses, dorsum of hand, a frequent site. (Courtesy of Dr. Axel W. Hoke.)

Salasche SJ, et al: Cutaneous manifestations of chronic solar exposure. J Assoc Milit Dermatol 1985, 11:3.

Smith JG Jr: The dermal elastoses. Arch Dermatol 1963, 88:382.

Warin AP: The ultraviolet erythemas in man. Br J Dermatol 1978, 98:473.

Weiss JS, et al: Topical tretinoin improves photoaged skin. JAMA 1988, 259:527.

Winton GB, et al: Dermabrasion of the scalp as a treatment for actinic damage. JAAD 1986, 14:661.

CHRONIC ACTINIC DERMATITIS

In parallel with chronic actinic damage (v.s.) but independent of it is a spectrum of disorders, chiefly UVA-induced, beginning with *photoallergic dermatitis* and progressing through *persistent light eruption* to *actinic reticuloid.* Soter spoke on this entity at the 1989 meeting of the American Dermatological Association.

Soter NA: Chronic actinic dermatitis. Paper read before the annual meeting of the American Dermatological Association, 1989.

EPHELIS (Freckle)

Freckles are yellowish, brownish, or black macules that occur in profusion on the sun-exposed skin of the face, neck, shoulders, and backs of the hands. They become prominent during the summer when exposed to sunlight and subside, sometimes completely, during the winter when there is no exposure. Blonds, redheads, and mulattoes are especially susceptible to the disorder.

Ephelides may be genetically determined and may recur in successive generations in similar locations and patterns. There may be a delay in their appearance after birth till about the seventh year of life.

Ephelis (freckle) must be differentiated from lentigo simplex. The lentigo is a benign discrete hyperpigmented macule appearing at any age and on any part of the body, including the mucosae. The intensity of the color is not dependent on sun exposure. The senile lentigo (frequently called "liver spot") is clinically the same but appears at a later age, mostly in persons long exposed to the sun. The backs of the hands and the face (especially the forehead) are favorite sites. Ordinary freckles develop in childhood, are lighter in color, and become more pronounced during the summertime when there is increased exposure to sunlight.

Histologically, the ephelis shows increased production of melanin pigment by a normal number of melanocytes. Otherwise the epidermis is normal, whereas the lentigo has elongated rete ridges which appear club-shaped. The amount of melanin is increased in the melanocytes.

The preventive treatment is similar to that for sunburn, but far less effective.

Azizi E, et al: Skin type, hair color, and freckles are predictors of decreased minimal erythema ultraviolet radiation dose. JAAD 1988, 19:32.

Wilson PD, et al: Experimental induction of freckles by ultraviolet B. Br J Dermatol 1982, 106:401.

XERODERMA PIGMENTOSUM

CLINICAL MANIFESTATIONS. Xeroderma pigmentosum (XP), first described by Kaposi in 1870, is a rare pigmentary and atrophic disease that begins in childhood and progresses to the early development of senile changes in the sun-exposed skin, which consist of ephelides, lentigenes, telangiectases, keratoses, papillomas, carcinoma, and melanoma.

The main feature of this disease is sensitivity to light with wavelengths of 280 to 340 nm. The regions most often affected are the sun-exposed areas such as the face, neck, hands, and arms, although a few lentigines may appear on other areas. The lesions are worse on the face, particularly about the nose and eyes. The earliest manifestation of XP is often an acute sunburn after a small amount of sun exposure. As a rule, owing to coalescence of the freckles, the entire face is dappled with pigmented spots of various tints of brown, mingled with white atrophic patches and telangiectases. Actinic keratoses, vascular tumors, basal and squamous cell carcinomas, and melanomas complete the picture. These tumors are usually ulcerated or crusted.

The monumental landmark review article by Kraemer et al in 1987 reviewed 830 cases published in 297 articles from 1874 to 1982. Space prevents even a summary of it here, but 152 had neurologic abnormalities, including low intelligence, areflexia, impaired hearing, and abnormal speech. Twelve cases were accompanied by malignancy elsewhere than the skin.

The effects of the disease on the eyes are most distressing. Photophobia and lacrimation are early symptoms; keratitis and resulting corneal opacities and tumors of the lids generally supervene and cause a loss of vision, so that schooling and even simple games are impossible and the child becomes pitiably withdrawn.

Numerous concomitant diseases may be associated with xeroderma pigmentosum. Lynch and his associates reported a family in which five of the seven siblings were affected; four of the five had congenital ichthyosis and two of these had malignant melanoma. Porphyria and lupus erythematosus have been reported to be present in some cases.

Cases have been divided into 10 "complementation groups" (A through I, plus "Variant") on the basis

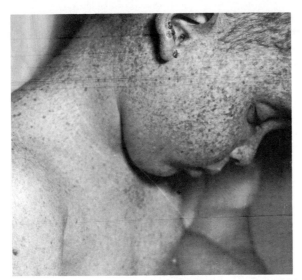

Figure 3–10. Early xeroderma pigmentosum in a 4-year-old boy.

of each group's separate defect in the ability to repair damaged DNA. Groups A, C, Variant, and D comprise over 90 per cent of all cases. XP Variant, or "pigmented xerodermoid," has a later onset of disease manifestations and defective postreplication DNA repair. In two complementation groups, types B and H, there has been coexistent Cockayne's syndrome.

DeSanctis-Cacchione Syndrome. This syndrome consists of xeroderma, microcephaly, mental deficiency, dwarfism, and gonadal hypoplasia. Reed and his associates reported four such cases.

ETIOLOGY AND PATHOGENESIS. Xeroderma pigmentosum is an autosomal recessively inherited familial disease with an altered reaction of the epidermis to light. The main biochemical defect is a failure to repair UV-induced DNA damage. Cleaver has shown the presence of genetically determined biochemical mechanisms that repair sunlight-dam-

aged DNA. In xeroderma pigmentosum the sunlight-damaged DNA strands in the skin cells cannot be repaired because of a deficiency of DNA endonuclease, the enzyme that paves the way for DNA polymerase to repair the rungs in the DNA "ladder."

TREATMENT. Exposure to sunlight should be strictly avoided. The actinic keratoses should be treated thoroughly before malignant degeneration takes place; 5-fluorouracil has been especially helpful. Carcinomas and melanomas should be removed in their early stages. Kraemer et al documented in 1988 that high-dose isotretinoin prevents skin cancer in these patients.

PROGNOSIS. There are varying degrees of severity. Mild forms of the disease that give no serious trouble are occasionally seen; however, death often occurs early in adulthood, mainly from metastasis of the malignant lesions. Prenatal diagnosis of XP has been determined by Ramsay and his associates.

Carter VH, et al: Xeroderma pigmentosum. Arch Dermatol 1968, 98:526.

Cleaver JE: Defective repair replication of DNA in xeroderma pigmentosum. Nature, London 1968, 218:652.

Idem: DNA damage and repair in light-sensitive human skin disease. J Invest Dermatol 1970, 54:181.

Idem: Xeroderma pigmentosum: Genetic and environmental influences in skin carcinogenesis. Int J Dermatol 1978, 17:435.

Kraemer KH, et al: Xeroderma pigmentosum. Arch Dermatol 1987, 123:241.

Idem: Prevention of skin cancer in xeroderma pigmentosum with the use of oral isotretinoin. N Engl J Med 1988, 318:1633.

Lynch HT, et al: Xeroderma pigmentosum. Arch Dermatol 1977, 113:193.

Ramsay CA, et al: Prenatal diagnosis of xeroderma pigmentosum. Lancet 1974, 2:1109.

Reed WB, et al: Xeroderma pigmentosum. JAMA 1969, 207:2073.

Robins JH: Xeroderma pigmentosum. JAMA 1988, 260:384.

COLLOID DEGENERATION

Also known as **colloid milium** and **colloid pseudomilium**, three types of colloid degeneration are recognized. One of these occurs in children and spontaneously disappears as they reach maturity.

The commonest type of colloid degeneration occurs in adults who have been exposed to strong sunlight. It is relatively common in the tropics. Firm, discrete, close-set, flat-topped papules occur on the forehead, cheeks, and backs of the hands. They are exquisitely discrete because each occupies a dermal papilla. The rete ridges prevent them from coalescing.

Nodular colloid degeneration presents with either a single large facial nodule or multiple nodules on the face, chin, or scalp. In some instances, lesions are limited to the trunk, suggesting that sun exposure is not essential in the pathogenesis of this entity.

The exact nature of "colloid" is unknown, except that it shows considerable resemblance to amyloid. In juvenile colloid milium the colloid is derived from the epidermis. Adult colloid is a structureless, amorphous substance on electron microscopic examination and nodular colloid is similar.

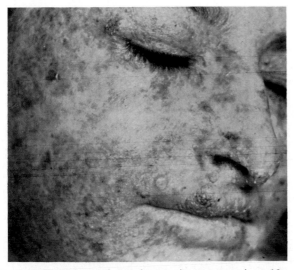

Figure 3–11. Advanced xeroderma pigmentosum in a 10-year-old girl, with basal and squamous cell carcinomas.

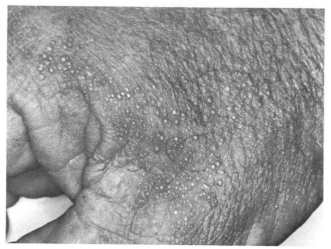

Figure 3–12. Colloid milium on dorsum of hand, a frequent site, in an oil well worker from Texas. (Courtesy of Dr. P. C. Holzberger.

The cause of colloid degeneration is unknown, but there is evidence that it is provoked by long exposure to sun.

Colloid degeneration of the skin is to be differentiated from milium, syringoma, steatocystoma multiplex, and lichen amyloidosis.

Agius JRG: Colloid pseudomilium. Br J Dermatol 1963, 75:55.
Hashimoto K, et al: Colloid milium. Arch Dermatol 1972, 105:684.

PHOTOSENSITIVITY

A number of substances known as photosensitizers may induce an abnormal reaction in skin exposed to sunlight or its equivalent. Contact of the skin with these substances may be external, or internal by enteral or parenteral administration, or by host synthesis of photosensitizers in response to an administered drug. The result may be either a markedly increased sunburn response without prior allergic sensitization (phototoxicity) or actual allergic sensitization triggered by sunlight, produced either internally (photoallergic dermatitis, photodrug reaction) or by external contact (photocontact dermatitis).

Drugs associated with photosensitivity (photosensitizers), according to Baer and Harber, are usually resonating compounds with a gram-molecular weight of less than 500. Absorption of radiant energy (sunlight) by the photosensitizer produces an excited state, which then reacts to dissipate itself through fluorescence, phosphorescence, charge transfer, heat, or free radical formation. Each photosensitizing substance absorbs only a specific wavelength of light. Depending upon the cellular localization of the photosensitizer, primary damage may occur in the nucleus, cytoplasmic organelles, or cell membrane.

A representative list of photosensitizers in man is shown in Table 3–2.

Action Spectrum. The specific wavelengths of light required to evoke a photosensitive drug reaction are known as the action spectrum. This action spectrum is approximately the same as the absorption spectrum of the photosensitizing substance.

The action spectrum for photoallergy is mostly in the long ultraviolet (UVA) (320 to 425 nm) region and may extend into the visible light region.

Apparatus. Various types of apparatus are available to produce these specific wavelength radiation ranges. The fluorescent sunlamp tube (Westinghouse) has a range between 285 and 350 nm. The fluorescent black light tube (Westinghouse tube, GE, Sylvania) has a 320 to 450 nm range. Other light sources that may also be of use in eliciting photosensitivity reactions include the high-pressure mercury-vapor lamp (hot-quartz), carbon arc, and an intense Wood light (Black-Ray B-100 A).

Types of Photosensitivity. In order that a photosensitivity reaction may occur, several factors must be present. The photosensitizing substance must be in or on the skin and exposed to specific wavelengths of light characteristic of the absorption spectrum of the photosensitizer. The prime factors determining the magnitude of a cutaneous photosensitivity response are the concentration of the photosensitizer and the intensity of the light absorbed.

Adverse photosensitivity may occur through diverse mechanisms. Three major pathways are phototoxic, photoallergic, and enzyme-induced photosensitization.

Phototoxic Reaction. A phototoxic reaction is a nonimmunologic reaction that develops within two to six hours after the skin has been exposed to a photosensitizing substance and light of the proper wavelength and intensity. There is a sunburn-type of reaction, with erythema occurring only on the sun-exposed parts. This type of reaction can be elicited in many persons who have no previous history of sensitivity to that particular substance: individual susceptibility varies widely. To elicit a phototoxic reaction a considerably greater amount of the photosensitizing substance is necessary than in the case of the photoallergic reaction. The erythema begins (like any sunburn) within a few hours, but worsens for 48 to 96 hours before beginning to subside. In severe cases, nails may be involved (photo-onycholysis).

Photoallergic Reaction. After exposure of the photosensitizing substance on the skin to a suitable light source, a clinical response is elicited in 24 to 48 hours. There is a papulovesicular, eczematous, or exudative dermatitis that occurs chiefly on the light-exposed areas; in addition, the eruption may extend onto other parts of the body. This type of reaction occurs only in the previously sensitized person.

The reaction may be produced with only small amounts of the photosensitizing substance. However, there is evidence to suggest that a sufficiently high concentration of the particular substance will also show phototoxic attributes.

Table 3–2. COMMON PHOTOSENSITIZERS

Inducers of Phototoxicity

Oral	*Topical*

Antimicrobials
  Demeclocycline (Declomycin)
  Tetracycline (rarely)
  Sulfonamides
  Nalidixic acid (NegGram)
  Griseofulvin (infrequently)
	Coal Tar Derivatives
	  Acridine
	  Anthracene
	  Phenanthrene
	  Pyridine
	  Crude coal tar

Furocoumarins (psoralens)
  Methoxsalen (Oxsoralen)
  Trimethylpsoralen (Trisoralen)
	Furocoumarins (psoralens)
	  Methoxsalen (8-MOP) in lime, rue, orange, celery, dill,
	    anise, or mokihana berry.
	  Bergapten (5-methoxypsoralen) in oil of bergamot

Dyes
  Acridine
  Eosin	

Calcium cyclamate	

Inducers of Photoallergy

Oral ("Photodrug")	*Topical ("Photocontact")*

Diuretics
  Chlorothiazides (Diuril, Hydrodiuril)
  Quinethazine (Hydromox)
	Antimicrobials
	  Bithionol
	  Sulfathiazole
	  Halogenated salicylanilides
	    and carbanilides
	  Hexachlorophene (usually only
	    secondary sensitizer)

Hypoglycemics
  Chlorpropamide (Diabinese)
  Tolbutamide (Orinase)	

Phenothiazines
  Chlorpromazine (Thorazine)
  Promazine (Sparine)
  Perchlorperazine (Compazine)
  Promethazine (Phenergan)
  Trifluoperazine (Stelazine)
	Antihistamines
	  Diphenhydramine? (Benadryl)

Enzyme-Induced Photosensitivity. Some drugs taken internally may act upon the metabolism systemically to induce changes in enzyme activity. In response to these enzymes the host manufactures the photosensitizer, such as tetrapyrroles, which figure prominently in the porphyrias. The drugs producing exacerbations in acute porphyria increase the delta aminolevulinic acid synthetase in hepatic cells and increase tetrapyrrole (porphyrin) synthesis.

This type of photosensitivity may be induced by estrogens, Sedormid ([2-isopropyl-4 pentenoyl] urea), barbiturates, and griseofulvin. Similar abnormalities have been noted in thousands of people who developed porphyria from the ingestion of cereals sprayed with hexachlorobenzene. In addition, alcohol (chlorinated phenols) may alter enzyme activity. This photosensitivity is an expression of a phototoxic reaction to a porphyrin produced by the host as a result of an ingested drug or chemical.

PHOTOTOXICITY

Phototoxic dermatitis usually occurs with the first exposure to the photosensitizing substance, when it is in a high cutaneous cellular concentration and is followed by exposure to sunlight. Prior sensitization is not required.

As already noted, the dermatitis occurs upon the sun-exposed areas within a few hours after exposure. Clinically the most common finding is the sunburned appearance of the skin, followed later by hyperpigmentation. Sometimes bullae develop.

The action spectrum is usually in the 285 to 450 nm range. The phototoxic substances causing this type of dermatitis usually absorb radiation in the ultraviolet or visible light range and have a gram-molecular weight of 500 or less.

Phototoxic Tar Dermatitis. Coal tar, creosote, crude coal tar, or pitch, in conjunction with sunlight exposure, may induce a sunburn reaction with episodes of severe burning sensation. This is followed by hyperpigmentation, which may persist for years, especially in those whose occupations involve constant exposure to sunlight.

Coal tar or its derivatives may be found in cosmetics, drugs, dyes, insecticides, and disinfectants. In the Goeckerman therapy of psoriasis, the phototoxic effect is utilized to advantage by making the skin more susceptible to ultraviolet light.

Phytophotodermatitis. The phototoxicity-inducing furocoumarins in many plants may bring about phytophotodermatitis when these plants come in contact with moist skin which is then exposed to sunlight. Several hours after exposure to the plant a burning erythema occurs, followed by edema and the devel-

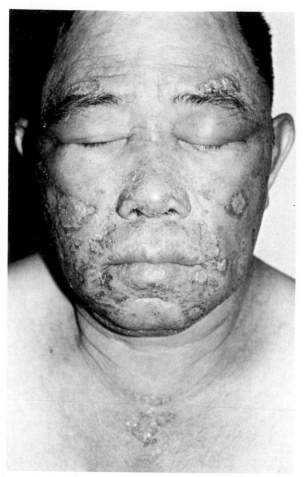

Figure 3–13. Phototoxic dermatitis. (*Courtesy of Dr. Axel W. Hoke.*)

opment of small vesicles. The following day the small blisters coalesce into large bullae. This is followed by involution and then by an intense residual hyperpigmentation that may persist for weeks or months.

The hyperpigmentation is the postinflammatory type. It is epidermal as well as dermal, i.e., increased melanin within keratinocytes and also in dermal histiocytes, and is only very slowly reversible with time.

Phytophotodermatitis is believed to be caused mostly by plants containing furocoumarin (psoralen, 8-methoxypsoralen and 5-methoxypsoralen), which are primarily in the families of the Umbelliferae, Rutaceae (rue), Compositae, Papilionaceae, and Moraceae.

Plants known to cause phytophotodermatitis include the fig, cowslip, garden and wild parsnip, fennel, dill, parsley, wild carrot, garden carrot, masterwort, atrillal, angelica, common rice, gas plant, lime bergamot, lime, Persian lime, buttercup, mustard, blind weed, agrimony, yarrow, goose foot, bavachi, and St. John's wort. In Hawaii the anise-scented *mokihana* berry (*Pelea anisata*) was known to natives for its phototoxic properties (the "mokihana burn"). Like the lime, it is a member of the rue family.

Occupational disability from exposure to the pink rot fungus (*Sclerotinia sclerotiorum*) present on celery roots, which occurs in celery farmers in upper Michigan and Florida, has been reported by Birmingham. However, disease-resistant celery of high quality contains furanocoumarins and was the probable source of phytophotodermatitis in an epidemic studied by Berkley et al in 1984.

Phytophotodermatitis must be differentiated from vesicles and bullae due to poison ivy dermatitis. The vesicles and bullae of poison ivy are not necessarily limited to the sun-exposed areas. Itching is the most prominent symptom in poison ivy dermatitis, whereas there is burning in phytophotodermatitis.

Treatment of a severe, acute reaction is wet compresses (1:5000) for 20 to 30 minutes daily, and topical applications of Sarna lotion, Acid Mantle Creme, bland or corticosteroid cream, lotion, or ointment. Calamine lotion is a popular layman's remedy.

Berloque (Berlock, Perfume) Dermatitis. In 1916 Freund described a peculiar artificial discoloration of the skin that appeared with the use of eau de Cologne during sunbathing. Clinically this pigmentary disturbance is characterized by lavalliere (hanging drop)-

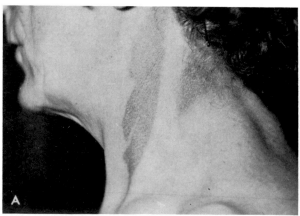
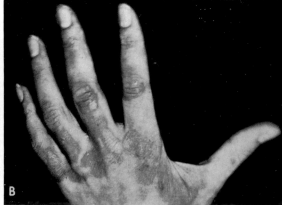

Figure 3–14. A, Berloque dermatitis on the side of the neck from perfume, and B, on the hand from handling limes, with subsequent sunlight exposure.

shaped pigmented patches. The word for pendant in French is berloque, and in German it is Berlocke. Other patches may be quadrilateral or occur in streaks of erythema or pigmentation.

This dermatitis is seen most frequently on the sides of the neck and in the retroauricular areas of women. In addition, the shoulders, breasts, face, and other areas may be involved. When men have this type of dermatitis, it is usually on the bearded area and is caused by bergamot oil or related substances in aftershave lotion.

The chief cause, oil of bergamot, contains a furocoumarin (5-methoxypsoralen), a potent photosensitizer. However, such compounds have been removed from most perfumes and lotions, and berlock dermatitis is rarely seen anymore.

Treatment consists of stopping the use of furocoumarin preparations. Benoquin, though a fairly effective bleach, is a potential sensitizer and should seldom be used unless total depigmentation (in nearly universal vitiligo) is being attempted. An effective, safe bleach which may be used is a modification of Kligman's formula: 5 per cent hydroquinone, 0.1 per cent retinoic acid, and 0.1 per cent dexamethasone in hydrophilic ointment rubbed in daily.

Azelaic acid cream may also be effective.

Dermatitis Bullosa Striata Pratensis (Grass or Meadow Dermatitis). This is a phytophotodermatitis with an eruption consisting of streaks and bizarre configurations with vesicles and bullae that heal with residual hyperpigmentation.

Sunbathing in the fields with exposure to furocoumarin-containing plants is the cause of this unusual dermatitis. Treatment is that recommended for any phytophotodermatitis.

Photosensitivity in Tattoo. Yellow cadmium sulfide, a known photosensitizer, has been incorporated into red mercuric sulfide pigment to produce a brighter red color. Bjornberg has reported extensively on the photosensitivity in tattoos due to the yellow pigment of cadmium sulfide. Goldstein has reported swollen erythematous verrucose lesions in the red parts of tattoos, containing cadmium sulfide, after exposure to sunlight. The other colors do not produce this disorder.

Either the tattooed person must avoid sunlight exposure or the red part of the tattoo must be removed.

PHOTOALLERGY

Photoallergic dermatitis is an allergic dermatitis caused by a photosensitizing substance plus sunlight exposure in a sensitized person. If the photosensitizer acts internally, we speak of a *photodrug dermatitis* or *reaction*; if it acts externally, of *photocontact dermatitis*.

The clinical and histopathologic findings of this type of dermatitis are similar to those in allergic contact dermatitis. It differs only in that sunlight

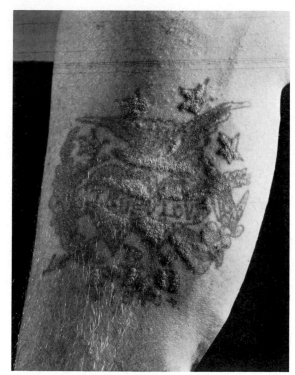

Figure 3–15. Cadmium sulfide photosensitivity in red portions of tattoo done with red mercuric sulfide "brightened" with cadmium sulfide. Note rough inflammatory crusts from the eczematous reaction. (Courtesy of Dr. H. Shatin.)

must be present to induce the reaction. The nature of the allergenic substances is similar in that both types are low-molecular-weight compounds. However, in photoallergic dermatitis light photochemically alters the hapten. This newly created hapten (like urushiol) then reacts with cutaneous protein (carrier protein) to form a complete antigen. The remainder of the reaction is similar to other types of delayed immunologic hypersensitivity.

S. Epstein has described the histologic picture in *phototoxic* contact dermatitis as that of epidermal necrosis with vacuolation, pyknosis, and a slight infiltration of the dermis. The *photoallergic* reaction is an allergic contact dermatitis with spongiosis, vesiculation, and a pronounced lymphocytic infiltrate in the dermis.

PHOTOSENSITIZING SUBSTANCES

Phenothiazine and Related Compounds. Phenothiazine used as an insecticide, chlorpromazine (Thorazine) handled by medical personnel for injection, and promethazine (Phenergan) may produce allergic reactions. Sometimes substances such as Thorazine and Phenergan may produce both phototoxic and photoallergic reactions.

Sulfonamides. Sulfanilamide may produce both phototoxic and photoallergic reactions. The former reaction is elicited when the sulfanilamide is taken internally. The other sulfonamides such as sulfadiazine and sulfathiazole rarely produce photosensitivity reactions.

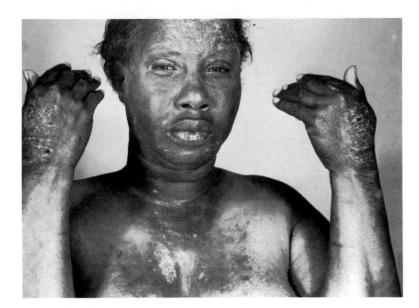

Figure 3–16. Photoallergic dermatitis on the sun-exposed areas. (Courtesy of Dr. C. Ames.)

The hypoglycemic sulfonamides (chlorpropamide and tolbutamide) may produce photoallergic reactions. In a similar way the thiazides, such as chlorothiazide and hydrochlorothiazide, may produce photoallergic reactions and cross sensitization.

Other Photosensitizers. Starke reported photosensitization to oil of sandalwood, a common ingredient in aftershave lotions. Other ingredients in cosmetics, notably the fragrance musk ambrette, can cause photoallergic dermatitis as well as persistent light reaction. Sunscreening agents containing PABA esters, the cinnamates, and digalloyl trioleate may produce photoallergy. Quinidine may produce photoallergic dermatitis as well as an unusual photosensitive livedo-reticularis–like eruption. Zelickson reported photosensitization to nalidixic acid, a urinary antimicrobial.

Photosensitive Dermatoses. Photosensitivity may be seen as a component of many skin diseases, including xeroderma pigmentosum, porphyria cutanea tarda, erythropoietic protoporphyria, pellagra, lupus erythematosus, dermatomyositis, albinism, piebaldism, vitiligo, keratosis follicularis, Rothmund-Thompson syndrome, Bloom's syndrome, Cockayne's disease, Hartnup disease, pityriasis rubra pilaris, and atopic dermatitis.

Gross has shown that the Koebner phenomenon may be produced in certain skin diseases by exposure to light, and Pascher has shown that **purpura solaris** is a true entity. Individuals may be sensitized only to certain wavelengths. Not only do ultraviolet, infrared, and other forms of light induce sensitization, but the reactions to light are of a very diverse character.

TESTING FOR PHOTOSENSITIVITY. Although there are numerous techniques suitable for photopatch testing, the most practical for an office procedure is essentially that described by S. Epstein.

Each of the suspected photosensitizers is applied in duplicate to two symmetrical sites on the lumbar area which have not been exposed to sunlight. The usual concentration used for the patch test is 1 per cent in petrolatum. After 48 hours one set is removed and noted for reactions as a contactant without exposure to light. Then the site is exposed to 5 to 15 joules/m² long wave ultraviolet above 320 nm and covered with opaque material.

Again after 48 hours the irradiated site is compared to the other patch test site, which has not been exposed to light.

When both sites are equally positive there is contact sensitivity. When both sides are negative there is no contact sensitivity or photocontact sensitivity. When the irradiated site alone is positive there is only photocontact sensitivity. When the irradiated site is more positive than the unirradiated site, there is both contact and photocontact dermatitis.

TREATMENT. Both acute and chronic photosensitivity are treated similarly to any other inflammatory dermatitis, such as with topical corticosteroids. In addition, efforts should be concentrated on recognition of the photosensitizer and its elimination from the patient's environment. Sun exposure must be avoided as much as possible. Protective clothing and the use of topical sunscreens, such as Photoplex, are mandatory.

Addo HA, et al: Thiazide-induced photosensitivity: Study of 33 subjects. Br J Dermatol 1987, 116:749.

Berkeley SF, et al: Dermatitis in grocery workers associated with high natural concentrations of furocoumarins in celery. Ann Intern Med 1986, 105:351.

Birmingham DJ, et al: Phototoxic bullae among celery harvesters. Arch Dermatol 1961, 88:73.

Bjornberg A: Reactions to light in yellow tattoos from cadmium sulfide. Arch Dermatol 1963, 38:267.

Blank H, et al: Photosensitivity studies with demethylchlortetracycline and doxycycline. Arch Dermatol 1968, 97:1.

Bruce S, et al: Quinidine-induced photosensitive livedo-reticularis–like eruption. JAAD 1985, 12:332.

Epstein JH: Phototoxicity and photoallergy in man. JAAD 1983, 8:141.

Epstein S: Chlorpromazine photosensitivity. Arch Dermatol 1968, 98:354.

Fisher AA: Contact Dermatitis. Philadelphia, Lea and Febiger, 1986.

Giovinazzo VJ, et al: Photoallergic contact dermatitis to musk ambrette. JAAD 1980, 3:384.

Goldstein N: Mercury-cadmium sensitivity in tattoos. Ann Intern Med 1967, 67:984.

Harber LC, et al: Photosensitivity Diseases, Philadelphia, WB Saunders Co., 1981.

Kaidbey KH, et al: Clinical and histologic study of coal tar sensitivity in humans. Arch Dermatol 1977, 113:592.

Lang PG: Quinidine-induced photodermatitis confirmed by photopatch testing. JAAD 1983, 9:124.

Magnus IA: Dermatologic Photobiology. New York, Blackwell Scientific Publications, 1976.

Menz J, et al: Photopatch testing. JAAD 1988, 18:1044.

Regan JD, et al: The Science of Photomedicine, New York, Plenum Press, 1982.

Shelley WB, et al: Naproxen photosensitivity demonstrated by challenge. Cutis 1986, 38:169.

Sommer RG, et al: Phytophotodermatitis (solar dermatitis from plants). N Engl J Med 1967, 276:1481.

Starke JC: Photoallergy to sandalwood oil. Arch Dermatol 1965, 96:62.

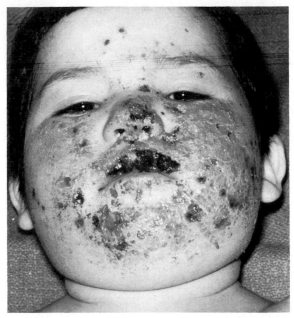

Figure 3–17. Hereditary polymorphous light eruption in American Indian boy. (Courtesy of Dr. A. R. Birt.)

POLYMORPHOUS LIGHT ERUPTION

Various eruptions on sun-exposed areas of the skin have been noted in which no other etiologic agent could be incriminated except sunlight. The eruptions assume various forms. There are the vesicular, the papular (prurigo aestivalis), the plaque type (in which the scaling, telangiectatic, indurated plaque suggests lupus erythematosus), and the eczematous and erythematous forms. There is no scarring or atrophy in these forms.

The lesions appear one to four days after exposure to sunlight. They may involve the face, the V area of the chest, the neck, and the arms. The lips are usually involved in Canadian Indian cases but are typically spared in most cases. Usually the eruption is present during the summertime, subsiding during the winter when there is less sun exposure. Most frequently light-complexioned adults are affected.

Dover et al have recently reported seven cases with childhood onset of severe pruritus from exposure to sunlight: polymorphous light eruption *sine eruptione.* Two of them later developed ordinary polymorphous light eruption.

The **etiologic agent** is ultraviolet light. The wavelengths which are responsible for inducing this eruption are a subject of controversy. J. Epstein states that the action spectrum is in the UVB range. Holzle et al report only 5 to 10 per cent success in reproducing PMLE lesions with UVB, but a 50 to 90 per cent positive response to high-dose UVA. Visible light does not induce these lesions.

The cause of the sensitivity is unknown, but Arnold in 1975 reported cases occurring simultaneously in blond identical twin sisters, each of whom had had similar attacks for three successive summers, when each was at a different southern resort. The fourth attack was the first they had had together. It seems that a genetic factor may be operative in some cases.

The **diagnosis** can be made by exposing a small unaffected area to graded amounts of ultraviolet light below 320 nm. Repeated exposures over 10 to 14 days may be necessary, as outlined by J. Epstein. Some 48 hours after exposure the lesions typical of those elsewhere on the body will appear at the test site and persist for about two weeks. Holzle et al reported a high rate of reproduction of lesions using 50–100 joules/m^2 of UVA.

In the **differential diagnosis** the following should be considered: lupus erythematosus, lymphocytic infiltration of Jessner, mycosis fungoides, prurigo nodularis, contact dermatitis, and photosensitive

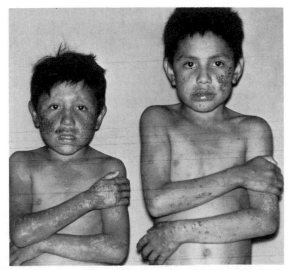

Figure 3–18. Hereditary polymorphous light eruption in American Indian brothers. (Courtesy of Dr. A. R. Birt.)

contact dermatitis. It is to be noted that lesions appear only on sun-exposed areas of the skin. Histopathologic examination and direct immunofluorescence are helpful in distinguishing the above diseases.

Treatment is mostly symptomatic. For the severe pruritus the antihistaminics (e.g., Periactin) used orally are helpful. Corticosteroids applied topically in creams are also effective. Corticosteroids given internally may be necessary in severe attacks. Hydroxychloroquine sulfate (Plaquenil), 200 to 400 mg daily, is frequently effective. Antimalarial drug toxicity should be kept in mind when using the chloroquine compounds, but retinopathy due to 200 mg of Plaquenil daily for a year or two is extremely rare. A morbilliform drug eruption is uncommon but not rare.

Birt and Davis had favorable response in 30 American Indians treated with Trisoralen. Of the 23 children treated, 6 had complete remission; however, all 30 patients had marked improvement while on Trisoralen therapy.

Sunscreens should be used topically, preferably one that protects against UVA as well as UVB, such as Photoplex. Tanning does not protect against attacks induced by UVB; attacks induced by UVA, however, may be prevented very well by PUVA therapy. Gschnait's study (1983) should be referred to as well as those by Murphy et al (1987) and Addo et al (1988). UVB therapy may also be effective, as these studies demonstrate.

Addo HA, et al: Actinic prurigo—a specific photodermatosis? Photodermatology 1984, 1:119.
Idem: UVB photochemotherapy and phototherapy in the treatment of PMLE and solar urticaria. Br J Dermatol 1987, 116:539.
Birt AR, et al: Hereditary polymorphic light eruption of American Indians. Int J Dermatol 1975, 14:110.
Dover JS, et al: Polymorphous light eruption *sine eruptione*. Br J Dermatol 1985, 113 (supp 29):12.
Epstein JH: Polymorphous light eruption. JAAD 1980, 3:329.
Gschnait F, et al: Treatment of polymorphous light eruption. Arch Dermatol Res 1984, 275:379.
Holzle E, et al: Polymorphous light eruption. JAAD 1982, 7:1110.
Jansen CT: Hereditary polymorphous light eruption. Arch Dermatol 1978, 114:188.
Idem: Natural history of PMLE. Arch Dermatol 1979, 115:165.
Murphy GM, et al: Prophylactic PUVA and UVB in PMLE. Br J Dermatol 1987, 116:531.
Idem: Hydroxychloroquine in PML. Br J Dermatol 1987, 116:379.

Actinic Prurigo

Onset in childhood, frequent appearance of small vesicles, occasional pitted scarring, and frequent personal or family history of atopy distinguish this sometimes severe dermatosis from ordinary polymorphous light eruption, according to Addo and Frain-Bell. We believe it to be a subset of that disorder, occurring in atopic patients.

PERSISTENT LIGHT REACTOR SYNDROME

Men over 40 are sometimes afflicted with severe, intractable, extremely photosensitive dermatitis which ranges from simple eczematization of exposed surfaces to the thickened, hyperpigmented plaques of *actinic reticuloid*. Sunscreens affording total block may be helpful in milder cases, but in severe involvement, as Leigh and Hawk showed, azathioprine should be tried, 100–200 mg daily. If there is intolerance to it, PUVA may be tried; Robinson et al found it effective. Should it fail, the extreme photosensitivity and disabling discomfort justify systemic steroid therapy, but in so chronic a disorder oral prednisone is likely to be dangerous, and triamcinolone acetonide (Kenalog) intramuscularly is the preferred steroid. It usually takes 60 mg monthly to control it, and occasional doses of 80 mg may be required.

There is often a history of having taken a photosensitizing drug prior to the onset of this syndrome, or having been sensitized topically by halogenated salicylanilides. Sulfanilamide, chlorpromazine, musk ambrette, and thiazide derivatives have also been implicated.

SOLAR URTICARIA

Urticarial reactions to sunlight are seen rarely. Typical cases occur in otherwise healthy patients who suddenly develop stinging and pruritic hives on skin areas that are exposed to sunlight. In most cases this reaction may be induced even through window glass. Systemic reactions, with chills, fatigue, syncope, and abdominal cramps, may be concomitant. The symptoms subside in several hours. Solar urticaria most often occurs in female children and adolescents.

Harber and his associates have classified solar urticaria into six types, depending upon the action spectrum. Some are sensitive to the 280 to 320 nm spectrum, others to the 280 to 500 nm, and still others to 400 to 500 nm. One type is a manifestation of erythropoietic protoporphyria.

Sams and his associates used passive transfer tests, both direct and reverse, 48/80-induced histamine depletion, exhaustion response, and chemical and physical blocking methods in the study of this interesting urticarial reaction. Passive transfer and reverse passive transfer can be positive in some patients with solar urticaria.

Chloroquine 250 mg daily or Plaquenil 200 mg daily is beneficial in increasing the tolerance to sunlight exposure to the point that the patient may have normal exposure to sunlight even during the summertime. Both of these substances may induce retinopathy, but rarely, if ever, at 250 mg a day for less than two years.

For relief of the urticaria antihistaminics are usually effective. UVB and PUVA may also be helpful, as shown by Addo et al (1987).

Addo HA, et al: UVB . . . in treatment of PMLE and solar urticaria. Br J Dermatol 1987, 116:539.

Epstein JH, et al: Solar urticaria. Arch Dermatol 1963, 88:135.

Harber LC, et al: Immunologic and biophysical studies in solar urticaria. J Invest Dermatol 1963, 41:439.

Horio T, et al: Solar urticaria. Arch Dermatol 1977, 113:157.

Idem: Augmentation spectrum in solar urticaria. JAAD 1988, 18:1189.

Sams WM Jr, et al: Solar urticaria. Arch Dermatol 1969, 99:390.

Warin RP, et al: Urticaria. London, WB Saunders Co, Ltd, 1974, p 151.

DISSEMINATED SUPERFICIAL ACTINIC POROKERATOSIS

BRACHIORADIAL SUMMER PRURITUS

Waisman described and named this lichenified intermittently itchy disorder of the skin overlying the brachial nerves and the brachial muscle at the elbow-bends in 1968. Heyl reported it from South Africa in 1983, and Walcyk and Elpern reported 42 cases seen in Hawaii over a two-year period, in 1986. Heyl suspected nerve damage from cervical spine disease, but 60 per cent of Walcyk and Elpern's patients under age 50 had no cervical abnormality by x-ray, and they point out that the lesions are limited to a much smaller area than that served by any nerve.

All cases have been reported from the subtropics. All patients in Walcyk's series had lived in Hawaii for at least one year. They consider it, as Waisman did, a result of chronic sunlight exposure. Treatment with topical corticosteroids and photoprotection helps the condition to resolve.

Arnold considered it—erroneously—a variant of neurodermatitis and omitted it from the seventh edition of this text.

Heyl T: Brachioradial pruritus. Arch Dermatol 1983, 119:115.

Waisman M: Solar pruritus of the elbows (brachioradial summer pruritus). Arch Dermatol 1968, 98:481.

Walcyk PJ, Elpern DJ: Brachioradial summer pruritus: A tropical dermopathy. Br J Dermatol 1986, 115:177.

HYDROA VACCINIFORME

CLINICAL SIGNS. Also known as hydroa aestivale, summer prurigo of Hutchinson, and hydroa puerorum, hydroa vacciniforme is a vesicular and bullous disease that tends to recur each summer during childhood on skin areas exposed to sunlight. Deep, pitted scars may remain at the sites of healed lesions, although there is contention that hydroa aestivale does not produce scars. The lesions appear mostly on the face and the extensor aspects of the extremities and are arranged symmetrically chiefly over the nose, cheeks, ears, and dorsal surfaces of the hands. Itching and burning, as well as mild constitutional symptoms, may precede the outbreak of skin lesions in crops. The vesicles and bullae dry up in the course of three or four days with the formation of adherent brown crusts. Each lesion is surrounded by a mildly inflammatory zone so that the appearance simulates a vaccination vesicle. The itching may lead to lichenification that persists through the winter.

Sonnex et al (1988) implicated UVA and were able to elicit new lesions with broad-spectrum UVA radiation.

Recent well-documented reports indicate both sexes are affected nearly equally. It is believed to be transmitted as a genetic recessive trait. It begins during the first four years of life and generally disappears after puberty, although it may persist into the third decade of life.

The porphyrin metabolism is normal in hydroa vacciniforme and exclusion of porphyria via skin biopsy for routine histology and direct immunofluorescence, and erythrocyte protoporphyrin analysis, is necessary. Erythropoietic protoporphyria and polymorphous light eruption are the disease entities most important to differentiate.

Treatment is principally the avoidance of sunlight exposure and the use of sunscreens, such as Photoplex, that block in the UVA range. The intermittent low-dosage treatment with antimalarials has been helpful. Potential ocular toxicity should always be kept in mind when prescribing synthetic antimalarials. Topical and systemic corticosteroids may be indicated.

Goldgeier MH, et al: Hydroa vacciniforme. Arch Dermatol 1982, 118:588.

Halasz CLG, et al: Hydroa vacciniforme: Induction of lesions with ultraviolet A. JAAD 1983, 8:171.

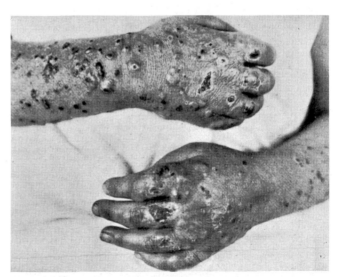

Figure 3–19. Hydroa vacciniforme. The face was also involved. Note almost pathognomonic sparing of the two distal phalanges of each finger, on which the sun never shines. (Courtesy of Dr. B. M. Kesten.)

McGrae JD Jr, et al: Hydroa vacciniforme. Arch Dermatol 1963, 87:618.

Sonnex T, et al: Hydroa vacciniforme. Br J Dermatol 1988, 118:101.

ACTINIC GRANULOMA

O'Brien described this granuloma-annulare–like lesion, occurring in sun-damaged skin, in 1975; and in 1985 he could say, with reason, that "it seems to be surviving a rather difficult birth." Ragaz and Ackerman regard it as simply granuloma annulare occurring in elastotic skin. Cases have been reported, however, from widely scattered sources, and the concept has been broadened to include necrobiotic, histiocytic, and sarcoid variants. We are not persuaded that it is an entity *sui generis*.

McGrae JD: Actinic granuloma. Arch Dermatol 1986, 122:43.

O'Brien JP: Actinic granuloma: An annular connective tissue disorder affecting sun- and heat-damaged (elastotic) skin. Arch Dermatol 1975, 111:460.

Idem: Actinic granuloma: The expanding significance: analysis of its origin in elastotic ("aging") skin and a definition of its necrobiotic (vascular), histiocytic, and sarcoid variants. Int J Dermatol 1985, 24:474.

Ragaz A, et al: Is actinic granuloma a specific condition? Am J Dermatopathol 1979, 1:43.

RADIODERMATITIS

The effects of ionizing radiation on the cells depend upon the amount of radiation, its intensity (exposure rate), and the characteristics of the individual cell. In small amounts the effect is insidious, and cumulative. When the dose is large, cell death results. When it is sublethal, many changes occur. Mitosis is arrested temporarily, with consequent retardation of growth. In the chromosome, "stickiness" occurs as a result of breaks. The exposure rate affects the number of chromosome breaks. The more rapid the delivery of a certain amount of radiation, the greater is the number of chromosome breaks. The number of breaks is increased also by the presence of oxygen.

Ionizing radiation interferes with the enzymes synthesizing chromosomal deoxyribonucleic acid (DNA). These effects and many other complex reactions result in at least a temporary halt of the normal cell cycle.

When an "erythema dose" of ionizing radiation is given to the skin there is a *latent period* of several hours to several days before visible erythema appears. After this initial reaction subsides there is another latent period, lasting several years, after which late radiation sequelae may appear.

TYPES

Acute Radiodermatitis. The skin, when exposed to a large amount of ionizing radiation, will sustain a violent reaction whose extent will depend considerably on the amount, quality, and duration of exposure. Such radiation reaction occurs in the treatment of malignancy and in accidental overexposure.

The reaction is manifested by erythema, vesiculation, edema, and ulceration, accompanied by severe pain. This type of radiation injury may subside in several weeks to several months, again depending upon the amount of radiation exposure.

Chronic Radiodermatitis. Chronic exposure to "suberythema" amounts of ionizing radiation over a prolonged period will produce varying degrees of damage to the skin and its underlying parts after a variable latent period of time from several months to several decades. In the past this type of radiation reaction occurred most frequently in roentgenologists and radiation technicians who were constantly exposed to ionizing radiation. It may also occur through overtreatment of various dermatoses with ionizing radiation and through excessive use of fluoroscopy and roentgenography for diagnostic purposes.

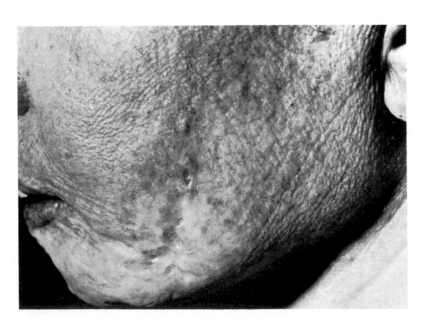

Figure 3–20. Chronic radiodermatitis in a woman, 60, given an unknown amount of x-radiation for the removal of superfluous hair.

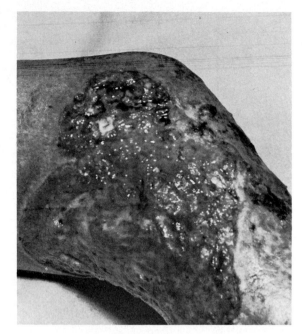

Figure 3–21. Squamous cell carcinoma in chronic radiodermatitis on the knee of a 60-year-old woman.

After a latent period, telangiectasia, atrophy, and freckling may appear. The skin becomes dry, thin, smooth, and shiny. The nails may become striated, brittle, and fragmented. Growth is slowed. The hair becomes brittle and sparse. In the more severe cases these chronic changes may be followed by actinic keratoses, ulcerations, and carcinoma.

Radiation Cancer. After a long latent period, usually years after the radiation injury, various malignant neoplasms may form. Most frequent is the squamous cell carcinoma, followed by basal cell carcinoma. Still other changes may be Bowen's disease, angiosarcoma, malignant fibrous histiocytoma, sarcoma, pseudosarcoma, osteosarcoma, and anaplastic carcinoma. The incidence of malignant neoplasms increases with the passage of time.

The induction of leukemia, lymphoma, or carcinoma of the breast or thyroid as a result of mutations caused by repeated minute (millirem) exposures of scattered radiation to the bone marrow, thyroid, or breast, especially in children, must be taken into account. With appropriate shielding and modern-day equipment this risk is small. In any case, genetic damage from scattered radiation reaching the gonads does not threaten the offspring of the patient at all. It merely is additive to the background radiation to which the population pool (to which the patient belongs) is subject, and affects future generations only.

TREATMENT. Radiodermatitis without carcinoma requires little or no attention except protection from sunlight and the extremes of heat and cold. Careful cleansing with mild soap and water, the use of emollients, and, on occasion, corticosteroid ointments, especially the hydrocortisone types, are the only requirements for good care.

The early removal of keratoses and ulcerations, both precancerous in nature, is helpful in reducing the incidence of metastasizing cancers. For the actinic or radiation keratoses, treatment with cryosurgery is an excellent method.

When the keratosis appears to be somewhat infiltrated, a biopsy is indicated, and usually a deep shave biopsy is adequate. This may then be followed by cryosurgery or curettage and fulguration, if indicated.

Topical fluorouracil (5-FU) applications are not as effective as the two mentioned modalities mainly because of the long time necessary for applications and the frequent recurrences.

Radiation ulcerations should be studied by biopsy if they have been present for three or more months. When feasible, excision and grafting should be done.

For radiation carcinomas, biopsies should confirm the diagnosis. This is followed by excision, and grafting if required.

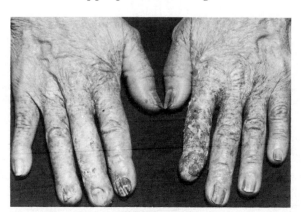

Figure 3–22. Chronic radiodermatitis with actinic keratoses and basal and squamous cell carcinomas.

Cipollaro AC, Crossland PM: X Rays and Radium in the Treatment of Diseases of the Skin, 5th ed., Philadelphia, Lea and Febiger 1967, pp 357–374.

Goette DK, et al: Post-irradiation angiosarcoma. JAAD 1985, 12:922.

Idem: Post-irradiation malignant fibrous histiocytoma. Arch Dermatol 1985, 121:535.

Goldschmidt H, et al: Reactions to ionizing radiation. JAAD 1980, 3:551.

James WD, et al: Late subcutaneous fibrosis following megavoltage radiotherapy. JAAD 1980, 3:616.

MECHANICAL INJURIES TO THE SKIN

Various mechanical factors may induce distinctive skin changes. Pressure, friction (such as rubbing), and the mechanical introduction of foreign substances (such as injections) are some of the means by which skin injuries may occur.

CALLUS

Callus is a nonpenetrating circumscribed hyperkeratosis produced by pressure. It occurs on parts subject to intermittent pressure, particularly on the palms and soles, more especially over the bony prominences of the joints.

The callus on the sole may be the site of plantar warts; as a result, it may at times be difficult to detect the latter.

Ronchese has demonstrated that those engaged in various sports and certain occupations develop callosities of distinctive size and location as stigmata of their occupation.

The callus differs from the clavus in that it has no penetrating central core and is a more diffuse thickening. It tends to disappear spontaneously when the pressure upon the skin is removed. Most problems are encountered with calluses on the soles. Ill-fitting shoes and orthopedic problems of the foot caused by aging (bunions, exostoses) are some of the etiologic factors to be considered in painful callosities of the feet.

Padding to relieve the pressure, paring of the thickened callus, and the use of keratolytics such as 40 per cent salicylic acid plasters are some of the effective means of relieving painful callosities.

They may also be softened by moistening them nightly with two parts propylene glycol to one part water under snug plastic occlusion (a plastic "baggie" and a sock will do). This is especially effective with fissured calluses of the heels.

CLAVUS (Corn)

Corns are circumscribed, horny, conical thickenings with the base on the surface and the apex pointing inward and pressing upon subjacent structures. There are two varieties: the *hard corns*, which occur on the dorsa of the toes, or on the soles, and the *soft corns*, which are present between the toes and are softened by the macerating action of sweat. In the hard corn, the surface is shiny and polished and, when the upper layers are shaved off, a core is noted in the densest part of the lesion. It is this core that causes the dull boring, or sharp lancinating pain by pressing on the underlying sensory nerves in the papillary layer. Frequently a bony spur or exostosis is present beneath both hard and soft corns of long duration, and unless this exostosis is removed cure is unlikely. The soft interdigital corn usually occurs in the fourth interdigital space of the foot. Frequently

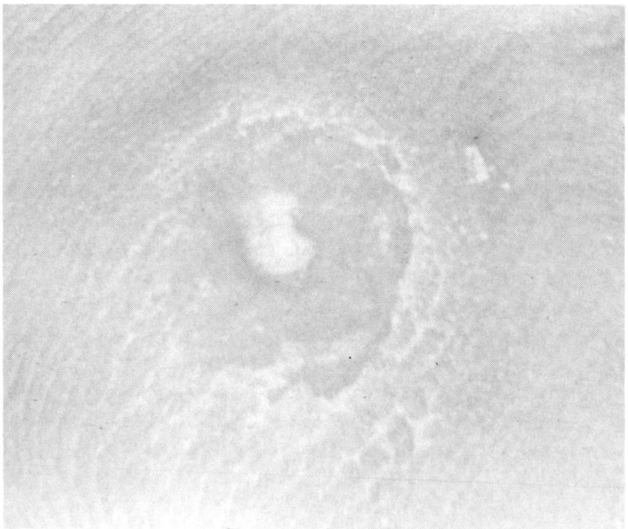

Figure 3–23. White keratinous core deep in a plantar corn, exposed by shaving. (Courtesy of Dr. Axel W. Hoke.)

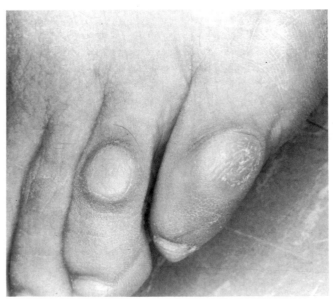

Figure 3–24. Hard corns.

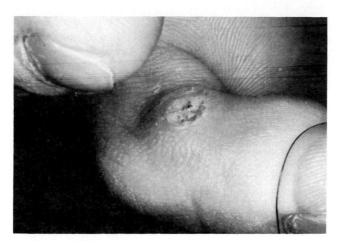

Figure 3–25. Soft corn on side of toe. (Courtesy of Dr. Axel W. Hoke.)

there is an exostosis at the metatarsal-phalangeal joint that causes pressure on the adjacent toe. These are soft, soggy, and macerated so that they appear white. Meltzer reports successful treatment by simple excision.

Plantar corns must be differentiated from plantar warts, and in most cases this can be done with confidence only by paring off the surface keratin until either the pathognomonic elongated dermal papillae of the wart with its blood vessels, or the clear horny core of the corn, can be clearly seen.

Corns arise at sites of friction or pressure, and when these causative factors are removed they may spontaneously disappear.

TREATMENT. The relief of pressure or friction by corrective footwear is of first importance; however, this step alone frequently does not cure the corns. Salicylic acid and dichloracetic acid have been favorite methods of treatment, and are successful when carefully and diligently used. In the case of the soft corn it may be necessary to remove the underlying exostosis, if present.

After careful paring of the corn with emphasis on removing the center core, 40 per cent salicylic acid plaster is applied. After 48 hours the plaster is removed, the white macerated skin is rubbed off, and a new plaster is reapplied. This is continued until the corn is gone.

Sometimes it is more feasible to use a salicylic acid–lactic acid in collodion (Duofilm) rather than the plaster. The collodion medication is carefully painted on the pared site of the corn and allowed to dry. This is done daily for seven days, when the foot is soaked for a half hour and the collodion peeled off the corn site. This process is continued weekly until healing occurs. This treatment is especially effective for the interdigital soft corns; however, it may be necessary to remove the underlying exostosis at the site of the soft corn.

Soaking the feet in hot water and paring the surface by means of a razor, pumice stone, or sharp knife, followed by the application of a ring of soft felt wadding around the region of the corn, will often bring a good result by relieving all friction and pressure in the area. The base should then be painted with 10 per cent silver nitrate solution. This should be repeated once a week. In these manipulations it is imperative that the instruments employed be aseptic.

If causative factors cannot be identified and removed, in the case of plantar corns, deep paring (pinching the corn up between thumb and finger to raise it) followed by vitamin A orally in a single daily dose of 300,000 to 500,000 units for two or three months, will usually prevent rekeratinization and recurrence—which are otherwise inevitable within a month at most. The prescription label should bear the warning "STOP IF HEADACHE OCCURS," lest pseudotumor cerebri be induced. Only very rarely indeed will adults develop the anorexia, dry lips, or breakage of hair that signal systemic vitamin A toxicity over and above the suppression of keratinization which is the purpose of this large dose. Arnold has not seen them occur in adults. Although it does not seem to have been tried, isotretinoin used for 2 or 3 months would seem likely to be similarly effective in preventing recurrence.

The pain of a corn on the dorsum of a toe may be greatly alleviated by the injection just under it of 0.01 to 0.02 ml of triamcinolone suspension, 40 mg per ml.

POROKERATOSIS PLANTARIS DISCRETA

Montgomery emphasizes the occurrence of the porokeratotic plug, mostly in the metatarsal area. This plug resembles a plantar corn 1 to 3 mm in diameter that is painful and frequently is confused with a plantar wart. Taub and Steinberg call attention to the histologic similarity to porokeratosis of the usual kind.

SURFER'S NODULES

Nodules 1 to 3 cm (rarely as much as 5 or 6 cm) in diameter, sometimes eroded or even ulcerated, may develop on the tops of the feet or over the tibial tubercles of surfboard riders who paddle their boards in a kneeling position, as is customary in the cold water off the California coast. In warmer waters, as in Hawaii, the prone position is customary and such nodules seldom occur.

These nodules are hyperplastic granulomas that slowly involute over the months when there is no surfing. They respond readily to intralesional corticosteroid injections.

CORAL CUTS

A severe type of skin injury may rarely occur from the cuts of coral skeletons. The abrasions and cuts are painful, and local therapy may sometimes provide little or no relief. Healing may take months. As a rule, if secondary infection is guarded against, such cuts heal as well as any others.

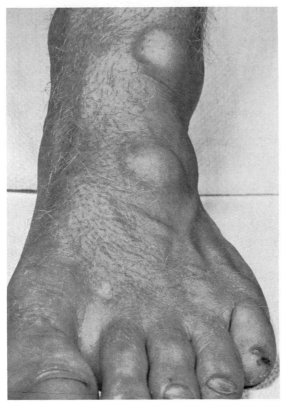

Figure 3–26. Surfer's nodules on instep and ankle, over bony prominences. (Courtesy of Dr. E. A. Taylor.)

DECUBITUS ULCER

The bedsore or decubitus is an ulcer produced anywhere on the body by prolonged pressure. The bony prominences of the body are the most frequently affected sites. The ulcer usually begins with erythema at the pressure point; in a short time a "punched-out" ulcer develops. Most frequently this occurs on the back over the sacrum, buttocks, backbone, and heels. Necrosis with a grayish pseudomembrane is seen, especially in the untreated ulcer.

The pressure sore is caused by ischemia of the underlying structures of the skin, fat, and muscles as a result of sustained and constant pressure. Usually it occurs in chronically debilitated persons who are unable to change position in bed.

Treatment consisting of relief of the pressure on the affected parts by frequent change of position, meticulous nursing care, and an alternating air-circulating mattress are especially helpful.

In some cases, 20 per cent benzoyl peroxide gel has been extremely beneficial in promoting healing. The surrounding area is ringed with petrolatum; the gel is applied to the ulcer and covered with petrolatum gauze. It is redressed daily.

Debrisan (dextranomer) may be applied several times daily. Occlusive dressings such as Op-Site, Vigilon or Duo-Derm may be helpful. Surgical debridement with reconstructive procedures are necessary at times.

FRICTION BLISTERS

The formation of vesicles or bullae may occur at sites of combined pressure and friction and may be enhanced by heat and moisture. The feet of military recruits in training and the palms of the oarsman who has not yet developed protective calluses are examples of those at risk. The size of the bulla depends upon the site of the trauma. If the skin is tense and uncomfortable, the blister should be drained, but the roof should not be completely removed as it may act as its own dressing.

SCLEROSING LYMPHANGITIS

Fiumara has reported a cordlike structure encircling the coronal sulcus of the penis, or running the length of the shaft, which he attributes to trauma during vigorous sexual play. It is produced by a sclerosing lymphangiitis. Treatment is not necessary as it follows a benign, self-limiting course.

BLACK HEEL

Synonyms: talon noir, calcaneal petechiae, *chromidrose plantaire.*

A sudden shower of minute black punctate macules, most often on the posterior edge of the plantar surface of one or both heels, but sometimes on the distal planta of one or more toes, black heel is often seen in basketball, volleyball, tennis, or lacrosse players. Seeming confluence may lead to mimicry of melanoma. Wilkinson recently pointed out that the bleeding is caused by shearing stress of sports activities. Treatment is unnecessary.

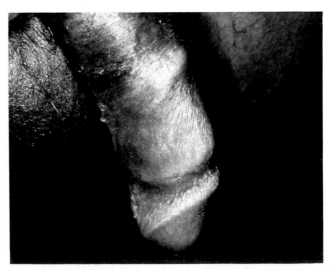

Figure 3–27. Firm linear cord of sclerosing lymphangitis in coronal sulcus of penis. (Courtesy of Dr. Axel W. Hoke.)

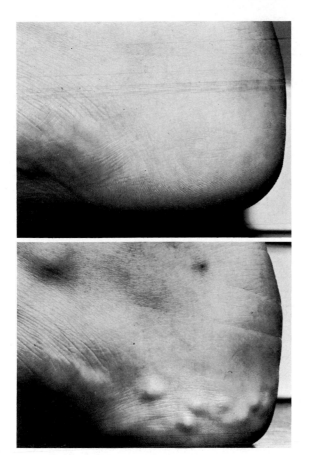

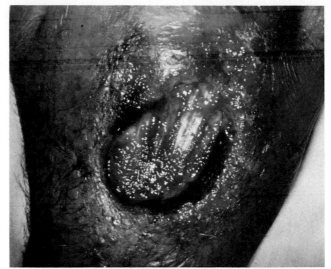

Figure 3–29. *Narcotic dermopathy: ulcer from extravascular injection of "speed" (amphetamine). (Courtesy of Dr. Axel W. Hoke.)*

Figure 3–28. *Fat herniation. Papules appear as pressure is put on heel ("piezogenic"). (Shelley WB, et al, JAMA 205:308, 1968.)*

PAINFUL FAT HERNIATION

Also called **painful piezogenic pedal papules,** this has been described by Shelley and Rawnsley as an unusual cause for painful feet in the form of fat herniations through thin fascial layers of the weight-bearing parts of the heel. These dermatoceles become apparent when weight is placed on the heel and disappear as soon as the pressure is removed. The extrusion of the fat tissue together with its blood vessels and nerves initiates pain on prolonged standing. Avoidance of standing for a long time is the only means of obtaining relief from this pain. These fat herniations may be present in many people without symptoms.

NARCOTIC DERMOPATHY

Heroin (diacetylmorphine) is the narcotic most frequently used by addicts, according to Minkin and Cohen. It is prepared for injection by dissolving the heroin powder in boiling water and then injecting it with a needle and syringe or with a medicine dropper.

The favored route of administration is intravenous, known among addicts as "mainlining." This results

in thrombosed, cordlike, thickened veins at the sites of injection.

Subcutaneous injection ("skin popping") is resorted to only when mainlining is no longer feasible. Multiple, scattered, discrete atrophic scars result.

Ulcerating nodules may also occur in just a few hours after injection; these are attributed to an idiosyncrasy to one of the adulterants used to dilute the heroin before it reaches the user. Foreign body granulomas may present as firm, movable nodules on the upper extremities which may develop months to years after their last injection. These are most likely talc granulomas.

Paregoric addicts favor the jugular vein in the

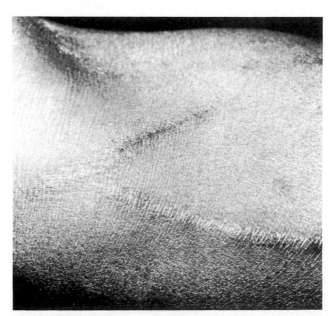

Figure 3–30. *Narcotic dermopathy: "tracks"—from phlebitis following intravenous injections of heroin. (Courtesy of Dr. Axel W. Hoke.)*

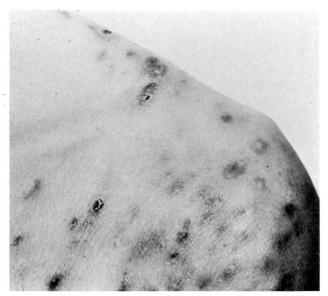

Figure 3–31. Narcotic dermopathy: scars from "skin popping"—injecting deliberately darkened heroin intracutaneously. (Courtesy of Dr. Axel W. Hoke.)

supraclavicular area; therefore, scars seen in that area may be due to this type of addiction. Abscesses due to infection are also frequently seen.

Weidman and Fellner have reported the various cutaneous manifestations of addiction to heroin and other addictive drugs. Some of these are camptodactylia, edema of the eyelids, persistent nonpitting edema of the hands, urticaria, abscesses, atrophic scars, and hyperpigmentation. Intramuscular pentazocine abuse leads to a typical clinical picture of tense, woody fibrosis, irregular punched-out ulcerations, and a rim of hyperpigmentation at the sites of injections.

In recent years it has been established that male users of intravenous drugs with unsterile needles are two to four times as likely to acquire AIDS as female users; the overall incidence of HIV infection in intravenous drug users in New York City was 50 per cent.

FOREIGN BODY REACTIONS

Tattoo. Tattooing is the introduction of insoluble pigments into the skin to produce permanent inscriptions and figures. Pigment is applied to the skin and then needles pierce the skin to force the material into the cutis. The pigments inserted may be carmine, indigo, vermilion, India ink, chrome green, manganese, Venetian Red, titanium or zinc oxide, lead carbonate, logwood, cobalt blue, cinnabar (mercuric sulfide), and cadmium sulfide. The latter, used for yellow color or to brighten the cinnabar red, causes photosensitive reactions. (See p. 37.)

In addition to the photosensitivity that may develop from tattoos, numerous other reactions can occur. Kirsch reported malignant melanoma occurring many years after tattooing. Unsanitary tattooing

methods have resulted in inoculation of syphilis, infectious hepatitis, tuberculosis, AIDS, and leprosy. Occasionally the tattoo marks may become keloidal. Accidental tattoo marks may be induced by narcotic addicts who sterilize the needles for injection by flaming the needle with a lighted match. The carbon formed on the needle is then "tattooed" into the skin as the needle is inserted. Discoid lupus erythematosus has been reported by Lerchin and associates occurring in the red pigmented portion of tattoos. Also sarcoid nodules in tattoos have been reported by Farzan. Granuloma-annulare-like lesions have also been seen.

Treatment for the removal of tattoo marks is usually unsatisfactory. Excision is the most satisfactory when the lesions are small enough and situated so that ellipsoid excisions are feasible.

Relatively superficial dermabrasion, either with the usual instrument or by vigorous rubbing with a paste of wet table salt, has been fairly successful. The pigment is discharged into the dressings, a little each day, until the residual amount is negligible. Clabaugh has described his 5-year experience with dermabrasion.

Laser treatment of tattoos has been successfully performed by Goldman and his associates. Its action is on the dark dye particles; intense heat selectively burns out the tattoo. Clabaugh has described a five-year experience with this procedure.

Paraffinoma. At one time the injection of paraffin into the skin for cosmetic purposes, such as the smoothing of wrinkles and the augmentation of breasts, was popular. Injection of oils such as paraffin, camphorated oil, cottonseed or sesame oil, and beeswax may produce plaquelike indurations with ulcerations after a time lapse. Another reaction may be inflammatory, with mild erysipeloid attacks and marked tenderness. *Human adjuvant disease*, which

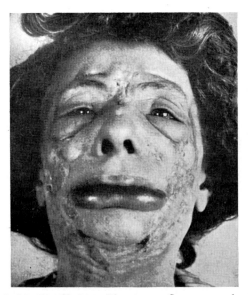

Figure 3–32. Paraffinoma. The masses fluoresce under Wood's light.

usually presents with scleroderma-like findings, may also occur, as reported by Kumagai et al.

Present treatment methods are unsatisfactory. When these tumors are treated surgically it is necessary to remove them widely and completely.

Mercury Granuloma. Lupton et al recently reviewed these lesions, which occur as foreign-body giant cell granulomas. Systemic toxicity may develop from cutaneous injury and may result in death.

Beryllium Granuloma. This is seen as a chronic, persistent, granulomatous inflammation of the skin with ulceration which may follow accidental laceration by an old-fashioned broken fluorescent light bulb coated with zinc beryllium silicate. Modern bulbs do not contain beryllium.

Zirconium Granuloma. This papular eruption involving the axillae is sometimes seen as an allergic reaction in those shaving their armpits and using a deodorant containing zirconium lactate. It may also be seen following the application of various poison ivy lotions containing zirconium compounds. The lesions are brownish red, dome-shaped, shiny papules suggestive of sarcoidosis.

This is an acquired, delayed-type, allergic reaction resulting in a granuloma of the sarcoidal type; in many respects it mimics the course of a Kveim reaction.

After many months the lesions involute spontaneously.

Silica Granuloma. Automobile and other types of accidents may propel the victim along the ground, thereby producing accidental tattooing of dirt (silicon dioxide) into the skin to induce silica granulomas. These are usually black or blue papules or macules arranged in a linear fashion and are extremely unsightly, especially on the face. At times the granulomatous reaction to silica may be delayed for years, until sensitization develops, and the ensuing dermatitis may be both chronic and disfiguring. They may be caused by amorphous or crystalline silicon dioxide (quartz), by magnesium silicate (talcum), or by complex polysilicates (asbestos). Talcum granulomas of the skin and peritoneum may develop after surgical operations from the talc powder used on surgical gloves.

The removal of these granulomas is fraught with difficulties. Dermabrasion is a satisfactory method for the removal of dirt accidentally embedded into the skin of the face or scalp.

Carbon Stain. Discoloration of the skin from embedded carbon usually occurs in children from the careless use of firearms or firecrackers or from a puncture wound by a pencil, which may leave a permanent black mark of embedded graphite, easily mistaken for a metastatic melanoma. The carbon is deposited at various depths to produce a connective tissue reaction and even keloids.

Carbon particles may be removed immediately after their deposition by the use of a toothbrush and forceps. This expeditious and meticulous early care results in the best possible cosmetic result. If the particles are left in place long enough, they are best removed by the use of skin punches 2 mm in diameter. Under local anesthesia the skin is put under tension and the punch is rotated into the skin to the depth of the imbedded powder. The corelike bit of skin is then lifted, the powder particle cut off with small curved scissors, and replaced. Alternative procedures are dermabrasion and use of the carbon dioxide laser.

Silicone Granuloma. Liquid silicones, composed of long chains of dimethyl siloxy groups, are biologically inert, and have been used for the correction of wrinkles, for the reduction of scars, and for building up of atrophic depressed areas of the skin. However, for chin or breast or other augmentation procedures of any great extent, it is now almost always used in silastic implants, which completely confine it. If trauma causes rupture of the bag, subcutaneous fibrotic nodules may develop. Human adjuvant disease after such events has been reported by Spiro.

Winer and his associates reported three cases of reactions to liquid silicone typical of foreign body granulomas. We have observed several cases of granulomatous reactions at the site of silicone injections for erasure of wrinkles. Chemically pure medical grade silicone, though not yet approved by the FDA and therefore not available through the usual channels, seems to be free of this fault, and may safely be injected in small amounts. For an extensive and excellent review concerning silicone injections into the skin, consult the paper of Selmanowitz and Orentreich.

Zyderm Collagen Granulomas. Barr and Stegman recently reviewed the granulomatous type of response one may encounter with injectable enzyme-digested purified bovine collagen solution (Zyderm). The major histologic differential diagnosis is granuloma annulare.

Lipoatrophy. Atrophy of the subcutaneous fat tissue is being seen more frequently, owing to the increased use of corticosteroid for repository injections and intralesional therapy. This type of reaction may develop even two months after injection. Such reaction is rarely seen after injections of other medications such as penicillin and insulin.

Treatment is not necessary since after several months the depressed area fills out and assumes its normal contours.

Dermoepidermal Atrophy. Depigmentation, thinning, and atrophy with depression of the epidermis, dermis, and even the panniculus, will occur if too much or too strong a corticosteroid preparation is injected intradermally or subcutaneously. Judicious choice of the right concentration, the right amount, and the right site will usually (but not invariably) prevent this very undesirable result. Most such lesions return to normal within a few months to a year or two at most. For **treatment** on the face, 2.5 to 5 mg per ml is a strong enough suspension of triamcinolone. For most other areas, 5 to 10 mg per ml is permissible. For keloids, 40 mg per ml is usually

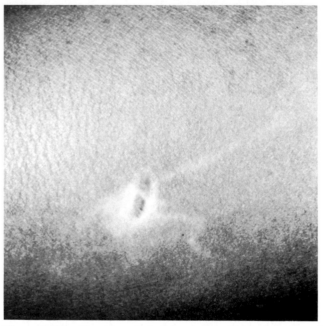

Figure 3–33. Atrophy and depigmentation due to intradermal injection of triamcinolone acetonide. (Courtesy of Dr. Axel W. Hoke.)

required. This concentration should never be injected into the arm for systemic therapy, however, but only deeply into the gluteus maximus, with a needle at least 3.5 cm long, to prevent a deep dimple from forming. Such dimples almost always fill in and disappear in 8–18 months and should not be excised.

Alper JC, et al: Use of vapor-permeable membrane for cutaneous ulcers: Details of application and side effects. JAAD 1984, 11:858.

Barr RJ, et al: Delayed skin test reaction to injectable collagen implant (Zyderm). JAAD 1984, 10:652.

Idem: Necrobiotic granulomas in bovine collagen test injection sites. JAAD 1982, 6:867.

Bito L, et al: Unusual complications of mercurial (cinnabar) tattoo. Arch Dermatol 1967, 96:165.

Clabaugh WA: Tattoo removal by superficial dermabrasion: Five-year experience. Plast Reconstr Surg 1975, 55:401.

Erickson JG, et al: Surfer's nodules and other complications of surfboarding. JAMA 1967, 201:134.

Farzan S: Sarcoidal reaction in tattoos. NY State J Med 1977, 77:1477.

Fiumara NJ: Nonvenereal sclerosing lymphadenitis of the penis. Arch Dermatol 1975, 111:902.

Friedman SJ, et al: Management of leg ulcers with hydrocolloid occlusive dressings. Arch Dermatol 1984, 120:1329.

Gibbs RC, et al: Abnormal biomechanics of the feet and the cause of hyperkeratoses. JAAD 1982, 6:1061.

Goldman L, et al: Laser treatment of tattoos. JAMA 1967, 201:841.

Horn RT, et al: Circular indurated lymphangitis of the penis. J Assoc Milit Dermatol 1980, 6:11.

James WD, et al: Allergic contact dermatitis from compound tincture of benzoin. JAAD 1984, 11:847.

Idem: Treatment of wounds received during live fire exercises. J Assoc Milit Dermatol 1984, 10:32.

Kirsch N: Malignant melanoma developing in a tattoo. Arch Dermatol 1967, 99:596.

Krull E: Chronic cutaneous ulcerations and impaired healing in human skin. JAAD 1985, 12:394.

Lerchin E, et al: Discoid lupus erythematosus occurring in red pigment of tattoos. J Assoc Milit Dermatol 1976, 1:19.

Lupton GP, et al: Cutaneous mercury granuloma. JAAD 1985, 12:296.

Meltzer L: Surgical correction of intertriginous soft corns. J Dermatol Surg 1976, 2:135.

Minkin W, et al: Dermatologic complications of heroin addiction. N Engl J Med 1967, 277:473.

Montgomery RM: Porokeratosis plantaris discreta. Cutis 1977, 20:711.

Padilla RS, et al: Cutaneous and venous complications of pentazocine abuse. Arch Dermatol 1979, 115:975.

Posner DI, et al: Cutaneous foreign body granulomas associated with intravenous drug abuse. JAAD 1985, 13:869.

Pucevich MV, et al: Widespread foreign body granulomas and elevated angiotensin-converting enzyme. Arch Dermatol 1982, 119:229.

Schlappner OLA, et al: Painful and nonpainful piezogenic pedal papules. Arch Dermatol 1972, 106:729.

Selmanowitz VJ, et al: Medical grade silicone: A monographic review. J Dermatol Surg Oncol 1977, 3:597.

Shelley WB, et al: The pathogenesis of silica granulomas in man. J Invest Dermatol 1960, 34:107.

Weidman AI, et al: Cutaneous manifestations of heroin and other addictive drugs. NY State J Med 1971, 71:2643.

Wilkinson DS: Black heel: A minor hazard of sport. Cutis 1977, 20:393.

HEMODIALYSIS

With the increased use of hemodialysis for many end-stage kidney problems, various untoward skin reactions have been reported.

Gilchrest and her associates have reported a bullous dermatosis appearing as subepidermal bullae on the backs of the hands in five patients undergoing weekly hemodialysis for chronic renal failure. Neither sun, porphyrias, nor drugs could be implicated in their production.

Gilkes and his associates reported that in renal failure, poor renal catabolism of melanocytic-stimulating hormone appears to account for the hyperpigmentation so often seen in patients on long-term hemodialysis. The plasma concentration of MSH correlates well with the duration of hemodialysis.

Perforating disorders, most commonly Kyrle's disease, have been increasingly reported in patients on hemodialysis. These occur as 2 to 15 mm, elevated, flesh-colored or hyperpigmented nodules with a central keratin plug. These cases have been reviewed by Hood et al and Patterson et al.

Gilchrest B, et al: Bullous dermatosis of hemodialysis. Ann Intern Med 1975, 83:480.

Gilkes JJH, et al: Plasma immunoreactive melanotrophic hormones in patients on maintenance hemodialysis. Br Med J 1975, 1:656.

Hood AF, et al: Kyrle's disease in patients with chronic renal failure. Arch Dermatol 1982, 118:85.

Patterson JW: The perforating disorders. JAAD 1984, 10:561.

4

Pruritus and Neurocutaneous Dermatoses

PRURITUS

Pruritus, commonly known as itching, is a sensation exclusive to the skin. It may be defined simply as that sensation which produces the desire to scratch. It has been determined that there are no specific anatomic fibers for each of the cutaneous sensations but rather that itch, touch, temperature (hot and cold), and pain sensations are all mediated by the same receptors. These sensations arise in fine unmyelinated C nerve fiber endings in the subepidermal area and are transmitted via the lateral spinothalamic tract to the thalamus and sensory cortex.

Itching may be elicited by many normally occurring stimuli such as light touch, temperature change, and emotional stress. Chemical, mechanical, thermal, and electric stimuli may also elicit itching. Pruritus is mediated by the release of chemical substances such as histamine, kinins, and proteases. When histamine mediates itching it is usually associated with urticaria.

Pruritus is modulated by other factors. Prostaglandin E lowers the threshold for histamine-induced pruritus, while enkephalins, pentapeptides which bind to opiate receptors in the brain, modulate pain centrally.

Patterns of Itching. There are great variations from person to person; indeed, in the same person there may be a variation in reactions to the same stimulus. Psychic trauma, stress, absence of distractions, anxiety, and fear may all enhance itching. It is apt to be most severe at the time of undressing for bed.

Variations also occur according to regions of the skin. The ear canals, eyelids, nostrils, and perianal and genital areas are especially susceptible to pruritus.

Denman ST: A review of pruritus. JAAD 1986, 14:375.

PAROXYSMAL PRURITUS

Severe, persistent, or recurrent pruritus, with or without prior skin lesions, is often paroxysmal in character: sudden in onset, irresistibly severe, frequently awakening the patient, and stopping instantly and completely as soon as pain is induced by scratching. The pleasure of scratching is so intense that the patient—despite his realization that he is damaging the skin—is unable to stop short of inflicting such damage.

Why is no pain but only intense pleasure felt while the fingernails are digging right into the dermis? It seems possible that Wolff's theory of antidromic impulses passing outward over sensory nerves, and thus temporarily incapacitating them, could account for such a bizarre sensory aberration. The instant that a pain impulse reverses this flow, pain replaces the itching, and there is no itching until the injuries have healed.

In a number of more or less dramatic instances, we have seen the sudden recall of a powerful but completely suppressed emotional reaction stop such pruritus immediately and completely, even when it had occurred daily for many years. When itching stops, scratching stops. The "habit" of scratching is a myth—at least in such cases.

Itching of this distinctive character is never seen as a result of dermatitis venenata, or tinea, or scabies. It is characteristic of only a few dermatoses: lichen simplex chronicus, atopic dermatitis, nummular eczema, dermatitis herpetiformis, neurotic excoriations, and prurigo nodularis. Only in these does pruritus regularly induce scratching of such violence as to induce bleeding and leave hyperpigmentation or scarring, or both.

Such itching is often a result not of feeling emotional tension but of rejecting and suppressing it. In cases of very recent onset the victim may rarely, by patient questioning, be enabled to recall an emotionally traumatic incident that happened on the day the itching began—and be dramatically cured thereby. But, as a rule, the cause is too deeply buried to be found; and, indeed, it may be such a traumatic event that the patient is better off with the neurodermatitis than with the knowledge of its cause. It may be "too hot to handle."

Arnold HL Jr: Paroxysmal pruritus. JAAD 1984, 11:322.

INTERNAL CAUSES OF PRURITUS

Itching as a symptom may be present in a number of internal disorders. The degree of intensity and the duration of itching vary from one disease to another.

Among the most frequent internal disorders causing itching are malignant lymphoma, uremia, diabetes mellitus, malignancies, obstructive biliary disease, intestinal parasitosis, polycythemia vera, hypo- and hyperthyroidism, carcinoid, multiple sclerosis, and myeloma.

In Hodgkin's disease itching is usually continuous and at times accompanied by severe burning. The incidence of pruritus is between 10 and 25 per cent and Amblard found it to be the first symptom of this disease in 7 per cent of 94 patients. Its cause is unknown.

The pruritus of leukemia has a tendency to be more generalized and less severe than in Hodgkin's disease.

It has been reported that internal cancer may be found in between 3 and 47 per cent of patients with generalized pruritus unexplained by skin lesions. However, Paul et al have lately confirmed the finding of Kantor et al, that no significant overall increase of malignant neoplasms is to be expected in patients with pruritus, and no general efforts at cancer screening are warranted. A suggested workup for chronic generalized pruritus is a complete history and physical; CBC and differential; thyroid, liver, and renal panels; chest x-ray, and fasting blood sugar.

Kantor GR, et al: Generalized pruritus and systemic disease. JAAD 1983, 9:375.

Paul R, et al: Itch and malignancy prognosis in generalized pruritus: A 6-year follow-up of 125 patients. JAAD 1987, 16:1179.

Peterson AO, et al: Pruritus and nonspecific nodules preceding myelomonocytic leukemia. JAAD 1980, 2:496.

Biliary Pruritus. Chronic liver disease with obstructive jaundice may cause severe generalized pruritus. Twenty to 50 per cent of patients with jaundice have pruritus.

Freedman showed that serum conjugated bile acid levels were not correlated with pruritus. Bile acids on the skin surface are primarily of the unconjugated dihydroxy variety. These are effective pruritogens and may be involved in causing pruritus in these patients, as Garden et al stated in their review. Whatever the cause, bile-salt–containing cholestyramine is an effective antipruritic in cholestatic disease.

Primary Biliary Cirrhosis. This type of cirrhosis occurs almost exclusively in women over 30 years of age. Itching may begin insidiously; with time, extreme pruritus develops. This almost intolerable itching is accompanied by jaundice and a striking melanotic hyperpigmentation of the entire skin; the patient may turn almost black, except for a hypopigmented "butterfly" area in the upper back. Reynolds first called attention to this in 1973, and Goldman et al reemphasized it in 1983. At the sites of extreme pruritus, mottled vitiliginous spots may be observed. In addition, xanthomatosis in the form of plane xanthomas of the palms, xanthelasmas, and tuberous xanthomas over the joints may be seen.

Dark urine, steatorrhea, and eventual decalcification of bone may frequently be recognized. The serum bilirubin, alkaline phosphatase, serum phospholipids, and cholesterol values are increased. Serum transaminases are also elevated. The antimitochondrial antibody test is positive.

The disease is usually relentlessly progressive with the development of hepatic failure and esophageal varices. The latter may produce hemorrhage and

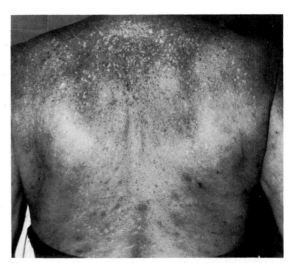

Figure 4–1. Melanotic pigmentation and depigmentation, and excoriations, due to intractable generalized pruritus from primary biliary cirrhosis, in a 50-year-old woman.

even death. Several cases have been accompanied by scleroderma.

Treatment is directed against the extreme pruritus. At the present the most effective therapy is the continual use of cholestyramine resin.

Duncan JS, et al: Treatment of pruritus due to chronic obstructive liver disease. Br Med J 1984, 289:22.
Freedman WR, et al: Pruritus in cholestasis. Am J Med 1981, 70:1011.
Garden JM, et al: Pruritus in hepatic cholestasis. Arch Dermatol 1985. 121:1415.
Goldman RD, et al: The "butterfly" sign. Arch Dermatol 1983, 119:183.
Perlson SM: Phototherapy for primary biliary cirrhosis. Arch Dermatol 1981, 117:608.
Person JR: Ultraviolet A and cholestatic pruritus. Arch Dermatol 1981, 117:684.

Pruritus of Anemia. Iron deficiency anemia was implicated by Lewiecki and Rahman as a cause of chronic generalized pruritus in a 62-year-old woman. Ferrous sulfate orally corrected the anemia and stopped the pruritus; other causes were excluded. Vickers and Valsecchi et al have made similar reports.

Valsecchi R, et al: Generalized pruritus: A manifestation of iron deficiency. Arch Dermatol 1983, 119:630.
Vickers CF: Iron deficiency and the skin. Br J Dermatol 1973, 89 (Suppl 9):10.

Uremic Pruritus. Chronic renal failure is the commonest internal systemic cause of pruritus. Gilchrest found that 77 per cent of patients with chronic renal failure had experienced it at some time, though only 37 per cent (of 237 patients) were having prolonged bothersome itching at the time of questioning. Two-thirds of those with pruritus said it was worst at the time of hemodialysis. Almost all were relieved by UVB treatment: 32 of 38 patients treated by Gilchrest et al responded.

Gilchrest BA, et al: Ultraviolet phototherapy of uremic pruritus. Ann Intern Med 1979, 91:17.
Idem: Clinical features of pruritus among patients undergoing maintenance hemodialysis. Arch Dermatol 1982, 118:154.
Pederson JA, et al: Idiopathic generalized pruritus in dialysis patients treated with activated oral charcoal. Ann Intern Med 1980, 93:446.
Schultz BC, et al: Uremic pruritus treated with ultraviolet light. JAMA 1980, 243:1836.
Silverberg DS: Cholestyramine in uremic pruritus. Br Med J 1977, 1:752.

Polycythemia Vera. Over one-third of these patients experience pruritus, usually induced by temperature changes. Antiserotonin treatment is helpful, but there is danger of gastric bleeding from aspirin. Swerlick reported a good response to PUVA. Antihistamines are usually ineffective.

Swerlick RA: Photochemotherapy treatment of pruritus associated with polycythemia vera. JAAD 1985, 13:675.

TREATMENT OF PRURITUS

Pruritus is frequently difficult to control, be it paroxysmal pruritus, a symptom complex of some internal disorder, or a symptom of a definite dermatosis. There are only a few pruritic dermatoses in which specific medication is available. Dapsone (Avlosulfon) and sulfapyridine are specific for dermatitis herpetiformis. Cholestyramine provides almost complete relief for the severe itching of primary biliary cirrhosis. UVB therapy for uremic pruritus is effective in the vast majority treated. Scabicides are specific for scabies.

Since the number of dermatoses for which we have specific treatment for causes is small, general measures are important. Removal of the cause and breaking of the habit of scratching are extremely desirable. Emotional tension is extremely conducive to paroxysms of pruritus. Stimulants such as caffeine and theobromines, which are abundant in coffee, tea, chocolate, and cola drinks, may aggravate itching, as may alcohol. As a rule the skin should be protected against external irritants such as wool.

Various lubricants in the bath water and afterwards emollients to the entire body are helpful, especially in senile pruritus, winter itch or xerotic eczema, and the pruritus associated with hyperthyroidism.

Corticosteroids, internally or topically, are effective in the control of pruritus, especially when it is due to inflammation or lichenification. Topical corticosteroids are available in the form of sprays, ointments, creams, and lotions. Intralesional injection of triamcinolone suspension (Kenalog) is extremely effective.

Internal remedies against itching are the antihistaminics, especially promethazine (Phenergan), trimeprazine (Temaril), diphenhydramine (Benadryl), methdilazine (Tacaryl), and azatadine maleate (Optimine). Two third-generation, non-sedating H_1 antagonists are terfenadine and astemizole. The antiserotonin drug cyproheptadine (Periactin) may be effective. Hydroxyzine (Atarax or Vistaril) is helpful in the urticarial types of pruritus and is especially effective in cholinergic urticaria and dermatographia. Amitriptyline (Elavil) is effective, especially in paroxysmal pruritus. The tricyclic antidepressants are highly potent H_1 antagonists. Doxepin (Sinequan) is usually helpful in the treatment of chronic urticaria.

The relief of pruritus with topical remedies is accomplished by numerous medications. The application of an ice bag or the opposite, a hot water bottle, to the affected area is primitive but sometimes effective, especially when nothing else is available. Phenol incorporated into lotions and ointments with a concentration varying from 0.5 to 1 per cent is helpful. Bernstein et al studied topically applied tricyclic antidepressants (doxepin and amitriptyline) and found them partially effective.

The "caine" preparations such as benzocaine, procaine, and lidocaine (Xylocaine) 5 per cent ointments are excellent antipruritics, but prolonged usage may produce contact sensitization.

Liquor carbonis detergens, 2 to 10 per cent in alcohol, thymol, 0.5 per cent in lotions, tincture of benzoin, chloral, resorcin, olive oil, alcohol, and acetic acid are other topical antipruritics.

Arnold AJ, et al: Suppression of histamine-induced pruritus by hydroxyzine and various neuroleptics. JAAD 1979, 1:509.
Bernstein JE, et al: Inhibition of histamine-induced pruritus by topical tricyclic antidepressants. JAAD 1981, 5:582.
Boss M, et al: Lack of effect of the antihistamine drug clemastine on the potentiation of itch by prostaglandin E. Arch Dermatol 1981, 117:208.

PRURITIC DERMATOSES

Itching is the most common symptom of skin diseases. The reactivity of certain cutaneous diseases varies. One of the most pruritic dermatoses is dermatitis herpetiformis, but others may be just as severe, depending mostly on the degree of involvement and the susceptibility of the patient.

Some of these, in addition to dermatitis herpetiformis, are insect bites, scabies, pediculosis, atopic dermatitis, contact dermatitis, psoriasis, nummular eczema, lichen chronicus simplex, prurigo nodularis, and generalized neurodermatitis. Because of the distinctiveness of each of these diseases, they are readily recognized.

Vigorous and persistent scratching and rubbing in an effort to relieve the tormenting symptoms may produce objective signs such as scratch marks, erythema, fissures, ulcers, wheals, and pigmentation. The most common effect of chronic, paroxysmal pruritus is *lichenification*, which is leathery thickening of the skin resulting from prolonged rubbing and

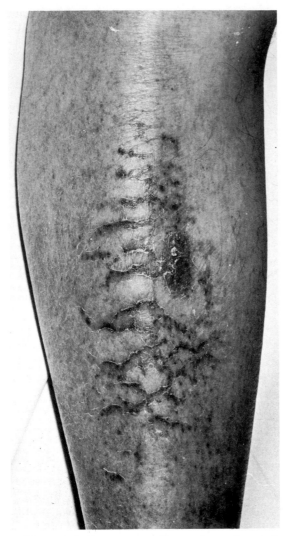

Figure 4–3. Eczema craquelé, weeping and crusted.

scratching well beyond the degree which would be possible with a normal pain threshold.

Winter Itch

Asteatotic eczema, eczema craquelé, pruritus hiemalis, and xerotic eczema are some other names given to this pruritic condition. It is characterized by generalized body pruritus which is usually most severe on the arms and shins. The skin is dry and fine flakes are seen over the entire skin. In severe cases eczematization may occur on the shins. The disease is known as eczema craquelé because the skin exhibits fine cracks in the eczematous area, which resemble the cracks in old porcelain dishes.

Frequent and lengthy bathing with plenty of soap during the wintertime is the most frequent cause. This is especially prevalent in the elderly, whose skin tends to have decreased sebum secretion. Low humidity in overheated rooms during cold weather contributes to this condition.

Treatment consists of educating the patient regarding the above factors; using soap only in the armpits and crotch area; and lubrication of the skin immedi-

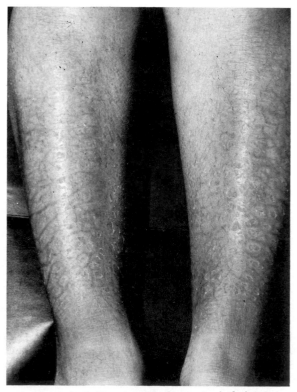

Figure 4–2. Eczema craquelé in a typical site.

ately after bathing, with bath oil such as Alpha Keri. Mineral oil (Albolene is very good), Eucerin, and lactic acid preparations such as ammonium lactate lotion (Lac-Hydrin) are very helpful after-bath applications. In severe cases soaking in salt water, a cupful in a tub, or the addition of mineral oil to the bath water may be helpful.

Dahl MV, et al: 12 per cent Lactate lotion for the treatment of xerosis. Arch Dermatol 1983, 119:27.
Griest MC, et al: Cimetidine-induced xerosis and asteatotic dermatitis. Arch Dermatol 1982, 118:253.

Pruritus Ani

The anal area is a common site of eroticism. Itching symptoms are often centered in the anal or genital area (very rarely both) with little or no pruritus elsewhere. Many cases are psychogenic in nature.

Anal neurodermatitis is characterized by paroxysms of violent itching, at which time the patient may tear at the affected area until bleeding is induced. Manifestations are identical with those of lichen chronicus simplex elsewhere, as in neurodermatitis of the ear canals. Not all cases of pruritus ani are due to psychogenic causes; therefore, a thorough search for other etiologic factors should always be made.

Mycotic pruritus ani is characterized by fissures and white sodden epidermis. Scrapings from the anal area examined directly with potassium hydroxide mou fungi. Cultures for fungi are also taken. *Candida albicans, Epidermophyton floccosum,* and *Trichophyton rubrum* are frequent causative fungi in this area. Other sites of fungus infection such as the groins, toes, and nails should also be investigated. Erythrasma in the groins and perianal region may also occasionally produce pruritus. The diagnosis is established by pinkish or coral red fluorescence under the Wood's light. Baral has found *Staphylococcus aureus* present in many cases of pruritus ani, which cleared upon appropriate antibiotic therapy.

Anal psoriasis may also cause itching. The perianal lesions are usually sharply marginated, and psoriatic lesions may be present on other parts of the body. Other frequent favorite sites for psoriasis may show lesions. Sometimes the diagnosis of psoriasis is made by observing the characteristically pitted or spotted fingernails of the patient as he pulls his buttocks apart.

Seborrheic dermatitis of the anal area may also cause pruritus ani. It also involves other areas such as the groins, scalp, chest, and face. Similarly, lichen planus may involve the perianal region.

Allergic contact dermatitis from local anesthetics used in suppositories for hemorrhoids, or irritational contact dermatitis from gastrointestinal contents such as hot spices, cathartics, or failure to adequately cleanse the area after bowel movements may be causes. Tetracyclines may cause pruritus ani, most often in women, by inducing candidiasis.

Pruritus ani caused by *pinworm infestation*, especially in children and sometimes in their parents, is not too uncommon. Nocturnal pruritus is most prevalent. Other intestinal parasites such as *Taenia solium, T. saginata,* and *Strongyloides stercoralis* may produce pruritus. Intestinal amebiasis may also cause pruritus. Pediculosis pubis may cause anal itching; however, attention is focused by the patient on the pubic area where itching is most severe.

Physical changes such as *hemorrhoids, anal tags, fissures,* and *fistulas* may aggravate or produce pruritus. *Anal warts* and *condyloma latum* (syphilis) may be causative agents, though these rarely itch. Anal gonorrhea, especially in men, is frequently overlooked when pruritus is the only symptom.

Thorough examination for malignancies should be made. Extramammary Paget's disease is easily overlooked in women.

TREATMENT. Except in psychogenic pruritus ani, once the etiologic agent has been found, a rational and effective treatment regimen may be started such as antifungals and anthelmintics for fungal and helminthic disease respectively.

Topical corticosteroids are most effective for the nonfungal types of pruritus ani. Intralesional injections with a syringe with a 30 gauge needle of triamcinolone suspension into the perianal area after careful cleansing with hexachlorophene are extremely beneficial in many instances. (*Caution:* even with most careful asepsis, intralesional injections in the groin and perianal region may produce abscesses.) Pramoxine hydrochloride, a nonsteroidal topical anesthetic, is effective. In Pramosone lotion it is combined with hydrocortisone.

Meticulous toilet care should be followed no matter what the cause of the itching. After defecation the anal area should be cleansed with soft cellulose tissue and, whenever possible, washed with mild soap and water. Cleansing with wet toilet tissue after dry is advisable in all cases. Medicated cleansing pads such as Tucks should be used regularly. An emollient lotion, Balneol, is helpful for cleansing without producing irritation.

Baral J: Pruritus ani and *Staphylococcus aureus.* JAAD 1983, 9:962.
Bowyer A, et al: Erythrasma and pruritus ani. Acta Dermatol 1971, 51:444.

Pruritus Vulvae

The vulva is also a common site for pruritus of different causes. Psychogenic pruritus vulvae is the counterpart of pruritus scroti in men, and the same neurogenic mechanisms may be responsible for the symptoms.

Vaginal candidiasis is one of the most frequent physical causes of pruritus vulvae. This is true especially during pregnancy and when tetracyclines are taken by mouth. The inguinal and perineal and perianal areas may also be involved.

Microscopic examination of the secretions for the presence of *Candida albicans* as well as cultures for fungus should be taken.

Trichomonas vaginitis may also cause vulvar pruritus. For the detection of *Trichomonas vaginalis* a cotton-tipped applicator is inserted into the vagina before any other examination is made. The applicator is then rinsed off in 1 cc of normal saline solution. A drop of this is placed on a hanging drop slide and examined under the dry high-power objective. The organism, if present, will be readily recognized by its motility, its size (somewhat larger than a leukocyte), and its piriform shape.

Contact dermatitis may also cause pruritus vulvae. Sanitary pads, contraceptives, douche solutions, and partner's condoms are some of the causative agents.

Urinary incontinence and diabetes mellitus should also be kept in mind as possible causes.

Lichen sclerosus et atrophicus is one of the frequent causes of pruritus in the genital area in middle-aged and elderly women.

Within this differential diagnosis is *essential vulvodynia,* which is a painful burning sensation in the vulva with no objective dermatologic or gynecologic abnormalities. In a recent review McKay discussed vulvodynia in all its subsets. Extramammary Paget's disease should be considered.

Extramammary Paget's disease has already been mentioned under pruritus ani and pruritus vulvae.

TREATMENT. Candidiasis is treated best with miconazole (Monistat Derm) or with nystatin vaginal suppositories.

Trichomonas infection is best treated with metronidazole (Flagyl) by mouth and also vaginal inserts. Lichen sclerosus et atrophicus responds best to topical testosterone, or Deladumone. Topical steroids

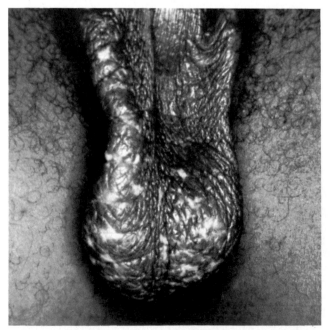

Figure 4–4. Pruritus scroti, analogous to pruritus vulvae in a woman.

may be used in psychogenic pruritus or irritant or allergic reactions. Topical lidocaine or Pramoxine or oral tricyclic antidepressant may be helpful.

Pruritus Scroti

The adult scrotum, like the adult scalp, is virtually immune to dermatophyte infection, but it is a favorite site for circumscribed neurodermatitis (lichen simplex chronicus). Pruritus of the scrotum is seen less frequently than pruritus ani and pruritus vulvae.

Psychogenic pruritus is probably the most frequent type of itching seen. Lichenification may result, be extreme, and persist for many years despite intensive therapy. Topical corticosteroids are the mainstay in controlling most cases.

Itchy Points (Puncta Pruritica)

Noxon Toomey described this entity, recently confirmed by Crissey, in 1922. It consists of one or two intensely itching spots in clinically normal skin, sometimes followed by the appearance of seborrheic keratoses at exactly the same site. Curettage, cryosurgery, or punch biopsy of the itching point usually cures the condition.

Crissey JT: Puncta pruritica. Internat J Dermatol (in press).
Toomey N: Itchy points (puncta pruritica). Arch Derm are
    5:744.   nts for fun
                                                             albicans,

Hereditary Localized Pruritus

The members of a large family afflicted with this unusual itch have themselves named it *hereditary itch.* It was early thought to be a hereditary form of localized pruritus occurring in the third decade of life. Comings and Comings reported eight of the 15 members of several generations affected. Seven of the eight were women. The area was a 7 × 12 cm patch on the inner lower right scapular area. The scratching frequency was four to eight times daily. Subsequent reports and our own observations indicate that some cases were and are examples of *macular amyloidosis* without lichenification.

Most of these patients are unaware of the familial nature of this condition. The diagnosis is easily established by its typically unilateral appearance on the scapular or interscapular area.

Intralesional injections of corticosteroid suspension give prompt relief from the nagging and persistent pruritus for several months. Eventually the patient returns for more injections. Repeatedly rubbing dimethyl sulfoxide (DMSO) into the area for several weeks has provided considerable relief to three patients treated by Arnold.

Comings DE, et al: Hereditary localized pruritus. Arch Dermatol 1965, 92:236.

Aquagenic Pruritus

Steinman et al and Kligman et al have described this condition, in which there is severe, prickling discomfort within minutes of exposure to water, or on cessation of exposure to water. There is often a family history of similar symptoms. Either UVB therapy or antihistamines may be helpful. Patients should be checked for polycythemia vera, as it may rarely present in this fashion. Wolf et al describe baking soda in the bath water as helpful.

Bircher AJ, et al: Aquagenic pruritus. Arch Dermatol 1988, 124:84.
Kligman AM, et al: Water-induced itching without cutaneous signs. Arch Dermatol 1986, 122:183.
Steinman HK, et al: Aquagenic pruritus. JAAD 1985, 13:91.
Wolf R, et al: Variations in aquagenic pruritus and treatment alternatives. JAAD 1988, 18:1081.

Scabies

One of the most frequent pruritic dermatoses encountered by the physician is scabies. Generalized itching with lesions in typical locations should suggest scabies in the differential diagnosis of pruritus. Mention of scabies is made here to emphasize the importance of pruritus in this dermatosis.

Pruritus of Scalp

Pruritus of the scalp, especially in the elderly, is rather common. When excoriations, scaling, or erythema are not found, seborrheic dermatitis, psoriasis, or nodular neurodermatitis cannot be diagnosed. The cause of this is unknown in most cases.

Topical treatment with tar shampoos, salicylic acid sprays, and corticosteroid topical gels, and in severe cases the intralesional injection of corticosteroid suspension will bring relief. Cyproheptadine (Periactin) or trimeprazine (Temaril) internally may occasionally be helpful.

CUTANEOUS NEUROSES

Under the heading of functional disorders and psychosomatic dermatoses are included a great many diseases. Many have studied the influence of the psyche on the skin and the influence of the skin on the psyche. There are those dermatoses that are purely psychic in origin, such as acarophobia, parasitophobia, neurotic excoriations, and trichotillomania. In other dermatoses psychic factors have a more or less prominent role. Dermatitis factitia, psychogenic pruritus, neurodermatitis, exudative chronic discoid and lichenoid dermatitis, and hyperhidrosis are included in this group in which *stress*, *tension*, and *anxiety* are essential factors.

LICHENIFICATION

As a result of long-continued rubbing and scratching, more vigorously than a normal pain threshold would permit, the skin becomes thickened and leathery. The normal markings of the skin become exaggerated, so that the striae form a criss-cross pattern, and between them there is produced a mosaic composed of flat-topped, shiny, smooth, quadrilateral facets. This change, known as lichenification, may originate upon seemingly normal skin, or may develop upon skin that is the site of another disease, such as eczema or ringworm. Paroxysmal pruritus is the main symptom. This is known as *lichen simplex chronicus (neurodermatitis circumscripta)*.

Lichen Simplex Chronicus

CLINICAL FEATURES. Also known as **neurodermatitis circumscripta,** this circumscribed, lichenified, pruritic patch may develop on any part of the body. However, the disease has a predilection for the back and sides of the neck, and the extremities—especially the wrists and ankles. At times the eruption is decidedly papular, resembling lichen planus; in other instances the patches are excoriated, slightly scaly or moist, and rarely nodular.

Several distinctive types are recognized. **Lichen simplex nuchae** occurs on the back of the neck. It is not unusual to find this area excoriated and bleeding.

Nodular neurodermatitis of the scalp of Ayres consists of multiple pruritic and excoriated papules. It may be called prurigo of the scalp. The nodules or papules may ooze and form crusts and scales.

The vulva, the scrotum, and the anal area can be sites of severe neurodermatitis. Seldom, however, as Rees has pointed out, are genital and anal areas involved at the same time. An upper eyelid, the orifice of one or both ears, or a palm or sole may also be involved, and the ankle flexure is a favorite site as well.

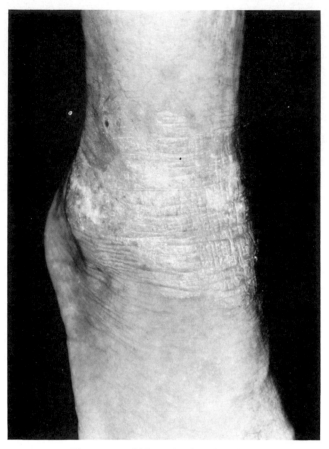

Figure 4–5. Lichen simplex chronicus.

It is not known by what mechanism the act of tearing through the epidermis with the fingernails, or burning the skin with painfully hot water, is made not merely painless but exquisitely and irresistibly pleasurable. But that is what happens, and virtually every patient with the disorder experiences this mysterious hallucination. The same phenomenon is encountered in atopic dermatitis, dermatitis herpetiformis, and prurigo nodularis.

ETIOLOGY. To what extent mechanical trauma plays a role in producing the original irritation is not known. The onset of this dermatosis is usually insidious, developing gradually. Scratching of a localized area on a chronic basis is a response to unknown factors; however, stress and anxiety have long been thought important.

TREATMENT. The primary consideration is the control of the pruritus, which is accomplished by no other means so effectively as by intralesional injections of triamcinolone suspension, using a concentration of 5 or (with caution) 10 mg per ml. Superficial injection invites the twin risks of epidermal and dermal atrophy and depigmentation, which may last for many months. Injection should not be made into infected or even excoriated or eroded lesions, for fear of causing abscesses. In such cases it is better to give 40 to 60 mg of triamcinolone acetonide intramuscularly instead initially to gain control, and perform the

intralesional injections later, when the lesions first recur.

Superficial x-ray or even grenz ray therapy, though effective, has been virtually completely superseded by therapy with topically applied corticosteroids. These are today the mainstay of therapy. High potency agents such as clobetasol propionate (Temovate) or betamethasone dipropionate (Diprolene) cream or ointment should be used initially, but not indefinitely; within weeks to months, they may cause epidermal and even dermal atrophy, with hypopigmentation, and before this a milder steroid should be substituted for them. Occlusion may rarely be required. If lichenification is well established, it is better not to waste time with topical applications but to resort immediately to intralesional triamcinolone injections.

Essentially, cessation of pruritus is the goal. Recurrences are frequent even after most thorough treatment. There are instances when the clearance of one lesion will see the onset of another elsewhere.

Distinctive Exudative Discoid and Lichenoid Dermatitis (DEDLE)

Sulzberger and Garbe in 1937 reported a psychosomatic disease encountered mostly in middle-aged or older patients of Jewish heritage, commonly called *"oid-oid"* disease. Since then it has been seen frequently by some observers (Knox) and not at all by

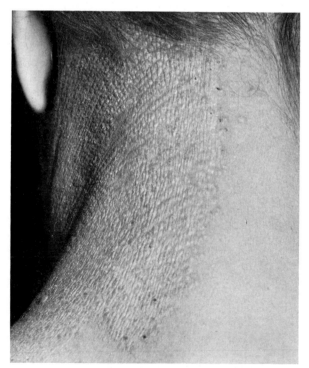

Figure 4–6. Neurodermatitis (lichen simplex chronicus) of the nape, a characteristic site.

others (Arnold), and its existence has been questioned. Recently two cases were reported in one issue of the *International Journal of Dermatology*, and Frank discussed its checkered career.

CLINICAL FEATURES. The eruption often begins on the penis or the bridge of the nose and persists there after other manifestations have disappeared. The onset is usually sudden, with a severely itching discoid plaque that later becomes a widespread dermatitis. Intractable and uncontrollable itching, with nocturnal accentuation and frequent crises, is the outstanding symptom. The lesions are sharply demarcated oval and discoid plaques showing rapid variations in consistency and appearance; they are at times flat and scaly, elevated, and edematous or oozing and crusting, and pass speedily through many of the clinical stages considered characteristic of eczematous lesions. Distinct clinical vesiculation and true herpetiform lesions are uniformly absent. The general lack of distinct and persistent vesicles and complete absence of bullae are emphasized, for these are important points in differentiating the findings in this dermatosis from characteristic findings in dermatitis herpetiformis, dermatophytids, and acute contact dermatitis. Sulzberger emphasized the constancy of penile involvement as an essential diagnostic criterion.

The significant histologic findings are a dilatation and thickening of the arterioles and a swelling of the nuclei in the intima. The entire dermis is edematous. An infiltrate of polymorphonuclear leukocytes, eosinophils, and many plasma cells forms a mantle about the blood vessels. Epidermal changes are variable degrees of acanthosis. Direct immunofluorescence has only very rarely been performed.

TREATMENT. The disease is usually refractory to treatment, most patients requiring prolonged care. Rest in the sunshine of warm southern climates with salt-water bathing was reported to be helpful.

The disease is benefited by corticosteroids. Intralesional injections of triamcinolone suspension have been the most effective treatment. Tranquilizers and the antihistaminics have a definite place in treatment of this disease. Cyproheptadine is frequently helpful. Tar baths are useful. The disease may have a self-limited course; however, usually it has been a persistent problem, affected mainly by the emotional status of the patient.

Baughman RD: Distinctive exudative discoid and lichenoid dermatosis. In Clinical Dermatology, Vol. 3, Unit 13–16, Demis DJ (ed). Philadelphia, Harper & Row, 1987.

Frank SB: EDLCD: does it exist or should it be discarded? Int J Dermatol 1989, 28:59 (letter).

Rebetti A: Sulzberger-Garbe disease in Europe. Int J Dermatol 1989, 28:22.

Rongioletti F: EDLCD: a fictional disease? Int J Dermatol 1989, 28:40.

Sulzberger MB, et al: Nine cases of a distinctive exudative discoid and lichenoid chronic dermatosis. Arch Derm Syph 1937, 36:247.

Idem: Distinctive exudative discoid and lichenoid dermatosis. Ztschr Haut Gesch Krankh 1959, 17:233.

Idem: DEDLCD (Sulzberger and Garbe) re-examined 1978. Br J Dermatol 1979, 100:13.

PRURIGO NODULARIS

SIGNS AND SYMPTOMS. Prurigo nodularis is a disease with multiple itching nodules situated chiefly on the extremities, especially on the anterior surfaces of the thighs and legs. A linear arrangement is common. The individual lesions are pea-sized or larger, firm, and erythematous or brownish. When fully developed they become verrucous, or fissured. The course of the disease is chronic and the lesions evolve slowly. Itching is always severe but is confined to the lesions themselves. Bouts of extreme pruritus occur when these patients are under stress. Prurigo nodularis is one of the disorders in which the pruritus is characteristically paroxysmal: intermittent, unbearably severe, and only relieved by scratching to the point of damaging the skin, usually inducing bleeding and often scarring.

King et al reported a case in which unilateral pruritus and prurigo nodularis—also unilateral—associated with diminished touch, pain, temperature, and position, followed surgical repair of a cerebral aneurysm.

ETIOLOGY. The etiology is unknown. The disease

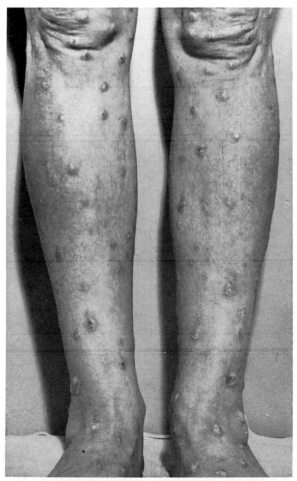

Figure 4–7. Prurigo nodularis.

is regarded as an atypical nodular form of neuro-dermatitis circumscripta.

Some clinical resemblance to dermatitis herpetiformis is by no means rare—with similarly severe and paroxysmal pruritus, similar hyperpigmentation, and similar remissions and recurrences. Occasionally *pemphigoid* may present as the so-called *prurigo nodularis variant,* which was reviewed by Roenigk et al. Half of 46 patients reviewed by Payne et al had potential metabolic causes of pruritus, and an additional 37 per cent had focal causes. Psychosocial factors were considered relevant in one-third of the cases.

HISTOPATHOLOGY. The histologic findings are irregular acanthosis and abundant hyperkeratosis, degenerated nerve fibers and hyperplasia of Schwann cells, and dilated blood vessels surrounded by lymphocytes and occasional mast cells.

TREATMENT. The lesions respond readily if only temporarily to intralesional injections of triamcinolone. Thalidomide was tried successfully in 1979 by van den Broek, and its effectiveness was confirmed by Winkelmann et al in 1984. The dose was 100 mg twice a day. Relief was noted in two or three weeks, and treatment continued for three months. The safety of thalidomide is still in doubt; chronic neuropathy has been observed after long use.

Cryotherapy has also been used successfully, as reported by Waldinger et al.

Jorizzo JL, et al: Prurigo: A review. JAAD 1981, 4:723.
King CA, et al: Unilateral neurogenic pruritus. Ann Intern Med 1982, 97:222.
Payne CMER, et al: Nodular prurigo. Br J Dermatol 1985, 113:431.
Roenigk RK, et al: Bullous pemphigoid and prurigo nodularis. JAAD 1986, 14:944.
Stoll DM, et al: Treatment of prurigo nodularis. J Dermatol Surg Oncol 1983, 9:11.
Van Den Broek H: Treatment of prurigo nodularis with thalidomide. Arch Dermatol 1980, 116:571.
Waldinger TP, et al: Cryotherapy improves prurigo nodularis. Arch Dermatol 1984, 120:1598.
Winkelmann RK, et al: Thalidomide treatment of prurigo nodularis. Acta Dermatovener 1984, 64:412.

MORBUS MONILIFORMIS

SYNONYMS: Morbus moniliformis lichenoides, lichen ruber moniliformis.

CLINICAL FEATURES. This extremely rare disorder simulates some of the manifestations of lichen planus clinically but shows none of its characteristics microscopically. The elementary lesions consist of 1- to 3-mm, round, dome-shaped, waxy papules, which may be dark or bright red. Another type has waxy, yellow, milialike papules. They are usually keloidal in consistency, often forming a moniliform pattern to give an impression of keloidal bands running parallel to the axis of the limb. At other times there is a conspicuous beaded arrangement without the keloidlike strands. Moderate itching is present, especially in warm weather.

The eruption may be generalized, with the excep-

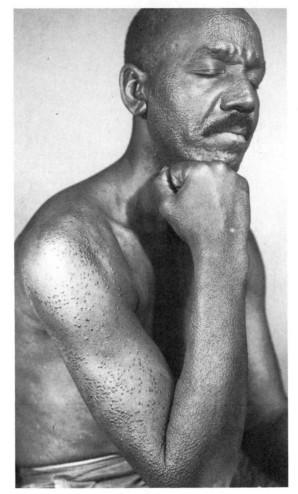

Figure 4–8. Morbus moniliformis.

tion of the cheeks and nose, subclavicular area, interscapular area, glans penis, palms and soles, nails, and the visible mucosae. It may be conspicuous on the forehead, below the ears, the neck, antecubital areas, axillae, lower back, lower legs, backs of the hands, and the insteps.

ETIOLOGY. Morbus moniliformis was originally described by Kaposi, who believed it to be a form of lichen planus, a concept now thought to be erroneous. Clinical and histologic variations from case to case cast doubt about this being a definite entity.

HISTOLOGY. In early lesions the pathology consists of a moderate exudative inflammatory reaction with degeneration of the vessel walls in the upper dermis. Later there are profound degenerative changes in the vessel walls. Edema, collagen degeneration, and in some areas necrobiosis ensue.

TREATMENT. Topical applications of tar and corticosteroids are helpful. Intralesional injections of triamcinolone are also beneficial.

McFarland ER: Morbus moniliformis lichenoides. Arch Dermatol Syph 1947, 60:674.
Pinkus H: Lichen ruber moniliformis. Arch Dermatol Syph 1946, 54:472.

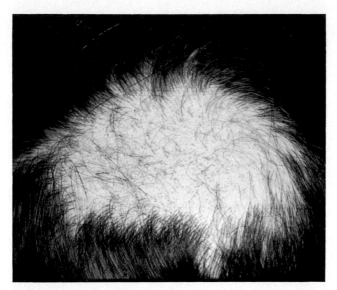

Figure 4–9. Trichotillomania. (Courtesy of Dr. Axel W. Hoke.)

TRICHOTILLOMANIA

Trichotillomania is a neurosis characterized by an abnormal urge to pull out the hair. The sites involved are generally the frontal region of the scalp, the eyebrows, and the beard. These are irregular areas of hair loss, which may be linear or bizarrely shaped. Hairs are broken and show differences in length. The nails may show evidence of onychophagy (nail biting) but no pits are present. The disease is seven times more common in children than in adults, and in Oranje et al's series girls were affected 2.5 times more often than boys.

This disease often develops in the setting of psychosocial stress in the family, which may revolve about school problems, sibling rivalry, moving to a new house, the hospitalization of a mother, or a disturbed mother-daughter relationship.

Differentiation from alopecia areata is possible because of the varying lengths of broken hairs present, the absence of nail pitting, the microscopic appearance of the twisted or broken hairs as opposed to the tapered club hairs of alopecia areata, and if necessary by biopsy.

One should address the diagnosis openly, and referral to a child psychiatrist may be beneficial. In adults with the problem psychiatric impairment may be severe.

Greenberg HR, et al: Trichotillomania. Arch Gen Psychiat 1965, 12:482.

Oranje AP, et al: Trichotillomania in childhood. JAAD 1986, 16:614.

DERMATOTHLASIA

Dermatothlasia is a cutaneous neurosis characterized by an uncontrollable desire to rub or pinch oneself to form bruised areas on the skin, sometimes as a defense against pain elsewhere.

SYPHILOPHOBIA

Syphilophobia is an abnormal fear or belief on the part of the patient that he is afflicted with syphilis. This neurosis is not uncommon and is, as a rule, an expression of guilt regarding some sexual act. The belief is generally but not invariably amenable to informative and argumentative methods of treatment.

BROMIDROSIPHOBIA

Bromidrosiphobia is a neurosis in which there is the conviction that the sweat has a repugnant odor that keeps other people away. It is one of three conditions referred to as monosymptomatic hypo-

Figure 4–10. Bruises resulting from dermatothlasia. The patient produced one of these lesions as a defense against ulcer pain. (Courtesy of Dr. Axel W. Hoke.)

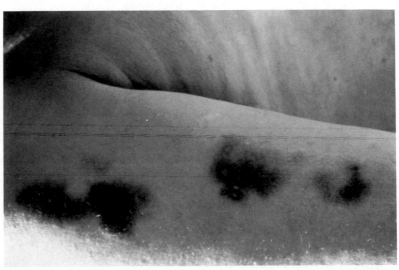

chondriacal syndromes: bromidrosis, delusions of parasitosis, and delusions of dysmorphosis (the erroneous belief that one is misshapen or unattractive). The patient is unable to accept any evidence to the contrary. Three-fourths of patients with bromidrosiphobia are males with an average age of 25. Littler found pimozide effective in one patient. It may be an early symptom of schizophrenia.

ACAROPHOBIA

Acarophobia is an unreasoning fear of insects or other parasites. Regardless of advice to the contrary and of repeated examinations with negative results, the abnormal fear persists. Patients are usually very secretive about the matter and will not consult their local physicians concerning it, but instead will travel great distances to seek the advice of strangers. Most are married women with an average age of 55 years. Many times their beliefs are shared or introduced by others, in which case it is referred to as *folie à deux* or *trois*. This disorder is part of a psychosis and is rarely amenable to medical treatment.

However, Frithz had extremely encouraging results with injections of Prolixin (fluphenazine) decanoate, 7.5 mg subcutaneously, increased by 2.5 mg every three weeks until complete remission or a maximum dose of 25 mg is reached. Tardive dyskinesia, with warning symptoms in the form of fine vermicular movements of the tongue, is a not uncommon side effect about which the patient should be warned. Frithz has not found it a problem.

Pimozide has also been reported to be effective by Duke.

Bishop ER Jr: Monosymptomatic hypochondriacal syndromes in dermatology. JAAD 1983, 9:152.
Duke EE: Clinical experience with pimozide. JAAD 1983, 8:845.
Frithz A: Delusions of infestation: Treatment by depot injections of neuroleptics. Clin Exp Dermatol 1979, 4;485.
Idem: Personal communication, 1989.
Littler CM: Pimozide for delusions of bromosis. JAAD 1986, 15:1303.
Idem: Delusions of parasitosis. JAAD 1983, 8:895.

CUTANEOUS BEHAVIOR DISORDERS

The skin is a frequent target for the release of emotional tension. Self-injury by the same prolonged compulsive repetitious acts may produce various mutilations, depending upon the act and the site of injury. Several reviews have been published by Koblenzer, Rasmussen, and Medansky et al.

Self-biting may be manifested by biting the nails (onychophagia), by skin-biting (most frequently the forearms, hands, and fingers) and by lip-biting; all are signs of anger and frustration.

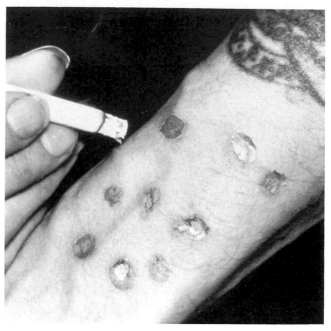

Figure 4–11. *Self-inflicted cigarette burns, done as a means of self-discipline. (Courtesy of Dr. Axel W. Hoke.)*

Bumping of the head produces lacerations and contusions.

Compulsive repetitive hand-washing may produce an irritant dermatitis of the hands.

Bulimia, with its self-induced vomiting, results in crusted papules on the dorsa of the dominant hand from cuts by the teeth.

Clenching of the hand produces swelling and ecchymosis of the fingertips and subungual hemorrhage.

Self-inflicted lacerations are frequently of suicidal intent. They are sometimes seen in adolescents who are trying to demonstrate their bravery.

Licking of the lips produces increased salivation and thickening of the lips. Eventually the perioral area becomes red and produces a distinctive picture resembling the exaggerated mouth make-up of a clown. Thomas et al and Crotty et al have reviewed this type of factitious cheilitis.

Pressure produced by binding the waistline tightly with a cord will eventually lead to atrophy of the subcutaneous tissue.

DELUSIONS OF PARASITOSIS

Delusions of parasitosis are firm fixations in a person's mind that he suffers from a parasitic infestation of his skin. The belief is so fixed that he may pick small pieces of epithelial debris from the skin and bring them to be examined, always insisting that the offending parasite is contained in such material.

Probably the only symptom will be pruritus with some nondescript excoriations. In any event, examination of the skin should be thorough lest an actual parasitic infestation be overlooked.

Frequently these patients have paranoid tendencies. These are usually middle-aged or elderly people who are conscientious, high-principled, and fairly well-educated, with little to show in the way of mental changes except the delusion of parasitosis. Tullett charged such patients with "monosymptomatic hypochondriasis occurring in an obsessional personality."

Management of this difficult problem varies. Most frequently the patient will reject suggestions to seek psychiatric help. Various prescriptions are accepted, but there is little or no improvement of symptoms when the medication is used. Usually there is some deep-rooted psychosis which is kept suppressed by this convenient delusion of parasitosis. Uncovering or digging into the deep-seated problem may have more grave consequences than those incurred by allowing the patient to endure the stigma of (imaginary) parasitosis.

NEUROTIC EXCORIATIONS

Many persons have unconscious compulsive habits of picking at themselves, and at times the tendency is so persistent and pronounced that excoriations of the skin are produced. The lesions are caused by picking, digging, or scraping, and they usually occur on parts readily accessible to the hands. As a rule the action is unconscious. However, it may be done deliberately, in the belief that it corrects some abnormality of the skin.

The excavations are superficial or deep, and are often linear. The bases of the ulcers are clean or covered with a scab. Right-handed persons tend to produce lesions on their left side and left-handed

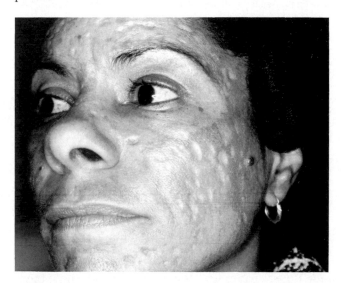

Figure 4–12. Neurotic excoriations produced to relieve suppressed hostility toward an alcoholic husband. (Courtesy of Dr. Axel W. Hoke.)

persons on the right side. Many people will persistently pluck at an area until they can pull a "thread" from it. There is evidence of past healed lesions, usually with linear scars, or rounded hyper- or hypopigmented lesions, in the area of the active excoriations. Senear and Shellow showed that many such "threads" are cutaneous nerve fibers.

The face is the favorite site for these excoriations. Sometimes this aggravates acne, producing acne excoriée. The upper arms are also commonly involved.

Most of these people are otherwise healthy adults. They usually lead normal lives; however, there is a greater tendency for single persons to be afflicted with this problem.

FACTITIOUS DERMATITIS
(Dermatitis Artefacta)

Factitious dermatitis is the term applied to self-inflicted skin lesions made consciously and often with the intent to elicit sympathy, escape responsibilities, or collect disability insurance. The subjects are psychiatrically impaired and most commonly hysterical young women, although men are by no means free from the condition.

The skin lesions are provoked by mechanical means or by the application of chemical irritants and caustics. The lesions may simulate other dermatoses but usually have a distinctive, clear-cut, bizarre appearance. Frequently the shape and arrangement are such as are not encountered in any other affection. The lesions are generally distributed on parts easily reached by the hands and have a tendency to be linear and arranged regularly and symmetrically. They are rarely seen on the right hand or right wrist or arm unless the patient is left-handed.

When chemicals are used, one may often see red streaks or guttate marks beneath the principal patch, where drops of the chemical have accidentally run or fallen upon the skin. According to the manner of production, the lesions may be erythematous, vesicular, bullous, ulcerative, or gangrenous. The more common agents of destruction used are the fingernails, pointed instruments, hot metal; chemicals such as carbolic, muriatic, nitric, or acetic acid; caustic potash or soda, turpentine, and table salt. The lesions are likely to appear in crops.

At times the disorder is manifested only by the indefinitely delayed healing of an operative wound, which is purposely kept open by the patient.

Proof of diagnosis is sometimes difficult. Occlusive dressings may be necessary to protect the lesions from ready access by the patient. It is usually best not to reveal any suspicion of the cause to the patient and to establish the diagnosis definitely without the patient's knowledge. If the patient is hospitalized a resourceful, cooperative nurse may be useful in helping to establish the diagnosis. When injection of foreign material is suspected, examination of biopsy

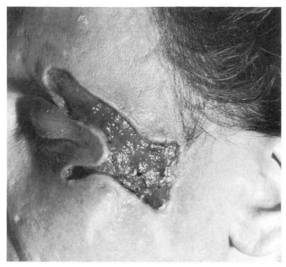

Figure 4–13. Dermatitis artefacta, produced by acid, self-applied.

material by spectroscopy may reveal talc, as shown by Robert Jackson et al.

Shelley in 1981 opened the door to what may well be a simple, if hard to prove and rarely encountered, explanation of dermatitis artefacta: induction of it by one of the patient's multiple personalities. The dermatitis of his patient's left arm was being induced by one of the patient's "other" selves, a belligerent, macho Marine, by rubbing it with poison ivy leaves—an act of which the patient was completely unaware. In *The Three Faces of Eve* one of Eve's personalities would deliberately dress in nylon hose, which made this personality (to whom she would then deliberately change) itch unbearably. The reader should read Shelley's paper.

Sneddon believes that dermatitis artefacta encompasses three specific syndromes of self-inflicted injury. These are dermatitis artefacta, Munchausen's syndrome, and true malingering. He also believes that dermatitis artefacta is a manifestation of emotional instability.

Treatment should ideally involve psychotherapy, but most frequently the suggestion is promptly rejected. The patient goes to another physician to seek a new round of treatment. It is best for the dermatologist to maintain a close relationship with the patient and provide symptomatic therapy and non-judgmental support.

Pimozide (Orap) has been used with success. However, its many potential side effects lead us to recommend one use this only in concert with a psychiatrist. Lindskov et al reported improvement within two to four weeks in all but one of 14 patients, with doses of up to 4 mg daily. There was lasting relief in seven and recurrence on stopping medication in three; only four were not relieved.

Arnold HL Jr: Stress dermatoses. Arch Dermatol 1953, 67:566.

Crotty CP, et al: Factitious lip crusting. Arch Dermatol 1981, 117:338.

Fabisch W: Psychiatric aspects of dermatitis artefacta. Br J Dermatol 1980, 102:29.

Fisher BK, et al: Dermatitis artefacta. Cutis 1977, 19:665.

Frankel EB: Treatment of delusions of parasitosis. JAAD 1983, 9:772.

Gould WM, et al: Delusions of parasitosis. Arch Dermatol 1976, 112:1745.

Gupta MA, et al: Psychotropic drugs in dermatology. JAAD 1986, 14:633.

Jackson RM, et al: Factitial cutaneous ulcers and nodules. JAAD 1984, 11:1065.

Koblenzer CS: The dysmorphic syndrome. Arch Dermatol 1985, 121:780.

Idem: Psychosomatic concepts in dermatology. Arch Dermatol 1983, 119:501.

Lindskov R, et al: Delusions of infestation treated with pimozide: A follow-up study. Derm Venereol 1985, 65:267.

Lyell A: Cutaneous artifactual disease. JAAD 1979, 1:391.

Medansky RS, et al: Dermatopsychosomatics. JAAD 1981, 5:125.

Rasmussen SA: Obsessive-compulsive disorder in dermatologic practice. JAAD 1985, 13:965.

Schwartz BK, et al: A cutaneous sign of bulimia. JAAD 1985, 12:725.

Shelley WB: Dermatitis artefacta induced in a patient by one of her multiple personalities. Br J Dermatol 1981, 105:587.

Sneddon IB: Dermatitis artefacta. Proc Roy Soc Med 1977, 70:754.

Thomas JR, et al: Factitious cheilitis. JAAD 1983, 8:368.

Weber PJ, et al: Notalgia paresthetica. JAAD 1988, 18:25.

NEUROCUTANEOUS DERMATOSES

HYPERESTHESIA

Hyperesthesia is the word for increased sensitivity of the skin to light touch—as compared to its sensitivity nearby. It is characteristically present throughout the involved neurotome in herpes zoster before the rash appears.

It is also an inherent part of the syndrome of causalgia (see below).

BURNING TONGUE
(Glossodynia; Burning Mouth Syndrome)

Postmenopausal women are particularly prone to a feeling of burning of the tongue or mouth or both, with no objective findings. It varies in severity, but is more or less constant. It has been blamed on deficiency of B_{12}, iron, or folate; on hypoestrogenism, diabetes, local trauma, and psychological disturbance. Grushka found a veritable potpourri of immunologic abnormalities in eight men and 19 women with this complaint: 60 per cent had some deviation from normal. Whether this is indicative of a link to the connective tissue diseases, or of an emotional impact ("immunomodulation" is the new term for it) on the immune system, is not at all clear. The First International Workshop on Immunomodulation was held at the National Institutes of Health in 1984. There seems to be no effective treatment.

MERALGIA PARESTHETICA
(Roth-Bernhardt Disease)

This affection is a variety of paresthesia, there being persistent numbness, with periodic transient episodes of burning or lancinating pain, on the anterolateral surface of the thigh. This area is innervated by the lateral femoral cutaneous nerve. The disease occurs most frequently in middle-aged obese men. Aranoff et al report alopecia localized to the area innervated by the lateral femoral nerve to be a sign of this disease. Arthritis of the lumbar vertebrae, a herniated disc, pregnancy, or rarely a retroperitoneal tumor may cause this.

Three well-known students of leprosy—T. F. Davey, H. W. Wade (long-time editor of the *International Journal of Leprosy*), and H. L. Arnold, Jr.—all had the disease, and each initially believed it to be early leprosy. None was obese.

There is no reliable therapy.

Aranoff SM, et al: Alopecia in meralgia paresthetica. JAAD 1985, 12:176.

CAUSALGIA

The syndrome of burning pain, hyperesthesia, and trophic disturbances resulting from injury to a peripheral nerve is called causalgia or reflex sympathetic dystrophy. It usually occurs in one of the upper extremities, the commonest symptom being burning pain aggravated by movement or friction. The skin of the involved extremity becomes shiny, cold, profusely perspiring, and frequently cracked, and there is usually hyperesthesia and radiographic evidence of decalcification.

The intensity of the pain varies from trivial burning to a state of torture accompanied by extreme hyperesthesia and frequently hyperhidrosis. The part is not only subject to an intense burning sensation, but a touch or a tap of the finger causes exquisite pain. Exposure to the air is avoided with a care that seems absurd, and the patient walks carefully, carrying the limb tenderly with the sound hand. The patients are tremulous and apprehensive, and keep the hand

constantly wet, finding relief in the moisture rather than in the temperature of the application.

A condition resembling permanent chilblains or even trophic ulcers may be present, or there may be diffuse osteoporosis of the digits as a result of reflex sympathetic dystrophy. Ingram et al reported a case of reflex sympathetic dystrophy occurring as a complication of nail biopsy.

Treatment should be started before central nervous system changes occur and narcotic addiction develops. Consultation with a neurologist or neurosurgeon is generally advisable. Paravertebral block or sympathectomy is most effective. Defalque also recommends an axillary block with lidocaine and hyaluronidase, rather than stellate ganglionic block, to eliminate the risk of pneumothorax. Tolazoline (Priscoline) may be administered cautiously. Trifluoperazine (Stelazine), diazepam (Valium), or chlordiazepoxide (Librium) is an effective conservative measure for treatment.

TRIGEMINAL TROPHIC LESIONS

A few weeks or months following rhizotomy (or more commonly, alcohol injection) for tic douloureux, a slowly enlarging uninflamed ulcer may appear on the cheek beside the ala nasi. It may infrequently occur elsewhere upon the face, or after other surgery: Weintraub et al reported a case occurring after removal of a cerebellopontine-angle meningioma.

Self-inflicted trauma to the anesthetic skin is believed to be the cause, and the appropriate treatment is to prevent this by persuasion or coercion. It is usually successful, but scarring may be severe.

In addition, the following complications may occur after operation for trigeminal neuralgia: herpes simplex, neuropathic keratitis, corneal ulcer, iritis, conjunctivitis, paresthesias, facial paralysis, and dryness of the nasal mucous membrane.

Postencephalitic Trophic Ulcer. Ulceration of the nose similar to the trigeminal trophic ulcer has been reported following epidemic encephalitis.

MALUM PERFORANS PEDIS

Also known as perforating ulcer of the foot and neurotrophic ulcer, malum perforans is a chronic, trophic, and ulcerative disease seen on the sole in the denervating diseases, particularly tabes dorsalis, leprosy, arteriosclerosis, or diabetes, resulting from loss of pain sensation at a site of constant trauma. The primary cause of the trouble is either in the posterolateral tracts of the cord (in tabes and arteriosclerosis) or the lateral tracts (in syringomyelia) or in the peripheral nerves (in diabetes or leprosy).

In most cases, malum perforans begins as a circumscribed hyperkeratosis, usually on the ball of the foot. This lesion becomes soft, moist, and malodor-

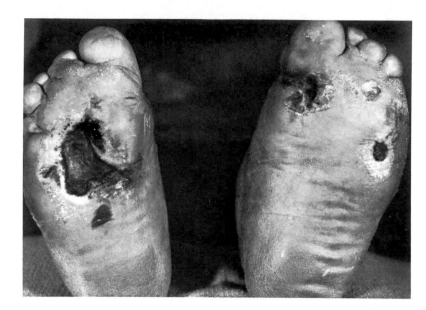

Figure 4–14. Malum perforans of the feet in a 65-year-old woman with lepromatous leprosy.

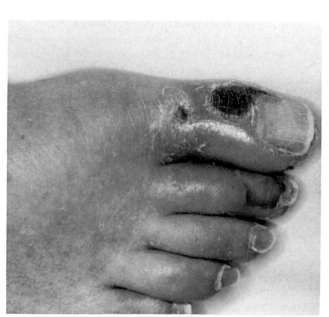

Figure 4–15. Early diabetic gangrene.

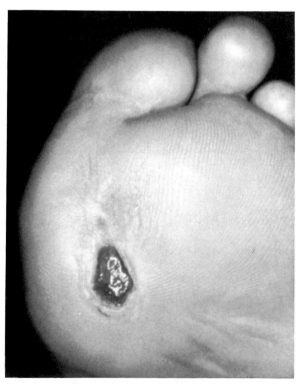

Figure 4–16. Diabetic foot ulcer.

ous, and later exudes a thin purulent discharge. A slough slowly develops and there is left an indolent, necrotic, usually painless but sometimes painful ulcer, which lasts indefinitely. Deeper perforation and secondary infection often lead to osteomyelitis of metatarsal or tarsal bones. The process must be differentiated from ulcers due to suppurating corns and from the ordinary type of diabetic gangrene.

Treatment should consist of relief of pressure on the ulcer by padding and by keeping the patient off his feet as much as possible. Antibiotics locally and sometimes internally are most helpful.

SCIATIC NERVE INJURY

Serious sciatic nerve injury, especially in infants, can result from improperly performed injections into the buttocks. A paralytic foot drop simulating poliomyelitis is the most common finding. There is sensory loss and absence of sweating over the distribution of the sciatic nerve branches.

The skin of the affected extremity becomes thin, shiny, and often edematous.

The midanterior or midlateral thigh is recommended as the preferable site for intramuscular injections in infants and young children.

FAMILIAL DYSAUTONOMIA
(Riley-Day Syndrome)

This syndrome, first recognized by Riley in 1949, has features of defective lacrimation, excessive sweating, drooling, and transient erythema, predominantly on the trunk. In addition, there may be acrocyanosis, especially of the hands.

Attention is called to two interesting features. One is the absence of fungiform and circumvallate papillae of the tongue and the other is the sensation of tickling of the scalp experienced when the head is stroked lightly.

There is an overactivity of acetylcholine secretion at the nerve endings. The disease is probably inherited as an autosomal recessive trait, most often in Jewish families.

The Schirmer test for lacrimal dysfunction is positive. The intradermal histamine test shows a diminished flare, and immersion of the hands in water 40°C causes erythematous mottling of the hands.

No satisfactory treatment is available. Dryness of eyes may be relieved by artificial tears.

SYRINGOMYELIA

Also known as **Morvan's disease,** syringomyelia results from progressive expansion of the central canal of the spinal cord, compressing the lateral tracts especially and producing sensory and trophic changes on the upper extremities, particularly in the fingers. The disease begins insidiously and gradually causes muscular weakness, hyperhidrosis, and sensory disturbances, especially in the thumb and index and middle fingers. The skin changes are characterized by dissociated anesthesia with loss of pain and temperature sense but with retention of tactile sense. Burns are the most frequent lesions noted. Bullae, warts, and trophic ulcerations occur on the fingers and hands, and ultimately there are contractures and gangrene. The disease must be differentiated chiefly from leprosy. Unlike leprosy, syringomyelia does not interfere with sweating or block the flare around a histamine wheal.

CONGENITAL SENSORY NEUROPATHY

Recurrent acral ulcers from birth on characterize this sensory neuropathy occurring on the hands and feet. Repeated injuries to the hands produce these ulcers because of trophic disturbances. There may be decreased acral pain perception; however, the sense of touch is present. Complete anhidrosis was reported by Person and his associates in their patient with this disorder.

Treatment of this disorder is symptomatic. Care should be taken to avoid burning, scratching, and the various other traumatic events that can happen in ordinary living.

Combes MA, et al: Sciatic nerve injury in infants. JAMA 1960, 173:1336.

Defalque RJ: Treatment of causalgia. JAMA 1969, 209:259.

Fellner MJ, et al: Manifestations of familial autonomic dysautonomia. Arch Dermatol 1964, 89:190.

Grushka M: Immunologic aspects of "burning mouths." JAMA 1983, 249:1151.

Howell JB: Neurotropic changes in trigeminal territory. Arch Dermatol 1962, 86:442.

Ingram GJ, et al: Reflex sympathetic dystrophy following nail biopsy. JAAD 1987, 16:253.

Ishii N, et al: Congenital sensory neuropathy and anhidrosis. Arch Dermatol 1988, 124:564.

Kleinert HE, et al: Post-traumatic sympathetic dystrophy. Orthop Clin N Am 1973, 4:917.

Marx JL: The immune system "belongs in the body." Science 1985, 227:1190.

Person JR, et al: Congenital sensory neuropathy. Arch Dermatol 1977, 113:954.

Spiegel IJ, et al: Causalgia. JAMA 1945, 127:9.

Weintraub E, et al: Trigeminal trophic syndrome. JAAD 1982, 6:52.

5

Atopic Dermatitis; Eczema; Noninfectious Immunodeficiency Disorders

ATOPIC DERMATITIS

Atopic dermatitis is also known as atopic eczema, infantile eczema, flexural eczema, disseminated neurodermatitis, and *prurigo diathésique* (Besnier).

In 1925 Coca introduced the term *atopy*, meaning "out of place" or "strange," to signify the hereditary tendency to develop allergies to food and inhalant substances, as manifested by eczema, asthma, and hay fever. In 1933 Wise and Sulzberger detailed the diagnosis of—and named—atopic dermatitis.

The tendency to develop atopic dermatitis is inherited, probably in a polygenic fashion strongly modulated by environmental factors. Above one fourth of offspring of atopic mothers develop atopic dermatitis in the first three months of life. If one parent has allergies, over half the children develop allergic symptoms by two years of age. The incidence rises to 79 per cent if both parents have allergic symptoms.

Much effort has been put into the study of allergens which may cause or exacerbate atopic dermatitis. Identification of these allergens, their elimination, or hyposensitization to them have been a principal method of study and management of this disease. In practice, this approach has been remarkably unrewarding.

The entity undergoes a clinical and histologic evolution from an acute eczematous eruption in early life to a characteristic lichenified dermatitis seen in older patients.

Atopic dermatitis may be divided into three stages, namely: *infantile atopic dermatitis*, occurring from two months to two years of age; *childhood atopic dermatitis*, from two to 10 years; and the *adolescent* and *adult stage of atopic dermatitis*.

INFANTILE ATOPIC DERMATITIS

Eczema in infancy usually begins as an itchy erythema of the cheeks between two months and two years of age. In the erythematous patches minute epidermal vesicles develop, rupture, and produce moist crusted areas. The eruption may rapidly extend to other parts of the body, chiefly the scalp (cradle cap), the neck, the forehead, the wrists, and the extremities. The buttocks and diaper area are often involved. The eruption may become generalized, with erythroderma and considerable desquamation.

This *moist type* is the most common. The lesions show polymorphism. Exudation may be marked, and there are many secondary effects from scratching, rubbing, and infection: crusts, pustules, and infiltrated areas. The infiltrated patches eventually take

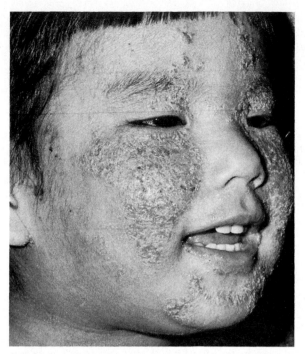

Figure 5–1. Infantile atopic dermatitis of the face. Note perioral sparing, a frequent feature.

on a characteristic lichenified appearance. Itching is severe and is the main symptom.

In the *dry type* there is excessive dryness, and xerosis, which with pruritus predisposes to eczematization. This is seen especially in older children in whom the antecubital and popliteal fossae are involved.

In most infants who suffer from this disease, the skin symptoms disappear toward the end of the second year or sometimes before. The patients are able to eat, without bad effect, foods that previously seemed to cause disturbances; they seem to outgrow their sensitive phase. Exacerbations are often observed after immunizations. Colds are often followed by flare-ups. Partial or even complete remission of the dermatitis in summer and relapse in winter seem almost the rule in cases aggravated by wool irritation and low humidity.

The role of food allergy in infantile and childhood atopic dermatitis has been debated for years. Recent work by Sampson et al has helped to define its relative importance. In a prospective study of 132 patients with severe atopic dermatitis, 59 per cent experienced at least one positive food challenge, and 85 per cent of positive challenges were associated with cutaneous symptoms. Foods most commonly testing positive were egg, peanut, milk, wheat, fish, soy, and chicken. The positive challenges correlated with a rise in plasma histamine. If the implicated food was withheld, the patients did better clinically and had a decrease in serum IgE, and 45 per cent lost their reactivity to the food over a one-to-two-year period. A negative skin prick test was a reliable indicator of nonsensitivity; a positive test was less

reliable. The RAST (RadioAllergoSorbentTest) had no advantages over the prick test. Food allergy, then, may play a significant role in a selected population of young atopic patients.

CHILDHOOD ATOPIC DERMATITIS

Throughout childhood less acute lesions in the same areas may recur. Such lesions as occur are apt to be less exudative, drier, and more papular. The classic locations are the antecubital and popliteal spaces, the wrists, eyelids, and face, and in a collarette about the neck. Other areas are frequently affected, however, and quite often lichenified, slightly scaly, or infiltrated patches intermingled with isolated, excoriated papules are widely scattered over the exposed parts.

Pruritus is a constant feature, and many of the cutaneous changes are secondary to it, for scratching induces lichenification and secondary infections. A vicious cycle is established, for the itching leads to scratching, and the scratching causes thickening of the skin and secondary changes that in themselves cause itching. The scratching impulse is usually beyond control of the patient and the various forms of local treatment must aim primarily to reduce the itching to the point at which the patient is able to

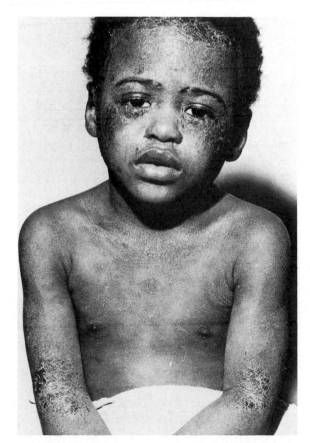

Figure 5–2. Childhood atopic dermatitis. Lichenification and some scarring have occurred.

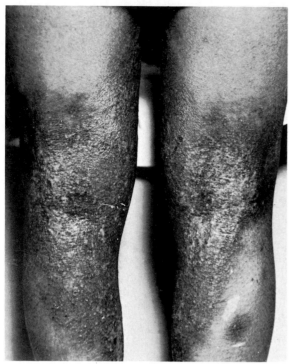

Figure 5–3. Heavy eczematization with lichenification, the adolescent-adult pattern in the popliteal spaces. (Courtesy of Dr. R. Feinstein.)

restrain himself. The itching is of exactly the same compelling, paroxysmal type, with inability to feel pain during the paroxysms, that was described under circumscribed neurodermatitis. Indeed, Brocq called atopic dermatitis "*neurodermite disseminée.*"

During childhood there is a decrease in the frequency of sensitization to egg, wheat, and milk and an increase in sensitization to noningested substances, particularly wool, cat hair, dog hair, and pollens.

Wool irritation appears as pruritus and eczema on the neck, face, hands, wrists, and legs. It is worse every winter and almost disappears during the summer. Feather sensitivity also has its onset in childhood during the second year but is more common in adults. All feather-containing objects, feather comforters, or feather pillows in the house must be discarded or kept out of rooms the child frequents. Sensitivity to cat and dog hair or to lacquer paint on toys may exacerbate eczema in children.

Sensitivity to nickel, neomycin, and ragweed oleoresin occurs more frequently in atopics than in normal persons. This is an exception to the rule that atopics have diminished ability to acquire delayed hypersensitivity. Möller et al have shown that, despite a clinical history of nickel sensitivity, patch tests may be negative.

ATOPIC DERMATITIS IN ADOLESCENTS AND ADULTS

The disease in adults may occur as localized erythematous, scaly, papular, or vesicular patches, or in the form of pruritic, lichenified patches. Usually the eruption involves the antecubital and popliteal fossae, the front and sides of the neck, the forehead, and the area about the eyes.

The hands, including the wrists, are frequently involved. Hand dermatitis occurs more frequently in atopic individuals, and eczematous lesions of the dorsum are usual. But the palms may be involved as well, either by an ironing-out of the fingerprint ridges such as is seen in inverse psoriasis, or by hyperlinearity. However, this hyperlinearity, though long thought to be a marker for atopy, has lately been recognized both by Lobitz and by Uehara and associates in Japan to be a manifestation of ichthyosis vulgaris, which accompanies atopic dermatitis in 30 to 40 per cent of cases. Fifty per cent of patients with ichthyosis have a personal or family history of atopic dermatitis. At times the eruption is generalized, being most severe in the flexures. It consists mostly of lichenification. The essential lesions are dry, slightly elevated, flat-topped papules that tend to coalesce to form lichenified, slightly scaly plaques, which are nearly always excoriated. The plaques are often somewhat erythematous and hyperpigmented. As a result of trauma from scratching, the plaques may become exudative and crusted or infected. The skin, in general, is usually dry and has a tendency to become thickened, and in the widespread type of involvement (disseminated neurodermatitis) there is a leathery quality with exaggerated markings.

Pruritus is commonly the symptom that causes the skin changes. It usually occurs in crises or paroxysms, often nocturnal or triggered by acute emotional upsets, and it may be absent in the intervals between them. Sweat retention may be an important factor. Atopic dermatitis typically becomes less severe as the patient grows older, and is uncommon after middle life. Triggering factors may be rough clothing, wool irritation, foods, or tension.

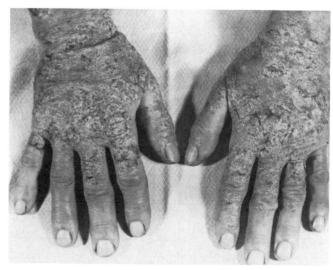

Figure 5–4. Atopic dermatitis of backs of hands, a frequent location.

Associated Features

CUTANEOUS STIGMATA. A linear transverse fold just below the edge of the lower eyelids, known as the Dennie-Morgan fold, is widely believed to be indicative of the "atopic diathesis," i.e., a tendency to, or a family history of, atopic dermatitis, asthma, or hay fever. A study by Uehara of 300 atopic dermatitis cases and 11 cases of contact dermatitis showed the fold in 25 per cent of the former and 70 per cent of the latter. He regarded it as a nonspecific consequence of any dermatitis of the lower lids.

Keratosis pilaris, horny follicular lesions of the outer aspects of the upper arms and legs, is commonly associated with atopic dermatitis. It is discussed in Chapter 26.

Thinning of the lateral eyebrows, *Hertoghe's sign*, is sometimes present. Keratosis punctata palmaris et plantaris is a condition seen chiefly in black atopics. In a prospective study of 573 patients Anderson et al found that of 11 affected patients 9 (82 per cent) had atopy or a family history of atopy. Clover et al described reticulated pigmentation of the neck as an adjunctive sign.

VASCULAR STIGMATA. Atopic individuals are prone to cold hands. There often exists perinasal and periorbital pallor ("headlight sign"); indeed, there may be generalized pallor.

White dermographism (white line, *tâche blanche*) is blanching of the skin at the site of stroking with a blunt instrument. It is best elicited on the brow of an adult with atopic dermatitis. This reaction differs from the triple response of Lewis in that the third response (flaring) is replaced by a blanching to produce a white line. Blanching is due to the local accumulation of edema, which obscures the color of underlying vessels.

When 0.1 ml of a 1:100,000 solution of histamine is injected intradermally the flare phase of the triple response is absent or diminished. There is also an increase in skin temperature at sites of predilection for atopic dermatitis, on intramuscular injection.

In atopic dermatitis, 0.1 ml of 1:10,000 acetylcholine injected intradermally will produce in 70 per cent of subjects a delayed blanch phenomenon lasting for some 20 minutes after the injection; moreover, there is increased whealing in response to acetylcholine in atopic dermatitis as well as in those with hay fever or asthma without dermatitis.

PERSONALITY TRAITS. Nervous tension has been shown to be an important factor in atopic dermatitis, especially in the adult. A characteristic psychosomatic relationship is present in many patients who have atopic dermatitis, asthma, or hay fever. Many have a suppressed feeling of resentment and are born battlers. They are sensitive, easily depressed, tense, intolerant, and overactive.

Aggressiveness and hypochondriasis are common. Such patients must be taught to relax mentally and to avoid emotional strain and nervous tension.

OPHTHALMOLOGIC ABNORMALITIES. Cataracts may be an associated finding. Approximately 8 per cent of patients with atopic dermatitis develop lens opacities. It is most frequent in women during the third decade. Cases have been reported, however, at all ages and in males as well as females. The opacities are unilateral in about half the cases, and the posterior cortex is twice as often involved as the anterior cortex.

Keratoconus is an uncommon entity which occurs in approximately 1 per cent of atopic patients. Contact lenses may be of benefit in treating this condition, which is an elongation of the corneal surface.

SUSCEPTIBILITY TO INFECTION. Superimposed infections such as verrucae vulgares, molluscum contagiosum, and widespread dermatophytosis are common. In atopic patients, *Staphylococcus aureus* is present abundantly and dominates the skin flora. Over 90 per cent of chronic eczematous lesions contain *Staphylococcus aureus*, oftentimes in large numbers. Antistaphylococcal IgE antibodies have been documented in some atopic individuals, resulting in the hypothesis that staphylococcal infection may lead to histamine release and flare of disease. Atopics are prone to upper respiratory infections. There is a history of pneumonia in 10 to 15 per cent of patients with atopic dermatitis.

There is increased susceptibility to generalized herpes simplex or vaccinia virus infections to produce *Kaposi's varicelliform eruption*. This is seen frequently in young children and one or more of the siblings may have this infection. Vaccination against smallpox is dangerous and is contraindicated in persons with atopic dermatitis, even in remission. Fortunately, vaccination against smallpox is rarely done today and exposure to vaccinia virus is highly unlikely.

IMMUNOLOGY. Frequent immunologic peculiarities are elevated serum IgE (80 per cent of patients), decreased ability to be sensitized to DNCB or bacterial or fungal antigens, decreased T suppressor cells, decreased NK cell activity, decreased antibody-dependent cellular cytotoxicity, decreased T cytotoxic cells, decreased chemotaxis and activation of polymorphonuclear leukocytes, and decreased cytotoxicity and chemotaxis of monocytes. How all these abnormalities relate to the disease and whether they are primary or secondary changes is as yet unresolved.

Atopic patients are susceptible to recurrent type I herpes simplex infections and show decreased sensitivity to topically applied antigens. Toxicodendron sensitivity occurs in only 15 per cent of individuals with atopic dermatitis as compared to 61 per cent of nonatopic controls. Despite the depression in circulating T cells, these patients do not show an increased incidence of cancer. Rola-Pleszczynski and Blanchard confirmed a negative correlation of suppressor cell function with IgE levels.

There appears to be an easy releasability of histamine from mast cells. The beta-adrenergic theory postulates that there is a reduced response of cAMP to beta-adrenergic stimulation. This decreased cAMP would lead to increased histamine release from mast cells.

DIAGNOSIS. This summary of diagnostic criteria for atopic dermatitis, after Hanifin and Lobitz, is valuable:

Must have each of the following:
1. Pruritus
2. Typical morphology and distribution:
   a. Flexural lichenification in adults
   b. Facial and extensor involvement in infancy
3. Tendency toward chronic or chronically relapsing dermatitis, plus either

Two or more of the following features:
1. Personal or family history of atopic disease (asthma, allergic rhinitis, atopic dermatitis)
2. Immediate skin test reactivity
3. White dermographism or delayed blanch to cholinergic agents
4. Anterior subcapsular cataracts, or else

Four or more of the following features:
1. Xerosis/ichthyosis/hyperlinear palms
2. Pityriasis alba
3. Keratosis pilaris
4. Facial pallor/infraorbital darkening
5. Elevated serum IgE
6. Keratoconus
7. Tendency to nonspecific hand dermatitis
8. Tendency to repeated cutaneous infections

DIFFERENTIAL DIAGNOSIS. The typical atopic dermatitis is not difficult to diagnose because of its predilection for symmetrical involvement of face, neck, and antecubital and popliteal fossae. Dermatoses resembling atopic dermatitis may be seborrheic dermatitis, irritant or allergic eczematous contact dermatitis, nummular dermatitis, scabies, psoriasis (especially palmoplantar), dermatitis herpetiformis, or keratosis follicularis (Darier's disease). In infants, certain immunodeficiency syndromes must be kept in mind: Wiskott-Aldrich syndrome, ataxia-telangiectasia, and Swiss-type agammaglobulinemia. Histiocytosis X (Letterer-Siwe or Hand-Schüller-Christian disease) and phenylketonuria may at times also resemble atopic dermatitis.

HISTOPATHOLOGY. There are hyperkeratosis, parakeratosis, and acanthosis. The essential features are intercellular edema and resultant spongiosis in the epidermis, with migration of leukocytes into the epidermis and the formation of small vesicles. The capillaries are dilated, and there is some edema of the dermis. There is a perivascular infiltrate in the upper part of the dermis composed of various types of cells that include eosinophils, lymphocytes, and histiocytes. When there is lichenification, as in disseminated neurodermatitis, the acanthosis is marked. These changes resemble those seen in psoriasis, but there is more edema and not the clubbing of the rete ridges.

GENERAL MANAGEMENT IN INFANCY AND CHILDHOOD. Any external irritation may precipitate an attack of eczema—sudden change of temper

ature, excessive bathing, vigorous rubbing, chafing; unduly heavy, tight or soiled clothing; insufficient cleanliness especially in the diaper region, local infections, irritating secretions, or even medicated baby oils. Attacks may be induced by teething. One of the first considerations is the protection of the affected parts from scratching, and mechanical restraints may be resorted to, such as cardboard splints over the elbows to prevent the infant's hands from reaching his face.

As soap and water may aggravate the disease, olive oil on absorbent cotton may be used with gentle patting for cleansing to avoid rubbing the affected parts. Particular attention should be given the genitals and buttocks, and the diapers should be changed whenever they are soiled, fresh ones being applied after the parts have been cleansed with vegetable or mineral oil and powdered with cornstarch.

Antihistaminic drugs are moderately helpful especially if given at night, when the accompanying sedative effects may be helpful. The dosage must be adequate and regular.

In cases where specific food allergies are implicated, dietary restrictions are in order. Those foods should be avoided. Food substitutes for wheat are oats (oatmeal, oatmeal crackers), rice (puffed rice, boiled rice), barley, corn (cornstarch, cornmeal, cornflakes), soybean flour, sobee sticks, and rye (Rykrisp). When milk is eliminated, soybean emulsion gives adequate nourishment. These may be used when prick testing is positive for these items and specific challenge is not done.

Eliminating the foods on a trial basis for several weeks is an alternative to food challenge. The challenge may induce anaphylaxis and is not an outpatient procedure. A general restriction diet for infantile eczema which avoids most of the commonly implicated foods is prune juice, boiled rice, puffed rice, rice flakes for cereal; Ry-krisp for breadstuff; soybean emulsion substitute for milk; preserved apples or pears, mashed banana; margarine; baked potato, peas, lima beans; broiled beef and lamb.

Williams in 1949 reported on two groups of children with atopic dermatitis matched by sex and age. One group was treated by orthodox dermatologic procedures and medications. The other was managed solely by intensive efforts to make their mothers more demonstratively warm and affectionate. Improvement was about equal in the two groups, but it occurred much sooner in the latter!

GENERAL MANAGEMENT IN ADULTS. It is important to have the patient be aware that emotional stress is an important factor in causing exacerbations. Atopics should avoid extremes of cold and heat. Xerotic skin tends to be worse in the winter and should be hydrated by avoiding soaps and greases and using hydrophilic creams and lotions. Humidifiers in rooms are helpful. The patient should not wear wool, because its fibers are irritating.

TREATMENT

Internal Treatment. Limiting the use of coffee, tea,

cola beverages, chocolate, and other stimulants is desirable.

The antihistaminics may be used to aid in the relief of the severe pruritus. Hydroxyzine (Atarax or Vistaril) is of value for suppression of pruritus. Doxepin (Sinequan) is often helpful, in doses of about 25 mg t.i.d. in adults.

Staphylococcus aureus has long been known to be a frequent resident of both normal and involved skin in atopic dermatitis. Most patients benefit from more or less prolonged courses of erythromycin, even when clinical evidence of infection is lacking.

Corticosteroid therapy is the dominant method of treatment for adult atopic dermatitis. In localized cases topical therapy may be adequate, whereas in more generalized involvement, internal therapy may be hard to avoid.

Oral prednisone or prednisolone has been the standard preparation for many years. We have had enough experience with it now to advise against it. A safe dose level can rarely be found; but if control is achievable at 5 to 10 mg a day, especially if treatment is not continued for more than a few months, harm is not likely to result. At 10 to 15 mg a day or more, moon face, thinning of the skin, osteoporosis, posterior subcapsular cataracts, and hypertension are likely to occur. Alternate-day dosage is not known to reduce the risk of occurrence of any of these.

Far safer is triamcinolone acetonide suspension by intramuscular injection. Initially the patient may require treatment every four weeks, but this later may be increased to longer intervals. With this treatment method, there is usually recovery from any adrenal suppression before the subsequent dose is given. This method puts the therapy completely under the control of the therapist, and decreases the possible side effects by reducing total corticosteroid intake. Also, treatment is not continued during remissions, as it is with oral prednisone. This therapy has not found favor among academic dermatologists, few of whom have had any experience with it.

Nonsteroidal Internal Therapy. A careful double-blind study was done in 99 patients with atopic dermatitis who were given large oral doses of evening-primrose seed oil (180 mg gamma-linolenic acid minimum, 540 mg maximum, for adults; 90 to 180 mg in children). They gave 2 to 12 capsules of Efamol daily, and the higher dose gave the most improvement in itching, scaling, and overall severity.

Rudolf Baer has called attention to the usefulness of papaverine, 100 mg 4 to 6 times a day, a therapy he has been using for 40 years. He also uses timed-release capsules, 150 mg 2 to 3 times daily as needed. Side effects have been limited to occasional nausea or drowsiness, and one instance of acute urticaria. In his experience it controls itching so well that he has rarely resorted to systemic steroids.

Sodium cromoglycate orally has been generally disappointing and is little used nowadays. A subgroup of patients in whom it may be useful, however, is children whose atopic dermatitis is exacerbated by foods. Businco et al in a double-blind trial found it useful in many such cases.

Topical Treatment. For the acute weeping eczematous dermatitis, wet compresses of Burow's solution are the treatment of choice. Burow's solution is available in powder form: Domeboro packets and Aluwets. Alibour's solution and potassium permanganate (1:5000) solution are also effective when applied for 20 to 30 minutes several times daily. Acid Mantle Cream is applied after compressing.

The corticosteroid topical applications have almost completely supplanted all other medications. They are available in creams, ointments, sprays, and lotions manufactured by many pharmaceutical firms. Continued use of these medications without improvement should make one think of preservative sensitivity such as paraben in the base. Neomycin sensitivity also occurs and should be kept in mind. Another severe side effect of long-continued topical fluorinated corticosteroid therapy is the development of telangiectasia and connective tissue atrophy.

For the hydration of xerotic skin of atopic dermatitis 10 per cent urea in a hydrophilic cream, Eucerin cream, Lac-hydrin, Moisturel, or 1 per cent hydrocortisone in 10 per cent urea cream have been gratifying and effective creams to use.

Topical or systemic antistaphylococcal antibiotics such as Bactroban topically or erythromycin orally may help to decrease pruritus and infectious complications, such as the distal phalangeal osteomyelitis recently reported by Boiko et al.

Tar is still effective in ointments. Crude coal tar 1 to 5 per cent in white petrolatum or hydrophilic ointment USP is helpful. Estar Gel and Psorigel are 5 per cent tar preparations in a soluble gel which are esthetically nice to apply. Wright's liquor carbonis detergens 5 to 10 per cent in hydrophilic ointment USP is also helpful.

Leyden has determined that lesions of atopic dermatitis are irritated by frequent washing with soap. Least irritating, he found, are AlphaKeri, Dove, Basis, Neutrogena, and Emulave.

Scholtz reported decades ago a treatment method that preserves the existing natural surface lipid film and copes with the sweat retention problem. All stimuli that might induce sweating are avoided. Likewise, all greases, soaps, and ointments are interdicted. The treatment consists of discontinuation of internal corticosteroids as well as bathing and washing in the usual manner; however, ocean bathing is allowed. The skin is cleansed daily with Cetaphil lotion, a lipid-free cleanser. Soap and water may be used only to cleanse the skin folds of axillae, groins, and perianal region. Erythromycin is taken for any secondary infection of the skin, and corticosteroid creams (or preferably fluocinolone acetonide 0.01 per cent in propylene glycol—Synalar Solution) is rubbed in with the finger tips, using not more than 15 ml daily. A daily dose of 50,000 units of vitamin A is taken for six months and 30 to 60 mg of desiccated thyroid, or Euthroid-1, one tablet, is taken daily if well tolerated. Antihistaminics, phenobarbital, and ataractic agents are given as needed, especially in the beginning, when all internal corticosteroid therapy is stopped. Excellent results are occasionally seen, with amelioration of symptoms and the lichenification in a few weeks and the return of normal skin with a normal sweat pattern in six weeks.

The Scholtz regimen has few enthusiastic proponents; the majority of dermatologists appear to have found it disappointing.

PUVA Therapy. Psoralen (methoxsalen, 20 mg) followed by UVA, as given for psoriasis, is often helpful in severe atopic dermatitis. Midelfart has recently studied the effect of UVB combined with UVA in severe atopic dermatitis in Norway. The combination was superior, producing complete clearing in half the patients with a 40 per cent lower dose than UVB alone.

Abramson JS, et al: Antistaphylococcal IgE in patients with atopic dermatitis. JAAD 1982, 7:10.

Anderson WA, et al: Keratosis punctata and atopy. Arch Dermatol 1984, 120:884.

August PS: House dust mite causes atopic eczema. Br J Dermatol 1984, 111(supp 26):10.

Ayres S Jr.: Atopic dermatitis: Response to Scholtz regimen. Aust J Dermatol 1984, 25:131.

Baer RL: Papaverine therapy in atopic dermatitis. JAAD 1985, 13:806.

Boiko S, et al: Osteomyelitis of distal phalanges in 3 children with severe atopic dermatitis. Arch Dermatol 1988, 124:418.

Businco L, et al: Double-blind crossover trial with oral sodium cromoglycate in children with atopic dermatitis due to food allergy. Ann Allergy 1986, 57:433.

Clover GB, et al: The "dirty neck." Clin Exp Dermatol 1987, 12:1.

Dahl MV: Some aspects of atopic dermatitis. Arch Dermatol 1982, 119:237.

Idem: Staphylococcus aureus and atopic dermatitis. Arch Dermatol 1983, 119:840.

Frosch PJ, et al: A double-blind trial of H_1 and H_2 receptor antagonists in the treatment of atopic dermatitis. Arch Dermatol Res 1984, 276:36.

Garrity JA, et al: Ocular complications of atopic dermatitis. Can J Ophthalmol 1984, 19:21.

Graham P, et al: Hypoallergenic diets and oral sodium cromoglycate in the management of atopic eczema. Br J Dermatol 1984, 110:457.

Hanifin JM: Diet, nutrition, and allergy in atopic dermatitis (editorial). JAAD 1983, 8:5.

Idem: Basic and clinical aspects of atopic dermatitis. Ann Allergy 1984, 52:386.

Idem: Atopic dermatitis. J Allergy Clin Immunol 1984, 73:211.

Idem: Atopic dermatitis. JAAD 1982, 6:1.

Hanifin JM, et al: Immunopharmacology of the atopic diseases. J Invest Dermatol 1985, 85:161s.

Idem: Newer concepts of atopic dermatitis. Arch Dermatol 1977, 113:663.

Hannuksela M, et al: Ultraviolet therapy in atopic dermatitis. Acta Derm Venereol (Stockh) 1985, 114:137.

Midelfart K, et al: UVB and UVA phototherapy of atopic dermatitis. Dermatologica 1985, 171:95.

Norris PG, et al: Screening for cataracts in patients with . . . atopic eczema. Clin Exp Dermatol 1987, 12:21.

Platts-Mills TAE, et al: The role of dust mite allergens in atopic dermatitis. Clin Exp Dermatol 1983, 8:233.

Roberts DLL: House dust mite avoidance and atopic dermatitis. Br J Dermatol 1984, 110:735.

Rola-Pleszczynski M, et al: Abnormal suppressor cell function in atopic dermatitis. J Invest Dermatol 1981, 76:279.

Sampson HA: Role of immediate food hypersensitivity in the pathogenesis of atopic dermatitis. J Allergy Clin Immunol 1983, 71:473.

Idem, et al: Comparison of results of skin test, RAST, and double-blind, placebo-controlled food challenge in atopic dermatitis. J Allergy Clin Immunol 1984, 74:26.

Idem: Increase in plasma histamine following food challenge in children with atopic dermatitis. N Engl J Med 1984, 311:372.

Idem: Food hypersensitivity and atopic dermatitis. J Pediatr 1985, 107:669.

Scholtz JR: Management of atopic dermatitis. Calif Med 1965, 102:210.

Seta O: Hyperlinear palms: Association with ichthyosis and atopic dermatitis. Arch Dermatol 1981, 117:490.

Soppi E, et al: Cell-mediated immunity in PUVA-treated and untreated atopic dermatitis. J Invest Dermatol 1982, 79:213.

Uehara M: Infraorbital fold in atopic dermatitis. Arch Dermatol 1981, 117:627.

Vickers CFH: The natural history of atopic eczema. Acta Dermatovener 1980, 72:1135.

Wright S, et al: Oral primrose-seed oil improves atopic eczema. Lancet 1982, 2:1120.

ECZEMA

The word eczema seems to have originated in A.D. 543 and is derived from the Greek word "ekzein" meaning "to boil out" or "to effervesce." This word probably has been applied to more skin diseases than any other term, with the possible exception of the term dermatitis. Baer describes "eczema" as "a pruritic papulovesicular process which in its acute phase is associated with erythema and edema and which in its more chronic phases, while retaining some of its papulovesicular features, is dominated by thickening, lichenification, and scaling."

Ackerman points out that the word refers to a group of diseases with no common denominator, and calls for its elimination from the dermatologist's vocabulary. Morris Leider has published a rebuttal.

The important thing to realize is that it is a symptom only, and in no sense of the word a disease. As a symptom, it is an indispensable word.

Histologically, the hallmark of all eczematous eruptions is a serous exudate between cells of the epidermis (spongiosis), together with an inflammatory infiltrate in the dermis. Spongiosis is very prominent in acute dermatitis of the atopic, infectious eczematoid, dyshidrotic, and contact types and often manifests macroscopic as well as microscopic vesiculation. A scale or crust composed of serous exudate, acute inflammatory cells, and keratin corresponds to the honey-colored crust noted clinically. The dermal infiltrate is usually lymphocytic in nature.

Spongiosis and a mixed-cell inflammatory infiltrate

are likewise prominent in nummular eczema, which also shows psoriasiform epidermal hyperplasia. Xerotic eczema is characterized by minimal spongiosis, a scant lymphocytic inflammatory infiltrate, and a change in the appearance of the keratin layer from the normal "basketweave" pattern to a compact one.

Eczema, regardless of etiology, will manifest similar histologic changes if allowed to persist chronically. These features, which correspond clinically to lichen simplex chronicus, include hyperkeratosis, irregular acanthosis (hyperplasia) of the epidermis, and thickening of the collagen bundles in the papillary portion of the dermis. The development of lichen simplex chronicus is directly related to persistent rubbing and scratching of the skin.

As knowledge of skin diseases has been gained over the centuries new entities have emerged from this all-inclusive designation of eczema. Some of the factors or conditions that react in the form of eczema will be discussed.

Emotional factors and psychologic stress exacerbate all forms of eczema. A similar effect is produced by stimulants, which may be psychic (excitement) or gustatory (coffee, tea, chocolate, tobacco, alcohol). Fatigue from lack of sleep or overexertion produces a similar effect. Often a patient who is consuming 10 cups of coffee and smoking many cigarettes a day shows improvement of the eczema after stopping use of these excitants.

In these reactions severe pruritus is a common and often the most prominent symptom. The degree of irritation at which itching begins (the itch threshold) is lowered by stress.

REGIONAL ECZEMAS

Ear Eczema

Eczema of the ears or otitis externa may involve the helix, postauricular fold, and the external auditory canal. By far the most frequently affected site is the external canal, where many mechanisms join to protect the delicate structures of the internal ear from contamination. Secretions of the ear canal derive from the apocrine and sebaceous glands, which form cerumen. Traumatization of the ear canal by rubbing, wiping, scratching, and picking induces edema and infection with inflammation. Seborrheic dermatitis, psoriasis, or atopic dermatitis may also initiate otitis of the external canal. Infection is most frequently caused by staphylococci, streptococci, and *Pseudomonas aeruginosa*; rarely, fungus or *Corynebacterium diphtheriae* may be responsible. Contact dermatitis to neomycin, benzocaine, and the parabens may follow remedies used to treat these conditions. Earlobe dermatitis signals nickel allergy.

Treatment should be directed to removal of causative agents such as those already mentioned. Scales and cerumen should be removed by lavage with an ear syringe. Frequent instillation of antibiotic-corticoid preparations, such as Cortisporin, Terra-Cortril, or topical steroid creams or solutions with or without 5 per cent liquor carbonis detergens, are favored for effective treatment.

Eyelid Dermatitis

Dermatitis of one eyelid is most frequently caused by nail polish. When both eyelids are involved, then one must suspect mascara, eye shadow, eyelash cement, or eye liner. Hair dye, rinse, tint, lacquer, and hair spray must also be considered. More infrequently "blush-on" rouge, fluoridated toothpaste, perfumes, and after-shave lotions may also cause this. Many of these substances are transferred by the hands to the eyelids.

Volatile gases such as insect sprays, lemon peel oil, benzalkonium chloride and thimerosal in the rinsing solution used in connection with contact lenses, or plastics in spectacle frames containing ethylene glycol monomethyl ether acetate (EGMEA) may all cause eyelid dermatitis.

Any sensitizer or irritant on the palms or fingers may cause dermatitis of the eyelids long before it affects any other parts of the face. Thus, mango dermatitis often appears only on the eyelids, initially.

Breast Eczema (Nipple Eczema)

Eczema of the breasts may affect the nipples, the areolae, the skin, or the folds beneath. Usually eczema of the nipples is of the moist type with oozing and crusting. Painful fissuring is frequently seen, especially in nursing mothers.

Psoriasis, seborrheic dermatitis, circumscribed neurodermatitis, and contact dermatitis must be considered in the differential diagnosis. Nipple eczema may be an isolated manifestation of atopic dermatitis.

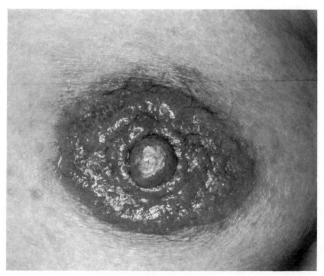

Figure 5–5. Nipple eczema.

In those patients in whom the eczema of the nipple or areola has persisted for over three months, especially if it is unilateral, a biopsy is mandatory to rule out the possibility of Paget's disease of the breast.

Topical or intralesional corticosteroids are effective in the treatment of non-Paget's eczema of the breast.

Diaper (Napkin) Dermatitis

Dermatitis of the diaper area in infants is perhaps the most common cutaneous disorder in this age group. When due to irritation and friction, as it most commonly is, it is an erythematous and papulovesicular dermatitis distributed over the lower abdomen, the genitals, the thighs, and the convex surfaces of the buttocks. The folds remain unaffected, since they are not in direct contact with the diaper. Erythematous patches sometimes spread to the legs from contact with the wet diaper. In some instances the eruption has well-demarcated, often polycyclic, and elevated psoriasiform patches with micaceous scales. In severe cases there may be superficial erosion. The tip of the penis may become irritated and crusted, with the result that the baby urinates frequently and spots of blood appear on the diaper. The condition occurs most frequently in infants whose diapers are not changed all night.

Diaper dermatitis of this type has been attributed to the alkaline irritative effects of ammonia formed in the wet diaper by the splitting of urea by the ammonia-forming bacillus in feces. Experimental work suggests, however, that this may not be the case. Leyden and his associates' studies do not support the notion that ammonia is a primary factor in common diaper dermatitis.

Diaper dermatitis must also be differentiated from intertriginous fungous infection due to *Candida albicans*, intertrigo, inverse psoriasis, and seborrheic dermatitis. In these cases, in contrast to diaper dermatitis, the inguinal and suprapubic folds are involved early. Letterer-Siwe disease, allergic contact dermatitis, and congenital syphilis should be included in the differential diagnosis.

Treatment is closely connected with prophylactic measures. The frequent changing of diapers is the best measure. Disposable diapers, especially those with synthetic liners, tend to minimize contact of the skin with urine. Topical hydrocortisone applied lightly at the time of diaper change is effective and safe since there is little internal absorption.

For those who want to avoid use of corticosteroids completely, 1–2–3 ointment is excellent:

℞ Burow's solution	1 part
Anhydrous lanolin	2 parts
Lassar's paste without salicylic acid	3 parts
Dispense 120 grams	
M Sig: Apply when changing diapers.	

Acid Mantle Creme, A and D ointment, and zinc oxide ointment are excellent substitutes for 1–2–3 ointment.

Hand Eczema

The hands may be remarkably involved with various dermatoses both obscure in their etiology and resistant to treatment.

In addition to the irritant hand eczema described here that involves only the hands, other dermatoses must be kept in mind that may occur on other parts of the body also. These, described elsewhere in the text, are: atopic dermatitis, allergic contact dermatitis, nummular eczema, tinea manus, lichen simplex chronicus, dermatitis repens, id reactions, pustular bacterid, psoriasis, and scabies.

IRRITANT HAND DERMATITIS

Housewife's Eczema

CLINICAL SIGNS. This type of hand eczema is a common disease frequently seen in housewives, due to or at least aggravated by excessive and prolonged exposure to soaps or detergents and water. The eruption usually begins with dryness and redness of the fingers. Dry scales with peeling are evident at the tips of the fingers, "chapping" is seen on the backs of the hands, and erythematous hardening of the palms with fissures develops. Frequently, dermatitis appears around and under rings, especially wedding bands that are not removed when using soap and water.

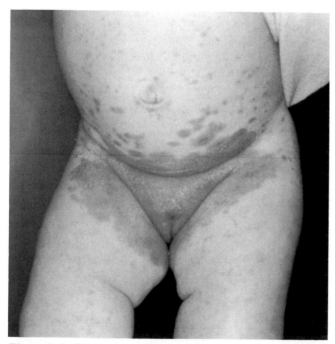

Figure 5–6. Diaper dermatitis, sometimes referred to as napkin psoriasis.

The defatting action and maceration produced by prolonged immersion or frequent washing of the hands may be seen in many other types of workers such as bartenders, food handlers, chefs, physicians, dentists, and nurses, all of whom wash their hands frequently.

Irritant hand dermatitis is also frequently seen in occupations in which there is exposure to chemicals, solvents, acids, or alkalis. Friction and cold or dry air are other factors which irritate the skin of the hands.

Numerous things may complicate irritant hand dermatitis. Allergic reactions may develop. In housewives, there may be allergic sensitization to such foodstuffs handled in the kitchen as garlic, onion, carrot, tomato, spinach, grapefruit, orange, radish, fig, parsnip, or cheese. Some foods may produce a contact urticaria type of dermatitis. These include potatoes, flour, fish, shellfish, and cheese. There may be sensitization to rubber gloves, plastic articles, or house plants such as the philodendron; to metals such as nickel; to dyes such as paraphenylenediamine, and numerous other allergenic contactants. In other occupations the relevant exposures to potential allergens should be ascertained by history. Candidiasis may develop, especially in the finger webs. Secondary bacterial infection, especially with *Staphylococcus aureus*, may occur in the fissured areas.

DIAGNOSIS. Diagnosis of hand eczema should be made by exclusion of other disorders with which it may be confused, notably nummular eczema, patchy pompholyx, or volar (inverse) psoriasis. Pitting of the nails may occur in all three of these but is characteristic of psoriasis, especially in the absence of nail fold involvement. Palmar tinea is likely to be unilateral and keratolysis exfoliativa symmetrical and superficial.

Atopic dermatitis as a primary disorder of the hands is an important consideration. In addition, this disease, or a genetic predisposition to it, is frequently present in many patients with irritant hand dermatitis. It is important when considering psoriasis and atopic dermatitis to take a family history, and a personal history of previous related problems, and to examine the entire cutaneous surface. The feet should always be examined in evaluating any hand dermatitis.

Allergic reactions should be considered in the differential diagnosis, again either as a primary disease or as a complicating factor of irritant hand dermatitis. Exposures to potential allergens at the workplace, at home, or during hobbies or sports should be sought by a thorough history. Also topical medicaments, either over-the-counter or by prescription, may sensitize. Patch testing should be done if the history or morphology suggests allergic reactions, in recalcitrant or long-standing disease, or in occupationally related hand dermatitis which fails to clear promptly. Materials for this should be obtained directly from the workplace: the patch test tray may be inadequate.

TREATMENT. Alleviation of hand dermatitis will, at times, tax the ingenuity of the patient and the physician to the limit. In most cases it is impossible for the patient, especially the young mother, to discontinue soap and water exposure. Frequently a halt in the use of chlorine bleaches and ammonia water may bring about remarkable improvement. Vinyl or latex gloves should be worn, especially when strong detergents are used. This avoids the possibility of the development of sensitivity to the rubber in rubber gloves. The patient should try to avoid wearing vinyl gloves for more than a few minutes because of the macerating action of the accumulated perspiration in the glove. If white cotton gloves can be worn, the patient is deterred from frequent wetting of the hands. This is almost always impractical, however.

The various corticosteroid creams are beneficial; they should be applied lightly every two to three hours. Many cases of hand dermatitis will respond to hydrocortisone-containing preparations in a lubricating base applied frequently. Encouragement for use after each hand washing can be accomplished by having the patient keep a container of the lubricant medication at each sink in the house and workplace. For many cases application of a stronger steroid ointment under occlusion at night provides a period during which a thicker, greasier preparation may be applied and also provides better long-term penetration of the antiinflammatory component.

For the acutely inflamed, swollen, oozing, and weeping dermatitis, compresses of ice cold milk or Burow's 1:20 solution (Domeboro packets or tablets) applied for 20 minutes every four hours will relieve the acute symptoms. This is usually needed only for a day or two. If continued too long it may cause dryness and cracking. After the compresses, corticosteroid creams in an emollient base should be applied. Potent topical steroids such as betamethasone dipropionate (Diprolene) or clobetasol propionate (Temovate) may be necessary for the effective control of severe hand eczema. In persistent cases, rather than continue potent topical corticosteroids to the point of producing side effects, it may be advisable to resort to the use of systemic steroids: triamcinolone acetonide (Kenalog-40) intramuscularly, repeated every four weeks or longer as required. It has less risk of side effects than even medium-potency topical steroids.

PUVA therapy has been reported effective in hand eczema by Tegner et al and by Rosen et al.

Dyshidrotic Eczema
POMPHOLYX (DYSHIDROSIS)

CLINICAL FEATURES. Pompholyx (meaning bubble) is also known as cheiropompholyx. It is a vesicular eruption of the palms and soles characterized by eczematous, weeping patches containing intraepidermal vesicles, infrequently by hyperhidro-

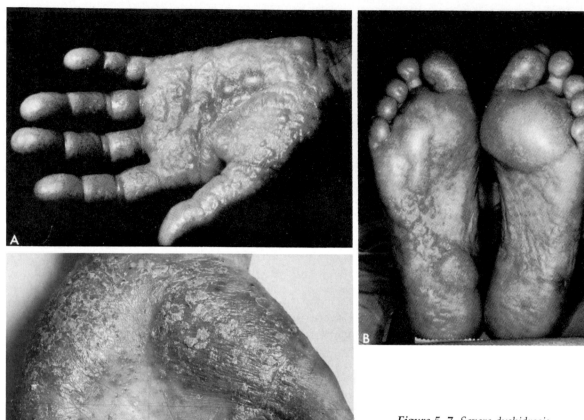

Figure 5–7. Severe dyshidrosis.

sis, and often by burning or itching. There is a tendency for the pruritic 1- to 2-mm vesicles to be most pronounced at the sides of the fingers. The application of the term "pompholyx" is limited to those typical eruptions that have small deep-seated vesicles resembling "sago grains," occurring only on the palms, soles, and interdigits, accompanied by itching or burning and excessive perspiration, in which examination fails to reveal fungi or external chemical cause. In long-standing cases the nails may become damaged. It is also discussed in Chapter 10.

The distribution of the lesions is, as a rule, bilateral and roughly symmetric. Sometimes they are arranged in groups. By coalescence of several contiguous vesicles, bullae may be formed. The contents are clear and colorless but may later become straw-colored or purulent. Attacks generally last a few weeks, but because of the tendency to relapses the condition may persist for long periods. The lesions involute by drying up rather than by rupturing.

ETIOLOGY. The etiology of dyshidrosis is unknown; however, chronic emotional stress may be one prominent predisposing factor. Hyperhidrosis of the palms and soles may be associated with it. Sweat glands and ducts are not connected with the vesicles. Pompholyx must be differentiated from an id reaction due to active fungus infection of the soles. Contact dermatitis must also be differentiated from pompholyx, as must tinea manuum.

Christensen and Moller have reported nickel dermatitis of the pompholyx type. Ingestion of nickel in food may play a role in the chronicity of this dermatitis.

HISTOPATHOLOGY. The sweat ducts are not involved. Pinkus and Mehregan state, "The sweat ducts thread their way between the vesicles." Spongiotic vesicles are found in the epidermis with lymphocytic exocytosis.

DIFFERENTIAL DIAGNOSIS. Vesicular eruptions of the palms and soles closely resemble each other, so that the clinical features may not be enough to arrive at a diagnosis. Dermatophytid, atopic dermatitis, contact dermatitis (primary), drug eruption (penicillin), pustular psoriasis of the palms and soles, psoriasis, acrodermatitis continua, and pustular bacterid are some dermatoses to be kept in mind. Localized bullous pemphigoid has recently been reported to initially manifest in this way.

TREATMENT. Topical application of high-potency corticosteroid creams and ointments, 5 per cent salicylic acid in alcohol and 3 per cent vioform cream may be used. Soaking of the hands and feet in potassium permanganate solution (1:5000) for one half hour is still helpful. Burow's solution compresses are more esthetic to use. Intramuscular injection of triamcinolone suspension (Kenalog) 40 mg or short courses of oral prednisone are valuable in clearing and inducing remissions in the more severe or recalcitrant cases.

Previously, x-ray therapy has been widely used. It is still effective, but today radiation therapy is rarely used. When other methods are ineffective or steroids cannot be used, 75 rads of superficial x-rays to the palms at weekly intervals for a total of not more than 300 rads will be extremely (though temporarily) helpful. Oral psoralen plus ultraviolet A light (PUVA) has been reported to be effective, but in view of its cost and inconvenience and potential for side effects (as compared to a single injection of triamcinolone acetonide intramuscularly), it seems difficult to justify its use.

Keratolysis Exfoliativa
LAMELLAR DYSHIDROSIS

Lamellar dyshidrosis (dyshidrosis lamellosa) is a superficial exfoliative dermatosis of the palms and soles characterized by the absence of inflammatory changes and by small patches with peripheral white scaling that gradually extend peripherally, while at the same time the stratum corneum in the central part becomes ruptured and peels off. The disorder spreads, new desquamating areas developing, and eventually by coalescence the entire part may show flaky scales. The disease usually affects only the palms and soles. The involvement is bilateral, and it can occur in association with dyshidrosis, although at times no cause can be ascertained.

The disorder must be differentiated from dermatophytosis.

Treatment is difficult for this mild malady, but spontaneous involution occurs usually in a few weeks. Tar (Zetone cream) usually produces satisfactory results. Five per cent tar in gel (Estar Gel) is an excellent preparation to use. A mild emollient, however, may suffice. Lac-Hydrin Lotion is often effective. A small dose, 20 or 30 mg, of triamcinolone acetonide (Kenalog) intramuscularly will often terminate a prolonged attack and induce a remission lasting one or several months. Arnold would sometimes use this in severe cases; Odom and James would not. Keratolytic emollient creams and lotions are helpful.

AUTOSENSITIZATION DERMATITIS

When a person's skin becomes sensitized to a substance elaborated in or on his body from his own tissue proteins, autosensitization dermatitis may develop. Whitfield first in 1921 reported two patients in whom generalized toxic eruptions developed 10 days after they had large hematomas caused by trauma. Since then generalized acute vesicular eruptions associated with chronic eczema of the legs with or without ulceration, generalized exfoliative dermatitis subsequent to local dermatitis, id eruptions due to distant foci which provoke sensitization to a combination of the patient's own protein and staphylococcus toxin, and various other instances of apparent autosensitization have been noted.

It is well established that the ordinary cutaneous bacterial flora may, in the presence of a relatively minor dermatitis, especially if there is exudation, suddenly be transformed so that a previously harmless saprophytic staphylococcus, streptococcus, or *Candida albicans* assumes a pathogenic role and literally covers the body surface with its growth within a day or two. This may be due to greater availability of bacterial adherence factors, such as fibronectin. Such cases are called infectious eczematoid dermatitis.

Cunningham et al recently studied a patient with autoeczematization and found an elevated ratio of T helper cells to T suppressor cells, as well as increased circulating activated T cells. They hold this as evi-

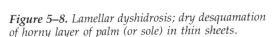
Figure 5–8. Lamellar dyshidrosis; dry desquamation of horny layer of palm (or sole) in thin sheets.

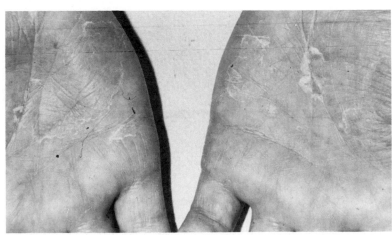

dence to support Whitfield's original hypothesis that this disease represents a cellular immune response to a cutaneous autoantigen.

Infectious Eczematoid Dermatitis

The eruption may be vesicular, pustular or crusted, dry and scaly, or multiform. It is invariably pruritic and may be accompanied by factitious urticaria. Linear lesions are often present. The disease has a predilection for regions easily accessible to the patient's fingers. In mild cases and in the subsiding stages of the more severe cases the patches may be dry, scaly, and fissured. In the severe types of the disease there is marked edema, especially of the face and extremities, accompanied by large vesicles and pustulation. The exudation may be extreme and the skin is easily irritated by mild remedies.

Infectious eczematoid dermatitis is regarded as an example of autosensitization. The disease spreads from a local site by peripheral extension. Often it develops about a discharging abscess, sinus, or ulcer. It may develop from chronic otitis media, a bedsore, a fistula, or from discharges from the eyes, nose, or vagina. Eczematous eruptions during the acute stages of radiodermatitis and about chronic x-ray and radium ulcers belong in this category.

Important considerations in the therapy of this recalcitrant dermatitis are the removal of the focus and antibiotic treatment. Cultures should be made and tested for antibiotic sensitivity. Potassium permanganate or Burow's solution baths, containing 1 pint of liquor alumini acetatis to one third of a tub of water, are helpful. Acute extensive weeping eczematous eruptions also respond to Aveeno meal baths by drying out the "weeping." Topical applications of aqueous solution of gentian violet 1 per cent and antibiotic lotions or ointments are used as indicated, although other ointments and pastes should be avoided. Appropriate antibiotics may also be given orally or parenterally. Topical antibiotic/corticosteroid creams or ointments or systemic corticosteroids are usually beneficial.

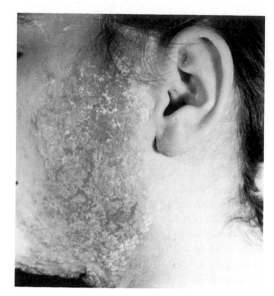

Figure 5–10. Infectious eczematoid dermatitis. (Courtesy of Dr. F. Daniels, Jr.)

Circumileostomy Eczema

Eczematization or autosensitization of the surrounding skin frequently occurs after ileostomy. It is estimated that some 75 per cent of ileostomy patients have some postoperative sensitivity. This is due to the leakage of intestinal fluid onto the unprotected skin. As the consistency of the intestinal secretion becomes viscous the sensitization subsides. Proprietary medications containing karaya powder have been found to be helpful. Rodriguez reported in 1976 that 20 per cent cholestyramine (an ion exchange resin) in Aquaphor promptly alleviated the condition in all of eight children in whom it was used.

Juvenile Plantar Dermatosis

This eczematous plantar disorder of children, first described by Enta and Moller in 1972, and named juvenile plantar dermatosis by Mackie in 1976, was reviewed by Ashton et al in 1985 in a study of 56 cases. It usually begins as a patchy, symmetrical, smooth, red, glazed macule on the great toes, sometimes with fissuring and desquamation, in children aged 3 to 13. Toewebs are rarely involved; fingers may be.

Histologically there is psoriasiform acanthosis and a sparse, largely lymphocytic infiltrate in the upper dermis, most dense around sweat ducts at their point of entry into the epidermis. Spongiosis is commonly present.

The diagnosis may be apparent on inspection, especially if there is a family or personal history of atopy and the toewebs are spared. Shoe dermatitis and dermatophytosis should be considered in the differential diagnosis.

Treatment may consist of bed rest in the most severe cases. Cotton socks may be helpful. Topical

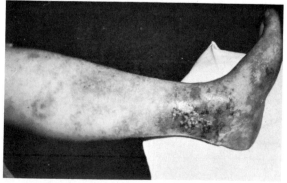

Figure 5–9. Infectious eczematoid dermatitis, which started in an ulcer on the ankle.

steroids are of value. Urea preparations may help. Most cases clear within four years of diagnosis.

Based on a (presumably, in retrospect, erroneous) diagnosis of plantar psoriasis, Arnold has treated it since about 1965 with 5–20 mg of triamcinolone acetonide intramuscularly every four to eight or more weeks, with gratifying success and complete absence of side effects. Injections are given only as required by symptoms.

XEROTIC ECZEMA

Xerotic eczema is also known as xerosis, winter itch, winter dry skin, eczema craquelé, and asteatotic eczema.

These vividly descriptive terms are all applied to dehydrated skin showing redness, dry scaling, and fine crackling that may resemble crackled porcelain. These changes usually occur in patches over many parts of the skin; however, they are seen most frequently on the extremities, especially on the shins of the elderly. These changes are seen most frequently during wintertime when there is low humidity in the air of excessively heated rooms.

This xerosis is similar to that seen in chapped hands when there is excessive water loss from the stratum corneum of the skin. Blank has shown that the water content of the horny layer of the skin is also determined by the relative humidity of the environment.

TREATMENT. Bathing dries the skin. However, with the limitation of the use of soap to only the apocrine-bearing areas (axilla and groin) all but the most severe cases may continue to bathe. The use of bath oils in the bath water or applied to the hydrated skin is recommended. The use of humidifiers is to be encouraged.

The relief and prevention of dryness of the skin is centered around the maintenance of proper hydration of the stratum corneum. The rate of water loss from this layer may be impeded by using emulsions of oil and water. The residual film of oil on the skin prevents or at least impedes evaporation from the surface of the skin and soothes the skin surface to prevent fissuring.

Emollients such as lanolin and glycerin are hydrophilic and not only hydrate the skin but at the same time form an occlusive film that decreases evaporation. Hydrophilic ointment USP, cold creams, vanishing creams, moisturizing creams, and lubricating creams are all effective in hydration.

Extremely effective are the modern emollients such as Aquacare HP cream or lotion containing 10 per cent urea, Carmol Ten lotion also containing 10 per cent urea, Lacti-care lotion containing 5 per cent lactic acid, Keri lotion or cream, and Lubriderm. Lac-Hydrin (12 per cent ammonium lactate) is a highly effective lotion in the management of xerosis.

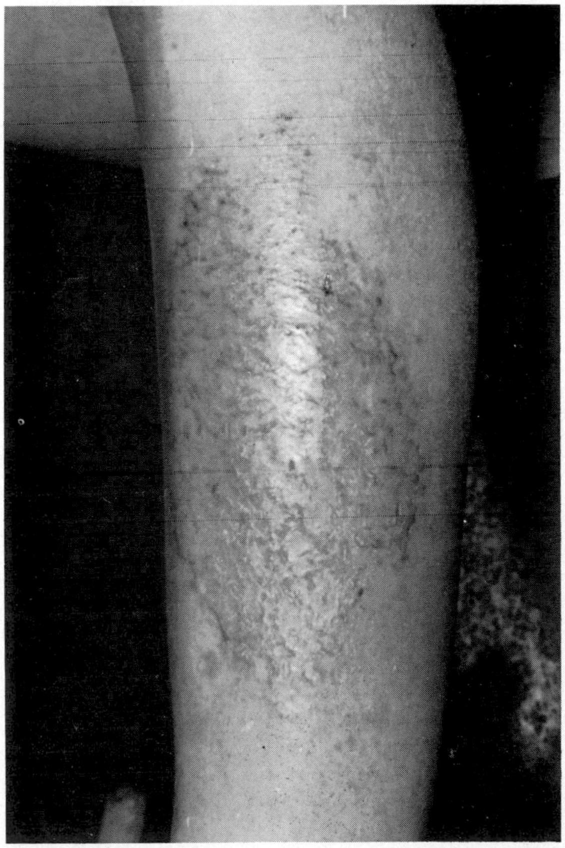

Figure 5–11. Winter eczema—another cause of eczema craquelé.

NUTRITIONAL DEFICIENCY ECZEMA

This type of eczema is apt to occur in alcoholics and in those who have been on restricted diets for years because of chronic gastrointestinal complaints or in efforts to avoid obesity or because of living alone. The skin lesions are localized, thickened, scaling patches that have some characteristics of nummular eczema, seborrheic dermatitis, and neurodermatitis. There may be keratotic papules and thickening of the palms and soles. The distribution on the elbows, about the neck, and on the lower back may suggest pellagra or psoriasis. Frequently the eruption is generalized but spares the face.

The tongue may be smooth and bright red, having a glazed, beefy appearance, or may be purplish; aphthae or swollen gums may be present. In women the vulva may show kraurosis. Examination should be made for anemia and candidiasis, which may accompany the deficiency.

Various factors such as deficiency of fatty acids, amino acids, trace metals, or vitamins may be the cause of such eruptions, though this is often difficult to document.

Proper and effective treatment consists of a liberal diet of fresh fruits, vegetables, milk, eggs, and meat, particularly liver. Multiple vitamins should be taken regularly. Improvement is usually accompanied by considerable gain in weight, increased vigor, and disappearance of the eczema.

NUMMULAR ECZEMA
(Nummular Neurodermatitis)

The condition usually begins upon the dorsa of the hands, extensor surfaces of the arms, legs, thighs, shoulders, buttocks, breasts, or nipples, and consists of discrete, coin-shaped, erythematous, edematous, vesicular, and crusted patches from 5 to 50 or more mm in diameter, but most often about 20 to 40 mm wide. Linear (Koebner) streaks may be present. In advanced cases the condition may become greatly aggravated and spread into palm-sized or larger patches in which papules or papulovesicles and exudation occur. The plaques sometimes ooze and become thickened and scaly. Although the patches are usually coin-sized, an extensive area may become covered by a single patch and, in time, such a lesion may become thickened into a solid plaque about which may be satellites of papulovesicular and crusted lesions. Pruritus is usually severe and of the same paroxysmal, compulsive quality and nocturnal timing seen in circumscribed neurodermatitis. Francis Lynch called it nummular neurodermatitis.

Emotional stress is usually present in patients with nummular eczema, and some of the worst cases are seen in alcoholics.

Histologically, the most distinctive feature of nummular eczema is spongiosis, associated with the features suggesting psoriasis.

Initial treatment consists of potent topical steroid creams applied once or twice daily, oral erythromycin 250 mg four times daily for 10 days, and hydroxyzine hydrochloride (Atarax) 25 mg three times daily. If this regimen is ineffective, management consists of intralesional or systemic corticosteroids. In cases too extensive for intralesional injections, Arnold considers triamcinolone acetonide intramuscularly the treatment of choice. A patient of Arnold's who had been

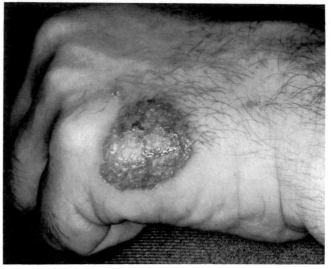

Figure 5–13. Coin-shaped lesion of nummular eczema.

maintained by almost-monthly 40-mg doses for over seven years (with no detectable side effects!) divorced his wife at that point and never required another dose during a four-year follow-up. He then relapsed.

Mild sedatives and tranquilizers may help in this treatment regimen. Superficial x-ray therapy in fractional doses has been of definite value but is now not recommended if steroid therapy is possible.

AUTOIMMUNE PROGESTERONE DERMATITIS

This is an autosensitive dermatitis from progesterone that may appear as urticaria, a vesicobullous eruption, or erythema multiforme. The eruption typically appears 5 to 10 days before menses and spontaneously clears following menstruation, only to return in the next menstrual period.

When urticaria is the predominant skin lesion, there is a generalized distribution. It may be severe

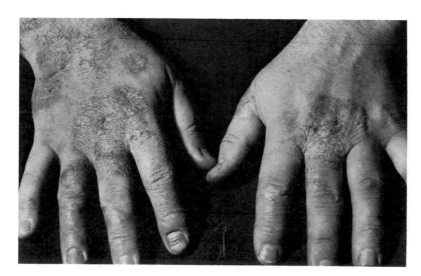

Figure 5–12. Nummular eczema of the backs of the hands.

enough to produce laryngeal spasms that require epinephrine medication. When vesicles and bullae predominate, the lesions are extremely pruritic and commonly occur on the hands and feet in a dyshidrosiform pattern. They may occur on the oral mucosa, chest, back, and arms. Usually erythema multiforme is accompanied by a vesicobullous eruption on the palms and soles. Target lesions on the legs and trunk with erosions on the mucous membranes complete the picture.

In 14 cases reviewed in the literature, each patient gave a typical history of the onset of dermatitis prior to menses and clearing afterward. Intradermal tests with progesterone may show an urticarial response within a few minutes after injection and a positive delayed hypersensitivity reaction in 48 hours. Aqueous progesterone suspension containing 100 mg/ml is diluted to 0.1 mg/ml with normal saline. A provocative test injection of 25 mg progesterone intramuscularly may produce the pruritic lesions almost immediately.

It is believed that sensitivity to one's own progesterone is the cause of this dermatitis. There is a marked rise in progesterone levels prior to ovulation, and it reaches its peak a few days before onset of menses. Six of the seven cases in one series had had exogenous progesterone at some time before onset of their dermatitis.

Effective treatment has been achieved with the use of estrogens to inhibit ovulation. Estinyl estradiol 0.02 mg t.i.d. from the fourth to the twenty-fourth day effectively inhibits ovulation. Conjugated estrogen (Premarin) 1.25 mg/day for 21 days of each cycle also is effective.

Ackerman AB, et al: A plea to expunge . . . "eczema" from the lexicon of dermatology. Am J Dermatopathol 1982, 4:315.

Ashton RE, et al: Juvenile plantar dermatosis: A clinicopathologic study. Arch Dermatol 1985, 121:225.

Borglund E, et al: Classification of peristomal skin changes in patients with urostomy. JAAD 1988, 19:623.

Christensen OB, et al: Nickel allergy and hand eczema. Contact Dermatitis 1975, 2:353.

Cowen MA: Nummular eczema. Acta Derm Venereol (Stockh) 1961, 41:253.

Cunningham MJ, et al: Circulating activated T lymphocytes in a patient with autoeczematization. JAAD 1986, 14:1039.

Epstein E: Hand dermatitis: Practical management and current concepts. JAAD 1984, 10:395.

Feingold DS: Bacterial adherence, colonization, and pathogenicity. Arch Dermatol 1986, 122:161.

Jones SK, et al: Juvenile plantar dermatosis. Clin Exp Dermatol 1987, 12:5.

Leider M: Eczema: Consulting editor's reply. Am J Dermatopathol 1983, 5:411.

Leyden JJ, et al: Role of microorganisms in diaper dermatitis. Arch Dermatol 1978, 114:56.

Mackie RM: Juvenile plantar dermatosis. Semin Dermatol 1982, 1:67.

Moller P, et al: Cholestyramine ointment . . . [for] perianal irritation after ileal anastomosis. Dis Colon and Rectum 1987, 30:106.

Nilsson E, et al: Density of microflora in hand eczema before and after . . . use of a topical corticosteroid. JAAD 1986, 15:192.

Okazaki M, et al: Radiodermatitis. J Dermatol 1986, 13:356.

Pegum S, et al: Diaper dermatitis. Arch Dermatol 1978, 114:1552.

Rebora A: Sulzberger-Garbe disease in Europe. Int J Dermatol 1989, 28:22.

Rietschel RL, et al: Nonatopic eczemas. JAAD 1988, 18:569.

Rodriguez JT: Treatment of skin irritation around colostomies with cholestyramine. J Pediatr 1976, 88:659.

Rosen K, et al: Chronic eczematous dermatitis of the hands. Acta Derm Venereol (Stockh) 1987, 67:48.

Rothstein MS: Dermatologic considerations of stomal care. JAAD 1986, 15:411.

Shelley WB, et al: Chronic hand eczema strategies. Cutis 1982, 29:569.

Sinha SM, et al: Vegetables responsible for contact dermatitis of the hands. Arch Dermatol 1977, 113:776.

Warin A: Eczema craquelé as a presenting feature of myxedema. Br J Dermatol 1973, 89:289.

Ziboh VA, et al: Biologic significance of polyunsaturated fatty acids in the skin. Arch Dermatol 1987, 123:1686a.

IMMUNODEFICIENCY SYNDROMES

Many of the immunodeficiency syndromes have cutaneous manifestations associated with other disorders. The most common of these skin diseases are bacterial or fungal infections (especially mucocutaneous candidiasis), LE-like syndromes, and atopic dermatitis. The primary immunodeficiencies may be classified as those of impaired humoral antibody (B cell) production, impaired cell-mediated antibody (T cell) formation, and combined B and T cell deficiencies.

Some of the many immunodeficiencies with cutaneous involvement are presented in this section.

X-LINKED AGAMMAGLOBULINEMIA

Also known as Bruton's syndrome and sex-linked agammaglobulinemia, this rare hereditary immunologic disorder usually becomes apparent at around six months of age, with great susceptibility to gram-positive pyogenic infections such as *Pneumococcus* and *Streptococcus*. Persistent viral and parasitic infections occur often despite normal cell mediated immunity. There is an increased tendency to develop atopic dermatitis, diffuse vasculitis, dermatomyositis, urticaria, or viral hepatitis.

IgA, IgM, IgD, and IgE are virtually absent from the serum, although IgG may be present in small amounts. Isohemagglutinins and C1q may also be absent. The spleen and lymph nodes lack germinal centers and plasma cells are absent from the lymph nodes, spleen, bone marrow, and connective tissues.

Cell-mediated immunity is intact. The T lymphocytes are normal in number, function, and proportion, but B cells are usually completely lacking. Current evidence indicates that the defect lies in a maturation block in pre-B-cell to B-cell differentiation.

Treatment with gamma globulin is helpful, but it does not completely control the disease. Progressive fatal encephalitis may develop. Respiratory disease with pulmonary fibrosis is also frequently seen, as there is no means of restoring secretory IgA to mucous membrane surfaces. Lymphoreticular malignancy, especially leukemia, may develop.

ISOLATED IgA DEFICIENCY

An absence or marked reduction of serum IgA occurs in approximately 1 in 700 people in the general population. Most such persons are entirely well. Of the symptomatic group, half have repeated infections and one quarter have autoimmune or collagen vascular disease. Allergies such as anaphylactic transfusion reactions, asthma, and atopic dermatitis are common in the symptomatic group, and Arnold has seen a case in which classic dermatitis herpetiformis occurred in adult life. There is an increased association of celiac disease, ulcerative colitis, and regional enteritis. Systemic lupus erythematosus, dermatomyositis, thyroiditis, rheumatoid arthritis, and Sjögren's syndrome have all been reported to occur in these patients. Ten to 15 per cent of clinically serious immunodeficiency cases occur in patients with symptomatic IgA deficiency.

It is believed that these patients have a maturation defect of the B lymphocyte as it transforms into an IgA-producing plasma cell. The defect is transmitted as an autosomal recessive trait. It may also be an acquired deficiency, induced by certain drugs, such as phenytoin.

Recently there have been reports of associated IgG2 and IgG4 deficiency, as well as decreased levels of IgE, in these patients. The abnormality may be more generalized in symptomatic cases. Patients with associated IgG abnormalities may benefit from immunoglobulin replacement, but over 40 per cent of these patients have antibodies to IgA, and gamma globulin may cause allergic reactions.

ISOLATED PRIMARY IgM DEFICIENCY

Eczematous dermatitis is present in about one fifth of the cases with this abnormality. The other immunoglobulins are usually present in normal amounts. Isohemagglutinins are absent. Affected persons are predisposed to severe infections, especially those due to meningococci, pneumococci, and Hemophilus influenzae. Verrucae vulgares may occur in great numbers. Thyroiditis, splenomegaly, and hemolytic anemia may occur. Patients with mycosis fungoides and gluten-sensitive enteropathy may have a secondary IgM deficiency.

This disease is probably also due to a defect in the maturation of IgM-producing plasma cells.

THYMIC HYPOPLASIA

Congenital thymic hypoplasia, also known as DiGeorge syndrome and as III and IV pharyngeal pouch syndrome, is a sporadic disorder characterized by a distinctive facies: notched, low-set ears, shortened philtrum, and hypertelorism.

The syndrome includes congenital absence of the parathyroids and thymus, and an abnormal aorta. Neonatal tetany is usually the first sign of the disease. Aortic and cardiac defects are the most common cause of death. T-cell defects are present, and cell-mediated immunity is absent or depressed. Fungous and viral infections commonly occur despite usually normal immunoglobulin levels.

SEVERE COMBINED IMMUNODEFICIENCY DISEASE (SCID)

This disease, which is usually fatal by age two, may have various cutaneous manifestations. These include a simple morbilliform eruption, seborrheic dermatitis, and necrolysis. In addition severe recurrent infections may occur, due to *Pseudomonas, Staphylococcus,* Enterobacteriaceae, or *Candida.* Moniliasis of the oropharynx and skin, intractable diarrhea, and pneumonia are the triad of findings which commonly lead to the diagnosis of SCID. Overwhelming viral infections are the usual cause of death.

SCID is characterized by deficiency or total absence of circulating lymphocytes. Mature T cells are almost invariably absent, but B cells are greatly reduced too, and immunoglobulin levels are consistently very low. The thymus is very small, and its malformed architecture at autopsy is pathognomonic.

The inheritance may be autosomal dominant or X-linked. About half the autosomal recessive cases have a deficiency of adenosine deaminase. In these cases there is a gene defect on chromosome 20. There is a rib cage abnormality resembling the rachitic rosary, as well as many other skeletal abnormalities.

Both these forms of SCID have been reported to respond to bone marrow transplantation.

LYMPHOPENIC AGAMMAGLOBULINEMIA

Also known as "Swiss Type," or hereditary thymic dysplasia, this is inherited as an autosomal recessive trait. Affected infants do poorly and fail to thrive. They are susceptible to mucocutaneous candidiasis as well as bacterial and virus infections.

This is a subset of the severe combined immunodeficiency syndrome. There is a decrease in both T and B cells and both cell-mediated and antibody-mediated immunity are deficient. The presumed level of the basic cellular defect is in the lymphopoietic stem cell, which fails to differentiate into lymphoid cells. Lymphoid tissue in the body is usually absent.

One patient with deficient thymus function treated with daily intramuscular injections of thymosine (an immunologically active thymus hormone) had a complete return of the lymphocytes, increased appetite, decreased diarrhea, and weight gain.

ATAXIA-TELANGIECTASIA
(Louis-Bar Syndrome)

Distinctive telangiectasia in the bulbar conjunctiva and the flexural surfaces of the arms develops during the fifth year of age. Later, telangiectases appear on the butterfly area of the face, the palate, the ears and exposed surfaces of skin. Café-au-lait patches, graying hair, and progeria may also be present. Cohen et al also listed vitiligo, impetigo, recurrent herpetic gingivostomatitis, hirsutism, and lipoatrophy among cutaneous problems associated with this disease.

Cerebellar ataxia is the first sign of this syndrome. It begins in the second year of life, usually after the child starts walking. An awkward swaying gait develops, and becomes progressively worse. Choreic and athetoid movements are usually present.

The ovaries and testicles do not develop normally. There is deficient thymus development, with absence of Hassall's corpuscles, and a lack of T helper cells. Suppressor T cells are normal. In 80 per cent of cases, IgA is absent or deficient, in 75 per cent absent or deficient IgE is seen, and in 50 per cent IgG is very low. Persistently elevated levels of alpha-fetoprotein and carcinoembryonic antigen occur. These may be useful in early establishment of the diagnosis.

The syndrome is transmitted as an autosomal recessive trait. Swift et al reported in 1987 that heterozygous carriers of the gene have an excess risk of cancer, especially breast cancer.

In culture, ataxia-telangiectasia fibroblasts are three times more sensitive to killing by ionizing radiation, but not to ultraviolet light. It appears to be a heterogeneous disease: five different complementation groups have been described. Heterozygous carriers share the defective repair of radiation-induced damage, and there is a fivefold higher risk for development of neoplasms in presumed heterozygotes under age 45, according to Swift et al.

Severe pulmonary infections and progressive bronchiectasis occur in most patients. Malignancies, predominantly lymphoreticular, are the commonest cause of death.

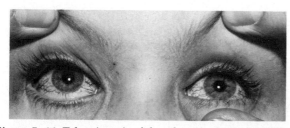

Figure 5–14. Telangiectasia of the sclerae in ataxia-telangiectasia.

WISKOTT-ALDRICH SYNDROME

This rare syndrome, seen exclusively in young boys, consists of a triad: chronic eczematous dermatitis resembling atopic dermatitis; increased susceptibility to recurrent infections, such as pyoderma or suppurative otitis media; and thrombocytopenic purpura, with hepatosplenomegaly. Death occurs usually by age six, from either infection, or, less often, bleeding. Only a few patients have been able to survive to adulthood. They are prone to develop lymphoreticular malignancies. Ormerod published a valuable review in 1985.

There is accelerated synthesis of IgA, IgM, and IgE; however, accelerated catabolism of all of them usually results in low levels of IgM, and low or normal levels of IgG and elevated levels of IgA and IgE remain. There seems to be an intrinsic platelet abnormality. T cells progressively decline in numbers and activity.

Treatment with platelet transfusions, antibiotics, immune globulin, and splenectomy is in order. Parkman et al in 1978 reported complete restoration of platelet production and immunologic functions by allogeneic marrow transplantation, and Kapoor et al confirmed their results in 1981. Ochs et al also reported using this approach successfully. A thought-provoking result of this therapy is that patients exhibited improvement or clearing of their eczematous dermatitis after successful transplantation.

THYMOMA WITH IMMUNODEFICIENCY

This disorder, also known as Good's syndrome, occurs in adults in whom hypogammaglobulinemia, deficient cell-mediated immunity, and benign thymoma may develop almost simultaneously. Recurrent abscesses and pyoderma develop. There is a striking deficiency of B and pre-B cells. Lymphopenia, eosinopenia, thrombocytopenia, anemia, or pancytopenia may occur.

Thymectomy does not affect the immunodeficiency.

THYMIC DYSPLASIA WITH NORMAL IMMUNOGLOBULINS
(Nezelof Syndrome)

In Nezelof syndrome there is faulty development of the thymus gland. Onset is in early infancy, with severe recurrent candidiasis, severe varicella, recurrent bacterial infections of skin and lungs, or diarrhea.

It is an autosomal recessive disorder. Serum immunoglobulins are normal or increased, but cell-mediated immunity is lacking. The syndrome differs from DiGeorge syndrome in that the thymus is present but underdeveloped, and there are no cardiac abnormalities. One patient was reconstituted to normal immune function by bone marrow transplantation.

Some authors regard purine-nucleotide phosphorylase deficiency as a subset of this condition. This enzyme defect leads to greatly reduced T cells and depressed cell-mediated immunity, but intact B cells and antibody formation. Patients usually die from overwhelming viral infections.

CHRONIC GRANULOMATOUS DISEASE (CGD)

Clinically, CGD is characterized by recurring purulent and granulomatous infections involving long bones, lymphatic tissue, liver, skin, and lungs. It occurs most frequently in boys (because of X-linked inheritance), who have eczema of the scalp, backs of the ears, and face. Ulcerative stomatitis, furunculosis, subcutaneous abscesses, and suppurative lymphadenopathy may occur.

There is decreased ability to destroy catalase-positive bacteria. These organisms destroy any hydrogen peroxide they generate, thus leaving the CGD phagocytes, which have defective ability to generate hydrogen peroxide, without full antimicrobial killing ability. *Staphylococcus aureus* infection is most frequently seen; infections by streptococci and pneumococci are uncommon. In addition, IgG, IgM, and IgA hyperglobulinemia, neutrophile leukocytosis, and an abnormally low reduction of NBT to blue formazan occur. The X-linked form appears to be due to a lack of cytochrome b 558.

Female carriers have intermediate NBT reduction, no increase in infections, discoid-lupuslike skin lesions, and often aphthous stomatitis. A few autosomal recessive cases have been reported. Kragballe et al reported that two of 10 unselected women with discoid LE were shown to be carriers.

Treatment of infections, according to Dahl, should be early, aggressive, and prolonged; and though he counsels against prophylactic treatment, trimethoprim-sulfamethoxazole prophylaxis significantly prolongs disease-free intervals. Gallin et al recently reviewed many of the newly recognized cellular defects and therapeutic interventions. Bactroban ointment should be useful. Ezekowitz et al reported several patients whose granulocyte-bactericidal activity was corrected by subcutaneous injections of gamma interferon.

CHEDIAK-HIGASHI SYNDROME

This is a progressively degenerative fatal familial disease in young children, characterized by partial oculocutaneous albinism, cutaneous and intestinal infections early in childhood, and leukocytes with very large azurophilic granules. The hair is blond and sparse. The ocular albinism is accompanied by nystagmus and photophobia.

This syndrome is transmitted by an autosomal recessive gene. Consanguineous marriages are frequent in the family.

A generalized lysosomal structural defect involving all lysosomal granule–containing cells is associated with this syndrome, producing increased susceptibility to infections, especially those of enteric bacterial origin. There is a neutropenia and the abnormal neutrophils do not phagocytose normally. The immunoglobulins are present in normal amounts. Chemotaxis is usually decreased.

Early death usually occurs, most frequently due to malignant lymphoma or other forms of cancer.

HYPERIMMUNOGLOBULINEMIA E SYNDROME

This immunodeficiency consists of atopiclike eczematous dermatitis, recurrent pyogenic infection (frequently in the lungs and skin), high values of serum IgE, elevated IgD levels, IgE antistaphylococcal antibodies, and eosinophilia. The eczematous eruption, seen in over 80 per cent of patients, is typically found in the sites of predilection for atopic dermatitis. The face is consistently involved: over 80 per cent of patients manifest this condition. It is chronic and begins early in life (age two months to two years). Many of the lesions resemble papular prurigo, and there may be keratoderma of the palms and soles. Ichthyosis, urticaria, asthma, and chronic mucocutaneous candidiasis may also occur. The hands and feet may have lesions suggestive of contact dermatitis.

Furuncles, carbuncles, and abscesses are present in varying degrees of severity. Chronic nasal discharge and recurrent otitis media are common.

The serum shows an extremely high concentration of IgE (over 10,000 IU/ml), and eosinophilia is present, with diminished local resistance to staphylococcal infections. Chemotaxis of neutrophils and monocytes is impaired.

"Job's syndrome" is similar to hypergammaglobulinemia E syndrome, but the inflammatory response is much less severe, so that cold abscesses are formed. This syndrome occurs mainly in girls with red hair, freckles, blue eyes, and hyperextensible joints.

COMPLEMENT DEFICIENCY

The complement system is an effector pathway of inflammation involving the progressive activation of plasma proteins, resulting in three basic types of biologic activity: membrane damage, membrane alteration, and mediator functions such as anaphylatoxin or chemotactic activity.

In the "classic" complement pathway, complement is activated by an antigen-antibody reaction involving IgG and IgM. Each component of complement has a specific biologic function in the induction of inflammation and maintenance of host resistance. The classic pathway of complement starts with C1q and the "alternative" (or "alternate") pathway with C3; and through numerous consecutive steps, complement finally exerts its effects.

Guenther, who reviewed the hereditary deficiencies of complement components in 1983, lists a complete chart of associated abnormalities. In general, deficiencies of the early components of the classic pathway result in connective tissue disease states; deficiency of C3 results in recurrent infections by encapsulated bacteria such as pneumococcus, *Hemophilus influenzae*, and *Streptococcus pyogenes*; and deficiencies of the late components of complement lead to recurrent Neisserial sepsis. Properdin dysfunction, inherited as an X-linked trait, predisposes to fulminant meningococcemia. Patients deficient in C9 have been identified, but they do not have these problems.

Among the complement deficiencies, C2 deficiency is most frequently seen. Most of these patients are healthy. Diseases that occur with increased frequency in persons deficient in C2 are SLE, SLE-like syndrome, frequent infections, anaphylactoid purpura, lethal dermatomyositis, vasculitis, DLE, and cold urticaria.

Inherited deficiencies of complement are usually inherited in autosomal recessive pattern, except for C1 inhibitor deficiency and possibly C5 dysfunction, which are inherited in an autosomal dominant manner. Deficiencies of all 11 components of the classic pathway, as well as two inhibitors of this pathway, have been described. Genetic deficiency of the C1 inhibitor results in hereditary angioedema. C3 inactivator deficiency, like C3 deficiency, results in recurrent pyogenic infections. A defective opsonization capacity associated with C5 dysfunction, known as Leiner's disease, has been described. These infants have generalized erythroderma, diarrhea, and failure to thrive.

When complement deficiency is suspected, a useful screening test is a CH50 (total hemolytic complement level in serum) determination, because deficiency of any complement component higher in the chain will nearly always result in CH50 levels that are markedly reduced, or zero. The important exceptions are C9 deficiency, C5 dysfunction, and C1 inhibitor deficiency. The screening laboratory test of choice when the latter is suspected is a serum C4 level.

GRAFT-VS-HOST DISEASE

Graft-versus-host disease (GVHD) occurs when immunocompetent cells are introduced as a graft or blood transfusion into an antigenically foreign host

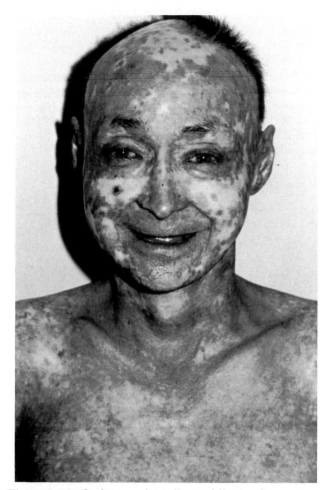

Figure 5–15. Graft-versus-host disease following bone marrow transplantation for aplastic anemia, showing alopecia, dyspigmentation, and scleroderma. (Courtesy of Dr. Axel W. Hoke.)

who is unable to reject the graft, because he is not immunocompetent. There are two forms: an acute form with cutaneous, hepatic, and gastrointestinal manifestations, and a chronic form with manifestations similar to a collagen vascular disorder.

In the acute form the cutaneous eruption begins between the fifth and forty-seventh day, most often between the fourth and fifth weeks. It is characterized by an erythematous maculopapular eruption of the face and upper trunk, which may become confluent and result in exfoliative erythroderma.

While up to 80 per cent of bone marrow transplantations may be followed by acute GVHD, only 30 per cent of long-term survivors develop chronic GVHD. In this a lichen-planuslike eruption may occur at three to five months after grafting, usually beginning on the hands and feet. Progressive sclerosis develops, which may remain localized, but more often is generalized, with attendant dyspigmentation and alopecia. There may be a "parrot-beak" deformity of the nose.

Since GVHD occurs so frequently after bone-marrow transplantation, and after transfusions given to immunocompromised patients, efforts have been made to prevent it by giving methotrexate, or, more recently, cyclosporin A, with limited success. Hypertrichosis occurs in 80 per cent of patients given cyclosporin A, but is slowly reversible after the drug is withdrawn. Five of 67 patients given cyclosporin A developed "capillary leak" syndrome, and three of them died. Prevention of posttransfusion GVHD is most safely achieved by irradiating the blood with 1500–2000 rads of x-rays before transfusing it, according to Leitman and others.

Ammann AJ: New insight into the cause of immunodeficiency disorders. JAAD 1984, 11:653.

Cohen LE, et al: Common and uncommon cutaneous findings in patients with ataxia-telangiectasia. JAAD 1984, 10:431.

Colten HR: Hereditary angioneurotic edema. N Engl J Med 1987, 317:43.

Cooper MD, et al: Developmental immunology and the immunodeficiency diseases. JAMA 1982, 248:2658.

Ezekowitz RAB, et al: Partial correction of . . . chronic granulomatous disease by interferon gamma. N Engl J Med 1988, 319:146.

Frank MM: Complement in the pathophysiology of human disease. N Engl J Med 1987, 316:1525.

Gallin JI, et al: Recent advances in chronic granulomatous disease. Ann Intern Med 1983, 99:657.

Guenther LC: Inherited disorders of complement. JAAD 1983, 9:815.

Haeney MR, et al: Recurrent bacterial meningitis [and] defects . . . of complement components. Clin Exp Immunol 1980, 40:16.

Harper JI, et al: Dermatological aspects of the use of cyclosporin A for prophylaxis of graft-versus-host disease. Br J Dermatol 1984, 110:469.

Hershfield MS, et al: Treatment of adenosine deaminase deficiency with polyethylene glycol modified adenosine deaminase. N Engl J Med 1987, 316:589.

Hymes SR, et al: Methoxsalen and ultraviolet A radiation in treatment of chronic cutaneous graft-versus-host reaction. JAAD 1985, 12:30.

Hirschhorn R: Therapy of genetic disorders (editorial). N Engl J Med 1987, 316:623.

James WD, Odom RB: Graft-versus-host disease. Arch Dermatol 1983, 119:683.

Jordon RE: The complement system and the skin. Arch Dermatol 1982, 118:359.

Kapoor N, et al: Reconstitution of megakaryocytopoiesis and immunologic functions in Wiskott-Aldrich syndrome by marrow transplantation following myeloablation and immunosuppression with busulphan and cyclophosphamide. Blood 1981, 57:692.

Kragballe, et al: Relation of monocyte and neutrophile oxidative metabolism to skin and oral lesions in carriers of chronic granulomatous disease. Clin Exp Immunol 1981, 43:390.

Lehrer RI, et al: Neutrophils in human disease. Ann Intern Med 1988, 109:127.

Leitman SF, et al: Irradiation of blood products. Transfusion 1985, 25:293.

Malech HC, et al: Neutrophils in human disease. N Engl J Med 1987, 317:687.

Matsuoka LV: Graft versus host disease. JAAD 1981, 5:595.

Miller ME: Cutaneous infections and disorders of inflammation. JAAD 1980, 2:1.

Ochs HD, et al: Bone marrow transplantation in Wiskott-Aldrich syndrome: Complete hematological and immunological reconstitution. Transplantation 1982, 34:284.

Ormerod AD: The Wiskott-Aldrich syndrome (review). Int J Dermatol 1985, 24:77.

Parkman R, et al: Complete correction of the Wiskott-Aldrich syndrome by allogeneic bone marrow transplantation. N Engl J Med 1978, 298:921.

Paslin D, et al: Atopic dermatitis and impaired neutrophil chemotaxis in Job's syndrome. Arch Dermatol 1977, 113:801.

Rodu B, et al: Oral manifestations of the graft-versus-host reaction. JAMA 1983, 249:504.

Rosen FS, et al: The primary immunodeficiencies. N Engl J Med 1984, 311:235, 300.

Ross SC, et al: Complement deficiency states and infection. Medicine 1984, 63:243.

Royer HD, et al: T lymphocytes. N Engl J Med 1987, 317:1136.

Sjöholm AG, et al: Dysfunctional properdin in a family with meningococcal disease. N Engl J Med 1988, 319:33.

Spitler LE, et al: Wiskott-Aldrich syndrome: results of transfer factor therapy. J Clin Invest 1972, 51:3216.

Swift M, et al: Breast and other cancers in families with ataxia-telangiectasia. N Engl J Med 1987, 316:1289.

Von Fliedner V, et al: Graft-versus-host reaction following blood product transfusion. Am J Med 1982, 72:951.

Waldmann TA, et al: Ataxia-telangiectasia. Ann Intern Med 1983, 99:367.

Wolff JA: Wiskott-Aldrich syndrome with partial response to transfer factor. Br J Dermatol 1978, 98:567.

Yount WJ: IgG2 deficiency and ataxia-telangiectasia (editorial). N Engl J Med 1982, 306:541.

6

Contact Dermatitis; Drug Eruptions

CONTACT DERMATITIS

Generally there are two types of dermatitis caused by substances coming in contact with the skin. These are irritant dermatitis and allergic contact dermatitis. Irritant dermatitis was previously known as—and is still often called—"primary" irritant dermatitis. Irritant dermatitis is due to a nonallergic reaction in the skin resulting from exposure to an irritating substance. Allergic contact dermatitis is due to acquired sensitivity to various substances that produce inflammatory reactions in those, and only those, who have been previously exposed to the allergen.

IRRITANT DERMATITIS

There are many substances, acting as irritants, that will produce a nonallergic inflammatory reaction of the skin. This type of dermatitis may be induced in any person if a sufficiently high concentration is used. No previous exposure is necessary, and the effect is evident within minutes, or a few hours at most.

The only variation in the severity of the dermatitis from person to person, or from time to time in the same person, is due to the condition of the skin at the time of exposure to a given concentration of the irritant. The skin may be more vulnerable by reason of maceration from excessive humidity, or exposure to water, heat, cold, pressure, or friction. Dry skin is less likely to react to contactants. Thick skin is less reactive than thin.

Repeated exposure to some of the milder irritants may, in time, produce a "hardening" effect. This process makes the skin more resistant to the irritant effects of the given substance.

ALKALIS

Irritant dermatitis is often produced by alkalis such as soaps, detergents, bleaches, ammonia preparations, lye, drain pipe cleaners, toilet bowl cleansers, and oven cleansers.

Alkalis penetrate and destroy deeply because their compounds dissolve keratin. Strong solutions are corrosive, and immediate application of a weak acid such as vinegar, lemon juice, or 0.5 per cent hydrochloric acid solution will lessen their effects.

The principal compounds are sodium, potassium, ammonium, and calcium hydroxides. Occupational exposure is frequent among workers in soap manufacture and oil handlers such as oilers and those using oil to cool and lubricate metal-cutting tools.

Sodium silicate (water glass) is a caustic used in soap manufacture and paper sizing and for the preservation of eggs. Alkaline sulfides are used as depilatories. Calcium oxide (quicklime) forms slaked lime when water is added. Severe burns may be caused in plasterers.

Alkalis in the form of soaps, bleaching agents, detergents, and most household cleansing agents figure prominently in the etiology of hand eczema.

ACIDS

The powerful acids are corrosive, whereas the weaker ones are astringent. *Hydrochloric acid* produces burns that are less deep and more liable to form blisters than injuries from sulfuric and nitric acids. Hydrochloric acid burns are encountered in those who handle or transport the product, and in plumbers and those who work in galvanizing or tin-plate factories. *Nitric acid* is a powerful oxidizing substance that causes deep burns, the tissue being stained yellow. Such injuries are observed in those who manufacture or handle the acid or use it in the making of explosives in laboratories. *Sulfuric acid* produces a brownish charring of the skin, beneath which is an ulceration that heals slowly. Sulfuric acid is used more widely than any other acid in industry, being handled principally by brass or iron workers or by those who work with copper or bronze. It is the weapon of so-called vitriol throwers.

Oxalic acid may produce paresthesia of the finger tips, with cyanosis and gangrene. The nails become discolored yellow. Oxalic acid is best neutralized with lime water or milk of magnesia to produce precipitation.

Hydrofluoric acid may act insidiously at first, starting with erythema and ending with vesiculation, ulceration, and, finally, necrosis of the tissue. It is one of the strongest inorganic acids, and dissolves glass.

Phenol (carbolic acid) is a protoplasmic poison which produces a white eschar on the surface of the skin. It can penetrate deeply into the tissue. If a large surface of the skin is treated with phenol for cosmetic peeling effects, the absorbed phenol may produce glomerulonephritis and arrhythmias. Locally, temporary anesthesia may also occur. Phenol is readily neutralized with 65 per cent ethyl or isopropyl alcohol.

Other strong acids that are irritants include acetic, arsenious, chlorosulfonic, chromic, fluoroboric, hydriodic, hydrobromic, iodic, perchloric, phosphoric, salicyclic, silicofluoric, sulfonic, sulfurous, tannic, and tungstic acid.

Treatment of these acid burns consists of immediate rinsing with copious amounts of water and alkalization with sodium bicarbonate, calcium hydroxide (lime water), or soap solutions.

Some chemicals require unusual treatment measures. *Fluorine* is best neutralized with magnesium oxide. Periungual burns should be treated intralesionally with 10 per cent calcium gluconate solution, which deactivates the fluoride ion and averts more tissue damage. Hydrofluoric acid is used widely in

rust remover, in the semiconductor industry, and in germicides, dyes, plastics, and glass etching. *Phosphorus* burns should be rinsed off with water followed by application of copper sulfate to produce a precipitate.

Titanium hydrochloride is used in the manufacture of pigments. Water application to the site of the exposed part will produce severe burns. Treatment consists only of wiping away the noxious substance.

OTHER IRRITANTS

Some metal salts which act as irritants are the cyanides of calcium, copper, mercury, nickel, silver, and zinc, and the chlorides of calcium and zinc. Bromine, chlorine, iodine, and fluorine are also irritants. Herzemans-Boer et al reported six patients occupationally exposed to methyl bromide who developed erythema and vesicles in the axillary and inguinal areas.

Chloracne. Workers in the manufacture of chlorinated compounds may develop chloracne, with small black follicular plugs and papules, chiefly on the malar crescent and retroauricular areas. Another characteristic site is the scrotum. Machinists' use of chlorinated compounds in cutting oils predisposes them to the development of chloracne on their thighs.

The synthetic waxes chloronaphthalene and chlorodiphenyl used in the manufacture of electric insulators and in paints, varnishes, and lacquers similarly predispose to chloracne workers engaged in the manufacture of these synthetic waxes. Taylor has reported chloracne in 41 patients as a result of direct contact with 3,4,3',4',tetrachloroazo-oxybenzene, which occurs as an unwanted intermediate in the manufacture of a pesticide. Exposure to 2,6-dichlorobenzonitrile, encountered in the manufacture of a herbicide, may also produce chloracne. Tindall has recently reviewed chloracne and the effects of exposure to the dioxin compounds during the Vietnam War.

Insecticides as Irritants. Various insecticides may act as irritants.

Flea-collar Dermatitis. This is an interesting example reported by Cronce and Alden. Dog collars containing an insecticide, 2,2-dichlorovinyl dimethyl phosphate (Vapona), an irritant, have caused dermatitis resembling toxicodendron dermatitis in some of those who handled dogs wearing such collars. This insecticide is also used in roach powder and hang-up fly repellents and killers.

Hunan Hand: The irritation produced by capsaicin in hot peppers used in Korean and North Chinese cuisine may be severe and prolonged. Cold water is not much help: capsaicin is insoluble in it. Acetic acid, 5 per cent (white vinegar), may completely relieve it even if applied an hour or more after the contact (Vogl). Soaking should be continued until the area can be dried without return of the discomfort.

DERMATITIS DUE TO DUSTS AND GASES

Some dusts and gases may irritate the skin in the presence of heat and moisture such as perspiration. The dusts of lime, zinc, and arsenic may produce folliculitis. Dusts from various woods such as teak may incite itching and dermatitis. Dusts from cinchona bark, quinine, and pyrethrum produce widespread dermatitis.

Tobacco dust in cigar factories, powdered orris root, lycopodium, and dusts of various nutshells may cause swelling of the eyelids and dermatitis of the face, neck, and upper extremities. Dusts formed during the manufacture of high explosives may cause erythematous, vesicular, and eczematous dermatitis that may lead to generalized exfoliative dermatitis.

Tear Gas Dermatitis. Lacrimators such as chloroacetophenone in concentrated form may cause dermatitis, with a delayed appearance some 24 to 72 hours after exposure. Irritation or sensitization, with erythema and severe vesiculation, may result.

Treatment consists of lavage of the affected skin with sodium bicarbonate solution and instillation of boric acid solution into the eyes. Contaminated clothing should be removed.

Mace. This is a mixture of tear gas (chloroacetophenone) in trichloroethane and various hydrocarbons resembling kerosene. Frazier has reported contact allergy in a prison guard from contact with a can of Mace, which he wore on his belt.

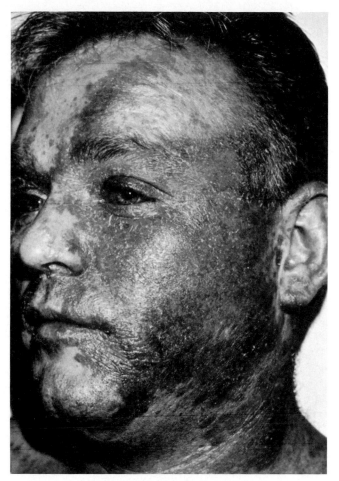

Figure 6–1. Dermatitis due to mace.

DERMATITIS DUE TO VARIOUS HYDROCARBONS

Many hydrocarbons produce skin eruptions. Crude *petroleum* causes generalized itching, folliculitis, or acneiform eruptions. Irritant properties of petroleum derivatives are directly proportional to fat-solvent properties and inversely proportional to viscosity. Oils of the naphthalene series are more irritating than those of the paraffin series.

Lubricating oils and *cutting oils* are causes of similar cutaneous lesions. Water-soluble cutting oils rarely cause dermatitis, whereas chlorinated cutting oils (not water-soluble) are very irritating. They represent a frequent cause of occupational dermatoses in machine tool operators, machinists, layout men, instrument makers, and set-up men. They were major causes of occupational *chloracne*, but these have now been eliminated; the insoluble cutting oils are still responsible for a follicular acneiform eruption on the dorsa of the hands, the forearms, face, thighs, and back of the neck. Scrotal cancer has been found to occur in those exposed to cutting oils.

Knox has recently described eight cases of an acquired perforating disease in oil field workers. The patients developed tender umbilicated papules of the forearms which microscopically showed transepidermal elimination of calcium. The drilling fluid was found to contain calcium chloride.

Refined fractions from petroleum are less irritating than the unrefined products, although *benzene, naphtha,* and *carbon disulfide* may cause a mild dermatitis.

Coal briquette makers develop dermatitis as a result of a tarry residue from petroleum used in their trade. Workers in *paraffin* show an irritation of the skin that leads to pustules, keratoses, and ulcerations.

Shale oil workers develop an erythematous, follicular eruption that eventually leads to keratoses, which may become the sites of carcinoma. It is estimated that 50 per cent of shale oil workers suffer from skin troubles.

Impure and low grade *paraffins* and *mineral oils* cause similar skin eruptions. The skin changes at first are similar to chloracne. In due time a diffuse erythema with dappled pigmentation develops. Gradually keratoses appear, and after many years some of these are the sites of carcinoma. **Melanoderma** may occur from exposure to mineral oils and lower grade petroleum, from *creosote, asphalt,* and other *tar* products. Photosensitization may play a role. Creosote is a contact irritant, a sensitizer, and a photosensitizer. Allergy is demonstrated by patch testing with 10 per cent creosote in oil.

Petrolatum dermatitis may appear as a verrucous thickening of the skin caused by prolonged contact with impure petroleum jelly or, occasionally, lubricating oil. A follicular type occurs in which erythematous horny nodules are present, usually on the anterior and inner aspects of the thighs. There are no comedones and the lesions are separated by apparently normal skin.

Acne cornée, another dermatitis, consists of follicular keratosis and pigmentation due to crude petroleum, tar oils, and paraffin. Chiefly involved are the dorsal aspects of the fingers and hands, the arms, the legs, the face, and the thorax. The lesions are follicular, horny papules, often black, and are associated at first with a follicular erythema and later with a dirty brownish or purplish spotty pigmentation, which in severe cases becomes widespread, being especially marked about the genitals. This syndrome may simulate pityriasis rubra pilaris or lichen spinulosus.

Mule spinners' cancer of the scrotum, formerly an important problem in the cotton industry in England, was caused by certain lubricating oils no longer used. Castiglione recently reported such a case. Coal tar and pitch and many of their derivatives produce photosensitization and an acneiform folliculitis of the forearms, legs, face, and scrotum.

Follicular keratoses (pitch warts) may develop and later turn into carcinoma. *Naphthalene, creosote, anthracene,* and related products are also responsible for skin eruptions.

Soot, lamp black, and *peat* produce dermatitis of a dry, scaly character, which in the course of time forms warty outgrowths and cancer. **Chimney sweep's cancer** was the first described in England by Pott in 1790. The cancer occurs under a soot wart and is usually located on the scrotum, where soot, sebum, and dirt collect in the folds of the skin. This form of cancer has virtually disappeared. *Asbestos* workers develop *asbestos warts,* but the known carcinogenicity of asbestos has not been described in the skin.

ALLERGIC CONTACT DERMATITIS

Allergic contact dermatitis is probably more exactly termed **allergic eczematous contact dermatitis,** but it is also known as **dermatitis venenata, contact eczema,** and **industrial dermatitis.**

Allergic contact dermatitis results when an allergen comes into contact with previously sensitized skin. Allergic contact dermatitis results from a specific acquired hypersensitivity of the delayed type, also known as cell-mediated hypersensitivity or immunity. Occasionally dermatitis may be induced upon a sensitized area of skin when the allergen is taken internally; this occurs, for example, with substances such as the antihistaminics or sulfonamides, and is called an anamnestic reaction. Persons may be exposed to allergens for years before finally developing hypersensitivity. One attack, however, seems to predispose the involved area so that subsequent outbreaks may result from extremely slight exposure. The sensitized area, although usually generalized, may be strictly localized.

The allergens are extremely varied and may be nonprotein in nature. Many substances, such as dyes and their intermediates, oils, resins, coal tar derivatives, chemicals used for fabrics, rubbers, cosmetics, insecticides, the oils and resins of woods and plants, as well as the products or the substances of bacteria, fungi, and parasites, are proven allergens. These sensitizers do not cause demonstrable skin changes on first contact but may produce specific changes in the skin when the patient is reexposed to the allergen a second, third, or fourth time.

Such allergens possess little capability of acting as antigens that stimulate antibody production. No transferable sensitizing antibodies have been demonstrated in the blood serum in most of these eruptions; however, they sensitize lymphocytes, after processing and presentation by Langerhans cells, which are then responsible for the delayed type of hypersensitivity. In those instances of wheal-reacting allergies known as contact urticaria, which may lead to a chronic eczema, IgE antibodies have occasionally been demonstrated. At times passive tranfer experiments have been positive.

Prunieras suggested that the Langerhans cells might play a major role in the pathogenesis of contact allergy, but how they might act was not known until Silberberg, Baer, and Rosenthal showed in 1976 that, in both guinea pigs and humans, during challenge with contact allergens, there is direct apposition of mononuclear cells to the dendrites of the Langerhans cells, followed by damage to the latter. Langerhans cells in the dermis are more numerous after such challenges, and they are also found in lymph nodes.

Bergstresser has recently reviewed the accumulating evidence that Langerhans cells play a critical role in the induction of contact hypersensitivity and that specific T-helper cells play a major role in the elicitation of the inflammatory response.

One must distinguish the eczematous type of reaction, as exemplified by contact dermatitis, hand eczema, and the patch test, from the urticarial type of reaction *(contact urticaria),* present with urticaria, asthma, and hay fever, and in scratch, intracutaneous, and passive transfer tests. One must also keep in mind, however, that persons who exhibit the latter type of reaction, which is chiefly vascular, may concomitantly have epidermal sensitization and eczema from the same allergen.

Odom and Maibach reported true allergic contact urticaria, mediated by IgE through immediate-type hypersensitivity. Such reactions have been described from contact with potato, mechlorethamine (nitrogen mustard), and diethyltoluamide (an insect repellent), among many other materials. In suspected cases, an open patch test should be performed and watched for half an hour.

Immunologically speaking, then, contact dermatitis is one thing; atopic dermatitis is another; and urticaria, hay fever, and all such immediate wheal-reacting allergies are another. They may and do exist side by side in the same person, especially in infants and children.

Although these eruptions involute spontaneously upon identification and removal of the cause, some cases prove difficult because the identity of the allergen is not easily ascertained. Typical cases of dermatitis of external origin with erythema, vesiculation, and linear lesions within scratch marks, occurring upon exposed parts, occasionally defy the skill of the dermatologist and require prolonged observation before the causative factor is isolated. In other instances, as in painters, plasterers, and dentists, the cause of the dermatitis may be obvious because of known exposure to specific sensitizing substances.

In some instances impetigo, pustular folliculitis, and irritations or allergic reactions from applied medications are superimposed upon the original dermatitis. The cutaneous reaction also may provoke a hypersusceptibility to various other previously innocuous substances, which continue the inflammation indefinitely as eczema.

Very rarely, allergic contact sensitivity to corticosteroids may be acquired. Tegner's prospective study concluded there was a 1 per cent incidence of such sensitivity to at least one corticosteroid. Guin stated that the usual clinical situation in which an allergic reaction to topical corticosteroids should be suspected is one in which a chronic eczema fails to heal. He felt a pragmatic screen was a patch test to 0.5 per cent triamcinolone acetonide ointment or 0.05 per cent fluocinolone ointment.

FREQUENT SENSITIZERS

In his excellent and recommended textbook on contact dermatitis, Alexander Fisher states that the most common causes of contact dermatitis are the following: toxicodendrons (poison ivy, oak, or sumac), paraphenylenediamine, nickel, rubber compounds, ethylene diamine, potassium dichromate, and thimerosal.

The Patch Test

The patch test is used to detect hypersensitivity to a substance which is in contact with the skin. In this manner the allergen may be determined and corrective measures taken. There are so many allergens causing allergic contact dermatitis that it is impossible to test a person for all of them; rather, one must be reasonably sure that the given case of dermatitis is of the allergic contact type. In addition, a good history and observance of the pattern of the dermatitis, its localization on the body, and its state of activity are all helpful in determining the etiology. The patch test is confirmatory and diagnostic but only within the framework of the history and findings; it is rarely helpful if it must stand alone.

The patch test consists of the application to the intact skin, in nonirritating concentration, of substances suspected to be causes of the contact dermatitis. Although the patches may consist of adhesive bandages with the testing substance applied to the gauze portion, a superior patch test cover has been developed. These are aluminum chambers (Finn chambers) mounted on Scanpor tape.

Test substances on the test strips are applied usually to the upper back, although if only one or two are applied, the arm may be used. Each patch should be numbered to avoid confusion.

The patches are removed after 48 hours (or less if itching or burning occur at the site). The patch sites are observed 24 hours later, and again at 72 hours, as positive reactions may not appear earlier.

Excited Skin ("Angry Back") Syndrome. Strong patch test reactions may induce a state of hyperirritability ("angry back") in which negative tests appear as weakly positive. Since the phenomenon is not limited to the back, Bruynzeel et al have suggested that it be called the "excited skin" syndrome. They concluded that weakly positive tests in the presence of strong ones do not prove sensitivity.

A positive reaction consists of marked pruritus, erythema, and edema (often intensified at the follicles, or small vesicles). Reactions are graded as follows: 1+, weak (nonvesicular; erythema, edema, possibly papules); 2+, strong (vesicular); 3+, maximum (bullous); and −, negative.

There is wide variation in the ability of the skin and mucous membranes to react to antigens. The oral mucosa is more resistant to primary irritants and is less liable to be involved in allergic reactions. This may be because of the keratin layer of the skin which may contain proteins which more readily combine with haptens to form allergens. Also the oral mucosa is bathed in saliva, which cleanses and buffers the area, and dilutes irritants.

The ability of the skin to react to allergens also depends upon the presence of functional antigen-presenting cells, the Langerhans cells. Potent topical steroids, ultraviolet light, and the acquired immunodeficiency syndrome all have been reported to interfere with the number and function of these key cells.

Open Test. This is used to test liquids, gels, and creams that are irritants if tested under occlusion. Substances such as plant oleoresins, shampoos, perfumes, nail polish, hair sprays, and skin fresheners are applied undiluted to normal skin of the outer aspect of the arm above the elbow twice a day for two days. The reading is the same as with the closed patch test.

Provocative Use Test. This is used to confirm positive closed patch test reactions to ingredients of a substance, such as a cosmetic. The material is rubbed onto normal skin of the antecubital fossa twice daily for one week, or until a reaction is seen.

Pustular Patch Test. Occasionally patch tests to potassium iodide, nickel, arsenic, or mercury will produce pustules at the site of the test application. Usually no erythema is produced; therefore, the reaction has no clinical significance.

Photo-Patch Test. This is to test for contact photo-allergy to such substances as sulfonamides, phenothiazines, para-aminobenzoic acid, 6-methyl coumarin, musk ambrette, or tetrachlorsalicylanilide. A standard patch test is applied for 48 hours; this is then exposed to 5 to 15 joules/m^2 of UVA and read after another 48 hours. A duplicate set of nonirradiated patches is used in testing for the presence of routine delayed hypersensitivity reactions. Also a site of normal skin is given an identical dose of UVA to test for increased sensitivity to light without prior exposure to chemicals.

Regional Predilection

Familiarity with certain contactants and the typical dermatitis they elicit on specific parts of the body will assist in diagnosis of the etiologic agent.

Head and Neck. The scalp is relatively resistant to the development of contact allergies; however, involvement may be due to hair dye, hair spray, shampoo, or permanent-wave solutions. The surrounding glabrous skin including the ear rims and backs of the ears may be much more inflamed and suggestive of the cause. Persistent otitis of the ear canal may be caused by sensitivity to the neomycin that is an ingredient of most aural medications. The forehead of a man may be the site of a hatband dermatitis. One eyelid is the most frequent site for nail polish dermatitis. Volatile gases, false-eyelash cement, mascara, and eyeshadow cosmetics are also frequently implicated. Perioral dermatitis may be caused by dentifrices, bubble gum, or ordinary chewing gum. Perfume dermatitis may cause redness just under the ears. Nickel sensitivity may be noted at the clasp site of necklaces or earrings. Photocontact dermatitis may involve the entire face and may be sharply cut off at the collar line or extend down onto the sternum in a V shape. In both cases there is a typical clear area under the chin where there is little or no exposure to sunlight. In men, in whom shaving lotion fragrances are often responsible, the left cheek and left side of the neck (from sun exposure while driving a left-hand drive car) may be the first areas involved. Berloque dermatitis is frequently seen on the preauricular areas and sides of the neck.

Trunk. The trunk is an infrequent site; however, the dye or finish of clothing may cause dermatitis. The axillae may be the site of deodorant and clothing-dye dermatitis. Involvement of the axillary vault suggests the former; of the axillary folds, the latter. In women brassieres frequently cause dermatitis either from the material itself or from elastic or metal snaps, which seem invariably to be nickel-plated.

Arms. The wrists may be involved because of jewelry or the backs of watches and clasps, all containing nickel. Wrist bands made of leather are a source of chrome dermatitis.

Hands. Innumerable substances may cause contact dermatitis of the hands. Dermatitis venenata typically occurs on the backs of the hands and spares the palms. Poison ivy and other plant dermatitides frequently occur on the hands and arms. Rubber glove sensitivity must be kept constantly in mind.

Abdomen. The abdomen, especially the waistline, may be the site of rubber dermatitis from the elastic in pants. The metallic rivets in blue jeans may lead to periumbilical dermatitis in nickel-sensitive patients.

Groin. The groin is usually spared, but the buttocks and upper thighs may be sites of dermatitis due to dyes. The penis is frequently involved in poison ivy dermatitis. Condom dermatitis may also occur. The perianal region may be involved from the "caine" medications in suppositories.

Lower Extremities. The shins may be the site of rubber dermatitis from elastic stockings. Feet are sites for shoe dermatitis, most often attributable to rubber sensitivity, chrome-tanned leather, or adhesives.

Adams RM: Patch testing—a recapitulation. JAAD 1981, 5:629.

Arndt KA: Cutting fluids and the skin. Cutis 1969, 5:143.

Bergstresser PR: Contact allergic dermatitis. Arch Dermatol 1989, 125:276.

Bruynzeel DP, et al: Excited skin syndrome (angry back). Arch Dermatol 1986, 122:323.

Castiglione FM, et al: Mule spinner's disease. Arch Dermatol 1985, 121:370.

Fisher AA: Contact Dermatitis, 3rd ed. Philadelphia, Lea & Febiger, 1986.

Idem: Contact dermatitis from topical medicaments. Semin Dermatol 1982, 1:49.

Idem: The persulfates: a triple threat. Cutis 1985, 27:25.

Idem: Allergic stomatitis from dental impression compounds. Cutis 1985, 27:295.

Fischer T, et al: Easier patch testing with the TRUE test. JAAD 1989, 20:447.

Guin J: Contact sensitivity to topical corticosteroids. JAAD 1984, 10:773.

Harber LC, Bickers DC: Photosensitivity Diseases, 1st ed. Philadelphia, W. B. Saunders Co., 1981.

Herzemans-Boer M, et al: Skin lesions due to methyl bromide. Arch Dermatol 1988, 124:917.

Iverson RE, et al: Hydrofluoric acid burns. Plast Reconstr Surg 1971, 48:107.

Jolly HW: Tear gas dermatitis. JAMA 1968, 203:808.

Knox JM, et al: Acquired perforating disease in oil field workers. JAAD 1986, 14:605.

Larsen WG: Perfume dermatitis. Arch Dermatol 1977, 113:623.

Leyden JJ, et al: Urinary ammonia and ammonia-producing microorganisms in infants with and without diaper dermatitis. Arch Dermatol 1977, 113:678.

Markovitz SS, et al: Occupational acroösteolysis. Arch Dermatol 1972, 106:219.

Perry HO, et al: Atypical gingivostomatitis. Arch Dermatol 1973, 107:872.

Roper S, et al: A new look at conditioned hyperirritability. JAAD 1982, 7:643.

Samitz MH: Effect of metal-working fluids on the skin. Progr Dermatol 1974, 8:11.

Silberberg I: Apposition of mononuclear cells to Langerhans cells in contact allergic reactions: An ultrastructural study. Acta Derm Venereol 1973, 53:1.

Idem, et al: The role of Langerhans cells in allergic contact hypersensitivity. J Invest Dermatol 1976, 66:210.

Smith JD, et al: Contact urticaria from cobalt chloride. Arch Dermatol 1975, 111:610.

Tindall JP: Chloracne and chloracnegens. JAAD 1985, 13:539.

Vogl TP: Treatment of Hunan hand. NEJM 1982, 306:178.

DERMATITIS DUE TO PLANTS

A large number of plants including trees, grasses, flowers, vegetables, fruits, and weeds are potential causes of dermatitis, formerly usually called *dermatitis venenata*. Eruptions from them vary considerably in appearance but are usually vesicular and accompanied by marked edema. After previous exposure and sensitization to the active substance in the plants, the typical dermatitis may result from contact. The onset is sudden, a few hours or days after exposure, with involvement of the face, legs, wrists, and hands. The linear grouped lesions which are so characteristic are probably produced by brushing the skin with a leaf-edge or a broken twig or by carriage of the allergen under a nail or nails. Contrary to general belief, the contents of vesicles are not capable of producing new lesions.

Toxicodendron Dermatitis (Poison Ivy Dermatitis)

Toxicodendron *(Rhus)* dermatitis includes dermatitis from *poison ivy, poison oak,* and *poison sumac,* as well as the Japanese lacquer tree, *Toxicodendron vernicifera,* and the lacquer manufactured from it; also the ginkgo, *Ginkgo biloba,* cashew, mango, Brazilian pepper, rengas tree, and Indian marking nut, whose antigens (and the dermatitis they cause) are nearly identical.

CLINICAL SIGNS. Toxicodendron dermatitis appears within 48 hours after exposure of a previously sensitized person to the plant. It usually begins upon the backs of the fingers, the interdigital spaces, the wrists, and the eyelids, although it may begin upon the ankles or other parts that have been exposed. Marked pruritus is the first symptom; then inflammation, vesicles, and bullae may appear. The vesicles are usually grouped and often linear. Large bullae may be present, especially on the forearms. The eyelids are puffy, being worst in the morning and improving as the day progresses. Pruritus ani and

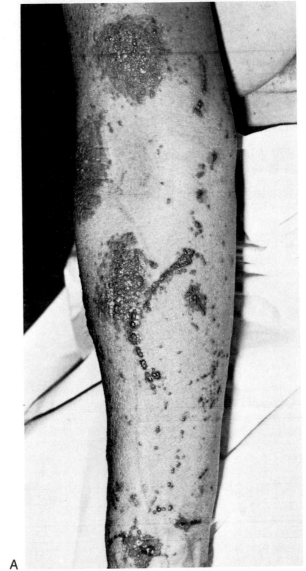

A

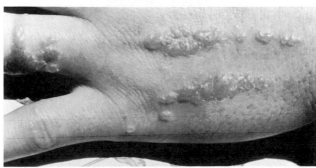

B

Figure 6–2. A and B, *Rhus dermatitis with characteristic linear groups of vesicles. (B, Courtesy of Dr. Axel W. Hoke.)*

involvement of the genital areas occur frequently. A black lacquer deposit may occur in which the sap of the plant has been oxidized after being bound to the stratum corneum.

The allergen is transferred by the fingers to other parts, especially the forearms and the male prepuce,

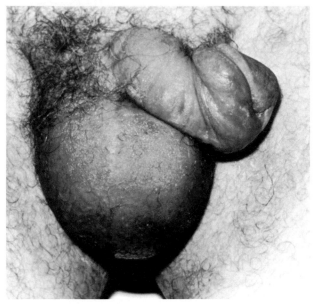

Figure 6–3. Rhus dermatitis in a common site. (Courtesy of Dr. Axel W. Hoke.)

which become greatly swollen. However, once the causative oil has been washed off, there is no spreading of the allergen and no further spread of the dermatitis. Some persons are so susceptible that direct contact is not necessary, the allergen apparently being carried by the fur of their pets or by the wind. It can also be acquired from golf clubs or fishing rods, or even from furniture which a dog or cat might have occupied after exposure to the catechol.

Repeated attacks do not confer immunity, though a single severe attack may achieve this by what has been called "massive-dose desensitization." The attacks usually last two to three weeks, during which time the patches become crusted and dry.

ETIOLOGY. Toxicodendron dermatitis is caused by an oleoresin known as urushiol, of which the active principle is pentadecylcatechol. This antigen is present not only in poison ivy but also in poison oak and poison sumac. This catechol can produce cross reactions with other plants belonging to the Anacardiaceae family. These are the Japanese lacquer trees, which can produce lacquer dermatitis, cashew oil from the cashew nutshell, the ginkgo fruit pulp from the ginkgo tree, the black marking ink, *dhobie* (or washerwoman's) ink, derived from an Indian nut tree, and the rind, leaves, or sap of the mango.

DIAGNOSIS. The most striking diagnostic feature is the linearity of the lesions. It is rare to see vesicles arranged in a linear fashion except in plant-induced dermatitis. The history of exposure in the country or in the park to plants that have shiny leaves in groups of three, followed by the appearance of vesicular lesions within two days, usually establishes the diagnosis.

A most complete summary on poison ivy derma-

titis and related dermatitides is given by Guin (see References).

PROPHYLAXIS. Persons with known susceptibility not only should avoid touching plants having grouped "leaves-of-three" but, in addition, should exercise care in handling articles of clothing, tools, toys, and pets that have come in contact with such plants.

Innumerable attempts have been made to immunize against poison ivy dermatitis by ingestion of the leaves, by oral administration of the tincture, or by subcutaneous injections of oily extracts. To date, no accepted method of immunization has evolved. Protective creams containing silicone and other substances are ineffective.

Continued work to refine polyamine salts of a linoleic acid dimer reported by Orchard et al to prevent poison ivy patch test reactions offers one hope for the future.

Injectable Toxicodendron extracts are, according to William Epstein, a "safe placebo." The dose that can be given is too small to help. A diacetylated urushiol was no better, and those that were helped were helped for only three months. In a 1982 study 15 of 21 subjects were successfully orally hyposensitized; 18 experienced vesicular or urticarial rashes or pruritus ani. Hyposensitization lasted at least three months. Sheard reported the case of a woman who had suffered annual attacks of poison ivy dermatitis for many years, but had none after she began chewing six raw cashew nuts daily from February to November.

Plants growing in frequented places should be eradicated by spraying with 2,4 dichlorophenoxyacetic acid (Dow Chemical) or with Weed-No-More (Sherwin-Williams). These compounds kill most broad-leaved plants including Rhus.

TREATMENT. When the diagnosis is clear, and the eruption severe or extensive, systemic steroids should be started without delay: either 40 to 80 mg of prednisone orally in a single oral dose daily, tapered off over a 3-week period, or a single intramuscular injection of triamcinolone acetonide (Kenalog)—or in a young woman, the diacetate (Aristocort, to obviate the potential problem of polymenorrhea) is an alternative treatment. Betamethasone sodium phosphate and acetate (Celestone Soluspan), 12 mg IM, is more rapidly effective but must be repeated in five to seven days as a rule. Improvement should be so rapid that there is seldom any need for wet dressings or hospitalization. Several very hot showers a day are also said to relieve itching and expedite healing.

When the eruption is limited in extent and severity, the local application of topical corticosteroid creams, lotions, or aerosol sprays is superior to any other local application. The time-honored calamine lotion without phenol is helpful and does no harm. Antihistaminic ointments should be avoided because of their sensitization possibilities. This also applies to the local application of the "caine" topical anesthetics.

Toxicodendron-Related Dermatitis

Lacquer dermatitis is caused by a furniture lacquer made from the Japanese lacquer tree, used on furniture, jewelry, or bric-a-brac. Antique lacquer is harmless, but lacquer less than a year or two old is highly antigenic. Cross sensitivity with Toxicodendrons is complete.

Cashew nutshell oil is extracted from the nutshells of the cashew tree (*Anacardium occidentale*). This vesicant oil contains cardol, a phenol similar to urushiol in poison ivy. The liquid has many commercial applications such as the manufacture of brake lining, varnish, synthetic glue, paint, and sealer for concrete.

Mango dermatitis is uncommon in natives of mango-growing countries (Philippines, Guam, Hawaii, Cuba) never exposed to contact with Toxicodendron species. Many persons who have been so exposed, however, whether they had dermatitis from it or not, are sensitized by one or a few episodes of contact with the peel of the mango fruit. Since the palms are contaminated from the first, the eyelids and the male prepuce are often early sites of involvement. Sponging all contaminated or itchy areas meticulously and systematically with equal parts of ether and acetone at the outset will often remove the oleoresin and prevent any worsening of the dermatitis, which can be treated just as outlined above.

Ginkgo tree dermatitis simulates *Toxicodendron* dermatitis with its severe vesiculation, erythematous papules, and edema. Sowers and his associates described an epidemic of contact dermatitis resulting from trampling on the fallen fruit of a large female ginkgo tree. The causative substances were ginkgolic acid and bilobol from the fruit pulp of the ginkgo tree.

Dermatitis Due to Flowers and House Plants

Philodendron. Among the more common house plants, the velvety-leaved philodendron, *P. crystallinum* (and its several variants) is known in India as the money plant. It is a frequent cause of contact dermatitis. The eruption is often seen on the face, especially the eyelids, carried there by hands that have watered or cared for the plant. Patch tests readily reveal its antigenicity.

English Ivy. English ivy follows philodendron in frequency of cases of occult contact dermatitis.

Primrose. Primrose dermatitis affects the fingers, eyelids, and neck with a punctate or diffuse erythema and edema. It is frequently encountered in Europe. *Primin*, a quinone, is the causative oleoresin abounding in the glandular hairs of the plant *Primula obconica*.

Chrysanthemum. Among the many flowers, the chrysanthemum causes dermatitis most frequently. The eyelids are frequently involved. Florists are most commonly affected. The α-methylene portion of the sesquiterpene lactone molecule is the antigenic site, as it is in the other genera of the Compositae family.

Prairie Crocus. A severe inflammatory reaction with bulla formation, reported by Aaron and Muttit, was caused by the prairie crocus (*Anemone patens L.*), the floral emblem of the Province of Manitoba.

Grevillea. An ornamental "bottle brush" from Queensland, *Grevillea banksii*, was found to be a source of dermatitis from touching the blossoms, (Arnold), but the leaves were not sensitizing. However, Menz, in Australia, has found both the flower and the leaf of both *G. banksii* and *G. Robyn Gordon* to be sensitizing.

Parthenium. *Parthenium hysterophorus*, a photosensitizing weed, was accidentally introduced into India in 1956 and has spread over most of the country; it is also spreading in Australia, China, and Argentina.

Dieffenbachia. This common, glossy-leaved house plant's well-deserved reputation for harmfulness rests on the high content of calcium oxalate crystals in its sap, which burn the mouth and throat severely if any part of the plant is chewed or swallowed. Severe edema of the oral tissues may result in complete loss of voice, hence its common nickname, "dumb cane." It does not appear to sensitize.

Alstroemeria. Florists handling the increasingly popular Peruvian lily were reported by Marks to have become sensitized to tuliposide A, the allergen in this plant. It penetrated through vinyl gloves but not through nitrile gloves.

Castor Bean. The castor bean, seed of *Ricinus communis*, contains ricin, a poisonous substance

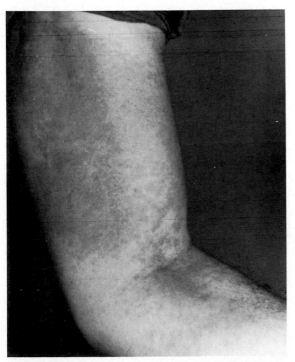

Figure 6–4. Cashew nutshell oil dermatitis resembling poison ivy dermatitis.

(phytotoxin). Its sap contains an antigen that may cause anaphylactic hypersensitivity and also dermatitis. The plant itself is harmless.

Other Flowers and House Plants. Contact dermatitis may be caused by handling many other flowers, such as the geranium, scorpion flower (*Phacelia crenulata* or *campanularia*), creosote bush (*Larvia tridentata*), *Heracula*, daffodil, foxglove, lilac, lady slipper, and magnolia, and tulip and narcissus bulbs. Poinsettia and oleander almost never cause dermatitis, despite their reputation for it (Arnold, Fisher). Treatment of all these plant dermatitides is the same as that recommended for Toxicodendron dermatitis.

Dermatitis Due to Vegetables

Many vegetables may cause contact dermatitis, including the following: tomato, carrot, mushroom, onion, garlic, asparagus, cucumber, cow-parsnip, Indian bean, turnip, parsley, and celery. Onion, among other vegetables, has been incriminated in the production of contact urticaria as well.

Dermatitis Due to Trees

Some of the trees whose timber and sawdust may produce contact dermatitis are the following: cedar, pine, mahogany, myrtle, teak, cocobolo, elm, maple, mesquite, Kentucky coffee tree, ash, *koa*, *milo*, mango, and birch. The latex of the fig and rubber trees may also cause dermatitis, usually of phototoxic (berloque) type.

Dermatitis Due to Tree-Associated Plants

Foresters and lumber workers can be exposed to allergenic plants other than trees.

Lichens are a group of plants composed of symbiotic algae and fungi. Foresters and wood choppers exposed to these lichens growing on trees may develop severe allergic contact dermatitis. Exposure to the lichens may occur from firewood, funeral wreaths, and so forth. Hypersensitization is produced by the d-usnic acid contained in lichens.

The leafy *liverwort (Frulliana nisquallansis)*, a forest epiphyte growing on tree trunks, has produced allergic dermatitis in forest workers, as reported by Mitchell and associates. The eruption is commonly called "cedar poisoning." It resembles Toxicodendron dermatitis, with its attacks being more severe during wet weather. The allergen is sesquiterpene lactone.

Dermatitis Due to Pollens and Seeds

The pollens in ragweed are composed of two antigens. The protein fraction causes the respiratory symptoms of asthma and hay fever and the oil-soluble portion causes contact dermatitis.

Ragweed Oil Dermatitis. Ragweed oil dermatitis is a seasonal disturbance seen mainly during the ragweed pollination season beginning around August 15 and ending with the first frost. Contact with the plant or with wind-blown fragments of dried plants produces the typical dermatitis. Controversy exists whether airborne pollen may do so, however, Fisher believes it does. The oil causes swelling and redness of the lids and entire face and a red blotchy eruption on the forearms that, after several attacks, may become generalized, with lichenification; it closely resembles chronic atopic dermatitis, with lichenification of the face, neck, and major flexures, and severe itching. The distribution mimics that of photodermatitis with the differentiating point being that in ragweed dermatitis there is involvement of the upper eyelids and the retroauricular and submental areas. Chronic cases may continue into the winter. However, signs and symptoms are most severe at the height of the season. Sesquiterpene lactones are the cause. Coexistent sensitization to pyrethrum may account for prolongation of ragweed dermatitis. Men sufferers far outnumber women. Farmers outnumber patients of all other occupations.

Sesame Seed Dermatitis. Hypersensitivity reactions to sesame seeds have been noted. Generalized erythema, oral pruritus, wheezing, and shock may be induced. Sesame oil, containing the allergens sesamine and sesamolin, may cause contact urticaria when used on stasis dermatitis.

Dermatitis Due to Marine Plants

Numerous aquatic plants are toxic or produce contact dermatitis. Algae seem to be the worse offenders. Fresh-water plants are rarely of concern.

Seaweed Dermatitis. Seaweed dermatitis is a type of swimmer's eruption produced by contact with a marine blue-green alga that has been identified as *Lyngbya majuscula* Gomont. An outbreak was reported in 1961 by Grauer and Arnold off Oahu in Hawaii. The onset is within a few minutes after leaving the ocean, with severe itching and burning, followed by dermatitis, blisters, and deep and painful desquamation that affects the areas covered by the bathing suit (in men, especially the scrotum, perineum, and perianal areas; occasionally, in women, the breasts under tight-fitting brassieres). Patch tests with the alga are neither necessary nor helpful, since it is a potent irritant. The dermatitis may be prevented by bathing within 10 or 15 minutes after leaving the ocean. Seaweed dermatitis must be differentiated from swimmer's itch produced by sensitization to schistosomes in the cercarial stage. Their appearances are entirely dissimilar.

Bermuda Fire Sponge Dermatitis. Yaffee and Stargardter reported erythema multiforme from contact with the Bermuda fire sponge.

Dogger Bank Itch. Trawler fishermen in the Dogger Bank area of the North Sea develop allergic dermatitis after contact with *Alcyonidium hirsutum.* This is a seaweedlike animal colony, which comes up in the fishermen's net and produces erythema, edema, and lichenification on the hands and the wrists.

Plant-Associated Dermatitis

Phytophotodermatitis. Mention has previously been made concerning the role of sunlight-producing photosensitivity contact dermatitis. The furocoumarins (psoralens) in certain plants will produce a phototoxic reaction in individuals with the plant substance on their skin who are exposed to the sunlight. The UVA spectrum of light is responsible for producing the phototoxic eruption. This is known as phytophotodermatitis.

Some of the furocoumarin-containing plants that can produce phytophotodermatitis are dill, parsley, parsnip, celery, lime bergamot, lime, fig, mustard, St. John's wort, meadow grass, and mokihana *(Pelea anisata)* berries. Plants of the Umbelliferae family are the most frequent cause of this eruption.

Meadow grass *(Agrimonia eupatoria)* produces *dermatitis bullosa striata pratensis.* It occurs on the hands and legs as irregularly shaped bullae, which heal with pigmented streaks.

Insecticides. The residua of various insecticides on plants may also produce dermatitis. This is especially true of arsenic- and malathion-containing sprays.

Herbicides. Randox(2-chloro-N,N-diallyl-acetamide) has been reported by Spencer as the cause of hemorrhagic bullae on the feet of farmers. Numerous types of weed killers are used, but little is known of their sensitizing potential.

Mechanical Irritations. Barbs, bristles, spines, thorns, spicules, and cactus needles are some of the mechanical accessories of plants that may produce dermatitis.

Sabra dermatitis is an occupational dermatitis resembling scabies. It is seen among pickers of the prickly pear cactus plant. It also occurs in persons handling Indian figs in Israel, being seen from July to November. Banerjee believes that it is also prevalent in India. It is caused by the penetration of minute, invisible thorns into the skin.

Dermatitis Due to Tobacco Tars and Smoke

Weary and Wood described allergic contact dermatitis of the fingers and arms due to tobacco smoke residues that were trapped on the internal portion of the filters of smoked cigarettes. Unconfirmed (but abundant) anecdotal evidence suggests that both Toxicodendron and mango dermatitis can be caused by smoke of the burning plant material, though experimental attempts to reproduce it have been unsuccessful.

Dermatitis Due to Plant Derivatives

The sensitizing substances derived from plants are found in the oleoresin fractions which contain camphors, essential oils, phenols, resins, and terpenes.

The chief sensitizers are the essential oils. They may be localized in certain parts of the plant, such as in the peel of citrus fruits, the leaves of the eucalyptus tree, and the bark of the cinnamon tree.

Cinnamon oil (cassia oil) is a common flavoring agent, especially in pastries. Hand dermatitis in pastry bakers is often due to cinnamon. It is also used as a flavor for lipstick, bitters, alcoholic and nonalcoholic beverages, and chewing gum. Perioral dermatitis may be caused from cinnamon in chewing gum. A 5 per cent cinnamon solution in olive oil is used for patch testing.

Eugenol, clove oil, and *eucalyptus oil* are used by dentists, who may acquire contact dermatitis from them. Patch testing is done with 25 per cent eugenol in petrolatum, 1 per cent oil of clove in olive oil, and 1 per cent eucalyptus in alcohol.

Anise, peppermint, and *spearmint oils* may cause sensitization.

Lemon oil from lemon peel or lemon wood may cause sensitization in the various handlers of these substances. *Citric acid* may cause dermatitis in bakers. *Lime oil* in lime shaving cream or lotion may cause photoallergy.

Balsam of Peru contains numerous substances, among which are essential oils similar to the oil of the lemon peel. Balsam of Peru is known to cross-react with vanilla and cinnamon, among many others.

Vanillin is derived from the vanilla plant and frequently produces contact dermatitis, *vanillism,* in those connected with its production and use.

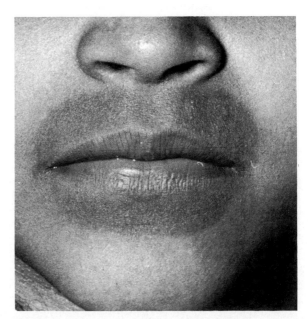

Figure 6–5. Perioral hyperpigmentation following dermatitis caused by cinnamon in bubble gum.

Turpentine frequently acts as an irritant and as an allergic sensitizer (carene). It is contained in paints, paint thinners, varnishes, and waxes.

Testing for Plant Allergies

The method of testing for plant hypersensitivity is the application of the plant leaf or substance as a covered patch test. A 1 cm square leaf is left on the skin for 48 hours. A test should be done on several controls also to make sure that the leaf is not an irritant.

It must be remembered that some of the plants are photosensitizers. Test sites to these must be done in duplicate, with one set kept covered and the other exposed to artificial light or sunlight for the detection of photosensitivity.

Becker LE, et al: Ginkgo tree dermatitis, stomatitis and proctitis. JAMA 1975, 231:1162.

Drach G, et al: Toxicity of the common houseplant Dieffenbachia. JAMA 1963, 184:1047.

Epstein WL: Poison oak and poison-ivy dermatitis as an occupational problem. Cutis 1974, 13:544.

Idem, et al: Induction of antigen-specific hyposensitization to poison oak in sensitized adults. Arch Dermatol 1982, 118:630.

Fisher AA: Erythema multiforme-like eruptions due to exotic woods and ordinary plants. Cutis 1986, 37:101, 158, 262.

Guin J: Recognizing the *Toxicodendrons*. JAAD 1981, 4:95.

Idem: Compositive dermatitis in childhood. Arch Dermatol 1987, 123:50.

Mallory SB, et al: Toxicodendron radicans dermatitis with black lacquer deposit on the skin. JAAD 1983, 6:363.

Marks JG Jr, et al: Dermatitis from cashew nuts. JAAD 1984, 10:627.

Idem: Oral hyposensitization to poison ivy and poison oak. Arch Dermatol 1987, 123:476.

Idem: Allergic contact dermatitis to Alstroemeria. Arch Dermatol 1988, 124:914.

Menz J: Contact dermatitis from plants of the Grevillea family. Austral J Dermatol 1985 26:74.

Mitchell JC, et al: Diagnosis of contact dermatitis from plants. Semin Dermatol 1982, 1:25.

Newhouse ML: Dogger Bank itch. Proc Roy Soc Med 1966, 59:1119.

Orchard SM, et al: Poison ivy/oak dermatitis. Arch Dermatol 1986, 122:783.

Sheard C: Poison oak/ivy desensitization by chewing raw cashew nuts. The Schoch Letter, 1987, item 5, May.

Stoner JG: Plant dermatitis. JAAD 1983, 9:1.

DERMATITIS DUE TO CLOTHING

A predisposition to contact dermatitis from clothing occurs in persons who perspire freely, or who are obese and wear clothing that tends to be tight in the seams. Depending upon the offending substance, various regions of the body will be affected. Regional location is helpful in finding the sensitizing substance. The axillary folds are commonly involved; the vaults of the axillae are usually spared. Sites of increased perspiration and sites where perspiration is impeded, such as the intertriginous areas, will tend to leach dyes from fabrics to produce dermatitis.

Secondary changes of lichenification and infection occur frequently because of the chronicity.

Cotton, wool, linen, and silk fabrics were used exclusively prior to the advent of synthetic fabrics. Most materials are now blended in definite proportions with synthetics to produce superior lasting and esthetic properties.

Cotton. Dermatitis from cotton is virtually nonexistent. Only the sizing used in cotton to stiffen or glaze the material may sensitize the skin to produce dermatitis.

Wool. In most instances there is no true sensitization to wool. Wool acts as an irritant, due to the barbs on its fibers. These barbs may produce severe pruritus at points of contact with the skin, especially in the intertriginous areas. In sensitive-skinned persons such as those with atopic dermatitis the use of wool is not advisable because of its mechanical irritative properties. When a positive patch test to wool is elicited, it is usually due to dye or other chemicals rather than the wool itself.

Silk. Silk is a sensitizer but rarely; the nature of the allergen is not known.

Synthetic Fibers. Numerous types of synthetic fibers are now available for clothing and accessory manufacture, all of which again are remarkably free of sensitizing properties. Only the dyes and finishes of these fabrics cause dermatitis. Some of the synthetic fibers are acetates, such as rayon; acrylics such as Orlon and Acrilan; modacrylics such as Dynel, nylon; metallic yarns, olefin, and polyesters such as Dacron, Fortrel, Kodel, Mylar, and Vycron.

Polyvinyl Resins. These are the plastics that are used in such wearing apparel as raincoats, rainhoods, wristbands, suspenders, plastic mittens, and gloves. These again are only infrequently found to be causes of contact dermatitis.

Workers engaged in cleaning the vats used in producing polyvinyl chloride from vinyl chloride may develop acroösteolysis (bone destruction of the hands and forearms), preceded by Raynaud's phenomenon, and thickening and tightening of the hands. Markowitz has reported this.

Spandex. This nonrubber (but elastic) polyurethane fiber is widely used for garments such as girdles, brassieres, and socks. Dermatitis from Spandex has been reported only with brassieres. It was found that Spandex containing mercaptobenzothiazole produced the contact dermatitis. Spandex manufactured in the United States does not contain this and, therefore, does not produce allergic contact dermatitis.

Clothing Dyes. Aniline and the azo dyes are used in textile dyeing. When properly manufactured and used for this purpose, they produce little contact dermatitis; however, cross sensitization may occur in persons sensitive to paraphenylenediamine or other members of the "para" group such as para-aminobenzoic acid, benzocaine, procaine, and sulfonamides.

Paraphenylenediamine is used in wearing apparel

only in fur pieces. However, it is tolerated by patients allergic to this chemical, because it is in the fully oxidized form.

Clothing dye dermatitis usually occurs when the patient is subject to hyperhidrosis, which "bleeds" dye from fabrics. However, this bleeding process is extremely rare in today's fabrics because of the superior methods of fixing the dyes. It is usually the various other chemicals used in conjunction with the dyes that cause sensitization.

In patch testing for dye sensitivity Fisher recommends that the test fabric be soaked in 1 ml of water with a drop or two of vinegar for 24 hours, and the solute be applied as a patch test for 48 hours. In testing for axillary dermatitis, the suspected fabric is soaked in 250 ml of water to which a drop of 20 per cent sodium hydroxide has been added and then applied to the skin for 48 hours. Hatch and Maibach have recently reviewed this.

Fabric Chemical Finishes. Fabric finishes are used to improve the durability, appearance, and feel of a material. Antiwrinkling and crease-holding chemicals are mostly resins, which are incorporated into the fibers as they are being manufactured or applied to the completed (finished) fabric. These resins are cured or polymerized. Properly prepared resins do not produce dermatitis; however, faulty manufacture may.

Formaldehyde and Formaldehyde Resins. Not only are free formaldehyde and formaldehyde resins used extensively in the preparation of fabrics, but they are used in the manufacture of toilet paper, facial tissues, and various other papers to increase their tensile strength. Fabrics are treated with the formaldehydes to make them less vulnerable to the effects of perspiration and of ironing. Clothing may be treated with these substances to make them wrinkle free and to make them dry rapidly after washing. They are used to make clothing fabrics shrink-resistant and water-repellent as well as stain-repellent. When all these uses are taken into consideration, the low incidence of dermatitis from these formaldehyde-treated materials is remarkable. Improved finishing agents are becoming available which do not release formaldehyde at all. The incidence of formaldehyde allergy secondary to the wearing of treated clothing is diminishing rapidly.

The mere presence of free formaldehyde in clothing does not establish the diagnosis of formaldehyde-caused contact dermatitis. A 2 per cent formaldehyde patch test and a positive patch test with the suspected material must also be demonstrated. Also, wearing of the fabric must induce contact dermatitis.

Formaldehyde resins, melamine formaldehyde and urea formaldehyde, are the most commonly used finishes. Patients suspected of formaldehyde resin hypersensitivity should be tested with 2 per cent formaldehyde in water, 10 per cent urea formaldehyde in petrolatum, 10 per cent melamine formaldehyde in petrolatum, and the material itself.

Trousers that are crease-resistant and drip-dry may

produce this type of dermatitis. The inner thighs and popliteal spaces are especially involved. Patch testing is done with 2 per cent formaldehyde solution ("formalin" is a 10 per cent solution). Higher concentrations may cause irritant reactions. Medical personnel may be so sensitive to formaldehyde that even a 0.1 per cent formaldehyde solution patch test will produce a positive reaction.

Malten calls attention to textile finishes causing contact dermatitis in some cases in which formaldehyde in the wearing apparel is implicated. He believes this may represent a cross reaction between the ureas and melamine formaldehyde.

Treatment is the same as for other types of contact dermatitis—the avoidance of exposure of the skin to formaldehyde resin and free formaldehyde. This is, however, most difficult. New clothes should be thoroughly washed before wearing the first time. Clothes should be thoroughly aired.

Fisher AA: Hypoallergenic surgical gloves and gloves for special purposes. Cutis 1975, 15:797.
Hatch K, et al: Textile dye dermatitis. JAAD 1985, 12:1079.
Jordan WP Jr, et al: Allergic contact dermatitis to underwear elastic chemically transformed by laundry bleach. Arch Dermatol 1975, 111:595.
Schorr WF, et al: Formaldehyde allergy. Arch Dermatol 1974, 110:73.

Shoe Dermatitis

Footwear dermatitis may begin on the dorsal surfaces of the toes and may remain localized to that area indefinitely. There are erythema and lichenification and, in severe cases, weeping and crusting. Secondary infection is frequent. In severe cases an id reaction may be produced on the hands similar to the reaction from fungus infection of the feet. A diagnostic point is the normal appearance of the skin between the toes, which has no contact with the offending substance. In fungus infections the toe webs are usually involved. Another pattern seen commonly today is involvement of the sole with sparing of the instep and flexural creases of the toes.

Shoe dermatitis is most frequently caused by the rubber accelerators, mercaptobenzothiazole and tetramethylthiuram disulfide; by the adhesives used; and by the dichromates in leather. Other causative agents are felt, cork liners, formaldehyde, dyes, asphalt, and tar.

Patch testing to determine the offending substance may be helpful in securing footwear made without sensitizing substances.

Chromate sensitivity is due to the chrome tanning process most frequently used for tanning leather to make it more resistant to the stresses to which leather is subject. The prevalence of chrome allergy is decreasing in North America, probably as a result of better fixation of chrome to leather. Chromate sensitivity is commonly seen in those with hyperhidrosis of the feet.

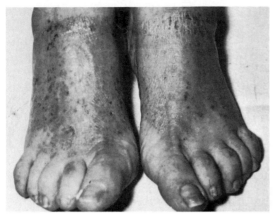

Figure 6–6. Shoe dermatitis produced by chrome tanning of leather.

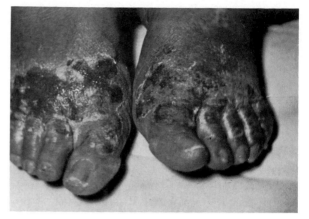

Figure 6–7. Contact dermatitis caused by rubber box toes of shoes.

Aldehydes are used for tanning of white leather. Sensitivity to white shoe leather may be due to formaldehyde.

Tannin is derived from various trees around the world. Vegetable tanning is still used for tanning shoe sole leather, but not for the shoe uppers, which makes it difficult for those sensitive to dichromates.

Patients with shoe dye sensitivity should avoid redyed shoes because of the usually inadequate binding of the dye with the leather. Artificial leather, synthetic leather, and Corfam materials are excellent substitutes; however, the linings of such shoes may be chrome-tanned and may contain dyes and formaldehyde, which can continue to cause hypersensitivity. A. Fisher lists shoe companies where special shoes are available.

Shoes free of dichromates and rubber cement are obtainable from the Alden Shoe Co., Taunton St., Middleborough, Massachusetts, 02346, manufacturers of Derma-Pedic shoes.

For women the company is U.S. Shoe, One Eastwood Drive, Cincinnati, Ohio 45227, and for children McMahan Shoes, 505 Courtland St NE, Augusta, Georgia 30308.

Shoes may be ordered containing no rubber cement or other sensitizing materials from the Foot-So-Port Shoe Division of the Musebeck Shoe Co., Inc., Oconomowoc, Wisconsin 53066.

Mali JWH, et al: Allergy to chromium. Arch Dermatol 1966, 93:41.
Nater JP: Possible causes of chromate eczema. Dermatologica 1963, 126:160.
Slog E: Sensitization to p-phenylenediamine. Arch Dermatol 1965, 92:276.
Storrs FJ: Dermatitis from clothing and shoes. In Contact Dermatitis, 3rd ed. Fisher AA (ed). Philadelphia, Lea & Febiger, 1986.

DERMATITIS DUE TO METALS AND METAL SALTS

Metal dermatitis is most frequently caused by nickel, chromates, and mercury. Usually, with the exception of nickel, the pure metals do not cause hypersensitivity; it is only when they are incorporated into salts that they cause reactions. Patch test reactivity to an aqueous solution of the metallic salt does not usually indicate sensitivity to the pure metal.

Most objects containing metal or metal salts are combinations of several metals, some of which may have been used to plate the surface, thereby enhancing its attractiveness, durability, or tensile strength. For this reason suspicion of a metal-caused dermatitis should be investigated by doing patch tests on several of the metal salts. Fisher recommends the following in water solutions:

> Nickel sulfate 5%
> Mercury bichloride 0.05%
> Cobalt sulfate 2%
> Ferric chloride 2%
> Zinc chloride 2%
> Gold chloride 1%
> Copper sulfate 5%
> Aluminum chloride 2%
> Platinum chloride 1%
> Sodium arsenate 10%
> Silver nitrate 2% (open test only)

The following should be tested in petrolatum:

> Potassium dichromate 0.5%
> Manganese chloride 10%

Nickel sulfate (5%) and cobalt sulfate (1%) may also be tested in petrolatum.

Black Dermatographism

Black or greenish staining under rings, metal wristbands, bracelets, and clasps is due to the abrasive effect of cosmetics or other powders containing zinc or titanium oxide on the gold jewelry. This skin discoloration is always black due to the deposit of metal particles upon skin that has been powdered and that has metal, such as gold, silver, or platinum, rubbing on it. Abrasion of the metal is due to the fact that some powders are hard (zinc oxide) and are capable of abrading the metal.

Nickel Dermatitis

Since we are all constantly exposed to nickel, nickel dermatitis is a frequent occurrence, especially among women. Nickel produces more cases of allergic contact dermatitis than all other metals combined. Erythematous and eczematous eruptions, sometimes with lichenification, appear beneath earrings, bracelets, hairpins, rings, wristwatches, clasps, eyelash curlers, metallic spectacle frames, brassiere cups, and blue-jeans buttons. Dermatitis stemming from coins containing nickel has always been rare; more common is dermatitis from handles of doors, handbags, faucets, and so forth. Nickel dermatitis is seen most frequently on the earlobes of women. Piercing the ears with nickel-plated instruments or wearing nickel-plated jewelry readily induces nickel sensitivity, Fisher points out. Ears should be pierced only with stainless steel instruments, and only stainless steel earrings should be worn until the ears have healed.

Exposure to the metal may not be readily apparent most of the time. Even in gold jewelry the clasps and the solder may contain nickel. The nickel object may be plated with chrome and yet cause nickel dermatitis through the "leaching out" of some of the nickel through the small pores of the chromium plating.

Nickel oxides occurring in green paints may also produce nickel dermatitis. Sweat, containing sodium chloride, may combine with nickel to form nickel chloride. This affects the degree of nickel dermatitis, it being more severe in persons who perspire profusely. Prevention of sweating may help to prevent the areas exposed to nickel from developing dermatitis or may at least attenuate the affliction.

The diagnosis is established by a positive reaction to a 5 per cent nickel sulfate solution patch test. A U.S. nickel coin may be used as a patch test. However, it must be the older nickel coin that has an Indian head on one side and a buffalo on the other. Fisher states that nickel may be detected by applying a freshly prepared 1 per cent alcoholic solution of dimethylglyoxime and a freshly prepared 10 per cent aqueous solution of ammonia separately in equal amounts to the test object. In the presence of nickel,

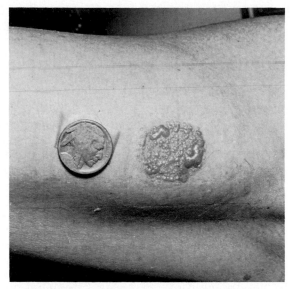

Figure 6–9. "Money dermatitis." Nickel dermatitis: 3-plus reaction to the application of an Indian head nickel.

the object will turn orange-pink. A positive test always means nickel is present, but a negative test does not eliminate it. Katz and Samitz have pointed out that sweat, blood, or saline may leach nickel from stainless steel, even though Fisher's test is negative.

Prophylactic measures should include the reduction of perspiration in those sensitive to nickel. Fisher suggests application of Decadron aerosol spray prior to exposure to nickel, such as before putting on a brassiere or wristband. Clasps and other objects are now available in plastic material so that at least some of the exposure to nickel may be decreased. Polyurethane varathane 91 (Flecto) applied in three coats will give protection for several months.

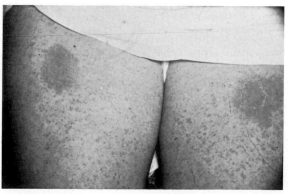

Figure 6–8. Allergic contact dermatitis from nickel in garters.

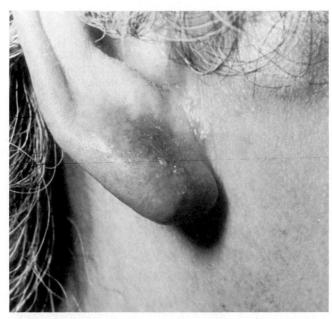

Figure 6–10. Dermatitis of earlobe caused by nickel-containing earrings. (Courtesy of Dr. John R. T. Reeves.)

Treatment of nickel dermatitis consists of the application of topical corticosteroid creams, sprays, or lotions.

Chromium Dermatitis

The chromates are strongly corrosive and irritating to the skin; they may act as primary irritants or as sensitizers to produce allergic contact dermatitis. Aside from occurrence among employees in chromate works, chrome dermatitis is encountered among tanners, painters, dyers, photographers, French polishers, welders, aircraft workers, Diesel engine workers, and those concerned with the bleaching of crude oils, tallows, and fats. Traces of dichromates in shoe leather and gloves may cause eczema of the feet and hands. Many zippers are chromium-plated, and the nickel underneath the plate may be the causative agent. Chromium metal and stainless steel do not produce contact dermatitis.

Zinc chromate paint is a common source of dermatitis. Matches, hide glues, chrome alloys, cigarette lighters, leather hatbands, and leather sandals or camera cases may cause chrome dermatitis. Anticorrosion solutions used for refrigeration and other recirculation systems often contain chromates that produce dermatitis.

Most of those in the cement industry suffering from *cement eczema* show patch tests positive to dichromates. Cement eczema is often a primary irritant dermatitis complicated by allergic contact dermatitis to the hexavalent chromates. Nickel, arsenic, and cobalt are also in cement.

The skin changes are multiform, ranging from a mild follicular dermatitis to widespread nodular and crusted eruptions, all being worse upon exposed parts. Often they are slow to clear up, lasting from a few weeks to six months after contact has ceased.

Heavy exposure of industrial workers to chromates may produce *chrome ulcers* ("chrome holes") upon the backs of the hands and forearms, usually beginning around a hair follicle or in the creases of the knuckles, or in the finger webs. The hole begins as a small abrasion that deepens and widens as its edges grow thick, eventually forming a conical indolent ulceration. Chrome ulcers may also arise on—and perforate—the nasal septum.

Diagnosis of chrome sensitivity is made by a positive patch test to 0.5 per cent potassium dichromate in petrolatum. Although it is believed that the hexavalent chrome compounds cause chrome dermatitis, there is evidence that, rarely, trivalent chrome may also be a causative factor.

Prophylaxis for nonindustrial workers should consist mainly of avoidance of contact with the chromate. Some recommend even the avoidance of contact with chrome-plated metal objects; on the other hand, based on negative patch tests to metallic chrome, Fisher believes that touching or handling chrome objects will not cause dermatitis. However, the chromate-sensitive person should avoid zinc chromate paints, chrome-tanned leather, glue, and other chromate-containing objects.

Mercurial Dermatitis

The mercurials may not only act as irritants but also as sensitizers. Dermatitis may be caused by the local application of *calomel* (mercurous chloride) or other *mercurial remedies* (mercurochrome and ammoniated mercury), or by their internal use. *Mercuric chloride*, even in weak solutions (1:1000), is irritating, causing dermatitis chiefly among surgeons, nurses, taxidermists, and those using insecticides; 1:2000 is not irritating. *Phenylmercuric salts* are used as weed killers as well as agricultural fungicides and insecticides. Phenylmercuric salts have wide usage in industrial materials (gelatin waving solutions, glue, sizing, starch pastes, bentonite gels, mildew-proofing). They are also used as preservatives in cosmetic creams, suppositories, nasal jellies, eyewashes, and throat tablets. Sensitization dermatitis may appear at the site of exposure to the phenylmercuric salts, on the legs after exposure to weed killers, and also on the hands.

Nitrate of mercury produces irritation. The eruptions are encountered among felt-hat workers and those who do etching, embossing, or art metalwork. The manufacturing of thermometers and barometers, the handling of furs, the use of amalgams by dentists, fire gilding, and solder used for dry batteries are all common sources of contamination with mercury, causing various eczematous eruptions.

Among the organic mercurial compounds, Merthiolate may be implicated in sensitization reactions.

Skin previously sensitized to mercury may react severely when the sensitized person receives a mercurial compound systemically. Occasionally, free mercury may be released from an amalgam filling and produce dermatitis not in the mouth but on the skin; such a case was reported by Feuerman from Israel in 1975.

Patch testing for diagnosis is done with 0.05 (1:2000) per cent mercuric bichloride in aqueous solution.

Cobalt Dermatitis

Cobalt is frequently combined with nickel as a contaminant. They have similar properties but do not produce cross reactions. Cobalt dermatitis may occur in those involved in the manufacture of polyester resins and paints, in the manufacture of hard metal used for cutting and drilling tools, and in the manufacture and use of cement. Cobalt dermatitis may also occur in producers of pottery, ceramics, metal alloys, glass, carbides, and pigments. One may be exposed to cobalt in hair dye, flypaper, and vitamin B_{12}. Blue tattoo pigment contains cobalt oxide.

For patch testing a 2 per cent cobalt sulfate solution is used. Rarely, cobalt chloride may cause nonimmunologic local release of vasoreactive materials, with a local urticarial response, as described by Odom and Maibach.

Arsenical Contact Dermatitis

Arsenic is one of the most common chemical causes of dermatitis in those who mine copper and arsenical ores, and in those coming into contact with the artificial dyes used in wallpaper, flowers, and chalk. Arsenical compounds are used in dyeing fabrics and domestic articles, for the preservation of animal skins and hides, and for embalming. Arsenic is an ingredient of some disinfectants and weed exterminators. It is used in sheep dips and in the making of flypaper. It is encountered in the manufacture of insecticides, in chemical factories for the manufacture of sulfuric and other acids, in printing establishments where gilt or bronze powder is used, and in farming and gardening.

Among those who may incur this disease in the course of their occupation are glucose and candy factory workers, those who use sizing and dextrin, bookbinders, fruit handlers, furriers who handle raw furs, machinists, and metal workers who handle brass, copper, and zinc.

The dermatitis caused by the arsenicals is frequently a folliculitis with secondary pyoderma. Furunculosis is also common. Ulcerations on the extremities and nasal perforation similar to chrome ulcers may occur.

Patch testing is done with a 10 per cent solution of sodium arsenate.

Dermatitis Due to Other Metals

Most of the other commonly used metals are not important in causing contact dermatitis.

Gold dermatitis may rarely occur from the wearing of gold jewelry. It is the gold salts that are allergenic. Patch testing is done with 1 per cent gold chloride solution.

A number of cases of dermatitis due to gold jewelry, especially gold rings, contaminated with radon and its decay products, have been reported. This may eventuate in radiation dermatitis and squamous cell carcinoma of the finger. Evidently the source of the contaminated gold for the rings had been reclaimed decayed radon gold seeds.

Platinum dermatitis may occur from exposure to platinum salts and sprays in industry. Platinum rings, earrings, white gold spectacles, clasps, and other jewelry cause eruptions resembling those caused by nickel. Patch testing is with 1 per cent platinum chloride solution.

Zinc, aluminum, copper sulfate and *antimony dermatitis* rarely occur; they frequently act as irritants.

Contact Stomatitis

Contact stomatitis may be seen in cases of sensitivity to metals used in dental fillings and prostheses and to topical therapeutic drugs. Some of these metals known to produce stomatitis include mercury, bismuth, chromium, nickel, gold, copper, and zinc. Muniz and Berghman reported contact stomatitis to lithium carbonate tablets used in therapy for schizophrenia, and Hogan et al reported lichenoid stomatitis with ulceration in a man taking 1500 mg of lithium carbonate daily for depression. Chewing gums and dentifrices may also produce contact stomatitis. Ingredients thought to be responsible for this are hexylresorcinol, thymol, dichlorophene, oil of cinnamon, and mint.

Clinical signs may be bright erythema of the tongue and buccal mucosa with scattered erosions. Angular cheilitis may also develop.

Edwards EK Jr, et al: Allergic contact dermatitis (due) to lead acetate in a hair dye. Cutis 1982, 30:629.
Emmett EA, et al: Allergic contact dermatitis to nickel. JAAD 1988, 19:314.
Feuerman EJ: Recurrent contact dermatitis caused by mercury in amalgam dental fillings. Int J Dermatol 1974, 14:657.
Fisher AA: Detection of nickel by dimethyl glyoxime spot test. JAMA 1975, 234:429.
Idem: Nickel dermatitis. Dermatology 1981, Dec, p 19.
Idem: Allergen replacement in allergic dermatitis. Int J Dermatol 1977, 16:319.
Idem: Contact stomatitis, glossitis, and cheilitis. Otolaryngol Clin N Am 1974, 7:827.
Idem: Allergic stomatitis from dental impression compounds. Cutis 1985, 36:295.
Ho VC, et al: Nickel dermatitis in infants. Contact Dermatitis 1986, 15:270.
Lupton GP, et al: Cutaneous mercury granuloma. JAAD 1985, 12:296.
Mountcastle EA, et al: Mucosal allergy to dental impression material. JAAD 1986, 15:1055.
Muniz CE, et al: Contact stomatitis and lithium carbonate tablets. JAMA 1978, 239:2759.
Schubert H, et al: Epidemiology of nickel dermatitis. Contact Dermatitis 1987, 16:122.
Slater DN: Aluminium hydroxide granulomas: light and electron microscopic studies and x-ray microanalysis. Br J Dermatol 1982, 107:103.
Smith JD, et al: Contact urticaria from cobalt chloride. Arch Dermatol 1975, 111:1610.
Stutzman CD, et al: Squamous cell carcinoma from wearing radioactive gold rings. JAAD 1984, 10:1075.
Veien NK, et al: Aluminum allergy. Contact Dermatitis 1986, 15:295.
Watts TL: Nickel earlobe dermatitis. Arch Dermatol 1968, 98:155.

RUBBER DERMATITIS

Rubber dermatitis generally occurs on the hands from wearing rubber gloves (surgeons, nurses, houseworkers). The eruption is usually sharply limited to the gloved area but may spread up the forearms. Rubber dermatitis also develops in the axillae from the use of rubber dress shields. Rubber girdles and panties cause pruritus and dermatitis of the areas covered by the girdle, especially the groins

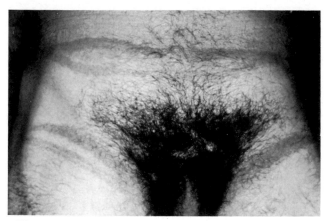

Figure 6–11. Dermatitis caused by rubber in jockey shorts.

and sides of the hips. Antiwrinkle bands may cause dermatitis of the submental region or forehead. Worn cloth coverings, allowing the rubber within to protrude and touch the skin, may explain rubber dermatitis caused by a garment worn for years without trouble.

Infants may develop dermatitis of the diaper region from rubber panties, or eczematous eruptions on other areas from lying on rubber sheets. Wearers of goggles, gas masks, respirators, and other rubber goods sometimes develop rubber dermatitis.

Prepatellar dermatitis may be caused by rubber kneeling pads. Rubber sheeting used as bed underpads may cause bizarre eruptions on the trunk. Dermatitis of the glans penis from rubber condoms and vaginitis from pessaries or diaphragms may occur.

Natural and synthetic rubbers are used separately or in combination to make the final rubber product. Natural rubber does not cause sensitization, rather it is the chemicals added in the manufacturing process, most importantly the accelerators and antioxidants, that cause allergic contact dermatitis. A frequent antioxidant sensitizer, propyl paraphenylenediamine,

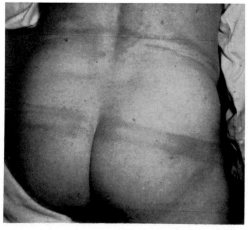

Figure 6–12. Contact dermatitis due to rubber elastic band of athletic supporter.

is used in tires, heavy-duty rubber goods, girdles, boots, and elastic underwear. Jordan and Bourlas have shown that elastic in underwear is chemically transformed by laundry bleach, such as Clorox, into a potent sensitizing substance. The offending garments must be thrown out and the use of bleaches interdicted.

Accelerators. During the manufacturing process, chemicals are used to hasten the vulcanization of rubber. Among the numerous chemicals available tetramethylthiuram disulfide, mercaptobenzothiazole, and diphenylguanidine are frequently used. Tetramethylthiuram disulfide and its analogues, known as *disulfiram* and *thiuram*, may produce contact dermatitis when moist skin is exposed to the finished rubber product.

Antioxidants. In order to preserve rubber, antioxidants are used. Among the antioxidants the amine type such as phenyl-alpha-naphthylamine is most effective. Hydroquinone antioxidants may cause depigmentation of the skin as well as allergic contact dermatitis. The use of vinyl plastic gloves or other rubber substitutes may be the only solution to the problem.

Fisher AA: Condom dermatitis in either partner. Cutis 1987, 39:281.

ADHESIVE DERMATITIS

Adhesive dermatitis may be caused by cements, glues, and gums. Most of these adhesives are now made of synthetic material, but some may still contain rubber with its accompanying allergenic substances. Formaldehyde resin adhesives contain free formaldehyde, naphtha, glue, and disinfectants. Synthetic resin adhesives contain plasticizers; hide glues may contain chromates from the tanned leather while other glues incorporate preservatives such as formaldehyde.

Vegetable gums such as gum tragacanth, gum arabic, and karaya may be used in denture adhesives, hair wave lotions, topical medications, toothpastes, and depilatories, and many cause contact dermatitis.

Resins are used in adhesive tapes and in various adhesives such as tincture of benzoin. Compound tincture of benzoin may be a potent sensitizer when applied under occlusion. Turpentine is frequently found in rosin; abietic acid in the rosin is the causative sensitizer.

An ethyl cyanoacrylate adhesive ("Krazy Glue") used on the fingernails produced an extensive eruption of scaling plaques misdiagnosed as parapsoriasis en plaques; there were vesicular patch test reactions to both Krazy Glue and 5-Second Nail Glue, as reported by Dorinda Shelley.

Many adhesive tape reactions are due to the irritative effects of the "adhesiveness" upon the skin.

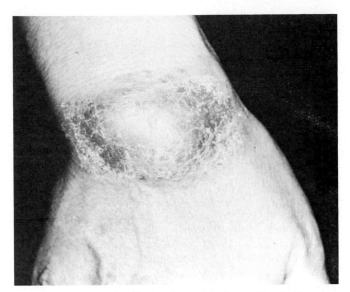

Figure 6–13. Adhesive dermatitis due to Band-aid.

Allergic reactions to adhesive tape itself are due to the rubber components, to accelerators, to antioxidants, and to various resins or turpentine.

Some adhesive tapes contain acrylate polymers rather than rubber adhesives; Dermicel, Micropore Surgical Tape, and Steri Strip are among these. These acrylates may cause allergic contact dermatitis. Pressure-sensitive adhesives are in widespread use in the tape and label industries. Allergens present in these adhesives include rosin, rubber accelerators, antioxidants, acrylates, hydroquinones, lanolin, thiourea compounds, and N-dodecylmaleamic compounds.

James WD: Allergic contact dermatitis to colophony. Contact Dermatitis 1984, 10:6.
Shelley ED, et al: Chronic dermatitis simulating small-plaque parapsoriasis due to cyanoacrylate adhesive. JAMA 1984, 252:2455.

SYNTHETIC RESIN DERMATITIS

The many varieties of synthetic resins preclude adequate discussion of each. The reactions incurred during the manufacture of these substances are more frequent than those encountered in their finished state.

Epoxy Resin. The epoxy resins in their liquid form may produce severe dermatitis, especially during the manufacturing process. Nonindustrial exposure is usually to the epoxy resin glues, to nail lacquers, and to artificial nails. Epoxy resins are used in the home as glues and paints (bathtub and refrigerator). Artists and sculptors frequently use epoxy resins.

Epoxy resins consist of two or more components, the resin and the curing agent. There are numerous curing agents such as the amines, phenolic compounds, peroxides, and polyamides. These may be irritants or allergens or both. The resin, based on an acetone and phenol compound known as bisphenol A, in its raw state may cause allergic contact dermatitis. One per cent epoxy resin in acetone is used for patch testing.

Epoxy resins are used also as stabilizers and plasticizers. Their use in the manufacture of polyvinyl chloride (plastic) film has caused dermatitis from plastic handbags, beads, gloves, and panties.

Polyester Resins. Ordinarily, completely cured or polymerized resins are not sensitizers. The unsaturated polyester resins are dissolved and later copolymerized with vinyl monomers. Such polyester resins are used for polyester plasticizers, polyester fibers (Dacron), and polyester film (Mylar).

The unsaturated polyester resins, on the other hand, will produce primary irritation in their fabrication. The dermatitis occurs typically as an eczematous eruption on the back of the hands, wrists, and forearms.

Polyester resins are commonly incorporated into other plastic material as laminates to give them strength; applications include boat hulls, automobile body putty, safety helmets, fuel tanks, lampshades, and skylights.

Acrylic Monomers. Multifunctional acrylic monomers may produce allergic or irritant contact dermatitis. Pentaerythritol triacrylate, trimethylolpropane triacrylate, and hexanediol diacrylate are widely used acrylic monomers. These are used in combination with ultraviolet light to cure epoxy resin. Printing presses and coating machines have the ultraviolet source incorporated into the printing press so that the photoengraving process is the modern printing technique for books, newspapers, and metal containers. In printing, the acrylates are applied to the printing plates and hardened with ultraviolet light to become the letters that were previously composed of lead.

This same technique is now used in dentistry where an acrylic monomer is applied to the teeth and then exposed to ultraviolet light to produce a superior dental sealant. Acrylic monomer–induced dermatitis is sometimes seen in dentists and dental technicians.

Nethercott has reported contact dermatitis in 18 cases of printers who handled multifunctional acrylic monomers in printing inks and acrylic printing plates. The clinical manifestations were an erythematous pruritic eruption, mainly of the hands and arms, swelling of the face, and involvement of the eyelids.

Orthopedic surgeons are experiencing contact dermatitis due to acrylic bone cement (methyl methacrylate monomer) used in mending hip joints. The sensitizer passes through rubber and polyvinyl gloves.

Benzoyl peroxide (Desquam-X, BenzaGel, Xerac, Panoxyl) is a popular acne remedy. It is also used for bleaching flour and edible oils and for curing plastics such as acrylic dentures. Infrequently an allergic contact dermatitis may be caused. Patch testing is done with 1 per cent in petrolatum.

Fisher AA: Epoxy resin dermatitis. Cutis 1976, 17:1027.
Gaul LE: Prevalence of epoxy resin dermatitis. Arch Dermatol 1967, 96:227.
James WD, et al: Allergic contact dermatitis due to compound tincture of benzoin. JAAD 1984, 11:847.
Nethercott JR: Skin problems associated with multifunctional acrylic monomers in ultraviolet curing inks. Br J Dermatol 1978, 98:541.
Shelley ED, et al: Dermatitis simulating small-plaque parapsoriasis, due to cyanoacrylate adhesive. . .on fingernails. JAMA 1984, 252:2455.

VINYL CHLORIDE DISEASE

Vinyl chloride disease presents with symptoms of Raynaud's phenomenon and acrosclerosis in industrial workers who are exposed to perchlorethylene, a widely used industrial solvent.

DERMATITIS DUE TO SOLVENTS

Alcohol. Allergic contact dermatitis due to alcohol is rarely encountered with lower aliphatic alcohols. Wasilewski reported a severe case of bullous and hemorrhagic dermatitis on the fingertips and on the deltoid region caused by isopropyl alcohol. Though rare, ethyl alcohol dermatitis may also be encountered. Gaul reported cetyl and stearyl alcohols provoking an urticaria-like dermatitis. "Solvent sniffers" may develop an eczematous eruption about the mouth and nose. There is erythema and edema. It is a direct irritant dermatitis caused by the inhaling of the solvent placed on a handkerchief.

FIBERGLASS DERMATITIS

Fiberglass dermatitis is seen after occupational or inadvertent exposure. The small spicules of glass penetrate the skin and cause severe irritation with tiny erythematous papules, scratch marks, and intense pruritus. Usually there is no delayed hypersensitivity reaction. Wearing clothes that have been washed together with fiberglass curtains, handling air conditioner filters, or working in the manufacture of fiberglass material may produce severe folliculitis, pruritus, and eruptions that may simulate scabies or insect or mite bites. Fiberglass is also used in thermal and acoustical installations, padding, vibration isolation, curtains, draperies, insulation for automobile bodies, furniture, gasoline tanks, and spacecraft.

A thorough washing of the skin after handling fiberglass is helpful against the itching. Talcum powder thoroughly dusted on the flexure surfaces of the arms makes the fibers slide off the skin.

Abel RR: The washing machine and fiberglass. Arch Dermatol 1966, 93:78.
Parlette HL: Fiberglass dermatitis. Bull Assoc Milit Dermatol 1974, 22:53.

PARAPHENYLENEDIAMINE DERMATITIS

Exposure to paraphenylenediamine (PPDA) figures frequently in the induction of allergic contact dermatitis. Those engaged in the manufacture of PPDA, furriers, hairdressers, and those in the photographic and rubber vulcanization industries develop eruptions at first on the backs of the hands, the wrists, the forearms, the eyelids, and the nose, consisting of an eczematous, erythematous, oozing dermatitis. In those whose hair has been dyed, sensitivity is manifested by itching, redness, and puffiness of the upper eyelids, tops of the ears, temples, and back of the neck. Lichenification and scaling are seen in the chronic type.

Both covered and open patch tests are recommended for demonstration of sensitization. The *covered patch test* is done with 2 per cent PPDA in petrolatum. The testing material should be stored in dark containers and made fresh at least yearly; if it blackens, new material should be prepared. The *open technique* consists of mixing five drops each from the two bottles in which the dye is supplied. The 10 drops of solution are allowed to stand for five minutes and then applied to a 2.5 cm area.

For the person sensitive to this type of hair dye, use of semipermanent dyes might be the solution. In the case of sensitivity to the latter, vegetable dyes such as henna should then be tried. Metallic dyes are usually not favored by women but are frequently used by men as "hair color restorers."

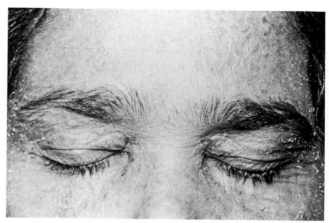

Figure 6–14. Dermatitis resulting from use of hair dye (paraphenylenediamine). Eyelid involvement is characteristic. (Courtesy of Dr. Axel W. Hoke.)

COSMETIC DERMATITIS

Cutaneous reactions to cosmetics may be divided into irritant, allergic hypersensitivity, and photosensitivity reactions. The leading cause of allergic contact dermatitis due to cosmetics is fragrances. Second is preservatives such as Bronopol (2-bromo-2-nitropropane-1-3-diol), Kathon CG Quaternium-15, and imidazolidinyl urea. Third is lanolin and the woolwax alcohols. Walter Larsen has recently reviewed the subject thoroughly. The following is a modified version of a tabulated list prepared by March and Fisher for the Committee on Cutaneous Health and Cosmetics of the American Medical Association.

Axillary Antiperspirants. The aluminum salts such as aluminum chloride and chlorhydroxide and the zinc salts such as zinc chloride act as primary irritants and may rarely produce a folliculitis. Aluminum chlorohydrate is considered to be the least irritating antiperspirant. Zirconium preparations, now removed from all antiperspirants, produced a granulomatous reaction. Quaternary ammonium compounds in some roll-on deodorants may produce allergic contact dermatitis.

Axillary Deodorants. The aluminum salts, such as those just mentioned, and the chlorinated phenols such as hexachlorophene rarely produce allergic sensitization; the latter may cause photosensitization. This is also true of bithionol. Neomycin is also used, and allergic contact dermatitis may be caused by this antibiotic.

Hair Dyes. Permanent type hair dyes incorporate paraphenylenediamine (PPDA), a popular but potent sensitizer that may cross-react with many chemicals.

In rinses and tints the azo dyes, acid violet 6B, water-soluble nigrosine, and ammonium carbonate may sensitize and cross-react with PPDA.

The currently popular metallic hair dyes (Grecian Formula, for example) may contain nickel, cobalt, chromium, or lead.

Hair Bleaches. The bleaches utilize peroxides, persulfates, and ammonia, which may act as primary irritants. Hair bleaches that contain ammonium persulfate, a primary irritant, may produce a local urticarial and a generalized histamine reaction, according to Calnan and Shuster.

Permanent Waves. The permanent wave preparations are rarely sensitizers and usually cause only hair breakage. The cold type uses thioglycolates; the hot type, alkaline sulfides. Storrs recently reported 12 cases of contact allergy to glyceryl monothioglycolate, first used in the U.S. in 1973. The compound is known as an "acid perm," and is far more sensitizing than the ammonium thioglycolate which was formerly used. Storrs listed 24 preparations that contain glyceryl monothioglycolate.

Hair Straighteners. The greases and gums are not sensitizers; however, the perfume incorporated in these preparations can be. Thioglycolates are also used, but hair breakage is the only untoward irritating reaction noted.

Hair Sprays. Shellac, gum arabic, and the synthetic

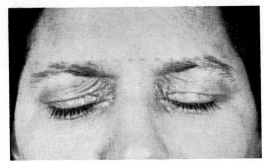

Figure 6–15. Nail polish dermatitis. (Courtesy of Dr. W. L. Dobes.)

resins are sensitizers, and allergic reactions occur infrequently. Lanolin is frequently incorporated into the aerosol sprays.

Depilatories. Calcium thioglycolate and the sulfides and sulfhydrates may cause primary irritation dermatitis. Mechanical hair removers are the mercaptans, waxes, and resins. The latter may produce allergic dermatitis.

Hair Tonics and Lotions. Tincture of cinchona produces allergic sensitization; tincture of cantharidin and salicylic acid, primary irritation. Resorcin, quinine sulfate, and perfumes such as bay rum are also sensitizers.

Nail Lacquers. These contain sulfonamide-formaldehyde resins and are the most frequent causes of eyelid and neck dermatitis.

Nail Polish Removers. These are solvents such as acetone, which can cause nail brittleness.

Artificial Nails. The acrylic monomers as well as the glue required to attach the prosthetic nail may produce allergic sensitivity.

Nail Hardeners. Formaldehyde and formaldehyde-releasing agents are the most common of nail hardeners and produce allergic sensitization. Paronychia, onycholysis, onychomadesis, and subungual hemorrhage may result from use of these hardeners.

Lipsticks. Di- and tetrabromofluorescein in the indelible dyes and the perfumes of the lipsticks may cause sensitization reactions. This reaction may be

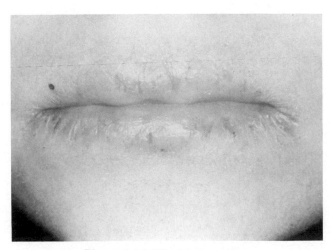

Figure 6–16. Lipstick dermatitis.

enhanced if allantoin compounds are also included in the lipstick formula.

Eye Make-up. This consists of mascara, eye shadow, and eye liners. The preservative, base wax, and perfumes are the components that may produce sensitization, but rarely.

Stephan Epstein called attention to false positive reactions to "automatic" mascaras when a closed patch test is used. This is due to the irritative qualities of the solvents. An open or nonocclusive patch test is recommended. A provocative use-test in the antecubital fossae may ultimately be necessary.

Sunscreens. Para-aminobenzoic acid and its esters, digalloyl trioleate, cinnamates and benzophenones are photosensitizers as well as sensitizers. Hydroquinone is also used not only as a sunscreen but also as a skin bleach.

Depigmenting Creams. Ammoniated mercury is a sensitizing agent formerly used in bleaching creams. Hydroquinones are also occasional sensitizers.

Lanolin. A fatty alcohol, lanolin is rarely a sensitizer on the normal skin, although Wereide found 7 per cent of 240 patients with eczema sensitive to wool fat. Patch testing must be done with 30 per cent wool wax alcohols in petrolatum.

Dentifrices and Mouthwashes. These contain sensitizers such as the essential oils used as flavoring agents and antiseptics.

Perfumes. Almost all cosmetic preparations contain perfumes. Even those labeled as nonscented often contain a "masking" fragrance which may be a sensitizer. Photoallergy is frequently reported. Almond oil may produce rhinitis and dermatitis. Other perfumes that may cause dermatitis are coriander, geraniol, heliotropine, hydroxycitronella, jasmine, linalool, lavender, lemon, lemongrass, neroli, origanum, oil of cloves, peppermint, spearmint, and wintergreen. Larsen found that cinnamic alcohol and aldehyde, hydroxycitronella, eugenol, and isoeugenol are the most common offenders.

Broeckx W, et al: Cosmetic intolerance. Contact Dermatitis 1987, 16:189.

Calnan CD, et al: Reactions to ammonium persulfate. Arch Dermatol 1963, 88:180.

deGroot AC, et al: The allergens in cosmetics. Arch Dermatol 1988, 124:1525.

Idem: Contact allergy to preservatives II. Contact Dermatitis 1986, 15:218.

Idem: Kathon CG. JAAD 1988, 18:350.

Eiermann HJ, et al: Prospective study of cosmetic reactions. JAAD 1982, 6:909.

Held JL, et al: Consort contact dermatitis due to oak moss. Arch Dermatol 1988, 124:261.

Larsen WG: Perfume dermatitis. JAAD 1985, 12:1.

Idem, et al: Fragrance contact allergy. Semin Dermatol 1982, 1:85.

Nakayama H, et al: Pigmented cosmetic dermatitis. Int J Dermatol 1984, 23:299.

Rothenberg HW, et al: Allergy to perfumes from toilet soaps and detergents in patients with dermatitis. Arch Dermatol 1968, 97:417.

Santucci B, et al: Contact dermatitis due to fragrances. Contact Dermatitis 1987, 16:93.

Storrs FJ: Permanent wave dermatitis: Contact allergy to glyceryl monothioglycolate. JAAD 1984, 11:74.

OCCUPATIONAL CONTACT DERMATITIS

Workers in various occupations are prone to contact dermatitis from primary irritants and allergic contactants. In certain occupations it is a common occurrence. Some causative agents are listed below according to occupations:

Agriculture: cement, cobalt in animal feed, pesticides, plants, rubber, wood preservatives, diesel oil, gasoline, disinfectants.

Airplane workers: glues, chromium; casein; phenol formaldehyde, urea formaldehyde, epoxy and polyester resins, dichromates.

Artists: synthetics such as acrylic and vinyl acrylic resins, epoxy and polyester resins; solvents such as carbon tetrachloride, benzene, toluene, acetone, turpentine; azo dyes; nickel and chromium pigments; clay, plaster.

Bakers: flour, cottonseed oil, potash (used in making pretzels), cardamom, cinnamon, benzoyl peroxide, persulfones.

Barbers: quinine, resorcin, mercury, nickel, paraphenylenediamine, capsicum, arsenic, sulfur.

Beekeepers: poplar resins in unpurified beeswax, cross reaction with balsam of Peru.

Carpenters and cabinetmakers: teak, mahogany, rosewood, glues, nickel, plastics, polishes, rubber, turpentine.

Chemists: innumerable.

Compositors: benzine, dichromates.

Cooks: soap, detergents; vegetables (such as onions, garlic, artichokes, carrots, potatoes), nickel, insecticides, ammonia.

Dentists: soaps and detergents; acrylic monomers; local anesthetics such as procaine (most frequently) and tetracaine of the para-aminobenzoic acid derivatives; topical anesthetics such as benzocaine and tetracaine (diclonine hydrochloride is recommended instead of these two "caines"); self-curing acrylic resins, essential oils such as eucalyptol, menthol, thymol, eugenol, and methylsalicylate; formaldehyde for disinfection of instruments; quaternary ammonium compounds such as Zephiran (benzalkonium chloride) and Phemerol (benzethonium chloride).

Diesel engine workers: dichromates, lubricating oils, nickel.

Dyers: sodium silicate.

Electroplaters: cyanide, various acids.

Exterminators: D.D.T., arsenic, formalin, sodium fluoride, formaldehyde, pyrethrum.

Foresters: poisonous shrubs; sprays containing arsenic and lead; lichens, moss, wood, oleoresins.

Furriers: arsenic, dyestuffs such as paraphenylenediamine.

Gardeners: plants, arsenic, insecticides, lime dust, fertilizers, formaldehyde, primula, chrysanthemum, tulip, narcissus, manure.

Hairdressers: paraphenylenediamine, soaps, peroxide, ammonium persulfate, glyceryl monothioglycolate, rubber, nickel, perfumes, acrylic plastics.

Jewelers: cyanide, nickel, metal polish.

Masons: chromates and cobalt in cement, leather goods, epoxy resin.

Metal polishers: oxalic acid, turpentine, dichromates.

Milliners: dyes, arsenic.

Newspaper production workers: tertiary butyl catechol in phototypesetting paper (Fardal).

Nurses: penicillin, streptomycin, codeine, morphine, bichloride formalin, medicated alcohol, lye, hexachlorophene, formaldehyde, chlorpromazine.

Painters: turpentine, varnish remover, arsenic, linseed oil, aniline dyes, paints, benzene, paint thinners, detergents, chromates (green, yellow), cobalt (dyes, driers), epoxy resin, formaldehyde, polyester resins.

Photographers: pyrogallol, metol, dichromates, sodium hydroxide, azo compounds, selenium, formaldehyde, used in color film processing.

Physicians: rubber gloves, soaps. (See Surgeons.)

Printers: arsenic, dichromates, nickel, hydrocarbons in ink, acrylic monomers.

Sculptors: woods such as satin wood, South American box wood, cocobolo, birch, pine, and beech; binders in synthetic materials such as urea, formaldehyde, alkyds, hexamethylenetetramine.

Soap workers: strong alkalis, perfumes.

Surgeons: antiseptics, iodine, mercurials, hexachlorophene, rubber gloves, glove powder, procaine, formaldehyde, acrylic polymers.

Tanners: dichromate, hydrochloric acid, vegetable tanning agents (glutaraldehyde), antimildew chemicals.

Management of Occupational Contact Dermatitis

Occupational contact dermatitis is managed by eliminating contact of the skin with irritating and sensitizing substances. The work environment should be carefully controlled, with use of all available protective devices to prevent accidental and even planned exposures. Personal protective measures such as frequent clothing changes, cleansing showers, protective clothing, and protective barrier creams should be used. Hand cleansing procedures should be thoroughly surveyed, with particular attention paid to the soaps available and also what solvents may be used.

Treatment of the dermatitis follows closely that recommended for Toxicodendron dermatitis. Topical corticosteroid preparations are especially helpful in the acute phase.

Skin Protective Preparations. When rubber and polyvinyl gloves are not feasible to use against irritant and allergenic substances, skin protective creams may offer a solution, although they are often impractical.

A wide variety are available. Two main types of protective creams are used. One is for "wet work": protective against acids, alkalis, water-base paints, coolants, and cutting oils with water. The other type is for "dry work," to protect against oils, greases, cutting oils, adhesive, resins, glues, and wood preservatives.

For industrial uses a thorough survey should be made of the various preparations available for the specific problem. Dimethyl and trimethyl phenyl polysiloxanes and dimethyl silicones are popular. Sources of protective ointments and barrier creams are Ayerst Laboratories, 685 Third Ave, New York, New York 10013; Zee Medical Products, 11800 Woodruff Avenue, Downey, California 90241; Calgon Corporation, 7501 Page Street, St Louis, Missouri 63133.

Adams RM: Occupational Skin Disease, 1st ed. New York, Grune and Stratton, 1983.

Fardal RW, et al: Phototypesetting paper as a cause of allergic contact dermatitis in newspaper production workers. Cutis 1983, 31:509.

Fisher AA: Allergic baker's dermatitis due to benzoyl peroxide. Cutis 1989, 43:128.

Markovitz SS, et al: Occupational acroösteolysis. Arch Dermatol 1972, 106:219.

Mathias GGT: Occupational dermatitis. JAAD 1988, 19:1107.

Nurse DS: Industrial dermatitis. Int J Dermatol 1987, 26:434.

TOPICAL DRUG CONTACT DERMATITIS

Drugs, in addition to their pharmacologic and possible toxic action, also possess sensitizing properties. This may not only occur from topical application but also from ingestion.

Some drugs may produce sensitization of the skin when applied topically; if the medication is later taken internally an acute flare at the site of the contact dermatitis may result. This so-called anamnestic (recalled) eruption can occur with antihistaminics, sulfonamides, and penicillin. The same is true of the local anesthetic ointments containing "caine" medications.

According to Fisher, four of the most frequent offenders are Mycolog cream, neomycin, Caladryl, and Merthiolate (thimerosal). Since Mycolog's reformulation, the number of sensitized persons has dropped.

Although it is impossible to mention all topical medications that cause irritation or allergic contact dermatitis, some are important enough to be dealt with individually.

Boric Acid Intoxication. In young children especially, anorexia, oliguria, albuminuria, central nervous system irritation, generalized dermatitis, and even toxic epidermal necrolysis may develop simply from the topical application of boric acid in powder form as incorporated into talcum powder and in compresses, especially when applied to the broken skin such as in oozing eczema. Chronic exposure to lower concentrations may lead to alopecia.

There is a failure of the urine to concentrate, specific gravity remaining in the 1.000 to 1.005 range, and creatinine clearance may be markedly decreased. Boric acid has an affinity for the brain, liver, and kidneys.

Some authorities believe that boric acid should be made unavailable because of its hazardous potentialities.

Only supportive measures are therapeutically feasible.

Hypersensitivity to Local Anesthetics. Physicians and dentists may develop allergic contact dermatitis from local anesthetics. In addition, the continued use of these local anesthetics as antipruritic ointments and lotions may cause sensitization of the skin. Benzocaine is a frequently used topical antipruritic.

Allergy to local anesthetics may induce edema and erythema (especially of the face), severe pruritus, urticaria, and even anaphylactic reaction a few minutes after injection.

Local anesthetics may be divided into two groups: the first includes the *para-aminobenzoic acid esters,* such as benzocaine, butethemine (Monocaine), chloroprocaine, procaine (Novocain), and tetracaine (Pantocaine); the second, which sensitizes much less frequently, includes the *amides,* such as dibucaine (Nupercainal), lidocaine (Lido-Mantle, Xylocaine) (least likely to sensitize), mepivacaine (Carbocaine), and prilocaine (Citanest). In addition, the preservative methylparaben, frequently found in these prepared solutions, may cause hypersensitivity reactions that can easily be attributed to the local anesthetics.

Benzocaine sensitivity is determined by a patch test of 5 per cent benzocaine in petrolatum. Patch testing with the remainder of the topically applied anesthetics is reliable. Intradermal tests are unreliable.

Topical Medication Vehicle and Preservative Sensitizers. Sensitization dermatitis can occur from various ingredients incorporated into the base of the topical agents. There are antioxidants, emulsifying agents, preservatives, and stabilizers. Some of these ingredients are the following:

Ethylenediamine. This is used as a stabilizer in medicated creams. This chemical became one of the most common sensitizers in the United States primarily because of the widespread exposure to Mycolog cream. Squibb has recently removed this (as well as neomycin and gramicidin) from the newly formulated Mycolog cream, Mycolog II. Ethylenediamine may cause contact dermatitis and cross-react with internally taken aminophylline, which consists of theophylline and ethylenediamine. In addition, the following medications should be avoided: Pyribenzamine, tagathen, antistine, pyna, and hydroxyzine (Atarax and Vistaril). Topical applications to be avoided are creams of Pyribenzamine, Surfadil, Allergen, and Preferin, Privine, and Vasocon-A eye drops. Patch tests are done with 1 per cent ethylenediamine in petrolatum.

Formaldehyde and Formaldehyde-releasing Agents. Formaldehyde itself is used in cosmetics primarily in shampoos. Since it is quickly diluted and washed away, sensitization through this exposure is rare. Formaldehyde releasers are polymers of formaldehyde which may release small amounts of formaldehyde under certain conditions. Allergy may be due to the formaldehyde-releasing preservatives (which act as antibacterial and antifungal agents in their own right), to the released formaldehyde, or both. Bronopol, Imidazolidinyl urea, and Quaternium-15 are examples found in current patch test kits.

Parabens. Allergic contact dermatitis may develop from parabens, which are also used in some cosmetics, foods, drugs, dentifrices, and suppositories. The paraben esters (methyl, ethyl, propyl, and butyl parahydroxybenzoates) are used in concentrations

below 0.3 per cent as preservatives. Parahydroxybenzoic acid (another paraben) has also been found to cause reactions.

Perpetuation of a dermatitis, despite effective topical medication, suggests the possibility of paraben sensitivity or corticosteroid sensitivity, or that another sensitizer may be present. The concentration of paraben (below 0.3 per cent) is too low in the various topical applications to produce a positive patch test to the medication; therefore, testing is done with a 12 per cent paraben mix (methyl, ethyl, propyl, and butyl, 3 per cent each) in petrolatum. Nagel and his associates found that parabens, frequently employed as bacteriostatic agents, are capable of producing immunologically mediated immediate systemic hypersensitivity reactions.

Para-chloro-metaxylenol (PCMX). This chlorinated phenol antiseptic is used in over 30 over-the-counter products including Absorbine Jr, Desitin Baby Powder, and Unguentine Spray.

Chloro-meta-cresol. Sensitization occurs primarily through exposure to betamethasone-containing cream.

Propylene glycol. This is widely used as a vehicle for topical medications, cosmetics, and various emollient lotions. It is used in the manufacture of automobile brake fluid and alkyd resins, as a lubricant for food machinery, and as an additive for food colors and flavoring agents. It is commonly used in antiperspirants. Fisher concludes that propylene glycol must be considered as a sensitizer able to produce contact dermatitis, and it can cause a flare of the contact dermatitis when ingested. It is tested as a 4 per cent aqueous solution.

Sorbic acid. A rare sensitizer, it is tested as 2 per cent in petrolatum.

Antibiotic Contact Dermatitis. Physicians, dentists, nurses, and other medical personnel, as well as patients, may develop contact dermatitis from various antibiotics.

Neomycin sensitivity. As a topical antibiotic, neomycin sulfate has been incorporated into innumerable ointments, creams, and lotions. It is present in such preparations as underarm deodorants and antibiotic creams and ointments available without prescriptions.

The signs of neomycin sensitivity may be those of a typical contact dermatitis but are often those of a recalcitrant skin eruption which has become lichenified and even hyperkeratotic. This picture may be seen in persistent external otitis, lichen simplex chronicus of the nuchal area, or dermatophytosis between the toes.

Patch testing is done with 20 per cent concentration of neomycin in petrolatum. After 48 hours the patch is removed, but it is observed for four to seven days more for possible delayed reactions.

Ghadially et al have reviewed gentamicin sensitivity.

Streptomycin. Allergic dermatitis of the fingertips due to streptomycin is most frequently encountered in nurses who prepare streptomycin for injection. The dermatitis may become chronic, with eczematization and fissuring. Others handling streptomycin may also develop dermatitis at the site of contact. Cross reactivity to neomycin and kanamycin may occur. Patch testing is with 2.5 per cent aqueous solution of streptomycin.

Bacitracin. Held et al have reviewed reports of sensitivity to this widely used antibiotic. Reactions to it are uncommon but not rare.

Penicillin. Hypersensitivity develops in many people exposed to contact with this substance, as in topical application of penicillin ointments or the handling of the material for injection. Anaphylactic reaction may occur upon exposure to topical penicillin, but usually it is only the delayed reaction which appears, as in the application of the ointment or powder for patch testing.

Antimicrobial Drugs. Hydroxyquinolones, Furacin, mercury compounds such as ammoniated mercury, thimerosal, and phenylmercuric acetate are sensitizers, as are the sulfonamides, resorcinol, and formaldehyde.

Phenothiazine Drugs. The handling of the injectable solutions and tablets may produce dermatitis in those sensitized to chlorpromazine and other phenothiazine derivatives. The reactions may be photoallergic or nonphotoallergic.

Coskey RJ: Contact dermatitis caused by diphenhydramine hydrochloride. JAAD 1983, 8:204.

Edwards EK Jr, et al: Allergic reaction to tertiary butyl alcohol in a sunscreen. Cutis 1982, 29:476.

Epstein E: The detection of neomycin sensitivity. Arch Dermatol 1965, 91:50.

Fisher AA: Contact dermatitis from topical medicaments. Semin Dermatol 1982, 1:49.

Ghadially R, et al: Gentamicin. JAAD 1988, 19:428.

Goh CL, et al: Contact sensitivity to topical medications. Int J Dermatol 1989, 28:25.

Grekin RC, et al: Local anesthesia in dermatology surgery. JAAD 1988, 19:599.

Guin J: Contact sensitivity to topical steroids. JAAD 1984, 10:773.

Held JL, et al: Allergic contact dermatitis from bacitracin. JAAD 1987, 17:592.

McBurney EI, et al: Contact dermatitis to transdermal estradiol system. JAAD 1989, 20:508.

Purcell SM, et al: Allergic contact dermatitis to dyclonine hydrochloride simulating extensive herpes simplex. JAAD 1985, 12:231.

Reitamo S, et al: Delayed hypersensitivity to topical corticosteroids. JAAD 1986, 14:582.

Schillinger BM, et al: Boric acid poisoning. JAAD 1982, 7:667.

Schorr WF: Paraben allergy: A cause of intractable dermatitis. JAMA 1968, 204:859.

Storrs FJ, et al: Allergic contact dermatitis to 2-bromo-2-nitropropine-1, 3-diol in a hydrophilic ointment. JAAD 1983, 8:157.

Trozak DJ: Delayed hypersensitivity to scopolamine delivered by a transdermal device. JAAD 1985, 13:247.

CONTACT URTICARIA SYNDROME
(Syndrome of Immediate Reactions)

Contact urticaria may be defined as a wheal and flare reaction occurring when a substance is applied to the intact skin.

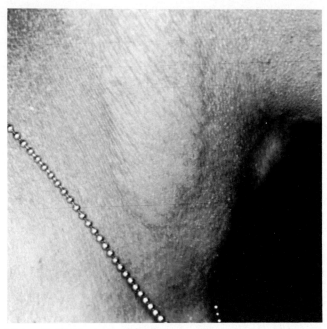

Figure 6–17. Contact urticaria due to cobalt chloride used to test for the ability to sweat.

It may be nonimmunologic (no prior sensitization), immunologic, or of unknown mechanism. The nonimmunologic type is the commonest, and may be due to direct release of vasoactive substances from mast cells. The allergic type may be the most severe, as anaphylaxis is possible. The third type has features of both. Elpern has reported on the syndrome.

Actually, as Elpern points out, urticaria is only one of a broad spectrum of immediate reactions, including pruritus, dermatitis, local or general urticaria, bronchial asthma, orolaryngeal edema, rhinoconjunctivitis, gastrointestinal distress, headache, or an anaphylactic reaction. Any combination of these is subsumed under the expression "syndrome of immediate reactions."

There are many different substances that can elicit such a reaction. It is seen in housewives and food handlers who handle raw vegetables, raw meats and fish, shellfish, and other foods. Raw potatoes have been shown to cause not only contact urticaria but also asthma at the same time. It has been seen in hairdressers who handled bleaches and hair dyes containing ammonium persulfate, in whom the contact urticaria was accompanied by swelling and erythema of the face followed by unconsciousness. Nettle rash (contact urticaria) may be experienced by those touching nettles. Caterpillars and moths may cause contact urticaria just by touching the skin.

Nonimmunologic Mechanism. This type of reaction is most frequent and may produce contact urticaria in almost all exposed individuals. Examples of this type of reaction are seen with nettle rash (plants), dimethyl sulfoxide (DMSO), cobalt chloride, and Trafuril.

Immunologic Mechanism. This reaction is of the immediate hypersensitivity type. The reaction may range from a localized urticaria to a generalized urticaria progressing to asthma. This has been seen to occur in the case of potatoes, as mentioned above, also to phenylmercuric propionate used as an antibacterial agent in laundering sheets, where not only contact urticaria occurred but also asthmatic attacks. Certain allergens have been shown to be IgE-mediated (see the article by Tuer et al).

Uncertain Mechanism. This type of reaction occurs with those agents that produce contact urticaria and a generalized histamine-type reaction but lack a direct or immunologic basis for the reaction.

Contact Urticaria–Causing Substances. A wide variety of substances can cause contact urticaria. Some are plants, nettles, caterpillars, moths, oatmeal, flour, meat, turkey skin, calf liver, banana, lemon, potato, monoamylamine, benzophenone, nail polish, tetanus antitoxin, phenylmercuric propionate, streptomycin, cetyl alcohol, stearyl alcohol, estrogenic cream, cinnamic aldehyde, sorbic acid, benzoic acid, castor bean, and lindane.

VonKrogh and Maibach list 80 substances that can produce contact urticaria. In addition to those mentioned above, they list carrots, spices, wool, silk, dog and cat saliva, dog hairs, horse serum, ammonia, sulfur dioxide, formaldehyde, acrylic monomers, and exotic woods. To these Fisher adds wheat, cod liver oil, and aspirin.

Testing. The usual closed patch tests do not show sensitivity reactions. Instead, open patch tests are performed for eliciting immediate type of hypersensitivity. The substance is applied to a 1 cm square area on the forearm and 20 to 30 minutes later erythema occurs that can evolve into a wheal and flare response. When foods are tested, a small piece of the actual food is placed upon the skin.

Scratch or intradermal testing is resorted to only when there are problems of interpretation of the open patch tests. These tests have produced anaphylactic reactions. The use of passive transfer test and compound 40–80 testing are of value but usually not feasible.

Elpern DJ: The syndrome of immediate reactivities (contact urticaria syndrome): An historical study from a dermatology practice. Hawaii Med J 1985, 44:426.
Fisher AA: Contact Dermatitis, 3rd ed. Philadelphia, Lea & Febiger, 1986, pp 686–709.
Okano M, et al: Anaphylactic symptoms due to chlorhexidine gluconate. Arch Dermatol 1989, 125:50.
Tanaka T, et al: Ulcerative contact dermatitis caused by sodium silicate: coexistence of primary irritant dermatitis and contact urticaria. Arch Dermatol 1982, 118:518.
Tuer W, et al: Contact urticaria to sodium-o-phenyl phenol. Ann Allergy 1986, 56:19.
Turjanmaak K, et al: Rubber contact urticaria. Contact Dermatitis 1988, 19:362.
VonKrogh G, et al: The contact urticaria syndrome. Semin Dermatol 1982, 1:59.
Winton GB, et al: Contact urticaria. Int J Dermatol 1982, 21:573.

DRUG REACTIONS

Eruptions produced by taking drugs or having them injected (dermatitis medicamentosa) may likewise be caused, in many cases, by local application of the same drug. Drugs, in addition to their pharmacologic and possible toxic action, also possess potential sensitizing properties. Sensitivity to drugs is produced by the covalent bonding of a chemical group component (hapten) with body protein to form an antigen. After the skin sensitization is manifest, the reaction time is shorter with subsequent use of the drug. The dose necessary to produce such symptoms is often below that required for the pharmacologic effect of the drug. Even minute amounts of a drug that previously has been well tolerated may suddenly produce severe symptoms. The eruption, once it has appeared, is likely to recur with the use of the particular drug (specific reaction) or those closely related (cross reaction), and sometimes even unrelated substances.

It is of the utmost importance to withdraw all potentially offending drugs immediately at the onset of an eruption which might be due to them. TEN or exfoliative dermatitis could supervene at any time and bring about a fatal outcome. Systemic steroids may be given in a short course to terminate the reaction quickly, in early cases.

It is impossible to give a complete list of all the drugs that cause eruptions; instead, reactions to a selected group of the more commonly used drugs are listed.

Acetanilide: cyanosis, erythema, fixed eruption.
Acetazolamide (Diamox): erythema multiforme bullosum, papules, hirsutism.
Acetphenetidin: fixed eruption, purpura, urticaria.
Acetylsalicylic acid (aspirin): anaphylactic reaction, anaphylactoid purpura, bullae (palms), erythema multiforme, erythema nodosum, hand dermatitis (vesicles), morbilliform erythema, scaling, angioedema, purpura, urticaria.
ACTH: anaphylactic reaction, pigmentation, purpura, urticaria.
Adriamycin: alopecia.
Aldactazide: photoallergic eruption.
Alkylating agents: erythema, urticaria.
Allopurinol: exfoliative dermatitis, morbilliform rash, purpura, urticaria.
Amethopterin: alopecia, stomatitis.
Aminopyrine: fixed eruption, toxic epidermal necrolysis.
Amiodarone: photosensitivity, toxic epidermal necrolysis, pigmentation.
Amitriptyline: urticaria, photosensitization, alopecia, jaundice.
Amodiaquin: dyschromia, nail hyperpigmentation.
Amoxicillin: Same as ampicillin.

Amphetamine: fixed eruption.

Ampicillin: discrete, bright pink, often itchy, morbilliform, sometimes maculopapular, eruption.

Antihistaminics: fixed eruption, urticaria.

Antimalarials: bizarre hyperpigmentation has been reported with these, and aggravation of porphyria by full doses of them is well recognized; quinacrine (Atabrine), though little used nowadays, turns the skin quite yellow on long continued use. All the antimalarials will frequently aggravate psoriasis, except in those cases aggravated by sunlight—who are often greatly benefited. Exfoliative dermatitis, fixed eruptions, and erythema annulare centrifugum have also occurred.

Antimony compounds (tartar emetic): erythema, fixed eruption, urticaria.

Antipyrine: bullae, erythema, erythema multiforme, fixed eruption, morbilliform erythema, pigmentation, pustular lesions, scaling, scarlatiniform erythema, Stevens-Johnson syndrome, stomatitis, urticaria.

Antituberculosis drugs: urticaria and morbilliform eruptions constitute about a third of the reactions to isoniazid, the others being fever, jaundice, and peripheral neuritis. Lupus erythematosus syndromes also occur, chiefly in slow acetylators. Some patients have had a severe acneiform eruption. Acanthosis nigricans may result.

Rifampicin reactions are in general infrequent and mild; flushing and pruritus have been seen and acneiform eruptions may occur. Drug eruptions occur more frequently in AIDS.

Less than 2 per cent of 2000 persons given ethambutol had reactions to it, and only one-fourth of these were cutaneous. PAS causes a wide spectrum of skin reactions in nearly 10 per cent of patients, usually about a month into therapy. Streptomycin causes skin reactions in about 5 per cent of patients, and a wide assortment of reactions is seen. Pyrazinamide causes a great deal of hepatic necrosis, but only a few cases of reddish brown discoloration in exposed skin. Ethionamide rarely produces skin reactions. Kanamycin and capreomycin rarely produce skin reactions, but viomycin has caused urticaria, purpura, or eczema in several instances.

Arsenic and arsenical salts: erythematous bullae, papular eruptions, exfoliative dermatitis, Bowen's disease; edema of feet, hands and eyelids; fixed eruption, palmar hyperhidrosis, arsenical keratoses of hands and feet, pigmented basal cell and basal cell carcinoma, epidermoid carcinoma, pigmentation.

Atenolol: Induction of psoriasis or pustular psoriasis.

Atropine: erythema, fixed eruption, pruritus.

Aurothioglucose: see *Gold.*

Bactrim: see *Trimethoprim.*

Barbiturates: aphthae, bullae, erythema (generalized), erythema multiforme, exfoliative dermatitis, morbilliform erythema, pruritus, purpura, scarlatiniform erythema, Stevens-Johnson syndrome, stomatitis, toxic epidermal necrolysis, urticaria.

Bendroflumethiazide: erythema, lichen-planuslike papules, papulovesicles, petechiae, purpura, vesicles.

Bishydroxycoumarin (Dicumarol): necrotizing angiitis.

Bleomycin: alopecia, mucocutaneous ulcerations, flagellare pigmentation, induratal erythema.

Bromides: acneiform eruption (most common), bullae, erythema multiforme, erythema nodosum, fungating tumors (pseudolymphoma), urticaria, vesicles.

Camoquin: melanosis, pigmentation.

Cancer chemotherapy agents: stomatitis and hair loss (breakage of the thin shafts at the surface) are common side effects, as is onychodystrophy; urticaria, exfoliative dermatitis, pigmentation of skin and nails, and volar erythema also occur. Bronner has reviewed this in some detail. Volar erythrodysesthesia has been reported.

Captopril: urticaria, angioedema, morbilliform, maculopapular, pityriasis rosea-like, lichenoid, pemphigus.

Carbromal: purpura.

Carisoprodol (Soma, Rela): fixed eruption, cross reaction with meprobamate.

Cephalosporin: maculopapular eruption, urticaria, pruritus.

Chloral hydrate: acneiform eruption, bullae, erythema, erythema multiforme, eczematous dermatitis, fixed eruption, purpura, urticaria.

Chloramphenicol (Chloromycetin): candidiasis, pruritus ani, urticaria, aplastic anemia, toxic epidermal necrolysis.

Chlordiazepoxide (Librium): edema, erythema, jaundice.

Chloroquine: achromotrichia, albinism, dyschromia, transient edema, exfoliative dermatitis, fixed eruption, lichenplanuslike dermatitis, photosensitization, pigmentation, exacerbation of psoriasis, porphyria, pruritus ani, retinopathy with blindness.

Chlorothiazide (Diuril): cutaneous vasculitis, erythema, lichen-planuslike papules, papulovesicles, petechiae, photoallergy, urticaria, purpura, thrombocytopenic purpura, vesicles.

Chlorpromazine (Thorazine): bullae, edema, exfoliative dermatitis, maculopapular or morbilliform erythema, petechiae, blue-gray slate-colored pigmentation of sun-exposed areas, photosensitivity, eye and skin pigmentation syndrome, stomatitis, urticaria.

Chlorpropamide: erythema multiforme, photoallergy, Stevens-Johnson syndrome, urticaria, lichenoid eruption.

Chlorthalidone: jaundice, purpura, toxic epidermal necrolysis, cutaneous vasculitis, photoallergy.

Cimetidine alopecia: Since its introduction the FDA has received over 60 case reports of alopecia associated with cimetidine administration. Khalsa et al have reviewed 21 cases within their own experience. The hair has usually resumed growing on stopping the drug.

Cinchophen: angioneurotic edema, bullae, erythema, fixed eruptions, scarlatiniform erythema, stomatitis.

Clindamycin: diarrhea, morbilliform rash, jaundice, *Clostridium difficile* colitis, leucocytoclastic angiitis.

Codeine: erythema, fixed eruption, pruritus, pruritus ani, scaling, urticaria.

Colchicine: alopecia.

Corticosteroids: ecchymosis, moon face, petechiae, purpura, striae, acneiform eruptions, thin fragile skin (subcutaneous atrophy), increased perspiration.

Corticotropin (ACTH): acneiform eruption, anaphylactic reaction (sensitivity to pork and beef), erythema, erythema multiforme, urticaria pigmentation.

Coumarin: alopecia, ecchymosis, gangrene, hemorrhagic bullae and necrosis, petechiae, purple toes, purpura, purpura fulminans, urticaria, vesicles.

Cyclamate, calcium (artificial sweetener): cold urticaria, photosensitization.

Cyclophosphamide: alopecia.

Dactinomycin: alopecia, stomatitis.

Dapsone: toxic epidermal necrolysis, fixed drug eruption, methemoglobinemic gray or slate-blue cyanosis, hemolysis, agranulocytosis, motor neuropathy.

Demethylchlortetracycline (Declomycin): photo-onycholysis, phototoxicity, photosensitivity.

Desacetyl methylcolchicine: alopecia.

Diaminodiphenylsulfone: see *Dapsone.*

Diethylstilbestrol: angioedema, exfoliative dermatitis, fixed eruption.

Digitalis: desquamation, erythema, fixed eruption, papular dermatitis, scarlatiniform erythema, urticaria.

Dilantin: see *Phenytoin.*

Diphenhydramine: anaphylactic reaction, contact dermatitis, necrotizing angiitis, papular dermatitis, pruritus, vasculitis.

Diphenylhydantoin hypersensitivity reaction. A macular purpuric rash with fever, facial edema, lymphadenopathy, leucocytosis, hepatitis, and sometimes nephritis may occur one to three weeks after starting the drug. A possible variant is seen in which lymph node enlargement with histologic atypia predominates, and skin symptoms are less marked. Sulfasalazine may do this too.

Gingival hyperplasia, which may be extreme, may be seen. Also seen are acne (papulopustular), bullae, edema (facial), exfoliative dermatitis, hypertrichosis, hypertrophic gingivitis, pseudolymphoma, SLE-like dermatitis, Stevens-Johnson syndrome, toxic epidermal necrolysis, methemoglobinemia.

Emetine hydrochloride: fixed eruption.

Ephedrine: eczema, erythema, fixed eruption, purpura, vasculitis, urticaria.

Ergot: bullae, fixed eruption, gangrene, pustules.

Erythromycin lauryl sulfate: jaundice, urticaria.

Ethchlorvynol: fixed eruption, urticaria, purpura.

Ethiodized oil: erythema of lower extremities.

Eucalyptus: erythema, urticaria.

Fowler's solution: see *Arsenic.*

Furosemide (Lasix): urticaria, rarely exfoliative dermatitis, bullous-pemphigoidlike eruption, erythema multiforme, pruritus.

Gold: morbilliform or lichenoid eruptions, pityriasis-rosealike eruptions, erythema nodosum, vaginal pruritus, and hyperpigmentation. Pruritus may be severe and intractable. Reinstitution of therapy at lower doses may be possible after a skin reaction.

Griseofulvin: angioedema, burning, cold urticaria, erythema multiforme, exfoliative dermatitis, morbilliform erythema, petechiae, photosensitivity, porphyria cutanea tarda, pruritus, SLE-like syndrome, urticaria.

Heparin: alopecia, intense pruritus, skin necrosis.

Hexachlorobenzene: porphyria cutanea tarda.

Hydantoin: see *Diphenylhydantoin.*

Hydralazine: erythema multiforme, fixed eruption, SLE-like dermatitis.

Hydrochlorothiazide: photoallergy, erythema, lichen-planuslike dermatitis, papules, papulovesicles, petechiae, purpura, thrombocytopenic purpura, vesicles.

Imipramine: petechiae, urticaria, photosensitization.

Insulin: lipodystrophy, morbilliform erythema, pruritus, urticaria.

Iodides: acneiform eruption, bullae, erythema multiforme, erythema nodosum, eyelid edema, fixed eruption, follicular pustules, fungating nodules (pseudolymphoma), furuncles, pruritus, purpura, urticaria.

Ipecac: fixed eruption.

Isonicotinic hydrazide (INH): acneiform eruption, erythema, purpura, urticaria.

Karaya gum: fixed eruption.

Levodopa: seborrheic dermatitislike rash, alopecia.

Lead: contact allergy (hair dye), pigmentation.

Lithium: acneiform eruption, aggravation of psoriasis.

Menthol: chronic urticaria.

Meperidine: urticaria.

Mephenytoin (Mesantoin): alopecia, edema, exfoliative dermatitis, gum hyperplasia, pseudolymphoma, morbilliform erythema, skin pigmentation, purpura, scarlatiniform erythema, Stevens-Johnson syndrome.

Mephenesin carbamate: lightens hair color.

Mephobarbital (Mebroin): gum hypertrophy, hirsutism, SLE-like dermatitis.

Meprobamate: anaphylactic reaction, angioedema, erythema, fixed eruption (cross reaction with carisoprodol), lichen-planuslike dermatitis, maculopapular morbilliform erythema, purpura, urticaria, vesicles.

Mercury: acrodynia, bullae, calomel disease, blotchy erythema, erythema multiforme, exfoliative dermatitis, fixed eruption, folliculitis, granuloma morbilliform erythema, erythredema, polyneuritis, painful edema of extremities, petechiae, pigmentation, scarlatiniform erythema, stomatitis, urticaria, vesicles.

Methenamine: fixed eruption.

Methimazole: urticaria.

Methotrexate: alopecia, stomatitis.

Methsuximide: SLE-like dermatitis.

Methyclothiazide: purpura, photosensitivity, urticaria, cutaneous vasculitis.

Minocycline: conjunctival, oral, cutaneous, nail, and dental pigmentation.

Morphine and opium: erythema, fixed eruption, morbilliform erythema, pruritus, scarlatiniform erythema, urticaria.

Nadisan: edema, erythema, papules, papulovesicles, photosensitivity.

Nafoxidine: maculopapular eruption.

Nalidixic acid: erythema, photoallergy, pruritus, urticaria.

Naproxen: phototoxic eruption.

Nicotinic acid: acanthosis-nigricanslike dermatitis, erythema.

Nitrofurantoin (Furadantin): alopecia, anaphylactic reaction, eczema, erythema, maculopapular erythema, pruritus, toxic epidermal necrolysis, urticaria, SLE syndrome.

Nonsteroidal antiinflammatory agents: urticarial and morbilliform eruptions, bullous fixed drug eruptions, bullous erythema multiforme, toxic epidermal necrolysis, vasculitis, and photosensitivity reactions.

Novobiocin: jaundice; morbilliform and scarlatiniform erythemas.

Para-aminosalicylic acid (PAS): anaphylactic reaction, jaundice, urticaria.

Paramethadione: acneiform eruption, alopecia, erythema multiforme, exfoliative dermatitis, SLE-like dermatitis.

Penicillamine: loss of taste, GI upsets, stomatitis, proteinuria, thrombocytopenia, leukopenia, morbilliform or urticarial rash, pruritus; purpura, acquired epidermolysis bullosa, elastosis perforans, pemphigus, SLE-like eruption.

Penicillin: anaphylactic reaction, angioedema, black hairy tongue, glossitis, ecchymosis, edema, erythema multiforme, erythema nodosum, exfoliative dermatitis, fixed eruptions, morbilliform erythema, papules, pruritus, purpura, scarlatiniform erythema, toxic epidermal necrolysis, urticaria, vesicles.

Pentaerythritol tetranitrate: fixed eruption.

Phenacetin: angioedema, erythema, fixed eruption.

Phenantoin: SLE-like dermatitis.

Phenazopyridine: yellowish pigmentation of the skin with acute renal failure.

Phenindione: exfoliative dermatitis, morbilliform erythema, stomatitis.

Phenobarbital: bullae on genitals, generalized erythema, erosive lesions in mouth, erythema multiforme, exfoliative dermatitis, fixed eruption, hyperpigmentation, jaundice, morbilliform erythema, pruritus, scarlatiniform erythema, Stevens-Johnson syndrome, stomatitis, urticaria.

Phenolphthalein: bullae, erythema multiforme bullosum, photoallergy, fixed eruption, pruritus, scarlatiniform erythema, stomatitis, toxic epidermal necrolysis.

Phenothiazine: erythema multiforme, exfoliative dermatitis, fixed eruption, hyperpigmentation and cataracts, photosensitivity, urticaria.

Phenylbutazone: generalized erythema, exfoliative dermatitis, fixed eruption, toxic epidermal necrolysis, urticaria.

Pilocarpine: erythema, urticaria.

Piroxicam: phototoxic eruption, vesiculobullous eruption, maculopapular dermatitis.

Pituitary extract (anterior lobe): anaphylactic reaction, morbilliform erythema.

Poliomyelitis vaccine (Salk): eczema, psoriasiform eruption, urticaria.

Polyvinylpyrrolidone (PVP): cutaneous storage disease (thesaurismosis).

Potassium chlorate: fixed eruption.

Potassium mercury iodide: hand dermatitis.

Potassium sulfocyanate: erythema, exfoliative dermatitis.

Practolol: corneal perforation, eczema, lichen-planuslike eruption, SLE syndrome, hyperkeratosis of palms and soles, psoriasis or pustular psoriasis.

Procaine: erythema multiforme, pruritus, urticaria.

Promazine: see *Phenothiazine.*

Promethazine: bullae, edema, maculopapules, morbilliform erythema, petechiae, urticaria.

Propantheline bromide: dryness of mouth, exfoliative dermatitis, maculopapular erythema, vesicles.

Propranolol: erythematous eruption, psoriasis or pustular psoriasis.

Quinacrine, quinidine, quinine: bullae, cocktail purpura, dyschromia, eczematous lesions, erythema, fixed eruption, gangrene, extensive lichen-planuslike eruption, nail fluorescence, golden yellow pigmentation, pruritus, photoallergy.

Quinidine: light-induced livedo reticularis, photodermatitis.

Reserpine: erythema, fixed eruption, petechiae, photoallergy, purpura, necrotizing angiitis, urticaria.

Saccharin: fixed eruption, urticaria.

Salicylates: erythema multiforme, erythema nodosum, fixed eruption, purpura, urticaria.

Scopolamine: acneiform eruption, allergic contact dermatitis, hallucinations.

Septra: see *Trimethoprim.*

Serum, animal: bullae, morbilliform and scarlatiniform erythema, eyelid edema, urticaria.

Silver, silver salts: argyria pigmentation.

Streptomycin: erythema, erythema multiforme, exfoliative dermatitis, fixed eruption, morbilliform erythema, pigmentation, pruritus, stomatitis, urticaria.

Succinylcholine: anaphylactic reaction.

Sulfadiazine: Stevens-Johnson syndrome, fixed drug eruption.

Sulfathiazole: erythema nodosum, Stevens-Johnson syndrome, toxic epidermal necrolysis.

Sulfbromophthalein: anaphylactic reaction.

Sulfonamides. Thiazide diuretics and antihypertensives are included, since they are substituted sulfonamides and

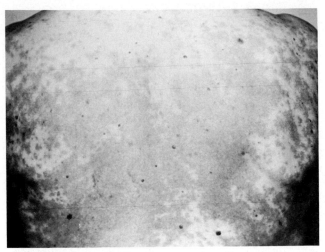

***Figure 6–18.** Morbilliform drug eruption due to sulfonamide. (Courtesy of Dr. Axel W. Hoke.)*

share many features with them. They can produce all the usual types of drug eruption, and in addition may cause photosensitivity reactions.

Sulfonylurea: photoallergy.

Tartar emetic: fixed eruption.

Tetracaine: anaphylactic reaction.

Tetracyclines: Ordinary drug eruptions are rare with these. However, vesicular fixed drug eruptions (often of the glans penis) and phototoxicity reactions, including photo-onycholysis, are relatively frequent, especially with demeclocycline (Declomycin) and doxycycline (Vibramycin). Pseudoporphyria (J. Epstein) has occurred. Permanent staining of teeth may occur if tetracyclines are taken before full adult dentition is achieved, and minocycline (Minocin) may pigment the oral mucosa, nails, gums, conjunctiva, areas of inflammation, sun-exposed areas, or scars.

Tetraethylthiuram: fixed eruption.

Tetraiodofluorescein: fixed eruption.

Thiamine chloride: erythema, pruritus, and dermatitis simulating scabies, urticaria.

Thiazide: lichen-planuslike eruption, purpura, photoallergy.

Thiouracil: erythema, exfoliative dermatitis, hair loss, jaundice, stomatitis.

Thiouracil derivatives: alopecia, jaundice, polyarteritis nodosa, pigmentation (yellowish hair), pruritus, urticaria.

Tiaprofenic acid: phototoxic eruption.

Tocopherol: folliculitis, dermatitis.

Tolbutamide: photoallergy, urticaria.

Triazinate (Antifol): acanthosis-nigricanslike pigmentation.

Trichlormethiazide: erythema, lichen-planuslike eruption, papules, papulovesicles, petechiae, purpura, vesicles.

Tridione: erythema multiforme, morbilliform erythema.

Triethylenemelamine: maculopapular erythema, pruritus.

Trimethadione: SLE-like dermatitis, Stevens-Johnson syndrome.

Trimethoprim-sulfamethoxazole: morbilliform rash, Stevens-Johnson syndrome, TEN, SLE-like syndrome; fever; leucopenia, hepatitis, thrombopenia. Incidence ×10 in AIDS.

Vermouth: fixed eruption.

Vinblastine: alopecia.

Vitamin E.: see *Tocopherol.*

DRUG ERUPTIONS ACCORDING TO REACTIONS

Acanthosis-nigricanslike eruption: isonicotinic hydrazide, nicotinic acid, triazinate (Antifol).

Acneiform eruption: bromides, chloral hydrate, corticotropin (ACTH), corticosteroids, iodides, isonicotinic hydrazide (INH), phenytoin, scopolamine, lithium.

Acrodynia: mercury.

Albinism: chloroquine, monobenzone (Benoquin).

Alopecia: chlorambucil, colchicine, coumarin, desacetylmethylcolchicine, gold, heparin, methotrexate, thallium, thiouracil derivatives, vitamin A.

Anaphylactic reaction: acetylsalicylic acid, ACTH, allergen extracts, aminopyrine, cephalosporins, chymotrypsin, furaltadone, meprobamate, mercurial diuretics, opiates, para-aminosalicylic acid, penicillin, pituitary extract, procaine, radiocontrast media, succinylcholine, sulfbromophthalein, tetracaine, tetracycline, thiouracil.

Angiitis, necrotizing: bishydroxycoumarin (Dicumarol).

Angioedema: cinchophen, meprobamate, penicillin, stilbestrol, sulfonamides.

Argyria: silver salts.

Arteritis: cyclobarbital, chlorpromazine, iodides, methyl thiouracil, phenylbutazone, phenytoin, poison ivy extract, sulfonamides, thiouracil.

Black hairy tongue: tetracycline, penicillin, methyldopa.

Bowen's disease: arsenic, Fowler's solution.

Bullae: acetylsalicylic acid, antipyrines, arsenic, barbiturates, bromides, chloral hydrate, chlorpromazine, cinchophen, coumarin, Dilantin, hydantoin derivatives, iodide, Mesantoin, phenobarbital, promethazine, sodium thiosulfate, sulfamethoxypyridazine, sulfonamides, tetracycline.

Burning: griseofulvin.

Candidiasis: tetracyclines.

Cocktail purpura: quinine water.

Cyanosis: acetanilide.

Depigmentation: chloroquine.

Dermatitis: benzocaine, chloral hydrate, methaminodiazepoxide, procaine.

Dermatomyositis: acetylsalicylic acid.

Dyschromia: amiodarone, amodiaquine, cancer chemotherapy regimens, chloroquine, estrogen, Minocin, quinacrine.

Dyshidrosis: acetylsalicylic acid, salicylates.

Ecchymosis: corticosteroids, coumarin, sulfamethoxypyridazine.

Edema: arsenic, chlorpromazine, nadisan, penicillin, phenytoin, promethazine.

Edema, transient: chloroquine.

Erythema: antipyrines, arsenic, aurothioglucose, barbiturates, bendroflumethiazide, chloral hydrate, chlorothiazide, chlorpropamide, cinchophen, codeine, corticotropin, gold, griseofulvin, hydrochlorothiazide, isonicotinic acid, meprobamate, methaminodiazepoxide, morphine, nadisan, nicotinic acid, opium, penicillin, phenobarbital, pilocarpine, quinacrine, quinidine, quinine, streptomycin, trimethoprim-sulfamethoxazole, thiamine chloride, tolbutamide, trichlormethiazide.

Erythema annulare centrifugum: cimetidine, chloroquine, estrogen, hydroxychloroquine, penicillin, piroxicam, progesterone, salicylates.

Erythema multiforme: acetazolamide, acetylsalicylic acid, amidopyrine, antihistaminics, antipyrines, barbiturates, bromides, chloral hydrate, griseofulvin, iodides, mercury, para-aminosalicyclic acid, penicillin, phenobarbital, phe-

nolphthalein, phenothiazine, phenylbutazone, procaine, rifampin, salicylates, sulfapyridine, trimethoprim-sulfamethoxazole, sulfonamides.

Erythema nodosum: acetylsalicylic acid, bromides, iodides, oral contraceptives, penicillin, salicylates, sulfathiazole.

Exfoliative dermatitis: allopurinol, actinomycin D, aminosalicylic acid, arsenicals, arsphenamine, aurothioglucose, barbiturates, bismuth, carbamazepine, chloroquine, chlorpromazine, gold, griseofulvin, iodides, mercury, mesantoin, penicillin, phenindione, phenobarbital, phenothiazines, phenylbutazone, phenytoin, potassium sulfocyanate, quinidine, quinacrine, sodium thiosulfate, stilbestrol, streptomycin, trimethoprim-sulfamethoxazole, sulfonamides, tetracycline, thiouracil, vitamin A.

Fixed eruption: acetaminophen, acetanilide, aminopyrine, amphetamines, anovulatory agents, antihistaminics, antimony compounds, antipyrines, arsenic, barbiturates, belladonna, bismuth, bromides, chloral hydrate, chlordiazepoxide, chloroquine, 8-chlorotheophylline, cinchophen, codeine, diaminodiphenylsulfone (dapsone), diethylstilbestrol, digitalis, emetine, ephedrine, ergot, ethchlorvynol, gold salts, hydantoin, hydralazine, iodides, ipecac, karaya gum, meprobamate, mercury, methenamine, morphine, nystatin, opium, para-aminosalicylic acid, penicillin, pentaerythritol tetranitrate, phenacetin, phenolphthalein, phenothiazine, phenobarbital, phenylbutazone, potassium chlorate, quinacrine, quinidine, quinine, rauwolfia, reserpine, saccharin, salicylates, streptomycin, sulfonamides, tartar emetic, tetracyclines, tetraethylthiuram, tetraiodofluorescein, vermouth.

Gangrene: coumarin.

Granulomas: injected DPT vaccines prepared with aluminum hydroxide; mercury.

Hair color changes: carbamate, chloroquine, chlorpromazine, mephenesin.

Hand dermatitis: acetylsalicylic acid.

Hemolysis. Dark urine, pallor, or weakness and dyspnea may herald a hemolytic reaction after a few days' use of sulfones (dapsone), sulfonamides, phenylhydrazine, acetanilide, p-aminosalicylic acid, acetylsalicylic acid, or nitrofurantoin. The reaction almost always occurs, and is most likely to be severe, in patients who have inherited a deficiency in glucose 6-phosphate dehydrogenase. This deficiency can be identified by a simple test, but its routine use has low cost-effectiveness, and small initial doses and close attention to the color of the urine will serve to nip the disorder in the bud. Persons of African or Mediterranean origin are most at risk, and it would be reasonable to limit testing to them.

Hirsutism: acetazolamide, cyclosporin.

Jaundice: aurothioglucose, erythromycin lauryl sulfate, novobiocin, para-aminosalicylic acid, phenobarbital, thiouracil.

Keratoderma: gold.

Keratoses: arsenic, Fowler's solution, gold.

Lenticular opacity: phenothiazine, trifluoperazine, steroids by mouth.

Leukokeratosis: gold.

Lichenoid eruption: beta blockers, captopril, chloroquine, chlorothiazide, gold, hydrochlorothiazide, meprobamate, para-aminosalicyclic acid, quinacrine, thiazides, trichlormethiazide, practolol.

Livedo reticularis, photosensitive: quinidine.

Maculopapular rash: allopurinol, chloroquine, meprobamate, penicillin, piroxicam, promethazine, streptomycin, trimethoprim-sulfamethoxazole.

Morbilliform erythema: acetylsalicylic acid, ampicillin,

barbiturates, benzodiazepines, bromides, chlorpromazine, erythromycin, gentamicin, griseofulvin, gold salts, insulin, meprobamate, novobiocin, penicillin, phenindione, promethazine, salicylates, streptomycin.

Nail changes: amodiaquin (hyperpigmentation), arsenic (transverse white stripes), argyria (dark blue nail bed), chloroquine (blue-black nail bed), 5-FU and other cancer chemotherapeutic agents (dark or white stripes or "shoreline" transverse grooves), minocycline (pigmentation), phenolphthalein (dark blue fixed eruption), tetracycline (yellow nail and yellow fluorescence), demethylchlortetracycline (phototoxic onychomadesis), Zidovudine.

Nodules: iodides.

Ochronosislike pigmentation: phenol, quinacrine, resorcin, hydroquinone.

Onycholysis: demethylchlortetracycline plus sunburn.

Papular dermatitis: acetazolamide, acetylsalicylic acid, arsenic, aurothioglucose, benzydroflumethazide, chlorothiazide, digitalis, hydrochlorothiazide, nadisan, penicillin, trichlormethiazide.

Papulovesicles: bendroflumethiazide, chlorothiazide, hydrochlorothiazide, trichlormethiazide.

Pemphigoidlike eruption: phenacetin, lasix, perhaps others.

Pemphigus, pemphigus erythematosus: penicillamine, captopril.

Petechiae: chlorpromazine, chlorothiazide, corticosteroids, coumarin, griseofulvin, hydrochlorothiazide, promethazine, reserpine, sulfonamides, trichlormethiazide.

Photoallergy: chlorothiazide, chlorpromazine, chlorpropamide, demethychlortetracycline, griseofulvin, nadisan, nalidixic acid, phenothiazine, piroxicam, promethazine, quinidine, reserpine, sulfonamides, sulfonylureas, tetracyclines, tolbutamide.

Phototoxicity: chlorpromazine, demethylchlortetracycline, griseofulvin, methoxsalen, nalidixic acid, naproxen, piroxicam, sulfonamides, tetracycline, tiaprofenic acid, trimethyl psoralen.

Pigmentation: ACTH, amiodarone, antimalarials, antipyrines, arsenic, bismuth (gums), camoquin, chlorpromazine (slate-colored), clofazimine, gold (melanoderma, chrysiasis), lead, mercury, minocycline, oral contraceptives, phenothiazine (slate-colored and purple), psoralens, silver (metallic blue), streptomycin, tetracyclines, thiouracil, triazinate (Antifol, Baker).

Pityriasis rosealike eruptions: arsenicals, barbiturates, bismuth, captopril, clonidine, gold, methoxypromazine, metronidazole, tripelennamine hydrochloride.

Polyarteritis nodosa (vasculitis): sulfonamides, thiouracil iodides.

Porphyria: barbiturates, chloroquine, estrogens, griseofulvin, hexachlorobenzene, barbiturates, estrogens.

Pruritus: atropine, aurothioglucose, barbiturates, belladonna, bismuth, codeine, coumarin, gold (intense), griseofulvin, heparin, insulin, iodide, morphine, penicillin, phenobarbital, procaine, quinacrine, streptomycin, tetracyclines, thiamine chloride, thiouracil.

Pruritus ani: chloroquine, codeine, liver extract, tetracyclines.

Purple toes: coumarin.

Purpura: ACTH, allopurinol, barbiturates, bendroflumethiazide, carbromal, chloroform, chlorothiazide, corticosteroids, coumarin, ephedrine, hydrochlorothiazide, iodide, meprobamate, mercury, penicillin, quinidine, quinine water, sodium thiosulfate, trimethoprim-sulfamethoxazole, sulfonamides, thiazides, trichlormethiazide.

Purpura fulminans: acetylsalicylic acid, coumarin, iodides.

Pustular psoriasis: acetylsalicylic acid, antimalarials, atenolol, poliomyelitis vaccine, propranolol.

Pustules: bromides, chloral hydrate, iodides.

Scaling patches: acetylsalicylic acid, codeine, gold, penicillin, quinine.

Scarlatiniform erythema: barbiturates, cinchophen, mercury, morphine, novobiocin, opium, penicillin, phenobarbital, pituitary extract, quinine, salicylates, streptomycin, sulfonamides.

Serum sickness: ATG, cephalosporins, dextrans, hydralazine, penicillins, phenylbutazone, sulfonamides, thiouracils.

"Shoreline nails": Severe drug eruptions caused by cefitoxin sodium (Mefoxin), dicloxacillin (Dynapen), allopurinol (Zyloprim, Lopurin), or codeine—or, presumably almost any drug—may cause transient arrest of nail growth, with resultant transverse bands of leuconychia followed by an irregular transverse rough ridge-and-groove to which the Shelleys have given the expressive name of "shoreline" nails.

SLE-like syndrome: chlorpromazine, griseofulvin, hydantoin, hydralazine, isoniazid, isonicotinic hydrazide, mephobarbital, methsuximide, paramethadione, penicillamine, phenantoin, phenytoin, procainamide, sulfasalazine, trimethoprim-sulfamethoxazole, tetracycline HCl (degraded), trimethadione.

Stevens-Johnson syndrome: amithiozone (thiacetazone), antipyrines, barbiturates, chloroquine, chlorpropamide, cough mixtures, lithium, meprobamate, phenacetin, phenobarbital, phenytoin, sulfadiazine, sulfadimethoxine, sulfamerazine, trimethoprim-sulfamethoxazole, sulfathiazole, sulfonamides, trimethadione.

Stomatitis: aurothioglucose, bismuth, chlorpromazine, cinchophen, Dilantin (gingivitis), fluorides, Mesantoin, methotrexate, phenobarbital, streptomycin, thiouracil.

Thesaurismosis: polyvinylpyrrolidine (PVP).

Thrombocytopenic purpura: chlorothiazide, hydrochlorothiazide, thiouracil.

Toxic epidermal necrolysis: acetazolamide, allopurinol, aminopyrine, antihistaminics, antipyrines, barbiturates, boric acid powder, brompheniramine, carbamazepine, chloramphenicol, dapsone, Fansidar, gold salts, methyl salicylate, nitrofurantoin, NSAIDs, penicillin, phenolphthalein, phenylbutazone, phenytoin, salicylates, polio vaccine, sulfonamides, tetracyclines, tolbutamide, trimethoprim-sulfamethoxazole.

Urticaria: acetylsalicylic acid (aspirin), allopurinol, aminoglycosides, antimony, antipyrines, barbiturates, blood products, chloral hydrate, chlorpromazine, corticotropin (ACTH), eucalyptus, fluorides, gold, griseofulvin (cold urticaria), hydantoins, hydralazine, insulin, iodides, menthol, meprobamate, mercury, morphine, NSAIDs, opium, para-aminosalicylic acid, penicillin, phenacetin, phenobarbital, phenylbutazone, pilocarpine, polio vaccine, potassium sulfocyanate, procaine, promethazine, quinidine, quinine, reserpine, saccharin, sulfonamides, thiamine chloride, thiouracil.

Vasculitis: allopurinol, chlorpromazine, cimetidine, clindamycin, cyclobarbital, methylthiouracil, penicillins, phenylbutazone, phenytoin, sulfonamides, thiouracil.

Vesicles: acetylsalicylic acid, aurothioglucose, bendroflumethiazide, bromide, chlorothiazide, hydrochlorothiazide, meprobamate, nadisan, piroxicam, trichlormethiazide.

Alanko K, et al: Topical provocation of fixed drug eruptions. Br J Dermatol 1987, 116:561.

Barnett JH, et al: Lichenoid reactions to chlorpropamide and tolazamide. Cutis 1984, 34:542.

Bencini PL, et al: Cutaneous lesions in 67 cyclosporin treated renal transplant recipients. Dermatologica 1986, 172:24.

Idem: Drug-induced cutaneous reactions. JAMA 1986, 256:3358.

Berger TG, et al: Quinidine-induced lichenoid photodermatitis. Cutis 1982, 29:585.

Bigby M, et al: Cutaneous reactions to nonsteroidal anti-inflammatory drugs. JAAD 1985, 12:866.

Idem: Drug-induced cutaneous reactions. JAMA 1986, 256:3358.

Bonner AK, et al: Cutaneous complications of chemotherapeutic agents. JAAD 1983, 9:645.

Brothers DM, et al: Conjunctival pigmentation associated with tetracycline. Ophthalmology 1981, 88:1212.

Bruce S, et al: Quinidine-induced photosensitive livedo-reticularis-like eruption. JAAD 1985, 12:232.

Chalmers A, et al: Systemic lupus erythematosus during penicillamine therapy for rheumatoid arthritis. Ann Intern Med 1982, 97:659.

Crider MR, et al: Chemotherapy induced acral erythema in patients receiving bone marrow transplantation. Arch Dermatol 1986, 122:1023.

Daniel F, et al: Captopril drug eruptions. Ann Dermatol Venereol 1983, 110:441.

Davis RL, et al: The "red man" syndrome and slow infusion vancomycin. Ann Intern Med 1986, 104:285.

Diffey BL, et al: Phototoxic reactions to prioxicam, naproxen, and tiaprofenic acid. Br J Rheumatol 1983, 22:239.

Foster CA, et al: Propranolol-epinephrine interaction. Plast Reconstr Surg 1983, 72:74.

Furness P, et al: Severe cutaneous reactions to captopril and enalapril. J Clin Pathol 1986, 39:902.

Gaspari AA, et al: Dermatologic changes associated with interleukin-2 administration. JAMA 1987, 258:1624.

Gordin FM, et al: Adverse reactions to trimethoprim-sulfamethoxazole in patients with AIDS. Ann Intern Med 1984, 100:495.

Granstein RO, et al: Drug- and heavy metal-induced hyperpigmentation. JAAD 1981, 5:1.

Greenspan AH, et al: Acanthosis nigricans-like hyperpigmentation secondary to Triazinate therapy. Arch Dermatol 1985, 121:232.

Guin JD: Complications of topical hydrocortisone. JAAD 1981, 4:417.

Hogan DJ, et al: Lichenoid stomatitis associated with lithium carbonate. JAAD 1985, 13:243.

Holdiness MR: Adverse cutaneous reactions to antituberculosis drugs. Int J Dermatol 1985, 24:280.

Insley BM, et al: Thallium poisoning in cocaine abusers. Am J Emerg Med 1986, 4:545.

Kashihara M, et al: Bullous-pemphigoid-like lesions induced by phenacetin. Arch Dermatol 1984, 120:1196.

Khalsa JH, et al: Cimetidine-associated alopecia. Int J Dermatol 1983, 22:202.

Korkij W, et al: Fixed drug eruption. Arch Dermatol 1983, 120:520.

Lambert WC, et al: Leucoytoclastic angiitis induced by clindamycin. Cutis 1982, 30:615.

Lasser EC, et al: Pretreatment with corticosteroids to alleviate reactions to intravenous contrast material. N Engl J Med 1987, 317:845.

Lokich JJ, et al: Chemotherapy-associated palmar-plantar dysesthesia syndrome. Ann Intern Med 1984, 101:798.

Marx JL, et al: Quinidine photosensitivity. Arch Dermatol 1982, 119:39.

Poliak SC, et al: Minocycline-induced tooth discoloration in young adults. JAMA 1985, 254:2930.

Reed BR, et al: Subacute cutaneous lupus erythematosus with hydrochlorthiazide therapy. Ann Intern Med 1985, 103:49.

Ridgway HA: Hyperpigmentation associated with oral minocycline. Br J Dermatol 1982, 107:95.

Rosen T, et al: Vesicular Jarisch-Herxheimer reaction. Arch Dermatol 1989, 125:77.

Sehgal VH, et al: Genital fixed drug eruptions. Genitourin Med 1986, 62:56.

Shelley WB, et al: Shoreline nails: Sign of drug-induced erythroderma. Cutis 1985, 27:222.

Silverman AK, et al: Cutaneous and immunologic reactions to phenytoin. JAAD 1988, 18:721.

Slagel GA, et al: Plaquenil-induced erythroderma. JAAD 1985, 12:857.

Stern RS, et al: An expanded profile of cutaneous reactions to nonsteroidal antiinflammatory drugs. JAMA 1984, 252:1433.

Stricker H, et al: Heparin-induced skin neurosis. Am J Med 1988, 85:721.

Strieker BHC, et al: Skin reactions to terfenadine. Br Med J 1986, 293:536.

VanArsdel PP Jr: Allergy and adverse drug reactions. JAAD 1982, 6:833.

Wintroub BU, Stern R: Cutaneous drug reactions: Pathogenesis and clinical classification. JAAD 1985, 13:167.

Yung CW, et al: D-penicillamine-induced pemphigus syndrome. JAAD 1982, 6:317.

Zamora-Quezada JC, et al: Muscle and skin infarction after freebasing cocaine. Ann Intern Med 1988, 108:564.

Acrodynia

Also known as calomel disease, pink disease, and erythredemic polyneuropathy, it is caused by mercury poisoning, usually in infancy.

The skin changes are outstandingly characteristic and almost pathognomonic. They consist of painful swelling of the hands and feet, sometimes associated with considerable itching of these parts. The hands and feet are also cold, clammy, and pink or dusky red. The erythema is usually blotchy but may be diffuse. Hemorrhagic puncta are frequently evident. Over the trunk a blotchy macular or papular erythema is usually present. Stomatitis and loss of teeth may occur. The review by Dinehart et al in 1988 was excellent.

Constitutional symptoms consist of moderate fever, irritability, marked photophobia, increased perspiration, and a tendency to cry most of the time. There is always moderate upper respiratory infection with soreness of the throat.

There may be hypertension, hypertonia, anorexia, and insomnia.

The diagnosis is made by finding over 0.001 mg of mercury per liter of urine. Albuminuria and hematuria are usually present.

The ingestion or inhalation of mercury used in some house paints has caused acrodynia. Calomel ingestion in prior times was a common cause. The use of mercury ointments and mercurial preparations has also been implicated. Acrodynia occurs in infants and children only.

Treatment is directed to the elimination of the mercury from the system. Hirschman and his associates reported excellent results with the use of N-acetyl-D,L-penicillamine. Javett also treated an eight-month-old child with D-penicillamine, with excellent results.

Dinehart SM, et al: Cutaneous manifestations of acrodynia (pink disease). Arch Dermatol 1988, 124:107.

Javett SN, et al: Acrodynia treated with penicillamine. Am J Dis Child 1968, 115:71.

Arsenism

Systemic exposure to inorganic pentavalent arsenic may result in acute or chronic arsenic poisoning.

The acute type is due to a hypersensitivity and may occur in a short time with only a minimal exposure.

Acute Arsenical Dermatitis. The signs and symptoms of acute arsenism are generalized erythematous papular, pustular, and bullous eruptions that may become erythema multiforme bullosum or exfoliative dermatitis. This type occurred frequently when organic arsenic (Mapharsen, arsphenamine) was used to treat syphilis.

Systemic involvement may be manifested by abdominal pain, diarrhea, painful extremities, fever, and edema of the eyelids, feet and hands.

Chronic Arsenism. When arsenic was taken in fairly small doses for months or years, as with Fowler's solution or Asiatic pills, the reaction did not become apparent clinically for a decade or more after stopping the drug.

The late lesions are due to the stimulation of epithelial hyperplasia, with the formation of *arsenical keratoses,* chiefly on the palms and soles but elsewhere too. Invasive or noninvasive basal or squamous cell carcinomas may also develop, either from the keratoses or from apparently normal skin. Pigmented basal cell carcinomas on covered areas are especially significant. The keratoses are especially

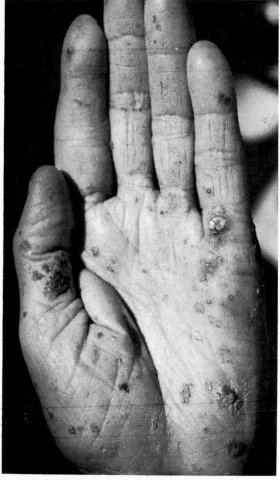

Figure 6–20. Arsenical keratoses on hands caused by inorganic arsenic in drinking water. (Courtesy of Dr. A. Kaminsky, Buenos Aires.)

prominent about sweat pores. Small, black, shiny pegs of keratin are mounted in the pores and, when picked out, leave pits.

When multiple basal cell carcinomas develop on the trunk there is a great likelihood of a history of arsenic ingestion. Many of the tumors are pigmented. Domonkos has removed 700 carcinomas in one patient who took Fowler's solution for his psoriasis for many years. He died from carcinoma of the gastrointestinal tract.

Arsenical carcinomas may develop not only in the gastrointestinal tract but also in the larynx and genitourinary system.

Arsenical melanosis is characterized by black, generalized pigmentation or by only a pronounced hyperpigmentation confined to the trunk, with depigmented scattered macules on the trunk that resemble raindrops. The hyperpigmentation is believed to be due to arsenic's combining with sulfhydryl groups in the epidermis, which simulates the oxidation of tyrosine to DOPA.

Transverse white striations in the fingernails (*Mee's lines*) may appear.

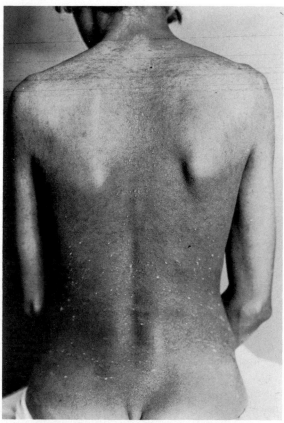

Figure 6–19. Acute arsenical dermatitis.

It is believed that only pentavalent inorganic arsenic is capable of producing chronic arsenism. This type of arsenic was used medicinally as Fowler's solution (solution of potassium arsenite) for the empirical treatment of psoriasis, epilepsy, asthma, hay fever, and atopic dermatitis.

Endemic arsenism occurs in several areas of the world where the drinking water supply and soil contain large quantities of arsenic, such as Cordoba, a region in Argentina, and the pampas. Another endemic area is on the southwest coast of Taiwan. In a population of 40,000, the skin cancer rate was 10 per 10,000. The drinking water is drawn from artesian wells with a high arsenic concentration.

Normal excretion of arsenic in the urine is in the range of 0.005 to 0.04 mg per day. Acute or subacute poisoning will produce an excess of 0.1 mg per day. The nails and hair tend to store arsenic. The normal amount in hair is about 0.008 to 0.025 mg per 100 gm, with 0.1 mg being indicative of the presence of excess arsenic.

Biagini RE: Chronic arseniasis from water and lung cancer. Arch Argent Dermatol 1966, 16:172.
Domonkos AN: Neutron activation analysis of arsenic in normal skin, keratoses, and epithelioma. Arch Dermatol 1959, 80:672.
Evans S: Arsenic and cancer. Br J Dermatol 1977, 97 (suppl 15):13.
Reymann JH, et al: Relationship between arsenic intake and internal malignant neoplasms. Arch Dermatol 1978, 114:378.

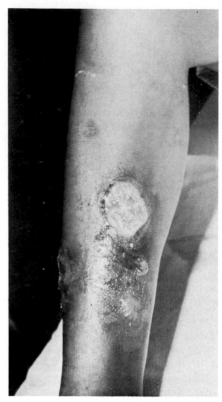

Figure 6–21. Bromide eruption on shin; bullae and granulomas.

Bromoderma

Bromides commonly produce distinctive follicular eruptions. The most common eruption is acneiform, with inflammatory pustules in the hairy parts of the body as well as on the butterfly area of the face, where it must be differentiated from rosacea.

Vesicular lesions and bullae are common in bromoderma. Nodular lesions with a violaceous color not infrequently are mistaken for a malignant lymphoma of the skin; indeed, the histopathologic findings of such lesions may also be suggestive of lymphoma. There is rapid involution of the lesions upon cessation of bromide ingestion. A thick inflammatory plaque, with pustules in its border, resembling blastomycosis, may also occur.

Bromoderma may occur after a small dose or after protracted use of bromides. A small child suffered fatal bromoderma as a result of one 50-mg dose of methacholine bromide by injection. Nursing mothers may transmit bromides in their milk.

Plasma bromide levels in bromoderma have been found to vary from 25 to 400 mg per 100 ml. A level of 75 mg per 100 ml is suggestive of bromism; however, no correlation seems to exist between plasma levels and the severity of cutaneous lesions.

Treatment of bromoderma is simply cessation of bromide ingestion. In acute intoxication 2 to 4 gm of sodium chloride by mouth, taken daily, rapidly replaces the bromide in body fluids. Ammonium chloride is also helpful. In severe cases of intoxication in which the patient is badly confused, ethacrynic acid rapidly decreases the bromide level, with clearing of the lesions.

Burnett JW: Iodides and bromides. Cutis 1989, 43:130.

Iododerma

Iodides cause a wide variety of skin eruptions. The most common type is the acneiform eruption with numerous acutely inflamed follicular pustules, each surrounded by a ring of hyperemia.

Bullous lesions are also common and may become ulcerated and crusted. Vegetative or fungating nodules typical of iodism are frequently mistaken for malignant lymphoma (pseudolymphoma) or even for basal cell carcinoma. Pruritus and urticaria may be the only manifestations of mild iodism. Purpura, furuncles, erythema multiforme, erythema nodosum, and polyarteritis nodosa may also occur. Swelling, redness, and scaling of the eyelids are frequently encountered.

Acne vulgaris and rosacea are unfavorably affected by iodides, which are commonly found in iodized

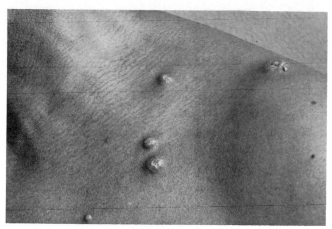

Figure 6–22. Iododerma.

salt and seafoods, especially shellfish. Hypersensitivity to iodides does not seem to be dose-dependent. Treatment is the same as for bromoderma.

Boudonlas O, et al: Iododerma occupying after orally administered topanic acid. Arch Dermatol 1987, 123:387.

Polyvinylpyrrolidone (PVP) Storage

Chapuis and his associates have reported cutaneous intracellular deposits of PVP resembling Letterer-Siwe reticulosis. A 45-year-old man with diabetes insipidus took an antidiuretic medication containing PVP for 14 years. The cutaneous manifestation consisted of a palm-sized pink plaque with a slightly elevated and infiltrated border. Histologically, there were large, oval cells suggestive of Letterer-Siwe reticulosis. In the middle dermis foamy Touton giant cells as well as empty cavities were

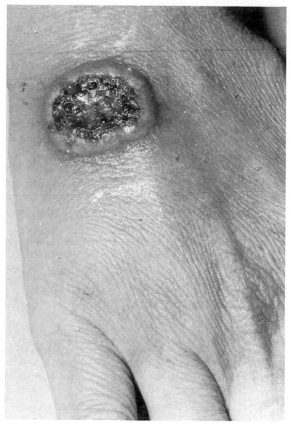

Figure 6–24. Iododerma. Only brief duration distinguishes it clinically from basal cell carcinoma.

found. The PVP in this tissue was demonstrated by impregnation with hemalumphloxine-safranin and staining with chlorazal-fast pink B, which gives a brown-violet stain.

Chloroquine

This antimalarial is prescribed extensively for lupus erythematosus, arthritis, and malaria, but it should be kept in mind that it has some serious side effects. Hydroxychloroquine (Plaquenil) is safer.

Keratopathy and Retinopathy. Eye changes may occur at any time during antimalarial therapy; indeed, retinopathy may begin months after the drug has been discontinued.

Some of the abnormal findings are photophobia (most frequent symptom), lens opacities, macular edema, arteriolar narrowing and retinal pigment clumping. The classic "bull's eye" appearance of the retina always indicates irreversible damage. Antimalarial keratopathy is virtually never serious, and usually does not even require stopping the drug. Retinopathy, though rare, does require that the drug be stopped.

Percival reports that it is possible to detect incipient maculopathy by testing central fields to red targets. In this manner retinopathy may be avoided or at least recognized at an early reversible stage by pre-

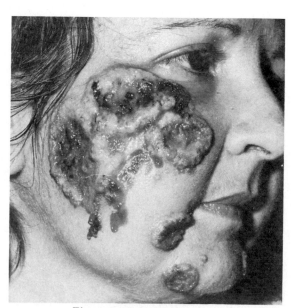

Figure 6–23. Iododerma.

treatment and serial ophthalmologic examinations at 4- to 6-month intervals. The administration of daily doses not to exceed 250 mg per day of chloroquine (or 400 mg per day of hydroxychloroquine) will also aid in prevention of retinopathy.

Hyperpigmentation. Bluish black hyperpigmented patches have appeared on the shins and on the hard palate following prolonged use of chloroquine. Melanosis of the face and subungual melanosis in patches may also occur. Tuffanelli and his associates reported that this type of localized hyperpigmentation occurred not only with chloroquine but also with quinacrine and hydroxychloroquine.

Hypopigmentation. Whitening of the scalp hair, beard, eyebrows, and eyelashes may occur. Fortunately the reaction is reversible, with a return to normal within six months after chloroquine has been stopped.

Dupré A, et al: Chloroquine-induced hypopigmentation of hair and freckles. Arch Dermatol 1985, 121:1164.
Koranda FC: Antimalarials. JAAD 1981, 4:650.
Olansky AJ: Antimalarials and ophthalmologic safety. JAAD 1982, 6:19.
Rees RB, et al: Chloroquine: A review of reactions and dermatologic indications. Arch Dermatol 1963, 88:280.
Tanenbaum L, et al: Antimalarial agents. Arch Dermatol 1980, 116:587.

Chlorpromazine

High-dose, long-term therapy with chlorpromazine may induce a skin-eye syndrome consisting of star-shaped opacities in the lens, corneal clouding, and a photosensitivity of the skin that causes a distinctive slate gray or violaceous pigmentation of

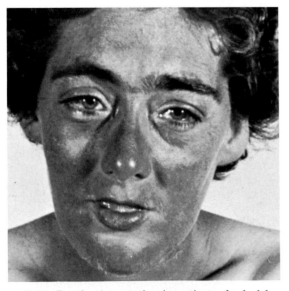

Figure 6–25. Purple pigmentation in patient who had been on high doses of chlorpromazine. Note sparing of deep creases on the face. (Satanove A: JAMA 191:263, 1965.)

the skin in the sun-exposed areas. A yellowish brown pigmentation may also appear on the exposed areas of the conjunctiva, the cornea, and even on the central portion of the anterior face of the lens. The majority of those afflicted are women.

The development of eye changes depends upon total dose and duration of administration.

Chelation therapy with 300 mg D-penicillamine four times daily for six days of each week for four weeks has been effective, with the disappearance of pigmentation and improvement of vision.

Aram H: Henoch-Schönlein purpura induced by chlorpromazine. JAAD 1987, 17:139.
Zelickson AS: Skin changes and chlorpromazine: Some hazards of long-term therapy. JAMA 1966, 198:341.

Penicillin Allergy

Penicillin allergy is responsible for a large number of allergic reactions. It manifests in a wide variety of morphologic patterns.

TYPES

Anaphylaxis. An immediate reaction to penicillin may occur within a few seconds to two hours after administration. This reaction is mediated by IgE antibodies. Itching of the scalp, flushing, tingling of the face and tongue, vague apprehension, weakness, and dyspnea due to bronchial obstruction or laryngeal edema may occur. Acute abdominal pain and a desire to urinate may be present. Angioedema of the face, sudden vascular collapse, respiratory compromise, and shock may be fatal.

Treatment consists of the following: When the penicillin has been given by injection, a tourniquet should be applied, if possible, proximal to the site of injection. This should be released for 1 to 2 minutes every 10 minutes. Epinephrine, 0.3 to 0.5 ml (1:1000) aqueous solution, is given subcutaneously or intramuscularly. This can be repeated in a few minutes if severe signs and symptoms do not begin to subside. The slow intravenous administration of 1:10,000 aqueous solution may be necessary in extreme cases. Cardiac arrhythmia and increased blood pressure and pulse rate are signs of overdosage of epinephrine.

Oxygen should be administered immediately when anaphylaxis occurs.

Soluble corticosteroids, as dexamethasone 4 mg or methyl prednisolone 40 to 80 mg, are given intramuscularly or intravenously, depending upon the gravity of the situation.

Antihistaminics, such as diphenhydramine hydrochloride (Benadryl) 25 to 50 mg intramuscularly are also advisable.

In the case of a severe respiratory reaction, 5 to 8 mgm per kilogram of aminophylline is given slowly over 15 to 20 minutes intravenously. Artificial respiration or even tracheostomy may be necessary. The possibility of myocardial infarction should alert one to monitor the cardiac status for the first 24 hours. Also, anaphylaxis may recur over the ensuing 24 hours, reinforcing the necessity for monitoring during this time period.

Morbilliform Eruption. This is the most common allergic reaction, and is seen most frequently with ampicillin or amoxicillin. It often begins 24 to 48 hours after taking penicillin, but it may be as much as five weeks after penicillin therapy has been started. It is estimated that 10 per cent of all patients taking ampicillin will develop this type of reaction. Susceptibility is higher in infectious mononucleosis. There is usually pruritus.

Corticosteroids, either in oral or intramuscular form, are effective. Antihistaminics may also be given.

Serum Sicknesslike Reaction (Delayed Reaction). After an incubation time of 5 to 21 days, urticaria appears, with arthralgia, lymphadenopathy, fever, proteinuria, angioedema (especially periorbital), and purpura. Urticaria is the most prominent manifestation in this delayed reaction. Again corticosteroids are effective and antihistaminics are helpful.

Other Reactions. Allergic reactions may also be manifested by an erythematous-vesicular or idlike eruption. This involves the palms and soles with deep-seated vesicles that dry and peel away.

Contact dermatitis to topical applications of penicillin caused this use to be abandoned years ago.

SLE-like syndrome may occur as an abnormal immunologic reaction. Purpura, fixed drug eruption, vasculitis, erythema multiforme, and toxic epidermal necrolysis may also stem from use of this antibiotic.

DETECTION OF PENICILLIN SENSITIVITY. As already mentioned, penicillin G (benzyl penicillin), a low molecular weight compound, is most commonly used. One of its degradation products, benzyl penicilloyl, is a hapten which reacts with serum or tissue proteins to form a complete antigen. This is believed to be the major antigenic determinant in penicillin hypersensitivity. Testing with dilute penicillin G misses many potential reactors and, moreover, may rarely produce a severe anaphylactic reaction.

Penicilloyl-polylysine Test. A skin test consisting of penicilloyl combined with polylysine, a polyfunctional hapten, has been developed. It is marketed by William H. Rorer, Inc., Fort Washington, Pennsylvania 19034 as Pre-Pen in 0.25 ml ampules. Intradermal injection of this will elicit a wheal and erythema response in 20 minutes in 75 per cent of sensitive persons.

Penicillin G (Benzyl Penicillin) Test. A freshly prepared saline solution of penicillin G in a dilution of 10,000 units per ml is used for scratch testing. If the scratch test is negative after 20 minutes, an intradermal injection of 0.02 ml of the solution is made and read. A positive reaction is indicated when a wheal of 5 mm is produced, with a flare and pseudopodia.

Minor Determinant Mix Test. Minor determinants of penicillin are benzyl penicilloate, crystalline benzyl penicillin, and a benzyl penicilloyl-amine. Clinical collaborative trials are in progress to assess the effectiveness of a minor determinant mix test as a predictor or an allergic reactor. It appears to be quite effective in identifying many of the remaining 25 per cent of patients who are not reactive to the penicilloyl-polylysine test.

Penicillin therapy is contraindicated when there is a history of previous penicillin reaction and a positive skin test. In these patients we believe that it is imperative to use alternative antibiotics.

Desensitization should be attempted only in the most extraordinary circumstances. Patients with a prior history of exfoliative dermatitis to penicillin should never be reexposed to it.

TREATMENT OF DELAYED REACTIONS. The severity varies in this type of reaction. Generally the use of antihistaminics and the judicious use of corticosteroids are effective in clearing the cutaneous lesions in a week or so. ACTH given twice weekly is also effective. Triamcinolone acetonide or diacetate intramuscularly is advisable in most cases; often a single 60-mg dose is all that is required, but in severe cases it should be repeated in three days if improvement is not noted by then. Oral prednisone, 40 to 60 mg every morning, is usually promptly effective; no tapering is needed if treatment lasts less than 3 or 4 weeks.

PROPHYLAXIS. Hidden penicillin contacts may produce continued urticaria for several months after the sensitization reaction has occurred. Beer should be avoided. Penicillin sprays may contaminate the air enough to produce reactions in the exquisitely sensitive person.

DeHaan P, et al: Onset of penicillin rashes. Allergy 1986, 41:75.
Fellner MJ: Penicillin allergy 1976. Int J Dermatol 1976, 15:497.
Sogn DD: Penicillin allergy. J Allergy Clin Immunol 1984, 74:589.
Voss H: Penicillin allergy. Curr Concepts Allergy Clin Immunol 1976, 5:1.

Immunologic Drug Reactions

Drugs often elicit an immune response but it is rare for symptoms to result. Topical skin application tends to induce sensitivity, mucosal application much less so; mucosal application may stimulate production of secretory immunoglobulins, IgA, and IgE or IgM. Infectious mononucleosis may alter the body's response so as to increase the frequency of ampicillin-induced morbilliform eruptions. Penicillin is the commonest cause of IgE-dependent reactions. Serum sickness is now more often caused by drugs than by serum, and the onset of symptoms six to nine days after first administration of the drug may be seen with penicillins, sulfonamides, thiouracils, gallbladder dyes, diphenylhydantoin, aminosalicylic acid, antithymocyte globulin (ATG), and streptomycin.

Nonimmunologic Drug Reactions

Wintroub and Stern suggest that many eruptions are caused by nonimmunologic activation of effector pathways—release of mast cell mediators by opiates, tubocurarine, polymyxin B, or radiopaque media; or release of complement; or release of prostaglandins from inhibition of cyclooxygenase, by aspirin or other nonsteroidal antiinflammatory agents. Other problems under this heading are overdosage, cumulative toxicity, side effects, ecologic disturbances, drug interactions, effects on nutrition or metabolism, and exacerbation of pre-existing diseases, as for example, psoriasis by lithium or beta-blockers, lupus by cimetidine, or rosacea by vasodilators.

Drug eruptions are distinguished clinically from dermatoses which they may simulate by their sudden appearance; by the typical symmetrical and widespread distribution; and by the comparatively extensive skin lesions, with little systemic disturbance. There is generally also the history of use of the drug shortly before onset, and an improvement of the skin lesions when its administration is stopped.

Photosensitizing Therapeutic Drugs. Light-induced reactions may occur on exposed surfaces of the body as a result of the use of various drugs. The term photosensitization dermatitis has been used to designate skin changes induced by light as a consequence of drug therapy. Since this term includes both phototoxic and photoallergic reactions, however, it is preferable to use one or the other of these terms if the nature of the reaction is known.

Shwartzman Reaction. It is possible that various cutaneous reactions such as hemorrhagic purpura may be explained by this phenomenon. The skin preparatory factor may be the toxins of an infecting agent such as staphylococci. The eliciting agent is the antigen-antibody complex of a drug to which the patient has already manifested an allergic sensitivity.

Herxheimer Reaction. Existing lesions may be exacerbated at the time when a highly effective drug is given to combat an infection. This reaction is exemplified in syphilis when penicillin is first given to the syphilitic. It has been extensively reviewed in a recent article by Rosen et al.

Cross Sensitization. In allergic cross sensitization a sensitization induced by one substance extends to one or more chemically related substances. This phenomenon helps explain why some drugs elicit an allergic response on the first exposure; why drug eruptions recur when there has been no exposure to the primary sensitizing drug; why some drug eruptions will persist over an interminable length of time; and why drugs of low sensitizing qualities will induce allergic reactions. An example is the cross reaction of sulfonamides with paraphenylenediamine and aniline dyes.

Skin Manifestations of Drug Reactions. Drug eruptions fall into several morphologic patterns and form characteristic lesions, depending to some degree on the type of reaction. Types of reaction may be vascular, eczematous, follicular, ulcerating, vegetating, and furunculoid.

The *acneiform eruption* consists of a papular, pustular, cystic, and furunculoid reaction that is distinguished by its sudden onset, usually well past the adolescent age. Oiliness of the skin is absent and the distribution of the lesions does not follow the pattern of seborrhea. Comedones are absent.

Morbilliform Drug Reactions. These, the commonest of drug reactions, consist of irregularly shaped small macules which may be edematous enough to be called papules. Palms, soles, and mucosal surfaces may be involved, and the resemblance to a viral exanthem often creates a problem in differential diagnosis. Ampicillin should be avoided in infectious mononucleosis, since either it or amoxicillin will induce such a rash in 50 to 80 per cent of patients. Morbilliform drug reactions are usually only mildly itchy, and most often begin within a week or two of starting therapy.

Erythema Multiforme. Generalized erythematous macules or bullae, with iris lesions, may occur especially with long-acting sulfonamides. Usually it appears after a week or two of therapy, and is often associated with fever. An abrupt onset with severe lesions of the mouth, conjunctiva, or os urethrae is known as Stevens-Johnson syndrome; and a rapidly spreading form with exfoliation of sheets of skin is called toxic epidermal necrolysis. Established lesions of any of these are affected little or not at all by steroids; but in the earliest stages, the entire process may be turned off and stopped by prompt systemic steroid therapy. Drugs that produce these reactions are sulfonamides, allopurinol, penicillins, diphenylhydantoin, and phenylbutazone.

Fixed Drug Eruptions. One or a few sharply defined round or oval red macules (or less often, vesicles), occurring suddenly within a few hours after ingestion of a drug, and recurring in exactly the same place or places on each subsequent dose, and leaving a little more pigment behind with each attack, is recognizable instantly as a fixed drug eruption. Pigment incontinence lends a bluish hue to lesions by

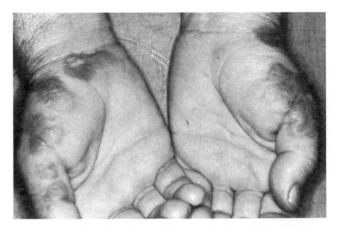

Figure 6–26. Fixed eruption due to phenolphthalein.

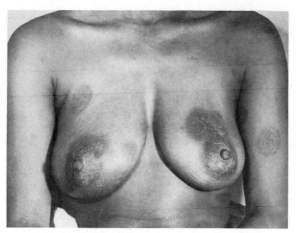

Figure 6–27. Fixed eruption due to phenolphthalein.

the time of the fourth or fifth attack. Korkij has reviewed a host of potentially causative drugs.

Palmar-Plantar Chemotherapy-Associated Dysesthesia Syndrome. Continuous infusion chemotherapy for extended periods is associated with a high incidence (probably 8 to 10 per cent) of tingling of the hands and feet, with progressive discomfort, then tenderness and swelling of the palms and soles. On stopping treatment, it resolves in a week, with desquamation and residual pigmentation. Fluorouracil and doxorubicin may both produce it.

Corticosteroid Reactions

Cutaneous corticosteroid reactions may result from topical, subcutaneous, or systemic applications.

Topical Application. The prolonged topical use of fluorinated corticosteroid preparations may produce distinctive changes in the skin. Atrophy, striae, telangiectasia, and purpura are the most frequent

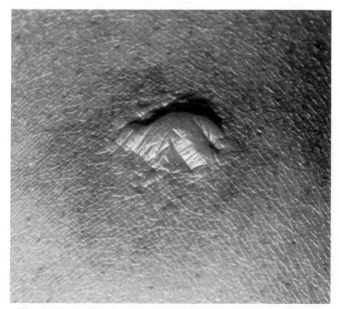

Figure 6–28. Fixed eruption due to sulfamethoxazole (Septra).

changes seen. The most striking changes of telangiectasia are seen in fair-skinned individuals who use fluorinated corticosteroids on the face.

The changes in the skin are enhanced by applying plastic film as an occlusive dressing over the fluorinated corticosteroids. Substitution of plain hydrocortisone topical preparations is indicated when continued topical corticosteroid preparations must be used. Usually the telangiectases disappear in a few months after corticosteroid applications are stopped.

When fluorinated corticosteroid preparations are applied to the face over a period of weeks or months, persistent erythema with telangiectases, and often small pustules, may occur. Perioral dermatitis is in some cases due to the prolonged use of topical corticosteroids. Although hydrocortisone does not usually produce such reactions, Guin recently reported such changes from long-term use of 1 per cent hydrocortisone cream. We have not encountered the problem with this preparation. Topical application of corticosteroids can also produce epidermal atrophy with hypopigmentation and, if used over large areas, has been known to induce not only hypercortisolism but also Cushing's syndrome.

Subcutaneous Injection. Good results have been obtained in many dermatoses by the intralesional injection of corticosteroids. The injection of corticosteroids either by syringe or by high-pressure air propulsion (Dermojet) may produce subcutaneous atrophy at the site of injection. The ill-advised injection of insoluble corticosteroids into the deltoid muscle sometimes causes subcutaneous atrophy. The patient becomes aware of the reaction by noticing depression and depigmentation at the site of injection. There is no pain, but it is bothersome cosmetically. The patient may be assured that this will fill out again, but that it may take as much as six months to two years to accomplish this.

Systemic Corticosteroids. The prolonged use of corticosteroids in dosages of over 20 to 25 mg prednisone equivalents a day may produce numerous changes of the skin.

Purpura or Ecchymoses. This is seen especially over the dorsal forearms in many patients over 50 who have had corticosteroid treatment monthly for several months. It is aggravation of solar purpura. Triamcinolone acetonide intramuscularly is even more prone to produce this side effect than oral prednisone is.

Cushingoid Changes. The most common change is probably the alteration in the fat distribution. Buffalo hump, facial and neck fullness, increased supraclavicular and suprasternal fat, gynecomastia, protuberant or pendulous abdomen, and flattening of the buttocks may occur.

Steroid Acne. Small firm follicular papules or the forehead, cheeks, and chest may occur after only a single dose—and after each subsequent one. These can persist as long as the corticosteroids are continued even in moderate doses (15 to 20 mg daily). They usually respond rapidly to vitamin A, 300,000 units daily in an adult. Tetracycline is also usually effective.

Striae. These may be widely distributed, especially over the abdomen, buttocks, and thighs. The lesions consist of wide violaceous lines sometimes as much as 30 cm long.

Other Skin Changes. There may be generalized skin dryness (xerosis); the skin may become thin and fragile; keratosis pilaris may develop; persistent erythema of the skin in sun-exposed areas may occur, and erythromelanosis may rarely occur.

Hair Changes. Hair loss occurs in about half of the patients on long-term corticosteroids in large doses. There may be thinning and brittle fracturing along the hairshaft. There may be increased hair growth on the bearded area and on the arms and back with fine vellus hairs. These changes are rare with triamcinolone injections.

Hypertension, cataracts, and *osteoporosis* are likely consequences of therapy with orally administered prednisone for periods of a year or more, in doses of 15 mg a day or greater. Triamcinolone acetonide (Kenalog), because it is effective in an intramuscular dose of 40 to 60 mg every four or five (or occasionally more) weeks, produces none of these; even moon face, if already induced by oral therapy, goes away if Kenalog is given intramuscularly instead.

Gallant C, et al: Oral glucocorticoids and their complications. JAAD 1986, 14:161.
Guin JD: Contact sensitivity to topical corticosteroids. JAAD 1984, 10:773.
Robertson DB, et al: Topical corticosteroids: Review. Int J Dermatol 1982, 21:59.
Storrs FJ: Use and abuse of systemic corticosteroid therapy. JAAD 1979, 1:95.
Tan PL, et al: Current topical corticosteroid preparation. JAAD 1986, 14:79.
Verbov J: The place of intralesional steroid therapy in dermatology. Br J Dermatol 1976, 94:51.

SLE-Like Syndrome

Also known as *drug lupus* and *hydralazine lupus syndrome*, drug-induced systemic lupus erythematosuslike syndrome (SLE-like syndrome) is a relatively benign form of lupus, which has a low incidence of skin, renal, and CNS abnormalities. That drug reactions could mimic SLE was not known until it was found that 10 per cent of adults treated for hypertension with hydralazine (Apresoline) developed a syndrome clinically and pathologically indistinguishable from SLE. The syndrome developed after therapy of long duration and high dosage.

Irias in 1975 reported the first such case in a child, a girl of eight with hypertension secondary to renal disease. Like most adults with this syndrome, she was a "slow acetylator" on testing with sulfamethazine. Other characteristics of hydralazine-induced

lupus are dosages which exceed 300 mg per day, a predominance of females, and an increased prevalence of the HLA-Dr4 phenotype.

Since then phenytoin, trimethadione, isonicotinic hydrazide, procainamide, isoniazid, and others have been shown to produce similar reactions. The serologic findings in the drug-induced SLE-like syndrome show a positive ANA with 90 per cent having antihistone antibodies. D-Penicillamine has unmasked what seems to be naturally occurring SLE with the full spectrum of SLE signs and symptoms, and unlike the disease induced by other drugs, has induced anti–double-stranded DNA antibodies. Subacute cutaneous lupus erythematosus has been reported by Reed et al to be induced by hydrochlorothiazide.

Most cases are mild and clear within three months after discontinuance of the drug; however, death may also occur, especially if lupus nephritis develops.

Drugs that have a connection with systemic lupus erythematosus are listed in Table 6–1.

Chalmers A, et al: Systemic lupus erythematosus during penicillamine therapy for rheumatoid arthritis. Ann Intern Med 1982, 97:659.
Hess E: Drug related lupus. N Engl J Med 1988, 318:1460.
Reed BR, et al: Subacute cutaneous lupus erythematosus with hydrochlorthiazide therapy. Ann Intern Med 1985, 103:49.

Toxic Epidermal Necrolysis (TEN)

Toxic epidermal necrolysis is a bullous drug eruption that is so severe that it has the appearance of a widespread scalding burn. Cases were described by Ruskin in 1948 and under various names by many others since then. In 1956 Lyell reported four osten-

Table 6–1. DRUGS THAT MAY INDUCE SLE

Proved	Possible
Hydralazine	Allopurinol
Isoniazid	Captopril
Procainamide	Chlorthalidone
	Cimetidine
Probable	Gold salts
Acetylprocainamide*	Griseofulvin
Chlorpromazine	Methysergide
Ethosuximide	Oral contraceptives
Lithium carbonate	Phenylbutazone
Mephenytoin	Practolol
Methylthiouracil	Other beta blockers
Nitrofurantoin	Reserpine
Penicillamine	Streptomycin
Phenytoin	Sulfonamides
Propylthiouracil	Tetracycline
Quinidine	
Trimethadione	

*Acetylprocainamide may safely be given to patients who have had procainamide-induced lupus syndrome. Blocking the amino group by acetylation appears to prevent the lupus-inducing effect. This drug is not yet available for use in the United States.

(From Dermatologic Capsule and Comment, February, 1986, p. 4.)

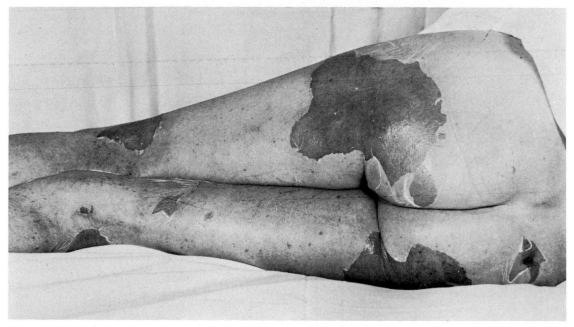

Figure 6–29. *Toxic epidermal necrolysis showing desquamation in sheets, leaving raw, red surface. (Courtesy of Dr. A. Lyell.)*

sible cases under the title *toxic epidermal necrolysis* (TEN).

It is mimicked closely in children by a quite different disease caused by *Staphylococcus aureus*, an epidermolytic enzyme of which splits the epidermis in the granular cell layer. In TEN the level of the split is below the epidermis, at the dermal-epidermal junction. The staphylococcal disease (which is milder and has a far better prognosis) is usually called "staphylococcal scalded skin syndrome" (SSSS) to distinguish it from its more serious drug-induced look-alike, TEN. Here we will concern ourselves only with TEN, due to drugs.

CLINICAL EVIDENCE. The onset is sudden, with an eruption of urticarial plaques and an erythema of the neck. Clear bullae appear and may become the size of a hand. Intense fatigue, diarrhea, angina, and vomiting are prodromal symptoms; within a few hours the condition becomes extremely grave. The patient may be comatose, there is fever, and the large flaccid bullae grow and become confluent, with extreme congestive erythema and purpura. The epidermis comes off in large sheets, leaving the raw, red dermis exposed to make the skin surface look scalded. A positive Nikolsky's sign is usually present. There may be fissures of the lips, erosions of the buccal mucosa, and conjunctivitis. The outcome may be fatal within the course of a few days. Bad prognostic factors include age, extent of necrolysis, and elevation of serum urea.

ETIOLOGY. The drugs implicated as causative agents have been enumerated already. Guillaume et al identified the culprit drugs in 67 cases: sulfonamides, anticonvulsants, and nonsteroidal anti-in

flammatory drugs were most frequently implicated. Cases caused by diphtheria inoculation, poliomyelitis immunization, and tetanus antitoxin have also been described. A fatal case of TEN caused by Fansidar prophylaxis in an HIV-infected patient was reported by Raviglione et al. However, in some cases it is not possible to obtain a history of any drug ingestion.

Toxic epidermal necrolysis is regarded by many as a confluent, acute-onset, severe form of Stevens-Johnson syndrome.

Neutropenia seems to be unusual in the experience of most, but lymphopenia is not unusual, and overall there may be moderate leucopenia. Westly et al thought granulocytopenia a bad prognostic sign.

HISTOPATHOLOGY. There is full-thickness epidermal necrosis, with separation of the entire epidermis by formation of a subepidermal bulla, as in erythema multiforme. More superficial separation, in the upper prickle or granular layer, means that the lesion is one of SSSS (staphylococcal scalded skin syndrome), not TEN.

TREATMENT. There is general agreement that corticosteroids should not be used in TEN that has progressed to involve 20 per cent or more of body surface. Still unproven is whether they may arrest the progression of TEN if given in the first 24 to 48 hours.

The treatment is that of extensive second-degree burns. The main problem is to relieve the pain caused by the absence of skin over large portions of the body. Continuous moist compresses of 0.5 per cent silver nitrate solution followed later by a dexamethasone-neomycin aerosol spray and cholesterinized petrolatum (Eucerin) has been recommended by Kob lenzer for local treatment. Silvadene (silver sulfadiazine) cream is also extremely effective, and far easier to use. However, if it is used over large areas or beneath pressure dressings, considerable absorption will occur, and it has been suggested that this may cause granulocytopenia in susceptible persons. Also, if sulfonamides are felt to be implicated as a cause of TEN, Silvadene should not be used. The incidence of mortality from TEN varies from 20 to 50 per cent, depending on the series.

Goldstein SM, et al: Toxic epidermal necrolysis. Arch Dermatol 1987, 123:1153.
Guillaume J-C, et al: The culprit drugs in 87 cases of toxic epidermal necrolysis. Arch Dermatol 1987, 123:1166.
Izumi AK, et al: Topical silver nitrate in toxic epidermal necrolysis–Lyell's disease. Cutis 1970, 6:865.
Lyell A: The staphylococcal scalded skin syndrome in historical perspective. JAAD 1983, 9:285.
Raviglione MC, et al: Fatal toxic epidermal necrolysis during prophylaxis with pyrimethamine and sulfadoxine in a human immunodeficiency virus-infected person. Arch Intern Med 1988, 148:683.
Revuz J, et al: Toxic epidermal necrolysis. Arch Dermatol 1987, 123:1160.
Revuz J, et al: Treatment of toxic epidermal necrolysis. Arch Dermatol 1987, 123:1156.
Roujeua J-C, et al: Granulocytes, lymphocytes, and toxic epidermal necrolysis (Letter). Arch Dermatol 1985, 121:305.
Siegel DM: (Letter). Arch Dermatol 1985, 121:305.
Westly ED, et al: Toxic epidermal necrolysis: Granylocytopenia as a prognostic factor. Arch Dermatol 1984, 120:721; 1985, 121:306.

7

Erythema and Urticaria

ERYTHEMA

The term *erythema* signifies redness—hyperemia—of the skin, either localized or widespread, due to the dilatation of the superficial blood vessels near the surface of the skin. It is usually transient and blanches momentarily under pressure of a finger. Erythema is the first and commonest objective skin reaction produced by an internal or external irritant.

TYPES

Flushing. Flushing is a transient diffuse redness of the face and neck, or adjacent trunk. If it is intense and frequent it may eventuate in rosacea. Vasomotor control in the face is achieved through a balance between vasoconstrictor and active vasodilator innervation. Alcohol provokes flushing, much more in Orientals than in Caucasians. In addition, alcohol flushing has been linked with a possible predisposition to alcoholism, to various disulfiramlike agents, or to neoplastic disease, including carcinoid. Diabetics receiving chlorpropamide (Diabinese) tend to flush after alcohol ingestion, unless their diabetes is insulin-dependent. This flush is blocked by the opiate antagonist naloxone, which also blocks the flushing reaction associated with the menopause. Nadolol (Corgard) blocks the flush associated with rosacea, as Wilkin recently reported. Mastocytosis may be associated with severe flushing. Wilkin (1981) has written a valuable review of flushing to which reference should be made.

Many descriptive names are attached to more persistent erythemas with different causes. **Erythema intertrigo** is an erythema of apposed skin surfaces, usually in the groins or axillae, or beneath pendulous breasts, due to friction, maceration, or infection (*Candida*). **Erythema solare** is redness caused by the sun's rays; **erythema caloricum** is redness produced by any kind of heat; **erythema pernio (chilblains)** is a purplish erythema on the acral parts of the body due to exposure to cold.

Erythema Palmare. This distinctive localized persistent erythema is usually most marked on the hypothenar areas. Palmar erythema may occur in carcinoma of the pancreas with metastasis to the liver. Cirrhosis may cause palmar erythema. Erythema palmare also may be associated with spider nevi; it frequently occurs in pregnancy. The common denominator in nearly all of these is an elevated level of circulating estrogen. Other causes include graft-versus-host disease and chemotherapy-induced acral erythema. **Erythema palmare hereditarium** may appear as a persistent erythema with no other changes. This type of erythema may also be the precursor to keratoderma palmare et plantare hereditarium.

Generalized Erythema. Generalized erythemas vary greatly in their appearance, extent, and distribution, being most marked on the chest, upper arms, thighs, and face. The eruption consists of pinhead-sized red macules blending into the surrounding macules to produce a diffuse rash that may cover the entire body. There is nearly always a tendency to involve the follicles. This may be due to a drug reaction, a virus infection, cancer, or an unknown cause.

Scarlatiniform Erythema. In some instances the eruption may resemble scarlet fever. The subjective symptoms are rarely pronounced but are most marked before the erythema appears, after which there is a gradual diminution. There may be itching, pricking, or burning, which may provoke scratching and secondary infections. Marked desquamation of the epidermis, defluvium of the hair, or changes in the nails may follow an attack. It is differentiated from scarlet fever by the absence of constitutional

131

symptoms. Usually the mouth remains normal, whereas in scarlet fever the tongue is coated, the papillae are red and enlarged, and the tonsils are inflamed, enlarged, and covered with an exudate. The Schultz-Charlton phenomenon is negative in nonbacterial scarlatiniform erythema. Rarely, *Staphylococcus aureus* may be the cause.

Morbilliform Erythema. Drug eruptions frequently react in this manner, with discrete red macules appearing first and then coalescing to form a diffuse erythema. Koplik's spots and eye symptoms of photophobia and burning are not present in nonviral morbilliform erythema.

Toxic Erythema. Generalized erythema is the usual manifestation of toxic erythema, a loose term frequently used, especially when the etiology is doubtful. It is usually caused by a hypersensitivity to certain foods or drugs, especially the sulfonamides, antibiotics, anticonvulsants, or nonsteroidal antiinflammatory agents. They produce erythemas as well as other types of eruptions which are discussed under dermatitis due to drugs. Frequently toxic erythemas develop in the course of systemic diseases such as typhoid fever, cerebrospinal meningitis, brucellosis, rheumatic fever, infectious mononucleosis, malaria, or pneumonia. When there is a streptococcal pharyngitis and a widespread morbilliform or scarlatiniform erythema, rheumatoid arthritis must be considered. This mode of onset is common in young people, especially when there is pain in the hands, knees, or other joints.

TREATMENT. Every effort should be made to determine the exact cause of these erythemas, and when discovered this should be eliminated or suitably treated. Idiosyncrasies to foods or drugs should be investigated. All internal medications should be avoided until the exact cause of the erythema is determined. Tepid baths containing starch, bran, or sodium bicarbonate are beneficial.

EXANTHEMATOUS ERYTHEMA

Several of the exanthems are characterized by the sudden and explosive appearance of erythema after prodromal symptoms. Many of these are of viral origin, or at least are believed to be of viral origin. Some of these are roseola infantum (exanthema subitum), erythema infectiosum (fifth disease), morbilli, and the echovirus exanthems. These are discussed in the chapter on viral diseases.

Bacterial infections may also be the cause of exanthems. **Erythema arthriticum epidemicum (Haverhill fever), scarlet fever,** and **brucellosis** are examples of bacterial exanthems.

Erythemas in epidemic forms are not uncommon. **Nonbacterial meningitis** with morbilliform erythema has occurred in Europe in epidemic form. Echovirus-caused epidemics of erythema, and erythema multiforme with gastrointestinal symptoms, are also seen occasionally.

Kasha EE, et al: Scombroid fish poisoning with facial flushing. JAAD 1988, 18:1363.

Martin-Ortesa E, et al: Acral erythema. Arch Dermatol 1987, 123:424.

Idem: Effect of nadolol on flushing in rosacea. JAAD 1989, 20:202.

Wilkin JK: Flushing reactions: Consequences and mechanisms. Ann Intern Med 1981, 95:468.

ERYTHEMA TOXICUM NEONATORUM

Erythema toxicum neonatorum is a patchy benign eruption of the newborn. The lesions consist of macules, papules, and pustules, sometimes accompanied by large patches of erythema, usually with a widespread distribution, but occurring only rarely on the soles or palms. There is no fever or other known cause. The eruption appears within the first three to four days of life and generally disappears by the tenth day.

Although the nature of the disease suggests a viral infection, no satisfactory etiologic agent has been found.

The pustules are filled with eosinophils and are follicular or perifollicular. In the erythematous macules there is a slight perivascular infiltration of eosinophils. It is differentiated from neonatal pustular pyoderma by the presence of eosinophils in the smears of the pustules; neutrophilic leukocytes are found in pyoderma.

Specific treatment is not indicated, since it involutes within a few days.

Carr JA, et al: Erythema and infant maturity. Am J Dis Child 1966, 112:129.

Freeman RG, et al: Histopathology of erythema toxicum neonatorum. Arch Dermatol 1960, 82:586.

Marino LJ: Toxic erythema at birth. Arch Dermatol 1965, 92:402.

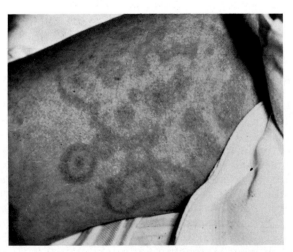

Figure 7–1. Erythema annulare. Iris lesions on inner thigh.

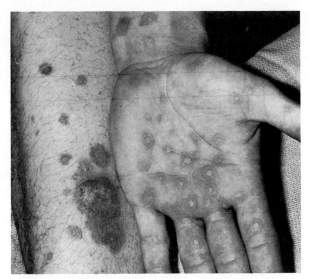

Figure 7–2. Erythema multiforme. Note the iris lesions on the palms.

ERYTHEMA MULTIFORME

HISTORY. In 1860 Hebra first described this as **erythema exudativum multiforme**; since then this description has gradually been expanded to distinguish several forms with numerous manifestations not only in the skin but also in the mucous membranes and in various internal organs. It is now viewed as a hypersensitivity syndrome. Various types of skin reactions may occur from the same causative agent and, conversely, many causative agents may induce the same cutaneous and mucous membrane reactions. The multiformity in its broadest sense is the characteristic feature of this disease.

In 1922 Stevens and Johnson described an acute form of this disease with severe eye manifestations. Since then there has been a tendency to regard most severe cases of erythema multiforme as Stevens-Johnson syndrome, especially when bullae on the skin and mucosal involvement are present.

CLINICAL FEATURES. There are many varieties of erythema multiforme, and these are named according to the more prominent features composing the eruption. The lesions may be macular, papular, nodose, vesicular, or bullous. They may be annular, circinate, or iris-shaped (target, bull's eye). They may be persistent, purpuric, or urticarial.

The main sites of predilection are the upper part of the face, the neck, the forearms, the legs, and the dorsal surfaces of the hands and feet. On the forearms the lesions are usually of the iris type and occur on the extensor surfaces. The mucous membranes are often involved. The trunk is mostly spared, in contrast to the distribution of pemphigus.

The evolution of the eruption is rapid, occurring over 12 to 24 hours. The attacks may be recurrent at more or less regular intervals, sometimes occurring each spring. Herpes simplex labialis often occurs seven to 10 days prior to the onset. When this happens, herpesvirus is considered to be the antigenic stimulus of erythema multiforme.

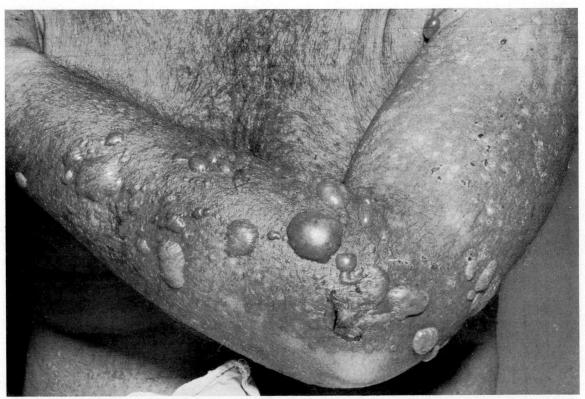

Figure 7–3. Erythema multiforme bullosum. Note predilection for the arms, sparing the trunk—unlike pemphigus.

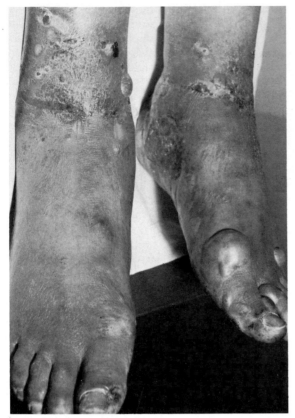

Figure 7–4. Erythema multiforme bullosum.

cyclic patches. Variegated tints may be a feature, particularly bluish and yellowish mixture with red. There may be annular, target-shaped lesions with central clearing. A special type, **erythema iris**, is characterized by concentric rings and is found chiefly on the dorsa of the hands and wrists and on the ankles.

The **bullous type** may show large hemorrhagic bullae on an erythematous base. The erythematous base and the sparing of the trunk are helpful in differentiating it from pemphigus. It is this severe bullous type that is frequently designated **erythema multiforme bullosum** or **Stevens-Johnson syndrome**. The palms and soles are sites of predilection, but other areas, particularly the buccal mucosa, conjunctiva, and glans penis, may be involved. Subungual hemorrhage is also reported. Pruritus is usually absent but may occasionally be a prominent symptom.

When the bullae are rapidly enlarging, reaching great size, flaccid, and desquamating, the process is referred to as toxic epidermal necrolysis (TEN). There may be difficulty in differentiating this from staphylococcal scalded skin syndrome (SSSS), but the desquamated skin in TEN is the entire epidermis, and in SSSS it is only the stratum corneum and stratum granulosum.

The internal manifestations of erythema multiforme may be many and varied. Loeffler's syndrome with eosinophilia occurs. Comaish and Kerr reported a series of five patients with erythema multiforme associated with albuminuria, hematuria, and elevated blood urea and sedimentation rate. Bluefarb and Szanto have reported acute tubular necrosis in an extensive and severe case of erythema multiforme with a history of aspirin ingestion six days before onset of illness.

The characteristic lesions of the **maculopapular type** are bright bluish red, well-defined macules or edematous flat-topped papules which have a tendency to spread peripherally and to fuse into poly-

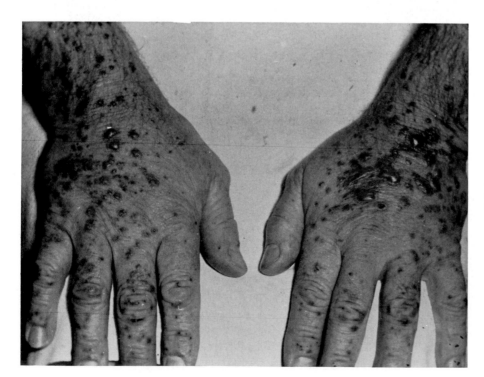

Figure 7–5. Erythema multiforme with large hemorrhagic bullae in a 47-year-old man. Cause undetermined.

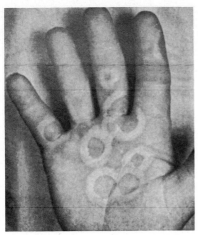

Figure 7–6. Erythema multiforme. Annular lesions.

ETIOLOGY. A complete listing of all etiologic associations mentioned in the medical literature is present in a review by Huff et al. Erythema multiforme may be a symptom complex of many infective processes.

Bacterial Infections. These may be brucellosis, diphtheria, erysipeloid, glanders, Yersinia infections, *Mycoplasma* pneumonia, psittacosis, tuberculosis, tularemia, lepromatous leprosy, or typhoid fever.

Viral Infections. This etiologic type may well be the most frequently encountered. As many as one third of all cases may be due to herpesvirus. Stevens-Johnson syndrome may occur in the initial stages of viral upper respiratory tract infection in viral pneumonia. It may occur with Asian flu, lymphogranuloma venereum, infectious mononucleosis, measles, milker's nodules, mumps, and smallpox vaccination. The coxsackie viruses, echoviruses, and poliomyelitis may induce it.

Kazmierowski et al have demonstrated herpes simplex virus in immune complexes isolated from patients with erythema multiforme. Shelley reproduced the characteristic lesions by skin testing with herpesvirus hominis, and in another case by skin testing with lipopolysaccharide W, an endotoxin common to numerous bacteria previously associated with erythema multiforme.

Mycotic Infections. Coccidioidomycosis and histoplasmosis may cause erythema multiforme bullosum.

Protozoan Infections. Malaria and trichomoniasis are also causative agents.

Collagen Diseases. Erythema multiforme has occurred in association with systemic and chronic discoid lupus erythematosus.

Drugs. Drugs often cause erythema multiforme exudativum, Stevens-Johnson syndrome, or TEN. Those indicted include allopurinol, antipyrine, arsenic, barbiturates, bromides, dapsone, digitalis, Dilantin, gold salts, hydralazine, iodides, mercurials, penicillin, penicillamine, phenytoin, phenobarbital, salicylates, sulfonamides, tetracycline, tolbutamide, and trimethoprim-sulfamethoxazole.

Vaccines. BCG, smallpox, diphtheria-tetanus toxoid, hepatitis B vaccine, measles-mumps-rubella vaccine, and poliomyelitis vaccines are possible causative agents.

Allergenic Skin Contactants. Bromofluorine, fire sponge *(Tedania ignis),* and *Toxicodendron* (3-pentadecylcatechol) may be causes. Fisher lists many others in his recent review of this subject.

Internal Malignant Disease. Carcinoma, Hodgkin's disease, lymphoma, myeloma, leukemia, and polycythemia may be accompanied by erythema multiforme.

Miscellaneous. Hormonal changes such as pregnancy and menstruation may also be causes of erythema multiforme. Hart described progesterone autosensitization erythema multiforme in 1977. Wojnarowska et al reported a case with pruritus from days 12–17 of each cycle and an eruption from day 20 to day 2 of the following cycle, which could be induced by 10 mg of either progesterone or medroxyprogesterone intramuscularly. Tamoxifen (Nolvadex), 20 and 10 mg on alternate days, completely suppressed it. Radiotherapy for malignant disease may also induce it.

Erythema multiforme may occur with Loeffler's syndrome, an eosinophilic pneumonopathy with an increase of the eosinophils in the blood and sputum, and only slight systemic symptoms.

The hops in beer have also been implicated, as has the ingestion of spoiled meat, fish, or shellfish.

PATHOGENESIS. In erythema multiforme the epidermal damage appears to be the primary process. It is hypothesized that foreign antigens are sequestered in the epidermis and are an immune stimulus for specific cytotoxic responses which lead to epidermal cell damage. While circulating immune complexes have been documented in some cases of erythema multiforme, and direct immunofluorescence may show vascular deposits of IgM and C3, vasculitis does not appear to be the primary process in the formation of skin lesions. Classic leucocytoclastic vasculitis is not seen histologically.

HISTOPATHOLOGY. The characteristic epidermal change is necrosis. When the epidermal involvement is mild, necrotic keratinocytes are scattered among normal-appearing keratinocytes. More marked necrosis is characterized by a homogeneous eosinophilic appearance to full-thickness epidermis. There is a prominent perivascular lymphocytic infiltrate in the upper third of the dermis. Edema of the papillary dermis leading to the formation of a subepidermal blister is characteristic of bullous lesions. The histopathologic changes, as noted above, are distinctive and of diagnostic significance.

DIFFERENTIAL DIAGNOSIS. Different varieties of erythema multiforme may simulate other dermatoses. The maculopapular type may be confused with the maculopapular syphilid and with urticaria. Many drugs will produce eruptions with the characteristics of erythema multiforme, and a complete drug history should be taken in all patients with this affliction.

Annular lesions of the disease may be confused with pityriasis rosea and ringworm. Vesicular and bullous types may be difficult to distinguish from dermatitis herpetiformis, pemphigus, bullous pemphigoid, herpes gestationis, and drug eruptions. Bullous contact dermatitis such as that induced by rhus (*Toxicodendron*) is localized to the areas which contact the oleoresin. Occasionally erythema multiforme produces slightly elevated, erythematous plaques on the nose and cheeks which simulate discoid lupus erythematosus. They are distinguished from the latter by the absence of atrophy or adherent scales with horny follicular plugs.

TREATMENT. The many possible causes of erythema multiforme preclude any specific treatment, except when the specific cause is known. Local treatment consists of measures to allay the symptoms of burning and itching. Antibacterial preparations are used for any secondary infection.

Systemic therapy should in general be limited to general supportive measures and systemic corticosteroids. All other drugs should be avoided since there may be cross reactivity if drugs are causing the eruption. *In early cases*, systemic treatment may arrest progression and in many cases will permit avoidance of hospitalization and lead to more rapid involution than the 2 to 3 weeks required in untreated cases.

Acyclovir, given to suppress outbreaks of recurrent herpetic disease, has been effective in eliminating recurrent erythema multiforme in some patients in whom this virus stimulates such attacks. Huff has recently reviewed these reports.

Finan MC, et al: Cutaneous immunofluorescence study of erythema multiforme: Correlation with light microscopic patterns and etiologic agents. JAAD 1984, 10:497.

Fisher AA: Erythema multiforme-like eruptions to contactants. Cutis 1986, 38:101.

Fitzpatrick JE, et al: Photosensitive recurrent erythema multiforme. JAAD 1983, 9:419.

Griffith RD, et al: Erythema multiforme following diphtheria and tetanus toxoid. JAAD 1988, 19:758.

Howland WW, et al: Erythema multiforme: Clinical, histopathologic, and immunologic study. JAAD 1984, 10:438.

Huff JC: Acyclovir for recurrent erythema multiforme due to herpes simplex. JAAD 1988, 18:197.

Idem et al: Erythema multiforme: A critical review of characteristics, diagnostic criteria and causes. JAAD 1983, 8:763.

Kazmierowski JA, et al: Herpes simplex antigen in immune complexes of patients with erythema multiforme. JAMA 1982, 247:2547.

Marvin JA: Improved treatment of Stevens-Johnson syndrome. Arch Surg 1984, 119:601.

Shelley WB: Bacterial endotoxin (lipopolysaccharide) as a cause of erythema multiforme. JAMA 1980, 243:58.

Wojnarowska F: Progesterone-induced erythema multiforme. J R Soc Med 1985, 78:407.

STEVENS-JOHNSON SYNDROME

CLINICAL FEATURES. Stevens-Johnson syndrome (ectodermosis erosiva pluriorificalis, erythema multiforme exudativum) is a severe, at times fatal variety of erythema multiforme. The disease has an abrupt onset manifested by a fever of 39 or 40°C, headache, malaise, and soreness of the throat and mouth. Soon the constitutional symptoms become severe, including rapid, weak pulse, rapid respirations, prostration, and joint pains. Stomatitis is an early and conspicuous symptom. It begins with vesicles on the lips, tongue, and buccal mucosa and later becomes more severe, with pseudomembranous exudation, salivation, and ulcerations, so that eating and drinking become difficult. Bilateral conjunctivitis, corneal ulcers, rhinitis with epistaxis, and crusting of the nares may develop. Erosive vulvovaginitis or balanitis may be severe. The anal mucosa may show involvement. Occasional cases present with no skin lesions, the patient showing only stomatitis, rhinitis, conjunctivitis, and sometimes urethritis, but in most cases, a vesicobullous or edematous erythematous eruption involves especially the face, hands, and feet.

Not infrequently bronchial pneumonia develops. There may be associated gastrointestinal disturbances. These patients are extremely ill. Arthritis, convulsions, coma, cardiac arrhythmia, pericarditis,

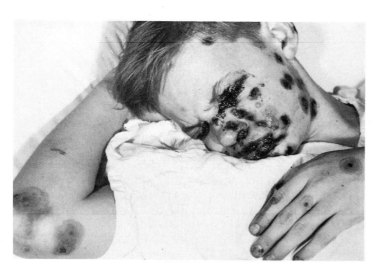

Figure 7–7. Stevens-Johnson syndrome. Severe involvement of orifices is characteristic.

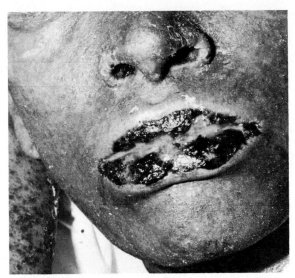

Figure 7–8. Stevens-Johnson syndrome. (Courtesy of Dr. F. Rosenberg.)

myositis, and hepatopathy may occur. In fatal cases septicemia is usually the cause of death.

Stevens-Johnson syndrome occurs mostly in children and in young men. Males outnumber females two to one. Most of the cases develop in the winter or spring. The disease may begin with herpes simplex lesions in or around the mouth, and in such cases herpesvirus is thought to be the cause of the disease.

The disease is sometimes fatal and not infrequently causes blindness. Costello reported 17 patients with a mortality of 18 per cent.

ETIOLOGY. See erythema multiforme.

PATHOGENESIS. See erythema multiforme.

HISTOLOGY. See erythema multiforme.

TREATMENT. Despite Rasmussen's study indicating little benefit from corticosteroid therapy, we believe that the treatment of choice is early, vigorous steroid therapy with 1.5 to 2 mg of prednisone per kg of body weight, in a single daily morning dose, or about 1 mg of triamcinolone acetonide per kg of body weight, in a single intramuscular dose, repeated after three or four days if there is a poor response.

Odom and James are concerned to exclude underlying disease (e.g., infection) which might be worsened by steroids, before giving triamcinolone. Arnold feels that infections are mitigated, not worsened, by parenteral triamcinolone, and that this step is unnecessary.

Toxic Epidermal Necrolysis

This serious disorder may occur as a primary dermatosis or as a complication of Stevens-Johnson syndrome, of which it is really an extensive, confluent, hyperacute variant. It was discussed in greater detail in Chapter 6.

Ruiz-Maldonado has categorized it as acute dis-

seminated epidermal necrosis (ADEN) and divided it into three types: type 1 corresponds to Stevens-Johnson syndrome, type 2 to transitional cases, and type 3 to toxic epidermal necrolysis. No type 1 cases died, but mortality was 37 per cent in type 2 and 60 per cent in type 3 (three of five patients). No steroids were used. Death occurred most often from septicemia, after cutaneous recovery. He suspects secondary immune depression, as described by Schwab.

Marvin et al reported successful use of porcine xenografts in five cases of "Stevens-Johnson syndrome" which appears actually to have been TEN.

Chan HL: Observations on drug-induced toxic epidermal necrolysis in Singapore. JAAD 1984, 10:973.

Goldstein SM, et al: Toxic epidermal necrolysis. Arch Dermatol 1987, 123:1153.

Nethercott JR, et al: Erythema multiforme (Stevens-Johnson). Dermatologica 1985, 171:383.

Revuz J, et al: Treatment of toxic epidermal necrolysis (International workshop report). Arch Dermatol 1987, 123:1156.

Ruiz-Maldonado R: Acute disseminated epidermal necrosis types 1, 2, and 3. Study of 60 cases. JAAD 1985, 13:623.

Westly ED, et al: Toxic epidermal necrolysis: Granulocytic leukemia as a prognostic indicator. Arch Dermatol 1984, 120:721.

Yetiv YZ, et al: Etiologic factors of the Stevens-Johnson syndrome. South Med J 1980, 73:599.

ERYTHEMA ANNULARE CENTRIFUGUM

Erythema annulare centrifugum is a disease characterized by polycyclic, erythematous, sometimes bizarre, ringed lesions that grow eccentrically over several weeks, break up, disappear, and are replaced by new elements that follow a similar course. It is not a severe eruption but is often chronic and recurrent. The disease occurs on the trunk and especially on the buttocks and inner thighs where it forms large pink rings with elevated borders in festoons or arcs. Annular and gyrate shapes are seen. Occasionally a new lesion or even a third lesion begins within a primary lesion and traverses the area that has been involved. Usually there is a trailing scale at the inner border of the annular erythema. Rarely it is steep, with a firm rubberlike induration, while the internal border presents a gentle slope. Typically the surface is devoid of crusts or vesicles, and there are no local or general symptoms. Atypical cases with telangiectasia and purpuric spots are described. Mucosal lesions do not occur.

On histologic examination, the epidermis may show mild spongiosis or parakeratosis focally but is generally normal. Within the superficial and at times deep dermis, lymphocytes tightly encircle blood vessels in a pattern referred to as a "coat-sleeve" arrangement.

The cause is unknown. Some cases have been associated with dermatophytosis, drug allergy, or internal cancer. In the majority of cases, however, a specific etiology is not uncovered, and an extensive workup for associated internal diseases is not warranted.

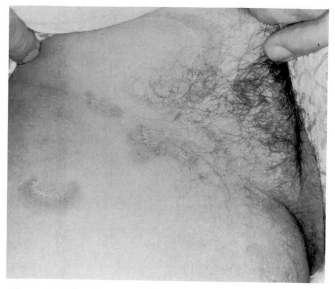

Figure 7–9. Erythema annulare centrifugum. (From Moschella SL, Pillsbury DM, Hurley HJ Jr: Dermatology. Philadelphia: WB Saunders, 1975.)

Shelley and Hurley reported a patient who was sensitive to her own cystic breast tissue. In another patient Shelley was able to show hypersensitivity to the *Penicillium* mold of blue cheese. Ashurst reported two cases resulting from the administration of hydroxychloroquine sulfate (Plaquenil) and one following use of chloroquine phosphate (Aralen).

Peterson and Jarratt (1981) reported a case of three months' duration in a six-month-old boy; lesions were transitory (36 to 48 hours), and the eruption stopped without treatment at age 11 months. They called it "annular erythema of infancy." A similar case, with more persistent lesions, was reported in a six-month-old girl by Toonstra and de Wit of Utrecht in 1984; it lasted 11 months, without treatment. Cox et al have reviewed this syndrome and believe their cases, and some earlier reported ones, to represent a separate entity.

Erythema annulare centrifugum tends to be persistent over several months to a few years, waxing and waning in severity. Most cases eventually subside spontaneously. While active, the eruption is responsive to topical steroids.

Cox NH, et al: Annular erythema of infancy. Arch Dermatol 1987, 123:510.

Hebert AA, et al: Annular erythema of infancy. JAAD 1986, 14:339.

Mahood JM: Erythema annulare centrifugum: Review of 24 cases with special reference to its associations with underlying disease. Clin Exp Dermatol 1983, 8:383.

Peterson AO Jr, et al: Annular erythema of infancy. Arch Dermatol 1981, 117:145.

Saurat JH, et al: Infantile epidermodysplastic erythema gyratum responsive to imidazoles. Arch Dermatol 1984, 120:1601.

Shelley WB: Erythema annulare centrifugum. Arch Dermatol 1964, 90:54.

Idem, et al: Unusual autoimmune syndrome: Erythema annulare centrifugum, generalized pigmentation and breast hypertrophy. Arch Dermatol 1960, 81:889.

Toonstra J, et al: 'Persistent' annular erythema of infancy. Arch Dermatol 1984, 120:1069.

ERYTHEMA MARGINATUM

Another of the figurate erythemas is this eruption, which is associated with rheumatic fever. Lesions are nonpruritic, rapidly spreading, annular or polycyclic, erythematous, and chiefly on the trunk. Like erythema annulare centrifugum, they wax and wane in severity, and may appear or disappear in a few hours. Troyer reported a case which histologically showed a perivascular infiltrate of polymorphonuclear leukocytes.

ERYTHEMA GYRATUM REPENS

A strikingly unusual pattern on the skin is characterized by undulating wavy bands of slightly elevated erythema over the entire body. Usually a manifestation of malignant disease, it has occurred with carcinoma of the breasts, lungs, pharynx, and ovaries. Most cases precede detection of the malignancy by one to 21 months. If the carcinoma is removed, the lesions clear.

Leavell and his associates summarized the reported cases of erythema gyratum repens associated with internal malignant disease and reported a case of their own. This was a 75-year-old man with an undifferentiated metastatic tumor of the brain with undetermined systemic malignancy. The skin lesions, accompanied by severe pruritus, disappeared for 25 days following craniotomy in which a large portion of the tumor was removed. Noteworthy was the overwhelming eosinophilia in the skin and blood, hyperpigmentation of the skin, and the appearance of the cutaneous eruption three years before the presence of the malignancy became apparent.

Holt and Davies studied one case with IgG and C3 present in the basement membrane zone of involved

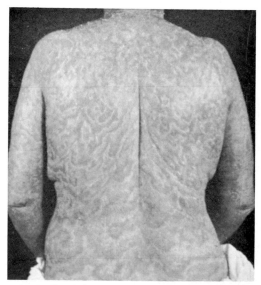

Figure 7–10. Erythema gyratum repens in association with bronchiogenic carcinoma. (Courtesy of Dr. John A. Gammel.)

and uninvolved skin; however, all other studies were unrevealing for the establishment of an immunologic pathogenetic mechanism. James has seen a case with similar immunofluorescent findings.

The histology is the same as that of erythema annulare centrifugum.

Langlois et al recently reported a case of erythema gyratum repens unassociated with internal malignancy and summarized the literature on this subject.

The disease is largely limited to adults, but in 1984 Saurat and Janin-Mercier reported a case with an unusual bowenoid histologic picture, in a 12-month-old girl, which persisted to age four after having responded very well to ketoconazole, 50 mg daily.

Holt PGA, et al: Erythema gyratum repens. Br J Dermatol 1977, 96:343.

Langlois JL, et al: Erythema gyratum repens unassociated with internal malignancy. JAAD 1985, 12:911.

Leavell UW Jr, et al: Erythema gyratum repens and undifferentiated carcinoma. Arch Dermatol 1967, 95:69.

Sholnick M, et al: Erythema gyratum repens with metastatic adenocarcinoma. Arch Dermatol 1975, 111:227.

Troyer C, et al: Erythema marginatum in rheumatic fever: Early diagnosis by skin biopsy. JAAD 1983, 9:724.

White JW Jr: The gyrate erythemas. J Assoc Milit Dermatol 1983, 9:13.

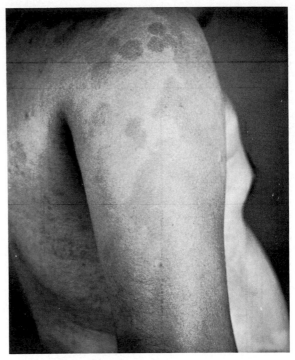

Figure 7–12. Erythema dyschromicum perstans. (Courtesy of Dr. F. Kerdel-Vegas.)

ERYTHEMA CHRONICUM MIGRANS

The recent discovery that this is caused by infection with a spirochete, *Borrelia burgdorferi*, has caused this to be discussed in Chapter 14 on bacterial diseases.

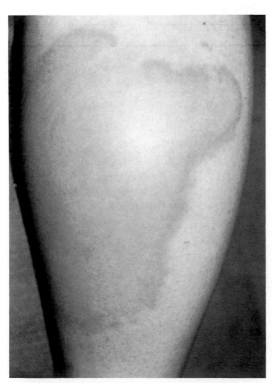

Figure 7–11. Erythema chronicum migrans.

ERYTHEMA DYSCHROMICUM PERSTANS

This is also known as **ashy dermatosis**. It was first described by Ramirez in 1957 as **dermatosis cinecienta**. In 1961 the first reports of this unusual dermatosis as erythema dyschromicum perstans were made by Convit and his associates.

Grayish, pigmented, ashy patches with some violaceous hues and a fine erythematous noninfiltrated or at most slightly infiltrated border may occur on the face, trunk, or extremities. Some of the patches are bandlike or orbicular, but always sharply demarcated. Growth is by centrifugal extension to bizarre polycyclic patterns.

In the acute phase, the characteristic histologic features are those of a lichenoid dermatitis with disruption of the basal layer of the epidermis and a bandlike inflammatory infiltrate in the superficial dermis. In the chronic phases, the histologic changes are those of postinflammatory pigmentation; the characteristic gray-blue skin hue reflects the presence of melanin-laden macrophages in the dermis. Immunofluorescence microscopy reveals numerous cytoid bodies, and Person and Rogers suggest that these are the result of apoptosis (individual cell death).

Clinically, only the distinctive, often slightly elevated, red margin permits this disorder to be distinguished from similar ashen gray pigmentation caused by noninflammatory irritative or allergic reactions to perfumes or fragrances.

There are no systemic manifestations. It can occur in all ages from five (Person and Rogers) through early adulthood, and it affects both sexes. It occurs mostly in Central America and Venezuela, although Stevenson, Knox and his associates, and Person et al have described cases occurring in the United States.

The cause of the eruption has not been identified. It is considered to be a form of erythema perstans.

Convit J, et al: Erythema dyschromicum perstans: Hitherto un-described skin disease. J Invest Dermatol 1961, 36:457.
Nelson BR, et al: Asymptomatic progressive hyperpigmentation in a 16-year-old-girl. Arch Dermatol 1988, 124:769.
Novick NL, Phelps R: Erythema dyschromicum perstans. Int J Dermatol 1985, 24:630.
Person JR, et al: Ashy dermatosis. Arch Dermatol 1981, 117:701.
Ramirez CO: The ashy dermatosis (erythema dyschromicum per-stans). Cutis 1967, 3:244.
Tschen JA: Erythema dyschromicum perstans. JAAD 1980, 2:295.
Venencie PY, et al: Erythema dyschromicum perstans following HIV seroconversion in a child with hemophilia B. Arch Dermatol 1988, 124:1013.

FAMILIAL MEDITERRANEAN FEVER

This genetic disorder, which is restricted to certain ethnic groups, is characterized by acute self-limited febrile episodes of 24 to 48 days' duration. An ery-sipelaslike erythema on the lower extremities accompanied by mild arthralgia may be the only manifestation of this irregularly occurring bout. Other infrequent skin lesions may be Henoch-Schönlein purpura, subcutaneous nodules, and herpes simplex labialis.

Recently Matzner and Brzezinski have found a deficiency of an inhibitor of anaphylatoxin C5a in the peritoneal fluid of patients with this disease. They postulate that its lack may have a role in the inflammatory attacks.

Colchicine is effective preventive therapy in most patients.

Azizi E, et al: Cutaneous manifestations of familial Mediterranean fever. Arch Dermatol 1976, 112:364.
Matzner Y, et al: $C_5\alpha$-inhibitor deficiency in peritoneal fluid from patients with familial Mediterranean fever. N Engl J Med 1984, 311:287.

ERYTHEMA ELEVATUM DIUTINUM

CLINICAL FEATURES. Erythema elevatum diutinum is characterized by persistent, elevated, erythematous, annular plaques. The infiltrated plaques may become nodular, varying from 0.5 to several centimeters in diameter, with a preference for location overlying the joints, especially those of the fingers, wrists, elbows, knees, ankles, and toes, and over the Achilles tendons. The calves, buttocks, and forearms may also be involved. The surface of the lesion is usually smooth but may be slightly verrucous. The lesions are usually painful rather than pruritic. It is a chronic and progressive disease that

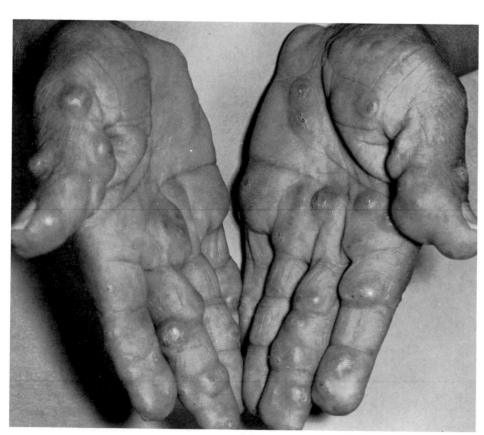

Figure 7–13. Nodules of erythema elevatum diutinum on the palms. (Courtesy of Dr. H. L. Hines.)

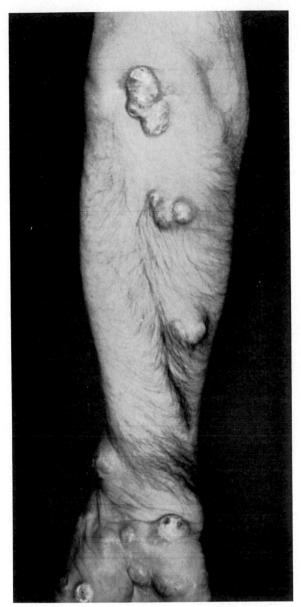

Figure 7–14. Erythema elevatum diutinum on the hand and arm. (Courtesy of Drs. J. P. Mraz and V. D. Newcomer.)

LABORATORY FINDINGS. Most patients have elevated erythrocyte sedimentation rates. IgA and IgG monoclonal gammopathies have been reported, as have occasional cases of myeloma.

DIFFERENTIAL DIAGNOSIS. Sweet's syndrome, xanthomas, granuloma annulare, granuloma faciale, and multicentric reticulohistiocytomas should be considered in the differential diagnosis.

TREATMENT. Steroids used topically or intralesionally produce but little amelioration. There is often a dramatic response with dapsone (Avlosulfon, Ayerst) within 48 hours after start of therapy. It is well to begin with 50 mg nightly for three or four days, increasing to twice daily; then if there is no response, three times daily on the seventh day, and four times daily on the tenth. Methemoglobinemia and hemolytic anemia must be watched for early, and leukopenia later. The course of the disease may extend many years.

Kohler and Lorincz reported a severe case with bullae, which responded to tetracycline and niacinamide and had excellent control from intermittent use of the latter alone, 100 mg t.i.d.

Extracellular Cholesterosis

Originally described by Urbach in 1932, extracellular cholesterosis is now regarded as erythema elevatum diutinum.

Fort SL, et al: Erythema elevatum diutinum. Arch Dermatol 1977, 113:819.

Katz SL, et al: Erythema elevatum diutinum: Skin and systemic manifestations, immunologic studies and successful treatment with dapsone. Medicine 1977, 56:443.

Kohler IK, et al: Erythema elevatum diutinum treated with niacinamide and tetracycline. Arch Dermatol 1980, 116:693.

may last for many years, with the involution of some lesions and the appearance of new ones. The purplish red and chilblainlike infiltrations on the thenar and hypothenar eminences, wrists, forearms, and ankles are characteristic. Vesicles may be present in many patients.

ETIOLOGY. This disease is considered to be a chronic vasculitis. Recurrent streptococcal infections occur in some of these patients, and streptococcal infections exacerbate the disease. Hypersensitivity to streptococcal cell products may induce an immune-complex disease state.

HISTOLOGY. There is a dense, diffuse infiltrate composed of neutrophils and eosinophils. There is vasculitis with leucocytoclasia and fibrinoid deposits.

ERYTHEMA BRUCELLUM (Contact Brucellosis)

Erythema brucellum is an erythematous eruption usually occurring in veterinary surgeons and cattlemen after attending cows infected with brucellosis. The eruption begins with itching and erythema of the upper extremities and sometimes also of the face and neck within a few hours after exposure. Soon the skin becomes thickened and covered with conical follicular papules, pustules, and brownish crusts; it finally heals in about two weeks. *Brucella abortus* has not been demonstrated in the lesions, suggesting that the disease is due to sensitization rather than infection.

White PC, et al: Brucellosis in a Virginia meat-packing plant. Arch Environ Health 1974, 28:263.

ERYTHEMA NODOSUM

CLINICAL FEATURES. The eruption consists of bilateral, tender nodules 1 to 5 cm in diameter on the shins. The skin over the nodules is red, smooth, and shiny. The individual lesions may coalesce to form sizable indurations, which lead to considerable edema of the affected parts. Ulceration does not occur. The lesions occur also on other parts of the extremities, on the buttocks, and rarely, on the face. The nodules last a few days or weeks, appearing in crops, and then slowly undergo involution. The disease occurs chiefly in young women during the spring or autumn.

The onset of an attack is ushered in by constitutional symptoms, which are usually mild. These consist of fever, malaise, and pains in the muscles and joints.

A chronic form of erythema nodosum, erythema nodosum migrans, is characterized by a persistent course, peripherally expanding lesions, a tendency to a unilateral distribution, and a lesser degree of tenderness.

ETIOLOGY. Erythema nodosum is considered a reactive process and is commonly associated with a streptococcal infection or a drug reaction. Streptococcal infections implicated may be rheumatic fever, streptococcal pharyngitis and tonsillitis, erysipelas, or scarlet fever.

Tuberculosis was at one time an important causa-

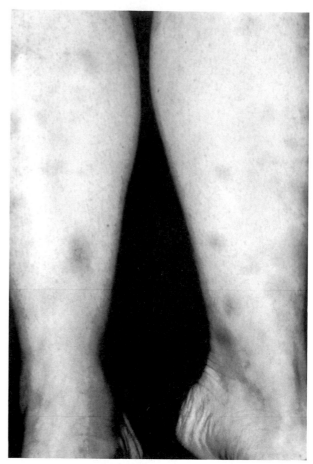

Figure 7–16. Erythema nodosum in sarcoidosis. (Courtesy of Dr. Axel W. Hoke.)

tive factor, especially in children. Erythema nodosum may occur in these children as frequently as pleurisy.

Sarcoidosis may present with fever, cough, joint pains, hilar adenopathy, and erythema nodosum. This symptom complex, known as Löfgren's syndrome, is especially common in Scandinavia.

Coccidioidomycosis, histoplasmosis, blastomycosis, American leishmaniasis, Trichophyton fungus infections, cat-scratch fever, leptospirosis, and lymphogranuloma venereum may be accompanied by erythema nodosum.

Erythema nodosum has been reported as the initial manifestation in a case of acute granulocytic leukemia. It has also occurred concomitantly with acute monocytic leukemia, chronic lymphocytic leukemia and chronic granulocytic leukemia.

Drugs may also induce erythema nodosum. The bromides, iodides, and sulfonamides were once the most frequent causative drugs. In recent years contraceptive pills have been implicated, and Bombardieri reported one patient who had erythema nodosum from the second to the fifth month in each of four pregnancies.

Erythema nodosum is sometimes seen in patients with inflammatory diseases of the bowel such as regional enteritis and ulcerative colitis. Tami reported a case in which attacks were chronologically related

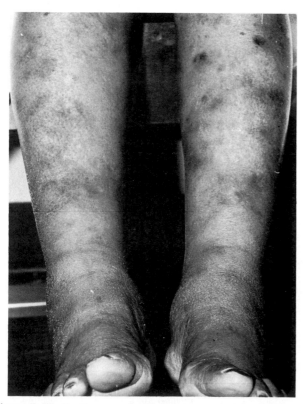

Figure 7–15. Erythema nodosum leprosum mimicking true erythema nodosum.

to a colitis caused by *Shigella flexneri*. Infectious diseases of the bowel such as that due to *Yersinia enterocolitica* and *Campylobacter jejuni* may be associated with erythema nodosum.

PATHOGENESIS. Erythema nodosum is an inflammatory disease in which delayed hypersensitivity reactions involve the large blood vessels of the skin and the fibrous septa of the subcutaneous tissue.

DIFFERENTIAL DIAGNOSIS. Early cases of erythema induratum may resemble erythema nodosum so closely that differential diagnosis is difficult, although the microscopic findings are of considerable assistance. Erythema induratum usually affects the calves alone and runs a slower course, with likelihood of ulceration. Syphilitic gummas, as well as the nodules of sporotrichosis, are, as a rule, unilateral. Weber-Christian disease, subcutaneous fat necrosis associated with pancreatitis, lipogranulomatosis subcutanea, and nodular vasculitis may also occur on the shins and must be differentiated from erythema nodosum. The classic picture of symmetrical tender nodules on the legs in a young woman usually offers no great difficulty in diagnosis.

HISTOLOGY. Erythema nodosum is a septal panniculitis; there is an inflammatory infiltrate principally involving the connective-tissue septa between fat lobules of the panniculus. The infiltrate may be composed of either acute or chronic inflammatory cells or it may be mixed. Histiocytes and multinucleate giant cells may predominate. Fat lobules are only secondarily affected by the inflammation. Classic leucocytoclastic vasculitis is not a histologic feature of erythema nodosum, although the vessels demonstrate endothelial proliferation and damage.

TREATMENT. The treatment of any underlying associated abnormality should be initiated promptly. In addition, salicylates and other nonsteroidal antiinflammatory agents are of value. Indomethacin (Indocin) 25 mg t.i.d. was reported effective by Barr, by Ubogy, and by Elizaga, and Lehman reported success with naproxen (Naprosyn) in a case that had persisted for two years. Corticosteroids or colchicine are often effective.

Schulz and Whiting had good results from treatment with potassium iodide, and this has been confirmed repeatedly since their report. Five drops t.i.d., increased gradually to 30 drops, is the usual dose; it may also be administered as a tablet, in which case 300 mg is given t.i.d. Induction of hypothyroidism by prolonged iodide therapy (the Wolf-Chaikoff effect) should be watched for, as pointed out by Johnson et al.

All therapy should be combined with rest in bed and supportive treatment of the affected parts.

PROGNOSIS. The prognosis usually is good, the disease running its course in a few weeks. Recurrences are extremely rare.

Badan HP, et al: Erythema nodosum from oral contraceptives. Arch Dermatol 1968, 98:634.
Bafverstedt B: Erythema nodosum migrans. Acta Derm Venereol (Stockholm) 1968, 48:381.

Barr WG, et al: Chronic erythema nodosum treated with indomethacin. Ann Intern Med 1981, 95:659.
Bombardieri S, et al: Erythema nodosum associated with pregnancy and oral contraceptives. Br Med J 1977, 1:1509.
Buckler JMH: Leptospirosis presenting with erythema nodosum. Arch Dis Child 1977, 52:418.
Elizaga FV: Erythema nodosum and indomethacin. Ann Intern Med 1982, 96:383.
Fine RM, et al: Chronic erythema nodosum: Form of allergic cutaneous vasculitis. South Med J 1968, 61:680.
Horio T, et al: Potassium iodide in erythema nodosum and other erythematous dermatoses. JAAD 1983, 9:77.
Johnson TM, et al: The Wolf-Chaikoff effect. Arch Dermatol 1988, 124:1184.
Katz BT, et al: Subcutaneous nodules in a man diagnosed as having tuberculosis. Arch Dermatol 1988, 124:121.
Lehman CW: Control of chronic erythema nodosum with naproxen. Cutis 1980, 6:66.
Rostas A, et al: Erythema nodosum migrans in a young woman. Arch Dermatol 1980, 116:325.
Shulz EJ, et al: Treatment of erythema nodosum and nodular vasculitis with potassium iodide. Br J Dermatol 1976, 94:75.
Sumaya CV, et al: Erythema nodosum-like lesions of leukemia. Arch Dermatol 1974, 110:415.
Tami LF: Erythema nodosum associated with Shigella colitis. Arch Dermatol 1985, 121:590.
Ubogy Z: Suppression of erythema nodosum by indomethacin. Acta Dermatovener (Stockh) 1982, 62:265.

Subacute Nodular Migratory Panniculitis

In 1956 Vilanova and Aguade described subacute nodular migratory panniculitis. This is now felt to be erythema nodosum migrans.

GLUCAGONOMA SYNDROME

Also known as **necrolytic migratory erythema**, this syndrome is characterized by eczematous and bullous dermatitis, stomatitis, elevated serum glucagon, abnormal glucose tolerance, weight loss, and anemia. Hypoaminoacidemia is a hallmark finding and hypocholesterolemia is frequent.

Erythematous plaques appear on the central face, perineum, and lower abdomen. Flaccid vesicles and bullae develop, rupture, and produce extensive erosions or exudative crusted plaques.

Histologically, there is irregular acanthosis with spongiosis, subcorneal and midepidermal clefts, fusiform keratinocytes with pyknotic nuclei, absence of acantholysis, and negative immunofluorescence findings. Ohyama has described the ultramicroscopic findings.

Etiologically, this syndrome occurs in association with a glucagon-secreting alpha-cell tumor of the pancreas. Over 80 per cent of tumors are malignant, and half have demonstrated metastases at surgery. Cases have been reported in which no glucagonoma was found, however.

In the differential diagnosis, toxic epidermal necrolysis, pemphigus foliaceus, acrodermatitis enteropathica, and erythema multiforme must be kept in mind.

The surgical removal of the primary pancreatic tumor produces complete clearing of the syndrome. Topical corticosteroids are helpful prior to removal of the tumor.

Machina et al reported that diphenylhydantoin (Phenytoin), 200 mg t.i.d., lowered the plasma glucagon level and abolished the effect of arginine on it, prior to removal of a glucagonoma.

When surgical removal is not feasible for any reason, dacarbazine (DTIC) should be tried. It was first reported to be effective by Kessinger et al in 1977. Most recently, van der Loos et al have reported a complete cure with two and a half-year follow-up in a case with hepatic metastases.

Dons RF, et al: Intertriginous rash responsive to topical or surgical therapy. Arch Dermatol 1988, 124:431.
Hashizume T, et al: Glucagonoma syndrome. JAAD 1988, 19:377.
Kessinger A, et al: The glucagonoma syndrome and its management. J Surg Oncol 1977, 9:419.
van der Loos TLJM, et al: Successful treatment of glucagonoma-related necrolytic migratory erythema with dacarbazine. JAAD 1987, 16:468.

NODULAR VASCULITIS

First described by Montgomery, O'Leary, and Barker, nodular vasculitis is characterized by recurrent slightly painful nodules located chiefly on the calves, and less often the shins, in women past their thirties. The nodules may or may not ulcerate, and heal with dyspigmentation and scarring. They may occur only on the feet. They do occur in men.

The etiology is unknown. Erythema nodosum is a clinically similar disorder, within which many include nodular vasculitis as a subset. Nodular vasculitis is not associated with tuberculosis and does not show caseation necrosis. We prefer to separate these entities.

Histologically, a vasculitis occurs with varying degrees of obliterative changes in the veins and arteries, fibrosis of the subcutaneous tissues, and fat necrosis. Pinkus and Mehregan aver that when a large artery or vein is the center of the infiltration reaction, a diagnosis of nodular vasculitis is appropriate.

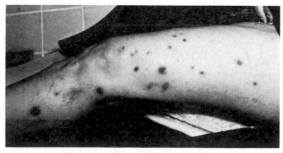

Figure 7–17. Nodular vasculitis.

In the differential diagnosis the following must also be considered: erythema induratum, erythema nodosum, Weber-Christian disease, erythema nodosum migrans, recurrent thrombophlebitis, and periarteritis nodosa.

Treatment is along the lines of possible etiology. Antibacterial and anti-inflammatory measures are important. Elastic bandages and bed rest are helpful. Systemic steroids or colchicine may be effective. One of us (HLA) had a patient, disabled by recurrent tender nodules in his feet, who recovered completely as soon as he stopped smoking.

Horio T, et al: Potassium iodide in erythema nodosum and other erythematous dermatoses. JAAD 1983, 9:77.

GRANULOMA ANNULARE

TYPES

Localized Granuloma Annulare. This peculiar, nodular, ringed eruption chiefly affects children. Females are affected two to one. It usually begins on the lateral or dorsal surfaces of the fingers or hands, wrists, ankles, and insteps as a white or pink flat-topped papule, which slowly spreads peripherally, at the same time undergoing central involution, so that roughly annular lesions are formed. Lesions may also occur on the scalp, arms, trunk, and legs and may be single or multiple, but are seldom over a half dozen in number. They may coalesce and sometimes form scalloped patterns or firm plaques. The lesions never ulcerate and on disappearing leave no trace. The disease develops slowly and involutes spontaneously. Wells reported 73 per cent of 115 patients

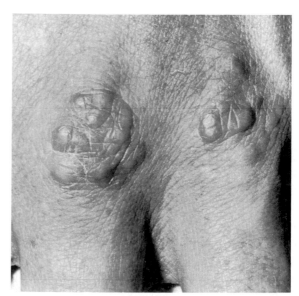

Figure 7–18. Granuloma annulare in a typical location on the knuckles.

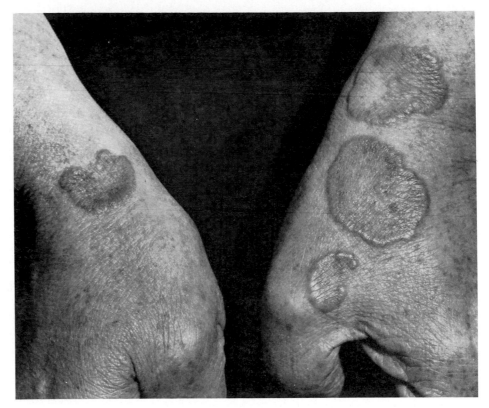

Figure 7–19. Granuloma annulare on wrists of a 57-year-old woman, which cleared with intralesional corticosteroid suspension injections. (Courtesy of Dr. Axel W. Hoke.)

had clearing within two years, but 25 per cent had no clearing in eight years.

Generalized Granuloma Annulare. This is characterized by a diffuse papular eruption involving the sun-exposed areas, especially the nape of the neck and the V area of the upper chest. Other involved areas may be the forearms and dorsa of the hands.

The face is usually spared despite the sun-exposure factor, but in 100 cases reviewed by Dabski et al, every location was found to be affected except the genital area. The disease affects mostly women past middle age. Diabetes has been reported to occur with this disease.

Sarcoidosis, lichen myxedematosus, cutaneous

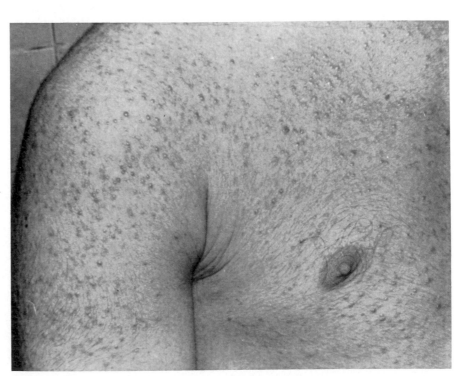

Figure 7–20. Generalized papular granuloma annulare over entire body.

amyloidosis, and lichen planus are to be considered in the differential diagnosis.

Complete spontaneous clearing has been known to occur in as early as four months, but eruptions persist for three to four years on the average. Some may last over a decade and relapse may occur. The excellent complete review by Dabski et al is highly recommended.

Macular Granuloma Annulare. Often the earliest lesions will be, especially on the feet and ankles, sharply defined brown oval macules, 1 to 4 cm in diameter.

Nodular Granuloma Annulare. Scalp lesions, especially in children, may be very deep-seated, even subcutaneous, nodules. Such deep nodules may also occur on the arms or legs. Superficial papular lesions are present in about one fourth of patients with this subcutaneous variety.

Perforating Granuloma Annulare. Allan Izumi in 1972 confirmed Owens and Freeman's report of perforating lesions of granuloma annulare: papules in which the granuloma had perforated through the epidermis.

Granuloma Multiforme (Leiker). This is a papular eruption that evolves into round or oval plaques up to 15 cm wide within a year's time. They may be elevated to as much as 4 mm in height and have a slightly depressed center.

Marshall and his associates found this type of granuloma annulare among the Tio people in Nigeria. No cause has been found.

PATHOGENESIS. Dahl and his associates found IgM and C3 in the blood vessels of the skin in 10 of 20 patients studied. In some, fibrinogen was found in the dermal-epidermal junction. These findings suggest to them an immunoglobulin-mediated vasculitis in the pathogenesis of granuloma annulare.

ETIOLOGY. The cause of the various forms of granuloma annulare is unknown. Ultraviolet light, insect bites, such as sandfly bites, and trauma have been postulated, but proof is lacking. Its occurrence in scars is well documented. Recent reports of its association with Epstein-Barr virus and HIV infection raise the possibility of a viral etiology.

HISTOPATHOLOGY. There is a palisading granuloma characterized by histiocytes and epithelioid cells surrounding a central zone of altered collagen in the mid- to upper dermis. In well-developed lesions, there is mucin deposition within the foci of altered collagen.

Necrobiosis lipoidica may histologically resemble granuloma annulare but it involves the deep dermis and subcutis as well and mucin is usually not present.

DIFFERENTIAL DIAGNOSIS. In the differential diagnosis the following must be considered: sarcoidosis, lichen planus, urticaria pigmentosa, and papular mucinosis.

TREATMENT. Various forms of treatment have been tried with indifferent success. It has been maintained that a biopsy of the lesion will cause its involution; however, these are anecdotal reports. The intralesional injection of triamcinolone suspension has been more effective for us than any other method. Sparrow and Abell, using intralesional steroids, reported success in 70 per cent of their cases, as opposed to 44 per cent of controls injected (by a jet injector) only with saline solution. Most relapsed within three to seven months.

In generalized eruptions, systemic steroids may be very effective, though the high dose required for the oral route makes this approach too dangerous. The risk with intramuscular triamcinolone acetonide is acceptably small. Spontaneous clearing does occur, although it may take several years.

Saied et al reported two cases, one of three years' duration, which recovered (apparently permanently) on dapsone, 100 mg once or twice daily. Steiner et al have recently confirmed the effectiveness of dapsone. It is worth a trial. Isotretinoin (Accutane) 80 mg daily was effective in a very refractory case treated by Schleicher et al. Niacinamide, 1.5 gm daily (900 mg was not effective), cleared a case treated by Ma et al. Gressel et al reported in 1979 that potassium iodide was effective, and Caserio et al confirmed this in 1984.

Caserio RJ, et al: Treatment of granuloma annulare with potassium iodide. JAAD 1984, 10:294.
Czarnecki DB, et al: The response of generalized granuloma annulare to dapsone. Acta Derm Venereol (Stockh) 1986, 66:82.
Dabski K, et al: Generalized granuloma annulare. JAAD 1989, 20:28, 39.
Freidman SJ, et al: Familial granuloma annulare. JAAD 1987, 16:600.
Ghadially R, et al: Granuloma annulare in patients with human immunodeficiency virus infections. JAAD 1989, 20:232.
Huerter CJ, et al: Perforating granuloma annulare in a patient with acquired immunodeficiency syndrome. Arch Dermatol 1987, 123:1217.
Izumi AK: Perforating granuloma annulare. Arch Dermatol 1973, 108:708.
Ma A, et al: Response of generalized granuloma annulare to high-dose niacinamide. Arch Dermatol 1983, 119:836.
Mahlbauer JE: Granuloma annulare. JAAD 1980, 3:217.
Marshall J, et al: Granuloma multiforme. (Leiker). Dermatologica 1967, 134:193.
McFarland JP, et al: Periorbital granuloma annulare. Arch Dermatol 1982, 118:190.
Schwartz ME: Necrobiosis lipoidica and granuloma annulare. Arch Dermatol 1982, 118:192.
Shelnitz LB, et al: Umbilicated papular eruption on the extremities of a child. Arch Dermatol 1986, 122:933.
Sparrow G, et al: Granuloma annulare and necrobiosis lipoidia treated by jet injector. Br J Dermatol 1975, 93:85.
Steiner A, et al: Sulfone treatment of granuloma annulare. JAAD 1985, 13:1004.
Wells RS, et al: The natural history of granuloma annulare. Br J Dermatol 1963, 75:199.

SWEET'S SYNDROME
(Acute Febrile Neutrophilic Dermatosis)

This is characterized by large, rapidly extending, tender, erythematous, painful, elevated plaques 2 to

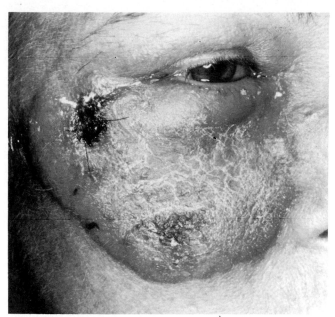

Figure 7–21. Sweet's syndrome. (Courtesy of Dr. Lewis Shapiro.)

10 cm in diameter appearing typically on the face, neck, and extremities. In about one third of cases the plaques become studded with pustules. The onset is typically one to three weeks after an upper respiratory infection; arthritis and iritis may accompany the eruption. Most of the reported cases have occurred in women.

There is fever and leukocytosis, with a high percentage of neutrophils in the blood.

Biopsy of the skin lesions usually shows dense infiltration of neutrophilic leukocytes in the upper and mid-dermis.

The differential diagnosis must distinguish this from erythema multiforme and erythema nodosum.

The etiology is considered to be a hypersensitivity reaction to a preceding upper respiratory infection in some cases. An association with the onset of leukemia, especially of the myelogenous types, has been reported. Caughman et al identified separate bullous and pustular plaques previously reported as bullous pyoderma gangrenosum and atypical Sweet's syndrome with leukemia as an entity called *neutrophilic dermatosis of malignancy*. They (and we) feel these neutrophilic reaction patterns are part of a continuum of inflammation that is reactive to underlying malignancy.

Treatment is with systemic corticosteroids. Doses of 40 to 60 mg of oral prednisone a day result in resolution of fever and lesions within days. Saxe has reported success with clofazimine (Lamprene), 100 mg t.i.d. Medication should be continued over an adequate length of time to prevent relapse, which occurs with some frequency. Horio et al used potassium iodide with excellent results, and Suehisa treated a case successfully with colchicine. Aram reported a chronic relapsing case, without fever, which cleared on dapsone, 100 mg twice a day. Colchicine and indomethacin have also been said to be effective in anecdotal case reports.

Bechtel MA, et al: Acute febrile neutrophilic dermatosis. Arch Dermatol 1981, 117:664.
Caughman W, et al: Neutrophilic dermatosis of myeloproliferative disease. JAAD 1983, 9:751.
Cohen PR, et al: Sweet's syndrome and malignancy. Am J Med 1987, 82:1220.
Cooper DH, et al: Acute febrile neutrophilic dermatosis and myeloproliferative disorders. Cancer 1983, 51:1518.
Idem: Subcutaneous neutrophilic infiltrate in acute febrile neutrophilic dermatosis. Arch Dermatol 1983, 119:610.
Going JJ, et al: Sweet's syndrome. J Clin Pathol 1987, 40:175.
Goette DK: Sweet's syndrome in subacute cutaneous lupus erythematosus. Arch Dermatol 1985, 121:789.
Gunawardena DA, et al: The clinical spectrum of Sweet's syndrome. Br J Dermatol 1975, 92:363.
Leibovici V, et al: Sweet's syndrome. Int J Dermatol 1987, 26:178.
Levin DL, et al: Sweet's syndrome in children. J Pediatr 1981, 99:73.
Perry AE, et al: Rapid onset of pustular plaques. Arch Dermatol 1987, 123:519.
Su WPD, et al: Diagnostic criteria for Sweet's syndrome. Cutis 1987, 37:167.

RHEUMATOID NEUTROPHILIC DERMATOSIS

Chronic urticaria-like plaques characterized histologically by a dense neutrophilic infiltrate, occurring in patients with debilitating rheumatoid arthritis, were described by Ackerman in his book. One of us (WDJ) has recently had such a patient, and the disorder seems to be clinically and histologically separable from Sweet's syndrome and erythema elevatum diutinum.

Ackerman AB: Histologic Diagnosis of Inflammatory Skin Disease, 1st ed. Philadelphia, Lea & Febiger, 1978, p 449.
Scherbenske JM, et al: Rheumatoid neutrophilic dermatosis. Arch Dermatol 1989, 125:1105.

URTICARIA

Synonyms: Hives, nettle rash, cnidosis.

CLINICAL FEATURES. Urticaria is a vascular reaction of the skin characterized by the appearance of wheals, which are elevated, whitish or reddish evanescent plaques, generally surrounded by a red halo or flare, and associated with severe itching, stinging, or pricking sensations. These wheals are caused by localized edema. The eruption may also consist of

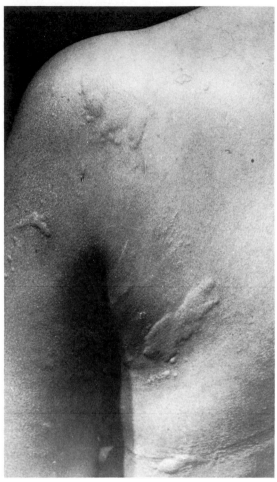

Figure 7–22. Urticaria. (Courtesy of Dr. I. Abrahams.)

macular erythema or papules and may be localized or generalized, the latter being the more common. Their size can vary from a small papule to the diameter of a large platter. The eruption usually favors the covered areas, such as the trunk, buttocks, or chest. The palms and soles are favorite sites for penicillin urticaria. Subcutaneous swellings (angioedema), especially of eyelids or lips, may accompany the wheals, or occur alone.

Tissues other than the skin may be involved, which gives rise to symptoms such as coryza, asthma, and abdominal pain. Laryngeal edema may occur with severe urticaria, and this may lead to a life-threatening situation, especially in familial cases (familial angioneurotic edema). Therefore, prompt treatment with subcutaneous injections of epinephrine is mandatory. Intravenous injections of diphenhydramine (Benadryl) or methylprednisolone succinate (Solu-Medrol) may be tried. Tracheostomy may become necessary.

Urticaria may be acute or chronic and also may have special forms.

Acute Urticaria. Acute hives are commonly experienced. Insect bites and stings are common urticaria inducers in many people. Food allergies, drugs such as penicillin and sulfonamides, or physical allergies may be the causes of acute urticaria. Often it is impossible to find the causative agent; however, if it can be found and removed, the hives involute rapidly.

Chronic Urticaria. When urticaria recurs daily over a six or more week period, it is termed "chronic" urticaria. Finding the cause challenges not only the physician but also the patients, who must search for a cause in their daily exposures and endure discomfort throughout efforts at testing for the cause and finding efficacious medication for the relief of symptoms.

Contact Urticaria. (See Syndrome of Immediate Reactivity, Chapter 6.) Odom and Maibach have described a half-hour open patch test for demonstrating either nonimmunologic or immunologic urticarial responses to a variety of substances.

ETIOLOGY. There are seemingly countless causes of urticaria. Food, drugs, and infections are the most frequent causes of chronic urticaria. Other factors will be treated in more detail under the discussions of the various types of urticaria.

Food. Varying opinions are held regarding the role of food allergens in chronic urticaria. In acute urticaria foods are frequently the cause, whereas in chronic urticaria food is a less frequent factor. The most allergenic foods are chocolate, shellfish, nuts, peanut butter, tomatoes, strawberries, melons, pork, cheese, garlic, onions, and spices. In addition to these there are many common foods to which a person may become allergic.

If the urticaria is acute and recurrent, food allergy may at times be diagnosed through the use of a diary kept by the patient, recording ingestants taken within 24 hours before each attack. The best method of determining a food allergy in chronic urticaria is by an elimination diet which allows only bland nonallergenic foods. Such a diet usually permits use of the following: lamb, beef, rice, potatoes, carrots, string beans, peas, squash, applesauce with tapioca, preserved pears, peaches, or cherries, Ry-Krisp, butter, sugar, tea without milk or lemon, and coffee without cream. This diet is followed for three weeks. If urticaria does not occur, then suspected foods are added one by one and reactions observed.

The use of scratch and intradermal tests is untrustworthy and uninformative. An offending food may give a negative response. Moreover, food additives and preservatives, as shown by Michaëlsson and Juhlin, may be responsible.

Drugs. Drugs are probably the most frequent causes of urticaria and angioedema. A list of urticariogenic drugs appears on page 119. Of these, probably penicillin is the most frequent causative agent; it is discussed separately on page 124. A frequently overlooked factor is that penicillin sensitivity may become so exquisite that reactions can occur from penicillin-contaminated milk. Penicillin is sometimes used for treating mastitis in cows, although this is forbidden by law. Beer may also produce hives because of penicillin in the fermentation products.

Aspirin. Michaëlsson and Juhlin have emphasized the high incidence of aspirin-caused urticaria. In addition, they have been able to demonstrate that aspirin-sensitized persons tend to have cross sensitivity with tartrazine, the yellow azo benzone dye, and other azo dyes, as well as benzoic acid and its derivatives. These are common food additives and preservatives with a high index of exposure in everyday eating.

Other common drugs that may cause hives are sulfonamides, narcotics, nonsteroidal antiinflammatory agents, vitamins, estrogens, insulin, quinine, phenylbutazone, salicylates, phenothiazine, probenecid, nitrofurantoin, bromosulphalein, procaine, thiouracil, and isoniazid.

Food Additives. Although foods may cause urticaria, the food additives are also important etiologic factors. Natural food additives are yeasts, salicylates, citric acid, egg, and fish albumin. In addition to these there are the synthetic additives. The most important are azo dyes, benzoic acid derivatives, and penicillin.

Yeast is widely used, and when it is suspected as the causative agent, bread and breadstuffs, sausages, wine, beer, grapes, cheese, vinegar, pickled foods, catsup, and yeast tablets should be avoided.

Azo dyes, particularly the yellow dye tartrazine, and the related green and red dyes should be avoided. Foods containing azo dyes and benzoic acid are the "penny" candies, soft drinks, jellies, marmalades, custards, puddings, various cake and pancake mixes, mayonnaise, ready-made salad dressings and sauces, packaged soups, anchovies, and colored toothpastes. There are undoubtedly many more and only by constant awareness in looking for these substances can one be reasonably sure that they are being avoided.

Infections. The role of chronic focal infections in urticaria is still undetermined. Nevertheless, the possibility of chronically infected tonsils, periapical infections, impacted wisdom teeth, or infected sinuses, gallbladder, or kidneys as causative factors may be investigated.

Urticaria may be associated with upper respiratory infections, and more especially with streptococcal etiology, according to Schuller et al, who found that 33 of 81 cases had evidence of streptococcal infection.

Emotional Stress. There is little doubt that persons under severe emotional stress will have more marked urticaria no matter what the primary cause may be. In cholinergic urticaria emotional stress is a particularly well-documented inciting stimulus.

Physical Factors. Various responses of the body to the same factor, such as cold, trauma, or sunlight, suggest that there may be various pathogenic mechanisms at work.

Cryoglobulins, cryofibrinogens, and cold hemolysins are cold-activated agents mediating the complement cascade (see later), in which urticaria may be but one of several manifestations.

Trauma such as stroking and pressure may also invoke urticaria. This is called dermatographia. (See below.)

Serum Sickness. Urticaria may be caused by the injection of serums or drugs. This form of hypersensitivity may be the forerunner of neuritis, hypersensitivity angiitis, polyarteritis nodosa, or anaphylaxis.

Menthol. This is a rare cause of urticaria; however, when it does occur, a number of different substances into which it is incorporated may elicit an urticarial response. Mentholated cigarettes, candy and mints, cough drops, aerosol sprays, and topical medications are among these.

Neoplasms. Urticaria has been associated with carcinomas and Hodgkin's disease. Cold urticaria with cryoglobulinemia has been reported associated with chronic lymphocytic leukemia.

Inhalants. Shelley and Florence have shown *Aspergillus flavus* was the causative agent in a woman with urticaria of seven years' duration. Grass pollens, feathers, formaldehyde, acrolein (produced when frying with lard or by smoking cigarettes containing glycerin as a hygroscopic agent), castor bean dust, cottonseed, animal dander, cosmetics, aerosols, pyrethrum, orris, and molds have been known to cause urticaria.

Hyperglobulinemia E syndrome may be accompanied by urticaria. There may be urticaria present in hypercatabolism C3.

Viruses. Serum hepatitis, infectious mononucleosis, and psittacosis have been shown to induce urticaria.

Parasites. Many of the helminthic infestations may be associated with urticaria. Among these are ascaris, ankylostoma, strongyloides, filaria, echinococcus, schistosoma, trichinella, toxocara, and liver fluke. Witkowski and Parish reported a case of scabies in which urticaria was the presenting complaint.

Alcohol. Elphinstone et al recorded a case in which urticaria was induced by the ingestion of ethyl alcohol in any form. The reaction could not be blocked by sodium cromoglycate, indomethacin, chlorpheniramine, cimetidine, or naloxone.

INCIDENCE. Two reports have helped in gaining knowledge regarding the frequency of occurrence of various causes of urticaria. Miller and his associates reported on a series of 50 hospitalized patients with chronic urticaria, in 37 of whom they were able to find the cause. There were five patients whose urticaria was caused by drugs; 11, by inhalants; two, by food; six, by infection; nine, by cholinergics; and four, by physical agents.

Tas also surveyed 100 hospitalized patients and found 25 with chronic urticaria due to fungi, seven due to parasites, eight due to drugs, 10 due to focus of infection, and three due to house dust.

Jacobson et al studied 125 patients with chronic urticaria with an extensive battery of laboratory tests and x-rays; 3.5 per cent of laboratory tests were abnormal, but 17 per cent of dental x-rays and 16 per cent of sinus x-rays were abnormal; and treatment of the abnormality relieved the urticaria.

Data from other large series, such as those of Green et al and Champion et al, depict a truer picture of the usual results in identifying underlying causes in chronic urticaria. In only 20 per cent of the cases, on the average, does one identify a cause, if one eliminates the physical urticarias.

PATHOGENESIS. The urticarial wheal results from increased capillary permeability, which allows proteins and fluids to extravasate. The capillary permeability results from the increased release of histamine from the mast cells situated around the capillaries.

The mast cell is probably the chief factor in all urticarial reactions. The mast cell granules containing heparin and histamine disappear or almost disappear during the whealing and the mast cells are said to be "degranulated."

Other substances besides histamine may cause vasodilation and capillary permeability and thereby may possibly become mediators of urticaria and angioedema. These are serotonin, slow-reacting substances (leukotrienes), prostaglandins, proteases, bradykinin, and various other kinins. The role of these substances in the pathogenesis of human urticaria is still speculative.

The major basic protein of eosinophil granules is abnormally high in the blood of over 40 per cent of patients with chronic urticaria even when peripheral blood eosinophil counts are normal, and there are extracellular deposits of it in the skin in about the same proportion.

HISTOPATHOLOGY. The histopathologic changes are not dramatic. The epidermis is normal. Collagen bundles in the reticular dermis are separated by edema and there is a perivascular lymphocytic inflammatory infiltrate. Mast cells may be increased in number.

DIAGNOSIS. Urticaria is usually easily diagnosed by the presence of transitory wheals. These may occur with overlapping, some forming and some involuting at the same time. Atypical forms may be mistaken for the erythemas, such as erythema nodosum, systemic lupus erythematosus, and Henoch-Schönlein syndrome. The latter may combine erythema and urticaria with arthralgia, abdominal pain, and purpura.

TREATMENT. When the etiology in acute urticaria is not yet established and a food allergy is suspected, certain foods should be avoided entirely, particularly fish, shellfish (shrimp, lobster, crab, scallops, oysters, clams), turtle, pork, garlic, onions, mushrooms, tomatoes, pickles and relishes, melons, strawberries, citrus fruits, nuts, peanut butter, and cheese. Depending upon the response, further elimination of foods that may be causative should be instituted as necessary.

In chronic urticaria determination of an offending food is often difficult. If a food substance is implicated as a possible cause, suspected foods are eliminated from the diet for three weeks and then resumed one by one. In this manner it may be possible to determine the offending substance or substances or whether there are any such.

Antihistaminics are effective, but the doses must be adequate. The commonly written dose, "t.i.d.,"

is almost always too much or too little. Write, instead, "One now, one whenever hives return, and repeat any dose after one half hour if hives are not relieved." The patient should be warned about driving an automobile because of the tendency to drowsiness following their use. In new-onset, daily urticaria, one of us (WDJ) likes to start with 25 (or if it is ineffective, 50) mg of hydroxyzine (Atarax) h.s. for seven to 14 days; if there has been relief, it is stopped and restarted if necessary. This single nighttime dose is sufficient in some cases. Greene et al compared the effects of diphenhydramine (Benadryl) and doxepin (Sinequan, or Adapine) and found seven times as many patients were relieved by doxepin, with only half as many experiencing sedation.

Cerio and Lessof found in a double-blind crossover study that terfenadine (Seldane) was highly effective against chronic urticaria and caused no sedation at all. However, Monroe has recently reviewed and compared the properties of the newer nonsedating H_1 antihistamines and feels loratadine is superior to terfenadine, astemizole, and cetirizine.

Epinephrine 1:1000 in sterile water solution is given in doses of 0.3 to 1.0 ml in emergencies such as laryngeal edema. Sus-phrine (epinephrine suspension), 0.1 to 0.3 ml, may be injected subcutaneously for more prolonged action.

Kennes and associates reported success with terbutaline (Brethine), a beta$_2$-adrenergic agent, in urticaria, giving 1.25 mg t.i.d., with an extra 2.5 mg when an attack occurred.

In stubborn cases the combination of H_1 and H_2 antihistamines, e.g., hydroxyzine and cimetidine or ranitidine, may be effective. Cimetidine or ranitidine should not be used alone for urticaria. Harvey et al compared a placebo, terbutaline (Brethine), cyproheptadine (Periactin), chlorpheniramine (Chlortrimeton), cimetidine (Tagamet), and a combination of the last two. In 23 refractory cases, 58 per cent preferred the H_1–H_2 combination, and it gave the greatest wheal suppression.

Corticotropin (Acthar Gel) in 20 to 40 mg doses intramuscularly also gives prompt relief in most cases. Corticosteroids orally or parenterally are also generally effective in giving temporary relief.

Wernsdörfer recommended long-term treatment with corticosteroids as a satisfactory method for chronic urticaria of unknown origin. Mikhail and his associates suggest triamcinolone acetonide in 40 mg doses intramuscularly at four-week or longer intervals.

For local treatment, tepid or cold tub baths or showers may be freely advocated. Their efficacy is increased by the addition of starch, sodium bicarbonate, menthol, or magnesium sulfate. For soothing colloid baths, Aveeno Colloidal Oatmeal or Aveeno Oilated may be used for relief.

Local antipruritic lotions containing phenol (1–2 per cent) and menthol (1/2 per cent) give relief. Sarna lotion contains menthol, phenol, and camphor, and Prax lotion contains pramoxine hydrochloride, an antipruritic.

SOME TYPES OF URTICARIA

Angioedema

This was previously known as angioneurotic edema. Other synonyms are Quincke's edema and giant urticaria. It is a subcutaneous variant of urticaria.

Angioedema is an acute, evanescent, circumscribed edema that usually affects the most distensible tissues, such as the eyelids, the lips, the lobes of the ears, and the external genitals (the prepuce is a frequent site) or the mucous membranes of the mouth, tongue, or larynx. The swelling occurs in the deeper parts of the skin or in the subcutaneous tissues, and, as a rule, is only slightly tender, with the overlying skin unaltered, edematous, or, rarely, ecchymotic. On the hands, forearms, feet, and ankles a diffuse swelling may take place. Frequently the condition begins during the night and is found upon awakening. Urticaria is frequently concomitant with angioedema. *Cryoglobulins* may be present. Owing to the action of histamine or similar substances there is a vasomotor lability, which leads to sudden transudation of fluids from the vessels into the loose tissues.

Angioedema has been reported in association with encephalopathy; Sunder et al reported two cases in boys, and reviewed 19 cases from the literature. Seizures and headaches are the commonest symptoms, but a wide variety of focal and generalized deficits have occurred.

The etiology of angioedema is as varied as that of urticaria. Phenothiazine intolerance has been known to cause angioedema of the tongue and laryngeal edema.

The treatment is similar to that described for urticaria. Antihistaminic remedies may be given intravenously and orally. They must be given in fairly large doses to effectively counter the large amount of histamine being released. ACTH and cortisone are temporarily effective.

Freed et al produced complete remission of attacks in four patients by the use of antiproteases such as aminocaproic acid (Amicar), tranexamic acid, or aprotinin. Withdrawal of tranexamic acid maintenance therapy resulted in relapse. Gleich reported four cases with fever, weight gain, and eosinophilia, and elevated eosinophil major basic protein. There was no underlying disease. A similar case was recently reported by Wolf et al. This subset of patients appears to have a clinically unique syndrome, now known as *episodic angioedema with eosinophilia.* Treatment was with hydroxyzine (Vistaril) and (if needed) prednisone orally.

A solution of epinephrine 1:1000 (0.2 to 0.5 ml) may be given subcutaneously and Sus-phrine, 0.1 to 0.3 ml, may be injected subcutaneously for more prolonged action. Ephedrine sulfate, 25 mg, may be given orally three or four times a day. When the larynx is affected and breathing is obstructed, epinephrine is given as soon as possible. In minor cases the sucking of ice is recommended. Laryngotomy may be necessary.

Hereditary Angioedema. Also known as chronic familial giant urticaria, this was originally described and named by Osler in 1888.

Hereditary angioedema characteristically appears in the second to the fourth decade. Sudden attacks of angioedema occur, as frequently as every two weeks throughout the patient's life, and last for one to three days. Swelling is typically asymmetric, and urticaria, or itching, rarely occurs. There is little response to antihistamines, epinephrine, or steroids. Gastrointestinal edema is a frequent accompaniment, along with pharyngeal and laryngeal edema. The mortality rate is high and death is often caused by laryngeal edema. Gastrointestinal edema is manifested by nausea, vomiting, and severe colic, and it may simulate appendicitis so closely that appendectomy is mistakenly performed.

Van Dellen and Myers reported a case who developed gross hematuria at ages 16, 20, and 36 because of raised hemorrhagic lesions in the bladder wall, with normal mucosa on biopsy. The hemorrhage stopped when the angioedema was better controlled.

Hereditary angioedema is transmitted in an autosomal dominant pattern.

In hereditary angioedema, C1 inhibitor levels are either markedly reduced (Type I disease), or (in about 20 per cent of cases) the levels are normal but the protein is nonfunctional. The screening test of choice is a C4 level, it being low as a result of continuous activation and consumption. The factors that may mediate the deficiency may be minor trauma, sudden changes of temperature, or sudden emotional stress.

Stoppa-Lyonnet and her associates in 1987 reported identifying a cluster of four distinctive DNA restriction sites, indicating a genetically heterogeneous defect for patients with deficient C1 inhibitor.

There is also an acquired form of this disorder,

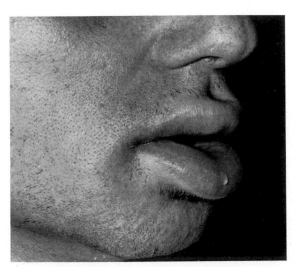

Figure 7–23. Angioedema of the lips.

which occurs most often in patients with lymphoproliferative disorders. In addition to depressed C1 inhibitor and C4 levels, these patients also have low C1, C1q, and C2.

Alsenz reported in 1987 a second form of acquired angioedema without associated disease in which anti-C1 inhibitor antibodies enabled activated C1s to inactivate C1 inhibitor. Papadoulos and Frank report that serum protein electrophoresis, detecting paraproteins in the acquired type, is a simple screen for distinguishing acquired from hereditary angioedema.

Treatment is preferably with danazol, an ethinyl testosterone derivative (Danacrine, Winthrop). The dose is 200 mg q.i.d. for acute episodes and 200 mg q.d. for prevention. Epinephrine should be readily available. The patient should be taught self-administration of the drug. Birth control pills do not exacerbate the disease as long as danazol is being given concomitantly. Epsilon aminocaproic acid (EACA) may inhibit the sequence of events leading to C1 activation. Tranexamic acid, a drug related to epsilon aminocaproic acid, is given in smaller doses with fewer side effects; however, it is not yet available in this country.

Gadek et al prepared a C1-inhibitor concentrate from pooled human plasma by chromatography, concentration, and lyophilization, and were able to control the disease with it in five cases.

In 25 per cent of the cases death is due to laryngeal edema.

Vibratory Angioedema

This has been described as a familial variety of physical urticaria, but Wener et al reported a case acquired after some years of work as a metal grinder. Attacks could be induced by light pressure with a laboratory vortexer. Plasma histamine rose from 1 to 18 ng/ml after five minutes of vibration, and returned to normal in 14 minutes.

Facial Edema and Eosinophilia

Songsiridej et al reported two patients with episodic facial edema and eosinophilia, in whom the granule major basic protein was deposited in the tissue. Both responded well to oral prednisone 30 mg daily.

Dermatographia (Factitious Urticaria)

Also known as dermographism, this is a sharply localized edema or wheal with a surrounding erythematous flare occurring within seconds after the skin has been stroked. This differs from the normal physiologic reaction by an exaggerated response to a much less intense stimulus. When this hypersensitive state is present, a scratch may provoke a linear, raised,

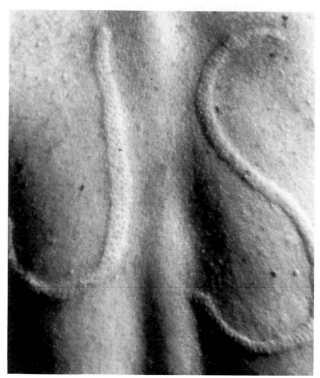

Figure 7–24. Dermatographism.

pale streak bordered on each side by a hyperemic line, so that it is possible to write upon the skin by scratching it with a dull instrument. Minor trauma or pressure such as that produced by tight belts or brassieres may also produce urticaria. Dermatographism may also arise spontaneously after drug (penicillin)-induced urticaria and persist for months. It may also occur in hypo- and hyperthyroidism, infectious diseases, diabetes mellitus, and during onset of menopause. Wong et al have recently reviewed the various kinds of dermographism.

Hydroxyzine is effective as a suppressor of this reaction, but there is no effective treatment. Probably doxepin (Sinequan), terfenadine (Seldane), or astemizole should be tried. Kaur et al got better results using chlorpheniramine (Chlortrimeton) and cimetidine (Tagamet) in combination than with either alone, or a placebo. Deutsch found phenylpropanolamine hydrochloride and chlorpheniramine maleate (Ornade spansules) initially helpful, and later a combination of cimetidine and hydroxyzine virtually curative, in one case.

Pressure Urticaria

This is characterized by the development of severe swelling with deep pain occurring three to 12 hours after local pressure has been applied. This occurs most frequently on the feet after walking, and on the buttocks after sitting. It is unique in that there may be a latent period of as much as 24 hours before the pressure urticaria develops. The pain and swelling last for some eight to 24 hours.

There is no explanation for the cause of this phenomenon.

Systemic corticosteroids control this disease when it is so severe that this course of action is justified. Antihistaminics are ineffective. Ketotifen is reported by Huston et al to be effective in some types of physical urticaria, including pressure, cholinergic, and exercise induced.

Aquagenic Pruritus

Greaves et al reported in 1981 three subjects in whom intense itching was evoked by contact with water at any temperature. They found increased degranulation of mast cells, and increased concentration of histamine and acetylcholine in the skin after contact with water. Lotti et al reported a similar case in which cutaneous fibrinolytic activity was abnormally high before contact with water, and about the same after. They hypothesized that this elevation of CFE might explain the absence of any wheal despite elevation of histamine and acetylcholine in the involved area.

Aquagenic Urticaria

Shelley and Rawnsley first described urticaria elicited by water or seawater at any temperature in 1964, and 19 cases have been reported so far, according to Czarnetzki. Using extracts of callus, Czarnetzki et al found that two women with this disorder reacted to them with burning pain (absent in controls) and with degranulation of basophils in vitro. They concluded that water produces urticaria in these patients by acting as a carrier for a soluble epidermal antigen.

Cholinergic Urticaria

This form of urticaria is also known as **heat-induced** or **stress-induced urticaria**.

Cholinergic urticaria, produced by the action of acetylcholine upon the mast cell, is characterized by minute, highly pruritic, punctate wheals or papules 1 to 3 mm in diameter surrounded by areas of erythema and associated with extreme pruritus. These lesions occur primarily on the trunk and face. It spares the palms and soles. The lesions are actually follicular hives, which persist from 30 to 90 minutes and are followed by a refractory period of several hours.

The lesions may be induced in the susceptible patient by exercise, emotional stress, increased environmental temperature, or intradermal injection of nicotine picrate or methacholine.

Treatment with antihistaminics is effective provided there is adequate dosage. Hydroxyzine is the

drug of choice. An initial high dosage may be necessary for control of symptoms, but later only a low maintenance dose is required. There is no cure, but spontaneous recovery in a few months or years is the rule.

Sometimes an attack may be aborted by rapid cooling of the body, such as taking a cold shower. A refractory period with no lesions is developed for some 24 hours after an attack.

Simple attention to any psychologic factors present is usually very helpful.

Adrenergic Urticaria

The Shelleys reported in 1985 two cases of urticaria attributable to norepinephrine. Both were characterized by an eruption of small (1–5 mm) red macules and papules with or without a pale halo, appearing within 10–15 minutes after emotional upset, or coffee or chocolate, in one case. Serum catecholamines, noradrenalin and adrenalin, rose markedly during attacks, while histamine, dopamine, and serotonin remained normal. Lesions were experimentally induced by 3–10 ng of noradrenalin intradermally. Propranolol (Inderal), 10 mg four times a day, was effective; atenolol (Tenormin) was ineffective.

Cold Urticaria

Exposure to cold may cause a hypersensitivity reaction that is manifested by edema and whealing on the exposed areas. The face and hands are the common sites. In severe cases other parts of the body may also be involved. The urticaria does not develop during the chilling but upon rewarming. Symptoms of headache, hypotension, laryngeal edema, and

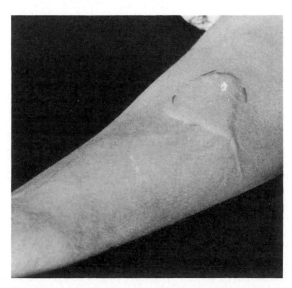

Figure 7–25. Cold urticaria after ice cube had been applied to site for 3 minutes.

even syncope are common. Fatal shock may occur when these sensitive persons go swimming in cold water or take cold showers. This type of cold urticaria usually begins in adulthood.

Neittaanmäki studied 220 patients with cold urticaria of 1 month to 37 years' duration. A third also had other types of urticaria: dermographism in 21 per cent, cholinergic urticaria in 8 per cent, chronic urticaria in 2 per cent. One fourth of the patients were atopic. In 90 per cent, 20 minutes' contact with an ice cube gave a positive reaction; in the remainder, immersion of a forearm for 5 to 15 minutes in water at 0° to 8°C or exposure in a cold room (4°C) was necessary.

Histamine is the mediator of cold urticaria; however, the cause of the hypersensitivity is not known. Kinins may also be mediators. Passive transfer of the thermolabile serum factor in cold urticaria has been demonstrated.

Another form of cold hypersensitivity is a secondary reaction to cold hemolysins, cryoglobulins, or cryofibrinogens. This form causes occlusive vascular changes in the skin evident as ulcers, purpura, acrocyanosis, and Raynaud's phenomenon. There may be a biologic false positive reaction for syphilis. This may be associated with multiple myeloma, leukemia, kala-azar, SLE, or malignancy.

Cold urticaria must be differentiated from cryoglobulinemia, cold hemagglutinins, and syphilitic paroxysmal cold hemoglobinuria.

The treatment of cold urticaria with antihistamines has been found to be mostly ineffective. Cyproheptadine (Periactin, Merck) is useful in 4-mg doses three times daily. Wanderer and associates confirmed reports dating back to 1964 of the efficacy of cyproheptadine in cold urticaria: chlorpheniramine was as ineffective as the placebo control. Sigler et al confirmed the effectiveness of cyproheptadine again in 1980. Corticosteroids are ineffective.

Desensitization by repeated increased exposures to cold has been effective in some cases. Leigh and his associates report a successful desensitization in an 18-year-old lad with severe cold urticaria. They induced tolerance in a small area of the skin by repeated applications of an ice cube at 30-minute intervals for seven hours. This was followed by forearm immersion in cold water hourly for four hours. The other limbs were then treated one at a time, and finally the trunk. After a week, he was able to tolerate whole-body immersion in cold water for five minutes without urticaria. He maintained this "desensitization" by a five-minute cold shower every 12 hours. He was free from urticaria for six months, continuing his daily cold showers.

There is a tendency for this type of hypersensitivity to disappear after months or years.

Familial Cold Urticaria. Familial cold hives are observed by the fourth month of life. The lesions produce a burning sensation rather than itching. Chills, fever, joint pains, and headaches are usually present with the appearance of urticaria after exposure to cold. A prominent feature is the leucocytosis that is the first observable response to cold. Inheritance is of the autosomal dominant pattern.

Urticarial Leucocytoclastic Vasculitis With Cold Urticaria. Wanderer et al reported a case of this combination, and consider it a new subset of urticarial vasculitis. Hypocomplementemia, leucocytoclastic vasculitis on biopsy, arthritis, purpura, and GI symptoms were manifested.

Solar Urticaria

This type of urticaria appears soon after the exposure of unshielded skin to sunlight. This can be a relatively benign type of erythema and pruritus or it may cause severe urticaria, malaise, and shock. Several types of solar urticaria occur. These have been described in Chapter 3.

Heat Urticaria

Within five minutes after the skin has been exposed to heat above 43°C, the exposed area begins to burn and sting, and it becomes red, swollen, and indurated.

This rare type of urticaria may also be generalized and is accompanied by cramps, weakness, flushing, salivation, and collapse. Acetylcholine is probably the mediator of this type. The mecholyl test is positive.

There is evidence that the alternate pathway of complement is activated. At the time of activity, C3 and properdin factor B fall to almost undetectable levels.

Exercise-Induced Urticaria

Lewis et al studied six patients with exercise-induced urticaria by exercising them until profuse sweating occurred; five of the six then developed giant and cholinergic urticaria and angioedema. Anaphylaxis may occur in such individuals.

There is a high incidence of atopy in these patients. In some, food ingestion around the time of exercise is a necessary additive factor for this reaction, as recounted by Silverstein et al.

Papular Urticaria

Papular urticaria, also known as **lichen urticatus**, is a common disease of infancy and childhood. Small, pruritic papules are distributed mostly on the arms and legs, especially on the extensor surfaces, but also occur on the face and neck and usually least on the trunk. The individual fresh lesions are small urticated papules that become rubbed, excoriated, and secondarily infected or lichenified, sometimes with impetiginous crusts or ecthymatous ulcers.

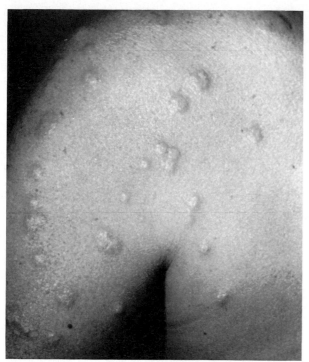

Figure 7–26. Papular urticaria. (Courtesy of Dr. Axel W. Hoke.)

The lesions recur in crops, usually at night. Each lesion may persist for two to 12 days. All stages of development and regression of the papules may be noted at the same time. The attack may persist for months or years. Frequently the attacks are seasonal. Usually there are no palpable lymph nodes and no constitutional symptoms.

Papular urticaria has been proved to be due to hypersensitivity to bites of fleas, gnats, mosquitoes, mites, and most frequently, bedbugs. The latter probably cause about 90 per cent of the cases.

Alexander found mites to be an important etiologic factor: he found over 1000 dead mites per gram of dust in one third of the homes with pet birds and animals of patients with papular urticaria. The most common mite was *Dermatophagoides pteronyssinus.*

The histologic changes resemble an arthropod bite reaction. There is a superficial and deep perivascular infiltrate composed of lymphocytes, histiocytes, and eosinophils.

Treatment should begin with elimination of the insects to which the child may be exposed, especially cat and dog fleas, human fleas, and bedbugs. The sleeping quarters of the pets should be thoroughly treated with insecticides. The baseboards, corners, rugs, and furniture in all the rooms of the home should be treated with insect sprays such as Gulf-spray twice weekly. Infested sandboxes, cellar debris, and theater seats as well as neighbors' homes may also be sources of infestation.

Antipruritic lotions are used topically. Corticosteroid creams are applied several times daily. Antihis-taminics by mouth also give relief from frenzied itching.

Agneilo V, et al: Partial genetic deficiency of the C4 component of complement in discoid lupus erythematosus and urticaria/angioedema. JAAD 1983, 9:894.

Alsenz J, et al: Autoantibody-mediated acquired deficiency of C1 inhibitor. N Engl J Med 1987, 316:1360.

Bernhard JD, et al: Ultraviolet A phototherapy in the prophylaxis of solar urticaria. JAAD 1984, 10:29.

Black JT: Amyloidosis, deafness and limb pains: A hereditary syndrome. Ann Intern Med 1969, 70:989.

Breathnach SM, et al: Symptomatic dermographism: Natural history, clinical features, laboratory investigations, and response to therapy. Clin Exp Dermatol 1983, 8:463.

Brickman M, et al: Hereditary angioedema. Int J Dermatol 1983, 22:141.

Casale TB, et al: Guide to physical urticarias. J Allergy Clin Immunol 1988, 82:758.

Cerio R, et al: Treatment of chronic idiopathic urticaria with terfenadine. Clin Allergy 1984, 14:139.

Champion RH, et al: Investigation and management of chronic urticaria and angioedema. Clin Exp Dermatol 1982, 7:291.

Cicardi M, et al: Hereditary angioedema: An appraisal of 104 cases. Am J Med Sci 1982, 284:2.

Colten HR: Hereditary angioneurotic edema (editorial). N Engl J Med 1987, 317:43.

Commens CA, et al: Tests to establish the diagnosis in cholinergic urticaria. Br J Dermatol 1978, 98:47.

Czarnetzki BM, et al: Morphology of the cellular infiltrate in delayed pressure urticaria. JAAD 1985, 12:253.

Idem: Evidence that water acts as a carrier for an epidermal antigen in aquagenic urticaria. JAAD 1986, 15:623.

Idem: Clinical, pharmacological, and immunological aspects of delayed pressure urticaria. Br J Dermatol 1984, 111:315.

Dennehy JJ: Hereditary angioneurotic edema. Ann Intern Med 1970, 73:55.

Deutsch PH: Dermographism treated with hydroxyzine and cimetidine and Ranitidine. Ann Intern Med 1984, 101:524.

Dover JS, et al: Delayed pressure urticaria. JAAD 1988, 18:1289.

Duschet P, et al: Solar urticaria: Treatment by plasmapheresis. JAAD 1986, 15:712.

Elphinstone PE, et al: Alcohol-induced urticaria. J R Soc Med 1985, 78:340.

Estes SA, et al: Delayed pressure urticaria: An investigation of some parameters of lesion induction. JAAD 1981, 5:25.

Faek DK: Pulmonary disease in idiopathic urticarial vasculitis. JAAD 1984, 11:346.

Frank MM, et al: Hereditary angioedema: The clinical syndrome and its management. Ann Intern Med 1976, 84:580.

Fredriksson T, et al: Terfenadine in chronic urticaria: A comparison with clemastine and placebo. Cutis 1986, 35:128.

Freed DLJ, et al: Angioedema responding to antiprotease treatment but without abnormalities of the complement system. Clin Allergy 1980, 10:21.

Gadek J, et al: Replacement therapy in hereditary angioedema. N Engl J Med 1980, 10:542.

Gange RW: Solar urticaria. Arch Dermatol 1985, 121:475.

Geha RS, et al: Acquired C1-inhibitor deficiency associated with antiidiotypic antibody to monoclonal immunoglobulins. N Engl J Med 1985, 312:534.

Gleich GJ, et al: Episodic angioedema associated with eosinophilia. N Engl J Med 1984, 310:1621.

Goldstein DJ, et al: A case of episodic flushing and organic psychosis: reversal by opiate antagonists. Ann Intern Med 1983, 98:30.

Grant JA, et al: Familial exercise-induced anaphylaxis. Ann Allergy 1985, 54:35.

Greene SP, et al: Double-blind crossover study comparing doxepin with diphenhydramine for the treatment of chronic urticaria. JAAD 1985, 12:669.

Harris A, et al: Chronic urticaria in childhood: Natural course and etiology. Ann Allergy 1983, 51:161.

Harto A, et al: Doxepin in the treatment of chronic urticaria. Dermatologica 1985, 170:90.

Harvey RP, et al: A controlled trial of therapy in chronic urticaria. J Allergy Clin Immunol 1981, 68:262.

Hasei K, et al: Solar urticaria, determinations of action and inhibition spectra. Arch Dermatol 1982, 118:346.

Highet S, et al: Treatment of cold urticaria. Br J Dermatol 1979, 51:161.

Hirschmann JV, et al: Cholinergic urticaria. Arch Dermatol 1987, 123:462.

Horio T, et al: Production and inhibition of solar urticaria by visible light exposure. JAAD 1984, 11:1094.

Hosea SW, et al: Long-term therapy of hereditary angioedema with danazal. Ann Intern Med 1980, 93:809.

Huston DP, et al: Preventing mast-cell degranulation by ketotifen . . . Ann Intern Med 1986, 104:507.

Ichihashi M, et al: Solar urticaria: Further studies on the role of inhibition spectra. Arch Dermatol 1985, 121:503.

Jacobson KW, et al: Laboratory tests in chronic urticaria. JAMA 1980, 243:1644.

Jorizzo JL: Cholinergic urticaria. Arch Dermatol 1987, 123:455.

Idem: The physical urticarias. Arch Dermatol 1982, 118:194.

Juhlin L, et al: Urticaria and asthma induced by food and drug additives in patients with aspirin hypersensitivity. J Allergy Clin Immunol 1972, 50:92.

Juhlin L: Recurrent urticaria: Clinical investigation of 330 patients. Br J Dermatol 1981, 104:369.

Kailasam V, et al: Controlled clinical assessment of astemizole in the treatment of chronic idiopathic urticaria and angioedema. JAAD 1987, 16:797.

Kaplan AP, et al: Exercise-induced anaphylaxis as a manifestation of cholinergic urticaria. J Allergy Clin Immunol 1981, 68:319.

Idem: Identification of a new physically induced urticaria: Cold-induced cholinergic urticaria. J Allergy Clin Immunol 1981, 68:438.

Idem: Exercise-induced hives. J Allergy Clin Immunol 1984, 73:704.

Kauppinen K, et al: Urticaria in children: Retrospective evaluation and follow-up. Allergy 1984, 39:469.

Kaur S, et al: Factitious urticaria (dermographism): Treatment by cimetidine and chlorpheniramine in a randomized double-blind study. Br J Dermatol 1981, 104:185.

Keahey TM, et al: Cold urticaria: Dissociation of cold-evoked histamine release and urticaria following cold challenge. Arch Dermatol 1980, 116:174.

Kojima M, et al: Solar urticaria, relationship of photoallergen and action spectrum. Arch Dermatol 1986, 122:550.

Krause LB, et al: A comparison of astemizole and chlorpheniramine in dermographic urticaria. Br J Dermatol 1985, 112:447.

Kushimoto H, et al: Masked type I wheat allergy: Relation to exercise-induced anaphylaxis. Arch Dermatol 1985, 121:355.

Lawrence CM, et al: Cholinergic urticaria with associated angioedema. Br J Dermatol 1981, 105:543.

Ledo A, et al: Doxepin in treatment of chronic urticaria. JAAD 1985, 13:1058.

Lewis J, et al: Exercise-induced urticaria, angioedema, and anaphylactoid episodes. J Allergy Clin Immunol 1981, 68:432.

Leznoff A, et al: Association of angioedema and urticaria with thyroid autoimmunity. Arch Dermatol 1983, 119:636.

Maibach HI, et al: Contact urticaria syndrome. Arch Dermatol 1975, 111:726.

Massa MC, et al: An association between C1 esterase inhibitor deficiency and lupus erythematosus: Report of two cases and review of the literature. JAAD 1982, 7:255.

Matthews CNA, et al: The effect of H1 and H2 histamine antagonists on symptomatic dermographism. Br J Dermatol 1979, 101:57.

McLelland J: Mechanism of morphine-induced urticaria. Arch Dermatol 1986, 122:138.

Miller DA, et al: Chronic urticaria—a clinical study of 50 patients. Am J Med 1968, 44:68.

Monroe EW, et al: Urticaria. Arch Dermatol 1977, 113:80.

Idem: Chronic urticaria: . . .nonsedating H₁ antihistamines . . . JAAD 1988, 19:842.

Monroe EW: Combined H1 and H2 antihistamine therapy in chronic urticaria. Arch Dermatol 1981, 117:404.

Natbony SF, et al: Histologic studies of chronic idiopathic urticaria. J Allergy Clin Immunol 1983, 71:177.

Neittaanmaki H, et al: Cold urticaria: Clinical findings in 220 patients. JAAD 1985, 13:636.

Idem: Comparison of cinnarizine, cyproheptadine, doxepin, and hydroxyzine in treatment of idiopathic cold urticaria: Usefulness of doxepin. JAAD 1984, 11:483.

Ostrav MR: Dermographism. A critical review. Ann Allergy 1967, 25:591.

Papadopoulos NM, et al: Electrophoretic differentiation of acquired from hereditary angioedema. Clin Chem Acta 1987, 163:231.

Peters MS, et al: Neutrophilic urticaria. Br J Dermatol 1985, 113:25.

Idem: Extracellular deposition of eosinophil granule major basic protein in pressure urticaria. JAAD 1987, 16:513.

Ravits M, et al: Solar urticaria, clinical features and wavelength dependence. Arch Dermatol 1982, 118:228.

Ros AM, et al: Follow-up study with recurrent urticaria. Br J Dermatol 1976, 95:19.

Rosen FS, et al: The "neurotic edema" (hereditary angioedema). N Engl J Med 1969, 280:1356.

Saihan EN: Ketotifen and terbutaline in urticaria. Br J Dermatol 1981, 104:205.

Sanchez NP, et al: Clinical and histopathologic spectrums of urticarial vasculitis: Study of 40 cases. JAAD 1982, 7:599.

Schewach-Millet M, et al: Urticaria and angioedema due to topically applied chloramphenicol ointment. Arch Dermatol 1985, 121:587.

Schuller DE, et al: Acute urticaria associated with streptococcal infection. Pediatrics 1980, 65:592.

Sheffer AL, et al: Exercise-induced anaphylaxis. J Allergy Clin Immunol 1980, 66:106.

Idem: Exercise-induced anaphylaxis. Clin Allergy 1983, 13:317.

Idem: Hereditary angioedema. J Allergy Clin Immunol 1987, 80:855.

Shelley WB, et al: Adrenergic urticaria: A new form of stress-induced hives. Lancet 1985, 1:1031.

Idem: Aquagenic urticaria. JAMA 1964, 189:895.

Shelley WB: Commentary: Antihistamines and treatment of urticaria. Arch Dermatol 1983, 119:442.

Sigler RW, et al: The role of cyproheptadine in the treatment of cold urticaria. J Allergy Clin Immunol 1980, 65:309.

Silverstein SR, et al: Celery-dependent exercise-induced anaphylaxis. J Emerg Med 1986, 4:195.

Simons FER, et al: The pharmocokinetics and antihistaminic of the H1 receptor antagonist hydroxyzine. J Allergy Clin Immunol 1984, 73:69.

Small P, et al: Chronic urticaria and vasculitis. Ann Allergy 1982, 48:172.

Songsiridej V, et al: Facial edema and eosinophilia. Ann Intern Med 1985, 103:503.

Sørensen HT, et al: . . .Followup of children with urticaria. Scand J Prim Health Care 1987, 5:24.

Soter NA, et al: Release of mast-cell mediators and alterations in lung function in patients with cholinergic urticaria. N Engl J Med 1980, 302:604.

Steinman HK, et al: Aquagenic pruritus. JAAD 1985, 13:91.

Stoppa-Lyonnet D, et al: Altered C₁ inhibitor genes in . . . hereditary angioedema. N Engl J Med 1987, 317:1.

Sunder HR, et al: Neurological manifestations of angioedema. JAMA 1982, 247:2005.

Sussman GL, et al: Delayed pressure urticaria (DPU). J Allergy Clin Immunol 1982, 70:337.

Tas J: Chronic urticaria: Surgery of 100 hospitalized cases. Dermatologica 1967, 135:90.

Tatnall FM, et al: Localized heat urticaria and its management. Clin Exp Dermatol 1984, 9:367.

Thompson JS: Urticaria and angioedema and deficiency of C1 esterase inhibitor in a 61-year-old woman. Ann Intern Med 1969, 71:353.

Tindall JP, et al: Familial cold urticaria. Arch Intern Med 1964, 124:129.

Ting S, et al: Nonfamilial, vibration-induced angioedema. J Allergy Clin Immunol 1983, 71:546.

Vaida GA, et al: Testing for hepatitis B virus in patients with chronic urticaria and angioedema. J Allergy Clin Immunol 1983, 72:193.

Van Dellen RG, et al: Bladder involvement in hereditary angioedema. Mayo Clin Proc 1980, 55:277.

Von Krogh G, et al: The contact urticaria syndrome—an updated review. JAAD 1981, 5:328.

Wanderer AA, et al: Primary acquired cold urticaria; double-blind comparative study with cyproheptadine, chlorpheniramine and placebo. Arch Dermatol 1977, 113:1375.

Idem: Urticarial leukocytoclastic vasculitis with cold urticaria. Arch Dermatol 1983, 119:145.

Warin RP: Role of trauma in spreading wheals of hereditary angioedema. Br J Dermatol 1983, 108:189.

Wener MH, et al: Occupationally acquired vibratory angioedema with secondary carpal tunnel syndrome. Ann Intern Med 1983, 98:44.

Witkowski JA, et al: Scabies: A cause of generalized urticaria. Cutis 1984, 33:277.

Wolf C, et al: Episodic angioedema with eosinophilia. JAAD 1989, 20:21.

Wong RC, et al: Dermographism: A review. JAAD 1984, 11:643.

Prurigo

The problem of prurigo was met head on by Kocsard in 1962 when he pointed out the confusing interpretations offered by various authors. The following is essentially Kocsard's classification and presents his views on this subject.

Prurigo is characterized by the lesion known as the *prurigo papule*. It is dome-shaped and topped with a small vesicle. The vesicle is usually present only momentarily because of its immediate removal by scratching, so that a crusted papule is more frequently seen. Lichenification is only secondary in true prurigo.

TYPES. Kocsard classifies prurigo into two main groups: prurigo simplex and the pruriginous dermatoses.

Prurigo Simplex. The prurigo papules are present in various stages of development and are seen mostly in middle-aged persons of both sexes. The trunk and extensor surfaces of the extremities are favorite sites. The face and scalp may also be involved, alone or with the other locations, and the lesions usually appear in crops, so that papulovesicles and the late stages of scarring may be seen at the same time.

Several variations of prurigo have been described. **Melanotic prurigo of Pierini and Borda**, occurring in middle-aged women, has been described under pruritus associated with primary biliary cirrhosis. These lesions consist of reticulated hyperpigmentation, appearing most markedly on the trunk, with extreme and seemingly unbearable itching.

Prurigo of the scalp may occur alone or in association with prurigo lesions elsewhere. This is considered to be different from *nodular neurodermatitis* of the scalp.

Pruriginous Dermatoses. In this group the prurigo papules occur with urticarial wheals, pyogenic infection, scratch marks, lichenification, and eczematization. Additionally included is **prurigo of Hebra**, occurring commonly in childhood. This is known as

prurigo mitis and is probably *papular urticaria*. A more severe form is *prurigo agria* or *ferox* which persists into adulthood and is now probably known as *atopic dermatitis*.

Prurigo mitis begins in early childhood and is characterized by the uniform type of the primary lesion (the prurigo papules topped by a vesicle), and by chronicity, severity, scars, lichenification, and eczematization. The prurigo papules at first are easier to palpate than to see, but later become small, rounded, extremely pruritic, skin-colored or reddish elevations. The lesions are symmetrically distributed and may be few or very profuse. As time progresses the urticarial element is less noticeable but the extreme pruritus persists and leads to even greater secondary changes. The excoriations, lichenification, and eczematization become more and more pronounced and are accompanied by enlarged nodes and associated constitutional symptoms.

In *prurigo agria* the hard, excoriated prurigo papules and lichenification are completely predominant, the urticarial elements being sparse or absent. Incessant scratching causes pitted scars and pustulation. The adenopathy is pronounced in the groins and axillae, which are free from skin lesions. The hair is lusterless. The blood shows eosinophilia. There is usually a family history of allergenic reactions, and skin tests reveal multiple sensitizations.

Prurigo Nodularis. (See p. 59.)

ETIOLOGY. The external causes of prurigo and the pruriginous dermatoses may be heat, cold, light, insect bites, ectoparasites, and allergic contactants of the skin. The internal causes have been attributed to the intestinal parasites that produce oxyuriasis, ascariasis, and taeniasis. Echinococcosis may also cause prurigo. Other causes may be internal foci of infec-

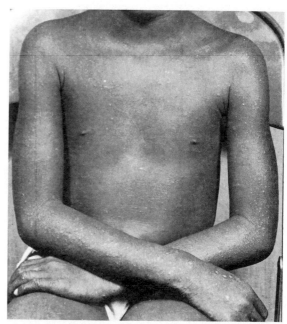

Figure 7–27. Prurigo mitis. (Courtesy of Dr. F. Daniels, Jr.)

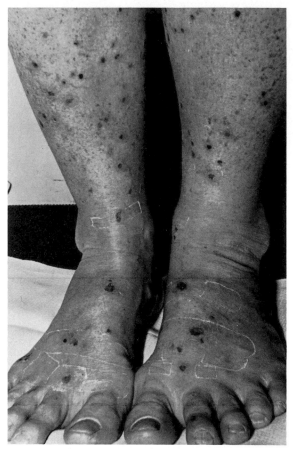

Figure 7–28. Prurigo mitis in a 25-year-old woman.

upper dermis, are frequently found. In addition, an inflammatory perivascular infiltrate is usually found in the upper dermis.

Marked proliferation of Schwann cells and nerve filaments in the dermis has recently been confirmed by electron microscopy.

DIFFERENTIAL DIAGNOSIS. Probably the most difficult dermatosis to differentiate is dermatitis herpetiformis. The tendency for grouping and the presence of neutrophilic microabscesses in the papillae in dermatitis herpetiformis are helpful. Prurigo of the scalp must be differentiated from nodular neurodermatitis of the scalp; this latter is lichenified, whereas prurigo may be accompanied by the typical vesicle and prurigo papules elsewhere on the body. In acne necrotica miliaris of the scalp the lesions are at the margins of the scalp only.

TREATMENT. Most frequently, recourse must be made to symptomatic treatment of the prurigo. Locally the antipruritic, emollient, or ordinary corticosteroid preparations are virtually useless unless the steroid is combined with lactic acid or retinoic acid to enhance penetration. Temovate cream 0.05 per cent may be effective. Intralesional injections of triamcinolone acetonide suspension (Kenalog, Squibb) are far more effective. In extensive, profuse eruptions Oliver found intramuscular triamcinolone (Kenalog), 40 to 60 mg monthly or less often, effective and far more practical. Local anesthetics such as the "caines" inevitably produce sensitization and are mentioned to warn against their use.

Administration of antihistaminics, cyproheptadine, or tranquilizers is of moderate benefit in allaying the symptoms.

tion such as colitis or infected tonsils. Endocrine factors may cause this problem, as seen in prurigo gestationis or prurigo simplex. Ovarian dysfunction may cause prurigo simplex; it responds to progesterone therapy. Food and drug allergies, malignant lymphomas, malignant tumors, and polycythemia (**prurigo polycythaemica Kocsard**) are additional etiologic agents.

Psychogenic factors exert an important influence upon this most severe and frustrating dermatosis. They may be the primary cause.

HISTOPATHOLOGY. The histologic changes are nonspecific. Acanthosis, hyperkeratosis, and parakeratosis, with edema in the lower epidermis and

Aronson IK, et al: Thalidomide-induced peripheral neuropathy in prurigo nodularis. Arch Dermatol 1984, 120:1466.

Barnhill RL, et al: Thalidomide: Use and possible mode of action in reactional lepromatous leprosy and in various other conditions. JAAD 1982, 7:317.

Boer J, et al: Nodular prurigo-like eruptions induced by etretinate. Br J Dermatol 1987, 116:271.

Clemmensen OJ, et al: Thalidomide neurotoxicity. Arch Dermatol 1984, 120:338.

Griether A: On the different forms of prurigo. Curr Probl Dermatol 1970, 3:1.

Jorizzo JL: Prurigo: A clinical review. JAAD 1981, 4:723.

Kocsard E: The problem of prurigo. Aust J Dermatol 1962, 6:156.

Oliver PR (Harare, Zimbabwe): Personal communication to the senior author.

Waldinger TP, et al: Cryotherapy improves prurigo nodularis. Arch Dermatol 1984, 120:1598.

8

Connective Tissue Diseases

The classification by Klemperer of lupus erythematosus, dermatomyositis, scleroderma, rheumatoid arthritis, rheumatic fever, and polyarthritis as collagen disease, or more correctly connective tissue disease, is based on the widespread fibrinoid degeneration of the collagen fibers occurring in the mesenchymal tissues.

Several other syndromes, some newly described, are included in our concept of connective tissue diseases. They include Sjögren's syndrome, eosinophilic fasciitis, mixed connective tissue disease (MCTD), and relapsing polychondritis. Basic to them all, we now know, is a complex array of autoimmune responses.

Callen JP, Provost TT, Tuffanelli DL: Periodic synopsis on collagen vascular disease. JAAD 1985, 5:809.
Kohler PF, et al: The autoimmune diseases. JAMA 1982, 248:2646.

LUPUS ERYTHEMATOSUS (LE)

LE is manifested in many forms and may involve any organ of the body. It used to be considered that there were two forms: discoid lupus erythematosus (DLE) of the skin, and systemic lupus erythematosus (SLE), in which constitutional symptoms and visceral lesions predominate but skin lesions are also often present.

Utilizing important recent advances by Provost, Sontheimer, Gilliam, Tuffanelli, and Callen, we now modify the classification of cutaneous LE in the following way:

1. Chronic cutaneous LE.
   a. Discoid LE, localized (head and neck) or generalized ("disseminated") discoid LE.
   b. Verrucous (hypertrophic) LE (Bechet).
   c. Palmoplantar erosive discoid LE (lichen planus–lupus erythematosus overlap).
   d. Chilblain LE.
   e. Lupus panniculitis (LE profundus).
      (1) With discoid LE.
      (2) With systemic LE.
   f. Discoid LE with systemic involvement (relatively benign subset).
2. Subacute cutaneous LE.
   a. Morphologic types.
      (1) Papulosquamous.
      (2) Annular.
   b. Syndromes commonly exhibiting this morphology.
      (1) Neonatal LE.
      (2) Complement deficiency syndromes.
3. Acute cutaneous LE (systemic LE with skin lesions) localized or generalized erythema or bullae.

Systemic lupus erythematosus will be discussed separately, reviewing selected internal manifestations as well as the many dermatologic findings that are disease related and should suggest the diagnosis of systemic connective tissue disease, but are not specific to LE.

Discoid Lupus Erythematosus (DLE)

The cutaneous findings in DLE are characterized by dull red macules with adherent scales extending into patulous follicles, telangiectases, and atrophy. The macule may be 1 cm or more in diameter. Removal of the scale shows its under surface to be covered with the horny plugs which filled the follicles, resembling "carpet tacks" or *langue au chat* ("cat's tongue").

The patches tend to heal centrally first, with atrophy, scarring, dyspigmentation, and telangiectasia.

Some discoid lesions are very superficial, resembling mild seborrheic dermatitis. Others may be brightly erythematous or even urticarial, suggesting dermatitis due to a drug or contactant, or even erythema multiforme. On the other hand, erythema may be minimal, and the patch merely hyperkera-totic, dark gray, and centrally depressed, suggestive of a solitary lesion of lichen planus or a carcinoma. Indeed, very small lesions of discoid LE are easily mistaken, both clinically and histologically, for actinic keratoses.

TYPES

Localized DLE. These patients have discoid lesions localized above the neck. This form is far more

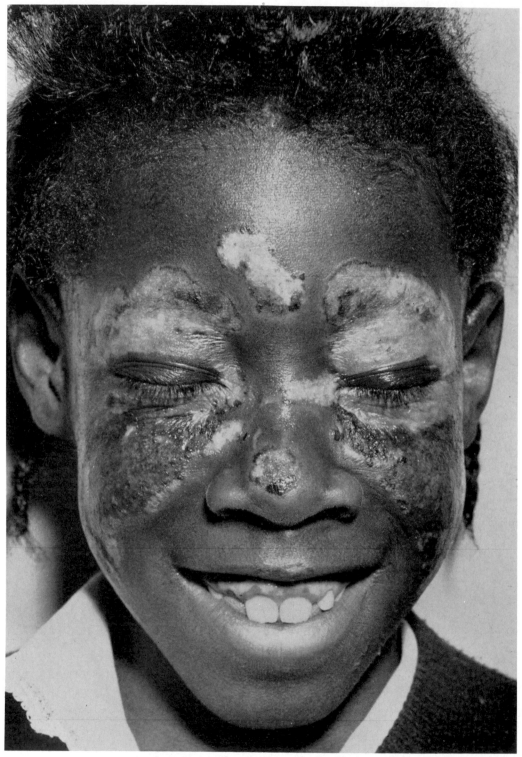

Figure 8–1. Discoid lupus erythematosus with typical butterfly distribution, atrophy, and depigmentation of skin. (Courtesy of Dr. L. Schweich.)

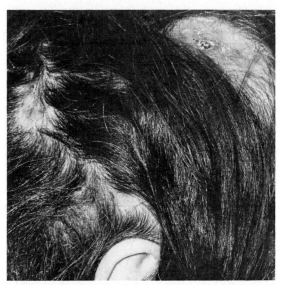

Figure 8–2. Discoid lupus erythematosus on the scalp, a typical site. (Courtesy of Dr. L. Lewis.)

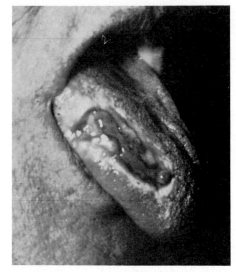

Figure 8–4. Lupus erythematosus of tongue.

common than the generalized form. Favored sites are the bridge of the nose, the malar areas, the lower lip, and the ears.

On the scalp the scars are more sclerotic and depressed than on other areas, and are apt to be hairless. Dilated follicles, with or without horny plugs, are usually seen. Itching may rarely be severe.

On the lips or in the mouth the patches are grayish and hyperkeratotic; they may be eroded, and are usually surrounded by a narrow red inflammatory zone.

Generalized DLE. This is usually superimposed on a localized discoid case. All degrees of severity are encountered. Most often the thorax and upper extremities are affected, in addition to the usual sites for localized DLE. The scalp may become quite bald, and diffuse scarring may involve the face and upper extremities. In Callen's series, laboratory abnormalities such as an elevated sedimentation rate, elevated antinuclear antibodies, or leucopenia were more common with this form of LE than with localized DLE.

The course of DLE is variable, but 95 per cent of

cases confined to the skin at the outset will remain so. Progression from chronic cutaneous (discoid) LE to SLE is uncommon. Fever may signal its occurrence, but laboratory tests (elevation of ANA, leucopenia, hematuria, or albuminuria) are a more sensitive indicator. If no abnormalities are found, reassurance is advised; if two or three criteria are present, careful reevaluation should be carried out at regular intervals, with rest, aspirin, perhaps diphenhydramine, and close observation. If four or more criteria for SLE (p. 167) are met, one may make the diagnosis of SLE.

Spontaneous involution, with scarring, is common. Calcific nodules may develop in affected sites. Deposits of mucin may occur. Relapses are common. Rarely basal or squamous cell carcinoma may occur, often in scars, and often aggressive. Several recent reports document this in the lower lip of black patients with the hypopigmented scars of DLE.

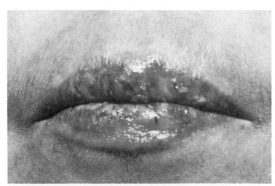

Figure 8–3. Discoid lupus erythematosus of lips.

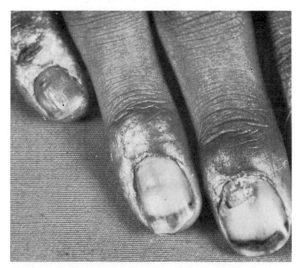

Figure 8–5. Lupus erythematosus affecting distal phalanges of fingers. (Courtesy of Dr. A. Bensel.)

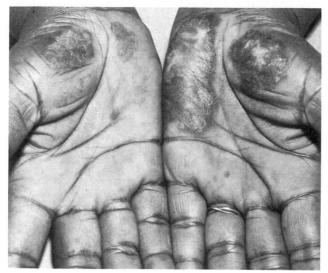

Figure 8–6. Discoid lupus erythematosus of the palms.

Verrucous DLE. In some cases of DLE on the face, hyperkeratotic nonpruritic papulo-nodular lesions may occur on the arms and hands, resembling keratoacanthoma or hypertrophic lichen planus. Uitto and his associates found the histology of these lesions similar to that of DLE. Callen recently confirmed the clinical findings of Uitto et al and found no serologic or HLA correlates in this subgroup.

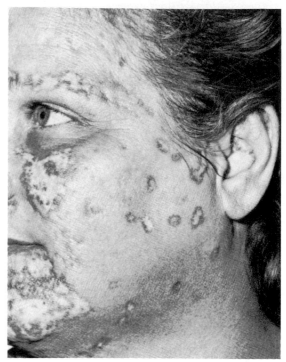

Figure 8–8. Disseminated discoid lupus erythematosus.

Treatment with intralesional injections of triamcinolone acetonide is usually feasible and almost invariably effective. Recently success has been reported with isotretinoin alone or in combination with hydroxychloroquine.

LE–Lichen Planus Overlap Syndrome. The lesions are usually large atrophic hypopigmented patches and plaques, with a bluish red color. Fine telangiectasia and scaling are usually present. The extensor aspects of the extremities are a site of election, and palmoplantar involvement is common. The histology

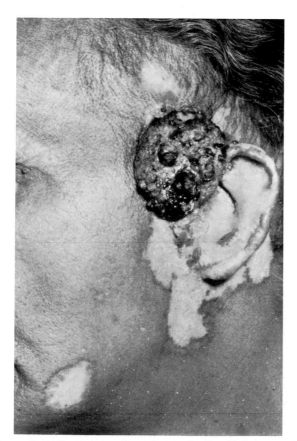

Figure 8–7. Squamous cell carcinoma in discoid lupus erythematosus. (Courtesy of Dr. F. Kerdel-Vegas.)

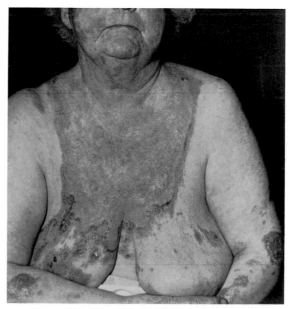

Figure 8–9. Disseminated lupus erythematosus.

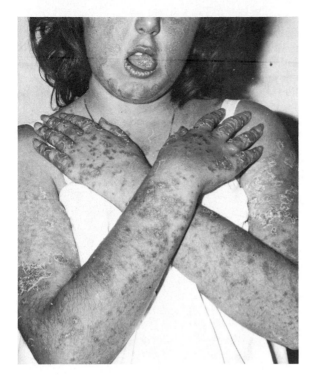

Figure 8–10. Disseminated discoid lupus erythematosus. (Courtesy of Dr. J. Kroll.)

The histology shows lymphocytic panniculitis, hyaline degeneration of the fat, hyaline papillary bodies, and dense, sharply circumscribed lymphocytic nodules in the lower dermis and fat. The overlying epidermis may show basal liquefaction and follicular plugging, or may be normal.

In seven of nine cases reviewed by A. K. Izumi, direct immunofluorescence showed granular deposition of immunoglobulin and C3 at the dermoepidermal junction.

Treatment with antimalarials is, as a rule, dramatically successful. An initial dose of hydroxychloroquine, 200 mg twice a day, reduced as soon as a

has features of either lichen planus or LE, or both. Direct immunofluorescence usually suggests the former. The lupus band test may be positive. Response to treatment is poor, though dapsone may be effective.

Chilblain Lupus Erythematosus. Chilblain LE (Hutchinson) is a chronic, unremitting form of LE with acral distribution: fingertips, rims of ears, calves, and heels, especially in women. It is usually preceded by DLE on the face. Systemic involvement is sometimes seen. Mimicry of sarcoidosis may be striking. The chilblain lesions themselves are due to cold injury to the microvasculature, for which the usual LE treatment modalities are ineffective. Allegue et al reported a case associated with antiphospholipid antibody.

LE Panniculitis ("LE Profundus"). In this type of LE, deep dermal or even subcutaneous nodules 1 to 3 or 4 cm in diameter, rubbery-firm, sharply defined, and nontender, occur, most often beneath normal skin of the head, face, or upper arms. The chest, buttocks, and thighs may also be involved. This form of LE is characteristically chronic, and occurs most often in women between the ages of 20 and 45. Partly because the diagnosis is more likely to be made if it is known that the patients have LE, most patients have DLE at other sites, or less typically in the overlying skin. The lesions heal with deep depressions from loss of the panniculus, which may take years to fill in. Paul Bechet's "lupus hypertrophicus et profundus," with its severe distortions of surface contour, usually of the cheek or chin, may have been what we would now call verrucous DLE (above). It was certainly not LE panniculitis.

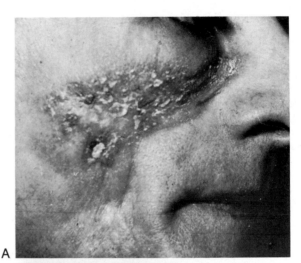

A

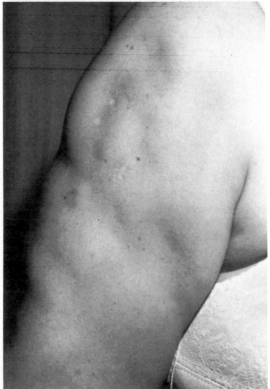

B

Figure 8–11. A and B, LE panniculitis. (B, Courtesy of Dr. Axel W. Hoke.)

response is achieved, is believed to be very safe even if it has to be continued for a year or two, which is rarely the case. Intralesional triamcinolone acetonide is also extremely effective.

Childhood DLE. There is nothing distinctive about DLE in childhood, clinically or in the histology. It is uncommon to see involvement of this age group.

HISTOLOGY. The epidermis is usually thin and there is loss of the normal rete ridge pattern. Hyperorthokeratosis and parakeratosis, with follicular plugging, occur. Hydropic degeneration of the basal layer results in transfer of melanin to melanophages in the papillary dermis. A primarily lymphocytic focal inflammatory infiltrate occurs in the superficial dermis, especially around follicles. The superficial dermis may be edematous, and mucin is often present.

Chronic, inactive lesions show atrophy, with post-inflammatory pigmentation. Dermal fibrosis may be present. The basement membrane zone is generally thickened. Inflammatory infiltrate is sparse to absent. Pilosebaceous units, except for arrector muscles, are destroyed.

Direct immunofluorescence test of lesional skin is positive in over 75 per cent of cases, with immunoglobulin and complement located at the dermoepidermal junction, usually in a granular or particulate pattern. Early lesions (under eight weeks) may have negative immunofluorescence, especially if on covered skin areas, and uninvolved skin is negative.

DIFFERENTIAL DIAGNOSIS. Chronic cutaneous LE (DLE) must often be differentiated from seborrheic dermatitis, rosacea, lupus vulgaris, sarcoid, drug eruptions, Bowen's disease, lichen planus, lupoid sycosis, tertiary syphilis, polymorphous light eruption, actinic keratosis, and lymphocytic infiltration (Jessner). Immunoglobulin deposits distinguish DLE from the latter condition. Seborrheic dermatitis does not show atrophy, alopecia, or dilated follicles and has greasy yellowish scale without follicular plugs, and involvement of other sites of election for seborrheic dermatitis—eyebrows, eyelids, nasolabial angles, ears, or sternal and axillary areas—in most cases.

In rosacea, atrophy does not occur and pustules are nearly always found. Apple-jelly nodules are seen in lupus vulgaris. Sunlight-sensitizing agents such as sulfonamides may produce lesions similar to lupus erythematosus. It may be necessary to differentiate syphilis and sarcoid by biopsy and FTA-ABS test. It is difficult to exclude LE in cicatricial alopecia of the scalp; indeed, many such cases are due to LE. Direct immunofluorescence is especially useful in diagnosing these cases. Polymorphous light eruption offers considerable difficulties. The absence of scarring and the presence of edematous plaques may help in the diagnosis.

TREATMENT. Certain general measures are important. The patient should avoid exposure to strong sunlight, to excessive cold, to heat, and to localized trauma. Exposure to sunlight should be at a minimum and sunscreen lotion should be used to protect against burning and tanning.

Local Treatment. The application of corticosteroid creams and ointments (e.g., Temovate) has merit. Aerosol spray preparations (Kenalog Aerosol, Squibb) have also proved effective.

The best local treatment is the injection of corticosteroids into the lesions. Triamcinolone, 2.5 mg/cc in suspension, is infiltrated into the lesion through a 30-gauge needle at intervals of four to six weeks. We prefer to use not more than 40 mg of triamcinolone at one time. With the exception of one case of localized urticarial reaction, no side effects have been experienced by our patients except occasional localized transient atrophy at the sites of injection.

Internal Treatment. The safest and most beneficial internal treatment is antimalarials. Hydroxychloroquine (Plaquenil), 200 mg twice or once daily, is the preferred antimalarial. If no response occurs after three months at the higher dose, a switch to chloroquine (Aralen) is advised, in a dose of 250 mg a day. If response is still incomplete, quinacrine (Atabrine), 100 mg a day, may be added, as this probably entails no increased risk of retinal toxicity. Sometimes this is necessary during the summer months, but may be reduced or stopped during the winter.

Relapses are frequent even with the antimalarials, and long-term therapy is frequently necessary. Patients should be watched closely for possible side effects, especially ocular toxicity. Ophthalmologic consultation should be obtained before, and at four- to six-month intervals during, treatment. In a review of 99 patients taking hydroxychloroquine over a seven-year period, Tobin found only one instance of side effects: a 5° constriction of visual fields to a red object in a man who had taken 444 gm of chloroquine in 36 months. Vision was 20/20 throughout and he was normal 18 months later. Rynes later found, in 99 patients taking 400 mg of hydroxychloroquine a day for over one year, two with paracentral scotomas, two with slight visual field constrictions, and one with pigmentation of the retina; all changes were transitory. There were no cataracts. The finding of any visual field defect or pigmentary abnormality is an indication to stop antimalarial therapy.

There may be eruptions of erythema multiforme, purpura, urticaria, nausea, vomiting, nervousness, tinnitus, abducens nerve paralysis, toxic psychoses, leukopenia, and thrombocytopenia. Antimalarials, except in very small doses, will exacerbate porphyria cutanea tarda and most cases of psoriasis (except the few that are exacerbated by sunlight). They may also produce maculopapular and light-sensitivity eruptions, and bleach the hair. Chloroquine toxicity may be explained by its tendency for binding to melanin for a long time, with insufficient excretion.

From quinacrine (Atabrine) the skin and conjunctivae become yellow. Bullous erythema multiforme, lichen-planuslike lesions, and gastrointestinal symptoms of nausea, vomiting, anorexia, and diarrhea may develop. Aplastic anemia has also been noted in long-term therapy. Patients with brown or red hair may turn light blond. Quinacrine has been known to produce blue-black pigmentation of the hard palate, nail beds, cartilage of the ears, alae nasi, and sclerae.

Systemic corticosteroids for widespread or disfiguring lesions are effective; however, treatment should be limited to a maximum of four to six weeks. It may be useful to use this for initial quick control while antimalarial therapy is being initiated.

Newton et al reported nine patients with chronic or subacute cutaneous LE who responded to 16 weeks of isotretinoin therapy. Dapsone, clofazimine, acetretin, auranofin (oral gold), and thalidomide have all been reported to favorably affect DLE, and one of us (WDJ) has seen several dramatic responses to isotretinoin; however, these agents have not had widespread use and they must still be regarded as experimental. Likewise, though gold and bismuth injections were frequently used in the past, they are generally not recommended today.

Subacute Cutaneous Lupus Erythematosus (SCLE)

Sontheimer, Thomas, and Gilliam described in 1979 a clinically distinct subset of cases of LE to which they gave this name. The patients are most often white women aged 15 to 40. These make up approximately 10 to 15 per cent of the LE population. Lesions are scaly papules, which evolve into either a psoriasiform or a polycyclic annular lesion. The scale is thin and easily detached, and telangiectasia and dyspigmentation are nearly always present. Follicles are not involved and there is no scarring. Lesions tend to occur on sun-exposed surfaces of the upper trunk and arms; inner arms, axillae and flanks, and knuckles are spared. Photosensitivity occurs in about half, as does alopecia. The hard palate is involved in 40 per cent, and concomitant DLE is present in 20 per cent.

Given these cutaneous parameters, and considering that three fourths have arthralgia or arthritis, 20 per cent have leukopenia, and 80 per cent have a positive ANA, it is not surprising that (despite the name) at least half meet the 1982 revised American Rheumatism Association criteria for a diagnosis of systemic LE (SLE). The disease generally runs a mild course, however, and renal, central nervous system, or vascular complications are unusual.

HISTOPATHOLOGY. Histologic changes are similar to those of DLE, except that follicular plugging, hyperkeratosis, and lymphocytic infiltration are less marked. Direct IF is positive in lesions in 60 per cent.

Over 60 per cent of cases have antibodies to Ro/SSA antigen, and a comparable number are HLA-Dr3–positive.

Hydrochlorothiazide has recently been reported to have induced this type of LE.

TREATMENT. Treatment is primarily with antimalarials (see above under DLE). Low-dose systemic steroids and photoprotection are helpful. McCormack et al recently reported good results in two cases treated with dapsone.

NEONATAL LUPUS ERYTHEMATOSUS

Annular scaling erythematous macules may appear on the head and neck within the first few weeks of life in babies born to mothers with LE, rheumatic disease, or other collagen disorders, although half the mothers are asymptomatic. The children's lesions usually resolve spontaneously by six months of age, and heal without scarring. Photosensitivity may be

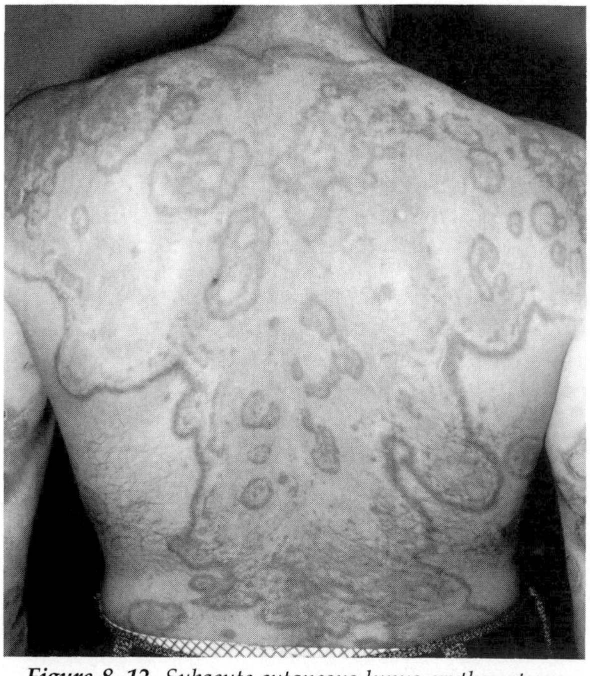

Figure 8–12. Subacute cutaneous lupus erythematosus.

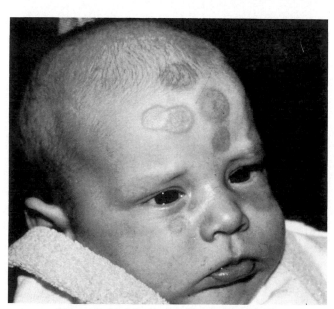

Figure 8–13. Neonatal lupus erythematosus.

prominent. Histopathology and immunopathology are characteristic of LE. Seventy-five per cent of cases are girls.

Though the skin lesions are transient, there is often an associated isolated congenital heart block, usually third degree, which is permanent. Some infants have only this manifestation of LE, and for heart lesions alone, there is no female predominance.

As with other forms of SCLE, there is a strong Ro/SSA antibody association. Nearly all mothers, and hence nearly all infants, are positive for this antibody. There is also a gene linkage to HLA-Dr3 in the mother. Lee has reported that most asymptomatic mothers will eventually have symptoms, that the risk that a second child will have LE is less than 50 per cent, and that the outlook for the infants is good. Occasional cases have been associated with U₁RNP antibodies.

McCune et al reported in 1987 that 18 of 21 mothers of children with neonatal LE—half of whom were initially asymptomatic—developed LE or Sjögren's syndrome during a follow-up period of 0.25 to 9.5 years.

COMPLEMENT DEFICIENCY SYNDROMES

While deficiency of many complement components may be associated with LE-like conditions, deficiencies of the early components, especially C2 and C4,

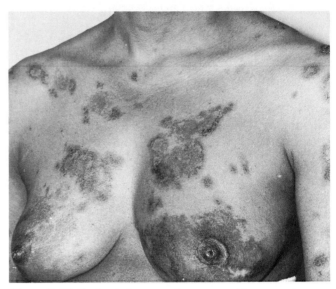

Figure 8–15. *Systemic lupus erythematosus. (Courtesy of Dr. P. Salinger.)*

are most characteristic. Many such cases are being found to have photosensitivity, annular SCLE lesions, and Ro/SSA antibody formation.

The common denominators of this clinical subset of patients are the clinical lesions, the photosensitivity, and the Ro/SSA antibody formation. Norris has found that Ro antigen is expressed on the cell membranes of keratinocytes after ultraviolet light exposure. This could lead to autoantibody formation with resultant cell damage by the mechanism of antibody-dependent cellular cytotoxicity.

Acute Cutaneous Lupus Erythematosus

The characteristic butterfly facial erythema seen in patients with SLE is the common manifestation of this type of cutaneous LE. There may be associated edema. The eruption may last from a day to a month, and resolves without scarring. There may be more widespread erythema in some cases.

Bullous lesions represent a newly defined subgroup of acute "cutaneous" LE, again typically systemic (SLE). These occur as single or grouped vesicles or bullae, often widespread, with a predilection for sun-exposed areas. They may rarely itch. Histologically there is a subepidermal bulla containing neutrophils. Granular fluorescence with IgG, IgM, IgA, or C3 is seen in the lamina densa on immunoelectron microscopy. Epidermolysis bullosa acquisita has been suggested in some bullous LE lesions by indirect immunofluorescence, by protein precipitation, and by the fact that in both diseases there are circulating antibodies against Type VII collagen. Most of these patients are HLA-DR2 positive. The separation of this subset as a distinct one is perhaps made most clear, however, by its dramatic therapeutic response to dapsone, which is ineffective against epidermolysis bullosa acquisita.

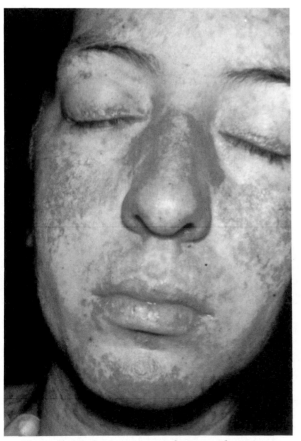

Figure 8–14. *Acute cutaneous lupus erythematosus.*

Systemic Lupus Erythematosus (SLE)

Middle-aged women are predominantly affected, with a wide range of symptoms and signs either somatic (e.g., profound weakness and fatigability, or fever of undetermined origin) or cutaneous (simple erythema or purpura, butterfly erythema; or at the other extreme, fulminating toxemia with widespread erythema or purpura and high fever). Skin involvement occurs in 80 per cent of cases, but this is partly because it is likely to be helpful in arriving at a diagnosis. Its importance is suggested by the fact that four of the American Rheumatism Association's 11 criteria for the diagnosis are cutaneous findings.

1982 Revised American Rheumatism Association Criteria for the Diagnosis of SLE.
1. Malar erythema.
2. Discoid LE.
3. Photosensitivity.
4. Oral ulcer(s).
5. Nonerosive arthritis.
6. Serositis (pericarditis or pleurisy).
7. Nephropathy (albuminuria or cellular casts).
8. CNS disorder (unexplained seizures or psychosis).
9. Hematologic disorder (hemolytic anemia with reticulosis, or leucopenia below 4000 on two occasions, or lymphopenia below 1500 on two occasions).
10. Immunologic disorder: positive LE-cell preparation, or antibody to native DNA or SM antigen, or false positive STS.
11. Antinuclear antibody in abnormal titer, unexplained.

For identification of patients in clinical studies, a patient may be said to have SLE if four or more criteria are satisfied, serially or simultaneously.

SLE may easily go undiagnosed during years of invalidism manifested by prolonged irregular hectic or intermittent fever with weight loss and ease of fatigue, and recurrent involvement of various organs.

CUTANEOUS MANIFESTATIONS. In acute cutaneous LE, the eruption usually begins on the malar areas and the bridge of the nose, its configuration often suggesting a butterfly. The ears and V of the chest may also be the site of early lesions. Discoid LE may precede SLE in as many as one fourth of cases.

A variety of vascular lesions occur in 50 per cent of cases, which, while not specific for SLE, suggest underlying connective tissue disease. Often the fingertips or toe tips show suggestive puffiness, erythema, or telangiectasis. The palms, soles, elbows, knees, or buttocks may become persistently erythematous or purplish. Minute telangiectases appear in time on the face or elsewhere, and flat telangiectases commonly appear about the nail folds. Petechiae or aphthae may occur in the mouth.

Alopecia areata or diffuse hair loss, nonscarring, is common. Scarring hair loss occurs in healed discoid lesions of the scalp. Short broken-off hairs in the frontal region as a result of increased fragility are referred to as "lupus hairs."

Mucous membrane lesions are seen in 10 to 15 per cent of SLE patients. Conjunctivitis is common. Oral mucosal hemorrhages, erosions, shallow ulcerations with surrounding erythema, and gingivitis occur commonly. Erythema, petechiae, and erosions may occur on the hard palate.

Lin et al reported three cases of SLE in which *multiple dermatofibromas* supervened, 120 in one case. They suggest that 15 should be the lower limit of "multiple."

Leg ulcers, typically deeply punched out, very indolent, and little-inflamed, are seen with some frequency on the pretibial or malleolar areas particularly. Vasculitis or thrombosis due to the presence of an antiphospholipid antibody may cause them. Cryoglobulinemia or livedo reticularis may also be present. Gangrene of the toes is a rare event.

Bullae may be primary or secondary to the occurrence of other bullous diseases, such as porphyria, dermatitis herpetiformis, bullous pemphigoid, or acquired epidermolysis bullosa.

Cutaneous angiitis shown by petechiae, papulonodules, livedo reticularis, and superficial ulceration may be an initial manifestation of SLE, as reported by Tuffanelli and Dubois.

SYSTEMIC MANIFESTATIONS. Most organs can be involved; the symptoms and findings are primarily due to vasculitis. The earliest changes noted may be transitory or migratory arthralgia, often with periarticular inflammation and thrombophlebitis. Fever, weight loss, pleurisy, adenopathy, or acute abdominal pain may occur.

Thrombosis in vessels of various size, and thromboembolism, may be a recurring event, and it is attributed to a plasma constituent paradoxically called "lupus anticoagulant factor" (LA). Thrombocytopenia, a false positive STS, livedo reticularis, neurologic disorders, and a high incidence of obstetric complications further characterize these patients. No treatment diminishes LA except plasmapheresis, steroid pulse therapy, and (in at least two cases) splenectomy. An excellent editorial review by Sontheimer is recommended (see below).

Renal involvement may be of either nephritic or nephrotic type, leading in either case to chronic renal insufficiency with proteinuria and azotemia. Hypercholesterolemia and hypoalbuminemia may occur. Immunoglobulin and complement components have been found localized to the basement membrane of glomeruli, where vasculitis produces the characteristic "wire-loop" lesion.

Orth reported five women and one man with *lupus cystitis*, every one of whom had marked frequency and oliguria. All four of his own cases had severe gastrointestinal symptoms during the period of bladder symptoms. Four had ureterectasis and three had frank hydronephrosis. Resolution under therapy was achieved in only two.

Myocarditis is indicated by cardiomegaly and gallop rhythm, but the electrocardiographic changes are usually not specific. *Pericarditis* (the most frequent cardiac manifestation) and endocarditis also occur fairly frequently. Purpura, often thrombocytopenic, may occur, with ecchymoses. Raynaud's phenomenon occurs in about 15 per cent of patients; these individuals have less renal disease and consequently lower mortality.

The *central nervous system* may be involved with vasculitis, manifested by hemiparesis, convulsions, epilepsy, diplopia, retinitis, choroiditis, psychosis, and other personality disorders. Livedo reticularis is a marker for patients at risk for CNS lesions. Mental depression, cephalalgia, peripheral neuritis, mental confusion, and loss of memory may also be present.

Idiopathic thrombocytopenic purpura is occasionally the forerunner of SLE. Avascular bone necrosis may occur. Coombs-positive hemolytic anemia, neutropenia, and lymphopenia are other hematologic findings.

Lupus hepatitis is now believed to be an LE response of serologic antibodies to chronic active hepatitis. LE cells have also been demonstrated. This serious liver disease is frequently combined with ulcerative colitis, and resembles chronic viral hepatitis. The prognosis is grave.

Gastrointestinal involvement may produce symptoms of nausea, vomiting, and diarrhea. Frequently the intestinal wall and the mesenteric vessels show vasculitis.

Pulmonary involvement with pleural effusions, interstitial lung disease, and acute lupus pneumonitis may be present.

Sjögren's syndrome (keratoconjunctivitis sicca) and *Hashimoto's thyroiditis* are associated with SLE with some frequency. This suggests that similar autoimmune mechanisms may be causing these diseases. Sjögren's syndrome more often occurs independently of SLE.

Muscular atrophy may accompany extreme weakness so that dermatomyositis may be suspected. Myopathy of the vacuolar type may produce muscular weakness, myocardial disease, dysphagia, and achalasia of the esophagus. Tsokos and associates at the NIH reported 17 women and one man with myositis, among 228 patients with SLE (8 per cent), and found the myositis mild, and the serum aldolase level (but not creatine phosphokinase) frequently elevated.

Arthralgia is often the earliest abnormality and may remain the sole symptom for some time at the onset of SLE. Ninety-five per cent of SLE patients will manifest this symptom. Arthralgia, deforming arthropathy, and acute migratory polyarthritis resembling rheumatoid arthritis may all occur in conjunction with or as manifestations of SLE. Avascular necrosis of the femoral head has been observed. Although this has been known to occur during corticosteroid therapy, it has occurred also in patients with SLE who never have had corticosteroids and in

patients who have never had SLE. The evidence that it is caused by steroids is inconclusive.

A history of exposure to sunlight prior to the onset of the disease or prior to an exacerbation is sometimes obtained. Some patients may suffer from mild constitutional symptoms for weeks or months, and immediately after exposure to strong sunlight may develop the facial eruption and a severe relapse. In other cases, no history of exposure to sunlight can be elicited.

TYPES

Childhood SLE. The onset of childhood SLE occurs between the ages of three and 15 years, with girls outnumbering boys by four to one. The skin manifestations may be the typical butterfly eruption on the face. In addition, there may be morbilliform, bullous, purpuric, ulcerating, or nodose lesions. The oral mucosa is frequently involved.

The skin eruptions may be associated with joint, renal, neurologic, and gastrointestinal disease. Weight loss, fatigue, and fever are other manifestations.

The indirect fluorescent antibody test for antinuclear antibodies is usually positive, according to Meislin and Rothfield, who also suggest that SLE should be considered in children with hepatosplenomegaly and lymphadenopathy, a frequent occurrence in children with SLE.

Familial SLE. Familial SLE has been found to be associated with hereditary hyperglobulinemia and with a high incidence of rheumatic disorders and other "collagen diseases" in family members of those with SLE. Concordance in monozygotic twins is 70 per cent. Lahits et al reported four kindreds with 22 members, of whom 10 had clearcut SLE; nine of the 10 were male. Several other family members had intermittent symptoms, including tenosynovitis and positive ANA tests.

Pregnancy and SLE. Women with LE may have successful pregnancies, although there might be difficulty in becoming pregnant, and miscarriages may occur with greater frequency. The course of pregnancy may be entirely normal, with remission of the LE, or the symptoms of LE may become worse. Female patients without renal involvement usually may safely become pregnant during periods of remission. Risk of fetal death is increased in women with SLE. It is in the postpartum period that the risk to the patient is highest; the pregnancy itself is usually well tolerated. For the patient with anticardiolipin antibodies, however, the risk of intrauterine death and spontaneous abortion is significantly increased.

Evidence that estrogen-containing contraceptives can aggravate SLE is scanty and unconvincing, but Jungers et al have at least shown that progesterone does *not* have this effect.

ETIOLOGY. As previously discussed, genetic factors may play a role in predisposing first-degree relatives of patients with SLE to the development of this disease. The prevalence of SLE in this group is

1.5 per cent. SLE occurs predominantly in females in the reproductive years, perhaps because sex hormones may potentiate SLE. Multiple abnormal immune responses are present, which may be responsible for many of the manifestations. The possible linkage to an infectious agent, especially a virus, has been hypothesized for many years, but remains unproved. An abnormal response to sunlight, both UVB and, as recent evidence suggests, UVA, exists. That these factors contribute to the clinical disease manifestations is evident. Their exact interaction and relative importance are not as yet understood.

Drugs such as hydralazine, the sulfonamides, penicillin, anticonvulsants, tetracycline, and procainamide have precipitated or unmasked SLE. Though many such cases run a relatively benign course, with clearing and recovery within a few weeks or months after discontinuation of the drug, some patients continue to be gravely ill, or have repeated relapses, and seem to develop true SLE.

Acetylprocainamide may safely be given to patients who have had procainamide-induced lupus syndrome. Blocking the amino group by acetylation appears to prevent the lupus-inducing effect. This drug is not yet available for use in the U.S.

Hydralazine gradually induces a positive ANA reaction in about 10 per cent of treated patients. HLA-Dr4 individuals who are slow acetylators, taking 300 mg a day for three months or more, are predisposed to develop a drug-induced SLE syndrome. The risk is even higher with procainamide, which induces a positive ANA in about 50 per cent of treated patients. Antibody to the histone complex H2A-H2B is closely associated with symptomatic disease. There is a 20 per cent incidence of this with isoniazid taken for a year or more. In all these, over 90 per cent of the positive ANAs are directed against histone. An exception is penicillamine-induced cases, which seem to have native disease, with anti-dsDNA antibodies. Hydrochlorothiazide, however, has been implicated in production of SCLE.

Drug-induced SLE is typically mild, with skin, renal, and CNS manifestations being unusual as compared to naturally occurring disease. Skin lesions do occur in about 18 per cent of cases.

Several aspects of the altered immune response are worth particular attention. T–suppressor-cell function is reduced. The resulting overproduction of gamma globulins by B cells causes overresponsiveness to endogenous antigens. The immune complexes thus produced may induce complement-mediated tissue damage. Reduced clearance of immune complexes by the reticuloendothelial system aggravates matters. Also, as mentioned above, there is evidence for externalization of cellular antigens, such as Ro/SSA, in response to sunlight. This may lead to cell injury by way of antibody-dependent cellular cytotoxicity.

DIAGNOSIS. The 11 criteria proposed by the American Rheumatism Association, and modified in 1982 (p. 167), should be consulted. If four criteria are met, consecutively or simultaneously, over any period of time, the diagnosis of SLE may be made with confidence.

LABORATORY FINDINGS. Albumin, red blood cells, and casts are the most frequent findings in the urine.

Many varied findings are found in SLE. There may be hemolytic anemia, thrombocytopenia, lymphopenia, antiphospholipid antibody, or leukopenia; the erythrocyte sedimentation rate is usually markedly elevated, Coombs test may be positive, and there is a biologic false positive test for syphilis in about 20 per cent. Unexplained fever, weakness, and easy fatigability are common. The rheumatoid factor may be present. Protein electrophoresis and immunoglobulin tests often show levels of IgG greater than 2000 mg per cent. The albumin:globulin ratio is usually reversed. The serum globulin is increased, especially the gamma globulin or alpha$_2$ fraction. The LE factor is a gamma globulin protein.

The specific frequencies of each of these findings, and those that follow, are listed in Tan's article defining these criteria.

IMMUNOLOGIC FINDINGS

1. *ANA (antinuclear antibody) test.* Positive in about a third of all connective tissue disorders, but in 95 per cent of cases of SLE. Hep-2 tumor cell line is the most sensitive substrate.

2. *LE cell test.* Specific but not very sensitive. Little used.

3. *"dsDNA"*: anti–double-stranded DNA; tested with kinetoplast of *Crithidia luciliae.* Specific, not very sensitive. Indicates high risk of renal disease.

4. *Anti-SM antibody.* Sensitivity only 20–40 per cent, but has highest specificity of any test.

5. *Antinuclear ribonucleic acid* protein (anti-nRNP). Indicates low risk of renal disease, and a good prognosis. Seen in mixed connective tissue disease as well as in SLE.

6. *Anti-La antibodies.* Found in only 10–15 per cent of SLE cases and 30 per cent of cases of Sjögren's syndrome. Hence sometimes referred to as SSB.

7. *Anti-Ro antibodies.* Found in about one fourth of SLE and 40 per cent of Sjögren's cases: antigen found in both cytoplasm and nucleus. Photosensitivity may be striking.

8. *Serum complement.* Low levels indicate disease activity. Immunodiffusion for C3 and C4 is most useful for following patients.

9. *Lupus band test.* Direct cutaneous immunofluorescence. Granular deposits of immunoglobulins and complement along the dermoepidermal junction occur in over 75 per cent of lesions of DLE and SLE, and in normal skin in SLE only (where it is twice as common in sun-exposed as in protected skin). A positive test in protected skin correlates well with the presence of anti-dsDNA antibodies and renal disease, and hence with a poor prognosis.

10. *Anti-ssDNA antibody.* Sensitive but not specific. Many are photosensitive. An IgM isotype seen in DLE may identify a subset of patients at risk for developing systemic symptoms.

11. *ANA patterns. Peripheral,* SLE-specific (anti-

DNA); in some patients antibodies to lamin B may be present when this pattern is present. *Homogeneous* (least specific) histone determinants.

Good recent reviews by Provost, Sams, and Tan are recommended for more detailed discussion.

DIFFERENTIAL DIAGNOSIS. SLE mimics many diseases and is known as the great imitator, probably exceeded in this reputation only by syphilis, and possibly drug eruptions. SLE must be differentiated from dermatomyositis, toxic erythema multiforme, polyarteritis nodosa, acute rheumatic fever, rheumatoid arthritis, pellagra, pemphigus erythematosus (Senear-Usher syndrome), drug eruptions, hemolytic anemia, hyperglobulinemic purpura, Sjögren's syndrome, necrotizing angiitis, and myasthenia gravis.

SLE may be differentiated by several factors. In SLE there are usually fever, arthralgia, weakness, lassitude, skin lesions suggestive of LE, increased sedimentation rate, a leukocyte count of less than 4000, proteinuria, "band" immunoglobulin deposition at the dermal-epidermal junction, and positive LE cell, ANA, or DNA complement fixation tests. Biopsies of skin lesions, kidney, or liver are also useful adjuncts in doubtful cases.

TREATMENT. Many cases run a relatively benign course, with perhaps mild rheumatoid-arthritislike symptoms requiring only bed rest and salicylates. Salicylates may produce dramatic relief of musculoskeletal symptoms. If salicylates are not tolerated, ibuprofen (Motrin, Advil), 1200 to 3200 mg daily, or other nonsteroidal antiinflammatory medications may be substituted.

Antimalarials. The various antimalarials (atabrine, chloroquine, and hydroxychloroquine) are effective in the treatment of SLE. These may be used also in conjunction with the corticosteroids. Dosage and side effects of the antimalarials are discussed in the treatment section of DLE, above.

Corticosteroids. In moderately severe cases in which the diagnostic criteria of the American Rheumatism Association are satisfied, corticosteroids have proven to be effective and to prolong survival rates. In moderately severe cases with renal or neurologic involvement, corticosteroids should be administered. Lange has shown that it is advantageous to monitor complement determinations (CH_{50}) frequently and adjust the steroid dose as indicated.

Just enough therapy to ensure a good response should be given. The aim should be to control the symptoms with acetylsalicylic acid. If this is not enough, antimalarials should be given. Urman and Rothfield reported a group of 156 patients in which corticosteroid dosage was determined by the disease activity as measured by the serum C3 complement levels and the antibody to native DNA titers determined at each patient visit to the clinic. They believe that this is a more exact control of dosage and it may be an important factor in achieving a longer survival rate in these patients. Their 5- and 10-year survival rates were 93 per cent and 84 per cent, respectively.

Ponticelli and his associates in 1977 confirmed that 1000 mg of methylprednisolone intravenously daily for three days, followed by oral prednisone, 0.5 to 1 mg per kg daily, reverses most clinical and serologic signs of activity of lupus nephritis. The effect on long-term prognosis remains to be assessed.

Immunosuppressive Therapy. This has become widespread because of a number of reports describing its efficacy in conjunction with corticosteroids. These medications (e.g., azathioprine) are often employed to allow reduction of the dose of systemic steroids, the so-called steroid-sparing effect.

Renal Dialysis. In severe lupus nephritis Roenigk and his associates reported successful renal dialysis and kidney transplantation in two patients in the terminal stages. Kimberly et al reported on 41 patients followed for 12 years, 17 of whom recovered and could stop dialysis. For one subset of patients, distinguished by recent onset and rapid decline of renal function, dialysis is not the end of the road.

Two interesting reports of therapies not recommended by the authors follow.

Psychoimmunomodulation. Kirkpatrick in 1981 reported a moderately severe case with renal involvement in which, when sustained high-dose prednisone and cyclophosphamide were recommended, the patient elected to return to her native village, from which she returned three weeks later perfectly well and entirely off medication. The village witch doctor had removed the curse placed on her by a former suitor!

Acupuncture. Feng et al treated 25 patients with systemic lupus erythematosus with acupuncture three times a week for three to seven weeks and followed them for six months or more. Eight of the 10 who had received no steroid therapy improved in all respects by six weeks, clinically and immunologically; nine of the 15 who had had steroid therapy—for nephrotic syndrome in 12—were likewise improved. Corticosteroid dosage was much reduced in all cases.

Ahmed AR, et al: Coexistence of lichen planus and systemic lupus erythematosus. JAAD 1982, 7:478.

Allegue F, et al: Chilblain LE and antiphospholipid antibody syndrome. JAAD 1988, 19:908.

Bangert JL, et al: Subacute cutaneous lupus erythematosus and discoid lupus erythematosus: Comparative histologic findings. Arch Dermatol 1984, 120:332.

Beaufils M, et al: Clinical significance of anti-Sm antibodies in systemic lupus erythematosus. Am J Med 1983, 74:201.

Bernstein HM: Ophthalmological considerations and testing in patients receiving long-term antimalarial therapy. Am J Med 1983, 75(1A):25.

Brown MM, et al: Skin immunopathology in systemic lupus erythematosus. JAMA 1980, 243:38.

Burnham TK: Antinuclear antibodies: Prognostic significance . . . Arch Dermatol 1975, 111:203.

Callen JP: Chronic cutaneous lupus erythematosus. Arch Dermatol 1982, 118:412.

Idem et al: Hypertrophic lupus erythematosus. J Invest Dermatol 1986, 86:467.

Idem: Systemic lupus erythematosus in patients with chronic cutaneous (discoid) lupus erythematosus. JAAD 1985, 12:278.

Idem: Serologic and clinical features of patients with discoid lupus erythematosus. JAAD 1985, 13:748.

Idem: Systemic LE in patients with discoid LE. JAAD 1985, 12:278.

Camisa C: Vesiculobullous SLE. JAAD 1988, 18:93.

Idem, et al: Vesiculobullous systemic lupus erythematosus. JAAD 1983, 9:924.

Carette S, et al: Controlled studies of oral immunosuppressive drugs in lupus nephritis. Ann Intern Med 1983, 99:1.

Caruso WR, et al: Skin cancer in black patients with DLE. J Rheumatol 1987, 14:156.

Chalmers A, et al: Systemic lupus erythematosus during penicillamine therapy for rheumatoid arthritis. Ann Intern Med 1982, 97:659.

Coplon NS, et al: The long-term clinical course of systemic lupus erythematosus in end-stage renal disease. N Engl J Med 1983, 308:186.

Dahl MV, ed.: Usefulness of direct immunofluorescence in patients with lupus erythematosus. Arch Dermatol 1983, 119:1010.

Dalziel K, et al: Oral gold in DLE. Br J Dermatol 1986, 45:211.

Davis BM, et al: Prognostic significance of the lupus band test in systemic lupus erythematosus: A 10-year longitudinal study. J Invest Dermatol 1982, 78:360. Dermatologic Capsule & Comment, August 1982.

Doré N, et al: Antinuclear antibody determinations in Ro(SSA)-positive, antinuclear antibody–negative lupus and Sjögren's syndrome patients. JAAD 1983, 8:611.

Dubois EL: Antimalarials in the management of discoid and systemic lupus erythematosus. Semin Arthritis Rheum 1978, 8:33.

Idem (ed.): Lupus Erythematosus, A Review, 2d ed. University of Southern California Press, 1976.

Felson DT, et al: Evidence for the superiority of immunosuppressive drugs and prednisone over prednisone alone in lupus nephritis. N Engl J Med 1984, 309:1528.

Fine LG, Moderator: Systemic lupus erythematosus in pregnancy. Ann Intern Med 1981, 94:667.

Fine RM: Thromboembolism in patients with the lupus anticoagulant factor. Int J Dermatol 1984, 23:545.

Fox JN, et al: Lupus profundus in children: Treatment with hydroxychloroquine. JAAD 1987, 16:389.

Idem: Lupus profundus in children. JAAD 1987, 16:839.

Gammon WR, et al: HLA-DR2 in patients with autoantibodies to EBA antigen. J Invest Dermatol 1988, 91:228.

Gastineau DA, et al: Lupus anticoagulant. Am J Hematol 1985, 19:265.

Gilliam JM, Chmn, et al: Subsets of lupus erythematosus. Proc XVI Internat Congr Dermatol, Tokyo, 1983, p 237.

Green SG, et al: Successful treatment of hypertrophic lupus erythematosus with isotretinon. JAAD 1987, 17:364.

Grob JJ, et al: Cutaneous manifestations associated with the presence of the lupus anticoagulant. JAAD 1986, 15:211.

Halberg P, et al: The lupus band test as a measure of disease activity in systemic lupus erythematosus. Arch Dermatol 1982, 118:572.

Hall RP, et al: Bullous eruption of systemic lupus erythematosus: Dramatic response to dapsone therapy. Ann Intern Med 1982, 97:165.

Harrist TJ, et al: The specificity and clinical usefulness of the lupus band test. Arthritis Rheum 1980, 23:479.

Herrero C, et al: SCLE. JAAD 1988, 19:1057.

Hess E: Drug related lupus. N Engl J Med 1988, 318:1460.

Hymes SR, et al: The anti-Ro antibody system. Int J Dermatol 1986, 25:1.

Izumi AK, et al: Lupus erythematosus panniculitis. Arch Dermatol 1983, 119:61.

Jungers P, et al: Influence of oral contraceptive therapy on the activity of systemic lupus erythematosus. Arthritis Rheum 1982, 25:618.

Kale SA: Drug-induced systemic lupus erythematosus. Postgrad Med 1985, 77:231.

Kephant DC, et al: Neonatal lupus erythematosus: New serologic findings. J Invest Dermatol 1981, 77:331.

Kettler AH, et al: SLE presenting as a bullous eruption in a child. Arch Dermatol 1988, 124:1083.

Kimberly RP, et al: Reversible "end-stage" lupus nephritis: Analysis of patients able to discontinue dialysis. Am J Med 1983, 74:361.

Kirkpatrick RA: Witchcraft and lupus erythematosus. JAMA 1981, 245:1937.

Kluher J, et al: Acetylprocainamide therapy in patients with previous procainamide-induced lupus syndrome. Ann Intern Med 1981, 95:18.

Lahits RG, et al: Familial systemic lupus erythematosus in males. Arthritis Rheum 1983, 26:39.

Lange K: Treatment of systemic lupus erythematosus (letter). JAMA 1981, 245:822.

Lassoued K, et al: Antinuclear autoantibodies specific for lamins. Ann Intern Med 1988, 108:829.

Lee LA: AntiRo (SSA) and AntiLa (SSB) antibodies in Lupus erythematosus and in Sjögren's syndrome. Arch Dermatol 1988, 124:61.

Lee LA, et al: Immunogenetics of the neonatal lupus syndrome. Ann Intern Med 1983, 99:592.

Idem: New findings in neonatal lupus syndrome. Am J Dis Child 1984, 138:233.

Leib RC: Lupus nephritis: The dogma deliberated. Southern Med J 1983, 76:490.

Lerner EA, et al: Whither the ANA? Arch Dermatol 1987, 123:638.

Lin RY, et al: Multiple dermatofibromas and systemic lupus erythematosus. Cutis 1986, 37:45.

Lindskov R, et al: Dapsone in the treatment of chronic lupus erythematosus. Dermatologica 1986, 172:214.

McCormack LS, et al: Annular subacute cutaneous lupus erythematosus responsive to dapsone. JAAD 1984, 11:397.

McCune AB, et al: Prognosis for fetal outcome and mothers' and children's health in neonatal lupus families. J Invest Dermatol 1986, 86:493.

Idem: Maternal and fetal outcome in neonatal lupus erythematosus. Ann Intern Med 1987, 106:518.

McCune WJ, et al: Clinical and immunological effects of monthly administration of IV cyclophosphamide in severe SLE. N Engl J Med 1988, 318:1423.

Meislin AG, et al: Systemic lupus erythematosus in childhood. Pediatrics 1968, 42:37.

Millard LE, et al: Chilblain lupus erythematosus (Hutchinson). Br J Dermatol 1978, 98:497.

Moreley KD, et al: Systemic lupus erythematosus: Causative factors and treatment. Drugs 1982, 23:481.

Newton RC, et al: Electron microscopic and immunohistologic assessment of isotretinoin in cutaneous LE. J Invest Dermatol 1985, 85:333.

Norris DA, et al: Antibody-dependent cellular cytotoxicity and skin disease. J Invest Dermatol 1985, 85:165.

Orth RW: Lupus cystitis: Primary bladder manifestations of systemic lupus erythematosus. Ann Intern Med 1983, 98:323.

Plotnick H, et al: Lichen planus and coexisting lupus erythematosus versus lichen-planus–like lupus erythematosus. JAAD 1986, 14:931.

Provost TT: Neonatal lupus erythematosus (Commentary). Arch Dermatol 1983, 119:619.

Idem: The neonatal lupus syndrome associated with U₁RNP (nRNP) antibodies. N Engl J Med 1987, 316:1135.

Idem: Lupus band test. J Invest Dermatol 1981, 20:475.

Idem: Nucleoprotein autoantibodies in lupus erythematosus. J Invest Dermatol 1981, 20:475.

Idem: The relationship between anti-Ro(SSA) antibody positive Sjögren's syndrome and anti-Ro(SSA) antibody positive lupus erythematosus. Arch Dermatol 1988, 124:63.

Prystowky S, et al: Chronic cutaneous lupus erythematosus (DLE). Medicine 1976, 55:183.

Reed BR, et al: Subacute cutaneous lupus erythematosus associated with hydrochlorothiazide therapy. Ann Intern Med 1985, 103:49. Dermatol Capsule & Comment, October 1985.

Reeves WH, et al: Lamin B autoantibodies in sera of certain patients with SLE. J Exp Med 1987, 165:950.

Ruzicka T, et al: Efficiency of acitretin in the treatment of cutaneous lupus erythematosus. Arch Dermatol 1988, 124:897.

Rynes RI: Ophthalmologic safety of long-term hydroxychloroquine sulfate treatment. Am J Med 1983, 75(I A):35.

Sams WM, et al: Practical management of cutaneous lupus erythematosus, vasculitis, and erythema multiforme. Prog Dermatol 1984, Dec.

Sanchez NP, et al: The histopathology of lupus erythematosus panniculitis. JAAD 1981, 5:673.

Santa Cruz DJ, et al: Verrucous lupus erythematosus. JAAD 1983, 9:82.

Shelley WB: Chloroquine-induced remission of nodular panniculitis present for 15 years. JAAD 1981, 5:168.

Smith D, et al: The clinical utility of the lupus band test. Arthritis Rheum 1984, 26:382.

Sontheimer RD, et al: Serologic and HLA associations in subcutaneous LE. Ann Intern Med 1982, 97:664.

Idem: Subacute cutaneous lupus erythematosus. Arch Dermatol 1979, 115:1409.

Idem: Antinuclear and anticytoplasmic antibodies: Concepts and misconceptions. JAAD 1983, 9:335.

Idem: The anticardiolipin syndrome. Arch Dermatol 1987, 123:590.

Tan M: Autoantibodies to nuclear antigens: Their immunobiology . . . Adv Immunol 1982, 33:167.

Idem, et al: The 1982 revised criteria for the classification of SLE. Arth Rheum 1982, 25:1271.

Idem: Systemic lupus erythematosus with vesiculobullous lesions. Arch Dermatol 1984, 120:1497.

Tobin DR, et al: Hydroxychloroquine: Seven-year experience. Arch Ophthalmol 1982, 100:81.

Totoritis MC, et al: Association of antibody to histone complex H2A-H2B with symptomatic procainamide-induced lupus. N Engl J Med 1988, 378:1413.

Triplett DA, et al: The relationship between lupus anticoagulants and autoantibodies to phospholipid. JAMA 1988, 259:550.

Tsokos GC, et al: Muscle involvement in systemic lupus erythematosus. JAMA 1981, 246:766.

Tuffanelli DL: Lupus erythematosus. JAAD 1981, 4:127.

Idem: Lupus erythematosus panniculitis (profundus): Clinical and immunologic studies. Arch Dermatol 1971, 103:231.

Idem: Connective tissue disease. Year Book of Dermatology, 1978. Chicago Year Book Medical Publishers, Inc, 1978. pp 9–36.

Idem: Antinuclear antibody subsets: clinical and prognostic features. Dermatol Clinics 1984, 1:517.

Vandersteen PR, et al: C2-deficient systemic lupus erythematosus: its association with anti-Ro (SSA) antibodies. Arch Dermatol 1982, 118:584.

Varner NW, et al: Pregnancy in patients with SLE. Am J Obst Gynecol 1983, 145:1025.

Wallace DJ, et al: Systemic lupus erythematosus, survival patterns: Experience with 609 patients. JAMA 1981, 245:394.

Wechsler HL, et al: Systemic lupus erythematosus with anti-Ro antibodies: Clinical, histologic and immunologic findings. JAAD 1982, 6:73.

Weigand DA: Lupus band test. JAAD 1986, 14:426.

Weinstein CL, et al: Severe visceral disease in subacute cutaneous lupus erythematosus. Arch Dermatol 1987, 123:638.

Idem: Livedo reticularis associated with increased titers of anticardiolipin antibodies in SLE. Arch Dermatol 1987, 123:596.

Weiss RA, et al: Diagnostic tests and clinical subsets in SLE. Ann Allergy 1983, 51:135.

Weston WL: Significance and character of SSA and SSB antigens. J Invest Dermatol 1985, 84:85.

Winkelmann RL: Panniculitis in connective tissue disease. Arch Dermatol 1983, 119:336.

Winton GB: Skin diseases aggravated by pregnancy. JAAD 1989, 20:1.

Yasue T: Livedo vasculitis and central nervous system involvement in systemic lupus erythematosus. Arch Dermatol 1986, 122:66.

DERMATOMYOSITIS

Dermatomyositis (polymyositis) is an inflammatory myositis characterized by vague prodromata followed by edema, dermatitis, and multiple muscular inflammation and degeneration. Erythema, telangiectasia,

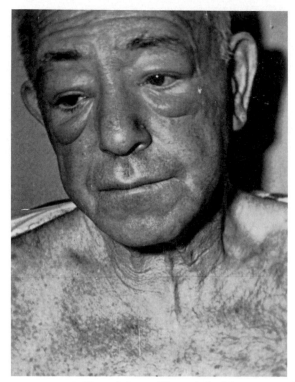

Figure 8–16. Swelling of the eyelids typical of dermatomyositis. (Courtesy of Dr. P. Gross.)

pigmentation, and interstitial calcinosis may also be present. Acute, subacute, and chronic forms occur. Muscle involvement without skin changes is called polymyositis. With or without skin lesions, weakness of proximal muscle groups is characteristic.

CLINICAL FEATURES. Usually the disease begins with erythema and swelling of the face and eyelids, sometimes extending to other regions. Usually the eyelids are first involved. They become swollen and pinkish violet (heliotrope) and may be tender to the touch, owing to involvement of the *orbicularis oculi*. Minute telangiectases on the eyelids may be seen with a magnifying glass.

This phase may last for months but is succeeded

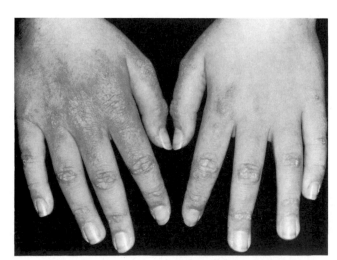

Figure 8–17. Gottron's papules of dermatomyositis.

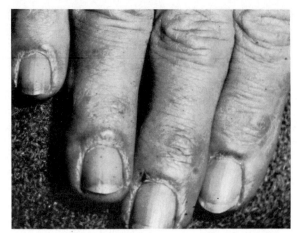

Figure 8–18. *Paronychial telangiectasia in dermatomyositis.*

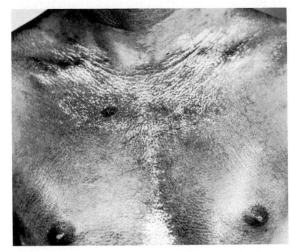

Figure 8–20. *Dermatomyositis with scleroderma in a 37-year-old man. (Courtesy of Dr. H. Shatin.)*

by more persistent cutaneous changes resembling lupus erythematosus and spreading from the face to the neck, thorax, shoulders, arms, and elsewhere.

Telangiectatic vessels cause an erythematous line or spots upon the fingernail folds. Enlarged capillaries of the nail fold appear as sausage-shaped loops, similar to those changes observed in scleroderma. A reddish purple scaling eruption occurs over the knuckles and over the knees and elbows. Ulceration of the fingertips may occur. Flat-topped violaceous papules over the knuckles (Gottron's sign) are thought to be pathognomonic of dermatomyositis. An intermittent fever, malaise, anorexia, and marked weight loss are usually found at this stage.

The skin changes occur early in the disease and may be puffy, edematous swellings of the lids, or erythematous or urticarial patches. The upper portion of the face and the extremities are favorite locations for the skin eruptions and for deep tenderness. Firm, slightly pitting edema occurs, especially over the shoulder girdle, arms, and neck. In unusual cases the characteristic skin signs may be present without evidence of myositis ever developing.

Many have subcutaneous calcified nodules in later stages of the disease. These are frequently located on the elbows, but the knees and other acral parts may also be affected. Such nodules are more prevalent in childhood dermatomyositis.

Vasomotor disturbances (Raynaud's phenomenon) occur in about 30 per cent of the patients. Alopecia of the scalp may be noted as well as hypertrichosis of the body.

Other lesions, seen less frequently, include urticaria and erythema multiforme. Photosensitivity may occur. When there is regression of the disease, a hyperpigmentation develops that simulates the bronze discoloration of Addison's disease. Telangiectasia and erythematous patches on the face and upper chest may persist for months or years, with periodic flare-ups, eventually being replaced by brown pigmentation. In some cases poikiloderma eventually develops.

There may be calcium deposits in the skin and muscles in more than half of the child patients; this also occurs rather frequently in adults. The skin, subcutaneous, and muscle involvement occurs mostly on the upper half of the body around the shoulder girdle, elbows, and hands. Ulcerations and cellulitis are frequently associated with this debilitating and disabling complication of dermatomyositis.

Childhood Dermatomyositis. Several features differ from the adult form. Two childhood variants

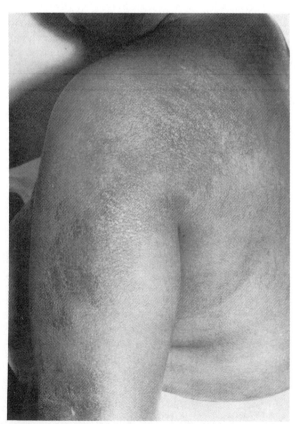

Figure 8–19. *Dermatomyositis. Poikiloderma-like lesions.*

exist. The more common Brunsting type has a slow course, progressive weakness, calcinosis, and steroid responsiveness. Calcinosis may be subcutaneous and acral (elbows, knees, fingers) as in adults, or the "classical" form involving intermuscular fascial planes. The second type, the Banker type, is characterized by a vasculitis of the muscles and gastrointestinal tract, by a rapid onset of severe weakness, steroid unresponsiveness, and death. This type is uncommon. Internal malignancy is seldom seen with either type.

Treatment has been high-dose corticosteroid therapy until remission has been achieved, then long-term low-dose therapy. A unique steroid-responsive type of dermatomyositis, with rash, weakness, tenderness of the proximal muscles, and a good prognosis, has been described in children under eight years of age by Carpenter and others.

Muscle Changes. In severe cases early and extensive muscular weakness occurs, with acute swelling and pain. The muscle weakness is seen symmetrically, most frequently involving the shoulder girdle and sometimes the pelvic region, as well as the hands. The patients may notice difficulty in lifting even the lightest objects. They may be unable to raise their arms to comb their hair. Patients often complain of pain in the legs when standing barefoot. Difficulty in swallowing, talking, and breathing, due to the weakness of the involved muscles, may be noted early in the disease. The voice may be nasal. Later there are atrophy and arthritic changes leading to ankylosis. Cardiac involvement with cardiac failure may be the terminal phase of the disease.

In summary, the following criteria are used to define dermatomyositis/polymyositis: 1) Symmetric weakness of limb girdle muscles and anterior flexors of the neck; 2) Elevated creatine phosphokinase, transaminases, lactic dehydrogenase, and aldolase; 3) Abnormal electromyogram; 4) Myositis by biopsy; and 5) The typical dermatologic features. Two of these criteria (in addition to dermatologic features) make dermatomyositis probable (if rash is present); three permit a diagnosis.

Eye Changes. Ophthalmoscopic examinations may show areas of cotton wool patches of exudate, and hemorrhages in the retina about the disk and at the macula.

Associated Diseases. Dermatomyositis may be associated with or complicated by other diseases. Localized sclerodermatous changes have been noted in chilblain dermatomyositis. This is called *sclerodermatomyositis*. Hardening of the skin, especially the arms, with acrosclerosis, may occur. Rheumatoid arthritis, lupus erythematosus, and Sjögren's syndrome may occur concomitantly. Quinones and his associates called attention to the carpal tunnel syndrome's being associated with dermatomyositis. Sandbank and his associates reported dermatomyositis associated with subacute pulmonary fibrosis. The presence of anti–Jo-1 antibody correlates well with the development of pulmonary fibrosing alveolitis.

Carcinoma with Dermatomyositis. Malignant neoplastic disease in adults is frequently associated with dermatomyositis. Callen found that of 67 malignancies in 57 patients, cancer preceded dermatomyositis in 26 cases, occurred simultaneously in 18, and followed it in 23.

In dermatomyositis, malignancy is most frequently seen in patients in the fifth and sixth decades of life. The two entities occur together more often in women than in men. A search for malignancy, directed by historical and physical findings, is warranted in adults (especially those over 40) with dermatomyositis.

ETIOLOGY. Dermatomyositis belongs to the diseases of the connective tissue and as such shows some immunologic characteristics relevant to this group. Its relationship to malignancy in many cases suggests another intriguing autoimmune mechanism. A hereditary deficiency of C2 has been found in some cases. The question of an association of this disease with acquired toxoplasmosis continues to be investigated. The report of Bowles et al suggests another potential cause: Coxsackie virus infection.

INCIDENCE. Dermatomyositis is relatively rare. It is twice as prevalent in women as in men. The familial occurrence of dermatomyositis and associated connective tissue disorders with serum protein abnormalities such as elevated alpha$_2$ globulins and gamma globulins has been seen in rare instances.

HISTOPATHOLOGY. The histologic changes in dermatomyositis are similar to those of lupus erythematosus: thinning of the epidermis, hydrops of the basal layer, edema in the papillary dermis, and a perivascular lymphocytic infiltrate in the superficial dermis. Scattered melanophages are present. The infiltrate does not favor adnexal structures as it does in lupus erythematosus. The more characteristic changes are to be found in the muscles. The deltoid, trapezius, and quadriceps muscles seem to be almost always involved, and are good biopsy sites. Muscle biopsy is directed by those areas found to be most tender.

LABORATORY FINDINGS. Albuminuria and hematuria are frequently present. Although there are different opinions regarding its significance, urinary excretion of creatine is increased and the creatinine is decreased, especially when there is at least moderate muscle involvement.

There may be leukocytosis, anemia with low serum iron, and an increased sedimentation rate.

The serum levels of aldolase and creatinine phosphokinase are elevated. The serum alpha$_2$ and gamma globulin are also elevated. Rheumatoid factor is frequently present. The SGOT (serum glutamic oxaloacetic transaminase) is raised.

Direct immunofluorescence tests are positive in at least one third of the cases. Cytoid body staining is the usual type of reaction, with deposition of IgM, IgA, and C3 in large globules in the upper dermis.

X-ray studies with barium swallow may show weak pharyngeal muscles and a collection of barium in the pyriform sinuses and valleculae.

Electromyographic studies for diagnosis show spontaneous fibrillation, polyphasic potential with voluntary contraction, short duration potential with decreased amplitude, and salvos of muscle stimulation. The disease is usually symmetric, so that the muscle biopsy should be taken from the opposite corresponding site.

DIFFERENTIAL DIAGNOSIS. Dermatomyositis must be differentiated from erysipelas, SLE, angioedema, and erythema multiforme. In addition, scleroderma may be difficult to differentiate. Trichinosis may cause muscle weakness simulating dermatomyositis. Some others to be considered are myasthenia gravis, muscular dystrophy, and toxoplasmosis.

Aldosteronism, with adenoma of adrenal glands and hypokalemia, may also cause puffy heliotrope eyelids and face. Systemic sclerosis is frequently involved in the diagnosis of dermatomyositis since sclerodermatous changes frequently accompany it; however, systemic involvement is usually absent in dermatomyositis except for possible malignancy.

TREATMENT. Strictly enforced bed rest is essential during the acute phase of the disease. Acetylsalicylic acid is given regularly, 2 tablets four times daily.

Methotrexate, when given early in the course of the disease, will produce remission in most cases. Sokoloff and his associates noted definite improvement in five of the seven patients they treated with intravenous methotrexate, giving 0.8 mg per kg weekly for four to six weeks. Fischer et al confirmed the usefulness of this combination.

Prednisone or its equivalent is given in doses beginning with 60 mg daily until the severity decreases and muscle enzymes are almost normal. The dosage is reduced in line with clinical response. The SGOT and creatinine phosphokinase assume normal levels as remission occurs.

Combining azathioprine with oral prednisone improved the results in a Mayo Clinic series, according to Bunch. The antimalarials have also been used, with equivocal results. Woo et al found hydroxychloroquine greatly improved stubborn cutaneous lesions. This observation was confirmed by James et al.

Metzger and his associates treated 22 patients with combined prednisone and intravenous methotrexate when moderate or high-dose prednisone therapy was ineffective. They noted marked improvement in 17 of the 22 patients. Toxicity was minor and reversible. Dramatic success was also achieved by Jacobs in four of five cases, using biweekly intravenous methotrexate in addition to corticosteroids.

Testosterone propionate, 50 mg once weekly, may be given, especially in the convalescent stage.

G. Goldstein has treated dermatomyositis with 6-mercaptopurine (Purinethol—Burroughs-Wellcome), giving 100 mg daily for three weeks, then azathioprine (Imuran—Burroughs-Wellcome), 200 mg daily, with excellent improvement of muscle power. Cyclophosphamide was reported by Plowman and Stable-

forth to be effective after prednisone therapy was decreased. Improvement persisted on a daily regimen of 100 mg cyclophosphamide and 10 mg prednisone daily. Physiotherapy, consisting of whirlpool baths, warmth, and gentle massage, is helpful. Weng et al reported a patient with juvenile dermatomyositis with extensive calcinosis who responded remarkably to aluminum hydroxide therapy.

PROGNOSIS. Benvassat et al reviewed the course of 72 cases (and 20 possible cases) over age 20; major causes of death were cancer, ischemic heart disease, and lung disease. Independent risk factors were failure to induce clinical remission, white count above 10,000 and temperature 38°C at diagnosis, older age, shorter disease history, and dysphagia.

Spencer et al reported on the prognosis of juvenile dermatomyositis. Of 66 children with this disease, 8 per cent died within one year of diagnosis; of 32 patients followed for at least two years, only 25 per cent had resolution and 44 per cent had no response to continuous steroid therapy. The prognosis for children is considered guarded.

Dermatomyositis and pregnancy affect each other adversely. In half the patients who become pregnant the facial lesions and muscle weakness get worse, and fetal loss occurs in over half the patients.

Benvassat J, et al: Prognostic factors in polymyositis/dermatomyositis: A computer-assisted analysis of 92 cases. Arthritis Rheum 1985, 28:249.

Bohan A, et al: Polymyositis and dermatomyositis. N Engl J Med 1975, 292:344, 403.

Bowles NE, et al: Dermatomyositis, polymyositis, and Cocksackie-B virus infection. Lancet 1987, 1:1004.

Bunch TW: Prednisone and azathioprine for polymyositis: Long-term follow-up. Arthritis Rheum 1981, 24:45.

Callen JP: The value of malignancy evaluation in . . . dermatomyositis. JAAD 1982, 6:253.

Idem: Dermatomyositis. Dermatol Clinics 1983, 1:461.

Carpenter S, et al: Childhood dermatomyositis. Neurology 1976, 26:592.

Crowe WE, et al: Clinical and pathogenetic implications of histopathology in childhood polydermatomyositis. Arthritis Rheum 1982, 25:126.

DeVere R, et al: Polymyositis. Brain 1975, 98:367.

Fischer TJ, et al: Childhood dermatomyositis and polymyositis: Treatment with prednisone and methotrexate. Am J Dis Child 1979, 133:386.

James WD, et al: Plaquenil therapy for dermatomyositis. J Rheumatol 1985, 12:1214.

Magid SK, et al: Serologic evidence for acute toxoplasmosis in polymyositis/dermatomyositis. Am J Med 1983, 75:313.

Malleson P: Juvenile dermatomyositis: A review. J R Soc Med 1982, 75:33.

Metzger AL, et al: Polymyositis and dermatomyositis. Am Intern Med 1974, 81:182.

Minkin W, et al: Office nailfold capillary microscopy using an ophthalmoscope. JAAD 1982, 7:190.

Pachman LM, et al: Juvenile dermatomyositis: A clinical and immunologic study. J Pediatr 1980, 96:226.

Pearson CM, et al: The spectrum of dermatomyositis and polymyositis. Med Clin N Am 1977, 61:439.

Philips TS, et al: Dermatomyositis and pulmonary fibrosis associated with anti-Jo-1 antibody. JAAD 1987, 17:381.

Plowman PN, et al: Treatment of dermatomyositis. Proc Roy Soc Med 1977, 70:738.

Sams WM Jr: Chloroquine: Its therapeutic use in photosensitive eruptions. Int J Dermatol 1978, 15:99.

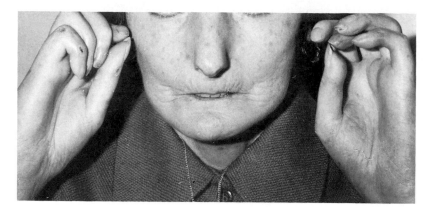

Figure 8–21. Scleroderma.

Spencer CH, et al: Course of untreated juvenile dermatomyositis. J Pediatr 1984, 105:399.

Tymms KE, et al: Dermatomyositis and other connective tissue diseases. J Rheumatol 1985, 12:1140.

Weng WJ, et al: Calcinosis cutis in juvenile dermatomyositis. Arch Dermatol 1988, 124:1721.

Winkelmann RK: Dermatomyositis in childhood. JC Dermatology 1979, 18:13.

Winton GB: Skin diseases aggravated by pregnancy. JAAD 1989, 20:1.

Woo TY, et al: Cutaneous lesions of dermatomyositis are improved by chloroquine. JAAD 1984, 10:592.

SCLERODERMA

Scleroderma is sclerosis of the skin characterized by the appearance of circumscribed or diffuse, hard, smooth, ivory-colored areas that are immobile upon the underlying tissues and give the appearance of hide-bound skin.

Scleroderma occurs in both systemic and localized forms. *Progressive systemic sclerosis* and the Thibierge-Weissenbach syndrome (commonly referred to as the CREST syndrome) are the two types of systemic scleroderma. Localized lesions may be categorized as *morphea* (localized, guttate, generalized, profunda, and pansclerotic forms) or *linear scleroderma* (with or without melorheostosis or hemiatrophy).

SYSTEMIC TYPES

Progressive Systemic Sclerosis (PSS). This is a generalized disorder of connective tissue in which there is fibrous thickening of the skin combined with fibrosis and vascular abnormalities in certain internal organs. *Raynaud's phenomenon* is frequently the first manifestation of PSS. It is nearly always present. The heart, lungs, gastrointestinal tract, kidney, and other organs may be involved. Women are affected three times more commonly than men, with an increasing incidence with age, peaking in the 65-and-over age group.

CREST Syndrome. Systemic sclerosis may be limited to the hands, or sometimes the hands and lower face, for months to years. During this time it is often called acrosclerosis. If it is associated with calcinosis, Raynaud's phenomenon, esophageal dysmotility, sclerodactyly (always present), and telangiectasia, it is called CREST syndrome. This form of scleroderma is not as severe as PSS.

Immunologically, anticentromere antibody appears to be highly specific for the CREST syndrome, being positive in 50 to 90 per cent of cases and in only 2 to 10 per cent of patients with progressive sclerosis.

This variant of systemic scleroderma has the most favorable prognosis, owing to the usually limited systemic involvement.

Vinyl Chloride Disease. Acrosclerosis and Raynaud's phenomenon have been observed in workers in charge of cleaning vinyl chloride polymerization reactors. There is acroösteolysis of the central portion of the shafts of distal phalanges. Pulmonary fibrosis and angiosarcoma of the liver are sometimes associated.

LOCALIZED TYPES

Localized Scleroderma (Morphea). This form of scleroderma is twice as common in women as in men. Progressive systemic sclerosis or even acrosclerosis rarely develop from it. It occurs in childhood as well as in adult life.

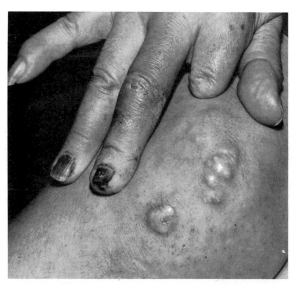

Figure 8–22. CREST syndrome on the knee and fingers of a 60-year-old woman. Note calcium nodules over the patella, telangiectasia over the upper knuckles, amputation of the forefinger due to gangrene, and Raynaud's phenomenon of the fingertips.

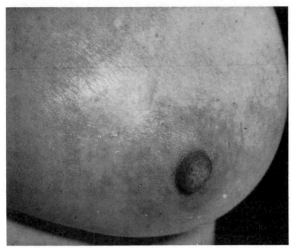

Figure 8–23. Morphea. Note fine crinkling of skin on the upper part of the lesion.

It occurs most often in macules or plaques a few centimeters in diameter but also may occur in bands or spots, or in guttate lesions. Rose or violaceous macules may appear first, followed by smooth, hard, somewhat depressed yellowish white or ivory-colored lesions. They are commonest on the trunk but also occur on the extremities.

This type of scleroderma, except for the linear and profuse, extensive forms, tends to slowly involute over a three- to five-year period.

The margins of the areas are generally surrounded by a light violaceous zone or by telangiectases. Within the patch the elasticity of the skin is lost, and when it is picked up between the thumb and index finger it feels rigid. The follicular orifices may be unusually prominent, leading to a condition that resembles pigskin. Such localized lesions generally spread a little but remain circumscribed, or even remain stationary, or spontaneously involute, with few or no sequelae or with atrophy.

Guttate Morphea. Multiple small, chalk-white, flat or slightly depressed macules may occur in large numbers over the chest, neck, shoulders, or upper back. These are not very firm or sclerotic and are difficult to separate with confidence from lichen sclerosus et atrophicus.

Generalized Morphea. Widespread involvement by indurated plaques with hypo- (less often hyper-) pigmentation characterizes this variety. Muscle atrophy may be associated. There is no systemic involvement.

Pansclerotic Morphea of Children. This variant, described by Diaz-Perez et al, is manifested by sclerosis of the dermis, panniculus, fascia, muscle, and at times bone. There is disabling limitation of motion of joints. It is also called *morphea profunda*.

Linear Scleroderma. These linear lesions may extend the length of the arm or leg, beginning most often in the first decade of life. They may also occur para-sagittally on the frontal scalp and extend part way down the forehead (*en coup de sabre*). The Parry-

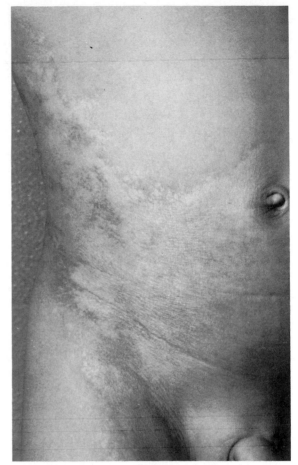

Figure 8–24. Extensive morphea.

Romberg syndrome, which manifests progressive facial hemiatrophy, epilepsy, exophthalmos, and alopecia, may be a form of linear scleroderma. When the lower extremity is involved, there may be spina bifida, or faulty limb development, hemiatrophy, or

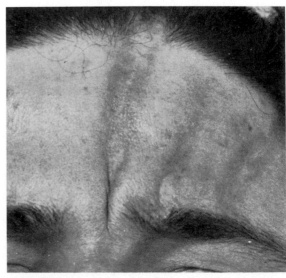

Figure 8–25. Scleroderma (morphea) en coup de sabre on mid forehead.

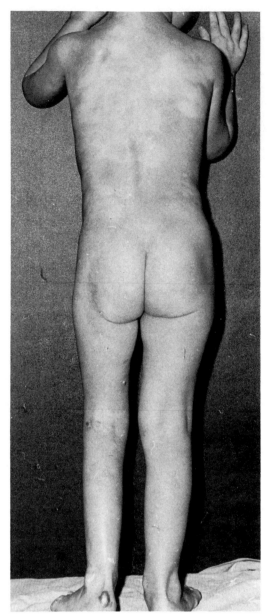

Figure 8–26. Scleroderma in a 3-year-old boy. (Courtesy of Dr. H. Jacobs.)

flexion contractures. Melorheostosis, seen in roentgenograms as a dense linear cortical hyperostosis, may occur.

CLINICAL FEATURES. In the earlier phases of scleroderma the affected areas are erythematous and swollen, but sclerosis soon supervenes. The skin becomes smooth, yellowish, and firm and shrinks so that the underlying structures are bound down. The earliest changes often occur insidiously upon the face and hands, and in more advanced stages these parts become hide-bound, so that the face is expressionless and the hands are clawlike (sclerodactylia). The skin of the face appears drawn, stretched, and taut, but not hard, with loss of lines or expression. There is difficulty in opening the mouth. The lips are thin, contracted, and radially furrowed, the nose appears

sharp and pinched, and the chin may be puckered. In this type, vasomotor disturbances and Raynaud's disease are nearly always associated.

The disease may remain localized to the hands and feet for long periods ("acrosclerosis"). The fingers become semiflexed, immobile, and useless, the skin over them being hard, inelastic, incompressible, and pallid. The terminal phalanges are boardlike and indurated. Trophic ulcerations and gangrene may occur on the tips of the fingers and knuckles, which may be painful or insensitive, usually the latter. Dilated, irregular nail fold capillary loops are present in 75 per cent of PSS patients. There is a progressive increase in induration from the forearm and hand to the fingertips.

Although similar changes occur in the feet and toes, they are seldom as severe as in the hands. Keloidlike nodules may develop on the extremities or the chest and there may be a widespread diffuse calcification of the skin as shown by radiographs. A diffuse involvement of the chest may lead to a cuirasslike restraint of respiration. Late in the course of the disorder, hyperpigmented or depigmented spots or a diffuse bronzing may be present, and the affected areas become hairless. Jawitz et al reported the finding of pigment retention over superficial blood vessels of the forehead within a wider field of depigmentation. Atrophy may be associated with telangiectasia. Bullae and ulcerations may develop, especially on the distal parts of the extremities. Partial alopecia and decreased sweat gland activity are frequently found.

Sclerodermatous skin changes may be associated with porphyria cutanea tarda, primary systemic amyloidosis, Sjögren's syndrome, Werner's syndrome, POEMS syndrome, carcinoid syndrome, phenylketonuria, progeria, ataxia telangiectasia, Hurler's syndrome, or congenital poikiloderma. They may also be associated with the other connective tissue diseases such as SLE, dermatomyositis, and rheumatoid arthritis. Chemicals such as vinyl chloride, bleomycin, silica, epoxy resins, hydrocarbons, pentazocine, and chlorethylene may induce sclerodermalike thickening of the skin. All of these except bleomycin and pentazocine may occur through occupational exposure.

Spiera reported scleroderma occurring after augmentation mammoplasty. Phelps et al reviewed the scleroderma-like illness in persons in Spain who ingested industrial oil when it was sold as olive oil.

Internal Involvement. Progressive systemic sclerosis may involve most of the internal organs. Fibrosis, loss of smooth muscle of the internal organs, and progressive loss of visceral function characterize this disorder. Most frequently the gastrointestinal tract is involved, followed by the lungs, then the cardiovascular-renal system. The central nervous system and the musculoskeletal system are less frequently involved. Esophageal involvement (chiefly atony) is seen in over 90 per cent of patients. The distal two thirds is affected, leading to dysphagia and reflux esophagitis. Small intestinal atonia may lead to constipation, malabsorption, or diarrhea.

In pulmonary involvement there may be pulmonary fibrosis with arterial hypoxia, dyspnea, and productive cough. Progressive nonspecific interstitial fibrosis, with bronchiectasis and cyst formation, is the most frequent pathologic change.

The cardiac involvement produces dyspnea, palpitation, and other symptoms of congestive heart failure. Sclerosis of the myocardium produces conduction changes. There may also be pericarditis. Death usually occurs from cardiac or renal failure.

Acute renal disease in late scleroderma produces azotemia and proteinuria. Hypertension and retinopathy may be present.

The skeletal manifestations are first noted by articular pain, swelling, and inflammation. Polyarthritis may be the initial symptom in systemic sclerosis. There is limitation of motion, due to skin tautness, followed by ankylosis and leading to severe contractural deformities. The hand joints are involved most frequently, and there may be resorption and shortening of the phalanges, changes in the small joints, and narrowing of the joint spaces. Osteoporosis and sclerosis of the bones of the hands and feet may occur, as well as decalcification of the vault of the skull. Muscular involvement, with myosclerosis and calcium deposits in the muscles, is common.

Childhood PSS has identical cutaneous manifestations to those in adults. Raynaud's phenomenon is less frequent, while cardiac wall involvement is more common and is responsible for half the deaths. Renal disease is unusual.

Familial scleroderma rarely occurs but has been documented by both Burge and Greger.

Systemic sclerosis may be associated with Hashimoto's thyroiditis, Sjögren's syndrome, dermatomyositis, congenital hypogammaglobulinemia, myasthenia gravis, mycosis fungoides, muscular dystrophy, urticaria pigmentosa, hyperthyroidism alopecia, vitiligo, pretibial myxedema, and melanoderma.

The course of PSS is variable. Prognostic information may be gained from antinuclear antibody testing. The nucleolar pattern, which is highly specific for scleroderma, occurs chiefly in patients with diffuse skin involvement but limited internal disease. A thready pattern, as defined by Burnham, indicates a subgroup with a high incidence of pulmonary disease. Negative tests for antinuclear antibody may be associated with more severe systemic disease. The true speckled or anticentromere pattern is associated with the CREST variant, as described below. Overall, the 10-year survival rate for PSS may be approximately 50 per cent. The prognosis is worse in men and in patients with renal involvement.

ETIOLOGY. The cause of scleroderma is not known, but it has been suggested that an autoimmune mechanism is concerned. Vascular changes—vasospasm, sclerosis, or toxic damage—may be involved. The occasional onset after trauma,

head injury, or emotional shock suggests the possibility of a trophoneurosis. Certainly this is not incompatible with an autoimmune mechanism. Chemicals may induce sclerodermalike changes: drugs such as bleomycin or pentazocine, or occupational exposure to vinyl chloride, hydrocarbons, or trichloroethylene. Silica dust is accepted in East Germany as a potential cause of systemic scleroderma. Haustein reported that of 86 men with scleroderma, 77 per cent had been exposed to silica dust, 45 per cent had silicosis, and 22 per cent had proven progressive systemic sclerosis at autopsy. The relationship of infection with *Borrelia burgdorferi* and the development of morphea or scleroderma are discussed in Chapter 14.

The onset of scleroderma immediately following a severe emotional shock, especially an event which gravely threatens the patient's security, such as an unexpected demand for a divorce, has been documented repeatedly. There is increasing evidence that scleroderma, like Raynaud's disease, is in some cases a manifestation and result of a psychosomatic disturbance that causes vascular spasm. Kobayashi's demonstration of striking perineural thickening of deep dermal nerves beneath lesions of morphea is suggestive objective evidence of a possible relationship.

LABORATORY FINDINGS. In a series of 413 patients with scleroderma, Clark and his associates found 66 per cent had a sedimentation rate of 40 mm or higher; rheumatoid factor was present in 35 per cent of 265 patients. Serologic tests for syphilis were positive in 5 per cent of 363 patients. The IgG was increased in 26 per cent. LE cell tests were only rarely demonstrable (four of 413).

Antinuclear antibodies are present in nearly all PSS patients; the majority are anticentromere in type in the CREST variant. A special antibody called Scl-70 is seen in 20 per cent of PSS patients. There is a high incidence of anti-ssDNA in linear scleroderma.

PATHOGENESIS. The theories center about vascular damage as a primary disorder and autoimmune mechanisms. These might be interrelated. Skin ischemia is a prominent feature of scleroderma. A toxic substance, perhaps some autoimmune factor, may promote or cause endothelial cell damage. Stimulated T cells and macrophages might then release lymphokines and monokines, which stimulate fibroblast migration and proliferation and collagen synthesis. The stimulated B cells could elaborate antibodies against the centromere, centriole, nucleolus, Scl-70 protein, and other nonspecific proteins. Recently the role of the mast cell and its proteolytic enzymes in the promotion of fibrosis has been the subject of much study. All this is speculation: the mechanisms and interactions of these factors have yet to be elucidated.

HISTOLOGY. Generalized scleroderma and morphea, generalized or localized, show identical histologic changes. In the acute phase there is a periadnexal lymphocytic infiltrate. The epidermis is normal except for increased pigmentation, which may be present. Collagen bundles appear swollen and the total thickness of the dermis is increased. Eccrine glands and coiled ducts, instead of being located at the junction of the dermis and subcutis, are found in the midportion of the thickened dermis. The subcutaneous fat is quantitatively reduced.

In more advanced lesions, the inflammatory infiltrate may be minimal. Pilosebaceous units are absent, and eccrine glands and ducts are compressed by surrounding collagen.

Since the thickness of the dermis normally depends upon the anatomic site, biopsy specimens from suspected cases of scleroderma (or morphea) must include the subcutis and, if possible, a control site from adjacent normal skin should be submitted as well.

Kobayashi et al reported finding remarkable thickening and lack of basal lamina in perineural cells in the deep dermis in five of 15 cases of morphea. They suggested an essential involvement of perineural cells in the sclerotic process.

RADIOGRAPHIC FINDINGS. The gastrointestinal tract is commonly involved. The esophagus may have decreased peristalsis and dilatation, causing dysphagia, heartburn, and regurgitation of liquids. Esophagogram with ciné studies should be performed in these cases; however, scleroderma is most easily recognized by esophageal manometry. The stomach may be dilated and atonic, resulting in delayed emptying time. Involvement of the small intestine may cause constipation alternating with diarrhea and distention. The extreme dilatation of the duodenum and jejunum produces a characteristic roentgenographic picture of persistently dilated intestinal loops long after the barium has passed through. The colon is only rarely involved.

In early esophageal involvement, a barium swallow in the usual upright position may be reported as normal. If the patient is supine, however, barium will often be seen to pool in the flaccid esophagus.

DIFFERENTIAL DIAGNOSIS. The diffuse variety of scleroderma must be distinguished from myxedema, scleredema, and scleromyxedema, in which the parts are softer, edematous, and not atrophic. Sclerodactylia may be confused with leprosy and syringomyelia. Dermatomyositis and lupus erythematosus sometimes resemble the progressive generalized type of scleroderma.

Eosinophilic fasciitis, described by Shulman and by others, is a benign, steroid-responsive disorder simulating some features of scleroderma. The skin is thickened, edematous, and erythematous, and has a coarse *peau d'orange* appearance, as opposed to its sclerotic, taut appearance in scleroderma. The hands and face are usually spared in eosinophilic fasciitis.

In vitiligo the depigmentation is the sole change in the skin, other features present in scleroderma being absent. Scleroderma in the atrophic stage may so closely resemble acrodermatitis chronica atrophicans that differentiation is impossible. The subject is discussed at greater length under the latter disease. Morphea may resemble vitiligo, lichen sclerosus et atrophicus, cicatrix, and epithelioma, but careful examination can easily establish its identity.

TREATMENT. In all varieties treatment is unsatisfactory, but spontaneous recovery is not uncommon, especially in children. Often in localized scleroderma an end point is reached beyond which the disease does not progress.

Well-planned daily general exercise is an important therapeutic measure. Regular massage, warmth, and protection from trauma are advised. Exposure to cold is to be avoided, and smoking is forbidden.

Vasospasm resulting in Raynaud's phenomenon may be treated in a variety of ways. Vasoactive drugs such as dibenzyline, 10 mg three times daily initially and then increased as tolerance permits, are worth trying. Winkelmann and his associates have found phenoxybenzamine and tolazoline, 30 to 60 mg daily in divided doses, to be best tolerated.

Prazosin (Minipress), 1 mg t.i.d. orally, was found by Surwit et al, in a double blind study, to be effective in reducing the frequency and severity of vasospastic attacks in two men and 18 women suffering from scleroderma with Raynaud's phenomenon.

Alpha-methyldopa, 1 to 2 gm daily, has been used by Varadi and Lawrence for inhibition of Raynaud's phenomenon. Nicotinic acid and intravenous procaine are also helpful.

Three separate studies have documented the usefulness of the calcium channel blocker nifedipine (Procardia), 10 mg four times daily, in reducing the frequency of vasospastic episodes. Ketanserin, a serotonin agonist, was effective at a dose of 20 mg twice a day.

Subcutaneous calcinosis with ulceration was successfully treated by Hazen et al with intralesional injections of triamcinolone acetonide, 20 mg/ml every four to eight weeks for over a year.

Antiinflammatory therapy has relied mostly on immunosuppressives or corticosteroids, or both. Greer reported improvement in several severe cases with azathioprine or cyclophosphamide. Jansen and his associates obtained improvement in half of 16 patients treated with azathioprine (Imuran).

Corticosteroid therapy does not offer any lasting benefit; however, the patient feels better and the joint symptoms may be ameliorated when prednisone is taken, 10 to 15 mg daily. Corticosteroids are beneficial when there is real evidence of inflammatory myositis.

Malabsorption, a common occurrence in gastrointestinal sclerosis, is effectively controlled with tetracyclines, as shown by Cliff and his associates.

Reversal of the vascular and renal crises by oral angiotensin-converting–enzyme blockade, with captopril (Capoten) and other antihypertensive agents, has dramatically improved the outlook in this situation, as reported by Lopez-Ovejero et al and Zawada et al.

Therapy for the fibrosis is the subject of much clinical research, yet no effective therapy is available.

D-Penicillamine in high doses was used by Fulghum and Katz in the treatment of five patients, with no improvement noted. Steen et al in a retrospective study found evidence of its effectiveness, however. The difference of opinion awaits a double-blind study for its resolution. There was a significant problem with side effects of D-penicillamine.

Neldner reported success in four cases of circumscribed and linear scleroderma with phenytoin (Dilantin), 100 mg one to three times a day. Morgan confirmed his report.

Dimethyl sulfoxide (DMSO) was used in the treatment of 24 patients by Tuffanelli. No improvement was noted. However, soaking in DMSO was found at Cleveland Clinic to be highly beneficial for hands with ulceration secondary to Raynaud's syndrome.

Asboe-Hansen G: Scleroderma. JAAD 1987, 17:102.

Atkins FM, et al: Mast cells and fibrosis. Arch Dermatol 1987, 123:191.

Brozena SJ, et al: Human adjuvant disease following augmentation mammoplasty. Arch Dermatol 1988, 124:1383.

Burge KM, et al: Familial scleroderma. Arch Dermatol 1969, 99:681.

Catoggio LJ, et al: Serological markers in progressive systemic sclerosis: Clinical correlations. Ann Rheum Dis 1983, 42:23.

Clark JA, et al: Serologic alterations in scleroderma and sclerodermatomyositis. Mayo Clin Proc 1971, 46:406.

Connolly SM: Scleroderma: Therapeutic options. Cutis 1984, 34:724.

Czarnecki DB, et al: Generalized morphea successfully treated with salazopyrine. Acta Dermatovener (Stockh) 1981, 62:81.

Diaz-Perez JL, et al: Disabling pansclerotic morphea in children. Arch Dermatol 1980, 116:169.

Falanga V, et al: Antinuclear and anti-single-stranded DNA antibodies in morphea and generalized morphen. Arch Dermatol 1987, 123:350.

Fleischmajer R, et al: Scleroderma. Arch Dermatol 1983, 119:957.

Gershwin ME: Slow progress with scleroderma. Ann Intern Med 1982, 97:776.

Greer KE: Newer therapies for the sclerodermas. Dermatol Clin 1983, 1:505.

Greger RE: Familial progressive systemic scleroderma. Arch Dermatol 1976, 111:81.

Haustein UF, et al: Pathogenesis of progressive systemic sclerosis. Int J Dermatol 1985, 24:147.

Idem: Pathogenesis of progressive systemic sclerosis. Int J Dermatol 1986, 25:286.

James WD, et al: Nodular (keloidal) scleroderma. JAAD 1984, 11:1111.

Jansen GT, et al: Generalized scleroderma. Treatment with an immunosuppressive agent. Arch Dermatol 1968, 97:696.

Jawitz JC, et al: A new skin manifestation of progressive systemic sclerosis. JAAD 1984, 11:625.

Kleinsmith d'AM, et al: Antibody markers . . . and characteristics of scleroderma. Arch Dermatol 1982, 118:88.

Kobayashi T, et al: Nerve changes in morphea. Proc XVI Int Cong Dermatol, Tokyo, 1983.

Krieg T, et al: Systemic scleroderma. JAAD 1988, 18:457.

Larrègue M, et al: Systemic scleroderma in childhood. Ann Dermatol Venereol 1983, 110:317.

Lopez-Ovejero JA, et al: Reversal of vascular and renal crises of scleroderma by oral angiotensin-converting enzyme blockade. N Engl J Med 1979, 300:1417.

McGregor AR, et al: Familial clustering of scleroderma spectrum disease. Am J Med 1988, 84:1023.

Morgan RJ: Scleroderma: Treatment with diphenylhydantoin. Cutis 1971, 8:278.

Neldner KH: Treatment of localized linear scleroderma with phenytoin. Cutis 1978, 22:659.

Phelps RG, et al: Clinical, pathologic, and immunologic manifestations of the toxic oil syndrome. JAAD 1988, 18:313.

Powell C, et al: The anticentromere antibody: Disease specificity and clinical significance. Mayo Clin Proc 1984, 59:700.

Rodeheffer RJ, et al: Controlled double-blind trial of nifedipine in Raynaud's phenomenon. N Engl J Med 1983, 308:880.

Rowell NR: The prognosis of systemic sclerosis. Br J Dermatol 1976, 95:57.

Spiera H: Scleroderma after silicone augmentation mammoplasty. JAMA 1988, 260:236.

Stáva Z, et al: Salazopyrin in the treatment of scleroderma. Br J Dermatol 1977, 96:451.

Steen VD, et al: D-Penicillamine therapy in progressive systemic sclerosis: A retrospective analysis. Ann Intern Med 1982, 97:652.

Idem: Clinical and laboratory association of anticentromere antibody in patients with progressive systemic sclerosis. Arthritis Rheum 1984, 27:125.

Stratham BN, et al: Quantification of nail field capillary abnormalities in systemic sclerosis and Raynaud's phenomenon. Acta Derm Venereol (Stockh) 1986, 66:139.

Surwit RS, et al: A double-blind study of prazosin in the treatment of Raynaud's phenomenon. Arch Dermatol 1984, 120:329.

Tan EM, et al: Diversity of antinuclear antibodies in progressive systemic sclerosis. Arthritis Rheum 1980, 23:617.

Torök E, et al: Morphoea in children. Am Exp Dermatol 1986, 11:607.

Tuffanelli DL, et al: Anticentromere and anticentriole antibodies in the scleroderma spectrum. Arch Dermatol 1983, 119:560.

Velayos EE, et al: The CREST syndrome. Ann Intern Med 1979, 139:240.

Zawada ET Jr, et al: Clinical course of patients with scleroderma: Renal crisis treated with captopril. Nephron 1981, 27(2):74.

MIXED CONNECTIVE TISSUE DISEASE (MCTD)

Tuffanelli prefers LeRoy's expression, *undifferentiated connective tissue disease* (UCTD), to "mixed" connective tissue disease.

Sharp and his associates described a disease that has overlapping features of scleroderma, SLE, and dermatomyositis. In a series of 25 patients, 21 were women who had severe arthralgia, swelling of the hands and tapered fingers, Raynaud's phenomenon, abnormal esophageal motility, pulmonary fibrosis, muscle pain and tenderness, and weakness of the muscles. Hyperglobulinemia and lymphadenopathy were present in some cases.

The fluorescent antinuclear antibody (FANA) test is an important diagnostic procedure in MCTD. The speckled pattern of nuclear fluorescence, and the dilution titer of the serum to produce fluorescence, are used in the evaluation of this disease. In addition, particulate epidermal nuclear IgG deposition on direct immunofluorescence study of skin is a distinctive finding in MCTD. MCTD patients have high titers of ribonucleoprotein (RNP) antigen, which persist through periods of remission.

Gratifying improvement has been achieved by the use of a corticosteroid (prednisone) at a daily dose of 1 mg/kg of body weight.

Generally, the prognosis is good, with long periods of remission. Sharp and Anderson found that the LE features of MCTD were most likely, and the scleroderma features the least likely, to improve. In a long-term evaluation of Sharp's original study patients, Nimelstein et al found that the inflammatory components became less frequent with time, while the sclerodermatous features persisted.

Callen JP: Systemic LE in patients with discoid LE. JAAD 1985, 12:278.

Gilliam JN, et al: Mixed connective tissue disease syndrome. Arch Dermatol 1977, 113:583.

Gladman DD: So you suspect mixed connective tissue disease (MCTD): Which tests to perform? Int J Dermatol 1985, 24:392.

Grant KD, et al: Mixed connective tissue disease: A subset with sequential clinical and laboratory features. J Rheum 1982, 8:587.

Minikin W, et al: Mixed connective tissue disease. Arch Dermatol 1976, 112:1535.

Nimelstein SH, et al: Mixed connective tissue disease: A subsequent evaluation of the original 25 patients. Medicine 1980, 59:239.

Rasmussen EK, et al: Clinical implications of ribonucleoprotein antibody. Arch Dermatol 1987, 123:601.

Sharp GC, et al: Mixed connective tissue disease—an apparently distinct rheumatic disease syndrome associated with a specific antibody to an extractable nuclear antigen. Am J Med 1972, 52:148.

Idem: Current concepts in the classification of connective tissue diseases: Overlap syndrome and mixed connective tissue disease (MCTD). JAAD 1980, 2:269.

Winkelmann RK, et al: Direct immunofluorescence in the diagnosis of scleroderma syndromes. Br J Dermatol 1977, 96:231.

SJÖGREN'S SYNDROME
(Sicca Syndrome)

Sjögren (Syur-gren) described in 1933 a triad of keratoconjunctivitis sicca, xerostomia, and rheumatoid arthritis. In the syndrome the last disease may be replaced by other connective tissue disorders such as scleroderma, mixed connective tissue disease, polyarteritis nodosa, polymyositis, or SLE.

Xerostomia (dryness of the mouth) may produce difficulty in speech and eating, increased tooth decay, and decreased taste acuity (hypogeusia). Rhinitis sicca (dryness of the nasal mucous membranes) may induce nasal crusting and decreased olfactory acuity (hyposmia). Vaginal dryness and dyspareunia may develop.

Fatigue is a prominent symptom.

Skin manifestation is purpura of the legs, which is usually palpable. This is indistinguishable from Waldenström's benign hypergammaglobulinemic purpura. Other cutaneous manifestations are urticaria and erythema multiforme. Eccrine sweating may be decreased. Histologically leucocytoclastic vasculitis, or less often mononuclear vasculitis, is found; and 80 per cent of such patients have anti-Ro/SSA antibodies; half as many have anti-La/SSB antibodies. Alexander and Provost have reviewed this in detail (1983).

In addition there may be laryngitis and achylia gastrica. Thyroid enlargement resembling Hashimoto's thyroiditis, malignant lymphoma, thrombotic thrombocytopenic purpura, necrotizing angiitis, and splenomegaly are some of the associated manifestations. On the other hand, the sicca syndrome may show only keratoconjunctivitis, drying of the conjunctiva, and xerostomia unassociated with the other disorders. This is called *sicca complex*. It is seen most frequently in women in their fifties.

Labial salivary gland biopsy is regarded by many as the most definite diagnostic test for xerostomia. Typically, there is a dense lymphocytic infiltrate with many plasma cells and fewer histiocytes in aggregates of small foci. More than one focus should be present per 4 square mm of the tissue biopsy. The biopsy is taken from inside the lower lip.

Diminished glandular secretion from the lacrimal glands is measured by the Schirmer test.

The diagnosis is made when there is objective evidence for two of the three major criteria: 1) xerophthalmia, 2) xerostomia, and 3) an associated autoimmune, rheumatic, or lymphoproliferative disorder.

Primary Sjögren's syndrome, or the sicca complex, may be distinguished from a secondary form that occurs with rheumatoid arthritis. The primary form is more closely associated with SLE; extraglandular and lymphocyte-aggressive phenomena are more common; and the ocular and oral involvements are more severe. Anti-Ro/SSA and anti-La/SSB occur in higher frequency in the primary form, while rheumatoid factor positivity is more often present in the secondary type.

Numerous serologic abnormalities are frequently found associated with the sicca syndrome. The rheumatoid factor is usually positive, with elevated serum globulin and C-reactive proteins, and high titers of IgG, IgA, and IgM. Cryoglobulins may be demonstrated at times.

Patients with Sjögren's syndrome appear predisposed to the development of lymphoreticular malignancies such as non-Hodgkin's lymphoma. A nonmalignant, extraglandular lymphoproliferative process may also occur. This produces pseudolymphoma, with a potential for regression.

Specific treatment is not yet available for Sjögren's syndrome, and should be directed against the various manifestations of connective tissue disease. Artificial lubricants for oral, nasal, and vaginal dryness may be used, as may artificial tears for eye symptoms.

Alexander EL, et al: Cutaneous manifestations of primary Sjögren's syndrome: A reflection of vasculitis and association with anti-Ro (SSA) antibodies. J Invest Derm 1983, 80:386.

Idem: Sjögren's syndrome: Cutaneous vasculitis and CNS disease. Arch Dermatol 1987, 123:801.

Idem: Sjögren's syndrome. Arch Dermatol 1987, 123:801.

Chudwin DS, et al: Spectrum of Sjögren's syndrome in children. J Pediatr 1981, 98:213.

Fox RI, et al: Primary Sjögren syndrome: Clinical and immunologic features. Semin Arthritis Rheum 1984, 14:77.

Greenspan JS, et al: Histopathology of Sjögren's syndrome in labial salivary gland biopsies. Oral Surg Med Pathol 1974, 37:217.

Lee LA: AntiRo(SSA) and antiLa(SSB) antibodies in lupus erythematosus and in Sjögren's syndrome. Arch Dermatol 1988, 124:61.

Moutsopoulos HM, moderator, et al: Sjögren's syndrome (sicca syndrome): Current issues. Ann Intern Med 1980, 92:212.

Provost TT, et al: The relationship between antiRo(SSA) and antibody-positive Sjögren's syndrome and antiRo(SSA)-antibody–positive lupus erythematosus. Arch Dermatol 1988, 124:63.

RHEUMATOID ARTHRITIS

The skin manifestations of rheumatoid arthritis have been the subject of an extensive recent review by Jorizzo and Daniels. Most are produced by the cutaneous vasculitis associated with rheumatoid arthritis. There may be annular erythemas, purpura, bullae, shallow ulcers, and gangrene of the extremities. Many diseases have been reported to occur in association with rheumatoid arthritis, such as erythema elevatum diutinum, pyoderma gangrenosum, Felty's syndrome, Sjögren's syndrome, bullous pemphigoid, and yellow nail syndrome.

Rheumatoid Nodules. Subcutaneous nodules are seen in 20 to 30 per cent of the patients. They may arise anywhere on the body but most frequently are found over the bony prominences, especially on the extensor surface of the forearm just below the elbow. These are 2-mm to 2.5-cm, nontender, firm, skin-colored, round nodules, which may or may not be attached to the underlying tissue. Frequently they are attached to the fibrous portions of the periarticular capsule, or they may be free in the subcutaneous tissue.

Pseudoxanthomatous rheumatoid nodules have been described by Watt and Baumann. These can easily be mistaken for xanthomas.

Rheumatoid nodules are differentiated from Heberden's nodes, which are tender, hard, bony proliferations on the dorsolateral aspects of the distal interphalangeal joints. Osler's nodes are pea-sized and somewhat larger reddish swellings with white centers. The nodes are located on the pads of the fingers, the thenar and hypothenar eminences, and the toes. They last for a day or two and fade away. They are probably due to embolism arising during the course of subacute bacterial endocarditis. Nodules or tophi of gout are characterized by masses of crystals of urates surrounded by a chronic inflammatory cellular infiltrate containing foreign body giant cells.

Histologic examination of the rheumatoid nodule shows dense foci of fibrinoid necrosis with basophilic streaks and granules surrounded by histiocytes in palisade arrangement. The upper dermis may show a perivascular inflammation.

Rheumatoid nodules also occur in 5 to 7 per cent of patients with SLE, especially around small joints of the hands; rheumatoid factor may or may not be present.

Rheumatoid Vasculitis

Peripheral vascular lesions appear as typical features of rheumatoid arthritis. These are localized purpura, cutaneous ulceration, and gangrene of the distal parts of the extremities. The majority of patients with vasculitis have rheumatoid nodules. The rheumatoid factor is present. Peripheral neuropathy is frequently associated with the vasculitis.

The presence of rheumatoid nodules may help to distinguish these lesions of vasculitis from SLE, polyarteritis nodosa, Buerger's disease, and the dysproteinemias.

Therapy for these lesions consists of the salicylates and antimalarials such as chloroquine. The corticosteroids should be used in the severe cases only. Dapsone or methotrexate may be effective.

Juvenile Rheumatoid Arthritis

Also known as *Still's disease*, this arthritis shows skin manifestations in some 40 per cent of young patients ranging in age from seven to 25 years. The eruption consists of evanescent, nonpruritic, salmon-pink, macular or papular lesions on the trunk and extremities, which may precede the onset of joint manifestations by many months. Urticaria may also occur.

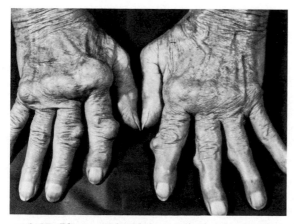

Figure 8–27. Rheumatoid nodules on the hands over the metacarpal-phalangeal joints and several Heberden's nodes on the distal interphalangeal joints. (Courtesy of Dr. C. Ames.)

Calabro JJ, et al: Rash associated with juvenile rheumatoid arthritis. J Pediatr 1968, 71:611.

Jorizzo JL, et al: Dermatologic conditions reported in patients with rheumatoid arthritis. JAAD 1983, 8:439.

Sibbitt WL Jr, et al: Cutaneous manifestations of rheumatoid arthritis. Int J Dermatol 1982, 21:563.

Upchurch KS, et al: Low-dose methotrexate therapy for cutaneous vasculitis of rheumatoid arthritis. JAAD 1987, 17:355.

Vollersten RS, et al: Rheumatoid vasculitis. Medicine (Baltimore) 1986, 65:365.

Weinblatt ME, et al: Methotrexate in rheumatoid arthritis. JAAD 1988, 19:126.

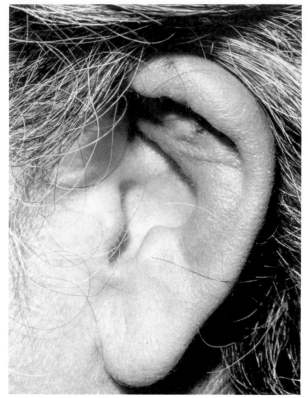

Figure 8–28. Relapsing polychondritis. (Courtesy of Dr. Axel W. Hoke.)

EOSINOPHILIC FASCIITIS

Lawrence Shulman described in 1974 a disorder that he called diffuse eosinophilic fasciitis. Classically, patients have been engaging in strenuous muscular effort for a few days or weeks before the acute onset of weakness, fatigability, and pain and swelling of the extremities, soon followed by severe induration of the skin and subcutaneous tissues of the forearms and legs. Both flexion and extension of the limbs are soon limited. The skin is edematous and erythematous, with a coarse *peau d'orange* appearance, most noticeable inside the upper arms or thighs, or in the flanks. The contrast to scleroderma, where the skin is smooth and taut, is quite striking. The hands and face are usually—but not always—spared. Patients are often unable to stand fully erect. Raynaud's phenomenon is usually absent.

Biopsy shows patchy lymphocytic and plasma-cell infiltrate in the muscle and great thickening, 10 to 50 times normal, of the fascia. Blood eosinophilia of 10 to 40 per cent is usual. The sedimentation rate is increased. Hypergammaglobulinemia is common, and serum eosinophilic chemotactic activity is increased. Patients have been reported to develop pancytopenia, anemia, thrombocytopenia, lymphadenopathy, and pernicious anemia. Two cases have had antibody-mediated hemolytic anemia, Sjögren's

syndrome has occurred, and cardiac involvement, usually pericardial effusion, has been reported.

The response to steroids, orally or intramuscularly, is often excellent. Complete recovery is usual within one to three years.

One man, unable to reduce the prednisone dose that had virtually cleared his fasciitis, and having postprandial epigastric pain, was given cimetidine, and had dramatic resolution of his fasciitis. Stopping it led to a return of symptoms.

Patients with a prolonged course unresponsive to systemic steroids are being recognized with increasing frequency.

Botet MV, et al: The fascia in systemic scleroderma. JAAD 1980, 3:36.

Cramer SF, et al: Eosinophilic fasciitis. Arch Pathol Lab Med 1982, 106:85.

Doyle JA: Eosinophilic fasciitis: Extracutaneous manifestations and associations. Cutis 1984, 34:259.

Idem, et al: Cutaneous and subcutaneous inflammatory sclerosis syndromes. Arch Dermatol 1982, 118:886.

Falanga V, et al: Frequency, levels, and significance of blood eosinophilia in systemic sclerosis, scleroderma, and eosinophilic fascitis. JAAD 1987, 17:648.

Jarratt M, et al: Eosinophilic fasciitis: An early variant of scleroderma. JAAD 1979, 1:221.

Michet Jr, et al: Eosinophilic fasciitis: Report of 15 cases. Mayo Clin Proc 1981, 56:27.

Rosenthal J, et al: Diffuse fasciitis and eosinophilia with symmetric polyarthritis. Ann Intern Med 1980, 92:507.

Shulman LE: Diffuse fasciitis with hypergammaglobulinemia and eosinophilia: A new syndrome. Abstracted, J Rheumatol 1974, 1 (suppl 1):46.

Solomon G, et al: Eosinophilic fasciitis responsive to cimetidine. Ann Intern Med 1982, 97:457.

Wassermann SI, et al: Serum eosinophilotactic activity in eosinophilic fasciitis. Arthritis Rheum 1982, 25:1352.

RELAPSING POLYCHONDRITIS

Relapsing polychondritis is characterized by intermittent episodes of inflammation of the articular and nonarticular cartilage eventuating in chondrolysis, dystrophy, and atrophy of the involved cartilage. There may also be dissolution of the cartilage of the ears and nose and of the respiratory tract. The "beefy red" involvement of the ears is confined to the pinnae, while the ear lobes remain conspicuously normal. The affected areas are swollen and tender. There may be conductive deafness as a result of the obstruction produced by the swollen cartilage. The nasal septal cartilage is similarly involved to produce rhinitis, with crusting and bleeding and possibly saddle-nose. The involvement of the bronchi produces hoarseness, coughing, and dyspnea. Migratory arthralgia is often present. Ocular disease most often presents as conjunctivitis, scleritis, or iritis.

Autoimmune mechanisms appear to be responsible for this disease. Cell-mediated immunity to cartilage has been demonstrated in vitro, with a degree of response correlated with disease activity. IgG anti–type-II-collagen antibodies have been documented in these patients, again in titers corresponding with disease activity—and steroid therapy lowers them. The course of the disease is chronic and variable, with episodic flares.

Histologically, chondrolysis with associated perichondritis occurs.

Dapsone, 100 mg once or twice a day (after 50 mg a day initially) may clear the condition in a couple of weeks. A maintenance dose is usually continued for four to six asymptomatic months. Systemic corticosteroids have also been effective, and indomethacin and salicylates have been used with some success.

Cohen PR, et al: Relapsing polychondritis. Int J Dermatol 1986, 25:280.

Estes SA: Relapsing polychondritis. Cutis 1983, 32:471.

Foidart JM, et al: Antibodies to type I collagen in relapsing polychondritis. N Engl J Med 1978, 299:1203.

9

Mucinoses

The mucinoses or mucoid states are characterized by a deposition of mucin, either discretely or diffusely throughout the dermis.

The connective tissue system is composed of fibers set in a matrix known as ground substance. This ground substance is composed largely of mucopolysaccharides, which are long-chain forms of a basic disaccharide. The fibroblast is believed to be responsible for the production of acid mucopolysaccharides (glycosaminoglycans) in the ground substance; in some diseases fibroblasts are induced to produce abnormally large amounts of acid mucopolysaccharides in the forms of hyaluronic acid, chondroitin sulfate, and heparin. As a result the acid mucopolysaccharides (mucin) accumulate in large amounts in the dermis.

Diseases belonging to the cutaneous mucinoses are myxedema, pretibial myxedema, lichen myxedematosus, follicular mucinosis, plaque-like cutaneous mucinosis, self-healing juvenile cutaneous mucinosis, cutaneous mucinosis of infancy, cutaneous focal mucinosis, and scleredema. Mucin may also accumulate in the skin as a secondary phenomenon, such as when it is present in connective tissue disease, Degos's disease, granuloma annulare, or cutaneous tumors, or after therapies such as PUVA or etretinate. The mucopolysaccharidoses, in which there is a primary accumulation of mucin, are discussed in Chapter 25.

Schermer enumerated the *mucin stains* for the demonstration of the various mucins:

Acid mucopolysaccharide: Blue-green with colloidal iron; blue with alcian blue; red with mucicarmine; metachromatic with methylene blue, toluidine blue, and thionine.

Sulfated mucopolysaccharide (chondroitin sulfate and heparin): Aldehyde-fuchsin stains mucin violet.

Neutral mucopolysaccharide: Periodic acid–Schiff reagent (PAS) with diastase does not stain acid mucopolysaccharides or mucin.

Truhan AP, et al: The cutaneous mucinoses. JAAD 1986, 14:1.

MYXEDEMA

Myxedema is produced by a functional insufficiency of the thyroid gland, resulting in deficiency of thyroid hormone.

In adults the onset is slow, with gradual development of mental and physical sluggishness, gain in weight, asthenia, anemia, subnormal body temperature, drowsiness, intolerance of cold, hypohidrosis, and lowered basal metabolic rate. It is seen mostly in persons who have had surgical thyroidectomy or radioiodine therapy for hyperthyroidism or have developed Hashimoto's autoimmune thyroiditis. The skin becomes puffy about the eyes and on the cheeks and there is a typical dull and expressionless facies, with a broad, thick nose, and fat lips. There is no pitting upon pressure in the edematous areas. The hands and ankles may be swollen. The skin generally is dry, waxlike, translucent, and firm, with more or less fine scaling.

The hair disappears from the outer part of the eyebrows and universally becomes sparse, dry, and thin. The nails are brittle and show longitudinal and transverse striations. Rolls of fat develop on the shoulders. The tongue and oral mucous membranes are sometimes so thickened that speech is slow, hoarse, and labored. Pigmentation of the skin may be greatly increased from a slight yellowish tinge to the point of a general bronzing. Keratotic lesions may occur on the knees, elbows, and buttocks, resembling the lesions of vitamin A deficiency.

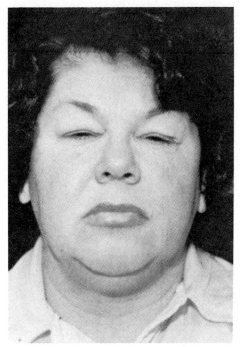

Figure 9–1. Myxedema.

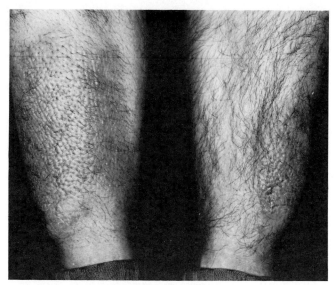

Figure 9–2. Pretibial myxedema.

The extreme form of the disease, congenital hypothyroidism, is called *cretinism*. Children may be born with little or no thyroid gland. These children are dwarfed and stocky, and have wide-set eyes, thick lips, macroglossia, and pale, mottled, edematous skin. There is a characteristic hoarse cry, and a pot belly. There is mental retardation.

Subclinical hypothyroidism may be identified by finding early morning temperatures below 97.5°F (36.5°C).

Histologically, the epidermis shows some hyperkeratosis with keratotic plugs in the hair follicles and sweat ducts. In the dermis there are edema and basophilic degeneration of the collagen. Mucin is widely distributed throughout the dermis and subcutaneous tissue. There is sometimes thickening with obliterative changes in the smaller vessels.

Myxedema responds to treatment with desiccated thyroid, L-thyroxine (Synthroid), L-triiodothyronine (Cytomel), or liotrix (Euthroid). Patients should be started with a low dose, which is then gradually increased to the limit of tolerance. Mental retardation results from congenital hypothyroidism unless the diagnosis is made and hormone replacement begun prior to four months of age.

Pretibial Myxedema

The lesions occur most frequently on the lower shins as bilateral, plaquelike, round or oval swellings, which are firm and do not pit on pressure. They have also occurred on the scalp, ears, and upper trunk. The overlying epidermis is stretched thin and may have a "pigskin" appearance, being brownish and slightly erythematous with depressed follicular orifices; this is also known as *peau d'orange*. Although these lesions are found most frequently on the shins, they may extend about the legs to produce a "shin-guard" appearance, with heavy masses of uneven contour. There may be increased sweating and hair growth in the affected areas.

Cutaneous Focal Mucinosis With Hypothyroidism. Jakubovic et al reported a 54-year-old woman with myxedema who had hundreds of discrete mucinous cystic papules, scattered all over, which had disappeared almost completely by the time she became euthyroid, two to three months later.

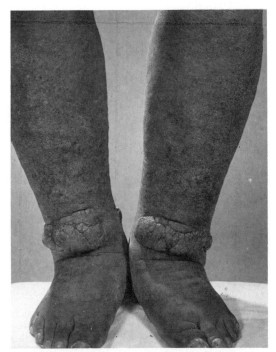

Figure 9–3. Severe pretibial myxedema. (Courtesy of Dr. H. Shatin.)

There may be hypertrichosis, thyroidectomy scar, a diffusely enlarged goiter, significant levels of long-acting thyroid stimulator (when associated with Graves's disease), thyrotoxic exophthalmos, and thyroid acropachy (clubbing of fingers and toes due to hypertrophic osteoarthropathy). The incidence of pretibial myxedema in Graves's disease is estimated to be between 1 and 10 per cent.

The histologic findings are similar to those in generalized myxedema although the quantity of mucin within the dermis is generally greater. Mucin deposition in pretibial skin must be interpreted with caution, since its presence in small quantities is not abnormal.

Treatment with triamcinolone intralesionally has been quite effective. Improvement occurs over several months with repeated monthly injections. Occlusive dressings of polyethylene film (Saran Wrap) over topical corticosteroids have been helpful.

Caron GA: Pretibial myxedema and LATS. Arch Dermatol 1968, 98:310.

Jakubovic HR, et al: Multiple cutaneous focal mucinoses with hypothyroidism. Ann Intern Med 1982, 96:56.

Jones BE, et al: Topical fluocinolone with occlusion in pretibial myxedema. Arch Dermatol 1964, 90:305.

Lang PJ Jr, et al: Intralesional triamcinolone therapy for pretibial myxedema. Arch Dermatol 1975, 111:197.

Noppakun N, et al: Unusual locations of localized myxedema in Graves's disease: Report of 3 cases. Arch Dermatol 1986, 122:85.

Paver WKA: The treatment of pretibial myxedema and cutaneous myxoid cysts. Cutis 1977, 18:144.

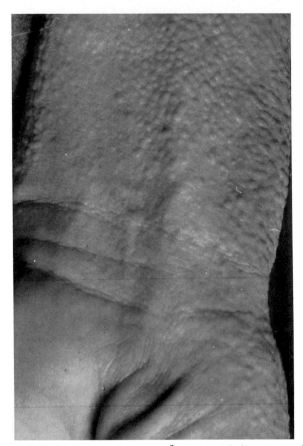

Figure 9–5. Papular mucinosis on the wrist with discrete papules and diffuse erythematous infiltration of the skin. (Courtesy of Dr. J. R. Haserick.)

PAPULAR MUCINOSIS

Papular mucinosis, also known as **lichen myxedematosus** and **scleromyxedema**, occurs either as a widespread symmetric or generalized lichenoid papular eruption; as more or less localized papular, nodular, annular, or discoid lesions; or as discrete lichenoid, at times urticarial, plaques. Some 100 cases have been reported.

Sometimes the lesions are arranged in a linear or patchy manner; they have a predilection for the face and the extensor surfaces of the extremities. In some of the reported cases, the infiltration has caused an exaggeration of the skin folds of the face, with marked furrowing and tightness of the mouth.

Scleromyxedema, a term frequently used synonymously with lichen myxedematosus or papular mucinosis, is characterized by diffuse or limited infiltration of the skin in addition to the papules on the skin. This infiltration is most noticeable on the forehead, where it accentuates the folds and creases and forms a vertical swelling at the root of the nose. A woody, fibrous sclerosis of the skin is characteristic. Mild pruritus may be present.

The general health is usually not affected.

Laboratory studies reveal normal thyroid tests. The elevated erythrocyte sedimentation rate (ESR) and albuminuria are frequent nonspecific early findings. There may be leukocytosis.

Cellulose acetate electrophoresis frequently shows an abnormal homogeneous basic M-type protein. The M-protein is identified as IgG. This was first demonstrated by McCarthy and subsequently has been corroborated by others.

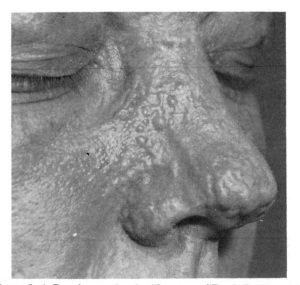

Figure 9–4. Papular mucinosis. (Courtesy of Dr. J. R. Haserick.)

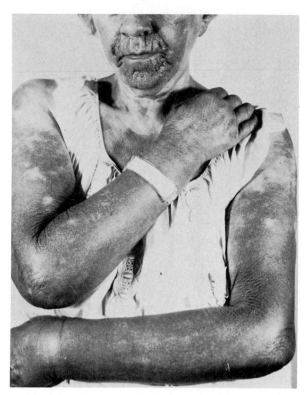

Figure 9–6. Papular mucinosis with widespread lichenoid papules over the arms, legs, and face. (Courtesy of Dr. M. H. Slatkin.)

A bone marrow biopsy may reveal aggregates of plasma cells.

The *etiology* of this disorder is unknown. A serum factor has been identified that stimulates human fibroblasts in vitro. This factor is not the abnormal IgG.

The *histologic features* of papular mucinosis include a prominent increase in the number of fibroblasts, and deposits of mucin between collagen bundles.

Papular mucinosis must be differentiated from unusual forms of scleroderma, nodular urticaria pigmentosa, dermatomyositis, amyloidosis, colloid degeneration, malignant lymphoma, lichen planus, epithelioma adenoides cysticum, and syringoma.

Treatment has been unsatisfactory. Steroids are not helpful. Brenner reported a 45-year-old man with severe scleromyxedema who did not respond to combined melphalan-steroid therapy but was treated successfully with etretinate because of a strong family history of psoriasis. Plastic surgery or dermabrasion may rarely be helpful for disfiguring lesions. If features of a plasma-cell dyscrasia are present, it may be appropriate to try cyclophosphamide (Cytoxan), with which Howsden et al had success in a dose of 200 mg a day (lowered gradually to 50 mg) for six months. Some cases have improved with L-phenylalanine mustard (melphalan, Alkeran) therapy. Farr and Ive reported success with PUVA therapy. Systemic steroids and electron beam therapy have also been successful at times. Milam et al reviewed reported treatments and their relative benefits and risks in 1988.

Abulafia J, et al: Cutaneous mucinosis with special reference to papular mucinosis, and a new dermatosis; generalized mucoid granulomatous papulosis. Arch Argent Dermatol 1961, 11:1.
Brenner S, et al: Treatment of scleromyxedema with etretinate. JAAD 1984, 10:295.
Farmer ER, et al: Papular mucinosis: A clinicopathologic study of four patients. Arch Dermatol 1982, 118:9.
Farr PM, et al: PUVA treatment of scleromyxedema. Br J Dermatol 1984, 110:347.
Lai RFM, et al: Scleromyxedema (lichen myxedematosus) associated with paraprotein IgG, of type kappa. Br J Dermatol 1973, 88:107.
Lowe NJ, et al: Electron-beam treatment of scleromyxedema. Br J Dermatol 1982, 106:449.
McCarthy JT, et al: An abnormal serum globulin in lichen myxedematosus. Arch Dermatol 1964, 89:446.
Milam CP, et al: Scleromyxedema. JAAD 1988, 19:469.
Truhan AP, et al: Lichen myxedematosus. Int J Dermatol 1987, 26:91.

Plaquelike Cutaneous Mucinosis

(Reticular Erythematous Mucinosis, REM Syndrome.) In this syndrome lesions are large plaques, several centimeters in diameter, on the upper trunk. Three such cases were reported by Perry et al in 1960. Steigleder et al described another plaquelike form in 1974, which they called reticular erythematous mucinosis; it appears to be the same disease.

A circumscribed sheetlike or reticulated erythema appears initially on the chest, and then may spread to the upper abdomen and middle back. It evolves slowly, sometimes taking two years to develop. Photosensitivity is common: lesions have been induced by phototesting with UVB.

Histologically there are varying degrees of lymphocytic infiltration around vessels, and deposits of mucin in the dermis. Treatment with antimalarials is successful in most cases.

Bleehen SS, et al: Reticular erythematous mucinosis. Br J Dermatol 1982, 106:9.
Braddock SW, et al: Reticular erythematosus mucinosis and thrombocytopenic purpura. JAAD 1988, 19:859.

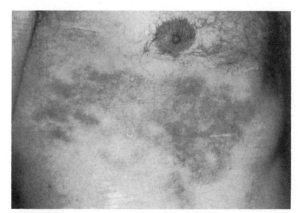

Figure 9–7. REM syndrome. (Courtesy of Dr. E. Kocsard, Australia.)

Butler DF, et al: Reticular erythematous mucinosis. J Assoc Milit Dermatol 1984, 10:24.

Kocsárd E, et al: Reticular erythematous mucinosis of Steigleder. Australas J Dermatol 1978, 19:121.

Perry HO, et al: A plaquelike form of cutaneous mucinosis. Arch Dermatol 1960, 82:980.

Idem: Diseases that present as cutaneous sclerosis. Austral J Derm 1982, 23:45.

Quimby SR, et al: Plaque-like cutaneous mucinosis: Its relationship to reticular erythematous mucinosis. JAAD 1982, 6:856.

Steigleder GK, et al: REM syndrome: A new entity. Br J Dermatol 1974, 91:191.

Self-Healing Juvenile Cutaneous Mucinosis

Bonerandi et al reported in 1980 a case of circumscribed lesions of cutaneous mucinosis on the face, trunk, and joint areas of a child, associated with hypertension and arthralgia. It healed spontaneously in a few weeks. Pucevich reported a very similar case in 1984, differing only in being normotensive, having persistent arthralgia, and having a dermal mucin, hyaluronic acid, instead of sialomucin.

Pucevich MV, et al: Self-healing juvenile cutaneous mucinosis. JAAD 1984, 11:327.

Cutaneous Mucinosis of Infancy

Lum reported in 1980 a 16-month-old girl with symmetric, densely grouped 1-to-2-mm, firm, opalescent papules on the elbows, which histologically showed accumulations of hyaluronic acid. McGrae reported a second case in 1983.

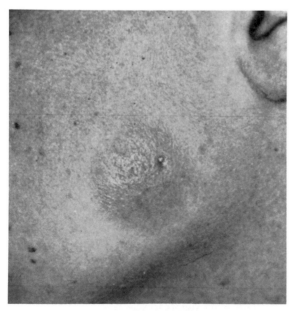

Figure 9–8. Follicular mucinosis. Cleared entirely within one year. (Courtesy of Dr. J. Bembenista.)

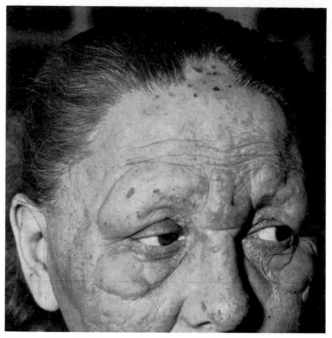

Figure 9–9. Malignant lymphoma of the skin with alopecia mucinosa on the anterior scalp line for one year. Note alopecia of eyebrows and plaques of infiltration around eyes, glabella, and forehead, producing a leonine facies and accompanied by universal intensely pruritic, excoriated nodules.

Lum D: Cutaneous mucinosis of infancy. Arch Dermatol 1980, 116:198.

McGrae JD: Cutaneous mucinosis of infancy. Arch Dermatol 1983, 119:272.

FOLLICULAR MUCINOSIS (Alopecia Mucinosa)

In 1957 Pinkus applied the name *alopecia mucinosa* to cases of peculiar inflammatory plaques with alopecia characterized histologically by mucinous deposits in the outer root sheaths of the hair follicles. The plaques may be simply hypopigmented or erythematous and scaly, eczematous, or composed of flesh-colored, follicular papules, or there may be a solitary nodule. These are firm and coarsely rough to the palpating finger. They are distributed mostly on the face, neck, and scalp but may appear on any parts of the body. Snyder et al reported a case of diffuse alopecia in normal-appearing skin. Itching may or may not be present.

Sensory dissociation, with dysesthesia to cold, has been reported in some lesions, with a resultant misdiagnosis of leprosy in some instances. Matuska recently reported a case with anesthesia to light touch.

Alopecia occurs regularly in lesions on the scalp and frequently in lesions located elsewhere. Some papules show a black central dot that corresponds to a hair broken off at the skin surface. These may cause the surface of a patch to look like keratosis pilaris.

Three categories of patients have been identified. One is younger patients with few lesions confined to the head and neck, or upper arms. This, the commonest kind, resolves spontaneously in two months to two years. The second group, somewhat older, has larger, more numerous, and more widespread lesions, and resolution may take several years. The third group, still older, has widespread lesions, most commonly as a result of mycosis fungoides.

Anesthesia to cold or touch occurs in many cases. Serious confusion with leprosy is possible, as Fan and associates pointed out.

A variant that is quite common in girls between six and 20 years of age (and sometimes in boys) shows round or oval clusters, 1 to 6 cm in diameter, of hypopigmented follicular macules, from which most or all of the vellus hairs have been shed. The outer aspects of the upper arms are by far the commonest area involved. Triamcinolone acetonide, 20 or 30 mg, given intramuscularly, permits repigmentation within three or four weeks and rarely requires repetition in less than three to six months. If lesions are not large or numerous, intralesional steroids may be used.

Follicular mucinosis may appear in idiopathic alopecia mucinosa, in reticulosis or lymphoma with symptomatic follicular mucinosis, and rarely in cases that progress from idiopathic alopecia mucinosa to mycosis fungoides with persisting follicular mucinosis.

Histologically, alopecia mucinosa is characterized by large collections of mucin within cells of the sebaceous gland and outer root sheath. An associated dermal infiltrate of atypical cells is prominent when the condition occurs in association with mycosis fungoides (T-cell lymphoma).

Spontaneous involution may occur. Some cases have benefited from fractional x-ray therapy. Corticosteroids externally and internally have produced varying degrees of improvement. Dapsone and PUVA have been effective.

Arnold HL Jr: Dysesthesia in alopecia mucinosa: A possible diagnostic sign. Arch Dermatol 1962, 85:409.
Fan J, et al: Alopecia mucinosa simulating leprosy. Arch Dermatol 1967, 95:354.
Ferreira-Marques J: Sensory imbalance in alopecia mucinosa. Arch Dermatol 1961, 84:170.
Gibson LE, et al: Follicular mucinosis. JAAD 1989, 20:441.
Lancer HA, et al: Follicular mucinosis. JAAD 1984, 10:760.
Matuska MA, et al: Anesthesia in alopecia mucinosa. Cutis 1987, 40:46.
Nickoloff BJ, et al: Benign idiopathic vs mycosis-fungoides–associated follicular mucinosis. Pediatr Dermatol 1985, 2:201.
Pinkus H: Alopecia mucinosa (Commentary). Arch Dermatol 1983, 119:698.
Schwartz BK, et al: Indurated facial plaques in a young man. Arch Dermatol 1987, 123:939.

Cutaneous Focal Mucinosis

Focal mucinosis is characterized by a solitary nodule or papule of fibroblastic proliferation. Johnson and Helwig have used the term "cutaneous focal mucinosis" since 1961. The solitary, flesh-colored lesion occurs in adulthood mostly. Generally it is a smooth-surfaced, asymptomatic lesion appearing on the head, neck, trunk, or extremities, but not over the joints of the hands.

Histologically, the lesion is characterized by a loose dermal stroma containing large quantities of mucin together with numerous dendritic-shaped fibroblasts. There is no evidence of a well-formed cystic space.

The clinical appearance is not distinctive and may at times be suggestive of a cyst. Histologically, it may closely resemble a myxoma, a myxoid cyst, a ganglion, or alopecia mucinosa.

Treatment of choice is simple excision.

Hazelrigg DE: Cutaneous focal mucinosis. Cutis 1974, 14:241.

SCLEREDEMA

Scleredema, also known as *scleredema adultorum*, was first described by Piffard in 1886, but first reported by Buschke in 1902. It is characterized by a stiffening and hardening of the subcutaneous tissues, as if they were infiltrated with paraffin. The tissues on the back of the neck feel woody or cartilaginous. The onset is so gradual that it may not be noticed by the patient. Erythema of the upper back may be an early sign, as reported by Millns and others; it occurred in two of the 33 cases reviewed by Venencie et al.

The nonpitting, solid edema frequently begins on the head, neck, or upper back, and spreads rapidly to involve large areas, advancing from the neck over the face and downward over the trunk, but usually leaving the hands (and always the feet) free. It fades out gradually on the distal extremities.

The induration may be marked on the face, causing a masklike expression due to the inflexibility of the skin. The overlying skin cannot be wrinkled and shows no inflammation, atrophy, loss of hair, or pigmentary changes. A blotchy erythema is rarely seen.

There may be systemic involvement. The tongue may be swollen and make swallowing difficult. Ocular involvement may restrict eye and eyelid movement. There may be pleural, pericardial, or peritoneal effusion. Electrocardiographic changes may occur.

In one subset of the disease the induration spreads for two to six weeks. After a period of one to two years, resolution may take place without sequelae, but recurrent attacks at intervals of several years are common. Persistence of induration beyond two years appears to be more common in this group of patients than previously appreciated.

In this subset of patients, the disease occurs in adults and children following one of the exanthemata or some respiratory infection such as scarlet fever, measles, influenza, or tonsillitis; but it may develop after other local or general infections, mostly of streptococcal origin. In a series of 223 patients reported by Graff and Perry, 29 per cent were children.

The laboratory findings are normal, with the exception of the antistreptolysin (ASO) titer, which may be elevated, and monoclonal gammopathy of IgG type, which was present in eight cases reviewed by Kövary et al.

In the second, larger group, there is an association with insulin-dependent diabetes, especially in older men. These lesions are of insidious onset and long duration. At least 10 adult patients with scleredema have had an associated paraproteinemia. In adults it must be differentiated from scleroderma, scleromyxedema, myxedema, and lymphedema. Scleroderma may be difficult to rule out at first, but in scleredema the fingers are spared.

Histologically, the epidermis shows no important changes. There may be slight hyperkeratosis, particularly at the follicles. In the mid- and deep dermis, the collagen is swollen, homogenized, and broken up by clear spaces. The elastic tissue shows no changes. There is a slight perivascular infiltration, but the blood vessels show no obliterative alterations.

The diagnosis histologically or histochemically may be made by the demonstration of increased amounts of acid mucopolysaccharides. This is shown more easily when a special fixative such as cetylpyridinium chloride is used.

There is no specific or effective treatment. Massage, warm baths, systemic corticosteroids, methotrexate, and penicillamine have all proved useless.

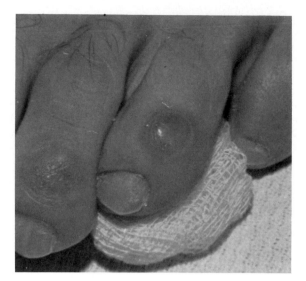

Figure 9–11. Synovial (myxoid) cyst of toe.

Kövary PM, et al: Monoclonal gammopathy in scleredema. Arch Dermatol 1981, 117:536.

McFadden N, et al: Scleredema adultorum associated with a monoclonal gammopathy and generalized hyperpigmentation. Arch Dermatol 1987, 123:629.

Millns JL, et al: Scleredema and persistent erythema. Arch Dermatol 1982, 118:296.

Olita A, et al: Paraproteinemia in patients with scleredema. JAAD 1987, 16:96.

Venencie PY, et al: Scleredema: review of 33 cases. JAAD 1984, 11:128.

SYNOVIAL "CYSTS"
(Myxoid Cysts)

Synovial "cysts" are focal accumulations of mucin in the dermis of the dorsal aspect of the distal phalanges or proximal nail folds of the fingers, or less often the toes. They are usually but not necessarily solitary. After Johnson showed that they had no cyst wall, it was generally accepted that they should be called "myxoid" rather than "synovial."

Then it was shown that they always have a connection with the synovial space of the distal interphalangeal joint, both by surgical dissection and by injection of methylene blue into either the "cyst" or the joint space and observing its appearance in the other. It seems most appropriate to call them synovial "cysts."

They are usually about 5 to 7 mm in diameter, opalescent, shiny, perhaps slightly reddened, dome-shaped, and smooth-surfaced. They are quite often painful. When they are punctured there exudes a clear, nearly colorless, viscid fluid composed of mucin and containing hyaluronic acid. Later the cyst may refill and produce the same lesion as previously. It is more often complained of by women than by men, and it occurs most frequently in patients over 40.

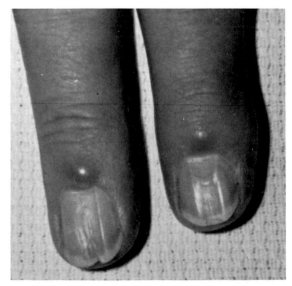

Figure 9–10. Distortion of nails distal to synovial cysts on two fingers.

The nail distal to the cyst often shows longitudinal grooving. It is not unusual to mistake this grooving for fungus infection, dystrophia unguium mediana canaliformis, or other nail dystrophies.

Treatment of these synovial "cysts" is frequently disappointing; they may recur regardless of the method of therapy.

Ernst Epstein achieved a 70 per cent cure rate by teaching the patient to puncture the cyst repeatedly and express the contents. Salasche reported a method of excision for these cysts.

One of us (HLA) has had success with a method taught him by J. Warren White, a distinguished orthopedist: splinting the distal i-p joint with a small splint for four to eight weeks. The cyst cannot undergo replenishment of its contents, and simply disappears. But it frequently recurs.

Electrofulguration is often effective. The lesion is first drained and then fulgurated. A variation of this method is to remove the roof with fine scissors under local anesthesia; the gelatinous material is removed, and the base is touched with bichloracetic acid. Healing takes place in a month.

Meticulous excision of "the cyst and its stalk" was successful in 11 cases reported by Nasca et al; there were no recurrences.

Epstein E: A simple technique for managing digital mucous cysts. Arch Dermatol 1979, 115:1315.

Johnson WC, et al: Cutaneous myxoid cyst. JAMA 1965, 191:15.

Nasca RJ, et al: Mucous cysts of the digits. Southern Med J 1983, 76(9):1142.

Salasche SJ: Myxoid cysts of the proximal nail fold: a surgical approach. J Dermatol Surg Oncol 1984, 10:35.

10

Seborrheic Dermatitis, Psoriasis, Recalcitrant Palmoplantar Eruptions, and Erythroderma

SEBORRHEIC DERMATITIS

Synonyms: Seborrheic eczema, seborrheide.

CLINICAL FEATURES. Seborrheic dermatitis is a chronic superficial inflammatory disease of the skin, with a predilection for the scalp, eyebrows, eyelids, nasolabial creases, lips, ears, sternal area, axillae, submammary folds, umbilicus, groins, and gluteal crease. The disease is characterized by scanty, loose, dry, moist, or greasy scales, and by crusted, pinkish or yellowish patches of various shapes and sizes; by remissions and exacerbations; and more or less by itching. For the sake of clarity the different expressions of seborrheic dermatitis will be considered topographically.

On the *scalp* the least severe but by far the commonest phase—**pityriasis sicca**, or **dandruff**—manifests itself as a dry, flaky, branny desquamation, beginning in small patches and rapidly involving the entire surface, with a profuse amount of fine powdery scales commonly called "dandruff." An oily type, **pityriasis steatoides**, at times accompanied by erythema and an accumulation of thick crusts, is also encountered.

Other types of seborrheic dermatitis on the scalp are more severe and are manifested by greasy, scaling, configurate patches or psoriasiform eruptions, exudation, and thick crusting. The disease frequently spreads beyond the hairy scalp to the forehead, ears, postauricular regions, and neck. On these areas, the patches have convex borders and a reddish yellow or yellowish color. In extreme cases the entire scalp is covered by a greasy, dirty crust with an offensive odor. In infants, yellow or brown scaling lesions on the scalp with accumulated adherent epithelial debris are called **cradle cap**.

On the *supraorbital regions*, flaky scales are seen in the eyebrows, and the underlying skin is erythematous and pruritic or may show yellowish scaling patches. The edges of the *lids* may be erythematous and granular (**marginal blepharitis**). The *conjunctivae* are at times injected. The lids may show yellowish pink, fine scales, the borders of which are usually indistinct. Pruritus may be present. If the *glabella* is involved, there may be cracks in the skin in the wrinkles at the inner end of the eyebrow accompanying the fine scaling on an erythematous patch. In the nasolabial creases and on the *alae nasi*, there may be yellowish or reddish yellow scaling macules, sometimes with fissures. In men, folliculitis of the upper *lip* may occur.

On and in the ears, seborrheic dermatitis is frequently mistaken for otitis externa due to fungus infection (*otomycosis*). There is scaling in the aural canals, around the *auditory meatus*, and in the postauricular region, or under the lobe. In these areas

194

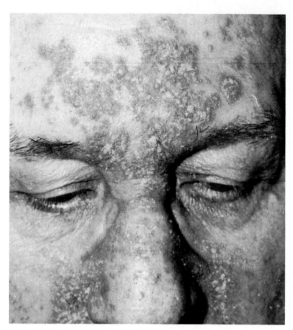

Figure 10–1. Severe seborrheic dermatitis.

the skin often becomes red, fissured, and swollen. Serous exudation, puffiness of the ears and surrounding parts, and regional adenopathy occur less frequently. Examination for fungus is invariably negative for hyphae.

Cortisporin otic suspension, a polymyxin B–hydrocortisone suspension, 4 drops in the auditory meatus, usually brings about prompt clearing. Tridesilon Otic Lotion, 0.5 per cent desonide and 2 per cent acetic acid, is also effective.

Seborrheic dermatitis of the face may also be manifested by a papular eruption on the *cheeks, nose,* and *forehead.* Persistent erythema in the alar-malar angle areas is called **dyssebacea.** Sodium sulfacetamide, which may be applied in 10 per cent strength in any convenient cream such as desonide (Tridesilon), is almost a specific for dyssebacea. Rees B. Rees cured it permanently in one of us (HLA) with this some 25 years ago.

The *lips* and mucosae are not usually involved, but sometimes the changes on the lips are pronounced, resulting in **cheilitis exfoliativa.** The vermilion surfaces may be persistently dry, red, scaly, and fissured.

In the *axillae* the eruption begins in the apices, bilaterally, and later progresses to neighboring skin. The involvement may vary from simple yellowish erythema and scaling to more pronounced petaloid or discoid patches with fissures.

The areolae of the *breasts,* the inframammary folds, especially when the breasts are pendulous, and the *umbilicus* may be involved. The presternal area is a favored site on the trunk.

Seborrheic dermatitis is common in the *groins* and *gluteal crease,* where its appearance may closely sim-

ulate ringworm, psoriasis, or candidiasis. The patches, however, are more finely scaly with less definite borders and are more likely to be bilateral and symmetrical and of the typical color. In these locations fissures often occur and there may be psoriasiform patches with thick scales in severe cases.

The lesions may be generalized, with erythema, scaling, oozing, and pruritus. Often, however, the eruption remains localized in one area, such as the scalp, ears, sternal region, or umbilicus. In the acute stages the inflammation may be intense, with moist exudation from the scalp and ears and papulovesicles on the palms and soles. Secondary infections, impetiginization, or furunculosis may ensue.

Seborrheic dermatitis may progress to a generalized exfoliative state. In the newborn this type of severe and generalized seborrheic dermatitis is known as **erythroderma desquamativum.** Generalized eruptions may be accompanied by adenopathy and may simulate mycosis fungoides and leukemic or psoriatic erythroderma.

Seborrheic dermatitis may be associated with or accentuated by several internal diseases. In Parkinson's disease a severe seborrheic dermatitis involving the scalp and face, with waxy, profuse scaling and usually little erythema, is sometimes seen. A unilateral injury to the innervation of the face may lead to an ipsilateral localized seborrheic dermatitis. Patients with the acquired immune deficiency syndrome, and to a lesser degree those with the related complex, have a markedly increased incidence of seborrheic dermatitis. Diabetes mellitus, especially in obese persons; sprue; malabsorption disorders; epilepsy; and reactions to arsenic and gold have all produced seborrheic dermatitis–like lesions.

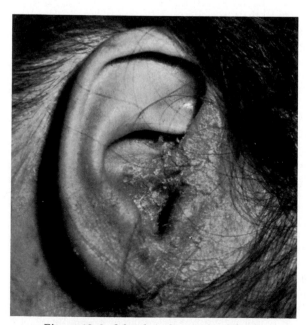

Figure 10–2. Seborrheic dermatitis of the ear.

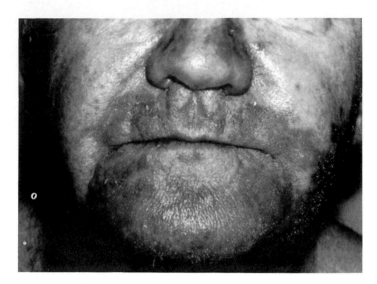

Figure 10–3. Seborrheic dermatitis of the face.

ETIOLOGY AND PATHOGENESIS. The etiology of this common disorder remains unresolved. This is a dermatitis that affects areas with many sebaceous glands; however, recent evidence indicates that hypersecretion of sebum was not present in a group of affected patients when compared with a control group. A hormonal influence should be postulated, since the disease is generally not seen before puberty. There is evidence that this is a hyperproliferative state, but the cause remains obscure.

Investigations have confirmed the presence of a lipophilic, pleomorphic fungus, *Malassezia ovalis* (*Pityrosporum ovale*), in profuse numbers in the scalp lesions. Rosenberg et al have lately shown that 2 per cent ketoconazole cream sharply reduces the numbers of yeast organisms in lesions of hairy or glabrous skin, at the same time clearing the seborrheic dermatitis. The argument that the yeast is the cause of the dermatitis is a persuasive one. However, others have demonstrated that *P. ovale* may be abundant on the scalps of patients who have no clinical signs of the disease.

It is made worse by conditions that increase perspiration. Emotional stress has been found to influence its course unfavorably. Neuroleptic drugs that may induce parkinsonism, such as haloperidol, may also induce seborrheic dermatitis.

HISTOLOGY. The epidermis is acanthotic. There is overlying parakeratosis, and neutrophils are present within the stratum corneum and upper stratum malpighii. The dermis contains a perivascular mixed cell inflammatory infiltrate. Pinkus's "spurting papilla" is almost as characteristic of seborrheic dermatitis as of psoriasis, but Munro abscesses are not seen. Seborrheic dermatitis is often hard to distinguish from eczema or other low-grade inflammations.

DIFFERENTIAL DIAGNOSIS. Some cases of seborrheic dermatitis bear such a close clinical resemblance to psoriasis that there is some justification for thinking that their etiologies must be similar.

Indicative of psoriasis are erythema; heavy scales, whose removal discloses bleeding points; strong predilection for involvement of the frontal scalp margin; and resistance to treatment. Absence of itching is also suggestive. Characteristic psoriasis elsewhere (nail pitting, balanitis) may resolve the question. Impetigo of the scalp, especially when associated with pediculosis and even more so when the eyelashes and eyebrows are involved, may cause difficulty in differentiation. Inverse psoriasis of the intertriginous areas is also frequently mistaken for seborrheic dermatitis. The jocular coinage "seborrhiasis" sometimes seems more appropriate than either psoriasis or seborrheic dermatitis.

Other diseases to be differentiated are otitis externa, blepharitis, perleche, tinea corporis, and pityriasis rosea.

TREATMENT. The scalp should be shampooed several times per week. Selenium sulfide (Selsun or Exsel lotions), tar, zinc pyrithionate, and resorcin

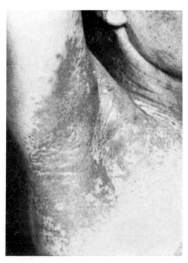

Figure 10–4. Seborrheic dermatitis affecting the axilla. (Courtesy of John T. Ingram and Br J Dermatol.)

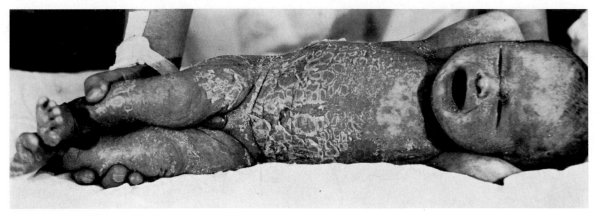

Figure 10–5. Erythroderma desquamativum in a 6-week-old neonate. (Courtesy of Drs. E. Liebner and E. Florian, Budapest.)

shampoos are all excellent. Priestley et al showed in 1980 that zinc pyrithione is not antimitotic to keratinocytes, but it is 100 times more toxic to them than zinc oxide or zinc sulfate. Valisone (betamethasone 17-valerate) lotion applied twice daily to the scalp is very effective. Corticosteroid solutions such as Synalar or Fluonid, corticosteroids in combination with crude coal tar (Zetone lotion) or with iodochlorhydroxyquin (Vytone cream, Vioform-Hydrocortisone lotion or Cor-tar-quin lotion) are all effective. Skinner et al showed in a double-blind study in 1985 that ketoconazole topically in a 2 per cent cream is effective. Several studies have confirmed this and shown a lower relapse rate after its use.

The most efficacious agents on glabrous skin are the corticosteroid creams (the trade names are too numerous to list); in severe cases in which bacterial infection is prominent, the corticosteroids combined with antimicrobial preparations are extremely beneficial. Generally, nonfluorinated topical steroid preparations are adequate.

Topical steroids should not be used for blepharitis, as steroid preparations used in this area may induce

glaucoma and cataracts. Daily debridement with a cotton-tipped applicator and baby shampoo, sometimes combined with a topical antibiotic ointment, is recommended.

Before the advent of the corticosteroids and antibiotics, topical preparations containing iodochlorhydroxyquin 1 to 3 per cent, crude coal tar 1 to 5 per cent, ammoniated mercury 5 to 10 per cent, and sulfur 2 to 15 per cent were used.

In generalized or severe cases, systemic corticosteroids, and even antibiotics, for secondary infection, may be necessary and effective.

Shohat et al reported in 1987 that a 2 per cent aqueous solution of eosin was as effective as topical corticosteroids in 30 infants, half treated with flumethasone pivalate 0.02 per cent and half with the eosin.

ERYTHRODERMA DESQUAMATIVUM

Erythroderma desquamativum was originally described by Leiner in the early 1900s as a disease occurring chiefly in nursing infants from the ages of six to 20 weeks as a generalized exfoliative dermatitis with marked erythema and scaling, usually suggesting a severe type of seborrheic dermatitis.

The disease usually begins in the perianal and inguinal areas, then appears on the scalp, intertriginous areas (particularly the anogenital region), trunk, and extremities. At first there is a diffuse inflammatory erythema, which may cover the whole body. Later the skin becomes covered with grayish white scales, which may be fine and branny. In fact, as the process develops there may be general exfoliation, cracking, and thickening of the skin. The scalp is always thickly crusted and the nails are damaged. There is glandular enlargement. Nikolsky's sign is absent.

Affected infants are usually in poor general condition. Diarrhea, wasting, and intercurrent infection are the rule. Since the original description of this disease antedated the appreciation of several nutri-

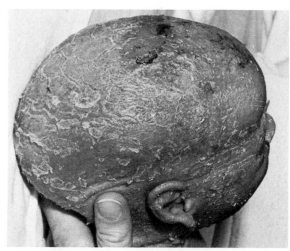

Figure 10–6. Leiner's disease.

tional diseases that may have a similar appearance, such as zinc-deficient acrodermatitis enteropathica, free fatty acid deficiency, and biotin-responsive multiple carboxylase deficiency, many reported cases may have represented other, now more precisely defined, entities.

A small subset of the cases reported with this clinical syndrome have been reported to have a dysfunction of the fifth component of complement, with decreased opsonic activity present. This defect does not result in an abnormal level of CH50, and requires detailed laboratory confirmation to affirm the diagnosis. It appears to be of autosomal dominant inheritance. The specific defect and the disease manifestations may be ameliorated by infusions of fresh frozen plasma.

Bennetblanc JM, et al: Benzoyl peroxide in seborrheic dermatitis. Arch Dermatol 1986, 122:752.

Berger RS, et al: Cutaneous manifestations of early HIV exposure. JAAD 1988, 19:298.

Binder RL, et al: Seborrheic dermatitis in neuroleptic-induced Parkinsonism. Arch Dermatol 1983, 119:473.

Boyle J, et al: Topical lithium succinate for seborrheic dermatitis. Br Med J 1986, 292:28.

Burton JL, et al: Seborrhea is not a feature of seborrheic dermatitis. Br Med J 1983, 286:1169.

Carr MM, et al: Treatment of seborrheic dermatitis with ketoconazole. Br J Dermatol 1987, 116:213.

Coldiron BM, et al: . . .skin disease in patients infected with HIV. Arch Dermatol 1989, 125:357.

Faergemann J: Seborrheic dermatitis and *P. orbiculare*. Br J Dermatol 1986, 114:695.

Ford GP, et al: The response of seborrheic dermatitis to ketoconazole. Br J Dermatol 1984, 111:603.

Fox BJ, et al: Papulosquamous diseases. JAAD 1985, 12:597.

Green CA, et al: Treatment of seborrheic dermatitis with ketoconazole. Br J Dermatol 1987, 116:217.

Mathes BM, et al: Seborrheic dermatitis in patients with AIDS. JAAD 1985, 13:947.

Priestley GC, et al: Acute toxicity of zinc pyrithione to human skin cells in vitro. Acta Dermatovener (Stockh) 1980, 60:145.

Sheth RA, et al: Dandruff: Assessment and management. Int J Dermatol 1983, 22:511.

Shohat M, et al: Efficacy of topical corticosteroids compared with eosin in infants with seborrheic dermatitis. Cutis 1987, 40:67.

Shuster S: The aetiology of dandruff and the mode of action of therapeutic agents. Br J Dermatol 1984, 11:235.

Skinner RB Jr, et al: The pathogenic role of microbes in seborrheic dermatitis. Arch Dermatol 1986, 122:16.

Idem: Double-blind treatment of seborrheic dermatitis with 2% ketoconazole cream. JAAD 1985, 12:852.

Idem: Seborrheic dermatitis and AIDS (letter). JAAD 1986, 14:147.

Soeprano FF, et al: Seborrheic-like dermatitis of AIDS. JAAD 1986, 14:242.

Yates VM, et al: Early diagnosis of infantile seborrheic dermatitis and stopic dermatitis—clinical features. Br J Dermatol 1983, 108:633.

PSORIASIS

CLINICAL FEATURES. Psoriasis is a common, chronic, recurrent, inflammatory disease of the skin characterized by rounded, circumscribed, erythematous, dry, scaling patches of various sizes, covered by grayish white or silvery white, imbricated, and lamellar scales. The lesions in ordinary cases have a predilection for the scalp, nails, extensor surfaces of the limbs (especially the shins), the elbows, the knees, and the sacral region. The eruption is usually symmetrical and may vary from a solitary macule to countless patches. The eruption usually develops slowly but may be exanthematous, with the sudden onset of numerous guttate lesions, or may consist of a few inveterate patches. Subjective symptoms such as itching or burning may be present and may cause extreme discomfort.

The early lesions are guttate erythematous macules, which from the beginning are covered with

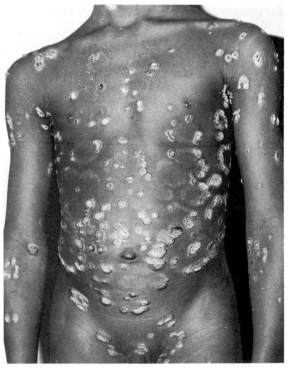

Figure 10–8. Ostraceous psoriasis, relapsing.

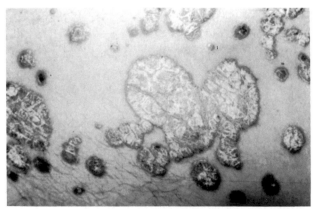

Figure 10–7. Psoriasis. The silvery scaling, serpiginous outlines, confluence, erythema beyond the scaling area, and varied size of lesions are well illustrated.

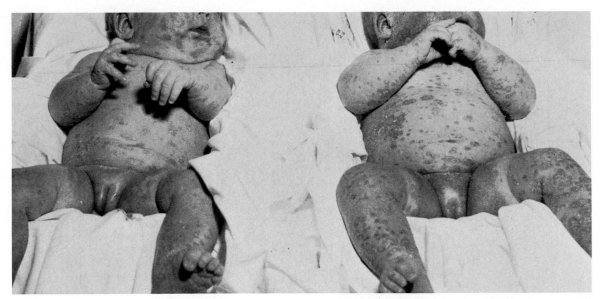

Figure 10–9. Psoriasis in 5-month-old twins. Onset was simultaneous. Note that folds are involved: "inverse" distribution.

dry, silvery scales, which typically do not extend all the way to the edge of the erythematous area. By peripheral extension and by coalescence, the patches increase in size and, through the accumulation of scales, become thicker. Nummular (coin-sized) lesions are common. In this variety certain distinctive

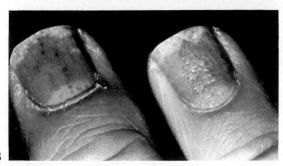

Figure 10–10. A, Onycholysis with psoriatic nails. Note "oil spot" on thumb. B, Pitting, distal onycholysis, and "oil spots" in psoriatic nails. (Courtesy of Dr. Axel W. Hoke.)

features may be easily demonstrated: the scales are micaceous and are looser toward the periphery of the patch, although adherent at its center; upon removal of the scales, bleeding points appear (Auspitz's sign). When the patches reach a diameter of about 5 cm, they may cease spreading and undergo involution in the center, so that annular, lobulated, and gyrate figures are produced.

Old patches may be thickened and tough and covered with lamellar scales like the outside of an oyster shell (**psoriasis ostracea**). Various other descriptive terms have in the past been applied to the diverse appearances of the lesions: **psoriasis guttata**, in which the lesions are the size of water drops; **psoriasis follicularis**, in which tiny scaly lesions are located at the orifices of the pilosebaceous follicles; **psoriasis figurata, psoriasis annulata,** and **psoriasis gyrata**, in which curved linear patterns are produced by central involution; **psoriasis discoidea**, in which central involution does not occur and solid patches persist; **psoriasis rupioides**, in which crustaceous lesions occur resembling syphilitic rupia. The term **plaque psoriasis** is often applied to other than guttate or inverse varieties. **Psoriasis flexura**, better known as **inverse psoriasis**, is found in intertriginous areas. On palms or soles it is called **volar psoriasis**.

COURSE. The course of psoriasis is inconstant. It usually begins on the scalp or on the olecranons, and may remain localized in the original region for an indefinite period, or completely disappear, recur, or spread to other parts. It may first be seen over the sacrum, where the patch slowly extends to form an inveterate lesion. This may easily be confused with fungus infection. At other times the onset is more sudden and widespread, as already described; in still other cases the first lesions may be limited to the fingernails.

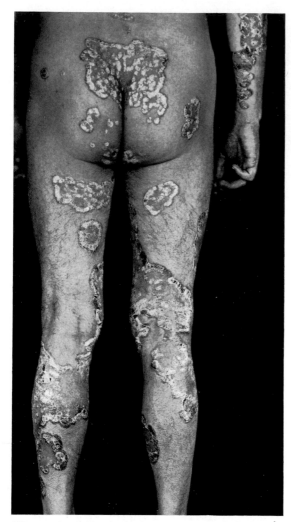

Figure 10–11. Psoriasis. (Courtesy of Dr. H. Shatin.)

Two of the chief features of psoriasis are its tendency to recur and to persist. Rarely, however, psoriatics may remain completely free of the disease for years and may be considered, in at least a practical

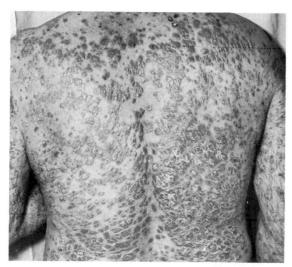

Figure 10–12. Generalized nummular psoriasis.

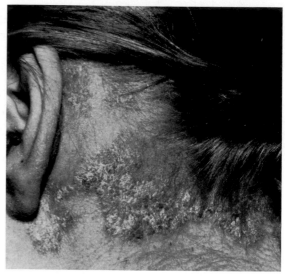

Figure 10–13. Psoriasis on back of neck and scalp.

sense, cured. On the scalp it rarely causes loss of hair. The lesions—even the chronic ones—are sometimes easily irritated, and when this takes place they are liable to spread by the development of satellites, or new spots in other regions. In acute guttate or spreading nummular eruptions, if irritating remedies or physical agents are applied, a generalized exfoliative dermatitis may result.

The isomorphic response, commonly known as the **Koebner reaction**, is the appearance of typical lesions of psoriasis at sites of even trivial injuries. This characteristic feature of the disease accounts for the frequent appearance of typical psoriatic patches on scars and at sites of scratches, eruptions, and burns. In the presence of early lesions, new lesions can be produced by scratching the skin. The Koebner response occurs in many other skin diseases, such as lichen planus, lichen nitidus, infectious eczematoid dermatitis, and nummular eczema.

The **Auspitz sign** is pinpoint bleeding when a psoriatic scale is forcibly removed. This occurs only in psoriasis. It occurs because of the severe thinning of the epidermis over the tips of the dermal papillae.

The **Woronoff ring** is concentric blanching of the erythematous skin at or near the periphery of a healing psoriatic plaque. It does not redden with ultraviolet-induced erythema or under anthralin therapy, which Gupta et al suggest implies a more complex cause than lowered levels of a single prostaglandin.

On the *scalp* the lesions are often nummular patches, but at times there is a bandlike patch along the anterior hair line, or a palm-sized patch on the occiput, which may be thickened and pruritic so that alone it might be mistaken for seborrheic dermatitis with lichenification. In other cases, profuse scaling may be the only sign. Absence of itching or hair loss, marked predilection for the frontal scalp margin, deep erythema, and resistance to effective therapy (for seborrheic dermatitis) all suggest psoriasis. In

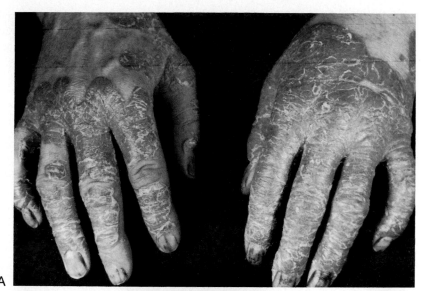

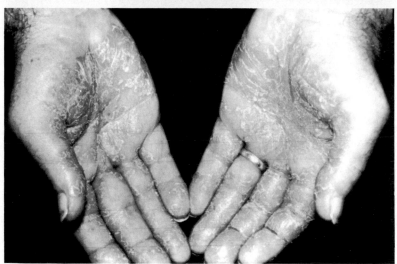

Figure 10–14. A, *Psoriasis of backs of hands. B, Psoriasis of palms. (B, Courtesy of Dr. Axel W. Hoke.)*

A

B

psoriasis the lesions are well demarcated. Associated with the scalp involvement, there are often fissuring of the superior and posterior auricular folds and erythematous scaling patches about the external auditory meatus. Nail pitting may also confirm a suspicion of psoriasis, as may a hyperkeratotic macule on the glans penis.

On the *face* (which is generally entirely spared except for the upper edge of the forehead) chiefly guttate lesions are seen, especially in acute widespread eruptions, although some patients with inveterate patches of the trunk may develop a few on the face. Larger lesions, particularly the discoid variety, commonly have the appearance of seborrheic dermatitis or lupus erythematosus.

The *palms* and *soles* are often, sometimes exclusively, affected, showing discrete erythematous, dry, scaling patches, or circumscribed verrucous thickenings, sometimes linear. Pustular psoriasis of the palms and soles, as described by Barber and Ingram, is considered in detail elsewhere. Briefly, the patches begin on the middle portions of the palms or on the

soles, and, with recurring crops of small pustules, eventually form exfoliative areas in which the pustules, though more evident at the edges, are often observed throughout. The pustules sometimes fuse to form so-called **lakes of pus**. The condition is extremely resistant to all methods of treatment that are usually beneficial in psoriasis, except PUVA, intralesional steroids, etretinate, and sometimes dapsone.

The *axillae, submammary folds, pubis, genitalia, groins,* and *gluteal crease* may be affected. "Flexural" or inverse psoriasis is not uncommon in seborrheic subjects. It shows the typically salmon-red, demarcated plaques that frequently become eczematized, moist, and fissured; there is little scaling. Lesions in these locations, owing to perspiration, maceration and friction, may become extensive, sodden patches that burn and itch.

Numerous cases of psoriasis of the *mucous membranes* have been reported. The buccal mucosa, the tongue, and especially the lips may be involved. Hubler reported the association of geographic tongue

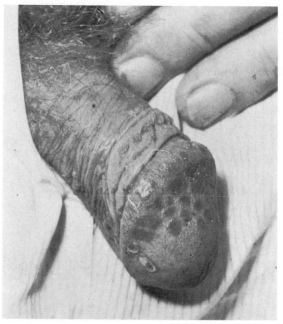

Figure 10–15. Psoriasis of penis. Predilection for the glans is characteristic, as is scantiness of scale.

and fissured tongue in generalized pustular psoriasis. Hietanen et al studied the oral mucosa in 200 consecutive psoriatic patients. They found histologically proven oral psoriasis in 2 per cent of patients.

Both the *fingernails* and *toenails* may be attacked. The characteristic changes are numerous pits 1 mm or so in diameter, like dents made with a ball-point pen; tan oval spots 2 to 4 mm in diameter ("oil spots"); onycholysis; uplifting of the distal portion from the nailbed; cracking of the free edges; and heaped-up crusts accumulated beneath them.

ETIOLOGY. The cause of psoriasis is still unknown. It is apparent that heredity is of decisive

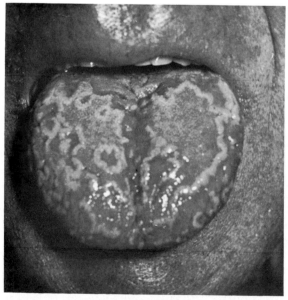

Figure 10–16. Psoriasis of tongue, glossitis annularis migrans.

significance. In a large study of psoriasis in monozygotic twins, Brandrup et al found heritability high and environmental influence low. A multifactorial inheritance is felt to be operating. There was a concordance rate of 65 per cent in the twins they studied.

INCIDENCE AND PREVALENCE. Psoriasis occurs with equal frequency in both sexes. Farber et al have shown that the onset of psoriasis is at a mean age of 27 years, but the range is wide, from a few months to the seventies. Some 36 per cent of 2144 patients knew of relatives who also had psoriasis. Hot weather improved psoriasis in 77 per cent, cold weather in 12 per cent, and sunlight in 78 per cent of patients.

Severe emotional stress tended to aggravate psoriasis in 40 per cent, and worry made psoriasis worse in 37 per cent; there was no definitive reaction in 42 per cent. There was arthritic involvement in 25 per cent of the patients. Complete periodic disappearance of psoriasis during its course was experienced by 39 per cent.

It has been shown that 1 to 2 per cent of the population has psoriasis. It occurs less frequently in the tropics. It is uncommon in blacks. American Indians and native Fijians do not have psoriasis. The correlation with certain HLA tissue genotypes is useless in assessment of individual cases.

In pregnancy there is a distinct tendency for improvement or even temporary disappearance. After childbirth there is a tendency for exacerbation of lesions. However, the psoriasis may behave differently from one pregnancy to another in the same patient. During menopause lesions may change for better or worse, with no set pattern of behavior.

PATHOGENESIS. Accelerated epidermopoiesis has been considered to be the fundamental pathologic event in psoriasis. The transit rate of psoriatic keratinocytes is increased and the deoxyribonucleic acid synthesis time is decreased. It has been suggested that it is the heightened proportion of epidermal cells participating in the proliferative process, rather than the actual rate of epidermopoiesis, that is the basic fault in psoriatic lesions. The result in either case is greatly increased production of keratin.

Ragaz and Ackerman have studied the histologic changes from the earliest erythematous macule through the mature hyperkeratotic plaque. The earliest change was an inflammatory perivascular upper dermal infiltrate, with only epidermal acanthosis and parakeratosis after the transformation of the lesion into a scaly papule. According to Farber et al, in the symptomless skin of the psoriatic, a similar upper dermal perivascular infiltrate is sometimes seen.

Voorhees has shown that polyamines are significantly increased in psoriatic lesions. There is an increased production of the leukotrienes and 12-hydroxy-eicosatetraenoic acid, both of which are chemotactic for polymorphonuclear leukocytes.

The Arachidonic Acid Cascade. The complexity of the pattern of inducers of inflammation is nowhere better shown than in the production of leukotrienes, prostaglandins, and eicosatetraenoic acid from arach-idonic acid. Arachidonic acid is obtained from dietary sources: membranes of red meat, green leafy vegetables, and corn and safflower oils. Its products are central to the aggravation of psoriasis by trauma, and to the pathogenesis of psoriatic lesions. It explains the aggravation of psoriasis by indomethacin (it enhances leukotriene formation) and its amelioration by benoxaprofen (which inhibits leukotriene production). And it leads to a helpful supportive treatment: eating more fish and less red meat (or none), and taking evening-primrose oil (to provide linolenic and gamma-linolenic acid). Benoxaprofen would help enormously; unhappily, strong suspicion of side effects has forced its withdrawal from the market. This cascade is reviewed in detail in an editorial by Voorhees and more recently by Ziboh.

Psoriasis is associated with different HLA antigens. They are B13, B17, Cw6, Bw16, and Bw37. It is believed that any individual who has B13 or B17 has a fivefold risk of developing psoriasis. In pustular psoriasis HLA-B27 may be seen, whereas B13 and B17 are increased in guttate and erythrodermic psoriasis. In palmoplantar pustulosis, there is an increased proportion of persons having HLA-B8, -Bw35, -Cw7, and -DR3.

Henseler and Christophers found HLA-Cw6 in 85.3 per cent of patients whose psoriasis began before age 30, and in less than 15 per cent of patients with onset after 30. In early-onset psoriasis, immediate family members were far more likely to be affected; disease tended to be widespread and frequently relapsing; and nail involvement was much more common.

Farber affirms an abnormal nucleoprotein metabolism in the incomplete keratinization process in psoriasis. In the stratum corneum the free amino acids are low, with an accumulation of mucopolysaccharides and of free and esterified choline. DNA and RNA accumulate, and pentose, purines, uracil, and organic phosphates are also increased.

There is a prominent neutrophil response in psoriatic lesions. How this relates to findings of increased plasminogen activator activity in psoriatic skin, or to the enhanced physiologic functions that have been attributed to psoriatic polymorphonuclear leukocytes, or to the immunologic findings of IgG and complement in the stratum corneum, is not yet known. Two other immunologic associations bear mentioning. Both psoriasis and Reiter's disease occur with increased frequency in patients with AIDS, as Onvic et al report. Also, interleukin-2 therapy for malignancy may induce psoriasis, by what mechanism is not clear.

Stress. Seville studied the relapse rate in 51 psoriatics who could recall stress as an aggravating factor in their disease. At three years after clearing under treatment, 83 per cent had relapsed; only 47 per cent of 81 cases who recalled no stress had relapsed. He compared the course of 31 patients with insight, under therapy: at three months, all had cleared (and

only 47 per cent of 30 patients without insight); at a year 93 per cent were still clear (and 33 per cent of those without insight); at three years, 74 per cent were clear (and 20 per cent of those without insight). He concluded that repression of emotional problems led to chronicity.

Weddell showed that there is a profuse hyperplasia of nerve endings beneath and into the lesions of psoriasis, just as there is in prurigo nodularis.

Farber et al have postulated that the regularity with which some cases of psoriasis are aggravated by emotional stress and the quite extraordinary symmetry of lesions suggest a neurogenic factor in pathogenesis. They implicate a neuropeptide, "substance P," in the process.

Drug-induced Psoriasis. Psoriasis may be induced by many drugs: beta blockers, lithium, antimalarials, and some nonsteroidal antiinflammatory agents, among others.

PATHOLOGY. The histologic changes in psoriasis are usually diagnostic. There is regular epidermal hyperplasia with long, test-tube-shaped rete ridges. There is atrophy over the dermal papillae, thus explaining Auspitz's sign. The granular layer is thin or absent, and there is overlying parakeratosis. Small collections of neutrophils (Munro microabscesses) may be present in the stratum corneum. The dermal papillae are prominent and contain ectatic vessels. There is a perivascular mononuclear cell infiltrate.

Lesions of guttate psoriasis are less characteristic histologically, and clinical-pathologic correlation is often necessary for determining the correct diagnosis.

HISTOLOGIC DIFFERENTIAL DIAGNOSIS. Psoriasis may be distinguished from eczema by the paucity of edema, the absence of spongiosis and vesicle formation, the clubbing of the papillary bodies, and the tortuosity of the capillary loops. In psoriasiform syphiloderm, the panarteritis and the plasma cell infiltration are characteristic; and in psoriasiform lesions of mycosis fungoides the infiltrate is composed of many different types of cells. The microabscesses of Darier and Pautrier in mycosis fungoides contain lymphocytes and monocytes, whereas the microabscesses of Munro in psoriasis contain polymorphonuclear leukocytes.

Hashimoto and Lever report that the electron microscopic findings in the epidermis of the psoriatic skin consist of dilatation of the intercellular spaces in the basal layer, decreased tonofilament formation within the basal cell layers, absence of keratohyaline granules, increased intracytoplasmic corpuscles (membrane-coated granules) in the stratum spinosum and stratum granulosum, and numerous lipoid bodies in these strata.

DIFFERENTIAL DIAGNOSIS. Psoriasis must be differentiated from seborrheic dermatitis, pityriasis rosea, lichen planus, eczema, the psoriasiform syphilid, and lupus erythematosus. The distribution in psoriasis is on the extensor surfaces, especially of the elbows and knees, and on the scalp, whereas in seborrheic dermatitis, although the scalp is involved, there is a predilection for the eyebrows, nasolabial angle, the ears, the sternal region, and the flexures. The scales in psoriasis are dry, white, and shiny, whereas those in seborrheic dermatitis are greasy and lusterless. On removal of the scales in psoriasis there is an oozing of blood from the capillaries (Auspitz's sign), whereas this does not occur in seborrheic dermatitis.

In pityriasis rosea the eruption is located on the upper arms, trunk, and thighs, and the duration is a matter of weeks. There are oval, fawn-colored patches that centrally show a crinkling of the epidermis and an almost imperceptible scaling, often of collarette type. The onset with the herald patch, and the tendency of the subsequent lesions to arrange themselves so that their long diameters are parallel to the direction of the rib, helps to distinguish between pityriasis rosea and psoriasis.

Lichen planus affects chiefly the flexor surfaces of the forearms and wrists, and the shins and ankles. The patches are pruritic and thickened. Often the violaceous color is pronounced, but at other times the patches are a dirty brown color and are then only distinguished from psoriasis by close examination, which reveals that the scaling is not at all micaceous, but scanty and tightly adherent, and that there are lichen papules at the edge of the patch. The scalp is much less frequently involved, and the nails are not pitted as in psoriasis, but longitudinally ridged and thickened, with pterygium a characteristic finding.

In atopic dermatitis the distribution is usually not on the extensor surfaces of the elbows and knees, and exudation and a slight grayish scaling, accompanied by severe itching, are present.

The psoriasiform syphilid has infiltrated patches of copper-colored papules, often arranged in a configurate manner. The scales are brownish and sparse. Serologic tests for syphilis are positive; a general adenopathy, and often mucous patches, condylomas, and other symptoms of late secondary syphilis are present. Itching is usually absent.

In lupus erythematosus, the lesions are discrete plaques, usually on the face and scalp, associated with atrophy, scaling, and alopecia. Rarely is the face affected by psoriasis. The scales of lupus erythematosus are grayish and adherent. Upon removal of the scale the undersurface is seen to be papillose due to the projecting follicular plugs. There is a psoriasiform subset of subacute cutaneous LE that may be distinguished by its location on the upper trunk, arms, and face and by other signs of LE such as photosensitivity.

Psoriatics are not immune to other diseases, however; psoriasis, elicited by a Koebner response, may accompany other diseases, or follow them when they subside. This is of great practical importance in relation to neurodermatitis circumscripta, seborrheic dermatitis, drug eruptions, scarlatina or other exanthems, and palmoplantar pompholyx.

Psoriasis and Skin Cancer. For years it was believed that patients with psoriasis enjoyed particular freedom from skin cancer. However, Halprin et al in 1982 found in 150 psoriatics who had never been treated with PUVA that the incidence of skin cancer (basal and squamous cell combined) was 1.96 per year—three times that of a control group of diabetics. Stern emphasized a caveat mentioned by Halprin: that psoriatics have often been exposed to carcinogens (UVR); topical nitrogen mustard was mentioned, but surely few psoriatics have had it used on them. Bias is introduced because skin cancer might result in admission to hospital, and because psoriatics' skin is subject to more careful examination than diabetics'. In response, Halprin agreed completely, but added that—whatever the causes—psoriatics do have more skin cancer than nonpsoriatics. Pittelkow et al detailed the follow-up for 25 years of a group of psoriatics who were treated with UV radiation and coal tar (the Goeckerman regimen). They found that there was no appreciable increase of skin cancer above that in the general population.

TREATMENT. The lesions may disappear spontaneously or as the result of therapy, but recurrences are almost certain, and there is a tendency for each remedy to lose its effectiveness gradually. Treatment methods will vary according to the site, severity, duration, previous treatment, and the age of the patient. In some instances treatment may be solely topical, or it may be systemic, or a combination of both.

Topical Treatment. In many patients topical applications alone will suffice to keep psoriasis under control. Numerous local medications are available.

Corticosteroids. Topical application of corticosteroids in creams, ointments, lotions, and sprays is the most frequent therapy. The most potent topical steroid is clobetasol propionate. Van Scott suggests up to three separate two-week courses, with two weeks' rest between. On the scalp corticosteroids in propylene glycol or a gel base are used; the creams are preferred in the intertriginous areas and in exposed areas. With all corticosteroids, ointments are more effective than creams of the same strength (Stoughton).

To augment effectiveness of the topical corticosteroids, a corticosteroid cream or ointment is applied to the lesion; this is then followed by an occlusive dressing of a polyethylene film (Saran Wrap), which remains in place for 12 to 24 hours at a time. A prompt response is usually noted. Unfortunately there is recurrence of the lesions within a short time with this type of therapy. It is not so much an effective treatment as a way of life. Moreover, side effects (miliaria, pyoderma, epidermal atrophy) may be troublesome and even serious.

Intralesional corticosteroid suspensions of triamcinolone are frequently used, either by intralesional injections with the hypodermic needle or by the dermajet, which injects the medication by air pressure. The authors use triamcinolone acetonide (Kenalog) suspension 10 mg per ml, which may be diluted with distilled sterile water to make a concentration of 5 mg per ml or even 2.5 mg. A 30-gauge needle and a 1-ml disposable plastic tuberculin syringe are strongly recommended. There is (except in premenopausal women not on contraceptive pills) no reason to limit the dose thus injected to less than 60 mg in any one session, or in any one month.

This is an excellent method for treating small lesions of psoriasis. Usually one injection produces clearing at the site of insertion. Good results are also obtained in the treatment of psoriatic nails by injecting triamcinolone into the region of the matrix and the lateral nail folds. Injections are given once a month. The intertriginous areas such as the inframammary, inguinal, and perianal regions are effectively treated with the corticosteroid creams or aerosol sprays. Irritation is thereby eliminated.

It should be remembered that intralesional therapy may cause atrophy of the subcutaneous tissue at the site of injection. Usually the depression will disappear in a few months.

Of all localized methods, intralesional steroid therapy is the most ideal because of its prompt and effective action, and because of its long-acting benefit. The only untoward side effect is thinning, paling, and depression of the treated area, which may be severe enough to be unsightly and even create a medicolegal problem. Pyoderma may occur after treatment of lesions on the foot or ankle. The method deserves more frequent use, tedious though it is when lesions are numerous or large.

Tars. The staining property and odor of the tars may hinder the use of these otherwise effective topical medications. Several tar ointments from which the staining properties have been removed are now available. One is Tarstill (Gorga), available in lotion or 2 per cent ointment forms. Another is Estar Gel (Westwood). Coal tar solution or liquor carbonis detergens is applied to the lesions before ultraviolet treatment in the Goeckerman method. It is also incorporated into liquid soap solutions to be used for a tar bath. Oil of cade (pine tar) or birch tar in concentrations of 5 to 10 per cent may be incorporated into ointments.

For severe psoriasis of the scalp a combination of 20 per cent oil of cade, 10 per cent sulfur, and 5 per cent salicylic acid in hydrophilic ointment is effective. Another, somewhat pleasanter regimen is the use of Keralyt (salicylic acid) Gel, Topsyn (betamethasone) Gel, and Estar Gel, either together or consecutively, as suggested by Rees.

Iodochlorhydroxyquin (Vioform). This has also been used frequently. A 3 per cent ointment or cream rubbed in several times daily is moderately helpful.

Dihydroxyanthralin (Anthralin). This has been extensively used for over 50 years, and is of unquestionable effectiveness. But it is highly irritating, and stains skin, clothing, and bedding. To avoid these drawbacks, lower concentrations (0.01–1 per cent) have been used, and Pearlman et al tried anthralin "soft paste" (0.1–0.2 per cent with 0.2 per cent salicylic acid, with 2.5 per cent hard paraffin in equal parts ZnO paste and petrolatum), or "stiff paste" (anthralin 0.2–0.8 per cent with 0.4–0.8 per cent salicylic acid, in 5 per cent hard paraffin in zinc oxide paste), occluded with adhesive paper tape. Treatment was carried out only at night; it was wiped off

with mineral oil in the morning. Irritation was negligible and results were very good.

Studies using anthralin in a short contact time have shown good results, especially when a 0.5 to 3.0 per cent concentration is applied for 10 to 30 minutes and removed.

Retinoic Acid. Retinoic acid has been used in 0.05 per cent concentration in ointment form (Retin-A). It acts like anthralin. Frequently a moderately severe reaction is induced at the site of application and it is therefore contraindicated in generalized psoriasis.

Salicylic Acid. Usually a 3 to 5 per cent concentration is incorporated into cold cream or hydrophilic ointment. Keralyt Gel, 6 per cent salicylic acid in a gel base, is an excellent formulation. Ross compared Keralyt-Estar-Topsyn in combination with 10 per cent salicylic acid in Sofsyn oil and in plain mineral oil; they were equally effective.

Ultraviolet Light. In most instances strong sunlight improves psoriasis remarkably. However, sudden burning of the untanned skin may cause a Koebner phenomenon and an exacerbation.

Artificial ultraviolet light (UVB) is frequently used as a substitute. In persistently recurring cases it is often advisable for the patient to own an ultraviolet lamp and to expose himself daily to this form of therapy. A General Electric or Westinghouse sunlamp is inexpensive. Daily exposures should be regulated so as not to produce burns but only a mild transient erythema. A fixed treatment distance such as three feet should be used. The time of exposure can be slowly increased by a few seconds daily, starting with an exposure of two minutes. Tar applications or baths prior to UVB have been credited with enhancing its effect, but Stern et al studied 22 patients with respect to halves of the body treated with UVB alone, and tar oil followed by UVB and found a maximum of 9 per cent reduction in clearing time after use of the tar oil.

Using a monochromator, Parrish and Jaenicke found that wavelengths of 254, 280, and 290 nm were ineffective; at 296, 300, 304, and 313 nm, there was clearing, with the lowest total dose achieved by fixed daily doses, not by an incrementally increased daily dose.

For widespread and recalcitrant psoriasis ultraviolet therapy combined with tar or anthralin applications is the basis for the Goeckerman and Ingram treatment techniques. Recent studies indicate that an emollient followed by suberythemogenic doses of UVB gives results comparable to those with the use of a tar followed by UVB. In a recent study it was shown that maintenance UVB phototherapy after clearing contributes to the duration of remission and is justified for many patients.

GOECKERMAN TECHNIQUE. This is an effective and frequently gratifying method of treatment, and despite the popularity of PUVA treatment, the Goeckerman treatment with its many modifications continues to be popular. The technique has been modified, simplified, and changed, but basically the principles are the same as originally described. Essentially a 2 to 5 per cent tar preparation such as Zetar, ichthammol, Balnetar, or liquor carbonis detergens is applied to the skin several times daily and a tar bath is taken at least once daily. Daily the excess tar is removed with mineral or vegetable oil and ultraviolet light is applied. Petrozzi et al find 1 per cent crude coal tar in hydrophilic ointment still the most effective. Diette et al have shown UVA added to UVB does not add significant benefit to the Goeckerman regimen.

Menter and Cram reported the results of Goeckerman therapy in two day-care centers, in a population of 300 severe resistant cases; they cleared in an average of 18 days, and 75 per cent remained free of disease for more than 1 year. Muller and Perry have lately reviewed the Mayo Clinic experience of 60 years of Goeckerman therapy, and found it good. Remission may be speeded and prolonged if 60 mg triamcinolone acetonide is given intramuscularly before the Goeckerman regimen is started. This was Pillsbury's customary routine. Horwitz et al showed that the addition of a topical hydrocortisone cream to the Goeckerman regimen shortened the time required for remission.

The role of coal tar in this regimen was questioned by LeVine and Parrish in 1980 and again by Belsito and Kechijian in 1982, who confirmed the finding of the former that the ointment base alone (plus UVR) was as effective as crude coal tar ointment against psoriasis, in a Goeckerman regimen. Eells et al in 1983 confirmed this; they found not only no advantage in the preliminary use of coal tar, but also no advantage in pushing the dose of UVR to an erythemogenic level. Halprin also found a constant low dose of UVR as effective as a progressively increasing one.

Ingram Technique. The Ingram method consists of a daily coal tar bath in a solution such as 120 ml liquor carbonis detergens to 80 liters of warm water. This is followed by exposure to an ultraviolet light for daily increasing periods. An anthralin paste is then applied to each psoriatic plaque. Talcum powder is sprinkled over the lesions and stockinette dressings are applied.

The method requires close attention to details and personal supervision; if properly used, it is very effective.

PUVA Therapy. Parrish and Fitzpatrick in 1974 reported that high-intensity longwave ultraviolet radiation (UVA) preceded by two hours by a phototoxic enhancing dose of 10 to 30 mg of 8-methoxypsoralen (Oxsoralen), and given two or three times a week, would completely clear almost every patient with severe psoriasis in 20 to 25 treatments. It induces no remissions: maintenance treatment must be continued indefinitely, usually about once a week. A new dosage form of methoxsalen with greater bioavailability, Oxsoralen-Ultra, is now standard. Tables in the package insert (or the PDR) should be referred to for the dose. The risk of enhanced carcinogenesis is now proven, with a reversal of the usual ratio of squamous cell carcinomas to basal cell carcinomas. Accelerated actinic elastosis, melanocyte dysplasia,

the potential for eye damage, and the deleterious effects on lymphocytes all remain areas of concern when deciding whether to recommend this to any patient. One of us (Arnold) has never employed it. Great care in quantitating the doses of psoralen (P) and light (UVA) is essential.

Boer et al in the Netherlands compared UVB and PUVA and found that, in patients with less than 50 per cent of the skin surface affected, UVB was as good as PUVA or better. In more extensive cases, PUVA required less frequent maintenance therapy.

X-Ray Treatment. Although effective, ionizing radiation should be used very rarely if at all in the treatment of psoriasis. The many hazards of overtreatment far outweigh the temporary beneficial results achieved by either the superficial x-rays or the low-voltage grenz rays.

Because of the overpublicized and largely unwarranted fear of x-ray therapy in benign skin diseases producing cancer of the thyroid gland and breasts, we have completely abandoned the use of all forms of x-ray therapy in psoriasis, and in almost all other benign skin conditions as well.

Surgical Treatment. Though no one seriously embraces it as an acceptable therapy, denervation by surgery has long been known to abolish psoriatic plaques, and in 1985 Jette et al reported that surgical excision in 24 patients of a psoriatic plaque to the depth of the reticular dermis, with a dermatome, completely abolished the lesion for 3 to 36 months in 17 and required only re-excision of minor recurrences in the other seven.

Hyperthermia. Twenty-two chronic psoriatic plaques in nine patients were heated to 42–45° C with ultrasound for 30 minutes three times a week for four to 10 treatments, by Orenberg et al, and 15 completely cleared; only two remained unchanged. They relapsed within three months. Urabe et al carried out various conventional therapies on one side of the body in 22 patients with plaque psoriasis, and heated the opposite half of the body with exothermal pads continuously for five weeks. Skin lesions disappeared from the heated side in 19 patients.

Methotrexate. This drug penetrated the stratum corneum poorly and was considered ineffective topically until Weinstein et al found that in a base containing 3 to 7 per cent laurocapram (Azone), 0.1 to 1 per cent methotrexate temporarily cleared psoriatic plaques. The benefit was, mysteriously, not dose related.

Occlusive Treatment. Shore reported clearing of psoriatic lesions by occluding them with tape. Friedman showed that hydrocolloid occlusion (with Actiderm) had a similar effect on small lesions.

Internal Treatment. In some instances psoriatic involvement may be so extensive and recalcitrant that systemic treatment is necessary.

Corticosteroids. The hazards of the injudicious use of oral corticosteroids must be emphasized. The side effects of orally administered prednisone are so dangerous that its use should be limited to patients who are in great distress and who do not respond to other measures. There is great risk of "rebound" or induction of pustular psoriasis when it is stopped.

However, the much smaller and far safer total dose made possible by the use of intramuscularly injected triamcinolone acetonide, and the absence of any rebound at all following its use, make it a highly satisfactory treatment *for some responsive patients.* A trial may be made, and patients who have good clearing and long remissions, so that they require retreatment only every nine to 10 weeks or longer, may be safely controlled with it for very long periods. Cataracts, osteoporosis, hypertension, and impairment of carbohydrate metabolism do not occur.

Cyclosporine. This relatively new T-helper–cell suppressant, which has many serious side effects, may rarely have a place in the treatment of psoriasis. It is marketed as Sandimmune in an intravenous and a liquid oral form. Van Hooff et al, Wentzell et al, and others have reported on its use in psoriasis.

Voorhees has established its effectiveness, and freedom from side effects for the one-month study period, in a preliminary study; relapses occurred in two weeks to three months. Doses as low as 3 to 6 mg/kg/day—which are virtually free of side effects even for long periods—may be therapeutically effective. It is not yet approved for use in psoriasis, but it is available.

Methotrexate. This folic acid antagonist, used as an antimitotic agent, is currently one of the most effective and safest medications for the treatment of extensive and severe psoriasis. Methotrexate has a greater affinity for dihydrofolic acid reductase than has folic acid. The synthesis of deoxyribonucleic acid is blocked when dihydrofolic acid reductase is bound and thereby cell division is thwarted; in psoriasis the greatly increased epidermal cell turnover rate is slowed.

Numerous treatment schedules have evolved. Of these the ones recommended are either three divided oral doses (12 hours apart) weekly, weekly doses orally, or single weekly intravenous or intramuscular injections.

The weekly oral dose—2.5 to 7.5 or rarely even 10 mg at 12-hour intervals for three doses, one day each week—is the most widely used. One of us (HLA) has used it for 30 years without seeing a single example of a serious side effect.

Before treatment is started it is important to make sure that the patient has no history of liver or kidney disease. Other contraindications are alcohol abuse, severe illness, debility, pregnancy (or nursing), male or female fertility, leucopenia, thrombocytopenia, active infectious disease, immune deficiency, anemia, or colitis. Blood urea nitrogen (BUN), serum glutamic oxaloacetic transaminase, serum glutamic pyruvic transaminase, bilirubin, creatinine, alkaline phosphatase, chest x-ray, complete blood count, thrombocyte count, and urinalysis should all be done before starting treatment. In addition, a liver biopsy is advised by many authorities, though many do not insist upon it. One of us (HLA), during 30 years' use of the drug in a great many cases, made it a practice to insist on liver biopsy only when there was some contraindication present indicative of liver damage. Exceptions to requiring liver biopsy may include obesity, age, or illness such as pustular psoriasis, or the anticipated short-term use of the drug.

The most frequent side reactions in our experience have been anorexia, headache, and nausea and vomiting. Other toxic effects are leukopenia and thrombocytopenia. Gastrointestinal ulceration, hepatotoxicity with degenerative changes, and hepatic necrosis or cirrhosis may occur. Several deaths have been reported. Ongoing monitoring during therapy should include a leukocyte count and platelet count every one to four weeks; hemoglobin, urinalysis, creatinine, SGOT, SGPT, and alkaline phosphatase every four months; and creatinine clearance and chest x-ray once yearly. Liver biopsy after each 1500 mg of the drug has been recommended.

Zachariae et al did 764 liver biopsies in 328 patients using divided weekly doses of methotrexate; cirrhosis occurred in 21, after 590 to 8105 (average, 2200) mg of methotrexate, and without any abnormal liver function tests. Five of the eight patients with cirrhosis had a history of arsenic treatment *and* had only taken 590 to 1585 mg of methotrexate. Continuation of methotrexate did not increase the degree of cirrhosis in the few patients in which it was done. Nyfors found cirrhosis in 14 (21 per cent) of 68 psoriatics whose mean total dose had increased from 3 to 4 gm over a period of about 5½ years. Alcohol intake, age, and obesity were factors favoring development of cirrhosis. Cirrhosis occurred in only 1 of 92 patients after a mean methotrexate dose of 2287 gm.

Voorhees has looked for chromosomal damage subsequent to methotrexate treatment of psoriasis. No increase in chromosomal abnormalities was found.

Psoriasis treated with methotrexate follows a variable course. The early, sometimes spectacular improvement is frequently followed by a sluggish response, even to increased amounts of methotrexate. In other cases the psoriasis is kept under control with only infrequent treatment; however, lasting remissions are exceptional. Topical methotrexate, recently reported by Weinstein et al, holds some promise of being helpful.

Three decades of experience, according to Farber and associates, have given us no indication of any enhancement of carcinogenesis as a result of methotrexate therapy. Updated guidelines for methotrexate use were reported by Roenigk et al in 1988.

Diet. Ever since psoriasis became known as an entity there have been frequent dietary restrictions imposed upon the unfortunate psoriatic patient. The dietary fads have come and gone and psoriasis is still rampant. Zackheim and Farber have concluded after controlled studies that various dietary restrictions, especially those of low protein intake, cause no appreciable difference in the course of psoriasis. Ziboh has reviewed the theoretical benefits of increased vegetable or fish oil content of the diet. This is unproved to date as a practical measure.

Oral Antimicrobial Therapy. Rosenberg has published extensively on the aggravation of psoriasis by activation of the alternate pathway of complement by *Malassezia ovalis*, or by intestinal yeasts, or by endotoxins produced by gram-negative bacteria in the gut. He believed this helps to explain the following:

1. Seborrheic localization (*M. ovalis* effect).
2. Poststreptococcal flares.
3. Diaper area lesions (*C. albicans*).
4. Precipitation by typhoid vaccine (which contains endotoxin).
5. Improvement during imprisonment and relapse when Enterobacteriaceae return to the gut on resumption of a "good" Western diet.
6. Severity of psoriasis in alcoholics, who are not well protected against release of endotoxins into the circulation by their damaged Kupffer cells.

Crutcher has confirmed the beneficial effect of oral nystatin, 1,000,000 units three times a day, reported earlier by Baker, and by Rosenberg himself, and observed by one of us (HLA). Rosenberg has achieved good results with oral ketoconazole.

Relevant are reports of the beneficial action of metronidazole (Flagyl) in acute flares of plaque psoriasis.

Combination Chemotherapy. Alper et al combined 5-FU with either methotrexate or triacetyl-azauridine in nine patients, most of whom did well and tolerated the treatment well. It is a potential alternative therapy in recalcitrant cases. Pearlman et al reported some success on localized lesions using 5-FU topically or intralesionally.

Peritoneal Dialysis. In the treatment of severe, intractable psoriasis peritoneal dialysis may yield impressive results. Side effects may be the development of hernias and peritonitis in some 18 per cent of the cases. Rappaport et al, in a double-blind crossover study of seven very severe cases of psoriasis, used peritoneal dialysis and observed no improvement whatever. Whittier et al compared "real" peritoneal dialysis with sham dialysis of their own devising in five patients with severe, extensive plaque psoriasis; two cleared, and two markedly improved (one did not respond) on "real" dialysis; none improved on sham dialysis. Rasmussen reported a severe case of some years' duration in a 13-year-old girl that cleared completely without any therapy at all two weeks after investigations had shown she was not, after all, a suitable candidate for dialysis. Hemofiltration was employed by Steck et al weekly for four weeks in 11 patients with severe psoriasis; six cleared substantially; the other five, though they were not much improved, were later cleared easily and rapidly by topical therapy (which had previously been ineffective). Cuprophan (Travenol Laboratories), Polyacrylonite (Hospital Medical Corp.), and polysulfone (Amicon Corp.) were the membranes used. No adverse effects were seen. The method is still experimental.

Retinoic Acid. Treatment internally with 13-cis-retinoic acid has been reported by G. L. Peck of NIH to produce good results. The dosage used was 0.5 to 7.4 mg/kg/day from one to 55 weeks. Side effects are cheilitis, conjunctivitis sicca, facial dermatitis, xerosis, rhinitis sicca with nose bleed, and skin fragility. It is still experimental.

Klaus Wolf has combined this retinoic acid derivative with photochemotherapy. In this manner he has been able to reduce the amount of UVA given during the course of treatment by 75 per cent.

The aromatic retinoid ethylester, etretinate, appears to be far more effective in generalized pustular psoriasis, at a dose level of 1 mg/kg/day. Its effects in psoriatic erythroderma are also impressive. Wolska and Jablonska reported their results in a double-blind study; it is the treatment of choice in pustular psoriasis. Roenigk et al reported 12 patients treated for three years, with four liver biopsies each; there was no evidence of hepatotoxicity in any of them. Kaplan et al treated 20 patients with 0.75 mg/kg/day and all but one noted marked improvement to clearing in six months' time. Psoriatic arthritis improved significantly in four of seven patients. Side effects of dry lips, skin, and nasal mucosa; hair loss; and skin fragility were observed. Triglycerides were elevated in 11 patients. Remission lasted about eight weeks, and maintenance therapy was required, usually 20 to 60 mg/day. All retinoids are teratogenic, and etretinate is stored in the fat for years.

Lowe et al reviewed the status of etretinate in psoriasis. It is especially useful in plaque disease in combination with anthralin, UVB, PUVA, or topical steroids.

Acitretin was found by Gollnick et al to be as effective as etretinate. It has a very much shorter half-life in the body.

Dapsone. A controlled study by Corrales-Padilha showed that dapsone in a dose of 100 mg twice a day for three weeks and 100 mg daily for one week was three times as effective as a placebo and yielded only one fourth as many failures. However, dapsone is not well tolerated and side effects may be serious. Its usefulness in psoriasis is limited largely to palmoplantar pustulosis.

Somatostatin. Weber observed complete or partial remission in 22 of 26 psoriatics given somatostatin (an inhibitor of human growth hormone) by intravenous drip. Joint pains in the four with arthropathic psoriasis responded as well.

Vitamin D. Morimoto et al in 1989 reviewed experience with vitamin D_3 in psoriasis. Several studies have reported success with both topical and oral regimens. It holds some hope.

Types of Psoriasis

Seborrheic-like Psoriasis. In some cases of psoriasis prominent features of seborrheic dermatitis may occur not only in the typical sites of psoriasis vulgaris but also in the flexural areas such as the

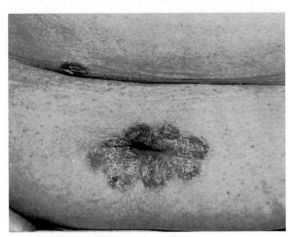

Figure 10–17. Seborrhea-like psoriasis of the umbilicus.

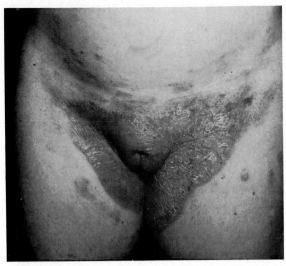

Figure 10–19. Psoriasis (inverse psoriasis) in inguinal region of a 5-year-old girl.

antecubital areas, axillae, under the breasts, groins, and intergluteal areas. The lesions are moist and erythematous with minimal amount of greasy and soft scales rather than dry and micaceous. This pattern of eruption is also known as **inverse psoriasis** (see below). Terms such as **seborrhiasis** and **seborrheic psoriasis** may be heard in these unusual cases.

Inverse Psoriasis. Also known as **flexural psoriasis** or (on palms or soles) **volar psoriasis**, this form is so called because it selectively and often exclusively involves folds, recesses, and flexor surfaces: ears, axillae, groins, inframammary folds, navel, intergluteal crease, glans penis, lips, and above all, the palms, soles, and nails. The scalp quite often participates as well. In the involved nail (or more often, nails), simple onycholysis may be seen, or there may be more diagnostic pitting. "Oil spots," round or oval areas of onycholysis 2 to 6 mm in diameter in the nail bed, not extending to the free distal border, are more characteristic and diagnostic than the more commonly seen distal onycholysis. Nail pitting is even more common. In such cases, a characteristic lesion elsewhere or a positive family history may help confirm the diagnosis. Pillsbury has called inverse psoriasis one of the most underdiagnosed of dermatologic entities, and we strongly agree.

"Napkin" Psoriasis. Diaper dermatitis, caused by the irritative effects of urine in the wet diaper area, may imitate a psoriasiform eruption. In addition, there is commonly infection with *C. albicans*, as shown by cultures for fungus. On the other hand, napkin psoriasis, or psoriasis in the diaper area, may also be seen in infants between two and eight months of age. A diagnosis of true psoriasis must be extremely guarded unless typical psoriatic lesions are present in other sites of predilection for psoriasis.

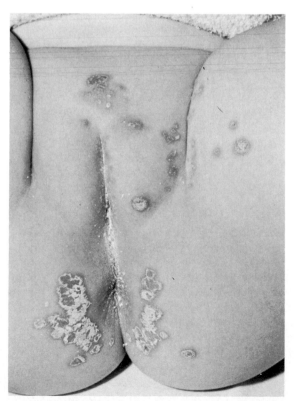

Figure 10–20. Napkin psoriasis, from which Candida albicans *was cultured, in a 7-month-old child.*

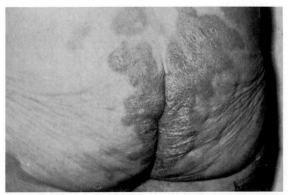

Figure 10–18. Intertriginous psoriasis (inverse psoriasis) extending onto buttocks.

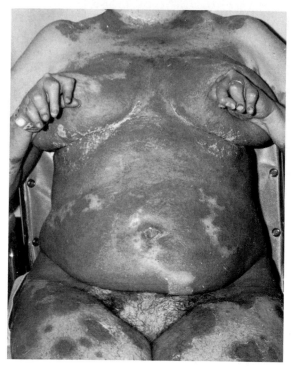

Figure 10–21. Psoriatic arthritis. Notice the claw hands.

Lichen-Planuslike Psoriasis. In some cases of psoriasis many of the individual papules and small patches may have the characteristics of lichen planus and at the same time resemble psoriasis. The areas affected tend to be those favored by lichen planus, i.e., the inner thighs, both flexor and extensor surfaces of the upper extremities, and the lower legs.

Psoriatic Arthritis. The incidence of psoriasis is 10 times greater in persons with seronegative arthritis than in persons without arthritis. Five clinical patterns occur:

1. Asymmetric distal interphalangeal joint involvement with nail damage (16 per cent of cases).
2. Arthritis mutilans with osteolysis of phalanges and metacarpals (5 per cent).

3. Symmetric polyarthritislike rheumatoid arthritis, with claw hands (15 per cent).
4. Oligoarthritis with swelling and tenosynovitis of one or a few hand joints (70 per cent).
5. Ankylosing spondylitis alone or with peripheral arthritis (5 per cent).

In most cases radiographic findings are the same as in rheumatoid arthritis; suggestive of psoriasis, however, are erosion of terminal phalangeal tufts (acroösteolysis); tapering or "whittling" of phalanges or metacarpals; "cupping" of proximal ends of phalanges; bony ankylosis; osteolysis of metatarsals; predilection for DIP and PIP joints and relative sparing of MCP and MTP joints; paravertebral ossification; asymmetric sacroiliitis; and rarity of "bamboo spine" when the spine is involved. Nearly half the patients with psoriatic arthritis have HLA-B27; in any individual case, therefore, a flipped coin would provide an equally valuable diagnostic criterion, and cost less.

Rest, splinting, passive motion, and aspirin or indomethacin are appropriate. Methotrexate, chrysotherapy, etretinate, and intramuscular triamcinolone are all likely to help both the psoriasis and the arthritis.

Guttate Psoriasis. In this distinctive form of psoriasis typical lesions are the size of water drops, 2 to 5 mm in diameter. This type usually occurs as a severe eruption following some acute infection, such as a streptococcal pharyngitis. Whyte and Baughman found abnormal antistreptolysin (ASO) titers in 17 of their 20 patients with acute guttate psoriasis. In all 20 patients, severe upper respiratory infection preceded the onset of the psoriasis by one to two weeks.

We have seen guttate psoriasis mostly in patients under 30. Recurrent episodes are likely, because of pharyngeal carriage of the responsible streptococcus. If penicillin or cephalosporin fail to eradicate it, rifampin should be tried: it has been successful in many cases.

Generalized Pustular Psoriasis (von Zumbusch). This severe and sometimes even fatal form of psoriasis with pustular involvement is known as generalized pustular psoriasis of von Zumbusch. It is

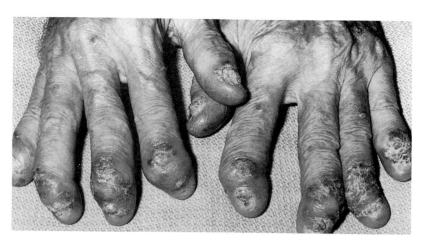

Figure 10–22. Psoriatic arthritis. (Courtesy of Dr. R. Hochman.)

of pustules, then there are flare-ups of fever and pustules, and finally continuous fever, erythroderma, and cachexia.

Although the etiology of this type is not any better known than that of psoriasis vulgaris, Shelley has shown that iodides and salicylates may trigger the attacks. There is usually a strong familial history of psoriasis. Ogawa et al reported it as having been evoked by the topical use of crude coal tar.

Its incidence in Japan closely parallels the use of oral systemic steroids in the treatment of psoriasis, and a causal relationship is suspected. We have not observed its occurrence during therapy with intramuscular triamcinolone.

Generalized pustular psoriasis may occur in infants and in children. Beylot et al cite 48 cases in which the peaks of onset were at the ages of one and five years. Fifty per cent were of the Zumbusch type. It may occur as an episodic event punctuating the course of localized acral pustular psoriasis. Rarely, it may be familial. Hubler reported such a kindred, in which three siblings had chronic localized acral-pustular psoriasis with episodes of generalized pustular psoriasis.

Histologic examination shows a characteristic spongiform pustule in the upper epidermis. The pustule is lined with swollen epidermal cells and contains polymorphonuclear leukocytes. Spongiform pustules are also seen in acrodermatitis continua of Hallopeau, impetigo herpetiformis, and keratosis blennorrhagica (Reiter's syndrome).

Etretinate is the drug of choice in this severe disease. Response is rapid and predictable. Isotretonoin is inferior. Cyclosporin and acitretin are alternatives.

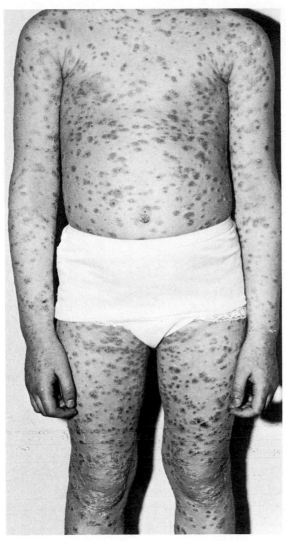

Figure 10–23. Guttate psoriasis. (Courtesy of Dr. R. Feinstein.)

considered the most severe type of psoriasis, with serious systemic involvement such as hepatitis. Typical patients have had psoriasis and psoriatic arthritis.

The onset is sudden, with formation of lakes of pus periungually, on the palms, and in psoriatic plaques. Erythema occurs in the flexures before the generalized eruption appears. This is followed by a generalized erythema and more pustules. Pruritus and intense burning cause extreme discomfort. There is fever, and a fetid odor develops. The pustules dry up to form yellow-brown crusts over a reddish brown, shiny surface. Some of the lesions are patches of typical psoriasis vulgaris.

Mucous membrane lesions are common on the tongue and in the mouth. There are red scaling of the lips and superficial ulcerations of the tongue and mouth. Hubler has reported three families in which five examples of geographic tongue and fissured tongue, along with pustular psoriasis, occurred.

Zumbusch psoriasis may go through several stages. There is the exanthematous febrile eruption

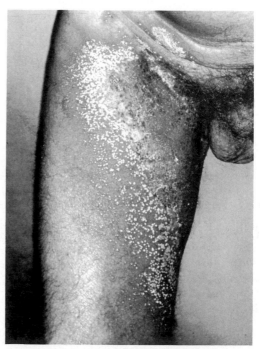

Figure 10–24. Pustular psoriasis.

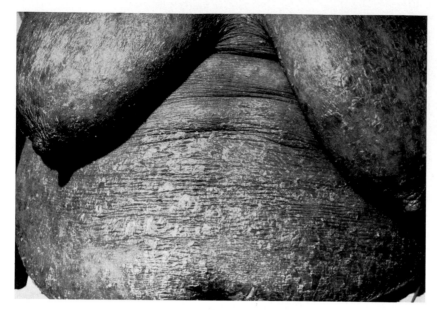

Figure 10–25. Generalized pustular psoriasis, exfoliative stage. *(Courtesy of Dr. J. Teich.)*

Methotrexate is also effective in carefully selected cases and, in a patient with an uncompromised liver, appears to be safer by far than systemic corticosteroids.

Sometimes dapsone (Avlosulfon, Ayerst) is effective. The dose is 50 mg daily and then increased. MacMillan and Champion reported successful suppression in one man for over an 18-month period starting with 300 mg dapsone daily.

The differential diagnosis of pustular psoriasis should include subcorneal pustular dermatosis and eosinophilic pustular folliculitis.

Subcorneal Pustular Dermatosis. Sanchez et al suspect that this disease, which was described by Sneddon and Wilkinson in 1956, is "strongly associated biologically, clinically, and histopathologically with psoriasis, and that continued observation of the clinical course may . . . substantiate this relationship in many cases." Many of their cases, however, were not associated with psoriasis, indicating subcorneal pustular dermatosis may develop sui generis. This disease will be discussed in more detail in Chapter 21.

Eosinophilic Pustular Folliculitis (Ofuji's Syndrome). This name has been given to spreading red macules with follicular pustules in their periphery. There is little or no spongiosis, and eosinophils are numerous. All immunofluorescent stains are negative. Degos and Braun-Falco believe it is atypical psoriasis. Ofuji originally believed it to be a variant of subcorneal pustular dermatosis. Its exact etiology is as yet unknown. It responds well to steroids, oxyphenbutazone, and dapsone. Colton et al recently reviewed the literature on this subject, which will be more fully discussed in Chapter 21.

Ise S, et al: Subcorneal pustular dermatosis: A follicular variant? Arch Dermatol 1965, 92:169.

Nunzi E, et al: Ofuji's disease: High titers of IgG and IgM directed to basal cell cytoplasm. JAAD 1985, 12:268.

Vakilzadeh F, et al: Eosinophilic spongiosis with pemphigus-like antibody. Dermatologica 1981, 106:347.

PSORIASIS

Abel EA, et al: Epidermal dystrophy and actinic keratoses in psoriasis patients following oral psoralen photochemotherapy (PUVA). JAAD 1982, 7:333.

Idem: Drugs exacerbating psoriasis. JAAD 1986, 15:1007.

Alper JC, et al: Rationally designed combination chemotherapy for the treatment of patients with recalcitrant psoriasis. JAAD 1985, 13:567.

Anderson PC: Dialysis treatment of psoriasis. Arch Dermatol 1981, 117:67.

Anderson TF, et al: UV-B phototherapy. Arch Dermatol 1984, 120:1502.

Idem: Metabolic aspects of psoriasis: The basis for specific therapy. Postgr Med 1980, 67:135.

Armstrong RB, et al: Modified Goeckerman therapy for psoriasis. Arch Dermatol 1984, 120:313.

Ashton RE, et al: Anthralin: Historical and current perspectives. JAAD 1983, 9:173.

Idem: Complications in methotrexate therapy of psoriasis with particular reference to liver fibrosis. J Invest Dermatol 1982, 79:229.

Brandrup F, et al: Psoriasis in monozygotic twins. Acta Derm-Venerol (Stockh) 1982, 62:229.

Comaish S: Ingram method of treating psoriasis. Arch Dermatol 1965, 92:56.

Corrales-Padilha H: Avlosulfon in psoriasis. Dermatologia, Revista Mex 1966, 10:270.

Cram DL: Psoriasis: Current advances in etiology and treatment. JAAD 1981, 4:1.

Crutcher N, et al: Oral nystatin in the treatment of psoriasis (letter). Arch Dermatol 1984, 120:435.

Diette KM, et al: Role of ultraviolet A therapy for psoriasis. JAAD 1984, 11:441.

Duvic M, et al: AIDS-associated psoriasis and Reiter's syndrome. Arch Dermatol 1988, 123:1622.

Economidou J, et al: HLA A, B, and C in Greek patients with psoriasis. JAAD 1985, 13:578.

Eells LD, et al: Comparison of euberythemogenic and maximally aggressive ultraviolet therapy for psoriasis. JAAD 1984, 11:105.

Ellis CN, et al: Cyclosporine improves psoriasis. JAMA 1986, 256:3110.

Farber EM, et al: Psoriasis: Questionnaire survey of 2,144 patients. Arch Dermatol 1968, 98:248.

Idem: Current status of oral PUVA therapy for psoriasis. JAAD 1979, 1:106.

Idem: Current status of oral PUVA therapy for psoriasis; Eye protection revisions. JAAD 1982, 6:851.

Idem: Recent advances in the treatment of psoriasis. JAAD 1983, 8:311.

Idem: Long-term risks of psoralen and UV-A therapy for psoriasis. Arch Dermatol 1983, 119:426.

Idem: Psoriasis: A disease of the total skin. JAAD 1985, 12:150.

Idem: Stress, symmetry, and psoriasis: Possible role of neuropeptides. JAAD 1986, 14:305.

Fraki JE, et al: Correlation of epidermal plasminogen activator activity with disease activity in psoriasis. Br J Dermatol 1983, 108:39.

Friedman SJ: Management of psoriasis with a hydrocolloid dressing. Arch Dermatol 1987, 123:1046.

Gold MH, et al: Beta blockers and psoriasis. JAAD 1988, 19:458.

Goldfarb MT, et al: Acitretin improves psoriasis . . . in dose-dependent fashion. JAAD 1988, 18:655.

Gollnick H, et al: Acitretin vs etretinate in psoriasis. JAAD 1988, 19:458.

Gottlieb AB: Immunologic mechanisms in psoriasis. JAAD 1988, 18:1376.

Idem: Psoralen photochemotherapy. JAAD 1987, 17:1703.

Gupta AK, et al: Woronoff ring during anthralin therapy for psoriasis. Arch Dermatol 1986, 122:248.

Halevy S, et al: Dialysis therapy for psoriasis. Arch Dermatol 1981, 117:69.

Halprin KM, et al: Cancer in patients with psoriasis. JAAD 1982, 7:633.

Idem: Constant low-dose ultraviolet light therapy for psoriasis. JAAD 1982, 7:614.

Hammershoy O, et al: A retrospective study of cataract formation in 96 patients treated with PUVA. Acta Dermatovenereol 1982, 62:444.

Hanno R, et al: Methotrexate in psoriasis. JAAD 1980, 2:171.

Harber LC, et al: Preliminary report: Modified Goeckerman therapy for hospitalized patients: Ambulatory day care center and improved quantitative dosimetry. J Invest Dermatol 1981, 77:162.

Harper JI, et al: Cyclosporin for psoriasis. Lancet 1984, 2:981.

Heng MCY, et al: Beta-adrenoceptor-antagonist-induced psoriasiform eruption. Int J Dermatol 1988, 27:619.

Henseler T, et al: Psoriasis of early and late onset: Characterization of two types of psoriasis vulgaris. JAAD 1985, 13:450.

Hietanen J, et al: Study of oral mucosa in 200 consecutive patients with psoriasis. Scand J Dent Res 1984, 92:50.

Horwitz SN: Addition of topically applied corticosteroid to a modified Goeckerman regimen. JAAD 1985, 13:784.

Hubler WR Jr: Familial juvenile generalized pustular psoriasis. Arch Dermatol 1984, 120:1174.

Idem: Lingual lesions of generalized pustular psoriasis: Report of 5 cases and review of the literature. JAAD 1984, 11:1069.

Kaplan RR, et al: Etretinate therapy for psoriasis: Clinical responses, remission times, epidermal DNA and polyamine responses. JAAD 1983, 8:95.

Kavli G, et al: Psoriasis. Br Med J 1985, 291:999.

Kemmett D, et al: Histocompatibility antigens in plaque psoriasis and palmoplantar pustulosis. Br J Dermatol 1984, 113:(supp. 29)40.

Kiil J, et al: Surgical treatment of psoriasis. Lancet 1985, 2:116.

Kocsard E: The rarity of actinic keratoses in psoriasis patients: Preliminary report. Austral J Dermatol 1976, 17:65.

Kouskoukis CE, et al: Psoriasis of the nails. Cutis 1983, 31:169.

Lanse SB, et al: Low incidence of hepatotoxicity associated with long-term, low-dose oral methotrexate in treatment of refractory psoriasis, psoriatic arthritis, and rheumatoid arthritis: An acceptable risk-benefit ratio. Dig Dis Sci 1985, 30:104.

Lassus A, et al: The effect of etretinate compared with different regimens of PUVA in treatment of persistent palmoplantar pustulosis. Br J Dermatol 1985, 112:455.

Lee RE, et al: Interleukin-2 and psoriasis. Arch Dermatol 1988, 124:1811.

Leibiger C, et al: Pustular psoriasis of von Zumbusch type in childhood. Hautarzt 1967, 18:168.

Lowe NJ, et al: Coal tar therapy for psoriasis reevaluated. JAAD 1983, 8:781.

Idem: Anthralin for psoriasis. JAAD 1984, 10:69.

Idem: Etretinate. Arch Dermatol 1988, 124:527.

Lyons JH III: Generalized pustular psoriasis. Int J Dermatol 1987, 26:409.

MacMillan AL, et al: Generalized pustular psoriasis treated with dapsone. Br J Dermatol 1973, 88:183.

Marisco AR, et al: Ultraviolet light and tar in Goeckerman treatment of psoriasis. Arch Dermatol 1976, 112:1249.

Marks R: Surgery for psoriasis (letter). Lancet 1985, 2:335.

Marley WM, et al: Effectiveness of low-strength anthralin in psoriasis. Arch Dermatol 1982, 118:906.

Melski JW, et al: Oral methoxsalen photochemotherapy for psoriasis . . . J Invest Dermatol 1977, 68:328.

Idem: The Koebner (isomorphic) response in psoriasis. Arch Dermatol 1983, 119:655.

Menter A, et al: The Goeckerman regimen in two psoriasis day-care centers. JAAD 1983, 9:59.

Milliard LG, et al: Is methotrexate safe for the treatment of psoriasis? Br J Dermatol 1979, 101:14.

Morimoto S, et al: Psoriasis and vitamin D_3. Arch Dermatol 1989, 125:231.

Morison WL, et al: Combined methotrexate-PUVA therapy in the treatment of psoriasis. JAAD 1982, 6:46.

Muller SA, et al: The Goeckerman treatment of psoriasis: Six decades of experience at the Mayo Clinic. Cutis 1984, 34:265.

Nyfors A: Methotrexate therapy of psoriasis: Effect and side effects, with particular reference to hepatic changes. A survey. Laegeforenigens Forlag, Copenhagen, 1980.

Orenberg EK, et al: Response of chronic psoriatic plaques to localized heating induced by ultrasound. Arch Dermatol 1980, 116:893.

Parker F: Psoriatic arthritis, lecture, American Academy of Dermatology, 1984.

Parrish JA, et al: Photochemotherapy of psoriasis with oral methoxsalen and long-wave UVL. N Engl J Med 1974, 291:1207.

Idem: Action spectrum for phototherapy of psoriasis. J Invest Dermatol 1981, 76:359.

Peachey RDG, et al: Treatment of psoriatic nail dystrophy with intradermal steroid injections. Br J Dermatol 1976, 95:75.

Pearlman DL, et al: Paper-tape occlusion of anthralin paste. Arch Dermatol 1984, 120:625.

Idem: Weekly pulse dosing schedule of fluorouracil. JAAD 1986, 15:1247.

Idem: Weekly psoriasis therapy using fluorouracil. JAAD 1987, 17:78.

Petrozzi JW, et al: Comparison of once-daily and twice-daily ultraviolet radiation treatments in psoriasis. Arch Dermatol 1981, 117:695.

Piamphongsant T, et al: Treatment of generalized pustular psoriasis. Clin Exp Dermatol 1985, 10:552.

Picascia DD, et al: Treatment of severe resistant psoriasis with systemic cyclosporine. JAAD 1987, 17:408.

Pittelkow MR, et al: Skin cancer in patients with psoriasis treated with coal tar. Int J Dermatol 1981, 117:465.

Rapaport M: Dialysis and psoriasis (letter). JAAD 1984, 8:425.

Rasmussen JE: Clearing of psoriasis after threatened dialysis (letter). Arch Dermatol 1980, 116:752.

Robinson JK, et al: Methotrexate hepatotoxicity in psoriasis. Arch Dermatol 1980, 116:413.

Roenigk HH Jr, et al: Serial liver biopsies in psoriatic patients receiving long-term etretinate. Br J Dermatol 1985, 112:77.

Idem: Methotrexate in psoriasis. JAAD 1988, 19:145.

Rook AJ, et al: Psoriasis. Semin Dermatol 1985, 4:271.

Rosenberg EW, et al: Microbial factors in psoriasis (letter). Arch Dermatol 1982, 118:143.

Idem: Koebner phenomenon and the microbial basis of psoriasis. Arch Dermatol 1987, 123:151.

Ross SD, et al: Randomized comparison of three modes of treatment of psoriasis of the scalp. Cutis 1981, 28:438.

Sanchez NP, et al: Subcorneal pustular dermatosis and psoriasis. Arch Dermatol 1983, 119:715.

Schwartz T, et al: Anthralin minute entire skin treatment. Arch Dermatol 1985, 121:1512.

Seville RH: Psoriasis and stress I & II. Br J Dermatol 1977, 97:297 and 98:151.

Shore RN: Clearing psoriasis lesions under tape. N Engl J Med 1985, 312:246.

Skott A, et al: Exacerbation of psoriasis during lithium treatment. Br J Dermatol 96:445, 1977.

Steck WD, et al: Hemofiltration treatment of psoriasis. JAAD 1982, 6:346.

Stern RS: Bias in assessment of skin cancer risk in patients with psoriasis. JAAD 1982, 7:639.

Idem: Contribution of topical tar oil to UVB phototherapy of psoriasis. JAAD 1986, 14:742.

Idem: The effect of continued UVB therapy on the duration of remission of psoriasis. JAAD 1986, 115:546.

Idem, et al: Heart disease, cancer, and cause of death in psoriasis. J Invest Dermatol 1988, 91:197.

Idem: Nonmelanoma skin cancer after PUVA. J Invest Dermatol 1988, 91:120.

Stevens DM, et al: On the concept of bacterids (pustular bacterid, Andrews). Am J Dermatopathol 1984, 6:281.

Urabe H, et al: Hyperthermia in the treatment of psoriasis. Arch Dermatol 1981, 117:770.

Vanderveen EE, et al: Methotrexate and etretinate as concurrent therapies in severe psoriasis. Arch Dermatol 1982, 118:660.

Van Hoff JP, et al: Cyclosporin and psoriasis. Lancet 1985, 1:335.

Van Scott EJ: Lecture. American Academy of Dermatology, 1985.

Voorhees JJ: Leukotrienes and other lipoxygenase products in the pathogenesis and therapy of psoriasis and other dermatoses (editorial). Arch Dermatol 1983, 119:541.

Ward JM, et al: A double-blind trial of clomocycline in palmoplantar pustulosis. Br J Dermatol 1976, 95:317.

Weber G, et al: Treatment of psoriasis with somatostatin. Arch Dermatol Res 272:31, 1982.

Weinstein GD: Three decades of folic acid antagonists in dermatology. Arch Dermatol 1983, 119:525.

Idem, et al: Topical methotrexate for psoriasis. Arch Dermatol 1989, 125:227.

Wentzell JM, et al: Cyclosporin in psoriasis. Arch Dermatol 1987, 123:163.

White SW: Palmoplantar pustular psoriasis provoked by lithium therapy. JAAD, 1982, 7:660.

Whittier FC, et al: Peritoneal dialysis for psoriasis: A controlled study. Ann Intern Med 1983, 99:165.

Whyte HJ, et al: Acute guttate psoriasis and streptococcal infection. Arch Dermatol 1964, 89:350.

Wolska H, et al: Etretinate in severe psoriasis: Results of double blind study . . . in pustular psoriasis. JAAD 1983, 9:883.

Ziboh VA: Implication of dietary aids and polyunsaturated fatty acids in management of cutaneous disorders. Arch Dermatol 1989, 125:241.

Recalcitrant Palmoplantar Eruptions

Recalcitrant pustular eruptions of the hands and feet—palmoplantar pustulosis—have been studied intensively during the past 50 years. However, the entire subject has become more involved because of the introduction of a variety of new ideas that are still in dispute. The various diseases have so many characteristics in common that it is difficult to divide them definitely into separate entities. These eruptions are currently divided into acrodermatitis continua (dermatitis repens), pustular psoriasis of the hands and feet, and pustular bacterid. All of these have palmoplantar pustulosis, and—for those who retain their belief in pustular bacterid—similar features. This fact does not belittle their importance. The task is chiefly the unraveling little by little of the vagaries of these recalcitrant acropustuloses, most of which seemingly have close connections with psoriasis.

Recalcitrant pustular eruptions of the hands and feet are often examples of inverse psoriasis, and a search for lesions elsewhere (scalp, ears, nails, glans penis, etc.) or for a positive family history will many times confirm this suspicion.

Dermatitis Repens. Dermatitis repens, also known as **acrodermatitis continua** and **acrodermatitis perstans**, is a chronic inflammatory disease of the hands and feet. It usually involves the extremities but in rare cases may become generalized. The disease usually begins on the extremity of a digit, either as an infected ulcer, or a pustule, or as a paronychia. Thus, at the beginning it is unilateral and localized. At the edge of this, the epidermis is cast off, leaving

a red surface, from which a clear or slightly turbid fluid oozes. An irregular ring of loose, sodden epidermis remains about the denuded areas. Extension takes place by the further detachment of the epidermis as the result of continued exudation, or there may be fresh pustules just beyond the border, which break down and add another denuded area to the original adjacent one. Crusted, eczematoid, and psoriasiform lesions may be observed, and there may be moderate itching. The disease is essentially unilateral in its beginning and asymmetric throughout its entire course. Although new foci may thus be formed locally, the disease seldom becomes generalized or spreads to distant parts.

The parts involved are the hands and feet and occasionally the mucous membranes, particularly of the mouth. The nails are often affected, causing paronychia. As the disease progresses, one or more of the nails may become dystrophic or be destroyed. The lesions cause atrophy of the skin with underlying soft tissue sclerosis, which may lead to resorption of bone or entire digits. The process generally remains limited to these parts. Involvement of the mucous membranes may occur even when the eruption of the skin is localized. Painful, circular, white plaques surrounded by inflammatory areolae are found on the tongue and may form a diphtheritic membrane; fissures have been described. In the generalized cases there may be gross sepsis in the mouth.

Histologically, the primary lesion is found in the epidermis, where the intraepithelial spongiform pustule is formed by infiltration with vast numbers of

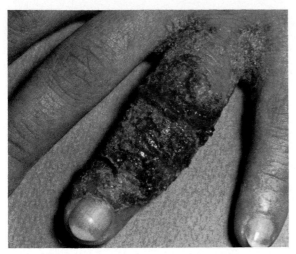

Figure 10–26. Dermatitis repens.

polymorphonuclear leukocytes. This abscess dries up and is exfoliated together with the overlying parakeratotic horny layer.

Lever calls attention to the epidermal changes, which are similar to those seen in psoriasis, such as parakeratosis and elongation of the rete ridges. He also points out that, basically, pustular psoriasis of Zumbusch, acrodermatitis continua (Hallopeau), and impetigo herpetiformis represent the same disease process. Histologically, the characteristic spongiform pustule of Kogoj is present in all three diseases.

The onset and evolution of the eruption and the results of bacteriologic and serologic investigations point to the fact that dermatitis repens may be complicated by invasion of the skin, and often of the mucous membranes, by *Staphylococcus aureus* and *Pseudomonas aeruginosa*.

Dermatitis repens responds slowly and poorly to internal and local use of antibiotics. Corticosteroids orally provide improvement, but upon withdrawal of the drug there is usually a severe exacerbation. The oral route is therefore not satisfactory: the intramuscular route, using triamcinolone acetonide, should be used from the beginning, to keep the total dose at a safely low level and to obviate "rebound." One or two 60-mg doses two to five weeks apart frequently suffice, and often—mysteriously—there is not even a relapse. Pearson et al reported a case that responded to etretinate, and as experience with this and acitretin grows, these are becoming the therapy of choice—at least for cases unresponsive to injected triamcinolone. Arnold has never seen one, however.

Palmoplantar Pustulosis (Pustular Psoriasis of the Extremities). Pustular psoriasis of the extremities, according to Barber, in contradistinction to dermatitis repens, is essentially a bilateral and symmetric dermatosis from which cultures are sterile. The favorite locations are the thenar or hypothenar eminences or the central portion of the palms and soles. The patches begin as erythematous areas in which minute intraepidermal pustules form. At the beginning these are pinhead-sized; then they may enlarge and coalesce to form small lakes of pus that are not at all or only slightly elevated above the skin surface. As a rule these pustules do not rupture but in the course of a week or two tend to dry up, leaving punctate brown scabs that eventually are exfoliated. Stages of quiescence and exacerbation characterize the condition. Medications, such as lithium, which aggravate psoriasis, have also been reported to induce palmoplantar pustular psoriasis. Before the brown scabs of preceding lesions are gone, crops of fresh pustules often appear either within the scaly patch or beyond its edge.

Through the repetition of these attacks, in the course of time a patch is produced that is deeply erythematous and markedly exfoliative and in which the pustules are more evident at the edges but also are observed throughout. The scales are large and tenacious, usually being adherent at one edge so that it is difficult or impossible to pull them off without causing pain and bleeding.

The fully developed patches clinically resemble psoriasis. The nails are often affected, becoming malformed, ridged, stippled, pitted, and discolored. Both generalized eruptions of pustular psoriasis and pustular psoriasis limited to the hands and feet may be associated with typical psoriasis vulgaris.

The disease is extremely resistant to most treatments. Etretinate (the aromatic retinoid) is reported to be extremely effective, in a dose of 1 mg/kg/day; in so chronic a disease, however, one might want to use a drug with less potential for side effects.

In that event, one may have recourse to triamcinolone acetonide, either intralesionally (as Goette has shown) or intramuscularly, 40 to 60 mg every four

Figure 10–27. Acrodermatitis continua.

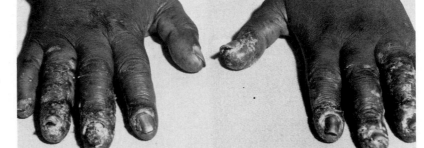

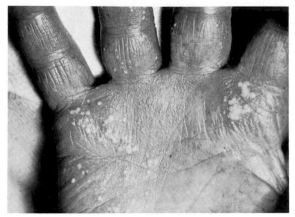

Figure 10–28. *"Lakes of pus" on palms in psoriasis of Zumbusch type.*

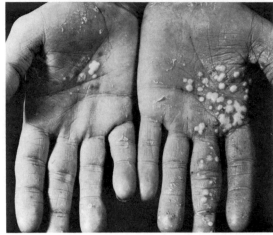

Figure 10–29. *Pustular psoriasis of palms. (Courtesy of Dr. H. Shatin.)*

to six weeks (or longer if remissions last longer). An occasional patient may be so tolerant of dapsone, and so responsive to it, that this can be used instead, with the hope of longer remissions than can be expected with triamcinolone. Methotrexate is usually ineffective and is not recommended. Oral 8-methoxypsoralen and high-intensity UVA irradiation is effective, and superior to topical psoralen applications followed by UVA light. Occlusive polyethylene gloves under which fluocinolone or other corticosteroid has been placed are also helpful; however, the beneficial effects are usually short-lived.

Colchicine has been employed with success in some cases. The dose is 1 to 2 mg daily, reduced to 0.5 to 1 mg daily for maintenance. Nausea or diarrhea may occur.

Ägren-Jonsson S, et al: PUVA for palmoplantar pustulosis. Acta Derm Venereol (Stockh) 1985, 65:531.

Foged E, et al: Randomized trial of etretinate in palmoplantar pustulosis. Dermatologica 1983, 166:220.

Goette DK, et al: Treatment of palmoplantar pustulosis with intralesional triamcinolone . . . Arch Dermatol 1984, 120:319.

Jurik AG, et al: Arthro-osteitis in pustulosis palmoplantaris. JAAD 1988, 18:666.

Lassus A, et al: Efficacy of etretinate in clearing and prevention of relapse of palmoplantar pustulosis. Dermatologica 1983, 166:215.

Paul R, et al: Suppression of palmoplantar pustulosis . . . with oral 8-MOP and high-intensity UVA radiation. Dermatologica 1983, 167:283.

Pearson LH, et al: Acrodermatitis continua of Hallopeau. JAAD 1984, 11:755.

Rosen K, et al: PUVA, etretinate, and PUVA-etretinate for pustulosis palmoplantaris. Arch Dermatol 1987, 123:885.

Takigawa M, et al: Pustulosis palmaris et plantaris treated with oral colchicine. Arch Dermatol 1982, 118:458.

Thestrup-Pedersen K, et al: Treatment of pustulosis palmaris et plantaris with colchicine. Acta Dermatovener 1984, 64:76.

Uehara M: Pustulosis palmaris et plantaris: Evolutionary sequence from vesicular to pustular lesions. Semin Dermatol 1983, 2:51.

White SI, et al: Etretinate in pustular psoriasis of palms and soles. Br J Dermatol 1985, 113:581.

Pustular Bacterid. Pustular bacterid was first described by George Andrews. It is characterized by a

symmetric, grouped vesicular or pustular eruption on the palms and soles marked by exacerbations and remissions over long periods of time.

The basic lesions are pustules. At the beginning it is possible that they are vesicles that become rapidly purulent. Tiny hemorrhagic puncta intermingled with the pustules are frequently seen. When lesions are so numerous as to coalesce, they form a honeycomblike structure in the epidermis.

The disease usually begins on the midportions of the palms or soles, from which it spreads outward until it may eventually cover the entire flexor aspects

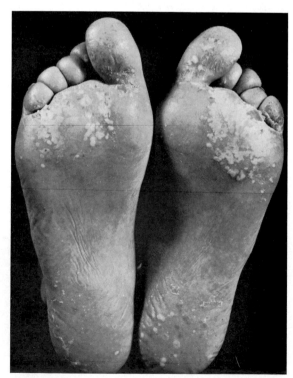

Figure 10–30. *Pustular psoriasis of soles. (Courtesy of Dr. H. Shatin.)*

of the hands and feet. There has not been any involvement of the webs of the fingers or toes, or in the flexion creases of the toes, as in ringworm.

When the eruption is fully developed, both palms and soles are completely covered, and the symmetry is pronounced. During fresh outbreaks, the white blood count may show a leukocytosis that ranges from 12,000 to 19,000 cells with 65 to 80 per cent polymorphonuclears. As a rule scaling is present and the scales are adherent, tough, and dry. During exacerbations, crops of pustules or vesicles make their appearance, and there is often severe itching of the areas and sometimes swelling, pain, and infiltration. From day to day fresh crops of lesions appear. Then the number of new lesions gradually diminishes and the condition subsides to a quiescent stage.

Andrews regarded the discovery of a remote focus of infection, and cure upon its elimination, as crucial to the diagnosis, and one of us (HLA) has observed this sequence of events in a few cases. One of us (HLA) also has seen a typical case, fully controlled by 0.5 gm of sulfamerazine t.i.d. at the onset of each recurrent attack, in a young man whose slowly worsening seborrheic dermatitis of the scalp was transformed into typical plaque psoriasis over a period of a few months—by which time his palmar lesions had entirely ceased to recur.

The integrity of this entity as a distinctive disease is questioned by many. The occasional observation of typical cases that respond to antibiotic or antimicrobial medication or irradiation or removal of a focus of infection leads us to include this entity as a distinct

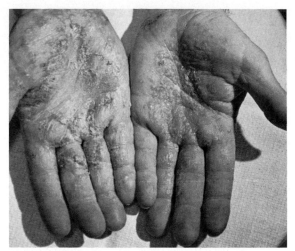

Figure 10–32. Pustular bacterid. Notice small pustules, especially on the left palm.

disease. We suspect, however, that it is a variant of psoriasis, and perhaps Rosenberg's observations explain its unpsoriasislike behavior.

Andrews GG, et al: Pustular bacterids and allied conditions. South Med J 1941, 34:1260.

INFANTILE ACROPUSTULOSIS

Jarratt and Ramsdell, and Kahn and Rywlin, in 1979, simultaneously described infantile acropustulosis (acropustulosis of infancy), an intensely itchy vesicopustular eruption of the hands and feet, beginning at any age up to 10 months, clearing in a few weeks, and recurring repeatedly until final subsidence at 6 to 36 months of age. Jennings and Burrows reported four more cases in 1983. They did not give dapsone, though Kahn and Rywlin had reported that it was effective at 2 mg/kg/day. Potent topical steroids are reported to afford symptomatic relief. There is speculation that in some cases this may be a persistent remnant of prior scabies. One of us (WDJ) has seen such a sequence of events in a black infant.

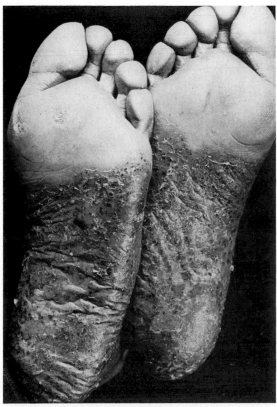

Figure 10–31. Pustular bacterid.

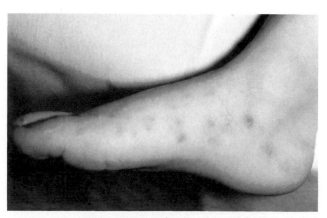

Figure 10–33. Infantile acropustulosis.

Findlay RJ, et al: Infantile acropustulosis. Am J Dis Child 1983, 137:455.
Jarratt M, et al: Infantile acropustulosis. Arch Dermatol 1979, 115:834.
Jennings JL, et al: Infantile acropustulosis. JAAD 1983, 9:733.
Kahn G, et al: Acropustulosis of infancy. Arch Dermatol 1979, 115:831.
Vignon-Pennamen D-D, et al: Infantile acropustulosis. Arch Dermatol 1986, 122:1155.

STERNOCLAVICULAR HYPEROSTOSIS

Association with persistent palmoplantar pustulosis in over half the cases characterizes this seronegative rheumatoid syndrome, first reported by Sonozaki et al from Japan in 1974 and most recently reported by Resnik et al, who reviewed the literature, in 1987. It manifests as pain and swelling of one or both sternoclavicular joints and often the sternomanubrial and upper costochondral junctions as well. There is shoulder, neck, and back pain, and limitation of motion of the shoulders and neck is common. Brachial plexus neuropathy and subclavian vein occlusion may occur. The lumbar spine and sacroiliac joints are usually spared. Chronic multifocal osteomyelitis in children may be a pediatric variant of the same syndrome.

Treatment with nonsteroidal antiinflammatory drugs and aspirin is only moderately effective. Dapsone, colchicine, and triamcinolone IM would appear to be worth trying.

Resnik CS, et al: Sternoclavicular hyperostosis: Rheumatologic, radiologic, and dermatologic considerations. South Med J 1987, 80:577.
Sonozaki H, et al: Four cases with symmetrical ossifications between the clavicles and first ribs of both sides. Kanto J Orthop Trauma 1974, 5:244.

POMPHOLYX (Dyshidrosis)

CLINICAL FEATURES. Pompholyx (meaning bubble) is also known as dyshidrosis and was once called cheiropompholyx. It is a vesicular eruption of the palms and soles characterized by spongiotic intraepidermal vesicles, and often by burning or itching. Hyperhidrosis may be present too. The application of the term "pompholyx" is at present limited to those typical eruptions that have small deep-seated vesicles resembling "sago grains" occurring only on the palms, soles, and interdigits, accompanied by itching or burning, in which examination fails to reveal fungi or external chemical cause.

The distribution of the lesion is, as a rule, bilateral and roughly symmetric. Sometimes the vesicles are arranged in groups. By coalescence of several contiguous vesicles, bullae may be formed. The contents are clear and colorless but may later become straw-colored or purulent. Attacks generally last a few weeks, but, because of the tendency to relapse, the condition may persist for long periods. The lesions involute by drying up and desquamating rather than by rupturing.

ETIOLOGY. Pompholyx occurs chiefly in individuals who are subject to much emotional stress. Probably hyperhidrosis of the palms and soles is not one of the causative factors. Sweat glands and ducts are not connected with the vesicles. Pompholyx must be differentiated from an id reaction due to active fungus infection of the soles. Contact dermatitis must also be differentiated from pompholyx, as must tinea manuum.

HISTOPATHOLOGY. The sweat ducts are not involved. Pinkus and Mehregan state, "The sweat ducts thread their way between [or even, rarely, through!] the vesicles." Spongiotic vesicles are found in the epidermis, usually without inflammatory changes.

Christensen and Moller have reported nickel dermatitis of the pompholyx type. Ingestion of nickel in food may play a role in the chronicity of this dermatitis.

DIFFERENTIAL DIAGNOSIS. Vesicular eruptions of the palms and soles closely resemble each other, so that the clinical features may not be enough to arrive at a diagnosis. Dermatophytid, contact dermatitis (allergic), atopic dermatitis, drug eruption (penicillin), pustular psoriasis of the palms and soles, acrodermatitis continua, and pustular bacterid are some dermatoses to be kept in mind. Localized bullous pemphigoid has recently been reported to initially manifest in this way.

TREATMENT. Topical application of high-potency corticosteroid creams, 5 per cent salicylic acid in alcohol, and 3 per cent vioform cream may be used in mild cases. Soaking of the hands and feet in potassium permanganate solution (1:5000) for one half hour is still helpful. Burow's solution compresses are more esthetic to use. Triamcinolone acetonide intramuscularly or a short course of oral prednisone is rapidly effective, often inducing remissions of a month or two.

Previously, x-ray therapy has been widely used. Today, if steroid therapy is possible, x-ray therapy is contraindicated. When other measures are ineffective, or steroids cannot be used, 75 rads of superficial x-rays to the palms at weekly intervals for a total of not more than 300 rads will be extremely (though temporarily) helpful. Oral psoralen plus ultraviolet A light (PUVA) has been reported to be effective, but in view of its cost and inconvenience, and potential for side effects (as compared to a single injection of triamcinolone acetonide intramuscularly), it seems difficult to justify its use.

Christensen OB, et al: Nickel allergy and hand eczema. Contact Dermatitis 1975, 2:353.
Levine MJ, et al: Oral methoxsalen phototherapy of dyshidrotic eczema. Acta Derm Venereol 1981, 61:570.
Young E: Dyshidrotic (endogenous) eczema. Dermatologica 1964, 129:306.

LAMELLAR DYSHIDROSIS (Keratolysis Exfoliativa)

Lamellar dyshidrosis (dyshidrosis lamellosa) is a superficial exfoliative dermatosis of the palms and sometimes soles characterized by the absence of inflammatory changes and by pinhead-sized white spots that gradually extend peripherally, while at the same time the horny layer in the central part becomes ruptured and peels off. The disorder spreads, new desquamating areas developing, and eventually by coalescence the entire part may show flaky scales. The involvement is bilateral, and it can occur in association with dyshidrosis, although at times no cause can be ascertained. It may represent a disorder of cohesion of the stratum corneum.

The disorder must be differentiated from dermatophytosis.

Treatment is difficult for this mild malady but spontaneous involution occurs usually in a few weeks. Tar creams (Zetone cream) usually produce satisfactory results. Five per cent tar in gel (*Estar Gel*) is an excellent preparation to use. A mild emollient, however, may suffice. Lac-Hydrin Lotion is often effective. A small dose, 20 or 30 mg, of triamcinolone acetonide (Kenalog) intramuscularly will often terminate a prolonged attack, and induce a remission lasting one or several months. Arnold would sometimes use this in severe cases; Odom and James would not. Keratolytic emollient creams and lotions are helpful.

PALMOPLANTAR KERATODERMA

Keratoderma is frequently used synonymously with hyperkeratosis, keratosis, and tylosis. Palmoplantar keratoderma is characterized by excessive formation of keratin on the palms and soles. The acquired and the congenital varieties may be present alone or they may accompany other diseases or be a part of a syndrome.

The most important features in classification of the palmoplantar keratodermas include the specific morphology and distribution of the hyperkeratosis, evidence for genetic transmission and particular inheritance pattern, presence of skin lesions on areas other than palms and soles, other ectodermal or systemic abnormalities, age at onset of the keratoderma, severity and prognosis of the disease process, and histopathologic findings.

The acquired types include keratoderma climactericum, arsenical keratoses, corns, calluses, porokeratosis plantaris discreta, porokeratotic eccrine ostial and dermal duct nevus, glucan-induced keratoderma in AIDS, keratosis punctata of the palmar creases, and many skin disorders that are associated with palmoplantar keratoderma such as psoriasis, cancer-associated paraneoplastic disorders, pityriasis rubra pilaris, lichen planus, and syphilis.

The hereditary types include hereditary palmoplantar keratoderma (Unna-Thost), punctate palmoplantar keratosis punctata, Papillon-Lefèvre syndrome, mal de Meleda, familial keratoderma with carcinoma of the esophagus (Howell-Evans), acrokeratoelastoidosis, focal acral hyperkeratosis, and several inherited disorders that have palmoplantar keratoderma as an associated finding, such as pachyonychia congenita, tyrosinema II (Richner-Hanhart), basal-cell nevus syndrome, Darier's disease, and dyskeratosis congenita.

The acquired types will be discussed first. Many of these disorders are presented in other chapters under the primary cutaneous diagnosis, such as lichen planus or pityriasis rubra pilaris. Three diseases will be discussed here: keratosis punctata of the palmar creases, porokeratosis plantaris discreta, and keratoderma climactericum.

Keratosis Punctata of the Palmar Creases

This common disorder occurs most often in black patients. The primary lesion is a 1- to 2-mm depression filled with a conical keratinous plug, primarily in the creases of the palms or fingers, and occasionally on the soles. Lesions are multiple. Friction aggravates the lesions and often causes them to become verrucoid or surrounded by callus. The tenderness on pressure may be relieved by lifting out the horny plug. At times only conical depressions are noted.

Anderson et al reported 31 cases. They found an incidence of nearly 2 per cent among 573 consecutively examined black patients. Thirteen per cent had foot lesions. It was highly associated with a personal or family history of atopy.

Porokeratosis Plantaris Discreta

This entity occurs in adults, with a 4:1 female preponderance. It is characterized by a sharply marginated, rubbery, wide-based papule, which on blunt dissection reveals an opaque plug without bleeding on removal. Lesions are multiple, painful, and usually 7 to 10 mm in diameter. They are usually confined to the weight-bearing area of the sole, beneath the metatarsal heads.

Treatment may be begun with fitted foot pads to redistribute the weight. Surgical excision or blunt dissection by electrocautery may be done. Limmer found cryotherapy successful in a high percentage of cases.

Keratoderma Climactericum

This is characterized by hyperkeratosis of the palms and soles (especially the heels) beginning at about the time of the menopause. The discrete, thickened hyperkeratotic patches are most pronounced at sites of pressure such as around the rim of the sole. Fissuring of the thickened patches may be present.

Histologically, there is extensive parakeratosis, without microabscesses such as are found in psoriasis, which it resembles clinically. Therapy consists of keratolytic ointments such as 10 per cent salicylic acid ointment, 6 per cent salicylic acid gel (Keralyt,

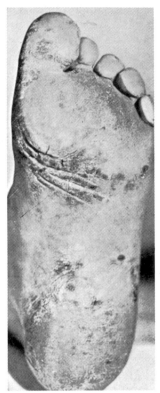

Figure 10–34. Keratoderma climactericum. (Courtesy of Dr. P. Gross.)

Westwood), 20 to 30 per cent urea mixtures, or 0.25 per cent anthralin ointment. Etretinate is more effective than Accutane. Steroid therapy is ineffective.

The hereditary syndromes are discussed below.

Again, many disorders that have palmoplantar keratoderma as a feature, such as pachyonychia congenita, Darier's disease, and tyrosinemia II, will be discussed in other chapters.

Hereditary Palmoplantar Keratoderma

Hereditary palmoplantar keratoderma (Unna-Thost) is characterized by a dominantly inherited, marked, congenital thickening of the epidermal horny layer of the palms and soles, usually symmetric and affecting all parts to an equal degree. At times the thickening extends to the lateral or dorsal surfaces, especially over the knuckles. When the keratoderma is on the soles, the arches are generally not involved. The epidermis becomes thick, yellowish, verrucous, and horny. Striate and punctate forms occur. In the ordinary variety the uniform thickening forms a rigid plate, which ends with characteristic abruptness at the periphery of the palm, usually without any contiguous inflammatory margin. There is frequently hyperhidrosis, which causes a sodden appearance. Occasionally there are associated changes in the nails, which become thickened, opaque, and malformed.

Local medications are rarely of value. Five per cent salicylic acid is helpful, but 6 per cent salicylic acid in a propylene glycol gel (Keralyt Gel) is probably the most effective local remedy. Twelve per cent ammonium lactate lotion (Lac-Hydrin) may be tried. Thirty per cent urea solution soaks are sometimes beneficial. Ten per cent sodium chloride in hydrophilic ointment has also been recommended. Etretinate or Accutane may be considered.

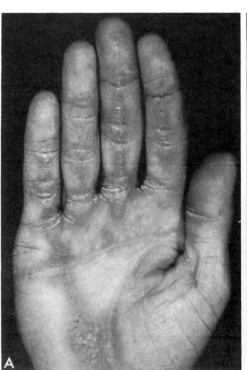
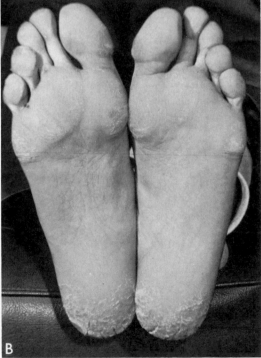

Figure 10–35. Hereditary palmoplantar keratoderma.

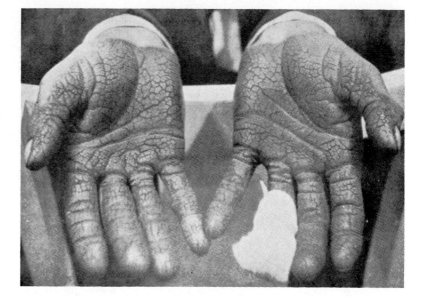

Figure 10–36. Keratosis palmaris. Seven members of family show same condition: father, grandfather, great grandfather, three brothers and one sister. Soles similarly affected. (Courtesy of Dr. S. T. Millard.)

Howell-Evans reported a diffuse, waxy keratoderma of the palms and soles occurring as an autosomal dominant trait associated with esophageal carcinoma.

Mutilating Keratoderma of Vohwinkel

Vohwinkel described this palmoplantar hyperkeratosis of the honeycomb type, associated with starfishlike keratoses on the backs of the hands and feet, linear keratoses of the elbows and knees, and annular constriction (pseudoainhum) of the digits, which may progress to autoamputation.

Gibbs and Frank emphasize that this keratoma is familial, being autosomal dominantly inherited and occurring early in life.

Reddy et al reported a case without alopecia, hearing defects, mutism, or plantar bullae, in which only the feet were affected, and in which the disease did not become manifest until the age of 18.

Rivers et al reported four cases, all family members, spanning three generations. There was marked improvement of the hyperkeratosis, as well as the pseudoainhum, with etretinate therapy.

Olmstead syndrome should be included in the differential diagnosis. Poulin et al reported a patient who had the distinctive features of this syndrome, which include a congenital sharply marginated palmoplantar keratoderma, constriction of the digits, linear keratotic streaks on the flexural aspects of the wrists, onychodystrophy, and periorificial keratoses. The latter feature may cause confusion with acrodermatitis enteropathica.

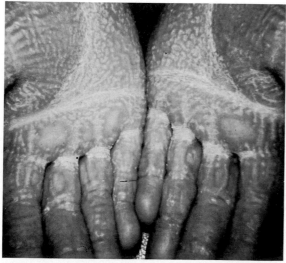

Figure 10–37. Mutilating keratoderma of Vohwinkel: diffuse honeycomb hyperkeratoses of the palms. (From Gibbs RC, Frank SB: Arch Dermatol 1966, 94:619–625.)

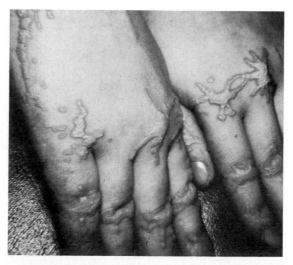

Figure 10–38. Mutilating keratoderma of Vohwinkel: "starfish" hyperkeratosis on backs of hands. (From Gibbs RC, Frank SB: Arch Dermatol 1966, 94:619–625.)

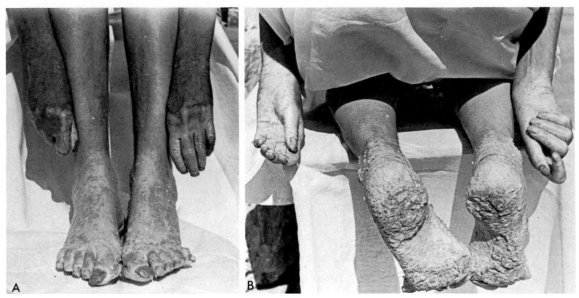

Figure 10–39. Mal de Meleda. (Courtesy of Dr. Mladen Filiporic, Split, Yugoslavia.)

Keratosis Punctata Palmaris et Plantaris

This autosomal dominantly inherited disorder is characterized by discrete, firm, slightly elevated papules on the palms and soles. They are usually quite numerous and are commonly asymptomatic on the palms, but may be quite tender on the soles. Bennion et al reported a large family in which this condition was associated with carcinoma of the alimentary tract, chiefly the colon.

Acrokeratoelastoidosis of Costa

This autosomal dominantly inherited condition is commonest in women. Costa described small, round, firm papules occurring over the dorsal hands, the knuckles, and the lateral margins of the palms and soles. The lesions appear in early childhood and progress slowly. They are asymptomatic. Histologic features include dermal elastorrhexis.

Focal Acral Hyperkeratosis

Dowd et al described this disease, which, while it closely resembles acrokeratoelastoidosis, shows no elastorrhexis on biopsy. Twelve of 15 patients were female, and 14 were black. All had papules on the medial and lateral edges of the hands and feet, developing at about age 20, and half had a family history of the disorder.

Papillon-Lefèvre Syndrome

Palmoplantar hyperkeratosis and periodontosis may occur in childhood after the eruption of the deciduous teeth.

Common cutaneous changes include well-demarcated, erythematous, hyperkeratotic lesions on the palms and soles, which may extend to the dorsal hands and feet. These changes often start in early childhood and may also be present on the elbows, knees, and Achilles tendon areas. Transverse grooves of the fingernails may occur. In most cases the cutaneous changes appear concomitantly with the odontal change; however, in some cases, skin changes precede the dental change. In several of the cases reported, Bach and Levan call attention to the presence of asymptomatic ectopic calcification in the choroid plexus and tentorium. It is believed that this is an autosomal recessive disorder. Therapy may retard both the dental and skin abnormalities. Nazzaro et al reported such a response in four siblings treated with acetretin.

The stocking-glove distribution of the hyperkeratosis is similar to that seen in *mal de Meleda*, an autosomal recessive disorder seen in individuals from the island of Meleda. No dental abnormalities are present in this syndrome, and there are often associated keratotic lesions of the groin and axilla. Bergfeld et al reported successful treatment with isotretinoin. El Darouti et al reported three cases responding well to etretinate.

Anderson WA, et al: Keratosis punctata and atopy. Arch Dermatol 1984, 12:884.

Bennion SD, et al: Keratosis punctata palmaris et plantaris and adenocarcinoma of the colon. JAAD 1984, 10:587.

Bergfeld WF, et al: The treatment of keratosis palmaris et plantaris with isotretinoin. JAAD 1982, 6:727.

Blum SL, et al: Hyperkeratosis papular in the hands and feet. Arch Dermatol 1987, 123:1225.

DeSchamps P, et al: Keratoderma climactericum (Haxthausen's Disease). Dermatologica 1986, 172:258.

Dowd PM, et al: Focal acral hyperkeratosis. Br J Dermatol 1983, 109:97.

Duvic M, et al: Glucan-induced keratoderma in AIDS. Arch Dermatol 1987, 123:751.

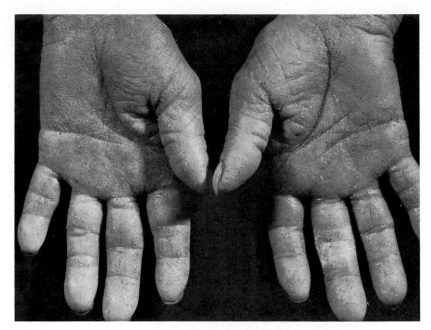

Figure 10–40. Keratosis punctata palmoplantaris. (Courtesy of Dr. H. Shatin.)

El Darouti MA, et al: Papillon-Lefèvre syndrome: Successful treatment with retinoids in 3 patients. Int J Dermatol 1988, 27:63.

Friedman SJ, et al: Punctate porokeratotic keratoderma. Arch Dermatol 1988, 124:1678.

Highet AS, et al: Acrokeratoelastoidosis. Br J Dermatol 1982, 106:337.

Kore A, et al: Acrokeratoelastoidosis of Costa in North America. JAAD 1985, 12:832.

Limmer B: Cryotherapy of porokeratosis plantaris discreta. Arch Dermatol 1979, 115:582.

Mandojana RM, et al: Porokeratosis plantaris discreta. JAAD 1984, 10:679.

Moreno A, et al: Porokeratotic eccrine ostial and dermal duct nevus. J Cutan Pathol 1988, 15:43.

Murrata Y, et al: Acquired diffuse keratoderma of the palms and soles with bronchial carcinoma. Arch Dermatol 1988, 124:497.

Nazzaro V, et al: Papillon-Lefèvre syndrome. Arch Dermatol 1988, 124:533.

Ortega M, et al: Keratosis punctata of the palmar creases. JAAD 1985, 13:381.

Poulin Y, et al: Olmstead syndrome. JAAD 1984, 10:600.

Rivers JK, et al: Etretinate: Management of keratoma hereditaria mutilans in four family members. JAAD 1985, 13:43.

Rubenstein DJ, et al: Punctate hyperkeratosis of the palms and soles. JAAD 1980, 3:43.

Sybert VP, et al: Palmo-plantar keratoderma. JAAD 1988, 18:75.

EXFOLIATIVE DERMATITIS
(Erythroderma)

Synonyms: Dermatitis exfoliativa, pityriasis rubra (Hebra), erythroderma (Wilson-Brocq).

CLINICAL FEATURES. Although the clinical picture is similar in most patients, there are many etiologic factors in this disease. Exfoliative dermatitis is characterized by a universal or very extensive obstinate scaling and itching erythroderma, often associated with loss of hair. The disease starts with erythematous swollen patches, which spread rapidly until the whole integument is involved. The onset is often accompanied by symptoms of general toxicity. The skin becomes scarlet and swollen and may ooze a straw-colored exudate. Desquamation is evident after a few days.

The scales are of various kinds, in some cases being small and thin and, in others, large sheets. The latter are often seen on the palms and soles. On the scalp thick crusts are formed, combined with sebum and products of secondary infection. The conjunctivae and the mucous membrane of the upper respiratory tract may be affected by desquamation. Secondary infections by pyogenic organisms often complicate the course of the disease in the absence of treatment.

There is a vivid widespread erythema, particularly on the face and extremities, and ultimately the entire body surface is dull scarlet and covered by small laminated scales that exfoliate profusely. Vesiculation and pustulation are usually absent. Pruritus is usually present and may be almost intolerable. Chilliness is a constant complaint owing to the patients' inability to constrict cutaneous blood vessels; there is severe heat loss.

The prognosis in generalized exfoliative dermatitis is grave. One attack may follow another every month or so. The course of the disease may be very protracted, lasting over a period of years, or it may simply persist and resist therapy.

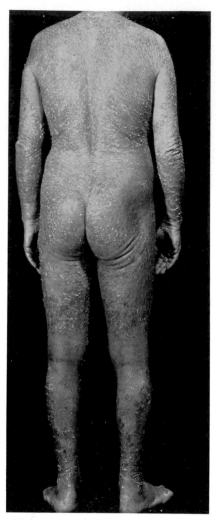

Figure 10–41. Psoriatic erythroderma.

Drug Allergy. Among the drugs that may cause a generalized erythroderma are allopurinol, sulfa drugs, gold, phenytoin, phenobarbital, isoniazid, and iodine. These drugs may also produce both morbilliform and scarlatiniform eruptions. Exfoliative dermatitis (sometimes fatal if not promptly dealt with) may supervene in any case of drug eruption if the drug is continued after the eruption starts.

Pityriasis Rubra Pilaris (PRP). Even the most severe or generalized PRP will have clear and normal-appearing "islands" of skin. These are pathognomonic of PRP. The thickened, hyperkeratotic, and shiny palms and the "nutmeg grater" follicular papules on the dorsum of the fingers are helpful in differentiating this from the other forms of erythroderma.

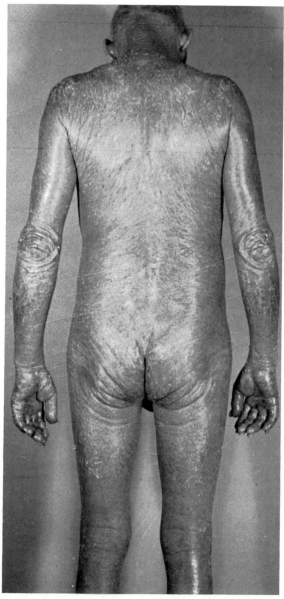

Figure 10–42. Generalized exfoliative dermatitis: "red man" syndrome.

ETIOLOGY. The original picture of exfoliative dermatitis may be considerably influenced by the causative factor. Both benign and malignant forms occur. Adam, in a review of 176 patients, found 36 per cent with a previous history of psoriasis, atopic dermatitis, or seborrhea; 10 per cent due to malignancy, and 11 per cent to drugs. There may be no history of previous skin disease; in some large series the idiopathic type is the most frequent category. The following are some of the known causes:

Psoriasis. Psoriatic erythroderma is one of the commonest precursors of exfoliative dermatitis. The histologic picture can be that of psoriasis with perhaps more edema and spongiosis; nevertheless, atopic dermatitis and pityriasis rubra pilaris and other diseases may show psoriasiform histologic changes. Pruritus and lymphadenopathy are usually minor features in this type of exfoliative dermatitis.

Eczema, Neurodermatitis. Exfoliative dermatitis is often preceded by the typical lesions of atopic dermatitis or other forms of eczema. Pruritus is intense, with great discomfort.

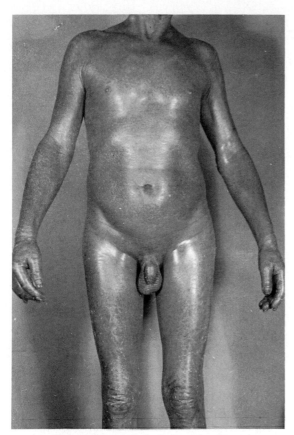

Figure 10–43. Universal erythroderma.

Seborrheic Dermatitis. Only rarely does generalized seborrheic dermatitis occur. It resembles psoriatic erythroderma. Usually seborrheic dermatitis has typical sites of predilection such as the scalp, ears, backs of the ears, alae nasi, midline of the chest, axillae, and inguinal regions.

Other Dermatoses. Streptobacillary fever, erythema multiforme, internal malignancies, generalized lichen planus, pemphigus foliaceus, generalized dermatophytosis, and even Norwegian scabies may show the picture of generalized exfoliative dermatitis.

Malignant Lymphoma. Among the malignant lymphomas, Hodgkin's disease may show generalized exfoliative dermatitis most frequently. It is estimated that 25 per cent of patients with Hodgkin's disease have cutaneous manifestations. Some of these are exfoliative dermatitis, severe pruritus, intracutaneous nodules, alopecia, and herpes zoster. Lymphadenopathy is usually present; splenomegaly and hepatomegaly are also frequently present in this group. The erythrocyte sedimentation rate is elevated in most of these patients.

Mycosis fungoides may have several cutaneous forms. A generalized exfoliative dermatitis may be present with poikiloderma as a part of the erythrodermic eruption. With it pigmentation and even infiltrated tumors may be present.

Malignant reticulemic erythroderma (Sézary's syndrome) consists of generalized exfoliative dermatitis with intense pruritus, leonine facies, alopecia, palmoplantar hyperkeratosis, and onychodystrophy. The presence of Sézary cells in the peripheral blood is diagnostic of this disease.

Leukemia may also present with generalized exfoliative dermatitis. Erythroderma occurs most frequently in lymphocytic leukemia, in both the acute and chronic forms. Splenomegaly and lymph node enlargement are early signs in leukemia.

Dermatogenic Enteropathy. Protein-losing enteropathy has been demonstrated in erythroderma by Shuster. A high incidence of steatorrhea was found in patients with exfoliative dermatitis, especially in psoriatic erythroderma. It is believed that the exfoliative dermatitis causes the enteropathy, not vice versa.

Unknown causes of exfoliative dermatitis may represent as many as 50 per cent of the cases. The signs and symptoms may be present for years before the etiology becomes apparent; even death may occur without discovery of the cause.

HISTOPATHOLOGY. Exfoliative dermatitis, regardless of its cause, tends to retain the histologic features of the original disease process. This applies to postpsoriatic and other inflammatory types, as well as to the lymphomatous types of generalized erythrodermas and exfoliative dermatitis. The papillae are elongated and thickened. In the epidermis there are acanthosis (particularly in the interpapillary portions) and marked parakeratosis. The granular layer is usually absent. In places there are leukocytes that have invaded the epidermis. There may be some atrophy and pigmentation in long-standing cases. Edema and parakeratosis are often more intense in the neighborhood of the hair follicles. Dilatation of the vessels is evident. Interstitial and parenchymatous edema of the upper part of the dermis and of the epidermis occurs. There is a perivascular infiltrate of both lymphocytes and polymorphonuclears.

TREATMENT. The varying degrees of involvement in this disease preclude any set methods for treatment. One of us (Arnold) has had successful results for some 30 years with systemic steroids—triamcinolone acetonide intramuscularly. The initial dose should be generous: 80 mg, repeated in four or five days if the response is disappointing, or in a week or 10 days if not much progress has been made. Thereafter treatment is gauged by the symptomatic need for it. Hospitalization and topical therapy are frequently not required: one of us (HLA) has not hospitalized a patient because of it for 30 years. The patient should have soothing inunctions of various emollients and starch or oatmeal baths. Corticosteroids internally are life-saving in severe involvement. Immunosuppressives such as azathioprine, methotrexate, and cyclophosphamide may occasionally be necessary.

Etretinate is useful in psoriatic erythroderma, and

isotretinoin in erythroderma due to PRP. Specific modes of therapy useful for the lymphomas and leukemias are indicated in those disorders. Discontinuance of the offending drug in drug-induced cases is, of course, mandatory.

Abrahams I, et al: 101 cases of exfoliative dermatitis. Arch Dermatol 1963, 87:96.

Frost M, et al: Acral hyperkeratosis with erythroderma. Arch Dermatol 1988, 124:123.

Hasan T, et al: Erythroderma. JAAD 1983, 8:836.

King LE, et al: Erythroderma. South Med J 1986, 79:1210.

Nicholis GD, et al: Exfoliative dermatitis. Arch Dermatol 1973, 108:788.

Sehgal VN, et al: Exfoliative dermatitis. Dermatologica 1986, 173:278.

Thestrup-Pedersen K, et al: The red man syndrome. JAAD 1988, 18:1307.

Winkelmann RK, et al: Pre-Sezary syndrome. JAAD 1984, 10:992.

11

Parapsoriasis, Pityriasis Rosea, Pityriasis Rubra Pilaris

PARAPSORIASIS

The term "parapsoriasis" was applied by Brocq (1902) to a group of maculopapular scaly eruptions of slow evolution, whose marked chronicity, resistance to treatment, and absence of subjective symptoms are characteristic features. Although the eruptions are psoriasiform and lichenoid, the diseases do not correspond to psoriasis, lichen planus, or other recognized dermatoses, and although the details of the eruptions do not harmonize, there is sufficient essential conformity to justify placing them in a distinct group.

Now we divide them into **pityriasis lichenoides chronica, parapsoriasis en plaques,** and **pityriasis lichenoides et varioliformis acuta**.

Pityriasis Lichenoides Chronica

In this disease erythematous, yellowish, scaly macules and lichenoid papules appear insidiously. They persist indefinitely with little change, chiefly on the sides of trunk, thighs, and upper arms. From time to time the eruption may be augmented by the development of a few new lesions. Several patients have been reported to have scaly, hypopigmented, guttate macules, which, on biopsy, revealed the findings of pityriasis lichenoides chronica. The disease may be confused with psoriasis and with secondary syphilis.

The histologic features of pityriasis lichenoides chronica are not specific. Focal parakeratosis, acan-

thosis, and even spongiosis may be present. There is an infiltrate of lymphocytes in the superficial dermis. These findings may be difficult to distinguish from those of guttate psoriasis, pityriasis rosea, and certain types of drug eruptions.

Treatment with ultraviolet light is beneficial; however, intensive doses may be necessary for good results. PUVA has also been reported to be effective, but should be limited in use owing to adverse long-term effects.

Piamphongsant treated 13 cases with oral tetracycline. Five were completely cured. The addition of an antihistamine enhanced the beneficial effects in one case.

Pityriasis lichenoides chronica is a benign disease that clears spontaneously in a few months or years.

Pityriasis Lichenoides et Varioliformis Acuta

This form has also been known as **parapsoriasis lichenoides, Habermann's disease, Mucha-Habermann disease,** and **parapsoriasis varioliformis acuta**.

Pityriasis lichenoides et varioliformis acuta (PLEVA) occurs with the sudden appearance of a polymorphous eruption composed of macules, papules, and occasional vesicles. It may run an acute, subacute, or chronic course. The papules are usually yellowish or brownish red rounded lesions, which tend to crusting, necrosis, and hemorrhage. Vesicular lesions are not common but are of great diagnostic importance. Upon close examination the vesicles are

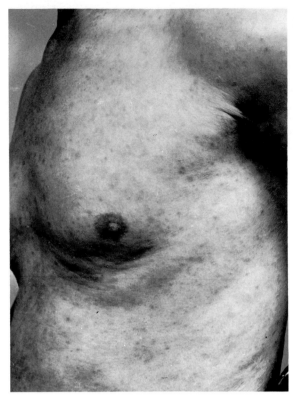

Figure 11–1. Pityriasis lichenoides chronica. *(Courtesy of Dr. R. Clayton, London.)*

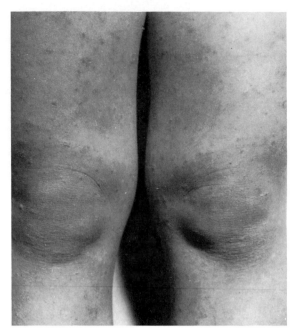

Figure 11–3. Pityriasis lichenoides et varioliformis acuta.

Almost the entire integument is uniformly involved, favorite sites being the anterior trunk, the flexor surfaces of the upper extremities, and the axillary regions. The palms and soles are infrequently involved but the mucous membranes are not.

found to be deep-seated and varicelliform. Papulonecrotic lesions with blackish brown crusts and hemorrhagic excoriations are evident. The exanthem then heals, leaving smooth, pigmented, depressed, varioliform scars. By this time, however, a new crop of lesions has usually appeared.

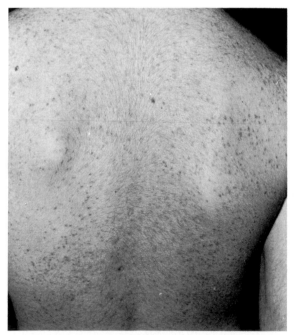

Figure 11–2. Pityriasis lichenoides et varioliformis acuta.

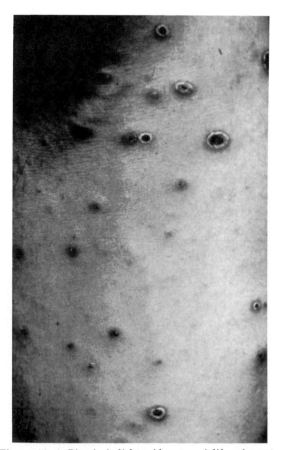

Figure 11–4. Pityriasis lichenoides et varioliformis acuta.

The general health is not affected, but generalized lymphadenopathy has been noted. The manifestations of the exanthem vary considerably. An unusually severe form characterized by large ulceronecrotic skin lesions with high fever has been reported.

The disorder must be differentiated from leucocytoclastic angiitis, papulonecrotic tuberculid, psoriasis, lichen planus, varicella, pityriasis rosea, drug eruptions, maculopapular syphilid, some forms of viral and rickettsial diseases, and most of all, lymphomatoid papulosis.

The course of the disease extends from four weeks to six months, or rarely for many years.

The etiology has not been determined.

Histologically, PLEVA is characterized by epidermal necrosis, together with prominent hemorrhage and primarily a dense perivascular infiltrate of lymphocytes in the superficial dermis. The absence of neutrophils simplifies the distinction from leucocytoclastic angiitis, which PLEVA may clinically resemble. Lymphomatoid papulosis differs histologically by the presence of large, atypical mononuclear cells in the dermal infiltrate.

IgM and C3 have been observed on direct immunofluorescence of fresh lesions by Clayton and Haffenden in 72 per cent of 43 cases. The fluorescence noted in the walls of superficial dermal vessels is nonspecific and its absence does not exclude PLEVA.

No one treatment is reliably effective. Tetracycline and erythromycin have both been reported to be effective and are worth trying. UVB and PUVA have both recently been reported to be effective.

Methotrexate, 2.5 to 7.5 mg every 12 hours for three doses on one day each week, has been reported effective. Several serious reactions, a few of them fatal, have been reported from the simultaneous administration of methotrexate and nonsteroidal antiinflammatory drugs. Katoh and Tanabe reported success with dapsone in three cases. Pentoxifylline (Trental), 400 mg twice daily, was effective in two cases reported by Sauer.

Parapsoriasis en Plaques

The division of parapsoriasis en plaques into small-plaque and large-plaque types, as proposed by Lambert and Everett, is helpful clinically and in prognosis. *Small-plaque parapsoriasis* is characterized by nonindurated brownish or yellowish red scaling patches, round to oval, with sharply defined, regular borders. Most lesions occur on the trunk and most of the lesions are between 1 and 5 cm in diameter. The eruption may be mildly itchy or asymptomatic. The patches may persist for years to decades and do not progress to lymphoma.

Large-plaque parapsoriasis has patches 5 to 10 or 15 cm in diameter, but similar in other respects to those of the small-plaque type. The prognosis, especially if pruritus is severe, is less benign: 10 per cent may eventuate in T-cell lymphoma. Ominous signs are the development of indurated areas within the patches, and at times the development of intense erythema.

Some degree of epidermal atrophy is present in many cases of either type, and poikiloderma is not uncommon in the large-plaque type. This change is particularly prominent in the retiform subtype, which is characterized by a netlike distribution of red to brownish red, flat-topped, scaling papules over the trunk and proximal extremities. This subtype carries the poorest prognosis: many cases progress to mycosis fungoides.

The histologic findings of small-plaque parapsoriasis are characterized by a dense infiltrate in the superficial dermis composed predominantly of lymphocytes. Lymphocytes are also found within the epidermis, which is otherwise unremarkable except

Figure 11–5. Parapsoriasis en plaques of 35 years' duration in a 64-year-old man.

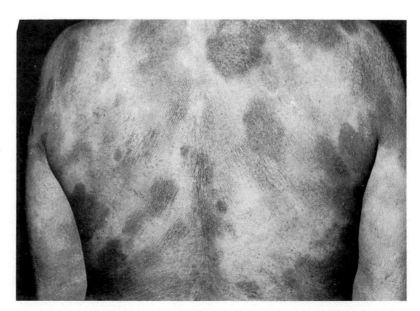

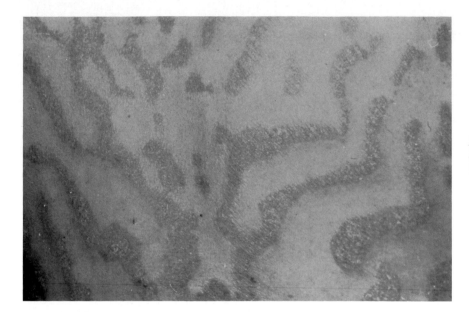

Figure 11–6. Parapsoriasis variegata on the back. (Courtesy of Dr. A. Johnson, Australia.)

for focal parakeratosis and mild acanthosis. Large-plaque parapsoriasis is distinguished from mycosis fungoides by the absence of cytologically atypical lymphocytes and the absence of Pautrier microabscess formation (i.e., collections of atypical lymphocytes in the epidermis). Large-plaque parapsoriasis may be indistinguishable from the above described changes. Atypical lymphocytes, however, may appear (particularly within the epidermis) in those lesions that progress to lymphoma.

The treatment of choice is ultraviolet radiation, either natural or in UVB units. Lubricants are helpful. Topical steroids are useful. UVA—long-wave ultraviolet radiation—with or without preliminary 8-methoxy psoralen is effective but should be used only if UVB is ineffective. The use of PUVA or high-potency topical steroids in the small-plaque type should be restricted, owing to their adverse long-term effects. The large-plaque variant's potential to develop lymphoma justifies more intense therapeutic endeavors.

Canizares suggested supplementation of this with vitamin D_2, 250,000 units in a single daily dose for two to four months. One of us (HLA) has achieved half a dozen apparent cures by means of vitamin D_2, including one case already histologically identifiable as mycosis fungoides, in complete remission for 31 years after only three months' treatment. Intake of milk should be restricted to prevent hypercalcemia.

Cañizares O: Parapsoriasis: Its treatment with calciferol. AMA Arch Dermatol 1952, 65:625.
Clayton R, et al: An immunofluorescence study of pityriasis lichenoides. Br J Dermatol 1978, 99:491.
Idem: Pityriasis lichenoides chronica presenting as hypopigmentation. Br J Dermatol 1979, 100:297.
Cornelison RL Jr, et al: Methotrexate for Mucha-Habermann disease. Arch Dermatol 1972, 106:507.
Everett MA: Lymphomatoid papulosis (editorial). JAAD 1986, 15:507.
Hood AF, et al: Histopathologic diagnosis of pityriasis lichenoides

et varioliformis acuta and its clinical correlation. Arch Dermatol 1982, 118:478.
Horowitz DC, et al: Parapsoriasis (Mucha-Habermann): Success with methotrexate. Cutis 1973, 12:401.
Katoh T, et al: Pityriasis lichenoides et varioliformis acuta: Dramatic response to sulfone. Jap J Clin Dermatol 1971, 25:145.
Lambert WC, et al: The nosology of parapsoriasis. JAAD 1981, 5:373.
LaVine MJ: Phototherapy of pityriasis lichenoides. Arch Dermatol 1983, 119:378.
Lindae ML, et al: Poikilodermatous mycosis fungoides and atrophic large-plaque parapsoriasis exhibit similar abnormalities of T-cell antigen expression. Arch Dermatol 1988, 124:366.
Longley J, et al: Clinical and histologic features of pityriasis lichenoides et varioliformis in children. Arch Dermatol 1987, 123:1335.
Marks R, et al: Pityriasis lichenoides: A reappraisal. Br J Dermatol 1972, 86:215.
Muhlbauer JE, et al: Immunopathology of pityriasis lichenoides acuta. JAAD 1984, 10:783.
Osmundsen PE: Parapsoriasis en plaques. Acta Dermatovener (Stockh) 1968, 48:345.
Piamphongsant T: Tetracycline for pityriasis lichenoides. Br J Dermatol 1974, 91:319.
Powell FC, et al: PUVA therapy of pityriasis lichenoides. JAAD 1984, 10:59.
Sauer GC: Pentoxifylline (Trental) therapy for vasculitis of pityriasis lichenoides et varioliformis. Arch Dermatol 1985, 121:487.
Shavin JS, et al: Mucha-Habermann disease in children: Treatment with erythromycin. Arch Dermatol 1978, 114:1679.
Tham SN: UVB phototherapy for pityriasis lichenoides. Austral J Dermatol 1985, 26:9.
Truhan AP, et al: Pityriasis lichenoides in children; therapeutic response to erythromycin. JAAD 1986, 15:66.
Warshauer BL, et al: Febrile ulceronecrotic Mucha-Habermann disease. Arch Dermatol 1983, 119:597.

PITYRIASIS ALBA

This dermatosis has a plethora of names: **pityriasis streptogenes, furfuraceous impetigo, pityriasis simplex, pityriasis sicca faciei,** and **erythema streptogenes.**

Pityriasis alba is characterized by hypopigmented, round to oval, scaling patches on the face, upper

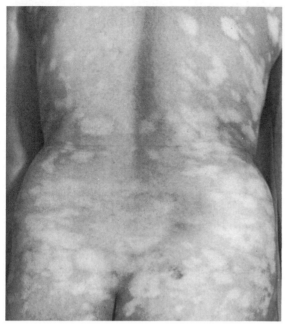

Figure 11–7. Atypically extensive example of pityriasis alba. (Courtesy of Dr. F. Kerdel Vegas.)

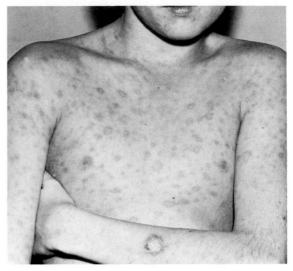

Figure 11–8. Pityriasis rosea with the herald patch on the forearm. (Courtesy of Dr. C. F. Burgoon, Jr.)

arms, neck, or shoulders. The patches vary in size, being usually a few centimeters in diameter. The color is white (but never actually depigmented) or light pink. The scales are fine and adherent. Usually the patches are sharply demarcated; the edges may be erythematous and slightly elevated. The lack of any early specifically follicular localization helps greatly to distinguish the lesions from those of follicular mucinosis. Vellus hairs are not lost in pityriasis alba, nor does hypesthesia to cold occur, as often happens in follicular mucinosis. As a rule, pityriasis alba is asymptomatic; however, there may be mild pruritus. The disease occurs chiefly in children and teenagers.

The cause is unknown. Excessively dry skin following exposure to strong sunlight appears to be contributory. However, since the patches are visible only in contrast to dark skin or a sun tan, it seems possible that sunlight merely makes them more apparent. Efforts to isolate an infectious agent, either bacterial, viral, or fungal, have been unsuccessful.

We have found 0.5 per cent hydrocortisone and 1 per cent crude coal tar in a cream base (Zetone cream), half-strength Pragmatar ointment, Lac-Hydrin, 2 per cent Zetar in Cordran cream, or 1 per cent Vioform cream to be helpful.

The prognosis is good. There is usually spontaneous healing within several months to a few years.

Bassaly M, et al: Studies on pityriasis alba. Arch Dermatol 1963, 88:272.

Bowen JH: Pityriasis alba. Cutis 1974, 14:745.

Wells BY, et al: Pityriasis alba: 10-year survey and review. Arch Dermatol 1960, 82:183.

Zaynoun ST, et al: Extensive pityriasis alba. Br J Dermatol 1983, 108:83.

Idem: Oral methoxsalen photochemotherapy for extensive pityriasis alba. JAAD 1986, 15:61.

PITYRIASIS ROSEA

CLINICAL FEATURES. Pityriasis rosea is a mild inflammatory exanthem of unknown origin, characterized by salmon-colored papular and macular lesions that are at first discrete but may become confluent. The individual patches are oval or circinate and covered with finely crinkled, dry epidermis, which often desquamates, leaving collarette scaling. The disease usually begins with a single **herald** or **mother patch**, usually larger than succeeding lesions, which may persist a week or more before others appear. By that time involution of the herald patch has begun. The efflorescence of new lesions spreads rapidly, and after three to eight weeks they usually disappear spontaneously.

The incidence is highest between the ages of 15 and 40 years, and the disease is most prevalent in the spring and autumn. Women are more frequently affected.

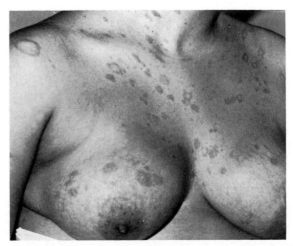

Figure 11–9. Pityriasis rosea. Herald patch on right shoulder with central clearing.

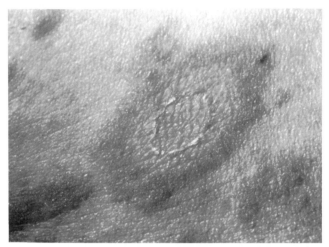

Figure 11–10. Pityriasis rosea. Note orientation of lesions along cleavage lines. (Courtesy of Dr. Axel W. Hoke.)

The fully developed eruption has a striking appearance because of the distribution and definite characteristics of the individual lesions. These are arranged so that the long axis of the macules runs parallel to the lines of cleavage. The eruption is usually generalized, affecting chiefly the trunk, and sparing sun-exposed surfaces. At times it is localized to a certain area, such as the neck, thighs, groins, or axillae. In these regions confluent circinate patches

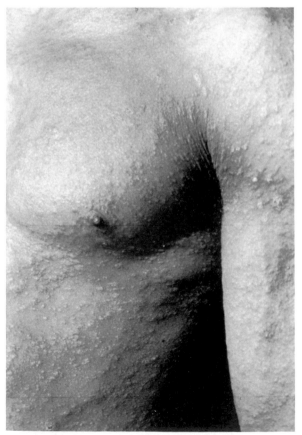

Figure 11–11. Pityriasis rosea, papular type. (Courtesy of Dr. Axel W. Hoke.)

with gyrate borders may be formed; these may strongly resemble tinea corporis (tinea circinata). Rarely, the eyelids, the scalp, or the penis may be involved. Sometimes involvement of the scalp is encountered. Occurrence on the oral mucous membranes has been noted.

Moderate pruritus may be present, particularly during the outbreak, and there may be mild constitutional symptoms prior to the onset.

Variations in the mode of onset, course, and clinical manifestations are extremely common. An unusual form, common in children under five, is that of **papular pityriasis rosea**, occurring in the typical sites and running a course similar to that of the common form of pityriasis rosea. Black children are particularly predisposed to this papular variant. An inverse distribution, sparing covered areas, is unusual but not rare. It is common in papular cases. Relapses and recurrences are observed infrequently.

Oral lesions are relatively uncommon. They are asymptomatic erythematous macules with raised borders and clearing centers. An aphthous ulcerlike appearance has recently been reported by Kay et al. They involute simultaneously with the skin lesions.

ETIOLOGY. The etiology of pityriasis rosea remains unknown. A virus infection is most frequently suggested but remains unproven. It does not occur in epidemic forms. The formation of a herald patch, the self-limited course, the seasonal preponderance, and rare recurrence are all suggestive of a virus infection. On the other hand, cases only rarely occur either together or consecutively in the same household.

A pityriasis rosealike eruption may occur as a reaction to captopril, arsenicals, gold, bismuth, clonidine, methoxypromazine, tripelennamine hydrochloride, or barbiturates.

HISTOLOGY. The histologic features of pityriasis rosea include mild acanthosis, focal parakeratosis, and extravasation of erythrocytes into the epidermis. Spongiosis may be present in acute cases. A mild perivascular infiltrate of lymphocytes is found in the dermis. Histologic evaluation is especially helpful in excluding the conditions with which pityriasis rosea may be confused.

DIFFERENTIAL DIAGNOSIS. Pityriasis rosea may closely mimic seborrheic dermatitis, tinea circinata, the macular syphilid, drug eruption, viral exanthema, and psoriasis. In seborrheic dermatitis the scalp and eyebrows are usually scaly and there is a predilection for the sternal and interscapular regions, and the flexor surfaces of the articulations, where the patches are covered with greasy scales. Tinea corporis is rarely so widespread, and some of the lesions in such an extensive eruption present the typical vesiculation at the borders. The fungus may be demonstrated. Pityriasis versicolor may also closely simulate pityriasis rosea. A positive KOH examination serves well to differentiate these last two. In the macular syphilid the lesions are of a uniform size and soon assume a brownish tint. Scaling and itching are absent or slight, and there are generalized adenopathy, mucous membrane lesions, palmoplantar lesions, a positive STS, and often the remains of a chancre. Scabies and lichen planus may be confused with the papular type.

TREATMENT. Treatment is symptomatic. The duration may be notably reduced by appropriate treatment.

Ultraviolet B in erythema exposures should be used to expedite the involution of the lesions after the acute inflammatory stage has passed. The erythema produced by ultraviolet treatment is succeeded by superficial exfoliation. Plemmons has reported unilateral clearing after unilateral ultraviolet radiation, and Arndt et al have reported beneficial results in a large study using five consecutive daily erythemogenic exposures.

Pruritus may uncommonly be intense and lead to eczematization and secondary infection due to scratching. Corticosteroid lotions, creams, or sprays give immediate relief. Antihistamines by mouth are also beneficial. For severe generalized forms a short course of systemic corticosteroids or one intramuscular injection of triamcinolone diacetate or acetonide, 20 to 40 mg, may be in order. For dryness and irritation, simple emollients are advised.

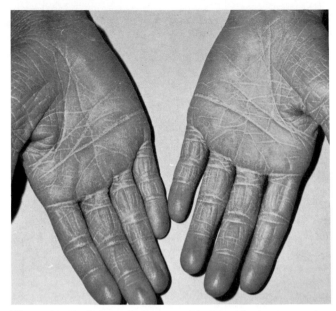

Figure 11–12. Palms of a 10-year-old girl with pityriasis rubra pilaris. (Courtesy of Dr. L. Dantzig.)

Aiba S, et al: Immunohistologic studies in pityriasis rosea. Arch Dermatol 1985, 121:761.

Arndt KA, et al: Treatment of pityriasis rosea with UV radiation. Arch Dermatol 1983, 119:381.

Chuang T, et al: Pityriasis rosea in Rochester, Minnesota, 1969–1978. JAAD 1982, 7:80.

Fox BJ, et al: Papulosquamous diseases: A review. JAAD 1985, 12:597.

Hudson LD, et al: Pityriasis rosea. JAAD 1981, 4:544.

Kay MH: Oral lesions in pityriasis rosea. Arch Dermatol 1985, 121:1449.

Parson JM: Pityriasis rosea update 1986. JAAD 1986, 15:159.

Wilkin JK, et al: Pityriasis rosea–like rash from captopril. Arch Dermatol 1982, 118:186.

PITYRIASIS RUBRA PILARIS

CLINICAL FEATURES. Pityriasis rubra pilaris (PRP) is a chronic skin disease characterized by small follicular papules, disseminated yellowish pink scaling patches, and, often, solid confluent palmoplantar hyperkeratosis. The papules are the most important diagnostic feature, being more or less acuminate, reddish brown, about pinhead size, and topped by a central horny plug. In the horny center a hair, or part of one, is usually embedded. The disease generally manifests itself first by scaliness and erythema of the scalp. The eruption is limited in the beginning, having a predilection for the sides of the neck and trunk and the extensor surfaces of the extremities, especially the backs of the first and second phalanges. Then, as new lesions occur, extensive areas are converted into sharply marginated patches of various sizes, which look like exaggerated goose-

flesh and feel like a nutmeg grater. Any portion of the body area or the entire surface may be affected.

The involvement is generally symmetric and diffuse, with, however, characteristic small islands of normal skin within the affected areas. There is a hyperkeratosis of the palms and soles, with a tendency to fissures. On the soles especially, the hyperkeratosis typically extends up the sides, and is so

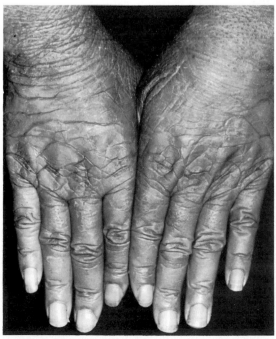

Figure 11–13. Pityriasis rubra pilaris. Note the horny plugs on the backs of proximal phalanges and on the wrists. (Courtesy of Dr. L. Fragola.)

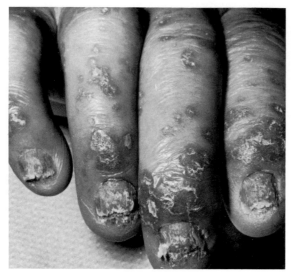

Figure 11–14. Nail changes in pityriasis rubra pilaris. (Courtesy of Dr. L. Dantzig.)

solid that it has been called a "sandal." The nails may be dull, rough, thickened, brittle, and striated, and are apt to crack and break. They are rarely if ever pitted, however; in the study by Sonnex et al, no pits were seen in the nails of 24 adult patients with PRP, but pits were found in 97 per cent of psoriasis patients. The exfoliation may become generalized and the follicular lesions less noticeable, finally disappearing and leaving a widespread dry, scaly erythroderma. The skin becomes dull red, glazed, and atrophic, sensitive to slight changes in temperature, and, over the bony prominences, subject to ulcerations.

There are no subjective symptoms except itching in some cases. The general health is not affected. The Koebner phenomenon may be present.

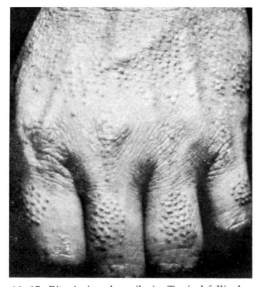

Figure 11–15. Pityriasis rubra pilaris. Typical follicular papules on backs of proximal phalanges.

PRP may be classified in respect to familial or acquired types and in respect to the onset of the disease in childhood or in adulthood. Griffith's classification is useful in this regard. Type I, the classic adult type, is seen most commonly and carries the best prognosis, with 80 per cent involuting over a three-year period. Three types of juvenile-onset forms account for up to 40 per cent of cases, with a poor prognosis for involution. Accordingly, the highest incidence is during the first five years of life or between 51 and 55 years of age.

ETIOLOGY. The etiology is unknown. The tendency to this disease is usually transmitted as an autosomal dominant characteristic in juvenile-onset PRP. Either sex may be attacked, with equal frequency. Both clinically and histologically, the disease has many features that suggest it is a vitamin deficiency disorder, particularly of vitamin A. Some reports of patients with low serum levels of retinol-binding protein have appeared, but this is not a reproducible finding.

HISTOLOGY. There is hyperkeratosis, follicular plugging, and focal parakeratosis at the follicular orifice. The inflammatory infiltrate in the dermis is composed of mononuclear cells and is generally mild. Specimens should be obtained from skin sites where hair follicles are numerous. Although there may be difficulty in making an unequivocal histologic diagnosis of pityriasis rubra pilaris, one can at least rule out the diagnosis of psoriasis, which is the most common clinical entity in differential diagnosis.

DIAGNOSIS. The diagnosis of fully developed PRP is rarely difficult because of its distinctive features, such as the peculiar orange or salmon-yellow color of the follicular papules, containing a horny center, on the backs of the fingers, sides of the neck, and extensor surfaces of the limbs; the thickened, rough, and slightly or moderately scaly, harsh skin; the sandal-like palmoplantar hyperkeratosis; and the islands of normal skin in the midst of the eruption. It is distinguished from psoriasis by the scales, which in the latter are silvery, light, and overlap like shingles, and by the papules, which extend peripherally to form patches. Lichen planus has characteristics such as shiny plaques of a violaceous or dark red hue and flattened, angular, shiny papules that rarely involve the face, scalp, and palms. Phrynoderma due to vitamin A deficiency gives a somewhat similar appearance to the skin, as may also eczematous eruptions due to deficiency of vitamin B.

TREATMENT. The management of pityriasis rubra pilaris has changed markedly in recent years; however, symptomatic treatment is still important.

Topical applications of bland emollients are recommended. Lac-Hydrin is particularly helpful.

Isotretinoin (Accutane) is the treatment of choice in adult-onset PRP. A several-month course in doses of 1 to 2 mg/kg/day may induce prolonged remissions or cures. Goldsmith et al detail these results. Etretinate has been reported to be effective also. Vitamin A in doses of 300,000 to 500,000 units daily, with the possible addition of vitamin E, 400 units two or three

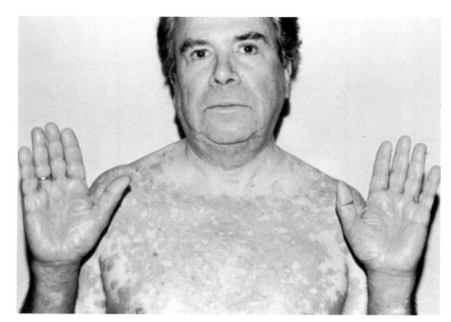

Figure 11–16. Pityriasis rubra pilaris. Note sparing of "islands of normal skin." (Courtesy of Dr. Axel W. Hoke.)

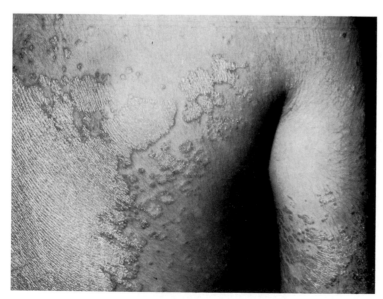

Figure 11–17. Pityriasis rubra pilaris on the scapular area.

times daily, is often effective and well tolerated by adults, but the synthetic retinoids are preferable.

Topical corticosteroids are variably, and as a rule not very, effective. Oral prednisone is not recommended, because of the availability of better therapeutic options, and because of the necessity for prolonged therapy, with the associated side effects. Intramuscular Kenalog, 60 to 80 mg, every four or five weeks, always helps and may be very effective.

Methotrexate therapy has been used by Brown and Perry, and by Chernosky, with good results. They gave methotrexate 2.5 mg orally alternately one day with 5 mg the next. A continuous daily regimen was far superior, in Chernosky's opinion, to the one-day-a-week approach. Hunter and Forbes reported cures in four of five cases treated with Imuran (azathioprine). Again, with the retinoids, these more toxic alternatives are no longer recommended.

Davison CL Jr, et al: Pityriasis rubra pilaris. Arch Dermatol 1969, 100:175.

Dicken CH: Isotretinoin treatment of pityriasis rubra pilaris. JAAD 1987, 16:297.

Fleissner J, et al: Etretinate in the treatment of juvenile pityriasis rubra pilaris. Arch Dermatol 1981, 117:749.

Goldsmith LA, et al: Pityriasis rubra pilaris: Response to 13-cis retinoic acid. JAAD 1982, 6:710.

Griffiths A: Pityriasis rubra pilaris. JAAD 1984, 10:1086.

Griffiths WAD: Pityriasis rubra pilaris: Clinical features and natural history in a study of 93 patients. Br J Dermatol 1977, 97(suppl.15):18.

Gross DA, et al: Pityriasis rubra pilaris. Arch Dermatol 1969, 99:710.

Hunter GA, et al: Treatment of pityriasis rubra pilaris with azathioprine. Br J Dermatol 1972, 87:46.

Knowles WR, et al: Pityriasis rubra pilaris: Prolonged treatment with [daily] methotrexate. Arch Dermatol 1970, 102:603.

Sonnex TS, et al: The nails in adult type 1 pityriasis rubra pilaris. JAAD 1986, 15:956.

12

Lichen Planus and Lichenoid Eruptions

LICHEN PLANUS

CLINICAL FEATURES. Lichen planus is an inflammatory pruritic disease of the skin and mucous membranes, characterized by distinctive papules with a predilection for the flexor surfaces and trunk. The eruption occurs especially on the volar aspects of the wrists and medial sides of the thighs, where the lesions tend to be grouped into irregular, annular, and linear patches. The shins, the backs of the hands, and the glans penis are also sites of election. The face is only rarely involved, and when it is, lesions are apt to be confined to the eyelids or lips, or both. The diagnostic papules are small, flat, polygonal, glistening facets of a characteristic violet color lying between and defined by the natural lines of the skin. Their surface is dry and shiny, with scanty, adherent scales.

The elementary lesion is almost pathognomonic. It is an angular papule about the size of a pinhead, with a flat, smooth, glistening surface, and is only slightly raised. On close examination a slight depression (umbilication) or a small horny plug at the site of a pore may be seen toward the center of the papule. With a lens one can make out grayish puncta or streaks (*Wickham's striae*), which form a network on the surface of the papule; these become more visible if the horny layers are rendered transparent by application of aniline oil. The color varies from red to purple but most commonly is lavender or "violaceous."

After the lichen planus lesions have disappeared, deep pigmentation may persist for several months. The pigmentation is often so intense that a diagnosis of the antecedent disease can be made from its distribution. Less often, depigmented atrophic spots remain.

The mucous membranes of the mouth are frequently affected. The lesions are usually located on the inner sides of the cheeks, and consist of pinhead-sized, silvery-white papules that form annular or linear patterns or appear as discrete puncta, or, more commonly, aggregations of them form irregular reticulated or lacelike patterns. Similar lesions may occur on the palate, lips, and tongue. In the last two locations they are less characteristic and may be mistaken for leukoplakia, except for the mosaic, reticulated appearance and tiny white or bluish white dots, often arranged in interlacing wavy lines or circles. On the lips the papules are more often annular, and there is an adherent scaling similar to that seen in lupus erythematosus. Vesicular lesions

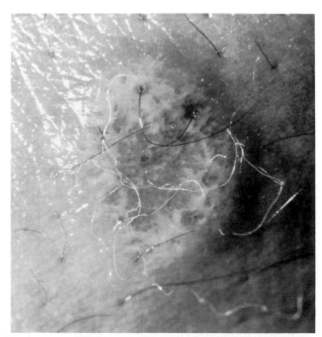

Figure 12–1. Wickham's striae in lichen planus. (Courtesy of Dr. Axel W. Hoke.)

237

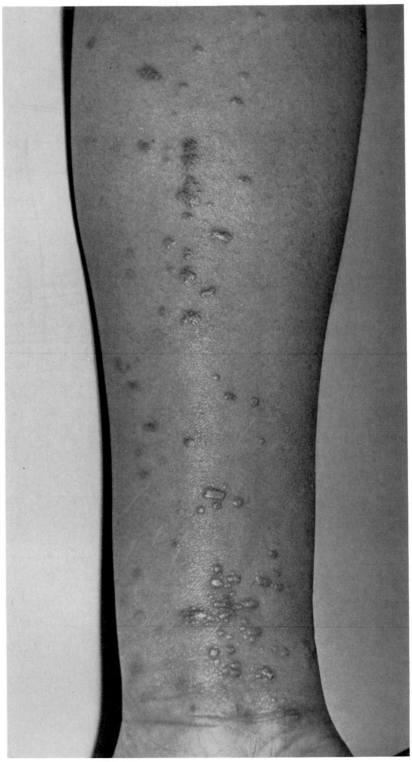

Figure 12–2. Lichen planus on forearm.

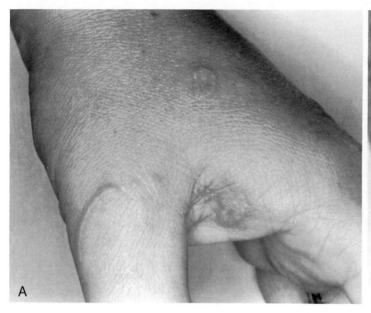

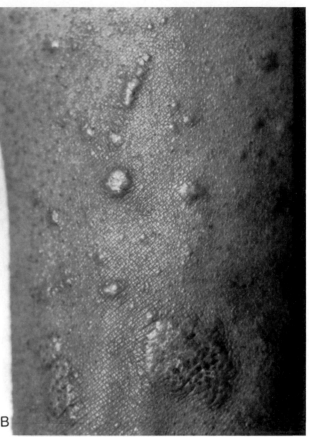

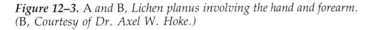

Figure 12–3. A *and* B, *Lichen planus involving the hand and forearm.* (B, *Courtesy of Dr. Axel W. Hoke.*)

have been observed on the palate also. Mucosal lesions may ulcerate. Ulcerative oral lichen planus is an uncommon, chronic, painful condition, often seen without associated skin lesions.

Carcinoma may rarely develop, especially at the site of ulcerations. Any part of the mouth may be involved. Grinspan and his associates found eight carcinomas developing in 65 patients with mucous membrane lichen planus. The tumors were located on the lower lip, tongue, and buccal mucosa. Koberg and his associates reported 51 cases of squamous cell carcinoma occurring in patients with lichen planus of the mouth. Carcinoma occurs only after a long time lapse following the development of the initial lesions. They also cited carcinoma occurring rarely in hypertrophic lichen planus and in lichen planus of the vulva. Bart and Kopf found 100 reported cases of carcinoma in oral lichen planus, and six cases with skin lesions only.

On the glans penis the lesions consist of flat polygonal papules, which may be arranged in rings. On the labia and anus similar lesions are observed; they are generally whitish, owing to maceration.

The disease may appear on any part of the body, but rarely on the face, except for the upper eyelids and the vermilion of the lower lip. One should always look for mucous membrane lesions, which are present in at least two thirds of patients. Not infrequently the lesions are limited to the mouth

without any skin lesions. The palms and soles may be found studded with acuminate papules forming a fairly hard mass. Diffuse palmoplantar lesions may occur. In a case of Arnold's, lichen planus of the dorsal hands shaded into typical pompholyx of the palms.

Nail changes are present in approximately 5 to 10 per cent of patients. Subungual papules may cause a thickening and malformation of the nails with tumefaction of the matrix regions. Pterygium formation is distinctive in lichen planus of the nails (see Chapter 32, Appendages). This occurs because the nail matrix is replaced by fibrosis. Thus the proximal nail fold fuses with the proximal portion of the nail bed. Involvement of the entire matrix may lead to obliteration of the whole nail. Longitudinal grooving, ridging, and splitting and a peculiar midline fissure are some of the manifestations of lichen planus of the nails. Twenty-nail dystrophy of childhood revealed lichen planus in one patient who was biopsied. Scher and Ackerman reviewed lichen planus of the nails and concluded that onychorrhexis was the most common manifestation. They described also (for the first time) proximal onycholysis occurring in lichen planus.

The scalp lesions are patches of scarring alopecia. The lesions may resemble the atrophic patches of lupus erythematosus. The resulting permanent patchy alopecia, because it resembles alopecia areata

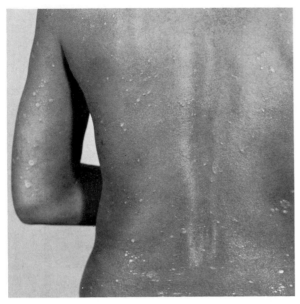

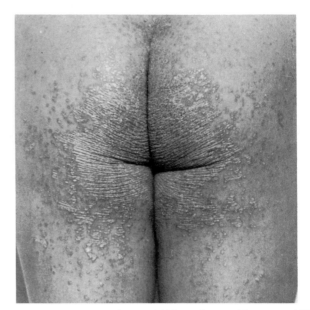

Figure 12–4. Acute widespread lichen planus resembling pityriasis rosea. (Courtesy of J. L. Miller.)

Figure 12–5. Acute widespread lichen planus. (Courtesy of Dr. L. Schweich.)

("*pelade*," in French), is called *pseudopelade*. (See the discussion on lichen planus follicularis, Chapter 32, Appendages).

Koebner's isomorphic phenomenon, as in psoriasis, occurs regularly in lichen planus. By physical trauma, such as scratching, skin lesions are produced in the scratch marks identical to those already on the patient's skin. Lichen planus may occur in healed lesions of herpes zoster or within sites of healing toxicodendron allergic contact dermatitis, a Koebner-like effect.

Pruritus is generally an outstanding symptom in lichen planus. It is often almost intolerable in acute cases. The pruritus occurs in spasms and causes frenzied itching that lasts for minutes to hours and then gradually subsides. Most patients react to the itching of lichen planus by rubbing rather than scratching and consequently scratch marks are usually not discernible.

A wide variety of skin manifestations may occur in lichen planus. The following are some of those more frequently seen.

Acute Widespread Lichen Planus. The acute exanthem most commonly begins on the inner surfaces of the arms and spreads rapidly, involving large areas of the body, with a predilection for the abdomen, lower back, thighs, and forearms. The acute outbreak may be preceded by one or two small patches of the disease for months or years. In severe cases the papules erupt so densely that the skin becomes diffusely erythematous and edematous. Vesicopapules and even bullae may be rarely observed, especially in the generalized cases, demonstrating that the severity of the inflammation plays an important role. Widespread eruptions of lichen planus persist for a few months and then tend to

subside spontaneously. Not infrequently a few hypertrophic patches may remain as a localized chronic variety, the shins being a favorite location for such lesions. Itching is typically severe. Sometimes at the beginning the eruption in the widespread type is vesicular and eczematous, and a definitive morphologic pattern does not appear for several weeks.

Chronic Localized Lichen Planus. The chronic type of the disease is of more common occurrence and its course is characterized by periodic exacerbations, during which new lesions appear and the eruption spreads. The areas involved are comparatively limited. The disease usually undergoes some involution after persistence for several months or years, or the lesions may become hypertrophic.

Hypertrophic Lichen Planus (Lichen Planus Verrucosus). The hypertrophic variety of the disease occurs most commonly on the shins, though it may be situated anywhere. The patches consist of verrucous plaques covered with fine adherent scales. At the edges of the patches, small, flat-topped polygonal papules may be discovered upon careful search, but superficial inspection of the lesion often suggests psoriasis rather than lichen planus. The patches usually are palm-sized or larger, but may be nummular. The clinical diagnosis is made from the bluish color of the patches, their thickening and small adherent scales, the itching, and the symmetric location on the shins, usually without any other skin lesions.

Lichen Planus Atrophicus. This is characterized by atrophy in the center of the papules so that, ultimately, atrophic spots are present. In this type the papules are usually flat and difficult to find. Close inspection will usually reveal their angular outlines, with often a prominent central umbilication. Aggre-

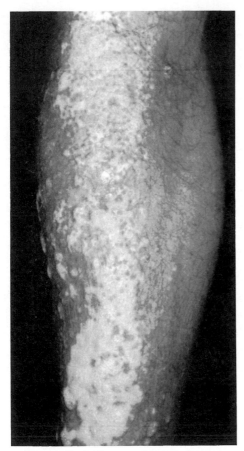

Figure 12–6. Hypertrophic lichen planus.

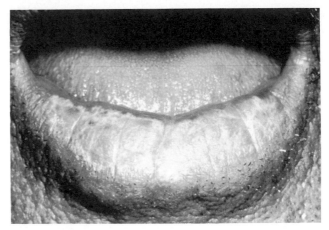

Figure 12–7. Lichen planus of the lips. (Courtesy of Dr. Axel W. Hoke.)

gations of these lesions form small ivory or violet-colored patches, around which there may be a zone of erythema. These may simulate morphea guttata and lichen sclerosus et atrophicus. When this atrophic variant occurs on skin with a black or olive complexion, the center may be hyperpigmented. There may be deep pigmentation centrally with only a rim of purple annular lesions. In rare cases the atrophy may be extensive, and ulcerations may develop (*lichen planus atrophicus et exulcerans*) that persist for years, with carcinoma developing in the ulcers.

Erosive and Bullous Oral Lesions of Lichen Planus. These may be difficult to diagnose when the classic lacy network of white lesions is absent. The erosive lesions occur with some frequency, especially on the sides or dorsum of the tongue and on the buccal mucosa, where they are extremely painful, but the diagnosis can be confirmed only by histologic examination. Shklar describes the histologic features as hyperkeratosis or parakeratosis, infiltration of the upper corium with a broad band of lymphocytes, and liquefaction degeneration of the basal layer. In the differential diagnosis pemphigus vulgaris, lupus erythematosus, mucous membrane (cicatricial) pemphigoid, and erythema multiforme must be considered. Herpetic stomatitis and herpes zoster should also be considered.

Ulcerative Lichen Planus. Cram and his associates

described an unusual syndrome of lichen planus confined to the feet and toes and manifested by bullae and ulcerations, permanent loss of the toenails, and cicatricial alopecia of the scalp. There was also involvement of the buccal mucosa. The chronic ulcerations on the feet were painful and disabling. In two of their patients skin grafting of the soles produced successful results. They reviewed the literature and found nine similar cases, mostly in women. Crotty et al reported two similar cases from the Mayo Clinic in 1980, and Zijdenbos et al another in 1985.

Hepatitis-Associated Lichen Planus. Primary biliary cirrhosis and lichen planus may coexist, as reported by Powell et al and Graham-Brown et al. Patients with this liver abnormality have a marked propensity to develop a lichenoid eruption while on D-penicillamine therapy.

Rebora et al have reported that nine of 11 patients with erosive lichen planus and 13.5 per cent of their patients with nonerosive lichen planus had evidence of chronic active hepatitis with negative hepatitis B surface antigen studies. Korkij et al found a similar

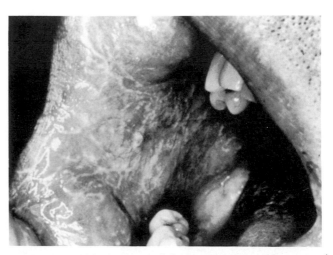

Figure 12–8. Lichen planus of the buccal mucosa. (Courtesy of Dr. Axel W. Hoke.)

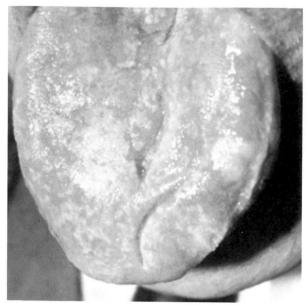

Figure 12–9. Lichen planus of the tongue.

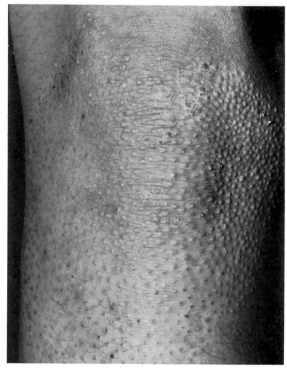

Figure 12–10. Lichen planopilaris on the knee of a 14-year-old boy.

incidence of documented liver disease, significantly higher than their control population. Two other studies have not confirmed these findings. One should be receptive to signs or symptoms of liver disease when evaluating patients with lichen planus.

Lichen Planus–Lupus Erythematosus Overlap. Over 20 cases have been reported of discoid lesions with central atrophy and hypopigmentation outlined by a reddish purple periphery, which are fixed, have a predilection for acral areas, and are poorly responsive to conventional therapy. Histologically and immunopathologically the diagnosis of lichen planus is supported. Often there are coexistent findings to support the diagnosis of lupus erythematosus.

Lichen Planus Erythematosus. This rare variant of lichen planus was originally described by Crocker in 1891. The deep crimson-colored papules are soft to the touch and are more erythematous than the ordinary lichen planus. The individual lesions vary from 5 to 10 mm in diameter and blanch on pressure; they are discrete and occur singly on the trunk. Mucosal and nail changes are usually absent. Tanenbaum et al reported one case, as did one of us (HLA).

Follicular Lichen Planus (Lichen Planopilaris). Follicular lichen planus produces a patchy eruption of spiny follicular papules, indistinguishable from those of lichen spinulosus. These may be mixed with flat papules. Sometimes the projecting horny filaments are extremely delicate. The eruption is usually not pruritic. Follicular lichen planus must be differentiated from Darier's disease, keratosis pilaris, and lichen scrofulosorum. This type of lichen planus occurs mostly on the scalp, with scarring alopecia ensuing in the affected areas. This produces irregularly shaped bald patches that usually persist permanently.

Graham Little–Piccardi–Lassueur Syndrome. This syndrome is characterized by patchy cicatricial alopecia of the scalp and by patches of follicular spinous papules involving the trunk, the upper parts of the arms and legs, and the scalp. There may be typical oral or cutaneous lichen planus. In addition, there may be patches of alopecia (noncicatricial-appearing) in the axillae and pubic areas. This syndrome with its many variants has received innumerable names,

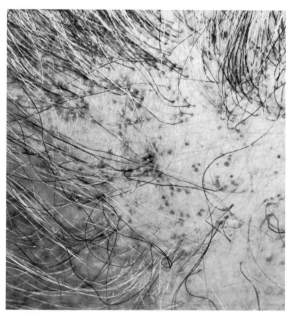

Figure 12–11. Graham-Little syndrome on scalp consisting of acuminate follicular papules, alopecia, and lichen planus. (Courtesy of Dr. D. Torre.)

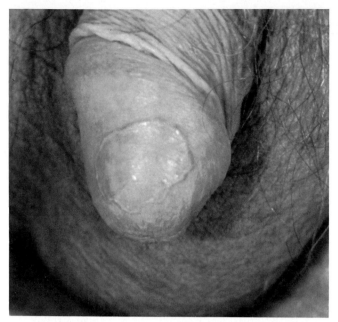

Figure 12–12. Annular lichen planus on glans penis.

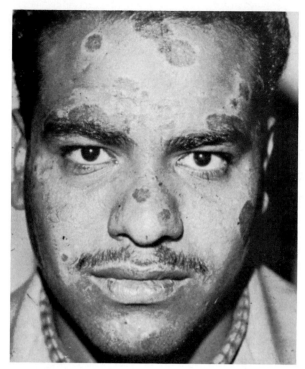

Figure 12–13. Lichen planus tropicus. (Courtesy of Dr. M. El-Zawahry, U.A.R.)

but there is agreement that it is a variant of follicular lichen planus.

Horn et al reported a case of typical lichen planopilaris and a case of Graham Little–Piccardi–Lassueur syndrome in which the clinical overlap and similarity of immunofluorescence findings supported the concept that both conditions are follicular variants of lichen planus.

Annular Lichen Planus. Most frequently annular configurations of lichen planus are located on the penis or lips, although they may be found scattered on the skin or, more frequently, in the mouth. The ringed edges are composed of small papules. The rings are often about 1 cm in diameter. They may coalesce to form polycyclic figures. Less often annular lesions may result from central atrophy in a flat papule.

Lichen Planus Tropicus (Subtropicus). This condition has been variously named *lichen planus actinicus, actinic lichen planus,* and *summertime actinic lichenoid eruption.* El-Zawahry has called attention to this variety of lichen planus, which favors the sun-exposed parts of the body such as the face (forehead, cheeks, and lips), the V area of the chest, the backs of the hands, and the lower forearms. The extremely pruritic lesions are typical lichen planus papules, which frequently show annular configuration and the distinctive violaceous coloration.

Lichen planus tropicus is elicited by long exposure to sun, particularly in the cases of adolescents and young adults who work all day in the fields. El-Zawahry estimates that 40 per cent of all cases of lichen planus in the United Arab Republic are of this variety. Constant exposure to heat also promotes the development of these lesions. Sixteen cases were reported by Salman et al in 1989 in young adults in

Lebanon; two had deposits of mucin in the reticular dermis. They estimated these cases to account for 14 per cent of the cases they saw.

Isaacson et al reported a case from the United States and van der Schroeff documented one from the Netherlands. Both were successfully induced by phototesting with UVB.

Lichen Planus Pemphigoides. These patients usually have typical lichen planus lesions that, two to six weeks later, erupt with bullae, which also may

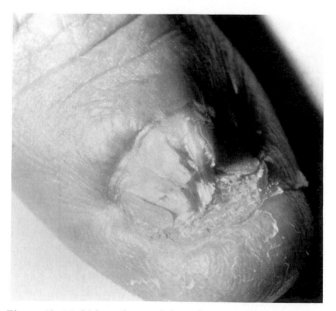

Figure 12–14. Lichen planus of the nails—pterygium formation. (Courtesy of Dr. Axel W. Hoke.)

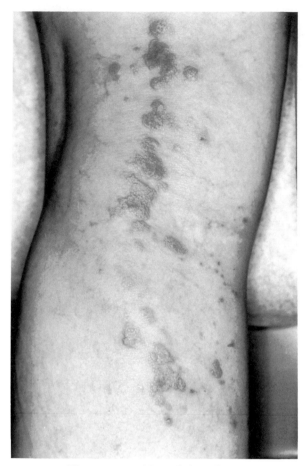

Figure 12–15. Linear lichen planus.

arise on normal skin. These cases should be separated from those patients in whom blisters erupt only within lesions of lichen planus, as blisters occur at times in lesions with severe inflammation.

The histopathology of the bullae may be that seen with bullous pemphigoid, and the immunopathology may reveal IgG and C3 in a linear pattern at the basement membrane zone. These deposits were seen to be present in the lamina lucida in a case reported by Hinter et al. Circulating anti-BMZ IgG antibodies may be present. In one case investigated by immunoprecipitation, bullous pemphigoid antigen was not identified. Whether this disease is coexistent lichen planus and bullous pemphigoid, or lichen planus and another as yet to be identified bullous disorder, or (as is most likely) is heterogeneous in nature, remains to be elucidated.

Erythema Dyschromicum Variants. Hermann Pinkus suggested that erythema dyschromicum perstans (EDP) was one of Gougerot's *lichens atypiques ou invisibles* revealed by pigmentation, and Naidorf and Cohen reported the case of a woman who had EDP for two years before developing annular lichen planus with pigmentation.

ETIOLOGY. The cause of lichen planus remains unknown. Evidence points to the possibility that an alteration of epidermal cell antigens induces a cell-mediated immune response similar to that seen in graft-versus-host disease. The type of infiltrate seen and its association with primary biliary cirrhosis and graft-versus-host disease support this.

Several recent reports document that lichen planus may be familial, and may occur in monozygotic twins. These familial cases occur at an early age and are chronic.

Drugs may induce lichenoid reactions. Medications commonly associated with the development of this type of response are penicillamine, the antimalarials, arsenic, gold, quinidine, thiazide derivatives, methyldopa, chlorpropamide, and phenothiazine derivatives. Propranolol, spironolactone, and naproxen are other drugs recently described to have induced this reaction.

INCIDENCE AND COURSE. Lichen planus is rare in children. Any that occurs is usually of the diffuse widespread variety. The familial cases are diffuse, chronic, and severe. The eruptive cases that occur in adults tend to involute after several months to a year. Oral lesions, especially of the ulcerative variety, are chronic, with little tendency for remission. The hypertrophic and linear varieties may persist indefinitely in spite of therapeutic measures.

HISTOLOGY. The histologic features of lichen planus are distinctive. There is a "saw-tooth" pattern of epidermal hyperplasia together with orthokeratosis and hypergranulosis. There is vacuolar alteration of the basal layer of the epidermis. Necrotic keratinocytes are present in the basal layer. In the superficial dermis there is a dense, bandlike infiltrate composed of lymphocytes, histiocytes, and melanophages. "Civatte bodies," often present in the infiltrate, represent necrotic keratinocytes that have descended into the dermis. Drug-induced lichenoid eruptions may have a considerable number of eosinophils in the infiltrate. Hypertrophic lichen planus shows the histologic features of lichen simplex chronicus superimposed upon those of lichen planus.

Pinkus (1973) has described the lichenoid tissue reaction in detail, and his classic article is worth studying.

On direct immunofluorescence, clumps of IgM and less frequently IgA, IgG, and C3 are commonly present subepidermally, corresponding to the colloid bodies. These do not occur in oral lesions, but instead oral biopsies show a fibrillar band of fibrinogen at the basement membrane zone. Lichen planopilaris and Graham Little–Piccardi–Lassueur syndrome show findings similar to those of lichen planus, except that involvement is in the superficial follicular epithelium. Duschet et al reported that 86 per cent of cases of lichen planus biopsied on the upper trunk had positive immunofluorescent findings, while only 50 per cent of lesions on the lower extremities were positive.

DIFFERENTIAL DIAGNOSIS. Lichen planus has so many manifestations that it must be differentiated from a number of diseases. Scabies, pediculosis corporis, pityriasis rosea, psoriasis guttata, the small-papular or lichenoid syphilid, and pityriasis lichenoides et varioliformis acuta are dermatoses that may resemble generalized lichen planus. Mucous membrane lesions may be confused with leukoplakia, lupus erythematosus, mucous patches of syphilis, candidiasis, cancer, and traumatic stomatitis. On the scalp the atrophic lesions may be mistaken for lupus erythematosus, folliculitis decalvans, and cicatrices.

The follicular type must be differentiated from lichen spinulosus, which usually occurs only in children, so that the diagnosis of "lichen spinulosus" in an adult generally means lichen planus. In lichen spinulosus, horny filiform papules appear in crops in symmetrically arranged patches over the trunk and limbs. In keratosis pilaris, the onset is insidious, with horny follicular papules the color of normal skin or slightly gray occurring chiefly on the lateral aspects of the arms and thighs, without itching.

The atrophic type of lichen planus may be difficult to distinguish from lichen sclerosus et atrophicus and morphea guttata.

The hypertrophic type may simulate psoriasis, Kaposi's multiple hemorrhagic sarcoma, and lichen amyloidosis. Isolated patches of lichen planus may resemble neurodermatitis circumscripta or, if heavily pigmented, may suggest a fixed drug eruption.

There is a striking similarity between lichen planus and lichenoid dermatitis due to contact with color film developer chemicals.

Annular lichen planus, especially on the extremities, may resemble granuloma annulare.

TREATMENT. Treatment is symptomatic and depends mostly upon the administration of corticosteroids. They should always be used intralesionally when feasible, but of course in most cases lesions are either too large or too numerous. Topical steroids are rarely effective, and though the newer high-potency ones such as Temovate might be effective, their potential for side effects is heightened too, and it would be safer to use intramuscularly injected triamcinolone, 60 mg, in most situations. The potent steroids in Orabase may be useful for oral lesions. Generally if lichen planus is eruptive or generalized, systemic steroids are needed. Oral prednisone should be avoided if possible, because of side effects, but if it is unavoidable, a dose of 40 to 60 mg daily is suggested, tapering off over 2 to 3 months.

Snyder et al reported a man with generalized lichen planus in whom low-to-intermediate–dose oral and intramuscular steroids as well as griseofulvin and methotrexate had failed, but who responded well to intermittent megadose IV ("pulse") therapy with methylprednisolone, 1 gm daily for three days, each month for three months.

Dapsone induced complete healing of oral and palmoplantar ulcerations in a case reported by Falk et al, and isotretinoin, 10 mg a day, cleared a case of

erosive oral lichen planus of 14 years' duration reported by Staus and Bergfeld. Woo also reported success with oral isotretinoin in two patients with erosive oral lesions. Giustina and associates reported improvement from topical isotretinoin gel in 20 cases.

Mahrle and associates reported their experience with etretinate. Twenty-six patients were given a starting dose of 1 mg/kg (75–100 mg) a day, tapered to a maintenance dose of 25 to 50 mg every other day after two to five weeks. All of four exanthematous eruptive patients responded. The overall response in classic lichen planus was 46 per cent "good to excellent"; it was less effective in cases with oral lesions.

Gonzalez et al have reported on the use of PUVA for lichen planus. Five of 10 patients cleared completely and needed no maintenance treatment; three others improved at least 50 per cent. Two patients were made worse.

Paslin reported success in three cases with cyclophosphamide, 50 mg a day, after failure or transitory success with a variety of agents, including grenz radiation, chlorambucil, amitriptyline, and others. Resolution of lesions was complete in a few weeks, and lasting.

Metronidazole (Flagyl) has been reported effective in 29 cases of erosive oral lichen planus, and Shelley et al saw an initial eruption and two relapses of lichen planus respond to metronidazole (given for resistant cystitis) after successive two-week trials of ampicillin, erythromycin, ketoconazole, and cholestyramine had failed to help. They also saw it succeed dramatically in a nine-year-old boy who was given it for giardiasis: his hitherto unresponsive lichen planus cleared in two weeks.

Tranquilizers and antipruritic drugs such as the antihistamines and cyproheptadine (Periactin) may be helpful in selected cases.

Levy et al in Israel reported complete healing in 80 to 90 per cent of 26 cases of lichen planus treated with griseofulvin, 125 mg twice daily for three to six months.

Altman J, et al: Variations and course of lichen planus. Arch Dermatol 1961, 84:179.
Arnold HL Jr: Lichen planus erythematosus. Arch Dermatol 1961, 84:83.
Ayala F, et al: Oral erosive lichen planus and chronic liver disease. JAAD 1986, 14:139.
Brice SL, et al: Childhood lichen planus: A question of therapy. JAAD 1980, 4:370.
Camisa C, et al: Bullous lichen planus. JAAD 1986, 14:464.
Caro I: Familial lichen planus (letter). Arch Dermatol 1984, 120:577.
Clover GB, et al: Is childhood idiopathic atrophy of the nails due to lichen planus? Br J Dermatol 1987, 116:709.
Copeman PWM: Familial lichen planus. Arch Dermatol 1981, 117:189.
Cram DL, et al: Ulcerative lichen planus of the feet. Arch Dermatol 1966, 93:692.
Crotty CP, et al: Ulcerative lichen planus. Arch Dermatol 1980, 116:1252.
Daniels TE, et al: Direct immunofluorescence in oral mucosal disease; a diagnostic analysis of 130 cases. Oral Surg 1981, 54:38.

Domonkos AN: Hypertrophic lichen planus treated by local injections of prednisolone. Arch Dermatol 1957, 75:264.

Duschet P, et al: Effect of anatomic location on immunofluorescence in lichen planus. JAAD 1985, 13:1057.

El-Zawahry M: Lichen planus tropicus. Dermatol Int 1965, 4:92.

Falk DK, et al: Dapsone in the treatment of erosive lichen planus. JAAD 1985, 12:567.

Feuerman EJ, et al: Lichen ruber planus beginning as a dyshidrosiform eruption. Cutis 1982, 30:401.

Fulling HJ: Cancer development in oral lichen planus. Arch Dermatol 1973, 108:667.

Gibstine CF, et al: Lichen planus in monozygotic twins (letter). Arch Dermatol 1984, 120:580.

Giustina TA, et al: Isotretinoin gel improves oral lichen planus. Arch Dermatol 1986, 122:534.

Gonzalez E, et al: Bilateral comparison of generalized lichen planus treated with psoralens and ultraviolet A. JAAD 1984, 10:958.

Gougerot MH: Lichens atypiques ou invisibles pigmentogènes revelés par des pigmentations. Bull Soc Fr Dermatol Syph 1935, 42:792.

Graham Brown RAC, et al: Lichen planus and primary biliary cirrhosis. Br J Dermatol 1982, 106:699.

Heymann WR, et al: Naproxen-induced lichen planus (letter). JAAD 1984, 10:299.

Horn RT, et al: Immunofluorescent findings and clinical overlap in two cases of follicular lichen planus. JAAD 1982, 7:203.

Isaacson D, et al: Summertime actinic lichenoid eruption (lichen planus actinicus). JAAD 1981, 4:404.

Johnson FR, et al: Ultrastructural observations on lichen planus. Arch Dermatol 1967, 95:596.

Karvonen J, et al: Topical trioxsalen PUVA in lichen planus and nodular prurigo. Acta Dermatol Venereol (Stockh) 1985, 120:53.

Kechijian P: Twenty-nail dystrophy of childhood: A reappraisal. Cutis 1985, 35:38.

Korkij W, et al: Liver abnormalities in . . . lichen planus. JAAD 1984, 11:609.

Lang PF Jr, et al: Coexisting lichen planus and bullous pemphigoid, or lichen planus pemphigoides? JAAD 1983, 9:133.

Levy A, et al: Treatment of lichen planus with griseofulvin. Int J Dermatol 1986, 25:405.

Magnusson N: Lichen ruber bullosus and tumors in internal organs. Dermatologica 1967, 134:166.

Mahood JM: Familial lichen planus: 9 cases from 4 families. Arch Dermatol 1983, 119:292.

Idem: Familial lichen planus. Arch Dermatol 1983, 119:292.

Mahrle G, et al: Oral treatment of keratinizing disorders . . . with etretinate. Arch Dermatol 1982, 118:97.

Mora RG: Lichen planus pemphigoides . . . JAAD 1983, 8:331.

Moss ALH, et al: Surgery for painful lichen planus of the hand and foot. Br J Plastic Surg 1986, 39:402.

Naidorf KF, et al: Erythema dyschromicum perstans and lichen planus. Arch Dermatol 1982, 118:683.

Nelson BR, et al: Asymptomatic progressive hyperpigmentation in a 16-year-old girl. Arch Dermatol 1988, 124:769.

Paslin DA: Sustained remission of generalized lichen planus induced by cyclophosphamide. Arch Dermatol 1985, 121:236.

Pinkus H, in discussion of Knox JM, et al: Erythema dyschromicum perstans. Arch Dermatol 1968, 97:270.

Idem: Lichenoid tissue reactions. Arch Dermatol 1973, 107:840.

Plotnick H, et al: Lichen planus and coexisting LE vs. lichen planus–like LE. JAAD 1986, 14:931.

Powell FC, et al: Primary biliary cirrhosis and lichen planus. JAAD 1983, 9:540.

Rebora A, et al: Chronic active hepatitis and lichen planus. Acta Dermatovener (Stockh) 1982, 62:351.

Idem: In reply to Monk B: Lichen planus and the liver (letter). JAAD 1985, 12:122.

Salman SM, et al: Actinic lichen planus mimicking melanoma. JAAD 1988, 18:275.

Idem: Actinic lichen planus: Clinicopathologic study of 16 patients. JAAD 1989, 20:226.

Samman PD: Lichen planus: Analysis of 200 cases. Trans St Johns Hosp Dermatol Soc 1961, 46:36.

Schafer JR, et al: Lichen planus–like lesions caused by penicillamine in primary biliary cirrhosis. Arch Dermatol 1981, 117:140.

Scher RK, et al: Lichen planus [of nails]. Am J Dermatopathol 1983, 5:375.

Shelley WB, et al: Urinary tract infection as a cause of lichen planus: Metronidazole therapy. JAAD 1984, 10:905.

Shiohara T: The lichenoid tissue reaction. Am J Dermatopathol 1988, 10:252.

Idem: Lichenoid skin disease: Immunopathologic study. JAAD 1988, 18:67.

Shklar G: Erosive and bullous oral lesions of lichen planus. Arch Dermatol 1966, 97:411.

Silverman D Jr, et al: Followup study of 570 patients with oral lichen planus. Oral Surg 1985, 60:30.

Snyder RA, et al: Intermittent megadose corticosteroid therapy for . . . lichen planus. JAAD 1982, 6:1089.

Staus ME, et al: Treatment of lichen planus with low-dose isotretinoin (letter). JAAD 1984, 11:527.

Stillman MA, et al: Squamous cell carcinoma . . . in oral lichen planus. Cutis 1973, 11:484.

Tanenbaum MH, et al: Lichen planus erythematosus. Arch Dermatol 1964, 90:91.

Van der Schroeff JG, et al: Induction of actinic lichen planus with artificial UV sources. Arch Dermatol 1983, 119:498.

Van Hecke E, et al: A lichenoid eruption induced by penicillamine. Arch Dermatol 1981, 117:676.

Venencie PY, et al: Erythema dyschromicum perstans following HIV seroconversion in a child with hemophilia B. Arch Dermatol 1988, 124:1013.

Voron D, et al: Annular lichen planus. Cutis 1973, 11:635.

Woo TY: Systemic isotretinoin treatment of . . . lichen planus. Cutis 1985, 33:385.

Zijdenbos LM, et al: Ulcerative lichen planus with associated sicca syndrome and good . . . result of skin grafting (letter). JAAD 1985, 13:667.

KERATOSIS LICHENOIDES CHRONICA

This chronic dermatosis is considered by some to be a variant of lichen planus, but will be discussed here separately. It is characterized by erythema, scaling, and telangiectasia of the face and purplish papulonodular lesions of the extremities and buttocks. The hyperkeratotic lesions may be manifested by a linear configuration of warty lichenoid lesions, by yellow keratotic patches, or by raised papules with keratotic plugs. Nail changes, including thickening of the nail plate, longitudinal ridging, onycholysis, hyperkeratosis of the nail bed, paronychia, and warty lesions of the periungual areas, have been described by Baran et al. They have not seen pterygium, pitting, or pustulosis.

Histologically there is irregular acanthosis; a lichenoid infiltrate consisting of lymphocytes, histiocytes, and plasma cells; and at times areas of liquefactive degeneration.

This condition is unresponsive to corticosteroid therapy and persists for many years.

Baran R, et al: The nails in keratosis lichenoides chronica. Arch Dermatol 1984, 120:1471.

Margolis MH, et al: Keratosis lichenoides chronica. Arch Dermatol 1972, 105:739.

Nabai H, et al: Keratosis lichenoides chronica. JAAD 1980, 2:217.

LICHEN NITIDUS

CLINICAL FEATURES. Lichen nitidus is a chronic inflammatory disease characterized by minute, shiny, flat-topped, pale, reddish, yellowish red, or flesh-colored, exquisitely discrete, uniform papules, rarely larger than the head of a pin. Usually there is no itching. Linear arrays of papules (Koebner phenomenon) are common, especially on the forearms. Both psoralens and ultraviolet A, and oral etretinate, have recently been reported to clear individual patients.

At the beginning lesions are localized and often remain so, in such cases being limited to a few areas, chiefly the penis and lower abdomen, the inner surfaces of the thighs, and the flexor aspects of the wrists and forearms. Weiss and Cohen described two cases, and reported eight others, in which the palms and soles were involved.

In other cases the disease assumes a more widespread distribution and the elementary papules become fused into erythematous, finely scaly patches. The reddish color varies with tints of yellow, brown, or violet. This generalized type of lichen nitidus affects chiefly the groins and thighs, ankles and wrists, feet and hands, the submammary region in women, the folds of the neck, and the extensor surfaces of the elbows. Minute, grayish, flat papules on the buccal mucous membrane have been described.

The course of lichen nitidus is slowly progressive, with a tendency to remissions. The lesions may

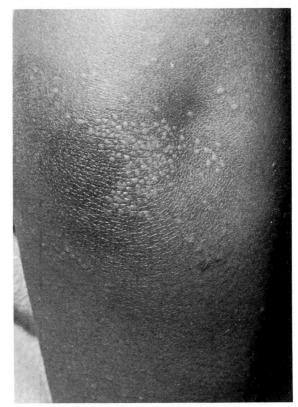

Figure 12–17. Lichen nitidus on knee. Note coalescence of lesions from the Koebner phenomenon.

remain stationary for years, but sometimes disappear spontaneously and entirely.

ETIOLOGY. The cause of lichen nitidus is unknown. Some observers (ourselves not included) believe it is merely a variety of lichen planus. On the basis of the absence of immunoglobulins at the dermal-epidermal junction, Waisman and associates concluded that there is no relationship between lichen nitidus and lichen planus. Clausen et al found,

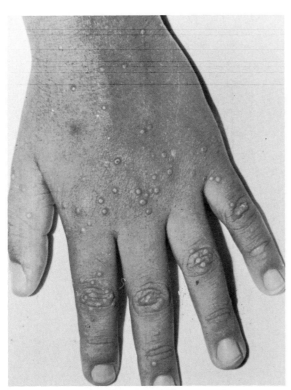

Figure 12–16. Lichen nitidus—clinically, highly suggestive of molluscum contagiosum. (Courtesy of Dr. V. Torres-Rodriguez.)

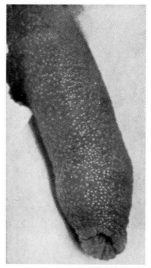

Figure 12–18. Lichen nitidus, in a typical site.

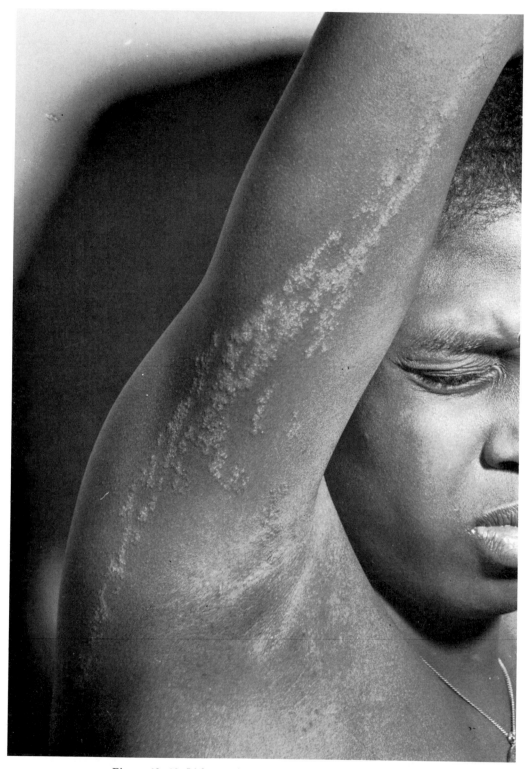

Figure 12–19. Lichen striatus. (Courtesy of Dr. E. Juhlin.)

however, no ultrastructural changes that would permit differentiation between lichen nitidus and lichen planus.

HISTOLOGY. Lichen nitidus has a characteristic histologic appearance. Solitary dermal papillae are widened and contain a dense, discrete infiltrate composed of lymphocytes, histiocytes, and melanophages. Multinucleate giant cells are often present, imparting a granulomatous appearance to the infiltrate. The epidermal rete ridges on either side of the papilla form a clawlike collarette. The overlying epidermis is attenuated and there is usually vacuolar alteration of its basal layer. Banse-Kupin et al confirmed Bardach's earlier report of transepidermal elimination of the dense inflammatory infiltrate in the dermal papilla in a case of perforating lichen nitidus.

DIFFERENTIAL DIAGNOSIS. Lichen nitidus is differentiated from flat warts by the small size, the greater number, and the distribution of the lesions; from lichen planus by the absence of itching, the color, and the distribution; and from lichen scrofulosorum by the darker coloring and follicular character of the papules in lichen scrofulosorum, and by the fact that in lichen nitidus the histologic changes occur immediately beneath the epidermis and show no basal inflammation.

TREATMENT. Little if any treatment is necessary. Topical application of corticosteroids is distinctly helpful if pruritus is severe. As mentioned earlier, PUVA and etretinate have both been reported to be effective. Ocampo et al reported success with astemizole, an H_1-blocking antihistamine, in two patients. Systemic steroids are rarely used but may be helpful in widespread cases.

Banse-Kupin L, et al: Perforating lichen nitidus. JAAD 1983, 9:452.
Bardach H: Perforating lichen nitidus. J Cutan Pathol 1981, 8:111.
Clausen J, et al: Lichen nitidus: Electron microscopic and immunofluorescence studies. Acta Dermatovener (Stockh) 1982, 62:15.
Eisen RF, et al: Lichen nitidus with plasma cell infiltrate. Arch Dermatol 1985, 121:1193.
Francoeur CJ Jr, et al: Generalized pinhead-sized papules in a child. Arch Dermatol 1988, 124:935.
Lapins NA, et al: Lichen nitidus: Study of 43 cases. Cutis 1978, 21:634.
Natarajan S, et al: Lichen nitidus; nail changes. Int J Dermatol 1986, 25:461.
Ocampo J, et al: Generalized lichen nitidus. Int J Dermatol 1989, 28:49.
Randle HW, et al: Treatment of generalized lichen nitidus with PUVA. Int J Dermatol 1986, 25:330.
Waisman M: Immunofluorescent studies in lichen nitidus. Arch Dermatol 1973, 107:200.
Weiss PM, et al: Lichen nitidus of palms and soles. Arch Dermatol 1971, 104:538.
Wright S: Successful treatment of lichen nitidus. Arch Dermatol 1984, 120:155.

LICHEN STRIATUS

Lichen striatus is a unilateral, linear eruption that suddenly appears as an irregular, proximally extending streak 1 to 3 cm wide, either continuous or interrupted, located chiefly on the extremities and sides of the neck, but capable of appearance in any region. It occurs mainly in children but may affect adults also. There is at least a 2 to 1 female to male sex predilection. Itching is usually absent but may be moderate or, rarely, severe.

The earliest lesions are grouped papules, which tend to coalesce and form a linear plaque.

They may extend along the ramus of the jaw or run around the trunk, but usually they extend along the arm, between neurotomes C4 to C7 laterally and C8 to T2 mesially, or down the back of the leg along the mesial or lateral border of the S1 to S3 neurotomes. The papules vary in appearance. Often they are flat-topped and lichenoid; they may be euchromic, or red or purple; they are often shiny, angular, and covered with a grayish scale. In blacks the lesion may be hypopigmented in contrast to the neighboring skin. After onset, several days or weeks may pass before the plaque reaches its full development. It has a prolonged course, sometimes lasting a year or rarely two before spontaneous involution occurs. Recovery is complete.

The histologic features of lichen striatus are not diagnostic and may be quite variable. Biopsy is generally most useful in excluding other conditions with which it may be clinically confused, notably nevus unius lateris and linear lichen planus.

The differential diagnosis is not easy. Linear lichen planus, psoriasis, neurodermatitis, inflammatory linear verrucous epidermal nevus, nevus unius lateris, and verruca plana must be excluded. Whereas some histologic similarities to lichen planus exist in lichen striatus, the perivascular infiltrate affects some papillae and the overlying epidermis more than others in the same papule (in contrast to lichen planus). Psoriasis presents a clear-cut, typical histologic picture, as does nevus unius lateris, in which hyperkeratosis is prominent around the hair follicles, with acanthosis and papillomatosis. In verruca plana there is a basket-weave pattern in the horny layer and vacuolation of the cells in the granular layer. Nevus unius lateris usually shows little or no cellular infiltrate histologically, and as a rule appears before age two.

No treatment is necessary, except reassurance.

Charles CR, et al: Lichen striatus. J Cutan Pathol 1974, 1:265.
Staricco RG: Lichen striatus. Arch Dermatol 1959, 79:311.
Toda K, et al: Lichen striatus. Int J Dermatol 1986, 25:584.

13

Acne

ACNE VULGARIS

CLINICAL FEATURES. Acne vulgaris is a chronic inflammatory disease of the pilosebaceous follicles, characterized by comedones, papules, pustules, cysts, nodules, and often scars, chiefly in certain sites of predilection, namely, the face, neck, upper trunk, and upper arms. It is a disease of the adolescent, with some 90 per cent of all teenagers being involved to some degree; however, the dermatosis may begin in the twenties or thirties, or may persist in adults for many years. As a rule, there is involution of the disease before age 20.

Acne vulgaris occurs primarily in the oily (seborrheic) areas of the skin. On the face it occurs most frequently on the cheeks, and in lesser degree on the nose, forehead, and chin. The ears are frequently involved, with large comedones in the concha, cysts in the lobes, and sometimes retroauricular comedones and cysts. On the neck, especially in the nuchal area, large cystic lesions may predominate. These may later become keloidal.

The comedo, commonly known as the blackhead, is the basic lesion in acne. It is produced by hyperkeratosis of the lining of the follicles, with retention of keratin and sebum. The plugging produced by the comedo dilates the mouth of the follicle, and papules are formed by inflammation around the comedones.

Superficial small cysts, pustules, or papules may form around the site of the comedones. According to the degree of involvement, not only pustules and small cysts but nodules, deep granulomatous infiltrations, scars, and keloids may also be seen.

In typical mild acne vulgaris the comedones predominate, with but occasional pustules. In more severe cases pustules and papules may predominate. These heal with scar formation, if the lesions are deep-seated. In moderately severe cases, cystic lesions occur. In acne conglobata the suppurating cystic lesions predominate, and severe scarring results.

Acne vulgaris appears in many clinical varieties. In the mild case the eruption is composed almost entirely of comedones on an oily skin: *acne comedo*. Another variety, *papular acne*, has numerous inflammatory papules; this is the type most common in young men with coarse, oily skin. *Atrophic acne* is characterized by tiny residual atrophic pits and scars. Quite the opposite of these are the elevated hypertrophic or sometimes keloidal scars seen not only in blacks but also, to lesser extent, in whites. They frequently appear in adult black men on the bearded region.

Papular acne often progresses into an indurated type, *acne indurata*. The lesions, deep-seated and destructive, produce severe scarring.

Corticosteroid "acne." When medium or high doses of corticosteroid are taken for as short a time as three to five days a distinctive eruption may occur, known as "steroid acne." It is a sudden out-cropping of inflamed papules, most numerous on the upper trunk and arms, but also seen on the face. The lesions present as papules rather than comedones; they are not follicular. Tretinoin (Retin-A) 0.05 per cent in a vanishing cream applied once or twice daily may clear the lesions within one to three months despite the continuation of high doses of corticosteroid. Irritation is a problem, however.

ETIOLOGY. Multiple factors cause acne vulgaris. There is undoubtedly a hereditary factor. Several members of the same family may be affected with severe scarring acne.

Basically, however, the primary defect in acne is the formation of a keratinous plug in the lower infundibulum of the hair follicle. Two major factors in the formation of these plugs are: androgentic stimulation of sebaceous glands, and colonization of follicles by *Propionibacterium acnes*, which metabolizes

250

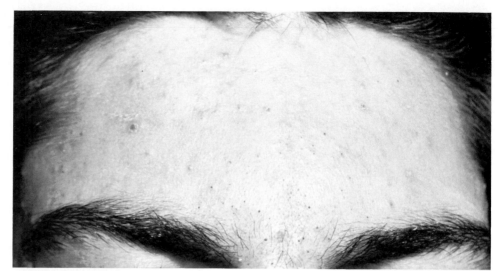

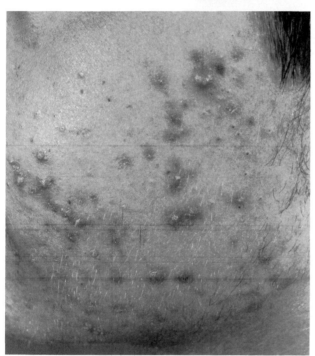

Figure 13–1. Acne vulgaris with comedones on the forehead.

Figure 13–2. Acne vulgaris, with papules and pustules, on the cheek.

Figure 13–3. Acne pits: "ice pick" scars.

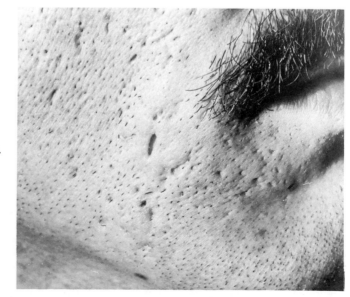

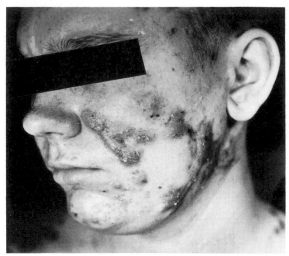

Figure 13–4. Severe cystic acne.

sebum to produce free fatty acids. The occurrence of androgen secretion at the onset of puberty explains the usual onset of acne at that age. Much evidence suggests that liberation of free fatty acids by the metabolic activity of *P. acnes* is a major factor in the genesis of acne papules and pustules.

PATHOGENESIS. Acne vulgaris is mostly a disease of the adolescent; it occurs with greatest frequency between the ages of 15 and 18 in both sexes. Nevertheless, acne may occur in prepubertal youngsters. It is also true that acne may first appear in women over 21 years of age and persist for many years. When acne persists in men after 21 years of age, it is often acne conglobata. The back is the usual major site of involvement in such cases.

Acne vulgaris is exclusively a follicular disease, with comedo formation produced by the impaction and distension of the follicles with tightly packed

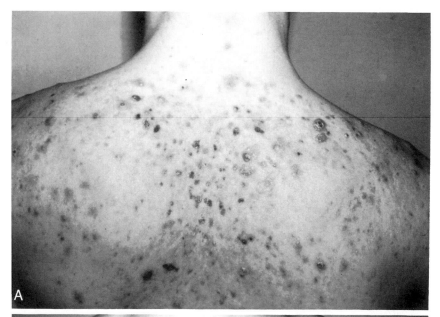

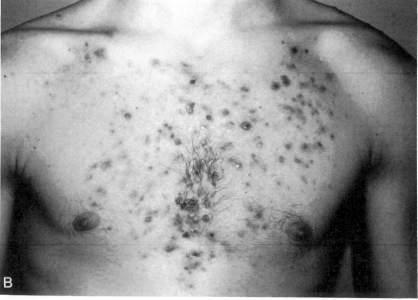

Figure 13–5. A *and* B, *Severe pustulocystic acne. (Courtesy of Dr. Axel W. Hoke.)*

horny cells. This leads to a disruption of the follicular epithelium, permitting discharge of the follicular contents into the dermis. This, in turn, causes the formation of inflammatory papules, pustules, and nodulocystic lesions.

As mentioned, comedo formation is caused by "stickiness" of the horny cells, which fail to be properly discharged at the follicular orifice. As the retained cells block the follicular opening, the lower portion of the follicle is dilated by entrapped sebum. Bacterial lipase acts on the sebum to produce free fatty acids. Largely because it is so abundant, the bacterium most responsible for this enzymatic reaction is *Propionibacterium acnes*. Leyden et al showed that the ratio of *P. acnes* counts in patients with acne, and without acne, is very high—15,000:0 from age 11 to age 15, and 85,000:590 from age 16 to 20. Above age 21 the ratio is 1:1—there is no difference between those with acne and those without.

Free fatty acids are chemotactic to the components of inflammation: if the follicle dilates sufficiently to rupture, these and other irritants are released into the dermis, where inflammation ensues. The beneficial effects of tetracycline, first reported by Andrews and Domonkos, are chiefly obtained by the consequent reduction of the free fatty acids.

Tetracyclines, clindamycin, or erythromycin applied topically can reduce the number of *P. acnes*. Kligman stresses that antibiotics do not produce involution of the inflammatory lesions present but rather inhibit the formation of new lesions. Topical retinoic acid acts by its influence on keratinization, causing horny cells to lose their stickiness.

Androgens (such as testosterone) affect the sebaceous glands by inducing enlargement and thereby increasing sebum production. Several recent studies disclose that women with acne can show biochemical hyperandrogenism. In one such study by Marynick et al, 91 patients with resistant cystic acne were found to have dehydroepiandrosterone sulfate elevated in both men and women, and testosterone and luteinizing hormone elevated in women and higher 17-hydroxyprogesterone levels in men; sex-hormone–binding globulin was decreased in both sexes. Other studies continue to confirm increases in various androgen blood levels in acne patients, especially older women; however, the exact androgenic substances reported to be elevated vary from study to study. There is also evidence for increased peripheral metabolic conversion of testosterone to dihydrotestosterone at the level of the skin in acne patients.

Emotional factors have long been believed to influence acne, and they continue to be regarded as a probable influence. The mechanism is presumed to be the increased production of adrenal androgens when the patient is under stress. This leads to increased seborrhea.

PATHOLOGY. This disease is characterized by a perifollicular inflammation around comedones, which are composed of sebum and keratin as well as parakeratotic cells, located in the pilosebaceous follicles. In pustular cases there are abscesses surrounded by a dense inflammatory exudate of lymphocytes and polymorphonuclear leukocytes. Indolent lesions frequently show, in addition to these findings, plasma cells, foreign body giant cells, and proliferation of fibroblasts. In the larger lesions the sebaceous gland is partly or completely destroyed, sometimes with the formation of large cysts. Epithelial-lined sinus tracts may form.

TREATMENT. Depending upon the degree of involvement, treatment varies from topical application of mild lotions to systemic therapy with antibiotics or retinoids.

Diet. There is no evidence that dietary habits influence acne; therefore elimination diets are not indicated, and no foods are explicitly forbidden.

Systemic Treatment. In the more severe cases, especially those with pustulation, treatment with antibacterials produces gratifying results.

Antibacterials

TETRACYCLINE. Tetracycline has been the preferred antibiotic since 1951, when Andrews and Domonkos first reported the use of tetracyclines and estrogens in the treatment of acne vulgaris. It is the safest, the cheapest, and usually a very effective choice. The usual dosage of tetracycline is 250 mg three or four times daily initially, with gradual reduction of the dose, depending upon clinical response. It is best to take tetracycline on an empty stomach, at least one-half hour before meals, so that it will be absorbed before it can combine with calcium or iron in the stomach. These combinations may reduce absorption by as much as half.

Tetracycline acts by killing *P. acnes* and thus reducing the concentration of fatty acids in the sebaceous follicles. Intermittent therapy may sometimes be necessary for several months or years. Lane and Williamson, in a double-blind study of 51 acne patients, showed a positive response in 73 per cent to oral tetracyclines as sole treatment. Wong et al in a prospective study of 68 patients showed that ibuprofen (Motrin, Advil) 600 mg daily and tetracycline 250 mg four times daily were over twice as effective as either drug alone. The addition of a nonsteroidal antiinflammatory may be of use in antibiotic-resistant cases who are unable to tolerate isotretinoin, or should not be given it.

Vaginitis or perianal itching may result from the tetracycline therapy in about 5 per cent of patients. *Candida albicans* may sometimes be cultured from the involved site. After several months, resumption of tetracycline may no longer cause these symptoms. The only other common side reactions may be gastrointestinal symptoms such as nausea, and staining of growing teeth, which precludes its use in pregnant women and in children under nine or 10.

Although Fox reported tetracycline toxicity manifested as a multisystem disease in 1976, and phototoxicity may occur infrequently as a result of its use, an ad hoc committee of the American Academy of Dermatology found it almost as safe as erythromycin, not requiring monitoring of laboratory parameters during long-term use. Sauer found no deleterious effects in 325 patients who took tetracyclines for three years or longer, except for one instance of transient hyperbilirubinemia with mild jaundice while taking 500 mg tetracycline daily. Tanzman in 1988 reported that routine monitoring of laboratory parameters was not done by nearly two thirds of college health services and found that only four instances of significant side effects had been reported in 70,297 treated patients. She advised such tests only on symptomatic or high-risk patients.

It may take three to four weeks of tetracycline therapy before a significant response is noted. This is because its action is preventive, and lesions present at the outset of therapy require their usual time to resolve.

Baer reported success in very severe, refractory acne by giving 1 gm of tetracycline twice daily for four to 15 months, in 27 of 33 patients in whom it was tried. Side effects were common but trivial.

MINOCYCLINE. Minocin is an even better antibiotic. Hubbell et al, in a randomized double-blind prospective study, showed that 100 mg a day of minocycline was superior to 500 mg of tetracycline. Its absorption is less affected by milk and food than tetracycline's is. Staining of teeth and pigmentation, chiefly in lesions, may rarely be seen, and should be watched for. Pigmentation of oral tissues and in a generalized pattern has also been seen. These pigmentary changes usually slowly clear once minocycline is discontinued.

CLINDAMYCIN. This is an excellent antibiotic for the treatment of acne; however, the development of pseudomembranous colitis in rare instances has limited its use. Cunliffe found that diarrhea occurred in nine of 70 patients receiving clindamycin, but no pseudomembranous colitis was seen. On the other hand, Besler found diarrhea very rare in patients receiving clindamycin for acne. The Academy's ad hoc committee endorsed clindamycin, with slight reservations, as second-choice antibiotic. However, because of its potential for colitis and the availability of retinoids, its use should be limited. The dose is 150 mg three times a day initially, reduced gradually as control is achieved.

ERYTHROMYCIN. For those who can't take tetracycline because of side effects, erythromycin is a satisfactory substitute, and the dosage is the same. Side effects are mostly nausea and an upset stomach; vaginal itching is a rare occurrence. The estolate may cause jaundice (cholestatic) more often than other forms, and should not be used for treatment of acne. The dose is 250 mg three to four times a day initially, reduced gradually after control is achieved.

Gammon et al, using erythromycin base (E-Mycin) 333 mg t.i.d. for four weeks and once a day for eight weeks, found it as effective as 500 mg of tetracycline. ERYC, 250 mg, is a pelletized, enteric-coated for-

mulation. Erythromycin is less likely than tetracycline to interfere with the action of contraceptive pills.

SULFONAMIDES. These are also prescribed. Sulfisoxazole or sulfamethoxazole is taken in 2-gm daily doses until a good response is elicited; then 1-gm maintenance dosage is followed. Trimethoprim-sulfamethoxazole (Bactrim, Septra) is also effective in many cases unresponsive to antibiotics, although drug eruptions from it are relatively frequent and often severe. Dapsone may be used in severe acne conglobata.

BACTERIAL RESISTANCE. Though it had long been believed that antibiotic resistance was a rare exception, Leyden et al were able to show close correlation between an unchanging or worsening clinical condition and a high mean minimum inhibitory concentration requirement for both erythromycin and tetracycline against *P. acnes*. The antibiotic resistance was lost over a period of one or two months after withdrawal of the antibiotic.

Hormones. Andrews and Domonkos first reported the effectiveness of diethylstilbestrol in 1951; however, the sequential anovulatory forms of medication have been highly effective and have superseded other estrogens. Improvement is usually noted some six weeks after therapy is begun. Strauss and Pochi believe that stimulation of sebum secretion in women is due mostly to the secretion of androgens from the ovary and that estrogen inhibits the activity of the ovarian androgen. They also found that with estrogen therapy the sebum production is markedly decreased (sometimes as much as 40 per cent) by the end of three months of oral contraceptive medication. Estradiol suppresses the uptake of testosterone by the sebaceous glands; it also inhibits its conversion into hydrotestosterone.

In general, contraceptive pills containing 100 mcg mestranol or ethinyl estradiol are more effective than those containing only 50 mcg. It appears that side effects from contraceptive pills are dose-related. Beneficial effects may be noted only after some three months of therapy.

Oral contraceptives containing androgenic progesterones may trigger or exacerbate acne in women. Three currently available oral contraceptives containing no androgenic progesterone are Enovid-E, Demulen, and Ovulen (Searle). These tablets are taken in the same way as those containing androgenic progesterone.

Both the physician and the patient should be familiar with the adverse reactions that may be caused by this type of medication. Its use is contraindicated in patients with a history of thrombophlebitis, thromboembolic disorders, cerebral apoplexy, liver disorders, and undiagnosed abnormal vaginal bleeding. Some of the disorders which have been traced to the use of anovulatory drugs have been thrombophlebitis, optic neuritis, cerebrovascular disorders, retinal thrombosis, pulmonary embolism, and erythema nodosum.

Anovulatory drugs may cause nausea, vomiting,

abdominal cramps and bloating, breakthrough bleeding, edema, melasma, breast tenderness, weight increase, cholestatic jaundice, or mental depression. In general, these drugs should rarely be given just for acne.

Corticosteroids. Though steroids may produce steroid "acne," they are also effective antiinflammatory agents in severe and intractable acne vulgaris. In severe acne cystica and acne conglobata, corticosteroid treatment is effective; however, the side effects of this medication should restrict its use to antiinflammatory dosages, and courses of at most a few weeks, in all but the most unusual circumstances.

Dexamethasone in doses from 0.125 mg to 0.5 mg given once at night to reduce androgen excess and alleviate cystic acne may at times be useful. Marynick et al found elevated levels of dehydroepiandrosterone sulfate (DHEA-S) and lowered sex-hormone-binding globulin levels, and clinical improvement on correcting these, in both men and women with severe cystic acne. One conclusion was that serum levels of DHEA-S could be used to monitor the efficacy of dexamethasone therapy.

Vitamin A. In stubborn cases unresponsive to the usual modalities, when the lesions are dry, hyperkeratotic, little-inflamed, and not pustular, vitamin A orally may be dramatically effective. It is the initial toxic side effect—suppression of keratinization—that is sought. The smallest effective dose is around 300,000 units a day according to Kligman (with whom we agree), although doses as low as 100,000 units a day are anecdotally reported to be of value. Toxicity in adults is certainly extremely rare at either dose level. With the availability of isotretinoin, the use of vitamin A in acne therapy is largely of historical interest.

Isotretinoin (Accutane). Though no comparison studies have been done, this retinoid exerts much the same effects as large doses of vitamin A, and is a reliable remedy in all forms of acne. The dose is 1 to 2 mg/kg/day in one or two doses, for 15 to 20 weeks. In practice, most patients (because of the high cost) are given 40, 80, or 120 mg daily. The smaller dose is very nearly as effective as the larger: its disadvantage is that it is unlikely to produce a prolonged remission even after 20 weeks of treatment. This is the major advantage of isotretinoin: it is the only acne therapy that is not open-ended, i.e., that leads to a remission, which may last as long as two years or even more. Nearly every patient will be clear long before 20 weeks.

Its most serious drawback is the virtual certainty that **it will severely damage a fetus** if it is given during pregnancy; it is of the utmost importance that a woman who *could* become pregnant follow closely the recommendations clearly outlined by the company in the patient package insert. The company now supplies consent forms and contraception education. Documentation of the absence of pregnancy by a blood or urine test is mandatory prior to treatment.

Side effects, apart from this, are not serious; the most important is, in some patients, progressive hyperlipidemia, usually easily controlled by a diet low in saturated fat. Dry skin, lips, eyes, and nose occur in up to 80 per cent of patients. This dryness of the nasal mucosa leads to *Staphylococcus aureus* colonization in 80 to 90 per cent of treated subjects. This may lead to skin abscesses, staphylococcal conjunctivitis, and folliculitis. This colonization may be treated by the use of 2% mupirocin ointment applied to the anterior nares twice daily for 5 to 7 days. Drinking six extra glasses of water daily is a useful precaution against dryness.

It is advisable to have every patient given Accutane read the package insert carefully twice, and be sure it is understood.

The drug is approved only for severe cystic acne; however, it is now common practice to use it in less severe forms of acne, in order to prevent continuous morbidity and the repeated office visits that some patients require.

Many patients experience worsening of the acne some time in the first month of treatment. This does not require any reduction of dose. Arthralgia may occur, but like other side effects, it does not require interruption of therapy, unless severe.

It is recommended that before therapy, at three weeks, at six weeks, and at the conclusion of treatment, cholesterol and triglyceride levels be checked. A complete blood count, and hepatic and renal function tests should be checked also at all but the third week. A urinary pregnancy test prior to the initiation of therapy is required, as stated earlier.

Hoffman-LaRoche will furnish patient-information brochures; write to them at Nutley, New Jersey 07110.

Zinc. Results with zinc sulfate are not reliably good, and the place of zinc in acne therapy is still unsettled. With the many excellent effective medications we have today, it is rarely used.

Topical Treatment. *Benzoyl Peroxide.* This is now chiefly used in gels or creams in 5 and 10 per cent concentrations; Benzagel, Desquam-X, Xerac, Panoxyl Gels, Persadox, Benzac. The 5 per cent strength should be used initially. The water-based formulation is less irritating. Some companies have a 2.5 per cent preparation available for sensitive patients.

Benzoyl peroxide has a potent antibacterial effect, suppressing *P. acnes* and consequently reducing free fatty acids in the follicles. Some studies have shown it to be comedolytic also.

These gels may also irritate the skin and produce peeling. In that case the frequency of application should be lessened to once daily or every other day, or Desquam-X Wash may be tried instead.

Retinoic Acid. Tretinoin (Retin-A) may be used as a solution, cream, or gel. It is available in 0.01, 0.025, 0.05, and 0.1 per cent concentrations. A popular form is 0.05 per cent tretinoin in a vanishing cream base. This is especially effective against comedones too small to express. It is less effective for the treatment of pustular and cystic acne. Retinoic acid may produce severe irritation or erythema at the onset of treatment; if it does, it should be used only once daily or even every other day until the skin becomes tolerant.

Therapy is generally started with daily application of the 0.05 per cent cream. It may take eight to 12 weeks before marked improvement occurs. In cases slow to respond to topical retinoic acid cream, swabs moistened with retinoic acid solution may be necessary. Its ability to profoundly affect follicular keratinization makes this an excellent comedolytic medication.

Topical Antibacterials. In addition to the benzoyl peroxide already mentioned above, the antibiotics are effective in reducing the levels of free fatty acids in the comedonic follicle.

CLINDAMYCIN. Cleocin T Topical Solution gel, and lotion, 1 per cent clindamycin, are in a "roll-on" dispenser, or a 1 per cent solution in 70 per cent alcohol. Their use is the same as that of tetracycline and erythromycin. Of these three antibiotics, clindamycin is believed to be the most effective in decreasing the count of *P. acnes*. Stoughton found it was the only antibiotic that actually sterilized the follicles. There is considerable difference of opinion regarding the efficiency of these lotions in the treatment of acne vulgaris. It is mostly effective against pustules and small papulopustular lesions, but has little effect on cystic lesions and comedones.

ERYTHROMYCIN. Staticin Lotion, Erygel, Erymax, Erycette, and A/T/S are available. Thomas et al conducted a double-blind study comparing topical erythromycin 1.5 per cent with topical clindamycin 1.0 per cent and found the two equally effective: two thirds of the patients had a good or excellent response in 12 weeks. Shalita et al confirmed this finding in 1984.

MECLOCYCLINE. One per cent meclocycline sulfosalicylate cream (Meclan) is another topical antibacterial agent for acne. It is applied twice daily.

SULFUR. Although benzoyl peroxide, retinoic acid, and antibiotic topical lotions have largely supplanted the older medications, sulfur, resorcin, and salicylic acid preparations are still useful and moderately helpful.

Some of the more elegant preparations available are Dermik's Klaron Acne Lotion, containing 2 per cent salicylic acid and 5 per cent colloidal sulfur; Rezamid lotion, containing 1 per cent resorcinol and 5 per cent sulfur; and Sulfacet-R lotion, containing 10 per cent sodium sulfacetamide and 5 per cent sulfur. Westwood produces Fostril lotion, containing 2 per cent sulfur and 6 per cent laureth-4, and Transact, containing 2 per cent sulfur and 6 per cent laureth-4 in a medical gel.

Azelaic Acid. Newest drug on the topical acne therapy scene is this dicarboxylic acid, believed to be the agent responsible for the hypopigmentation induced by pityriasis versicolor. Nazzaro-Porro has worked with it for several years. It is remarkably free from adverse actions of any kind, and its effect on all forms of acne is good, in a 15 per cent cream. It has the intriguing property of gradually destroying malignant melanocytes, as well. A double-blind comparison with vehicle study is needed to better assess efficacy.

Abrasive Cleansers. Despite the therapeutic claims made for abrasive cleansers, Fulghum et al were able to show no difference between lesion counts using a cleanser with and without abrasives, over an eight-week period.

Surgical Treatment. Local surgical treatment is helpful in bringing about quick resolution of the comedones and pustules as well as the cysts. The edge of the follicle is nicked with a sharp pointed number 11 Bard-Parker scalpel blade and the contents of the comedo are expressed with a comedo extractor. Several types of this instrument are available. Scarring is not produced by this procedure.

Intralesional Corticosteroids. This type of treatment is especially effective in reducing inflammatory papules, pustules, and smaller cysts. Kenalog-10 (triamcinolone acetonide 10 mg per ml) is best diluted with sterile normal saline solution to 5 or 2.5 mg per ml (or even, as Levine et al showed, 1.5 or 0.75 mg/ml) in order to safeguard against atrophy and hypopigmentation at the site of injection. Levine also tried betamethasone (Celestone) by the intralesional route and found it wholly ineffective even at 3 mg/ml concentration. After triamcinolone injections, no recurrence of lesions was seen at one month.

A disposable 30-gauge half-inch needle on a disposable 1-ml tuberculin luer syringe should be used. The injection should be made near the surface, again to avoid atrophy at the site of injection. These injections largely obviate the need for incision and expression of most small acne lesions. Do not dilute the Kenalog suspension with Xylocaine or other anesthetics—it is not helpful and indeed will cause the otherwise painless injections to be painful.

Cryotherapy. Hyperemia and peeling may be produced by solid carbon dioxide slush. Solid carbon dioxide is finely powdered by placing it into a strong canvas bag, such as a bank money bag, and pulverizing it with a mallet. The powdered dry ice is placed onto four layers of 8-inch square gauze. The corners are gathered together and a rubber band used to secure the dry ice into a ball. Using the gathered corners as a handle, the ball of carbon dioxide is dipped into a cup containing just enough acetone to moisten it. The bag is then gently rubbed over the treatment site, care being exercised to avoid overtreatment, since severe burns may be caused. This treatment causes some inflammatory reaction, with edema followed by desquamation. It may be repeated once each week.

Mopping the face repeatedly for a few minutes with large fluffy cotton applicators dipped in liquid nitrogen is a much more convenient way of achieving the same result. It seems especially valuable for reducing oiliness, if repeated about every two weeks. Cryosurgical units with special equipment for spraying acne lesions have been designed.

Ultraviolet Light Treatment. If ultraviolet-induced peeling of the skin is of value in acne vulgaris, it is when comedones are profuse and when there are superficial acutely inflamed papules and nodules.

In ultraviolet therapy pronounced local effects are desirable. Each exposure should produce marked erythema, which will be followed by a fine dry exfoliation of the epidermis. Before any treatment is given, the patient should be informed of the inevitable erythema and carefully acquainted with its duration and the subsequent peeling. The dose given is governed somewhat by the patient's acquiescence to the concomitant discomforts.

At the time of treatment the eyes are shielded with goggles or, better yet, water-moistened pledgets of cotton. Ultraviolet is usually given at a fixed distance such as 30 inches, and the treatment time is gradually increased in successive treatments. Each exposure should be long enough to produce erythema of the skin.

X-ray Therapy. Because of the efficacy of oral antibiotics, retinoids, and intralesional triamcinolone acetonide, x-ray treatment of acne is only rarely used. Because of the general disrepute into which x-ray therapy has fallen, x-ray therapy is now given only in extremely severe cases of cystic acne in men and women in their twenties or older in whom all other methods, including oral prednisone or triamcinolone acetonide intramuscularly, and Accutane orally, have failed. The patient should be completely aware of the alleged hazards of x-ray therapy that are being publicized today. For the technique of x-ray therapy for acne, reference should be made to the seventh edition of this book (p. 259).

Scar Removal. After acne vulgaris has cleared, particularly the indurated and cystic types, profuse pitted scarring may be an unfortunate disfigurement. Although there is no method by which all scars may be removed, several means are used to relieve scarring.

Dermabrasion. Also known as skin planing, this is a useful and effective method for removing or improving postacne scars. It is done with rotating motor-driven steel wire brushes or diamond fraises. The eyes are protected with gauze pads during the spraying of the refrigerant. An area of about 15 sq cm is frozen with an aerosol spray of fluorethyl or dichlorotetrafluoroethane such as Frigiderm. Immediately after the freezing, the eye pads and other gauze pads are removed from around the treatment site to avoid entanglement with the high-speed rotating brush. The frozen skin is then removed with long even strokes of the brush. As soon as thawing occurs, the area is refrozen if more dermabrasion is intended at the site. Moderate bleeding is mopped with sponges, and the next area is treated similarly. When the treatment is completed, the bleeding is stopped by pads in about 15 minutes. Nonadherent dressing pads (Telfa pads) are placed on the wound and then bandaged.

The next day the bandages are removed and frequent cold normal saline compresses are applied throughout the following week. At night the face is rebandaged for comfort during sleep. Heavy crusts are formed, which may be lessened by the frequent use of the cold compresses. In about a week all the crusts fall off, leaving a shiny, reddened, smooth treatment site. This is just one of several postoperative methods used. The patient is instructed to avoid exposure to sunlight for six to eight weeks in order to reduce the incidence of hyperpigmentation. The most common permanent complication is hypopigmentation of dermabraded areas, unhappily a fairly common result in Oriental patients especially. The practice of planing a small test area several months prior to complete dermabrasion will allow identification of some patients at risk for this complication.

Some patients develop numerous milia in the three weeks following the planing. These may be incised and expressed; however, if left alone there will be spontaneous involution.

Planing should be done only on the face. On the neck, trunk, and arms, severe scarring may be produced even by moderate dermabrasion.

Ayres S Jr, et al: Acne vulgaris: Therapy directed at pathophysiologic defects. Cutis 1981, 28:41.

Bigby M, et al: Adverse reactions to isotretinoin. JAAD 1988, 18:543.

Blandon PT, et al: Topical azelaic acid in acne. Br J Dermatol 1986, 114:493.

Breathnach AS: Azelaic acid. Br J Dermatol 1984, 111:115.

Bruno NP, et al: Adverse effects of isotretinoin therapy. Cutis 1984, 33:484.

Burket JM: Nodulocytic infantile acne . . . in a kindred of steatocystoma. Arch Dermatol 1987, 123:242.

Campbell JP, et al: Retinoid therapy is associated with excess granulation tissue responses. JAAD 1983, 9:708.

Cunliffe WJ: . . . strategy for treatment of acne. JAAD 1987, 16:591.

Cunningham WJ, et al: Clinical aspects of the retinoids. Semin Dermatol 1983, 2:145.

Darley CR: Recent advances in the hormonal aspects of acne vulgaris. Cutis 1984, 23:539.

Exner JH, et al: Pyogenic-granuloma-like acne lesions during isotretinoin therapy. Arch Dermatol 1983, 119:808.

Friedman SJ, et al: Solid facial edema as a complication of acne vulgaris. JAAD 1986, 15:286.

Fulton JE Jr, et al: Comedogenicity of current therapeutic products, cosmetics, and ingredients in the rabbit ear. JAAD 1984, 10:96.

Fulghum DD, et al: Abrasive cleansing in the management of acne vulgaris. Arch Dermatol 1982, 118:658.

Gammon WR, et al: Comparative efficacy of oral erythromycin versus oral tetracycline in the treatment of acne vulgaris: A double-blind study. JAAD 1986, 14:183.

Hubbell CG, et al: Efficacy of minocycline compared with tetracycline in the treatment of acne vulgaris. Arch Dermatol 1982, 118:989.

Kligman AM, et al: Oral vitamin A in acne vulgaris. Int J Dermatol 1981, 20:278.

Lammer EJ, et al: Retinoic acid embryopathy. N Engl J Med 1985, 313:834.

Levine RM, et al: Intralesional corticosteroids in the treatment of nodulocystic acne. Arch Dermatol 1983, 119:480.

Leyden JJ: Absorption of minocycline hydrochloride: effect of milk, food, and iron. JAAD 1985, 12:308.

Idem, et al: Tetracycline and minocycline treatment: Effects on skin-surface lipid levels and *Propionibacterium acnes*. Arch Dermatol 1982, 118:19.

Idem: *Propionibacterium acnes* resistance to antibiotics in acne patients. JAAD 1983, 8:41.

Idem: Retinoids in acne. JAAD 1988, 19:164.

Idem: Erythromycin gel compared with clindamycin solution in acne vulgaris. JAAD 1987, 16:822.

Idem: *Staphylococcus* complicating isotretinoin therapy. Arch Dermatol 1987, 123:606.

Marynick SP, et al: Androgen excess in cystic acne. N Engl J Med 1983, 308:17.

Mills OH, et al: Comparing 2.5%, 5%, and 10% benzoyl peroxide in . . . acne vulgaris. Int J Dermatol 1986, 25:664.

Idem: Isotretinoin guidelines in females. JAAD 1988, 19:920.

Muhlemann MF, et al: Oral spironolactone. Br J Dermatol 1986, 115:227.

Nazzaro-Porro M, et al: Beneficial effect of 15% azelaic acid cream on acne vulgaris. Br J Dermatol 1983, 109:45.

Poliak SC, et al: Minocycline-associated tooth discoloration in young adults. JAMA 1985, 254:2930.

Pochi PE: Acne: endocrinologic aspects. Cutis 1982, 30:212.

Idem: Endocrinology of acne (editorial). J Invest Dermatol 1983, 81:1.

Idem: Hormones, retinoids, and acne. N Engl J Med 1983, 308:1024.

Rothman KF, et al: [Treatment of] acne in pregnancy. JAAD 1988, 19:431.

Sauer G: Prospective study on the safety of long-term tetracycline therapy for acne. Cutis 1981, 27:492.

Shalita AR, et al: Topical erythromycin vs clindamycin therapy for acne. A multicenter double-blind comparison. Arch Dermatol 1984, 120:351.

Idem: Acne vulgaris. JAAD 1987, 16:410.

Idem: Isotretinoin revisited. Cutis 1988, 42:1.

Silverman AK, et al: Hypervitaminosis A. JAAD 1987, 16:1027.

Solotoff SA: Pitted scars. J Dermatol Surg 1986, 12:1079.

Stern RS, et al: Isotretinoin and pregnancy. JAAD 1984, 10:851.

Strauss JS, et al: Isotretinoin therapy for acne: Results of a multicenter dose-response study. JAAD 1984, 10:490.

Tanzman ES: Long-term tetracycline use in treatment of acne—the role of routine laboratory monitoring. J Am Coll Health 1988, 36:272.

Thomas DR, et al: Comparison of topical erythromycin versus topical clindamycin in the treatment of acne vulgaris. Cutis 1982, 29:624.

Tindall JP: Chloracne and chloracnegens. JAAD 1985, 13:539.

Valentic JP, et al: Inflammatory neovascular nodules associated with oral isotretinoin treatment of severe acne. Arch Dermatol 1983, 119:871.

Vergani C, et al: Low levels of HDL in severe cystic acne. N Engl J Med 1982, 307:1154.

Winton GB, et al: Wound dressings for dermatologic surgery. JAAD 1985, 13:1026.

Wong RC, et al: Oral ibuprofen and tetracycline for the treatment of acne vulgaris. JAAD 1984, 11:1076.

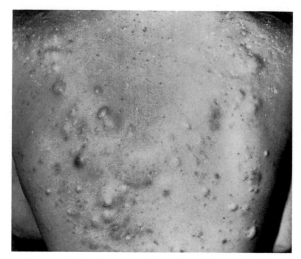

Figure 13–6. Acne conglobata in a 17-year-old boy.

ACNE CONGLOBATA

Cystic acne is the mildest form of **acne conglobata** (conglobate: shaped in a rounded mass or ball), an unusually severe form of acne. This not too rare form is characterized by numerous comedones (many of which are double or triple), large abscesses with interconnecting sinuses, cysts containing a clear viscid fluid, and grouped inflammatory nodules. Suppuration is characteristic of acne conglobata, but in simple cystic acne it is usually slight or absent.

Pronounced scars remain after healing. These are frequently keloidal and produce an unsightly appearance. The cysts are distinctive since they occur most frequently on the forehead, cheeks, and anterior neck. They contain a thick, yellowish, viscid, stringy, blood-tinged fluid. After incision and drainage of the cyst there is frequently prompt refilling with the same type of material. These cysts are suggestive of the type found in hidradenitis suppurativa.

This severe and distinctive disease occurs most frequently in young men around 16 years of age; it may extend and persist into adulthood and even into the fifth decade of life, especially on the posterior neck and back. Women have this severe and painful disease less frequently.

The therapy of choice in all but earliest lesions is isotretinoin, 2 mg/kg/day for five months, with a second course if resolution does not occur after a rest period of two months.

Ellis BI, et al: Acne-associated spondyloarthropathy. Radiology 1987, 162:541.

Goldschmidt H, et al: Acne fulminans. Arch Dermatol 1977, 113:444.

Kelly AP, et al: Acute febrile ulcerative conglobate acne with polyarthralgia. Arch Dermatol 1971, 104:182.

Warshaw T: Conglobate acne vulgaris. J Med Soc New Jersey 1967, 64:218.

HIDRADENITIS SUPPURATIVA

Suppurative hidradenitis is a chronic suppurative and cystic disease of the apocrine gland–bearing areas of the skin: axillae, groins, and perianal area. Obesity and a genetic tendency to acne, especially

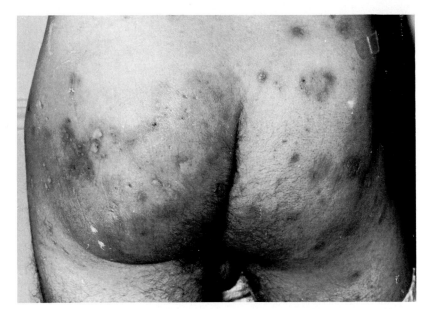

Figure 13–7. Acne conglobata: end stage.

acne conglobata, seem to be predisposing factors. It is often treated as furunculosis, which it superficially resembles; but the primary lesions are not infections—they are deep, aggressive, sterile lesions of cystic acne occurring in apocrine gland-bearing areas. Comedones in apocrine sites (including the retroauricular areas) are an important clue to early diagnosis. The most useful and effective therapy in early cases is not antibiotics, but steroids—intralesional or systemic: intramuscular triamcinolone acetonide.

In more chronic cases, antibiotics are helpful: Clemmensen showed in a double-blind study that topical clindamycin was highly effective in treating abscesses, inflammatory nodules, and pustules. Oral tetracycline and erythromycin are both useful in cases with draining sinuses. Excision of individual abscesses is often helpful, especially in the axillae.

Surgical extirpation of cyst-bearing tissues is a last resort: it is effective, but hard to bear.

Isotretinoin was used in eight cases by Dicken et al; one case cleared and two almost cleared; one got worse.

Ten patients with hidradenitis suppurativa or acne conglobata who had developed spondyloarthropathy were identified retrospectively by Rosner et al. Rheumatoid factor was negative in all. They thought it was reactive to chronic cutaneous infection.

Brown SWC, et al: . . . perianal hidradenitis suppurativa . . . Br J Surg 1986, 73:978.
Clemmensen OJ: Topical treatment of hidradenitis suppurativa with clindamycin. Int J Dermatol 1983, 22:325.
Dicken CH, et al: Evaluation of isotretinoin treatment of hidradenitis suppurativa. JAAD 1984, 11:500.
Highet AS, et al: Bacteriology and antibiotic treatment of hidradenitis. Arch Dermatol 1988, 124:1047.
Jemec GBE: Effect of local surgical excisions in hidradenitis. JAAD 1988, 18:1103.
Mortimer PS, et al: Androgens in hidradenitis. Br Med J 1986, 292:245.
O'Loughlin S, et al: Hidradenitis suppurativa. Arch Dermatol 1988, 124:1043.

Rosner IA, et al: Spondyloarthropathy associated with hidradenitis suppurativa and acne conglobata. Ann Intern Med 1982, 97:520.
Silverberg B, et al: Hidradenitis suppurativa. Plast Reconstr Surg 1987, 79:555.

ACNE FULMINANS

Acne fulminans is a rare form of extremely severe cystic acne occurring in teenage boys. It is characterized by highly inflammatory nodules and plaques which undergo swift suppurative degeneration leaving ragged ulcerations, mostly on the chest and back. The face is usually less severely involved. Fever and leukocytosis are common.

Polyarthralgia and polymyalgia, destructive arthritis, and myopathy have been reported in association with it. Actual focal lytic bone lesions were reported

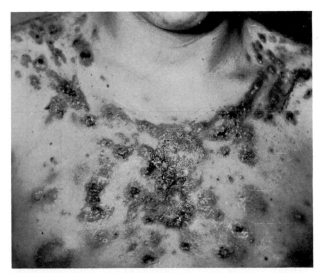

Figure 13–8. Severe acne conglobata with cystic and necrotic lesions.

by Hault et al. McCauley et al reported a case in a 29-year-old man which began simultaneously with the onset of Crohn's disease. For topical medication Vleminckx compresses are advisable. Large cysts should be opened and the contents expressed through a hole made with a 2-mm biopsy punch or a fine electrodesiccating needle on a high setting, so that it will not promptly heal and permit the cyst to refill.

It appears from a case reported by Wolf et al that the most effective therapy may be high-dose steroids, and we would suggest either 40 mg prednisone a day, or 60 mg of Kenalog (triamcinolone acetonide) IM. The addition of isotretinoin may aid in limiting the time of therapy by inducing remission of the disease.

Lorincz reported success with dapsone, but only in toxic doses: 100 mg three or four times daily, with close observation for hemolysis, methemoglobinemia, and neutropenia.

Tropical acne is merely unusually severe acne occurring in the tropics during the seasons when the weather is hot and humid. Nodular, cystic, and pustular lesions occur chiefly on the back, buttocks, and thighs. Characteristically, the face is spared from lesions. Conglobate abscesses occur often, especially on the back. Comedones are sparse.

Acne tropicalis usually occurs in older patients who may have had acne vulgaris at an earlier age. This is especially true of those in the armed forces stationed in the tropics and carrying back packs.

Treatment is that of cystic acne, but it is usually futile until the patient moves to a cooler and less humid climate.

Premenstrual Acne. A significant percentage of women patients with acne note a premenstrual exacerbation of papulopustular lesions. Usually five to ten lesions will appear a week or so before menstruation. There is some evidence that progesterone mediates premenstrual acne. Frequently, estrogen-dominant contraceptive pills will diminish or prevent premenstrual flares of acne.

Preadolescent Acne. Preadolescent acne can be subdivided into neonatal, infantile, and childhood acne.

Neonatal acne (acne neonatorum) is a common condition which by definition is limited to the neonatal period or the first four weeks of life. It develops a few days after birth, has a male sex preponderance, and is characterized by transient facial papules or pustules, which usually clear spontaneously in a few days or weeks. This type of acne is attributed to the stimulation of neonatal sebaceous glands by circulating maternal progesterone.

Infantile acne includes those cases which persist beyond the neonatal period or have an onset after the first four weeks of life. The acne process can extend into childhood, puberty, or adult life.

Childhood acne may result from persistent infantile acne or onset after age two. It is uncommon and has a male predominance. Grouped comedones, papules,

pustules, and cysts can occur alone or in any combination, usually limited to the face. The duration is variable, from a few weeks to several years, and occasionally extends into a more severe pubertal acne. Often there is a strong family history of moderately severe acne.

Preadolescent acne is a syndrome of multifactoral etiology. Acne neonatorum and the accompanying "mini-puberty" result from circulating maternal hormones, whereas acne extending or developing after the neonatal period may be a form of acne cosmetica, acne venenata, drug-induced acne, or part of an endocrinological disorder.

In the absence of any of the mentioned etiologies, one could postulate qualitative or quantitative alterations of cutaneous androgen synthesis or metabolism or increased end-organ sensitivity as pathogenetic mechanisms for preadolescent acne.

Acne Venenata. Contact with a great variety of acnegenic chemicals can produce comedones and result in acne venenata. Cosmetics, toiletries, and grooming agents cause the most common types. The most extensive and worst cases are seen in the industrial setting. The better known acnegens of occupational acne venenata are chlorinated hydrocarbons (chloracne), cutting oils, petroleum oil, and coal tar and pitches. Treatment consists of stopping the exposure to causative chemicals, and topical application of tretinoin.

Acne Cosmetica. A persistent low-grade acne manifested by closed comedones and papulopustules occurring on the chin and cheeks of adult women, presumably due to acnegenic cosmetics, has been described. The cosmetics which induce this condition are usually facial creams, but some sunscreens may be impugned. Avoidance of comedogenic cosmetics is curative, but it may take several months for complete clearing.

Pomade Acne. Pomade acne is a variety of acne cosmetica occurring almost exclusively in blacks, especially males, who apply various greases and oils to scalp hair and the face as a grooming aid. The lesions are usually closed comedones on the forehead, temples, cheeks, and chin. Comedogenicity of various pomades has been documented. Mineral oil is a very weak comedogenic agent and can be recommended for those who do not wish to avoid pomades altogether.

Acne Detergicans. This type of acne may develop in acne patients who overwash with soaps that contain comedogenic substances. These patients facewash at least four times daily. Closed comedones are the principal lesions seen. Few ordinary soaps are comedogenic. Unsaturated fatty acids and bacteriostatic substances probably contribute to the comedogenicity of soap.

Acne Aestivalis. Also known as Mallorca acne, this rare form of acne starts in the spring, progresses during the summer, and resolves completely in the fall. It affects almost exclusively women between the ages of 25 and 40. Dull red, dome-shaped, hard, small papules, usually not more than 3 to 4 mm in size, develop on the cheeks and commonly extend onto the sides of the neck, the chest, the shoulders, and characteristically the upper arms. Comedones and pustules are notably absent or sparse. Acne aestivalis does not respond to antibiotics but is benefited by application of retinoic acid.

Acne Mechanica. Many types of mechanical forces including various pressures, tensions, frictions, stretchings, rubbings, pinchings, and pullings can aggravate existing acne. The key feature is an unusual distribution pattern of the acne lesions. Provocative factors include chin straps, violins, hats, collars, surgical tape, orthopedic casts, chairs, and seats. Prophylactic measures against various mechanical forces are beneficial.

Excoriated acne, also known as *picker's acne*, is a term derived from the French *acne excoriée des jeunes filles*. It is seen in girls with a superficial type of acne in which the primary lesions are trivial or even nonexistent, but in which the compulsive neurotic habit of picking the face and squeezing minute comedones produces secondary lesions which may even leave scars. Often the lesions are too small to be seen by the naked eye, and the patient resorts to the use of a magnifying mirror. Eventually scabs and crusts form, and scarring with atrophy results.

Many of these patients tend to be meticulously clean, to be proper in their habits and appearance, and to pick nervously at their lesions.

Practical assistance to such patients might include suggestions to refrain from unreasonable efforts at cleanliness, to eliminate the use of a magnifying mirror for close observation of the skin, and to forego long fingernails.

Albrecht H, et al: Acne excoriée des jeunes filles—psychiatrically considered. Arch Klin Exp Dermatol 1965, 223:509.
Hault P, et al: Acne fulminans with osteolytic lesions. Arch Dermatol 1985, 121:662.
Hjorth N, et al: Acne aestivalis—Mallorca acne. Acta Derm Venereol 1972, 52:61.
Jemec GBE, et al: Bone lesions of acne fulminans. JAAD 1989, 20:353.
Kligman AM, et al: Acne cosmetica. Arch Dermatol 1972, 106:843.
Leiferman K, et al: Acne fulminans and myositis. Cutis 1984, 34:249.
Mills OH, et al: Acne aestivalis. Arch Dermatol 1975, 111:891.
Idem: Acne detergicans. Arch Dermatol 1975, 111:65.
Idem: Acne mechanica. Arch Dermatol 1975, 111:481.
Plewig G, et al: Pomade acne. Arch Dermatol 1970, 101:580.
Stevanovic DV: Acne in infancy. Austral J Dermatol 1960, 5:224.
Traupe H, et al: Acne of fulminans type following testosterone therapy in 3 excessively tall boys. Arch Dermatol 1988, 124:414.
Tromovitch TA, et al: Acne in infancy. Am J Dis Child 1963, 106:230.
Wolf R, et al: Acne with acute systemic reaction (acne fulminans?). Cutis 1981, 28:210.

GRAM-NEGATIVE FOLLICULITIS

This disease occurs in patients who have had moderately inflammatory acne for long periods and have been treated with long-term antibiotics, mainly tetracyclines. While on antibiotic treatment, patients develop either superficial pustules 3 to 6 mm in diameter flaring out from the anterior nares, or fluctuant, deep-seated nodules. Culture of these lesions usually reveals a species of Enterobacter, Klebsiella, or, from the deep cystic lesions, Proteus.

With long-term, broad-spectrum antibiotic therapy the anterior nares may become colonized with these gram-negative organisms. As the use of long-term antibiotic therapy declines (as it has done since the introduction of isotretinoin) this disease is becoming less common.

Isotretinoin is marvellously effective and is the treatment of choice in this disease. James and Leyden have shown that this treatment not only clears the acne component of the disease but also eliminates the colonization of the anterior nares with gram-negative organisms. If Accutane cannot be tolerated, or is contraindicated, amoxicillin, Augmentin, or trimethoprim-sulfamethoxazole may be effective in suppressing the disease.

James WD, et al: Treatment of gram-negative folliculitis with isotretinoin. JAAD 1985, 12:319.
Leyden JJ, et al: Gram-negative folliculitis—a complication of antibiotic therapy in acne vulgaris. Br J Dermatol 1973, 88:533.

ACNE KELOIDALIS

This is also known as *keloidal acne* and *folliculitis keloidalis*. An older obsolete name was *dermatitis papillaris capillitii*, the capillitium being the suboccipital portion of the scalp. This is a type of acneiform

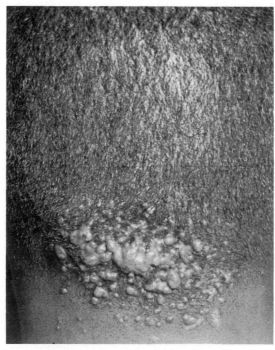

Figure 13–9. Acne keloidalis nuchae.

disease in which secondary pyogenic infection in and around pilosebaceous structures ends in keloidal scarring.

It is a persistent folliculitis and perifolliculitis of the back of the neck associated with an occlusion of the follicular orifices, leading to keloidal thickening and cicatrization. At times sinus tract formation results.

Acne keloidalis nuchae is most frequently encountered in black or Oriental men who otherwise are in excellent health. No cause has been found for this type of hypertrophic scarring.

Histologically, acne keloidalis is a folliculitis of the hair follicle that progresses into a perifolliculitis with an infiltrate consisting of polymorphonuclears, lymphocytes, plasma cells, mast cells, and even foreign-body giant cells. The normal connective tissue is eventually replaced by hypertrophic connective tissue that becomes sclerotic to form the hypertrophic scar or actual keloid.

Treatment consists of triamcinolone acetonide by intralesional injection, using Kenalog-10 in the inflammatory follicular lesions and Kenalog-40 in the hypertrophic scars and keloids.

Antibacterials are taken on a long-term basis. The sulfonamides, the tetracyclines, and erythromycin may all be helpful.

Treatment with roentgen rays—should intralesional steroids fail—reduces the fibrous thickening and produces epilation of the infected hairs. Good results are accomplished with unfiltered x-rays generated at 100 kV, 100 rads being given weekly, or 300 rads every three weeks for a total of 800 to 1000 rads. If the keloidal masses are hard and elevated considerably above the skin level, it is desirable to remove the projecting portions by cutting them off with a razor blade before starting the x-ray therapy. Equal parts of 2 per cent Xylocaine and 0.5 per cent triamcinolone suspension are used for anesthesia. It is believed that this reduces the incidence of subsequent keloid formation.

Kantor et al reported gratifying results in eight consecutive cases using the carbon dioxide laser to excise the involved plaques. Two of three patients in whom vaporization of lesions was employed experienced recurrences within eight and nine months, respectively, and they consider this method to be contraindicated.

The technique of McMullan and Zeligman used in the treatment of perifolliculitis capitis abscedens et suffodiens (see next section) may also be applied in this disease.

PERIFOLLICULITIS CAPITIS ABSCEDENS ET SUFFODIENS

Also known as *dissecting cellulitis of the scalp*, this is a rare chronic suppurative disease of the scalp in which there are numerous follicular and perifollicular inflammatory reactions with the formation of nod-

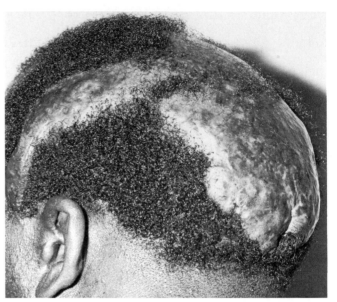

Figure 13–10. *Perifolliculitis capitis abscedens et suffodiens: end stage, with scarring.*

ules. These nodules suppurate and become undermined in the tissue to form intercommunicating sinuses. These sinuses, as long as 5 cm, can be easily traced by a probe. Scarring and alopecia ensue, although seropurulent drainage may last indefinitely.

The primary lesions are apparently large comedones about which the abscesses develop as a reaction of the tissues against foreign bodies. It is believed that this disease process is a variant of acne vulgaris; it closely resembles acne conglobata and hidradenitis suppurativa. Coagulase-positive *Staphylococcus aureus* and hemolytic *Staph. albus* may be found in the lesions. McMullan and Zeligman found *S. aureus* most frequently in their patients.

Histologically, the disease is an occluded folliculitis with keratinous debris and a perifolliculitis resulting from the occlusion and secondary infection. The usual inflammatory reaction is similar to that of acne keloidalis.

Treatment is varied and generally unsuccessful unless the most vigorous procedures are followed. The surgical approach is most feasible in the early stages of the disease. Antibacterial medication is given by mouth and the lesions are incised and drained. It is often possible to pass a probe through burrows of interconnecting pustular nodules. These intercommunicating sinuses should be slit wide open. The surface is cauterized to destroy the epithelium lining the sinuses. A similar situation is frequently encountered in hidradenitis suppurativa.

Moschella and his associates have reported successful results from removal of the entire scalp with subsequent grafting.

We have experienced excellent results using the technique of x-ray epilation recommended by McMullan and Zeligman. After the scalp is shaved as closely as possible, an epilating dosage of x-rays using the Kienböck five-point equidistant technique is administered. To all the five points 365 rads at 80 kV, 5 to 10 ma, 25 cm TSD, unfiltered, is given. Nineteen days later an adhesive tape cap is applied to the entire scalp and then removed after 48 hours with all the loosened hairs adhering to it. Good results have been achieved and one of our patients has gone five years with no evidence of the severe disease he had for several years prior to epilation.

There is no report of failure of regrowth of hair after such epilation.

Moschella SL, et al: Perifolliculitis capitis abscedens et suffodiens. Arch Dermatol 1967, 96:195.

ROSACEA

CLINICAL FEATURES. Rosacea, formerly called **acne rosacea**, is a chronic inflammatory eruption of the flush areas of the face and especially the nose. It is characterized by erythema, papules, pustules, and telangiectasia and, often, by hypertrophy of the sebaceous glands. The latter condition, known as rhinophyma, will be discussed subsequently.

Usually the mid-face is involved and most frequently the nose and cheeks, with the brow and chin also affected at times. The eyelids and eyes may be involved to produce *ocular rosacea*. Rosacea may be superimposed upon seborrhea. Rosacea occurs most

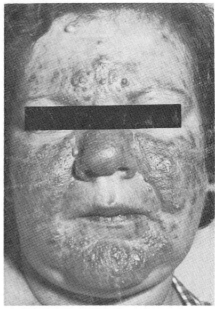

Figure 13–12. Severe rosacea, with acne-like pustules in typical butterfly distribution on cheeks. (Courtesy of Dr. A. Silva.)

often in middle-aged women; the most severe cases, however, are seen in men.

In the mild form of rosacea there is but slight flushing of nose and cheeks and possibly the forehead and chin. The conjunctivae may be affected. As the process becomes more severe, the lesions become a deeper red or purplish red with chronic dilatation of the superficial capillaries (telangiectasia) and inflammatory acneiform pustules.

In the most severe form lesions develop, which are deep-seated indolent pustules, furuncles, or cystic nodules that may resemble acne conglobata with large abscesses, discharging sinuses, and keloidal scarring. The eyelids may become involved, with blepharitis and conjunctivitis. The eye itself may be affected, with keratitis, iritis, and episcleritis.

Granulomatous Rosacea. Mullanax and Kierland have called attention to a distinctive form of papular rosacea designated as granulomatous rosacea. This type of rosacea is found not only on the butterfly areas but also on the lateral areas and periorally. The discrete papules appear as yellowish brown nodules upon diascopy and as noncaseating epithelioid cell granulomas resembling sarcoidosis, tuberculosis, or other granulomas histologically.

ETIOLOGY. A number of factors seem to be concerned with the etiology of rosacea.

The disease occurs most frequently between the ages of 30 and 50 and mostly in women. There is a suggestion of endocrine factors, especially menopausal; one definite type begins at menopause.

Another factor is that of vasomotor lability, which is especially pronounced in menopause and may be closely connected with the pathogenesis of rosacea. Traditionally, caffeine-containing beverages—tea and coffee—have been proscribed on the ground that

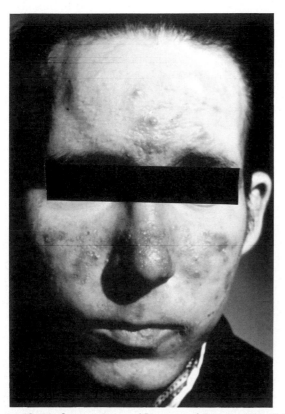

Figure 13–11. Severe rosacea. (Courtesy of Dr. Axel W. Hoke.)

since both cause flushing, and both contain caffeine, caffeine must be responsible. Wilkin showed that this is not the case: it is *heat* that is the common and responsible cause. Hot water, even if merely held in the mouth and not swallowed, causes the same degree of flushing as hot coffee; cold coffee, and caffeine (200 mg), cause no flushing at all. Alcohol is well known as an inducer of facial flushing, of course.

The continued application of fluorinated corticosteroids may induce a rosacealike syndrome consisting of severe erythema with telangiectases and pustules. This may also be seen in perioral dermatitis.

Demodex folliculorum is frequently found in the expressed contents of an inflamed pustular follicle of the nose in cases of rosacea. Its pathogenicity has been controversial for many years. The consistent demonstration of numerous demodices in the inflamed pustules of acute rosacea is suggestive of a pathogenetic factor. In pustular acne vulgaris we are usually unable to demonstrate demodices.

Daniels has postulated *infectious gingivitis* as an etiologic factor, and points to the fact that both diseases are responsive to metronidazole and tetracycline, and both occur in the same age group. Gingivitis should be looked for in cases of rosacea: treatment for either may help the other.

HISTOLOGY. The histologic changes vary according to the stage of the process. Usually there is disorganization of the upper dermal connective tissue, with edema, disruption of fibers, and often severe elastosis.

The inflammatory phase is marked by the presence of lymphocytes, histiocytes, polymorphonuclears, plasma cells, and foreign-body-type giant cells. *D. folliculorum* is frequently found in the follicles.

DIFFERENTIAL DIAGNOSIS. Rosacea is simulated by acne vulgaris, lupus erythematosus, bromoderma, iododerma, and papular syphilid.

Haber's syndrome is a genodermatosis characterized by a rosacealike facial dermatosis and multiple verrucous lesions on nonsun-exposed skin. The onset of the facial lesions is in the first two decades of life, in contrast to the later onset of rosacea.

TREATMENT. The treatment of choice is long-term oral administration of tetracycline, on a minimum maintenance dose basis. It is usually highly effective, although, as Knight and Vickers showed, it is only suppressive, not curative. Saihan and Burton reported in 1980 that metronidazole (200 mg b.i.d.) was just as effective as tetracycline, 250 mg b.i.d. It is, however, not as safe when given on a chronic basis. Metronidazole cream, however, appears to be both safe and effective, and MetroGel (metronidazole 0.75 per cent gel), approved and marketed late in 1988, may be even better.

Isotretinoin (Accutane) produces dramatic improvement even in treatment-resistant cases, but relapse in a few weeks or months is the rule. Schmidt et al, however, confirmed Nikolowski and Plewig's good results and saw no relapse in two of three female patients and in two of seven men after two

years; three men had numerous papular recurrences within one to nine months.

Topical therapy is helpful; however, like other forms of treatment for rosacea (with the occasional exception of isotretinoin) it is only suppressive and must be used on a long-term, daily basis. If they are prescribed, topical medications should be similar to those used in acne vulgaris. In addition, corticosteroid lotions and creams of the nonfluorinated type may be used when inflammation predominates. Ice cold boric acid compresses or Vleminckx compresses are also effective when inflammation and pustules are present. If *D. folliculorum* is present we find that a lotion containing 5 per cent benzoyl peroxide and 5 per cent precipitated sulfur (Sulfoxyl) is helpful.

Topical antibiotics such as erythromycin have shown promise in the management of this recalcitrant disease.

In the menopausal age estrogens have been found to be effective in some women with severe rosacea.

Topically, 5 per cent sulfur ointment or cream applied twice daily may be satisfactory. The use of corticosteroid creams, which are helpful, should be restricted to hydrocortisone or desonide because of the inherent danger of producing telangiectases and erythema with prolonged use of the fluorinated corticosteroid creams. Vioform with hydrocortisone is frequently effective. The use of Tridesilon (0.05 per cent desonide) one or more times daily, with Quinolor compound on alternate days, and tetracycline by mouth, has been recommended by Rees. Benzoyl peroxide gel, 5 per cent, once daily till any irritation subsides and then twice daily, was shown by Montes et al to be highly effective at four and eight weeks. Irritation and burning were common side effects.

Bleicher PA, et al: Topical metronidazole therapy for rosacea. Arch Dermatol 1987, 123:609.
Godbold RL, et al: Granulomatous rosacea. Cutis 1972, 9:513.
Hoting E, et al: Treatment of rosacea with isotretinoin. Int J Dermatol 1986, 25:660.
Kikuchi I, et al: Haber's syndrome. Arch Dermatol 1981, 117:321.
Kligman AM, et al: Rosacea. Dermatology 1978, 1:27.
Lowe NJ, et al: Topical metronidazole for severe and recalcitrant rosacea. Cutis 1989, 43:283.
Montes LF, et al: Topical treatment of acne rosacea with benzoyl peroxide acetone gel. Cutis 1983, 32:185.
Nikolowski J, et al: Rosazea. Oral Behandlung mit 13-cis-Retinsäure. Hautarzt 1980, 1981, 31:660, 32:575.
Pochi P: Talk given at the American Academy of Dermatology, 1985.
Rosen T, et al: Acne rosacea in blacks. JAAD 1987, 17:70.
Saihan EM, et al: A double-blind trial of metronidazole vs oxytetracycline treatment for rosacea. Br J Dermatol 1980, 102:443.
Schewach-Millet M, et al: Granulomatous rosacea. JAAD 1988, 18:1362.
Schmidt JB, et al: 13-cis-retinoic acid in rosacea. Acta Derm Venereol (Stockh) 1984, 64:15.
Idem: Rosacea. Int J Dermatol 1983, 22:393.

RHINOPHYMA

Rhinophyma consists of hypertrophic, hyperemic, large nodular masses centered around the distal half

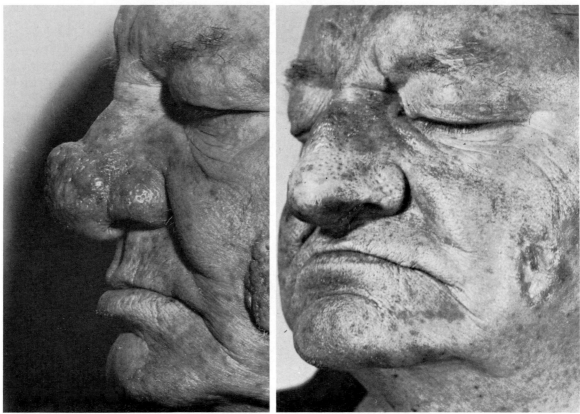

Figure 13–13. Rhinophyma before and after surgical ablation.

of the nose. Rhinophyma is seen almost exclusively in men over 40 years of age. The tip and wings of the nose are usually involved by large lobulated masses, which may even be pendulous. The hugely dilated follicles contain long vermicular plugs of sebum and keratin.

The cause of rhinophyma is unknown. It is usually associated with a long history of rosacea.

The histologic features are epidermal epithelial hyperplasia and pilosebaceous gland hyperplasia with fibrosis, inflammation, and telangiectasia.

Treatment of this disfigurement is simple and most effective. Isotretinoin, though surprisingly helpful, is hardly worth giving because the benefit is so temporary. Rhinophyma is best treated by surgical ablation, electrosurgery (surgical cutting current) laser surgery, or wire-brush surgery.

For anesthesia a bilateral infraorbital nerve block just below the notch in the maxilla on both sides and a ring of 2 per cent Xylocaine in the skin around the nose produce complete anesthesia. Often the latter is sufficient. The needle is introduced opposite each ala and the injection is made upward toward the bridge of the nose. If a needle 1½ inches long is used, the two injections will meet on the bridge of the nose. If the needle is partially withdrawn and then reintroduced along the upper lip horizontally, a complete ring of anesthesia is given through the same puncture wound. In addition, it is advisable to withdraw the needle partially again and then to make an injection downward toward the corner of the mouth.

Surgical ablation of redundant grapelike masses and of the bulbous swollen tip of the nose is easily done with a razor blade, though the invention of the Shaw scalpel, a decade or so ago, has superseded it. This instrument has a copper- and Teflon-coated standard scalpel blade with a thermostatically controlled heating element that heats it to 110–270° C, which provides hemostasis. Tromovitch et al reported on its use in 1983, and Eisen et al in 1986. Stegman still prefers it to the cutting loop. The excessive tissue is shaved off in successive layers until the desired amount has been removed. Bleeding ceases after a few minutes with application of pressure. If an artery is cut, a suture should be passed around it and tied. When oozing persists, Oxycel gauze may be applied. Wire-brush surgery (dermabrasion) is useful for mild cases. If there are pendulous redundant masses, these should first be cut off with scalpel or with surgical cutting current. Dermabrasion may then be used to remove any objectionable remnants.

Although the bipolar electrical cutting current is perfectly satisfactory, "brushing" with an electrode shaped like a small hockey stick is even better because it sears the tissues just enough to stop all bleeding, which may be troublesome with the bipolar cutting current and with plastic surgery. This brushing action is obtained by using a cutting current without the indifferent electrode, i.e., as if it were a "unipolar" current. After the operation, the nose is dressed with a nonadherent dressing such as a Telfa pad. This type of treatment produces the best results of any of the treatment modalities mentioned above.

The carbon dioxide laser has been used to excise redundant tissue, and the argon laser may ameliorate the vascular component of rosacea.

Acker DW, et al: Rhinophyma with carcinoma. Arch Dermatol 1967, 95:250.
Eisen RF, et al: Surgical treatment of rhinophyma with the Shaw scalpel. Arch Dermatol 1986, 122:307.
Fisher WJ: Rhinophyma: Its surgical treatment. Plast Reconstr Surg 1970, 45:466.
Greenbaum SS, et al: Comparison of CO$_2$ laser and electrosurgery in the treatment of rhinophyma. JAAD 1988, 18:363.
Pochi P: Talk given at the American Academy of Dermatology, 1985.
Simpson GT, et al: Rhinologic laser surgery. Otolaryngol Clin North Am 1983, 16:829.
Tromovitch TA, et al: The Shaw scalpel. J Dermatol Surg Oncol 1983, 9:316.

PYODERMA FACIALE

O'Leary and Kierland described this disease, which occurs on the face. It consists of an intense reddish or cyanotic erythema, combined with superficial and deep abscesses and cystic lesions. Some cysts are connected by communicating channels or sinus tracts. Some contain greenish or yellowish purulent material. Older cysts contain an oily substance. The condition occurs mostly in postadolescent girls, and is distinguished from acne by the absence of comedones, the rapid onset, the fulminating course, and the absence of acne on the back and chest.

A Mayo Clinic series of 29 patients, all women, ranged from 19 to 59 years old; only two were over 40. Late-onset acne preceded pyoderma faciale by from 7 to 20 years. None had gram-negative organ-

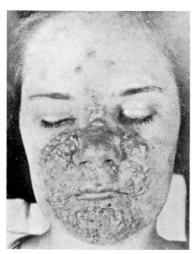

Figure 13–14. Unusually extensive pyoderma faciale. (Courtesy of Dr. M. J. Costello.)

isms, only two had staph; most had the usual acne pathogens.

Treatment is similar to that of pustular rosacea: chiefly, tetracycline or doxycycline orally. Massa and Su recommend choosing the antibiotic on the basis of results of cultures. They used intralesional, but not systemic, triamcinolone. They believe Vleminckx's solution packs are helpful.

Markson VJ, et al: Pyoderma faciale. JAAD 1987, 17:1062.
Massa MC, et al: Pyoderma faciale: A clinical study of 29 patients. JAAD 1982, 6:84.

ACNEIFORM ERUPTIONS

Acneiform eruptions are characterized by papules and pustules resembling acne lesions, not necessarily confined to the usual sites of acne vulgaris. The eruptions are distinguished by their sudden onset, usually in a patient well past adolescence.

Most of the acneiform eruptions originate from skin exposure to various industrial chemicals. Some eruptions may come from oral medications.

Acneiform eruptions may be induced by exposure of the skin to the fumes generated in the manufacture of chlorine and its by-products. These chlorinated hydrocarbons may cause *chloracne*, consisting of cysts, pustules, folliculitis, and comedones. The most potent acneiform-inducing agents are the polyhalogenated hydrocarbons, notably dioxin (2,3,7,8 tetrachlorobenzodioxin).

Cutting oils, lubricating oils, crude coal tar applied to the skin for medicinal purposes, heavy tar distillates, coal tar pitch, corticosteroids applied to the skin under occlusive dressings, and asbestos are known substances that may produce acneiform eruptions. Although commonly called "trade acne," "bromine acne," and "chloracne," they are not a true acne, even though they are often ushered in by open comedones.

Some of the acneiform eruptions are induced by medications such as iodides in vitamins with mineral supplement, and bromides in drugs such as propantheline bromide (Pro-Banthine), and corticosteroids (see Chapter 7).

Massive keratinization-suppressing doses of vitamin A, 300,000 units daily, or better, 150,000 units enhanced by 400 I.U. of vitamin E twice a day, may often clear steroid reactions rapidly, and smaller doses may be used even to prevent them in patients with this idiosyncrasy. More often used are topical retinoids, such as Retin-A cream or gel, or even oral Accutane, which may be considered in some cases. Most patients recover within two years after exposure has been stopped.

Hitch JM: Acneiform eruptions induced by drugs and chemicals. JAMA 1967, 200:879.
Tindall JP: Chloracne and chloracnegens. JAAD 1985, 13:539.

PERIORAL DERMATITIS

This common perioral papulosquamous eruption consists of discrete papules and vesicopustules on an erythematous and scaling base. It is a distinctive dermatitis confined symmetrically around the mouth with a clear zone of some 5 mm between the vermilion border and the affected skin. There is no itching; however, an uncomfortable burning sensation may be present. It occurs almost exclusively in women between 23 and 35.

The histopathology, according to Ramelet et al, is essentially the same as that of rosacea: edema and vasodilatation in the papillary dermis, and a mixed cellular inflammatory infiltrate, with occasional leucocytoclastic vasculitis. Wilkinson espouses the English view that since only 5–8 per cent of patients deny using strong corticosteroid creams, they must be the cause. Fluoridated dentifrices have been suspected, but not incriminated conclusively. Demodex has been suspected, and when it has been found, benzoyl peroxide lotion has often been effective.

Tetracycline, 1000 mg by mouth daily, should be used for pustular lesions, with dosages decreased as control is attained. It is believed by Sneddon and others that tetracycline is the most important treatment in rosacealike dermatitis even when it is steroid-induced.

Bikowski reported great success in six cases with the use of hydrocortisone valerate cream (Westwood) and topical erythromycin solution (Staticin–Westwood), but he believes oral tetracycline with topical steroids is the treatment of choice.

Periorbital Dermatitis. In A. A. Fisher's recent report of this, the same disease occurs in a distribution around the lower eyelids and skin adjacent to the upper and lower eyelids. All three of his patients had been using a "strong" fluorinated topical steroid cream for over a year, and all three responded promptly to 250 mg of tetracycline four times a day, with hydrocortisone topically. Periorbital dermatitis was first described by E. B. Smith et al in 1976.

Bikowski JB: Topical therapy for perioral dermatitis. Cutis 1983, 31:678.

Fisher AA: Periocular dermatitis akin to the perioral variety. JAAD 1986, 15:642.

Mellette JR, et al: Perioral dermatitis. Bull Assoc Military Dermatol 1983, 9:1:3.

Ramelet AA, et al: Histopathological study of perioral dermatitis. Dermatologica 1981, 163:361.

Smith EB, et al: Periorbital dermatitis. Arch Dermatol 1976, 112:563.

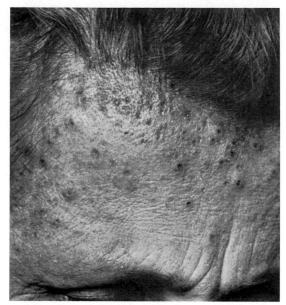

Figure 13–15. Acne varioliformis. (Courtesy of Dr. H. Müller, Germany.)

Wilkinson D: What is perioral dermatitis? Int J Dermatol 1981, 20:485.

ACNE MILIARIS NECROTICA
(Acne Varioliformis)

Acne miliaris necrotica consists of follicular vesicopustules, frequently solitary, usually very itchy, which appear anywhere in the scalp or adjacent areas, rupture early, and dry up after a few days. If they leave large scars the name acne varoliformis is used; they are probably not separate diseases.

Anecdotal reports of success with Vleminckx's solution, ketoconazole, Quinolor ointment, colchicine, dapsone, Keflex, culture-directed antibiotic therapy, papaya tablets, Augmentin, and even destruction by laser, have been seen; but the most hopeful would seem to be isotretinoin (Accutane). In so stubborn and itchy a disease, it seems justifiable.

Kossard S, et al: Necrotizing lymphocytic folliculitis: The early lesion of acne necrotica. JAAD 1987, 16:1007.

What to do for acne miliaris necrotica. The Schoch Letter 1985, 35:45.

Upton GL: Augmentin for acne miliaris necrotica. The Schoch Letter 1986, 36:5.

14

Bacterial Infections

Bacterial infections in the skin often have distinct morphologic characteristics which should alert the clinician that a potentially treatable and reversible condition exists. These cutaneous signs may be an indication of a generalized systemic process or simply an isolated superficial event.

Congenital agammaglobulinemia, primary acquired agammaglobulinemia, Wiskott-Aldrich syndrome, atopic dermatitis, ataxia telangiectasia, and the acquired immunodeficiency syndrome (AIDS) are often associated with pyogenic infections and should be thought of when severe or persistently recurrent examples of these are seen. Disorders in which neutrophil function is impaired should also be thought of: chronic granulomatous disease of childhood or Chédiak-Higashi disease.

The categorization of these infections will be first those diseases due to gram-positive bacteria, then those caused by gram-negative bacteria, and finally several miscellaneous diseases caused by the rickettsiae, chlamydiae, mycoplasmas, and spirochetes.

1985 STD Treatment Guidelines JAAD 1986, 14:707.
Bisno AL: Cutaneous infections. Am J Med 1984, 76(5A):172.
Feingold DS: Bacterial adherence, colonization, and pathogenicity. Arch Dermatol 1986, 122:161.
Idem: Bacterial infections of the skin. JAAD 1989, 20:469.
Hirschmann JV: Topical antibiotics in dermatology. Arch Dermatol 1988, 124:1691.
Leyden JJ: Infections in the immunocompromised host. Arch Dermatol 1985, 121:854.
Idem, et al: Skin microflora. J Invest Dermatol 1987, 88:65s.
Mandell GL, et al (eds): The Principles and Practice of Infectious Diseases. 2nd ed. New York, John Wiley and Sons, 1985.
Medical Letter: The choice of antimicrobial drugs. Vol 30 (Mar 25, 1988).
Percival A (ed): Quinolones: Their Future in Medical Practice. Int Congress and Symposium Series. London, Royal Society of Medical Services, 1985.
Roth RR, James WD: Microbiology of the skin: Resident flora, ecology, infection. JAAD 1989, 20:367.
Sheagren JN: Skin and skin structure infections in the patient at risk. Am J Med 1984, 76(A):191.

INFECTIONS DUE TO GRAM-POSITIVE ORGANISMS

STAPHYLOCOCCAL SKIN INFECTIONS

The skin lesions induced by this gram-positive coccus appear usually as simply pustules, furuncles, or erosions with honey-colored crusts; however, bullae, widespread erythema and desquamation, or vegetating pyodermas may also be indicators of *Staphylococcus aureus* infection. Purulent purpura may indicate bacteremia or endocarditis due to *S. aureus*, or, in immunocompromised patients, *S. epidermidis*.

Approximately 20 per cent of adults have *S. aureus* as a normal inhabitant of the anterior nares. These nasal carriers are particularly prone to infections with this bacterium because of its continuous presence on the skin and nasal mucosa.

SUPERFICIAL PUSTULAR FOLLICULITIS
(Impetigo of Bockhart)

Bockhart's impetigo is a superficial folliculitis with thin-walled pustules at the follicle orifices. Favorite

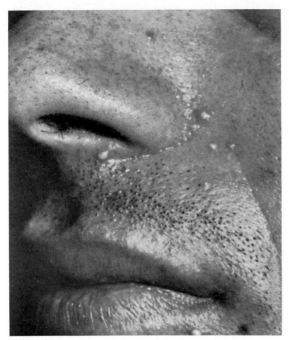

Figure 14–1. Impetigo of Bockhart (note superficial, persistent pustules).

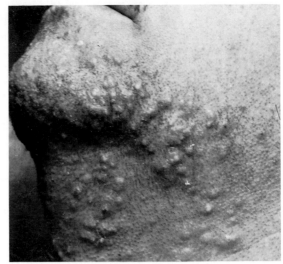

Figure 14–2. Sycosis vulgaris. (Courtesy of Dr. A. Kaminsky, Argentina.)

locations are the extremities and scalp, although it is also seen on the face, especially periorally. These fragile, yellowish white-domed pustules develop in crops and heal in a few days.

Staphylococcus aureus is the most frequent cause. The infection may result from scratches, insect bites, or other skin injuries.

Treatment consists of thorough cleansing of the affected areas with an antibacterial soap and water twice daily. Following this, an antibiotic ointment, preferably Bactroban (mupirocin), is applied; cloxacillin or erythromycin should be taken internally, especially in recalcitrant and recurrent cases.

SYCOSIS VULGARIS (Sycosis Barbae)

CLINICAL FEATURES. Sycosis vulgaris, formerly known as "barber's itch," is a perifollicular, inherently chronic, pustular staphylococcal infection of the bearded region, characterized by the presence of inflammatory papules and pustules, and a tendency to recurrence.

The disease begins with erythema and a burning or itching, usually on the upper lip near the nose. In a day or two one or more pinhead-sized pustules, pierced by hairs, develop. These rupture after shaving or washing and leave an erythematous spot, which is later the site of a fresh crop of pustules. In this manner the affection persists and gradually spreads. With the formation of pus about the hairs they become loose and can be readily epilated. Marginal blepharitis with conjunctivitis usually is present in severe cases of sycosis.

Staphylococcal folliculitis may affect other areas, such as the eyebrows, eyelashes, axillae, pubis, and

thighs. On the pubis it may be transmitted among sexual partners, and mini-epidemics of folliculitis and furunculosis of the genital and gluteal areas may be considered a sexually transmitted disease.

Sycosis Lupoides. This is a staphylococcic infection that, by peripheral extension and central scar formation, forms a patch somewhat resembling lupus vulgaris, hence the name. The hairless atrophic area is usually bordered by pustules and crusts.

ETIOLOGY. *Staphylococcus aureus* from the nasal cavity or from colonized skin often acts as a reservoir. Direct inoculation from shaving may cause the disease.

PATHOLOGY. It is a pyogenic folliculitis and perifolliculitis, with the infection extending deep into the follicles. Inflammatory changes with vascular dilatation and cellular infiltration are present, with edema and infiltration of neutrophils, and plasma cells.

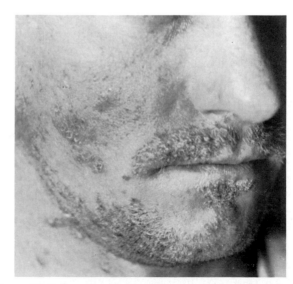

Figure 14–3. Sycosis vulgaris. (Courtesy of Dr. F. Daniels, Jr.)

DIFFERENTIAL DIAGNOSIS. Sycosis vulgaris is to be distinguished from tinea, contact dermatitis, seborrheic dermatitis, lupus erythematosus, pseudofolliculitis barbae, and herpetic sycosis. Tinea barbae rarely affects the upper lip, which is a common location for sycosis. In tinea barbae the involvement usually is in the submaxillary region or on the chin, and spores and hyphae are found in the hairs. In contact dermatitis the patches are vesicular and crusted and there are no follicular pustules. In seborrheic dermatitis the patches are symmetrical, occurring particularly along the hairline and eyebrows, as well as on the nasolabial angle and ears. Lupus erythematosus is not follicular and there is no pustulation. Pseudofolliculitis barbae manifests torpid papules at the sites of ingrowing beard hairs, in black men. In herpes simplex the duration is usually only a few days and even in persistent cases ("herpetic sycosis") there are vesicles, which help to differentiate the disease from sycosis.

TREATMENT. Bactroban (mupirocin) ointment topically is advised. If it fails, erythromycin, a cephalosporin, or a penicillinase-resistant penicillin such as oxacillin, cloxacillin, or dicloxacillin, is indicated. When the inflammation is acute, hot wet packs of Burow's solution diluted 1:20 (Domeboro) are beneficial. An anhydrous formulation of aluminum chloride (Drysol, Xerac-AC) has been reported by Shelley and Hurley to be effective when used once nightly for chronic folliculitis, especially of the buttocks. Antibiotic ophthalmic ointments are used for the blepharitis.

FURUNCULOSIS

CLINICAL FEATURES. A *furuncle* or *boil* is an acute, round, tender, circumscribed, perifollicular staphylococcic abscess which generally ends in central suppuration. A *carbuncle* is merely two more confluent furuncles, with separate "heads."

The lesions begin, as a rule, in a hair follicle, and often continue for a prolonged period by autoinoculation. Some lesions disappear before rupture, but most undergo central necrosis and rupture through the skin, discharging purulent, necrotic debris. Sites of predilection are the nape, the axillae, and the buttocks, but boils may occur anywhere.

ETIOLOGY. The integrity of the skin surface may be impaired by irritation, pressure, friction, hyperhidrosis, dermatitis, dermatophytosis, or shaving, among other factors. This may provide a portal of entry for the ubiquitous *S. aureus*. Compromised local integrity predisposes to infection. The proximate cause is either contagion, or autoinoculation from a carrier focus, usually in the nose or crotch.

Certain systemic disorders may predispose to furunculosis: alcoholism, malnutrition, blood dyscrasias, disorders of neutrophil function, iatrogenic or other immunosuppression, including AIDS, and diabetes. Atopic dermatitis, which predisposes to the

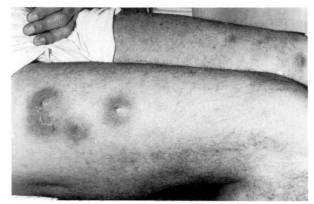

Figure 14–4. Furunculosis. (Courtesy of Dr. J. Knoll.)

S. aureus carrier state, increases the incidence of infections.

Hospital Furunculosis. Epidemics of staphylococcal infections occur in hospitals. Marked resistance to antibacterial agents in these cases is commonplace. Attempts to control these outbreaks center around meticulous handwashing. In nurseries, Seeberg et al achieved a dramatic fall in neonatal colonization and infections with *S. aureus* and non–group A streptococci by using a 4 per cent solution of chlorhexidine for skin and umbilical cord care.

HISTOPATHOLOGY. There is a deep abscess with both lymphocytes and neutrophils, and in longstanding cases, plasma cells and foreign-body giant cells.

TREATMENT. Warm compresses and antibiotics taken internally may arrest early furuncles. A penicillinase-resistant penicillin, erythromycin, or a cephalosporin should be given orally in a dose of 1 to 2 gm per day according to the severity of the case.

When the lesions are incipient and acutely inflamed, incision should be strictly avoided and moist heat employed. When the furuncle has become localized and shows definite fluctuation, free incision, with drainage, should be made without delay. The cavity should be packed with a rubber dam or iodoform or Vaseline gauze.

Special Locations. In boils of the *external auditory canal*, irrigations and early incisions should not be attempted. An antibiotic ointment (Bactroban) should be applied and antibiotics should be given internally. Heat should be applied to the auricle and the side of the face.

Nasal furuncles should be treated in the early stages by the application of hot saline solution compresses inside and outside the nostril, until softening occurs. They should not be incised but steamed. Antibiotics should be given internally and applied locally.

On the *upper lip* and *nose*, great care must be exercised and immediate energetic treatment instituted because of the dangers of sinus thrombosis, meningitis, and septicemia developing from boils on these parts. Trauma must be prevented by the use of an adequate dressing; local and general treatment should be followed in accordance with the principles already described; adequate doses of systemic antibiotics are essential. Incision should not be made unless all other treatments fail.

Chronic Furunculosis. Despite treatment, recurrences of some boils may be anticipated. Usually no underlying disease is present to predispose to this; rather, autoinoculation and intrafamilial spread among colonized individuals is responsible.

One of the most important factors in prevention is to avoid autoinoculation. Truman Nelson emphasized the nasal carrier state, which predisposes to chronic furunculosis. In addition, the hazard of contamination from the perianal and intertriginous areas is to be considered. Routine precautions to be taken in attempting to break the cycle of recurrent furunculosis should be the use of an antibacterial soap or chlorhexidine daily, with special attention to the axillae and crotch, laundering of bedding and clothing daily initially, and frequent handwashing.

Additionally, the daily application of an antibiotic ointment twice daily to the nares of patients and family members every fourth week has been found to be effective by Hedström. Wheat et al reported the efficacy of rifampin 600 mg daily for 10 days combined with cloxacillin, 500 mg four times daily, in eradicating the nasal carriage state. One of us (WDJ) has had success in several patients using this oral antibiotic combination. Recently low-dose (150 mg/day) clindamycin for three months was reported to be effective by Klempner et al.

The use of bacitracin or mupirocin ointment inside the nares twice daily throughout the course of Accutane therapy eliminates, or markedly reduces the risk of inducing, nasal carriage of *S. aureus*, and hence staphylococcal infections, after its use.

Bacterial interference treatment of recurrent and chronic furunculosis has been reported to be effective by several authors since the original work was done by Shinefield et al. Maibach et al, and more recently Steele, have had success by giving 1 gm of cloxacillin daily for two weeks, using antibacterial soaps, and applying bacitracin ointment inside the nostrils twice a day. This is done to clear the patient of carriage of *S. aureus*. A nonpathogenic strain of *S. aureus* (502A) is then introduced into the nares and other skin sites. As long as the nose carried this strain, no furuncles occurred.

PYOGENIC PARONYCHIA

Paronychia is an inflammatory reaction involving the folds of the skin surrounding the fingernail. It is characterized by acute or chronic purulent, tender, and painful swellings of the tissues around the nail, caused by an abscess in the nail fold. When the infection becomes chronic, horizontal ridges appear at the base of the nail. With recurrent bouts new ridges appear.

The primary disorder is separation of the eponychium from the nail plate. The separation is usually

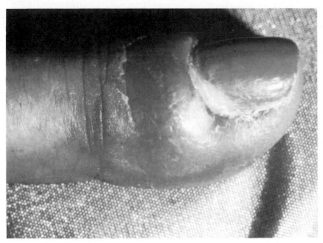

Figure 14–5. Paronychia due to Staphylococcus aureus.

caused by trauma as a result of moisture-induced maceration of the nail folds from frequent wetting of the hands. The relationship is close enough to justify treating chronic paronychia as work-related in bartenders, waitresses, nurses, and others who often wet their hands. The moist grooves of the nail and nail fold become secondarily invaded by pyogenic cocci and yeasts. The yeast-caused paronychia is discussed later. The pathogenic yeast is most frequently *Candida albicans*. In addition, the saprophytic fungi may also be involved. Wilson cites also the saprophytic fungi *Geotrichum, Mucor, Rhodotorula, Cryptococcus,* or *Saccharomyces* as possible secondary invaders.

The causative bacteria are usually *Staphylococcus, Pseudomonas aeruginosa,* or *Streptococcus.*

Treatment of pyogenic paronychia consists mostly of protection against trauma and studious, concentrated efforts to keep the affected fingernails meticulously dry. Rubber or plastic gloves over cotton gloves should be used whenever the hand must be placed in water. Incision and drainage should be done on the acutely inflamed pyogenic abscesses. The abscess may often be opened by pushing the nail fold away from the nail plate. For chronic paronychia a fungicide and bactericide such as Neosporin solution, Vioform, or 2 per cent thymol in chloroform or ether may be used. Castellani paint, which should be applied several times daily regularly for several months, is effective, and with the omission of the acid fuchsin, the colorless preparation does not stain the lesions or clothing. In acute suppurative paronychia, especially if stains show pyogenic cocci, erythromycin or cloxacillin should be given orally. Rarely, long-term antibiotic therapy may be required.

BOTRYOMYCOSIS

Botryomycosis is an uncommon, chronic, nodular, crusted, purulent disease characterized by sinuses discharging sulfur granules. These heal with atrophic scars. The granules yield most commonly *S. aureus* on culture, although cases due to *Pseudomonas aeruginosa*, *E. coli*, *Proteus*, *Bacteroides*, and *Streptococcus* have been reported. It occurs frequently in patients with altered immune function, such as patients with neutrophilic defects, as in the case reported by Leibowitz et al, or as in a patient reported by Patterson et al who had the acquired immunodeficiency syndrome (AIDS). Several studies have documented neutrophil defects in AIDS. Appropriate antibiotics, surgical drainage, and surgical excision are methods used to treat this chronic, indolent disease.

PYOMYOSITIS

S. aureus abscess formation within the deep large striated muscles usually presents with fever and muscle pain. It occurs most commonly in children and the most frequent site is the thigh. Maddox et al reported a case which presented with a purplish discoloration of the lower extremity. Occasionally erythema or yellow discoloration develops, but these are late findings. Drainage of the abscess and appropriate systemic antibiotics are required.

STAPHYLOCOCCAL IMPETIGO

Also known as **bullous impetigo** or impetigo neonatorum, this variety of impetigo occurs characteristically in newborn infants, though it may occur at any age. The *neonatal type* is highly contagious and is a constant threat in nurseries. In most cases the symptoms begin between the fourth and tenth days of life with the appearance of bullae, which may come out on any part of the body but are apt to occur on the face or hands and areas not covered by clothing. Constitutional symptoms are at first absent,

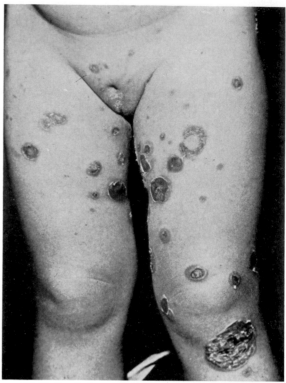

Figure 14–7. Staphylococcal (bullous) impetigo. Annular lesions are characteristic. Note collarette scale.

but later weakness and fever or a subnormal temperature may be present. Diarrhea with green stools frequently occurs. Bacteremia, pneumonia, or meningitis may develop rapidly, with fatal termination.

In warm climates particularly, adults may have

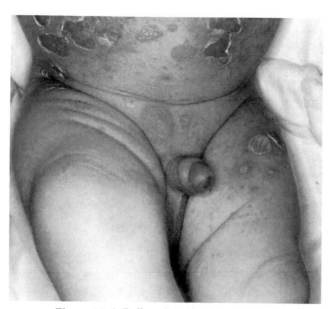

Figure 14–6. Bullous impetigo in a neonate.

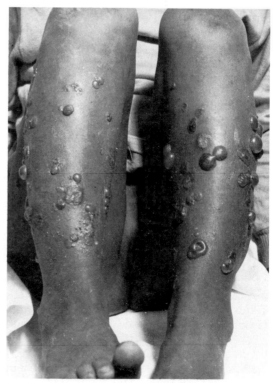

Figure 14–8. Staphylococcal (bullous) impetigo.

bullous impetigo, most often in the axillae or groins, or on the hands. Usually no scalp lesions are present. The lesions are strikingly large, fragile bullae, suggestive of pemphigus. When these rupture they leave circinate, weepy, or crusted lesions, and in this stage it may be called *impetigo circinata*. Children with bullous impetigo may give a history of an insect bite at the site of onset of lesions. Dillon found in a study of 31 patients, that the majority were caused by phage type 71 coagulase-positive *S. aureus*, or a related group 2 phage type.

STAPHYLOCOCCAL SCALDED SKIN SYNDROME (SSSS)

Staphylococcal scalded skin syndrome is a generalized, confluent, superficially exfoliative disease, occurring most commonly in neonates and young children. It was known in the past as Ritter's disease or dermatitis exfoliativa neonatorum. It has been reported to occur rarely in adults, as in Richard et al's patient, an immunosuppressed homosexual. When it does occur in an adult, usually either renal compromise or immunosuppression is a predisposing factor.

It is a febrile, rapidly evolving, generalized, desquamative infectious disease, in which the skin exfoliates in sheets. It does not separate at the dermoepidermal junction, as in toxic (drug-induced) epidermal necrolysis (TEN), but immediately below the granular layer. The lesions are thus much more superficial and less severe than in TEN, and healing is much more rapid. They also extend far beyond areas of actual staphylococcal infection, by action of the epidermolytic toxin, exfoliatin, elaborated by the staphylococcus in remote sites. Usually the staphylococci are present at a distal focus such as the

pharynx, nose, ear, or conjunctiva. Septicemia or cutaneous infection may also be the causative focus.

Its clinical manifestations begin abruptly with fever, skin tenderness, and erythema involving the neck, groins, and axillae. There is sparing of the palms, soles, and mucous membranes. Nikolsky's sign is positive. Generalized exfoliation follows within the next hours to days, with large sheets of epidermis separating.

Staphylococcus aureus of Group 2, most commonly phage type 71, has been the causative agent in most cases. If cultures are taken (which is not necessary) they should be obtained from the mucous membranes because the skin erythema and desquamation is due to the distant effects of the exfoliative toxin, unlike the situation in bullous impetigo, where *S. aureus* is present in the lesions.

Rapid diagnosis can be made by examining frozen sections of a blister roof and observing that the full thickness of the epidermis is not necrotic as in TEN but rather is cleaved below the granular layer.

Treatment of choice is a penicillinase-resistant penicillin such as cloxacillin or dicloxacillin, or erythromycin, combined with fluid therapy and general supportive measures. The prognosis is good, and corticosteroids are contraindicated.

TOXIC SHOCK SYNDROME (TSS)

This acute, febrile, multisystem illness has as one of its major diagnostic criteria a widespread macular erythematous eruption. It is caused by toxin-producing strains of *S. aureus*, most of which have been isolated from the cervical mucosa in menstruating young women. However, there are now several reports of a very similar syndrome in which the cause was streptococci.

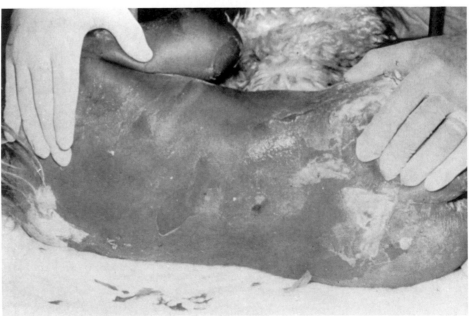

Figure 14–9. Staphylococcal scalded skin syndrome ("SSSS"), once regarded as a variety of toxic epidermal necrolysis.

The Center for Communicable Diseases (CDC) case definition of TSS includes the following: a temperature of 38.9° C or higher, an erythematous eruption, desquamation of the palms and soles one to two weeks after onset, hypotension, and involvement of three or more other systems—*gastrointestinal* (vomiting, diarrhea), *muscular* (myalgias, increased creatinine phosphokinase level), *mucous membrane* (hyperemia), *renal* (pyuria without infection or raised creatinine or blood urea nitrogen levels), *hepatic* (increased bilirubin, SGOT, or SGPT), *hematologic* (platelets less than 100,000/mm^3), or *central nervous system* (disorientation). In addition, serologic tests for Rocky Mountain spotted fever, leptospirosis, and rubeola, and cultures of blood, urine, and cerebrospinal fluid should be negative. Bach emphasized bulbar conjunctival hyperemia and palmar edema as two additional clinical clues.

Ninety per cent of cases occur in young women between the first and sixth days of a menstrual period. During the initial outbreak, between 1979 and 1982, the majority were using a "superabsorbent" tampon. Cases have now been reported in women using contraceptive sponges, in patients with nasal packing after rhinoplasty, and in patients with staphylococcal infections of bone, lung, or soft tissue. Huntley et al reported a case which occurred as a complication of dermatologic surgery. The offending *S. aureus* strain produces one or more exotoxins.

Histologic findings delineated by Hurwitz and Ackerman are spongiosis, neutrophils scattered throughout the epidermis, individual necrotic keratinocytes, perivascular and interstitial infiltrates composed of at least lymphocytes and neutrophils, and edema of the papillary dermis. These findings can help in the differentiation of toxic shock syndrome (TSS) from other diseases which can closely mimic its cutaneous presentation, such as viral exanthems, Kawasaki's disease, scarlet fever, drug eruptions, systemic lupus erythematosus, toxic epidermal necrolysis, and staphylococcal scalded skin syndrome.

Treatment consists of systemic antibiotics such as nafcillin, 1 to 1.5 gm intravenously every four hours, vigorous fluid therapy to treat shock, and drainage of the *S. aureus*–infected site.

Anderson KE, et al: Black and white human skin differences. JAAD 1979, 1:276.

Bach MC: Dermatologic signs of toxic shock syndrome. JAAD 1983, 8:343.

Bartter T, et al: Toxic shock syndrome. Arch Intern Med 1988, 148:1421.

Bronstein SW, et al: Bullous dermatosis caused by *Staphylococcus aureus* in locus minoris resistentiae. JAAD 1984, 10:259.

Chesney PJ, et al: Clinical manifestations of toxic shock syndrome. JAMA 1981, 246:741.

Cole GW, et al: The adherence of *Staphylococcal aureus* to human corneocytes. Arch Dermatol 1986, 122:166.

Cone LA, et al: Clinical and bacteriologic observations of a toxic shock–like syndrome due to *Streptococcus pyogenes*. N Engl J Med 1987, 317:146.

David TJ, et al: Bacterial infection of atopic eczema. Arch Dis Child 1986, 61:20.

Davis JP, et al: Toxic-shock syndrome. N Engl J Med 1980, 303:1429.

Diamond RL, et al: Staphylococcal scalded skin syndrome. Br J Dermatol 1977, 98:483.

Dillon HC: Treatment of staphylococcal skin infections. JAAD 1983, 8:177.

Duvic M: Staphylococcal infections and the pruritus of AIDS-related complex. Arch Dermatol 1987, 123:1599.

Elias PM, et al: Bullous impetigo. Arch Dermatol 1976, 112:856.

Idem: Staphylococcal scalded skin syndrome. Arch Dermatol 1977, 113:207.

Elias PM: Staphylococcal toxic epidermal necrolysis. J Invest Dermatol 1975, 65:501.

Ellis M, et al: Impaired neutrophil function in patients with AIDS or AIDS-related complex. J Invest Dis 1988, 158:1268.

Epstein EH Jr, et al: Adult toxic epidermal necrolysis with staphylococcal septicemia. JAMA 1974, 229:425.

Eykyn SJ: Staphylococcal sepsis. Lancet 1988, 1:100.

Faich G, et al: Toxic shock syndrome and the vaginal contraceptive sponge. JAMA 1986, 255:216.

Feldman SR, et al: Botryomycosis caused by *Moraxella nonliquefaciens*. Cutis 1989, 43:140.

Findlay RF, et al: Toxic shock syndrome. Int J Dermatol 1982, 21:117.

Garbe PL, et al: *Staphlococcus aureus* isolation from patients with nonmenstrual toxic shock syndrome. JAMA 1985, 253:25.

Goldberg NS, et al: Staphylococcal scalded skin syndrome mimicking acute graft-vs-host disease in a bone marrow transplant recipient. Arch Dermatol 1989, 125:85.

Gorden DM, et al: Staphylococcal folliculitis of the nose. JAMA 1988, 260:2915.

Graham ML, et al: Isotretinoin and *Staphylococcus aureus* infection. Arch Dermatol 1986, 122:815.

Hedström SP: Treatment and prevention of recurrent staphylococcal furunculosis. Scand J Infect Dis 1985, 17:55.

Huntley AC, et al: Toxic shock syndrome as a complication of dermatologic surgery. JAAD 1987, 16:227.

James WD: *Staphylococcus aureus* and etretinate. Arch Dermatol 1986, 122:976.

Klempner MS, et al: Prevention of recurrent staphylococcal skin infection with low-dose oral clindamycin therapy. JAMA 1988, 260:2682.

Laber H, et al: Mupirocin and the eradication of *Staphylococcus aureus* in atopic dermatitis. Arch Dermatol 1988, 124:853.

Leibowitz MR, et al: Extensive botryomycosis in a patient with diabetes and chronic active hepatitis. Arch Dermatol 1981, 117:739.

Leyden JJ, et al: *Staphylococcus aureus* infection as a complication of isotretinoin therapy. Arch Dermatol 1987, 123:60s.

Maddox JS, et al: Pyomyositis in a neonate. JAAD 1984, 10:391.

Melish ME: The staphylococcal scalded-skin syndrome. N Engl J Med 1970, 282:114.

Patterson JW, et al: Cutaneous botryomycosis in a patient with acquired immunodeficiency syndrome. JAAD 1987, 16:238.

Pitlick S, et al: Cellulitis caused by *Staphylococcus epidermidis* in a patient with leukemia. Arch Dermatol 1984, 120:1099.

Richard M, et al: Staphylococcal scalded skin syndrome in a homosexual adult. JAAD 1986, 15:385.

Rosene KA, et al: Persistent neuropsychological sequelae of toxic shock syndrome. Ann Intern Med 1982, 96:865.

Schutzer SE, et al: Toxic shock syndrome and lysogeny in *Staphylococcus aureus* infection. Science 1983, 220:316.

Sheagren JN: Staphylococcal infections of the skin and skin structure. Cutis 1985, 36(5A):2.

Shelley WB, et al: Anhydrous formulation of aluminum chloride for chronic folliculitis. JAMA 1980, 277:1956.

Steele RW: Recurrent staphylococcal infection in families. Arch Dermatol 1980, 116:189.

Tanner MH, et al: Toxic shock syndrome from *Staphylococcus aureus* infection at insulin pump infusion sites. JAMA 1988, 259:394.

Thomas SW, et al: Toxic shock syndrome following submucous resection and rhinoplasty. JAMA 1982, 247:2402.

Todd JU: Toxic shock syndrome. Ann Intern Med 1982, 96:839.

Tofte RW, et al: Clinical and laboratory manifestations of toxic shock syndrome. Ann Intern Med 1982, 96:843.

Wheat LJ, et al: Prevention of infections of the skin and skin structure. Am J Med 1984, 76(5A):187.

STREPTOCOCCAL SKIN INFECTIONS

IMPETIGO CONTAGIOSA

Impetigo contagiosa is a primarily streptococcic, often later a combined staphylococcic and streptococcic, infection, characterized by discrete thin-walled vesicles which rapidly become pustular and then rupture. Impetigo occurs most frequently on the exposed parts of the body: the face, hands, neck, and extremities. Impetigo on the scalp is a frequent complication of pediculosis capitis.

The disease begins with 2-mm erythematous macules, which may shortly develop into vesicles or bullae. As soon as these lesions rupture, a thin, straw-colored, seropurulent discharge is noticed. The exudate dries to form loosely stratified golden yellow crusts, which accumulate layer upon layer until they are thick and friable.

The crusts can usually be removed readily, leaving a smooth, red, moist surface that soon collects droplets of fresh exudate again; these are spread to other parts of the body by fingers, towels, or household utensils. As the lesions spread peripherally and the skin clears centrally, large circles are formed by fusion of the spreading lesions to produce gyrate patterns that are called **gyrate impetigo**. In streptococcal-induced impetigo, regional lymphadenopathy is common, and not serious.

Group A beta-hemolytic streptococcal skin infections are sometimes followed by acute glomerulonephritis (AGN). Some types of nephritogenic streptococci are associated with **impetigo** rather than with upper respiratory infections. There is no evidence that AGN occurs with staphylococcal bullous impetigo. The important factor predisposing to AGN is the serotype of the streptococcus producing the impetigo. Type 49, 55, 57, and 60 strains and strain M-type 2 are related to **nephritis**.

The incidence of AGN with impetigo varies from about 2 to 5 per cent (10 to 15 per cent with nephritogenic strains of streptococcus) and occurs most frequently in childhood, generally under the age of six. The prognosis in children is mostly excellent; however, in adults the prognosis is not as good. Treatment, however early and however appropriate, is not believed to reduce the risk of occurrence of AGN.

ETIOLOGY. The causative organism is *Streptococcus pyogenes* (Group A beta-hemolytic streptococcus). Later during the course of the disease coagulase-positive *Staphylococcus aureus* may also be found in cultures, probably as a secondary invader. However, recent studies have found a higher incidence of staphylococci than streptococci, and it is possible that some cases are caused initially and solely by this organism. In a study of 497 patients with impetigo, 213 had pure cultures. Dillon found 74 per cent with group A streptococci, 22 per cent with coagulase-positive staphylococci, and 4 per cent with coagulase-negative staphylococci. In mixed cultures Group A streptococci and coagulase-positive staphylococci occurred most frequently. Group B streptococci are associated with newborn impetigo and Groups C and G are rarely isolated from impetigo, as opposed to the usual Group A.

Common sources of infection for children are pets, dirty fingernails, and other children in schools; for adults, barber shops, beauty parlors, Turkish baths, swimming pools, and infected children. The late Stephen Rothman once remarked that anyone who doubts that impetigo is contagious ought to watch it spread in a children's summer camp.

Impetigo often complicates pediculosis capitis, sca-

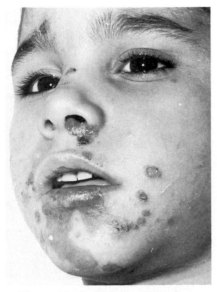

Figure 14–10. Impetigo contagiosa.

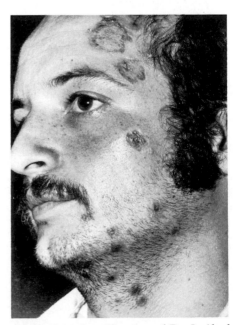

Figure 14–11. Impetigo. (Courtesy of Dr. I. Abrahams.)

bies, herpes simplex, insect bites, poison ivy, eczema, and other exudative, pustular or itching skin diseases.

INCIDENCE AND PREVALENCE. Impetigo occurs most frequently in early childhood, although all ages may be affected. It occurs, in the temperate zone, mostly during the summer months, in hot, humid weather.

HISTOLOGY. The histopathology in this disease is that of an extremely superficial inflammation about the funnel-shaped upper portion of the pilosebaceous follicles. A bulla or vesicopustule is formed, usually subcorneal, containing a few scattered chains of cocci, together with debris of polymorphonuclear leukocytes and epidermal cells. In the corium there is a mild inflammatory reaction—vascular dilatation, edema, and infiltration of polymorphonuclears.

DIFFERENTIAL DIAGNOSIS. Impetigo may simulate several diseases. The circinate patches are frequently mistaken for *ringworm*, but clinically are essentially different, being superficial, very weepy lesions covered by thick, bright yellow or orange crusts with loose edges, which do not resemble the scaling patches with slight peripheral vesiculation seen in tinea circinata.

Impetigo may be mistaken for *Toxicodendron* dermatitis, but it is more crusted and pustular, and more liable to involve the nostrils, the corners of the mouth, and the ears; it does not have associated with it the puffing of the eyelids and the linear lesions, or the itchiness, that are so often present in dermatitis due to poison ivy.

Ringed lesions on the face as in *syphilis* are an uncommon manifestation of either disease. Syphilis lesions are not moist; there are no vesicles, bullae, or cysts. They are dry and occasionally slightly scaly, and the rings are composed of fused papules that feel like a cord under the palpating finger.

In *varicella* the lesions are small, widely distributed, discrete, umbilicated vesicles that are usually also present in the mouth, a site rarely involved by impetigo.

In *ecthyma* the lesions are crusted ulcers, not erosions, and seldom occur anywhere but on the shins.

TREATMENT. Systemic antibiotics combined with topical therapy are advised. Penicillin, 250 mg four times daily (12.5 mg/kg/day divided into four daily doses for children), is effective if *Streptococcus* is known to be the cause; but in view of the recent apparent increase in cases caused by *Staphylococcus*, erythromycin in the same oral dose or cloxacillin or a cephalosporin is recommended. All treatment should be given for 7 to 10 days. It may be necessary to soak off the crusts once or twice a day, after which bacitracin or Polysporin ointment should be applied. Mupirocin ointment (Bactroban) has recently been shown to be as effective as oral antibiotics.

Maddox et al studied the effect of applying antibiotic ointment as a prophylactic to sites of skin trauma to prevent impetigo in a group of children at a rural day care center. Streptococci were frequently cultured from normal skin throughout the study and were regularly available to infect a traumatized site. Infections were reduced by 47 per cent with antibiotic ointment as compared with 15 per cent with a placebo.

ECTHYMA

Ecthyma is an ulcerative streptococcal pyoderma, nearly always of the shins or dorsal feet, caused by beta-hemolytic streptococci. The disease begins with a vesicle or vesicopustule, which enlarges and in a few days becomes thickly crusted. When the crust is removed there is a superficial saucer-shaped ulcer with a raw base and elevated edges.

The lesions tend to heal after a few weeks, leaving scars, but rarely may proceed to gangrene when the resistance is low. In fact, a debilitated condition and a focus of pyogenic infection precede the onset of ecthyma in many cases. Local adenopathy may be present. Uncleanliness, malnutrition, and trauma are predisposing causes.

Histologically, this dermatitis presents the picture of deep inflammation due to pyogenic cocci, associated with a pronounced polymorphonuclear infiltration, and abscesses, which begin around the pilosebaceous follicles as in impetigo but much more deeply.

Treatment is cleansing with soap and water, followed by the application of mupirocin ointment, twice daily. Penicillin, cloxacillin, or erythromycin *must* be given orally or parenterally.

SCARLET FEVER

Scarlet fever is a diffuse erythematous exanthem which occurs during the course of streptococcal phar-

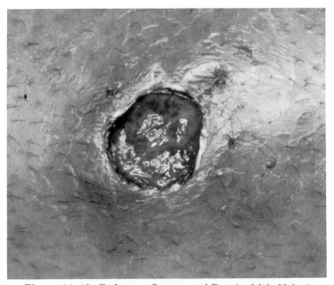

Figure 14–12. Ecthyma. Courtesy of Dr. Axel W. Hoke.)

yngitis. It affects primarily children, who develop the eruption 24 to 48 hours after the onset of pharyngeal symptoms. The tonsils are red, edematous, and covered with exudate. The tongue has a white coating through which reddened, hypertrophied papillae project, giving the so-called "white strawberry tongue" appearance. By the fourth or fifth day the coating disappears, the tongue is bright red, and the "red strawberry tongue" remains.

The cutaneous eruption begins on the neck, spreads to the trunk and finally the extremities. Within the widespread erythema are 1–2-mm papules, which give the skin a rough "sandpaper" quality. There is accentuation over the skin folds, and a linear petechial eruption, "Pastia's lines," is often present in the antecubital and axillary folds. There is facial flushing and circumoral pallor. A branny desquamation occurs as the eruption fades, with peeling of the palms and soles taking place about two weeks after the acute illness. The latter may be the only evidence that the disease has occurred, in subtropical climates.

The eruption is produced by erythemogenic toxin from group A streptococci. Cultures of the pharynx, or rarely a surgical wound or burn, will recover this organism. An elevated antistreptolysin O titer may provide evidence of recent infection if cultures are not taken early.

Penicillin, erythromycin, or cloxacillin treatment is curative, and the prognosis is excellent. A streptococcal vaccine is being developed, with Phase I trials soon to begin.

ERYSIPELAS

Also once known as St. Anthony's fire and *ignis sacer*, erysipelas is an acute beta-hemolytic group A streptococcic cellulitis of the skin involving the superficial dermal lymphatics. Occasional cases caused by streptococci of Group C or G are reported in adults, and Group B streptococcus may be the organism most often responsible in the newborn. It is characterized by local redness, heat, swelling, and a highly characteristic raised, indurated border. The onset is often preceded by prodromal symptoms of malaise for several hours, which may be accompanied by a severe constitutional reaction with chills, high fever, headache, vomiting, and joint pains. There is commonly a polymorphonuclear leukocytosis of 20,000 or more.

The skin lesions may vary from transient hyperemia followed by slight desquamation to intense inflammation with vesiculation and phlegmon. The eruption begins at any one point as an erythematous patch and spreads by peripheral extension. In the early stages the affected skin is scarlet, hot to the touch, brawny, and swollen. A distinctive feature of the inflammation is the advancing edge of the patch. This is raised, and sharply demarcated, and feels like a wall to the palpating finger.

In some cases the affected skin is the site of vesicles or bullae that contain seropurulent fluid and may result in local gangrene.

The face is the most frequent site affected. The inflammation generally begins on the cheek near the

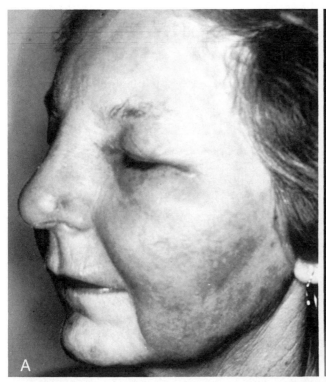
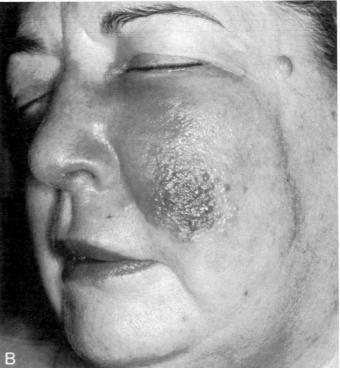

Figure 14–13. A and B, Erysipelas.

nose or in front of the lobe of the ear and spreads upward to the scalp, the hairline acting in some instances as a barrier against further extension. In severe cases the head, particularly the ears, may be tremendously swollen and distorted, and there may be associated delirium.

In severe cases, septicemia or deep cellulitis may occur as complications. These are more common in the newborn and following operations on the elderly.

Predisposing causes are operative wounds, or fissures in the nares, in the auditory meatus, under the lobes of the ears, on the anus or penis, and between or under the toes, usually the little toe. Any inflammation of the skin, especially if fissured or ulcerative, may provide an entrance for the causative streptococcus. Slight abrasions or scratches, accidental scalp wounds, unclean tying of the umbilical cord, vaccination, and chronic leg ulcers may lead to the disease.

The features of this disease microscopically are an intense edema, vascular dilatation, and a moderate collection of polymorphonuclear cells, lymphocytes, and streptococci in the enlarged lymphatic spaces about the vessels. The endothelial cells lining the lymphatic vessels are swollen. At times the edema is so intense that subepidermal collections of fluid form bullae.

Recognition of the disease is generally not difficult. It may be confused with dermatitis venenata from plants, drugs, or dyes, and with angioneurotic edema, in each of which, however, fever, pain, and tenderness are absent and itching is severe. In scarlet fever, there is a widespread punctate erythema, never localized and edematous as in erysipelas. A butterfly pattern on the face may mimic lupus erythematosus, and ear involvement may suggest relapsing polychondritis. Acute tuberculoid leprosy of the face may look exactly like erysipelas, but the absence of fever, pain, or leukocytosis is distinctive.

Oral, intramuscular, or intravenous penicillin is rapidly effective. Improvement in the general condition occurs in 24 to 48 hours, but resolution of the cutaneous lesion may require several days. Vigorous treatment with antibiotics should be continued for at least 10 days. Erythromycin is also efficacious. Locally, ice bags, cold compresses, and antibiotic ointments may be used.

CELLULITIS

Cellulitis is a suppurative inflammation involving particularly the subcutaneous tissue, caused most frequently by *Streptococcus pyogenes*. Usually, but not always, this follows some discernible wound. Mild local erythema and tenderness, malaise, and chilly sensations, or a sudden chill and fever may be present at the onset. The erythema rapidly becomes intense and spreads. The area becomes infiltrated and pits on pressure. Sometimes the central part becomes nodular and surmounted by a vesicle that ruptures and discharges pus and necrotic material. Streaks of lymphangitis may spread from the area to the neighboring lymph glands. Gangrene, metastatic abscesses, and grave sepsis may follow. These complications are unusual in immunocompetent adults; but children and compromised adults are at higher risk.

Spear et al reported—and many subsequent reports have confirmed it—14 children with perianal streptococcal cellulitis, which had led to painful defecation, anorectal bleeding, and tender erythema. One of us (WDJ) has seen two patients with similar perianal lesions caused by *Staphylococcus aureus*. Hurwitz et al reported streptococcal cellulitis occurring at the donor site in a patient who had undergone a coronary artery bypass graft.

Hook et al evaluated 50 patients with cellulitis

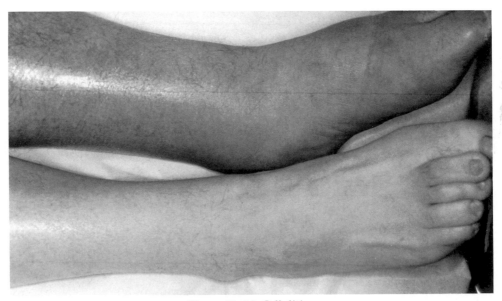

Figure 14–14. Cellulitis.

prospectively by culture of the primary site of infection (when one was present), and also by aspiration of the advancing edge, by skin biopsy, and by blood culture. In 24 the primary site was identified and in 17 beta-hemolytic streptococci were isolated, with *S. aureus* being present in 13. Other cultures were seldom positive and yielded no additional information. Bernard et al have used antigen detection by latex agglutination to identify the responsible organism.

Treatment, if *S. pyogenes* is isolated, is with penicillin or cefazolin or vancomycin. Arnold has found an intralesional injection of triamcinolone acetonide 1:10, without antibiotic "coverage," safe and effective treatment for early lesions.

CHRONIC RECURRENT ERYSIPELAS CHRONIC LYMPHANGITIS

Erysipelas (v.s.) is notorious for its tendency to recur. Recurrence may manifest itself within a few hours after apparently complete dissipation of the local signs and subsidence of fever, or it may come on a few days later, or after months or years. Recurrences may occur at certain times of the year.

Recurrence of erysipelas may cause local persistent lymphedema. This type of chronic lymphedema is the end result of recurrent bouts of bacterial lymphangitis and obstruction of the major lymphatic channels of the skin and the venous channels. The final result is a permanent hypertrophic fibrosis to which the term **elephantiasis nostras** has been given.

The recurrent bouts of erysipelas and lymphangitis produce chronic lymphedema, which must be differentiated from lymphangioma and chronic lymphedema caused by noninflammatory and noninfectious factors. These include neoplasms, syphilis, filariasis, and tuberculous lymphangitis.

During periods of active lymphangitis, antibiotics in large doses are beneficial and their use must be continued intermittently in smaller maintenance doses for long periods to get their full benefits. One such regimen is to give erythromycin, cloxacillin, or penicillin for one week in every four. Plastic surgery is recommended for persistent solid edema that does not respond to the above measures. Corticosteroid treatment is also sometimes beneficial.

Lymphangitis Dorsalis Penis. Nonvenereal sclerosing lymphangitis of the penis is a cordlike, cartilaginous, circumscribed hardness caused by fibrous thickening of a large lymph vessel. It may have a sudden onset and produce a wormlike, curved, firm, translucent lesion that almost encircles the penis. The condition is symptomless, and may be due to mechanical trauma. It resolves spontaneously in a week or so.

NECROTIZING FASCIITIS

Necrotizing fasciitis is an acute necrotizing process that involves the fascia of the skin and follows surgery or perforating trauma. Within 24 to 48 hours, redness, pain, and edema quickly progress to central patches of dusky blue discoloration, with or without serosanguineous blisters. By the fourth or fifth day, these purple areas become gangrenous. Many forms of virulent bacteria have been cultured from necrotizing fasciitis, including beta-hemolytic streptococci, hemolytic staphylococcus, coliforms, enterococci, *Pseudomonas,* and *Bacteroides.* Treatment should include early surgical debridement, intravenously administered antibiotics (penicillin, semisynthetic penicillin, gram-negative spectrum antibiotics), and supportive care. There may be a 20 per cent mortality even in the best of circumstances. Poor prognostic factors are age over 50, underlying diabetes, or atherosclerosis; delay of over seven days in diagnosis and surgical intervention, and infection on or near the trunk rather than the more commonly involved extremities.

BLISTERING DISTAL DACTYLITIS

Blistering distal dactylitis is characterized by tense superficial blisters on a tender erythematous base over the volar fat pad of the phalanx of a finger or thumb. The typical patient is between the ages of two and 16. It has been reported only in adults. A Group A beta-hemolytic streptococcus is the cause. It may be cultured from blister fluid and occasionally from clinically inapparent infections of the nasopharynx or conjunctiva. Benson et al reported this clinical entity in an adult diabetic, from whom a group B streptococcus was recovered. Oral penicillin or erythromycin, 250 mg four times daily for 10 days, is curative.

GROUP B STREPTOCOCCAL INFECTION

Streptococcus agalactiae is the major cause of bacterial sepsis and meningitis in neonates. It may cause orbital cellulitis or facial erysipelas in these patients. Up to 25 per cent of healthy adults harbor group B streptococcus in the genital or gastrointestinal tract. It has been reported by James and by Brook to cause

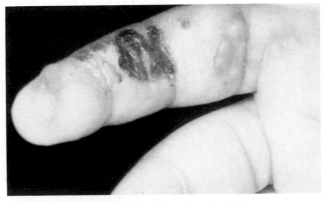

Figure 14–15. Blistering dactylitis.

balanitis. It may also cause cellulitis, recurrent erysipelas, or blistering dactylitis in adults, but nearly all adults with these manifestations have diabetes mellitus and peripheral vascular disease as predisposing factors.

Baker CJ, et al: Immunization of pregnant women with a polysaccharide vaccine of Group B streptococcus. N Engl J Med 1988, 319:1180.

Barton LL, et al: Impetigo. Pediatr Dermatol 1987, 4:185.

Benson PM, et al: Group B streptococcal blistering distal dactylitis in an adult diabetic. (In press)

Bernard P, et al: Early detection of streptococcal group antigens in skin samples by latex particle agglutination. Arch Dermatol 1987, 123:468.

Binnick AN, et al: Recurrent erysipelas caused by group B streptococcus organism. Arch Dermatol 1980, 116:798.

Brook I: Balanitis caused by group B B-hemolytic streptococci. Sex Transm Dis 1980, 7:195.

Coskey RJ, et al: Diagnosis and treatment of impetigo. JAAD 1987, 17:62.

Cupps TR, et al: Facial erysipelas in the immunocompromised host. Arch Dermatol 1981, 117:47.

Hanger SB: Facial cellulitis. Pediatrics 1981, 67:376.

Ho PWL, et al: Value of cultures in patients with acute cellulitis. South Med J 1979, 72:1402.

Hook EW, et al: Microbiologic evaluation of cutaneous cellulitis in adults. Arch Intern Med 1986, 146:295.

Hook EW III: Acute cellulitis. Arch Dermatol 1987, 123:460.

Horn RT, et al: Circular indurated lymphangitis of the penis. J Assoc Milit Dermatol 1980, 6:10.

Howard JB, et al: The spectrum of group B streptococcal infections in infancy. Am J Dis Child 1974, 128:815.

Hurwitz RM, et al: Streptococcal cellulitis proved by skin biopsy in a coronary artery bypass graft patient. Arch Dermatol 1985, 121:908.

James WD: Cutaneous group B streptococcal infection. Arch Dermatol 1984, 120:85.

Kohen GG: Necrotizing fasciitis. Arch Dermatol 1978, 114:581.

Kokx NP, et al: Streptococcal perianal disease in children. Pediatr 1987, 80:659.

Kranz DR, et al: Necrotizing fasciitis associated with porphyria cutanea tarda. JAAD 1986, 14:361.

Marks VJ, et al: Perianal streptococcal cellulitis. JAAD 1988, 18:587.

McCray MU, et al: Blistering distal dactylitis. JAAD 1981, 5:592.

Raymond CA: Group A streptococcus vaccine . . . JAMA 1988, 260:2778.

Rehder PA, et al: Perianal cellulitis. Arch Dermatol 1988, 124:702.

Rhyne L, et al: Necrotizing fasciitis. South Med J 1981, 74:1043.

Schachner L, et al: A therapeutic update of superficial skin infections. Pediatr Clin North Am 1983, 30:397.

Schneider JA, et al: Blistering distal dactylitis. Arch Dermatol 1982, 118:879.

Shama S, et al: Atypical erysipelas caused by group B streptococci in a patient with cured Hodgkins' disease. Arch Dermatol 1982, 118:934.

Spear RM, et al: Perianal streptococcal cellulitis. J Pediatr 1985, 107:557.

MISCELLANEOUS GRAM-POSITIVE SKIN INFECTIONS

ERYSIPELOID OF ROSENBACH

CUTANEOUS MANIFESTATIONS. The most frequent form of erysipeloid in man is usually manifested by a purplish, more or less marginated swelling on the hands, as originally described by Rosenbach. The first symptom is pain at the site of inoculation; this is followed by swelling and erythema. The most distinctive feature is the sharply marginated and often polygonal patches of bluish erythema. The erythema slowly spreads to produce a sharply defined, slightly elevated zone that extends peripherally as the central portion fades away. If the finger is involved the swelling and tenseness make movement difficult. Vesicles frequently occur.

Another characteristic of the disease is its migratory nature; new purplish-red patches appear at nearby areas. If the infection originally involved one finger, eventually all of the fingers and the dorsum of the hand, the palm, or both may become affected, the erythema appearing and disappearing; or extension may take place by continuity. The disease involutes without desquamation or suppuration.

A diffuse or generalized eruption in regions remote from the site of inoculation may occur, with fever and arthritic symptoms. Rarely, septicemia may eventuate in endocarditis, with prolonged fever and constitutional symptoms.

ETIOLOGY. The infection is caused by *Erysipelothrix insidiosa (rhusiopathiae)*.

INCIDENCE AND PREVALENCE. *E. insidiosa* is present on dead matter of animal origin. Swine are more frequently infected than any other animal. A large percentage of healthy swine are carriers of the organism. Turkeys are also often infected and the disease may arise from handling contaminated dressed turkeys.

The disease is widespread along the entire Atlantic seacoast among commercial fisherman who handle

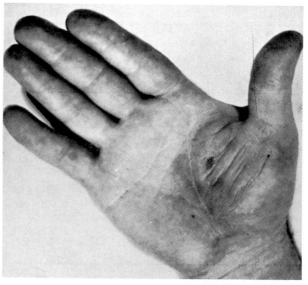

Figure 14–16. Erysipeloid.

live fish, crabs, and shellfish. The infection also occurs among veterinarians, and in the meat-packing industry, principally from handling pork products.

DIAGNOSIS. *Erysipelothrix insidiosa* is a rod-shaped, nonmotile, gram-positive organism which tends to form long branching filaments. The organism is cultured best on media fortified with serum, at room temperature.

TREATMENT. The majority of the mild cases of erysipeloid run a self-limited course of about three weeks. In some patients, after a short period of apparent cure, the eruption reappears either at the same area or, more likely, at an adjacent previously uninvolved area. Penicillin orally or intramuscularly is the best treatment, 2 million to 3 million units daily for seven to 10 days being required. If penicillin cannot be used, erythromycin, 250 mg every six hours for seven to 10 days, is effective.

Barnett JH: Erysipeloid. JAAD 1983, 9:116.

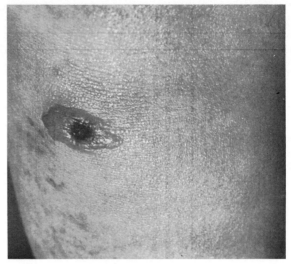

Figure 14–17. Anthrax on thigh. (Courtesy of Dr. A. Johnson, Australia.)

PNEUMOCOCCAL CELLULITIS

Reports have documented cases of periorbital cellulitis with fever in infants, caused by *Streptococcus pneumoniae*. These children presented with violaceous discoloration of the skin identical to that in cellulitis of *Haemophilus influenzae*. These reports emphasize the importance of obtaining cultures of the blood and soft tissue aspirate.

Rusonis PA, et al: Livedo reticularis and purpura. JAAD 1986, 15:1120.
Thiramoorthi MC, et al: Violaceous discoloration in pneumococcal cellulitis. Pediatrics 1978, 62:492.

ANTHRAX

Anthrax is an acute infectious disease characterized by a rapidly necrosing painless carbuncle with suppurative regional adenitis.

CLINICAL FEATURES. Three forms of anthrax occur in humans: *cutaneous*, accounting for 95 per cent of cases worldwide but nearly all U.S. cases; *inhalation*, known as *woolsorter's disease* (only twice reported in the U.S. in the past 20 years); and *gastrointestinal*, not yet reported in the U.S. The first clinical manifestation is an inflammatory papule, which begins a few hours or days after infection. The inflammation develops rapidly so that there is a bulla surrounded by intense edema and infiltration. Within a short time it ruptures spontaneously, the contents being purulent or sanguineous. A dark brown eschar is then visible surrounded by vesicles and pustules situated upon a red, hot, swollen, and indurated area. The regional lymph glands become enlarged and frequently suppurate.

In severe cases the inflammatory signs increase, there is extensive edematous swelling, other bullae and necrotic lesions develop, accompanied by a high temperature and prostration, terminating in death in a few days or weeks. This may occur in up to 20 per cent of untreated cases. In mild cases the constitutional symptoms are sometimes slight; the gangrenous skin sloughs, and the resulting ulcer heals. The lesion is neither tender nor painful. This is of diagnostic importance.

Internally, *inhalation anthrax* is manifested as a necrotizing hemorrhagic mediastinal infection. Anthrax spores involve the alveoli, then the hilar and tracheobronchial nodes. Bacteremia followed by hemorrhagic meningitis is the usual sequence of events, almost always ending in death. *Gastrointestinal anthrax* results when spores are ingested and multiply in the intestinal submucosa. A necrotic ulcerative lesion in the terminal ileum or cecum may lead to hemorrhage.

ETIOLOGY. The disease is produced by *Bacillus anthracis*, a large, square-ended, rod-shaped, gram-positive organism, which occurs singly or in pairs in smears from the blood or in material from the local lesion, or in long chains on artificial media, where it tends to form spores.

Human infection generally results from infected animals or the handling of hides or other animal products from stock that has died from splenic fever. Cattlemen, woolsorters, tanners, butchers, and workers in the goat-hair industry are most liable to infection. Human-to-human transmission has occurred from contact with dressings from lesions. One exotic case was that of a piano key maker who contracted anthrax from elephant tusks imported from Africa.

HISTOLOGY. There is loss of the epidermis at the

site of the ulcer, with surrounding spongiosis and intraepidermal vesicles. Leukocytes are abundant in the epidermis. The dermis is edematous and is infiltrated with abundant erythrocytes and neutrophils. Vasodilatation is marked. The causative organisms are numerous and are easily seen, especially with Gram's stain.

DIAGNOSIS. The diagnosis is made by the demonstration of the causative agent in smears and cultures of the local material. Since aerobic nonpathogenic bacilli may be confused with *B. anthracis*, a specific gamma bacteriophage may be used to identify the organism. All virulent strains are pathogenic to mice. A fourfold rise in the indirect hemagglutination titer in paired serum specimens confirms the diagnosis. The characteristic gangrenous lesion, surrounded by vesiculation, intense swelling and redness, lack of pain, and the occupation of the victim are accessory factors. Staphylococcal carbuncle is the most easily confused entity but here tenderness is prominent.

Early diagnosis and prompt treatment with penicillin G, 2 million units intravenously every six hours for four to six days, followed by a seven- to 10-day course of oral penicillin, is curative in the cutaneous form. Tetracycline is the preferred alternative in penicillin-allergic patients.

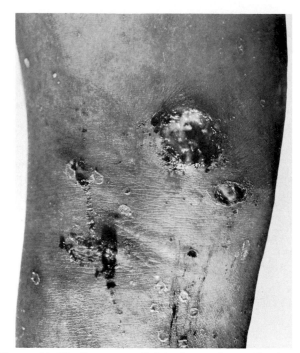

Figure 14–18. Cutaneous diphtheria on the popliteal space. (*Courtesy of Armed Forces Institute of Pathology.*)

Human cutaneous anthrax. Arch Dermatol 1988, 124:1324.
Tezer Kutluk M, et al: Cutaneous anthrax. Cutis 1987, 40:117.

Belsey MA, et al: *Corynebacterium diphtheriae* skin infections in Alabama and Louisiana. N Engl J Med 1969, 280:135.
Cameron JDS, et al: Cutaneous diphtheria in northern Palestine. Lancet 1942, 2:720.
Girdami M, et al: Tropicaloid ulcer. Dermatol Trop 1962, 1:75.
Karzon DT, et al: Diphtheria outbreaks in immunized populations. N Engl J Med 1988, 318:41.

CUTANEOUS DIPHTHERIA

The skin may become infected by the Klebs-Loeffler bacillus, *Corynebacterium diphtheriae*, in the form of ulcerations. The ulcer is punched-out and has hard, rolled, elevated edges with a pale blue tinge. Often the lesion is covered with a leathery grayish membrane. Regional lymph nodes may be affected.

Another type of skin involvement is that occurring in eczematous, impetiginous, vesicular, or pustular scratches, from which the *C. diphtheriae* may be recovered. Postdiphtherial paralysis not infrequently occurs.

Cutaneous diphtheria is common in tropical areas. Most of the cases occurring in the United States are in unimmunized migrant farm worker families and in elderly alcoholics.

Treatment consists of intramuscular injections of diphtheria antitoxin, 20,000 to 100,000 units, after skin tests have been performed to rule out hypersensivity to horse serum. An intracutaneous injection of 0.05 ml of a 1:20 dilution is made. If after 30 minutes there is no reaction the antitoxin is given. Penicillin is also given daily for 10 days to terminate the respiratory-tract–carrier state. Erythromycin is substituted for those who might be sensitive to penicillin.

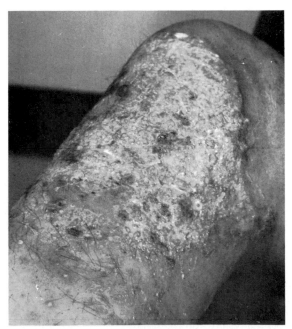

Figure 14–19. Cutaneous diphtheria on knee. (*Courtesy of Dr. F. Reiss.*)

CORYNEBACTERIUM GROUP JK SEPSIS

Jerdan et al in 1987 reported a case of *Corynebacterium* Group JK sepsis occurring in an immunosuppressed teenage boy. There was an extensive papular eruption, with effacement of eccrine glands by numerous pleomorphic bacilli, morphologically consistent with *Corynebacterium*, on biopsy.

Ticarcillin, nafcillin, and gentamicin (later changed to tobramycin) were ineffective; so was a combination of tobramycin, clindamycin, and trimethoprim-sulfamethoxazole. On the day the eruption appeared, vancomycin was begun, and from the fourth day on, no new lesions appeared. Vancomycin is the antibiotic of choice in this disease.

Jerdan MS, et al: Cutaneous manifestations of *Corynebacterium* Group JK sepsis. JAAD 1987, 16:444.

DESERT SORE

Also known as *veldt sore, septic sore, diphtheric desert sore,* and *Barcoo rot,* desert sore is an ulcerative disease that is endemic among bushmen and soldiers in Australia and Burma. The disease is characterized by the occurrence of grouped vesicles on the extremities, chiefly on the shins, knees, and backs of the hands. These rupture and form superficial indolent ulcers.

The ulcers enlarge and may attain a diameter of 2 cm. The floor of the ulcer may be covered by a diphtheritic membrane.

The original lesions may start as insect bites. Cultures show staphylococci, streptococci, and *Corynebacterium diphtheriae.*

Treatment of the desert sore is with diphtheria antitoxin if *C. diphtheriae* is present. Antibiotic ointments are used topically, and oral penicillin or erythromycin is the treatment of choice.

Bailey H: Ulcers of the leg and their differential diagnosis. Dermatol Trop 1962, 1:45.

TROPICAL ULCER

Synonyms: Tropical phagedena, Aden ulcer, Malabar ulcer, "jungle rot," also various native terms.
CLINICAL FEATURES. The disease occurs on exposed parts of the body, chiefly the legs and arms, frequently on preexisting abrasions or sores, sometimes beginning from a mere scratch. As a rule, only one extremity is affected and usually there is a single lesion, although it is not uncommon to find multiple ulcers upon both legs. Satellite lesions ordinarily occur as a result of autoinoculation.

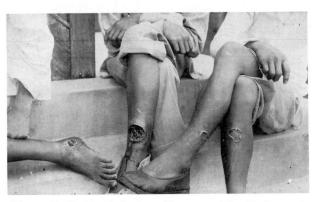
Figure 14–20. Tropical ulcer. (Courtesy of Dr. T. Corpus.)

The lesions begin with inflammatory papules that progress into vesicles and rupture with the formation of an ulcer. The ulcers vary in diameter and may, through coalescence, form extensive lesions. The lesions of some varieties are elevated or deeply depressed and generally the edges are undermined and either smooth or ragged.

At times the ulcers are covered by thick, dirty crusts or by whitish pseudomembranes. The edges are flat, without thickening, and around them there is a zone of inflammation characterized by redness, swelling, and some tenderness. Other than a slight itching, there is usually no distress.

The disease is most common in native laborers and in schoolchildren during the rainy season; it is probably caused in many instances by the bites of insects, filth, and pyogenic infection.

ETIOLOGY. Under the term "tropical ulcer" a variety of skin conditions have been described. Many of these have been due to syphilis or yaws or to the infection of abrasions by pyogenic organisms. Vincent has demonstrated the *Bacteroides fusiformis,* a fusiform bacillus, and *Borrelia vincenti,* the spirillum better known in connection with Vincent's angina, in smears from tropical ulcers, and in other lesions spirochetes of various forms have been found. Adriaans et al reviewed the infectious etiology with special reference to the role of anaerobic bacteria, especially fusobacteria and spirochetes, in 1987. They found anaerobic bacteria together with aerobes, some of them facultative anaerobes, were always present, especially in early lesions, suggesting that they were important in the pathogenesis of the lesions. Malnutrition appears to be a predisposing factor.

DIFFERENTIAL DIAGNOSIS. Since the concept of tropical ulcer is tenuous at best, various ulcers of known etiologies must be kept in mind. Some of these are the following:

The *septic desert ulcer* is superficial and shows *C. diphtheriae.*

The *gummatous ulcer* is punched out, with a sinking floor. Other signs of syphilis are present and the serologic test for syphilis is positive.

The *tuberculous ulcer* is undermined and usually not found on the leg. The mycobacterium can be isolated from the lesion.

The *mycotic ulcer* is nodulo-ulcerative, with demonstrable fungi both by direct microscopic examination and by culture.

The *frambesia ulcer* grows rapidly and yields *Treponema pertenue*.

The *Buruli ulcer* shows abundant *Mycobacterium ulcerans* in biopsies.

The *leishmania ulcer* contains *Leishmania tropica*; it is rarely found on the leg.

Carcinoma must be considered in any leg ulcer of long duration. A prompt biopsy is indicated.

The *arteriosclerotic ulcer* is seen in older people at sites of frequent trauma; it is deep and penetrates through the deep fascia to expose tendons.

The *hypertensive ischemic ulcer* is caused by thrombosis of the cutaneous arterioles. These painful ulcers are extremely shallow and usually bilateral and are seen most frequently on the mid and lower parts of the leg. Varicosities are usually absent.

The *varicose* or *venous ulcer* is shallow and has irregularly shaped edges. It is located typically on the lower half of the shins, mostly above and anterior to the medial malleolus along the course of the long saphenous vein.

The *ulcers of blood dyscrasias* are frequent in sickle-cell anemia, in hereditary spherocytosis, Mediterranean anemia, and Felty's syndrome. The diagnosis is aided by the fact that there is hypersplenism in each of these diseases.

The *ulcer of rheumatoid arthritis* occurs frequently in patients who have abundant concomitant subcutaneous nodules.

The *ulcer of Kaposi's sarcoma* frequently occurs on the lower extremities and is accompanied by a purpuric discoloration of the skin over the arches and by other violaceous nodules that may occur anywhere on the body. In the tropics it is endemic among the South African Bantus.

TREATMENT. Prevention of the disease is aided by protection from insect bites and from predisposing causes, such as debility, malnutrition, and filth. Topical and systemic antibiotic treatment is indicated in most patients.

Adriaans B, et al: The infectious aetiology of tropical ulcer—a study of the role of anaerobic bacteria. Br J Dermatol 1986, 116:31.

ERYTHRASMA

Erythrasma is characterized by sharply delineated, dry, brown, slightly scaling patches occurring in the intertriginous areas, especially the axillae, the genitocrural crease, and the webs between the fourth and fifth toes and, less commonly, between the third and fourth toes. There may also be patches in the intergluteal cleft and in the inframammary area. Rarely, widespread eruptions with lamellated plaques occur. As Negroni has shown, even the nails may be involved.

The lesions are asymptomatic except in the groins, where there may be some itching and burning. Patients with extensive erythrasma have been found to have diabetes mellitus or other debilitating diseases.

Erythrasma is caused by the diphtheroid, *Corynebacterium minutissimum*. Montes's electron-microscopic studies have confirmed *Corynebacterium* as the

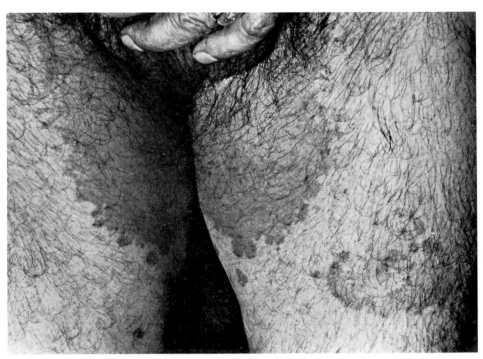

Figure 14–21. Erythrasma. (Courtesy of Dr. E. Florian, Budapest.)

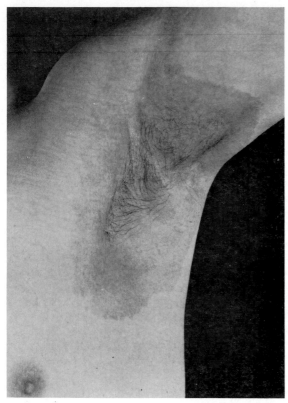

Figure 14–22. Erythrasma. (Courtesy of Dr. H. Shatin.)

causative organism of erythrasma. Two other diseases caused by a Corynebacterium, *pitted keratolysis* and *trichomycosis axillaris*, were reported to occur as a triad in two patients reported by Shelley et al.

The Wood's light is the diagnostic medium for erythrasma. The affected areas show a coral red fluorescence, which results from the presence of a porphyrin.

In the differential diagnosis, tinea cruris due to fungi, intertrigo, seborrheic dermatitis, inverse psoriasis, candidiasis, and lichen simplex chronicus must be considered. The Wood's light readily distinguishes erythrasma from the other diseases.

Treatment of choice is erythromycin, 250 mg four times daily for one week. Ayres and Mihan reported good results with tolnaftate solution applied twice daily for two to three weeks, and topical miconazole is equally effective. Topical erythromycin solution or topical clindamycin is easily applied and rapidly effective.

Montes LF, et al: Erythrasma and diabetes mellitus. Arch Dermatol 1969, 99:674.

Sarkany I, et al: Erythrasma. JAMA 1961, 117:130.

Shelley WB, et al: Coexistent erythrasma, trichomycosis axillaris, and pitted keratolysis. JAAD 1982, 7:752.

Sindhuphak W, et al: Erythrasma. Int J Dermatol 1985, 24:95.

Svejgaard E, et al: Tinea pedis and erythrasma in Danish recruits. JAAD 1986, 14:993.

INTERTRIGO

Intertrigo is a superficial inflammatory dermatitis occurring where two skin surfaces are in apposition. It is discussed here because of its clinical association with several diseases in this chapter.

As a result of friction (skin rubbing skin), heat, and moisture, the affected fold becomes erythematous, macerated, and secondarily infected. There may be erosions, fissures, and exudation, with symptoms of burning and itching.

Intertrigo is most frequently seen during hot and humid weather, chiefly in the obese. This type of dermatitis may involve the retroauricular areas, the folds of the upper eyelids, the creases of the neck, axillae, antecubital areas, fingerwebs, inframammary area, umbilicus; inguinal, perineal, and intergluteal areas; popliteal spaces; and toewebs.

As a result of the maceration, a secondary infection by bacteria (or fungi) is induced. The inframammary area in obese women is most frequently the site of intertriginous candidiasis. The groins are also frequently affected by fungal (yeast or dermatophyte) infection.

Bacterial infection may be caused by streptococci, staphylococci, pseudomonas, or corynebacteria.

In the differential diagnosis, seborrheic dermatitis typically involves the skinfolds. Intertriginous psoriasis and erythrasma are frequently overlooked, especially when the inguinal and the intergluteal areas or fourth toewebs are involved, as in erythrasma.

Treatment is directed toward the elimination of the maceration. Appropriate antibiotics or fungicides are applied locally. The apposing skin surfaces may be separated with gauze or other appropriate dressings. Benzoyl peroxide, 5 per cent cream, may be rapidly effective in such lesions, if tolerated. It may possibly sensitize, however, so beware of prolonged use. Castellani paint is also useful, as is Polysporin ointment.

PITTED KERATOLYSIS

This bacterial infection of the plantar stratum corneum was first named **keratoma plantare sulcatum** by Castellani in 1910, but was given its present name, **pitted keratolysis**, by Taplin and Zaias in 1967. The thick weight-bearing portions of the soles become gradually covered with shallow asymptomatic discrete round pits 1 to 3 mm in diameter, some of which become confluent, forming furrows. Men with very sweaty feet, during hot, humid weather, are most susceptible. Rarely, palmar lesions may occur. No discomfort is produced, though the lesions are often malodorous.

The causative infection is thought to be either a corynebacterium species or *Dermatophilus congolensis*. Recently Nordstrom et al have presented convincing evidence that its cause is *Micrococcus sedentarius*.

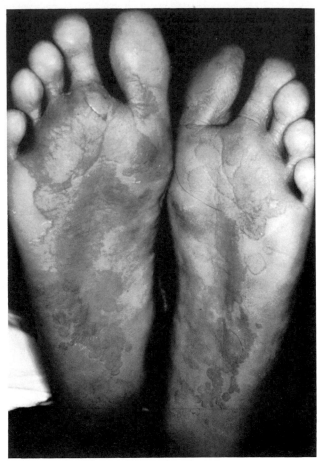

Figure 14–23. Pitted keratolysis.

However, clinical diagnosis is not difficult, based on its unique appearance.

Treatment by painting with 5 per cent formalin or 2 per cent buffered glutaraldehyde is rapidly effective and a 10 to 20 per cent solution of aluminum chloride may be curative. Also topical antibiotics such as erythromycin or clindamycin are curative. Miconazole or clotrimazole cream and Whitfeld's ointment are effective alternatives. Ely found 5 per cent benzoyl peroxide gel highly effective.

Gordon HH: Pitted keratolysis, forme fruste. Cutis 1975, 15:54.
Woodsyer AJ, et al: Isolation of *Dermatophilus congolensis* from two New Zealand cases of pitted keratolysis. Aust J Dermatol 1985, 26:29.
Zaias N: Pitted and ringed keratolysis. JAAD 1982, 7:787.

CLOSTRIDIAL INFECTIONS AND GANGRENE OF THE SKIN (Dermatitis Gangrenosa)

Gangrene of the skin results from loss of the blood supply of a particular area and, in some instances, from secondary bacterial invasion to promote necrosis and sloughing of the skin. Numerous causes are found for gangrene and the various forms of gangrene will be briefly mentioned here.

Gas Gangrene (Clostridial Myonecrosis). Gas gangrene is the severest form of infectious gangrene; it develops in deep lacerated wounds of muscle tissue. The onset is usually sudden, with an incubation period of only a few hours. The onset is accompanied by a chill, a rise in temperature, marked prostration, and severe local pain. Gas bubbles (chiefly hydrogen) produced by the infection cause crepitation when the area is palpated. A "mousy" odor is characteristic. Gas gangrene is caused by a variety of species of the genus Clostridium, most frequently *C. perfringens, C. oedematiens, C. septicum,* and *C. haemolyticum.* These are thick gram-positive rods.

A subacute variety occurs, which is due to an anaerobic streptococcus (peptostreptococcus). This nonclostridial myositis may be clinically similar, but with delayed onset (several days). The purulent exudate has a foul odor and gram-positive cocci in chains are present. It is important to distinguish these two entities, since involved muscle may recover in nonclostridial myositis, and debridement may safely be limited to removal of grossly necrotic muscle. Infections with Clostridia or anaerobic bacteria may also cause crepitant cellulitis, when the infection is limited to the subcutaneous tissue. Treatment of all clostridial infections is wide surgical debridement and intensive antibiotic therapy with intravenous penicillin G. Hyperbaric oxygen therapy may be of value if immediately available.

Hemolytic Streptococcus Gangrene (Necrotizing Fasciitis). This is a rapidly developing acute infection of the skin characterized by its rapid fulminant course, profound prostration, rapid appearance of bullae, and the absence of both lymphangitis and lymphadenitis. The infection starts from an abrasion, furuncle, or injury. Intense local heat, redness, swelling, fever, extreme apathy, and weakness occur. On the second, third, or fourth day the pathognomonic sign of a dusky bluish discoloration occurs at the inflamed site. Necrosis forms a gangrenous area of the skin. Treatment is prompt surgical therapy with wide incisions in the infected area and the immediate administration of penicillin.

The clinical syndrome of necrotizing fasciitis may also be due to a synergistic infection with facultative anaerobic bacteria.

Chronic Undermining Burrowing Ulcers (Meleney's Gangrene). This was first described by Meleney as *postoperative progressive bacterial synergetic gangrene.*

It usually follows drainage of peritoneal abscess, lung abscess, or chronic empyema. After one or two weeks the wound markings or retention suture holes assume a carbunculoid appearance, finally differentiating into three skin zones: outer, bright red; middle, dusky purple; and inner, gangrenous with a central area of granulation tissue. The pain is excruciating. In Meleney's postoperative progressive gangrene, the essential organism is a *microaerophilic nonhemolytic streptococcus* (peptostreptococcus) in the

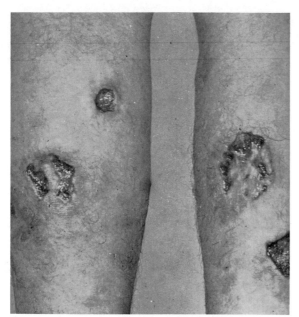

Figure 14–24. Meleney's ulcers. (Courtesy of Dr. S. F. Rosen.)

spreading periphery of the lesion, associated with *S. aureus* or Enterobacteriaceae in the zone of gangrene.

This disease is differentiated from *gangrenous ecthyma*, which begins as vesicles rapidly progressing to pustulation and gangrenous ulceration in debilitated subjects and is due to *Pseudomonas aeruginosa*. It is differentiated from *fusospirochetal gangrene*, which occurs from human bites. *Amebic infection with gangrene* usually follows amebic abscess of the liver. The margins of the ulcer are raised and everted and the granulations have the appearance of raw beef covered with shreds of necrotic material. Glairy pus can be expressed from the margins. *Pyoderma gangrenosum* occurs in a different setting, lacks the bacterial findings, and does not respond to antibiotic therapy.

Wide excision and grafting are primary therapy. Antimicrobial agents, penicillin, and an aminoglycoside should be given as adjunctive therapy.

Purpura Fulminans (Dermatitis Gangrenosa Infantum). This gangrenous disease may rarely develop during the course of varicella and other exanthemata, or independently. Cases are chiefly encountered in children under three years of age, especially girls. The lesions of the exanthem become erosive and pustular and progress into deep ulcerations surrounded by an inflammatory zone. At first these are small and multiple, but gradually they become larger and confluent so that extensive sloughs occur, usually worst over the lower back, buttocks, and upper and lower extremities.

Other infections associated with purpura fulminans include scarlet fever; pneumococcal, meningococcal, staphylococcal, and streptococcal bacteremias; Rocky Mountain spotted fever; leptospirosis; *Vibrio parahaemolyticus* sepsis; and *Haemophilus influenzae* type B sepsis. It is due to a consumptive coagulopathy which causes thrombotic occlusion of the vessels.

The prognosis in all varieties is grave. Treatment is by appropriate antibiotics, basic supportive measures, and intravenous heparin to prevent microthrombus formation.

Vaccinia Gangrenosa. This is discussed under virus diseases.

Gangrenous Balanitis. Gangrenous balanitis is a common form of *phagedena*. Clinically the disease is characterized by chronic painful destructive ulcers that begin on the prepuce or glans and spread by direct extension along the shaft of the penis, sometimes attacking the scrotum or pubes. The edges of the ulcer are likely to be elevated, firm, and undermined. The granulating base, which bleeds easily, is covered with a thick purulent exudate and dirty, necrotic detritus. The neighboring skin may be edematous and dusky red, and the regional lymph glands may be swollen, although this is not necessarily a marked feature. There is severe mutilation due to sloughing, without any evidence of spontaneous healing.

This type of phagedena (spreading and sloughing ulceration) is a rare complication of chancre and chancroidal infections together with another secondary bacterial infection.

Treatment is by the use of antibiotics locally and internally, directed against secondary bacteria, as well as the primary process, such as chancroid, syphilis, or granuloma inguinale, if present.

Fournier's Gangrene of the Penis or Scrotum. Fournier's syndrome is a malignant gangrenous infection of the penis, scrotum, or perineum, which may be due to infection with group A streptococci or a mixed infection with enteric bacilli and anaerobes. This is usually considered a form of necrotizing fasciitis, as it spreads along fascial planes. Peak incidence is between 20 and 50 years, but cases have

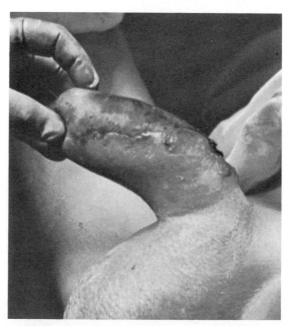

Figure 14–25. Gangrenous balanitis, with involvement of the whole penis.

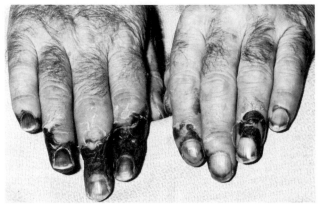

Figure 14–26. Gangrene of fingertips due to vasculitis.

been reported in children. Culture for aerobic and anaerobic organisms should be done, and appropriate antibiotics started; surgical debridement and general support should be instituted.

Vascular Gangrene. This is encountered mostly in those who have suffered from thrombophlebitis with systemic disorders or from localized inflammations. It may occur in those with arteriosclerosis, especially when associated with diabetes mellitus. In addition, gangrene may occur in polyarteritis, cryoglobulinemia, embolism, and Raynaud's phenomenon. It is usually of the dry form and is due to large-vessel blockage.

Diabetic Gangrene. Diabetic gangrene develops mostly in the diabetic past middle life; it affects chiefly the toes, although it may occur in any region. Usually there is a preceding trauma or local infection, and prior to the onset there may have been passive congestion, cyanosis, and numbness of the part. The gangrene develops suddenly and spreads rapidly, so that extensive destruction may result. It is usually of the wet variety, and is due to peripheral small-vessel disease. It often leads to putrefaction.

Treatment is largely directed against the essential disease, by diet and insulin. The condition of the cardiovascular system is also carefully controlled. Locally the treatment is surgical, often requiring amputation. Secondary infection is an important factor and should be treated by antibiotics orally or parenterally.

Benson PM, et al: Purpura and gangrene in a septic patient. Arch Dermatol 1988, 14:1851.

Bernstein SM, et al: Fournier's gangrene of the penis. South Med J 1976, 69:1242.

Feingold DS: Gangrenous and crepitant cellulitis. JAAD 1982, 6:289.

Hirschmann JV: Ischemic forms of acute venous thrombosis. Arch Dermatol 1987, 123:933.

Huntley AC: The cutaneous manifestations of diabetes mellitus. JAAD 1982, 7:427.

Hutchinson PE, et al: Postoperative progressive gangrene. Br J Dermatol 1976, 94:89.

Ratzer MA: Dermatitis gangrenosa infantum. Br J Dermatol 1963, 75:206.

Sussman SJ, et al: Fournier's syndrome. Am J Dis Child 1978, 132:1189.

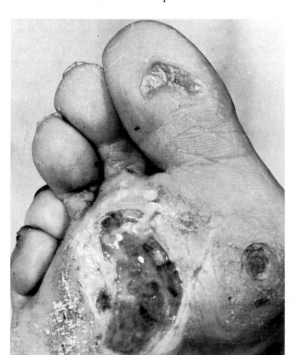

Figure 14–27. Diabetic malum perforans with gangrene. (Courtesy of Dr. F. Daniels, Jr.)

INFECTIONS DUE TO GRAM-NEGATIVE ORGANISMS

PSEUDOMONAS INFECTIONS

Ecthyma Gangrenosum. In the gravely ill patient opalescent, tense, grouped vesicles are surrounded by narrow pink to violaceous halos. The vesicles quickly become hemorrhagic and violaceous and rupture to become round ulcers with necrotic black centers. These lesions are usually on the buttocks and the extremities.

Ecthyma gangrenosum occurs in debilitated persons who may be suffering from leukemia, in the severely burned patient, and in pancytopenia, terminal carcinoma, or other severe chronic disease.

The classic vesicle suggests the diagnosis. In addition, the contents of the vesicle will show gram-negative bacilli and the blood culture will show *Ps. aeruginosa*.

Treatment is the immediate institution of intravenous anti-*Pseudomonas* medications. An aminoglycoside in combination with an antipseudomonal penicillin, such as piperacillin, is recommended. Greene et al found patients had a poor prognosis if there were multiple lesions, if there was a delay in diagnosis and institution of appropriate therapy, and if neutropenia did not resolve by the end of a course of antibiotics. Instrumentation or catheterization increased the risk of this infection.

Other lesions are also seen with *Pseudomonas* septicemia. These may be sharply demarcated areas of cellulitis, macules, papules, plaques and nodules, characteristically found on the trunk.

Green Nail Syndrome. This is characterized by onycholysis of the distal portion of the nail and a striking greenish discoloration in the separated areas. It is frequently associated with paronychia in persons whose hands are often in water. Soaking the affected finger in a 0.1 per cent polymyxin B and 1 per cent acetic acid solution twice daily for an hour has been found to be helpful. Trimming the onycholytic nail plate followed by twice daily application of neosporin solution is also effective.

Gram-Negative Toeweb Infection. This type of infection often begins with dermatophytosis. Prolonged immersion may also cause hydration and maceration of the interdigital spaces, with overgrowth of *Pseudomonas* organisms. Dermatophytosis may progress to a condition referred to by Leyden et al as dermatophytosis complex, where many types of gram-negative organisms may be recovered, and as inflammation, maceration, and inflammation progress, it is less often possible to culture dermatophytes. Gram-negatives dominate, with *Pseudomonas aeruginosa* being most prominent. Finally denudation with purulent or serous discharge and marked edema and erythema of the surrounding tissue may be seen. Again, as reported by Eaglstein et al, *Pseudomonas* predominates, but commonly a mixture of other gram-negative organisms such as *E. coli* and *Proteus* are present.

Early dermatophytosis, dermatophytosis simplex, may simply be treated with topical antifungals. However, once the scaling and peeling progress to white maceration, soggy scaling, bad odor, edema, and fissuring, treatment must also include topical antibiotics or acetic acid compresses. In this state systemic corticosteroids, briefly given, will produce more rapid resolution of the painful symptoms and will not aggravate the infection. Full-blown gram-negative toeweb infection with widespread denudation and erythema, purulence, and edema requires systemic antibiotics. Eaglstein et al recommend one week of intramuscular cefoperazone (cefobid); how-

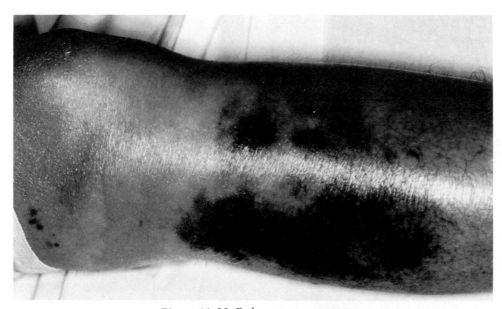

Figure 14–28. Ecthyma gangrenosum.

ever, an intravenous combination of an aminoglycoside and antipseudomonal penicillin is less painful and equally efficacious. A new class of oral antibiotics, quinolones, is effective orally against pseudomonas, and will be the drugs of choice. Parish has reviewed them.

Underlying *inverse psoriasis* (Waisman's "white psoriasis") should also be suspected, and may require treatment. Castellani paint is effective in the treatment of these lesions. Intramuscular injection of triamcinolone acetonide or diacetate (Kenalog or Aristocort), 40 to 60 mg, or of betamethasone salts (Celestone Soluspan) is likely to be extremely helpful in any event, and should be used almost routinely. It clears inverse psoriasis if that is present, and suppresses inflammation and exudation, and we have never seen any indication that it causes spread or aggravation of the infection.

Pseudomonas Aeruginosa Folliculitis (Hot Tub Dermatitis). Pseudomonas folliculitis is characterized by pruritic follicular, maculopapular, vesicular, or pustular lesions occurring within one to four days after bathing in a hot tub, whirlpool, or public swimming pool. Most lesions occur on the sides of the trunk, axillae, buttocks, and proximal extremities. The nipples and breasts are often involved. Associated complaints may include earache, sore throat, headache, fever, and malaise. Rarely, systemic infection may result; breast abscess and bacteremia were both reported by Goette et al.

Large outbreaks have occurred among scout troops, as reported by Fox et al and Thomas et al, or smaller groups of patients may be affected by an exposure to a health spa facility or their personal hot tub. A national survey of state epidemiologists in 1982 on outbreaks of nonresidential whirlpool spas reported 74 outbreaks in 49 states. Most occurred during the winter months. Most serotyped cases involve type 0-11.

The folliculitis involutes usually within seven to 14 days without therapy, although occasionally multiple prolonged recurrent episodes have been reported. Acetic acid compresses have been used. Preventive

measures have been water filtration, automatic chlorination to maintain a free chlorine level of 1 ppm, maintenance of water at pH 7.2 to 7.8, and frequent changing of the water.

External Otitis. Swelling, maceration, and pain may be present. In up to 70 per cent of cases *Pseudomonas aeruginosa* may be cultured. This is especially common in swimmers. Local applications of antipseudomonal Cortisporin Otic Solution or Suspension or 2 per cent acetic acid compresses will help clear this infection.

There is also a threat of this occurring after ear surgery. If the patient is a swimmer or diabetic, acetic acid compresses for a day or two before surgery may prevent this complication.

A more severe type, referred to as malignant external otitis, occurs in elderly diabetic patients. The swelling, pain, and erythema are more pronounced, with purulence and a foul odor. Facial nerve palsy develops in 30 per cent, and cartilage necrosis may occur. This is a life-threatening infection in these older, compromised individuals, and requires swift institution of appropriate systemic antibiotics.

Gram-negative Folliculitis. Although this is usually due to *Enterobacter, Klebsiella, Escherichia, Proteus,* or *Serratia,* occasional cases due to *Pseudomonas* have been seen, as reported by Leyden et al. They differed from the other types of gram-negative infection in acne patients in that the site of colonization of *Pseudomonas* was the external ear, and topical therapy alone to the face and ears was sufficient for cure.

Baze PE, et al: *Pseudomonas aeruginosa* 0-11 folliculitis. Arch Dermatol 1985, 121:873.

Chandrasekar PH, et al: Hot tub–associated dermatitis due to *Pseudomonas aeruginosa.* Arch Dermatol 1984, 120:1337.

Eaglstein NF, et al: Gram-negative bacterial toe web infection. JAAD 1983, 8:225.

Fanero US: Whirlpool spa-associated infections. Am J Public Health 1984, 74:653.

Fox AB, et al: Recreationally associated *Pseudomonas aeruginosa* folliculitis. Arch Dermatol 1984, 120:1304.

Goette DK, et al: Hot-tub-acquired pseudomonas septicemia. J Assoc Milit Dermatol 1984, 10:40.

Hall JH, et al: *Pseudomonas aeruginosa* in dermatology. Arch Dermatol 1968, 97:312.

Khabbaz RF, et al: *Pseudomonas aeruginosa serotype* 0:9. Am J Med 1983, 74:73.

King DF, et al: Importance of debridement in the treatment of gram-negative toe web infection. JAAD 1986, 14:278.

Leyden JJ, et al: Interdigital athletes foot. Arch Dermatol 1978, 114:1466.

Idem: *Pseudomonas aeruginosa* gram-negative folliculitis. Arch Dermatol 1979, 115:1203.

Merritt WT, et al: Malignant external otitis in an adolescent with diabetes. J Pediatr 1980, 96:872.

Parish LC, et al: The quinolones and dermatologic practice. Internat J Dermatol 1986, 25:351.

Roberts R, et al: Erysipelas-like lesions and hyperesthesia as manifestations of *Pseudomonas aeruginosa* septicemia. JAMA 1982, 248:2156.

Sausker WF, et al: Pseudomonas folliculitis acquired from a health spa whirlpool. JAMA 1978, 239:2362.

Scherbenske JM, et al: Acute pseudomonas infection of the external ear. J Dermatol Surg Oncol 1988, 14:165.

Schlossberg D: Multiple erythematous nodules as a manifestation of *Pseudomonas aeruginosa* septicemia. Arch Dermatol 1980, 116:446.

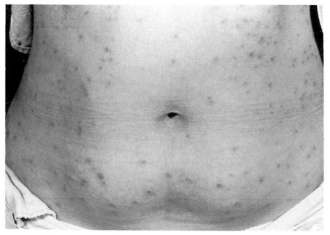

Figure 14–29. Pseudomonas "hot tub" folliculitis.

Silverman AR, et al: Hot tub dermatitis. JAAD 1983, 8:153.

Spitalny KC, et al: National survey on outbreaks associated with whirlpool spas. Am J Public Health 1984, 74:725.

Thomas P, et al: *Pseudomonas* dermatitis associated with a swimming pool. JAMA 1985, 253:1156.

Carter S, et al: Etiology and treatment of facial cellulitis in pediatric patients. Pediatr Infect Dis J 1983, 2:222.

Cochi SL, et al: Immunization of U.S. children with *Hemophilus influenzae* type B polysaccharide vaccine. JAMA 1985, 253:521.

Ginsburg CM: *Hemophilus influenzae* type B buccal cellulitis. JAAD 1981, 4:661.

Prevention of secondary cases of Haemophilus influenzae type B disease. MMWR 1982, 31:672.

Todd JK, et al: Severe *Hemophilus influenzae* infections. Am J Dis Child 1975, 129:607.

MALACOPLAKIA (Malakoplakia)

This rare granuloma, originally reported only in the genitourinary tract of immunosuppressed renal transplant recipients, may also occur in the skin and subcutaneous tissues of other patients with deficient immune responsiveness. Patients are unable to resist infections with *S.aureus, Ps. aeruginosa, and E.coli.* There is defective intracellular digestion of the bacteria once they have been phagocytized.

The granulomas may arise as yellowish red papules in the natal cleft, as in the case reported by Nieland et al, as draining sinuses in the vicinity of the urethra, as perianal ulcers, or as lesions on the uvula.

Histologically there are foamy eosinophilic histiocytes containing calcified, concentrically laminated, intracytoplasmic bodies called Michelis-Gutmann bodies. Scattered immunoblasts, neutrophils, and lymphocytes are found in the dermis.

Almagro UA, et al: Cutaneous malakoplakia: Report of a case and review of the literature. Am J Dermatopathol 1981, 3:295.

Arulk J, et al: Malakoplakia of the skin. Clin Exp Dermatol 1977, 2:131.

Helander I, et al: Lupus vulgaris with Michaelis-Gutmann–like bodies in an immunologically compromised patient: Cutaneous malakoplakia of tuberculosis origin? JAAD 1988, 18:577.

Nieland ML, et al: Cutaneous malakoplakia. Am J Dermatopathol 1981, 3:287.

Sian CS, et al: Malakoplakia of skin and subcutaneous tissue in a renal transplant patient. Arch Dermatol 1981, 117:654.

HAEMOPHILUS INFLUENZAE CELLULITIS

Haemophilus influenzae type B causes a distinctive bluish or purplish red cellulitis of the face accompanied by fever in children below the age of two years. The importance of recognizing the entity is related to the bacteremia which often accompanies the cellulitis. The bacteremia may lead to metastatic meningitis, osteomyelitis, or pyarthrosis. Cultures of the blood and needle aspirates of the cellulitis should yield the organism.

In a series of 72 cases reported by Ginsburg, 86 per cent had bacteremia, 68 per cent had had otitis media, and 8 per cent had meningitis. Cefuroxime intravenously, or a third-generation cephalosporin, or ampicillin with chloramphenicol is effective. In a family with children under four, the index case, both parents, and children at risk should be given rifampin to clear the nasal carriage state and prevent secondary cases. A vaccine is also available for children over 18 months old.

CHANCROID

CLINICAL FEATURES. Chancroid (*soft chancre*), uncommon in the U.S., is an infectious, contagious, ulcerative, sexually transmitted disease caused by the gram-negative bacillus *Haemophilus ducreyi* (the Ducrey bacillus). One or more deep or superficial tender ulcers on the genitalia, and painful inguinal adenitis in 50 per cent, which may suppurate, are characteristic of the disease.

Chancroid begins as an inflammatory macule or pustule one to five days—or rarely as long as two weeks—after intercourse. It generally appears on the distal penis (or perianal area) in men, or on the vulva, cervix, or perianal area in women. However, many cases of extragenital infection on hands, eyelid, lips, or breasts have been reported. Autoinoculation is frequent, and women are apt to have more numerous lesions.

The pustule ruptures early with the formation of a ragged ulcer that lacks the induration of a chancre, usually being soft with an indefinite inflammatory thickening. The ulcers appear punched-out or have undermined irregular edges surrounded by mild hyperemia. The base is covered with a purulent, dirty exudate. The ulcers bleed easily and are very tender.

A number of clinical variants have been described. Kraus and Werman et al have described lesions of chancroid resembling granuloma inguinale. Giant ulcers, serpiginous ulcers, transient chancroid, and follicular and papular variants have been described.

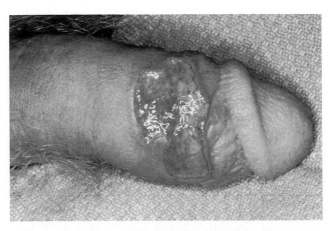

Figure 14–30. Chancroid with painful perforation of frenum, a common location.

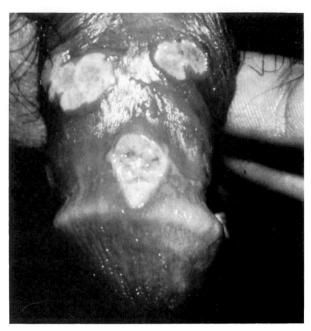

Figure 14–31. Chancroid.

Selective culture media now available make it possible to investigate the true incidence of such variants.

Only about half the cases of genital chancroid manifest inguinal adenitis. Suppuration of the bubo (inguinal lymph node) may be prevented by early antibiotic therapy. The lymphadenitis of chancroid, mostly unilateral, is tender and may rupture spontaneously. As a result of mixed infection, phagedenic and gangrenous features may develop. Left untreated, the site of perforation of the broken-down bubo may assume the features of a soft chancre (chancrous bubo). Many cases of primary extragenital involvement with lesions on the hands, eyelids, and other locations have been recorded.

ETIOLOGY. Chancroid is caused by the gram-negative bacillus *Haemophilus ducreyi*, and is sexually transmitted.

HISTOPATHOLOGY. The ulcer may include a superficial necrotic zone with an infiltrate consisting of neutrophils, lymphocytes, and red blood cells. Deep to this, new vessel formation is present, with endothelial proliferation and thrombosis. Deeper still is an infiltrate of lymphocytes and plasma cells. Ducrey bacilli may or may not be seen in the sections.

DIAGNOSIS. The diagnosis of chancroid has in the past been a clinical diagnosis, by exclusion of other clinically similar conditions. New solid-media culture techniques have made definitive diagnosis possible, and permit sensitivity testing. Specimens for culture should be taken from the purulent ulcer base without extensive cleaning. Cultures should be inoculated in the clinic, as transport systems have not been evaluated. The selective medium contains vancomycin and cultures are done in a water-saturated environment with 1 to 5 per cent carbon dioxide, at a temperature of 33° C.

Smears from the ulcer base may also be of benefit in diagnosis in the clinic. The lesion is cleansed with saline and dried.

In competent hands 50 per cent of the *H. ducreyi*–containing smears are positive. With the loop, material is gathered from the undermined border of the lesion and spread on a glass slide. The slide is permitted to dry and is flamed and stained with methyl green pyronine (Unna-Pappenheim stain). The organisms appear as red chains, the pus cells bluish green. The "school-of-fish" arrangement of the organisms is characteristic and is also visible in the methylene blue stain. Wright, Giemsa, and Gram stains may also be used.

DIFFERENTIAL DIAGNOSIS. Probably the disease for which chancroid is most frequently mistaken is *herpes progenitalis*. A history of recurrent grouped vesicles at the same site should quickly eliminate the chance of a misdiagnosis. Salzman et al recently reviewed this clinical differential.

Traumatic ulcerations should also be ruled out. These occur mostly along the frenulum or as multiple erosions on the prepuce. Adenopathy is absent and some degree of phimosis is present.

The clinical features that differentiate chancroid from syphilitic chancre are given in Chapter 18. However, the diagnosis of chancroid does not rule out syphilis. Either the lesion may be already a "mixed sore" or the subsequent development of syphilis should be anticipated, since the incubation period of chancre is much longer than that of chancroid. Repeated darkfield examinations for *T. pallidum* are necessary even in a sore where the diagnosis of chancroid has been established. Serologic tests for syphilis should be obtained initially, and monthly for the next three months. One may give 500,000 units of benzathine penicillin G intramuscularly, which will cure seronegative primary syphilis if it is present. For differential diagnosis from lymphogranuloma venereum see Chapter 20; from granuloma inguinale, page 294.

TREATMENT. The treatment of chancroid has been changed by the frequent isolation of sulfamethoxazole-and-tetracycline-resistant *H. ducreyi*. Erythromycin, 500 mg four times daily for seven days, is at present the treatment of choice; however, extending this treatment to 15 days will treat coexistent syphilis. Ceftriaxone, 250 mg intramuscularly in a single dose, or trimethoprim/sulfamethoxazole, one double-strength tablet twice daily for seven days, are alternative treatments. Sexual partners should be treated with a recommended regimen.

Phimosis that does not subside following irrigation of the preputial cavity may have to be relieved by a dorsal slit. Circumcision should be deferred for at least two or three months. Early doses of antibiotics prevent the formation of buboes. If frank pus is already present, repeated aspirations (not incisions) are indicated.

1985 STD treatment guidelines. JAAD 1986, 14:707.
Fitzpatrick JE, et al: Treatment of chancroid. JAMA 1981, 246:1804.

Fiumara NJ, et al: The diagnosis and treatment of chancroid. JAAD 1986, 15:939.

Kraus SJ, et al: Pseudogranuloma inguinale caused by *Haemophilus ducreyi*. Arch Dermatol 1982, 118:494.

McCurley ME, et al: Chancroid. JAAD 1988, 19:330.

Plummer FA, et al: Antimicrobial therapy of chancroid. J Infect Dis 1983, 148:726.

Ronald AR: Chancroid. Int J Dermatol 1986, 25:31.

Idem, et al: Chancroid and *Hemophilus ducreyi*. Ann Intern Med 1985, 102:705.

Salzman RS, et al: Chancroidal ulcers that are not chancroid. Arch Dermatol 1984, 120:636.

Werman BS, et al: A clinical variant of chancroid resembling granuloma inguinale. Arch Dermatol 1983, 119:890.

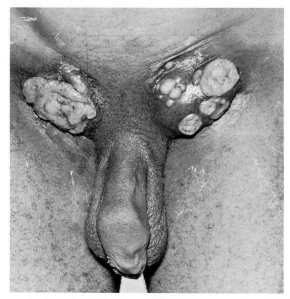

Figure 14–33. Granuloma inguinale. (Courtesy of Dr. H. Shatin.)

GRANULOMA INGUINALE
(Granuloma Venereum, Donovanosis)

CLINICAL FEATURES. Granuloma inguinale is a mildly contagious, chronic, granulomatous, locally destructive disease characterized by progressive, indolent, serpiginous ulcerations of the groins, pubes, genitalia, and anus.

The disease begins as single or multiple subcutaneous nodules, which erode through the skin to produce clean, granulomatous, sharply defined lesions, which are usually painless. Over 80 per cent of cases demonstrate hypertrophic, vegetative granulation tissue, which is soft, has a beefy-red appearance, and bleeds readily. Approximately 10 per cent of cases involve ulcerative lesions with overhanging edges and a dry or moist floor. A membranous exudate may cover the floor of fine granulations, and the lesions are moderately painful. Occasional cases have an array of presentations and are frequently misdiagnosed as carcinoma of the penis. The lesions enlarge by autoinoculation and peripheral extension with satellite lesions, and by gradual undermining of sound tissue at the advancing edge.

The genitalia are involved in 90 per cent of cases, the inguinal region in 10 per cent, the anal region in 5 to 10 per cent, and distal sites in 1 to 5 per cent. Lesions are limited to the genitalia in approximately 80 per cent of cases and to the inguinal region in less than 5 per cent. Unilateral lesions are more common than bilateral ones. In men, the lesions most commonly occur on the prepuce or glans, and in women, lesions on the labia are most common.

The incubation period is unknown; it may vary between eight and 80 days, with a two- to three-week period being most common. Zigos produced a lesion in his own thigh within nine days after inoculation with infective material.

Persisting sinuses and hypertrophic scars, devoid of pigment, are fairly characteristic of the disease.

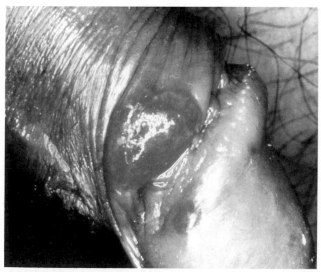

Figure 14–32. Early granuloma inguinale, showing beefy granulations.

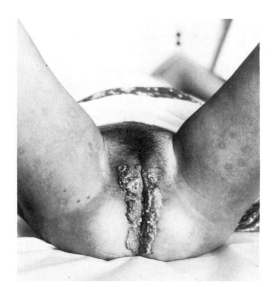

Figure 14–34. Granuloma inguinale. (Courtesy of Dr. Arturo L. Carrion.)

The regional lymph nodes are usually not enlarged. The lesions are not painful and produce only mild subjective symptoms.

In later stages, as a result of cicatrization, the lymph channels are sometimes blocked and pseudoelephantiasis of the genitals ("esthiomene") may occur. Mutilation of the genitals and destruction of deeper tissues are observed in some instances.

Dissemination from the inguinal region may be by hematogenous or lymphatic routes. There may be involvement of liver, other organs, eyes, face, lips, larynx, chest, and, rarely, bones. Hematogenous spread is believed to occur after pregnancy. During childbearing the cervical lesions may extend to the internal genital organs.

Epidermoid carcinoma may rarely supervene.

ETIOLOGY. Granuloma inguinale is caused by the gram-negative bacterium *Calymmatobacterium granulomatis*.

The exact mode of transmission of infection is undetermined. The role of sexual transmission is controversial, but several factors, including the genital location of the initial lesion in the majority of cases, the relationship of the first lesion to an incubation period following coitus, and the occurrence of conjugal infection in 12 to 52 per cent of marital or steady sexual partners, strongly favor sexual transmission. An unusual American epidemic reported by Rosen et al supports the venereal transmission of this disorder. Also, it has been speculated that *C. granulomatis* is an intestinal inhabitant which leads to granuloma inguinale through autoinoculation, or sexually through vaginal intercourse if the vagina is contaminated by enteric bacteria, or through rectal intercourse, heterosexual or homosexual. *C. granulomatis* probably requires direct inoculation through a break in the skin or mucosa to cause infection. Those affected are generally young adults.

PATHOLOGY. In the center of the lesion the epidermis is replaced by serum, fibrin, and polymorphonuclear leukocytes. At the periphery the epidermis is thickened. In the dermis there is a dense granulomatous infiltration composed chiefly of plasma cells and histiocytes, and scattered throughout are small abscesses containing polymorphonuclear leukocytes.

Characteristic pale-staining macrophages which have intracytoplasmic inclusion bodies are found. The parasitized histiocytes may measure 20 microns or more in diameter. The ovoid Donovan bodies measure 1 to 2 microns and may be visualized by using Giemsa or silver stains. The best method, however, is toluidine blue staining of semi-thin plastic-embedded sections. Crushed smears of fresh biopsy material stained with Wright or Giemsa stain permit the demonstration of Donovan bodies and provide rapid diagnosis.

DIFFERENTIAL DIAGNOSIS. Granuloma inguinale may be confused with ulcerations of the groin due to syphilis or carcinoma, but is differentiated from these diseases by its long duration and slow course, by the absence of lymphatic involvement, and, in the case of syphilis, by a negative test for syphilis and failure to respond to antisyphilitic treatment. It should not be overlooked that other venereal diseases, especially syphilis, often coexist with granuloma inguinale. Lymphogranuloma venereum at an early stage would most likely be accompanied by inguinal adenitis. In later stages when stasis, excoriations, and enlargement of the outer genitalia are common to granuloma inguinale and lymphogranuloma venereum, the absence of a positive lymphogranuloma venereum complement-fixation test and the presence of Donovan bodies in the lesions permit the diagnosis of granuloma inguinale.

TREATMENT. Tetracycline, 500 mg four times a day for three to four weeks, is preferred treatment, though doxycycline and minocycline have proved successful in some cases not responding to tetracycline. Rosen et al used twice daily oral trimethoprim-sulfamethoxazole tablets for two to four weeks and found it effective in all 20 patients treated.

Rosen T, et al: Granuloma inguinale. JAAD 1984, 11:433.
Sehgal NV, et al: Donovanosis. Int J Dermatol 1986, 25:8.

GONOCOCCAL DERMATITIS

Primary gonococcal dermatitis is a rare infection which occurs mostly as erosions that may be 2 to 20 mm in diameter.

A physician attending a patient with gonorrhea received a wound on his thumb followed 30 hours later by lymphangitis of the arm, with two small nodules on the thumb. The pus from the incised nodules showed grouped intracellular diplococci. The physician became severely ill and developed polyarticular gonococcal arthritis.

Gonococcal dermatitis has been reported as occurring on the median raphe without urethritis; Glicksman and his associates described a lesion as extragenital gonococcal ecthyma.

Scott et al reported a case of grouped pustules on an erythematous base on the finger, which simulated herpetic whitlow. Gonococcal scalp abscesses in infants secondary to direct fetal monitoring in mothers with gonorrhea have been reported, as well.

Treatment is the same as that of gonorrheal urethritis.

Gonococcemia

Gonococcemia is characterized by a hemorrhagic vesiculopustular eruption, bouts of fever, and arthralgia or actual arthritis of one or several joints.

The skin lesions begin as tiny erythematous macules that evolve into vesicopustules on a deeply erythematous base or into purpuric macules that may

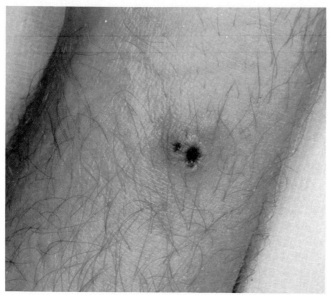

Figure 14–35. Hemorrhagic vesiculopustular lesion of gonococcemia.

Geelhoed-Duyrestiyir PHLM, et al: Disseminated gonococcal infection in elderly patients. Arch Intern Med 1986, 146:1739.

Goette DK: Gonococcal arthritis. Cutis 1973, 11:339.

Hansfield HH: Disseminated gonococcal infection. Clin Obstet Gynecol 1975, 18:131.

Holmes KK, et al: Disseminated gonococcal infection. Ann Intern Med 1971, 74:979.

Judson FN: Management of antibiotic-resistant *Neisseria gonorrhoeae*. Ann Intern Med 1989, 119:5.

Medical Letter: Treatment of sexually transmitted diseases. Vol 30 (Jan 15, 1988).

Rosen T: Unusual presentations of gonorrhea. JAAD 1982, 6:369.

Schroeter AL, et al: Gonorrhea. Ann Intern Med 1970, 72:553.

Strader KW, et al: Disseminated gonococcal infection caused by chromosomally mediated penicillin-resistant organisms. Ann Intern Med 1986, 104:365.

be as much as 2 cm in diameter. These purpuric lesions occur mostly on the palms and soles and over joints. It is accompanied by fever, chills, malaise, migratory polyarthralgia, myalgia, and tenosynovitis.

The vesicopustules are usually tender and sparse and occur principally on the extremities. Involution of the lesions takes place in about four days.

Many patients seen are women with asymptomatic anogenital infections in whom dissemination occurs during pregnancy or menstruation. Liver function abnormalities, myocarditis, pericarditis, endocarditis, and meningitis may complicate this infection.

The causative organism is *Neisseria gonorrhoeae*. These organisms can at times be demonstrated in the early skin lesion histologically, by smears, and by cultures. Gonococci may be found in the blood, the genitourinary tract, the joints, and the skin. If direct staining fails to show *Neisseria,* immunofluorescent staining should be done.

The skin lesions of gonococcemia may be identical to those seen in meningococcemia, nongonococcal bacterial endocarditis, rheumatoid arthritis, the rickettsial diseases, systemic lupus erythematosus, periarteritis nodosa, Haverhill fever, and typhoid fever.

The treatment of choice is ceftriaxone, 1 gm IV daily for seven days, and aqueous crystalline penicillin G, 10 million units IV daily for at least three days, followed by amoxicillin, 500 mg orally four times daily for four days. For the penicillin-allergic patient, doxycycline, 100 mg orally for two doses daily for at least seven days, is recommended. If penicillin or a cephalosporin is used, tetracycline should be given too, to treat coexisting chlamydial infection.

Ackerman AB, et al: Gonococcemia and its cutaneous manifestations. Arch Dermatol 1965, 91:227.

VIBRIO VULNIFICUS INFECTION

Infection with *Vibrio vulnificus*, a gram-negative rod of the noncholera group of vibrios, produces a rapidly expanding cellulitis or septicemia in patients who have been exposed to the organism, which occurs mainly along the Atlantic seacoast. It may be acquired via the gastrointestinal tract, where, after being ingested with raw oysters or other seafood, the bacterium enters the bloodstream at the level of the duodenum. Pulmonary infection by the aspiration of sea water has been reported. Localized skin infection may result after exposure of an open wound to sea water.

Skin lesions characteristically begin with localized tenderness followed by erythema, edema, and indurated plaques. A purplish discoloration develops centrally, which then undergoes necrosis and sloughs, leaving large ulcers. Other reported lesions include hemorrhagic bullae, as reported by Tyring et al; pustules, petechiae, generalized macules or papules, gangrene, and urticaria and erythema multiforme type lesions.

If the skin is invaded primarily, septicemia may not develop, but the lesions may be progressive and at times limb amputation may be necessary. With septicemia, cellulitic lesions are the result of seeding of the subcutaneous tissue during bacteremia. Patients with advanced liver disease are at particular risk for developing septicemia. Other predisposing disorders are immunosuppression, diabetes, renal failure, and iron-overload states such as hemochromatosis. The virulence of the bacterium is related in part to the production of exotoxin. The mortality in those with septicemia is over 50 per cent.

Treatment of this fulminant infection, which rapidly produces septic shock, includes antibiotics, surgical debridement, and appropriate resuscitative therapy. *Vibrio vulnificus* is sensitive to penicillins, cephalosporins, tetracyclines, cotrimoxazole, and chloramphenicol. Tetracycline is the drug of choice, with penicillin G as the alternative. Surgical debridement of necrotizing tissue is recommended.

Klontz KC, et al: Syndromes of *Vibrio vulnificus* infections. Ann Intern Med 1988, 109:318.

Morris JG Jr: *Vibrio vulnificus*—A new monster of the deep. Ann Intern Med 1988, 109:318.

Oliver JD: Highly invasive new bacterium isolated from U.S. East Coast waters. JAMA 1984, 251:323.

Tyring SK, et al: Hemorrhagic bullae associated with *Vibrio vulnificus* septicemia. Arch Dermatol 1986, 122:818.

Wickboldt LG, et al: *Vibrio vulnificus* infection. JAAD 1983, 9:243.

CHROMOBACTERIOSIS AND AEROMONAS INFECTIONS

Chromobacteria are a genus of gram-negative rods, which produce various discolorations on gelatin broth. They have been shown to be common water and soil saprophytes of the southeastern U.S. Several types of cutaneous lesions are caused by chromobacteria, ranging from fluctuating abscesses and local cellulitis to anthraxlike carbuncular lesions with lymphangitis and lymphadenopathy and fatal septicemia. *Chromobacterium violaceum*, the most common organism in this genus, produces a violet pigment.

Macher et al reviewed the 12 known cases of *C. violaceum* infection and found that all had been infected in Louisiana or Florida between June and September. Eight had had soil or ground-water contact before the onset, and 10 were seen with skin lesions. Sepsis, liver abscess, and death are frequent. Patients with chronic granulomatous disease may be at particular risk. Aminoglycosides systemically are indicated.

A gram-negative bacterium, *Aeromonas hydrophila*, another typical soil-and-water saprophyte, may cause similar skin infections manifesting as cellulitis, pustules, furuncles, gas gangrene, or ecthyma gangrenosumlike lesions, after water-related trauma and abrasions. Such a case was reported by Young et al. The treatment of choice is trimethoprim-sulfamethoxazole.

Macher AM, et al: Chronic granulomatous disease of childhood and *Chromobacterium violaceum* infections in the Southeastern United States. Ann Intern Med 1982, 97:51.

Young DF, et al: *Aeromonas hydrophila* infection of the skin. Arch Dermatol 1981, 117:244.

SALMONELLOSIS

Salmonellae are a genus of gram-negative rods that exist in man either in a carrier state or as a cause of active enteric or systemic infection. Most cases are acquired by ingestion of contaminated food or water. Poultry and poultry products are the most important sources, and are believed to be the cause in about one-half of common-source epidemics.

After an incubation period of one to two weeks, there is usually an acute onset of fever, chills, headache, constipation, and bronchitis. After seven to 10 days of fever, diarrhea and skin lesions appear: rose-colored macules or papules ("rose spots") 2 to 5 mm in diameter on the anterior trunk, between the umbilicus and the nipples. They occur in crops, each group of 10 to 20 lesions lasting three to four days, the total duration of the exanthem being two to three weeks in untreated cases. Rose spots occur in 50 to 60 per cent of cases. A more extensive erythematous eruption occurring early in the course, *erythema typhosum*, is rarely reported, as are erythema nodosum, urticaria, and ulcers or abscesses.

The diagnosis is confirmed by culturing the organism from blood, stool, skin, or bone marrow. If the organism is not grown on Shigella-Salmonella medium, or not analyzed correctly, it may be erroneously reported as a coliform.

The antibiotic of choice is chloramphenicol; ampicillin is the best alternative.

Hoffman TA, et al: Waterborne typhoid fever in Dade County, Florida. Am J Med 1975, 59:481.

SHIGELLOSIS

Shigellae are small gram-negative rods which cause bacillary dysentery, an acute diarrheal illness. Most cases are a result of person-to-person transmission; however, widespread epidemics have been due to contaminated food and water. Small blanchable erythematous macules on the extremities have been reported by Goscienski et al to have occurred in three children with shigellosis, and Barrett-Conner et al reported three patients with petechial or morbilliform eruptions. Recently Stoll reported a male homosexual who developed a 1-cm furuncle on the dorsal penile shaft from which a pure culture *S. flexneri* was grown. Shigellosis may then occur as a purely cutaneous form of sexually transmitted disease. Therapy with ampicillin or trimethoprim-sulfamethoxazole is curative.

Stoll DM: Cutaneous shigellosis. Arch Dermatol 1986, 122:22.

RHINOSCLEROMA

Rhinoscleroma is a chronic, inflammatory, granulomatous disease of the upper respiratory tract characterized by sclerosis, deformity, remission, and eventual debility. Death due to obstructive sequelae may occur. The infection is limited to the nose, the pharynx, and adjacent structures.

CLINICAL FEATURES. The disease begins insidiously with nasal catarrh, increased nasal secretion, and subsequent crusting. Gradually there ensues a nodular or rather diffuse sclerotic enlargement of the

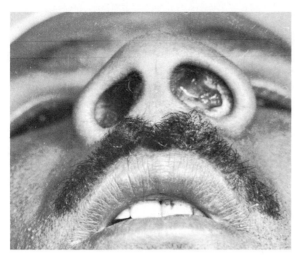

Figure 14–36. Early rhinoscleroma in the nose. (Courtesy of Dr. M. El-Zawahry, Egypt.)

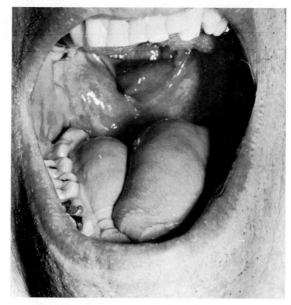

Figure 14–38. Rhinoscleroma on the palate and nasopharynx.

nose, upper lip, palate, or neighboring structures. The nodules at first are small, hard, subepidermal, and freely movable, but they gradually fuse to form sclerotic plaques that adhere to the underlying parts. Ulceration is common. The lesions have a distinctive, stony hardness, are quite insensitive, and are of a dusky purple or ivory color. Hyperpigmentation can be expected in dark-complexioned individuals.

In the more advanced stages of rhinoscleroma, the reactive growth produces extensive mutilation of the face and marked disfigurement. Complete obstruction of the nares, superficial breaking down, and seropurulent exudation may occur.

ETIOLOGY. A microorganism, *Klebsiella rhinoscleromatis*, first isolated by von Frisch, is the causative agent. The rhinoscleroma bacillus is a gram-negative rod, short, nonmotile, round at the ends, always encapsulated in a gelatinous capsule, and measuring 2.0 to 0.5 microns. It is found in the throats of scleroma patients only.

INCIDENCE AND PREVALENCE. The disease occurs in both sexes, and is commonest during the

third and fourth decades of life. Although endemic in Austria and southern Russia and occasionally found in Brazil, Argentina, Chile, Spain, Italy, Sweden, and the United States, it is especially prevalent in El Salvador, where many workers in the dye industry have been affected. It was first described by Hebra in 1870 and later by von Mikulicz, von Frisch, and others.

PATHOLOGY. In the primary stage of nasal catarrh, the histologic picture is that of a mild nonspecific inflammation. When proliferation and tumefaction develop, the granulomatous tumor is made up largely of plasma cells, Mikulicz cells, an occasional hyaline degenerated plasma cell (Russell body), a few spindle cells, and hypertrophic collagenous tissue.

The bacilli of rhinoscleroma are found within foamy macrophages known as Mikulicz cells. They are best visualized with the Warthin-Starry silver stain. It is fibrosis that is responsible for the hardness of rhinoscleroma.

DIFFERENTIAL DIAGNOSIS. Rhinoscleroma has such distinctive features that its diagnosis should not be difficult. The diagnosis depends on bacteriologic, histopathologic, and serologic tests. Heat-killed antigen gives a positive complement-fixation reaction with scleroma patients' serum. Titers run as high as 1:1280. Clinically, it can be confused with syphilitic gumma, sarcoid, leishmaniasis, frambesia, keloid, lepra, hypertrophic forms of tuberculosis, and rhinosporidiosis.

TREATMENT. This disease is usually progressive and extremely resistant to therapy. Kerdel-Vegas regards tetracycline, 2 gm a day in divided doses for six months, and 1 gm a day for six months, as the treatment of choice. In case of recurrence, he believes cephalexin should be tried at the same dose levels. Nasal packs of 2 per cent aqueous solution of acri-

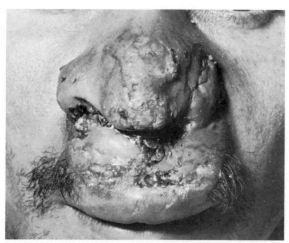

Figure 14–37. Rhinoscleroma. (Courtesy of Dr. F. Kerdel-Vegas.)

flavine, continued for eight weeks, are helpful. Streptomycin, 1 gm or more daily for two to three months, has been found to be effective. Corticosteroids are useful.

Convit J, et al: Rhinoscleroma: Arch Dermatol 1961, 84:55.
Kerdel-Vegas F: Rhinoscleroma. Clin Dermatol, Denis J, ed., 3:16–54, Philadelphia, Harper & Row, 1986.
Kraas EW, et al: Rhinoscleroma. J Assoc Milit Dermatol 1985, 11:64.
Tapia A: Rhinoscleroma: a naso-oral dermatosis. Cutis 1987, 40:101.

LISTERIOSIS

Listeria monocytogenes is a gram-positive bacillus with rounded ends, which may be isolated from soil, water, animals, and asymptomatic individuals. Human infection probably occurs via the gastrointestinal tract; however, in the majority of patients the portal of entry is unknown. Infections in man usually produce meningitis or encephalitis with monocytosis.

Cutaneous listeriosis is a rare disease. Owens reported a veterinarian who contracted cutaneous listeriosis from an aborting cow. The organism in the skin lesions was identical with that isolated from the fetus. The eruption consisted of erythematous tender papules and pustules scattered over the hands and arms. There were axillary lymphadenopathy, fever, malaise, and headache. Treatment with sulfonamides caused the disease to disappear within a few days.

Listeria also may cause a granulomatous disease of infants (**granulomatosis infanta peptica**). The endocarditis, meningitis, and encephalitis caused by listeria may be accompanied by petechiae and papules in the skin.

Burnett points out that cases of listeriosis may easily be missed on bacteriologic examination, because the organism produces few colonies on original culture and may be dismissed as a streptococcus or as a contaminant diphtheroid because of the similarity in gram-stained specimens. Serologic tests help to make the diagnosis.

Listeria monocytogenes is sensitive to most antibiotics. Ampicillin is probably the most effective, but tetracycline, penicillin, and erythromycin are also effective.

Ahlfors CE, et al: Neonatal listeriosis. Am J Dis Child 1977, 131:405.
Owens CR, et al: Case of primary listeriosis. N Engl J Med 1960, 262:1026.
Visintine AM: *Listeria monocytogenes* infection in infants and children. Am J Dis Child 1977, 131:393.

PASTEURELLOSIS

Primary cutaneous (ulceroglandular) infection due to *Pasteurella hemolytica* was reported by Muraschi, et al. It occurred in a woman who acquired numerous lacerations on the hands from berry bushes while hunting and later dressed a deer. The lacerations became inflamed, lymphangitis developed, and her axillary lymph nodes were enlarged. There was moderate fever. From the exudate of a papular lesion of the finger *P. hemolytica* was isolated in pure culture. *P. hemolytica* is a common pathogen of domestic animals, being associated with shipping fever in cattle and septicemia in lambs and newborn pigs.

Pasteurella Multocida Infections

Pasteurella multocida is a small, nonmotile, gram-negative, bipolar-staining bacterium known to be an animal pathogen. The most common type of human infection follows injuries from animal bites, principally cat and dog bites, but also cat scratches. Following animal trauma, erythema, swelling, pain, and tenderness develop within a few hours of the bite, with a gray-colored serous or sanguineopurulent drainage from the puncture wounds. There may or may not be regional lymphadenopathy or evidence of systemic toxicity such as chills and fever. Septicemia may follow the local infection in rare cases, and tenosynovitis and osteomyelitis appear with some frequency. It is recommended that all cat bites and scratches, all sutured wounds of any animal source, and any other animal injuries of an unusual type or source should be treated with systemic penicillin or tetracycline in addition to careful cleansing and tetanus prophylaxis.

Though a gram-negative bacillus, *P. multocida* is highly sensitive to penicillin.

Tindall JP, et al: *Pasteurella multocida* infections following animal injuries, especially cat bites. Arch Dermatol 1972, 105:412.

DF-2 SEPTICEMIA

DF-2, a newly identified gram-negative rod, is associated with severe septicemia after dog bites. Patients who have undergone splenectomy are at particular risk. A characteristic finding is a necrotizing eschar at the site of the bite. Fever, nausea, and vomiting occur abruptly within one to three days, and the eschar develops soon thereafter. Disseminated intravascular coagulation and extensive dry gangrene may complicate the course. DF-2 sepsis after a dog bite is another hazard splenectomized patients face in addition to their particular problems with pneumococcus, *Haemophilus influenzae* group B, babesiosis, *Neisseria meningitidis*, and group A streptococcus.

Westerink et al isolated DF-2 from the blood of a previously healthy man with fever, headache, rash, and thrombocytopenia in 1987. He had a false-positive latex agglutination test for cryptococcal antigen in the spinal fluid.

Treatment is with intensive intravenous antibiotics. DF-2 is reported to be susceptible to penicillin, clindamycin, cephalosporins, erythromycin, and tetracycline.

Kalb R, et al: Cutaneous infection at dog bite wounds associated with fulminant DF-2 septicemia. Am J Med 1985, 78:687.

Westerink JMA et al: Septicemia due to DF-2: Cause of a false-positive cryptococcal latex agglutination result. Am J Med 1987, 83:155.

CAT-SCRATCH DISEASE

CLINICAL FEATURES. *Localized cat-scratch disease* is characterized by a red papule appearing three to 12 days following a cat scratch, followed by the development of a single enlarged lymph node that is tender and may suppurate.

The primary red papule, vesicle, or pustule is found in 50 to 90 per cent of the patients. If inoculation is on the eyelids, palpebral conjunctivitis and preauricular adenopathy occur. This unusual presentation is called the *oculoglandular syndrome of Parinaud*. The primary lesion is noncrusted, and lymphangitis does not extend from the lesion. There is a resemblance to an insect bite; however, there is no itching. Healing of the single lesion (or at most several) usually occurs within two weeks without residual scarring.

Lymphadenitis is invariably present and is usually the presenting sign. The node enlargement occurs some 10 to 50 days after inoculation (average 17 days). The enlarged node may progress to suppuration (10 to 50 per cent of cases). There may be local redness and tenderness. Fifty per cent of adenopathy occurs from the upper extremity, 25 per cent from the neck or jaw, and 18 per cent from the leg. General lymphadenopathy does not occur; however, fever, malaise, and anorexia may be present.

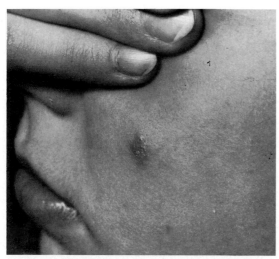

Figure 14–39. Disseminated cat-scratch disease.

Atypical manifestations of cat-scratch disease are oculoglandular syndrome of Parinaud, thrombocytopenic purpura, osteolytic lesions, pneumonitis, central nervous system involvement, and various skin lesions. The skin eruptions include erythema multiforme, erythema nodosum, and in 5 per cent of cases, an erythematous, nonpruritic, maculopapular generalized exanthem, which lasts for five to 14 days and involutes spontaneously.

Disseminated cat-scratch disease has been recognized recently. First named epithelioid hemangiomatosis because of the characteristic vascular proliferations, it is now known that the same organism causes both the localized and disseminated diseases.

Systemic toxicity, bone lesions, and friable exophytic angiomatous nodules 5 to 40 mm in diameter occur in immunocompromised patients. Occasionally there is a deep subcutaneous mass with skin changes resembling those seen in cellulitis. The article by Koehler et al includes a summary of reports to date.

LABORATORY FINDINGS. Routine laboratory tests are not usually helpful in establishing the diagnosis. Most patients have a positive skin test reaction to cat-scratch antigen (Hanger and Rose test). Skin testing should be performed at least one week following the appearance of adenitis: otherwise false negative tests are likely. Carithers reported 99 per cent positive skin tests in 1200 patients tested.

ETIOLOGY. In 1983 Wear et al reported finding pleomorphic gram-negative bacilli in 29 of 34 patients' lymph nodes. Margileth et al subsequently identified a similar bacterium in the primary lesions of three patients. Gerber et al have isolated an organism which they believe may be the same bacterium. Its classification is uncertain, but it may be *Rothia* spp. English et al were able to fulfill Koch's postulates in 1988, proving that this bacterium is the cause of cat-scratch disease.

EPIDEMIOLOGY. Most of the patients with localized disease are children and young adults. Although the disease has been reported after pin or splinter scratches, it is believed that contact with cats has preceded infection in most patients and that inoculation from other sources is experienced only rarely. Cat-scratch fever occurs throughout the world.

Although disseminated disease occurs chiefly in patients with AIDS, occasional cases have occurred in otherwise healthy individuals.

HISTOPATHOLOGY. The typical node contains multiple abscesses with necrotic centers surrounded by epithelioid cells, some giant cells, and eosinophils. The primary skin lesion, according to Johnson and Helwig, also has central necrosis surrounded by histiocytes, giant cells, and lymphocytes. The gram-negative organisms are best seen by the Warthin-Starry stain.

DIFFERENTIAL DIAGNOSIS. Localized cat-scratch disease lymphadenopathy differs from that of infectious mononucleosis and lymphoma by being unilateral. Other diseases with lymphadenitis that may require differentiation are suppurative bacterial lymphadenitis, atypical mycobacterial infection, tularemia, histoplasmosis, brucellosis, and mycotic infections such as sporotrichosis. Disseminated cat-scratch disease is primarily to be differentiated from Kaposi's sarcoma.

TREATMENT. Localized cat-scratch disease is a relatively benign disease, usually running its course in a few weeks with few or no symptoms. The administration of antimicrobials has no effect on the course of the illness. Fluctuant lymph nodes should be aspirated by a needle and syringe rather than incised.

Disseminated cat-scratch disease is cured rapidly by erythromycin, doxycycline, or antimycobacterial antibiotics.

Carithers HA: Cat-scratch disease. AJDC 1985, 139:1124.
Idem: Oculoglandular syndrome of Parinaud. Am J Dis Child 1978, 132:1195.
Cockerell CJ, et al: Epithelioid angiomatosis. Lancet 1987, 2:654.
Emmons RW: Cat-scratch disease. Ann Intern Med 1984, 100:303.
English CK, et al: Cat-scratch disease. JAMA 1988, 259:1347.
Gerber MA, et al: The aetiological agent of cat scratch disease. Lancet 1985, 1:1236.
Kitchell CC, et al: Bacillary organisms in cat-scratch disease. N Engl J Med 1985, 313:1090.
Knobler EH, et al: Unique vascular skin lesions associated with human immunodeficiency virus. JAMA 1988, 260:524.
Koehler JE, et al: Cutaneous vascular lesions and disseminated cat-scratch disease in patients with the acquired immunodeficiency syndrome and AIDS-related complex. Ann Intern Med 1988, 109:449.
LeBoit PE, et al: Epithelioid haemangioma-like vascular proliferations in AIDS. Lancet 1988, 1:960.
Margileth AM, et al: Cat scratch disease. JAMA 1984, 252:928.
Wear DJ, et al: Cat scratch disease. Science 1983, 221:1403.

GLANDERS

Once known as **equinia, farcy**, and **malleus**, glanders is a rare, usually fatal, infectious disease that occurs in man by inoculation with *Pseudomonas mallei*. It is encountered in those who handle horses, mules, or donkeys.

The distinctive skin lesion is an inflammatory papule or vesicle that arises at the site of inoculation, rapidly becomes nodular, pustular, and ulcerative, and forms an irregular excavation with undermined edges and a base covered with a purulent and sanguineous exudate. In the course of a few days or weeks other nodules (called "farcy buds") develop along the lymphatics in the adjacent skin or subcutaneous tissues; subsequently these break down. In the acute form the skin involvement may be severe and accompanied by grave diarrhea. In the chronic form there are few skin lesions and milder constitutional symptoms, but repeated cycles of healing and breakdown of nodules may occur for weeks.

The respiratory mucous membranes are especially susceptible to the disease. After accidental inhalation, first catarrhal symptoms are present and there may be epistaxis or a mucoid nasal discharge. The nasal discharge is a characteristic feature of the disease.

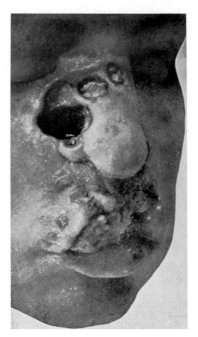

Figure 14–40. Human glanders; duration, 4 months. Note carbuncular lesion on upper lip and farcy buds. Patient was a groom. (Courtesy of Army Medical Museum.)

The diagnosis is established by finding the gram-negative *P. mallei* in this discharge or in the skin ulcers, and should be confirmed by serum agglutination. This organism has been fatal to many laboratory workers, but it is now rare in this country.

Treatment is chiefly by immediate surgical excision of the inoculated lesions and by streptomycin plus a tetracycline.

Howe C, et al: Human glanders. Ann Intern Med 1947, 26:93.

MELIOIDOSIS

Melioidosis (Whitmore's disease) is a specific infection caused by a glanderslike bacillus, *Pseudomonas pseudomallei*. The disease has an acute pulmonary and septicemic form with multiple miliary abscesses in the viscera and ends in early death. Less often it runs a chronic course, with subcutaneous abscesses and multiple sinuses of the soft tissues. Its clinical characteristics are similar to glanders disseminated fungal infections, and tuberculosis. Steck and Byrd have observed severe urticaria occurring with pulmonary melioidosis. The urticaria disappeared after one week of tetracycline therapy. Flemma and his associates reported 15 patients with positive cultures for *P. pseudomallei* who had suffered burns in Southeast Asia. About 80 per cent of these also had pulmonary melioidosis.

It is endemic in Southeast Asia and should be suspected in military and other personnel who have characteristic symptoms of a febrile illness and have been in that region.

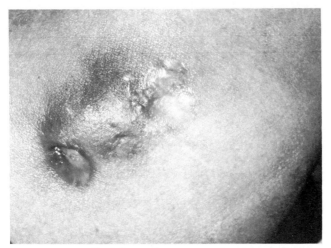

Figure 14–41. Draining subcutaneous abscesses and sinuses caused by melioidosis. (Courtesy of Dr. Axel W. Hoke.)

The diagnosis is made from the recovery of the bacillus from the skin lesions or sputum, and by serologic tests.

Effective therapy is determined by the antibiotic sensitivity of the specific strain. The majority of infections respond well to tetracyclines in doses of 2 to 3 gm daily for at least 30 days. Trimethoprim-sulfamethoxazole is also effective.

McDonnell F, et al: Melioidosis. JAMA 1947, 134:361.
Steck WD, et al: Urticaria secondary to pulmonary melioidosis. Arch Dermatol 1969, 99:80.

BARTONELLOSIS (Verruga Peruana)

Synonyms: Carrión's disease, Peruvian wart, Oroya fever, bartonelliasis, Guántara fever.

CLINICAL FEATURES. Verruga peruana is an infectious constitutional disease caused by *Bartonella bacilliformis*. The disease occurs in two stages.

Oroya fever, the acute febrile stage, has no cutaneous lesions other than the initial insect bite at the site of inoculation. This stage is followed by a delayed chronic stage, the chief feature of which is the verrucous cutaneous eruption known as verruga peruana (peruviana).

Oroya fever has an incubation period of 16 to 22 days, during which there is some malaise and mild fever. The onset is characterized by rapidly progressing hemolytic anemia, high fever, pains in the muscles, and weakness. Forty per cent of cases of untreated bartonellasis die in the anemic stage. The blood count may drop in three days from normal to 1,000,000 erythrocytes, and there may be either an increase or decrease in the leukocytes, together with the appearance of immature forms. Thrombocytopenic purpura may also occur. The majority of patients who recover from the febrile anemic stage of Oroya fever develop multiple, cherry-red, hard, verrucous lesions one to six months afterward.

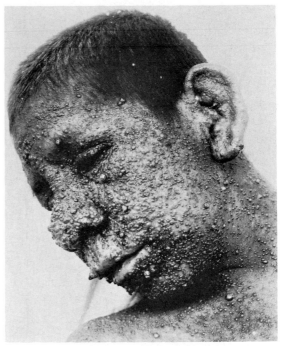

Figure 14–42. Verruga peruana showing small nodules that cover face and body. (Courtesy of Dr. P. Weiss.)

The *miliary lesions* are pinhead- to pea-sized and appear chiefly on the face and the extensor aspects of the extremities. The lesions are discrete and may be sessile or pedunculated; sometimes they are confluent. They are cherry-red and at first hard and shotty. After several months the lesions eventually disappear without a trace. Their clinical appearance resembles yaws, pyogenic granuloma, cherry angioma, or hemangiomas; it is frequently possible to identify lesions similar to each of these diseases on one patient.

The *nodular type* begins in the subcutaneous tissue over the elbows and knees, where it forms an ovoid growth that stretches the overlying skin, at times reaching a diameter of 1 or 2 cm. They are more chronic than the miliary lesions. The *mular* type may evolve from the nodular type. It is almost always associated with ulceration of the overlying skin, and has the appearance of an irregularly lobulated, highly vascular tumor, which occasionally may be as large as a small apple and bleed severely if traumatized. Such lesions usually heal in a few weeks, however, and this stage of the disease is rarely fatal. The eruption may involve all the mucous membranes, coming out in crops and at times causing severe hemorrhages.

ETIOLOGY. A gram-negative, rod-shaped organism, *Bartonella bacilliformis*, is the causative agent. It has been demonstrated in the blood during the preeruptive period and in the endothelial cells of the tumors. It was first cultivated by Battistini in 1925. By experimental inoculation in man and monkeys the disease has been reproduced in its two forms by *Bartonella* taken directly from the blood of patients, or from their skin nodules or from cultures.

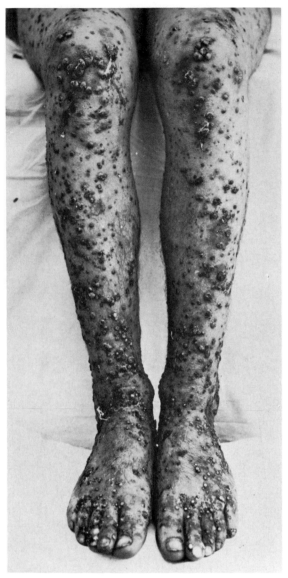

Figure 14–43. Verruga peruana showing verrucous nodules on legs. (Courtesy of Drs. O. Canizares and H. Fox.)

HISTOLOGY. The nodule is characterized by the formation of new blood vessels, proliferation of angioblastic cells, and an inflammatory infiltrate consisting of plasma cells, and leukocytes. The bacteria may be seen on Giemsa-stained sections in the cytoplasm of cells which line the vascular spaces.

DIAGNOSIS. In the preeruptive stage the diagnosis is established by the combination of fever, anemia, asthenia, joint pains, adenopathy, and the presence of the parasites in the blood. In the eruptive stage the manifestations are typical and, once seen, cannot be mistaken for any other eruption. Demonstration of the microorganisms on the surface of erythrocytes or in blood cultures confirms the diagnosis. The organisms can also be identified and cultured from the verruga.

TREATMENT. Prophylaxis is all-important. Spraying with insecticides, avoidance of sandfly-infested areas after sundown and at sunrise, and use of repellents and protective clothing are helpful measures. Because infection with *Salmonella* is a particularly common complication, chloramphenicol, which is effective against both *Bartonella* and *Salmonella*, is the antimicrobial of choice. The cutaneous lesions show a variable response with antibiotics, but eventual healing with fibrosis is the rule.

Reynafarje C, et al: The hemolytic anemia of human bartonellosis. Blood 1961, 17:562.
Ricketts WE: Clinical manifestations of Carrion's disease. Arch Intern Med 1949, 842:751.
Idem: Carrion's disease. Am J Trop Med 1947, 27:657.

The chief vectors are the sandflies *Phlebotomus noguchi* and *P. verrucarum,* which are active only in twilight. Man is probably the reservoir, since *B. bacilliformis* can be isolated from healthy adults or those who have recovered from infection. This carrier state is poorly understood.

INCIDENCE AND PREVALENCE. It is endemic in certain valleys in the central part of Peru, Ecuador, and Colombia, being strictly limited to the altitudes between 700 and 2500 meters. It occurs mostly toward the close of the rainy season, between January and April.

A lasting immunity is established by the disease. A mild attack in infancy or childhood gives permanent protection and probably accounts for the resistance to bartonellosis in the indigenous population. Outsiders who go to these valleys at night run grave danger.

PLAGUE

Plague normally involves an interaction among *Yersinia pestis,* wild rodents, and fleas parasitic on the rodents. Infection in humans with *Y. pestis* is accidental and presents usually as bubonic plague. Other clinical forms include pneumonic and septicemic plague.

In the milder form, the initial manifestations are general malaise, fever, and pain or tenderness in areas of regional lymph nodes, most often in the inguinal or axillary regions. In more severe infections, findings of toxicity, prostration, shock, and, occasionally, hemorrhagic phenomena prevail. Less common symptoms include abdominal pain, nausea, vomiting, constipation followed by diarrhea, generalized macular erythema, and petechiae. Rarely, vesicular and pustular skin lesions occur.

Plague is caused by a pleomorphic gram-negative bacillus, *Yersinia pestis.* The principal animal hosts involved have been rock squirrels, prairie dogs, chipmunks, marmots, skunks, deer mice, wood rats, rabbits, and hares. Transmission occurs through contact with infected rodent fleas or rodents, pneumonic spread, or infected exudates. *Xenopsylla cheopis* (Oriental rat flea) has traditionally been considered the vector in human outbreaks, but *Diamanus montanus*, *Chrassis bacchi*, and *Opisocrostis hirsutus* are species of fleas on wild animals responsible for spreading sylvatic plague in the U.S. Rodents carried home by dogs or cats are a potential source—and an important one in veterinarians—of infection. In the United States, 89 per cent of cases since 1945 have occurred in the Rocky Mountain states.

Blood, bubo or parabubo aspirates, exudates, and sputum should be examined by smears stained with Gram's stain or specific fluorescent antibody techniques, culture, and animal inoculation. A retrospective diagnosis can be made by serologic analysis.

The most effective drug against *Y. pestis* is streptomycin. It should be given in doses of 2 gm daily intramuscularly for 10 days. Other effective drugs include kanamycin, chloramphenicol, the tetracyclines, and certain sulfonamides. Nearly all cases are fatal if not treated promptly.

Finegold MJ: Pathogenesis of plague. Am J Med 1978, 45:549.
Scott DW, et al: Zoonotic dermatoses of dogs and cats. Vet Clin North Am 1987, 17:117.

RAT-BITE FEVER

This febrile systemic illness is usually acquired by direct contact with rats or other small rodents, which carry the gram-negative organisms *Spirillum minor* and *Streptobacillus moniliformis* among their oropharyngeal flora. *S. moniliformis* is the principal cause in the U.S., and bites of laboratory rats are an increasing source of infection. There is evidence that this disease has been known in India for two thousand years, and it is known throughout the world. Although the disease usually follows a rat bite, it may follow the bites of squirrels, cats, weasels, pigs, and a variety of other carnivores which feed on rats.

There are at least two distinct forms of rat-bite fever: 1) "sodoku," caused by *Spirillum minus* and 2) septicemia, produced by *Streptobacillus moniliformis*, otherwise known as epidemic arthritic erythema or Haverhill fever. This follows the bite of a rat, but other cases have been caused by contaminated milk (Haverhill fever). The clinical manifestations of these two infections are similar in that both produce a systemic illness characterized by fever, rash, and constitutional symptoms. However, clinical differentiation is possible.

In the streptobacillary form, incubation is brief, usually lasting 10 days after the bite, when chills and fever occur. Within two to four more days the generalized morbilliform eruption appears and spreads to include the palms and soles. It may become petechial. Arthralgia is prominent, and pleural effusion may occur. Endocarditis, pneumonia, and septic infarcts may occur, and 10 per cent of untreated cases may die from these causes.

While infection with *Sp. minor* also begins abruptly with chills and fever, the incubation period is longer, ranging from one to four weeks. The bite site is often inflamed and may become ulcerated, and lymphangitis occurs. The eruption begins with erythematous macules on the abdomen, resembling rose spots, which enlarge, become purplish red, and form extensive indurated plaques. Arthritis may rarely occur. Endocarditis, nephritis, meningitis, and hepatitis are potential complications. Six per cent of untreated cases die.

In both types of disease a leukocytosis of 15 to 30 thousand occurs, sometimes with eosinophilia. A biologic false-positive VDRL occurs in 25 to 50 per cent. The course without treatment is generally from one to two weeks, though relapses may occur for months.

The diagnosis is confirmed by culturing the causative organism from the blood or joint aspirate, or demonstration of an antibody response in the streptobacillary form.

Spirillum minus is demonstrable by animal inoculation with the patient's blood, usually in the guinea pig or mouse. Their blood will show large numbers of organisms in Wright-stained smears. Demonstration of *S. minus* in a darkfield preparation of exudate from an infected site establishes the diagnosis.

Rat-bite fever must be differentiated from erysipelas, pyogenic cellulitis, viral exanthems, gonococcemia, meningococcemia, and Rocky Mountain spotted fever.

Prompt cauterization of bites by nitric acid may prevent the disease. Cleansing of the wound, tetanus prophylaxis, and three days of penicillin (2 gm per day) are recommended for patients seen shortly after a bite. Both types respond readily to penicillin, tetracycline, or streptomycin therapy.

Cole JS, et al: Rat bite fever. Ann Intern Med 1969, 71:979.
Lambe DW, et al: *Streptobacillus moniliformis* isolated from a case of Haverhill fever. Am J Clin Pathol 1973, 60:854.
Portnoy BL, et al: Rat-bite fever misdiagnosed as Rocky Mountain spotted fever. South Med J 1979, 72:607.
Raffin BJ, et al: Streptobacillary rat bite fever. Pediatrics 1979, 64:214.

TULAREMIA

Synonyms: Ohara's disease, deerfly fever.

CLINICAL FEATURES. Tularemia is a febrile disease produced by *Francisella tularensis*; it is characterized by sudden onset, with chills, headache, and leukocytosis, after an incubation period of two to seven days. Its clinical course is divided into several general types.

The large majority are the **ulceroglandular type,** which begins with a primary papule or nodule that rapidly ulcerates at the site of infection, through contact with tissues or body fluid of infected mam-

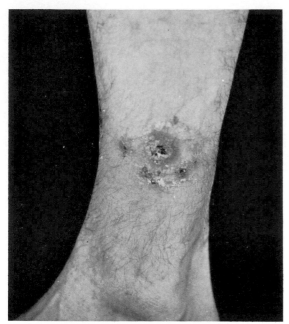

Figure 14–44. Tularemia above ankle: primary lesion. (Courtesy of Armed Forces Institute of Pathology.)

mals, via an abrasion or scratch, usually on the fingers, neck, or conjunctiva. The bites of a tick, *Dermacentor andersoni* or *Amblyomma americanum*, and of a deerfly, *Chrysops discalis*, transmit this type of disease also, in which case primary lesions are usually found on the legs or the perineum. The primary

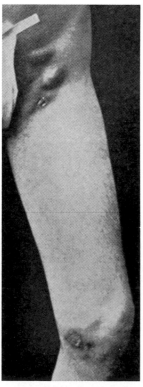

Figure 14–45. Tularemia following tick bite on left knee. Note enlargement of left inguinal glands. (Courtesy of Drs. T. B. Magath and W. M. Yater.)

ulcer is tender, firm, indolent, and punched-out, with a necrotic base that heals with scar formation in about six weeks. A lymphangitis spreads from the primary lesion; the regional lymph glands become swollen, painful, and inflamed, and tend to break down, forming subcutaneous suppurative nodules resembling those of sporotrichosis. The ulcers extend in a chain from the ulcer to the enlarged lymphatic glands.

The course of the ulceroglandular type is marked in the early stages by headache, anorexia, and vomiting, and by articular and muscular pains. The fever is at first continuous, varying between 102 and 104° F., and later shows morning remissions, and then falls by lysis to normal. Other skin lesions are encountered in the course of the disease, which are in no way characteristic and are probably of a toxic nature. A macular, papular, vesicular, or petechial exanthem may occur. Erythema multiforme and erythema nodosum often occur, as documented by Syrjälä et al. The clinical similarity of the primary ulcer of tularemia to a chancre of *sporotrichosis, cat-scratch disease,* or *Pasteurella infections* is important in differential diagnosis.

In the **typhoidal type** the site of inoculation is not known and there is no local sore or adenopathy. This form of the disease is characterized by persistent fever, malaise, gastrointestinal symptoms, and the presence of specific agglutinins in the blood serum after the first week.

In addition to these two types, there is the **oculoglandular type**, in which primary conjunctivitis is accompanied by enlargement of the regional lymph nodes.

The **pneumonic** form occurs rarely in laboratory workers, and is most severe. The **oropharyngeal** form may occur after ingestion of infected and inadequately cooked meat.

In the **glandular type** there is no primary lesion at the site of infection, but there is enlargement of the regional lymph glands. The glandular involvement may become general.

Several cases, mostly in children, have been acquired from cat bites, the cats having previously bitten infected rabbits.

ETIOLOGY. Tularemia is caused by *Francisella tularensis,* a short, nonmotile, nonsporeforming, gram-negative coccobacillus.

EPIDEMIOLOGY. The most frequent sources of human infection are the handling of wild rabbits and the bite of deerflies or ticks. No instance of the spread of the infection from man to man by contact has been reported; it is apparently noncontagious. Outbreaks of the disease occur chiefly at those times of the year when contact with these sources of infection is likely.

The disease occurs chiefly in the western and southern United States, although cases have been reported in almost all parts of the United States and in Japan. In Russia and other countries in the northern hemisphere the disease may be contracted from polluted water contaminated by infected rodent carcasses.

DIAGNOSIS. A definite diagnosis is made by staining the exudate smears with specific fluorescent antibody. *F. tularensis* can be cultured only on special media containing cystine glucose blood agar, or other selective media. Routine culture media do not support growth. The bacilli can be identified by inoculating guinea pigs intraperitoneally with sputum or with bronchial or gastric washings, exudate from draining lymph nodes, or blood.

Agglutination test is the most reliable diagnostic procedure. The titer becomes positive in the majority of patients after two weeks of illness. A fourfold rise in titer is diagnostic; a single convalescent titer of 1:160 or greater is diagnostic of past or current infection.

HISTOPATHOLOGY. The main histologic feature of tularemia is that of a granuloma; the tissue reaction consists primarily of a massing of endothelial cells and the formation of giant cells. Central necrosis and liquefaction occurs accompanied by polymorphonuclear leukocytic infiltration. Surrounding this is a tuberculoid granulomatous zone, and peripherally lymphocytes form a third zone. Small secondary lesions may develop. These pass through the same stages and tend to fuse with the primary one.

PROPHYLAXIS. All market men, hunters, cooks, and others who dress rabbits should wear rubber gloves when doing so. Thorough cooking destroys the infection in a rabbit, thus rendering an infected animal harmless as food. Ticks should be removed promptly, and tick repellents may be of value for people with occupations which require frequent exposure to them.

TREATMENT. Streptomycin, 0.5 gm intramuscularly every 12 hours for 10 days, is the treatment of choice. Obvious clinical improvement occurs after 48 hours, although the fever may persist for as long as a week after treatment is begun. Gentamicin is also effective, but the tetracyclines are useful only if given in doses of 2 gm daily for 15 days.

Gallivas MVE, et al: Fatal cat-transmitted tularemia. South Med J 1980, 73:240.
Kaiser AB, et al: Tularemia and rhabdomyolysis. JAMA 1985, 253:241.
Markowitz LE: Tick-borne tularemia. JAMA 1984, 254:2922.
Sanford JP: Tularemia. JAMA 1983, 250:3225.
Syrjälä H, et al: Skin manifestations of tularemia. Acta Derm Venereol (Stockh) 1984, 64:513.

BRUCELLOSIS (Undulant Fever)

Brucellae are gram-negative rods which produce an acute febrile illness with headache, or at times an indolent chronic disease characterized by weakness, malaise, and low-grade fever. It is acquired primarily by contact with infected animals or animal products. Primarily workers in the meat packing industry are at risk; however, veterinarians, pet owners, and travelers who eat unpasteurized milk or cheese may also acquire the disease.

Approximately 5 to 10 per cent of patients develop skin lesions. The variety of cutaneous manifestations reported is large, and has been reviewed by Berger et al. Erythematous papules, diffuse erythema, abscesses, erysipelaslike lesions, and erythema nodosum are some possible findings. Biopsy may reveal noncaseating granulomas.

Diagnosis is by culture of blood, bone marrow, or granulomas, and may be confirmed by a rising serum agglutination titer. Treatment with tetracycline or in combination with streptomycin results in prompt improvement.

Ariza J, et al: Characteristic cutaneous lesions of brucellosis. Arch Dermatol 1989, 125:380.
Berger TG, et al: Cutaneous lesions in brucellosis. Arch Dermatol 1981, 117:40.
Bertrand F, et al: Cutaneous manifestations of brucellosis. Sem Hôp Paris 1985, 61:881.
Yao JD, et al: Brucellosis and sinus histiocytosis with massive lymphadenopathy. Am J Med 1989, 86:111.

RICKETTSIAL DISEASES

It has been established that the rickettsiae are true bacteria. The natural reservoirs of these organisms are the blood-sucking arthropods; when transmitted to man through insect inoculation, the rickettsiae may produce disease. Most of the human diseases incurred are characterized by skin eruptions, fever, headache, malaise, and prostration. Those with skin manifestations are discussed here.

TYPHUS GROUP

Louse-borne **epidemic typhus** caused by *Rickettsia prowazekii*, and murine or cat or rat flea-borne **en**demic typhus, caused by *R. typhi* (formerly *R. mooseri*) constitute this group.

Epidemic Typhus

This is contracted by man from an infestation by body lice (*Pediculus humanus var. corporis*), which harbor the rickettsiae. *R. prowazekii* is not transmitted transovarially, as it kills the louse one to three weeks after infection. Until recently man was the only known vector, but several cases of sporadic disease have been reported in which there was direct or indirect contact with the flying squirrel, and a reservoir apparently exists in this animal. While the louse feeds on the man's skin, it defecates. The organisms in the feces are scratched into the skin. Some two weeks after infection the prodromal symptoms of chills, fever, aches, and pains appear. After five days a pink macular eruption appears on the trunk and axillary folds and rapidly spreads to the rest of the body, but usually spares the face, palms, and soles. These macules may later become hemorrhagic, and gangrene of the fingers, toes, nose, and ear lobes may occur. Mortality is from 6 to 30 per cent in epidemics, with the highest death and complication rates occurring in patients over 60.

Agglutinins for OX-19 and complement fixing antibodies are demonstrable after the eighth to twelfth day of illness.

Treatment is with tetracyclines. Doxycycline in a single dose of 100 mg orally is effective. Alternatively 25 mg/kg of oral tetracycline is given daily until three to four days after defervescence. Prophylaxis is by vaccination and delousing; people who succumb are usually living under miserable sanitary conditions such as occur during war and following natural disasters. Vaccination is suggested for only special high-risk groups.

Brill-Zinsser disease may occur as a recrudescence of previous infection, with a similar, but milder course of illness, which more closely resembles murine typhus.

Endemic Typhus

Endemic (murine) typhus is a natural infection of rats (and mice), sporadically transmitted to man by the rat flea, *Xenopsylla cheopis*. It has the same skin manifestations as epidemic typhus, but they are less severe, and petechiae and gangrene do not supervene. The OX-19 test is also positive and the complement fixation test helps in making the diagnosis. Fever and severe headache are suggestive early symptoms.

This disease occurs worldwide. In the United States the southeastern states and those bordering the Gulf of Mexico have been the commonest sites of incidence. It most often occurs in urban settings, with peak incidence in the summer and fall.

Treatment is the same as that of louse-borne (epidemic) typhus.

SPOTTED FEVER GROUP

To this group belong **Rocky Mountain spotted fever** caused by *R. rickettsii*; tick typhus such as Mediterranean (**boutonneuse**) fever and **South African tick-bite fever** caused by *R. conorii*; North Asian tick-borne **rickettsiosis** caused by *R. siberica*; Queensland **tick typhus** caused by *R. australis*; and **rickettsialpox** and Russian **vesicular rickettsiosis** caused by *R. akari*.

Rocky Mountain Spotted Fever

One to two weeks after the tick bite, there will be chills, fever, and weakness. An eruption appears, unlike typhus in that it begins on the ankles, wrists, and forehead rather than on the trunk. The initial lesions are small red macules, which blanch on pressure, and rapidly become papular in untreated patients.

A vasculitis of the skin is the pathologic process, and *Rickettsia rickettsii* can be found in these initial macules by applying a fluorescent antibody technique to frozen sections, as shown by Woodward et al. Oster found this a very specific, but not very sensitive, method.

In the 20 per cent or so of cases without a rash, the risk of a delay in diagnosis and a fatal outcome is greatest, with the case fatality rate rising precipitously if antibiotics are not initiated prior to the fifth day. Mortality in old persons approaches 60 per cent; it is far lower in young patients. Tetracycline or chloramphenicol, given early, is almost always effective. In all of the 10 fatal cases in the series reported by Walker and Mattern, multifocal perivascular interstitial nephritis was the principal pathologic lesion.

The causative organism, *R. rickettsii*, is spread by ixodid ticks, one or another species of which is found in all parts of the United States and in scattered pockets in Canada and Mexico. Principal offenders are the wood tick, *Dermacentor andersoni*, the dog tick, *D. variabilis*, and the Lone Star tick, *Amblyomma americanum*.

Antibodies to *Proteus* OX-2 and OX-19 become positive in the second or third week of illness, too late to be of help when the decision to institute therapy is necessary. This decision is usually made by clinical considerations.

The treatment is high doses of tetracycline, 25 to 50 mg/kg per day, or chloramphenicol, 50 mg/kg per day, with tetracycline being preferred. Medication should be continued for two to three days after the temperature returns to normal, the usual course being five to seven days.

Ehrlichiosis

A similar illness caused by a closely related rickettsia, *Ehrlichia canis*, but with only a 20 per cent incidence of an eruption, has been seen with increased frequency in the southeastern and south central U.S. It appears to be tick borne, is most common in men between 30 and 60, and is responsive to tetracycline.

Tick Typhus

This is a collective name for the varieties described previously. **Boutonneuse fever** or **Mediterranean fever** is an acute febrile disease endemic in southern

Europe and northern Africa and is the prototype of these diseases. It affects children mostly and is characterized by a sudden onset with chills, high fever, headache, and lassitude. The tick bite produces a small indurated papule known as *tache noir*, which becomes a necrotic ulcer. A macular or maculopapular eruption develops on the trunk and palms and soles.

The causative organism is *R. conorii*, transmitted by the dog tick, *Rhipicephalus sanguineus*.

Similar clinical manifestations are seen with the other diseases mentioned. All have type-specific antigens and can be identified by the complement fixation and neutralization tests. The OX-19 and OX-2 Weil-Felix reactions are positive.

Treatment with tetracycline or chloramphenicol is effective. Even without therapy the prognosis is good and complications are rare.

Rickettsialpox

First recognized in New York in 1946, rickettsialpox has been found in other cities of the United States and in Russia.

Rickettsialpox is an acute febrile disease characterized by the appearance of an initial lesion at the site of the mite bite about a week before the onset of the fever and by the appearance of a rash resembling

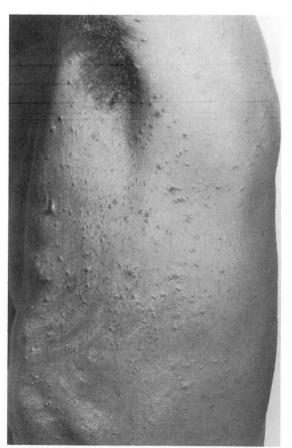

Figure 14–46. Rickettsialpox. (Courtesy of Dr. M. Liebman.)

varicella three or four days after the development of fever. The fever is accompanied by chills, sweats, headache, and backache. The fever is remittent and lasts for about five days. The initial lesions are firm, round or oval vesicles 5 to 15 mm in size. They are accompanied by a regional lymphadenitis. This initial lesion persists three to four weeks and leaves a small pigmented scar. The secondary eruption appears 24 to 96 hours after the fever begins and fades in about one week. Generalized lymphadenopathy and enlargement of the spleen may occur but are rarely encountered.

The causative organism, *R. akari*, is transmitted by the rodent mite, *Allodermanyssus sanguineus*. The house mouse (*Mus musculus*) is the reservoir. All cases have occurred in neighborhoods infested by mice, on which the rodent mite has been found.

Complement fixation tests demonstrate the antibodies of this disease. The Weil-Felix test is negative.

The disease is self-limited, and complete involution occurs in at most two weeks.

Tetracyclines are the agents of choice for treatment.

Burnett JW: Rickettsioses. JAAD 1980, 2:359.
D'Angelo J, et al: Rocky Mountain spotted fever in the United States. South Med J 1982, 75:3.
Durack DT: Spotted fever comes to town. N Engl J Med 1988, 318:1388.
Eubanks SW: The rickettsioses. J Assoc Milit Dermatol 1983, 9:32.
Harris RL, et al: Boutonneuse fever in travelers. J Infect Dis 1986, 153:126.
Hattwich MAW: Rocky Mountain spotted fever. Ann Intern Med 1976, 84:732.
Human ehrlichiosis. Arch Dermatol 1988, 124:993.
McDonald JC, et al: Imported Rickettsial disease. Am J Med 1988, 85:795.
Oster CN, et al: Laboratory-acquired Rocky Mountain spotted fever. N Engl J Med 1977, 297:859.
Raoult D, et al: Mediterranean spotted fever. Ann Dermatol Venereol 1983, 110:909.
Salgo MP, et al: A form of Rocky Mountain spotted fever within New York City. N Engl J Med 1988, 318:1345.
Walker DH, et al: The occurrence of eschars in Rocky Mountain spotted fever. JAAD 1981, 4:571.
Wong B, et al: Rickettsialpox. JAMA 1979, 242:1998.

SCRUB TYPHUS

Also known as tsutsugamushi fever, this disease is characterized by fever, chills, intense headache, skin lesions, and pneumonitis.

Some 10 days after a mite bite, fever, chills, and prostration develop and within five days thereafter pneumonitis and the skin eruption evolve. The erythematous macular eruption begins on the trunk, extends peripherally, and fades in a few days. Deafness and tinnitus occur in about a fifth of untreated cases.

An erythematous papule at the site of the bite becomes indurated and a multilocular vesicle rests on top of the papule. Eventually a necrotic ulcer with eschar develops and there is regional lymphadenopathy.

Scrub typhus is caused by *R. tsutsugamushi*. The vector is the trombiculid red mite (chigger) that infests wild rodents in scrub or secondary vegetation in transitional terrain between forests and clearings, in Far Eastern countries such as Japan, Korea, Southeast Asia, and Australia.

Antibodies to OX-K proteus antigen occur in 50 per cent of patients by the second week, and are rather specific for this disease, although cross reactivity does occur in leptospirosis. Treatment is as for other forms of rickettsiasis.

LEPTOSPIROSIS

Leptospirosis is also known as Weil's disease, pretibial fever, and Fort Bragg fever.

This is a systemic disease caused by many strains of the genus *Leptospira*. After an incubation period of eight to 12 days, **Weil's disease** (icteric leptospirosis) starts with an abrupt onset of chills, followed by high fever, intense jaundice, petechiae, and purpura on both skin and mucous membranes, and renal disease, manifested by proteinuria, hematuria, and azotemia. Death may occur in 5 to 10 per cent of cases, due to renal failure, vascular collapse, or hemorrhage. Leukocytosis of 15,000 to 30,000, and lymphocytosis in the spinal fluid, are commonly present.

Pretibial fever ("Fort Bragg fever," anicteric leptospirosis) has an associated acute exanthematous infectious erythema, generally most marked on the shins. It consists of 1–5 cm erythematous patches or plaques which histologically show only edema and nonspecific perivascular infiltrate. The erythema may become generalized. The eruption occurs during the immune (second) stage of this syndrome. High fever, conjunctival suffusion, nausea, vomiting, and headache characterize the septicemic first stage. This lasts three to seven days, followed by a one- to three-day absence of fever. During the second stage, when IgM antibody develops, headache is intense, fever returns, and ocular manifestations such as conjunctival hemorrhage and suffusion, ocular pain, and photophobia are prominent. At this time the eruption occurs. The skin lesions resolve spontaneously after four to seven days.

There may be different clinical manifestations from identical strains of leptospira.

Leptospira interrogans, serotype *icterohemorrhagiae*, has been the most common cause of Weil's disease, whereas pretibial fever is most commonly associated with serotype *autumnalis*. Humans acquire both types accidentally from urine or tissues of infected animals, or indirectly from contaminated soil or from drinking or swimming in contaminated water. In the continental U.S. dogs are the most common animal source; worldwide, rats are more often responsible. Leptospira enter the body through abraded or diseased skin, and the gastrointestinal or upper respiratory tract.

Leptospirosis may be diagnosed by finding the causative spirochetes in the blood by darkfield microscopy during the first week of illness, and by blood cultures, guinea pig inoculation, and the demonstration of rising antibodies during the second week of the disease. The genus-specific HA serologic test permits relatively early diagnosis.

Treatment with tetracyclines and penicillin shorten the disease duration if given early. Doxycycline, 100 mg daily for a week, has been shown by McClain et al to be effective in a controlled trial in anicteric patients. A dose of 200 mg once weekly will prevent infection while visiting a hyperendemic area.

Andrews ED, et al: Leptospirosis in New England. JAMA 1977, 238:2027.

Berman SJ, et al: Sporadic anicteric leptospirosis in South Vietnam. Ann Intern Med 1973, 79:167.

Edwards GA, et al: Human leptospirosis. Medicine 1960, 39:117.

Heath CW Jr, et al: Leptospirosis in the United States. N Engl J Med 1965, 273:857.

McClain JBL, et al: Doxycycline treatment of leptospirosis. Ann Intern Med 1984, 100:696.

Takafuji ET, et al: An efficacy trial of doxycycline chemoprophylaxis against leptospirosis. N Engl J Med 1984, 310:497.

BORRELIOSIS
(Erythema Chronicum Migrans)

Borrelia burgdorferi, a tick-borne spirochete, is the agent responsible for inducing Lyme disease. The characteristic cutaneous eruption which is the early

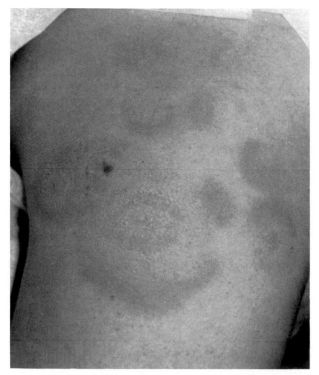

Figure 14–47. Erythema chronicum migrans.

manifestation of this systemic illness is erythema chronicum migrans (ECM). A late sequel of chronic infection is acrodermatitis chronica atrophicans (ACA).

Lyme disease. The *clinical features* typically begin with ECM and are often accompanied by an acute flulike illness. If it is untreated, chronic arthritis and neurologic and cardiac complications frequently develop.

As Shrestha et al have shown, diagnosing early Lyme disease depends upon recognition of the skin eruption. Twenty to 30 per cent of patients recall a tick bite, which leaves a small red macule or papule at the site. The areas most often involved are the thighs, groins, and axilla. Three to 32 (median: seven) days after the bite, there is gradual expansion of the redness around the papule. In one patient the peripherally expanding border migrated 1 cm per day. The advancing border is usually slightly raised, warm, red to bluish-red, and free of any scale. Centrally, the site of the bite may clear, leaving only a ring of peripheral erythema, or it may become indurated, vesicular or necrotic. The annular erythema usually grows to a median diameter of 15 cm, but may range in size from 3 to 68 cm. It is accompanied by a burning sensation in half the patients; rarely is it pruritic or painful.

Twenty-five to 50 per cent of patients will develop multiple secondary annular lesions, similar in appearance to the primary lesion, but without indurated centers, and generally of smaller size. They spare the palms and soles. Their number ranges from two to 100. Without treatment, ECM and the secondary lesions fade in a median of 28 days, although some may be present for months. Ten per cent of untreated cases experience recurrences of ECM over the following months.

Diffuse urticaria, malar erythema, and conjunctivitis may be present during this early period. Malaise, fever, fatigue, headaches, stiff neck, arthralgia, myalgia, lymphadenopathy, anorexia, and nausea and vomiting may accompany early signs and symptoms of *Borrelia burgdorferi* infection.

Ten per cent of patients eventually develop a chronic arthritis of the knees, which in half of these leads to severe disability. HLA-DRw2 positivity may predict this late arthritic complication. Cardiac involvement occurs most often in young men, with fluctuating degrees of atrioventricular block or complete heart block occurring over a brief time (three days to six weeks) early in the course of the illness. Neurologic findings include stiff neck, headache, and cranial and peripheral neuropathies.

LABORATORY FINDINGS. Nonspecific findings include an elevated sedimentation rate in 50 per cent, an elevated IgM level, mild anemia, and elevated liver function tests in 20 per cent.

ETIOLOGY. Burgdorfer et al isolated a spirochete from adult *Ixodes dammini* ticks in 1982, which were a known vector for Lyme disease. The spirochete was then identified by Warthin-Starry silver stain in skin biopsy specimens of ECM. Subsequently the spirochete, now designated *Borrelia burgdorferi*, has been cultured on artificial (modified Kelly's) medium from the blood, skin, and cerebrospinal fluid of patients with Lyme disease. Habicht et al have shown that lipopolysaccharide in the cell wall of the spirochete causes the release of interleukin-2, which triggers release of collagenase and prostaglandin.

EPIDEMIOLOGY. There is no male to female predominance, and the most common age range affected are adults, ages 20 to 50. Onset of this illness is generally between May and November, with over 80 per cent of cases identified in June, July, or August, in the northern hemisphere. In the U.S., Lyme disease occurs primarily in three geographic areas: the northeast, midwest, and west. Tick transmission has been proven, with large studies documenting spirochetes present in various members of the *Ixodes ricinus* complex. Specifically, *Ixodes dammini* is the vector in the northeast and midwest and *Ixodes pacificus* is incriminated in the west. *Amblyomma americana* has also been implicated.

Alzelius in Sweden described ECM in 1909. European cases are transmitted by the tick *Ixodes ricinus*. The spirochete causing ECM in Europe has some antigenic differences from that in the United States and this may account for the fact that the clinical illness resulting from infection is somewhat different from that seen in the United States. European ECM occurs more often in females; it is less likely to have multiple lesions; untreated lesions last longer; there are more laboratory abnormalities in Lyme disease; the arthritis symptoms are prominent in the U.S. but unusual in Europe; and the neurologic manifestations differ. In Europe, infection may lead to Bannwarth's syndrome, which is characterized by focal severe radicular pains, lymphocytic meningitis, and cranial nerve paralysis. Finally, acrodermatitis chronica atrophicans, and possibly linear morphea and lichen sclerosus et atrophicus, may eventuate as late cutaneous sequelae of *Borrelia burgdorferi* infection in Europe. Even lymphocytoma cutis is suspected of being associated with borreliosis, and a trial of penicillin therapy is worthwhile.

Schlesinger et al have documented transplacental transmission of *Borrelia*, resulting in infant death.

HISTOPATHOLOGY. There is a superficial and deep perivascular and interstitial mixed cell infiltrate. Lymphocytes, plasma cells, and eosinophils may be seen, the latter especially prominent when the center of the lesion is biopsied. Warthin-Starry staining may reveal spirochetes in the upper dermis. Park et al reported the use of a monoclonal antibody (H9724) directed against the axial filaments of *Borrelia* in an indirect immunofluorescence assay to identify the organism in tissue specimens.

DIAGNOSIS. The clinical finding of ECM is the most sensitive evidence of early infection. Serologic tests include the indirect immunofluorescence assay (IFA) and the enzyme-linked immunosorbent assay (ELISA). Titers of 1:256 or greater on IFA are regarded as evidence of Lyme disease. When ECM is present alone, 53 per cent have a positive IFA and 67 per cent a positive ELISA. Patients with rheumatologic, neurologic, or cardiac complications should have at least one positive test result, although Dattwyler et al have now reported seronegative Lyme disease, in which there is a specific T-cell blastogenic response but no antibody response. False positive tests occur in syphilis, pinta, yaws, leptospirosis, relapsing fever, infectious mononucleosis, and disease associated with antoantibody formation. The VDRL is negative in *Borrelia burgdorferi* infection. The organism may be cultured in modified Kelly's medium.

TREATMENT. Steere et al have shown that tetracycline, 250 mg four times a day for at least 10 days (and for up to 20 days if symptoms recur or persist), is the treatment of choice for early Lyme disease (ECM and associated symptoms). With this therapy ECM will resolve over several days and major late sequelae are prevented. Amoxicillin, 500 mg four times a day, combined with 500 mg of probenecid for 3 weeks or doxycycline, 100 mg twice daily for 3 weeks, is an alternative.

In established Lyme arthritis and Lyme meningitis, ceftriaxone, 2 gm once daily IV or IM for two weeks, is the treatment of choice, with intravenous penicillin G, 20 million units per day for 10 days, as an alternative. Fifty per cent of arthritis patients will not respond to penicillin therapy.

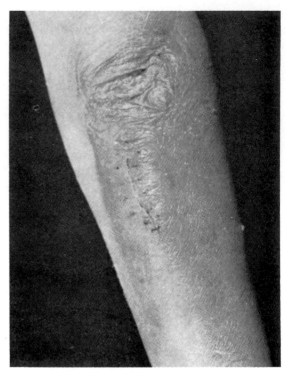

Figure 14–49. Ulnar band of acrodermatitis chronica atrophicans. (Courtesy of Dr. F. Daniels, Jr.)

Acrodermatitis Chronica Atrophicans (ACA)

Also known as primary diffuse atrophy, acrodermatitis chronica atrophicans is characterized by the appearance on the extremities of diffuse reddish or bluish red, paper-thin skin. The underlying blood vessels are easily seen through the wasted epidermis. It occurs almost exclusively in persons of European origin.

The disease begins on the backs of the hands and feet and then gradually spreads to involve the forearms, then the arms, and on the lower extremities, the knees and shins. Occasionally even the trunk may become involved.

In the beginning the areas may be slightly edematous and scaly, but generally they are level with the

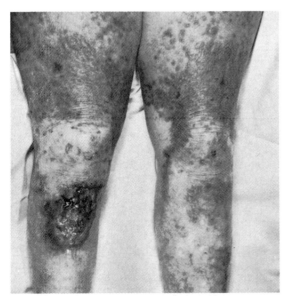

Figure 14–48. Acrodermatitis chronica atrophicans with severe ulceration. Note crinkled cigarette paper appearance of the skin at the knee. (Courtesy of Dr. R. Ames.)

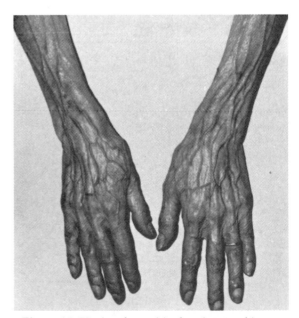

Figure 14–50. Acrodermatitis chronica atrophicans.

skin and smooth. After several weeks to months the skin has a smooth, soft, thin, velvety feel and may easily be lifted into fine folds. It may have a peculiar pinkish gray color and a crumpled cigarette-paper appearance.

Well-defined, smooth, edematous, bandlike thickenings may extend from a finger to the elbow (ulnar bands) or develop in the skin over the shins. With progression of the disease, marked atrophy of the skin occurs.

Subcutaneous fibrous nodules may form, chiefly over the elbows, wrists, and knees. They may be single or multiple, and are firm and painless. Diffuse extensive calcification of the soft tissues may be revealed by radiographic examination. Xanthomatous tumors may occur in the skin. Hypertrophic osteoarthritis of the hands is frequently observed. Occasionally atrophy of the bones of the involved extremities is encountered.

Ulcerations and carcinoma may supervene on the atrophic patches. The disease is slowly progressive and may remain stationary for long periods. Patches may change slightly from time to time, but complete involution never occurs.

Kraus and his associates, in a study of 42 women and one man, found cryoglobulins in 80 per cent. Serum electrophoresis showed an increase of alpha$_1$, alpha$_2$, and gamma globulins and a decrease in albumin.

ACA is a spirochetosis, thought to be a late sequel of infection with *Borrelia burgdorferi*. It is tick-transmitted by *Ixodes ricinus*. Nearly all patients with ACA have a positive test for antibodies to the spirochete, and Warthin-Starry stains demonstrate the organism in tissue in some cases. The organism has been cultured from skin lesions of ACA.

Some patients with ACA have had preceding ECM, and some have concurrent lichen sclerosus–type lesions. A study of 10 patients with chronic morphea by Aberer found positive antibodies to *Borrelia burgdorferi*, implicating this infection as a consideration for the etiology of lichen sclerosus et atrophicus and morphea. Studies from the U.S., however, have generally failed to confirm any link between morphea, LS&A, and *Borrelia* infection.

Histologically, there is marked atrophy of the epidermis and dermis without fibrosis. The elastic tissue is absent and the cutaneous appendages are atrophic. In the dermis a bandlike lymphocytic infiltration is seen, which varies in abundance according to the stage of the disease. The epidermis is slightly hyperkeratotic and flattened, and beneath it there is a distinctive narrow zone of connective tissue in which the elastic tissue is intact.

Four million units of penicillin G daily for two weeks effectively treats ACA in the early erythematous phase. Either tetracycline or erythromycin, 1 gm per day, is an alternative in penicillin-sensitive patients.

Aberer E: Is localized scleroderma a Borrelia infection? Lancet 1985, 2:278.

Åsbrink E: Erythema chronicum migrans Afzelius and acrodermatitis chronica atrophicans. Acta Dermato-Venereol (Stockh) 1985, Supp 118:1.
Idem, et al: Acrodermatitis chronic atrophicans—a spirochetosis. Am J Dermatopathol 1986, 8:209.
Berberian BJ: The usefulness of immunodiagnostic tests in the diagnosis of a case of Lyme disease. JAAD 1986, 15:302.
Berger BW: Erythema chronicum migrans of Lyme disease. Arch Dermatol 1984, 120:1017.
Idem, et al: Lyme disease is a spirochetosis. Am J Dermatopathol 1983, 5:111.
Idem: Isolation and characterization of the Lyme disease spirochete from the skin of patients with erythema chronicum migrans. JAAD 1985, 13:444.
Burgdorfer W: The enlarging spectrum of tick-borne spirochetoses. R. R. Parker Memorial Address. Rev Infect Dis 1986, 8:932.
Costello CM, et al: A prospective study of tick bite in an endemic area for Lyme disease. J Infect Dis 1989, 159:136.
Dattwyler RJ, et al: Seronegative Lyme disease. N Engl J Med 1988, 319:1441.
Fagrell B, et al: Acrodermatitis chronica atrophicans herxheimer can often mimic a peripheral vascular disease. Acta Med Scand 1986, 220:485.
Habicht GS, et al: Lyme disease. Sci Am 1987 (Sept), p. 78.
Hoesly JM, et al: Localized scleroderma (morphea) and antibody to *Borrelia burgdorferi*. JAAD 1987, 17:455.
Hovmark A, et al: The spirochetal etiology of lymphadenosis benigna cutis solitaria. Acta Dermato-Venereol (Stockh) 1986, 66:479.
Lastavica CC, et al: Rapid emergence of a focal epidemic of Lyme disease in coastal Massachusetts. N Engl J Med 1989, 320:133.
Metz LE, et al: Ticks, spirochetes and new diagnostic tests for Lyme disease. Mayo Clin Proc 1985, 60:402.
Park HK, et al: Erythema chronicum migrans of Lyme disease. JAAD 1986, 15:406.
Piesman J, et al: Duration of tick attachment and *Borrelia burgdorferi* transmission. J Clin Microbiol 1987, 25:557.
Schlesinger PA, et al: Maternal–fetal transmission of the Lyme disease spirochete. Ann Intern Med 1985, 103:67.
Shrestha M, et al: Diagnosing early Lyme disease. Am J Med 1988, 18:235.
Steere AC, et al: Diagnosing early Lyme disease. Ann J Med 1985, 78:235.
Idem: The spirochetal etiology of Lyme disease. N Engl J Med 1983, 308:733.
Idem: Chronic Lyme arthritis. Ann Intern Med 1979, 90:896.
Idem: Lyme carditis. Ann Intern Med 1980, 90:8.
Idem: Neurologic abnormalities of Lyme disease. Ann Intern Med 1983, 99:767.
Idem: Successful parenteral penicillin therapy of established Lyme arthritis. N Engl J Med 1985, 312:869.
Idem: Treatment of the early manifestations of Lyme disease. Ann Intern Med 1983, 99:22.
Waldo ED, et al: The spirochete in erythema chronicum migrans. Am J Dermatopathol 1983, 5:125.

MYCOPLASMA

Mycoplasmas are distinct from true bacteria in that they lack a cell wall and differ from viruses in that they grow on cell-free media. *Mycoplasma pneumoniae* (Eaton agent) is an important cause of acute respiratory disease in children and young adults. It has been estimated that in the summer it may account for 50 per cent of pneumonias.

Skin eruptions occurred during the course of infection in 17 per cent of patients in a large prospective study by Foy et al. According to Cherry et al the most frequently reported dermatologic manifestation is erythema multiforme, which may occur in the severe Stevens-Johnson form. Erythema nodosum has been occasionally reported. Of the various exanthems documented, they include urticarial, vesicular, maculopapular, scarlatiniform, and morbilliform lesions, distributed primarily on the trunk, arms and legs. Ulcerative stomatitis and conjunctivitis may be present. Ramilo et al reported a nine-year-old boy with fever and a petechial and purpuric eruption which resembled acute meningococcemia.

The diagnosis of *M. pneumoniae* infection is made in the acute situation by clinical means, but definitive diagnosis is made either by culture of the organism or by a rise in the specific antibody titer. The serologic procedures used are a complement fixation test and a sensitive ELISA test. Cold agglutinins with a titer of 1:128 or more are usually due to *M. pneumoniae* infection. Occasionally acrocyanosis may occur secondary to cold agglutinin disease, which clears with antibiotic therapy.

Treatment is with erythromycin, 500 mg three times daily, or tetracycline, 250 mg four times daily, both courses lasting a total of six to eight days.

Cherry JD, et al: *Mycoplasma pneumoniae* infections and exanthems. J Pediatr 1974, 87:369.
Foy HM, et al: *Mycoplasma pneumoniae* in an urban area. JAMA 1970, 214:1666.
Ramilo AL, et al: Mycoplasma infection simulating acute meningococcemion. Arch Dermatol 1983, 119:786.
Shelley WB, et al: Acrocyanosis of cold agglutinin disease successfully treated with antibiotics. Cutis 1984, 33:556.
Teisch JA, et al: Vesiculopustular eruption with mycoplasma infection. JAMA 1970, 211:1694.

CHLAMYDIAL INFECTIONS

Chlamydia species possess common characteristics, including particle size of 250 to 500 nm in diameter; obligatory intracellular parasitism with multiplication by means of a unique developmental cycle; production of characteristic cytoplasmic inclusions in susceptible host cells; susceptibility to antimicrobials such as sulfonamides, chloramphenicol, and tetracycline; and possession of group-specific, complement-fixing antigens. A typical cytoplasmic inclusion, which is pathognomonic of infection by *Chlamydia*, consists of a colony of small (elementary bodies) and large particles (reticulate bodies) in varying proportions. The chlamydial particles contain DNA, RNA, proteins, lipids, and carbohydrates. Peptidoglycan, a component characteristic of bacterial cell walls, is also found in *Chlamydia*. The *Chlamydia* are capable of synthesizing folic acid, lysine, and muramic acid, but are dependent on the host cell for an adequate supply of high-energy compounds to carry out biosynthetic processes. Two species of chlamydias, *C. trachomatis* and *C. psittaci*, have been recognized. The two species share a major common antigen, and there are numerous serotypes within each species. In man, *Chlamydia* cause trachoma, inclusion conjunctivitis, nongonococcal urethritis, cervicitis, epididymitis, proctitis, endometritis, salpingitis, pneumonia in the newborn, psittacosis (ornithosis), and lymphogranuloma venereum.

LYMPHOGRANULOMA VENEREUM (LGV)

LGV was formerly called lymphopathia venerea, climatic bubo, or lymphogranuloma inguinale. It is a sexually transmitted disease.

LGV is characterized by suppurative inguinal adenitis with matted lymph nodes, inguinal bubo with secondary ulceration, and constitutional symptoms.

CLINICAL FEATURES. After an incubation period of three to 20 days following exposure, a primary lesion consisting of a small (2 to 3 mm), herpetiform vesicle or erosion develops on the glans penis, the prepuce, the coronal sulcus, or at the meatus. In women it occurs on the vulva, vagina, or cervix. The lesion is painless and soon becomes a shallow ulceration.

Extragenital primary infections of LGV are rare. An ulcerating lesion may appear at the site of infection on the fingers, lips, or tongue.

In about two weeks after the appearance of the primary lesion enlargement of the regional lymph nodes occurs. Usually the lymph nodes are involved unilaterally. In one third of the cases, the lymphadenopathy is bilateral. In the rather characteristic inguinal adenitis of LGV, in men, the nodes in a chain fuse together into a large mass; the color of the skin overlying the mass usually becomes violaceous, the swelling is tender, and the bubo may break down with multiple fistulous openings. When the femoral nodes are involved as well as the inguinal nodes, a groove corresponding to Poupart's ligament separates the two to produce the characteristic "groove sign" considered to be pathognomonic of LGV. Along with the local adenitis there may be systemic symptoms of malaise, joint pains, conjunctivitis, loss of appetite, loss of weight, and fever, which may persist for several weeks. Cases with septic temperatures, enlarged liver and spleen, and even encephalitis have occasionally been observed.

Primary lesions of LGV have rarely been observed in female patients; women also have a lower incidence of inguinal buboes. Their bubo is typically pararectal in location. The diagnosis is recognized only much later when the patient presents an increasingly pronounced inflammatory stricture of the lower rectal wall, which may be annular or tubular. Since most of the lymph channels running from the vulva

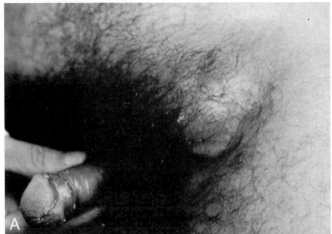

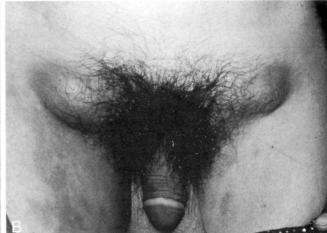

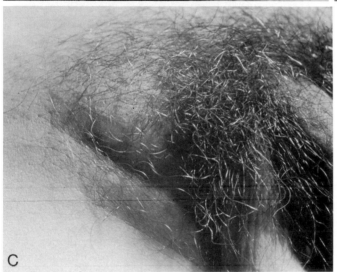

Figure 14–51. A, *Lymphogranuloma venereum with primary lesion.* B, *Bilateral lymphadenopathy of lymphogranuloma venereum.* C, *"Groove sign" of lymphogranuloma venereum. (C, Courtesy of Dr. Axel W. Hoke.)*

drain into the nodes around the lower part of the rectum, an inflammatory reaction in these nodes results in secondary involvement of the rectal wall. The iliac nodes may also be involved.

With or without rectal strictures, women may in later stages of the disease show elephantiasis of the genitals with chronic ulcerations and scarring of the vulva (esthiomene). Such a reaction is rare in men.

LGV may start in the rectum as proctitis, which may then progress to the formation of a stricture. The clinical hallmark is bloody, mucopurulent rectal discharge. The stricture can usually be felt with the examining finger 4 to 6 cm above the anus. Untreated rectal strictures of men and women may eventually require colostomy.

Cutaneous eruptions take the form of erythema nodosum, erythema multiforme, photosensitivity, and scarlatiniform eruptions. Arthritis associated with LGV involves finger, wrist, ankle, knee, or shoulder joints. Marked weight loss, pronounced secondary anemia, weakness, and mental depression are often encountered in the course of the anorectal syndrome. Colitis due to LGV is limited to the rectum

and rectosigmoid structures. Perianal fistulas or sinuses are often seen in cases of anorectal LGV.

Among the various extragenital manifestations which occur are glossitis with regional adenitis, unilateral conjunctivitis with edema of the lids due to lymphatic blockage with lymphadenopathy (Parinaud's oculoglandular syndrome), acute meningitis, meningoencephalitis, and pneumonia.

In LGV of long duration an active search for carcinoma of the bladder, the genitals, and the anus should be made.

LABORATORY FINDINGS. Marked hyperglobulinemia occurs, particularly in patients with chronic complications. A high sedimentation rate and biologic false positive tests for syphilis are also seen in chronic or early stages of the disease.

The pus from fistulas or draining buboes may be examined for organisms by inoculation into yolk sacs of embryonated eggs or brains of mice. This is very rarely done.

The complement fixation test is the most feasible and the simplest serologic test for detecting antibodies, which become detectable some four weeks after onset of illness.

Frei Test. The Frei test was an intradermal test for the diagnosis of LGV. It was troubled by low sensitivity and lower specificity. The antigen is no longer available commercially in the U.S.

ETIOLOGY. LGV is a sexually transmitted disease caused by microorganisms of the *Chlamydia trachomatis* group. Three serotypes, designated L_1, L_2, and L_3, are known for the LGV chlamydia. Characteristic surface antigens allow separation of the LGV chlamydias from the agents which cause trachoma, inclusion conjunctivitis, urethritis, and cervicitis, which also belong to the *C. trachomatis* group.

Although Wallace described the disease in 1833, the account of Durand, Nicolas, and Favre in 1913 is regarded as definitive. The causative agent was not cultured until 1940, when Rake and associates grew it in the yolk sac of chick embryos.

EPIDEMIOLOGY. LGV is contracted by heterosexual or homosexual sexual contact. It occurs in all races and is more common among the sexually promiscuous. The highest incidence is found in the 20–40-year-old group. Asymptomatic female contacts who shed virus from the cervix are an important reservoir of infection. The classic disease in men is declining in the United States, while anorectal LGV has been increasing in the homosexual population.

HISTOPATHOLOGY. The characteristic changes in the lymph nodes consist of an infectious granuloma with the formation of stellate abscesses. There is an outer zone of epithelioid cells with a central necrotic core composed of debris of lymphocytes, endothelial cells, and leukocytes. In lesions of long duration plasma cells may be present.

DIFFERENTIAL DIAGNOSIS

Chancroid. As opposed to LGV, with chancroid a primary chancre or multiple chancroidal ulcers are present and may permit the demonstration of *Haemophilus ducreyi*.

Granuloma Inguinale. The skin lesions are characteristic and usually much larger and more persistent than the primary lesion of LGV. Donovan bodies are demonstrable in granuloma inguinale. Inguinal adenitis is not a characteristic feature of granuloma inguinale. Esthiomene may also be a feature of granuloma inguinale.

Syphilis. If the primary lesion of LGV is well developed, it may be confused with the primary lesion of syphilis. In any genital lesion, darkfield examination for *Treponema pallidum* should be made. Syphilitic inguinal adenitis shows small, hard, nontender glands. It should be emphasized again that all venereal infections may be mixed infections and that observation for simultaneous or subsequent development of another venereal disease should be unrelenting. Late stages of LGV esthiomene with ulcerating and cicatrizing lesions will have to be differentiated from syphilis by search for spirochetes, the serologic tests for syphilis, and complement fixation tests.

Inguinal Lymphadenopathy. Lymphadenopathy may develop in traumatic lesions of the feet, in malignant genital, rectal, and abdominal diseases, in lymphoma, in the acquired immunodeficiency syndrome, and in blood dyscrasias. Determination of LGV-CFT is beneficial.

Balanitis. This may resemble the primary lesion of LGV. Subsequent inguinal adenopathy development and the result of LGV-CFT will help in differentiation.

Ulcerative Colitis. This may develop from LGV that is limited to the rectum and rectosigmoid structures. In other forms of ulcerative colitis LGV-CFT may be negative.

TREATMENT. The recommended treatment is doxycycline, 100 mg twice daily for three weeks. An alternative is erythromycin, 500 mg four times daily for 21 days. Sexual partners should also be treated.

The fluctuant nodules are aspirated through healthy adjacent normal skin to prevent rupture.

Becker LE: Lymphogranuloma venereum. Int J Dermatol 1976, 15:26.

Ellis RE: Chlamydial genital infections. South Med J 1981, 74:109.

McLelland BA, et al: Lymphogranuloma venereum. JAMA 1976, 235:56.

Schachter J: Chlamydial infections. N Engl J Med 1978, 298:428, 490, 540.

REITER'S SYNDROME

Reiter's syndrome is a characteristic clinical triad consisting of urethritis, conjunctivitis, and arthritis. There may also be other features that involve the skin, the mucous membranes, the gastrointestinal tract, and the cardiovascular system.

The disease occurs chiefly in young men of HLA-B27 genotype, although it may also occur in children and older men. It is rare in women.

SIGNS. Any one of the following triad signs may occur first, accompanied by fever, weakness, and weight loss.

Urethritis. A nonbacterial urethritis occurs, with painful and bloody urination and pyuria. Cystitis, prostatitis, and seminal vesiculitis may be accompaniments.

Conjunctivitis. When this occurs, which may be in about a third of the patients, the conjunctivitis may be bulbar, tarsal, or angular. Keratitis is usually superficial and extremely painful and may lead to corneal ulceration. Iritis is common, especially in recurrent cases.

Arthritis. Any synovial joint may be involved, but especially those which are weight-bearing. Its onset is sudden, with heat, tenderness, and swelling of the joints and a predilection for the knees, the ankles, the foot joints, and the wrists. Pain in one or both heels is a frequent symptom. Sacroileitis may develop in up to two thirds of patients, most of whom are of HLA-B27 type.

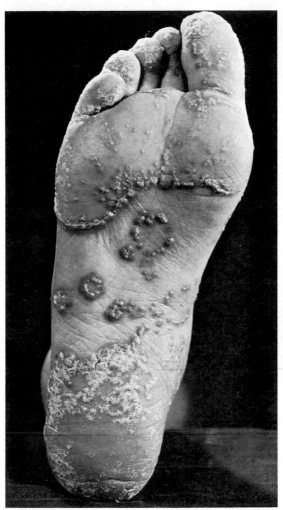

Figure 14–52. Reiter's syndrome. Note resemblance to volar psoriasis. (Courtesy of Dr. H. Shatin.)

of coalescence of the individual crusted lesions, so that the lesions have the appearance of a "relief map." Ultimately, the crusts and horny masses become detached and are shed, often leaving residual pigmentation.

Mucosal Lesions. The buccal, palatal, and lingual mucosa may show painless, shallow, red erosions, and severe stomatitis may ensue.

Cardiac Manifestations. Endocarditis, pericarditis, and myocarditis, as well as aortic insufficiency, occur in some patients.

ETIOLOGY. Reiter's syndrome has been attributed to many different agents such as *Shigella flexneri, Salmonella* spp., *Yersinia* spp., and *Campylobacter fetus,* which may be responsible for the infectious enteritis which precedes the onset in a small percentage of patients. In cases which follow infection of the genitourinary tract, *Chlamydia trachomatis* may be associated. The exact causative role of these or other infectious agents is still unclear.

Immunologically mediated tissue injury in a genetically predisposed patient is believed to be important. HLA-B27 positivity is present in 60 to 75 per cent of cases of Reiter's syndrome, rising to 90 to 100 per cent in patients with accompanying sacroileitis, uveitis, or aortitis. Because of this, some have linked psoriasis (pustular and spondylitic arthritis forms) and ankylosing spondylitis to Reiter's disease. The relationship of these diseases to one another is still unclear.

CLINICAL FEATURES

Skin Manifestations. The skin lesions start as multiple small yellowish vesicles which break, become confluent, and form superficial ulcers. They develop frequently on the genitals and the palms. The eruption on the glans penis occurs in 25 per cent of patients. Those on the soles are different: they start as pustules, which become very crusted or hyperkeratotic and are suggestive of rupial psoriasis. These are painless, occur approximately one month after the urethritis, and are present in about 10 per cent of patients. The eruption was formerly known as *keratoderma blennorrhagicum.* Later they may become deeply ulcerated.

The penile lesions, which are frequent, are characterized by perimeatal balanitis and vesicles, which become crusted and form circinate lesions. The nails become thick and brittle, and heavy keratotic deposits develop under them (subungual keratosis) not unlike those seen in severe nail involvement of psoriasis.

There is usually a thick, dry, horny crusting about the toes that spreads over the soles. This is the result

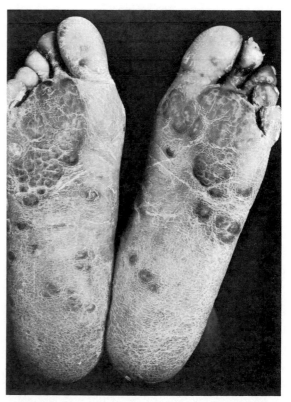

Figure 14–53. Keratoderma blennorrhagicum. (Courtesy of Dr. H. Shatin.)

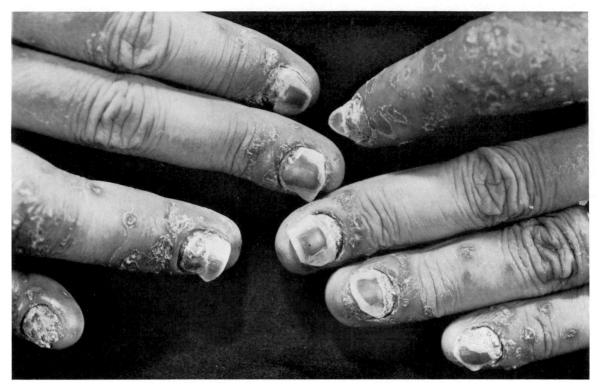

Figure 14–54. Reiter's syndrome. (Courtesy of Dr. H. Shatin.)

Duvic et al and Winchester et al have reported many cases of Reiter's disease and psoriasis occurring in patients with AIDS. What this means regarding the etiology of Reiter's disease or its relationship with psoriasis remains to be elucidated.

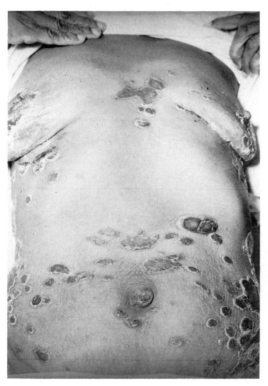

Figure 14–55. Reiter's syndrome. (Courtesy of Dr. F. Kerdel-Vegas.)

LABORATORY FINDINGS. No specific changes are characteristic of this syndrome. A leukocytosis of 10,000 to 20,000 and elevated sedimentation rate, depending upon the severity of the disease, are the most consistent findings. There is no specific test for Reiter's syndrome.

HISTOPATHOLOGY. The early lesion in the epidermis is a spongiform vesicopustule. In addition there are acanthosis and parakeratosis, and the interpapillary processes are elongated. Hyperkeratosis may be extreme. In the dermis the papillae are edematous, with dilated vessels and a perivascular infiltrate.

DIFFERENTIAL DIAGNOSIS. Reiter's disease may be confused with rheumatoid arthritis, ankylosing spondylitis, gout, psoriatic arthritis, gonococcal arthritis, acute rheumatic fever, and serum sickness.

TREATMENT. Therapy is centered mostly around palliative measures. The patient should have adequate rest and splinting of affected joints.

Usually the mucocutaneous lesions are self-limited and clear within a few months. Topical steroids may be helpful. For the joint disease, rest and nonsteroidal antiinflammatory agents should be used first. Indomethacin, 100 mg per day in two to four divided doses, and tolmetin, 400 mg three times a day, are often useful. Phenylbutazone is helpful but potential idiosyncratic bone marrow depression limits its usefulness. Methotrexate, 7.5 to 20 mg per week, may be tried in patients with severe, refractory joint disease, but it should not be used in an AIDS-related case. Etretinate is a better choice here. Arnold has had success—and no side effects—with Kenalog, 40 to 60 mg intramuscularly at monthly intervals or as needed, and believes it worth trying before methotrexate. Once the acute arthritis is controlled it is important to begin physical therapy to maintain joint mobility.

The course of Reiter's disease is characterized by exacerbations and remission in about one third of patients. A chronic deforming arthritis occurs in about 20 per cent of patients, with significant disability resulting, chiefly from foot deformities.

Callen JP: The spectrum of Reiter's disease. JAAD 1979, 1:75.

Duvic M, et al: Acquired immunodeficiency syndrome–associated psoriasis and Reiter's syndrome. Arch Dermatol 1987, 123:1622.

Felman YM, et al: Reiter's syndrome. Cutis 1983, 31:152.

Fox R, et al: The chronicity of symptoms and disability in Reiter's syndrome. Ann Intern Med 1979, 91:190.

Good AE: Reiter's disease. Cutis 1979, 24:514.

Jetton RL, et al: Treatment of Reiter's syndrome with methotrexate. Ann Intern Med 1969, 70:349.

Khan MA, et al: Diagnostic value of HLA-B27 testing in ankylosing spondylitis and Reiter's syndrome. Ann Intern Med 1986, 96:70.

Miller KA, et al: Family studies with HLA typing in Reiter's syndrome. Am J Med 1981, 70:1210.

Richman TB, et al: Reiter's syndrome. Arch Dermatol 1988, 124:1007.

Wilkens RF, et al: Reiter's syndrome. Arthritis Rheum 1981, 24:844.

Winchester R, et al: Reiter's syndrome and the acquired immunodeficiency syndrome. Ann Intern Med 1987, 106:19.

15

Diseases Due to Fungi and Yeasts

THE SUPERFICIAL MYCOSES

The skin constitutes the main site of recognizable fungal infections in man, and these infections can be conveniently divided into superficial and deep mycoses. When restricted to the skin, most mycotic infections are superficial and are limited to a depth of 1 or 2 mm. The fungi that usually cause only superficial infection on the skin are called *dermatophytes*. They are classified in three genera: *Microsporum*, *Trichophyton*, and *Epidermophyton*. They digest and live on keratin. Each species of dermatophyte tends to produce its own clinical picture, although several species may provoke identical eruptions. At other times the eruptions are so distinctive and characteristic that the species may be identified from the clinical findings. The skin appendages, namely, the hair and the nails, are also vitally involved in these infections.

The mycoses caused by dermatophytes are called **dermatophytosis, tinea**, or **ringworm**. On certain parts of the body tinea has certain distinctive features characteristic of that particular site. For this reason the tineas are divided into (1) **tinea capitis** (ringworm of the scalp and kerion), (2) **tinea barbae** (ringworm of the beard), (3) **tinea faciei**, (4) **tinea corporis**, (5) **tinea manus**, (6) **tinea pedis**, (7) **tinea cruris**, and (8) **onychomycosis** (fungus infection of the nails).

Superficial mycoses are also classified according to the causative dermatophyte. However, this is of largely epidemiologic interest. The management of such infections is only rarely assisted by the identification of the genus and species of the causative organism.

Andrews GC, et al: Griseofulvin in dermatomycoses. JAMA 173:1542, 1960.

Bogdanoff MD: Mycotic infections in man. Drug Therapy 1978, 8:31.

Dismukes WE: Azole antifungal drugs. Ann Intern Med 1988, 109:177.

Emmons CW, et al: Medical Mycology, 3rd ed. Philadelphia, Lea & Febiger, 1977.

Gray LD, et al: Laboratory diagnosis of systemic fungal diseases. Infect Dis Clin North Am 1988, 2:779.

Graybill JR: Therapeutic agents. Infect Dis Clin North Am 1988, 2:805.

Hazen EL, et al: Laboratory Identification of Pathogenic Fungi Simplified, 3rd ed. Springfield, IL, Charles C Thomas, 1970.

Holmberg L, et al: Diagnosis and treatment of local mycosis. Acta Derm Venereol (Stockh) 1986, 121:13.

Lesher JL, et al: Antifungal agents in dermatology. JAAD 1987, 17:383.

Macher AM, et al: AIDS and the mycoses. Infect Dis Clin North Am 1988, 2:287.

Rinaldi MG: Emerging opportunists. Infect Dis Clin North Am 1989, 3:65.

Rippon JW: New era in antimycotic therapy. Arch Dermatol 1986, 122:399.

TINEA CAPITIS

Synonym: Scalp ringworm.

CLINICAL FEATURES. Ringworm of the scalp is an infectious disease occurring chiefly in schoolchildren and less commonly in infants and adults. Boys have tinea capitis more frequently than girls; however, in epidemics caused by *T. tonsurans* there is often equal frequency in the sexes. The clinical types of infections can be conveniently divided into inflammatory and noninflammatory lesions. Tinea capitis can be caused by all the pathogenic dermatophytes with the exception of *Epidermophyton floccosum* and *Trichophyton concentricum*. In the United States, most cases are caused by *T. tonsurans* (which has displaced *M. audouinii* from first place) and *M. canis*.

M. audouinii infections present as the classic form of noninflammatory tinea capitis, characterized by multiple scaly lesions ("gray-patch"), stubs of broken hair, and a minimal inflammatory response. Occasionally the glabrous skin, eyelids, and eyelashes are involved. This infection sometimes is observed in epidemics in schools and orphanages. Over the past 20 years, *M. audouinii* infections gradually have been replaced by increasing numbers of cases of "black-dot" ringworm, caused primarily by *T. tonsurans* but occasionally by *T. violaceum*. *T. tonsurans* is the preponderant cause of tinea capitis in much of the United States. In one series of 30 black children (and one Oriental) in New York City, *T. tonsurans* was cultured from every case.

Not only has the incidence of *T. tonsurans* increased tremendously; that of *M. audouinii* has decreased. Since 1972 the average annual incidence at Cook

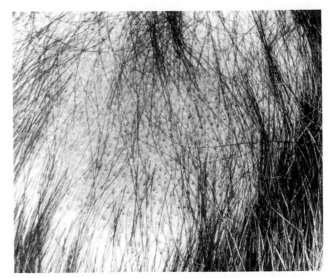

Figure 15–2. Tinea capitis. "Black dot" ringworm caused by Trichophyton tonsurans.

County Hospital in Chicago has been 1.5 cases per year; for nine years prior to that it was six cases; during comparable periods the incidence of *T. tonsurans* cases rose from seven a year to 36, as reported by Bronson et al. "Black dot" ringworm, as this infection is called, presents as multiple areas of alopecia studded with black dots representing infected hairs broken off at or below the surface of the scalp.

Inflammatory tinea capitis is usually caused by *M. canis* but can be caused by *T. mentagrophytes, T. tonsurans, M. gypseum,* or *T. verrucosum. M. canis* infections begin as scaly, erythematous, papular eruptions with loose and broken-off hairs, followed by varying degrees of inflammation, but in many cases it suddenly becomes severe. At times, a localized spot is accompanied by pronounced swelling, developing into boggy and indurated areas exuding pus, known as *kerion celsii*. This inflammatory reaction is felt to be a delayed type hypersensitivity reaction to fungal elements. If extensive lesions form, fever, pain, and regional lymphadenopathy may be present. Widespread "id" eruptions may appear concomitantly on the trunk and extremities. These are vesicular, lichenoid, or pustular. Kerion may be followed by scarring and permanent alopecia in the areas of inflammation and suppuration. Systemic steroids for a short period will greatly diminish the inflammatory response and reduce the risk of scarring. A single injection of Kenalog IM (1 mg/kg up to 40 mg) may suffice and obviate noncompliance as well as side effects.

Favus. This disease, very rare in the United States, appears chiefly upon the scalp, but may affect the glabrous skin and the nails. On the scalp, concave sulfur-yellow crusts form around loose, wiry hairs. Atrophy ensues, leaving a smooth, glossy, thin, paper-white patch. On the glabrous skin the lesions are pinhead to 2 cm in diameter with cup-shaped crusts called **scutulae**, usually pierced by a hair as

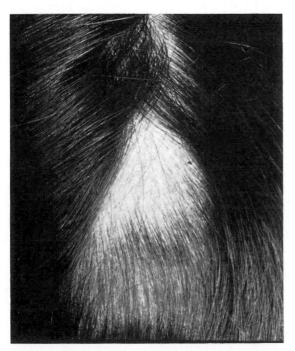

Figure 15–1. Tinea capitis, localized patch, caused by Trichophyton tonsurans.

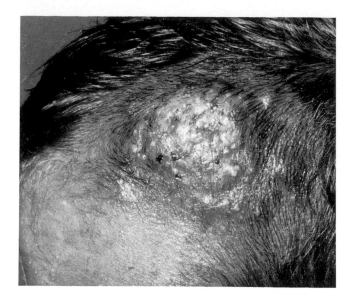

Figure 15–3. Kerion. Inflammatory reaction of tinea capitis frequently caused by M. canis *or* T. mentagrophytes. *(Courtesy of Dr. J. Penner.)*

on the scalp. The scutula have a distinctive mousy odor. When the nails are affected they become brittle, irregularly thickened, and crusted under the free margins.

Favus is not often seen in North America, although it has been reported in Kentucky and in the Gaspé peninsula of Canada by Beare. Favus among the Bantus in South Africa is called, in Afrikaans, **witkop** (whitehead). It is also prevalent in the Middle East, Southeastern Europe, and the countries bordering the Mediterranean Sea.

ETIOLOGY. Tinea capitis can be caused by any one of several of the dermatophytes. The most frequent causative fungi are *T. tonsurans, M. audouinii,* and *M. canis.* The first two spread from human to human, whereas the latter is caught from animals such as the kitten or dog. *M. ferrugineum* and *M. gypseum* species may occasionally cause ringworm of the scalp. Zaias et al have reported *M. rivalieri* in

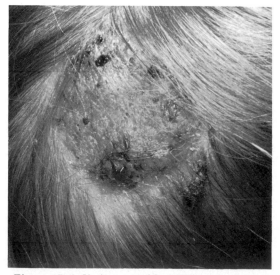

Figure 15–4. Kerion caused by Microsporum canis.

epidemic proportions in Florida; it had previously been reported only in Africa.

Among the trichophytons, endothrix types such as *T. tonsurans* (black-dot ringworm) and *T. violaceum,* are the most frequent invaders of the scalp. It is noteworthy that *T. tonsurans* alone affects adults (chiefly women) regularly; the others are almost always confined to children. The ectothrix fungi found most frequently on the scalp are *T. verrucosum* and *T. mentagrophytes;* less frequently seen is *T. megninii,* which is probably restricted to Southwest Europe.

INCIDENCE AND EPIDEMIOLOGY. Both *M. audouinii* and *M. canis* are endemic and infect mostly city children. *Trichophyton tonsurans* in 1978 was the major cause of tinea capitis in urban areas with a large Latin-American population. In the succeeding decade it has consolidated and extended its territory. It is difficult to diagnose clinically so it is probably far more widespread than is reported. *M. audouinii* is a human pathogen and can occur in epidemic proportions. The fungus has been found in barbers' brushes, and on the backs of theater seats and in caps and hats; however, transmission is probably from child to child. The same statements apply to *T. tonsurans. M. canis* is acquired from infected kittens or dogs; *T. mentagrophytes* is also transmitted by animals. *T. schoenleinii* and *T. violaceum* appear to be transmitted from human to human. In children up to 18 years of age, the latter occurs more frequently in boys than in girls; however, among adults the women greatly outnumber the men.

Geographic locations are important factors in the types of infection seen. *M. audouinii* and *M. canis* have been frequently noted fungi in the New York area; however, as noted before there has been a steady increase in *T. tonsurans.* This is now endemic in Latin and South America and Mexico; *T. violaceum* is prevalent in the U.S.S.R., Yugoslavia, and Spain; *T. schoenleinii* is rarely seen in the United States and

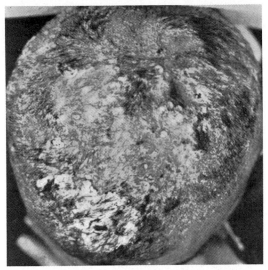

Figure 15–5. Favus of scalp, showing scutulae.

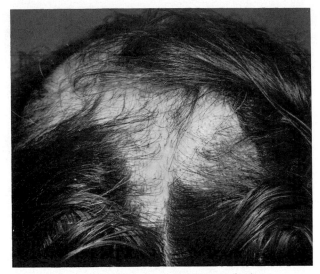

Figure 15–6. Scarring after favus infection.

usually only in immigrants, whereas it is predominant in the Middle East.

PATHOGENESIS. The incubation period lasts two to four days. The hyphae grow downward into the follicle, on the hair's surface, and the intrafollicular hyphae break up into chains of spores. There is a period of spread (four days to four months) during which the lesions enlarge and new lesions appear. At about three weeks hairs break off a few millimeters above the surface. Intrapilary hyphae descend to the exact upper limit of the keratogenous zone and here form "Adamson's fringe" about the twelfth day. The external portions of the intrapilary hyphae segment into chains of ectothrix spores. No new lesions develop during the refractory period (four months to several years). The clinical appearance is constant, with the host and parasite at equilibrium. This is followed by a period of involution in which the formation of ectothrix spores and intrapilary hyphae gradually diminishes.

Sharma et al have documented an asymptomatic carrier state among young black children. The frequency of this and its impact on disease spread and therapy have yet to be determined.

DIAGNOSIS. Vigne was the first to demonstrate ringworm by fluorescence.

Wood's Light. Ultraviolet of 365 nm wavelength is obtained by passing the beam through a Wood's filter composed of nickel oxide–containing glass. This apparatus, commonly known as Wood's light, is obtainable commercially. A simple form is the 125-volt purple bulb.

In a dark room the skin under this light fluoresces faintly blue; however, the infected hair fluoresces bright green, beads on the hairs contrasting strongly with the dark field. Bare scaly areas show a turquoise blue color. Fluorescent-positive infections are caused by *M. audouinii, M. canis, M. ferrugineum, M. distortum,* and *T. schoenleinii;* hairs infected with *T. tonsurans* and *T. violaceum* and others of the endothrix type

do not fluoresce. The fluorescent substance is a pteridine.

Microscopic Examination. For demonstration of the fungus, two or three loose hairs are removed from the suspected areas with epilating forceps. When the hairs are all broken off at the surface ("black-dot" ringworm), it is usually possible to tease a few out with a needle point. It is important to choose loose hairs taken from areas that fluoresce under the Wood's light. Bear in mind that hairs infected with *T. tonsurans* do not fluoresce. The hairs are placed on a slide and covered with a drop of a 10 to 20 per cent solution of potassium hydroxide. Then a coverslip is applied, and the specimen is warmed over a flame until the hairs are macerated. They are examined first with a low-power objective and then with a high-power objective for detail. Xylol is as satisfactory as KOH and need not be warmed. Scales or hairs cleared with it can still be cultured.

The fungus invades the hair shaft two ways, one being *ectothrix* involvement in which the hair is surrounded with a sheath of tiny spores. *Microsporum* species, as well as *T. mentagrophytes* and *T. verrucosum,* are ectothrix fungi. *T. verrucosum* is the fungus most frequently acquired by man from cattle and causes a severe inflammatory tinea barbae in men or tinea capitis in children. The other mode of fungus infection is the *endothrix* type in which the arthrospores are formed inside the hair shaft. This type is seen with *T. tonsurans, T. violaceum,* and *T. schoenleinii* infections.

The final and exact identification of the causative fungus may be determined by culture. It should be acknowledged, however, that such identification is of largely epidemiologic and academic interest; it makes little or no difference to the treatment of the patient. Several of the infected hairs are planted upon Sabouraud's glucose agar or Dermatophyte Test Medium (DTM). On the former a distinctive growth appears within one to two weeks. Most frequently

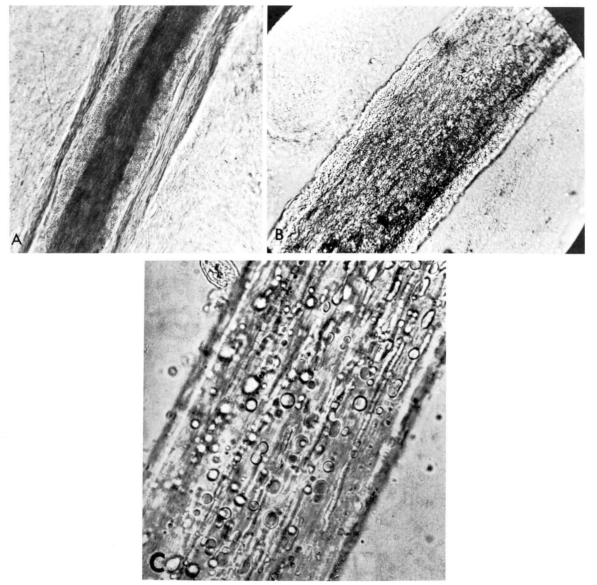

Figure 15–7. A, *Ectothrix type in* Microsporum canis. *Note the small spores surrounding the hair shaft.* B, *Endothrix spores in hair with* Trichophyton tonsurans. C, *Endothrix in* T. schoenleini *(favus) showing characteristic bubbles of air. (Courtesy of Dr. Lucille K. Georg.)*

the diagnosis is made by the gross appearance of the culture growth. In the case of an atypical growth and questionable identification the culture is examined under the microscope for characteristic morphologic forms. DTM not only contains antibiotics to reduce growth of contaminants but also contains a colored pH indicator to denote the alkali-producing dermatophytes. A few nonpathogenic saprophytes will also produce alkalinization and in the occasional case of onychomycosis of toenails caused by airborne molds, a culture medium containing an antibiotic may inhibit growth of the true pathogen.

T. tonsurans. This grows slowly in culture to produce a granular or powdery yellow to red, brown, or buff growth. Crater formation with radial grooves may be produced. Microconidia may be seen regularly. Diagnosis is confirmed by the fact that cultures grow poorly or not at all without thiamine. Cultures are best taken by rubbing the lesion vigorously with a sterile cotton swab moistened with sterile water and then streaked over the agar surface, as described by Head et al and by Rudolph.

T. mentagrophytes. Cultural growth is velvety or granular or fluffy, flat or furrowed, light buff, white, or sometimes pink. The back of the culture can vary from buff to dark red. Round microconidia borne laterally and in clusters confirm the diagnosis within two weeks. Spirals are sometimes present and macroconidia may be seen.

T. verrucosum. Growth is slow, and cannot be observed well for at least three weeks. The colony is compact, glassy, velvety, heaped or furrowed, and usually white, but may be yellow or gray. Chlamydospores are present in early cultures and microconidia may be seen.

M. audouinii. The gross appearance of the culture shows a slowly growing, matted, velvety colony with a light brown color, with the back of the colony reddish brown to orange in color. Under the microscope a few large multiseptate macroconidia (macroaleuriospores) are seen. Microconidia (microaleuriospores) in a lateral position on the hyphae are clavate. Racquet mycelium, chlamydospores, and pectinate hyphae are sometimes seen.

M. canis. The culture grossly shows profuse, fuzzy, cottony aerial mycelia tending to become powdery in the center. The color is buff to light brown. The back of the colony is lemon to orange-yellow in color. Microscopically, there are numerous spindle-shaped multiseptate microconidia and thick-walled macroconidia. Clavate microconidia are found along with chlamydospores and pectinate bodies.

DIFFERENTIAL DIAGNOSIS. Tinea capitis must at times be differentiated clinically from impetigo, pediculosis capitis, alopecia areata, psoriasis, seborrheic dermatitis, secondary syphilis, trichotillomania, lupus erythematosus, lichen planus, lichen simplex chronicus, and various inflammatory follicular conditions. Only uncommonly is ringworm of the scalp observed in patients over 15 years of age, and although favus can occur in adult life, it is more frequent in childhood. Alopecia areata, seborrheic dermatitis, psoriasis, lichen planus, and other inflammatory follicular conditions can occur at any age. The distinctive clinical features of tinea capitis are broken-off stumps of hairs, usually in rounded erythematous patches in which there are crusts or pustules and few hairs. The broken-off hairs are loose and when examined are found to be surrounded by, or contain, the fungus.

In alopecia areata the affected patches are bald and the skin is smooth and shiny without any signs of inflammation or scaling. Stumps of broken-off hairs are infrequently found, and no fungi are demonstrable. In seborrheic dermatitis the involved areas are covered by fine, dry, or greasy scales. In psoriasis, well-demarcated, sometimes diffuse, areas of erythema and white or silver scaling are noted. Lichen simplex chronicus frequently is localized to the inferior margin of the occipital scalp. In trichotillomania, as in alopecia areata, inflammation and scaling are absent. Circumscribed lesions are very rare. Serologic testing, scalp biopsies, and immunofluorescent studies may be indicated if the alopecia of secondary syphilis or lupus erythematosus is a serious consideration.

TREATMENT. Griseofulvin of ultramicronized form, 3.3 mg/lb, is the daily dose for children. Grifulvin V is the only oral suspension available for children unable to swallow tablets. The dose is 5 mg/lb/day. Treatment should continue for two to four months, or for at least two weeks after negative microscopic and culture examinations are obtained. Griseofulvin does not primarily affect the delayed type hypersensitivity reaction responsible for the inflammation in kerion. For this, systemic steroids, to minimize scarring, should be given concomitantly with the griseofulvin, or as a single IM dose of Kenalog (triamcinolone acetonide), which is effective for about four weeks and obviates the problem of compliance. There are no side effects from such treatment, apart from mild prolongation of the next menstrual period in about one woman in four.

Continuous and sustained griseofulvin therapy may be difficult in children, especially if the parents cannot be depended upon to carry it out. In this situation a single oral dose of 3 gm of griseofulvin (preferably micronized) is given. The crushed tablets may be taken in fluids, the whole tablets may be swallowed, or the griseofulvin may be suspended in a flavored syrup. Another 3-gm dose may be given three to seven days later. The criterion for cure is two negative cultures.

Barrett has shown that ultramicrosize griseofulvin (Gris-PEG, Fulvicin P/G, Grisactin Ultra) has so much greater bioavailability that 250 mg daily is equivalent to 500 mg of microsize griseofulvin, both in blood level obtained and in clinical response.

Herbert recommends culture of family members, caution regarding the sharing of potentially contaminated fomites, and simultaneous treatment of all persons infected clinically or by culture. Some advise keeping children out of school for a week or two, but we are not among them.

Allen et al have shown that selenium sulfide lotion used as a shampoo in patients receiving griseofulvin therapy resulted in negative cultures at two weeks in 15 of 16 patients; almost all using griseofulvin alone or with bland shampoos and topical clotrimazole had positive cultures as long as eight weeks later.

PROGNOSIS. Recurrence usually does not take place when adequate amounts of griseofulvin have been taken. As Herbert points out, exposure to infected persons, asymptomatic carriers, or contaminated fomites will increase the relapse rate. Without medication there is spontaneous clearing at about 15 years of age, except with *T. tonsurans*, which persists into adult life.

Dermatophytid

A generalized or localized skin reaction to fungal antigen is an "id" reaction, associated with some of the common dermatophytoses of the scalp, feet, and other sites. The primary site of infection is usually acutely inflamed, manifesting such lesions as kerion or bullous tinea pedis.

The most common type of "id" reaction is seen on the hands and sides of the fingers when there is an acute fungus infection of the feet. These lesions are mostly vesicular in reaction and are extremely pruritic and even tender. Secondary bacterial infection may occur; however, fungus is not demonstrable and should not be if it is a true dermatophytid.

The onset is at times accompanied by fever, anorexia, generalized adenopathy, spleen enlargement, and leukocytosis.

The dermatophytid may be an acute widespread eruption, usually follicular and lichenoid or decidedly scaly. The lesions are chiefly on the trunk, where there are pinhead-sized acuminate or flat-topped lichenoid papules, which are often grouped to form rings or scaly patches. Rarely the eruption may be morbilliform or scarlatiniform. This type of reaction is seen occasionally in tinea capitis with or without kerion reactions.

The histologic picture is characterized by spongiotic vesicles and a superficial, perivascular, predominantly lymphohistiocytic infiltrate. Eosinophils may be present.

Other reactive patterns have been noted, with speculation as to their true nature. These reactions may be in the form of *erythema nodosum, erythema annulare centrifugum, migratory thrombophlebitis, erysipelaslike reaction*, especially of the shin, and *urticaria*. However, very few of these eruptions occur secondary to a dermatophytosis. More commonly they are either idiopathic, or are reactions to drugs, carcinoma, or bacterial infections.

The erysipelaslike dermatophytid is most commonly seen on the shin, where it appears as an elevated, sharply defined, erysipelaslike plaque about the size of the hand, usually with toeweb tinea on the same side. It responds promptly to a few days of oral prednisone, or a single intramuscular injection of either 9–12 mg of Celestone Soluspan or 40–60 mg of Kenalog (triamcinolone acetonide). But streptococcal cellulitis has been reported in this situation as well, especially in patients who have had vein grafts taken from the affected leg; Greenberg et al and Baddour et al have both reported this sequence of events. Triamcinolone intramuscularly will not worsen, and usually ameliorates, erysipelas.

Diagnosis of a dermatophytid reaction is dependent upon the demonstration of a fungus at some site remote from the suspect lesions of the dermatophytid, the absence of fungus in the "id" lesion, and involution of the lesion as the fungus infection subsides. In addition, a skin test shows a positive reaction to trichophytin.

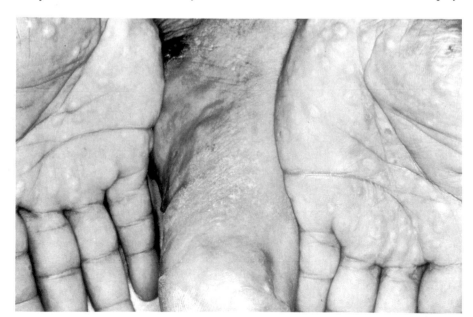

Figure 15–8. Dermatophytid due to bullous tineapedis. (Courtesy of Dr. Axel W. Hoke.)

Trichophytin. An antigen prepared from cultures of dermatophytes may produce reactions when injected intradermally into sensitized individuals with dermatophytosis. Wilson describes two types of reactions, the *immediate wheal reaction* and the *delayed tuberculin-type*. The delayed type of reaction to trichophytin is observed especially in acute kerion and dermatophytid reactions. The immediate reaction is seen commonly in chronic, noninflammatory infections with *T. rubrum*. Patients with atopic dermatitis and widespread tinea corporis form a significant portion of this subgroup. Lobitz has shown that the test may be positive in the erythematous portion of an annular dermatophytid and negative in the pale center of the same lesion. In general, the test is of negligible diagnostic value, and it is rarely performed in practice.

TINEA BARBAE

Synonyms: Tinea sycosis, barber's itch.
CLINICAL FEATURES. Ringworm of the beard is not a common disease. It occurs chiefly among those in agricultural pursuits, especially those in contact with farm animals. The involvement is mostly one-sided on the neck or face. Two clinical types are distinguished: deep nodular suppurative lesions; and superficial, crusted, partially bald patches with folliculitis.

The deep type of the disease develops slowly and produces nodular thickenings and kerionlike swellings, usually caused by *T. mentagrophytes* or *T. verrucosum*. As a rule the swellings are confluent and form diffuse boggy infiltrations with abscesses. The overlying skin is inflamed, the hairs are loose or absent, and pus may be expressed through the remaining follicular openings. Generally the lesions are limited to one part of the face or neck in men. The upper lip is not usually involved, although the mustache area may occasionally be the site of tinea barbae.

The superficial crusted type causes mild pustular folliculitis with broken-off hairs (*T. violaceum*) or without broken-off hairs (*T. rubrum*). The hairs affected are generally loose, dry, and brittle, and when extracted the bulb appears intact.

DIAGNOSIS. The clinical diagnosis is confirmed by the microscopic findings of the fungus and by standard culture techniques for dermatophyte infections.

Rarely, *E. floccosum* may cause widespread verrucous lesions known as *verrucous epidermophytosis*.

DIFFERENTIAL DIAGNOSIS. Tinea barbae differs from sycosis vulgaris by usually sparing the upper lip, and by often being unilateral. In sycosis vulgaris the lesions are pustules and papules, pierced in the center by a hair, which is loose and easily extracted after suppuration has occurred. Contact dermatitis and herpes infections are important differential diagnostic considerations. Careful history, patch testing, and appropriate cultures will resolve such possibilities.

TREATMENT. Micronized or ultramicronized griseofulvin orally in a dosage of 500–1000 mg or 350–700 mg, respectively, daily for adults will usually cure tinea barbae in four to six weeks. Topical antifungals, such as miconazole, clotrimazole, oxiconazole, sulconazole, econazole, ketoconazole, naftifine, or ciclopirox olamine (Loprox), are effective and should be applied from the beginning of treatment. The affected parts should be bathed thoroughly in soap and water, and the healthy areas that are not epilated may be shaved or clipped.

When kerion is present a short course of systemic steroid therapy may help reduce inflammation and the risk of scarring.

TINEA FACIEI

Fungus infection of the face (apart from the beard) is frequently misdiagnosed, since the typical ringworm is only uncommonly seen on the face. Instead, erythematous, slightly scaling, indistinct borders are usually seen.

The diagnosis is easily established by direct microscopic examination.

Most frequently tinea of the face is mistaken for seborrheic dermatitis, contact dermatitis, lupus ery-

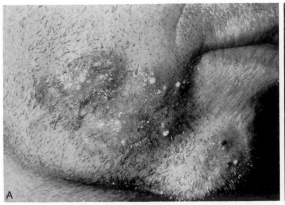
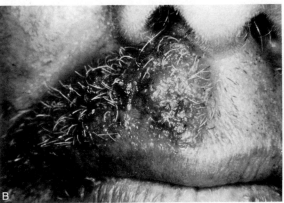

Figure 15–9. A *and* B, *Tinea barbae caused by* Trichophyton mentagrophytes.

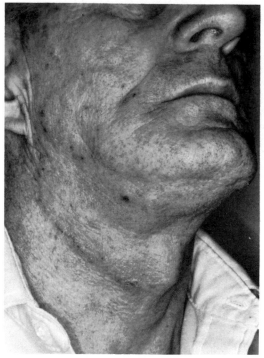

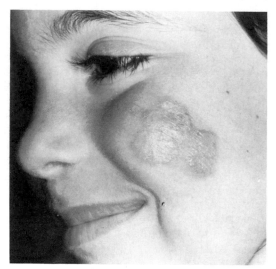

Figure 15–12. Tinea faciale (M. canis) *in a child.*

Figure 15–10. Tinea on the face and neck. Note arcuate margin.

(Nizoral), or sulconazole (Exelderm) usually bring about a prompt response. Oral griseofulvin is also administered for two to four weeks.

thematosus, or a photosensitive dermatosis, until the lack of response to various medication makes one think of fungus infection.

Usually the infection is caused by *T. rubrum, T. mentagrophytes,* or *M. canis.*

Topical applications of clotrimazole (Mycelex or Lotrimin), naftifine (Naftin), miconazole (Monistat or Micatin), ciclopirox olamine (Loprox) cream, econazole (Spectazole), oxiconazole (Oxistat), ketoconazole

TINEA CORPORIS (Tinea Circinata)

CLINICAL FEATURES. Tinea corporis includes all superficial dermatophyte infections of the skin other than those involving the scalp, beard, face, hands, feet, and groin. Sites of predilection are the neck, upper and lower extremities, and the trunk. It can be caused by any of the dermatophytes. This form of ringworm is characterized by one or more circular, sharply circumscribed, slightly erythematous, dry,

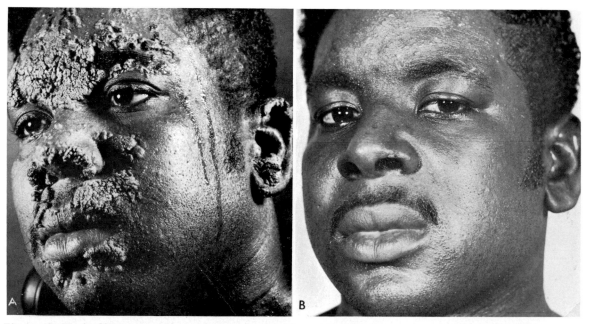

Figure 15–11. A, *Verrucous epidermophytosis from* Epidermophyton floccosum, *resistant to local therapy.* B, *Complete involution after 48 days of griseofulvin therapy. (Courtesy of Department of Dermatology, University of Miami Medical School.)*

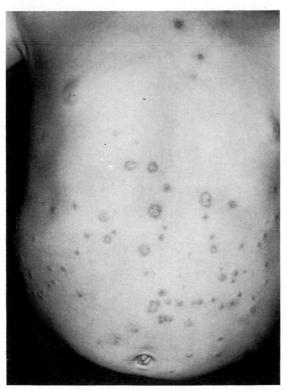

Figure 15–13. Tinea corporis in a child, caused by Microsporum canis.

scaly, usually hypopigmented patches. These lesions may be slightly elevated, particularly at the border, where they are more inflamed and scaly than at the central part. Progressive central clearing produces annular outlines which give them the name "ringworm." These lesions may widen to form rings many centimeters in diameter.

In some cases concentric circles form rings upon one another, making intricate patterns (tinea imbricata).

Multiple disseminated patches of both dry (macular) and moist (vesicular) types of tinea circinata are encountered in which most of the skin surface may be involved. Widespread tinea corporis may be the presenting sign of AIDS, the acquired immunodeficiency syndrome.

HISTOPATHOLOGY. Rarely the question of microscopic pathology may arise—rarely, because there are better ways to make the diagnosis than by histopathology. But if compact orthokeratosis is found in a section, a search should be made for fungal hyphae stained with hematoxylin. This, of course, is diagnostic; Ollague and Ackerman have reported on this subject.

ETIOLOGY. Various organisms may cause this type of fungus infection. Microsporum canis, T. rubrum, and T. mentagrophytes are frequently the causative organisms. T. tonsurans has experienced a dramatic rise as a cause of tinea corporis, as it has done for tinea capitis; it was the cause in 129 of 165 cases seen in the last six years at Cook County Hospital in Chicago. While this was no doubt largely the result

of heightened index of suspicion and new cases that might have been missed earlier, it surely represents a real increase as well. In children M. canis is the cause of the moist type of tinea circinata. Other causative organisms and their characteristic skin manifestations will be discussed under "Other Types of Tinea Corporis."

INCIDENCE. Tinea corporis is frequently seen in children, particularly those who are exposed to animals with ringworm (M. canis), especially cats, dogs, and less commonly, horses and cattle. In adults excessive perspiration is the most common predisposing factor. The incidence is especially high in hot and humid areas of the world.

DIAGNOSIS. The diagnosis is relatively easily made by finding the fungus under the microscope in skin scrapings. In addition, skin scrapings can be cultured on a suitable medium. Growth of the fungus on culture medium is apparent within a week or two at most and, in most instances, is identifiable by the gross appearance of the culture. Identification of the fungus, as stated above, is of epidemiologic interest, and is not helpful in managing the infection.

It is best not to rely routinely solely on cultures. Indeed, *cultures are most useful when—having been performed on lesions thought surely to be nonfungal—they surprise the physician by being positive.* Sterile cultures are frequently found in fungal lesions.

Other diseases which may closely resemble tinea corporis are pityriasis rosea, impetigo, nummular dermatitis, secondary and tertiary syphilids, seborrheic dermatitis, and psoriasis.

TREATMENT. When tinea corporis is caused by T. tonsurans, M. canis, T. mentagrophytes, or T. rubrum the treatment of choice is griseofulvin. The ultramicronized form (Fulvicin P/G, Grisactin Ultra, or GrisPEG) is used, and the usual dose is 350–750 mg once daily for four to six weeks. This dose may be increased to twice daily if necessary. Approximately 10 per cent of individuals will experience nausea with griseofulvin. These persons should stop therapy for three or four days and then resume to see if this pause will circumvent the unfavorable reactions. Other toxic reactions to griseofulvin are rare. However, headache, gastric upset, and infrequent and unusual skin eruptions with photosensitivity, glossitis, and stomatitis have been reported.

Apparent fungal resistance to griseofulvin is decidedly rare, and proven resistance rarer still; but if it seems that malabsorption can be excluded, or if griseofulvin is not tolerated, ketoconazole (Nizoral) is an effective alternative. It has potential for hepatotoxicity; but the incidence in one series was 1:15,000. The majority of these cases have occurred in women over 40 years of age, after two to six weeks of therapy with an average daily dose of 200 mg per day. It has also some potential for gynecomastia but the risk of this is low also. The dose of Nizoral is one 200-mg tablet daily, except in tinea versicolor, when the dose should be a single dose of 400 mg, as shown by Jacobs. The dose may be repeated after a

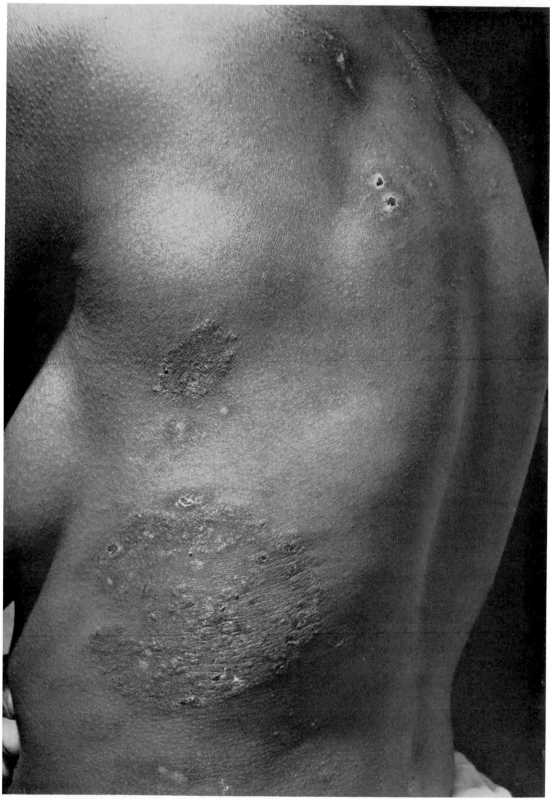

Figure 15–14. *Tinea corporis* (Trichophyton rubrum). *Note sharp margins, central clearing.*

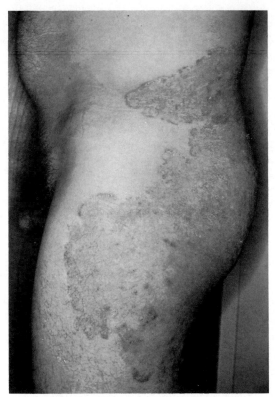

Figure 15–15. Trichophyton rubrum *infection of an American soldier in Vietnam.*

week. Newer azole derivatives such as itraconazole and other chemically diverse antifungals are being tested but are not available in mid-1989.

Ginsburg et al studied the absorption of griseofulvin in 23 children who were fed it either fasting or with a meal (milk) and found that levels were four-fold higher in the group that took it with milk. The only effective blood levels occurred in those taking 15/mg/kg/day, with milk.

When only one or two patches occur, topical treatment is sufficient. Sulconazole (Exelderm), oxiconazole (Oxistat), miconazole (Monistat cream or lotion, or Micatin cream), clotrimazole (Lotrimin or Mycelex cream), econazole (Spectazole), naftifine (Naftin), ketoconazole (Nizoral), or Loprox (ciclopirox olamine) are currently available and effective. Castellani paint (which is colorless if made without fuchsin) is very effective. Salicylic acid 3 to 5 per cent with precipitated sulfur 5 per cent, or half strength Whitfield's ointment, standbys 30 years ago, are little used today. The addition of a low-potency steroid cream during the initial three to five days of therapy will decrease irritation rapidly without compromising the effectiveness of the antifungal.

PROGNOSIS. When griseofulvin is well tolerated, there is rapid clearing within a week or two. Therapy is continued for two or three days to a week after clinical disappearance of the lesions, in order to avoid recurrence. Topical medication is effective only for small patches: recurrence is the rule for more generalized cases.

Other Forms of Tinea Corporis

Trichophytic Granuloma (Perifollicular Granuloma, Majocchi's Granuloma). Occasionally a deep pustular type of tinea circinata resembling a carbuncle or kerion is observed on the glabrous skin. It is a circumscribed, annular, raised, crusty, and boggy granuloma in which the follicles are distended with viscid purulent material. These occur most frequently on the shins or wrists. This type of lesion is a perifollicular granuloma caused by *T. rubrum* or *T. mentagrophytes* infecting hairs at the site of involvement. Early in its course, such a deep lesion may be a pale, circular edematous plaque, often KOH- and culture-negative.

Diagnosis is made by demonstration of the fungus by direct microscopic potassium hydroxide slide and by culture or by clinical suspicion. Occasionally the diagnosis is made on a biopsy specimen.

Treatment is the same as for tinea corporis, except that even for localized lesions oral therapy is necessary.

Tinea Imbricata (Tokelau). This is a superficial fungus infection limited to southwest Polynesia, Melanesia, Southeast Asia, India, and Central America. It is characterized by concentric rings of scales forming extensive patches with polycyclic borders. The eruption begins with one or several small rounded macules on the trunk and arms. The small macular patch splits in the center and forms large flaky scales attached at the periphery. As the resultant ring spreads peripherally, another brownish macule appears in the center and undergoes the process of splitting and peripheral extension. This is repeated over and over again. When fully developed the eruption is characterized by concentrically arranged rings or parallel undulating lines of scales overlapping each other like shingles on a roof (*imbrex* means shingle).

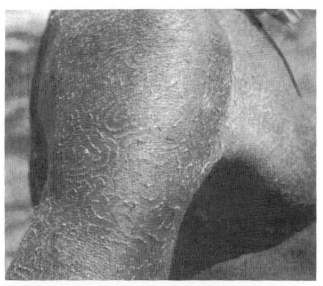

Figure 15–16. Tinea imbricata in New Guinea native. (Courtesy of Dr. J. C. Belisario.)

The causative fungus is *T. concentricum*. Microscopically, the scrapings show interlacing, septate, mycelial filaments that branch dichotomously. Polyhedral spores are also present.

Treatment of choice is griseofulvin, given in the same manner as for tinea corporis, or ketoconazole. There is a tendency for recurrence or reinfection when treatment is stopped. It may be necessary to give several courses of griseofulvin therapy and to remove the patient from the hot and humid environment.

TINEA CRURIS

Synonyms: Jock itch, crotch itch.

CLINICAL FEATURES. Tinea cruris occurs most frequently in men upon the upper and inner surfaces of the thighs, especially during the hot summer months if there is high humidity. It begins as a small erythematous and scaling or vesicular and crusted patch that spreads peripherally and partly clears in the center, so that the patch is characterized chiefly by its curved, well-defined border, particularly on its lower edge. The border may have vesicles, pustules, or papules. It may extend downward upon the thighs and backward on the perineum or about the anus. The penoscrotal fold or sides of the scrotum are seldom involved, and we have never seen involvement of the penis.

ETIOLOGY. Ringworm of the groin usually is caused by *T. rubrum*, *T. mentagrophytes*, or *Epidermophyton floccosum*. For description of the culture characteristics, see p. 323. *Candida albicans* infection may closely mimic tinea cruris; the most useful distinguishing features it possesses are the regular occurrence of small "daughter" macules, centrally desquamating to form collarette scales, and satellite

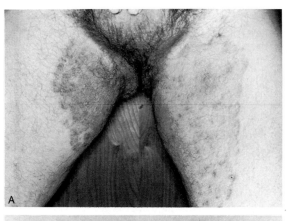
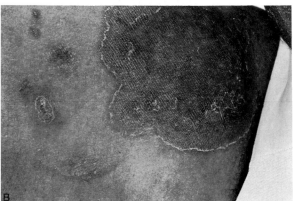
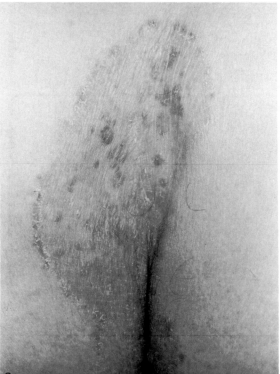

Figure 15–17. A, *Tinea cruris in a man.* B, *Tinea cruris in a woman.* C, *Tinea cruris of the buttocks.*

pustules, scattered along the periphery of the main macule.

INCIDENCE AND PREVALENCE. Heat and high humidity are the predisposing factors for the development of tinea cruris. Tight jockey shorts, which prevent evaporation of the increased perspiration produced during warm weather, may be an additional predisposing factor.

DIFFERENTIAL DIAGNOSIS. The crural region is not only a common site for tinea cruris infections but also for erythrasma, seborrheic dermatitis, pemphigus vegetans, and intertriginous psoriasis. Erythrasma is diagnosed by the Wood's light examination, which produces coral red fluorescence. When this fluorescence is found in the groin, examination should also be made of the axillae and the interdigital spaces of the toes, especially the fourth interspace. Demonstration of fungus by potassium hydroxide microscopic examination and culture establishes the diagnosis. As with dermatophytosis elsewhere, however, failure to demonstrate the fungus does *not* mean it is not there, and treatment should never be withheld in typical cases merely on this account.

TREATMENT. The reduction of perspiration and the enhancement of evaporation from the crural area are important prophylactic measures. The area should be kept as dry as possible by the wearing of loose underclothing and trousers. Plain talcum powder or antifungal powders are helpful.

Specific topical treatment is the same as that described earlier for tinea circinata.

The topical application of Castellani paint is an effective but messy method of treatment. The solution is painted on once daily, preferably at nighttime, for two weeks. Care is taken to prevent spillage. During the period of medication old underclothes are worn because of the inevitable staining if fuchsin is used.

Castellani paint:
℞ Fuchsin (may be omitted) 0.3
Ethyl alcohol 95% 10.0
Boric acid 1.0
Phenol liquef. 4.0
Acetone 5.0
Resorcinol 10.0
Aqua q.s. ad 100.0
Paint affected areas once daily.

Note: Omission of fuchsin diminishes the effectiveness only slightly and makes the paint colorless.

Whitfield's ointment, 2 per cent salicylic acid and 5 per cent precipitated sulfur in hydrophilic ointment, and iodochlorhydroxyquin 3 per cent creams, ointments, or lotions (Domeform HC, Vioform) may also be used.

Griseofulvin by mouth enhances the efficacy of the topical medications and, when well tolerated, 350–750 mg of the ultramicronized form should be taken daily.

TINEA OF HANDS AND FEET

CLINICAL FEATURES. Dermatophytosis of the feet, long popularly called athlete's foot, is by far the most common fungus disease. The primary lesions often consist of maceration, slight scaling, and occasional vesiculation and fissures between and under the toes. Any or all of the toe webs may be thus affected, although most often the third toe web is involved. The patient usually seeks relief because of itching or painful fissuring. If this condition is allowed to progress, there may be an overgrowth of gram-negative organisms. This may eventuate in an ulcerative, exudative process involving the toe webs, and at times the entire soles. It is discussed under intertrigo in Chapter 15, q.v.

Trichophyton mentagrophytes produces an acutely inflammatory condition. If the fungus invades the skin of the toes or of the soles, an acute vesicular or bullous eruption may occur.

The vesicular eruption tends to spread by extension and unless checked, may involve the entire sole. The vesicles are usually about 2 or 3 mm in diameter. They sometimes coalesce to form bullae of various sizes. They are firm to the touch and sometimes of a bluish tint. They do not rupture spontaneously but dry up as the acute stage subsides, leaving yellowish brown crusts. The burning and itching that accompany the formation of the vesicles may cause great discomfort, which is relieved by opening the tense vesicles. They contain a clear tenacious fluid of the consistency of glycerin. Extensive or acute eruptions on the soles may be incapacitating. The fissures between the toes as well as the vesicles may become secondarily infected with pyogenic cocci, which may

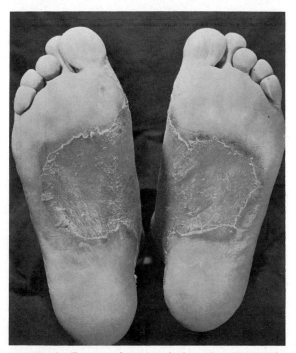

Figure 15–18. Dermatophytosis of the soles (Trichophyton mentagrophytes). *(Courtesy of Dr. H. Shatin.)*

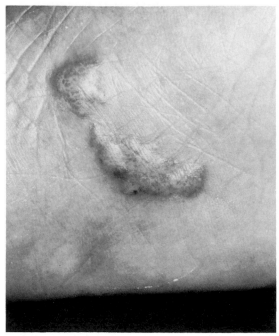

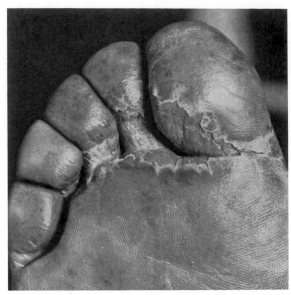

Figure 15–21. Tinea pedis showing interdigital scalping (Trichophyton mentagrophytes).

Figure 15–19. *Acute vesiculobullous eruption on sole caused by* Trichophyton mentagrophytes.

lead to recurrent attacks of lymphangitis and inguinal adenitis.

Hyperhidrosis is frequently present in this type of dermatophytosis. The sweat between the toes and on the soles has a high pH, and keratin damp with it is a good culture medium for the fungi.

Trichophyton rubrum, which causes the majority of cases, produces a relatively noninflammatory type of dermatophytosis characterized by a dull erythema and pronounced scaling that may involve the entire sole and the sides of the foot, giving a "moccasin" or "sandal" appearance. The eruption may, however, be limited to a small patch adjacent to a fungus-infected toenail, or to a patch between or under the toes, on a hand, or other part. Most frequently the involvement is bilateral, but it may be limited to one hand and both feet, an observation that is still awaiting an explanation. Sometimes an extensive patchy scaly eruption covers most of the trunk, buttocks, and extremities. Rarely there is a patchy hyperkeratosis resembling verrucous epidermal nevus.

Generally tinea infection of the hands is of the dry scaly and erythematous type that is suggestive of *T. rubrum* infection. Other areas are frequently affected at the same time. However, the moist, vesicular and eczematous type caused by *T. mentagrophytes,* which is seen more often on the feet, may at times occur on the hand. These two are the types of fungus involvement most frequently seen. Verrucous lesions on the hands resembling tuberculosis verrucosa cutis and caused by *T. rubrum* have been reported.

Occurring more frequently perhaps than true fungus infections, **dermatophytid** of the hands commonly begins with the appearance of groups of minute, clear vesicles on the palms and fingers. The itching may be intense. As a rule, both hands are involved and the eruption tends to be symmetrical; however, there are cases in which only one hand is

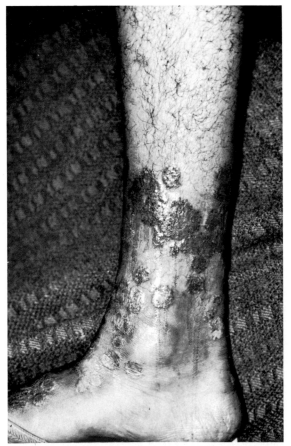

Figure 15–20. Trichophyton mentagrophytes *infection on lower leg of American soldier in Vietnam. (Courtesy of Drs. Blank, Taplin and Zaias.)*

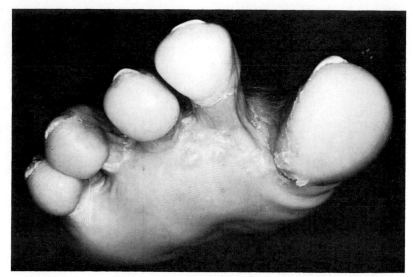

Figure 15–22. Interdigital scaling with vesiculation caused by Trichophyton mentagrophytes.

affected. As the disease becomes chronic the lesions take various forms—dry scaling patches; moist eczematoid areas, which tend to become crusted or thickened; and hyperkeratotic plaques, in which painful fissures are present. At times the patient complains only of the eruption on the hands, and examination of the feet is of utmost importance in these cases.

Dermatophytosis of the hands is frequently difficult to differentiate from allergic contact or irritant dermatitis, especially occupational, or from pompholyx, atopic dermatitis, or psoriasis. It may also resemble lamellar dyshidrosis. Eczematoid or dyshidrotic lesions of unknown cause on the hands call for careful search for clinical evidence of dermatophytosis of the feet and microscopic or cultural study of

suspected skin from the toe webs or nails. Although positive findings on the feet do not alone prove that the condition on the hands is dermatophytid, they do suggest a probable cause if no other findings are apparent. Bear in mind that negative findings do not rule out fungal causes!

If the feet get well but the hands do not, the condition may be pompholyx, or psoriasis, and may yield promptly to 40 mg of triamcinolone diacetate or acetonide intramuscularly—though it will usually recur in three to six weeks.

ETIOLOGY. *T. rubrum* is the most frequent causative fungus. Cultures of this organism are usually

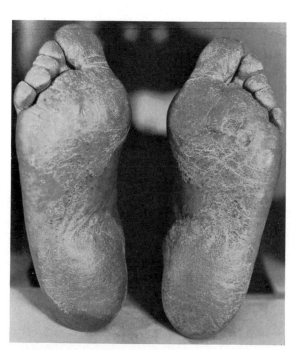

Figure 15–23. Tinea pedis (Trichophyton rubrum). (Courtesy of Dr. E. Florian, Budapest.)

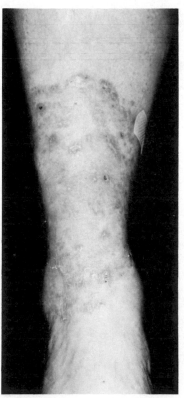

Figure 15–24. Trichophyton rubrum *infection of the lower leg.*

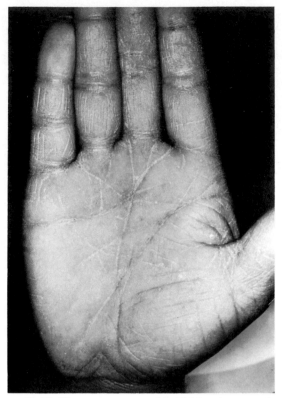

Figure 15–25. Tinea manus caused by Trichophyton rubrum.

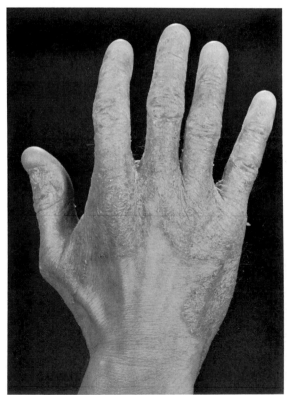

Figure 15–26. Tinea manus due to Trichophyton rubrum. *Note severe involvement of nail beds and sharp, arcuate margins. (Courtesy of Dr. H. Shatin.)*

fluffy, but they can be granular or folding. The backside of the culture is usually deep red; sometimes no color is produced. Microconidia are found in clusters and singly on the hyphae. Macroconidia, chlamydospores, coils, and racquet hyphae are rarely seen. Less frequent causes are *T. mentagrophytes* and *E. floccosum.*

DIAGNOSIS. Demonstration of the fungus by the microscopic examination of the scrapings taken from the involved site establishes the diagnosis. In addition, cultures made from the affected skin establish the identity of the fungus. However, failure to find the fungus does not rule out a fungal cause.

Tissue for examination is scraped off and placed on a glass slide. When the lesion is a vesicle, it is clipped off close to the margin by small pointed scissors; when dry or scaly, the material is scraped off with a scalpel or curet, an effort being made especially to obtain material from deep beneath the surface of chronic eruptions. A drop of a 10 to 20 per cent solution of potassium hydroxide is added to the material on the glass slide. A coverslip is placed over the specimen and pressed down firmly. Gentle heat is applied until the scales are thoroughly macerated. It is then ready for a thorough microscopic study. The mycelium may be seen under low power; but better observation of both hyphae and spores is obtained by the use of the high dry objective with reduced illumination. The lines of juncture of normal epidermal cells are hyaloid and greenish and may easily be mistaken for fungus structures. If you wonder whether it is really mycelium or not, it is not.

A rapid staining method was described by Burke et al, using 100 mg of chlorazol black E dye in 10 ml of DMSO (dimethyl sulfoxide) and adding it to 5 per

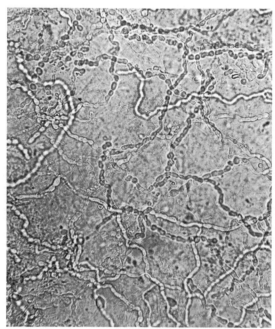

Figure 15–27. Fungus filaments under KOH mount, direct examination.

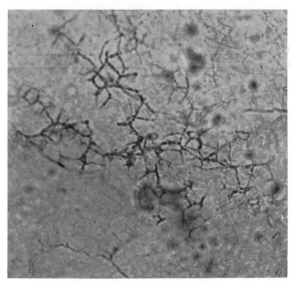

Figure 15–28. Mosaic fungus. (Courtesy of Dr. L. A. Fragola.)

cent aqueous solution of potassium hydroxide. The solution is then used in the same way as ordinary KOH solution, pressing coverglass and slide between pieces of filter paper. It is viewed under bright illumination; hyphae and spores are green against a gray background.

The other portion of the material is planted on Sabouraud's glucose agar or Mycosel agar and cultured at room temperature. Adequate growth for identification occurs in five to 14 days, depending upon the kind of fungus.

Taplin and his associates have devised a culture medium, **Dermatophyte Test Medium (DTM)**, for the diagnosis of dermatophytosis. The medium inhibits growth of bacterial and saprophytic contaminants. The alkaline metabolites of the dermatophytes change the color of the pH indicator in the medium from yellow to red, which distinguishes them from fungal contaminants and *Candida albicans*. If a dermatophyte is present, the medium will turn red. Saprophytes turn the medium green. *C. albicans* does not cause color changes, but produces a typical yeast colony.

Mosaic Fungus. In microscopic examination of the skin for fungi, one often finds the so-called mosaic fungus, which may closely resemble true hyphae. It is caused by overlapping cell borders. A positive potassium hydroxide preparation should reveal definite hyphal elements traversing several epidermal cells.

PROPHYLAXIS. Hyperhidrosis is a predisposing factor. As the disease often starts on the feet, the patient should be advised to dry the toes thoroughly after bathing. Dryness of the parts is essential if reinfection is to be avoided.

The use of a good antiseptic powder on the feet after bathing, particularly between the toes, is strongly advised for susceptible persons. Tolnaftate powder (Tinactin powder) or Zeasorb medicated powder are excellent dusting powders for the feet.

For prophylaxis the following formula has also been found useful:

Antiseptic dusting powder:
℞ Menthol 0.1
Thymol iodide 2.0
Zinc stearate 4.0
Magnesium carbonate 2.0
Boric acid 15.0
Talcum q.s. ad 100.0
Dispense in shaker-top container.

There are many commercially available fungicidal powders; however, the drying property may be the most effective aspect. Plain talc, cornstarch, or rice powder may be dusted into socks and shoes to keep the feet dry.

TREATMENT. Before the fungi can be actively attacked it is often necessary to employ mild soothing remedies on acutely inflamed or denuded areas of skin, or to relieve secondary pyogenic infection that has occurred through fissures or broken vesicles. Useful measures are wet dressings or soaks with such solutions as solution of aluminum acetate, one part to 20 parts of water, or daily soaks for 30 minutes in potassium permanganate solution 1:5000. The antiinflammatory effects of the corticosteroids are markedly beneficial. Topical antibiotic ointments, such as neosporin, polymyxin, or gentamicin (Garamycin), which are effective against gram-negative organisms, are helpful additions in the treatment of the moist type of interdigital lesions. In the ulcerative type of gram-negative toeweb infections, systemic cephalosporins are necessary. See Chapter 14, Gram-negative toeweb infections.

Clotrimazole (Lotrimin or Mycelex), miconazole, sulconazole, oxiconazole, ciclopirox, econazole, ketoconazole, and naftifine are effective fungicides and pleasant to use.

Salicylic acid has a keratolytic effect that is most important when the fungus is protected by a thick layer of overlying skin such as that on the soles. The strength used varies from 2 to 6 per cent, depending upon the degree of exfoliation required. The widely known Whitfield's ointment is still a very effective medication; however, this is too strong for all but very tough areas of skin. For tender areas, half-strength to quarter-strength is usually safe.

Whitfield's ointment:
℞ Acid salicylic 6.0
Acid benzoic 12.0
Lanolin 5.0
Vaseline q.s. ad 100.0
M. and S. Whitfield's ointment. Rub into affected areas morning and night.
Whitfield's solution:
℞ Acid salicyclic 3.0
Acid benzoic 6.0
Ethyl alcohol 70% q.s. ad 100.0
M. and S. Whitfield's solution. Apply twice daily.

Castellani's paint is very effective.
Treatment of fungus infection of the feet and hands with griseofulvin is effective when infection is caused by pathogens such as *T. mentagrophytes, T. rubrum,*

E. floccosum, and others. However, it is not effective in the treatment of *C. albicans* infections. Griseofulvin is only effective against dermatophytes. One of the major advantages of ketoconazole is that it is active against Candida as well.

When the fungus infection is due to *T. mentagrophytes* the acute inflammatory reaction is not decreased by griseofulvin; addition of a potent topical steroid will help. On the other hand, *T. rubrum* infections usually do not respond well to local treatment. In such cases, cessation of griseofulvin therapy may induce relapse.

Griseofulvin in ultramicronized particles is taken orally in doses of 350–750 mg daily. Dosage for children is 3.3 mg/lb/day. The period of therapy depends upon the response of the lesions. Repeated potassium hydroxide scrapings and cultures should be negative.

Griseofulvin should not be taken by persons with porphyria, hepatic dysfunction, or hypersensitivity to griseofulvin. During long-term therapy, observation should be made at intervals for hepatic, hematologic, and renal disorders. Patients on anticoagulant therapy should not receive griseofulvin, since hepatic enzymes activated by griseofulvin will also cause degradation of warfarin, and the increased dosage of warfarin required during concomitant griseofulvin treatment may prove excessive once griseofulvin is discontinued. One should not prescribe this medication during pregnancy.

The most common side effect of griseofulvin ingestion is gastrointestinal, with symptoms such as nausea, epigastric distress, and diarrhea. Some 10 per cent of those taking griseofulvin will experience gastric discomfort. A 48-hour cessation of therapy sometimes corrects this side effect. Other side effects may be fatigue, headache, dizziness, paresthesia, photosensitivity, urticaria, and mental confusion.

Jolly et al reported in a multicenter double-blind study that 200 mg of ketoconazole daily produced 61 per cent remissions, as compared to 39 per cent for griseofulvin, and the proportion of relapses in two

months was 9 per cent, compared to 43 per cent for griseofulvin. They observed no significant side effects. The warnings outlined previously in this chapter, regarding hepatic toxicity and gynecomastia with ketoconazole, apply here. We still prefer topical fungicides and, if systemic medication is needed, griseofulvin.

ONYCHOMYCOSIS (Tinea Unguium)

Onychomycosis is defined as the infection of the nail by fungus. Universally recognized as etiologic agents are species of *Epidermophyton*, *Microsporum*, and *Trichophyton* fungi. In addition to the accepted nail pathogens, there are a significant number of nondermatophytic fungi which have been reported to rarely cause onychomycosis. This type is usually a toenail problem, rarely seen in fingernails.

Frequently the clinical appearance of onychomycosis caused by one species of fungus is indistinguishable from that caused by any other species; however, there are various clinical clues which could allow one to speculate that an organism of a certain species is probably not responsible for a particular case of onychomycosis.

Zaias has outlined four classic types of onychomycosis: (1) Distal subungual onychomycosis primarily involves the distal nail bed and the hyponychium, with secondary involvement of the underside of the nail plate of fingernails and toenails. (2) White superficial onychomycosis (leukonychia trichophytica) is an invasion of the toenail plate on the surface of the nail. It is produced by *T. mentagrophytes*, species of *Cephalosporium* and *Aspergillus*, and *Fusarium oxysporum* fungi. (3) Proximal subungual onychomycosis involves the nail plate mainly from the proximal nail fold, producing a specific clinical picture. It is produced by *T. rubrum* and *T. megninii*. (4) *Candida* onychomycosis involves all the nail plate. It is due to *Candida albicans* and is seen only in patients with chronic mucocutaneous candidiasis.

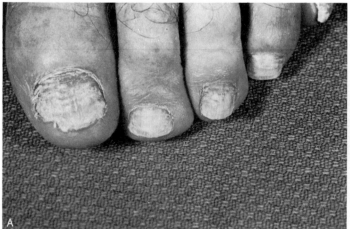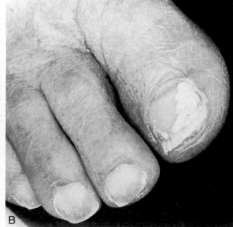

Figure 15–29. A, *Onychomycosis caused by* Trichophyton rubrum. B, *White superficial onychomycosis caused by* Trichophyton mentagrophytes.

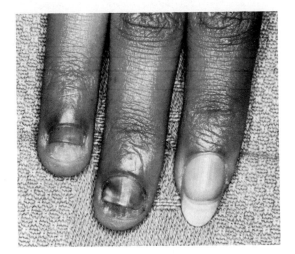

Figure 15–30. *Onychomycosis caused by* Trichophyton rubrum.

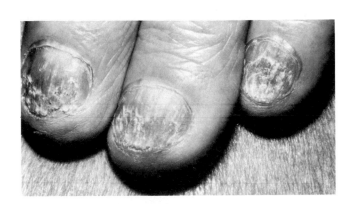

Figure 15–31. *Onychomycosis.*

Figure 15–32. *Onychomycosis caused by* C. albicans *in mucocutaneous candidiasis.*

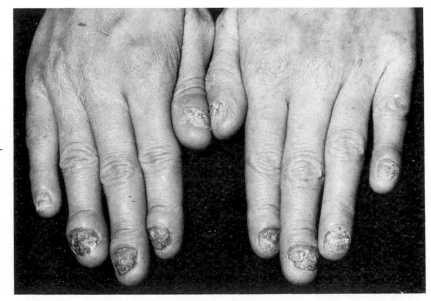

Onychomycosis caused by *T. rubrum* is usually a deep infection. The onset is slow and insidious, with little inflammatory reaction. The disease usually starts at the distal corner of the nail and involves the junction of the nail and its bed. First a yellowish discoloration occurs, which may spread until the entire nail is affected. Beneath this discoloration the nail plate comes loose from the nail bed. Gradually the entire nail becomes brittle and separated from its bed due to the piling up of subungual keratin; it may break off, leaving an undermined remnant that is black and yellow from the dead nail and fungi that are present. Fingernails and toenails present a similar appearance, and the skin of the toes or soles is likely also to be involved, with characteristic branny, scaling, erythematous, well-defined patches.

Onychomycosis caused by *T. mentagrophytes* is usually superficial and there is no paronychial inflammation. The infection generally begins with scaling of the nail under the overhanging cuticle and remains localized to a portion of the nail. In time, however, the entire nail plate may be involved. *Leukonychia trichophytica* is the name given to one type of superficial nail infection due to this fungus in which small chalky white spots appear on or in the nail plate. These may be multiple and variously shaped or just a single spot. They are so superficial that they may be easily shaved off.

However, white spots that resemble ordinary leuconychia may also occur, as Shelley and Wood showed, and they are an excellent "hunting ground" for hyphae lying well within the nail plate, so that overlying normal nail plate must be shaved away before a shaving of fungus-bearing nail plate can be removed. Shelley's method of shaving the nail, with half of a flexible Gillette Super Blue razor blade, is an excellent one.

In nail lesions due to *C. albicans* there is usually paronychia. The disease begins under the lateral or proximal nail fold and a small amount of pus may be expressed. The adjacent cuticle is pink, swollen, and tender on pressure. The neighboring portion of the nail becomes dark, ridged, and separated from its bed. Later the entire nail plate may separate. The fingernails are more commonly infected than the toenails; and it is encountered mostly in housewives, canners, and others who have their hands in water a great deal. In a candida infection the nail plate does not become friable, yellow, or white as in trichophyton infections, but remains hard and glossy as a normal nail plate; associated paronychia is a characteristic feature of this mycotic nail infection.

Scopulariopsis brevicaulis has been infrequently isolated from onychomycosis. Infection usually begins at the lateral edge of the nail, burrows beneath the plate, and produces large quantities of cheesy debris. *Hendersonula toruloidea* and *Scytalidium hyalinum* have been reported to cause onychomycosis, as well as a moccasin-type tinea pedis. In addition to the more common features of onychomycosis such as nail plate thickening, opacification, and onycholysis, features of infection with these fungi include lateral nail invasion alone, paronychia, and transverse fracture of the proximal nail plate. When these agents are suspected, culture must be done with a medium which does not contain cycloheximide. Oral ketoconazole and griseofulvin are not effective in treatment.

In addition to the already mentioned causative fungi, *T. violaceum*, *T. schoenleinii*, and *T. tonsurans* occasionally invade the nails.

In an inexplicable way, fungus infection may affect only some of the nails and leave the others completely free of any involvement. One hypothesis is that slower growing nails are more easily infected.

Usually onychomycosis is accompanied by infection in other sites. In tinea pedis, especially when the toewebs are affected, the nails may act as a reservoir from which reinfection may occur under proper environmental conditions. Infection of the great toenails is frequent in adults. Generally, there is only slight, or no, discomfort.

DIAGNOSIS. The demonstration of fungus is made by microscopic examination and by culture. Immediate examination may be made if very thin shavings are taken from the diseased portion of the nail and heated gently for a minute or so in a drop of potassium hydroxide solution—with or without chlorazol black E—under a coverglass. As the pieces of nail soften they may be pressed thin under the glass. The excess fluid should be removed by touching the sides of the coverglass with small squares of blotting paper. Similar thin shavings are inoculated into culture media such as Mycosel agar or DTM.

DIFFERENTIAL DIAGNOSIS. Numerous affections of the nails make a firm diagnosis of onychomycosis difficult unless fungi are actually demonstrated; therefore, great care should be exercised in the performance of the microscopic fungus examination. One is confronted most frequently with the fingernail problems of women. Allergic contact dermatitis due to nail polish is exceedingly difficult to distinguish from onychomycosis; one must resort to repeated fungus examination. Psoriasis may involve one nail by only a slight pitting, or onycholysis, or by heaped up subungual keratinization which eventually produces a moist oozing mass that separates the nail from its bed. Psoriasis, however, typically begins in the middle of the free edge of the nail rather than in a corner, and may, pathognomonically, begin proximal to the free edge ("oil spots"). Lichen planus is exceedingly difficult to differentiate, and again demonstration of the fungus is essential. Both psoriasis and lichen planus usually show other areas of skin involvement. Various nail dystrophies, such as those seen in Darier's disease, Reiter's disease, and hyperkeratotic ("Norwegian") scabies, should also be kept in mind.

TREATMENT. Ridding the nails of fungus still remains an extremely difficult task. For many years topical therapy, usually preceded by surgical avulsion, was the only means. Onycholysis due to *C. albicans* does not respond to griseofulvin, but fortunately responds fairly well to topical applications of haloprogin (Halotex), miconazole (Monistat-Derm, Micatin), naftifine (Naftin), ketoconazole (Nizoral), econazole (Spectazole), clotrimazole (Lotrimin or Mycelex), sulconazole (Exelderm), oxiconazole (Oxistat), or Castellani paint. Econazole nitrate (Spectazole) may offer enhanced penetration and some antibacterial activity against gram-positive bacteria. Trimming back the onycholytic portion of the nail is a prerequisite to the success of this therapy. At least 90 days of application are indicated, with expectation of fairly good results. Oral ketoconazole is effective against *C. albicans* and may be used in painful paronychias unresponsive to topical therapy.

Treatment for infection caused by dermatophytes poses many more problems. Local application of medication after thorough grinding down or scraping down of the nail offers some hope. Surgical avulsion of the nails, especially the fingernails, followed by topical medication and griseofulvin by mouth is probably the most successful method. However, since griseofulvin treatment is expensive and prolonged (at least six to 12 months), and reinfection is extremely likely to occur, the decision to treat should not be made lightheartedly. While ketoconazole may be effective in treating this condition, relapse is common, and the same drawbacks associated with griseofulvin therapy apply here. In addition, the risk of severe hepatic reactions, although it is only 1:15,000, should be weighed carefully. Risk-benefit considerations nearly always militate against use of this medication in tinea unguium.

Surgical removal of the nail can be done simply and painlessly in less than five minutes as follows: The patient thoroughly washes and dries his hands. An elastic band is placed about the proximal phalanx. The finger and nail are sterilized by scrubbing with soap and painting with tincture of iodine and alcohol, and then placed on a sterile towel.

With ethyl chloride, spray a small spot on the dorsolateral aspect just proximal to the nail to be anesthetized. Through this spot the needle of a hypodermic containing 2 per cent procaine or mepivacaine solution is introduced, the dorsal nail fold and lateral fold are injected, and 0.5 ml is placed deep laterally near the digital nerve. Another puncture is made on the other side and through this the other lateral nail fold is injected and 0.5 ml is injected near the other digital nerve. The entire tip of the finger is now numb.

A Bard-Parker No. 15 scalpel blade is inserted under the free margin of the nail, separating it from the bed. The loose nail is now grasped with a hemostat and lifted out. There is no bleeding. Now the really important part of the operation takes place. That is the meticulous removal under a magnifying glass of any fragments of nail or cuticle and the thorough scraping of the nail bed with the blade of the scalpel. There may be slight oozing. The elastic band is released. A large dressing is now applied and the patient is told to hold the finger upright. The patient dresses the finger himself daily, applying

an antibiotic ointment or griseofulvin powder as recommended by Demis and Brown. Oral griseofulvin is continued during regrowth.

The proportion of cures following this operation is a little better than 75 per cent. In case of failure it can be repeated. The results, as might be expected, seem to depend largely upon a bloodless field and the thoroughness of the removal of all infected tissue.

If the operation is not done, daily application of strong fungicides to the infected nails serves to destroy the organisms on the surface and to prevent spread of the infection to adjacent areas of skin and to nails that are not yet diseased. Of these, Castellani paint, Whitfield's ointment, or the following formula is recommended.

Nail paint:
  R Thymol 0.1
  Acid salicylic 6.0
  Tincture iodine strong 12.0
  Acetone 8.0
  Xylol 4.0
  Alcohol q.s. ad 100.0
  M. and S. Paint nails morning and night.

Nonsurgical Avulsion of the Nail. This method employs urea in 22 or 40 per cent formulations to allow easy removal of the nail plate in a variety of nail dystrophies and diseases, including mycotic nails.

Farber and South have recommended two formulations:

Compound A (22 per cent):
  Urea 22.25 per cent
  Anhydrous lanolin 22.25 per cent
  White wax 5.50 per cent
  White petrolatum 50.00 per cent

Compound B (40 per cent):
  Urea 40 per cent
  Anhydrous lanolin 20 per cent
  White wax 5 per cent
  White petrolatum 35 per cent

Cloth adhesive tape is used to cover the normal skin surrounding the affected nail plate after pretreatment with tincture of benzoin or Mastisol. Either Compound A or B is generously applied directly to the nail surface, which is then covered with a piece of plastic film wrap. This is covered either with adhesive tape alone or with a "finger" cut from a plastic glove held in place with adhesive tape.

The patients are instructed to keep the area completely dry. Plastic gloves or plastic booties can be dispensed for this purpose. The patients return after five to ten days and the treated nails are removed by either lifting the entire nail plate from the nail bed and cutting it behind the proximal nail fold, or by cutting away the abnormal portions using a bone spatula and nail cutter. This is followed by curettage until clinically normal nail is reached at all margins. Following nail avulsion, the patient is instructed to apply either antifungal agents or 3 per cent thymol in chloroform, or both, twice daily. Oral griseofulvin therapy must be administered concomitantly and for three to six months subsequent to avulsion.

The procedure is essentially painless, and apparently with little risk of infection or hemorrhage, making it the best option for treating patients with diabetes and others with vascular insufficiency and neuropathy of the digits.

Allen HB, et al: Selenium sulfide: adjunctive therapy for tinea capitis. Pediatrics 1982, 69:81.

Artis WM, et al: Griseofulvin-resistant dermatophytosis correlates with in vitro resistance. Arch Dermatol 1981, 117:16.

Bronson DM, et al: An epidemic of infection with *Trichophyton tonsurans* revealed in a 20-year survey of fungal infections in Chicago. JAAD 1983, 8:332.

Burke WA, et al: A simple stain for rapid office diagnosis of fungus infections of the skin. Arch Dermatol 1984, 120:1519.

Daily AD, et al: Econazole nitrate (Spectazole) cream, 1 percent: a topical agent for the treatment of tinea pedis. Cutis 1985, 33:278.

Eaglstein NF, et al: Gram-negative toeweb infection. JAAD 1983, 8:225.

Gentry RH, et al: Atypical dermatophytosis acquired in the tropics. J Assoc Milit Dermatol 1988, 14:17.

Ginsburg CM, et al: Effect of feeding on the bioavailability of griseofulvin in children. J Pediatr 1983, 102:309.

Goldsmith S: Vitamin E and onychomycosis (letter). JAAD 1983, 8:910.

Greenberg J et al: Vein-donor-leg cellulitis after coronary artery bypass surgery. Ann Intern Med 1982, 97:565.

Greer DL, et al: Tinea pedis caused by *Hendersonula toruloidea*. JAAD 1987, 16:1111.

Hanifin JM, et al: Itraconazole therapy for recalcitrant dermatophyte infections. JAAD 1988, 18:1077.

Hay RJ, et al: Clinical features of superficial fungus infections caused by *Hendersonula toruloidea* and *Scytalidium hyalinum*. Br J Dermatol 1984, 110:677.

Head ES, et al: The cotton swab technic for the culture of dermatophyte infections—its efficacy and merit. JAAD 1984, 11:797.

Herbert AA: Tinea capitis. Current concepts. Arch Dermatol 1988, 124:1559.

Jacobs AH, et al: Tinea in tiny tots. Am J Dis Child 1986, 140:1034.

Jolly HW Jr, et al: A multicenter double-blind evaluation of ketoconazole in the treatment of dermatomycoses. Cutis 1983, 31:208.

Joly J, et al: Favus. Arch Dermatol 1978, 114:1647.

Kearse HL, et al: Tinea pedis in prepubertal children. JAAD 1988, 19:619.

Keipert JA: Beneficial effect of corticosteroid therapy in *Microsporum canis* kerion. Austral J Dermatol 1984, 25:127.

Kligman AM, et al: Evaluation of ciclopirox olamine cream for tinea pedis. Clin Ther 1985, 7:409.

Lewis JH, et al: Hepatic injury from ketoconazole. Gastroenterology 1984, 86:503.

Leyden JJ, et al: Interdigital athlete's foot. Arch Dermatol 1978, 114:1466.

McLean T, et al: Ecology of dermatophyte infections in South Bronx, N.Y. 1969–1981. JAAD 1987, 16:336.

Ollague J, et al: Compact orthokeratosis as a clue to chronic dermatophytosis and candidiasis. Am J Dermatopathol 1982, 4:459.

Ravits MS, et al: Tinea capitis in the New York City area. Arch Dermatol 1983, 119:532.

Robinson HM Jr, et al: Tolnaftate: a potent topical antifungal agent. Arch Dermatol 1965, 91:372.

Roller JA, et al: *Microsporum nanum* infection in hog farmers. JAAD 1986, 15:935.

Rosen T, et al: Radiation port dermatophytosis. JAAD 1988, 19:1053.

Rudolph AH: Diagnosis and treatment of tinea capitis due to *Trichophyton tonsurans*. Int J Dermatol 1985, 24:426.

Serjeantson S, et al: Autosomal recessive inheritance of susceptibility to tinea. Lancet 1977, 1:13.

Sharma V, et al: Scalp colonization by *Trichophyton tonsurans* in an urban pediatrics clinic. Arch Dermatol 1988, 124:1511.

Shelley WB, et al: The white spot target for microscopic examination of the nails for fungi. JAAD 1982, 6:92.

Spiekermann PH, et al: Clinical evaluation of clotrimazole, a broad-spectrum antifungal agent. Arch Dermatol 1976, 112:350.

Taplin D, et al: Isolation and recognition of dermatophytes on a new medium (DTM). Arch Dermatol 1969, 99:203.

Zaias N: The Nail in Health and Disease. Jamaica, NY, Spectrum Publications, 1980.

CANDIDIASIS

Synonyms: Candidosis, moniliasis, thrush, oidiomycosis.

CLINICAL FEATURES. *Candida albicans* may cause different types of lesions of the skin, nails, mucous membranes, and viscera. It may be a normal inhabitant at various sites until there is some change in the state of the area; then it becomes a pathogen.

The intertriginous areas are frequently affected. Here warmth, moisture, and maceration of the skin permit the organism to thrive. The areas most often involved are the perianal and inguinal folds, the interdigital areas, the nail folds, and the axillae. There may be a generalized type in which not only most of the skin surface is involved but also the mucous membranes of the mouth and the gastrointestinal tract. Systemic forms may be superimposed upon cutaneous candidiasis.

Candida proliferates in both budding and mycelial forms in the outer layers of the stratum corneum where the horny cells are desquamating. The organism usually is found outside the living portion of the epidermis. It does not attack the hair, rarely involves the nail, and is incapable of breaking up the stratum corneum.

It is important to remember that *C. albicans* is very largely an opportunistic organism, able to behave as a pathogen for the most part only in the presence of impaired immune response, or in body folds (inframammary, axillary, nail, intercrural-inguinal, preputial, or vulvovaginal). Moisture also promotes its growth, as in moist lip corners (perleche).

DIAGNOSIS. The demonstration of the pathogenic yeast *C. albicans* establishes the diagnosis. Under the microscope the potassium hydroxide preparation may show spores and pseudomycelium. On Gram stain the yeast forms are dense, gram-positive, ovoid bodies, 2 to 5 microns in diameter. In culture *C. albicans* should be differentiated from other forms of *Candida* that are only rarely pathogenic, such as *C. krusei, stellatoidea, tropicalis, pseudotropicalis*, and *guillermondii*.

Culture on Sabouraud's glucose agar shows a growth of creamy, grayish, moist colonies in about four days. In time the colonies form small rootlike penetrations into the agar. Microscopic examination of the colony shows clusters of budding cells. When

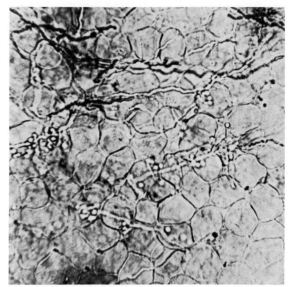

Figure 15–33. Mycelium and spores of Candida albicans *in a potassium hydroxide mount of skin scrapings.*

inoculated into corn meal agar culture, thick-walled, round chlamydospores characteristic of *C. albicans* are produced.

Oral Candidiasis (Thrush)

The mucous membrane of the mouth may be involved in the healthy newborn or the marasmic infant. In the newborn the infection may be acquired from contact with the vaginal tract of the mother. Grayish white membranous plaques are found on the surface of the mucous membrane. The base of these plaques is moist, reddish, and macerated. In its spread the angles of the mouth may become involved, and lesions in the intertriginous areas may occur, especially in marasmic infants.

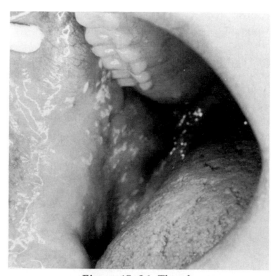

Figure 15–34. Thrush.

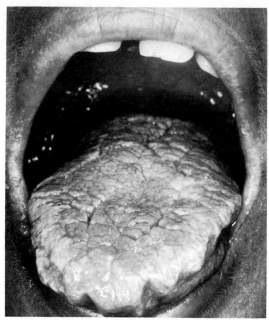

Figure 15–35. Candida albicans *infection of the tongue in chronic mucocutaneous candidiasis.*

The diaper area is especially susceptible to this infection. Most of the intertriginous areas and even the exposed skin may be involved, with small pustules that quickly turn into macerated and erythematous scaling patches.

In adults the buccal mucosa and the tongue may become involved. The papillae of the tongue are atrophied: the surface is smooth, glazed, and bright red. Sometimes there are small erosions on the edges. Frequently the infection extends onto the angles of the mouth to form perlèche.

This is seen in elderly, debilitated, and malnourished patients, and in diabetics. It is often the first manifestation of the acquired immunodeficiency syndrome, and is present in nearly all patients with fullblown AIDS. The observation of oral "thrush" in an adult with no known predisposing factors warrants a search for other evidence of infection with the human immunodeficiency virus (HIV), such as lymphadenopathy, leukopenia, or HIV antibodies in the serum. One predisposing factor to oral thrush is broad-spectrum antibiotics.

Successful treatment of oral candidiasis is not difficult. A baby with thrush may be allowed to suck on a clotrimazole suppository inserted into the slit tip of a pacifier four times a day for two or three days, as suggested by Montes. An adult can let tablets of clotrimazole or Mycelex troches dissolve in the mouth. In immunocompromised patients, however, oral ketoconazole is often necessary.

Perlèche

Perlèche or, more aptly, *angular cheilitis*, is a maceration with transverse fissuring of the oral commissures. The earliest lesions are ill-defined, grayish white, thickened areas with slight erythema of the mucous membrane at the oral commissure. When more fully developed this thickening has a bluish white or mother-of-pearl color and may be contiguous with a wedge-shaped erythematous scaling dermatitis of the skin portion of the commissure. Fissures, maceration, and crust formation ensue. Soft, pinhead-sized papules may appear. Involvement usually is bilateral.

Perlèche is regarded as a symptom, analogous to intertrigo elsewhere, that may come from infection by *C. albicans* (the patient may also have paronychia or interdigital erosions), by coagulase-positive *Staphylococcus aureus*, or from manifold other causes.

Although it has been regarded as an infectious disease, similar changes may occur in riboflavin deficiency. Iron deficiency anemia may be present.

Identical fissuring occurs at the mucocutaneous junction from drooling in persons with malocclusion due to ill-fitting dentures and in the aged in whom atrophy of the alveolar ridges, "closing" the bite, has caused the upper lip to overhang the lower at the commissures. There is sometimes a vertical shortening of the lower third of the face. Chernosky gives detailed instructions for measuring the face in the office to determine the degree of this shortening.

Perlèche may commonly be seen also in children who lick their lips, drool, or suck their thumbs.

Treatment of perlèche depends upon its cause. If due to *C. albicans*, Imidazole or naftifine creams are effective. Occasionally diabetes complicates this disease, which will persist unless the diabetes is brought under control. It may be seen in AIDS patients with or without thrush. Antibiotic topical medications are used when there is bacterial infection. If the perlèche is due to vertical shortening of the lower third of the face, dental or oral surgical intervention may be helpful. Injection of collagen into the depressed sulcus at the oral commissure may be beneficial.

In severe chronicity vegetative lesions with fissuring develop. These are best handled by the removal of the hyperkeratotic tissue by electrosurgery.

Candidal Vulvovaginitis

C. albicans is a common inhabitant of the vaginal tract, and, in some cases, it may cause severe pruri-

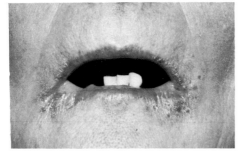

Figure 15–36. Perlèche. Candida albicans was present.

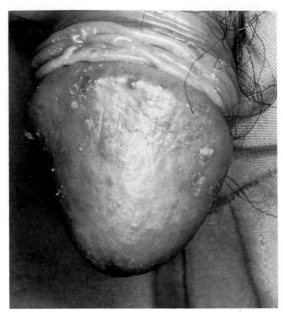

Figure 15–37. Candida balanitis.

tus, irritation, and extreme burning. The labia may be erythematous, moist, and macerated and the cervix hyperemic, swollen, and eroded, showing small vesicles on its surface. The vaginal discharge is not usually profuse but is frequently thick and tenacious.

Extreme hyperemia of the introitus is often present. This type of infection may develop during pregnancy, in diabetes, or secondary to therapy with broad-spectrum antibiotics. Candidal balanitis may be present in an uncircumsized sexual partner. If this is not recognized, repeated reinfection of a partner may result. It may also be precipitated by unrecognized emotional tension or any emotionally distressing experience.

Diagnosis is established by the clinical symptoms and findings as well as the demonstration of the fungus by potassium hydroxide microscopic examination and culture.

Treatment for this common vulvovaginitis is varied and many times disappointing because of frequent recurrences. Miconazole (Monistat cream), nystatin vaginal suppositories or tablets (Mycostatin), or clotrimazole (Gyne-Lotrimin or Mycelex G) vaginal tablets inserted once daily for seven days are usually very effective. The clotrimazole vaginal tablets may be employed successfully by inserting two tablets h.s. for three consecutive days. Oral ketoconazole is effective for chronic recurrent cases.

Swabbing with 1 per cent gentian violet solution is another of the many forms of therapy.

Candidal Intertrigo

The pruritic intertriginous eruptions caused by *C. albicans* may arise between the folds of the genitals, in groins or armpits, between the buttocks, under large pendulous breasts, under overhanging abdominal folds, or in the umbilicus. The pinkish intertriginous moist patches are surrounded by a thin overhanging fringe of somewhat macerated epidermis ("collarette" scale). Some eruptions in the inguinal region may resemble tinea cruris, but usually there is less scaliness and a greater tendency to fissuring. Persistent excoriation and subsequent lichenification and drying may, in the course of time, modify the original appearance. Often tiny superficial white pustules are observed closely adjacent to the patches.

Treatment with Castellani paint applied once daily for seven to 14 days is most effective. Clotrimazole (Lotrimin, Mycelex), miconazole (Monistat-Derm Lotion, Micatin), ketoconazole (Nizoral), econazole (Spectazole), oxiconazole (Oxistat), sulconazole (Exelderm), and naftifine (Naftin) preparations are effective.

Pseudo Diaper Rash

In infants C. albicans infection may gain a foothold on the skin in the diaper area, usually starting in the perianal region and spreading over the entire area. The dermatitis is enhanced by the maceration produced by the wet diapers. Scaly macules and vesicles with maceration in the involved areas cause burning, pruritus, and extreme discomfort.

The diagnosis of candidiasis may be suspected by the finding of involvement of the folds, and occurrence of many small erythematous desquamating "satellite" or "daughter" lesions scattered along the edges of the larger macules, and is usually easily confirmed by direct potassium hydroxide microscopic and culture examinations. Candida albicans is more consistently demonstrable by culture than by direct examination of smears. Swabbing is inadequate for making smears; one must scrape the surface to re-

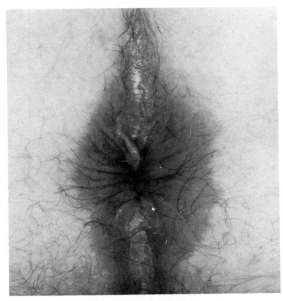

Figure 15–39. Perianal candidiasis.

move the horny material. The floor of opened pustules may be similarly scraped for specimens. However, such examinations are rarely needed.

Congenital Cutaneous Candidiasis

Infection of an infant during passage through a birth canal infected with C. albicans may lead to congenital cutaneous candidiasis. The eruption is usually noted within a few hours of delivery. Erythematous macules progress to thin-walled pustules, which rupture, dry and desquamate within a week or so. Lesions are usually widespread, involving the trunk, neck, and head, and at times the palms and soles, including the nail folds. The oral cavity and diaper area are spared, in contrast to the usual type of acquired neonatal infection.

Infants with candidiasis limited to the skin have favorable outcomes, in general; but if the birth weight is less than 1500 gm, or if there is early onset of severe respiratory symptoms, systemic disease is likely and a poor outcome is probable.

Perianal Candidiasis

When pruritus ani is present C. albicans infection should be suspected. Frequently the entire gastrointestinal tract is involved. This type of infection can be brought on by oral antibiotic therapy. There is perianal dermatitis with erythema, oozing, and maceration. Pruritus and burning can be extremely severe.

A psychogenic component is more frequent as a cause of pruritus ani than is candidiasis. Furthermore, psoriasis, seborrheic dermatitis, and contact dermatitis need to be ruled out as possible forms of perianal dermatitis.

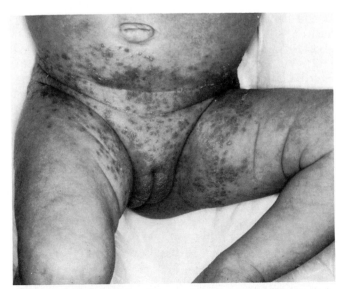

Figure 15–38. Candida albicans infection of the diaper area in an infant. Note characteristic "satellite pustules" and involvement of the folds.

In addition to the use of fungicides, other measures are essential. Meticulous cleansing of the perianal region after bowel movement must be practiced. The use of topical corticosteroids and antipruritic medications such as trimeprazine (Temaril) or hydroxyzine (Atarax) is helpful and may be indicated. The usual anticandidal imidazoles (see above) are recommended for this infection. Castellani paint, with or without the red dye, fuchsin, may still be useful in some cases.

Candidal Paronychia

Chronic inflammation of the nail fold produces occasional discharge of thin pus, cushionlike thickening of the paronychial tissue, slow erosion of the lateral borders of the nails, gradual thickening and brownish discoloration of the nail plates, and development of pronounced transverse ridges. Usually the fingernails only are affected, and frequently only one nail.

Chronic paronychia is caused by *C. albicans*, but at times there may be secondary mixed bacterial infection as well. Candidal paronychia is frequently seen in diabetics. Those whose hands are frequently in water or who handle moist objects are the prime sufferers from this type of disease; among them are food handlers, cooks, dishwashers, bartenders, nurses, canners, especially fruit canners using sugar syrup, and laundry workers. The diagnosis in such personnel is prima facie evidence of compensability under most Worker's Compensation laws. Manicuring the nails sometimes is responsible for mechanical or chemical injuries that lead to this infection. Candidiasis is often present in chronic paronychia caused by an ingrown toenail.

In those suffering from diabetes mellitus, one aspect of the treatment consists of bringing the diabetes under control. The avoidance of chronic exposure to moisture is also an important prophylactic measure. Solutions or creams of miconazole, clotrimazole, or

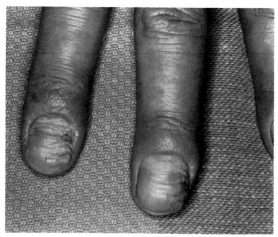

Figure 15–40. Paronychial infection and onychodystrophy caused by Candida albicans.

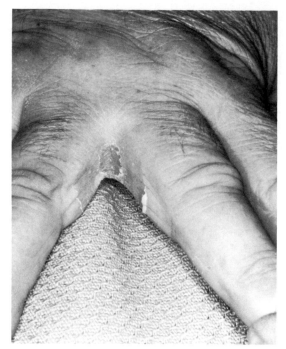

Figure 15–41. Erosio interdigitalis blastomycetica.

other imidazoles are the best topical therapy. Castellani paint is also very effective. Therapy must be continued for two to three months in order that there may be no recurrence.

In both acute and chronic cases, a single intramuscular injection of 40 mg of triamcinolone acetonide suspension is often extremely effective in bringing the condition under prompt control.

Erosio Interdigitalis Blastomycetica

This form of candidiasis is seen as an oval-shaped area of macerated white skin on the web between and extending onto the sides of the fingers. Usually at the center of the lesion there are one or more fissures with raw, red bases; as the condition progresses the macerated skin peels off, leaving a painful, raw, denuded area surrounded by a collar of overhanging white epidermis. It is nearly always the third web, between the middle and ring fingers, that is affected. The moisture beneath the rings macerates the skin and predisposes to infection. The disease is also seen in diabetics, in women who do housework, in laundresses, and in others whose skin is exposed to the macerating effects of water and strong alkalis.

Intertriginous lesions between the toes are similar. Usually the white, sodden epidermis is thick and does not peel off freely. On the feet it is the fourth interspace that is most often involved, but the areas are apt to be multiple. Clinically this may be indistinguishable from tinea pedis. Diagnosis is made by culture.

Treatment with clotrimazole, miconazole, or other imidazoles in cream or lotion, or Castellani paint, is effective.

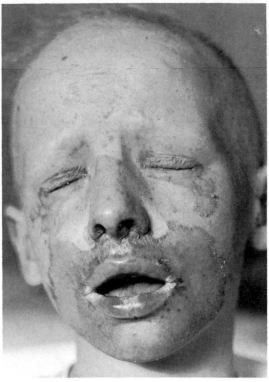

Figure 15–42. Candidiasis in an immunoincompetent patient.

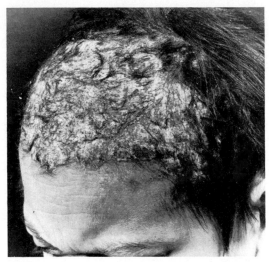

Figure 15–44. Candidiasis of the scalp. The patient has generalized mucocutaneous candidiasis. Nevertheless, note the striking resemblance to rupial psoriasis.

Chronic Mucocutaneous Candidiasis

This term designates a heterogeneous group of patients whose infection with *Candida* is chronic but superficial, never disseminating to deep structures. Onset is before age six as a rule; onset in adult life may herald the occurrence of thymoma. These cases may be either inherited, or sporadic; in the inherited types endocrinopathy is often found. Most cases have well-defined limited defects of cell-mediated immunity.

Oral lesions are diffuse, and perlèche and lip fissures are common. The entire thickness of the nail plates is invaded, and they become thickened and dystrophic. There is associated paronychia. Hyperkeratotic, hornlike, or granulomatous lesions are often seen.

Long-term therapy with ketoconazole is now the treatment of choice. Peterson et al reported good results and Hornsburgh et al confirmed their findings. However, cimetidine is worth trying: Jorizzo et al restored deficient cell-mediated immunity with it in four adults from one family, at a dose of 300 mg four times a day.

Systemic Candidiasis

Candida albicans is capable of causing a severe, destructive, disseminated disease, invariably when host defenses are compromised. Those who are at high risk include patients with malignancies, especially leukemias and lymphomas, in which there may be impaired immune defenses; the patients with AIDS (the acquired immunodeficiency syndrome); the debilitated and malnourished patient; patients with transplants requiring immunosuppressive drugs

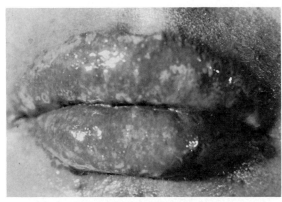

Figure 15–43. Candidiasis of the lips.

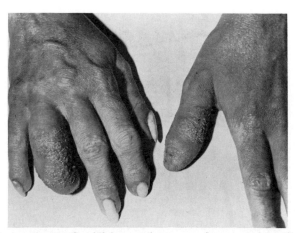

Figure 15–45. Candidal granulomas on fingers and candidal onychomycosis in a 34-year-old woman with generalized candidiasis for 30 years. Successfully treated with amphotericin B.

for prolonged periods; patients receiving oral cortisone; patients who have had multiple surgical operations, especially cardiac surgery; patients with indwelling intravenous catheters; and heroin addicts.

The initial sign of systemic candidiasis may be any of a number of clinical findings, such as fever of unknown origin, pulmonary infiltration, gastrointestinal bleeding, endocarditis, renal failure, meningitis, osteomyelitis, endophthalmitis, peritonitis, or a disseminated maculopapular exanthema. The cutaneous findings are erythematous macules which become papular, pustular, and hemorrhagic, and may progress to necrotic, ulcerating lesions resembling ecthyma gangrenosum. Deep abscesses may occur. The trunk and extremities are the usual sites of involvement. Proximal muscle tenderness is a common finding, and may be a valuable clue to the correct diagnosis.

The demonstration of microorganisms or a positive culture will substantiate a diagnosis of candidiasis only if the microorganism is found in tissues or fluids ordinarily sterile for *Candida* and if the clinical picture is compatible.

Amphotericin B is the mainstay of treatment in systemic candidiasis. A combination of amphotericin B and 5-fluorocytosine seems to produce an additive or synergistic effect. Ketoconazole (Nizoral) is fungistatic, rather than fungicidal like amphotericin B, and though it is effective in mucocutaneous candidiasis, it is not effective in systemic candidiasis in immunocompromised hosts.

Candidid

As in dermatophytosis with trichophytid, immunologically mediated lesions called candidids may develop secondary to *C. albicans* infection. They are much less common than the reactions seen with acute inflammatory dermatophytosis. The reactions, which have been reported to clear with treatment of candidal infection, are usually of the erythema annulare centrifugum or chronic urticaria type.

Antibiotic (Iatrogenic) Candidiasis

The use of oral antibiotics such as the tetracyclines and their related products may induce clinical candidiasis involving the mouth, the gastrointestinal tract, or the perianal area. In addition, vulvovaginitis may occur. The most frequent complaint is severe pruritus ani.

It has been suggested that perhaps the bacterial flora in the gastrointestinal system is changed by suppression of some of the antibiotic-sensitive bacteria, thereby permitting other organisms such as *Candida* to flourish.

Antifungal agents such as nystatin or amphotericin B have been combined with the tetracyclines to prevent this type of reaction. However, care to take tetracycline only on an empty stomach, and at least ½ to 1 hour before meals, suffices to prevent this complication in all but a few extremely susceptible persons.

Bennett JE: Flucytosine. Ann Intern Med 1977, 86:319.

Bielsu I, et al: Systemic candidiasis in heroin abusers. Int J Dermatol 1987, 26:314.

Chapel TA, et al: Congenital cutaneous candidiasis. JAAD 1982, 6:926.

Chernosky ME: Collagen implant in the management of perlèche. JAAD 1985, 12:493.

Crislip MA, et al: Candidiasis. Infect Dis Clin North Am 1989, 3:103.

Graybill JR, et al: Treatment of chronic mucocutaneous candidiasis with ketoconazole: Controlled clinical trial. Ann Intern Med 1980, 93:781.

Held JL, et al: Use of touch preparation for rapid diagnosis of disseminated candidiasis. JAAD 1988, 19:1063.

Honig P, et al: Amoxicillin and diaper dermatitis. JAAD 1988, 19:275.

Horsburg CH, et al: Long term therapy of mucocutaneous candidiasis with ketoconazole. Am J Med 1983, 75:23.

Jorizzo JC, et al: Cimetidine as an immunomodulator: chronic mucocutaneous candidiasis as a model. Ann Intern Med 1980, 92:192.

Mansour A: A new approach to the use of antifungal agents in infants with persistent candidiasis. J Pediatr 1981, 98:161.

Mobacken H, et al: Ketoconazole treatment of 13 patients with chronic mucocutaneous candidiasis. Dermatologica 1986, 173:229.

Montes LF, et al: Fungus-host relationship in candidiasis. Arch Dermatol 1985, 121:119.

Idem: Clotrimazole troches: a new therapeutic approach to oral candidiasis. Cutis 1976, 17:277.

Petersen EA, et al: Treatment of chronic mucocutaneous candidiasis with ketoconazole: controlled clinical trial. Ann Intern Med 1980, 93:791.

Sams WM Jr, et al: Chronic mucocutaneous candidiasis: immunologic studies of three generations of a single family. Am J Med 1979, 67:948.

Tanenbaum L, et al: A new treatment for cutaneous candidiasis: sulconazole nitrate cream 1%. Int J Dermatol 1983, 22:318.

GEOTRICHOSIS

Geotrichosis may produce symptoms of oral lesions of erythema, pseudomembranes, and mucopurulent sputum similar to that seen in thrush. The intestinal, bronchial, and pulmonary forms are similar to candidal infection.

The etiologic agent, *Geotrichum candidum*, is considered to be a pathogen only when it is repeatedly found at a diseased site. Its mere presence in undiseased sites is probably only as a saprophyte. In nature it is frequently found on fruit, tomatoes, in soil, and similar locations.

The diagnosis is made by the demonstration of the organism by potassium hydroxide microscopic examination and by its culture from sputum on Sabouraud's dextrose agar. Direct examination shows branching septate mycelium and chains of rectangular cells. In culture there is a mealy growth at room temperature. The hyphae form rectangular arthrospores.

Treatment is with potassium iodide or mycostatin suspension.

Chang WWL, et al: Disseminated geotrichosis. Arch Intern Med 1964, 113:356.
Webster BH: Bronchopulmonary geotrichosis. Review and report of 4 cases. Dis Chest 1959, 35:273.

TINEA NIGRA

This characteristic disorder manifests itself as one or several brown or black spots that resemble junction type nevi, melanoma, or silver nitrate or India ink stains, most frequently on the palms but also on the soles. The patches are not elevated or scaly. The fungus can easily be demonstrated and cultured. In appearance young colonies are glossy, black, and yeastlike, but older colonies are filamentous and grayish. Groups or chains of conidia, resulting from sporulation of the saprophyte *Exophiala phaeoannello-myces* (formerly *werneckii*), produce a melaninlike pigment.

Treatment is by the application of 40 per cent salicylic acid adhesive plaster or double-strength Whitfield's ointment. Topical imidazoles such as clotrimazole, miconazole, ketoconazole, sulconazole, and econazole are also effective; griseofulvin is not. Simply shaving away the superficial epidermis with a number 15 Bard-Parker blade is frequently effective therapy.

VanVelsor H, et al: Tinea nigra palmaris. Arch Dermatol 1964, 90:59.

PIEDRA (Trichosporosis)

In piedra, dark, pinhead-sized, gritty formations occur on the hairs of the scalp, brows, lashes, or beard. Minute, round or ovoid, hard nodules develop on the shaft of the hairs, not on the root. These nodules are distributed irregularly along the length of the shaft and are easily felt by palpation when too small to be recognized without close scrutiny.

Two varieties exist. **Black piedra**, caused by *Piedraia hortai*, occurs mostly in the tropics. It is frequently found in Brazil, Colombia, and other South American countries and in the Orient, or wherever the climate combines high temperature with high humidity. The nodelike masses in potassium hydroxide preparations show numerous oval asci containing two to eight ascospores and mycelium. Cultures produce black colonies composed of hyphae and chlamydospores.

White piedra, caused by *Trichosporon beigelii* (transiently named *T. cutaneum*), occurs commonly in temperate climates. The nodes are composed of hyphae and arthrospores. The culture shows cream-colored, soft colonies composed of blastospores and septate hyphae, which fragment into arthrospores.

Treatment is by cutting the hair. Spontaneous remissions were observed in some patients by Kalter et al.

Rarely, deep invasion and systemic dissemination may occur, as reported by Manzella et al in a patient with acute granulocytic leukemia.

Adam BA, et al: Black piedra in Malaysia. Austral J Dermatol 1977, 18:45.
Kalter DC, et al: Genital white piedra: epidemiology, microbiology, and therapy. JAAD 1986, 14:982.
LeBlond V, et al: Systemic infections with *Trichosporon beigelii* (cutaneum). Cancer 1986, 58:2399.
Londero AT, et al: White piedra of unusual localization. Sabouraudia 1966, 5:132.
Otsuka F, et al: Facial granuloma associated with *Trichosporum cutaneum* infection. Arch Dermatol 1986, 122:1176.
Walsh TJ: Trichosporonosis. Infect Dis Clin North Am 1989, 3:43.

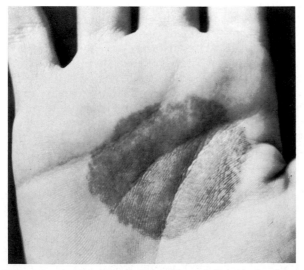

Figure 15–46. Tinea nigra. (*Courtesy of Dr. A. L. Carrion, Puerto Rico.*)

TINEA VERSICOLOR (Pityriasis Versicolor)

CLINICAL FEATURES. On the upper trunk and extending onto the upper arms, finely scaling, guttate or nummular patches appear, particularly on young adults who perspire freely. The individual patches are yellowish or brownish macules in pale skin, or hypopigmented macules in dark skin, with delicate scaling. Mild itching and inflammation about the patches may be present. In other instances a follicular tendency is a marked feature of the eruption. Sites of predilection are the sternal region and the sides of the chest, the abdomen, the back, the pubis, the neck, and intertriginous areas. The disease may even occur on the scalp, palms, and soles. Rarely, the face is involved, in which event the lesions resemble either chloasma or pityriasis alba. Facial lesions occur fairly commonly in infants and the immunocompromised. In the latter, penile lesions may occur as well.

In hypopigmented tinea versicolor, the fungus

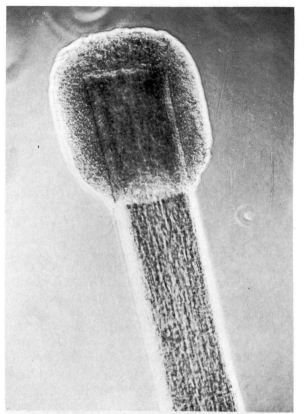

Figure 15–47. Nodule of white piedra resembling a match head at the end of the hair shaft. (Courtesy of Dr. A. T. Londero, Brazil.)

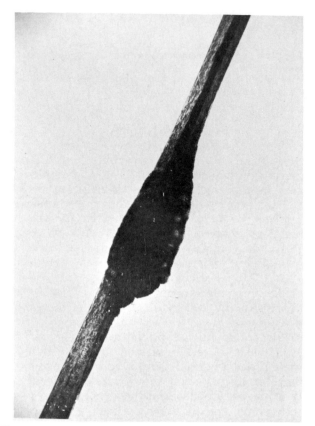

Figure 15–48. Nodule of black piedra on hair shaft. (Courtesy of Dr. A. T. Londero, Brazil.)

apparently compels the production of abnormally small melanosomes, which are not transferred to keratinocytes properly. This becomes conspicuous in dark-skinned people, on whom the white spots look

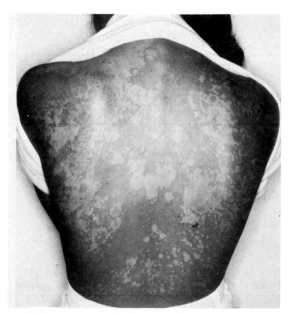

Figure 15–49. Tinea versicolor on the back of a 20-year-old man. Pale lesions on tan skin.

almost as pale as vitiligo. This hypopigmentation may persist for weeks or months after the fungus disease is cured unless an effort is made to regain the lost pigmentation through ultraviolet exposure.

This common disease is most prevalent in the tropics where there are high humidity and high temperatures and frequent exposure to sunlight.

ETIOLOGY. Tinea versicolor is due to *Malassezia furfur.* The yeast phase of this organism is classified as *Pityrosporum orbiculare.*

DIAGNOSIS. Lesions that are imperceptible or doubtful may be brought readily into view in a darkened room by use of the Wood's light. This causes fluorescence of the lesions, which appear yellowish or brownish; it also assists in determining the extent of involvement or the achievement of a cure.

Brown hyperpigmentation in tinea versicolor appears to arise from an increase in melanosome size and a change in their epidermal distribution pattern. On occasions, it is difficult to be certain whether the lighter or darker skin is the affected tissue. Generally, the skin involved by the fungus will produce moderate scaling when scratched with the fingernails or scraped with a blade, whereas uninvolved skin yields little or no scale if gently abraded. If the lesions have a convex border, the involved skin is usually inside the arc.

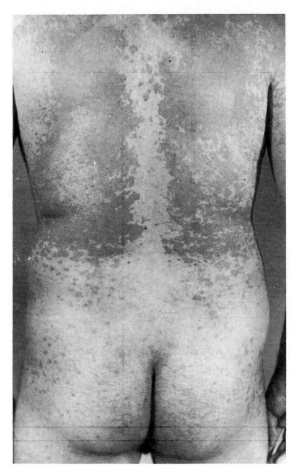

Figure 15–50. Hyperpigmented tinea versicolor. Tan lesions on pale skin.

The fungus is easily demonstrated in scrapings of the scales that have been soaked in 15 per cent solution of potassium hydroxide. Scales may also be removed by Scotch tape, which is examined directly. Microscopically, there are short, thick fungal hyphae

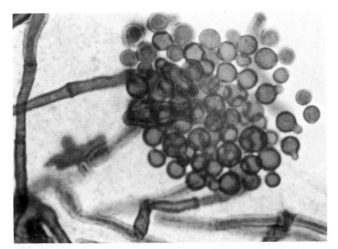

Figure 15–51. Malassezia furfur. Note blunt-ended hyphae and clusters of spores that form "spaghetti and meat balls" pattern. KOH mount.

and large numbers of variously sized spores. This combination of strands of mycelium and numerous spores is commonly referred to as "spaghetti and meat balls." Identification by culture is impractical and is not done to establish the diagnosis.

DIFFERENTIAL DIAGNOSIS. Tinea versicolor must be differentiated from seborrheic dermatitis, pityriasis rosea, pityriasis alba, leprosy, syphilis, and vitiligo. The diagnosis is generally easy because of the typical fawn color of the patches in tinea versicolor and their distribution on the upper trunk without involvement of the face or scalp, except occasionally by extension from the sides of the neck. The scalp is not visibly involved but it usually is affected, and provides a locus from which the upper back and shoulders can be rapidly reinfected. In seborrheic dermatitis the patches have an erythematous yellowish tint and the scales are soft and greasy, whereas in tinea versicolor the scales are furfuraceous. The macular syphilid consists of faint pink lesions, less than 1 cm in diameter, irregularly round or oval, which are distributed principally on the nape, the sides of the trunk, and the flexor aspects of the extremities. There may be general adenopathy. Serologic tests are positive in this phase of syphilis. The demonstration of this fungus also differentiates this disease from vitiligo and leprosy. It may be clinically indistinguishable from the latter.

TREATMENT. Successful treatment of tinea versicolor has been reported with clotrimazole cream or lotion, with selenium sulfide lotion shampoo, or the lather therefrom; with 50 per cent propylene glycol in water applied after baths; with topical benzoyl peroxide; with sulfur-salicylic acid in a shampoo or lotion; with 200 mg of ketoconazole daily for two weeks or for four weeks. But the best treatment appears to be 400 mg of ketoconazole in a single oral dose; Jacobs has established its effectiveness (200 mg did not work). Repeating the dose after a week has been advocated and is probably a good idea. One of us (WDJ) still prefers Selsun.

If patients are not warned that they must regain the lost tan in the lesions by sunbathing, they may think they have not been improved. Relapse after two to 12 months is likely if prophylactic doses are not given occasionally, but the question of maintenance therapy is unsettled.

Alternatively, in patients who cannot be given ketoconazole, a safe and effective medication which has been used for years is selenium sulfide 2.5 per cent suspension (Selsun Suspension or Exsel Lotion), commonly used as a shampoo. It may be applied directly, or as its own lather, and left on the skin for various lengths of time, and then washed off, or it may be applied daily after the shower, left on a few minutes, then rinsed off. One overnight application is usually curative, but shorter applications should be continued for two weeks.

Almost any modification of these may be used prophylactically to prevent recurrences, which are otherwise very apt to occur.

Albright SD III, et al: Rapid treatment of tinea versicolor with selenium sulfide. Arch Dermatol 1966, 93:460.

Allen HB, et al: Hyperpigmented tinea versicolor. Arch Dermatol 1976, 112:1110.

Bamford JTM: Treatment of tinea versicolor with sulfur-salicylic shampoo. JAAD 1983, 8:211.

Daneshvar SA, et al: An unusual presentation of tinea versicolor in an immunosuppressed patient. JAAD 1987, 17:304.

Faergemann J, et al: Propylene glycol in the treatment of tinea versicolor. Acta Dermatovener 1979, 60:92.

Gomez Urcuyo F, et al: Successful treatment of pityriasis versicolor by systemic ketoconazole. JAAD 1982, 6:24.

Klotz SA: Malassezia furfur. Infect Dis Clin North Am 1989, 3:53.

Prestia AE: Topical benzoyl peroxide for the treatment of tinea versicolor (letter). JAAD 1983, 9:277.

Rausch LJ, et al: Tinea versicolor: treatment and prophylaxis with monthly administration of ketoconazole. Cutis 1984, 34:470.

Savin RC: Systemic ketoconazole in tinea versicolor: a double blind evaluation and 1-year follow-up. JAAD 1984, 10:824.

Wurtz RM, et al: *Malassezia furfur* fungemia in a patient without the usual risk factors. Ann Intern Med 1988, 109:432.

Zimney ML, et al: Tinea versicolor. Arch Dermatol 1988, 124:492.

Pityrosporum Folliculitis

What used to be called a "follicular seborrheide" is apparently finding its place as pityrosporum folliculitis: a chronic, moderately itchy eruption of dome-shaped papules and tiny pustules involving the upper back and adjacent areas as far distant as the forearms, lower legs, face, and scalp, sometimes in association with either tinea versicolor or seborrheic dermatitis. Bäck et al collected 39 women and 12 men with the disease, and established it as an entity by biopsy, skin scrapings, and the response to selenium sulfide shampoo, 50 per cent propylene glycol in water, and topical econazole cream. Bufill et al described this occurring in marrow transplant patients. M. *furfur* may occasionally even cause fungemia in patients who have central arterial or venous catheters in place. Jillson has suggested that pityrosporum folliculitis may emerge when *Corynebacterium* acnes is suppressed by tetracycline therapy, and that it may be the same disorder as "acne estivalis." He suggested that it should respond well to ketoconazole.

Bäck O, et al: Pityrosporum folliculitis: a common disease of the young and middle-aged. JAAD 1985, 12:56.

Bufill JA, et al: Pityrosporum folliculitis after bone marrow transplantation. Ann Intern Med 1988, 108:560.

Jillson OF: Pityrosporum folliculitis. Cutis 1985, 33:226.

CONFLUENT AND RETICULATED PAPILLOMATOSIS

Gougerot and Carteaud in 1932 described three forms of papillomatosis, as follows: punctate pigmented verrucous papillomatosis, *confluent and reticulated papillomatosis*, and nummular and confluent papillomatosis. This disease begins in the intermammary region as punctate, verrucous, pigmented papules, which become generalized over the trunk. There may be severe itching and great discomfort. In time one can distinguish pale red macules and papules, reticulation, isolated circinate disks, and confluent, brownish, papillomatous surfaces. The changes show greatest intensity between the breasts and around the umbilicus.

Histologically, hyperkeratosis with thinning of the granular layer is seen. Acanthosis is a regular finding. The dermis shows edema and a perivascular infiltrate.

The principal differential diagnosis occurs between cutaneous papillomatosis and epidermodysplasia verruciformis, tinea versicolor, seborrheic keratoses, keratosis follicularis, and acanthosis nigricans.

There is controversy as to the etiology of this disease. Some authors feel it is an abnormal response to *Pityrosporum orbiculare* and have reported responses to selenium sulfide shampoo or ketoconazole. We feel this diagnosis should be reserved for cases in which no organism is demonstrable and therapy against tinea versicolor is ineffective.

Bruynzeel-Koomen et al reported a patient who was cleared by 50 mg of Tigason (etretinate) daily for four weeks. Nagy et al reported two cases in which they obtained moderate improvement from the use of topical Retin-A 0.01 per cent gel in one case, and keratolytic agents and 10 per cent urea cream in the other. Odom has experienced success with minocycline 100 mg twice daily.

Pseudo-atrophoderma colli occurs on the neck as a papillomatous and pigmented dermatosis with glossy lesions which produce a delicate wrinkling that can be obliterated by stretching the skin. There is a tendency to a vertical arrangement of the lesions. The light areas may suggest the appearance of vitiligo. Kesten and James reported nine cases in Caucasian women.

Bruynzeel-Koomen CAFM, et al: Confluent and reticulated papillomatosis successfully treated with the aromatic retinoid etretinate. Arch Dermatol 1984, 120:1236.

Friedman SJ, et al: Confluent and reticulated papillomatosis of Gougerot and Carteaud: Treatment with selenium sulfide lotion. JAAD 1986, 14:280.

Kellet JK, et al: Confluent and reticulated papillomatosis (letter). Arch Dermatol 1985, 121:587.

Nagy R, et al: Confluent and reticulated papillomatosis. Cutis 1982, 29:48.

Nordby CA, et al: Confluent and reticulated papillomatosis. Int J Dermatol 1986, 25:194.

Sau P, et al: Reticulated truncal pigmentation. Arch Dermatol 1988, 124:1271.

Yesudian P, et al: Confluent and reticulated papillomatosis (Gougerot-Carteaud): abnormal host reaction to *Malassezia furfur*. Acta Dermatovener 1973, 53:381.

THE DEEP MYCOSES

Most of the deep or systemic fungus infections come from inhalation of dust contaminated with the fungus, from droppings of animals infected by it, or from contamination from other sources. When primary infection is into the skin from puncture wounds, abrasions, or other trauma, a chancriform lesion is often produced and a secondary lymphangitis follows. In the absence of a chancriform lesion it is safe to say that other nodules and ulcerations of the disease, particularly bilateral ones, arise from an internal focus, usually pulmonary, or in the upper respiratory tract.

The outlook for spontaneous recovery is good when a chancriform lesion denotes primary cutaneous infection. The prognosis is, on the other hand, grave when the skin lesions result from dissemination of the disease from one or more visceral foci. In every case of deep mycotic infection except sporotrichosis, mycetoma, chromoblastomycosis, and phaeohyphomycosis, chest x-rays should be taken. Hermans and Keys have published a useful review of drugs currently available for the treatment of deep fungus infections.

Drouhet E, et al: Laboratory and clinical assessment of ketoconazole in deep-seated mycoses. Am J Med 1983, 71:30.

Hermans PE: Antifungal agents used for deep-seated mycotic infections. Mayo Clin Proc 1983, 58:223.

Sung P, et al: Intravenous and intrathecal miconazole therapy for systemic mycoses. West J Med 1977, 126:5.

Idem: Side effects of miconazole for systemic mycoses. N Engl J Med 1977, 297:786.

SPOROTRICHOSIS

CLINICAL FEATURES. Commonest and least serious of the deep mycoses, sporotrichosis is a chronic infectious disease caused by the fungus *Sporothrix schenckii*, a dimorphic fungus that grows in a yeast form at 37° C and in a mycelial form at room temperture. Human infection occurs accidentally at the site of some insignificant wound. The earliest manifestation may be a small nodule or ulcer, which may heal and disappear before the advent of further symptoms. In the course of a few weeks nodules generally develop along the draining lymphatics. These lesions are at first small, dusky red, painless, firm infiltrations. In time the overlying skin becomes adherent to them and may ulcerate, and may even show fistulous tracts or papillomatous vegetations. When the lesions occur near the eye, they may be confused with dacryocystitis. Sometimes the lesions heal spontaneously, but more often they progress slowly and persist indefinitely.

The disease, as a rule, is localized in the skin and the subcutaneous cellular tissues, and only exceptionally does it become disseminated. Regional lymphangitic sporotrichosis is the common type, causing first a primary sore, a sporotrichotic chancre, at the site of inoculation and then, in the course of a few days, weeks, or months, an ascending lymphangitis and multiple subcutaneous indolent painless granulomas, which soften and form cold abscesses and sometimes ulcers.

An unusual clinical pattern is a solitary ulcer without regional lymphangitis, or a rosacealike lesion of the face without regional adenopathy, as described by Day et al, and by Dellatorre et al. Such a lesion is produced by a strain of *Sporothrix* intolerant of warmth; it must be cultured at 25° C.

The disseminated type causes multiple cutaneous or subcutaneous abscesses on any part of the body. These are painless, tend to soften and form cold abscesses, ulcers, or fistulae. Friedman et al described 11 patients with extracutaneous infection, of knee

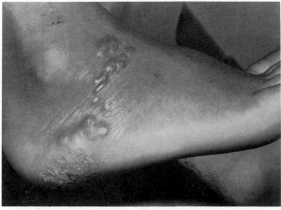

Figure 15–52. Sporotrichosis on the ankle. (Courtesy of Dr. V. M. Torres-Rodriguez.)

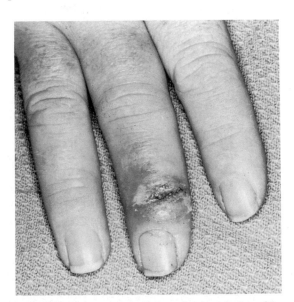

Figure 15–53. Sporotrichotic chancre. Primary lesion of 3 weeks' duration.

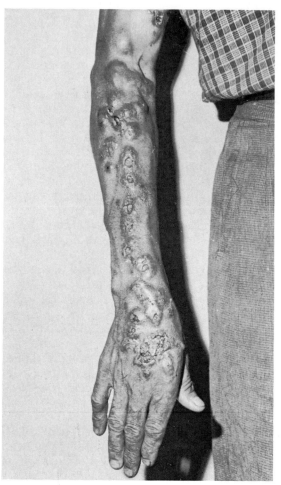

Figure 15–54. Sporotrichosis of 6 months' duration on arm of 45-year-old farmer. (Courtesy of Dr. A. T. Londero, Brazil.)

has been produced in many laboratory animals, and spontaneous cases have been observed in horses, mules, dogs, cats, mice, and rats. Several reports have documented the transmission of sporotrichosis from cats to humans. Dunstan et al reported five such cases. Carnations, rosebushes, barberry shrubs, and sphagnum moss are some of the sources from which inoculation into the skin takes place. High humidity and high temperature favor infection. An epidemic of sporotrichosis among South African miners was ascribed to inoculation of the organism by rubbing against the supporting wooden beams in the mines.

MYCOLOGY. *Sporothrix schenckii* is not often found in histologic tissue taken from the human lesion. Even with special stains it is difficult to recognize; however, when the organism-containing material is injected into a rat or mouse a great number of organisms may be seen. These are small, 3–5 μ, oval or elongated, budding cells, cigar-shaped, often called "cigar bodies." Fluorescent antibody staining of *S. schenckii* in cultures and clinical materials is a rapid method of identifying the organism. Asteroid bodies and mycelial elements are prevalent in regional lymphangitic sporotrichosis.

On Sabouraud's agar a moist white colony develops within three to seven days. The surface becomes wrinkled and folded. Later the culture turns tan and, ultimately, black. In slide culture preparations the colony shows septate mycelium that is branched. Conidia are found in clusters or in a sleevelike arrangement on delicate sterigmata. If the culture is grown at 37° C, grayish yellow, velvety colonies are produced. Cigar-shaped, round, oval and budding cells, hyphae, and conidia may be seen microscopically.

PATHOLOGY. The histologic changes are those of an infectious granuloma, with the formation of deep abscesses, sinuses, and ulcerations. Toward the center of a well-developed lesion are collections of polymorphonuclears, eosinophils, and macrophages. Between the central and the peripheral zones are numerous epithelioid cells and giant cells of the Langhans type, and the peripheral part is made up of plasma cells, lymphocytes, and connective tissue cells.

IMMUNOLOGY. Culture extracts from *S. schenckii*, known as sporotrichins, will produce a delayed tuberculin-type reaction in persons who have, or have had, sporotrichosis. The test is fairly reliable, but only indicates previous exposure. Agglutination is the most satisfactory test, and a titer of 1:80 or higher establishes the diagnosis.

DIFFERENTIAL DIAGNOSIS. The diagnosis is established by the history of the onset, the indolent character, and the linear distribution of the nodules along the lymphatic drainage of the area. The demonstration by culture clinches the diagnosis. Clinically, atypical mycobacteriosis (swimming pool granuloma), tuberculosis, syphilis, furunculosis, cat scratch disease, anthrax, tularemia, and the primary

and wrist joints, the mandible, and ethmoid sinuses; five had been on oral prednisone. At times the primary site may be indiscernible and only internal involvement, such as of the gastrointestinal system, lungs, central nervous system, or osteomyelitis, is apparent.

Systemic Visceral Sporotrichosis. Systemic invasion by an opportunistic infection with *S. schenckii* may produce cutaneous, pulmonary, or articular lesions, and may involve the central nervous system. Lynch et al have emphasized its striking similarities to other systemic fungal diseases.

The cutaneous lesions are reddish, tender nodules, which eventually suppurate. These are usually around arthritic joints and the face and scalp, but may occur anywhere on the skin. Arthritis or bone involvement occurs in most cases; lung involvement is much less frequent.

EPIDEMIOLOGY. There seems to be no geographic limitation to the occurrence of sporotrichosis. Most often the primary invasion is seen as an occupational disease in gardeners, florists, and laborers following injuries by thorns of plants or by straw. The pathogen commonly lives as a saprophyte on grasses, shrubs, and other plants. Experimentally it inoculation of several other deep fungal organisms, such as histoplasmosis, coccidioidomycosis, and North American blastomycosis, may resemble sporotrichosis, but differentiation is made without difficulty.

TREATMENT. Potassium iodide in doses of 2 to 6 gm daily is effective and should be continued for one month after apparent recovery to prevent recurrences. It is important to begin with 5 drops of the saturated solution in a little water or milk three times a day after meals. This dose should be gradually increased until 30 to 40 drops are taken thrice daily. Adverse effects of iodide therapy include nausea, vomiting, parotid swelling, acneiform rash, coryza, sneezing, swelling of the eyelids, and occasionally depression. Most of the side effects can be controlled by stopping the drug for a few days and reinstituting therapy at a slightly reduced dosage. In the severe disseminated cases in which patients do not tolerate iodides, amphotericin B is effective.

Amphotericin B in total doses of 0.75 to 3.0 gm produced apparent cure in all cases treated by Lynch and his associates.

Shelley and Sica reported a patient unresponsive to six months of iodide therapy and relapsing after amphotericin B, who was cured by six months of 5-fluorocytosine (Ancobon) 8 gm/day with a total of 4.8 gm of amphotericin B. The fluorocytosine was continued for a year, despite (as in Beardmore's case) development of severe photosensitivity.

Ketoconazole failed in a case of fixed cutaneous sporotrichosis reported by Day et al, but potassium iodide, 50 per cent, 10 drops t.i.d., was effective. The cases treated with ketoconazole usually, but not always, have had similarly poor results. Itraconazole, however, has been reported by Restrepo et al to be effective. It has to be given for 90 to 180 days.

Beardmore GL: Recalcitrant sporotrichosis: report of a patient treated with various therapies including oral miconazole and 5-fluorocytosine. Austral J Dermatol 1979, 20:10.

Coté TR, et al: Sporotrichosis in association with Arbor Day activities. N Engl J Med 1988, 319:1290.

Dahl BA, et al: Sporotrichosis in children. JAMA 1971, 215:1980.

Day TW, et al: Rosacea-like sporotrichosis. Cutis 1984, 33:549.

Dellatorre DL: Fixed cutaneous sporotrichosis of the face. JAAD 1982, 6:97.

Dunstan RW, et al: Feline sporotrichosis; report of 5 cases with transmission to humans. JAAD 1986, 15:37.

Friedman SJ, et al: Extracutaneous sporotrichosis. Int J Dermatol 1983, 22:171.

Itoh M, et al: Survey of 200 cases of sporotrichosis. Dermatologica 1986, 172:209.

Restrepo A, et al: Itraconazole therapy in lymphangitic and cutaneous sporotrichosis. Arch Dermatol 1986, 122:413.

Winn RE: Sporotrichosis. Infect Dis Clin North Am 1988, 2:899.

COCCIDIOIDOMYCOSIS

Synonyms: Coccidioidal granuloma, valley fever, San Joaquin valley fever.

CLINICAL FEATURES. Wilson et al classify this into primary pulmonary, disseminated (coccidioidal granuloma), and primary cutaneous coccidioidomycosis.

Primary Pulmonary Coccidioidomycosis. Inhalation of *Coccidioides immitis*, followed by an incubation period of 10 days to several weeks, produces a respiratory infection that may be mild, with only a low-grade fever resembling a flulike illness. Severe symptoms of chills, high fever, night sweats, severe headache, backache, and malaise may ensue. A large percentage of patients show lung changes upon roentgenographic examination. These may be due to a peribronchial infiltration or an infiltrate compatible with bronchopneumonia. At the time of onset a generalized maculopapular eruption may be present, which may be confused with a drug eruption, measles, or scarlet fever.

Within a few weeks the pulmonary symptoms subside. In about 30 per cent of women and in 15 per cent of men, allergic skin manifestations appear in the form of erythema nodosum over the shins and sometimes over the thighs, hips, and buttocks. These tender lesions may become confluent, gradually turn from purple to brown, and then disappear in about three weeks. This rarely occurs in blacks. Erythema nodosum is a favorable prognostic sign. Sometimes erythema multiforme may develop in a similar clinical setting.

Although valley fever is usually self-limited and the affected patients recover spontaneously, a small percentage steadily progress into the chronic progressive disseminated form, which carries a high mortality.

Disseminated Coccidioidomycosis (Coccidioidal Granuloma). From the localized pulmonary lesion dissemination may occur to the lungs, bones, joints, viscera, brain, meninges, and skin. A single organ or multiple organs may be involved.

The skin lesions are mostly subcutaneous abscesses that seem to remain localized for several years. They are indolent and eventually suppurate, with the formation of numerous sinuses that often resemble the more acute forms of cutaneous tuberculosis. Some of the lesions are not unlike those of mycosis fungoides. Other lesions such as the verrucous nodules and plaques simulate North American blastomycosis. The disease spreads slowly and causes considerable scarring.

Primary Cutaneous Coccidioidomycosis. This form rarely occurs since most of the lesions are attributable to dissemination from the primary lesion in the lung. A well-documented case of Wilson et al demonstrated the criteria of an acceptable case of primary coccidioidomycosis of the skin. The lesion, on the finger of an embalmer, was an indolent, indurated, ulcerated lesion resembling a chancre. Some time later nodules developed along the lymphatic vessels draining the site. Lymphangitis and lymphadenopathy were similar to those seen with sporotrichosis. Spontaneous healing occurred in sev-

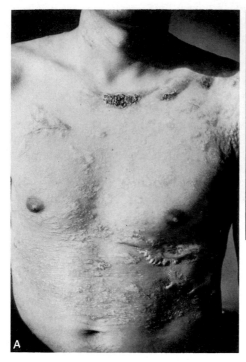

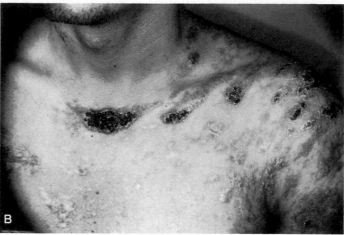

Figure 15–55. A, *Disseminated coccidioidomycosis.* B, *Close-up view. (Courtesy of Dr. Axel W. Hoke.)*

eral weeks, behaving in the same manner as the primary pulmonary form. Levan and Huntingdon reported two cases and Winn three more of primary cutaneous coccidioidomycosis.

ETIOLOGY. The causative organism is *Coccidioides immitis.* This fungus has been isolated from the soil, and from vegetation, especially fruit.

Emmons believes that the disease is endemic in rodents, especially those common to the southwestern states. Most infections are thought to occur through inhalation of dust laden with the organisms. It has been known to occur in laboratory workers; therefore, caution should be exercised when handling cultures.

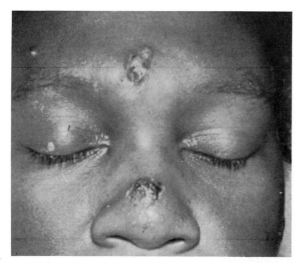

Figure 15–56. Disseminated coccidioidomycosis. (Courtesy of Dr. N. Levan.)

Coccidioides immitis is dimorphous, reproducing in tissue in an entirely different form from that seen in culture media. The parasite appears in tissues as a nonbudding, spherical, thick-walled structure 5–200 μ in diameter. This *spherule* contains numerous small *endospores.* These small rounded bodies are usually capsulated and range from 2–5 μ in diameter. At maturity the spherule ruptures, with release of the endospores.

Culture. The colonies appear in surface plants on Sabouraud's dextrose agar in from two to seven days as small, slightly raised disks penetrating the medium. Older cultures become covered with a dusty layer of aerial hyphae and assume a brownish color with age. In culture, spherical bodies throw out filaments of arthrospores that are branched and septate, and 2 to 8 μ in diameter.

EPIDEMIOLOGY. It is interesting to note that this disease occurs in limited areas in the Western Hemisphere. The original diagnosis was in a soldier from Argentina, where the disease is endemic in the Gran Chaco area. It is also endemic in northern Mexico, Venezuela, and in southwest United States, especially California (the lower Sonoran Life Zone). In the endemic areas most of the residents are infected and new residents have a good chance of becoming infected within six months. Its greatest prevalence is in the Philippine Islands (14,350 in 100,000 people in 1977).

PATHOLOGY. The histopathology is that of infectious granulomas. The essential lesions occur in the deep dermis, especially about the hair follicles and sweat glands, where there is a collection of neutrophils, plasma cells, and varying numbers of epithelioid and giant cells. The spherules occur free among the localized cellular collections and within the giant cells.

DIFFERENTIAL DIAGNOSIS. Clinically, it is extremely difficult to differentiate this disease from blastomycosis, which it closely resembles. Definite diagnosis depends upon the demonstration of C. immitis microscopically, culturally, or by animal inoculation. Guinea pigs inoculated with C. immitis die from the systemic infection, whereas no evidence of infection is apparent after inoculation with Blastomyces. Intradermal testing with coccidioidin is of value. A positive reaction of the delayed tuberculin type develops early and remains high in those who resist the disease well. A negative skin test does not exclude active disease. Negative tests may be the result of anergy, tolerance, impotent antigen, or administration before development of cell-mediated immunity.

Evaluation of skin lesions should include potassium hydroxide preparation and culture of available exudate. Tissue sections obtained by skin biopsy may reveal microorganisms when stained with hematoxylin-eosin; however, confirmation should be obtained by the use of special stains, such as the Gridley or Gomori methenamine silver stain.

IMMUNOLOGY. An extract prepared from a culture of C. immitis is used to perform the coccidioidin skin test. A tuberculin type of delayed response indicates present or past infection. A positive reaction usually appears several days after symptoms have developed. From date of exposure a positive reaction may occur within one to six weeks. Cross reactions with other fungus antigens may result in a false positive reaction. Smith et al found this to occur with antigens of histoplasmin, blastomycin, and paracoccidioidin.

In addition to this test, serologic tests have been developed. These are the precipitin, latex agglutination, immunodiffusion, and the complement fixation tests. The precipitin and latex agglutination tests indicate a very recent infection, since a maximum titer is reached in one to two weeks and then gradually falls and finally disappears. In later infections, the immunodiffusion test can be used for screening purposes. The complement fixation test is useful in diagnosing disseminated coccidioidomycosis since in primary coccidioidomycosis the titer is low, whereas in subsequent dissemination there is a rapid rise in titer.

TREATMENT. The only effective therapy available at present is intravenous administration of amphotericin B. In general, indications for intravenous amphotericin are threatened dissemination of coccidioidomycosis, disseminated disease, or exacerbation of pulmonary coccidioidomycosis.

Primary pulmonary coccidioidomycosis is usually a mild infection, which may heal without noticeable difficulty. In these patients no active therapy is indicated except that of good general care with adequate nourishing food, rest, and relaxation.

In coccidioidal meningitis, intrathecal and intravenous amphotericin therapy is indicated.

In primary cutaneous coccidioidomycosis, indications for amphotericin B therapy are the same as for the primary pulmonary form. A mild form usually does not require therapy.

An initial daily intravenous dose of 0.25 mg of amphotericin B per kg of body weight is given. This dosage should be increased gradually to between 0.5 and 1.0 mg/kg. Daily intravenous administration of 1.0 mg/kg appears to be the optimum dosage. However, since the individual tolerance to intravenous administration of amphotericin B varies considerably, dosages of 0.5 to 0.75 mg/kg daily have been used to good effect. Within this range, the largest possible dose failing to elicit toxic reactions should be administered daily, on alternate days, or every fourth day.

The initial intravenous administration of the antibiotic is usually associated with a febrile response, often combined with chills. These reactions tend to diminish with each succeeding infusion and may be limited by prophylactic oral administration of antipyretics or antihistaminics. During a febrile reaction, it is wise to halt therapy temporarily and to observe the patient. Headache, nausea, and vomiting are early toxic manifestations of the antibiotic, and the dose must be reduced to a level at which these side effects are absent. Toxic effects may also produce increase of blood urea nitrogen and creatinine; albumin casts, and red blood cells in the urine; and, less commonly, thrombocytopenia, anemia, hypokalemia, gastroenteritis, or polymyositis.

Phlebitis is a troublesome problem but may be alleviated by the use of small scalp vein needles, slow infusion of dilute solutions of amphotericin B, and the addition of 25–50 mg of heparin to the infusion bottle.

The length of therapy varies with the nature of the infection and is as yet not clearly defined, but significant clinical response has occurred after four to eight weeks of treatment. Treatment should be closely followed by laboratory tests for side effects on the kidneys, liver, and bone marrow.

Sung has reported miconazole orally to be an effective antifungal in the treatment of disseminated coccidioidomycosis, but it failed in five patients treated by Hoeprich et al, two of whom received presumably adequate total doses of 101 and 185 gm.

Ketoconazole has been reported to be effective in some cases of nonmeningeal and nonskeletal coccidioidomycosis and is an appropriate alternative medication when amphotericin B is contraindicated.

Carroll GF, et al: Primary cutaneous coccidioidomycosis. Arch Dermatol 1978, 113:953.

Hoeprich PD, et al: Treatment of coccidioidomycosis with ketoconazole. JAMA 1980, 243:1923.

Ingelman JD, et al: Persistent facial plaque. Arch Dermatol 1987, 123:937.

Knoper SR, et al: Coccidioidomycosis. Infect Dis Clin North Am 1988, 2:861.

Levan NE, et al: Primary cutaneous coccidioidomycosis in agricultural workers. Arch Dermatol 1965, 92:215.

Meyer RD, et al: Miconazole for disseminated coccidioidomycosis: unfavorable experience. Chest 1976, 73:825.

Stevens DA, et al: Experience with ketoconazole in three major manifestations of progressive coccidioidomycosis. Am J Med 1983, 74:58.

HISTOPLASMOSIS

CLINICAL FEATURES. Histoplasmosis is usually a systemic disease; dissemination to the skin is an infrequent occurrence. Even more infrequently, the primary lesion can be in the skin. Although no sharp delineation of the various manifestations of histoplasmosis can be made, it is possible to consider it in the following main forms.

Primary Pulmonary Histoplasmosis. This is usually a benign form of acute pneumonitis characterized by fever, malaise, night sweats, chest pain, cough, adenopathy, and weight loss. Resolution of the pneumonitis occurs rapidly, and the only residua may be calcifications in the lung and a positive skin test to histoplasmin. However, acute fatal pneumonitis due to histoplasmosis does occur. Such cases have been reported among the workers in guano caves in Mexico.

Progressive, Disseminated Histoplasmosis. Christie describes four main types of cutaneous or mucous membrane lesions.

Ulcerations and *granulomas* of the oronasopharynx are the most common lesions. Beginning as solid indurated plaques, they ulcerate and become deep-seated, painful, and secondarily infected.

Umbilicated nodules, papules, and *ulcers* appear on the skin. The ulcers have a punched-out appearance. They appear in crops and are extremely sensitive.

Abscesses, pyoderma, and *furuncles* may be the first lesions on the skin. Demonstration of the organisms is readily made in the histologic sections and cultures of the exudate.

The most common manifestation in children is *purpura.* Usually it appears a few days before death and is probably due to the severe involvement of the

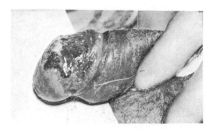

Figure 15–58. Histoplasmosis. (Courtesy of Drs. A. Amolsch and A. E. Palmer.)

reticuloendothelial system, with emaciation, chronic fever, and severe gastrointestinal symptoms.

Histoplasmosis affects both children (frequently infants) and adults, and the prognosis is equally serious in both.

Primary Cutaneous Histoplasmosis. This rare entity is characterized by a chancre-type lesion with regional adenopathy. This type has been reported as occurring on the penis.

African Histoplasmosis. This type is caused by *Histoplasma duboisii.* Its cutaneous manifestations are superficial cutaneous granulomas, subcutaneous granulomas, and osteomyelitic lesions with secondary involvement of the skin (cold abscesses). In addition, papular, nodular, circinate, eczematoid, and psoriasiform lesions may be seen. The granulomas are dome-shaped nodules, painless but slightly pruritic.

The reticuloendothelial system is frequently involved, inducing emaciation and chronic fever.

In this chronic type there may be skin and mucous membrane manifestations such as ulcerations of the nose, mouth, pharynx, genitals, and anus. These ulcers are chronic superficial lesions with no induration or noticeable inflammatory reaction. Erythema nodosum occurs frequently. Purpuric eruptions may also occur.

ETIOLOGY. Histoplasmosis was first discovered in Panama by S. T. Darling in 1906. It is caused by *Histoplasma capsulatum.* It is a dimorphic fungus that exists as a saprophyte in the soil; there are also tissue (yeast) and mycelial phases.

In tissue there are small oval bodies (1–5 μ) in large macrophages. Budding forms may be present. In direct examination the organism may be demonstrated in the peripheral blood, sputum, bronchial washings, spinal fluid, sternal marrow, lymph node touch smears, or ulcers when stained with Wright's, Giemsa, or periodic acid–Schiff stains. Gomori methenamine silver is the most reliable stain for showing microorganisms. In African histoplasmosis the ovoid bodies are large (10–13 μ in diameter).

The mycelial phase may be demonstrated on Sabouraud's dextrose agar, Mycosel medium, or brain-heart infusion agar to which blood has been added. A white fluffy colony is found, with microconidia and macroconidia.

If sputum is used for the culture, it should first be injected intraperitoneally into mice, to eliminate contamination with *Candida* and inhaled fungus spores.

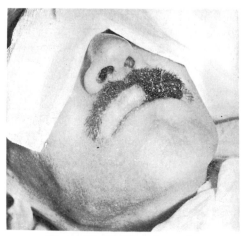

Figure 15–57. Histoplasmosis.

Four weeks later the mice should be killed and cultures should be made from the liver and spleen. Isolation of *H. capsulatum* from the acute benign form of the disease is best done by cultures of excised lymph nodes or from mice inoculated with sputum or stomach washings. Cultures should be kept at room temperature. One set of cultures should be inoculated at room temperature to demonstrate the mycelial phase and another at 37° C to produce the yeast phase.

EPIDEMIOLOGY. Although histoplasmosis occurs throughout the world, it is most frequent in North America, especially in the central states of the United States along the Mississippi River basin. Histoplasmosis is found frequently in river valley areas in the tropical and temperate zones. The Nile river valley seems to be one exception. Besides the Mississippi and Ohio river valleys, it has been found along the Potomac, Delaware, Hudson, and St. Lawrence rivers. It has been reported in the major river valleys of South America, Central Africa, and Southeast Asia.

Transmission of the disease does not occur between individuals; instead, the infection is contracted from the soil by inhalation of the spores, especially in a dusty atmosphere. Feces of birds and bats contain the fungus. The spores have been demonstrated in the excreta of starlings, chickens, and bats. The disease may be contracted by persons who enter caves inhabited by bats or birds. Epidemics have been reported from exposure to silos, abandoned chicken houses, and storm cellars. The infected people throughout the world number in the many millions.

In an outbreak occurring in Indianapolis in 1978, analyzed by Wheat et al, 120,000 residents were infected; 488 clinically recognized cases occurred, and 55 had disseminated disease; 19 died. None under one year old died. Fatal or disseminated infections occurred in 74 per cent of immunosuppressed persons, compared to 6.5 per cent of those without immunosuppression. Age over 54 was a worse prognostic factor than chronic lung disease in nonimmunosuppressed persons.

Disseminated histoplasmosis is seen as an opportunistic infection in HIV-infected individuals, reflecting impaired cellular immune function.

PATHOLOGY. Histologic examination shows a chronic granuloma containing innumerable intracellular oval bodies surrounded by a capsule which is an artifact produced by shrinkage of the cytoplasm away from the rigid cell wall. *H. capsulatum* has a predilection for the reticuloendothelial system. The fungus probably proliferates within the reticuloendothelial cells, which differentiates it from most fungi. The granulomatous nodule may show chiefly histiocytes, lymphocytes, plasma cells, epithelioid cells, giant cells, and the organism.

IMMUNOLOGY. Serologic testing for antibodies requires that the patient have normal immune responsiveness, and is further limited by a high rate of false positives and false negatives. Wheat et al reported in 1986 a radioimmunoassay to detect *H. capsulatum* antigen in serum or urine, which is rapid and reproducible and has adequate sensitivity and specificity for the early diagnosis of histoplasmosis.

TREATMENT. Prior to the introduction of ketoconazole (Nizoral), amphotericin B was the treatment of choice, with only the dubious alternative of sulfonamides for backup. A prospective multicenter clinical trial of Nizoral has shown that among 19 patients with chronic cavitary histoplasmosis treated six months or more, 400 and 800 mg/day were successful in 84 per cent. In 20 with localized or disseminated histoplasmosis treated six months or more, the low-dose regimen was more effective—100 per cent compared to 57 per cent. Side effects were twice as frequent with the high-dose regimen; gynecomastia occurred in six (14 per cent) at that level and in only one (1.4 per cent) with the lower dose. In the immunocompromised patient, amphotericin B remains the drug of choice. Itraconazole appears to hold great promise.

Cave-associated histoplasmosis. Arch Dermatol 1988, 124:994.

Hawkins SS, et al: Progressive disseminated histoplasmosis: Favorable response to ketoconazole. Ann Intern Med 1981, 95:446.

Johnson PC, et al: Progressive disseminated histoplasmosis in patients with acquired immunodeficiency syndrome. Am J Med 1988, 85:152.

Wheat LJ, et al: Risk factors for disseminated or fatal histoplasmosis. Ann Intern Med 1982, 96:159.

Idem: The diagnostic laboratory tests for histoplasmosis: analysis of experience in a large urban outbreak. Ann Intern Med 1982, 97:680.

Idem: Diagnosis of disseminated histoplasmosis by detection of *Histoplasma capsulatum* antigen in serum and urine specimens. N Engl J Med 1986, 314:83.

Idem: Histoplasmosis. Infect Dis Clin North Am 1988, 2:841.

NORTH AMERICAN BLASTOMYCOSIS

Synonyms: Gilchrist's disease, blastomycosis, blastomycetic dermatitis.

CLINICAL SIGNS. Cutaneous North American blastomycosis may appear in two forms. One is the rare primary cutaneous lesion characterized by the formation of a small primary nodule and subsequent small nodules along the draining lymphatics. This is similar to sporotrichosis. Healing takes place within several months.

The other form consists of chronic, slowly progressive, granulomatous lesions characterized by thick crusts, warty vegetations, discharging sinuses, and unusual vascularity. The lesions are often multiple and are located mostly on exposed parts, although they may occur anywhere on the integument. Papillomatous proliferation is most pronounced in lesions on the hands and feet, where the patches become very thick. There is a tendency for the patches to involute centrally and to form white scars while they spread peripherally. The crusts are thick

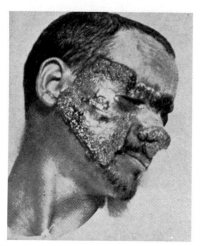

Figure 15–59. Blastomycosis. Note typical granular appearance.

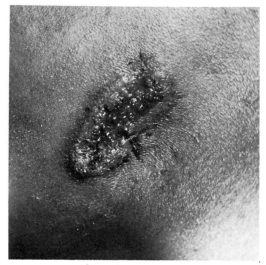

Figure 15–60. Blastomycosis on jaw.

and of a dirty gray or brown color. Beneath them there are exuberant granulations covered with a seropurulent exudate, which oozes out of small sinuses that extend down to indolent subcutaneous abscesses.

In this chronic cutaneous form, the infection is almost always primarily in the upper or middle lobes of the lungs, and the cutaneous lesions are disseminations from a primary pulmonary focus. The most frequent site of dissemination is the skin. It also frequently disseminates to the osseous system, especially the ribs and vertebrae. Other targets are the central nervous system, the liver and spleen, and the genitourinary system, especially the prostate, but rarely, if ever, the gastrointestinal tract.

ETIOLOGY. The fungus *Blastomyces dermatitidis* causes North American blastomycosis, which was first described by Gilchrist in 1894.

EPIDEMIOLOGY. North American blastomycosis is prevalent in the southeastern United States and the Ohio and Mississippi river basins, reaching epidemic proportions in the state of Kentucky. Furculow and his associates found in this area a male-female ratio of 6:1, most of the patients being over 60, and the white-black ratio 5:1. They found the most frequent sites of dissemination from the lung to be the skin and bones. Most common was the cutaneous form, occurring without known history of pulmonary lesions.

Blastomycosis has been reported from the bite of a dog suffering from pulmonary blastomycosis, by Gnann et al. Also there is a report of transmission occurring between men with prostatic involvement and their sexual partners.

Lasky and Sarsoi have reported apparent endogenous reactivation of the disease, with draining skin lesions in two patients and bone lesions in a third, four to 33 months after seeming spontaneous resolution of a pulmonary symptom complex.

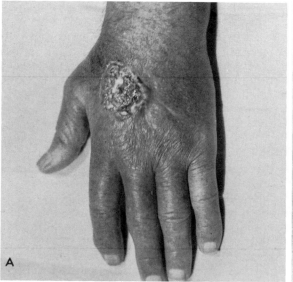

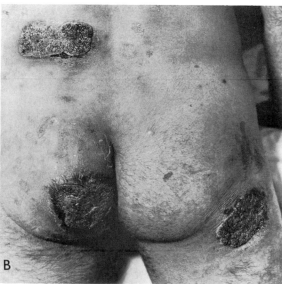

Figure 15–61. A and B, Blastomycosis.

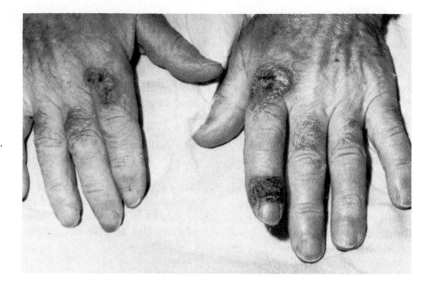

Figure 15–62. North American blastomycosis.

Klein et al investigated an outbreak of blastomycosis among children attending summer camp. They were able to culture *B. dermatitidis* from the soil in a beaver dam, which they concluded was the reservoir for human infection.

PATHOLOGY. The primary cutaneous blastomycosis consists of a polymorphonuclear infiltrate with many budding cells of blastomycetes. The lymph nodes may show marked inflammatory changes, giant cells, giant cells containing the organisms, lymphocytes, and plasma cells.

Various manifestations are present in the chronic disseminated-type skin lesion. The infiltrate of the verrucous lesion may show pseudoepitheliomatous hyperplasia. Microabscesses may abound in the epidermis, with giant cells, epithelioid cells, plasma cells, and lymphocytes in the cutis. A potassium hydroxide slide preparation containing a smear of pus from the lesion will show under the microscope single or budding spherical cells with refractile walls.

The lung involvement may show many changes that are suggestive of carcinoma or tuberculosis with tubercle formation. Purulent abscesses form not only in the lungs but also elsewhere when dissemination is taking place. The abscesses may break through to form draining abscesses and sinuses on the skin. There may be innumerable organisms in the pus.

MYCOLOGY. *Blastomyces dermatitidis* is a dimorphic fungus with a mycelial phase at room temperature and a yeast phase at 37° C. Direct microscopic examination of a potassium hydroxide slide of the specimen should always be made, since culture of the fungus is difficult. The specimen is cultured on Sabouraud's dextrose agar, mycosel, and brain-heart infusion agar to which blood has been added. Aerial mycelium will develop in 10 to 14 days, forming a white cottony growth that turns a tan color with age. The structures are septate mycelium and characteristic conidia on the sides of hyphae. The conidia are 3–5 μ and variously shaped from round to oval forms. Culture at 37° C produces a slow-growing, wrinkled yeast with spherules, single budding cells, and some abortive hyphae.

IMMUNOLOGY. The blastomycin test shows present or past infection of North American blastomycosis. Cross reactions may occur with histoplasmin and coccidioidomycin and therefore simultaneous testing to these various antigens should be done to detect the greatest sensitivity.

The complement fixation test is useful. With recovery there is regression of the titer. Cross reactions may also occur to the already mentioned antigens. The complement fixation reaction is usually negative in cutaneous blastomycosis except when the lesions are very extensive.

DIFFERENTIAL DIAGNOSIS. Blastomycosis may closely resemble tuberculosis verrucosa cutis, syphilis, granuloma inguinale, drug eruptions, trichophytic granuloma, and chronic serpiginous and gangrenous pyoderma. The similarity to tuberculosis verrucosa cutis is sometimes so close that one is unable to differentiate the two diseases by clinical examination without resort to laboratory procedures. The course of blastomycosis is more rapid, however; suppuration usually occurs early and involvement is more extensive than is common in the verrucous type of tuberculosis. Vegetative lesions of tertiary syphilis usually are accompanied by other signs of the disease and have a predilection for the scalp and the mucocutaneous junctions, areas not commonly affected by blastomycosis. Bromide and iodide eruptions are generally more acutely inflammatory and less purulent than blastomycosis. Sporotrichosis is characterized by subcutaneous abscesses distributed along lymphatic channels, the overlying skin becoming involved only secondarily.

Examination of the tissue or of smears from the exudate, together with the history, will determine the diagnosis. In deep trichophytic granuloma the duration is, as a rule, less than in blastomycosis, and the lesions are not so papillomatous. Microscopic demonstration of the causative fungi is conclusive.

TREATMENT. As in histoplasmosis, ketoconazole seems likely to replace amphotericin B as the drug of choice in immunocompetent, nonmeningeal cases of blastomycosis. It was curative in 35 of 44 patients treated by Bradsher et al for at least two weeks. Two relapsed despite six months' treatment with ketoconazole. Gynecomastia in four of 26 men taking 400 mg a day, and dysfunctional uterine bleeding in five of 20 women, were seen. The gynecomastia went away after treatment was stopped, and the bleeding stopped spontaneously after two months in three patients; two required reduction of dose to 200 mg/day. None had abnormal liver enzyme levels. Hudson and Callen reported a case which responded promptly to 400 mg of ketoconazole a day, with early reduction to 200 mg a day, which was continued for 15 months. There was no relapse within three months' follow-up. Amphotericin B is necessary for the immunocompromised host because ketoconazole is fungistatic at therapeutic levels, whereas amphotericin B is fungicidal.

Other drugs that may be useful are itraconazole, 5-fluorocytosine, and 2-hydroxystilbamidine. Side effects of 5-fluorocytosine include leukopenia, thrombocytopenia, liver toxicity, nausea, and vomiting. Potassium iodide is also helpful at times.

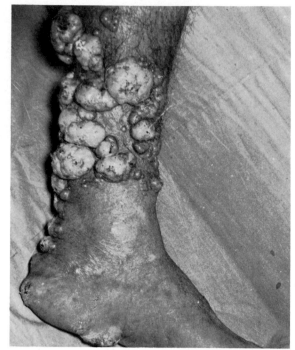

Figure 15–63. Keloidal blastomycosis. (Courtesy of Dr. J. Lobo, Brazil.)

Abadie-Kemmerly S, et al: Failure of ketoconazole treatment of *Blastomyces dermatitidis* due to interaction of isoniazid and rifampin. Ann Intern Med 1988, 109:844.

Bradsher RW: Blastomycosis. Infect Dis Clin North Am 1988, 2:877.

Idem, et al: Ketoconazole therapy for endemic blastomycosis. Ann Intern Med 1985, 103(6 pt 1):872.

Craig MW, et al: Conjugal blastomycosis. Am Rev Resp Dis 1970, 102:86.

Furculow ML, et al: North American blastomycosis. Trans NY Acad Sci 1973, 35:241.

Gnann JW Jr, et al: Human blastomycosis after a dog bite. Ann Intern Med 1983, 98:48.

Hudson CP, et al: Systemic blastomycosis treated with ketoconazole. Arch Dermatol 1984, 120:536.

Klein BS, et al: Isolation of *Blastomyces dermatitidis* from soil associated with a large outbreak of blastomycosis in Wisconsin. N Engl J Med 1986, 314:529.

Malak JA, et al: Blastomycosis in the Middle East. Br J Dermatol 1971, 83:161.

National Institute of Allergy and Infectious Diseases: Treatment of blastomycosis and histoplasmosis with ketoconazole: results of a randomized prospective clinical trial. Ann Intern Med 1985, 103 (6 pt 1):861.

Pirozzi DJ, et al: An unusual case of North American blastomycosis. Arch Dermatol 1978, 114:1370.

KELOIDAL BLASTOMYCOSIS
(Lobomycosis)

Keloidal blastomycosis was originally described by Jorge Lobo in 1931. All cases reported since then have occurred in countries in the tropical zone.

The disease may involve any part of the body. As the name implies, the lesions appear characteristically keloidal, with or without fistulas. The nodules increase in size gradually by invasion of the surrounding normal skin or through the superficial lymphatics. Long-standing cases involve the regional lymph nodes. A common location is the ear, which looks like the cauliflower ear of a boxer, with pseudokeloidal nodules and infiltrations of the helix. These are painless, violet to pink, and generally not associated with lymphadenopathy.

The fungus has not been found in nature. There are indications that snake or arthropod bites (tick, mosquito) may be the means of inoculation into the skin. Some 53 cases have been reported, with equal distribution between the sexes and the age of patients being between 30 and 80. Agricultural laborers have been most frequently affected.

Histologically, the epidermis is atrophic. In the

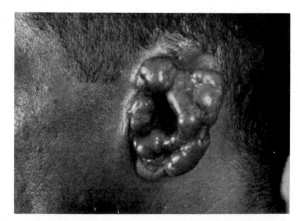

Figure 15–64. Keloidal blastomycosis in a typical location. (Courtesy of Dr. M. de Moraes, Brazil.)

dermis are seen numerous organisms with double-contoured walls. Refringent parasites are always conspicuous. The cellular infiltrate is composed of vacuolated histiocytes, giant cells, and parasites.

The organisms are thick-walled, refractile spherules larger than those of *Paracoccidioides brasiliensis*. One or two buds may be seen, but never multiple budding as in *P. brasiliensis*. It is difficult to obtain growth in any culture medium.

The causative fungus is a blastomyceslike organism called *Loboa loboi* (formerly *Glenosporella loboi*).

Surgical excision of the affected areas is usually unsuccessful, being followed by recurrence. No form of chemotherapy has produced any favorable results.

Bhawan J, et al: Lobomycosis: an electron microscopic, histochemical, and immunologic study. J Cutan Pathol 1976, 3:5.

Lobo J: Blastomicose Queloidiforme. Universidad de Recife, Imprensa Universitaria, 1963.

Idem: Keloidiform blastomycosis. Derm Ib Latin America 1967, 2:217.

SOUTH AMERICAN BLASTOMYCOSIS

Synonyms: Paracoccidioidal granuloma, paracoccidioidomycosis.

CLINICAL MANIFESTATIONS. The disease is almost always primary in the lungs. Some cases may arise from inoculation of the mucous membranes of the pharynx or other parts of the gastrointestinal tract. Lymph gland involvement is commonly present. Wide dissemination of the disease occurs to the skin and to all organs of the body, with a fatal termination unless treatment is instituted.

The *mucocutaneous type* usually begins in the region of the mouth, where small papules and ulcerations

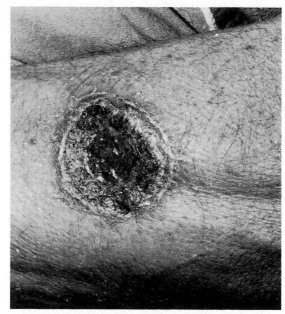

Figure 15–66. South American blastomycosis on forearm. (Courtesy of Dr. J. Kroll.)

appear. These spread, and ultimately extensive ulcerations destroy the nose, lips, and face. The skin lesions may show ulcerations, pseudoepitheliomatous hyperplasia, and microabscesses. In the latter the *P. brasiliensis* may be seen. This is a round cell, 10–60 μ in diameter, with multiple buds.

The *lymphangitic type* manifests itself by enlargement of the regional lymph nodes soon after the appearance of the initial lesions about the mouth. The lymphatic adenopathy may extend to the supraclavicular and axillary regions. Nodes may become greatly enlarged and break down with ulcerations that secondarily involve the skin, causing severe pain and dysphagia with progressive cachexia and death. It may closely simulate Hodgkin's disease, especially when the suprahyoid, preauricular, or retroauricular groups of lymph nodes are involved.

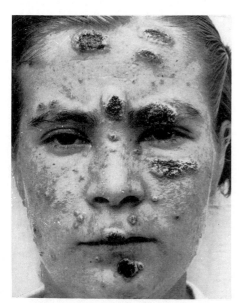

Figure 15–65. South American blastomycosis. (Courtesy of Dr. T. A. Furtado.)

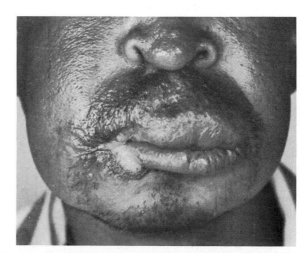

Figure 15–67. Paracoccidioidomycosis. (Courtesy of Dr. J. Convit, Venezuela.)

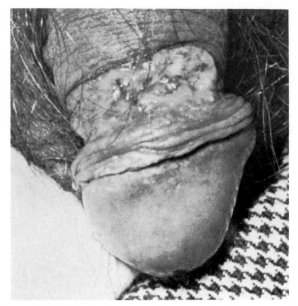

Figure 15–68. South American blastomycosis. (Courtesy of Dr. A. T. Londero, Brazil.)

There is a *visceral type*, due probably to hematogenous spread of the disease from the lungs to the liver, spleen, intestines, and other organs.

There is also a *mixed type* that has the combined symptomatology of the mucocutaneous, lymphangitic, and visceral types.

ETIOLOGY. South American blastomycosis was first described by Lutz in Brazil in 1908. It is caused by the fungus *Paracoccidioides brasiliensis.*

EPIDEMIOLOGY. This chronic granulomatous disease is endemic in Brazil and also occurs in Argentina and Venezuela. Occasional cases have been reported in the United States, Mexico, and Central America. The disease is generally found among laborers, mostly in men, and many are infected by picking the teeth with twigs or from chewing leaves. The fact that the disease is 15 times more common in men is of particular interest, since it has been shown that 17B-estradiol inhibits transition from the mycelial to the tissue-invasive yeast form. *P. brasiliensis* can lodge in periodontal tissues, and some cases start after extraction of teeth.

PATHOLOGY. An infectious granuloma occurs with abscess formation similar to that of blastomycosis.

MYCOLOGY. The causative fungus in tissue is a large thick-walled cell with multiple buds. In culture the colony is cream-colored, compact, and powdery. Chlamydospores are round or oval. Elongate lateral conidia may be present.

IMMUNOLOGY. Complement fixation tests are positive in 97 per cent of the severe cases and the titer rises as the disease becomes more severe. As improvement occurs the titer decreases.

TREATMENT. Amphotericin B is effective. The dosage schedule is similar to that described for coccidioidomycosis. Dillon et al reported that 400 mg of ketoconazole orally daily for one month, followed by 200 mg daily for 23 months, cured six patients completely and left three with only serologic evidence of infection. The only side effects were reversible elevations of serum transaminase, cholesterol, and triglycerides. Ketoconazole is becoming the drug of choice in the treatment of this disease.

Sulfamerazine or sulfadiazine gives good results. The usual treatment is 1 gm of either of these drugs every six hours until clinical cure is obtained, or approximately for two years. Recurrences are frequent upon cessation of therapy.

Dillon NL, et al: Ketoconazole treatment of paracoccidioidomycosis for . . . two years (Portuguese). An Brasil Dermatol 1985, 60:45.
Furtado T: Infection vs. disease in South American blastomycosis. Int J Dermatol 1975, 14:117.
Gimenez MF, et al: Langerhans cells in paracoccidioidomycosis. Arch Dermatol 1987, 123:479.
Linares G, et al: Paracoccidioidomycosis in the United States. Arch Otolaryngol 1971, 93:514.
Londero AT, et al: Paracoccidioidomycosis. Am J Med 1972, 52:771.
Santos Lima N, et al: Tratamento da blastomicose sulamericana pelo miconazole oral. Resultados satisfactorios in 5 casos. An Brasil Dermatol 1974, 49:245.
Stevens DA, et al: Paracoccidioidomycosis . . . treatment with miconazole. Am J Trop Med Hyg 1978, 27:801.
Sugar AM: Paracoccidioidomycosis. Infect Dis Clin North Am 1988, 2:913.

CHROMOBLASTOMYCOSIS

CLINICAL FEATURES. This disease usually affects one leg or foot. It begins as a small pink, scaly papule or warty growth, as a rule on some part of the foot, whence it slowly spreads by the growth of satellite lesions. The extremity is usually swollen and at its distal portion becomes covered with various nodular, tumorous, verrucous lesions that may resemble a cauliflower. The small lesions may resemble common warts. Plaquelike and cicatricial types of lesions also occur. The cicatricial types are formed by nodules and spread peripherally; healing with sclerosis takes place at the center, at times associated with keloid formation. Adenitis as a result of bacterial complications may occur. In rare instances the disease begins on the hand or wrist and involves the entire upper extremity. It may also begin on the nose. There is a slow progression of the disease and it may take many years to develop fully.

Usually the disease process remains localized to one lower extremity; however, there have been rare reports of central nervous system involvement both with and without associated skin lesions.

Metastases through the blood stream are rare, but there is no doubt that they can occur.

ETIOLOGY. Five dematiaceous fungi are the causative agents: *Cladosporium carrionii, Phialophora verrucosa, Fonsecaea pedrosoi (Hormodendrum pedrosoi), F. compacta (H. compactum),* and *Rhinocladiella aquaspersa.*

INCIDENCE AND PREVALENCE. It was first recognized in Brazil by Pedroso in 1911. Since then

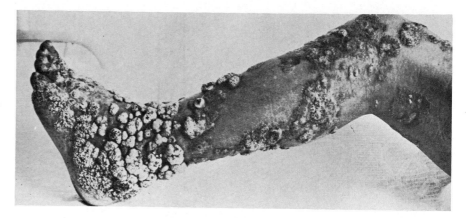

Figure 15–69. Chromoblastomycosis. (Courtesy of Dr. A. L. Carrion, Puerto Rico.)

it has been found in Cuba, West Indies, Madagascar, United States, Russia, and other countries. The distribution is predominantly among barefooted farm laborers. It occurs 20 times more commonly in men than in women, usually in the 20–50-year age range.

PATHOLOGY. The essential pathologic changes are characterized by a granulomatous reaction, with the formation of pseudotubercles containing giant cells, and a focal round cell infiltration in the superficial portions of the dermis. The fungus occurs in the form of brown, spherical cells with thick, dark cell walls and coarsely granular pigmented protoplasm. The fungi appear in clusters of spherical cells that reproduce by equatorial splitting, not by budding. Septate forms (Medlar bodies, "copper pennies") are occasionally encountered in the dermis, this being the characteristic tissue morphology of chromoblastomycosis, differentiating it from phaeomycosis.

MYCOLOGY. The cultural characteristics were extensively studied by Carrion. McGinnis has recently reviewed the nomenclature. The colonies produce black, slowly growing, heaped-up colonies. The three types differ according to the type of conidiophore produced; they are the *Phialophora*, the *Cladosporium*, and the *Acrotheca* types of sporulation.

TREATMENT. Chromoblastomycosis is best treated by surgical excision and grafting of the affected area if this is feasible. Application of heat has been reported effective, as it has with sporotrichosis and atypical mycobacterial infections. Kuttner recently described a case treated successfully with the carbon dioxide laser. Amputation may rarely be unavoidable.

The causative fungus is not killed by the concentrations of amphotericin B usually given intravenously, but may be killed by higher concentrations injected locally at the site of involvement. Costello suspended 40 mg of amphotericin B in 5 ml of 2 per cent procaine solution (8 mg per ml) and injected it into the lesions. This was repeated once weekly for three months. Complete clearing was obtained.

Ketoconazole, by itself, was effective in only about half the patients in whom it has been tried; but Silber et al found that in one patient in whom it had failed

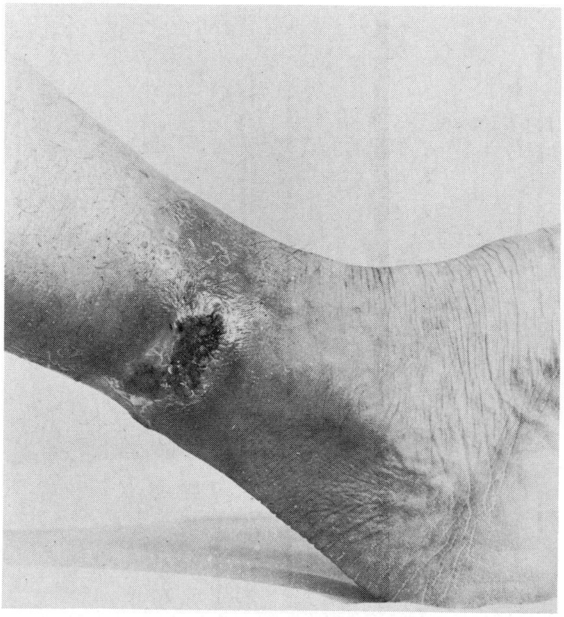

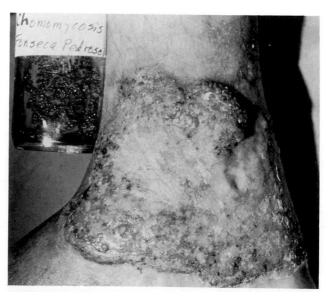

Figure 15–70. Early chromoblastomycosis. (Courtesy of Dr. A. L. Carrion, Puerto Rico.)

Figure 15–71. Chromomycosis. (Courtesy of Dr. Axel W. Hoke.)

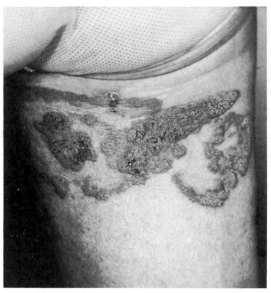

Figure 15–72. Chromoblastomycosis.

Bennett JE: Flucytosine. Ann Intern Med 1977, 86:319.

Borelli D: Diagnosis and treatment of chromomycosis. Arch Dermatol 1972, 106:419.

Carrion AL: Chromoblastomycosis and related infections. Int J Dermatol 1975, 14:27.

Fader RC, et al: Infections caused by dematiaceous fungi. Infect Dis Clin North Am 1988, 2:925.

Heyl T: Treatment of chromomycosis with itraconazole. Br J Dermatol 1985, 112:728.

Kuttner BJ, et al: Treatment of chromomycosis with a CO$_2$ laser. J Dermatol Surg Oncol 1986, 12:695.

McBurney EI: Chromoblastomycosis: treatment with ketoconazole. Cutis 1982, 30:746.

McGinnis MR: Chromoblastomycosis and phaeohyphomycosis. JAAD 1983, 8:1.

Perry AE, et al: Papules and nodules in a patient with sarcoidosis. Arch Dermatol 1987, 123:520.

Tagami H, et al: Topical heat therapy for cutaneous chromomycosis. Arch Dermatol 1979, 115:740.

Tschen JA, et al: Chromomycosis. Arch Dermatol 1984, 120:107.

Zaias N, et al: A simple and accurate diagnostic method in chromoblastomycosis. Arch Dermatol 1973, 108:545.

(even at 400 mg/day), when 5-fluorocytosine, 100 mg/kg/24 hours, was added, within a few weeks the lesions became flat and fibrotic, and at the end of one year, treatment was stopped. The organism was *Fonsecaea pedrosoi.* Itraconazole has been effective in some cases, but adequate trials have not yet been done.

Potassium iodide orally to highest tolerance, as given in sporotrichosis, has also been reported to occasionally be effective, given at times with vitamin D$_2$.

5-fluorocytosine (flucytosine, Ancobon), 37.5 mg/kg orally every six hours, is effective in some cases. Serum levels should be maintained between 50 and 100 μg for six weeks. Despite all these options, some lesions remain resistant, and amputation may be unavoidable.

Phaeohyphomycosis

This heterogeneous group of mycotic infections is caused by dematiaceous fungi whose morphologic characteristics in tissue include yeast-like cells, hyphae, pseudohypha-like elements, or any combination of these. This contrasts with chromomycosis in that the morphology in tissue appears as single, thick-walled, muriform fungal cells.

CLINICAL FEATURES. McGinnis et al have reviewed the many types of clinical lesions one may see with this histologic picture. They include superficial, cutaneous, subcutaneous, and systemic disease. Black piedra is an example of superficial infection. Cutaneous disease causes lesions similar to dermatophytosis. Noel et al recently reported three cases. Subcutaneous disease occurs most commonly as abscesses at the site of minor trauma, with *Exo-*

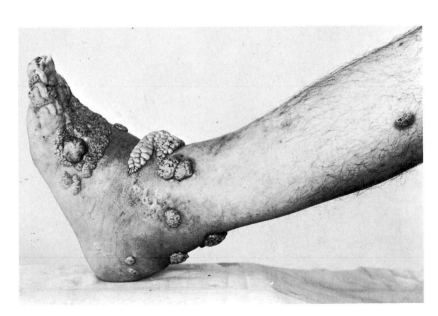

Figure 15–73. Chromoblastomycosis. (Courtesy of Dr. A. L. Carrion, Puerto Rico.)

phiala jeanselmi being the most common cause in temperate climates, although *Bipolaris* and *Exserohilum* genera are being more commonly recovered as causes of both subcutaneous lesions and systemic infections. Burges et al reviewed this recently. Finally, systemic phaeohyphomycosis is more frequently being reported as the population of immunocompromised patients increases.

ETIOLOGY. Over 30 agents are capable of causing phaeohyphomycosis. McGinnis in 1983 listed many of them and the subtype of disease they cause. Among them are *E. jeanselmi, Dactylaria gallopava, Phialophora parasitica, Phaeoannellomyces werneckii, Hendersonula toruloidea, Exserohilum rostratum, Bipolaris spicifera,* and *Xylopha bantiana.* Some fungi, such as *Phialophora verrucosa,* can cause both phaeohyphomycosis and chromoblastomycosis. Some fungi, such as *E. jeanselmi,* may cause mycetoma (characterized by granule formation) in some patients and phaeohyphomycosis in others.

TREATMENT. Cutaneous phaeohyphomycosis may respond to topical antifungal agents. Noel et al detail the options in their report. Other possibilities include excision, intralesional miconazole, griseofulvin, 5-flucytosine, systemic amphotericin B, ketoconazole, and, in one of their cases, fluconazole. Subcutaneous abscesses may be excised; however, systemic coverage with ketoconazole seems wise perioperatively. Systemic amphotericin B is recommended for systemic infection with these agents in the immunocompromised patient.

Burges GE, et al: Subcutaneous phaeohyphomycosis caused by *Exerohilum rostratum* in an immunocompetent host. Arch Dermatol 1987, 123:1346.
Duvic M, et al: Superficial phaeohyphomycosis of the scrotum in a patient with AIDS. Arch Dermatol 1987, 123:1597.
Ikai K, et al: Phaeohyphomycosis caused by *Phialophora richardsiae.* JAAD 1988, 19:478.
McGinnis MR: Chromoblastomycosis and phaeohyphomycosis. JAAD 1983, 8:1.
Idem, et al: Infections caused by black fungi. Arch Dermatol 1987, 123:1300.
Noel SB, et al: Primary cutaneous phaeohyphomycosis. JAAD 1988, 18:1023.

HYALOHYPHOMYCOSIS

This term complements phaeohyphomycosis and comprises those opportunistic mycotic infections caused by nondematiaceous molds whose basic form consists of hyaline hyphal fragments that are septate, branched or unbranched, or toruloid. It is not intended to replace such well-established names as aspergillosis or candidiasis but refers to infections caused by organisms such as *Fusarium, Penicillium,* and *Paecilomyces.*

These organisms are ubiquitous; they occur as saprophytes in soil or water or on decomposing organic debris. The generally do not cause disease except in immunocompromised patients. *Fusarium solani* (keratomycosis) and *F. oxysporum* (white superficial onychomycosis) are exceptions. There is no classic clinical morphology to the lesions, but keratotic masses, ulcerations, ecthyma gangrenosum–like lesions, erythematous nodules, and disseminated erythema have been described.

Most of the infections are treated with a combination of excision and amphotericin B. Success is generally low; Weitzman's excellent review should be consulted in individual cases.

Jade KB, et al: *Paecilomycelilacinus* cellulitis in an immunocompromised patient. Arch Dermatol 1986, 122:1169.
Matsuda T, et al: Disseminated hyalohyphomycosis in a leukemic patient. Arch Dermatol 1986, 122:1171.
Rinaldi MG: Emerging opportunists. Infect Dis Clin North Am 1989, 3:65.
Veglia KS, et al: *Fusarium* as a pathogen. JAAD 1987, 16:260.
Weitzman I: Saprophytic molds as agents of cutaneous and subcutaneous infection in the immunocompromised host. Arch Dermatol 1986, 122:1161.

ZYGOMYCOSIS
(Phycomycosis)

There are a number of important pathogens in the class Zygomycetes. The two orders within this class that cause cutaneous infection most often are the Mucorales and Entomophthorales. The Mucorales-caused disease mucormycosis is discussed in the next section.

CLINICAL FEATURES. Infections caused by the order Entomophthorales have been named entomophthoromycosis, rhinoentomophthoromycosis, conidiobolomycosis, or basidiobolomycosis. They occur usually in healthy individuals, unlike mucormycosis. The infections may be classified as cutaneous, subcutaneous, visceral, and disseminated.

Subcutaneous zygomycosis occurs in two basic types, each involving different anatomic sites. Well-circumscribed subcutaneous masses involving the nose, paranasal tissue, and upper lip, as in the case reported by Towersey et al, characterize one type. The second type occurs as indurated nodular subcutaneous lesions located on the extremities, buttocks, and trunk.

ETIOLOGY. *Conidiobolus coronatus* typically causes the perinasal disease, whereas *Basidiobolus ranarum* causes the type of subcutaneous disease seen off the face.

INCIDENCE. Occurrence is worldwide. It was first reported in Indonesia, where it is prevalent. Since then reports have come from Africa, Asia, and the Americas. Generally infection occurs in countries situated between 15° latitude North and 15° latitude South.

DIAGNOSIS. Isolation and identification of the causative fungus are fundamental to the diagnosis. Culture on Sabouraud's dextrose agar is made of nasal discharge, abscess fluid, or biopsy specimens. Biopsy specimens will show fibroblastic proliferation and an inflammatory reaction with lymphocytes, plasma cells, histiocytes, eosinophils, and giant cells. Broad, thin-walled hyphae with occasional septa, branched at right angles, are seen. The *Splendore-Hoeppli phenomenon* may be seen, in which an eosinophilic sleeve surmounts the hyphae.

TREATMENT. Potassium iodide has been the drug of choice. Sometimes combining this with trimethoprim-sulfamethoxazole improves results. Amphotericin B has also been effective in some cases. Several reports, including the one by Towersey et al, document a response to ketoconazole. Excision of small lesions is an alternative method of management.

Droubet DL, et al: Laboratory and clinical assessment of ketoconazole in deep-seated mycosis. Am J Med 1983, 74:30.

Rinaldi MG: Zygomycosis. Infect Dis Clin North Am 1989, 3:19.

Singh D, et al: Rhinoentomophthoromycosis. J Laryngol 1976, 90:871.

Towersey L, et al: *Conidiobolus coronatus* infection treated with ketoconazole. Arch Dermatol 1988, 124:1392.

MUCORMYCOSIS

This term refers to infections caused by the order Mucorales of the class Zygomycetes. They characteristically are acute, rapidly developing, often fatal, opportunistic infections of immunocompromised patients. Most occur in ketoacidotic diabetes, but leukemia, lymphoma, AIDS, iatrogenic immunosuppression, burns, and malnourishment all predispose to these infections.

CLINICAL FEATURES. The five major clinical forms (rhinocerebral, pulmonary, cutaneous, gastrointestinal, and disseminated) share features that include invasion of blood vessel walls by organisms. This leads to infarction, gangrene, and the formation of black, necrotic pus. Ulceration, cellulitis, ecthyma gangrenosum–like lesions, and necrotic abscesses comprise the usual cutaneous appearance. It may involve the skin through traumatic implantation or by hematogenous dissemination.

ETIOLOGY. The fungi that cause this infection are ubiquitous molds common in the soil, on decomposing plant and animal matter, and in the air. The pathogenic genera include *Absidia, Mucor, Rhizopus, Cunninghamella, Apophysomyces, Rhizomucor,* and *Saksenaea.*

DIAGNOSIS. Tissue obtained by biopsy or currettage is cultured. Prompt diagnosis by this method is essential in this rapidly fatal infection.

TREATMENT. Basic to effective therapy is gaining control of the underlying disease. A combination of excision of affected tissue with amphotericin B is necessary in addition.

Lehrer RI, et al: Mucormycosis. Ann Intern Med 1980, 93:93.

Mead JH, et al: Cutaneous *Rhizopus* infections as a postoperative complication associated with elasticized adhesive dressing. JAMA 1979, 242:272.

Meyer RD, et al: Cutaneous lesions in disseminated mucormycosis. JAMA 1973, 225:737.

Rinaldi MG: Zygomycosis. Infect Dis Clin North Am 1989, 3:19.

Rippon JW: Cutaneous and subcutaneous mucormycosis. Curr Concepts Skin Disord 1980, 1:8.

ASPERGILLOSIS

Formerly, this was known mainly as a pulmonary infection of pigeon and poultry handlers, and of penguins kept under crowded conditions. Aspergillus is one of the most frequently encountered fungi in the laboratory.

Aspergillosis is second only to candidiasis in frequency of opportunistic fungal disease in patients with leukemia and other hematologic neoplasia. Renal and heart transplant patients receiving immunosuppressive drugs may show aspergillosis at au-

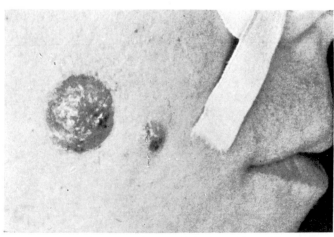

Figure 15–74. Cutaneous Mucor *infection of face. (Courtesy of Dr. J. L. Wade.)*

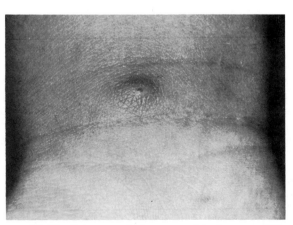

Figure 15–75. Cutaneous lesion on wrist of young girl with primary disseminated aspergillosis of the lungs. (Courtesy of Drs. J. Vedder and W. F. Schorr.)

topsy. Aspergillus infections may also complicate burn wounds and cause extensive local tissue destruction. Invasive aspergillosis is difficult to diagnose and is often lethal in the immunosuppressed host. Blood cultures and serologic tests are usually negative. Pulmonary involvement is usually present in invasive aspergillus disease, but skin lesions are infrequently reported.

Findlay et al grouped the skin lesions associated with systemic aspergillosis into five categories: the solitary necrotizing dermal plaque; the subcutaneous granuloma or abscess; persistent eruptive dermal spots or papules with suppurative, vegetating, or necrobiotic tendencies; miscellaneous erythemas and toxicodermas; and progressive confluent granulomas. *A. fumigatus* is the most common cause of disseminated aspergillosis with cutaneous involvement. It is imperative to obtain a cutaneous biopsy and culture of skin lesions when the clinical setting suggests the possibility of opportunistic fungal infections. Amphotericin B is the drug of choice in invasive aspergillosis and cutaneous infections in immunocompromised patients.

Primary Cutaneous Aspergillosis. This is a rare disease. Grossman et al's recent report of six children with hematologic malignancies who developed skin lesions at the site of intravenous cannulas typifies these cases. Hemorrhagic bullae, which progressed to necrotic ulcers, were present. All recovered when treated with intravenous amphotericin B.

Aspergillus species may involve the skin, mucous membranes, paranasal sinuses, conjunctiva, eyelids, and the orbit. Aspergillus is a frequent contaminant in cultures from thickened, friable, dystrophic nails. Various *Aspergillus* species have been reported to be etiologic agents in onychomycosis.

Otomycosis. A favorite site of infection is the ear canal, although its role as a pathogen has been questioned. Only erythema and scaling are present in the ear canal.

Aspergillus fumigatus, A. flavus, and *A. niger* are the most prevalent species found. They are composed of compact clusters of branching septate hyphae 4 to 6 μm in diameter.

Examination of a KOH wet slide shows densely packed hyphae. On Sabouraud's medium the black mold of *Aspergillus niger* grows.

There is always some doubt as to whether *A. niger* is the etiologic agent or is, rather, a contaminant. Pathogenic bacteria, especially *Pseudomonas aeruginosa*, are often found concurrently in otomycosis.

Treatment should be directed toward keeping the ear dry. Iodochlorhydroxyquin (Vioform, Ciba) is the treatment of choice. A 3 per cent lotion is applied to the canal three times daily. Neosporin otic lotion, 2 per cent gentian violet solution, and cresatin are also effective remedies.

Pulmonary Aspergillosis. The lungs are the most common site for aspergillosis, which occurs when there is some underlying disease that impairs the host's defense mechanisms. Bronchitis, pulmonary infiltrations, and pulmonary nodules known as "aspergillomas" may occur.

Aspergillosis of the lung is usually caused by *A. fumigatus*, which can be diagnosed by finding conidiophores in histologic sections. Direct examination of sputum and cultures from sputum and bronchial washings also aid in the diagnosis.

A case of nodular subcutaneous metastatic aspergillosis with pulmonary involvement was successfully treated with nystatin by inhalation therapy by Vedder and Schorr.

Keratomycosis. Ulceration of the cornea along with penetration into the deep stromal layers with an acute inflammatory reaction that may later progress into mycotic endophthalmitis may be a concomitant infection of the eye. Many different fungi, including *Aspergillus flavus*, may be the cause.

Allo MD, et al: Primary cutaneous aspergillosis associated with intravenous Hickman catheter. N Engl J Med 1987, 317:1105.

Cahill KM, et al: Primary cutaneous aspergillosis. Arch Dermatol 1967, 96:545.

Degregorio MW, et al: Fungal infections in patients with acute leukemia. Am J Med 1982, 73:543.

Grossman ME, et al: Primary cutaneous aspergillosis in six leukemic children. JAAD 1985, 12:313.

Levitz SM: Aspergillosis. Infect Dis Clin North Am 1989, 3:1.

Magid ML, et al: Violaceous nodules on the arm of a child with acute lymphocytic leukemia. Arch Dermatol 1988, 124:121.

McGonigle JJ, Jillson OF: Otomycosis: an entity. Arch Dermatol 1967, 95:45.

Prystowsky SD, et al: Invasive aspergillosis. N Engl J Med 1976, 295:655.

Vedder JS, et al: Primary disseminated and pulmonary aspergillosis with metastatic skin nodules. Successful treatment with inhalation nystatin therapy. JAMA 1969, 209:1191.

Weitzman I: Soprophytic molds as agents of cutaneous and subcutaneous infection in the immunocompromised host. Arch Dermatol 1986, 122:1161.

CRYPTOCOCCOSIS

CLINICAL FEATURES. Cryptococcosis is primarily an internal disease which most frequently involves the central nervous system. Wilson and Plunkett suggest that in this disease there is a primary pulmonary involvement from which dissemination occurs.

Primary pulmonary cryptococcosis infection may be so mild that the symptoms of fever, cough, and pain may be absent or present only mildly. On the other hand, some cases may be severe enough to cause death. X-ray studies will reveal disease at this stage.

When dissemination occurs the organism has a special affinity for the central nervous system. It is the most common cause of mycotic meningitis. All the symptoms of acute and severe involvement may be present. There may be restlessness, hallucinations, depression, severe headache, vertigo, nausea and vomiting, nuchal rigidity, epileptiform seizures, and symptoms of intraocular hypertension. Other

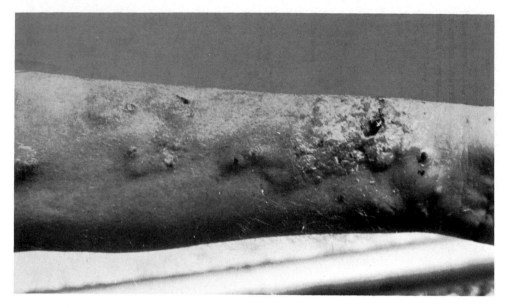

Figure 15–76. Cryptococcosis on the forearm in 28-year-old man with AV shunt for dialysis. (Courtesy of Dr. R. N. Buchanan, Jr.)

organs such as the liver, skin, spleen, myocardium, and skeletal system, as well as the lymph nodes, may be involved. Disseminated cryptococcosis can occur initially in other organ systems. Initial presentations with hepatitis, osteomyelitis, prostatitis, pyelonephritis, peritonitis, and skin involvement have all been reported. The incidence of skin involvement in cases of cryptococcosis is reported as being between 10 and 15 per cent, but may be even more common.

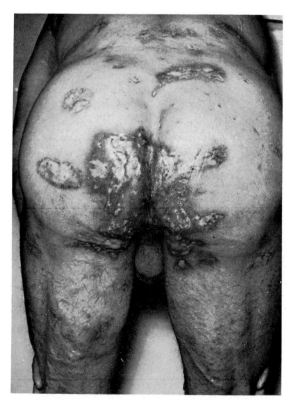

Figure 15–77. Cryptococcosis of 14 years' duration in a 42-year-old man. (Courtesy of Dr. E. Florian, Budapest.)

Skin infection with cryptococcosis has been reported to occur most frequently on the head and neck. A variety of morphologic lesions have been reported, including subcutaneous swellings, abscesses, tumorlike masses, molluscum-contagiosum–like lesions, draining sinuses, ulcers, granulomas, papules, nodules, pustules, acneiform lesions, plaques, and cellulitis. Wheeler et al have reported five cases in which skin lesions provided the first evidence of disseminated systemic cryptococcosis.

Primary inoculation of the skin is a very rare disease, if it occurs at all. For all practical purposes, identification of cryptococci in the skin indicates disseminated disease with a poor prognosis, and it requires prompt therapy.

ETIOLOGY. The causative organism is *Cryptococcus neoformans*.

EPIDEMIOLOGY. Cryptococcosis has a worldwide distribution and affects both man and animals. The organism has been recovered from human skin, soil, dust, and pigeon droppings. The latter, when deposited on window ledges in large cities, are a source of infection. Usually a concomitant debilitating disease such as AIDS, cancer, leukemia, lymphoma, severe diabetes mellitus, sarcoidosis, tuberculosis, or silicosis is present. Long-term oral prednisone or immunosuppressive therapy for chronic disease may also be a factor. The probable portal of entry is the lungs.

IMMUNOLOGY. Cryptococcin skin tests have been regarded as not very helpful in diagnosis. However, the latex slide agglutination test for specific antigen appears to be a sensitive and specific test. The complement fixation test for cryptococcal polysaccharide has also been found to be a sensitive test, and the indirect fluorescence test is also a valuable aid to diagnosis of cryptococcosis. The enzyme immunoassay for cryptococcal antigen detection is capable of detecting the presence of antigen earlier and at a lower concentration than other tests.

PATHOLOGY. Usually the organism is seen in great abundance in histologic sections of the lesion. *Cryptococcus neoformans* is an oval or rounded, thick-walled spherule measuring 5 to 20 μ in diameter. The organism is surrounded by a polysaccharide capsule that can be demonstrated by special staining such as methylene blue, Alcian blue, or mucicarmine stain. The latter method stains the budding cells and capsules brilliant carmine red.

MYCOLOGY. For direct examination, Margarita Silva-Hutner recommends placing a drop of serum or exudate on a slide and then covering it with a coverslip. If examination shows yeast, one drop of 10 per cent sodium hydroxide is added to one half of the coverslip and one drop of India ink to the other half to demonstrate the capsule.

The organism produces a moist, shiny, white colony on Sabouraud's dextrose agar. With aging the culture may turn to a cream and then a tan color. Subcultures from Sabouraud's may be made onto corn meal agar, and onto urea medium if it is desired to distinguish the yeast from *Candida* and other yeasts. The demonstration of pathogenicity in mice will differentiate the pathogenic from the nonpathogenic cryptococci in humans.

DIFFERENTIAL DIAGNOSIS. In regard to skin lesions, it is helpful to know that the lesions are indolent and nonspecific. Smears and cultures will easily demonstrate the causative organism.

TREATMENT. Amphotericin B is the drug of choice, and produces a 70 to 80 per cent cure rate. Bennett has recommended 5-fluorocytosine orally in a dose sufficient to keep serum levels between 50 and 100 μg/ml for six weeks. Ketoconazole has been successful and is an alternative drug in nonmeningeal cryptococcosis in immunocompetent patients.

Tagami et al reported complete cures in four women by the prolonged daily application of heat; one lesion went away in a month. The lesion was more susceptible than the culture of the organism.

Abdel-Fattah A, et al: Primary cutaneous cryptococcosis in Egypt. Int J Dermatol 1975, 14:606.

Bennett JE: Flucytosine. Ann Intern Med 1977, 86:319.

Carlson KC, et al: Cryptococcal cellulitis in renal transplant patients. JAAD 1987, 17:469.

Dismukes WE, et al: Treatment of systemic mycosis with ketoconazole. Ann Intern Med 1983, 98:13.

Granier F, et al: Localized cutaneous cryptococcosis successfully treated with ketoconazole. JAAD 1987, 16:243.

Hall JC, et al: Cryptococcal cellulitis with multiple sites of involvement. JAAD 1987, 17:329.

Kerkering TM, et al: The evolution of pulmonary cryptococcosis: clinical implications from the study of 41 patients with and without compromising host factors. Ann Intern Med 1981, 94:611.

Lerner EA, et al: Calf ulcer in immunocompromised host. Arch Dermatol 1988, 124:429.

Perfect JR: Cryptococcosis. Infect Dis Clin North Am 1989, 3:77.

Rico MJ, et al: Cutaneous cryptococcosis resembling molluscum contagiosum in a patient with AIDS. Arch Dermatol 1985, 121:901.

Schupbach CW, et al: Cutaneous manifestations of disseminated cryptococcosis. Arch Dermatol 1976, 112:1734.

ACTINOMYCOSIS

CLINICAL FEATURES. Actinomycosis is an anaerobic, gram-positive, bacterial infection, seen most often in the abdominal region, but also seen commonly on the cervicofacial and thoracic areas. Although it is bacterial, its clinical manifestations and long history of grouping with the deep fungi justify its placement here with them. The lesions are characteristic, being local dusky red swellings, firm fluctuating nodules, and sinuses exuding a purulent discharge. In this exudate may be whitish or yellowish granules, commonly known as *sulfur granules*, which are masses of microorganisms. The aggregate is usually surrounded by marked "wooden" induration which produces in the cervicofacial region a "lumpy jaw." The underlying jaw bone may be involved with periostitis and even osteomyelitis. When the gastrointestinal system is involved, the cecum and appendix are the more commonly affected organs, the gallbladder and the stomach less so. Extension into the abdomen and then the abdominal wall may produce draining sinuses on the abdominal skin. Abscesses may occur in the vertebrae, kidneys, ovaries, and urinary bladder.

The third most frequent site of involvement is the thoracic region, as a result of inhalation of the organism and infection of the lungs. Subsequent thoracic wall sinuses may form, and extension into the vertebrae and ribs ensues.

ETIOLOGY. Actinomycosis is caused in man by *Actinomyces israelii* and in animals by *Actinomyces bovis*. Human infections due to *A. bovis*, *A. naeslandii*, and *A. viscosus* have been documented.

DIAGNOSIS. On a microscope slide or Petri dish should be placed sputum; bronchial aspirates; pleural, joint, or pericardial fluid; pus; or biopsy specimens, which should be closely examined for sulfur-yellow granules measuring 1 to 5 mm in di-

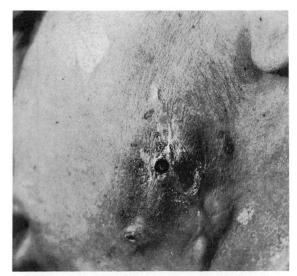

Figure 15–78. Actinomycosis ("lumpy jaw").

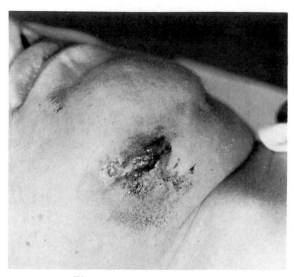

Figure 15–79. Actinomycosis.

ameter. Microscopic examination shows lobulated bodies consisting of delicate branching and intertwining filaments suggestive of clubs. These are best seen at the periphery of the sulfur granule body. They resemble rays; hence the name, *ray fungus (Actinomyces)*. Gram's stain on the crushed sulfur granule will show delicate, branching, intertwined gram-positive filaments.

The crushed granule is used for inoculating cultures containing brain-heart infusion blood agar, incubated under anaerobic conditions at 37° C.

PATHOGENESIS. Actinomycosis is believed to be acquired by endogenous implantation into deep tissues where anaerobic conditions prevail. Puncture wounds, dental extractions, or compound fractures are some of the routes of infection. *A. israelii* has been recovered from the normal mouth, from tonsils, and from carious teeth and is thought to be commonly present. The belief that infection is from

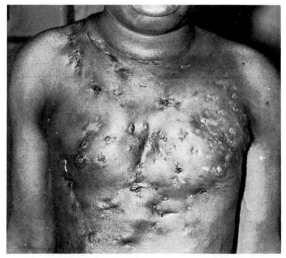

Figure 15–80. Actinomycosis of the skin with a primary lesion in the lung in a 25-year-old man. (Courtesy of Dr. El-Zawahry, U.A.R.)

endogenous sources is further confirmed by the fact that *A. israelii* has never been demonstrated in soil, in plants, or in any other object outside the body. Probably all cases of actinomycosis are closely connected with other contaminating bacterial infections.

PATHOLOGY. The histologic finding is that of an infective granuloma forming a deep nodular process, with granulation tissue, epithelioid cells, plasma and giant cells, and degenerative changes. Large and deep abscesses and sinuses are found, which contain polymorphonuclear leukocytes and miscellaneous debris, along with the ray fungus and its filaments.

DIFFERENTIAL DIAGNOSIS. Actinomycosis must be differentiated from scrofuloderma, which is likely to cause less infiltration and more corded and hypertrophic scars. Superficial examination may suggest sarcoma, carcinoma, blastomycosis, or tertiary syphilis, but these are readily excluded by a close study of the characteristics of the lesions. Positive diagnosis is made by a demonstration of the organism in the discharge or in scrapings from the edge of the lesions.

In addition to *A. israelii*, which is the most frequent cause of human actinomycosis, there are other closely related streptothrices that produce cutaneous and subcutaneous lesions similar to those encountered in this disease. In some cases of actinomycosis the characteristic granules cannot be found in the pus, and the cultures are repeatedly negative. As a result, diagnosis may be impossible, so persistent study and careful evaluation of the clinical manifestations are of utmost importance in the identification of this disease.

TREATMENT. Penicillin in large doses, ten to twenty million units daily for one month, followed by 4 to 6 gm of oral penicillin daily for another two months, may produce successful and lasting results. Arnold has had rapidly successful and lasting results with dapsone (Avlosulfon) 100 mg twice daily, as recommended 40 years ago by Latapi. Other effective medications have been erythromycin, tetracyclines, streptomycin, and sulfonamides. Chloramphenicol should be used only when all other medications have proved ineffective. Surgical incision, drainage, and excision of devitalized tissue is important in the treatment. If complete excision is possible, it is highly desirable—after a trial of dapsone.

PROGNOSIS. Of the three forms described, the cervical type usually responds best to treatment. Before the advent of penicillin the prognosis was poor. When surgical treatment is feasible and dapsone or penicillin therapy can be continued for a long time, a cure may be expected.

Arnold HL Jr, et al: Diasone therapy of actinomycosis of the jaw: case report. JAMA 1948, 138:955.
Katz BJ, et al: Subcutaneous nodules in a man diagnosed as having tuberculosis. Arch Dermatol 1988, 124:121.
Rogers RS, et al: Treatment of actinomycetoma with dapsone. Arch Dermatol 1974, 109:529.
Wallace RJ, et al: Actinomycosis: an update. Int J Dermatol 1977, 16:188.

NOCARDIOSIS

CLINICAL FEATURES. Nocardiosis usually begins as a pulmonary infection from which dissemination occurs. The clinical picture is not distinctive; however, weight loss, anorexia, night sweats, and cough symptoms similar to those of tuberculosis are frequently seen. In about one third of the patients there is central nervous system involvement. Symptoms are usually due to the formation of brain abscesses suggestive of brain tumors. Disseminated lesions may also involve the ribs, femurs, vertebrae, and pelvis. Multiple abscesses may develop in the skin. A generalized vesicular eruption may also occur. The skin lesions may be draining abscesses as an extension of the infective processes in the chest wall and lungs.

Nocardia asteroides, which is responsible for this disseminated form in most cases, occurs in association with debilitating disease such as Hodgkin's disease, periarteritis nodosa, leukemia, AIDS, organ transplants, or systemic lupus erythematosus.

Localized lymphocutaneous lesions in a sporotrichoid pattern occur after trauma to an extremity, usually the hand. A chancriform lesion develops with a proximal chain of nodules. This occurs usually in healthy individuals and is nearly always caused by *N. brasiliensis*.

ETIOLOGY. Nocardiosis is caused by *N. asteroides*, *N. caviae*, or *N. brasiliensis*, which are found in soil and may be inhaled in dust. Implantation from contaminated dust directly into the skin may also occur. A thorn prick by saw briar on which *N. brasiliensis* was residing has caused infections. The organisms have also been recovered from the noses and throats of normal individuals.

DIAGNOSIS. *N. asteroides* can be demonstrated in pus or sputum when stained with Gram's stain. These are gram-positive, partially acid-fast filaments measuring about 1 μ in diameter. Some are branched.

On Sabouraud's dextrose agar, without antibacterial additives, there are creamy or moist white colonies, which later become chalky and orange-colored.

Clinically, many cases resemble tuberculosis; however, the pulmonary form of nocardiosis should be considered, especially when abscesses and draining sinuses appear on the chest wall. When the central nervous system is involved, brain abscesses must be considered as the source of infection. Demonstration of the organism is helpful in all cases.

TREATMENT. Despite the availability of a vast array of modern medications, the mortality remains high. Trimethoprim-sulfamethoxazole (Bactrim, Septra) is the drug of first choice: 4 tablets twice daily. Sulfamethoxypyridazine, sulfamethoxine, and sulfadiazine are also used. Penicillin, chloramphenicol, tetracycline, and potassium iodide have been used also; however, none has been outstandingly effective. Dapsone, 100 mg twice daily, is frequently used for nocardiosis due to *N. brasiliensis*.

Kamalam A, et al: Nocardiosis. Austral J Dermatol 1972, 13:69.

Karassik SL, et al: Disseminated *Nocardia brasiliensis* infection. Arch Dermatol 1976, 112:370.

Nitidandhaprabhas P, et al: Treatment of nocardial mycetoma with trimethoprim and sulfamethoxazole. Arch Dermatol 1975, 111:1345.

Moeller CA, et al: Primary lymphocutaneous *Nocardia brasiliensis* infection. Arch Dermatol 1986, 122:1180.

Schreiner DT, et al: Disseminated *Nocardia brasiliensis* infection following cryptococcal disease. Arch Dermatol 1986, 122:1186.

Tsuboi R, et al: Lymphocutaneous nocardiosis caused by *Nocardia asteroides*. Arch Dermatol 1986, 122:1183.

MYCETOMA

Synonyms: Madura foot, maduromycosis. Mycetoma is a clinical entity but not an etiologic one. It comprises *actinomycetomas* caused by *Streptomyces*, *Nocardia*, or *Actinomyces* species, and *eumycetomas* caused by true fungi: *Madurella*, *Cephalosporium*, or *Pseudallescheria*.

CLINICAL MANIFESTATIONS. Mycetoma generally begins as a subcutaneous swelling, usually occurring on the instep or the toe webs. The tumor is 8 to 10 mm, painless, nontender, firm, and of rubbery texture. The overlying skin may be normal or attached to the underlying tumor. The mature, fully developed lesion is a tumefaction accompanied by the formation of nodules, tubercles, and draining sinuses, usually on the foot or ankle. The draining sinuses secrete microcolonies or grains of the causative organism. Not only the skin and subcutaneous tissues but also the underlying fascia and bone are usually involved. There is severe swelling, but pain may not be present. The lesion spreads by local

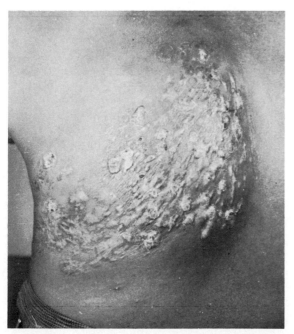

Figure 15–81. Nocardiosis cutis involving the left scapular area (Nocardia brasiliensis). (Courtesy of Dr. J. Convit, Venezuela.)

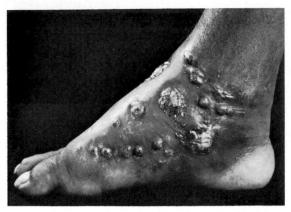

Figure 15–82. Mycetoma in typical location, caused by Nocardia brasiliensis. *(Courtesy of Dr. F. Latapi, Mexico.)*

extension, which may go on for decades before it interferes with local function.

Other parts of the body such as the hands, arms, chest, and buttocks may also be involved. Extensive osteomyelitis may be present. The progression of the disease is slow. As the foot enlarges, the leg atrophies from disuse. After decades the disease, if untreated, terminates in death due to sepsis and exhaustion.

ETIOLOGY. Palestine and Rogers have reviewed the causes of mycetoma in an article to which reference should be made. Etiologically, mycetoma is divided into eumycetoma, produced by true fungi, and actinomycetoma, produced by actinomycetes. Examples of eumycetomas are those caused by *Pseudallescheria boydii, Acremonium (Cephalosporium) falciforme, Acremonium recifei, Leptosphaeria senegalensis, Leptosphaeria tompkinsii, Madurella grisea, Madurella mycetomatis, Exophiala (Phialophora) jeanselmei* and *Pyenochaeta romeroi.* Examples of actinomycetomas are those caused by *Nocardia asteroides, Nocardia brasiliensis, Nocardia caviae, Actinomadura madurae (Nocardia madurae), Acremonium pelletieri (Streptomyces pelletieri, Nocardia pelletieri),* and *Streptomyces somaliensis. Actinomyces israelii,* an anaerobic species of Actinomycetales, is placed by some in the actinomycetoma group. Eubacteria, including staphylococcus and streptococcus, and various dermatophytes have also caused mycetoma. Grains, and bone involvement, are sufficient to justify the diagnosis of mycetoma.

INCIDENCE. Mycetoma occurs everywhere. In the Western Hemisphere the incidence is highest in Mexico, followed by Venezuela and Argentina. In Africa it is found most frequently in Senegal, Sudan, and Somalia.

PATHOGENESIS. Mycetoma is probably acquired from the soil by walking barefooted and sustaining some form of injury either by pricking or abrasion.

MYCOLOGY. No attempt is made to describe the various culture characteristics of the causative organisms. For true fungi (eumycetoma), cultures are made from the grains on Sabouraud's dextrose agar containing 0.5 per cent yeast extract and suitable antibiotics. Cultures should be incubated at 37° C and room temperature. For actinomycetes grains, culture

should be made in brain-heart infusion agar, incubated aerobically and anaerobically at 37° C, and on Sabouraud's dextrose agar with 0.5 per cent yeast extract incubated aerobically at 37° C and room temperature. The specimen for culture should be taken from a deep site, preferably from the base of a biopsy.

DIAGNOSIS. Mycetoma may be diagnosed by keeping in mind a triad of signs, namely: tumefaction, sinuses, and granules. Pus gathered from a deep sinus will show the granules when examined with the microscope. The slide containing the specimen should have a drop of 10 per cent sodium hydroxide added and a coverslip placed on top; the granule with the hyphae will be colored black, white, or red.

Grains may be light-colored (white, pearly, cream, sulfur), red or black, or dark-colored. Light-colored grains are caused by *Actinomyces israelii, Nocardia* sp., *Streptomyces somaliensis, Pseudallescheria boydii, Cephalosporium* sp., and *Neotestudina rosatii.* Red grains are produced only by *Streptomyces pelletierii.* Black or dark grains are produced by *Curvularia geniculata, Helminthosporium spiciferum, Leptosphaeria senegalensis, Madurella grisea* and *mycetomi, Exophiala (Phialophora) jeanselmii,* and *Pyrenochaeta romerai.*

Special stains for demonstration of fungi, such as PAS and Gomori's methenamine silver, will clearly show hyphae and other fungal structures within the grain. Hyphae 2–5 microns in thickness suggest true fungus mycetoma. Gram stain of an actinomycotic grain shows gram-positive thin filaments, 1–2 microns thick, embedded in a gram-negative amorphous matrix. Club formation in the periphery of a grain may be seen but is of limited value in the identification of the organism.

X-rays will show the bone involvement, and mycetoma can be diagnosed readily by expert radiologists.

TREATMENT. Patients in the early stage of mycetoma are successfully treated by thorough removal of the affected area by cautery. In the more advanced stages, especially of the eumycetomas, amputation is frequently necessary.

In *A. israelii* infection, dapsone (Avlosulfon) or penicillin in large doses by injection or phenoxymethyl potassium penicillin by mouth is curative. *Nocardia asteroides* should be treated with sulfonamides such as sulfadiazine in 3 to 8 gm daily doses. *Nocardia brasiliensis* responds favorably to prolonged treatment with dapsone as reported by Rogers et al, or sulfisoxazole (Gantrisin). Starting with 50 mg, the daily dose is increased to 200 mg and given well past the cure state. Rifampicin (Rifadin, Rimactane), 600 mg daily, is also effective in the actinomycetomas. Welsh et al reported a series of patients with actinomycotic mycetoma, in most caused by *N. brasiliensis,* who responded to amikacin, either alone or in combination with trimethoprim-sulfamethoxazole. Cases caused by the true fungi generally have not responded to systemic antifungal agents. However, in a series reported by Mahgoub et al, several responses were documented to ketoconazole, 400 mg a day, for extended periods (3 to 36 months), and one of us (WDJ) has observed a case with similar benefits. Other newer antifungals may also be effective and should be tried—for the only alternative is amputation, unfortunately a frequent outcome in the past.

Barneston RS, et al: Mycetoma. Br J Dermatol 1978, 99:227.
Mahgoub ES, et al: Ketoconazole in the treatment of eumycetoma due to *Madurella mycetomii* Trans R Soc Trop Med Hygiene 1984, 78:376.
McGinnis MR, et al: Mycetoma. Infect Dis Clin North Am 1988, 2:939.
Palestine RF, et al: Diagnosis and treatment of mycetoma. JAAD 1982, 6:107.
Rogers RS III, et al: Treatment of actinomycetoma with dapsone. Arch Dermatol 1974, 109:529.
Treatment of mycetoma (editorial). Lancet 1977, 2:23.
Welsh O, et al: Amikacin alone or in combination with trimethoprim-sulfamethoxazole in the treatment of actinomycotic mycetoma. JAAD 1987, 17:443.

RHINOSPORIDIOSIS

CLINICAL FEATURES. Rhinosporidiosis is a polypoid disease involving the nasal mucosa chiefly. The lesions begin as small papillomas and develop into pedunculated tumors with fissured and warty surfaces, on which there is a myxomatous material containing grayish white flecks or spots, which are large sporangia. The lesions are friable and may resemble a cauliflower. Bleeding occurs easily. Infection of the lacrimal sac, uvula, ears, vulva, vagina, or penis may occur. Conjunctival lesions begin as small pinkish papillary nodules. Later they become dark and lobulated. Penile lesions resemble venereal warts and may become cauliflowerlike vegetative growths. Rectal and vaginal lesions may have a similar appearance or may resemble condylomata or polyps. Widespread dissemination to all the viscera may occur.

ETIOLOGY. *Rhinosporidium seeberi* is the causative organism. In infected tissue the organisms are usually numerous and occupy much of the tissue. They appear as spores 7 to 10 μ in diameter, which are contained within large cystic structures, sporangia, that may be as large as 300 μ in diameter.

EPIDEMIOLOGY. The disease is endemic in Ceylon and India, but it also occurs in Argentina and Brazil. It has been seen in southern United States, England, Italy, Cuba, and Mexico.

Young adults and children are most frequently affected. It is more common in men than in women.

DIAGNOSIS. The demonstration of characteristic large sporangia in the polypoid mass is pathognomonic.

TREATMENT. Destruction of the involved area by electrosurgery is best. Chemotherapy is of no value.

Agrawal S, et al: Generalized rhinosporidiosis with visceral involvement. Arch Dermatol 1959, 80:22.
Levy MG, et al: Cultivation of *Rhinosporidium seeberi* in vitro. Science 1986, 234:474.
Rajam RV, et al: Rhinosporidiosis: fatal case with systemic dissemination. Indian J Surg 1955, 17:1.

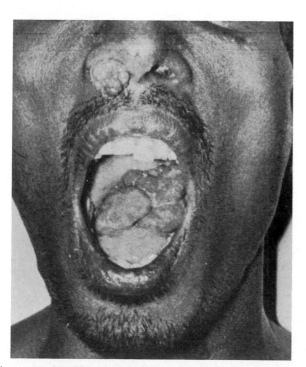

Figure 15–83. Rhinosporidiosis in the nasal mucosa and soft palate. (Courtesy of Dr. Kameswaran, Madurai, India.)

ALTERNARIOSIS

Alternaria is a genus of molds recognized as common plant pathogens but very rare causes of human infection. Most reported cases have occurred in immunocompromised patients. Cutaneous alternariosis usually presents as focal ulcerated papules and plaques on exposed skin of the face, forearms and hands, or knees. The course is chronic.

Mitchell et al have recently reviewed the literature on *Alternaria* infections and reported the first known case of infection by *Alternaria dianthicola*. A noncaseating, granulomatous, nodular lesion of the chest wall, at a site frequently traumatized by wooden stakes in the course of tobacco farming, was the lesion. Fusiform conidia 35 to 85 μ long were considered diagnostic. PAS-positive hyphae were most abundant at the deep border of the nodule. Surgical excision was curative. Iwatsu updated this literature review in 1988 while reporting a case caused by *A. tenuissima*. *A. alternata* is the cause in most cases. DeMoragas et al had success with intralesionally injected miconazole. Intralesional amphotericin B completely resolved the lesions in the patient reported by Iwatsu. Some isolates have been susceptible to ketoconazole.

DeMoragas JM, et al: Cutaneous alternariosis treated with miconazole. Arch Dermatol 1981, 117:292.
Iwatsu T: Cutaneous alternariosis. Arch Dermatol 1988, 124:1822.
Junkins JM, et al: Unusual fungal infection in immunocompromised oncology patient: Cutaneous alternariosis. Arch Dermatol
  1988, 124:1421.
Mitchell AJ, et al: Subcutaneous alternariosis. JAAD 1983, 8:573.

DISEASE DUE TO ALGAE (Protothecosis)

Protothecosis is a verrucous skin disease caused
by the *Prototheca* genus of saprophytic, achloric (nonpigmented) algae. These organisms reproduce asex-
ually via internal septation, producing autospores
identical to the parent cell. This reproductive
method, along with the absence of glucosamine and
muramic acid in the cell wall, separates the genus
from the bacteria and fungi. Five *Prototheca* species
are now recognized: *Pr. filamenta, Pr. moriformis, Pr.
stagnora, Pr. wickerhamii,* and *Pr. zopfi.* Stagnant water
and soil appear to be the source of infection in most
cases.

Skin lesions observed have now included papulonodular lesions, crusted papules with umbilication
and ulceration, and an extensive granulomatous
eruption. Protothecosis has usually occurred in
healthy individuals, but infections have been reported in patients receiving immunosuppressive
therapy, in renal failure, with widespread carcinomatosis, or with diabetes mellitus.

Prototheca species are easily recognized in PAS-
stained tissue specimens when the characteristic
endosporulating cells are visible. The organisms are
grown on most routine mycologic media; however,
cycloheximide, used to inhibit growth of saprophytic
fungi, will also suppress growth of *Prototheca* species.
Colonies on Sabouraud agar are smooth, creamy,
and yeastlike. The use of fluorescent antibody re-
agents makes possible the rapid and reliable identification of *Prototheca* species in culture and tissue.

Attempts to medically influence the course of the
cutaneous infection have, in general, proved unsuccessful. McAnally and Perry reported that a course
of amphotericin B combined with tetracycline, 250
mg four times a day, cured their patient. The drugs
are effective in vitro and appear to act in synergism.

Mars PW, et al: Protothecosis. Br J Dermatol 1971, 85 (Suppl 7):76.
Mayball CG, et al: Cutaneous protothecosis. Arch Dermatol 1976,
  112:1749.
McAnally T, et al: Cutaneous protothecosis presenting as recurrent
  chromomycosis. Arch Dermatol 1985, 121:1066.
Sudman MS: Protothecosis: a critical review. Am J Clin Pathol
  1974, 61:10.
Tindall JP, et al: Infections caused by achloric algae (protothecosis).
  Arch Dermatol 1971, 104:490.
Wolfe ID, et al: Cutaneous protothecosis in a patient receiving
  immunosuppressive therapy. Arch Dermatol 1976, 112:829.

16

Mycobacterial Diseases

TUBERCULOSIS

Tuberculosis of the skin may be divided into the localized forms and the exanthematous or hematogenous forms. The localized progressive forms are the *primary inoculation complex; lupus vulgaris; tuberculosis verrucosa cutis; scrofuloderma;* and *tuberculosis cutis orificialis.* The widespread, generalized, or exanthematous forms are *tuberculosis miliaris; tuberculous abscess; papulonecrotic tuberculid; lichen scrofulosorum (tuberculosis lichenoides).* Some cases of *erythema induratum (Bazin's disease)* meet the criteria for a tuberculid.

The cell-mediated immune response of the individual determines the form of development of the tuberculosis infection. Anergic nonresponses are of particular importance in certain types of cutaneous tuberculosis.

While cutaneous tuberculosis has become quite uncommon in North America, the advent of the acquired immunodeficiency syndrome (AIDS) and the growing problem of the homeless have reawakened awareness of this disease. Tuberculosis of the skin is a frequent presenting infection in certain HIV-infected populations such as Haitians in Florida and the inner-city minority of drug abusers. Pitchenik et al stress the high incidence of extrapulmonary tuberculosis. They also document that the response to therapy may be good, but treatment must be prolonged to prevent relapse. Some investigators feel it is the most treatable and curable pathogen of all those causing opportunistic infections in AIDS.

The separation and classification of various forms of cutaneous tuberculosis according to their reactivity to tuberculin is confusing and unreliable. Probably the most practical classification, despite its age, is that of Lewandowsky, which is followed approximately in this chapter.

Tuberculin Testing

The tuberculin test indicates sensitization to mycobacteria or their products. The test is the basic tool used to identify infected persons.

Cell-mediated immunity to mycobacteria can be detected by a variety of methods that introduce tuberculoprotein into the tissues of the test subject. The intradermal or Mantoux test is the standard and offers the highest degree of consistency and reliability. The standard dose for tuberculin surveys and for diagnostic purposes is 0.0001 mg (5 TU) of polysorbate-80–stabilized purified protein derivative (PPD). The test is read 48 hours after intradermal injection. Induration measuring 10 mm or more in diameter is considered positive; 5 to 9 mm induration, doubtful; and 0 to 4 mm induration, negative. This means that 10 mm or more induration most likely represents specific sensitivity to *M. tuberculosis;* as zones of induration become progressively smaller, the likelihood that they are due to *M. tuberculosis* infection decreases.

Reactivity to the tuberculin protein is impaired in certain medical conditions in which cellular immunity is impaired. Lymphoproliferative disorders, sarcoidosis, steroid therapy, miliary tuberculosis, overwhelming disease, immunosuppressive drugs, and numerous febrile illnesses are capable of diminishing tuberculin sensitivity. It is now well appreciated that a negative or doubtful reaction to PPD cannot exclude tuberculosis infection, particularly in the face of suggestive symptoms and signs.

Histopathology

The microscopic pathology of cutaneous tuberculosis differs from that in other tissues, in that the tubercles only occasionally undergo caseation, fibrosis, and calcification. Caseation necrosis is prominent in the primary inoculation complex and scrofuloderma, and moderate in tuberculosis verrucosa cutis. Erythema induratum undergoes caseation necrosis in 50 per cent of the cases. The cutaneous tubercle may be composed chiefly of epithelioid cells, although giant cells and lymphocytes are usually present. In other cases the tubercles are composed principally of lymphocytes, and in still others atypical nonspecific granulation tissue may be found in conjunction with tubercles. The epithelioid cell, so called from its resemblance to a keratinocyte, is an irregularly shaped, broad cell with a homogeneous cytoplasm and a large oval nucleus containing chromatin granules. The giant cells are usually of the Langhans type, with many nuclei arranged in an arc or in a ring near the periphery of the cytoplasm. The epithelioid and giant cells are usually surrounded by lymphocytes, and at the edge of the lymphocytic infiltration there may be found plasma cells, which have a tendency to be arranged along the blood vessels, the tubercle itself usually being avascular. The tubercles are frequently multiple and conglomerate.

BCG Vaccination

Bacillus Calmette Guérin (BCG) is a living attenuated bovine tubercle bacillus, used in many parts of the world to enhance immunity to tuberculosis. Vaccination is given only to tuberculin-negative persons. Once the patient has been vaccinated the tuberculin test becomes positive, and remains so for a variable length of time.

Dermatologic complications are but rarely seen. Dostrovsky and Sagher reported skin reactions in 27 patients among more than 200,000 vaccinated with BCG. Among reactions attributed to the vaccination were excessive lymphadenitis and scrofulosorumlike, lupus vulgarislike, and lichen nitidus lesions. Nonspecific reactions were noted in 33 patients. These included toxicoderma hemorrhagica, urticaria, erythema nodosum, erythema multiforme, and granuloma annulare. A progressive infectious granuloma may rarely occur; such a case was reported by Allan Izumi.

Factors responsible for these reactions are the strength and amount of the vaccine, the depth of the injection, and the patient's immune responsiveness.

LOCALIZED FORMS OF SKIN TUBERCULOSIS

PRIMARY INOCULATION TUBERCULOSIS (Primary Tuberculous Complex: Tuberculous Chancre)

Primary inoculation tuberculosis consists of the cutaneous reaction at the site of inoculation of tubercle bacilli into a tuberculosis-free individual, plus the involvement of regional lymph nodes. It occurs chiefly in children, although occasionally in adults with a prior negative tuberculin test, and affects the face or extremities. Usually the inoculation occurs in previously traumatized skin or mucosa. The site of entry may be a minor scratch, sore, hangnail, or puncture wound. Horney et al recently reported the development of this disease after tattooing. The earliest lesion is a brownish red papule which develops into an indurated nodule or plaque that may ulcerate. This is the *tuberculous chancre*. There is prominent regional lymphadenopathy. Primary tuberculous complex occurs on the mucous membranes in about one third of the patients.

It also may occur after BCG vaccination in tuberculin-negative children.

Healing takes place in several weeks; only the regional lymph node enlargement may be an indication of the previous infection.

Histologically there is a marked inflammatory response during the first two weeks, with many polymorphonuclear leukocytes and tubercle bacilli. During the next two weeks the picture changes. Lymphocytes and epithelioid cells appear and replace

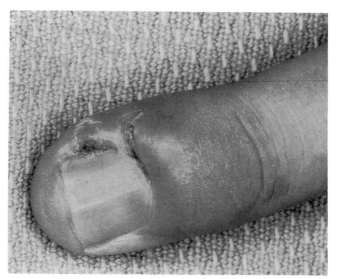

Figure 16–1. Primary inoculation tuberculosis in a 30-year-old pathologist.

the polymorphonuclear leukocytes. Distinct tubercles develop not only at the site of inoculation but also in the regional lymph nodes within three or four weeks after inoculation. Simultaneously with the appearance of epithelioid cells the number of tubercle bacilli decreases rapidly.

The differential diagnosis of primary inoculation tuberculosis extends over the spectrum of chancriform conditions of deep fungal or bacterial origin such as sporotrichosis, blastomycosis, histoplasmosis, coccidioidomycosis, nocardiosis, syphilis, leishmaniasis, yaws, tularemia, and atypical mycobacterial disease. Pyogenic granuloma and cat-scratch disease must also be considered. These conditions can be readily excluded by serologic studies, cultures, skin biopsies, tissue smears, and historical and physical findings.

The primary tuberculous lesion usually heals after a few months but the enlarged glands may persist and break down. These broken-down glands may require excision.

LUPUS VULGARIS

CLINICAL FEATURES. Lupus vulgaris is the most common type of cutaneous tuberculosis. It is so rare today in the U.S. that "lupus," unqualified, means lupus erythematosus (LE), not lupus vulgaris as it did 40 years ago. It is characterized by groups of reddish brown nodules which, when blanched by diascopic* pressure, have a pale brownish yellow or "apple-jelly" color. They tend to heal slowly in one area and progress in another. The nodules are minute, translucent, and embedded deeply and dif-

*A diascope is a glass plate or slide pressed against the skin to detect color changes other than those of congestion.

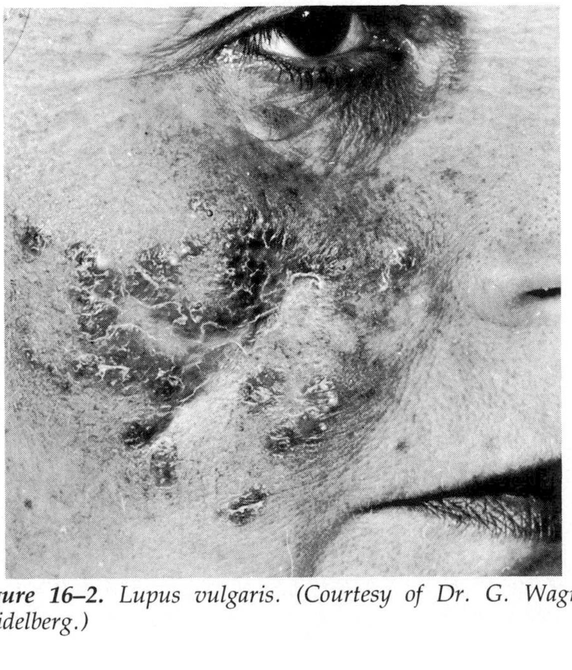

fusely in the infiltrated dermis, forming plaques by coalescence and by the development of new lupus nodules. The patches are slightly elevated and often are covered by adherent scales. The disease is destructive, frequently causes ulceration, and on involution leaves deforming scars as it slowly spreads peripherally over the years. Lupus vulgaris is most prevalent on exposed parts, especially the face.

At times in any type there may be edema, hypertrophy, or an associated lymphangitis or lymphadenitis. Patches on the face tend to involve the nose and the lobes of the ears, and after involution of the lesions these structures are shrunken and scarred, as if nibbled away. The tip of the nose may be sharply pointed and beaklike, or the whole nose may be destroyed and only the orifices and the posterior parts of the septum and turbinates visible. The upper lip, a site of predilection, may become diffusely swollen and thickened, with fissures, adherent thin crusts, ulcers, or granulations on the mucous aspect, and a tendency to bleed. On the trunk and extremities patches of the disease may be serpiginous or form gyrate patterns, and on the hands and feet and about the genitals or buttocks may cause mutilation due to destruction, scar formation, warty thickenings, and elephantiasic enlargement.

When the mucous membranes are attacked, the patches rapidly become papillomatous or ulcerative owing to the moisture and contamination with other microorganisms, and appear as circumscribed, grayish, macerated, or granulating patches, or on the tongue as irregular, deep, painful fissures, sometimes associated with great enlargement of the organ so that nutrition cannot be easily maintained.

The course of lupus vulgaris is so slow that a patch of the disease may remain limited to a small area for several decades, all the while showing signs of activity. A lupus patch may start in childhood and persist

Figure 16–2. Lupus vulgaris. (*Courtesy of Dr. G. Wagner, Heidelberg.*)

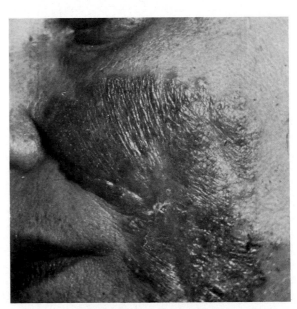

Figure 16–3. Lupus vulgaris.

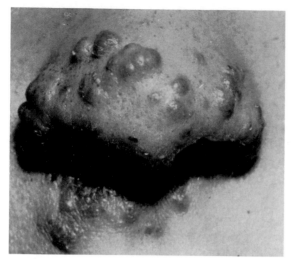

Figure 16–4. Lupus vulgaris with large apple jelly nodules on the nose and lip.

throughout a long lifetime. During this period it may slowly spread, or new patches may develop in other regions. In some cases considerable scarring may occur in the central part of the patch. In other cases, superficial or deep ulceration supervenes. Ulcers may be serpiginous, or arciform. In some instances the granulations become papillomatous, vegetative, fungoid, or thickly crusted so that they have a rupioid appearance.

In the severe cases on the face, where atrophy predominates, there is severe scarring that leads to the development of the "parrot-beak" nose. Ectropion and atrophied lips may eventuate in a werewolf appearance. This could be the reason for the term "lupus," which means wolf; or perhaps the name

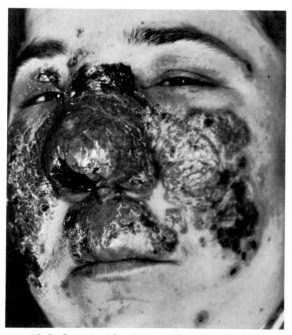

Figure 16–5. Lupus vulgaris, tumid type. (Courtesy of Dr. Simon, Szeged.)

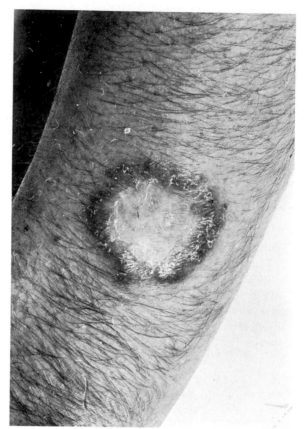

Figure 16–6. Lupus tumidus on the forearm. (Courtesy of Dr. G. Wagner, Heidelberg.)

alludes to the appearance of the face, as if it had been chewed by a wolf.

HISTOPATHOLOGY. In lupus vulgaris, acid-fast bacilli are almost never found in microscopic sections. Pinkus and Mehregan characterize the findings as "epithelioid cell nodules embedded in shells of lymphocytes." Langhans giant cells are present, whereas plasma cells, eosinophils, and polymorphonuclear leukocytes are absent or rare. Caseation necrosis is only slight in the center of the nodule. The epidermis is secondarily affected, sometimes flattened and at other times hypertrophic.

DIFFERENTIAL DIAGNOSIS. Typical "apple-jelly" (pale yellowish tan) nodules with scarring are distinctive. Sometimes colloid degeneration of the skin, acne vulgaris, sarcoidosis, or rosacea may simulate lupus vulgaris. Papular syphilids are monomorphic and bilateral, and spirochetes may be demonstrated in the serum from the lesions. Differentiation from the unilateral serpiginous forms of tertiary syphilid may be more difficult. The serpiginous lesions spread rapidly, with firm nodules rather than the soft apple-jelly nodules. Tuberculosis may recur in the scar; syphilis never does, because its scars are caused by an infarct. The underlying cartilage is not disturbed in the tertiary lesions. Lupus erythematosus may be more difficult to rule out, and only the presence of apple-jelly nodules—and biopsy—may eliminate LE.

TREATMENT. Of foremost importance is the

treatment of early lesions by surgical excision. Whenever feasible, this type of treatment yields most satisfactory results if it is thorough and complete. Before determining the extent of the surgical excision in any particular case, it is advisable to do a tuberculin test and to watch the local reaction in and about the lesion for an indication of the extent of the disease process. In advanced disease, the treatment of choice is systemic, and the local lesions are left alone except for ultraviolet therapy.

Isoniazid in combination with rifampin (Rifadin, Rimactane) is the initial treatment of choice. Isoniazid dosage is 300 mg a day for adults, and 10 mg/kg for children, or 15 mg/kg twice weekly if this seems preferable. The risk of hepatitis is less than 1 per 1000 up to age 20; 3 per 1000 up to age 35; 12 per 1000 between 35 and 50; 23 per 1000 for those age 50 to 64; and 8 per 1000 above that. Alcohol abusers are of course more susceptible. Serum aminotransferase levels should be checked occasionally in patients over 35. Only in drinkers, or others at increased risk, is there danger of pellagra from increased pyridoxine excretion, and 10 to 60 mg of pyridoxine may be given daily to prevent this. It may also prevent peripheral or optic neuritis, a rare side effect.

Rifampin, although very expensive, is standard concurrent treatment for pulmonary tuberculosis and worthwhile giving in cutaneous tuberculosis as well. It turns body fluids orange-pink, and patients should be warned of this. It is potentially hepatotoxic. It induces increased liver enzyme activity and thereby decreases blood levels of oral contraceptives, corticosteroids, warfarin, oral hypoglycemics, methadone, and digitalis derivatives.

Though nine months' treatment is standard for most cases of pulmonary tuberculosis, probably clinical recovery plus a reasonable margin is enough for lupus vulgaris.

Streptomycin, though potentially effective, is better avoided because of the risk of ototoxicity. Ethambutol, though it has essentially replaced paraaminosalicylic acid as a second or third drug in multiple drug regimens, is rarely used, because of its relatively weak antituberculous effect, and ocular toxicity. However, it may be advisable to include it in the initial regimen even if isoniazid resistance is only suspected. If isoniazid resistance is known, then the treatment should be rifampin and ethambutol, perhaps supplemented by pyrizinamide, for a minimum of 12 months. Details of treatment recommendations were updated in 1986 by the American Thoracic Society and have been well reviewed by Corsello, Jacobs et al, Bass et al, and Perez-Stable et al.

TUBERCULOSIS VERRUCOSA CUTIS

CLINICAL FEATURES. Tuberculosis verrucosa cutis is characterized by warty vegetations, which sometimes extend to form large plaques.

The *anatomist's wart*, which results from infection

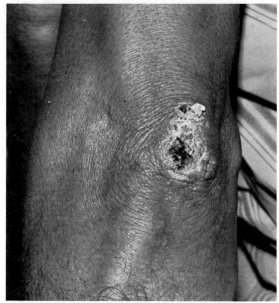

Figure 16–7. Originally called tuberculosis verrucosa cutis, this lesion on the left elbow of a 40-year-old Puerto Rican man was finally proved to be a case of atypical mycobacteriosis caused by M. marinum. (Courtesy of Dr. V. Torres-Rodriguez.)

arising from autopsies (*prosector's wart*) or the handling of tuberculous meat, is the prototype of tuberculosis verrucosa cutis. Heilman and Muschenheim reported a case infected by mouth-to-mouth resuscitation. Clinically this is usually a single hyperkeratotic, dull red lesion that persists harmlessly and indefinitely with very little growth; but at times it may be accompanied by tuberculous lymphangitis or adenitis, or by other serious developments such as erysipelas, generalized tuberculosis, or gangrene.

Frequent locations for tuberculosis verrucosa cutis are on the dorsa of the fingers and the hands, the ankles, and the buttocks. The lesions occur as dis-

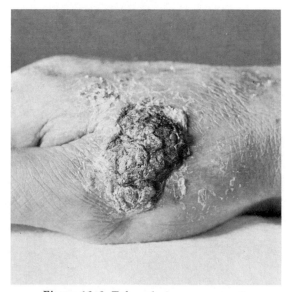

Figure 16–8. Tuberculosis verrucosa cutis.

coid, circumscribed, warty plaques of nummular or palm size, or even much larger; sometimes they are configurate. They may be single or multiple and may resemble blastomycosis, although they are generally drier and less inflammatory.

The growths are persistent, although usually superficial and limited in their extent. They may be separated by exudative or suppurative areas, but they seldom ulcerate and usually heal spontaneously. The disease is most common on the hands and other parts of the extremities, usually in adults, and is the reaction of a previously infected, highly resistant individual to external reinfection.

HISTOLOGY. In addition to the usual tubercle, there may be caseation, a considerable overgrowth of granulation tissue, and the formation of new blood vessels with predominating acanthosis and hyper-keratosis. Tubercle bacilli are present. Secondary infection may lead to miliary abscesses, ulcerations, or verrucous thickenings.

DIFFERENTIAL DIAGNOSIS. Tuberculosis verrucosa cutis is differentiated only by culture from atypical mycobacterial (swimming pool, or balnei) granuloma, due to *M. marinum*. It must also be distinguished at times from North American blastomycosis, tinea profunda (Majocchi's granuloma, trichophytic granuloma), chromoblastomycosis, verrucous epidermal nevus, hypertrophic lichen planus, iododerma, bromoderma, and even verruca vulgaris. This type of mycobacteriosis is but rarely seen now.

TREATMENT. Treatment for the prosector's wart is prompt surgical excision. If the excision is not prompt, treatment by isoniazid and rifampin is preferable to attempted removal.

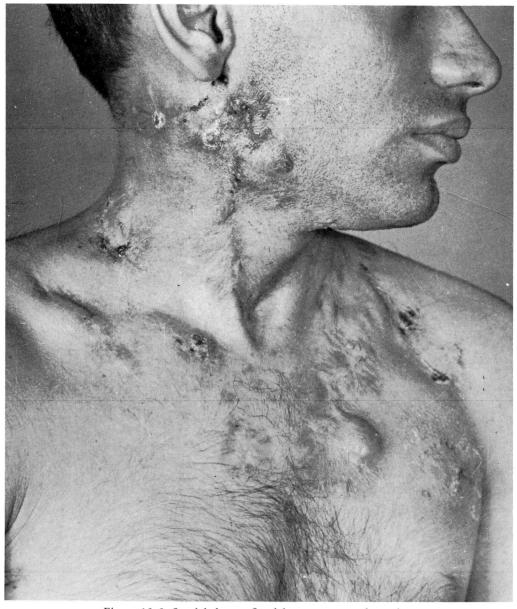

Figure 16–9. Scrofuloderma. Scrofulous gummas and scarring.

SCROFULODERMA
(Tuberculosis Cutis Colliquativa)

Scrofuloderma is a comprehensive term applied to tuberculous involvement of the skin by direct extension, usually secondary to underlying tuberculous lymphadenitis. It occurs most frequently over the cervical lymph nodes, but may occur over bone or about joints in children and young adults. Clinically the lesions are reddish granulations, edematous, exudative, and crusted, with small sinuses or ulcerations of various sizes. Undermined edges are usually present.

The process usually begins with a deep purplish induration of the skin overlying diseased lymphatic glands, which for months have been matted together and doughy. The glands tend to break down and the resulting purulent and caseous exudate stretches the superimposed skin and forms fistulas in it. Chronic discharging sinuses and oval or linear ulcerations, irregular pale granulations, bulky crusts, hypertrophic scars, and cicatricial bands result, and these combined conditions compose scrofuloderma.

Tuberculosis fistulosa subcutanea has been described by Simon. It is characterized by a chronic anal fistula in adults between 30 and 50 years of age. Involvement of the intestinal tract and especially the rectum is present in most of these cases. Anal strictures and involvement of the scrotum are frequently observed. The lesions consist of one or more fistulas extending into the deep tissue, infiltrated nodules, and swelling of the affected area. This entity is a form of tuberculosis colliquativa. Treatment with isoniazid has produced excellent results in this disease.

Histologically, in scrofuloderma the tuberculous process begins in the deep dermis with caseation necrosis and formation of a cavity filled with liquefied

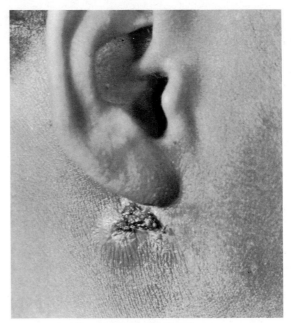

Figure 16–11. Scrofuloderma.

debris, the walls of which are formed by tuberculous granulation tissue. Ultimately there may be formation of sinuses that lead to the surface. Ulcers may develop with papillomatous proliferations. In the secondary type this process is generally associated with sinus formation, which has extended from tuberculous lymph nodes or tuberculous cystitis or osteomyelitis. Tubercle bacilli are present.

Scrofuloderma is to be differentiated from syphilitic gummas, which when ulcerated, form deep craters; sporotrichosis, which yields the typical fungus when cultured; and blastomycosis, as demonstrated by the presence of *Blastomyces dermatitidis*. Lymphogranuloma venereum is ruled out by a negative LGV complement fixation test. Lymphogranuloma venereum occurs most frequently in the inguinal and perineal areas. Scrofuloderma should also be differentiated from actinomycosis and tularemia by culture.

Treatment is with various antituberculous drugs described under lupus vulgaris.

TUBERCULOSIS CUTIS ORIFICIALIS

This form of localized cutaneous involvement in tuberculosis occurs at the mucocutaneous borders of the nose, mouth, anus, urinary meatus, and vagina, also on the mucous membrane of the mouth or tongue and occasionally on the skin itself. It is found usually in young adults with severe visceral tuberculosis, particularly of the larynx, palate, lungs, intestines, and genitourinary tract, and with failing resistance to the disease. It ulcerates from the beginning and extends rapidly, with no tendency to spontaneous healing. The ulcers are usually oval, shallow, and covered by crusts.

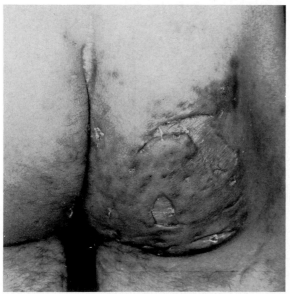

Figure 16–10. Tuberculosis colliquativa. (Courtesy of Dr. H. Shatin.)

Histologically, tubercles are usually not formed, but a severe inflammatory reaction is present.

In the differential diagnosis the general signs of advanced systemic illness are helpful in identifying this disease. Chancroid, lymphogranuloma vener-eum, syphilitic gummas, and ulcerated carcinoma are to be considered.

Treatment is the treatment of the underlying caus-ative tuberculosis.

GENERALIZED FORMS OF SKIN TUBERCULOSIS

TUBERCULOSIS MILIARIS DISSEMINATA

Tuberculosis miliaris disseminata is a rare form of tuberculosis that appears as an acute generalized eruption of indolent, brownish red, acuminate pap-ules which become necrotic and may form numerous minute ulcers. These ulcers are small and circular, with a dull red border and a pallid granulating base covered by a seropurulent exudate. Miliary tubercles may be present in the base or at the edge of the ulcer. Tubercle bacilli have been demonstrated in these lesions.

Exanthematous miliary tuberculosis usually occurs in infants following intercurrent illness which re-duces immunologic responsiveness, with subsequent embolism through the blood. It may also occur at the outset of an attack of general miliary tuberculosis, and, with a few exceptions, is fatal. Generally the patients have other unmistakable signs of severe miliary tuberculosis. Schumer and his associates have reviewed the literature on this now rare disease.

Metastatic Tuberculous Abscess

The hematogenous dissemination of mycobacteria from a primary focus may result in firm, nontender erythematous nodules which soften, ulcerate, and form sinuses. These are usually seen in patients who have impaired immune responsiveness, as in AIDS.

PAPULONECROTIC TUBERCULID

Darier designated as tuberculids a number of ap-parently dissimilar skin lesions supposedly caused by bacillary embolisms from lesions in the viscera. Cutaneous reactions may vary greatly according to the degree and kind of immune responsiveness pos-sessed by the individual and according to the atten-uation and amount of the bacterial material. The lesions are transient, bilateral, and symmetrical, and essentially are small indolent granulomas.

CLINICAL FEATURES. The eruption of papulo-necrotic tuberculid recurs in successive crops, usually on the extensor surfaces of the extremities, especially on the tips of the elbows, knees, and dorsal surfaces of the hands and feet, and also on the face and trunk, in children and young adults who have chronic tuberculosis elsewhere. The typical lesions vary in size from a pinhead to a pea, and are firm, isolated, follicular, brownish or bluish red papules or nodules, which undergo central necrosis and heal spontaneously with pitted scarring. Grouping and symmetry are clinically suggestive features.

There is a tendency for the lesions to run their course in four weeks to a few months and to be followed by fresh outbreaks, the disease lasting for years. Healing is by the formation of white punched-out scars. Tuberculids may appear in association with

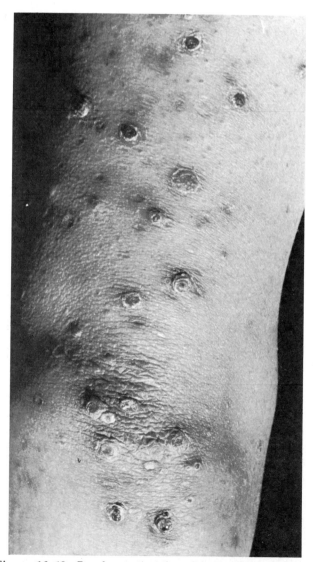

Figure 16–12. Papulonecrotic tuberculid on elbow and upper arm. Note new, active crusted lesions and scarring of old healed lesions. (Courtesy of Dr. A. Kaminsky, Argentina.)

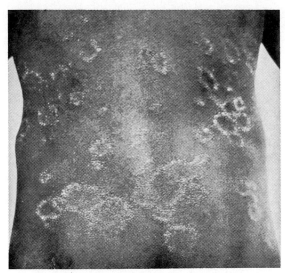

Figure 16–13. Lichen scrofulosorum.

other cutaneous manifestations of tuberculosis, particularly erythema induratum, lichen scrofulosorum, or scrofuloderma. Associated clinical phenomena have included tuberculous arteritis with gangrene and the development of lupus vulgaris from papulonecrotic tuberculids.

ETIOLOGY. Morrison and Fourie suggested that tuberculids begin as an Arthus reaction, which is followed by a delayed hypersensitivity response, arising from the intravascular release of *M. tuberculosis*. The latter response will prevent local proliferation of *M. tuberculosis* in most cases, but in rare cases local multiplication of the organisms may lead to the development of lupus vulgaris. At times, *M. tuberculosis* can be cultured from such lesions. These authors also demonstrated immune complexes in five cases of papulonecrotic tuberculid.

HISTOPATHOLOGY. Papulonecrotic tuberculid is a tuberculous manifestation with or without the formation of typical tubercles situated in the more superficial portions of the dermis and showing definite evidence of liquefaction necrosis, endarteritis, endophlebitis, and thrombosis of the vessels.

DIFFERENTIAL DIAGNOSIS. Papulonecrotic tuberculid is differentiated from acne varioliformis and papular syphilis by the absence of pustules and the stigmata of syphilis, respectively. Acne vulgaris must also be considered, but usually this is easily distinguished from the papulonecrotic tuberculid. Pityriasis lichenoides et varioliformis acuta should also be considered.

TREATMENT. Antituberculous therapy, as discussed under lupus vulgaris, is recommended.

LICHEN SCROFULOSORUM

Also known as tuberculosis cutis lichenoides, this eruption consists of groups of indolent, minute, keratotic, exquisitely discrete intrapapillary papules, scattered over the trunk or extremities. The lesions are pinhead-sized or smaller, being walled in by the rete ridges, and they are the color of normal skin or reddish brown. They are firm and flat-topped, or surmounted by a tiny pustule or thin scale. The lesions are arranged in nummular groups, usually on the trunk, where they persist unchanged for long periods and occasion no symptoms. There is no pruritus nor pain. They may slowly undergo spontaneous involution, followed at times by recurrences.

As a rule, they appear in children who have tuberculosis of the bones or lymph nodes. In lichen scrofulosorum the Mantoux reaction is always positive, by definition. Onset of the disease after injections of tuberculin is known to occur, especially in persons who are highly reactive to tuberculin.

The histopathology of lichen scrofulosorum shows definite small tubercles, situated just beneath the epidermis, usually surrounding hair follicles and sweat ducts. There is no caseation necrosis. Normally tubercle bacilli are not seen in the pathologic specimens, nor can they be cultured from biopsy material.

The treatment is systemic, with isoniazid.

ERYTHEMA INDURATUM

Erythema induratum (*Bazin's disease, tuberculosis cutis indurativa*) is a chronic benign vasculitis which causes soft recurrent nodules about the subcutaneous vessels of the lower calf. These may progress into deep-seated indurations, ulcers, and scarring. A subset of this clinical syndrome, unrelated to tuberculous infection, is discussed under nodular vasculitis. Erythema induratum connotes a tuberculous focus. Lebel recently reported two cases of this disease.

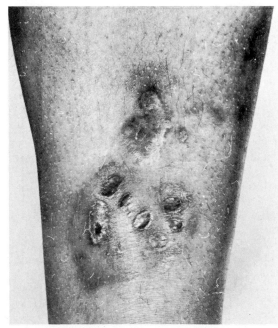

Figure 16–14. Erythema induratum on the shin. (Courtesy of Dr. G. Wagner, Heidelberg.)

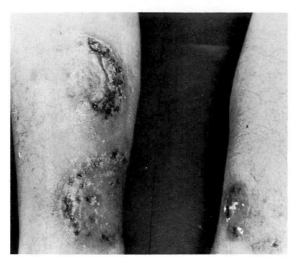

Figure 16–15. Erythema induratum on the shins. (Courtesy of Dr. F. Daniels, Jr.)

CLINICAL FEATURES. The lesions, like papulonecrotic tuberculids but larger, are usually symmetrical and indolent. They occur usually in young women who have tuberculosis and acrocyanosis. The calf is the preferred site. The nodules usually persist for three or four months, then tend to dry up and heal and then recur. In the period of evolution the lesions are slightly tender erythematous indurations that gradually become deep nodules. In the course of months the overlying skin assumes a dusky or bluish color, and on palpation some central softening is noted, which frequently progresses into ulceration.

The ulcers have irregular shapes and are deeply excavated, with steep or undermined edges. At times neighboring lesions coalesce. In any one case there are generally some depressed white scars from previous ulcers, as well as active lesions in all stages of evolution and involution, numbering anywhere from two to three up to a dozen or more. The lower calf is the favorite location on the leg; rarely, the disease may occur on the front of the leg, on the arms, or elsewhere. As the result of recurrences the disease may persist for years.

ETIOLOGY. Morrison and Fourie suggested that the pathogenesis of erythema induratum is similar to that of papulonecrotic tuberculid, but it occurs in larger vessels.

HISTOPATHOLOGY. The early manifestations consist of epithelioid cell tubercles originating in the deep dermis. There is a general thickening of the veins and arteries, which may be occluded by proliferation of the intima and become difficult to identify as a definite structure, appearing as an eosinophilic mass surrounded by lymphocytes. The elastic and collagenous tissues and fat cells in the zone of the infiltration are destroyed. Wucher atrophy (fat replacement atrophy) is in turn followed by fibrosis.

DIFFERENTIAL DIAGNOSIS. Care should be taken to distinguish erythema induratum from erythema nodosum, nodular vasculitis, the gummatous syphilid, and the nodose lesions caused by iodides

and bromides. Erythema nodosum is of relatively short duration and of rapid development and affects chiefly the shins instead of the calves. It produces tender, painful, scarlet nodules that appear simultaneously and do not ulcerate, whereas in erythema induratum the sensory symptoms are insignificant and the color is darker, and the lesions tend to evolve serially or in crops. Gumma is usually unilateral and single, or a small distinct group of lesions. Serologic, microscopic, and therapeutic tests are decisive. The lesions due to iodides and bromides resemble erythema nodosum or cause ulcers with vegetating bases. Nodular vasculitis is clinically and histologically quite similar, but there is no associated tuberculous infection and it does not respond to antituberculous therapy.

TREATMENT. Antituberculous therapy, as described under lupus vulgaris, is curative.

American Thoracic Society, Center for Disease Control: Treatment of tuberculosis infection in adults and children. Am Rev Respir Dis 1986, 134:355.

Bass JB Jr, et al: Drug resistant tuberculosis. Semin Respir Med 1988, 9:470.

Bishburg E, et al: Central nervous system tuberculosis with the acquired immunodeficiency syndrome. Ann Intern Med 1986, 105:210.

Brown FS, et al: Cutaneous tuberculosis. JAAD 1982, 6:101.

Chaisson RE, et al: Tuberculosis in patients with AIDS. Am Res Respir Dis 1987, 136:570.

Corsello BF: New approach to treatment of pulmonary and extrapulmonary tuberculosis. Int J Dermatol 1987, 26:185.

Dinning WJ, et al: Cutaneous and ocular tuberculosis: a review. J R Soc Med 1985, 78:756.

Dostrowsky A, et al: Dermatologic complications of BCG vaccination. Br J Dermatol 1963, 75:181.

Drugs for Tuberculosis, The Medical Letter 1986, 28:6.

Dutt AK, et al: Short-course chemotherapy for extrapulmonary tuberculosis. Ann Intern Med 1986, 104:7.

Feiwel M: Erythema induratum Bazin. Acta Dermatol 1968, 48:242.

Goette DK, et al: Primary inoculation tuberculosis of the skin. Arch Dermatol 1978, 114:567.

Gracey PR: Tuberculosis in the world today. Mayo Clin Proc 1988, 63:1251.

Harahap M: Tuberculosis of the skin. Int J Dermatol 1983, 22:542.

Heilman KM, et al: Primary cutaneous tuberculosis from mouth-to-mouth respiration. N Engl J Med 1965, 273:1035.

Helander I, et al: Lupus vulgaris with Michaelis-Gutman–like bodies in an immunocompromised patient. JAAD 1988, 18:577.

Horney DA, et al: Cutaneous inoculation tuberculosis secondary to "jailhouse tattooing." Arch Dermatol 1985, 121:648.

Iden DL, et al: Papulonecrotic tuberculid secondary to *Mycobacterium bovis*. Arch Dermatol 1978, 114:564.

Izumi AK, et al: BCG-vaccine–induced lupus vulgaris. Arch Dermatol 1982, 118:171.

Jacobs RF, et al: Tuberculosis in children. Semin Respir Med 1988, 9:474.

Lantos G, et al: Tuberculous ulcer of the skin. JAAD 1988, 19:1067.

Lao IO, et al: Lupus vulgaris. Cutis 1983, 21:177.

Lebel M, et al: Erythema induratum of Bazin. JAAD 1986, 14:738.

Minkowitz S, et al: Prosector's warts . . . in medical student. Am J Clin Pathol 1969, 51:260.

Morrison JGL, et al: The papulonecrotic tuberculide. Br J Dermatol 1974, 91:263.

Perez-Stable EJ, et al: Chemotherapy of tuberculosis. Semin Respir Med 1988, 9:459.

Pitchenik AE, et al: Tuberculosis, atypical mycobacteriosis, and the acquired immunodeficiency syndrome among Haitians and non-Haitians in south Florida. Ann Intern Med 1984, 101:641.

Reider HC: Tuberculosis verrucosa cutis. JAAD 1988, 18:1367.

Rongioletti F, et al: Papules on lower limbs of a woman with cervical lymphadenopathy, lichen scrofulosorum. Arch Dermatol 1988, 124:1421.

Selwyn PA, et al: A prospective study of the risk of tuberculosis among intravenous drug users with human immunodeficiency virus infection. N Engl J Med 1989, 320:545.

Smith NP, et al: Lichen scrofulosorum. Br J Dermatol 1976, 94:319.

Sunderam G, et al: Tuberculosis and HIV infections. Semin Respir Med 1988, 9:481.

VanScoy RE, et al: Antituberculous agents: isoniazid, rifampin, streptomycin, ethambutol, and pyrazinamide. Mayo Clin Proc 1983, 58:233.

Wilson-Jones E, et al: Papulonecrotic tuberculid. JAAD 1986, 14:815.

ATYPICAL MYCOBACTERIOSIS

For about a century infections with atypical mycobacteria have been known to occur in birds and cold-blooded vertebrates such as frogs, snakes, and fish. In 1954 Linell and Nordén first reported a peculiar form of verrucous granuloma caused by atypical mycobacteria following swimming pool injuries. Since then many hundreds of cases of skin infections due to atypical mycobacteria have been reported. In addition to the skin infections there are pulmonary infections, adenitis, osteomyelitis, and disseminated disease.

CLASSIFICATION OF MYCOBACTERIA. Runyon has classified the atypical mycobacteria into four groups.

Group I contains photochromogens. A yellow pigment on Löwenstein-Jensen culture medium is produced in 24 hours when exposed to light and cultured at 37° C. This group includes *M. kansasii, M. marinum (M. balnei), M. ulcerans,* and *M. simiae.*

Group II are the scotochromogens, which produce a yellow-orange pigment even when cultured in darkness. The main pathogen in this group is *M. scrofulaceum. M. szulgai* and *M. xenopi* also occasionally cause human disease, and *M. gordonae* has recently been reported to cause a hand infection.

Group III are the nonphotochromogens, which do not produce pigment. In this group are *M. avium-intracellulare* complex and *M. haemophilum.*

Group IV do not produce identifying pigment but are distinguished by their rapid growth rate of three to five days. The most important pathogens are *M. fortuitum* and *M. chelonae (M. abscessus).*

TUBERCULIN TESTING. Purified Protein Derivative (PPD-S) (human tuberculin), PPD-B (Battey strain), PPD-Y (photochromogen), PPD-G (scotochromogen), and PPD-F (rapid growers) are tested in the same manner as PPD. These antigens are of limited availability and limited usefulness in diagnostic clinical medicine, as cross reactivity is frequent. Culture is the only decisive diagnostic procedure.

SWIMMING POOL GRANULOMA
(Aquarium Granuloma)

An indolent granuloma usually starts about three weeks after injury as a small papule, characteristically located on the nose in Sweden (because Swedish swimming pools have a step between the shallow and deep ends). Elsewhere in the world it is usually on the knees, the elbows, or sometimes on the dorsa of the hands and feet. More infections are acquired from home aquariums than from swimming pools, and in such cases the fingers and hands are the site of the lesion.

A sporotrichoid pattern, with a succession of nodules ascending the arm, is common. The lesions may be erosions or verrucous papules or plaques. Multiple lesions occur infrequently. Usually there is no ulceration or necrosis. Synovitis, draining sinuses, bursitis, arthritis, and osteomyelitis may be seen, however.

This type of granuloma is caused by *M. marinum,* a group I photochromogen, growing optimally at 30° C in Löwenstein-Jensen medium, and very easily killed by warming to 35° or 36° C.

Histopathologically, there is at first an inflammatory type of reaction with hyperkeratosis and acanthosis. Later, epithelioid cell tubercles form in which Langhans giant cells are present. Central "fibrinoid"

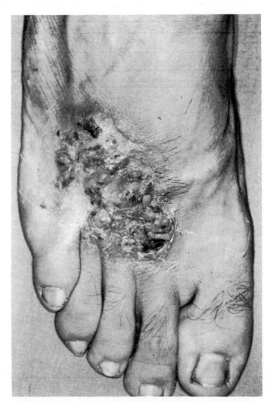

Figure 16–16. Swimming pool granuloma caused by Mycobacterium marinum.

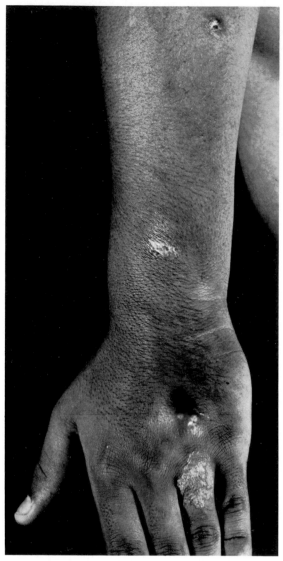

Figure 16–17. Sporotrichoid mycobacteriosis of the hand and forearm. (Courtesy of Drs. D. W. Owens and M. E. McBride.)

Langhans giant cells are present. Central "fibrinoid" necrosis may occur, but true caseation necrosis is rare. Acid-fast organisms may rarely be seen, especially within the histiocytes. The organisms are longer and thicker than *M. tuberculosis*.

The tuberculin reaction to *M. tuberculosis* usually becomes positive in those who have had *M. marinum* infection.

Excision of the lesion, when feasible, is effective. Minocycline, 100 mg twice daily, is effective in the majority of cases. Its use is documented in a large study from Japan by Arai. Tetracycline, 500 mg three or four times a day, may be effective, as advised by both Kim and Izumi; or trimethoprim and sulfamethoxazole (Bactrim, Septra), as suggested by Black and Eykyn. Bailey et al reported an *M. marinum* infection of the hand in a fish market employee which responded well to one year of treatment with 600 mg of rifampin and 1000 of ethambutol daily. Donta et al reported four patients who did not respond to tetracyclines, but cleared with either rifampin alone, or with rifampin plus ethambutol. Treatment is continued for at least 6 weeks but may be required for many months. No current recommendation for a drug of choice is available, and the clinician may choose from a number of effective options. Huminer et al provide an excellent review of these.

OTHER CUTANEOUS ATYPICAL MYCOBACTERIAL INFECTIONS

M. kansasii, a group I organism, occasionally involves the skin in a sporotrichoid pattern. Localized granulomatous lesions may also be seen. Inoculation is usually by minor trauma, and minocycline or antituberculous therapy may be effective if excision is impractical. Rosen reported isolating *M. kansasii* from a cellulitislike lesion of the leg which cleared under three months of treatment with rifampin, ethambutol, and kanamycin. Drabic et al reported perianal ulcerations due to this organism, and Hanke et al reviewed the literature of cutaneous infections with *M. kansasii*.

Group II organisms rarely involve the skin. *M. scrofulaceum* may produce a scrofulodermatous appearance. Shelley reported the first isolation of *M. gordonae*, from a nodule on the hand; it was sensitive only to rifampin and ethambutol, and resistant to isoniazid, streptomycin, and aminosalicylic acid. Tine test produced a true granuloma. The patient did not tolerate chemotherapy, but the lesion slowly regressed. Cross et al reported a case of *M. szulgai* infection of skin and bone which began during oral prednisone therapy for desquamative pneumonitis and responded well to combined therapy with isoniazid, ethambutol, and rifampin.

Group III organisms were uncommon causes of skin infection prior to the epidemic of the acquired immunodeficiency syndrome. Hawkins et al have recently reviewed their experience with 67 AIDS patients who developed disseminated *M. avium–intracellulare* complex infections, and Glassworth has reviewed the subject extensively. This condition may involve the skin by hematogenous dissemination. Friedman et al reviewed 11 cases of disseminated *M. avium-intracellulare* infection in non-AIDS patients. Most occurred in immunocompromised children with chronic pulmonary infections. It is generally unresponsive to therapy. Glassworth reviews factors affecting choice of drugs. Greene et al reported *M. avium-intracellulare* infection in five immunoincompetent men, all of whom died except one who was treated with multiple drugs starting two months before the infection was identified. Davis et al reported *M. hemophilum* granulomas of the leg in an immunosuppressed woman who responded well to isoniazid and rifampin, given for only six weeks.

Group IV organisms usually cause subcutaneous abscesses following trauma. These infections are commonly resistant to many antituberculous medications, so that excision is best for localized lesions, and wound debridement plays a role even in widespread disease. Amikacin, sulfonamides, erythromycin, and tetracyclines may be tried. Heironimus et al cured a man with *M. chelonae* abscess of the thigh following a thorn prick, with 2 gm a day of trisulfapyrimidines, later raised to 5 gm a day, for six months. Fenske et al reported a case of *M. chelonae* abscesses in which ethambutol with isoniazid, aminosalicylic acid, and several months of oral rifampin, followed by some months of minocycline, all failed; addition of Seromycin (cycloserine) helped but did not eradicate the infection. Cooper et al reviewed 10 renal transplant patients with *M. chelonae* infection. Seven had tender nodular lesions on the legs due to disseminated disease. An excellent review of the treatment of 123 patients with nonpulmonary Group IV infections, by Wallace et al, is recommended.

MYCOBACTERIAL ULCER

This is also known as *Buruli ulcer* and *Searl's ulcer*. The lesions begin as solitary, hard, painless, subcutaneous nodules that subsequently ulcerate and become undermined. There is a predilection for the occurrence of these ulcers on the extremities. *Mycobacterium ulcerans* produces a toxin that may be responsible for the extensive necrosis and ulceration seen in these infections.

Farber and Tsang described a case of a 20-year-old man whose entire foot was extensively involved; an amputation below the knee was necessary. The infection was incurred in Nigeria while he was wading in stagnant water building bridges.

Mycobacterium ulcerans has been identified in this type of ulceration. It is cultured in Löwenstein-Jensen medium at 33° C. This organism has been found to occur in Australia, Nigeria, Zaire, the Buruli district of Uganda, Mexico, and Malaysia.

Effective treatment is not available at present. When feasible, wide and deep excision is probably the best form of therapy. Hayman reported seven cases from the state of Victoria, east of Melbourne;

one responded to a combination of rifampicin and ethionamide, but two did not; excision of the ulcer was carried out in all. The ulcers are known locally as Bairnsdale ulcers. Koalas are afflicted with them as well, but no connection with human cases has been suggested.

Adams RM, et al: Tropical fish aquariums: a source of *M. marinum* infections resembling sporotrichosis. JAMA 1970, 211:457.

Arai H, et al: *Mycobacterium marinum* infection of the skin in Japan. J Dermatol 1984, 11:37.

Idem: Amikacin treatment for *Mycobacterium marinum* infection. J Dermatol 1986, 13:385.

Arnold HL Jr: Balnei granuloma in Hawaii (editorial). Hawaii Med J 1962, 21:422.

Bailey JP: *Mycobacterium marinum* infection: a fishy story. JAMA 1982, 247:1314.

Black MM, et al: Successful treatment of tropical fish-tank granuloma (*Mycobacterium marinum*) with co-trimoxazole. Br J Dermatol 1977, 96:689.

Cross GM, et al: Cutaneous *Mycobacterium szulgai* infection. Arch Dermatol 1985, 121:247.

Davis BR, et al: Skin lesions caused by *Mycobacterium hemophilum*. Ann Intern Med 1982, 97:724.

Denta ST, et al: Therapy of *M. marinum* infections. Arch Intern Med 1986, 146:902.

Drabic JJ, et al: Ulcerative perianal lesions due to *Mycobacterium kansasii*. JAAD 1988, 18:1146.

Fenske NA, et al: Resistant cutaneous infection by *Mycobacterium chelonae*. Arch Dermatol 1981, 117:151.

Fonseca E, et al: Nodular lesions in disseminated *Mycobacterium fortuitum* infection. Arch Dermatol 1987, 123:1603.

Freed JA, et al: Cutaneous mycobacteriosis. Arch Dermatol 1987, 123:1601.

Friedman BF, et al: *Mycobacterium avium-intracellulare*: Cutaneous presentations of disseminated disease. Am J Med 1988, 85:257.

Glassworth J: *Mycobacterium avium* complex in patients with AIDS. Semin Respir Med 1988, 9:486.

Grange JM: Mycobacteria and the skin. Int J Dermatol 1982, 21:497.

Hanke CW, et al: *Mycobacterium kansasii* infection with multiple cutaneous lesions. JAAD 1987, 16:1122.

Hawkins CC, et al: *M. avium* complex infections in patients with AIDS. Ann Intern Med 1986, 105:184.

Hayman J: Clinical features of *Mycobacterium ulcerans* infection. Austral J Derm 1985, 26:67.

Heironimus JD, et al: Cutaneous nonpulmonary *Mycobacterium chelonae* infection: successful treatment with sulfonamides in an immunosuppressed patient. Arch Dermatol 1984, 120:1061.

Hendrick SJ, et al: Giant *Mycobacterium fortuitum* abscess associated with SLE. Arch Dermatol 1986, 122:695.

Hirsh FS, et al: *Mycobacterium kansasii* infection: dermatologic manifestation. Arch Dermatol 1976, 112:706.

Hoy JF, et al: *Mycobacterium fortuitum* bacteremia in patients with cancer and long-term venous catheter. Am J Med 1987, 83:213.

Huminer D, et al: Aquarium-borne *Mycobacterium marinum* skin infection. Arch Dermatol 1986, 122:698.

Inman PM, et al: Outbreak of . . . *Mycobacterium* abscesses. Arch Dermatol 1969, 100:141.

Izumi AK, et al: *Mycobacterium marinum* infections treated with tetracycline. Arch Dermatol 1977, 113:1067.

Jolly HW, et al: Infections with *Mycobacterium marinum*. Arch Dermatol 1972, 106:32.

Loria PR: Minocycline hydrochloride . . . for atypical acid-fast infection. Arch Dermatol 1976, 112:517.

Maurice DPL, et al: *Mycobacterium avium-intracellulare* infection associated with hairy cell leukemia. Arch Dermatol 1988, 124:1545.

Maziary RT, et al: Reversal of infection with *M. avium-intracellulare* by treatment with alpha-interferon in a patient with hairy cell leukemia. Ann Intern Med 1988, 109:292.

Murray-Leisure KA, et al: Skin lesions caused by *Mycobacterium scrofulaceum*. Arch Dermatol 1987, 123:369.

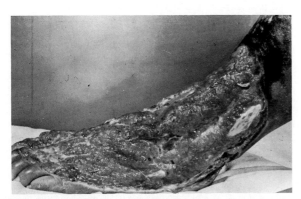

Figure 16–18. Mycobacterial (Buruli) ulcer on the foot of a 20-year-old man in The Peace Corps, contracted in Nigeria. (Courtesy of Dr. E. R. Farber.)

Owens DW: Atypical mycobacteria. Int J Dermatol 1978, 17:180.

Idem, et al: Sporotrichoid infections with *Mycobacterium kansasii.* Arch Dermatol 1969, 100:54.

Philpott JA Jr, et al: Swimming pool granuloma: study of 290 cases. Arch Dermatol 1963, 88:158.

Prevost E, et al: *Mycobacterium marinum* infections. South Med J 1982, 75:1349.

Radford AJ: Ulcerans ulcer: the sore that heals in vain. Int J Dermatol 1975, 14:422.

Raleigh JW: Disease due to *Mycobacterium kansasii.* Semin Respir Med 1988, 9:498.

Rosen T: Cutaneous *Mycobacterium kansasii* infection presenting as cellulitis. Cutis 1983, 31:87.

Safraneck TJ, et al: *Mycobacterium chelonae* wound infections after plastic surgery employing contaminated gentian violet skin-marking solution. N Engl J Med 1987, 317:197.

Shelley WB, et al: *Mycobacterium gordonae* infection of the hand. Arch Dermatol 1984, 120:1064.

Wallace RJ, Jr: Recent clinical advances in knowledge of the nonleprous environmental mycobacteria responsible for cutaneous disease. Arch Dermatol 1987, 123:337.

Idem: Treatment of nonpulmonary infections due to *Mycobacterium fortuitum* and *Mycobacterium chelonei* on the basis of in vitro susceptibilities. J Infect Dis 1985, 152:5001.

Wolinsky E: Nontuberculous mycobacteria and associated diseases. Am Rev Respir Dis 1979, 119:107.

17

Leprosy

Synonyms: Hansen's disease, hanseniasis, lepra.

DEFINITION. Leprosy is a chronic, systemic, infectious disease of man caused by *Mycobacterium leprae*. It manifests itself in the development of specific granulomatous or neurotrophic lesions in the skin, mucous membranes, nerves, anterior segment of the eye, bones, and viscera.

HISTORY. It is uncertain when leprosy first became known, since the disease has been called by many different names. Undoubtedly the early terms had a much wider meaning and included many more diseases than at present. There is evidence to indicate that the disease was known as early as 1500 B.C. and that it originated in India, Egypt, or the Sudan.

Around 100 B.C. it was known in Greece. The term "leprosy" is used in the New Testament, whereas it is designated as "zara'ath" in the Old Testament. The presence of leprosy was recorded in European countries, starting with Italy in 62 A.D., Germany in 180 A.D., Spain in 600 A.D., France in 800 A.D., and Ireland in 869 A.D. Later it spread to the remainder of the European countries. The disease reached its peak in the 1200s, then began to subside to the extent that in the 1600s small foci remained in the Scandinavian countries only, where it persisted until, by 1973, it had virtually disappeared. It remains in southern Europe still.

It is believed that it was introduced into the Western Hemisphere by Columbus, and later by slaves from West Africa. Foci of the disease in the United States are believed to come mostly from outside the country, possibly Puerto Rico, Cuba, and Mexico. It is found in the southern states of Florida, Louisiana, and Texas, and in California and Hawaii. It is prevalent in Central and South America, the Philippines, and Asia.

It was not until 1869 that the causative bacillus was reported by Dr. G. Armauer Hansen.

Classification of Leprosy

The classification of leprosy is based on the following criteria, listed in order of increasing importance: clinical, bacteriologic, immunologic, and histopathologic. The clinical manifestations of the cutaneous lesions and neurologic signs are of foremost importance. In addition to the clinical findings, the demonstration of bacilli in lepromatous or borderline lesions, either by skin scraping or by histologic examination of skin biopsy specimens, is indispensable. The immunologic status should be determined in each case with the lepromin test. As shown by Sehgal et al, the polar forms show good correlation in the results of histopathologic, bacteriologic, and immunologic testing. There is discordance in these findings in a large number of the borderline cases, because of the dynamic nature of this subset of patients.

At the Fifth International Congress of Leprosy, held in Havana, in 1948, the following classification was adopted: two fundamental stable "polar" (Rabello) types, the lepromatous or anergic, and the tuberculoid or hyperergic. An intermediate group, called *incaracteristico* or indeterminate, was established for cases that are neither lepromatous nor tuberculoid.

At the International Congress of Leprosy, in Madrid in 1953, a fourth clinical group was agreed upon. This newest type was named borderline, undifferentiated, or dimorphous. It is now known as borderline.

In 1966, Ridley and Jopling proposed a classification that recognizes the tuberculoid/lepromatous polarity to be, in essence, an indication of the immune status of the patient. They proposed that a spectrum of the disease exists which covers a particular patient's immunologic response. This spectrum ranges

Table 17–1. SPECTRUM OF HOST-PARASITE RESISTANCE

	High Resistance		Unstable Resistance		No Resistance
	Tuberculoid TT	Borderline Tuberculoid BT	Borderline BB	Borderline Lepromatous BL	Lepromatous LL
Lesions	one or two	few	few or many asymmetric	many	numerous and symmetrical
Smear for bacilli	0	1+	2+	3+	4+
Lepromin test	3+	2+	+	±	0
Histology	Epithelioid cells decreasing ⟶ Nerve destruction, sarcoid-like			increasing histiocytes, foam cells granuloma, xanthoma-like	

(Adapted from Dr. J. H. Pettit.)

between two poles: the tuberculoid (TT) and the lepromatous (LL). In the center is the borderline type (BB) with two subsidiary forms on each side of BB: borderline tuberculoid (BT) and borderline lepromatous (BL). There is a natural progression of the various features of leprosy along the spectrum. Table 17–1 demonstrates how the lepromin test is positive in TT and negative in LL, with a decreasing reaction from TT to LL. Other changing features throughout the spectrum are also demonstrated.

CLINICAL FEATURES. Usually the onset of leprosy is insidious.

Prodromal symptoms are generally so slight that the disease is not recognized until the appearance of a cutaneous eruption. Actually the first clinical manifestation in 90 per cent of patients is numbness, and years may elapse before skin lesions or other signs are identified. The earliest sensory changes are loss of senses of cold and light touch, most often in feet or hands.

The light touch of a wisp of cotton or even a fingertip may not elicit a response, whereas pinprick may be discerned. The bony prominences, namely the knuckles, elbows, patella, and malleoli, have a raised threshold of reaction. Sense of cold may be lost before pinprick sensibility. Such dissociation of sensibility is especially suspicious. The distribution of these neural signs and their intensity will depend upon the type of disease which is evolving.

Most often the first lesion noted is an ill-defined, hypopigmented macule which merges into the surrounding normal skin. This macule may have a pigskin appearance and may be a solitary lesion. Less often erythematous macules may be present. Such lesions may be located anywhere on the body, but have a predilection for the cheeks, upper arms, thighs, and buttocks. Usually there is but a solitary lesion. Usually no, or only a few, bacilli are seen on biopsy of this indeterminate form.

Few cases remain in this state; they evolve into lepromatous, tuberculoid, or borderline types, or (if immunity is good) may spontaneously resolve and never develop other signs or symptoms of leprosy. Browne, who recently reviewed this, feels that if on biopsy one finds abundant lymphocytes, evolution will be toward tuberculoid; if lymphocytes are scant, evolution will be toward lepromatous.

Tuberculoid Leprosy (TT). The typical lesion of tuberculoid leprosy is the large erythematous plaque with its sharply defined and elevated border that slopes down to a flattened atrophic center. As the lesions clear, they tend to become annular, arciform, or circinate, with borders of variable thickness.

A tuberculoid lesion is anesthetic and occurs commonly on the face, limbs, or elsewhere, with the exception of the scalp, axillae, groin, and perineum.

There are also the maculo-anesthetic or macular tuberculoid lesions, which tend to be large and asymmetrically positioned and are usually single or few in number. The macules are well defined and hypopigmented, usually dry and hairless. Anesthesia of the hypopigmented lesion is invariable, as is anhidrosis. Other heavily infiltrated prominent plaques occur. The plaques are erythematous and vary from a rose to a violaceous red color.

The evolution of the lesions is generally slow. The acute episodes that do occur are not associated with febrile systemic reactions, as happens in the lepromatous type. There is often spontaneous remission of the lesions in about three years, or remission may result sooner from treatment. Spontaneous involution may leave pigmentary disturbances and scars.

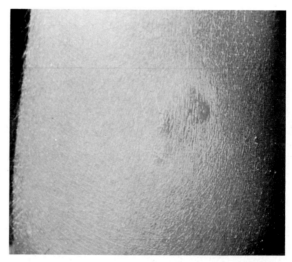

Figure 17–1. Early papular lesion of tuberculoid leprosy just below popliteal space. (Courtesy of Dr. J. Convit, Venezuela.)

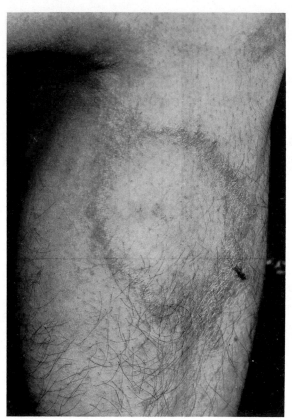

Figure 17–2. Tuberculoid (TT) leprosy on inner calf. (Courtesty of Dr. F. Reiss.)

The patient regularly reacts strongly to the lepromin test. There are few or no *M. leprae* in the lesions.

Neural Involvement in TT. Principal neural signs in leprosy are anesthesia, nerve enlargement, muscular weakness and wasting, and trophic manifestations.

In the tuberculoid type, invasion of the peripheral nerves leads very early to their tenderness, thickening, and loss of function, and to the development of the characteristic changes and deformities of neural leprosy. The great auricular nerve and the superficial peroneal nerve are often so large that they are plainly visible. The nerves may be thickened near the sites of the skin lesions. Nerve lesions become evident earlier, are more severe, and tend to be asymmetric in the tuberculoid type.

There may be atrophy of the interosseous muscles of the hand, wasting of the thenar and hypothenar eminences, contracture of the fingers, paralysis of the orbital and facial muscles, foot drop, and anesthesia.

Borderline Tuberculoid Leprosy (BT). These lesions are similar to TT lesions except that they are smaller and more numerous, there is less hair loss, and the nerves are only slightly enlarged.

Borderline Leprosy (BB). In BB leprosy, only the skin and nerves are clinically involved. Usually there are numerous bacilli on bacteriologic examination, and the lepromin reaction is generally negative or slightly positive. The cutaneous lesions are numerous and consist of red, irregularly shaped plaques. Small satellite lesions may be present. Their distribution may simulate that of the lepromatous type except that they are often asymmetric. The edges of lesions are not so well defined as the ones seen in the tuberculoid type. There may be regional adenopathy. Anesthesia is only moderate in these lesions.

Borderline Lepromatous Leprosy (BL). In this type, the lesions are usually numerous and may include macules, papules, plaques, and nodules. There may be a punched-out appearance of some plaques; in such annular lesions there is a sloping outer margin and a steep inner one, like an inverted saucer—the reverse of the configuration of an annular tuberculoid plaque. Nerve lesions appear late and patients usually show none of the lepromatous features, such as madarosis, keratitis, nasal ulceration, and leonine facies. Anesthesia is often absent.

Lepromatous Leprosy (LL). The cutaneous lesions of the lepromatous type consist mainly of pale lepromatous macules or lepromatous infiltrations, with numerous bacilli in the lesions. There is a negative reaction to lepromin, a typical histopathology, and a

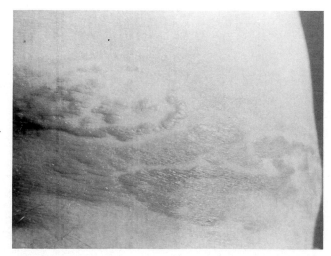

Figure 17–3. Borderline tuberculoid (BT) leprosy.

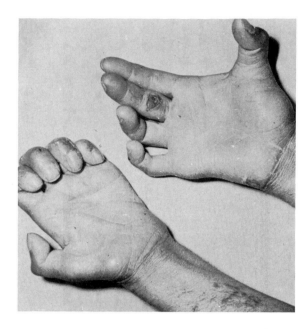

Figure 17–4. Muscle atrophy and claw hand with polyneuritis in tuberculoid leprosy. Note external rotation of thumbs ("ape" hand). (Courtesy of Dr. J. Convit, Venezuela.)

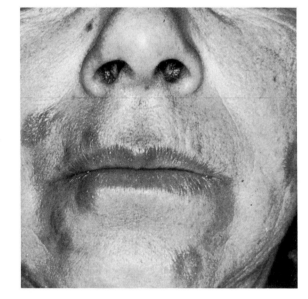

Figure 17–5. Borderline tuberculoid (BT) leprosy. (Courtesy of Dr. F. Latapí, Mexico.)

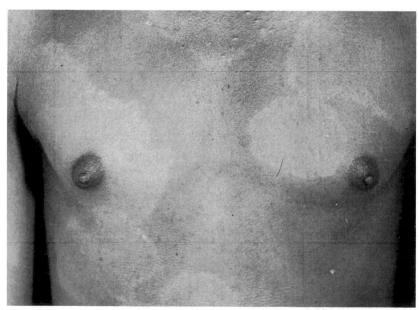

Figure 17–6. Borderline tuberculoid (BT) leprosy. Hypopigmented, anesthetic, anhidrotic patches on chest. (Courtesy of Dr. F. Kerdel-Vegas, Venezuela.)

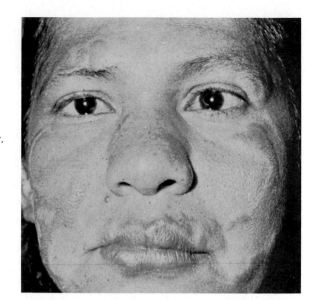

Figure 17–7. Annular infiltrations in borderline leprosy. (Courtesy of Dr. J. Convit, Venezuela.)

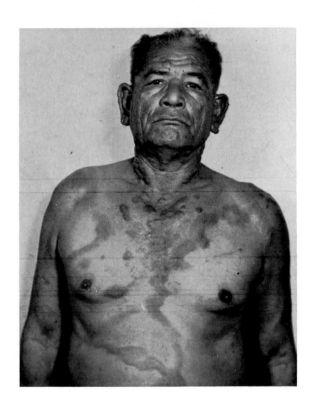

Figure 17–8. Borderline leprosy, showing nodules and bizarre erythematous-bordered plaques on chest. (Courtesy of Dr. J. Convit, Venezuela.)

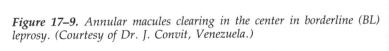

Figure 17–9. Annular macules clearing in the center in borderline (BL) leprosy. (Courtesy of Dr. J. Convit, Venezuela.)

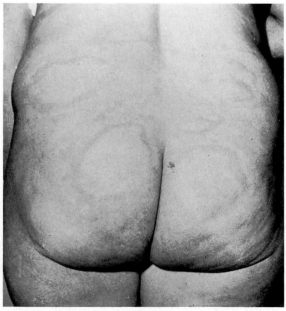

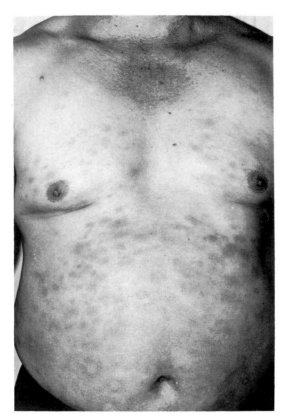

Figure 17–10. Borderline lepromatous leprosy, BB or BL.

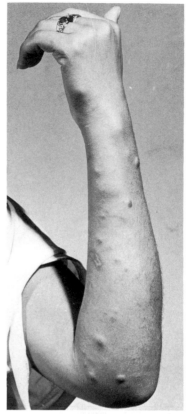

Figure 17–12. Nodules of lepromatous leprosy.

tendency for the disease to become progressively worse without treatment.

In *macular lepromatous leprosy* lesions are diffusely and symmetrically distributed over the body. Whereas tuberculoid macules are large and sparse,

lepromatous macules are small and numerous. The macules, ill-defined, show no change in skin texture. There is little or no loss of sensation; there is no nerve thickening; and there are no changes in sweating. A slow progressive loss of hair takes place from the outer third of the eyebrows, then the eyelashes and, finally, the body; however, the scalp hair usually remains unchanged, except in Japan, where alopecia of the scalp is not rare. There is, however, nearly always preservation of the hair overlying the major arteries of the scalp, where the skin is too warm for *M. leprae.*

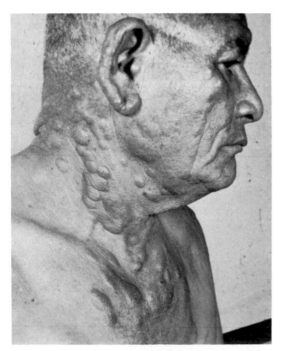

Figure 17–11. Nodular lesions of borderline (BB or BL) leprosy. (Courtesy of Dr. J. Convit, Venezuela.)

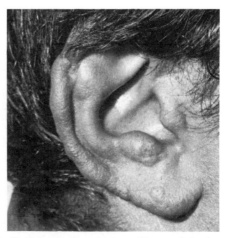

Figure 17–13. Leprosy, lepromatous. Note nodules in ear. (Courtesy of Dr. G. Salinger.)

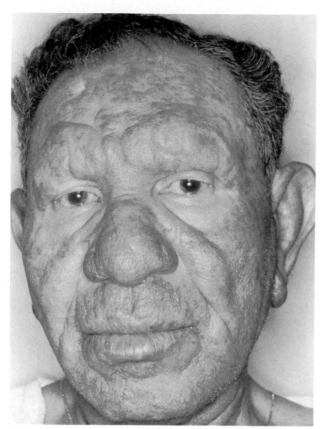

Figure 17–14. *Lepromatous leprosy—note loss of the eyebrows and eyelashes (madarosis).*

The *lepromatous infiltrations* may be divided into the diffuse, plaque, and nodular types. The diffuse type is characterized by the development of a diffuse infiltration of the face, especially the forehead, loss of the eyebrows (madarosis), and a waxy and shiny appearance of the skin sometimes described as a "varnished" appearance.

The infiltrations may be manifested by the development of nodules called *lepromas*. The early nodules are ill defined and occur most often in acral parts: ears, brows, nose, chin, elbows, hands, buttocks, or knees.

The lepromatous type either begins as such, or by transformation from borderline lesions. Usually it begins with macular lesions such as those described, but there is a lack of sharp demarcation at the periphery so that the edges merge into the normal skin. This characteristic helps to differentiate these lesions from similar ones seen in the tuberculoid and borderline types. Neuritic lesions invariably occur but they develop very slowly and are almost invariably bilaterally symmetrical, unlike those in TT leprosy.

Diffuse leprosy of Lucio is a striking cutaneous manifestation, rare except in Costa Rica and western Mexico, where it comprises nearly one third of lepromatous cases. This type is characterized by diffuse lepromatous infiltration of the skin: localized lepromas do not form. A unique complication of this subtype is the reactional state referred to as Lucio's phenomenon (erythema necroticans). Multiple areas of vasculitis occur with necrosis and resultant shallow ulcers that heal with scarring. This variety is endemic in Mexico, Cuba, Brazil, and Costa Rica, and occurs only rarely in the United States.

Piepkorn et al reported a case with the Lucio phenomenon in which auricular chondritis—not previously reported in this connection—occurred during therapy. Elevated circulating immune complexes declined after immunosuppressive therapy and plasmapheresis, concurrent with clinical improvement.

Histoid Leproma. During relapse, distinctive histoid lepromas may occur cutaneously or subcutaneously. These typical lepromas are yellowish red, shiny, large papules and nodules varying from 1 to 15 mm in diameter, scattered over the entire body.

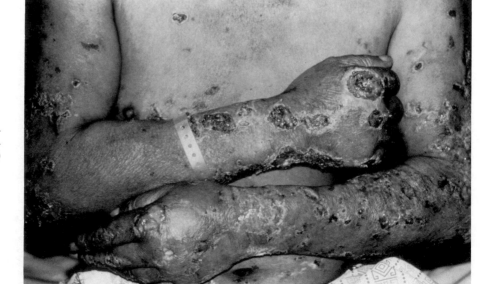

Figure 17–15. Diffuse leprosy, phenomenon of Lucio (erythema necroticans). (Courtesy of Dr. Axel W. Hoke.)

There is a predilection for cooler areas—buttocks, lower back, hands, and face. Histologically, there are characteristic spindle-shaped histiocytes arranged in whorls and containing numerous bacilli. Sehgal et al and Uyemura et al have recently reviewed the histoid pattern in leprosy.

Eye Involvement. In most lepromatous cases, the eyes become involved. Ffytche and McDougall have recently reviewed leprosy of the eye in some detail. In the eye, leprosy involves principally the distal hemisphere. Corneal erosions, exposure keratitis, and ulcerations may occur as a result of involvement of the seventh nerve.

Specific changes may include corneal opacity, avascular keratitis, pannus formation, interstitial keratitis, and corneal lepromas. The corneal opacities enlarge and finally form visible white flecks called "pearls." When (in BL or LL cases only) the iris and the ciliary body become involved, miliary lepromata (iris pearls), nodular lepromata, chronic granulomatous iritis, and acute diffuse plastic iridocyclitis may result.

Other Mucous Membrane Involvement. The mucous membranes may also be affected, especially in the nose, mouth, and larynx. By far the most common lesions in the nose are infiltrations and nodules. Perforation of the nasal septum may occur in advanced cases, with collapse of the nasal bridge. Nodules occurring on the vocal cords will produce hoarseness. Saddle-nose deformities and loss of the upper incisor teeth are some of the other changes.

Nerve Involvement. It is highly unusual to see advanced lepromatous leprosy of nerves with minimal skin involvement. All patients show nerve involvement to a greater or lesser degree. There are no "neural" cases from the clinical and histopathologic points of view, but leprous neuritis, lepromatous or tuberculoid, occurs as part of the disease. Symmetry

of nerve involvement is far more common in the lepromatous than in the tuberculoid type.

As already stated, the neural signs in leprosy are anesthesia, nerve enlargement, muscular weakness and wasting, and trophic changes. The lesions of the vasomotor nerves accompany the sensory disturbances or may precede them, as shown by the reaction to the histamine injection: loss of "flare."

Leprous anesthesia develops in a progressive manner. The first symptom is usually an inability to perceive a cold object as cold. Cold and warm objects are both called "warm" or elicit a "don't know" response. Subsequently the perception of light touch is lost, then that of pain, and lastly the sense of deep touch. At times the sensory changes in large patches are distributed irregularly because of variations in the involvement of the filaments supplying the area. The areas of anesthesia do not usually conform to the distribution of any particular nerve nor—except in lepromatous (LL) cases—are they symmetrical.

Nerve enlargement occurs chiefly in, and is of course most easily observed in, the more superficial nerve trunks, such as the ulnar, peroneal, median, radial, and especially the great auricular. Beaded enlargements, nodules, or spindle-shaped swellings are found, which at first may be tender. In the forearm they have been mistaken for sporotrichoid nodules along a lymphatic vessel. The ulnar nerve near the internal condyle of the humerus may be as thick as the little finger, round and stiff, and often easily felt several centimeters above the humeral pulley. As a result of the degeneration of the nerves, areas of anesthesia, paralyses, and trophic disorders in the peripheral parts of the extremities gradually develop.

Muscular paralysis and atrophy generally affect the small muscles of the hands and feet or some of the facial muscles, producing weakness and progressive

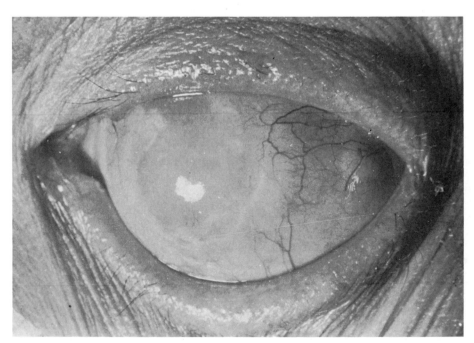

Figure 17–16. Leproma and a complete pannus in lepromatous leprosy. Courtesy of Dr. J. Convit, Venezuela.)

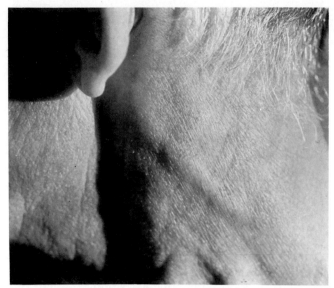

Figure 17–17. Enlargement of the greater auricular nerve in lepromatous leprosy. (Courtesy of Dr. Axel W. Hoke.)

atrophy. Deeper motor nerves are only rarely involved. One drooping lower eyelid, or one sagging oral commissure alone, strongly suggests leprosy. The fingers develop contractures, with the formation of the claw hand, and, as the result of concentric absorption of phalangeal shafts (which finally break), fingers and toes become shorter. Frequently a perforating ulcer develops on the ball or heel of the foot. Ptosis, ectropion, and a masklike appearance result from these changes.

Trophic changes consist of ulceration, disturbance of keratinization, bullae, alopecia, anhidrosis, and malum perforans pedis. There is concentric neurotrophic absorption of the shafts of the phalanges of fingers and toes, and the metatarsals; never, strangely, of the metacarpals, over the distal ends of which the fingernails often ultimately come to rest. The hardening and thickening of the nerves are most typical of leprosy and, since they are very rarely seen in any other affliction, are of diagnostic importance.

Internally, the lymph nodes, bone marrow, liver, spleen, and the testicles may be involved. Visceral affection is restricted mostly to the reticuloendothelial system, which is extensively involved, though visceral lesions reach the clinical horizon only in testicular atrophy with resultant gynecomastia. Amyloidosis may complicate this form of leprosy.

Indeterminate Leprosy. It is the classification, not the diagnosis, that is indeterminate. The cutaneous lesions consist of hypopigmented or, less often, erythematous macules. Plaques and nodules do not occur. Usually no or only a few bacilli are seen on biopsy, and only a simple lymphocytic infiltrate, rather than a granuloma. Sensory loss is seldom found.

Few cases remain in this state; the great majority evolve into lepromatous, tuberculoid, or borderline types. This is an ill-defined and unstable group. Pettit considers that the diagnosis of indeterminate leprosy should not be made. Browne, who recently reviewed the concept, says, "leprosy bacilli can always be demonstrated" (but may be very sparse). With abun-

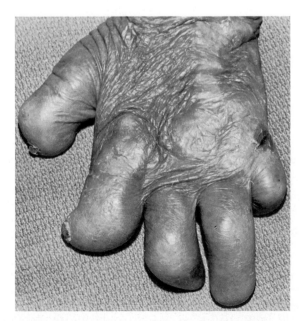

Figure 17–18. Shortening and contractures of the phalanges in a 60-year-old woman with lepromatous leprosy. (Courtesy of Dr. V. M. Torres-Rodriguez, Puerto Rico.)

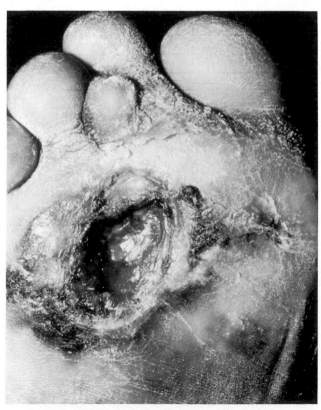

Figure 17–19. Trophic ulcer (malum perforans) caused by lepromatous leprosy. (Courtesy of Dr. Axel W. Hoke.)

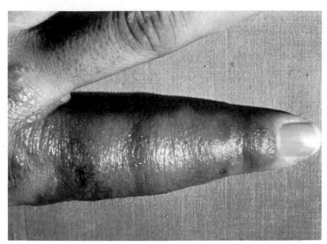

Figure 17–20. Dactylitis of leprosy.

dant lymphocytes, evolution toward a tuberculoid type is probable; with sparse, toward lepromatous.

ETIOLOGY. The causative organism, *Mycobacterium leprae*, is chiefly intracellular in habitat. It was first described by Hansen in 1869. It is a pleomorphic acid-fast bacillus, which varies from 2 to 7 µm in length and from 0.3 to 0.4 µm in breadth, usually straight or slightly curved, with parallel edges and rounded ends. It has a waxy capsule, and is scarcely distinguishable from *M. tuberculosis*. In the lesions of lepromatous leprosy the bacilli are present in enormous numbers, and in smears prepared in the usual manner many occur in round, bare globular masses called *globi*. Globi are largely intracellular, within histiocytes, but microcolonies lying free in tissue are found both in armadillos and in florid lepromatous lesions in human patients. The intracellular habitat is optional. Many also occur in bundles like bundles of cigars.

The bacilli are acid-fast, and though this quality is extractable with pyridine, as shown by Fischer (1971) and Convit (1972), Skinsnes et al (1975) showed that this is a characteristic of aging, nonviable bacilli, not a quality peculiar to *M. leprae*. Nevertheless, both Binford and Convit consider this an unsettled issue.

The bacilli are abundant in all lepromas, especially in the ear nodules and in the mucous membranes of the nose, eyes, and larynx. They may be identified in smears obtained by incising a lesion and curetting the edge of the cut.

The bacilli are less abundant in borderline forms, and in the tuberculoid form there are no, or at best only a few, bacilli.

The bacillus has been satisfactorily cultivated in the mouse footpad by Shepard. This is now being used as a source for bacilli to evaluate chemotherapeutic agents and to determine the efficacy of immunizing vaccines as well as the mechanism of drug resistance emergence. Even more importantly, it showed that bacilli which fail to stain solidly are dead bacilli, incapable of transmitting the disease,

and made possible the abolition of compulsory isolation of bacteriologically positive cases of leprosy.

Kirchheimer and Storrs reported in 1972 the induction of generalized progressive lepromatous leprosy in the nine-banded armadillo. It has been possible to make lepromin from such animals, and reactions to it are stronger than to human lepromin (Meyers et al and Millar et al, 1975). Studies of wild armadillos in Texas have revealed a prevalence rate of 4.7 per cent to 7.2 per cent.

The mangabey monkey has also been found to have naturally occurring disease. Experimental transmission of leprosy has been reported recently in three species of monkeys: the sooty mangabey, the rhesus, and the African green monkey. All developed lepromatous type disease.

The bacillus has not yet been acceptably cultivated. One significant advance, however, was the identification by Hunter et al in 1982 of a unique antigen found in *M. leprae*, phenolic glycolipid I. Using this antigen, an ELISA test has been produced and is presently being evaluated for its usefulness in identifying subclinical cases.

Skinsnes of Honolulu reported in 1976 that he had been able to cultivate *M. leprae* through successive generations in vitro, in an agar medium enriched with hyaluronic acid, and his work was successfully repeated in 1977 by Laszlo Kato of Montreal. Immunofluorescent and EM techniques have identified the organism as *M. leprae*, but its behavior, in the absence of all contact with human tissue, is sufficiently different to leave a few questions unanswered.

More recently Skinsnes et al have shown that 24 strains of supposed *M. leprae* cultured by himself, five strains cultivated by Kato, one strain cultured by Lapat, and two strains taken directly from tissue reacted strongly with lepromatous antibodies, while nine strains of *M. scrofulaceum*, four of *M. intracellulare*, and five of *M. avium* reacted not at all except for a single + + and 3 + reaction.

EPIDEMIOLOGY. It is estimated that there are about 15 million people in the world with leprosy. The highest prevalence rate is in Central Africa. Other areas in which the incidence is high are Asia, the Indian subcontinent, Brazil, Colombia, Venezuela, and the West Indies. Several other foci exist, such as the Baltic States, Spain and Portugal, Japan, the Philippines, Southeast Asia, and many islands of Melanesia and Polynesia.

Probably the most important factor in the epidemiology of leprosy has been the source of infection. It is believed that leprosy is transmitted from person to person. Transmission by contact with other afflicted members of a family is the most prevalent type. Lumpkin et al reported leprosy in five armadillo handlers who had no other identifiable risk factors for the disease.

The contagiousness of leprosy is substantiated by the fact that (1) healthy persons coming from a nonendemic area have acquired the disease after having moved into an endemic area; (2) patients with leprosy who have moved to places where leprosy does not exist have been responsible for epidemics, such as the one that occurred on Nauru Island; (3) epidemiologic studies reveal that the great majority of new cases are found among the contacts of open forms of leprosy. Lymphocyte transformation has been demonstrated in a majority of workers in a leprosarium during their first year there. While the majority of exposed individuals probably are transiently infected, relatively few manifest disease. An individual susceptibility, most likely through inheritance of an immunologic defect, determines who will manifest clinical disease.

The latent period between exposure and overt signs of the disease is usually from two to five years. Actually, the avenue by which the bacillus enters the body is not known, nor has a definite incubation period been determined. Children unquestionably are highly susceptible to infection and therefore the communicability of the disease within a family or household is high. It has been found in some leprosaria, where children are not separated from their parents or the group at birth, that nearly 50 per cent develop a positive lesion before the fifth year of life.

There have been several recent reports of young children with leprosy. Brubaker et al recently reviewed the world experience of leprosy occurring in children under one year of age. They were able to uncover 19 children, aged 2½ months to 12 months, who had clinical and histopathologic findings diagnostic of leprosy. In young children, the incubation period may be short. Of these 19, 14 had close family members with disease, usually of the lepromatous type.

Cochrane and Davey state that the greatest prevalence of leprosy has been in environments where the people are of low economic status, with inadequate housing, unsuitable sanitation, poor nutrition, and lack of education. However, a focus of the disease persisted for many years among only the more affluent residents of the state of Yucatan, in Mexico, to which the original victims had fled in order to escape compulsory isolation in Mexico City.

Among lepromatous cases, males outnumber females about 2:1 throughout the world. Tuberculoid cases are divided equally as to sex. Most cases occur in tropical climates.

Though it has long been suspected that transmission of leprosy may be by insects, this has not been shown to occur.

IMMUNE RESPONSE. Leprosy is a "spectrum" disease characterized by a variety of abnormal immune responses. The outcome of infection is dependent upon the integrity of the host's specific cellular immune response to *M. leprae*. An impaired response, perhaps genetically controlled, results in development of the lepromatous form; an intact response confers high resistance, reflected in the tuberculoid form. In an HLA study, van Eden et al demonstrated that while there was no inherited sus-

ceptibility to leprosy per se, the predilection to the development of a particular type (BL/LL or TT) is controlled by HLA-linked genes. They propose that an immune suppression gene might predispose to LL leprosy.

Nogueira et al found that 17 of 18 LL and BL patients produced no interferon in response to antigen, and did not respond to concanavalin A, despite a proliferative response to the mitogen. BT and TT patients had vigorous interferon production in response to both antigen and mitogen. Adding interleukin-2, 1–5 units/ml, in the presence of *M. leprae* antigen, significantly increased gamma interferon production.

Tausk et al have shown that erythrocytes from patients with lepromatous leprosy have decreased C3b receptors. This defect causes decreased clearance of immune complexes from the circulation. It is also a predictive marker for susceptibility to lepromatous leprosy.

Antibody responses are also abnormal in leprosy: specific antibody, usually of the IgG and IgA classes, directed against *M. leprae*, is correlated with antigenic load. As yet no protective role has been demonstrated.

Preliminary evidence suggests that erythema nodosum leprosum (ENL) represents an Arthus phenomenon. IgG and C3 deposits have been demonstrated in the vessel walls by immunofluorescent techniques. Circulating immune complexes have been found, as have elevated levels of serum complement components.

"Reversal" reactions are characterized by increased inflammation of existing skin lesions with histologic patterns of delayed hypersensitivity and clearance of organisms. Most evidence suggests that these reactions are associated with the rapid development of cell-mediated immunity to *M. leprae*.

Rea et al reported that their patients with lepromatous leprosy had normal immunologic responses to antigens other than lepromin. Mehta et al showed that a unique species of antigen present on *M. leprae*, phenolic glycolipid I, is capable of inducing suppression of mitogenic responses of lepromatous patients' lymphocytes in vitro. They also showed that suppressor T cells recognize the specific terminal trisaccharide moiety. Lim et al quantitated the T cell subsets in 20 patients with lepromatous leprosy and found T helper cells reduced by 96 per cent over controls; T suppressor cells were reduced by 47 per cent, and T rosette formers by 70 per cent. Modlin et al found lepromin-triggered T-suppressor activity in lepromatous patients, supporting the concept that the unresponsiveness of lepromatous patients to antigens of *M. leprae* is related to the prevalence of CD8-positive lymphocytes in lepromatous lesions and peripheral blood. Rea et al, using flow cytometry, found a deficiency in T helper cells in BL patients not in reaction, and in patients in reversal reaction. In active lepromatous leprosy, they did not observe any alteration in distribution.

HISTOPATHOLOGY. The tissues invaded by the lepra bacilli show two types of chronic inflammatory infiltrates: the simple inflammatory and the granulomatous.

The simple inflammatory infiltrate consists of lymphocytes with occasional histiocytes and fibrocytes localized around blood vessels, nerves, and glands of the skin. It is banal in character and it can be observed in many other disorders. In the *indeterminate group* it can be the only histopathologic finding for many years. This simple infiltrate is found in the skin, mucous membranes, nerves, and lymph glands.

In lepromatous lesions the granulomatous infiltrate is histiocytic, with acid-fast bacilli and, as Azulay showed, lipids, while in tuberculoid lesions it contains epithelioid-cell tubercles with no bacilli and no lipid.

Tuberculoid Type (TT). The histopathology reflects the high degree of resistance on the part of the host. There is a tuberculoid granuloma consisting of groups of epithelioid cells among which some giant cells are seen. The granuloma extends up to the epidermis, with no clear zone in between. Lymphocytes are found about the periphery. Acid-fast bacilli are rarely seen. The most important specific diagnostic feature, next to finding a bacillus, is selective destruction of nerve trunks. Bacilli are frequently found with comparative ease in sections of nerves, however. No fat is found in the epithelioid cells or elsewhere. The infiltrate contains predominantly T helper cells.

Borderline Tuberculoid (BT). The histopathology of this type is similar to that seen in the tuberculoid variety, but there are some vacuolated cells and a few bacilli. The most distinctive is the narrow clear subepidermal zone separating the granuloma from the epidermis. Some lipid may be found.

Borderline Leprosy (BB). Most characteristic is the diffuse spread of epithelioid cells throughout the granuloma. In addition, lymphocytes are not aggregated in zones. Langhans giant cells are absent, but acid-fast bacilli are typically numerous. Lipid is always present in fat-stained sections.

Borderline Lepromatous (BL). Histiocytes compose most of the granuloma, although there is a tendency for epithelioid cells to form. The histiocytes form foam cells. There is a dense lymphocyte infiltration. Perineural involvement with lymphocyte infiltration may be present. Lipid is abundant.

Lepromatous Type (LL). The granulomatous lesions in this type are composed chiefly of bacillus-laden histiocytes. These are the so-called *lepra cells* or *foam cells* of Virchow. The vacuoles contain lipids, fatty acids, and bacilli, which are either isolated or aggregated in globi. Between these foam cells are seen fibroblasts and a few lymphocytes, which become more abundant as the nodules or lesions become older. In the skin the infiltrate is localized in the dermis and is always separated from the epidermis by a well-defined clear grenz zone. Acid-fast bacilli are typically abundant. In the lepromatous type, degenerative changes with amyloid deposits may be seen in the liver, kidney, and spleen. The infiltrate contains predominantly T suppressor cells.

DIFFERENTIAL DIAGNOSIS. Fasal has called leprosy the "great imitator," since it has many atypical forms. When the differential diagnosis of the various forms is being determined, the following classification of Fasal may be considered:

Tuberculoid Type (TT). Tinea corporis, sarcoid, granuloma annulare, lichen planus, syphilis, drug eruptions, erythema multiforme, discoid lupus erythematosus, elastosis perforans, facial granuloma, lupus vulgaris, erythema nodosum, follicular mucinosis, and erythema induratum.

Borderline Type (BB). Pityriasis alba, tinea versicolor, seborrheic dermatitis, chloasma, berloque dermatitis, achromia perstans, and pellagra.

Lepromatous Type (LL). Mycosis fungoides, leishmaniasis, cystic acne vulgaris, Kaposi's sarcoma, neurofibromatosis, urticaria, lupus vulgaris, primary amyloidosis, gout, erythema dyschromicum perstans, yaws, and syringomyelia.

The coexistence of syphilis and leprosy, and of yaws and leprosy, has been difficult to determine since there is in lepromatous cases a high incidence, 30 to 60 per cent, of biologic false positive VDRL reactions. The TPI test and the FTA-ABS test are negative.

Lepra Reaction. During antileprosy treatment and also under other circumstances, reactions may occur. Three reactions are best known, namely, *acute exacerbation*, *reversal reaction*, and *erythema nodosum leprosum (ENL)*.

Acute exacerbation occurs at the sites of the largest and most active lesions. There is an exceptionally heavy bacterial load, and the histologic findings reveal a polymorphous infiltrate associated with mac-

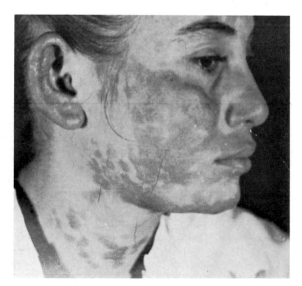

Figure 17–21. Acute erythema in lepra reaction in borderline (BL) leprosy.

rophage degeneration. This occurs only in lepromatous patients.

Reversal reactions may be of two types, one associated with increased cell-mediated immunity (upgrading) and the other with a decrease in cell-mediated immunity (downgrading). Upgrading consists of inflammation of existing lesions, often with ulceration. Neuritis may be severe and may lead to permanent scarring and loss of nerve function. Downgrading reactions lead to the appearance of new skin lesions, each less typically tuberculoid. Edema of the peripheral nerves may lead to sudden loss of function. A severe downgrading reaction occurring during griseofulvin therapy was reported by Shulman et al, who suggested that it might have been caused by the inhibition of polymorphonuclear chemotaxis by griseofulvin.

Erythema nodosum leprosum (ENL) is a lepra reaction which commonly shows a leucocytoclastic vasculitis. Its onset is commonly six months or more after treatment has been begun in lepromatous leprosy and in some instances of borderline leprosy. It may occur in untreated patients. The lesions are small erythematous nodules appearing in crops, which may leave the patient completely asymptomatic or may produce severe clinical expressions of fever, chills, malaise, myalgia, arthralgia, neuritis, and iritis. There may be visceral manifestations of hepatosplenomegaly, nephrosis, nephritis, orchitis, and pleuritis.

Pettit points out that in the past the sulfones have been implicated in eliciting ENL and that it has been mandatory to stop all antileprosy treatment. This view is no longer held, since ENL can occur prior to sulfone treatment; it does not occur until virtually all bacilli in the skin lesions are dead: the morphologic index (MI) is usually zero, and mouse footpad inoculation shows no viable organisms. The intensity of the reaction may vary from mild to severe and it may last from a few days to weeks, months, or even years.

The cause of acute exacerbation and ENL is attributed to a sensitization to the bacterial products released by the disintegration of the acid-fast bacilli in the host as a result of the development of immunity or of the bactericidal action of the sulfones.

Murphy et al studied four patients with ENL and found necrotizing vasculitis in all four, with electron-dense deposits in and around the basement membrane zone associated with circulating immune complexes.

The management of these reactions is with clofazimine, thalidomide, or corticosteroids. There is no indication for the cessation of antileprosy treatment.

DIAGNOSTIC PROCEDURES. Certain tests are helpful to the clinical findings for the diagnosis of leprosy. Most conclusive is the demonstration of acid-fast bacilli in smears from the skin lesions. Previously scrapings were also made from the nose; however, this is a reliable method only in experienced hands, since nonpathogenic acid-fast bacilli, difficult to distinguish from *M. leprae*, may be found in any nose. The bacterial index, or BI, determined from the tissue smear, indicates the abundance of organisms in a smear and is the mean score of the smears from a number of different lesions.

Tissue Smear. To make this test, cleanse the lesion with alcohol, dry, pinch the skin between the thumb and forefinger to blanch the area, and, maintaining pressure, make an incision of about 2 to 3 mm through the skin. With the scalpel at right angles to the cut, scrape the side to obtain a small specimen of fluid and cellular material. Spread this on a slide in a 1 cm diameter area, and dry the specimen in the air at room temperature. Place the slide in 10 per cent formalin for 15 minutes, then rinse in tap water.

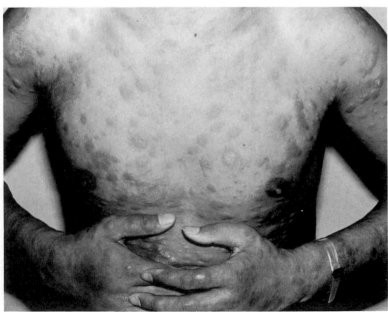

Figure 17–22. Erythema nodosum leprosum in a patient with "burned out" borderline lepromatous (BL) leprosy.

Stain in Ziehl-Neelsen's carbolfuchsin 20 minutes at room temperature, flooding the dye on the slide. Wash off excess dye in tap water and rinse in acid alcohol one minute; then rinse in tap water. Caution: *M. leprae* is destained much more readily than *M. tuberculosis*.

Counterstain in alkaline methylene blue for 10 seconds, rinse in tap water, dry in air. Use Permount and a coverslip for a permanent preparation.

Ziehl-Neelsen carbolfuchsin
    Basic fuchsin 0.4
    Phenol 5.0
    Alcohol 95 per cent 10.0
    Water q s ad 100.0

Acid alcohol
    Hydrochloric acid, conc. 2.0
    Alcohol 95 per cent q s ad 100.0

Alkaline methylene blue
    Sodium hydroxide 0.06
    Methylene blue 0.35
    Alcohol 95 per cent 16.0
    Water q s ad 100.0

Histamine Test. The histamine test is diagnostic of postganglionic nerve injury. A drop of 1:1000 solution of histamine diphosphate is put upon the skin of the test area, and another outside this area. A pin-prick is made through each drop. A wheal will form at each puncture, but the red flare that appears about the wheal in the unaffected area will not develop about the wheal in the test area if the intracutaneous nerves in it have been damaged. The flare may be difficult to see in dark-skinned people. In syringomyelia, the response is normal.

Methacholine Sweat Test. This test can be substituted in dark-skinned people in whom the histamine-induced flare cannot be seen. The sweat test demonstrates the absence of sweating in leprous lesions or, more importantly, its presence in nonleprous ones. In making this test, 0.1 ml of a 1 per cent solution of methacholine chloride (Mecholyl) is injected intradermally. The injections are made both inside and outside the test area, after the skin has been painted with Minor's solution (2 per cent iodine and 10 per cent castor oil in absolute alcohol). Powdered starch is then dusted over the parts. The starch granules are turned blue by the interaction of sweat and iodine. Methacholine and pilocarpine will not stimulate the denervated sweat glands in the skin lesions of leprosy; therefore, anhidrosis occurs, and there is no blue discoloration of the starch within the leprous lesions. In syringomyelia the sweat response is normal.

Skin Biopsy. This is the most important diagnostic procedure. A biopsy specimen which includes the entire dermis and the panniculus should be taken from the affected area and examined for morphology and for acid-fast bacilli. Bacilli are not usually seen in TT cases and are sparse in BT, but occasionally acid-fast granules are found.

The biopsy sections are also used to determine the *morphologic index* (MI) for evaluation of treatment efficacy. The MI is the number of viable bacilli (uniformly and solidly staining) per 100 bacilli found in leprous tissue. Dapsone is effective in the treatment, as Pettit points out, only if the MI becomes zero by the end of six months. If it is not, a sulfone-resistant infection is present and a change to a nonsulfone drug should be made. A successful drug substitution will be indicated by a rapid fall in the MI.

Skin Sensory Test. The entire skin area should be tested for the absence of tactile sense (anesthesia) and temperature sensations of heat and cold. In testing for anesthesia a wisp of cotton is used rather than a pin since it is touch and not pain that is to be tested. The patient closes his eyes and the cotton is touched lightly on various parts of his body. He responds by declaring that he feels the wisp touching his skin or, better yet, by pointing with his finger to the site that has been touched.

Temperature sensation is tested by touching the patient randomly in and outside of the lesions with warm and cold objects. In any TT or BT lesion, even a macule, the patient will regularly fail to identify the cold object correctly. In BL or LL cases, the lesions are seldom anesthetic but both feet, or hands and feet, may be.

Lepromin Test (Mitsuda Reaction). The lepromin test is an immunologic test indicative of host resistance to *M. leprae*. It is not a diagnostic test for leprosy, but rather is useful in estimating the resistance of the patient to the disease and in confirming the diagnosis of the *type* of the disease. It helps in this manner to predict the prognosis. It is used as a guide to treatment. If negative, the lepromin reaction suggests a lack of resistance to the disease; if positive, it indicates some degree of cell-mediated immunity, such as is seen in tuberculoid leprosy, and indicates a favorable prognosis. It should be noted that it is also positive in 50 to 90 per cent of normal persons over the age of 5 years.

Normally 0.1 ml of the bacillary suspension is injected intradermally into the forearm. The test is read after 48 hours for the early *Fernandez reaction* and again after three or four weeks for the delayed *Mitsuda reaction*. In over 90 per cent of patients with a positive Fernandez reaction, the Mitsuda reaction will be positive as well. However, 15 per cent of the negative early Fernandez reactions become positive by the late Mitsuda reaction.

A positive lepromin reaction is considered an index of resistance because the reaction is always negative in lepromatous leprosy. Patients with early disease showing a positive reaction have a favorable prognosis. Contacts with positive reactions usually do not acquire the disease and if they do it is likely to be of the tuberculoid type.

TREATMENT. Although the present treatment methods are not completely satisfactory, great strides have been made toward the development of effective antileprosy medication. Treatment is indicated in all forms of leprosy. There are six drugs or groups of drugs available to treat leprosy today.

DDS. Dapsone is the cornerstone of therapy, since it is effective, inexpensive, and relatively free of side effects in the doses given. The chief risks of sulfone therapy are methemoglobinemia, anemia, and leukopenia. The MI and BI are criteria used for determining the effectiveness of therapy. It is believed that the sulfones eliminate infectiousness after one to three months in patients with sensitive organisms. Because of the problem of dapsone-resistant organisms, combination drug therapy is standard; thus dapsone should always be given with the addition of at least one other drug. The dose is 100 mg daily in adults, from the start.

Rifampin. This drug is strongly bactericidal for *M. leprae* but should never be used as monotherapy, to avoid resistance. It has been shown to render LL cases noninfective for the mouse footpad by the seventh day of treatment. Untoward side effects are rarely encountered except in patients receiving concomitant therapy with ethionamide. Pattyn et al reported in 1984 that 4.5 per cent of a group of 596 patients with multibacillary leprosy who were given ethionamide, 500 mg daily, and rifampin, 600 mg daily, together with either clofazimine or dapsone, developed hepatitis, mostly with jaundice, in 5 to 186 days (mean 93, median, 76). Rifampin was given once weekly after the first two or eight weeks. Mortality was 26 per cent. The combination of rifampin with ethionamide was incriminated.

Clofazimine (Lamprene). This is a riminophenazine derivative which is bacteriostatic and antiinflammatory; thus it is useful both to treat the disease and in the management of reactive episodes. Lepromatous lesions in areas exposed to sunlight turn a red-brown to grayish blue color during therapy, and the color persists for months or years after treatment is stopped.

Ethionamide (Trecator-SC). This drug is intermediate in its bactericidal efficacy between rifampin and dapsone. It is used only as a combination drug, and side effects are common. They include gastrointestinal upset, hepatitis, hypotension, depression, and neuropathy.

Thiacetazone and the aminoglycosides are rarely used today, because of their toxicity.

MANAGEMENT. For paucibacillary cases—that is, patients with a BI of 1 + or 0 at all sites—the recommended therapy is dapsone, 100 mg daily, plus rifampin, 600 mg once monthly. This is continued for a minimum of six months. Many would treat for much longer periods, up to two to three years. For cases with known dapsone-resistant organisms, clofazimine, 100 mg daily, should be substituted for dapsone.

In multibacillary disease (with BI of 2 + or above at any site—BB, BL, or LL disease) dapsone, 100 mg daily, plus clofazimine, 50 mg daily, is given with rifampin, 600 mg once monthly. In dapsone-resistant cases the dapsone should be deleted. This should be given for a minimum of two years; however, many would treat for three to 10 years, with dapsone alone given by some for life.

These regimens are designed to give the patients at least two effective drugs. Ethionamide, 250 mg to 500 mg daily, may be substituted for clofazimine.

Several recent studies have investigated alternative therapies. Treatment of multibacillary leprosy with transfer factor, levamisole, BCG inoculation, transfusion of lymphocytes, and intravenous infusions of leukocytes has been tried. Martinez et al have reported dramatic success in two cases as a result of giving several intravenous infusions of leukocytes obtained by centrifuging one pint of whole blood, every week for 12 weeks. Both patients cleared clinically and improved in all objective parameters.

Zinc sulfate, 220 mg three times daily orally after meals, was given as an immunostimulant and antiinflammatory agent (together with dapsone) to 15 patients with multibacillary leprosy, and they all did decidedly better than controls receiving dapsone alone. Noteworthy was the benefit to patients with ENL.

Pure recombinant interferon-γ injected intradermally or intralesionally restored macrophage activity to normal at sites, and induced delayed-type hypersensitivity reactions, including diminution of bacillary load, in studies conducted by Nathan et al. These treatments are only of interest investigationally and are not recommended.

MANAGEMENT OF LEPRA REACTIONS. It is no longer regarded as necessary or even advisable to interrupt antileprosy medication because of lepra reaction. Reactions that begin soon after an increase of dosage of antileprosy drugs may be better managed if the dose is reduced somewhat, but in general one continues antileprosy treatment and manages the reaction in the usual ways.

Corticosteroids should be used in reversal reactions. They may be lifesaving in the severe cases. Therapy should be started with systemic steroids, either with triamcinolone acetonide intramuscularly (in the buttock), 60 mg once a week until control is achieved, and thereafter every four weeks if symptoms indicate that it is needed; or with prednisone given orally, 40 to 60 mg daily to start. Neuritis and eye lesions are urgent indications for systemic steroid therapy. Decrease or increase of this amount is determined by the clinical course of the reaction. Clofazimine is useful either as an alternative to corticosteroids or as a steroid-sparing drug. It is given in doses of 300 mg per day.

Thalidomide has been demonstrated to be uniquely effective against erythema nodosum leprosum and is the treatment of choice. Sheskin and Sagher have reported successful treatment in 91 per cent of 51 patients who experienced 173 episodes of lepra reaction. In a double-blind study Sheskin and Convit noted improvement in 92 per cent of the 59 patients they studied. Improvement was noted within eight to 48 hours, with only insignificant side effects. Dosage was 400 mg daily in patients over 50 kg of weight. In cases in which there is an acute episode of erythema nodosum leprosum the drug may be discontinued after two to three weeks. In chronic reactions, an attempt to discontinue the drug every six months should be made. Alternatively, corticosteroids, colchicine, or clofazimine may be used, but they are not as effective. Early results of trials with cyclosporin A have been encouraging, but the drug is still under investigation. Thalidomide is available only as an investigational drug in the United States because of its teratogenicity and neurotoxicity.

PROPHYLAXIS. Numerous workers have been concerned with preventive measures in leprosy. Several approaches have been made but none, including BCG vaccination, *M. leprae* bacterin vaccine, or prophylaxis with dapsone, is currently recommended.

Arnold HL Jr: Polar concept in leprosy (letter). Int J Lepr 1974, 42:459.

Idem: Differential diagnosis of leprosy. Cutis 1976, 18:53.

Baohong J, et al: The sensitivity and specificity of the fluorescent leprosy antibody absorption (FLA-ABS) test for detecting subclinical infection with *Mycobacterium leprae*. Lepr Rev 1984, 55:327.

Bechelli LM, et al: BCG vaccination of children against leprosy: 7-year findings of the controlled WHO trial in Burma. Bull WHO 1973, 48:323.

Binford CH, et al: Leprosy [comprehensive review]. JAMA 1982, 247:2283.

Browne SG: Indeterminate leprosy. Int J Dermatol 1985, 24:555.

Idem: Leprosy [comprehensive review]. Basle, Ciba-Geigy, 1984.

Brubaker ML, et al: Leprosy in children one year of age and under. Int J Lepr 1985, 53:517.

Duncan ME, et al: Clinical and immunologic study of 4 babies of mothers with lepromatous leprosy, two of whom developed leprosy in infancy. Int J Lepr 1983, 51:7.

Fasal P: But it was not leprosy! Cutis 1975, 15:499.

Fekete E, et al: Leprosy in 18-month-old children. Lepr Rev 1983, 54:61.

ffytche TJ, et al: Leprosy and the eye: a review. J R Soc Med 1985, 78:397.

Guillet G, et al: Leprosy in children. Ann Dermatol Venereol 1985, 112:353.

Haregewoin A, et al: T-cell–conditional media reverse T-cell unresponsiveness in lepromatous leprosy. Nature 1983, 303:342.

Hunter SW, et al: Structure and antigenicity of the major specific glycolipid antigen of *Mycobacterium leprae*. J Biol Chem 1982, 257:15072.

Jacobson RR: Hansen's disease drugs in use. The Star 1985, 44:1.

Jolliffe DS: Leprosy reactional states and their treatment. Br J Dermatol 1977, 97:345.

Karat ABA: Long-term follow-up of clofazimine (Lamprene) in management of reactive phases of leprosy. Lepr Rev 1975, 46:105.

Levinson AI, et al: Immunologic aspects of leprosy. Int J Dermatol 1977, 16:103.

Lim SD, et al: Leprosy CII. T cell subsets in lepromatous leprosy. Int J Dermatol 1982, 21:458.

Lumpkin LR III, et al: Leprosy in five armadillo handlers. JAAD 1983, 9:899.

Idem: Leprosy in armadillo handlers (letter). JAAD 1984, 10:1073.

Martinez MI, et al: Leprosy: weekly intravenous infusions of leukocytes. Int J Dermatol 1984, 23:341.

Mathur NK, et al: Oral zinc as an adjunct to dapsone in lepromatous leprosy. Int J Lepr 1984, 52:331.

Matsuo E, et al: Specific direct fluorescent antibody identification of *Mycobacterium leprae*. Int J Lepr 1975, 43:204.

Idem: Immunologic identification of *Mycobacterium leprae*: immunofluorescence and complement fixation. Int J Lepr 1976, 44:301.

Mehta V, et al: Lymphocyte suppression in leprosy induced by a unique *M. leprae* glycolipid. Nature 1984, 308:194.

Millikan LE, et al: Preliminary study of a *Mycobacterium leprae* bacterin in a human volunteer population in a nonendemic area. Int J Dermatol 1986, 25:245.

Modlin RL, et al: Leprosy: new insight into an ancient disease. JAAD 1987, 17:1.

Idem: Suppressor T lymphocytes from lepromatous leprosy skin lesions. J Immunol 1986, 137:2831.

Moschella SL: Leprosy today. Austral J Dermatol 1983, 24:47.

Murphy GF, et al: Erythema nodosum leprosum: nature and extent of the cutaneous microvascular alterations. JAAD 1986, 14:59.

Nathan CF, et al: Local and systemic effects of intradermal recombinant interferon gamma in lepromatous leprosy. N Engl J Med 1986, 315:6.

Nogueira N, et al: Defective gamma interferon production in leprosy: reversal with antigen and interleukin-2. J Exp Med 1983, 158:2165.

Pattyn SR, et al: Hepatotoxicity of rifampin-ethionamide in treatment of multibacillary leprosy. Int J Lepr 1984, 52:1.

Piepkorn M, et al: Auricular chondritis as a rheumatologic manifestation of Lucio's phenomenon: clinical improvement after plasmapheresis. Ann Intern Med 1983, 98:49.

Rea TH, et al: Lucio's phenomenon and diffuse non-nodular lepromatous leprosy. Arch Dermatol 1976, 114:1023.

Idem, et al: Immunologic responses in patients with lepromatous leprosy. Arch Dermatol 1976, 112:791.

Ridley DS, et al: Classification of leprosy according to immunity. Int J Lepr 1966, 34:255.

Ridley DS: Skin biopsy in leprosy. Basle, Ciba-Geigy Ltd, 1977.

Ridley MJ, et al: Immunopathology of erythema nodosum leprosum. Lepr Rev 1983, 54:95.

Saul A, et al: Medina's reaction. Rev Mex Dermatol 1967, 11:17.

Scharf MO, et al: Widespread eruption in a patient from Haiti. Arch Dermatol 1986, 122:1435.

Sehgal VN, et al: Histoid leprosy. Int J Dermatol 1985, 24:286.

Idem: Correlation of morphological, bacteriological, histopathological and immunological features of leprosy. J Dermatol 1985, 12:243.

Idem: Status of histoid leprosy. J Dermatol 1987, 14:38.

Sheskin J: Thalidomide in the lepra reaction. Int J Dermatol 1975, 14:575.

Shulman DG: Leprosy downgrading reaction associated with griseofulvin. Arch Dermatol 1982, 118:909.

Skinsnes OK, et al: Liberated intracellular pathogen—leprosy model. Acta Leprol 1984, 2:195.

Idem: In vitro cultivation of leprosy bacilli in hyaluronic acid based medium. Preliminary report. Int J Lepr 1975, 43:193.

Spickett SG: Genetics and epidemiology of leprosy. Lepr Rev 1962, 53:76.

Tausk F, et al: Leprosy: altered complement receptors in disseminated disease. J Invest Dermatol 1985, 85(Suppl):585.

Uyemura K, et al: Effect of cyclosporin A in erythema nodosum leprosum. J Immunol 1986, 137:3620.

VanEden W, et al: HLA-linked control of predisposition to lepromatous leprosy. J Infect Dis 1985, 151:9.

VanVoorhis W, et al: Cutaneous infiltrates of leprosy. N Engl J Med 1982, 307:1593.

Weddell AGMcD: New challenge to old concepts about leprosy. Med World News 1963, pp 101–103.

Wolf RH, et al: Experimental leprosy in three species of monkeys. Science 1985, 227:529.

Yawalkar SJ, et al: Monthly rifampin plus daily dapsone in initial treatment of lepromatous leprosy. Lancet 1982, I:1199.

18

Syphilis, Yaws, Bejel, and Pinta

SYPHILIS

Syphilis, once known as lues, is a contagious, sexually transmitted disease, leading to cutaneous and internal organic lesions; it is caused by the spirochete *Treponema pallidum*. Syphilis is a potentially lifelong disease. It is one of the chronic infectious granulomas. The infection enters through the skin or mucous membranes, on which the early manifestations are also observed. In congenital syph-ilis the treponeme crosses the placenta and infects the fetus.

With the advent of HIV-infected patients, many treatment recommendations have been altered. All patients with early syphilis should be tested for HIV infection because of their increased risk of exposure to the virus and because of their erratic serologic parameters and response to treatment.

STAGES IN THE DISEASE

Early syphilis, which lasts up to two years, comprises primary syphilis, secondary syphilis, and early latent syphilis.

Primary syphilis is manifest only as the chancre, or primary sore, which appears at the site of entry of the spirochete about three weeks after exposure, and the regional lymphadenopathy (bubo) which always accompanies it. The serologic test for syphilis (STS) usually becomes positive during this stage.

Secondary syphilis is characterized by a succession of increasingly conspicuous generalized eruptions, beginning usually three to six weeks after the chancre appears; they may overlap with it. There is accompanying generalized shotty lymphadenopathy, and mucosal lesions usually occur as well. The STS is invariably positive, in rapidly rising titer, except in HIV-infected patients, in whom the serologic response is unpredictable. Hicks et al reported seronegative secondary syphilis in such a patient; the diagnosis was made only by demonstrating *Trepo-*

nema pallidum in a biopsy from a characteristic lesion. Contagiousness is highest in this stage.

Throughout this early phase, moist lesions are infectious for others, and the potential for contagion is present even when lesions are not seen.

Latent syphilis is manifested solely by a positive STS, with no detectable clinical manifestations, and normal spinal fluid.

Late syphilis comprises late latent syphilis and tertiary syphilis.

Tertiary syphilis, occurring anywhere from three to 60 years after infection, manifests a wide spectrum of destructive lesions which have in common ischemic infarcts caused by syphilis of small blood vessels. In the skin, increasingly localized, asymmetrically distributed ulcers called *gummas* are produced; in the aorta, *aortitis* progressing to the point of producing an *aneurysm*; in the bones, *periostitis* and *osteomyelitis*; in the central nervous system, *gumma, asymptomatic neurosyphilis, meningovascular neurosyphilis, tabes dor-*

405

salis, or *paresis*; and so on. The VDRL slide test is positive in approximately 75 per cent of cases in this stage. Infectiousness is virtually nil, even for a fetus.

Progression to neurosyphilis may be rapid, over a few months, in HIV-infected patients.

The various stages may overlap somewhat, and are not perfectly mutually exclusive, but they are a useful clinical guide to the underlying pathologic processes. In fetal syphilis the timetable is compressed from years to months, roughly speaking.

Fetal infection with syphilis is probable if the mother acquires syphilis during pregnancy and remains untreated. Fetal infection may also occur if the mother was inadequately treated for early acquired syphilis. The newborn infected with syphilis may be symptomatic or stigmatized at birth or develop symptoms only later. An asymptomatic neonate with reactive serologic tests for syphilis may have incubating disease, may have been infected but treated in utero, or may have only passive transfer of maternal antibodies without infection. Neonates with signs such as rash, nasal discharge, hepatosplenomegaly, or sepsis may be suspected of having syphilis.

ETIOLOGY. *Treponema pallidum* was discovered by Schaudinn and Hoffman in 1905. It is a delicate spiral spirochete, which is actively motile. The number of spirals varies from four to 14 and the entire length is 5 to 20 μ. With high magnification, granules are clearly shown within the protoplasm and tufts of long flagella are seen.

It is usually demonstrated in wet preparations from fresh primary or secondary lesions by darkfield microscopy or by fluorescent antibody techniques. The motility is characteristic, consisting of three movements: a projection in the direction of the long axis, a rotation of the spiral on its long axis, and a bending or twisting from side to side. The precise uniformity of the spiral coils is not distorted during these movements. Nevertheless, it cannot be distinguished from *Treponema macrodentium* or *microdentium*, so that darkfield examination of mouth lesions is untrustworthy regardless of the result.

The electron microscope shows the organism to have an axial filament with several fibrils, a protoplasmic cylinder, and a thin membranaceous envelope called the periplast.

The organism is pathogenic for the anthropoid apes and produces a primary sore and secondary skin eruption closely simulating the disease in man. It is also pathogenic for rabbits.

INCIDENCE AND PREVALENCE. Syphilis is still a major problem throughout the world despite the great strides made in its control.

Various health departments have developed extensive and thorough case-finding methods. Their responsibilities consist of the investigation of sex contacts of patients who have recently acquired syphilis and also the investigation of other persons who have been discovered to have reactive tests for syphilis. It is estimated that 38 million serologic tests for syphilis are performed yearly in the United States. It is the task of health department workers to ferret out the sources of syphilis infections.

CUTANEOUS SYPHILIS

Chancre (Primary Stage)

CLINICAL FEATURES. The chancre is usually the first cutaneous lesion, appearing 18 to 21 days following infection. The typical incipient chancre is a small red papule or a crusted superficial erosion, which in the course of a few weeks becomes round or oval, decidedly indurated, and slightly elevated, with an eroded but not ulcerated surface which exudes a serous fluid. On palpation between two fingers, a cartilage-hard consistency is sensed. The lesion is usually—but not invariably—painless. This is an uncomplicated so-called *Hunterian chancre*. The regional lymph nodes on one or both sides are usually enlarged, firm, and nontender, the enlargement as a rule beginning a week or two after the appearance of the chancre. Being an erosion and not an ulcer, the Hunterian chancre leaves no scar when it heals.

Chancres generally occur singly, although they may be multiple; they vary in diameter from a few millimeters to several centimeters. In women the genital chancre is seldom observed because of its location within the vagina or on the cervix; when found, it is generally a small erosion. Extensive edema of the labia or cervix may occur. In men the chancre is common in the coronal sulcus or on either side of the frenum. A lesion at the frenum always strongly suggests a chancre. A chancre in the prepuce, being too hard to bend, will flip over all at once when the prepuce is drawn back, a phenomenon termed in New England a "dory flop," from the resemblance to the movement of a broad-beamed skiff or dory as it is being turned upside down.

Intraurethral primary lesions are not uncommon and may be found in early secondary cases when the chancre is not discovered. Intraurethral chancre gen-

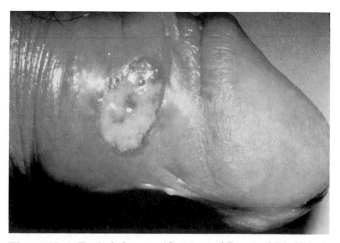

Figure 18–1. *Typical chancre. (Courtesy of Dr. Axel W. Hoke.)*

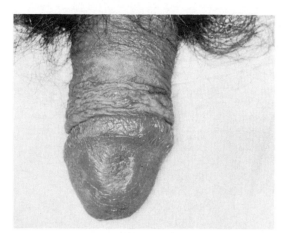

Figure 18–2. Chancre of glans penis.

erally causes a slight serosanguinous or purulent discharge at the meatus and an induration that may be palpated through the shaft of the penis.

Extragenital chancres are likely to be larger than those on the genitals. A frequent location of extragenital primary lesions is on the lips, where the inoculation has taken place through kissing or fellating an infected individual. They appear rarely in other locations, the most important sites being the tongue, tonsil, female breast, index finger and, especially in male homosexuals, the anus. Regional lymphadenopathy accompanies these chancres. When there is a florid secondary eruption, and no evidence of chancre, and the glands below Poupart's ligament are markedly enlarged, anal chancre should be strongly suspected. The presenting complaints for

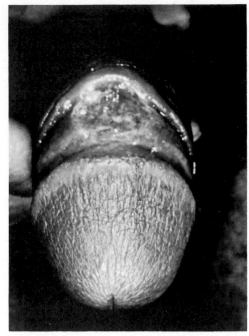

Figure 18–4. Chancre near coronal sulcus.

the chancre of the anal region are "lump" in the anus, "piles," irritation on defecation, "sore" on the anus, or bleeding.

VARIETIES OF THE CHANCRE. Simultaneous infection by a spirochete and some other microbial agent may produce an atypical chancre.

Mixed Chancre (Mixed Sore). Infection by the

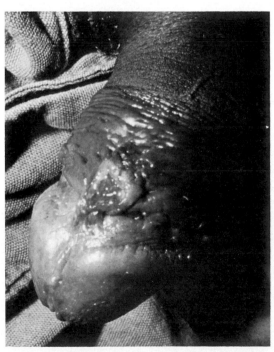

Figure 18–3. Chancre of frenulum. (Courtesy of Dr. Axel W. Hoke.)

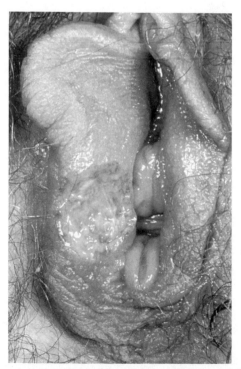

Figure 18–5. Chancre of labium minus. (Courtesy of Dr. Axel W. Hoke.)

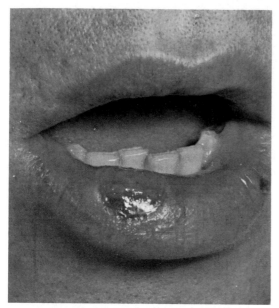

Figure 18–6. Chancre on lower lip.

Ducrey bacillus and *T. pallidum* at the same time will produce a "mixed sore," which runs a course different from either chancroid or primary syphilis alone. Such a sore begins a few days after exposure, as the incubation period for chancroid is short, and later the sore may become transformed into an indurated syphilitic lesion.

Phagedenic Chancre. The combination of the syphilitic chancre and contaminating cocci may cause severe tissue destruction. Such lesions are called phagedenic.

Multiple Chancres. These are uncommonly encountered. Parounagian exhibited a patient with 15 primary lesions.

Edema Indurativum. Marked solid edema of the labia or the prepuce and glans penis may accompany the chancre.

Chancre Redux. Because of insufficient treatment the chancre may relapse after partial disappearance; it is then accompanied by enlarged lymph nodes and the presence of numerous spirochetes at the site of recurrence. Such reappearance is termed *monorecidive* or chancre redux.

Pseudochancre Redux. This is a gumma occurring at the site of a previous chancre. It is distinguished from relapsing chancre chiefly by the absence of satellite glands and by a negative darkfield examination.

Syphilis d'emblée. Syphilis may begin without a chancre—syphilis *d'emblée.* Such cases usually arise from puncture wounds or from transfusion of infected blood. In women especially, it is not rare for a chancre to escape notice.

HISTOPATHOLOGY. From the beginning syphilis affects the blood vessels. The intima of the veins and arteries proliferates and thickens, as does the adventitia. In examining tissues for syphilis one studies the blood vessels first. The lesions tend to be "perivascular and very vascular."

The chancre is the prototype of other syphilitic lesions: it is characterized by a dense infiltration of round cells and plasma cells. An arteritis of the deep cutaneous vessels is present, which begins with the proliferation of the endothelial cells of the intima and progresses until all coats are involved and the vessel is obliterated. The infiltration is at first limited to the proximity of the vessels, forming collarettes about them. Later it becomes diffuse, filling the entire field in a uniform manner, except at the edges of the lesion, where it is chiefly perivascular. In the central portion of the lesion ulceration may occur, while at the margins there may be slight acanthosis.

IMMUNE RESPONSES. A broad-spectrum humoral immune response involving IgG and 19S IgM occurs early in the disease and operates at high titers, but is ineffective. In a carefully controlled study, Gschnait et al showed that regardless of the stage, leukocyte migration inhibition is absent, and remains absent until treatment is begun; within two days it begins, and rises to a maximum at one week.

DIAGNOSIS. In the patient who presents with an acute genital ulceration, a darkfield examination should be done if this investigation is available.

Does a positive finding establish the diagnosis? *T. pertenue,* which causes yaws, and *T. carateum,* which causes pinta, are both indistinguishable morphologically from *T. pallidum*; but the diseases that they produce are usually easy to recognize. Other spirochetes may be confused with *T. pallidum* in lesions about the mouth. *T. microdentium,* a common inhabitant of the mouth, is often indistinguishable from *T. pallidum* even by the most expert, but it is not found in genital or extragenital chancres, except those on the lips or mouth. A finding of typical *T. pallidum* by an experienced darkfield microscopist in a sore on the cutaneous surface establishes a diagnosis of syphilis beyond a reasonable doubt.

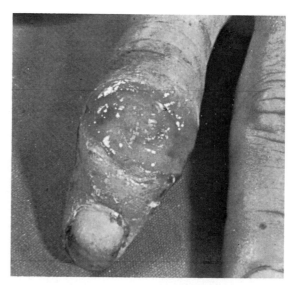

Figure 18–7. Chancre of finger. (Courtesy of Dr. S. Olansky.)

If the darkfield examination is negative or cannot be done, the clinical history and physical findings must be depended upon for diagnosis in the office. From an epidemiologic standpoint, treatment with 2.4 million units of benzathine penicillin G in suspected cases is indicated. The benefits and risks of this type of therapy need to be weighed relative to each individual patient from a practical standpoint. Biopsy findings and serologic testing may aid in the diagnosis.

Specimen. The lesion selected for examination is cleansed with water and dried. It is grasped firmly between the thumb and index finger and abraded sufficiently to cause clear or faintly blood-stained plasma to exude on squeezing. In case of an eroded chancre a few vigorous rubs with dry gauze are usually sufficient. If the lesion is made to bleed it is necessary to wait until free bleeding has stopped to obtain satisfactory plasma.

The surface of a clean coverslip is touched to the surface of the lesion so that plasma adheres. Then it is dropped on a thin clean slide and pressed down so that the plasma spreads out in as thin a film as possible.

Immunofluorescent Technique for Demonstrating T. pallidum. An alternative to darkfield microscopy is the direct fluorescent antibody test (DFATP) for the identification of *T. pallidum* in lesions. In this method, the lesion is prepared by removing tissue debris and cleansing with saline. After the area is dried, serum is obtained by abrading and squeezing the lesion. This serum is applied to a slide and allowed to dry, then stained with fluorescein-labeled antibody to *T. pallidum*. Fluorescence of a spirochete on the slide is judged to be a positive result. Since the antibody has been absorbed with nonpathogenic treponemes, the method is specific for *T. pallidum* and, unlike the darkfield examination, can be used for material from oral lesions.

The great advantage is that a chancre may be diagnosed by sending the exudate from the chancre to the laboratory, thus obviating the necessity of an immediate darkfield examination.

DIFFERENTIAL DIAGNOSIS. The chancre must be differentiated from *chancroid*. The chancre has an incubation period of three weeks; is usually a painless erosion, not an ulcer; has no surrounding inflammatory zone; and is round or oval in shape. The edge is not undermined. The surface is smooth and at the level of the skin. It has a dark, velvety red, lacquered appearance, is without a membrane, and is cartilage-hard on palpation. Lymphadenopathy is usually bilateral. It is usually a single lesion and the spirochete is demonstrable in the serum. Chancroid, on the other hand, has a short incubation period of one to three days; the ulcer is acutely inflamed, is extremely painful, and has a large surrounding inflammatory zone. The ulcer edge is undermined and the ulcer extends into the dermis. It has a yellowish red color, is covered by a membrane, and is soft to the touch. Lymphadenopathy is usually unilateral with severe inflammation, and the glands ulcerate. The lesions are usually multiple and extend into each other. The Ducrey bacillus is found in the smear.

However, since a combination of chancre and chancroid ("mixed sore") is indistinguishable from chancroid alone, appropriate direct and serologic testing should be done to investigate for the presence of syphilis.

The primary lesion of *granuloma inguinale* begins as an indurated nodule which erodes to produce hypertrophic, vegetative granulation tissue. It is soft, beefy-red and bleeds readily. A smear of clean granulation tissue from the lesion stained with Wright's or Giemsa's stain reveals Donovan bodies in the cytoplasm of macrophages.

The primary lesion of *lymphogranuloma venereum* is usually a small, painless, transient vesicle or superficial nonindurated ulcer, and most commonly occurs on the coronal sulcus, prepuce, or glans in men, or on the fourchette, vagina, or cervix in women. A primary genital lesion is noticed by about 30 per cent of infected heterosexual men, but less frequently in women. Primary lesions are followed in seven to 30 days by adenopathy of the regional lymph nodes. The LGV complement fixation test (LGV-CFT) is 90 to 95 per cent sensitive and can be titrated, which enhances its value.

Herpes simplex begins with grouped vesicles, often accompanied by burning pain. After rupture of the vesicles, lobulated irregular soft erosions form. Only rarely are the regional lymph nodes involved.

The extragenital chancre may be much more difficult to differentiate. The lip and tongue chancres strongly resemble *epidermoid carcinoma*.

When the female nipple is infected, *Paget's disease* must be considered. On the finger the chancre may resemble a pyogenic granuloma. A positive darkfield examination settles the question. A negative one should be followed by biopsy.

COURSE OF THE CHANCRE. If left untreated, the chancre tends to heal spontaneously in one to four months. About the time of its disappearance, or usually a little before, constitutional symptoms and objective signs of generalized (secondary) syphilis occur.

Syphilids

The skin manifestations of secondary syphilis are called *syphilids*. These occur in 80 per cent of cases. The early eruptions are symmetrical, more or less generalized, superficial, nondestructive, exanthematic, transient, macular roseolas; later they are maculopapular or papular eruptions, which are usually polymorphous, and less often scaly, pustular, or pigmented. The early manifestations are apt to be distributed over the face, shoulders, flanks, palms and soles, and anal or genital regions. The severity varies widely in different cases. The presence of

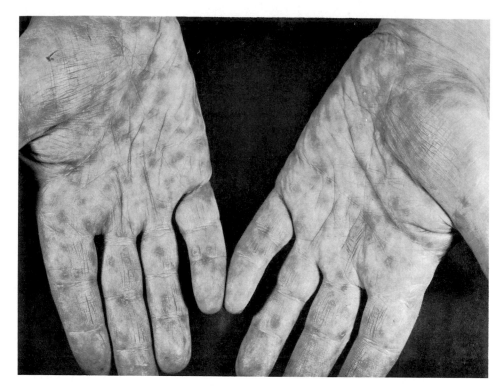

Figure 18–8. Typical palmar macules of early syphilis. (Courtesy of Dr. H. Shatin.)

lesions on the palms and soles is strongly suggestive. However, Baum et al reported four patients with a generalized syphilid which spared the palms and soles.

The individual lesions are generally less than a centimeter in diameter, except in the later secondary eruptions or in relapsing secondary eruptions. The macular lesions are characterized by a light pink color, which soon becomes brownish red, the tints being influenced by the amount of pigment and other qualities of the patient's skin. The color of the papular lesions has often been described as a *raw ham* color or a *coppery* tint.

MACULAR ERUPTIONS. The syphilids begin in sidiously with the appearance of an exanthematic roseola six to eight weeks after the development of the chancre, which may still be present or may have healed. The syphilitic exanthem extends rapidly, so that it is usually pronounced a few days after onset. It may be evanescent, lasting only a few hours or days, or it may last several months, or partially recur after having disappeared. This earliest eruption is macular and appears first on the sides of the trunk, about the navel, and the inner surfaces of the extremities. Of special importance is the appearance of slightly scaling "ham-colored" macules on the palms and soles.

The *roseola* consists of rounded indistinct macules

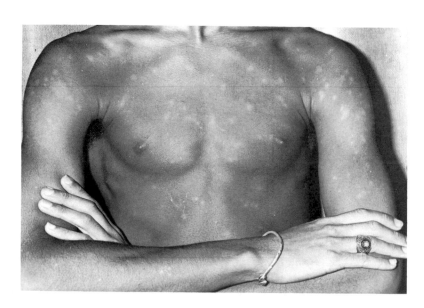

Figure 18–9. Early syphilis.

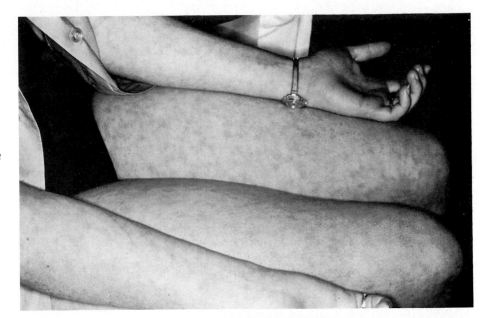

Figure 18–10. *Livedo reticularis as a manifestation of secondary syphilis.*

that are nonconfluent and may rarely be slightly elevated or urticarial. The color varies from a light pink, or old rose, to reddish brown. The macular eruption is seldom noticed in blacks and is so faint that it is frequently not recognized in others, although it is the commonest of the syphilids. The lesions are sometimes conspicuous, forming eruptions so characteristic that diagnosis is self-evident to even the casual observer. Pain, burning, and itching are usually absent, although recent reports indicate pruritus may be present in 10 to 20 per cent of cases. Simultaneous with the onset of the roseola there is a generalized shotty adenopathy most readily palpable in the posterior cervical, axillary, and epitrochlear areas. In men a primary lesion may be present.

The macular eruption may disappear spontaneously after a few days or weeks without any residuum, or may result in postinflammatory hyperpigmentation. After a varying interval the roseola may be followed by other eruptions.

Rarely, secondary syphilis may cause livedo reticularis.

Papular Syphilid. The papular types of eruption usually arise a little later than the macular. The most common and also the most easily recognized is the *lenticular papular syphilid.* The fully developed lesions are of a raw-ham or coppery shade, round, and from 2 to 5 mm or more in diameter. They are often only slightly raised, but a deep firm infiltration is palpable. The surface is smooth, sometimes shiny, at other times covered with a thick adherent scale. When this desquamates, it leaves a characteristic collarette of scales overhanging the border of the papule.

Papules are frequently distributed on the face and flexures of the arms and lower legs, but are often distributed all over the trunk. Palmar and plantar involvement characteristically appears as rather dusky yellowish red spots that on palpation are found to be deeply infiltrated. *Ollendorf's sign* is present: the papule is exquisitely tender to the touch of a blunt probe. As the infiltration and redness disappear they frequently leave pigmented spots which, especially on the palms and soles, may persist for weeks or months.

Split papules are hypertrophic and fissured papules that form in the creases of the alae nasi and at the oral commissures. These may persist for a long period.

The **papulosquamous syphilids** are lesions of somewhat the same character in which the adherent scales covering the lesions more or less dominate the picture, sometimes to the extent of producing a psoriasiform eruption.

Follicular or lichenoid syphilids occur much less

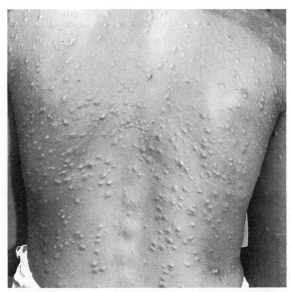

Figure 18–11. *Papular syphilid. (Courtesy of Dr. S. Olansky.)*

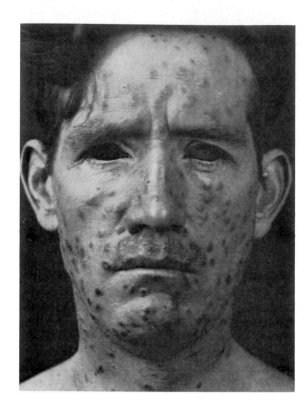

Figure 18–12. Large-papular syphiloderm.

Figure 18–13. Typical papulosquamous syphilid of the palms.

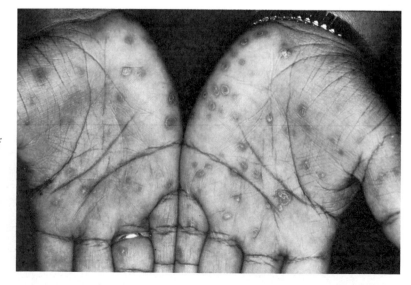

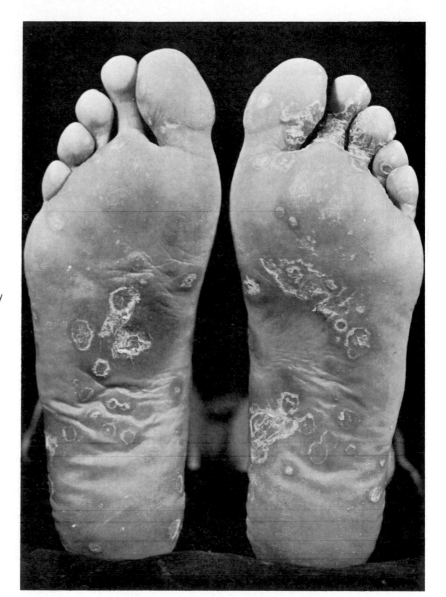

Figure 18–14. Papulosquamous syphilid in early syphilis. (Courtesy of Dr. H. Shatin.)

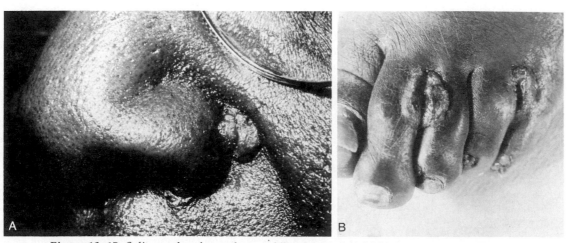

Figure 18–15. Split papules of secondary syphilis. A, nasolabial fold. B, interdigital lesions.

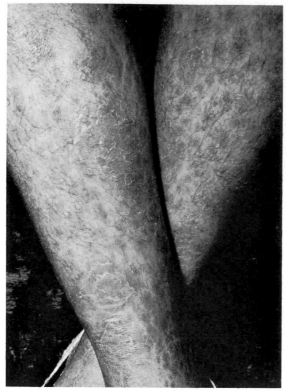

Figure 18–16. *Squamous lesions of early secondary syphilis on the legs of a 26-year-old woman.*

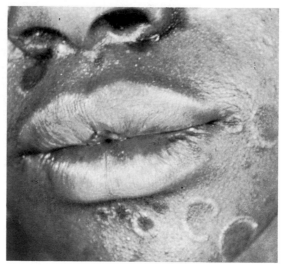

Figure 18–18. *Annular secondary syphilid of the face. Note the dryness and nonscaling nature distinguishing it from impetigo. (Courtesy of Dr. S. Olansky.)*

frequently and are more deceptive in appearance. They occur as minute scale-capped papules. If at the mouths of hair follicles, they are apt to be conical; elsewhere on the skin, domed. Often they are grouped to form scaling plaques, in which the minute component papules are still discernible.

Like the other syphilids, papular eruptions tend to be disseminated in the early course of the disease and later become more or less localized, often asymmetric, configurate, hypertrophic, or confluent. Grouping is a diagnostic aid of great value. The arrangement may be corymbose or in patches, rings, or serpiginous patterns.

The **annular syphilid**, like sarcoidosis, which it may mimic, is curiously common in blacks. It is often located on the cheeks, especially close to the angle of the mouth. Here it may form in circles and at

times in arcs and gyrate patterns of delicate, slightly raised, infiltrated, finely scaling ridges. The ridges are made up of minute flat-topped papules, the boundaries between which may be difficult to discern. An old term for annular syphilids was "nickels and dimes."

The **corymbose syphilid** is another infrequent variant, usually occurring late in the secondary stage, in which a large central papule is surrounded by a group of minute satellite papules.

The **pustular syphilids** are among the rarer manifestations of secondary syphilis. They occur widely scattered over the trunk and extremities, but usually

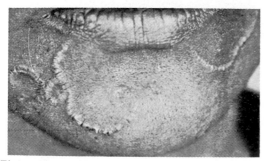

Figure 18–17. *Annular eruption in secondary syphilis.*

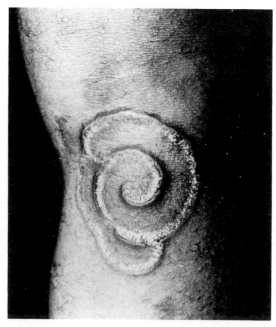

Figure 18–19. *An unusual morphologic lesion of secondary syphilis.*

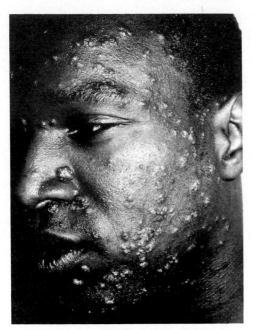

Figure 18–20. Pustular syphilid.

involve the face, especially the forehead. The pustule usually arises on a red, infiltrated base. Involution is usually slow, resulting in a small, rather persistent, crust-covered, superficial ulceration. Lesions in which the ulceration is deep are spoken of as ecthymatous. Closely related is the **rupial syphilid**, a lesion in which a relatively superficial ulceration is covered with a pile of terraced crusts resembling an oyster shell.

Lues maligna is a rare form of secondary syphilis with severe ulcerations, pustules, or rupioid cutaneous lesions. The skin and mucous membranes have irregularly distributed large pustules and deep ulcerations, accompanied by severe constitutional symptoms. Bahmer et al reported such a case, in which electronmicrographic studies showed a picture suggestive of an exaggerated immune response, rather than a deficient one.

Condyloma latum is a papular lesion, relatively broad and flat, located on folds of moist skin, especially about the anus and the genitals; it may become hypertrophic and, instead of infiltrating deeply, protrude above the surface, forming a soft, red, often mushroomlike mass 1 to 3 cm in diameter, and usually with a smooth, moist, weeping surface. It may be lobulated but is not covered by the digitate elevations characteristic of venereal wart (condyloma acuminatum). This latter lesion is a true verruca and is caused by the human papillomavirus.

Alopecia syphilitica of the eyebrows, beard, and scalp may occur with these cutaneous manifestations. Alopecia in the scalp is irregularly distributed so that the scalp has a *moth-eaten appearance*. The nails likewise may be involved, either from local inflammation due to the treponema, from suppuration, or from constitutional derangement.

Leukoderma colli may appear, especially in

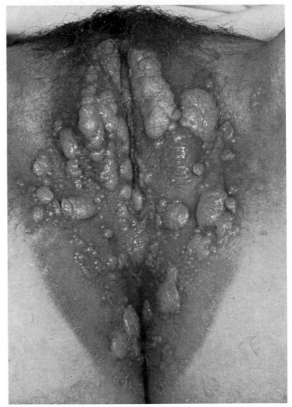

Figure 18–21. Condylomata lata on the labia. (Courtesy of Dr. S. Olansky.)

women, coincident with the appearance of the macular eruption or within several months following it on the chin, the sides and back of the neck, and, more rarely, on other parts. Most often there are variously sized, small, round or oval, ill-defined, depigmented spots surrounded by hyperpigmented areolae, so that a dappled appearance ("collar of pearls") results. Although of syphilitic causation, the

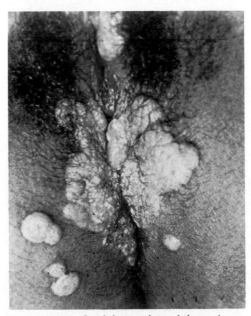

Figure 18–22. Condylomata lata of the perineum.

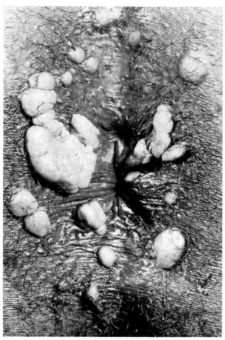

Figure 18–23. Perianal condylomata lata in early syphilis. (Courtesy of Dr. H. Shatin.)

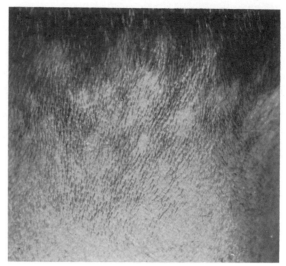

Figure 18–25. Moth-eaten alopecia of early syphilis. (Courtesy of Dr. F. Kerdel-Vegas, Venezuela.)

leukoderma is usually not responsive to antisyphilitic remedies and persists indefinitely.

Mucous membrane lesions are present in one third of patients with secondary syphilis. The most common mucosal lesion in the early phase is the **syphilitic sore throat**, a *diffuse pharyngitis* which may be associated with *tonsillitis* or *laryngitis*. Hoarseness and sometimes complete aphonia may be present. After the earliest generalized eruptions there may appear desquamating patches on the tongue analogous to the papular eruption on the skin. Such patches are usually on the dorsum near the median raphe and consist of one or several small or large, smooth, well-defined areas devoid of papillae.

The **mucous patch** is the best known and most characteristic mucous membrane lesion, which may accompany the eruptions of the intermediary period but is not observed in the early stages. Mucous patches, which are macerated papules, appear as flat, grayish, rounded erosions covered by a delicate, soggy membrane. These lesions are about 5 mm in diameter and teem with treponemata, so that they are very infectious. They occur on the tonsils, tongue, and pharynx and also on the gums, lips, and buccal areas, or about the genitalia, chiefly in women. In the latter location they are most common on the labia minora, the vaginal mucosa, and the cervix. Such mucous erosions are transitory and change from week to week, or even from day to day.

Ulcerations often occur on the tongue and lips during the late secondary period.

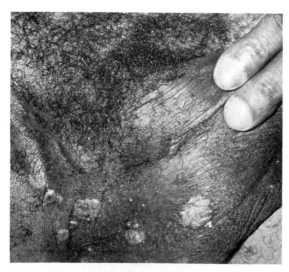

Figure 18–24. Condyloma latum of secondary syphilis on the scrotum.

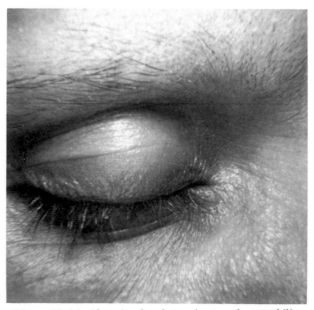

Figure 18–26. Alopecia of eyebrows in secondary syphilis.

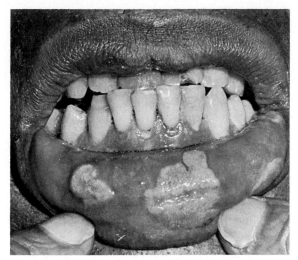

Figure 18–27. Mucous patches on inner lip.

The **lymphatic system** in secondary syphilis is characteristically involved. The lymph nodes most frequently affected are the inguinal, the posterior cervical, the postauricular, and the epitrochlear. The nodes are "shotty"—firm, very slightly enlarged, nontender, and discrete.

Fever of Unknown Origin. Rarely, fever of undetermined origin may occur as a manifestation of syphilis. Chung et al reported such a case, with an eight-month history of diarrhea, weight loss, nausea, and a generalized itchy papular rash sparing the palms and soles. The diarrhea responded to metronidazole, but only when a positive STS was discovered, and penicillin given, did the rest of the symptoms resolve.

Systemic Involvement. Acute membranous glomerulonephritis, gastropathy, proctitis, hepatitis, acute meningitis, sensorineural hearing loss, iritis, anterior uveitis, optic neuritis, Bell's palsy, multiple nodular infiltrates of the lung bases, periostitis, osteomyelitis, polyarthritis, or tenosynovitis may all be seen in secondary syphilis.

HISTOPATHOLOGY. The roseola and other cutaneous eruptions of the secondary stage show vary-

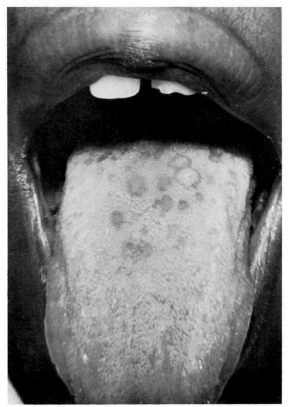

Figure 18–29. Mucous patches on the tongue. (Courtesy of Dr. S. Olansky.)

ing degrees of perivascular infiltration consisting chiefly of lymphocytes and plasma cells. Plasma cells are almost always present.

In the later secondary eruptions large multinucleated cells, as well as degenerative changes in the vessel walls, may be seen. The epidermal changes vary widely, particularly in late secondary lesions. The vessels are dilated and there is a panarteritis.

The papular lesions show superficial and deep vessel involvement, with endothelial swelling of the vessel wall and with a marked perivascular infiltrate. Direct fluorescent antibody staining (the Steiner stain) and Warthin-Starry silver stains will be positive and may serve to document the diagnosis in HIV-positive patients with an erratic serologic response, such as the patient reported by Hicks et al.

McNeely et al studied four patients with early secondary lesions and found evidence for circulating immune complexes in all four. Three showed a neutrophilic vascular reaction in early lesions; all had this histology after histamine injection into the skin.

DIAGNOSIS. A positive diagnosis of secondary syphilis is made when the *T. pallidum* can be demonstrated from the skin lesions. Most early lesions teem with spirochetes; however, the spirochetes can best be demonstrated from the moist lesions.

The STS is invariably strongly reactive. An exception occurs when very high titers of antibody are present. This may produce a false negative ("prozone") result. The true positivity of the serum is

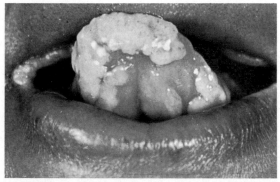

Figure 18–28. Condylomata lata of the tongue in secondary syphilis. These lesions may have started as mucous patches. (Courtesy of Dr. S. Olansky.)

detected upon dilutional testing. Also, Hicks et al documented a case of seronegative secondary syphilis in a patient with AIDS. HIV-infected patients have variable serologic responses. In addition to the lesions of the mucous membranes and the skin, there may be a history of a chancre, and signs and symptoms of the systemic illness. These contribute to the diagnosis, which is positively established by the demonstration of the spirochete under the darkfield microscope or by a positive STS, or both.

DIFFERENTIAL DIAGNOSIS. Syphilis has long been known as the "great imitator" because the various cutaneous manifestations may simulate almost any cutaneous or systemic disease.

Pityriasis rosea may be mistaken for secondary syphilis, especially since both begin on the trunk; however, the herald patch, the oval patches in the line of skin cleavage, the absence of lymphadenopathy, and infrequent mucous membrane lesions help to clinically distinguish pityriasis rosea from secondary syphilis. The presence of itching greatly favors pityriasis rosea.

Drug eruptions may produce a similar picture; however, they tend to be scarlatiniform or morbilliform. A history of drug intake may help to differentiate them from syphilis. Drug eruptions are often somewhat pruritic, as opposed to secondary syphilis.

Streptococcal pharyngitis may simulate secondary syphilis. The high fever, the diffuse and generalized scarlatiniform eruption, and the short and acute course without generalized adenopathy are suggestive of streptococcal infection.

Lichen planus may resemble papular syphilid. Of greatest importance is the recognition of the characteristic papule of lichen planus with its flat polygonal shape, the accompanying Wickham's striae, and the Koebner phenomenon. Pruritus is severe in lichen planus and rare in syphilis.

Other dermatoses to be kept in mind are pityriasis versicolor, pityriasis lichenoides chronica, pityriasis lichenoides et varioliformis acuta, macular and nodular leprosy, urticaria pigmentosa, the various forms of psoriasis, especially the guttate type, and sarcoid, which may be indistinguishable histologically, as Perry recently showed.

The differential diagnosis of mucous membrane lesions of secondary syphilis is of importance. Infectious mononucleosis may cause a biologic false positive test for syphilis and a high heterophile antibody titer.

Geographic tongue may be confused with the desquamative patches of syphilis or with mucous patches. Lingua geographica occurs principally near the edges of the tongue in relatively large areas, which are often fused and have lobulated contours; it continues for several months or years and changes in extent and degree of involvement from day to day. Aphthous stomatitis produces one or several painful ulcers, 1 to 3 mm in diameter, surrounded by hyperemic edges, which are distinctive features.

Relapsing Secondary Syphilis

The early lesions of syphilis undergo involution either spontaneously or under treatment, but relapses occur in about 25 per cent of untreated patients. Such relapses may take place at the site of previous lesions, on the skin or in the viscera. Sometimes after the disappearance of the typical macular eruption, especially in patients who have taken inadequate treatment, a relapsing macular eruption of somewhat different appearance is observed. The macules are larger and deeper red, and often form large rings with characteristically serpiginous margins. Cutaneous recurrences may be generalized eruptions in the form of large, sparse, lichenoid, annular, scaly, psoriasiform, or nodular lesions. In recurrent eruptions there is a distinct tendency toward increased configuration and infiltration, and the lesions are larger and separated by wider areas of healthy skin. For three to five years after the onset of the disease, recurrent nonulcerative lesions are infectious.

Latent Syphilis

After the lesions of secondary syphilis have involuted, a latent period occurs. This may last for a few months or continue for the remainder of the infected person's life. Sixty to 70 per cent of untreated infected patients remain asymptomatic in this latent form of disease for life. During this latent period there are no clinical signs of syphilis, but the STS is reactive. During the early latent period infectivity persists: for at least two years a woman with early latent syphilis may infect her unborn child.

Latent syphilis becomes late syphilis after two years, or earlier if gummatous lesions, cardiovascular syphilis, neurosyphilis, or other signs of late syphilis make themselves manifest, as may occur in HIV-infected patients. These may become overt in HIV-negative patients as soon as the third year, but usually do not appear for a longer period after syphilitic infection has occurred.

Tertiary Syphilis

Tertiary syphilids may occur as early as six months after infection but in general most often occur after three to five years. Sixteen per cent of untreated patients will develop tertiary skin lesions. Such lesions tend to be more localized, to occur in groups and patterns, and to be destructive. After the second year of the disease these characteristics become more common and pronounced. One generally considers as tertiary lesions those more localized and asymmetric in distribution, which are chronic and have a tendency to extend to surrounding areas of skin, acting in this way more as a local than a systemic

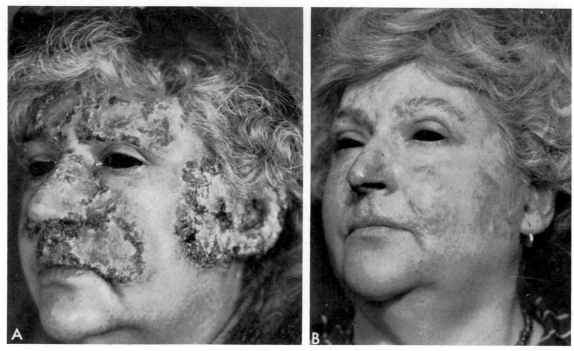

Figure 18–30. Tertiary syphilis. Before (A) and after (B) treatment.

infection. They are more infiltrated, usually destructive, and, when healed, leave scars.

Treponemata are usually not found by silver stains or darkfield examination, but may be demonstrated by using a modified indirect immunofluorescent technique, as shown by Handsfield et al. Lesions may be single or multiple, superficial or deep, and are characterized by indolence, painlessness, and a tendency to ulcerate with a punched-out appearance and by scar formation. The lesions are usually grouped and have a configurate arrangement.

TYPES. Two main types are recognized, the *nodulo-ulcerative syphilid* and the *gumma*, though the distinction seems unimportant and is sometimes difficult to make.

Nodular Syphilid. The nodular, nodulo-ulcerative, or tubercular type consists of reddish brown or copper-colored firm papules or nodules, 2 mm or larger. The individual lesions are usually covered with adherent scales or crusts. The lesions tend to form rings and to undergo involution as new lesions develop just beyond them, so that extraordinary and characteristic circular or serpiginous patterns are produced.

A distinctive and characteristic type is the kidney-shaped lesion. These frequently occur on the extensor surfaces of the arms and on the back of the trunk. Such patches are composed of nodules in different stages of development so that it is common to find

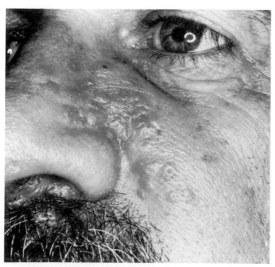

Figure 18–31. Tertiary syphilis, rosacea-like.

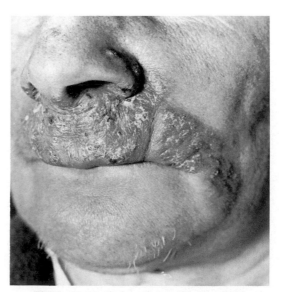

Figure 18–32. Tubercular tertiary syphilid.

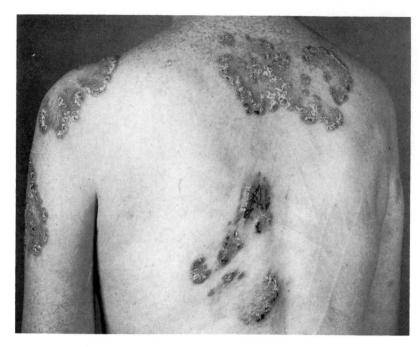

Figure 18–33. Tertiary nodulo-ulcerative syphilis. Note kidney-shaped lesions. (Courtesy of Dr. J. Lowry Miller.)

scars and pigmentation together with fresh and also ulcerated lesions. On the face the nodular eruption closely resembles lupus vulgaris. When the disease is untreated the process may last for years, slowly marching across large areas of skin. The process may leave barely perceptible scars, or may cause marked destruction, a loss of pigment, or subsequent hyperpigmentation.

The nodules may enlarge and eventually break down to form painless, rounded, smooth-bottomed, reddish ulcers a few millimeters deep. These punched-out ulcers arise side by side and form serpiginous syphilitic ulcers. They may be palm-sized and endure for many years, with only minimal healing and with scarring.

Gumma. Gummas may occur as unilateral, isolated, single or disseminated lesions or in serpiginous patterns resembling those of the nodular syphilid. They may be restricted to the skin or, originating in the deeper tissues, break down and secondarily involve the skin. The individual lesions, which begin as small nodules, slowly enlarge to several centimeters. Central necrosis is extensive and may lead to the formation of a deep punched-out ulcer with steep sides and a gummy base. Again, progression may take place in one area while healing proceeds in

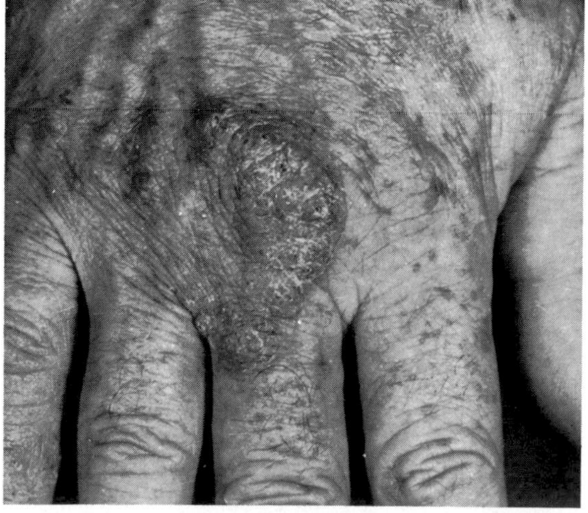

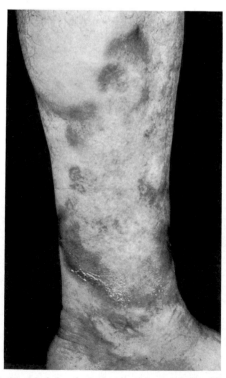

Figure 18–34. Late syphilis. Large annular patch of nodules. (Courtesy of Dr. F. Daniels, Jr.)

Figure 18–35. Nodulo-ulcerative tertiary syphilis. (Courtesy of Communicable Disease Center.)

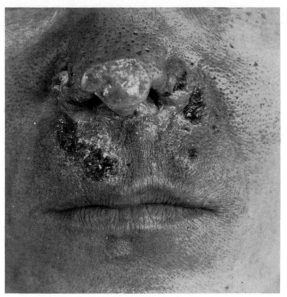

Figure 18–36. Gumma of tertiary syphilis.

another, and the resulting development of *kidney-shaped lesions* and *ulcerations* is characteristic. Perhaps the most frequent site of isolated gummas is the lower legs, where deep punched-out ulcers are formed, often in large infiltrated areas.

Deep Gummata. These may occur in muscle, bones, periosteum, lymph nodes, central nervous system, and the visceral organs. No part of the body seems to be exempt.

Histopathology of Gumma. Gummatous tertiary skin lesions show characteristic changes. A nodule composed of plasma cells, lymphocytes, epithelioid cells, and fibroblasts extends from the epidermis deep into the subcutaneous tissue. The number of giant cells varies greatly.

Within the gumma the blood vessels are affected in various degrees by obliterative endarteritis. The three coats of the vessel walls are thickened and the lumen is reduced. Frequently there is a marked fibrosis at the periphery of the infiltration. Usually the cellular elements gradually degenerate and caseation necrosis occurs. The epidermis may be thinned by pressure, or eroded, with the formation

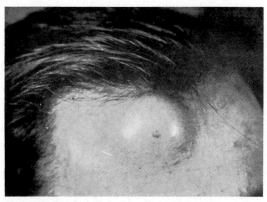

Figure 18–37. Gumma of forehead.

of an ulcer. Tertiary syphilis may produce, in addition to the gumma, a diffuse infiltration of the tissues with plasma cells and fibroblasts, forming syphilitic granulomas.

DIAGNOSIS OF TERTIARY CUTANEOUS SYPHILID

In addition to the typical and distinctive morphology of the skin lesions, much reliance is placed upon the serologic tests for syphilis. The nontreponemal tests, such as the VDRL and rapid plasma reagin (RPR), are positive in approximately 75 per cent of cases. The treponemal tests, such as the FTA-ABS, MHA-TP, and the TPI, are positive in nearly 100 per cent of patients. When there are mucous membrane lesions for which a diagnosis of carcinoma must also be considered, histologic examination is performed. Darkfield examination is not indicated, since it is always negative.

Differential Diagnosis of Nodular Syphilids and Gummas. When not ulcerated these syphilids must be distinguished from malignant tumors, leukemids, and sarcoidosis. Glanders and sporotrichosis may be distinguished by demonstration of the causative organisms.

The ulcerated syphilids must be differentiated from scrofuloderma, atypical mycobacterial infection, sporotrichosis, and blastomycosis. Mycosis fungoides is accompanied by eczematous changes and pruritus. Carcinoma and sarcoma have distinctive histologic findings.

Carcinoma is of first consideration for lesions occurring in the mouth. A biopsy is indicated in all cases. In addition, lichen planus, actinomycosis, tuberculosis, and periadenitis mucosa necrotica recurrens should be considered.

On the lower extremities gummas are frequently mistaken for erythema induratum and the various nonsyphilitic ulcers.

Mucous Membrane Lesions of Late Syphilis. In late syphilis the mucous membranes are attacked, the tongue being a favorite site. Gumma of the tongue usually involves the edge, toward the back, and rapidly breaks down to form a punched-out ulcer with irregular soft edges.

A *superficial glossitis* may cause irregular ulcers, atrophy of the papillae, and smooth shiny scarring, a condition known as *smooth atrophy.*

In *interstitial glossitis* there is an underlying induration due to sclerosis. In the advanced stages, tertiary syphilis of the tongue may lead to a diffuse enlargement (*macroglossia*).

Perforation of the hard palate from gummatous involvement is a characteristic tertiary manifestation. It generally occurs near the center of the hard palate. Destruction of the nasal septum may also occur.

Late syphilitic disease of the tongue must be differentiated from several other affections which it resembles closely. Gumma is differentiated from carcinoma in that the latter is invariably hard to palpation and often occurs in areas other than the tongue such as the floor of the mouth or the buccal mucosa. Other distinguishing features are the absence of pain and adenopathy in gumma, and their presence in cancer. Even in the presence of a positive STS, biopsy is essential. Scrotal tongue is a congenital anomaly in which uniformly arranged fissures radiate featherlike forward and outward from the median raphe without evidence of inflammation. In another anomaly, which is less conspicuous, the edges of the tongue apposed to the teeth have a markedly serrated contour. The atrophic glossitis associated with avitaminosis, chronic gastrointestinal disease, or anemia, and the infiltrations of the tongue that are observed in leukemia, Hodgkin's disease, mycosis fungoides, and leprosy should not lead to any difficulties in diagnosis.

Late Osseous Syphilis. Not infrequently gummatous lesions involve the periosteum and the bone. Skeletal syphilids occur most commonly on the head and face, then on the tibiae. Late manifestations of syphilis may produce periostitis, osteomyelitis, osteitis, and gummatous osteoarthritis. Osteocope—bone pain, most often at night—is a suggestive symptom.

Syphilitic joint lesions also occur, with the *Charcot joint* being the most prevalent manifestation. They are often associated with tabes dorsalis and occur most frequently in men. Although any joint may be involved, the knees and the ankles are the most frequently affected. There is hydrops, then loss of the contours of the joint, hypermobility, and painlessness. It is readily diagnosed roentgenologically.

Early Neurosyphilis. This is mainly meningeal, and spinal fluid abnormalities herald the early changes. The spinal fluid examination shows a positive STS and a high cell count with lymphocytosis. Biologic false positive serologic tests are rare.

Meningeal neurosyphilis manifests as meningitis, with headache, cranial nerve disorders, convulsions, and delirium, and with increased intracranial pressure indicated by papilledema.

This early type usually occurs within the first year after infection. Approximately 7 per cent of untreated patients will develop late neurosyphilis. Asymptomatic, meningeal and meningovascular, and parenchymatous forms exist; the parenchymatous forms (tabes dorsalis and paresis) predominate.

Meningovascular Neurosyphilis. This becomes manifest by the thrombosis of the various cerebral and spinal arteries. Hemiplegia, aphasia, hemianopsia, transverse myelitis, and progressive muscular atrophy may occur. Cranial nerve palsies such as eighth nerve deafness and eye changes may also occur. The eyes may show fixed pupils, Argyll Robertson pupils, or anisocoria.

Parenchymatous Neurosyphilis. This is manifested mainly in two ways: one is tabes dorsalis and the other paresis.

Tabes dorsalis is the degeneration of the dorsal roots of the spinal nerves and of the posterior columns of the spinal cord. The symptoms and signs are so numerous that only a partial listing is feasible here. Gastric crisis with severe pain and vomiting is the most frequent symptom. Some other symptoms are lancinating pains, urination difficulties, paresthesias (numbness, tingling, and burning), spinal ataxia, diplopia, strabismus, vertigo, and deafness. The signs that may be present are Argyll Robertson pupils, absent or reduced lower cord reflexes, Romberg sign, sensory loss (deep tendon tenderness, vibration, and position), atonic bladder, trophic changes, malum perforans pedis, Charcot joints, and optic atrophy.

Paresis has prodromal manifestations of headache, fatigability, and inability to concentrate. Later, personality changes occur, along with memory loss, dementia, and apathy. Grandiose ideas, megalomania, and delusions may develop. Hallucinations may also prevail and, finally, dementia sets in again.

Late Cardiovascular Syphilis. This occurs in about 10 per cent of untreated patients. Aortitis is the basic lesion of cardiovascular syphilis. From this, various forms emerge such as aortic insufficiency, coronary disease, and ultimately aortic aneurysm.

CONGENITAL SYPHILIS

Prenatal syphilis is acquired in utero from a mother with early syphilis. Infection through the placenta usually does not occur before the fourth month, so treatment of the mother prior to this time will almost always prevent infection in the fetus. If prenatal infection occurs soon after this, fetal death and miscarriage often result. During the remainder of the pregnancy, infection is at least equally likely to produce characteristic developmental physical stigmata, or, after the eighth month, active, infectious secondary syphilis ("bloody snuffles"). In utero infection of the fetus is rare when the pregnant mother has had syphilis for two or more years. Normal term birth may occur, with the development of active signs of syphilis a few weeks after birth, or the signs and symptoms of syphilis may not appear until puberty. For this reason, prenatal syphilis is divided into early and late congenital syphilis.

Early Congenital Syphilis

Cutaneous manifestations appear most commonly during the third week of life, but sometimes occur as late as three months after birth. The newborn is usually premature, marasmic, fretful, and dehydrated. The face is pinched and drawn, resembling that of an old man or woman. In severe cases there are secondary anemia and fever of varying degree. Many syphilitic infants, however, are well formed and of almost normal weight.

Snuffles, a form of rhinitis, is the most frequent and often the first specific finding. It blocks the nose, often with blood-stained mucus, and a copious mu-

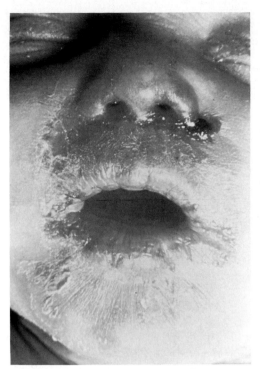

Figure 18–38. Snuffles. (Courtesy of Dr. Alagil.)

cous discharge runs down over the lips. The nasal obstruction often interferes seriously with the child's nursing. In persistent and progressive cases ulcerations develop, which may involve the bones and ultimately cause perforation of the septum or development of the saddle nose, which are important stigmata later in the disease.

The early skin eruptions are usually maculopapular, more rarely purely papular. The lesions are at first a bright or violaceous red, later fading to a coppery color. The papules may become large and infiltrated; scaling is frequently pronounced. Secondary pustule formation with crusting occurs, especially in lesions that appear a year or more after birth. The eruption shows a marked predilection for the face, arms, buttocks, legs, palms, and soles.

Important and characteristic lesions are infiltrations. These are present most frequently on the palms and soles, which are at first evenly and diffusely thickened and then desquamate, exposing a bright red, shiny surface. Similar infiltrations are found about the mouth, where they frequently develop deep fissures radiating from the borders and angles of the lips (*rhagades*). When healed, these often leave characteristic *radiating scars*, another important stigma of the disease. Similar infiltrations around the anus and vulva may result in similar scarring in these areas.

Syphilitic pemphigus, a bullous eruption, usually on the palms and soles, is a relatively uncommon lesion. The bullae quickly become purulent and rupture, leaving exuding areas. They are found also on the eponychium, wrists, ankles, and, infrequently, other parts of the body.

In the second or third year, recurrent secondary eruptions are apt to take the papulopustular form. Annular lesions similar to those in adults occur. Mucous patches in the mouth or on the vulva are seen infrequently. Condylomata, large moist hypertrophic papules, are found about the anus and in other folds of the body. They are more common after the first year than in the newborn.

Bone lesions are common in early congenital syphilis. *Syphilitic dactylitis* causes a diffuse, fusiform swelling of one or more fingers, sometimes with ulcerations. *Epiphysitis*, especially of the ulna, is common. A helpless condition of the involved extremity occurs, and the infant refuses to move, probably because of pain (*Parrot's pseudoparalysis*). Bone lesions in congenital syphilis during the first six months after birth are quite characteristic. The syphilitic changes occur chiefly at the epiphyseal ends of the long bones and are manifested first by an increased

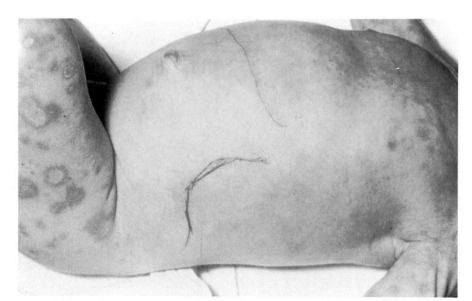

Figure 18–39. Early congenital syphilis. (Courtesy of Dr. Alagil.)

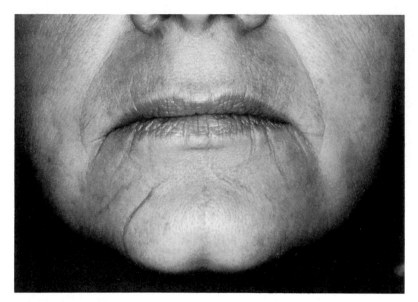

Figure 18–40. Rhagades.

and widened zone of calcification with a sawtoothed appearance. Later there develops a zone of decalcification.

The changes may be classified as *osteochondritis, osteomyelitis,* and *osteoperiostitis.* They can be demonstrated in the majority of syphilitic infants.

A general enlargement of the lymph nodes usually occurs, with enlargement of the spleen. Clinical evidence of involvement of the liver is rare, though *interstitial hepatitis* is a frequent finding at autopsy. The nephrotic syndrome and acute glomerulonephritis have been reported as complications of congenital syphilis.

Symptomatic or asymptomatic neurosyphilis as demonstrated by a positive spinal fluid serology may be present. Chronic meningitis, often simulating tuberculous meningitis, is also frequent. Hydrocephalus of some degree is present in one third of early cases of neurosyphilis. Optic atrophy may occur as early as two years after birth. Specific iritis may also occur in the first few months of the disease.

Late Congenital Syphilis

Although no sharp line can be drawn between early and late congenital syphilis, children who appear normal at birth and develop their first signs of the disease after the age of two years show a different clinical picture.

Lesions of the cornea, of the bones, and of the central nervous system are the most important. Of these, *interstitial keratitis,* beginning with intense pericorneal inflammation and persisting to characteristic diffuse clouding of the cornea without surface ulceration, is commonest. If persistent, it leads to permanent partial or complete opacity of the cornea, and was once a common cause of blindness, though it is rare today.

Interstitial keratitis must be differentiated from *Cogan's syndrome,* consisting of nonsyphilitic interstitial keratitis, usually bilateral, associated with vestibulo-auditory symptoms such as deafness, tinnitus, vertigo, nystagmus, and ataxia. It is congenital.

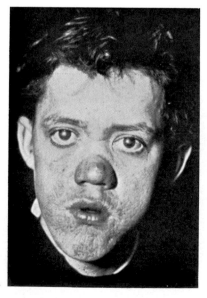
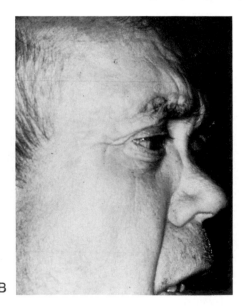

Figure 18–41. A, *Saddle nose in congenital syphilis, with interstitial keratitis and prominent rhagades radiating from mouth. (Courtesy of Dr. E. A. Oliver.)* B, *Frontal bossing, interstitial keratitis, and saddle nose in congenital syphilis.*

A   B

Periostitis, which affects the tibia with striking frequency, often confined to this one bone, is another frequent manifestation, causing an anterior bowing and thickening called *saber shin*.

Gummas may also be found in any of the long bones or in the skull. A less frequent lesion is an arthritis which usually manifests itself as a *bilateral effusion of the knee joints*. These swollen, slightly stiffened, but practically painless knees are characteristic and are known as *Clutton's joints*.

Ulcerating gummas are frequently seen. They probably begin more often in the soft parts or in the underlying bone than in the skin itself.

The lesions of the central nervous system in congenital syphilis may be classified, like the adult cases, as *meningeal*, *meningovascular*, and *parenchymatous* (tabes dorsalis and paresis), but the clinical pictures are rarely characteristic of those seen in adults. The meningovascular forms usually manifest themselves as paralyses of one or more extremities or one of the cranial nerves. Of these, involvement of the *eighth nerve*, leading to deafness, is not uncommon.

Of the lesions classed as parenchymatous, *optic atrophy* is the most frequent, but cases with ataxia, sensory disturbances, lightning pains, and visceral crises are occasionally encountered. The most serious

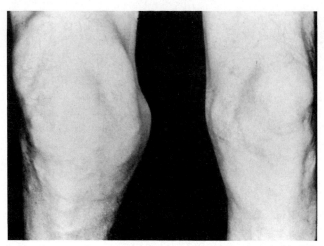

Figure 18–43. Charcot's joint. (Courtesy of Communicable Disease Center.)

cases are those of paresis. The characteristic early mental symptoms of adult paresis are seldom observed, but dementia or partial or complete lack of mental development is characteristic. *Epileptic attacks* are a frequent symptom in congenital cases.

CLINICAL FEATURES

Stigmata. The destructive effects of syphilis in young children often leave scars or developmental defects called "stigmata," which persist throughout life and enable one to make a diagnosis of congenital syphilis long after the infection has been cured or has ceased any activity. Hutchinson emphasized the diagnostic importance of changes in the incisor teeth, opacities of the cornea, and eighth nerve deafness, which have since become known as the *Hutchinson triad*. Hutchinson's teeth, corneal scars, saber shins, rhagades of the lips, saddle nose, and mulberry molars are of diagnostic importance.

Hutchinson's Teeth. A malformation of the central upper incisors appears in the second or permanent teeth, which are peg-shaped, barrel-shaped, and often notched. The characteristic teeth are cylindrical

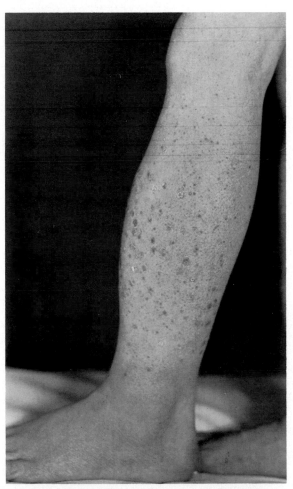

Figure 18–42. Saber shin in congenital syphilis.

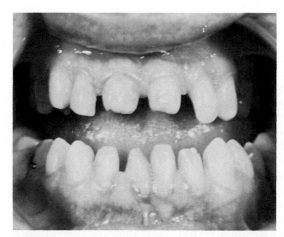

Figure 18–44. Hutchinson's teeth, upper central incisors peg-shaped and centrally notched.

rather than flattened, the cutting edge is narrower than the base, and in the center of the cutting edge a notch may develop. In characteristic form this type of tooth seems never to occur except in congenital syphilis and is considered a pathognomonic sign.

Mulberry Molar (Moon's Molars, Fournier's Molars). The mulberry molar (usually the first molar, appearing about the age of six years) is a hyperplastic tooth, the flat occlusal surface of which is covered with a group of little knobs representing abortive cusps.

Saddle Nose. The flattening of the nasal bones resulting in the so-called saddle nose is characteristic, but may result from other infections or from trauma.

Higoumenakis's Sign. The unilateral thickening of the inner third of one clavicle has been described by Higoumenakis as a hyperostosis resulting from syphilitic osteitis in those who have had late congenital syphilis. The lesion appears typically on the right side in right-handed persons and on the left side in left-handed persons.

DIAGNOSIS. All infants born to syphilitic mothers should be carefully examined for syphilis. At birth the newborn may have a high-titer STS from the mother's antibody; a rapidly decreasing titer in the first few weeks of the newborn's life confirms this finding. Maternal IgG antibody may be retained in the infant for as long as 100 days. However, if the newborn's titer is four times greater than the mother's, prompt treatment is indicated. The IgM-FTA-ABS test indicates active infection, because IgM antibody does not cross the placenta. It has proved less accurate than a positive VDRL test in rising titers.

Late congenital syphilis should be suspected in older children with "pink eye" (heralding interstitial keratitis), deafness, hydrarthrosis (Clutton's joints), osteomyelitis, or unusual tooth development.

TREATMENT. See p. 427.

SEROLOGIC TESTS FOR SYPHILIS (STS)

Serologic tests for syphilis reveal the individual's immunologic status, but not (unless in rising titer) whether the patient is currently infected.

Serum containing the antibody against *T. pallidum* forms aggregates with a cardiolipin-cholesterol-lecithin antigen which can be viewed directly in tubes or on cards or slides or can be examined in an autoanalyzer. Since these tests utilize lipoidal antigens, rather than *T. pallidum* or components of it, they are referred to as *nontreponemal antigen tests*. Most widely used is the VDRL (Venereal Disease Research Laboratory) slide test. It has replaced the Kahn, Kline, Eagle, Hinton, Mazzini, Laughlen, and other tests. It becomes positive as a rule within five or six weeks after infection, shortly before the chancre heals; is invariably strongly positive throughout the secondary phase, except in occasional HIV-infected patients, whose response is less predictable; and may become negative during therapy, especially

if therapy is begun within the first year. It may also become negative after a few decades even without treatment.

By diluting the serum serially, the strength of the reaction can be stated in dilutions or "dils," the number given being the highest dilution giving a positive test: 1:2, 2 dils; 1:16, 16 dils; and so on. In early infection the titer may be only 1:2; in secondary syphilis it is regularly high, 1:32 to 1:256 or so; in late syphilis, much lower as a rule, 1:4 or 1:8 perhaps. The rise of titer in early infection is of great potential diagnostic value, as is the fall after proper treatment, or the rise again in case of reinfection or relapse. Transient biologic false positive (BFP) reactions after viral infections or vaccination are almost invariably of low titer and tend to fall, though a chronic BFP test, as in lepromatous leprosy, may remain steady.

The Rapid Plasma Reagin (RPR) card test was introduced in 1962 as a simplified nontreponemal test for use in field or clinical settings. In performing the RPR test, modified VDRL antigen containing carbon particles and unheated serum are mixed on a plastic card. Because of the inclusion of the carbon particles in the antigen, flocculation can be determined with the naked eye. For screening purposes, the RPR card test is technically easier and has advantages over the VDRL test. However, any positive RPR test should be tested by VDRL, so that quantitative analysis may be performed and titer be determined.

Patients with very high antibody titers, as occur in secondary syphilis, may have a false negative result when undiluted serum is tested. This "prozone" phenomenon will be overcome by diluting the serum.

In order to improve sensitivity and specificity, tests have been devised using a treponemal antigen. Foremost among these is the FTA-ABS (fluorescent treponemal antibody absorption) test, which, like the others of this "treponemal" type, reliably identifies seroreactivity caused by treponemal diseases (syphilis, yaws, pinta, or bejel) from that caused by malaria, leprosy, or viral infections. Treponemal tests are negative in patients with Lyme disease, a spirochetal disease caused by *Borrelia burgdorferi*.

The treponemal tests become positive early, and remain so. Thus in late or latent disease they are most sensitive. Several variants exist, including the enzyme-linked immunosorbent assay (ELISA).

STS After Treatment

Quantitative VDRL testing should be performed on patients who are to be treated for syphilis, before therapy and then on several occasions during the next two years. The titer generally decreases by at least two dilutions within several months of adequate therapy for primary or secondary disease. Fiumara published in 1986 the last increment of a series of 588 patients with primary syphilis and 623 patients with secondary syphilis treated with two intramuscular injections of 2.4 million units of penicillin G benzathine a week apart, and found that they became seronegative within one and two years respectively. Brown et al calculated curves which describe the progressive decrease in VDRL titer after treatment. These may help early identification of treatment failures or reinfections. A stable or rising titer during this observation period may suggest inadequate therapy, reinfection, or a false positive serology. Patients treated for latent or late syphilis may be serofast, so that failure to observe a titer fall in these patients does not, in itself, indicate a need for retreatment.

The TPI and FTA-ABS tests tend to remain positive for life. This is not an indication for further treatment. In late syphilis 73 per cent have reactive cardiolipin tests, 90 per cent have reactive TPI, and 98 per cent reactive FTA-ABS tests. The titers of the cardiolipin tests often remain constant after treatment. A subsequent rise in titer of four dilutions, provided there is no laboratory error, indicates reinfection or relapse.

Biologic False Positive (BFP) Tests

This term is used to denote a positive STS (without laboratory error) in persons with no history or clinical evidence of syphilis. The reaction occurs in one of about every 4000 persons in the general population.

Acute BFP reactors are defined as anyone whose test reverts to normal in less than six months; those whose positive test persists for over six months are termed chronic BFP reactors. Some acute BFP reactions are due to recent vaccinations, the common cold, infectious mononucleosis, hepatitis, measles, typhoid, varicella, influenza, lymphogranuloma, malaria, pregnancy, or narcotic addiction. In autoimmune diseases, or suspected autoimmune diseases, the BFP may persist for six months or more. Such diseases include SLE (44 per cent have BFP), rheumatoid arthritis, Sjögren's syndrome, hemolytic anemia, thrombocytopenia, thyroiditis. It is to be remembered that the treponemal antigen tests are also positive in yaws, pinta, and bejel: such tests are true, not false, positive reactions.

Tuffanelli in a study of 103 patients with chronic BFP reactions showed an increased incidence of antinuclear antibodies, rheumatoid factor, hypergammaglobulinemia, and elevated IgG and IgM levels.

Serologic tests suspected of being false positive should be tested with the FTA-ABS procedure, which will rule out BFP in 98 per cent of the cases. When a negative FTA-ABS and a positive STS are found, a search for the underlying cause other than syphilis must be made. The BFP serologic tests have almost always a low titer, 1 to 4 or less.

False positive FTA-ABS reactions have been reported to occur in lupus erythematosus, drug-induced lupus syndrome, scleroderma, rheumatoid arthritis, smallpox vaccination, pregnancy, and genital herpes simplex infections. A pattern of beaded fluorescence associated with FTA-ABS testing may be found in sera of patients without treponemal disease who have systemic lupus erythematosus. The beading phenomenon is not specific for SLE or even for connective tissue disorders.

Spinal Fluid Examination

Examination of cerebrospinal fluid should be a routine procedure in almost every case of syphilis, especially if HIV disease is present. In early syphilis that has been promptly and adequately treated, a positive spinal fluid is unlikely; it is not so unlikely, however, in HIV-infected individuals. In them, moreover, it may be a matter of comparative urgency, because progression of disease may be more rapid, and therapy may be of reduced efficacy. A spinal fluid examination should be made about one year after treatment has been given if treatment with antibiotics other than penicillin has been used. If this is negative, no further spinal fluid examinations are required.

For untreated patients who have had syphilis of more than two years' duration, a spinal fluid examination should be performed before treatment is begun. If the result is negative, it need not be repeated, because any invasion of the cerebrospinal system occurs within the first two years of infection. If the initial spinal fluid test is positive, with an increased number of cells and elevated protein, lumbar puncture should be repeated annually for at least three years.

In late syphilis, when the spinal fluid STS is positive, titered spinal fluid tests for syphilis should be done routinely at six-month intervals for three years after treatment or until it becomes negative. Even after successful treatment the spinal fluid may be reactive for several years.

Active neurosyphilis is indicated by reactive spinal fluid reagin, pleocytosis, and increased protein. After vigorous treatment the cell count diminishes, then the protein, and, finally, the test for syphilis has a decreased titer. Colloidal tests are no longer considered to be of value in either the diagnosis or the treatment of neurosyphilis.

TREATMENT

At the outset it must be noted that treatment guidelines are in the process of change, particularly in relation to concurrent HIV infection. The most recent recommendations available are in the January, 1989, issue of the *Archives of Dermatology*, page 15, and in an article by Duncan and an editorial by Roth et al in the same issue.

Penicillin remains the drug of choice for treatment of all stages of syphilis. Patients with primary, secondary, or latent syphilis known to be of less than one year's duration can be treated effectively with a single intramuscular injection of 2.4 million units of penicillin G benzathine, or eight daily intramuscular injections of 600,000 units of penicillin G procaine.

In penicillin-allergic patients tetracycline or erythromycin orally in doses of 500 mg every six hours for 15 days is adequate therapy. Tetracycline is the more extensively studied of the two and is the preferential drug of second choice.

In latent syphilis of more than one year's duration penicillin G benzathine is increased to 2.4 million units intramuscularly weekly for three doses; penicillin G procaine to 600,000 units intramuscularly daily for 15 days; and tetracycline and erythromycin orally extended to 500 mg every six hours for 30 days. Again, tetracycline is the preferred alternative drug.

Recommended treatment regimens for neurosyphilis include penicillin G crystalline, 2 to 4 million units intravenously every four hours for 10 days followed by benzathine penicillin G, 2.4 million units intramuscularly weekly for three doses; penicillin G procaine, 2.4 million units intramuscularly daily plus probenecid 500 mg by mouth 4 times daily, both for 10 days, followed by benzathine penicillin G, 2.4 million units intramuscularly weekly for three weeks; or benzathine penicillin G, 2.4 million units intramuscularly weekly for three doses. Patients allergic to penicillin should have their allergy confirmed. If allergy exists, tetracycline or erythromycin, 500 mg orally every six hours for 30 days, may be effective. Concurrent AIDS, ARC, or even asymptomatic HIV infection may accelerate the development of neurosyphilis, and is an indication to treat more intensively, according to Johns et al. Benzathine penicillin alone should not be used to treat syphilis in an HIV-infected patient.

Infants with congenital syphilis should be given a single injection of 50,000 units/kg of penicillin G benzathine intramuscularly. If they have neurosyphilis, penicillin G crystalline, 50,000 units/kg, IM or IV twice daily for at least 10 days, or penicillin G procaine, 50,000 units/kg IM daily for at least 10 days, should be administered. If neurosyphilis cannot be excluded, one of the latter two regimens should be followed.

Pregnant women with syphilis should be treated with penicillin in doses appropriate for the stage of syphilis, and follow-up quantitative serologic tests should be performed monthly until delivery. Pregnant women allergic to penicillin should be given erythromycin in dosage schedules appropriate for the stage of syphilis as recommended for the treatment of nonpregnant patients. However, failures of the erythromycin regimen do occur. Tetracyclines given to pregnant women can cause staining of the teeth in the newborn.

Clinical and serologic follow-up is important for all patients after treatment for early syphilis.

Jarisch-Herxheimer Reaction. Also known as the Herxheimer reaction, this occurs after the initial dose of antisyphilitic treatment, such as penicillin, is given. It has been observed in about 60 per cent of

patients treated for seronegative primary syphilis, 90 per cent of those with seropositive primary or secondary syphilis, and 30 per cent of those with neurosyphilis. The reaction generally occurs six to eight hours after injection, but may not reach its height for several days, especially in osseous or neurologic involvement. The reaction consists of shaking chills, fever, malaise, sore throat, myalgia, headache, tachycardia, and exacerbation of the inflammatory reaction at sites of localized spirochetal infection.

Rosen et al recently described a vesicular reaction in four black patients, the mechanism of which is as yet unknown. Theories have included an endotoxic reaction, a circulating immune-complex reaction, complement mediation, a kinin-mediated reaction, and an endogenous opioid-mediated pathogenesis. Its importance lies in that a flare-up of a syphilitic inflammation in a vital structure may have serious consequences, as when there is an aneurysm of the aorta, or iritis. When there is involvement of the nervous system, special importance is attached to the avoidance of the Herxheimer reaction even though paralyses that may result are often transitory. Gumma of the brain or spinal cord should be treated surgically first, and for syphilis afterward.

It is also important to distinguish the Herxheimer reaction from a drug reaction to penicillin or other appropriate antibiotics. The reaction has also been described in other spirochetal diseases, such as leptospirosis and louse-borne relapsing fever.

Abortive Therapy. Schober et al recently reported that approximately 50 per cent of the contacts of infected patients developed syphilis. With this in mind, if there is known exposure, treatment with 2.4 million units of benzathine penicillin G intramuscularly may be given to abort disease, prior to onset of any signs and symptoms. Also, aqueous penicillin G procaine in the dosage of 2.4 and 4.8 million units is curative therapy for patients with gonorrhea with coexisting incubating syphilis. Every patient with syphilis requires epidemiologic follow-up with identification and treatment of contacts.

1985 STD treatment guidelines. JAAD 1986, 14:707.

Bahmer FA, et al: Ultrastructural features of malignant syphilis and demonstration of *Treponema pallidum*. Int J Dermatol 1983, 22:165.

Baum EW, et al: Secondary syphilis: still the great imitator. JAMA 1983, 249:3069.

Berry CD, et al: Neurologic relapse after benzathine penicillin therapy for secondary syphilis in a patient with HIV infection. N Engl J Med 1987, 316:1587.

Bos JD: Fluorescent treponemal antibody-absorption (FTA-ABS) test. Int J Dermatol 1982, 21:125.

Brown ST, et al: Serologic response to syphilis treatment. JAMA 1985, 253:1296.

Chapel TA: The variability of syphilitic chancres. Sex Transm Dis 1978, 5:68.

Chung WM, et al: Syphilis: a cause of fever of unknown origin. Cutis 1983, 31:537.

Drew FL, et al: False-positive FTA-ABS in pregnancy. JA Vener Dis Assoc 1975, 1:165.

Duffy J, et al: Serologic testing in Lyme disease. Ann Intern Med 1985, 103:458.

Duncan WC: Failure of erythromycin to cure secondary syphilis in a patient infected with HIV. Arch Dermatol 1989, 125:82.

Ewing CI, et al: Early congenital syphilis still ocurs. Arch Dis Child 1985, 60:1128.

Felman YM, et al: Syphilis serology today. Arch Dermatol 1980, 116:84.

Felman YM, ed: Dermatologic Clinics: Sexually Transmitted Diseases. Vol 1. Philadelphia, WB Saunders Co, 1983.

Fisher DA, et al: Lues maligna. Arch Dermatol 1969, 99:70.

Fiumara NJ: Treatment of primary and secondary syphilis: serologic response. JAAD 1986, 14:487.

Fiumara NJ, et al: Manifestations of late congenital syphilis. Arch Dermatol 1970, 102:78.

Foster JW, et al: The in vitro cultivation of *Treponema pallidum*. Corroborative studies. Br J Vener Dis 1977, 53:338.

Gelfand JA, et al: Endotoxemia associated with the Jarisch-Herxheimer reaction. N Engl J Med 1976, 295:211.

Gschnait F, et al: Laboratory evidence for impaired cellular immunity in different stages of syphilis. J Invest Dermatol 1982, 79:40.

Guinan ME: Treatment of primary and secondary syphilis: Defining failure at 3- and 6-month follow-up. JAMA 1987, 257:359.

Hager WD: Transplacental transmission of spirochetes in congenital syphilis—a new perspective (editorial). Sex Transm Dis 1986, 5:122.

Handsfield HH, et al: Demonstration of *Treponema pallidum* in a cutaneous gumma by indirect immunofluorescence. Arch Dermatol 1983, 119:677.

Harris WDM, et al: Congenital syphilis of the newborn. JAMA 1965, 194:1312.

Hicks CB, et al: Seronegative secondary syphilis in a patient infected with the human immunodeficiency virus (HIV) with Kaposi's sarcoma. Ann Intern Med 1987, 107:492.

Higoumenakis KG: Das Zeichen von Higoumenakis und seine Bedeutung für die Diagnose der angeborenen Syphilis. Derm Wschr 1968, 154:697.

Hira SK, et al: Clinical manifestations of secondary syphilis. Int J Dermatol 1987, 26:103.

Hooshmand H, et al: Neurosyphilis. JAMA 1972, 219:726.

Johns DR, et al: Alterations in the natural history of syphilis by concurrent infection with the human immunodeficiency virus. N Engl J Med 1987, 316:1569.

Jones RH, et al: Growth and subculture of pathogenic T. pallidum (Nichols strain) in BHK-21 cultured tissue cells. Br J Vener Dis 1976, 52:18.

Karayalcin G, et al: Monocytosis in congenital syphilis. Am J Dis Child 1977, 131:782.

Katz RA, et al: Multiple facial nodules in a young woman. Arch Dermatol 1987, 123:1707.

Kolar OJ, et al: Neurosyphilis. Br J Vener Dis 1977, 53:221.

Kraus SJ, et al: Atypical FTA-ABS test fluorescence in lupus erythematosus patients. JAMA 1970, 211:2140.

Lukehart SA, et al: Invasion of the central nervous system by *Treponema pallidum*. Ann Intern Med 1988, 109:855.

Mackey DM: Specificity of the FTA-ABS test for syphilis. JAMA 1969, 207:1683.

Mascola L, et al: Congenital syphilis revisited. Am J Dis Child 1985, 139:575.

McKenna CH, et al: The fluorescent treponemal antibody absorbed (FTA-ABS) test beading phenomenon in connective tissue diseases. Mayo Clin Proc 1973, 48:545.

McNeely MC, et al: Cutaneous secondary syphilis. JAAD 1986, 14:564.

McPhee SJ, et al: Secondary syphilis: uncommon manifestations of a common disease. West J Med 1984, 140:35.

Musher DM: How much penicillin cures early syphilis? Ann Intern Med 1988, 109:849.

Onoda Y: Clinical evaluation of amoxycillin (sic) in the treatment of syphilis. J Int Med Res 1979, 7:539.

Perry HO, et al: Secondary and tertiary syphilis presenting as sarcoidal reactions of the skin. Cutis 1984, 34:253.

Recommendations for diagnosis and treating syphilis in HIV infected patients. Arch Dermatol 1989, 125:15.

Rein MF: Treatment of neurosyphilis (editorial). JAMA 1981, 246:2613.

Robinson RCV: Congenital syphilis. Arch Dermatol 1969, 99:599.

Rolfs RT, et al: The perpetual lessons of syphilis. Arch Dermatol 1989, 125:107.

Rosen T, et al: Vesicular Jarish-Herxheimer reaction. Arch Dermatol 1989, 125:77.

Rudolph AH, et al: Treponemal infections. JAAD 1988, 18:1121.

Schober PC, et al: How infectious is syphilis? Br J Vener Dis 1983, 59:217.

Schroeter AL, et al: Therapy for incubating syphilis. JAMA 1971, 218:711.

Simon RP: Neurosyphilis. Arch Neurol 1985, 42:606.

Stokes JH, et al: Modern Clinical Syphilology, 2nd ed. Philadelphia, W.B. Saunders Company, 1945.

Tramont EC: Persistence of *Treponema pallidum* following penicillin G therapy. JAMA 1976, 236:2206.

Idem: Syphilis in the AIDS era (editorial). N Engl J Med 1987, 316:1600.

Triana AF, et al: Annular plaque on the shoulder. Arch Dermatol 1987, 123:1707.

Update: Lyme disease—United States. JAAD 1984, 11:517.

Wiesel J, et al: Lumbar puncture in asymptomatic late syphilis—an analysis of the benefits and risks. Arch Intern Med 1985, 145:464.

Wright JT, et al: False-positive FTA-ABS results in patients with genital herpes. Br J Vener Dis 1975, 51:329.

Wuepper KD, et al: Serologic tests for syphilis and the false-positive reactor. Arch Dermatol 1966, 94:152.

YAWS

Yaws is also known as *pian*, *boubas*, frambesia tropica, *dube*, and other native terms.

Yaws is an infectious systemic disease, caused by *Treponema pertenue*, which is endemic in many tropical regions. It usually begins in childhood and is characterized by frambesiform (raspberrylike) skin lesions; it has a disabling course, affecting the skin, bones, and joints. There is, however, freedom from involvement of the central nervous and cardiovascular systems. Yaws is not a sexually transmitted disease, but a childhood infection. It is divided into early and late disease.

EARLY YAWS

A primary papule or group of papules appears at the site of inoculation after an incubation period of several weeks, during which there may be headache, malaise, and other mild constitutional symptoms. The initial lesion becomes crusted and larger, and is known as the mother yaw (*maman pian*). The crusts are amber-yellow. They may be knocked off, forming an ulcer with a red, pulpy, granulated surface, but quickly reform so that the typical yaws lesion is

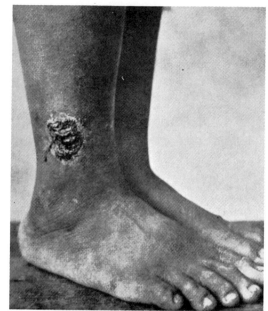

Figure 18–45. Yaws, primary stage. Note crusts around lesions. (Courtesy of Army Medical Museum.)

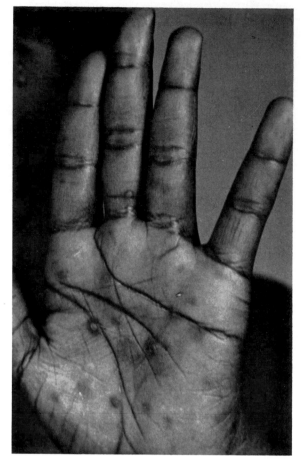

Figure 18–47. Palmar macules in secondary yaws.

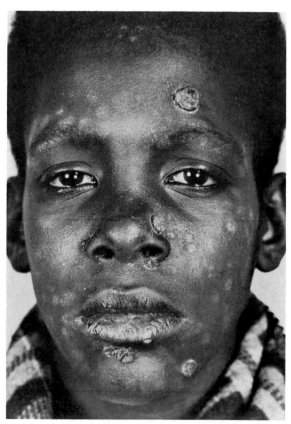

Figure 18–46. Secondary yaws in a 15-year-old boy.

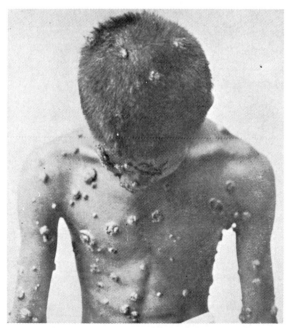

Figure 18–48. Yaws, secondary stage. Note typical raspberry-like lesions. (Courtesy of Army Medical Museum.)

crusted. The lesion is not indurated. There may be some regional adenopathy.

Exposed parts are most frequently involved—the extremities, particularly the lower legs, and the face—although the mothers' breasts and trunk may be infected by their children. The lesion is practically always extragenital, and when genital, is a result of accidental contact rather than intercourse. After being present a few months the mother yaw spontaneously disappears, leaving slight atrophy and depigmentation.

Bone lesions occur in the primary stage, especially in children. Osteoperiostitis of the long bones and of the face (*goundou*) and saber tibia are the manifestations.

Weeks or months after the primary lesion the secondary yaws appear. These lesions look like the mother yaw, but they are smaller. They are usually very profuse, particularly on the face and extremities, but it is common to see patients in whom there are only a few. The nodules are amber-yellow, crusted, soft, raspberrylike, granulomatous lesions, 1 cm or more in diameter. Sometimes the mother yaw may be absent and all the secondary lesions come out together. In the course of a few weeks or months the secondary lesions undergo spontaneous involution, leaving either no marks at all or whitish spots that later become hyperpigmented. However, the eruption may persist for many months as a result of fresh recurrent outbreaks. The course is slower in adults than in children, in whom the secondary period rarely lasts longer than six months.

In some sites, especially around the body orifices, the secondary lesions may coalesce and form rings (*ringworm yaws*), and in the armpits, groins, and

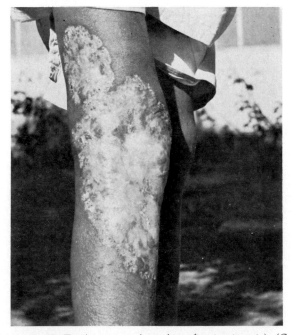

Figure 18–49. Tertiary yaws (scarring after treatment). (Courtesy of Drs. O. Reyes and F. Kerdel-Vegas, Venezuela.)

gluteal crease, condylomatous lesions may arise. On the dorsa of the feet verrucous changes are frequently seen. Crusted lesions of the eyelids are common and at times there is paronychia.

In yaws no macular eruption analogous to that seen in secondary syphilis occurs. Anemia may be present. In secondary yaws one frequently sees furfuraceous patches within which there are crops of miliary, reddish, slightly keratotic papules, some developing into typical crusted, granulomatous lesions. The papules at the periphery of the patch tend to be hyperpigmented. The miliary eruption that occurs in yaws may resemble lichen scrofulosorum.

After the secondary yaws have disappeared, or sometimes before the onset of the secondary eruption, keratotic lesions may develop on the palms and the soles. These are usually dry papules but sometimes, probably due to secondary infection, they become impetiginous and exudative. In Haiti the former are known as *dry crab* and the latter as *wet crab*, because of the crablike gait they provoke when plantar lesions are present.

LATE YAWS

The disease usually terminates with the secondary stage, but in some it may progress to a late *stage*, in which gummatous lesions occur. These are indolent ulcers with clean-cut or undermined edges, which tend to fuse to form configurate and occasionally serpiginous patterns clinically indistinguishable from those of tertiary syphilis. Upon healing, these sores cause scar tissue, leading to disfigurement. Similar processes may occur in the osseous system and other deep structures, leading to painful nodes on the bones, destruction of the palate and nasal bone (gangosa), and muscular contractures.

There may be periostitis, particularly of the tibia, epiphysitis, chronic synovitis, juxtaarticular nodules, and gummatous skin lesions.

In the later stages pigmented spots or marked hyperkeratosis may occur on the palms and soles. The hyperkeratosis may be diffuse or pitted as a result of the picking out of the central epithelial plug from the hard papules. This type of *keratodermia palmaris et plantaris* is highly diagnostic. Furtado found an incidence of 11 per cent in his studies.

ETIOLOGY. *Treponema pertenue* is identical morphologically with the *T. pallidum* of syphilis, being a slender spiral with six to 20 coils. In demonstrating *T. pertenue*, slides for darkfield examination should be prepared from the lesion after the crust has been removed.

Overcrowding, poverty, and poor hygiene predispose to yaws, which occurs chiefly in native children of both sexes in regions where it is endemic. The disease is usually acquired by human body contact. A break in the skin seems necessary for transmission, and frequently the disease begins upon preexisting ulcers or abrasions. There is no convincing evidence

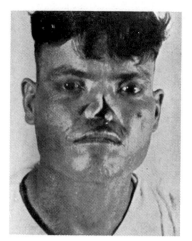

Figure 18–50. Gangosa.

of nonhuman vectors or reservoirs. Later, partial immunity becomes established, which is usually sufficient to prevent second infections. The disease is apparently not transmitted from mother to offspring and is uncommon during the first year of life.

HISTOPATHOLOGY. In the primary and secondary stages the epidermis shows elongation and a broadening of the interpapillary processes. The blood vessels are near the surface and predispose the lesions to ready bleeding. In the papillary and subpapillary layers an infiltration occurs, principally of plasma cells, mast cells, and small mononuclear cells. *Treponema pertenue* is usually demonstrable in the primary and secondary stages.

EPIDEMIOLOGY. Yaws is endemic in many tropical countries. It is common in parts of Africa and Southeast Asia.

There is a seasonal cycle of occurrence, with an increase in incidence during the rainy season. High humidity and high temperature are essential for the disease to thrive. Infection usually starts during the first five years of life. At present, approximately 50 million people live in areas where yaws is endemic, and it is estimated that cases of yaws still number in the thousands, although the disease is fast disappearing.

DIAGNOSIS. The diagnosis is established by the typical clinical appearance in a person living in an endemic zone. The presence of keratodermia palmaris et plantaris in such a person almost clinches the diagnosis. The darkfield demonstration of spirochetes in the early lesions and a reactive STS are the other criteria. The spirochetes may also be demonstrated by India ink preparations.

DIFFERENTIAL DIAGNOSIS. Differences between syphilis and yaws are evident in the mode of infection, the paucity of mucous membrane lesions during the secondary period of yaws, the absence of

congenital transmission of yaws, the lack of the late involvement of the central nervous and cardiovascular system in yaws, and the responsiveness of yaws to treatment.

TREATMENT. Treatment is with penicillin. Yaws responds to smaller doses than those used in syphilis. A single injection of 1.2 million units of benzathine penicillin G intramuscularly produces a dramatic response, with healing taking place in about one week. An alternative for penicillin-allergic patients is tetracycline, 2 gm daily for 10 days.

PROGNOSIS. Spontaneous cure (or permanent latency) may result after early disease. Others may suffer from anemia, weakness, and destructive tertiary bone and skin lesions. One attack confers immunity, which protects against future invasions. Yaws provides strong protection, if not total immunity, against sexually acquired syphilis.

Gangosa (rhinopharyngitis mutilans) is a mutilating rhinopharyngitis seen in the West Indies and endemic on the island of Guam. It is characterized by a progressive ulceration, which usually begins on the soft palate, pillars, or uvula and extends to the hard palate, nasal cavity, larynx, and face. The majority of cases occur in natives during the second and third decades, and it is a manifestation of the late stage of yaws.

The disease begins with a slight rise of temperature and the appearance of membranous sore throat followed rapidly by ulceration, which continues with alternate periods of activity and quiescence for several years, associated with a malodorous discharge and scarring. In children the process may be fulminating and lead to death, but in other cases it gives rise to no noticeable general symptoms. Penicillin is curative.

Goundou is a peculiar osteitis attributed to yaws. It is encountered in Africa, chiefly in the natives. It begins in childhood, with bony outgrowths on the sides of the nose, a nasal discharge, and headache. After a few months the discharge and headache disappear, but the tumors continue to grow and ultimately become like horns, leading to great distortion of the features and to destruction of the nose and orbit. Goundou may also occur as a proliferative osteitis in other parts of the body.

Browne SF: Yaws. Int J Dermatol 1982, 21:220.

Green CA, et al: Yaws. Clin Exp Dermatol 1986, 11:41.

Guthe TH: Clinical, serologic, and epidemiologic features of framboesia tropica (yaws) and its control in rural communities. Acta Dermatol Vener 1969, 49:343.

1984 International Symposium on Yaws and other Endemic Treponematoses. Rev Infect Dis 1985, 7(Suppl 2).

Nagreh DS: Yaws. Cutis 1986, 38:303.

Taneja BL: Yaws incidence and epidemiology. J Trop Med Hyg 1967, 70:215.

BEJEL

Bejel is a Bedouin term for nonvenereal treponematosis that closely resembles yaws with two exceptions, the rarity of an identifiable primary lesion, and the frequency of lesions in the mouth and nasopharynx. The late-stage lesions are indistinguishable. The etiologic agent of bejel is considered to be *Treponema pallidum*. The basic histologic changes of the mucosal lesions are virtually identical to those of venereal syphilis and the late lesions are pathologically not different from those seen in yaws. *Njovera* is a similar disease occurring in Zimbabwe.

Erdelyi RL, et al: Burned out endemic syphilis (bejel). Plast Reconstr Surg 1984, 74:589.
Pace JL, et al: Endemic non-venereal syphilis (bejel) in Saudi Arabia. Br J Venereal Dis 1984, 60:293.

PINTA

Pinta is also known as *mal del pinto, carate, cute,* or *cativi.*

Pinta, like yaws, is an infectious, nonvenereal, endemic treponematosis characterized by cutaneous lesions, whose marked pigmentary changes give the disease its name. The manifestations of pinta may be divided into primary, secondary, and tertiary stages.

PRIMARY STAGE

It is believed that the initial lesion appears seven to 10 days after inoculation. The lesion begins as a tiny red papule that becomes an elevated, ill-defined, erythematosquamous plaque in the course of two to three months. At five months this lesion becomes surrounded by satellite macules or papules that may fuse with it and form a configurate pattern. Ultimately it becomes impossible to distinguish the primary lesion from the secondary lesions. At no time is there erosion or ulceration such as occurs in the syphilitic chancre. Most initial lesions of pinta develop in natives on the legs and other uncovered parts. The STS is nonreactive in the primary stage. Darkfield examination may be positive.

SECONDARY STAGE

The secondary stage appears from five months to a year or more after infection. It begins with indeterminate erythematosquamous patches that may simulate psoriasis, ringworm, eczema, syphilis, or leprosy. They are located mostly on the extremities and face and frequently are somewhat circinate. The secondary eruption may be inconspicuous or absent in many patients. The STS is reactive in the secondary stage in about 60 per cent of patients. Darkfield examination from the patch may show spirochetes.

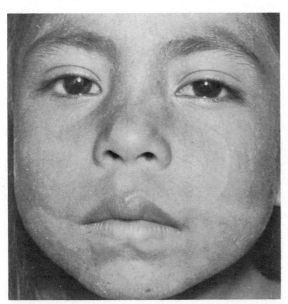

Figure 18–51. Primary lesion of pinta. (Courtesy of Dr. R. Medina, Venezuela.)

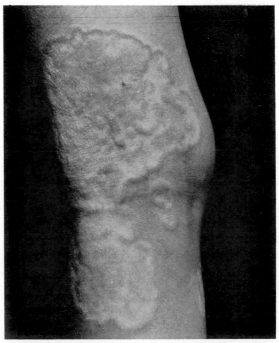

Figure 18–52. Primary lesion of pinta. (Courtesy of Dr. F. Latapí, Mexico.)

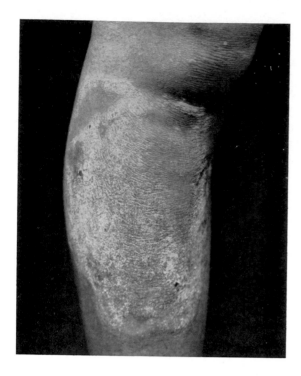

Figure 18–53. Early pinta on the shin. (Courtesy of Dr. B. S. Camacho, Mexico.)

LATE DYSCHROMIC STAGE

Until the 1940s the late pigmentary changes were the only recognized clinical manifestations of pinta. These have an insidious onset, usually in adolescents or young adults, consisting at first of localized, slate-blue pigmentation which after years becomes more widespread and gives way to depigmented spots resembling vitiligo. The lesions are located chiefly on the face, waistline, wrist flexures, and trochanteric region, although at times diffuse involvement occurs so that large areas on the trunk and extremities are affected.

At first the blue spots may have a stippled appearance or form discrete nummular or larger patches. The bluish patches occur chiefly on the head and neck, particularly on the nose and cheeks, the chin, lower part of the forehead, and also in the mouth or beneath the nails.

The lesions are symmetric in over one third of the patients. *Hemipinta* is a rare variety of the disease in which the pigmentary disturbances affect only one half of the body. Juxtaarticular nodules, like those in syphilis and yaws, are occasionally encountered.

In the late dyschromic stage of pinta, the STS is positive in nearly all patients. The spinal fluid is normal because this disease is limited to the skin.

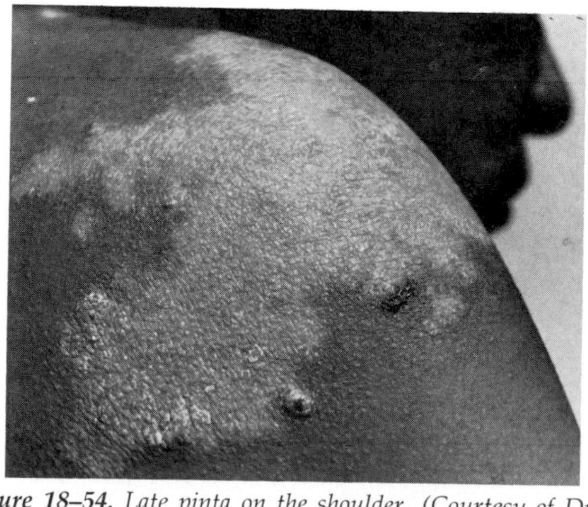

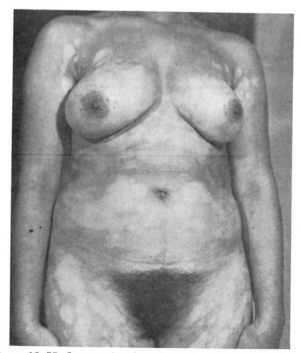

Figure 18–55. Symmetric achromic patches in late pinta. (Courtesy of Dr. F. Kerdel-Vegas, Venezuela.)

Figure 18–54. Late pinta on the shoulder. (Courtesy of Dr. R. Medina, Venezuela.)

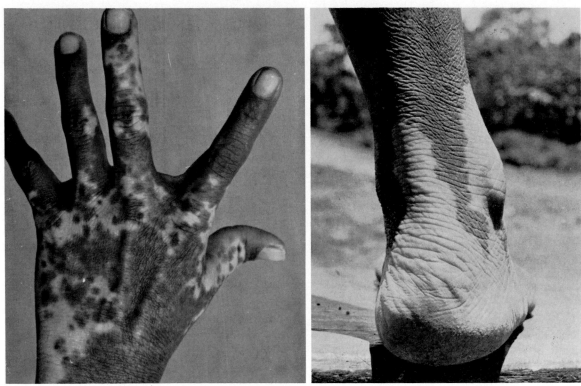

Figure 18–56. Pinta, showing achromic patches. (Courtesy of Dr. R. Medina, Venezuela.)

Spirochetes are demonstrable from all active skin lesions of pinta (not in the vitiliginous patches) by abrasion of the epidermis and examination of the serum thus obtained.

ETIOLOGY. Pinta is caused by a spirochete, *Treponemia carateum,* morphologically identical with *T. pallidum.* It was discovered in 1938 by the Cubans Saenz, Triana, and Armenteros. Pinta was first transmitted experimentally by the Mexican physicians Latapí and León y Blanco in 1939.

EPIDEMIOLOGY. The possible direct role of biting insects in the transmission of the disease has often been postulated, although never proved. The evidence seems to be compelling that household contact between persons with large areas of excoriated skin is the primary method of transmission. Superinfection or reinfection does not occur during the late pigmentary period of pinta but regularly occurs during the initial or spreading period. A first attack does not provoke lasting immunity. Contact with infective lesions should be avoided and precautions should be taken against the bites of flies and gnats. The inoculation studies of Herrejón showed that syphilitic infection, past or present, does not protect against pinta.

Pinta is indigenous in tropical and subtropical America. It is most prevalent in Mexico, Colombia, Venezuela, Ecuador, Peru, and Brazil. It is estimated that there are 600,000 cases in Colombia and 500,000 cases in Mexico. It also occurs in most of the other countries of Central America, West Indies, and the northern countries of South America.

HISTOPATHOLOGY. In blue pinta there are solid masses of melanophores in the papillary and subjacent layer with a mild inflammatory infiltration and no noteworthy changes in the epidermis. Spirochetes may be demonstrated in the epidermis by special stains. In white pinta there is an absence of spirochetes and of melanophores and scarcely any infiltration, and the epidermis is relatively thin. The rete cells are frequently vacuolated.

TREATMENT. The treatment of choice is benzathine penicillin G, 2.4 million units intramuscularly. Tetracycline and erythromycin, 2 gm daily for 10 days, are also effective. The STS becomes negative very slowly after treatment. The blue color gradually disappears, as do the areas that are partially depigmented. The vitiliginous areas, if present for more than five years, are permanent. The hyperkeratotic and desquamative lesions disappear, however.

Medina R: El carate en Venezuela. Dermatologia Venezolana 1962, 3:160.

Padilha-Gonçalves A: Immunologic aspects of pinta. Dermatologica 1967, 135:199.

19

Viral Diseases

Viral genomes are "elements of nucleic acid that replicate inside living cells, using the cellular synthetic machinery and causing synthesis of the specialized elements, the virions, that can transfer the genome to other cells." So said Luria and Darnell, in 1978. Viruses are obligatory intracellular parasites.

The structural components of a virus particle (virion) consist of a central core of nucleic acid (nucleoid); a protective protein coat (capsid); and (in certain groups of viruses only) an outermost lipoprotein membrane or envelope. The nucleoid and the capsid are often referred to as the nucleocapsid. Analysis of the structure of a virion shows three basic symmetries: cubic (icosahedral or spherical), helical, and complex. Nucleocapsid symmetry is important in the classification of viruses.

The capsid of the simplest viruses is made up of many identical polypeptides (structural units), which fold and interact with one another to form morphologic units (capsomeres). The number of capsomeres is believed to be constant for each virus with cubic symmetry, and it is an important criterion in the classification of viruses. The protein coat determines serologic specificity, protects the nucleic acid from enzymatic degradation in biologic environments, controls host specificity, and increases efficiency of infection.

Many larger viruses also contain internal proteins which have polymerase activity. Smaller viruses do not contain polymerases within the virion.

The outermost lipoprotein membrane of the enveloped viruses is essential for the attachment to, and penetration of, host cells. The envelope also contains important viral antigens.

Two main groups of viruses are distinguished: DNA and RNA. Viruses may be grouped according to the type of nucleic acid and according to the size,

shape, and substructure of the virus particle. Subgroups are also created on the basis of antigenic differences.

On the basis of physicochemical properties, viruses may be classified in the following groups: DNA viruses are parvovirus, papovavirus, adenovirus, herpesvirus, and poxvirus. RNA viruses are picornavirus, togavirus, reovirus, cornavirus, orthomyxovirus, retrovirus, arenavirus, rhabdovirus, and paramyxovirus. Five groups of viruses are distinguished by their mode of transmission: arthropod-borne viruses, respiratory viruses, fecal-oral or intestinal viruses, venereal viruses, and penetrating wound viruses. The cutaneous disorders caused by viruses will be presented in this chapter according to the above groups.

In some cutaneous disorders there are distinctive cellular changes in the specific lesions that are caused by the various viruses. In herpes simplex and varicella-zoster, these occur as *inclusion bodies*; in vaccinia and variola, as *Guarneri bodies*; in molluscum contagiosum, as *molluscum*, or *Henderson-Patterson*, *bodies*; and in warts, as *nuclear inclusions*. These unique intracellular bodies occur in the cytoplasm in the case of poxvirus infections or in the nucleus in the case of herpesvirus infections.

Androphy EJ, et al: Tumor viruses, oncogenes, and human cancer. JAAD 1983, 9:125.
Bryson YJ: Promising new antiviral drugs. JAAD 1988, 18:212.
Dorsky DL, et al: Drugs five years later: Acyclovir. Ann Intern Med 1987, 107:859.
Hermans PE, et al: Antiviral agents. Mayo Clin Proc 1983, 58:217.
Hirsch MS, et al: Resistance to antiviral drugs. N Engl J Med 1989, 320:313.
Luria SE, et al: General Virology. 3rd ed. New York, Wiley, 1978.
Robinson T: Antiviral agents and the skin. Semin Dermatol 1983, 2:130.

HERPESVIRUS GROUP

These medium-sized viruses contain DNA and replicate in the cell nucleus. They are characterized by the tendency to produce intermittently latent infections such as herpes simplex. Viruses constituting this group are varicella-zoster virus, cytomegaloviruses, Epstein-Barr virus, herpes simplex viruses 1 and 2, human herpesvirus-6 (HHV-6, HBLV), *Herpesvirus simiae* (B virus), and other viruses of animals.

HERPES SIMPLEX

Synonyms: Fever blister, cold sore, herpes febrilis, herpes labialis, herpes progenitalis.

CLINICAL FEATURES. Herpes simplex is characterized by an acute, self-limited eruption of grouped vesicles upon an erythematous base, occurring singly or severally, most frequently at or near the mucocutaneous junctures. The onset is usually preceded by localized itching, burning, and erythema of several minutes' or hours' duration. Rarely, neuralgic pain may precede, accompany, or follow (or any two, or all three) the eruption, as one expects with zoster. Formication, tingling, and pain may be severe. The sciatic nerve is often the site of such radiculopathy, as reported by Fisher.

The fully developed eruption consists of a cluster of pinhead-sized or slightly larger vesicles containing a clear exudate that later becomes seropurulent. In the course of a few days they rupture and the dried serum forms a flaky crust, beneath which epithelialization occurs. The neighboring lymph glands are sometimes enlarged and tender during the outbreak. Usually this common recurrent type of herpes runs its course in about a week. Spruance and associates in a fine prospective study found vesicles still present in only one fifth of cases after 48 hours. The lesions

tend to heal without scarring except where there has been an unusual amount of suppuration. On the mucous membranes or in other moist areas the patches rapidly become sodden.

The primary infection, upon initial exposure of an individual to the virus, is in the majority of cases asymptomatic. Only a small number manifest the systemic symptoms and severe local reactions seen in the primary inoculation complex. Herpes simplex in some individuals has a tendency to recur over and over again at the same location, *herpes recurrens*. After many recurrent attacks in the same location there may occasionally appear telangiectases, lymphedema of the hand after recurrent herpetic whitlow, depigmented spots, or scars. However, it usually clears without residua.

Although the lips are the most frequent site of the disorder, herpes may appear in any location. The nose, both outside and inside, is the next most common location, on the face, and not infrequently the cheeks and other parts of the face and the ears are involved. The genital region is also frequently involved, in both sexes. Rarely the lesions appear within the mouth, on the tongue or within the pharynx, and they have been described in the larynx and esophagus, where the eruption is generally accompanied by some constitutional symptoms. Herpes simplex lesions may be zosteriform and may be accompanied or preceded by severe pain and regional adenopathy.

Primary Inoculation Complex. The primary infection of herpes simplex may produce a violent systemic and local reaction in some young adults who for the first time experience an attack of the disease. All types of primary infection will be described; a discussion of the far commoner recurrent disease will follow. All primary infections result in latent disease, which may recur in a milder form.

Herpetic Gingivostomatitis. In less than 1 per cent of patients experiencing first-time exposure to herpes

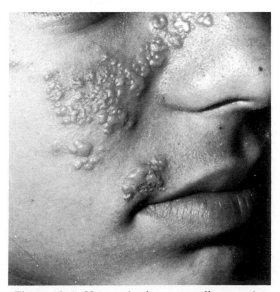

Figure 19–1. Herpes simplex, unusually extensive.

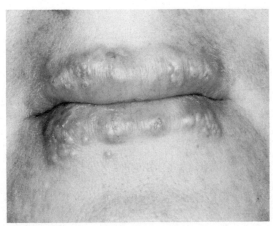

Figure 19–2. Herpes simplex. Note clusters of grouped vesicles.

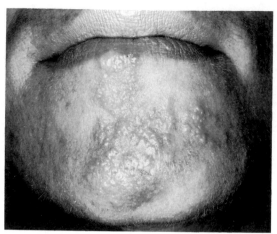

Figure 19–3. Herpes simplex on chin.

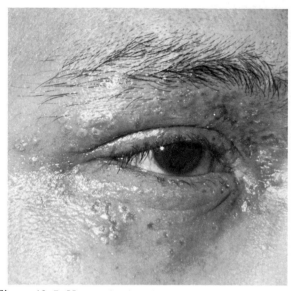

Figure 19–5. Herpes simplex of eyelids in a 27-year-old man.

simplex in the mouth, herpetic gingivostomatitis occurs, chiefly in children and young adults. The onset is often accompanied by high fever, regional lymphadenopathy, and malaise. The herpes lesions in the mouth are usually broken vesicles that show as white spots or ulcers. These may become widespread on the oral mucosa, tongue, and tonsils and produce pain, foul breath, and loss of appetite. In young children dehydration and acidosis may occur. It may cause pharyngitis, with ulcerative or exudative lesions of the posterior pharynx. The course of the disease runs one to two weeks. It must be differentiated from herpangina, streptococcal infection, infectious mononucleosis, thrush, erythema multiforme of the Stevens-Johnson type, and Behçet's syndrome. Oral vesicles may be caused by herpes zoster, pemphigus vulgaris, bullous pemphigoid,

stomatitis venenata, chickenpox, herpangina, and hand-foot-and-mouth disease.

Herpetic Vulvovaginitis. Vesicular lesions of the labia majora or minora, perianal area, or vaginal or cervical mucosa may appear three to seven days after exposure. They rupture to become erosions within 24 to 48 hours in the moist areas. Edema and erythema may be marked. Fever, headache, and malaise commonly occur. Pain and burning may be severe and urination may become difficult. The lesions usually heal spontaneously within two to six weeks. Men may experience similar systemic symptoms and a severe extensive local eruption on the penis and pubic area, easily misdiagnosed as staphylococcal folliculitis.

Herpes Gladiatorum. James and Rodman reported an epidemic of primary inoculation herpes simplex in a wrestling team and reviewed previous reports of this phenomenon. Skin-to-skin contact with a player with recurrent disease is responsible. Rugby players, especially the forwards who participate in the scrums, are also at risk. All reports of this not uncommon problem have implicated HSV Type 1 as the cause.

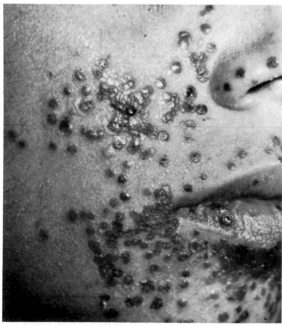

Figure 19–4. Severe hemorrhagic herpes simplex.

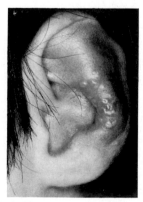

Figure 19–6. Herpes simplex of the external ear.

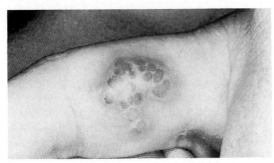

Figure 19–7. Primary herpes simplex of the finger.

Intrauterine and Neonatal Herpes Simplex. Herpesvirus contracted in utero can result in anomalies of the newborn. These cases usually occur in mothers who have acquired primary herpes simplex during pregnancy. The anomalies have included microcephaly, microphthalmos, encephalitis, chorioretinitis, and intracerebral calcifications, associated with vesicular skin lesions.

Maternal genital herpetic infections are associated with abortions, stillbirths, or premature delivery. Komorous et al proposed that intrauterine herpes simplex infections be termed "early" when there is evidence of disturbed embryogenesis, or "late" when development of the fetus seems to have been undisturbed. Glover et al reviewed cases of intrauterine infection. Widespread atrophic scars may be present at birth.

Seventy per cent of cases of neonatal herpes simplex are caused by HSV-2 and acquired as the child passes through an infected birth canal. Neonatal HSV-1 infections are usually acquired postnatally through contact with a person with oral–labial disease. The clinical spectrum of perinatally acquired herpes simplex in the neonate ranges from localized skin infection to severe disseminated disease with encephalitis, hepatitis, pneumonia, and coagulopathy. In 70 per cent of babies, skin vesicles are the presenting sign, and are the best hunting ground for virus retrieval. Because the incubation period may be as long as three weeks, the vesicles may not appear until the child has gone home. Central nervous system involvement may occur without skin lesions ever having been present.

The risk of infection of an infant delivered vaginally when the mother has active recurrent herpetic infection has been estimated to be 3 to 5 per cent, whereas it is 50 per cent if the maternal infection is a primary one. An epidemiologic study showed that the incidence of symptomatic maternal herpes simplex at the time of delivery was 1:1000, while the incidence of neonatal herpes simplex was 1:7500. Seventy per cent of mothers whose child gets neonatal herpes simplex are asymptomatic at the time of delivery and may have no history of recurrent herpes.

For the woman who is subject to recurrent genital herpes, the risk of exposure of the infant during labor is sufficient to require examination for herpetic lesions before delivery: if such are present, cesarean section should be done either before the membranes rupture, or within four hours. If no lesions are seen, viral culture should be taken prior to delivery, and followed by viral cultures from the baby's conjunctiva and nasopharynx at 24 and 36 hours. If the baby is premature, has underlying disease, or has been subject to prenatal instrumentation (monitoring electrodes, or intubation), or if there was early rupture of the membranes, and the mother's culture was positive, prophylactic acyclovir should be given. If the neonate's cultures are positive or any sign of disease develops, treatment is indicated.

This course of action is reasonable, but the rec-

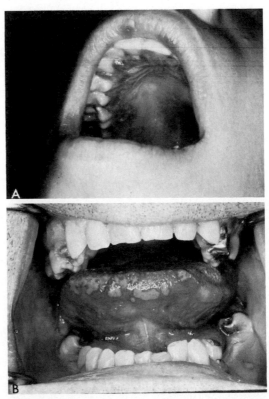

Figure 19–9. Herpetic gingivostomatitis. A, A 16-year-old boy, and B, a 51-year-old man.

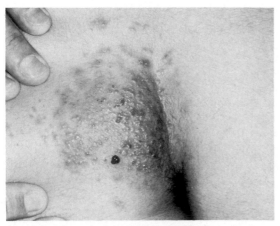

Figure 19–8. Herpes gladiatorum in a young male wrestler.

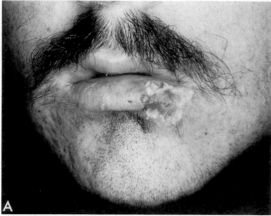

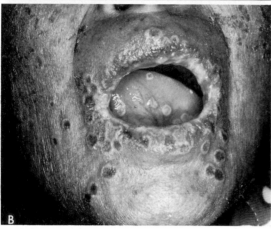

Figure 19–10. A, *Chronic herpes simplex in a young man with lymphosarcoma.* B, *Acute orocutaneous herpes simplex in a woman on high doses of prednisone with a severe drug reaction.*

three years of age, disseminated herpes simplex generally starts with a severe herpetic gingivostomatitis. Dissemination to the viscera, especially the liver, follows. Involvement of the lungs and a massive viremia may follow and produce gastroenteritis, encephalitis, and hepatic and adrenal dysfunction. Most deaths occur during the stage of severe viremia.

Severe disseminated herpes simplex occurs in the newborn, especially the premature (see Neonatal Herpes Simplex), and also in infants and malnourished persons such as those with kwashiorkor; in associated infections, particularly measles; in compromised hosts being treated with immunosuppressive drugs; with Hodgkin's and other related diseases; in the Wiskott-Aldrich syndrome; and in persons with the acquired immunodeficiency syndrome. See also Eczema Coxsackium.

Recurrent Herpes Simplex. Herpes simplex often recurs during some febrile diseases, such as pneumonia, influenza, malaria, and meningococcal meningitis. It may also accompany artificially induced fever. Recurrent disease usually occurs in the site of the primary infection.

Recurrent disease, compared to the primary inoculation complex, is characterized by fewer grouped localized lesions; few if any constitutional symptoms; and a shorter course, usually healing spontaneously within one week. Any blistering eruption which recurs at the same site should be suspected of being herpes simplex. It may occur at unusual sites such as vaccination scars, as reported by Mints in 1982.

Oral-facial Disease. The most common site is at or near the vermilion border, as grouped vesicles on an erythematous base. Spontaneous healing usually occurs in four to seven days.

Recurrent disease may be associated with neuralgia, especially in the buttocks area, and lead to the

ommendations given are not universally applied and are in a state of flux. The recent study by Probert et al indicates that most neonatal infections occurring at delivery from an asymptomatic mother are neither predictable nor preventable.

Disseminated Herpes Simplex Infection. A disease of children, usually between six months and

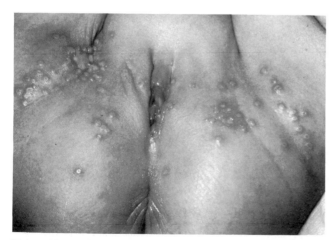

Figure 19–11. Primary herpes simplex in an infant. Sexual abuse was considered.

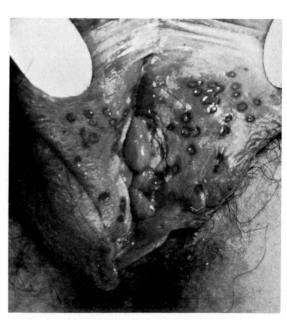

Figure 19–12. Herpes progenitalis on labia. (Courtesy of Dr. W. B. Hurlbut.)

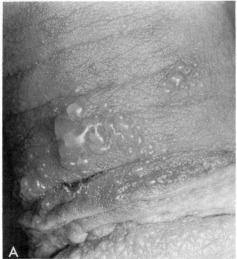

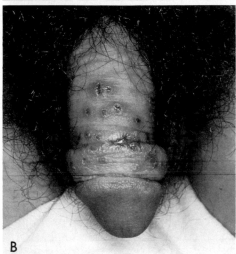

Figure 19–13. A, *Early stage herpes progenitalis.* B, *Late stage herpes progenitalis.*

erroneous diagnosis of herpes zoster. There is considerable risk of reactivation of herpes after decompressive surgery of the trigeminal nerve root, with dental extraction, and with dermabrasion or chemical peel. Intra-oral recurrences are unusual, and are likely to be limited to the attached tissues (hard palate and gingiva).

Genital Herpes (Herpes Progenitalis). More than 80 to 90 per cent of patients with first-episode HSV-2 infection have a recurrence within the first year. The 10 to 20 per cent of genital herpes which is due to HSV-1 recurs at a lower rate, about 55 per cent. Herpes progenitalis is about 10 times commoner than gonorrhea. Luby called it "a pervasive psychosocial disorder," because it frightens its victims so.

The lesions appear in men anywhere on the penis or occasionally in the urethra. Frequent sites in women are the labia, vulva, clitoris, and cervix. The vesicles appear singly or in clusters and rupture in a few days to form an erosion, with a nonindurated base. Inguinal lymphadenopathy may be present. Prodromal symptoms of localized burning or stinging

occur, usually 24 hours before the eruption, in over half of patients.

The recurrent infection usually runs its course within eight days. Healing usually occurs without scarring. Although epidemiologic evidence originally showed an association between HSV-2 infection and cervical carcinoma, a recent study in a large population by Vonka et al discounted any etiologic connection.

Genital herpes is easily mistaken for a syphilitic chancre or chancroid, especially when it occurs on the glans, prepuce, or shaft. Salzman recently reported a group of patients whose clinical "chancroids" grew out herpesvirus on culture in one half the cases.

Victims of herpes progenitalis are likely to have recurrent lesions at the same site as a result of some triggering mechanism such as menses, emotional stress, coitus, or trauma. Asymptomatic shedding of virus, in low titers, occurs intermittently in 1 to 5 per cent of patients.

Rectal and perianal recurrences are common in the homosexual population. Recurrent lesions of the sacral region or buttocks are seen frequently in women, possibly as a result of "spooning." Lafferty et al in a prospective study of 39 patients found a sixfold greater recurrence rate of genital HSV infections than of oral-labial ones.

Recurrent Erythema Multiforme. Recurrent erythema multiforme may be due to a recurrent herpes simplex infection. Shelley found in one case that there was in fact a hypersensitivity reaction to herpesvirus, and this is a common occurrence. Kazmierowski et al showed that these patients' serum contains immune complexes composed of antibody and HSV antigen. Such complexes may occasionally be found in patients with erythema multiforme of unknown cause.

This erythema multiforme was prevented by Lemak et al with prophylactic orally administered acyclovir. It can also be prevented, or aborted even after

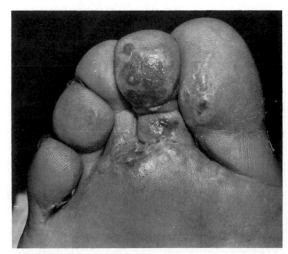

Figure 19–14. Herpes simplex eruption on toes, resembling acute dermatophytosis.

it has begun, by 60 mg of triamcinolone acetonide intramuscularly (Arnold).

Herpetic Sycosis. Following an attack of facial herpes simplex, the patient who shaves with a blade razor may experience a slowly spreading folliculitis of the beard, with a few isolated vesicles. Only its transient course, lasting two or three weeks, and the presence of vesicles, indicate that it is not ordinary sycosis vulgaris. Allan Izumi et al documented the features and the cause of this unusual form of herpes.

Herpetic Whitlow. Herpesvirus infection may rarely take the form of a felon, or whitlow: infection of the pulp of a fingertip. Such lesions are most often seen in dentists, dental hygienists, physicians, or nurses; but also, since there is no immune protection against autoinoculation, in patients with herpes elsewhere. Children may be thus superinfected while thumbsucking or nailbiting during an attack of herpes. Herpetic whitlow in a dental technician can readily be transmitted to patients. In a recent study, 37 per cent of patients thus exposed had contracted herpetic pharyngitis.

Eczema Herpeticum. Infection with herpesvirus in patients with atopic dermatitis may lead to spread of herpes simplex throughout the eczematous areas (Kaposi's varicelliform eruption). The same may occur in severe seborrheic dermatitis, impetigo, scabies, Darier's disease, pemphigus (foliaceus or vulgaris), or burns. Hundreds of umbilicated vesicles may be present at the onset, with fever and regional adenopathy. If this is the primary exposure to herpesvirus, hematogenous dissemination occurs as well, and any point of diminished resistance may develop viral disease. This has been reported in several cases of Wiskott-Aldrich syndrome. The more usual method of spread, however, is across abnormal skin surfaces, and while the resulting cutaneous eruption is alarming, the disease is often self-limited in healthy individuals.

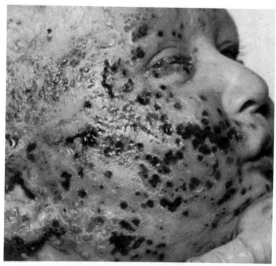

Figure 19–15. Eczema herpeticum. (From Moschella SL, Hurley HJ: Dermatology. 2nd Ed. Philadelphia, WB Saunders, 1985, p 677.)

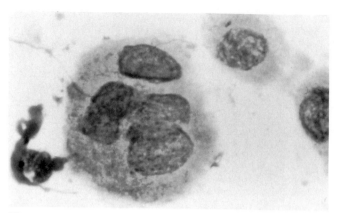

Figure 19–16. Multinucleated giant cell of herpes simplex (Tzanck smear).

Herpetic Keratoconjunctivitis. Herpes simplex infection of the eye is the most common cause of blindness in the United States. It occurs as a punctate or marginal keratitis, or as a dendritic corneal ulcer, which may cause disciform keratitis and leave scars that impair vision. Topical corticosteroids in this situation may induce perforation of the cornea. Vesicles may appear on the lids, and preauricular nodes may be enlarged and tender. Recurrences are common.

Immunocompromised Patients. When patients with underlying leukemia, lymphoma, or immunodeficiency disease such as AIDS develop recurrent herpes, it may become chronic. Slowly enlarging, nonhealing ulcerations develop in the perineum or on the face. Large eschars may cover the ulceration, Tzanck preparations are often negative, and the diagnosis may depend upon clinical suspicion, viral cultures, or biopsies. This disease may rarely occur in SLE or disseminated soft-tissue carcinomatosis. Symptomatic stomatitis associated with cancer chemotherapy is at times due to HSV infection. Acyclovir will induce healing of these chronic ulcerations in immunocompromised patients.

LABORATORY FINDINGS. The simplest yet most reliable finding is the demonstration of giant cells with multiple nuclei and acidophilic intranuclear inclusions in Giemsa- or Wright-stained cytologic (Tzanck) smears of scrapings from the base of the vesicles. Up to the time of crusting, the Tzanck smear was found positive in 60 to 70 per cent of cases by Solomon et al.

When submitting the vesicle fluid to a diagnostic virus laboratory, the vesicles should be cleaned with acetone (not ether), allowed to dry, and opened with a sharp needle or #11 blade. The vesicle fluid is collected, using the applicator, and transported to the laboratory in the tube provided in a Virocult collection and transportation system.

A rapid diagnosis may be made by direct fluorescent antibody (FA) technique using the fluid scraped from the base of the vesicle. Two drops of phosphate-buffered saline are placed on a slide containing the fluid; the material is mixed, dried in air, fixed and stained using rabbit antiherpetic serum and fluorescein-labeled antirabbit globulin. A positive fluorescence is noted. This test is virus-specific and is negative in varicella-zoster infections.

The tissue-culture method of recovery of virus from vesicles, blood, urine, spinal fluid, or biopsy material is considered a reliable diagnostic procedure. Electron microscopy demonstrates intracellular virions characteristic of herpetic infection in the affected tissue.

HISTOPATHOLOGY. The vesicles of herpes simplex are intraepidermal. The affected epidermis and the adjacent inflamed dermis become infiltrated with leukocytes, and a serous exudate containing dissociated cells collects beneath the stratum corneum to form the vesicle. There is ballooning degeneration of the epidermal cells to produce acantholysis.

Minute acidophil intranuclear bodies occur in the epithelial cells' nuclei. These small bodies increase in size, coalesce, and finally occupy the greater part of the nucleus to form the "inclusion body." It is eosinophilic and surrounded by a halo.

ETIOLOGY. The herpes infection is caused by *Herpesvirus hominis*, Type 1 or 2, which contains DNA and a protein coat with icosahedral symmetry. An envelope containing lipids encases the two elements. This enveloped form is 180 nm in diameter. The icosahedral capsid is made up of 162 capsomeres, which are hexagonal prism–shaped.

The initial attack is caused by direct contact with lesions in an infected person during the first five to eight days of an attack. Recurrent attacks are caused by virus returning to the skin from regional dorsal root ganglia, where it is sequestered between attacks. Specific immunoincompetence makes such recurrences possible though neutralizing antibody titer is high.

There are two serologically identified types of herpesvirus, Type 1 and Type 2. Most infections above the waist are due to Type 1; most below, to Type 2. However, as a result of oral-genital contact approximately 20 per cent of genital herpes simplex is due to HSV-1.

DIFFERENTIAL DIAGNOSIS. Herpes labialis must most frequently be differentiated from impetigo. The straw-colored serous fluid and the crusts of impetigo are distinctive; however, a mixed infection is not unusual. Herpes zoster presents with clusters of lesions along a nerve path.

Herpes progenitalis, especially on the glans or corona, is easily mistaken for a syphilitic chancre or chancroid. A darkfield examination and cultures for *Hemophilus ducreyi* on selective media will aid in making the diagnosis, as will smears for intranuclear inclusion bodies, the Tzanck preparation.

Herpetic gingivostomatitis is often difficult to differentiate from aphthosis, streptococcic infections, diphtheria, coxsackievirus infections, and Stevens-Johnson syndrome. Aphthae have a tendency to occur mostly on the buccal and labial mucosae. They are usually wider and form shallow, grayish erosions, generally surrounded by a ring of hyperemia. While these commonly occur on nonattached mucosa, recurrent viral disease of the oral cavity primarily affects the attached gingiva and palate.

Herpetic esophagitis may be the cause of severe retrosternal burning and dysphagia in patients with cancer, and when such pain is not relieved by mycostatin, fiberoptic esophagoscopy and brush cytology may permit a diagnosis of herpes simplex.

Grouped vesicles on an erythematous base located anywhere on the body always suggest herpes simplex (or if within one neurotome, and multiple, zoster).

TREATMENT. The treatment of herpes simplex infections has two aims: to shorten the current attack, and to prevent recurrences. There is no convincing evidence that any form of treatment other than acyclovir achieves either goal. Oral or intravenous acyclovir (Zovirax) is effective in all forms of primary herpes simplex infections, in prevention of recurrences, and in treatment of immunocompromised patients. Its topical use is not recommended. Acyclovir is an acyclic nucleoside analog of guanosine. It is a selective substrate for and inhibitor of herpesvirus DNA polymerase. Side effects are uncommon. The major route of elimination is via the kidney, therefore dose reduction is recommended in patients with impaired renal function.

Primary episodes of herpes genitalis are effectively treated with 200 mg orally five times daily for seven to ten days or by intravenous therapy, 5 mg/kg of body weight every eight hours for five to seven days. Neonatal herpes infections are preferentially treated with IV acyclovir 250 mg/m² every eight hours for seven days. This is due to greater ease of administration and lower toxicity than IV vidarabine, which is also effective. Acyclovir therapy is also recommended for disseminated herpes simplex (although there is currently no evidence that this will decrease mortality), herpetic whitlow, primary herpetic keratitis, and Kaposi's varicelliform eruption secondary to HSV. Oral acyclovir would be expected to be effective in the primary episodes of HSV proctitis, herpes gladiatorum, herpes labialis, and herpetic sycosis, but these manifestations have not yet been studied.

Immunocompromised patients with chronic ulcerative lesions usually respond well to 200 mg orally five times daily until healed; however, several recent reports document acyclovir-resistant HSV infections in AIDS patients. Foscarnet, trisodium phosphonoformate, has been an effective alternative.

Acyclovir is not recommended for routine use in recurrent episodes of herpes simplex infections except in the above lesions in immunocompromised patients. Occasional patients who experience prolonged episodes of two to three weeks' duration may benefit from patient-initiated treatment at the prodrome or earliest sign of disease.

In the patient who experiences frequent recurrences of herpes genitalis with short disease-free intervals, suppressive therapy with oral acyclovir 200 mg two to three times daily has been shown in several studies to reduce the frequency of reactivation disease. The longest studies to date are 24-month studies, so indefinite therapy cannot yet be recommended. Intermittent discontinuance of acyclovir is recommended to observe the recurrence pattern and determine if further therapy is needed. The studies done to date indicate there will be a return to the pretreatment recurrence pattern; however, this should be documented before reinitiation of suppressive therapy is considered.

Treatment (as opposed to prevention) of recurrent lesions is limited to drying agents such as compresses of dilute Burow's solution or hydrogen peroxide.

Shelley's treatment, a modification of Falk's recommendation to use simple curettage, consists of simple shallow excision of the lesion by sawing strokes with a flexible Gillette Super Blue razor blade, slightly bent between finger and thumb. His expressive name for this maneuver is "epidermal subsection." It has not been the subject of a comparative study and is not a widely accepted mode of therapy. When recurrence did occur it was more severe than prior to subsection. He has also used it for "farmyard pox," and in these nonrecurrent infections it may have a place in therapy.

The prevention of recurrences depends also upon discovery and avoidance of triggering causes. The history of each attack must be studied in detail, with careful examination made for disturbances that might have provoked the eruption. Trauma, sunburn, emotional stress, and menstruation are some factors that have appeared to trigger attacks. Dermabrasion, chemical peel, and trigeminal nerve decompression may precipitate attacks. Oral acyclovir may be used to prevent its occurrence.

The virus is transmitted by direct contact. Inoculation of any skin site or mucous membrane may result in recurrent disease at that site. This includes autoinoculation as well as superinfection from others. In genital disease, the use of condoms with the desired addition of spermicidal foams is necessary if there is sexual contact during active disease. Asymptomatic shedding occurs in men and women, and the patient should be aware of this. The sexual partner(s) of the patient may need medical care in the form of examination, treatment, or education. One area of cautious reassurance for female patients is that the potential risk of cervical cancer in women with genital herpes simplex infection, once felt to be higher than that of noninfected women, now is related to papillomavirus infection and unrelated to herpes simplex virus. However, the potential teratogenicity of acyclovir and the risk of transmitting herpetic infection to newborns remain hazards to infected women of child-bearing age.

Arndt KA: Adverse reactions to acyclovir. JAAD 1988, 18:188.
Arvin AM: Antiviral treatment of herpes simplex infection in neonates and pregnant women. JAAD 1988, 18:200.
Idem: Failure of antepartum maternal cultures to predict the infant's risk of exposure to herpes simplex virus at delivery. N Engl J Med 1986, 315:796.
Baringer JR: Recovery of herpes simplex virus from human sacral ganglions. N Engl J Med 1974, 291:828.
Barton SE, et al: Asymptomatic shedding and subsequent transmission of genital herpes simplex virus. Genitourin Med 1987, 63:102.
Behlmer SB, et al: Herpes simplex infections complicating parturition: Review. Int J Dermatol 1981, 20:242.
Bierman SM: A retrospective study of 375 patients with genital herpes simplex infections seen between 1973 and 1980. Cutis 1983, 31:548.
Binkin NJ, et al: Preventing neonatal herpes: the value of weekly viral cultures in pregnant women with recurrent genital herpes. JAMA 1984, 251:2816.
Blough HA: Topical 2-deoxy-d-glucose for herpes simplex (letter). JAAD 1983, 8:423.
Bork K, et al: Increasing incidence of eczema herpeticum. JAAD 1988, 19:1024.
Brown S, et al: Sensitivity and specificity of diagnostic tests for genital infection with herpesvirus hominis. Sex Transm Dis 1979, 6:10.
Bryson YJ, et al: Treatment of first episodes of genital herpes simplex virus infection with oral acyclovir. N Engl J Med 1983, 308:916.
Chang T-W: Herpes simplex virus infection. Int J Dermatol 1983, 22:1.
Chatis PA, et al: Successful treatment with foscarnet of an acyclovir-resistant mucocutaneous infection with herpes simplex virus in a patient with AIDS. N Engl J Med 1989, 320:279.
Conant MA: Prophylactic and suppressive treatment with acyclovir and the management of herpes in patients with AIDS. JAAD 1988, 18:186.
Idem: Herpes simplex virus transmission: condom studies. Sex Transm Dis 1984, 11:94.
Corey L, et al: Infections with herpes simplex viruses. N Engl J Med 1986, 314:686.
Idem: Part 2. N Engl J Med 1986, 314:749.
Idem: First-episode, recurrent, and asymptomatic herpes simplex infections. JAAD 1988, 18:169.
Idem: Genital herpes simplex virus infections. Ann Intern Med 1983, 98:958–973.
DiGiovanna JJ, et al: Failure of lysine in frequently recurrent herpes simplex infection. Arch Dermatol 1984, 120:48.
Douglas JM, et al: A double blind study of oral acyclovir for suppression of recurrences of genital herpes simplex virus infection. N Engl J Med 1984, 370:1551.
Erlich KS, et al: Acyclovir-resistant herpes simplex virus infections in patients with AIDS. N Engl J Med 1989, 320:293.
Feder HM Jr, et al: Herpetic whitlow. Am J Dis Child 1983, 137:861.
Fisher DA: Recurrent herpes simplex sciatica and its treatment with amantadine hydrochloride. Cutis 1982, 29:467.
Gill MJ, et al: Herpes simplex virus infection of the hand. Am J Med 1988, 84:89.
Glover MJ, et al: Congenital infection with herpes simplex virus type I. Pediatr Dermatol 1987, 4:336.
Goldberg LH, et al: Oral acyclovir for episodic treatment of recurrent herpes. JAAD 1986, 15:256.
Guinan ME: Oral acyclovir for treatment and suppression of genital herpes simplex virus infection (review). JAMA 1986, 255:1747.
Idem, et al: Topical ether and herpes simplex labialis. JAMA 1980, 243:1059.
Huff JC: Acyclovir for recurrent erythema multiforme caused by herpes simplex. JAAD 1988, 18:197.
James WD, et al: Herpes gladiatorum. J Assoc Milit Dermatol 1984, 10:4.
Jarratt M: Herpes simplex infection (editorial). Arch Dermatol 1983, 119:99.
Jawitz JC, et al: Treatment of eczema herpeticum with systemic acyclovir. Arch Dermatol 1985, 121:274.
Kazmierowski JA, et al: Herpes simplex antigen in immune complexes of patients with erythema multiforme: presence following recurrent herpes simplex infection. JAMA 1982, 247:2547.

Kibrick S: Herpes simplex infection at term: what to do with mother, newborn, and nursery personnel. JAMA 1980, 243:157.

Kurzrock R, et al: Cimetidine therapy of HSV infections in immunocompromised patients. Clin Exp Dermatol 1987, 12:326.

Lafferty WE, et al: Recurrences after oral and genital HSV infection. N Engl J Med 1987, 316:1444.

Laskin OL: Acyclovir and suppression of frequently recurring herpetic whitlow. Ann Intern Med 1985, 102:494.

Idem: Acyclovir. Arch Intern Med 1984, 144:1214.

Lemak MA, et al: Oral acyclovir for the prevention of herpes-associated erythema multiforme. JAAD 1986, 15:50.

Luby ED, et al: Genital herpes: a pervasive psychosocial disorder. Arch Dermatol 1985, 121:494.

Manzella JP, et al: An outbreak of herpes simplex virus type I gingivostomatitis in a dental hygiene practice. JAMA 1984, 252:2019.

McCune MA, et al: Treatment of recurrent herpes simplex infections with L-lysine monohydrochloride. Cutis 1984, 34:366.

Medical Letter, 1985: Oral acyclovir for genital herpes simplex infection. 27:41.

Mertz GJ, et al: Double-blind placebo-controlled trial of oral acyclovir in first-episode genital herpes simplex infection. JAMA 1984, 252:1147.

Mindel A, et al: Prophylactic oral acyclovir in recurrent genital herpes. Lancet 1984, 2:57.

Mintz L: Recurrent herpes simplex infection at a smallpox vaccination site. JAMA 1982, 247:2704.

Nerurkar LS, et al: Survival of herpes simplex virus in water specimens collected from hot tubs in spa facilities and on plastic surfaces. JAMA 1983, 250:3081.

Norris SA, et al: Severe, progressive herpetic whitlow caused by an acyclovir-resistant virus in a patient with AIDS. J Infect Dis 1988, 157:209.

Overall JC, et al: Prophylactic or anticipatory antiviral therapy for newborns exposed to herpes simplex infections. Pediatr Infect Dis 1984, 3:193.

Perna JJ, et al: Reactivation of latent herpes simplex virus infection by ultraviolet light. JAAD 1987, 17:473.

Prober CG, et al: Use of routine viral cultures at delivery to identify neonates exposed to herpes simplex virus. N Engl J Med 1988, 318:887.

Raab B, et al: Genital herpes simplex—concepts and treatment. JAAD 1981, 5:259.

Idem: Oral acyclovir for genital herpes—cautious optimism (editorial). JAAD 1985, 13:293.

Rand KH, et al: Cancer-chemotherapy–associated symptomatic stomatitis. Cancer 1982, 50:1262.

Reichman RC, et al: Treatment of recurrent genital herpes simplex infections with oral acyclovir. JAMA 1984, 251:2103.

Rozman TA, et al: Topical idoxuridine in the treatment of genital herpes (letter). JAMA 1983, 249:1826.

Salzman RS, et al: Chancroidal ulcers that are not chancroid. Arch Dermatol 1984, 120:636.

Sands M, et al: Herpes simplex lymphangitis. Arch Intern Med 1988, 148:2066.

Saral R, et al: Acyclovir prophylaxis of herpes-simplex–virus infection. N Engl J Med 1981, 305:63.

Shaw M, et al: Failure of acyclovir cream in the treatment of recurrent herpes. Br Med J 1985, 291:7.

Silverman AK, et al: Activation of herpes simplex following dermabrasion. JAAD 1985, 13:103.

Silvestri DL, et al: Ineffectiveness of topical idoxuridine in dimethyl sulfoxide for therapy of genital herpes. JAMA 1982, 248:953.

Skoldenberg B, et al: Acyclovir versus vidarabine in herpes simplex encephalitis. Lancet 1984, 2:707.

Solomon AR: New diagnostic tests for herpes simplex and varicella-zoster infections. JAAD 1988, 18:218.

Idem, et al: The Tzanck smear in the diagnosis of cutaneous herpes simplex. JAMA 1984, 251:633.

Spruance SL, et al: Acyclovir prevents reactivation of herpes simplex labialis in skiers. JAMA 1988, 260:1597.

Stagno H, et al: Herpes virus infections in pregnancy. N Engl J Med 1985, 313:1327.

Straus SE: Suppression of recurrent genital herpes: a placebo-controlled double-blind trial of oral acyclovir. N Engl J Med 1984, 310:1545.

Swart RNJ, et al: Treatment of eczema herpeticum with acyclovir. Arch Dermatol 1983, 119:13.

Taieb A, et al: Clinical epidemiology of symptomatic primary herpetic infection in children. Acta Pediatr Scand 1987, 76:128.

Vonderheid EC, et al: Chronic herpes simplex infection in cutaneous T-cell lymphoma. Arch Dermatol 1982, 116:1018.

Vonka V, et al: Epidemiological study on the relationships between cervical neoplasia and herpes simplex type-2 virus. Int J Cancer 1984, 33:49–66.

Westheim AI, et al: Acyclovir resistance in a patient with chronic mucocutaneous herpes simplex infection. JAAD 1987, 17:875.

Wheeler CE Jr: Herpes simplex. Vol 3, 14–2; 1–15, in Demis DJ, ed., Clinical Dermatology, Philadelphia, Harper & Row, 1985.

Idem: The herpes simplex problem. JAAD 1988, 163.

White WB, et al: Transmission of herpes simplex virus type-1 infection in rugby players. JAMA 1984, 252:533.

Whitley RJ, et al: The natural history of herpes simplex virus infection of mother and newborn. Pediatrics 1980, 66:489.

Idem: Vidarabine versus acyclovir therapy in herpes simplex encephalitis. N Engl J Med 1986, 314:144.

Yeager AS, et al: Reasons for the absence of a history of recurrent genital infections in mothers of neonates infected with herpes simplex virus. Pediatrics 1984, 73:188.

INFECTIOUS MONONUCLEOSIS

Also known as glandular fever, infectious mononucleosis is characterized by fever, adenopathy, splenomegaly, lymphocytosis with atypical lymphocytes, and the presence of heterophile antibodies.

After an incubation period of a few days to several weeks, bilateral lymph node enlargement of the cervical glands and possibly of the axillary and inguinal glands develops with accompanying fever as high as 40° C, malaise, and headache.

Pharyngitis is the most frequent sign. There is hyperplasia of the pharyngeal lymphoid tissue.

Cutaneous and mucous membrane lesions are present in about one third of patients. Edema of the eyelids and a macular or morbilliform rash may occur. The macular eruption is usually on the trunk and upper extremities. Scarlatiniform, herpetiform, erythema-multiforme–like, or Gianotti-Crosti–like eruptions, urticaria, and purpura are rare manifestations. One case of annular erythema of infancy was temporally related to EBV infection. The mucous membrane lesions consist of distinctive pinhead-sized petechiae, five to 20 in number, at the junction of the soft and hard palate.

The blood picture shows absolute lymphocytosis and monocytosis with abnormally large lymphocytes, which are basophilic and contain foamy cytoplasm and fenestrated nuclei. Atypical lymphocytes (Downey cells) usually represent at least 10 per cent of the total leukocyte count. The white blood cell count ranges from 10,000 to 40,000. The heterophile antibodies (agglutinins for sheep erythrocytes, or the Paul-Bunnell test) will be present in titers of 1:160 or higher. Antibodies reactive with Epstein-Barr virus develop regularly in patients with infectious mononucleosis and a rise in titer of EBV antibodies enables the diagnosis of infectious mononucleosis to be made. When hepatitis is present the SGOT and SGPT enzyme levels will be elevated.

IgM and IgG antibodies against the viral capsid antigen appear soon after infection, and shortly afterward, antibodies to the diffuse component of "early antigen" appear; these are referred to as "anti–early antigen." According to Jones et al, high titers of anti–early antigen antibody appear only during the initial infection, in abnormal responses to the primary exposure, or during prolonged or reactivated infections. Examples of the second category include ataxia-telangiectasia and the X-linked lymphoproliferative syndrome. The third category comprises patients with nasopharyngeal carcinoma or recurrent parotitis, immunosuppressed patients, some pregnant women, and persons of advanced age. Inexplicable or recurrent illness with symptoms which may include fatigue, headache, paresthesias, depression, pharyngitis, fever, lymphadenopathy, dyslogia, and weight loss is suggestive; rash and hepatomegaly occur in about 10 per cent. Spencer et al described a patient with this chronic illness who developed a granuloma annulare–like eruption. Atypical leucocytosis is uncommon. Four of nine patients with acute arthritis studied by Ray et al had evidence of Epstein-Barr virus infection; he suggests that EBV may cause acute rheumatic illnesses more commonly than is currently appreciated.

Infectious mononucleosis is caused by the Epstein-Barr (EB) virus, an antigenically distinct member of the herpesvirus group. The EB virus was originally observed in Burkitt lymphoma. Infection is transmitted by direct contact, usually intimate but not necessarily sexual.

Treatment is symptomatic; there is no specific therapy. Antimicrobial agents have no effect on uncomplicated cases of infectious mononucleosis. Patients with mononucleosis treated with ampicillin (for suspected streptococcal pharyngitis, usually) regularly develop a generalized, erythematous rash on about the seventh or eighth day of therapy. The discrete, itchy, 4–8-mm macules are distinctive.

During the acute febrile period, bed rest is advisable. Salicylates or other analgesics are usually sufficient to control the headache and sore throat. Gargling and irrigation with warm saline solution provide symptomatic relief of pharyngitis and stomatitis. If patients have severe pharyngeal involvement with encroachment on the airway, a short course of corticosteroids is useful to induce a prompt antiinflammatory effect.

Oral hairy leukoplakia, a poorly demarcated, corrugated white plaque seen on the lateral aspects of the tongue of patients with the acquired immunodeficiency syndrome, has been shown to contain the EBV genome. In 19 of 20 specimens tested, intense staining for viral capsid antigen of EBV was seen. Greenspan et al concluded that EBV replicates within the epithelial cells of hairy leukoplakia.

Several recent reports implicate EBV in the etiology of *Hodgkin's disease* and as the possible cause of many

transplant-related lymphomas or lymphomas associated with primary immunodeficiency disorders, such as AIDS-associated lymphoma. This last suggestion is as yet unconfirmed.

Cosky RJ, et al: Ampicillin sensitivity in infectious mononucleosis. Arch Dermatol 1969, 100:717.

Greenspan JS, et al: Replication of Epstein-Barr virus within the epithelial cells of oral hairy leukoplakia. N Engl J Med 1985, 313:1567.

Jaffe ES: The elusive Reed-Sternberg cell. N Engl J Med 1989, 320:529.

Jones JF, et al: Evidence for active Epstein-Barr virus infection in patients with persistent unexplained illnesses: elevated early-antigen antibodies. Ann Intern Med 1985, 102:1.

Kaplan LD, et al: AIDS-associated non-Hodgkin's lymphoma in San Francisco. JAMA 1989, 261:719.

Labbe A, et al: Gianotti-Crosti syndrome and Epstein-Barr virus infection. J Pediatr 1983, 102:1013.

Lowe NJ, et al: Gianotti-Crosti syndrome associated with Epstein-Barr virus infection. JAAD 1989 20:336.

Lupton GP, et al: Oral hairy leukoplakia. Arch Dermatol 1987, 123:629.

Mueller N, et al: Hodgkin's disease and Epstein-Barr virus. N Engl J Med 1989, 320:689.

Naparstek Y, et al: Rash and infectious mononucleosis. Ann Intern Med 1982, 97:284.

Ray CG, et al: Acute polyarthritis associated with active Epstein-Barr virus infection. JAMA 1982, 248:2990.

Spencer SA, et al: Granuloma annulare-like eruption due to chronic Epstein-Barr virus infection. Arch Dermatol 1988, 124:250.

Straus SE, et al: Persisting illness and fatigue in adults with evidence of Epstein-Barr virus infection. Ann Intern Med 1985, 102:7.

Weiss LM, et al: Detection of Epstein-Barr viral genomes in Reed-Sternberg cells of Hodgkin's disease. N Engl J Med 1989, 320:502.

ZOSTER

Synonyms: Shingles, herpes zoster.

CLINICAL FEATURES. Herpes zoster is characterized by several groups of vesicles on an erythematous and edematous base situated unilaterally within the distribution of a cranial or spinal nerve coming from one posterior ganglion, often with some overflow into the neurotomes above and below. The onset is rapid, with fever and neuralgic pain after an incubation period of seven to 12 days. In patients under 30, the pain may be minimal. The eruption appears in patches of various sizes, the larger ones as much as 8 cm in diameter. The early vesicles contain a clear serum, but after a few days the contents generally become purulent, and rupture produces crusts. Other vesicles dry up without rupturing; some become hemorrhagic or necrotic and ulcerate and slough, becoming gangrenous. Bullous lesions have been reported in patients suffering from malignancies. Chronic ecthymatous and verruciform lesions have been reported in AIDS patients.

The eruption is almost invariably unilateral, which is of diagnostic importance. The dermatomes most frequently affected are the thoracic (55 per cent), the cranial (20 per cent, with the trigeminal nerve being the most common single nerve involved), the lumbar

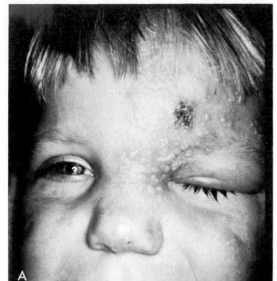

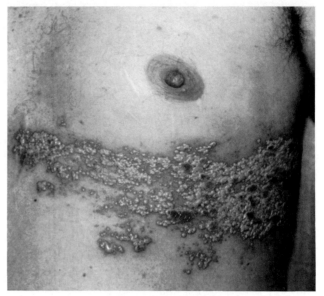

Figure 19–18. Herpes zoster.

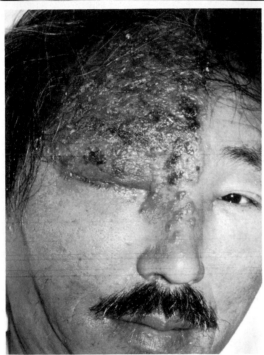

Figure 19–17. Herpes zoster ophthalmicus in A, a 5-year-old girl, and B, a man.

ceded by local itching, tenderness, or pain, which may radiate over the entire region supplied by the nerve. Hyperesthesia to light touch typically occurs throughout the involved neurotome, a little noted, but sometimes useful diagnostic sign. Sometimes the lesions appear without any prodromal symptoms; in other cases, in addition to the local symptoms already mentioned, there is enlargement of the neighboring lymph glands.

Herpes zoster generalisatus is a generalized varicelliform eruption accompanying the segmental eruption. It occurs chiefly in old or debilitated persons, especially sufferers from malignant lymphoma, AIDS, or myeloma. Mazur et al have shown that low levels of

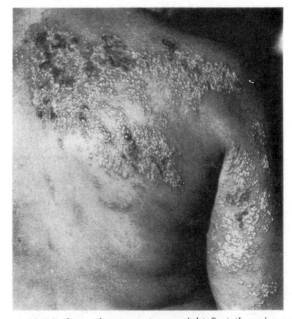

Figure 19–19. Severe herpes zoster on right first thoracic neurotome with spillover to C8 and T2 areas.

(15 per cent), and the sacral (5 per cent). Bilateral involvement and recurrence are rare, although in some cases there may be a few lesions on the opposite side of the midline owing to transverse nerve twigs. Zoster may even more rarely involve two widely separated regions at one time. This occurs more often in HIV-1 infection. With lesions of cranial nerve V or cervical nerve 2, in the scalp, alopecia may rarely occur and may lead to scarring. Lesions may develop on the mucous membranes within the mouth in zoster of the maxillary or mandibular division of the facial nerve, or in the vagina in zoster in the S2 or S3 neurotome.

The onset of the eruption is accompanied or pre-

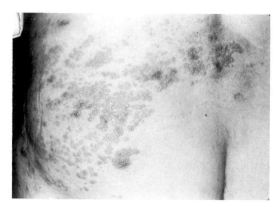

Figure 19–20. Herpes zoster.

serum antibody are a highly significant risk factor in predicting dissemination of disease. The zonal lesions are sometimes hemorrhagic or gangrenous. The outlying vesicles or bullae, which are usually not grouped, resemble varicella vesicles, and are often umbilicated. They may also be hemorrhagic. Fever, prostration, headache, and signs of meningeal irritation or viral meningitis may be present. Zoster encephalomyelitis may rarely follow and is often fatal. Pleocytosis in the spinal fluid helps in the diagnosis.

In *herpes zoster ophthalmicus* the ophthalmic division of the fifth cranial nerve is involved. If the long nasociliary branch participates, with vesicles on the side and tip of the nose (Hutchinson's sign), the eyeball may be involved, with vesicles on the cornea.

These change rapidly to ulcers, which may lead to scarring and loss of vision. Ophthalmologic consultation in advance of this event is advisable. Liesegang recently reviewed this subject.

Sacral Zoster. Izumi and Edwards reported in 1973 that neurogenic bladder is commonly present to some degree in patients with zoster of the S3 or less often S2 or S4 neurotome. Urinary hesitancy or actual urinary retention may occur. The prognosis is good for complete recovery. Systemic corticosteroids are advisable. In seven cases reported by Jellinek and Tullock, anal sphincter tone was also impaired. Recovery was complete.

Voluntary Muscle Weakness. Quadriceps weakness may occur with L2 involvement, and abdominal muscle weakness with involvement of T10 to L1. The result is a quite extraordinary protrusion of the abdomen on the affected side, which may last for some months. Rexinger reported such a case, and one of us (HLA) has seen two. O'Doherty et al reported a case of zoster at the C4 level with ipsilateral paralysis of the hemidiaphragm.

Ramsay Hunt Syndrome results from involvement of the facial and auditory nerves by V-Z virus. Herpetic inflammation of the geniculate ganglion is felt to be the cause of this syndrome. The presenting features include zoster of the external ear or tympanic membrane; herpes auricularis with ipsilateral facial paralysis; or herpes auricularis, facial paralysis, and auditory symptoms. Auditory symptoms include mild to severe tinnitus, deafness, vertigo, nausea and vomiting, and nystagmus. The risk that the facial palsy will persist is probably reduced, though not abolished, by early systemic steroid therapy.

Attacks vary widely in their intensity but rarely last more than three to four weeks. The pain may occur either before the onset, during the presence,

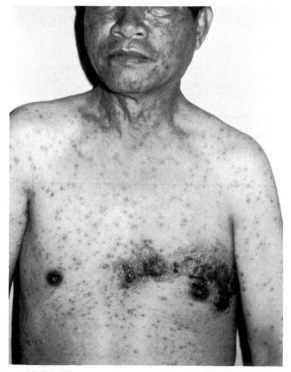

Figure 19–21. Herpes zoster generalisatus. (Courtesy of Dr. Axel W. Hoke.)

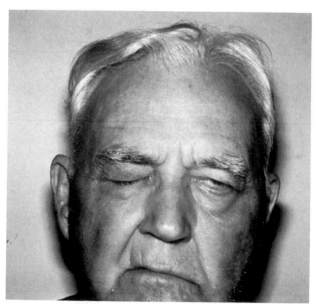

Figure 19–22. Ramsay-Hunt syndrome. (Courtesy of Dr. Axel W. Hoke.)

or after the disappearance of the skin manifestations. Pain may be entirely absent or very severe.

Postzoster Neuralgia. Severe postzoster neuralgia is seen in 10 to 25 per cent of older individuals who have not received systemic corticosteroid therapy early in their attack, but is rare in young persons and children. The pain is often severe, intractable, persistent, and exhausting. The sufferer is unable to focus his thoughts on anything except his malady. It is not unusual to see the neuralgia persist for six months or more after the attack, and it may last for years.

Zoster and Malignant Disease. Fueyo and Lookingbill concluded that herpes zoster should not be taken as a marker of malignancy, and that a screening malignancy workup is not indicated in patients with zoster. This fits with our personal experience.

On the other hand, patients with lymphoma (especially Hodgkin's disease and leukemia) are more prone to develop zoster than are their age-matched counterparts. Patients with deficient immune systems, such as those immunosuppressed for organ transplant or by carcinomatosis or connective tissue disease, also have a higher than normal incidence of zoster. Friedman-Kien showed that the occurrence of zoster prior to the age of 50 should prompt the suspicion of human immunodeficiency virus (HIV) infection in patients at risk for this.

Recurrent Zoster. Heskel and Hanifin aver that most if not all recurrent zosteriform eruptions are herpes simplex, and that a proved case of recurrent

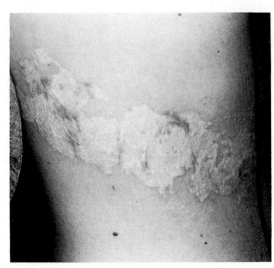

Figure 19–24. Post-herpes zoster scarring in a young man with Hodgkin's disease.

zoster has never been described. Viral culture, or demonstration of V-Z virus by indirect immunofluorescence in vesicle contents, is a minimum requirement for the diagnosis of recurrent zoster.

LABORATORY FINDINGS. The cytopathogenicity of the zoster virus may be demonstrated in tissue culture. Demonstration of antibodies in serum may be made by immunofluorescent techniques. The vesicle contains complement-fixing antigens. Tzanck smear shows multinucleated giant cells, as in herpes simplex and varicella. Electron microscopy has proved useful as a rapid (30 minutes) and reliable diagnostic procedure when available. Direct immunofluorescent antibody staining of infected cells is an effective and rapid aid in the diagnosis.

ETIOLOGY. The varicella-zoster virus causes both herpes zoster and varicella. The nucleic acid core is DNA and it is morphologically identical to the herpes simplex virus. It is an icosahedral virus containing 162 capsomeres surrounded by an envelope.

Its identity with the varicella virus has been demonstrated by the inoculation of zoster into the skin of children. Vesicles are produced in about 10 days at the site of inoculation. Patients who have not been infected with varicella, who are exposed to someone with zoster, regularly contract chickenpox. Conversely it is unusual, though occasionally seen, that someone exposed to varicella develops zoster, or exposure to a patient with zoster leads to a secondary case of zoster. A cross immunity is believed to exist between the two diseases. Children recovering from varicella are for a time immune to herpes zoster. Infants infected before the age of 2 months have a high risk of developing zoster after a relatively short latent period. The virus causing zoster is the varicella virus, which remains latent after an attack of varicella many years before. The eruption may be triggered by trauma or surgery.

An exception to the rule that zoster is caused by varicella virus, retained since the patient had varicella

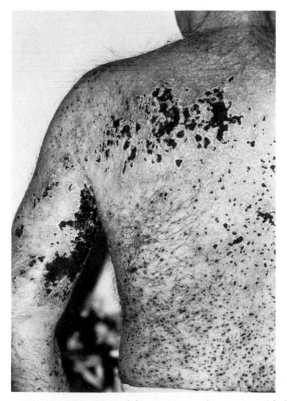

Figure 19–23. Disseminated herpes zoster in a man with lymphoma.

in childhood, is found in the rare cases of zoster following the administration of varicella vaccine: Williams reported such a case, occurring 22 months after vaccination; and virus grown from the zoster lesions was shown to be of vaccine type. It has also been seen in Japan. Lawrence et al have shown, however, that the incidence of zoster following immunization is no greater than that following natural varicella infection.

HISTOPATHOLOGY. As in the case of herpes simplex, the vesicles are intraepidermal. Within and at the sides of the vesicle are found large, swollen cells called "balloon cells," which are degenerated and swollen prickle cells. Acidophil inclusion bodies similar to those seen in herpes simplex are present in the nuclei of the cells of the vesicle epithelium. In localized dermatomal zoster these inclusions may be present in the dermal neurilemmal cells, whereas in disseminated zoster the inclusions may be seen in the connective tissue cells and the capillary endothelial cells of the dermis. In the vicinity of the vesicle there is marked intercellular and intracellular edema. In the upper part of the dermis, vascular dilatation, edema, and a perivascular infiltration of lymphocytes and polymorphonuclear leukocytes are present. An underlying leucocytoclastic vasculitis is not uncommonly seen in the dermis. Inflammatory and degenerative changes are also noted in the posterior root ganglia and in the dorsal nerve roots of the affected nerve. The lesions range closely to the areas of innervation of the affected nerve ganglion, with necrosis of the nerve cells.

DIFFERENTIAL DIAGNOSIS. The distinctive clinical picture permits a diagnosis with little difficulty. The unilateral painful eruption of grouped vesicles along a neurotome, with hyperesthesia and regional lymph node enlargement, is typical. Occasionally, segmental cutaneous paresthesias or pain may precede the eruption by four or five days. In such patients, prodromal symptoms are easily confused with the pain of angina pectoris, duodenal ulcer, biliary or renal colic, appendicitis, pleurodynia, or early glaucoma. The diagnosis becomes obvious once the cutaneous eruption appears. Herpes simplex infections may occasionally have a similar clinical presentation. Viral culture will distinguish them.

TREATMENT. Middle-aged and elderly people are urged to restrict their physical activities or even stay home in bed for a few days. Bed rest may be of paramount importance in prevention of neuralgia. Younger patients may usually continue with their customary activities. Local applications of heat, as with an electric heating pad or a hot water bottle, are recommended. Simple local application of gentle pressure, with the hand or with an abdominal binder, often gives great relief, as Tepperman reported. Topical anesthetics such as Quotane lotion, Lida-Mantle Cream, and Mantadil Cream are helpful in alleviating the surface discomfort.

Balfour et al showed that progression of zoster in immunocompromised patients is halted, and healing accelerated, by intravenously administered acyclovir (Zovirax), but neuralgia was not significantly lessened by the dose used (1500 mg/m^2 body surface per day, for five to seven days). It must be given slowly to avoid crystalluria and renal damage. Peterslund confirmed this, with somewhat better results in the relief of pain.

The use of oral acyclovir to treat healthy patients with zoster is controversial. McKendrick, giving 800 mg five times a day for a week, found it decreased acute pain and shortened healing time. If close attention is paid to hydration and renal function is unimpaired, we recommend this in severe cases. It is well tolerated.

The acute neuralgia of zoster can usually be relieved in young persons by analgesics such as aspirin or codeine. Riopelle et al investigated the effect of bupivacaine nerve block and found that immediate relief occurred, but there was no benefit in terms of preventing chronic neuralgia.

One of the most useful treatments for patients over 50 who have zoster neuralgia is systemic corticosteroid therapy. Since long-term therapy is not contemplated, oral prednisone is acceptable, but triamcinolone acetonide, 80 mg intramuscularly, repeated in four or five days if the response is disappointing, is often promptly effective. One of us (HLA), using this therapy almost routinely for over 22 years, has never seen the slightest suggestion that it altered the course of the skin eruption either for better or for worse, or caused any dissemination of the virus. It presumably suppresses the damaging inflammatory reaction in the affected ganglion and at least helps prevent further nerve damage.

The purpose of this therapy is to prevent postzoster neuralgia, and several studies have shown its efficacy in the older patients in whom this complication most often occurs. Other studies have questioned its value, and, although controversy exists, we recommend its use.

Cimetidine was dramatically effective in accelerating healing and relieving pain in four immunocompromised patients treated by Mavligit et al with 300 mg four times daily for seven days. A response occurred on the second day.

DeClercq et al reported immediate relief and healing in four patients (three of them immunocompromised) given (E)-5-(2-bromovinyl)-2'-deoxyuridine (BVDU) orally, three or four 125-mg capsules daily for five days. There were no side effects, discomfort, or toxicity. Other, newer antivirals holding promise are gancyclovir and cyclovir's predecessor, desciclovir.

Various tranquilizers may be helpful in the treatment of postzoster neuralgia. Taub reported in 1973 that amitriptyline in combination with perphenazine (Triavil; Trilafon, Etrafon), or with fluphenazine (Prolixin, Permitil), or thioridazine (Mellaril), almost completely relieved the pain of postherpetic neuralgia within one to two weeks. The dose of amitriptyline (ineffective alone in three of the five patients so treated) was 25 mg two or three times a day, or 50 to 75 mg h.s.; the usual dose range was used for the other drugs. Limbitrol may also be effective.

We have had dubious results in the treatment of postherpetic neuralgia following the suggestion of Epstein, who has recommended the intralesional injection of triamcinolone. Triamcinolone acetonide (Kenalog) 200 mg is diluted with 100 ml of 2 per cent procaine hydrochloride solution. This suspension is injected subcutaneously into the visible lesions and the symptomatic areas. A maximum of 15 ml is not exceeded at any one time. Epstein gives these injections daily. One or two injections should produce great relief from the neuralgic pain.

Arnold has seen complete relief of postzoster neuralgia of as long as 7 years' duration after an injection of 80 mg of triamcinolone acetonide intramuscularly; a man who had not known a night of sleep for 7 years slept all night for the next month, when he had a return of moderate pain and was given another dose of 60 mg. Topical inunction of capsaicin 0.025 per cent (Zostrix) has been reported effective by Bernstein et al. More documentation of its efficacy is necessary before we recommend it. There seems no doubt that it is worth trying, however.

Finally, Samuel Ayres, Jr., reported success in treating postzoster neuralgia with alpha-tocopherol acetate (vitamin E), 400 I.U. one to three times daily.

Alessi E, et al: Unusual varicella-zoster virus infection in patients with AIDS. Arch Dermatol 1988, 124:1011.

Baba K, et al: Increased incidence of herpes zoster in normal children infected with varicella zoster virus during infancy. J Pediatr 1986, 108:372.

Balfour HH Jr: Acyclovir therapy for herpes zoster: advantages and adverse effects (editorial). JAMA 1986, 255:387.

Ibid, et al: Acyclovir halts progression of zoster in immunocompromised patients. N Engl J Med 1983, 308:1448.

Bernstein JE, et al: Treatment of chronic post-herpetic neuralgia with topical capsaicin. JAAD 1987, 17:93; 1989, 21:265.

Cohen PR, et al: Disseminated herpes zoster in patients with HIV infection. Am J Med 1988, 89:1076.

DeClercq E, et al: Oral (E)-5-(2-bromovinyl)-2′-deoxyuridine in severe herpes zoster. Br Med J 1980, 281:1178.

Eaglstein WH, et al: The effects of early corticosteroid therapy on the skin eruption and pain of herpes zoster. JAMA 1970, 211:1681.

Epstein E: Treatment of herpes zoster and postzoster neuralgia by subcutaneous injection of triamcinolone. Int J Dermatol 1981, 20:65.

Esmann V, et al: Prednisolone does not prevent post-herpetic neuralgia. Lancet 1987, 1:126.

Friedman-Kien AE, et al: Herpes zoster. JAAD 1986, 14:1023.

Fueyo MA, et al: Herpes zoster and occult malignancy. JAAD 1984, 11:480.

Heskel NS, et al: "Recurrent herpes zoster": an unproved entity? JAAD 1984, 10:486.

Hira SK, et al: Cutaneous manifestations of human immunodeficiency virus in Lusaka, Zambia. JAAD 1988, 19:451.

Huff JC: Oral acyclovir in herpes zoster. Am Acad Dermatol, lecture, 1985.

Idem: Antiviral treatment in chickenpox and herpes zoster. JAAD 1988, 18:204.

Izumi AK, et al: Herpes zoster and neurogenic bladder dysfunction. JAMA 1973, 224:1748.

Janier M, et al: Chronic varicella zoster infection in AIDS. JAAD 1988, 18:584.

Jellinek EH, et al: Herpes zoster with dysfunction of bladder and anus. Lancet 1976, 2:1219.

Keczkes K, et al: Do corticosteroids prevent post-herpetic neuralgia? Br J Dermatol 1980, 102:551.

Lawrence R, et al: The risk of zoster after varicella vaccination in children with leukemia. N Engl J Med 1988, 318:543.

Liesegang TJ: The varicella-zoster virus: systemic and ocular features. JAAD 1984, 11:165.

Mavligit GM, et al: Cimetidine for herpes zoster. N Engl J Med 1984, 310:318.

McKendrick MW, et al: Oral acyclovir in acute herpes zoster. Br Med J 1986, 293:1529.

Novelli VM, et al: Oral acyclovir in immunocompromised children with varicella-zoster infections. J Infect Dis 1984, 149:478.

O'Doherty CJ, et al: Dermatologic dyspnea. Int J Dermatol 1986, 25:58.

Pahwa S, et al: Continuous varicella-zoster infection associated with acyclovir resistance in a child with AIDS. JAMA 1988, 260:2879.

Palmer SR, et al: An outbreak of shingles? Lancet 1985, 2:1108.

Peterslund NA, et al: Oral and intravenous acyclovir are equally effective in herpes zoster. J Antimicrob Chemother 1984, 14:185.

Post BT, et al: Do corticosteroids prevent post-herpetic neuralgia? JAAD 1988, 18:605.

Rexinger EL: Letter to the editor re abdominal zoster. Int J Dermatol 1983, 31:489.

Riopelle JM, et al: Chronic neuralgia incidence following local anesthetic therapy for herpes zoster. Arch Dermatol 1984, 120:747.

Sadick NS, et al: Comparison of detection of varicella-zoster virus by Tzanck smear, direct immunofluorescence with a monoclonal antibody, and virus isolation. JAAD 1987, 17:64.

Solomon AR, et al: Comparison of the Tzanck smear and viral isolation in varicella and herpes zoster. Arch Dermatol 1986, 122:282.

Stevens DA, et al: Zoster immune globulin prophylaxis of disseminated zoster in compromised hosts. Arch Intern Med 1980, 140:52.

Straus SE, et al: Varicella-zoster virus infections. Ann Intern Med 1988, 108:221.

Tepperman J: Symptomatic relief in herpes zoster (letter). N Engl J Med 1981, 306:1553.

Thiers BH: Unusual treatments for herpesvirus infections, II. Herpes zoster. JAAD 1983, 8:433.

Watson CP, et al: Amitriptyline versus placebo in postherpetic neuralgia. Neurology 1982, 32:671.

Weller TH: Varicella and herpes zoster. N Engl J Med 1983, 309:1362, 1434.

Williams DL, et al: Herpes zoster following varicella vaccine in a child with acute lymphocytic leukemia. J Pediatr 1985, 106:259.

VARICELLA

Varicella, commonly known as chickenpox, is an infection with the varicella-zoster virus, seen mostly in children. It is characterized by a vesicular eruption consisting of delicate "teardrop" vesicles on an erythematous base. The eruption starts with faint macules which develop into vesicles within 24 hours. Successive fresh crops of vesicles appear for a few days, mainly on the trunk, then on the face, and even on the mucous membranes of the mouth. Initially the exanthem may be limited to sun-exposed areas. The exanthem is therefore a polymorphous one. The incubation period is 14 to 21 days. Low-grade fever, malaise, and headache are usually present but slight. In AIDS patients the exanthem may become chronic and may be ecthymatous or even verruciform.

The diagnosis is easily made clinically. In atypical cases, a Giemsa-stained Tzanck smear from the floor of a vesicle will usually show typical varicella giant cells and cells with characteristic inclusion bodies, as in herpes zoster or simplex. Smallpox differs from varicella by critical defervescence on appearance of the exanthem; by a strong predilection for the sun-exposed areas; by a monomorphous eruption instead of a polymorphous one; and by absence of a vaccination scar.

Complications are rare. Encephalitis, pneumonia (uncommon in normal children but seen in 16 to 33 per cent of adults), and glomerulonephritis are those most frequently seen. Carditis, hepatitis, keratitis, vesicular conjunctivitis, orchitis, Reye's syndrome, arthritis, and splenic hemorrhage with rupture have also been reported. Symptomatic thrombocytopenia, with purpura and bleeding into mucous membranes, is a rare manifestation of varicella. Purpura fulminans represents a form of disseminated intravascular co-agulation with the clinical findings secondary to widespread arterial thrombosis or depression of clotting factors. Varicella is often extremely serious in patients with leukemia, lymphoma, or other disorders or treatment causing diminished cellular immunity. Maternal infection with V-Z virus during the first four months of gestation may result in a syndrome of congenital malformations as well as a life-threatening illness in the mother. Boyd et al documented the efficacy of intravenous acyclovir (10 to 18 mg/kg) intravenously in pregnant women with varicella. Manifestations of the congenital varicella syndrome may include low birth weight for gestational age, eye defects, encephalomyelitis, hypoplastic limbs, cutaneous scars, micrognathia, and pneumonitis. Overall the incidence of fetal mortality, or prematurity, is not significantly increased. Clinical congenital varicella—rash appearing within 10 days after birth—occurs in approximately 25 per cent of neonates whose mothers acquire varicella one to 16 days before delivery. The case fatality rate for neonates with rash developing between five and 10 days of life is approximately 20 per cent; deaths have not been reported in neonates whose rash began within

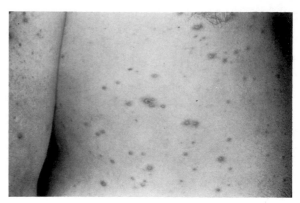

Figure 19–26. Varicella.

the first four days of life. This is probably because the infant has acquired maternal antibody. If the mother develops varicella within four days before delivery, or within 48 hours after delivery, varicella-zoster immune globulin (VZIG) and acyclovir should be given. Other criteria for the use of VZIG for the prophylaxis of varicella were reviewed by Liesegang. Occasionally, congenital varicella infection is subclinical and may be followed by the occurrence of herpes zoster later in infancy or childhood. Lasting immunity follows varicella. Zoster typically occurs some years after a varicella attack.

Varicella Vaccine. Live attenuated viral vaccine for varicella became available for testing in the United States in 1982; before that it had a good record of success in Japan. Asano et al in 1983 confirmed Arbeter's report in 1982 that the Oka strain was safe and effective. Weibel et al immunized 468 susceptible children, and gave a placebo to 446 others. No vaccinated child got varicella; 39 cases occurred among the controls. Long-term immunity and the effect on future zoster are being studied. Lawrence et al found that the incidence of zoster following vaccination is no higher than that after naturally acquired varicella.

Acyclovir should probably not be used in varicella uncomplicated by varicella pneumonia. Immunocompromised patients, however, should be treated with acyclovir to prevent visceral dissemination.

Arvin reported success with human leukocyte interferon. Adenine arabinoside, 15 mg/kg/day intra-

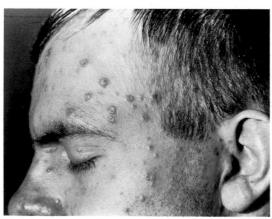

Figure 19–25. Varicella.

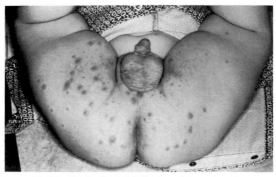

Figure 19–27. Varicella initially involving the diaper area.

venously for five and nine days respectively, was promptly effective in two cases of varicella with Wiskott-Aldrich syndrome, reported by Wade et al.

Acetaminophen (Tylenol)—not aspirin, as it may predispose to Reye's syndrome—is useful for control of fever, headaches, and myalgia. Trimming the fingernails and daily baths in tepid water with an antibacterial detergent help prevent secondary bacterial infection of lesions. Oral antihistamines are helpful in providing sedation and relief from pruritus. Calamine lotion and cornstarch or baking soda baths may relieve pruritus in mild cases.

Alessi E, et al: Unusual varicella zoster virus infection in patients with AIDS. Arch Dermatol 1988, 124:1011.

Arbeter AM, et al: Live attenuated varicella vaccine. Pediatrics 1982, 100:886.

Arvin AM, et al: Human leukocyte interferon for treatment of varicella in children with cancer. N Engl J Med 1982, 306:671.

Asano Y, et al: Five year follow-up study of recipients of live varicella vaccine. Pediatrics 1983, 72:291.

Baba K, et al: Increased incidence of herpes zoster in normal children infected with varicella zoster virus during infancy. J Pediatr 1986, 108:372.

Boyd K, et al: Acyclovir treatment of varicella in pregnancy. Br Med J 1988, 296:393.

Feder HM, et al: Varicella mimicking a vesiculobullous sun eruption. J Infect Dis 1988, 158:243.

Gilchrest B, et al: Photodistribution of viral exanthems. Pediatrics 1974, 54:136.

Glaser JB, et al: Varicella-zoster infection in pregnancy. N Engl J Med 1986, 315:1416.

Huff JC: Antiviral treatment in chickenpox and herpes zoster. JAAD 1988, 18:204.

Janier M, et al: Chronic varicella zoster infection in AIDS. JAAD 1988, 18:584.

Lawrence R, et al: The risk of zoster after varicella vaccination in children with leukemia. N Engl J Med 1988, 318:543.

Lipton SV, et al: Management of varicella exposure in a neonatal intensive care unit. JAMA 1989, 261:1782.

Myers JD: Congenital varicella in term infants: risks reconsidered. J Infect Dis 1974, 129:215.

Novelli VM, et al: Oral acyclovir in immunocompromised children with varicella-zoster infections. J Infect Dis 1984, 149:478.

Pahwa S, et al: Continuous varicella-zoster infection associated with acyclovir resistance in a child with AIDS. JAMA 1988, 260:2879.

Paryani SG, et al: Intrauterine infection with varicella-zoster virus after maternal varicella. N Engl J Med 1986, 314:1542.

Siegal M: Congenital malformations following chickenpox, measles and hepatitis. JAMA 1973, 226:1521.

Shulman ST: Acyclovir treatment of disseminated varicella in childhood malignant neoplasms. Am J Dis Child 1985, 139:137.

Straus SE, et al: Varicella-zoster virus infections. Ann Intern Med 1988, 108:221.

Wade NA, et al: Progressive varicella in three patients with Wiskott-Aldrich syndrome. Pediatrics 1985, 75:672.

Weibel RE, et al: Live attenuated varicella virus vaccine: efficacy in healthy children. N Engl J Med 1984, 310:1410.

Weller TH: Varicella and herpes zoster. N Engl J Med 1983, 309:1362, 1434.

Winkelmann RK, et al: Treatment of varicella-zoster pneumonia with transfer factor. Cutis 1984, 34:278.

CYTOMEGALIC INCLUSION DISEASE

Cytomegalovirus (CMV) infection is the most common viral infection of the newborn, with CMV excretion found in 0.5 to 2.0 per cent of them. Ninety per cent of these children are asymptomatic. The symptomatic neonate may have mild to severe disease; some die. The clinical manifestations in the infant may include jaundice, hepatosplenomegaly, interstitial pneumonitis, chorioretinitis, convulsions, cerebral (often paraventricular) calcifications, and microcephaly. Cutaneous manifestations may result from anemia and thrombocytopenia with resultant petechiae, purpura, and ecchymoses. A generalized maculopapular eruption may occur, and occasionally a generalized papulonodular eruption occurs, giving the "blueberry muffin baby" appearance. Most symptomatic cases occur within the first two months of life, with most survivors having neurologic impairment.

Symptomatic infection in adults is unusual, except in immunocompromised individuals. However, large-scale population studies have shown that 1.6 to 3.7 per cent of women acquire it for the first time during pregnancy, and in 30 to 40 per cent of such infections the virus is transmitted to the fetus. Pass et al reported in 1987 that in five families, infection could be traced to very young children who were shedding the virus. Quinnan et al documented CMV infection in all of 34 patients with AIDS. Many serious illnesses were attributable to CMV infection, with interstitial pneumonitis, chorioretinitis, and hepatic dysfunction being most common. CMV infection may occur in leukemia patients, as reported by Bodey et al, or following multiple blood transfusions, cardiopulmonary bypass, hemodialysis, or various types of primary or iatrogenic immunodeficiency states.

Feldman et al reported a patient with Hodgkin's disease who developed tender, hyperpigmented, indurated lesions of the thigh as the presenting sign of CMV infection. Inclusion bodies seen in the endothelial cells of the dermal capillaries led to the diagnosis. Bhawan et al reported a patient on immunosuppressive medications who developed hemorrhagic vesicles and bullae, which on Tzanck smear showed multinucleated giant cells. Diagnosis was based on histopathologic, electron microscopic, and culture findings. Immunocompromised patients with chronic ulcerative lesions have also been described.

The causative organism, cytomegalovirus (CMV), is morphologically indistinguishable from the herpesvirus and varicella-zoster viruses. It contains DNA. In tissue culture it grows best in fibroblasts. Antibodies to it are demonstrable by immunofluorescence. Documentation of its causative role requires demonstrating a rise in antibody titer, or demonstrating IgM antibodies in the newborn, or finding the virus in tissues or secretions. Intranuclear and intracytoplasmic eosinophilic inclusion bodies may be seen in histologic sections from infected sites; in the skin these are best seen in capillary endothelial cells.

No effective treatment is known: cytarabine, vidarabine, interferon, and transfer factor are not effective. Ganciclovir, a new antiviral agent used to treat life-threatening CMV infection in AIDS patients or transplant recipients, awaits licensing, but already reports of resistance to it have appeared. Foscarnet may be an experimental alternative.

Bhawan J, et al: Vesiculobullous lesions caused by cytomegalovirus infection in an immunocompromised adult. JAAD 1984, 11:743.

Erice A, et al: Progressive disease due to ganciclovir-resistant cytomegalovirus in immunocompromised patients. N Engl J Med 1989, 320:289.

Feldman PS, et al: Cutaneous lesions heralding disseminated cytomegalovirus infection. JAAD 1982, 7:545.

Hirsch MS, et al: Resistance to antiviral drugs. N Engl J Med 1989, 320:313.

Pass RF, et al: Young children as a probable source of maternal and congenital cytomegalovirus infection. N Engl J Med 1987, 316:1366.

Quinnan GV, et al: Herpesvirus infections in AIDS. JAMA 1984, 252:72.

Smith TF: Cytomegalovirus infection: current diagnostic methods. Mayo Clin Proc 1981, 56:767.

Walmsley SL, et al: Treatment of cytomegalovirus retinitis with trisodium phosphonoformate hexahydrate (Foscarnet). J Infect Dis 1988, 157:569.

HUMAN HERPES VIRUS 6 (HH6, HBLV)

Roseola Infantum (Exanthem Subitum, Sixth Disease)

This newly identified herpes virus is the sixth human virus in this category (EBV, CMV, V-Z, and herpes simplex 1 and 2 are the others). It was first described by Salahuddin et al in 1986. They isolated it from six patients with lymphoproliferative disorders and designated it HBLV. There has since been convincing evidence that it is the etiologic agent of roseola. This has been thoroughly reviewed by Hall.

Roseola infantum is a common cause of sudden unexplained high fever in babies and young children, most frequently between six and 36 months of age. Prodromal fever is usually high; convulsions and lymphadenopathy may accompany it. Suddenly on about the fourth day the fever drops by crisis and the child, who has been lethargic, sits up and commences to play. Coincident with the drop in temper-

ature a morbilliform erythema consisting of rose-colored discrete macules appears on the neck, trunk, and buttocks and, at times, on the face and extremities. The mucous membranes are spared. In one or two days complete resolution of the erythema occurs with no sequelae.

Breese BB Jr: Roseola infantum. NY State J Med 1941, 41:1854.

Briggs M, et al: Age prevalence of antibody to human herpesvirus 6. Lancet 1988, 1:1058.

Hall CB: The rash of roses. Arch Dermatol 1989, 125:196.

Salahuddin SZ, et al: Isolation of a new virus, HBLV, in patients with lymphoproliferative disorders. Science 1986, 234:596.

Yamanishi K, et al: Identification of human herpesvirus 6 as a causal agent for exanthem subitum. Lancet 1988, 1:1065.

Zahorsky J: Roseola infantilis. Pediatrics 1910, 22:60.

B VIRUS

B virus (*herpesvirus simiae*) is a herpes virus that infects macaque monkeys. Vesicular lesions similar to herpes simplex are seen on the oral mucosal surfaces as well as the lips or skin in these animals. Humans become infected after being bitten, scratched, or contaminated by an animal shedding B virus. Usually these patients are animal handlers or researchers. Benson et al recently reviewed the 22 reported cases of symptomatic human infection. Within a few days after the bite, a vesicular eruption may occur. However, it is the rapid progression to fatal encephalitis that is feared. Fifteen of the 22 reported cases have died, and all survivors suffered severe neurologic sequelae. Several anecdotal reports of the usefulness of acyclovir in this infection led Benson et al to early treatment of their patient, who survived without sequelae. However, the possibility that it may recur after a period of latency necessitates lifetime surveillance.

Benson PM, et al: B virus (herpesvirus simiae) and human infection. Arch Dermatol 1989, 125:1247.

Centers for Disease Control: B virus infections in humans. MMWR 1987, 36:289.

MANIFESTATIONS OF INFECTIOUS HEPATITIS

INFANTILE PAPULAR ACRODERMATITIS
Gianotti Disease (HBsAg present)
GIANOTTI-CROSTI SYNDROME
(no HBsAg)

"Gianotti-Crosti syndrome" has been expanded by Gianotti himself to include cases without hepatitis B surface antigen (HBsAg), resembling Gianotti disease (but with more conspicuous epidermal changes such as spongiosis and parakeratosis), usually idiopathic but sometimes with relationship to vaccinia, infectious mononucleosis, or coxsackie A-16 infection.

Gianotti applies the term *papulovesicular acrolocated syndrome* to these, reserving the term *papular acrodermatitis of childhood* for those cases associated with HBsAg.

CLINICAL FEATURES. These diseases are characterized by a monomorphous eruption of flat, nonpruritic, erythematous 1–5-mm papules suddenly erupting symmetrically over the face, buttocks, and limbs. The lesions develop over a few days' time, last for two or three weeks, and fade, with desquamation. The mucous membranes are spared. The typical eruption is generally found in children between two and six years of age.

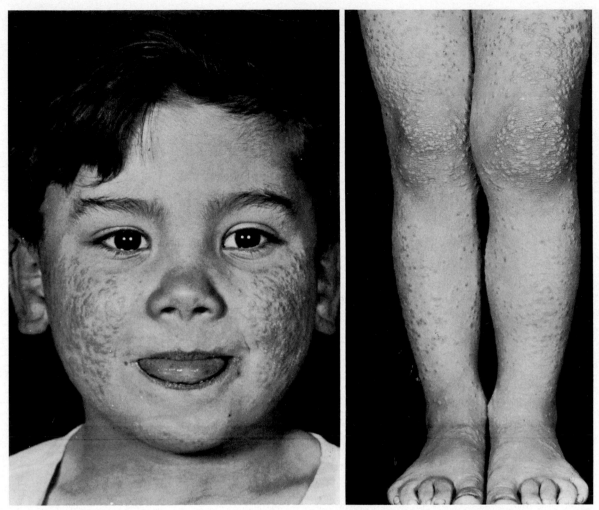

Figure 19–28. Gianotti-Crosti syndrome. (Courtesy of Dr. M. Eiloart.)

The lymph nodes, mainly the inguinal and axillary nodes, are moderately enlarged for two to three months. Splenomegaly, if present, is slight and rarely long-lasting. In those cases associated with HBsAg positivity, acute viral hepatitis occurs, beginning at the same time as, or one to two weeks after, onset of dermatitis. It is generally anicteric, but in some children jaundice may appear about 20 days after onset of the skin eruption. The liver usually remains moderately enlarged, but not tender, for one to two months. There are high serum levels of SGOT and SGPT, aldolase, LDH, and alkaline phosphatase; BSP retention is raised, but serum bilirubin is usually not increased except in icteric cases. Circulating monocytes are increased up to 20 per cent and are identical with those found in infectious mononucleosis and Turk's cells.

ETIOLOGY. Hepatitis B virus, subtype ayw (or occasionally adw or adr), is the cause of infantile papular acrodermatitis (Gianotti *disease*). This association has been common in Europe but is rarely encountered in the U.S. Gianotti-Crosti *syndrome* is a reactive process caused by many infections, among them Coxsackie A, respiratory syncytial virus, Epstein-Barr virus, rotavirus, vaccinia virus, poliovirus, BCG, streptococcus, or hepatitis A virus. The recent report by Draelos et al delineates this further. Infectiousness is very slight, though children with Down's syndrome are very susceptible. Gianotti reports that HBsAg may be detected from the tenth day of illness up to two months, or rarely as long as a few years by radioimmunoassay, and nearly always by immunodiffusion.

HISTOLOGY. There is a dermal infiltrate of lymphocytes, monocytes, and histiocytes around the blood vessels. Histiocytes are more prominent in Gianotti-Crosti syndrome; in papular acrodermatitis (Gianotti disease) dermal edema, and epidermal spongiosis and parakeratosis, are more conspicuous.

DIFFERENTIAL DIAGNOSIS. Papular pityriasis rosea, acute lichen planus, and drug eruption must be considered.

TREATMENT. No treatment appears to shorten the course of the disease, which in any case is self-limited.

PROGNOSIS. It should be noted that in long-term

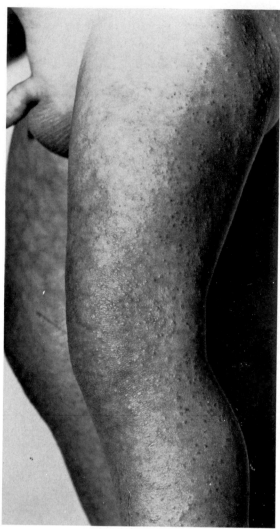

Figure 19–29. Gianotti-Crosti syndrome. (Courtesy of Dr. M. J. Woerdeman, Amsterdam.)

HEPATITIS B ANTIGENEMIA

Certain extrahepatic manifestations of hepatitis B virus infection ("serum" or "long incubation" hepatitis) appear to be related to circulating immune complexes consisting of hepatitis B surface antigen (HBsAg) and its antibody. Among the estimated 20 to 50 per cent of infected patients who have icteric hepatitis, 10 to 20 per cent have a serum-sicknesslike illness with a generalized morbilliform rash, urticaria, arthralgia, and occasionally arthritis, several days to weeks before the onset of clinically apparent liver disease. Immune complexes and low levels of complement have been seen in the serum, and in joint fluid. Polyarteritis nodosa may occur. Essential mixed cryoglobulinemia, erythema nodosum, and papular acrodermatitis (Gianotti disease) may also be seen in patients with hepatitis B infection. Martinez et al described a recurrent, asymptomatic erythematous papular eruption in chronic carriers of hepatitis B.

The prevention of hepatitis B requires protective gloves when performing even minor dermatologic surgery. Persons at extra risk from a needle-stick contact may be protected by an injection of 0.05–0.07 mg/kg of hepatitis B immune globulin immediately and again one month later. Lasting immunity may be conferred by three doses of hepatitis B vaccine: 1 ml twice one month apart, and 1 ml six months after the first. Three doses of the vaccine cost about $100, and immunity begins in three months and lasts at least five years. Injections should be given in the deltoid region. All dermatologists who have never had hepatitis B infection should be vaccinated against it. Leyden et al reported that a survey of 593 dermatologists found 15.4 per cent had evidence of previous infection by HBV.

follow-up, children with hepatitis B-associated disease develop the HBsAg carrier state and chronic liver disease, in a high proportion of cases.

Annalisa P, et al: Papular or papulovesicular syndromes. Arch Dermatol 1988, 124:1444.

Colombo M, et al: Immune response to hepatitis B virus in children with papular acrodermatitis. Gastroenterology 1977, 73:1103.

Draelos ZK, et al: Gianotti-Crosti syndrome associated with infections other than hepatitis B. JAMA 1986, 256:2386.

Gianotti F: The Gianotti-Crosti syndrome. JCE Dermatol 1979, 18:15.

Idem: Papular acrodermatitis of childhood: an Australia antigen disease. Arch Dis Child 1973, 48:794.

Ishimaru Y, et al: An epidemic of infantile papular acrodermatitis (Gianotti's disease) in Japan associated with hepatitis B surface antigen type AYW. Lancet 1976, 1:707.

James WD, et al: Gianotti-Crosti-like eruption associated with coxsackie A 16 infection. JAAD 1982, 6:862.

Lowe L, et al: Gianotti-Crosti syndrome associated with Epstein-Barr virus infection. JAAD 1989, 20:336.

Taieb A, et al: Gianotti-Crosti syndrome. Br J Dermatol 1986, 115:49.

Hepatitis A

Hepatitis A is caused by an RNA enterovirus, *Enterovirus 72*. Fowler and Callen reported a case of hepatitis associated with nodular panniculitis in a nonicteric man with a positive test for hepatitis A Ab. Hepatitis A is generally a benign asymptomatic disorder, which rarely becomes chronic or leads to cirrhosis or hepatoma.

Bastien MR, et al: Prevention of hepatitis B. Arch Dermatol 1989, 125:212.

Centers for Disease Control: Immune globulins for protection against viral hepatitis; Recommendations of the Immunization Practices Advisory Committee. Ann Intern Med 1982, 96:193.

Fowler JE Jr, et al: Panniculitis associated with hepatitis. Cutis 1983, 32:543.

Hoofnagle JH: Type D (delta) hepatitis. JAMA 1989, 261:1321.

Kutcher WL: The new hepatitis B vaccine: how, when, and why to use it. Postgrad Med 1983, 73:87.

Leyden JJ, et al: Serologic survey for markers of hepatitis B infection in dermatologists. JAAD 1985, 12:676.

Martinez MI, et al: Peculiar papular skin lesions occurring in hepatitis B carriers. JAAD 1987, 16:31.

McBurney EI: Protection from hepatitis B (letter). JAAD 1986, 13:909.

McElgunn PSJ: Dermatologic manifestations of hepatitis B virus infection. JAAD 1983, 8:539.

Segool RA, et al: Articular and cutaneous prodromal manifestations of viral hepatitis. J Pediatr 1975, 87:709.

Snydman DR, et al: Nosocomial viral hepatitis B: a cluster among staff with subsequent transmission to patients. Ann Intern Med 1976, 85:573.

POXVIRUS GROUP

The poxviruses belong to a large group of viruses with a high molecular weight. The nuclei contain DNA. The viruses are some 200 to 300 nm in diameter. They may be cultivated in chick embryos; however, the molluscum contagiosum virus has not been reproducibly propagated. Although it is sometimes difficult to do, the viral antibodies are demonstrable by complement fixation, precipitation, virus neutralization, and other methods.

VARIOLA MAJOR (Smallpox)

Smallpox, which was eradicated in 1977, has an incubation period of some 12 days, after which there is a sudden onset of fever and malaise, which cease abruptly and quite completely when the exanthem appears. The lesions, even when sparse, are distributed in a centrifugal pattern; the face, arms, and legs are more heavily involved than the trunk. Appearing as erythematous macules, the lesions become papular and evolve progressively through the vesicular and pustular stages to crusts in about two weeks. All lesions are in approximately the same stage of development. The crusts separate, leaving fresh scars, which are permanent in half the survivors.

A variety of complications occur, including pneumonitis, corneal destruction, encephalitis, joint effusions, and osteitis. The immunity following smallpox is, for practical purposes, lifelong. Depending upon the strain of infecting virus, the clinical form of the disease, and the age of the patient, the mortality rate may range from 5 to 40 per cent.

Prophylaxis of smallpox was for two centuries achieved by vaccination. It has now been officially abandoned virtually throughout the world, since smallpox has vanished. The last known cases were in Ethiopia and Somalia in 1977.

Glickman FS: "A ring around the rosie" (the rash that was). JAAD 1987, 16:1282.

VACCINIA

The vaccinia virus is an attenuated or modified cowpox virus that has been propagated in laboratories for immunization against smallpox. The present vaccinia virus is considered to be a distinctly different virus from that causing cowpox. Vaccinia virus–induced dermatoses result from complications of vaccination against smallpox. Vaccination is still being given to certain members of the military: thus complications are still occasionally seen in this setting.

Vaccination

The reactions to vaccination have been divided into three categories. *Primary response* occurs in the susceptible person some three days after vaccination. On the fifth day a papule appears that becomes a vesicle; on the ninth a maximal reaction appears, usually as a highly sensitive pustule with regional lymph node enlargement. The *accelerated response* (in the partially immune) consists of a small vesicle on the fifth day, which involutes by the tenth day. In immune persons the *immune* or *immediate reaction* occurs: a papule appears which involutes rapidly by the third day after vaccination.

Generalized Vaccinia. Some four to 10 days after vaccination a generalized vaccinia eruption may occur. The lesions are first papulovesicles that become pustules and involute in three weeks, although successive crops may occur within that time. Complications are ocular paralysis and postvaccinial retinitis.

Autoinoculation. Accidental inoculation of vaccinia may occur from contact with one's own vaccination or from contact with another person's vaccination site. This has recently been reviewed by James.

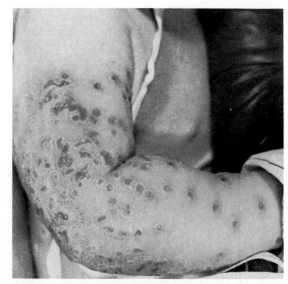

Figure 19–30. Vaccinia. (Courtesy of Dr. F. Daniels, Jr.)

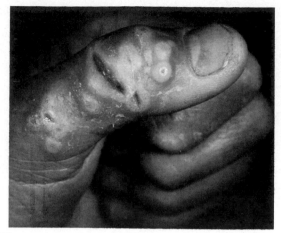

Figure 19–31. Autoinoculation from vaccinia vaccination.

Vaccinia Necrosum. Gangrenous vaccinia is rare, occurring principally in infants under six months of age who are unable to produce antibody, probably because of agammaglobulinemia or related disorders. The vesicular lesions involve the skin and mucous membranes and persist for months, becoming progressively gangrenous and nonhealing until death occurs. Metastatic necrotic lesions may occur throughout the body. Vaccinia immune globulin, which is available from the American Red Cross, should be used in these severe cases. Such a reaction was observed by one of us (WDJ) in a military recruit who had subclinical AIDS.

Roseola Vaccinia. Roseola vaccinia is characterized by an extensive and symmetrical eruption consisting of macules and papules which appear two weeks after a primary smallpox vaccination in young infants and children. In addition to the morbilliform eruption, the vaccination site contains a crust and is surrounded by a large erythematous halo. The indi-

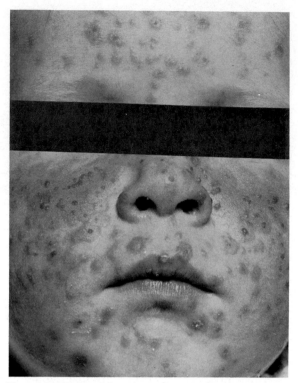

Figure 19–33. Roseola vaccinia; a monomorphic eruption.

vidual lesions are discrete and do not coalesce to form a scarlatiniform eruption. The infant is afebrile and no other signs or symptoms are present. Involution takes place in a few days.

Malignancies in Vaccination Scars. Marmelzat has reviewed the literature and described several of his cases in which malignant lesions have occurred with no history of trauma to the vaccination scar. Six cases of melanoma were reported occurring in vaccination scars, with the onset varying from three months to 41 years after vaccination. Thirteen cases of basal cell carcinomas with onset between two and 39 years after vaccination and five cases of squamous cell carcinoma with onset five weeks to 44 years after vaccination were also reported. Benign lesions with a tendency to occur in scars, such as sarcoidosis and granuloma annulare, are apt to occur in vaccination scars.

Eczema Vaccinatum. Eczema vaccinatum is an acute, eruptive, vesicular, febrile disease caused by vaccinia virus infection superimposed upon a chronic dermatitis, usually atopic dermatitis. It occurs most often in infants and children, but may develop in young adults.

The vesicles appear suddenly, mostly in eczematous areas, which become swollen. The lesions are sometimes umbilicated and appear in crops, resembling smallpox or chickenpox. The onset is sudden, and fresh vesicles appear for several days. Umbilicated vesicles surrounded by a ring of erythema rapidly appear on the face, head, neck, elbows, and wrists. Some become pustular and desiccated. Scarring is common. Often there is cervical adenopathy,

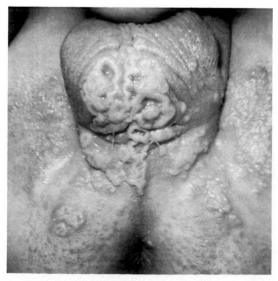

Figure 19–32. Heteroinoculation from mother's vaccinia vaccination.

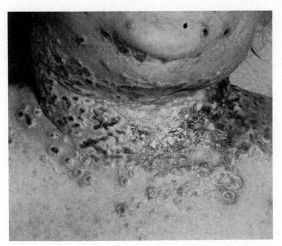

Figure 19–34. Eczema vaccinatum with multiple umbilicated lesions. (Courtesy of Dr. W. B. Muston, Australia.)

fever, and prostration, sometimes ending in death. Encephalitis and other neurologic disturbances are not uncommon.

The etiology of eczema vaccinatum is the vaccinia virus; however, the herpes simplex virus produces identical clinical manifestations known as eczema herpeticum. This type of eruption, previously known as **Kaposi's varicelliform eruption**, has as etiologic agents the *vaccinia virus, herpesvirus hominis,* or *coxsackie A16.* The etiologic virus is determined by the history of exposure to one of these viruses and confirmed by laboratory studies such as culture on chorioallantoic membrane of the chick embryo. See also Eczema Coxsackium.

It may also be identified by histologic examination of early vesicles. The inclusion bodies characteristic of herpes simplex (Lipschutz bodies) or of vaccinia (Guarnieri bodies) are the criteria used for identification.

Vaccination for smallpox should no longer be given except as determined by the armed forces. The complications reviewed above may occur, as may even more serious consequences. Lane and his associates reported 68 deaths in the United States from complications of smallpox vaccination from 1959 to 1968; 19 were attributable to vaccinia necrosum, 36 to postvaccinial encephalitis, 12 to eczema vaccinatum, and one to Stevens-Johnson syndrome.

James WD: Autoinoculation vaccinia. J Assoc Milit Dermatol 1984, 10:21.

Lane JM, et al: Complications of smallpox vaccination. N Engl J Med 1969, 281:1201.

Marmelzat WL: Malignant tumors in smallpox vaccination scars. Arch Dermatol 1968, 94:400.

Reed WB, et al: Malignant tumors as a late complication of vaccination. Arch Dermatol 1968, 98:132.

COWPOX

Jenner described two forms of infection that affect the teats and udder of the cow. One is the classic cowpox and the other is milker's nodules (paravaccinia, pseudocowpox).

Cowpox is an occupational disease affecting stockmen, milkers, and slaughterhouse employees who come into contact with cows affected with cowpox. The infected cows usually have vesicles on the teats. Natural cowpox is no longer present in the United States.

The inflammatory vesicles develop within a week after exposure and are usually localized on the fingers, although the virus may be implanted on other parts of the body, especially the face. The vesicles enlarge, become purulent, and usually form central umbilications in the largest lesions. Fever, regional lymphangitis, and adenitis may develop.

The cowpox virus, *Poxvirus bovis,* is in many ways similar to the vaccinia virus, *P. officinale,* but it is believed that the cowpox virus is distinct from the vaccinia virus. The cowpox virus is distinguished from the vaccinia virus by differences shown in cultures on the chorioallantoic membrane of the chick embryo.

Clinically cowpox is distinguished from milker's nodules and orf. The milker's nodules are smooth, brownish red, hemispheric nodules and are not umbilicated. The lesion is usually solitary, only rarely numbering two or three. It occurs most frequently on the radial aspect of the fingers and the palm.

FARMYARD POX

Milker's Nodules

Also known as paravaccinia or pseudocowpox, milker's nodules were described by Jenner as being contracted from the teats and udder of the cow. Milker's nodules are characterized by one or several brownish red, dome-shaped, smooth-surfaced or

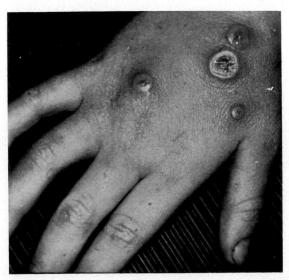

Figure 19–35. Eczema vaccinatum (Courtesy of Dr. J. Bembenista.)

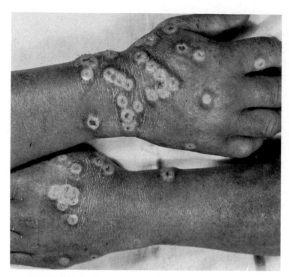

Figure 19–36. Typical cowpox on hands of an Australian dairy-man. Note umbilication. (Courtesy of Dr. A. Johnson, Australia.)

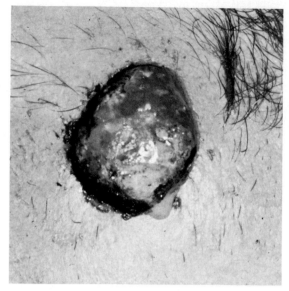

Figure 19–37. Orf. Ulcerated, weeping nodule resembling a pyogenic granuloma. (From Leavell U W, Jr: JAMA 204:657–664, 1968.)

slightly papillomatous vegetations which are generally confined to the hands and forearms. The incubation period is four to seven days. These usually start with a macule that progresses through a papular and then a vesicular stage to a nodule. The lesion may also be crusted. These lesions in some respects resemble those of pyogenic granulomas.

Schuler et al reported four patients who developed multiple lesions in burn sites. Indirect viral transmission, via contact with infected objects, was implicated.

Friedman-Kien and his associates in 1963 isolated the causative virus from a milker's nodule occurring in man. Its cytopathic effects are similar to the vaccinia virus, and the infected cells show metachromatic cytoplasmic inclusion bodies. The virions visible under the electron microscope are cylindrical.

Davis and Musil have demonstrated an easy method for the diagnosis of milker's nodule with electron microscopy. The suspected crusts and the dried vesicle fluid are used as specimens. The diagnosis can be established in an hour.

Histologically these nodules show a characteristic pseudoepitheliomatous hyperplasia with infiltrations of polymorphonuclears, eosinophils, and plasma cells in the papillary bodies and dermis. In the early stages eosinophilic inclusion bodies are seen in the cytoplasm. In some cases intranuclear inclusions may be present.

The differential diagnosis has been discussed under cowpox.

The disease is self-limited, clearing in about six weeks.

Orf

This is also known as ecthyma contagiosum, contagious pustular dermatosis, sheep pox, and infectious labial dermatitis. Orf is characterized by the occurrence of a single painless vesicle on the finger of a person exposed to sheep infected with sheep pox.

Orf passes through various stages in both sheep and man. According to Leavell the lesion begins as a papule, which then becomes a target lesion with a red center surrounded successively with a white ring and then a red halo. Next is the acute stage, a red and weeping nodule not unlike pyogenic granuloma. In a hairy area alopecia ensues. The nodule then becomes papillomatous and finally flattens to form a

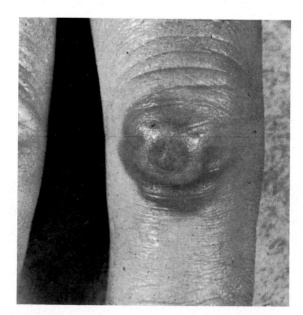

Figure 19–38. Orf on index finger of a 37-year-old woman, acquired through feeding "Bummer" lambs in Northern California. (Courtesy of Dr. R. C. Rucker.)

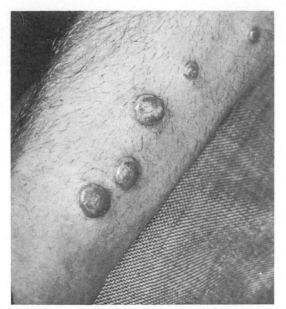

Figure 19–39. Orf on forearm. (Courtesy of Dr. B. Barrack, Australia.)

dry crust with eventual healing. As might be expected, the sites of predilection are the fingers, hands, wrists, and face. Mild swelling, fever, pain, and lymphadenitis may accompany the lesions.

The causative agent is the *orf virus*, an ether-sensitive DNA virus, which can be isolated on the chick chorioallantoic membrane. Eosinophilic inclusion bodies are but rarely seen and only during the early phase. They are most common in the cytoplasm, but also occur in the nucleus. The electron microscope shows an ovoid virion surrounded by characteristic tubules.

Orf commonly occurs in sheep and goats; human infection is acquired by contact with infected animals or laboratory material.

The incubation period lasts from a few days to one week. Transmission from man to man is not known. One attack gives lasting immunity.

It must be differentiated from cowpox, milker's nodules, pyogenic granuloma, and squamous cell carcinoma.

The disease is self-limited, the lesions reaching their maximum size in four to six weeks. After a crust appears, healing occurs in six to eight weeks, leaving only a slight scar.

In immunosuppressed patients the lesion may be progressive; Sacage et al reported such a case, in a patient with lymphoma, requiring amputation. Early surgical excision by Shelley's "subsection" would be desirable in such a case.

Bovine Papular Stomatitis

This disease of cattle has a cutaneous form in humans; Bowman et al described an outbreak of eight cases, all from handling cattle that were without

mucocutaneous lesions; the diagnosis was confirmed by isolation of bovine papular stomatitis virus. The incubation was five to eight days (24 days in one case), and the lesions were red nodules, often with characteristic white margins, lasting about three weeks. No treatment was given. The disease is self-limited.

Bowman KF, et al: Cutaneous form of bovine papular stomatitis in man. JAMA 1981, 246:2813.
Kennedy CTC, et al: Perianal orf. JAAD 1984, 11:72.
Leavell UW Jr, et al: Milker's nodules. Arch Dermatol 1975, 111:1307.
Idem: Orf: report of 19 human cases with clinical and pathologic observations. JAMA 1968, 204:657.
Rucker RC: Clinical picture of orf in northern California. Cutis 1977, 10:109.
Savage J, et al: "Giant" orf of finger in a patient with a lymphoma. Proc R Soc Med 1972, 65:766.
Schuller G, et al: The syndrome of milker's nodules in burn injury. JAAD 1982, 6:332.
Shelley WB: Razor blade surgery. In Epstein EH, Epstein EH Jr: Skin Surgery, 5th ed., Springfield, Illinois, 1982, p. 320.
Ibid: Surgical treatment of farmyard pox: Orf, milker's nodules, bovine papular stomatitis pox. Cutis 1983, 31:191.

MOLLUSCUM CONTAGIOSUM

Molluscum contagiosum is characterized by single, or much oftener multiple, rounded, dome-shaped, pink, waxy papules 2 to 5 mm (or rarely up to 1 cm) in diameter, which are umbilicated and contain a caseous plug. Lesions at first are firm, solid, and flesh-colored but upon reaching maturity become softened, whitish or pearly gray, and may suppurate. The principal sites of involvement are the face, hands, and through sexual transmission, the lower

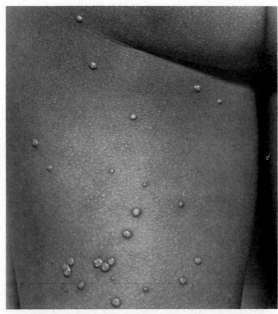

Figure 19–40. Molluscum contagiosum. (Courtesy of Dr. R. Walzer.)

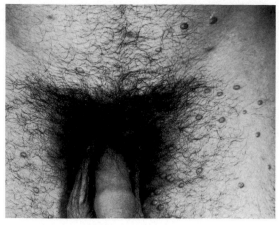

Figure 19–41. Molluscum contagiosum. Sexual transmission is probable. (Courtesy of Dr. H. Shatin.)

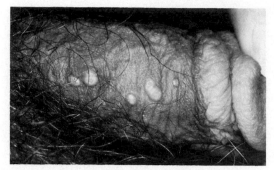

Figure 19–43. Molluscum contagiosum on penis.

abdomen and genitals. The papules are commonly found on other parts of the skin and at times are widely distributed. They may also occur on the mucous membranes of the lip, tongue, and buccal mucosa. The palms are spared, but solitary molluscum has been reported on the sole. Perilesional dermatitis and conjunctivitis may also be present and have been attributed to toxic substances produced by the virus or to a hypersensitivity reaction to the virus.

Rarely the molluscum lesions become horny. This type is called *molluscum contagiosum cornuatum*. Gigantic lesions 1 cm or more in diameter occur and may become inflamed from secondary infection. These are usually solitary lesions and can easily be confused with basal cell carcinoma, verruca vulgaris, keratoacanthoma, and various adenomata.

The electron microscope shows the molluscum bodies in the caseous core to be composed of virus particles shaped like the other pox viruses. They are oval or brick-shaped and measure 230 by 330 nm. The tendency of the virus to produce proliferation of the epidermal cells suggests that it provides a link between some pathogenic viruses and tumor-inducing agents.

The lesions are spread by autoinoculation and skin contact transmission. The incubation period varies from one to several weeks. The infectious nature of this disease, first demonstrated by Paterson (1841), has been amply confirmed. It is encountered chiefly among schoolchildren and among young adults. Hundreds of lesions may develop in intertriginous areas such as the axillae and intercrural region. Rosenberg and Yusk reported two cases of an extensive acute and florid eruption of hundreds of molluscum contagiosum lesions after patients received the immunosuppressive drugs prednisolone and methotrexate. Since then numerous other reports, reviewed by Redfield et al, attest to the occurrence of widespread molluscum lesions in immunosuppressed individuals. Widespread and persistent molluscum contagiosum may occur in patients with the acquired immunodeficiency syndrome, and may be the presenting complaint. Patients with atopic der-

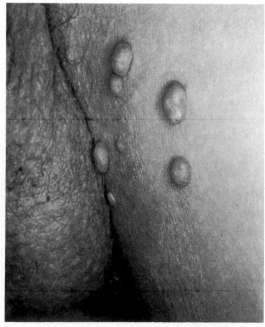

Figure 19–42. Molluscum contagiosum.

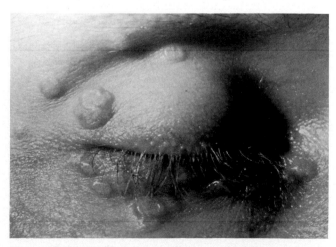

Figure 19–44. Multiple large molluscum contagiosum lesions in patient with AIDS. (Courtesy of Dr. Axel W. Hoke.)

matitis occasionally develop large numbers of lesions confined to areas of lichenified skin.

In sexually active individuals the lesions may be confined to such genital areas as the penis, pubis, and inner thighs. Lynch and Minkin reported 55 such cases and this type of venereal transmission is reviewed by Hook et al.

Molluscum contagiosum has a characteristic histopathology. It is essentially an acanthoma with a downward proliferation of the rete ridges and envelopment by the connective tissue to form a deep crater. In the cytoplasm of the prickle cells numerous small eosinophilic and later basophilic inclusion bodies, called molluscum bodies, or Henderson-Paterson bodies, are formed. Eventually their bulk compresses the nucleus to the side of the cell to form crescent-shaped nuclei. In the fully developed lesion a crater appears near the surface and gradually extends into each of the lobules. The crater contains the hyalinized molluscum bodies. Inflammatory changes are slight or absent.

The diagnosis is easily established in most instances because of the distinctive central umbilication of the dome-shaped lesion. If additional confirmation is desired, use Shelley's method of expressing the pasty core of a lesion, squashing it between two microscope slides (or a slide and a coverglass) and staining it for the particulate virions, as much as 0.3 micra in diameter, which are present in abundance. Firm compression between the slides is required to release the virions, with the stain in place. He prefers Sedi-Stain (Clay-Adams, Parsippany, NJ 07054: crystal violet, safranin, and ammonium oxalate in 10 per cent ethanol).

The best treatment is by curettage. Each lesion is sprayed with ethyl chloride until white freezing has occurred. The lesion is scraped away with a curette. When the lesions are on the eyelids, electrodesiccation under intradermally injected normal-saline anesthesia may be necessary. If the injection is performed by Dermojet, as described by Alexander, not only will children be more cooperative, but the pressure beneath lesions may extrude the core, or make it easy to remove by pressure with a comedo extractor. Other forms of treatment include applications of cantharidin, liquid nitrogen, or trichloracetic acid. Topical retinoic acid may induce enough irritant reaction to cause resolution. These methods have been less efficacious than curettage. Inosiplex, an immunomodulator, improved seven of nine children in whom it was used; however, this treatment is still experimental. Finally, spontaneous disappearance occurs, and treatment is not always necessary. One study showed that although lesions were present from six months to three years, a given lesion persisted for only two months.

In cases with numerous lesions, griseofulvin is worth trying; Ervin Epstein has described a dramatic cure with it.

Alexander AM: Molluscum contagiosum: The volcano phenomenon. Cutis 1979, 24:189.
Brown ST, et al: Molluscum contagiosum. Sex Transm Dis 1981, 8:227.
Epstein E: Treatment of molluscum contagiosum with griseofulvin. Schoch Letter 1989, 39:17.
Gross G, et al: Systemic treatment of mollusca contagiosum with inosiplex. Acta Derm Venereol (Stockh) 1986, 66:76.
Hook EW, et al: Sexually transmitted diseases in men. Med Clin North Am 1983, 67:235.
Mobacken H, et al: Molluscum contagiosum among cross-country runners. JAAD 1987, 17:519.
Postlethwaite R: Molluscum contagiosum. Arch Environ Health 1970, 21:432.
Redfield RR, et al: Severe molluscum contagiosum infection in a patient with human T-cell lymphotropic virus disease. JAAD 1985, 13:821.

HUMAN MONKEYPOX

In 1980, the World Health Association designated monkeypox the most important orthopox virus infection in humans in the era after smallpox eradication. Jezek et al reported an epidemiologic study of 2510 contacts of 214 patients with monkeypox in Zaire. They found that while most patients develop monkeypox from contact with wildlife sources, many cases of human-to-human transmission occur. The attack rate among unvaccinated household contacts was 12 per cent. Infection with this agent with its attendant umbilicated pustular eruption occurs mostly in children under 10, after an incubation period of seven to 24 days. In a follow-up study, Jezek et al reported the clinical features of the disease in 282 patients in Zaire in 1987. They found that early lymphadenopathy was the most important sign in differentiating human monkeypox from smallpox and chickenpox.

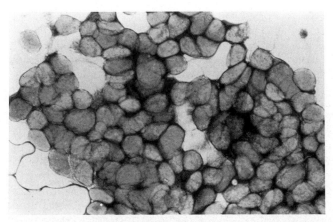

Figure 19–45. Microscopic appearance of molluscum bodies smeared on a glass slide and stained with methylene blue. (Courtesy of Dr. Axel W. Hoke.)

Jezek Z, et al: Human monkeypox. J Infect Dis 1986, 154:551.
Idem: Human monkeypox: Clinical features in 282 patients. J Infect Dis 1987, 156:293.

PICORNAVIRUS GROUP

Picornavirus designates viruses that were originally designated as *enterovirus*. A second important genus, *rhinovirus*, has been added. These two genera include the major human pathogens. There are three subclasses of *enteroviruses: polioviruses, coxsackieviruses*, and *echoviruses*. The first 67 enteroviruses identified were placed into the above subclasses. Newly identified enteroviruses are numbered under this genus, with the most recent four types designated *enterovirus* 68 through 72. Hepatitis A is *enterovirus* 72. The picornaviruses are small, RNA-containing, icosahedral viruses varying in size from 20 to 30 nm. They are resistant to lipid solvents.

The polioviruses causing poliomyelitis and the rhinoviruses causing the various upper respiratory infections are the most important in this group; however, dermatologically only the *coxsackieviruses*, the *echoviruses*, and enterovirus type 71, recently identified in epidemics of hand-foot-and-mouth disease, are significant.

COXSACKIEVIRUS INFECTIONS

The coxsackieviruses are identified by type-specific antigens and at present 23 group A and six group B viruses are identified. These type-specific antibodies appear in the blood about one week after infection has occurred and attain the maximum titer in three weeks. Neutralizing antibodies may be present afterwards for many years. The complement-fixing antibodies diminish after three months.

Coxsackie infection occurs most often in young children, especially during the summer. Many nonspecific exanthems and enanthems occurring during the summer and early fall are caused by coxsackie or echovirus. The exanthems may be diffuse macular or morbilliform erythemas, vesicular lesions, or petechial or purpuric eruptions. Each type of exanthem has been associated with many subtypes of coxsackie or echovirus, and specific clinical syndromes are only separated as listed below. Person-to-person transmission occurs by the intestinal-oral and possibly the respiratory routes.

Cases of Gianotti-Crosti syndrome and of dermatomyositis have been associated with coxsackie A16 and coxsackie B viruses.

Herpangina

This specific febrile disease of children is marked by the appearance of minute papular vesicles and ulcers in the pharynx. The onset is acute, with fever, headache, sore throat, dysphagia, anorexia, and sometimes stiff neck. The most significant finding, present in all cases, is the appearance in the throat of one or more yellowish white, slightly raised 2 mm vesicles, usually surrounded by an intense areola.

The lesions are found most frequently on the anterior faucial pillars, tonsils, uvula, or soft palate.

Only one or two lesions might appear during the entire course of the illness, or the entire visible pharynx may be studded with them. The lesions often occur in small clusters, which later coalesce. Most have a hyperemic border. Usually the individual or coalescent vesicles ulcerate, leaving a shallow, punched-out, grayish yellow crater 2 to 4 mm in diameter. Some lesions never ulcerate. The lesions disappear in five to 10 days, usually outlasting the fever, which may rise to 40° C. Usually the children do not appear very ill. Epidemics of herpangina have been reported in army camps. Such brief febrile attacks, including herpangina, may be the most common clinical manifestations of coxsackievirus infections.

Herpangina is caused by multiple types of coxsackie and echoviruses. The most commonly associated are nine types of coxsackie A (1, 2, 3, 4, 5, 6, 8, 10, and 22). Several other type A and some type B coxsackie as well as echovirus types 9, 16, and 17 have been recovered sporadically. The etiologic diagnosis is made by isolation of the causative organism from throat washings or feces through tissue culture or by inoculating suckling mice. Once the viral isolation has been made, serologic confirmation by neutralizing antibody, complement fixation, or hemagglutination inhibition tests is necessary. The acute-phase and convalescent blood specimens are taken several weeks apart.

Specimens for laboratory diagnosis should include pharyngeal and stool swabs and clotted blood.

Herpangina is to be differentiated from aphthosis and primary herpes gingivostomatitis by the acute febrile onset, the location of the lesions in the posterior oropharynx, and by culture of enterovirus.

Treatment is only symptomatic since the infection usually runs its course in about one week.

Hand-Foot-and-Mouth Disease

This striking disease, primarily affecting children, is characterized by vesicles on the hands and feet and in the mouth. The infection begins with a fever and mouth lesions consisting of small vesicles surrounded by red areolae on the buccal mucosa, tongue, soft palate, and gingivae.

The lesions on the hands and feet are red papules which quickly become small grayish vesicles surrounded by a red areola. They are often oval, linear, or crescentic, and run parallel to the skin lines on the fingers and toes. They are sparsely distributed on the dorsa of the fingers and toes and more frequently on the palms and soles. Vesicles and erythematous, edematous papules may occur sparsely on the buttocks. The infection is usually

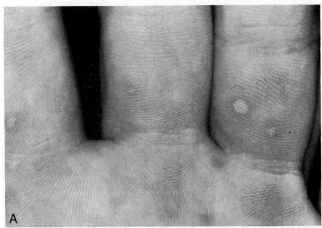

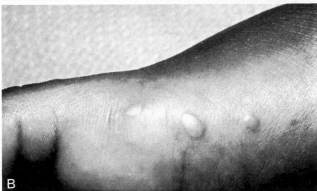

Figure 19–46. A, *Palmar lesions, and* B, *plantar lesions of hand-foot-and-mouth disease. (Courtesy of Dr. Axel W. Hoke.)*

mild, seldom lasting more than a week. The incubation period is three to five days.

Hand-foot-and-mouth disease is caused most commonly by the coxsackievirus A16, although A5 and A10 may cause it, and sporadic outbreaks have been seen due to coxsackie A7, A9, B1, B2, B3, or B5, and enterovirus 71.

The virus is recovered from rectal or pharyngeal swabs and from the ruptured vesicles on the hands and feet. A rising antibody titer is usually demonstrated.

Histopathologic findings are those of a nonspecific dermatitis without inclusion bodies or multinucleated giant cells.

Treatment is symptomatic. Some persons complain of inability to eat because of the severe mouth lesions. Xylocaine Viscous, Elixir of Benadryl, or Dyclone swirled in the mouth alleviates the severe pain, especially when done for a few minutes before eating.

The diagnosis includes differentiating the lesion from herpangina, which occurs typically in the throat area; from herpes simplex by its distinct oral lesions; and from erythema multiforme by the lack of iris lesions.

Eczema Coxsackium

Nahmias and his associates described a generalized vesicular exanthem, superimposed upon a preexist-ing atopic dermatitis, which resembled Kaposi's varicelliform eruption.

Serologic and cytologic studies confirmed the causative agent to be *coxsackievirus A16.* They suggest that this entity be called *eczema coxsackium* and that it be included with eczema herpeticum and eczema vaccinatum as a cause of Kaposi's varicelliform eruption.

ECHOVIRUS EXANTHEM

ECHO stands for Enteric Cytopathic Human Orphan, in reference to the identification of the virus before it was known to cause any disease.

The clinical manifestations, like those of the other enteroviruses, include constitutional, central nervous system, gastrointestinal, and respiratory manifestations, together with an exanthematous eruption of the skin.

Approximately one third of the ECHO infections have a rubelliform eruption consisting of discrete pinkish red macules noted early in the course of the disease. First the face and neck are involved, then the trunk and the extremities. Only occasionally is there an eruption on the palms and soles. The incubation period is usually three to five days, with fading of the lesions usually within four or five days. There may be involvement of the mucous membrane opposite the molars, resembling Koplik's spots. Fever is usually the initial sign. There may be gastrointestinal symptoms of anorexia, nausea, vomiting, and colicky abdominal pains. Respiratory symptoms of sore throat, cough, and conjunctivitis may be present. Aseptic meningitis may develop. Albuminuria and hematuria may be present.

Diagnosis is made by the isolation of the virus from the throat, stool, blood, or cerebrospinal fluid, and the demonstration of specific neutralizing antibodies in serum drawn during the first four days and then 14 to 21 days later.

The structure of the echoviruses is similar to that of the polioviruses. They are all RNA viruses and have been classified into 32 types. Type 9 is commonly found occurring with the rubelliform eruptions. Less frequently Type 4 and Type 16 are also found in this eruption. The echovirus is transitory in the human alimentary tract and occurs with a higher frequency in young children during the summer months. Dissemination takes place by means of the stool and by mouth secretions. The infection occurs in epidemics all over the world.

Meade and Chang reported a unilateral vesicular eruption, simulating herpes zoster, which was due to echovirus 6.

Boston Exanthem Disease

An epidemic in Boston was due to echovirus 16. In addition to the findings described previously, the lesions were sparsely scattered, pale red macules and papules. In severe cases the lesions were morbilliform and even vesicular. The eruption was chiefly on the face, chest, and back and in some cases on the extremities. On the soft palate and tonsils small ulcerations like those of herpangina were noted. There was little or no adenopathy. The incubation period was three to eight days.

The echovirus eruptions usually involute spontaneously in two to three weeks.

Bowles NE, et al: Dermatomyositis, polymyositis, and Coxsackie-B virus infection. Lancet 1987, 1:1004.

Cherry JD: Newer viral exanthems. Adv in Pediatrics: I, Schulman, ed., Chicago, Year Book Med Publ., Inc., 1969, pp. 233–286.
Duff ME: Hand-foot-mouth syndrome in humans. Br Med J 1964, 2:661.
Froeschle JE, et al: Hand, foot, and mouth disease (coxsackie virus A16) in Atlanta. Am J Dis Child 1967, 114:278.
James WD, et al: Gianotti-Crosti-like eruption associated with Coxsackie-A 16 infection. JAAD 1982, 6:862.
Meade RH, et al: Zoster-like eruption due to Echovirus 6. Am J Dis Child 1979, 133:283.
Miller GD, et al: Hand-foot-and-mouth disease. JAMA 1968, 203:827.
Wenner HA: Virus diseases associated with cutaneous eruptions. Progr Med Virol 1973, 16:269.

PARAMYXOVIRUS GROUP

The paramyxoviruses are the RNA viruses that have ether-sensitive envelopes and range from 100 to 300 nm in size. In this group the virus diseases of dermatologic interest are measles and German measles. Others in this group are mumps, parainfluenza, Newcastle disease, and respiratory syncytial disease.

MEASLES

Also known as *rubeola* and *morbilli*, measles is characterized by a maculopapular eruption over the body, upper respiratory infection, and conjunctivitis. The disease is seen chiefly in children. Confluence of the macules into small groups of irregular shape, 5 to 15 mm in diameter, is so characteristic that it has given us the word *morbilliform* to describe similar eruptions.

After an incubation period of some 10 days there are fever, malaise, headache, and muscular pains. Two or three days later there is a sudden appearance of conjunctivitis with distinctive redness of the sclera along with photophobia and burning. Simultaneously coryza appears, with running nose, pharyngitis, cough, and hoarseness. On the buccal mucosa nearest to the upper molars clusters of white papules on an erythematous base appear, which are pathognomonic (*Koplik's spots*).

Usually the macular or maculopapular eruption first occurs on the anterior scalp line, spreads quickly over the face, and then by the second or third day (unlike the rapid spread of rubella) extends down the trunk to the extremities. After some five days the exanthem clears, with the simultaneous subsidence of the high fever.

Complications may be otitis media, pneumonia, encephalomyelitis, and thrombocytopenic purpura.

The etiology of measles is the measles virus, an RNA virus 140 nm in diameter with a helical structure. Circulating antibodies are present two weeks after infection.

The diagnosis is established by the presence of a high fever, Koplik's spots, and the characteristic coryza and typical skin eruption. German measles,

scarlet fever, secondary syphilis, coxsackievirus and echovirus infections, and drug eruptions are to be considered in differential diagnosis.

Treatment is mostly symptomatic, with bed rest, analgesics, and antipyretics. These patients should be kept in darkened rooms because of photophobia.

Immune serum globulin may be given to exposed susceptible persons, especially infants under one, or older children who are immunocompromised and in whom live-virus vaccine is contraindicated, in order to prevent or modify the illness. Live attenuated measles virus vaccine is currently recommended as a part of the routine primary immunization series for all children at 15 months of age, or older. Older children and adults who have not had natural measles or the vaccine should also receive immunization. Even in mini-epidemics, it should rarely be given to

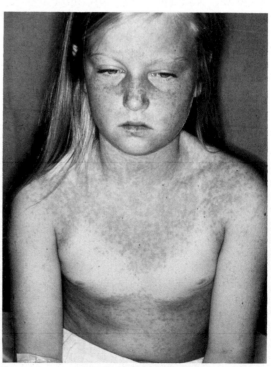

Figure 19–47. Rubeola.

younger infants, as it induces seroconversion in only 30 per cent at six months, less than 60 per cent at eight to nine months, and 72 per cent at 10–12 months (Krugman). More importantly, revaccination may fail to induce lasting immunity.

An interesting effect of vaccination has been a fourfold increase in the proportion of measles cases acquired in a medical setting, either the hospital or a doctor's waiting room. Davis documented this, and urged more attention to prevention in this situation. Bloch reported seven secondary cases from one case seen in an office, one of whom arrived an hour after the source patient had left.

Atypical Measles. This entity is seen in patients who received killed measles vaccine in the early to middle 1960s. The syndrome consists of fever, cough, headache, abdominal pain, myalgia, edema of extremities, pleural effusion, pneumonia, .and hilar adenopathy. In the skin, morbilliform lesions occur, occasionally with intermingled petechiae or vesicles, or both, beginning on the hands and feet and spreading centripetally. The main differential diagnosis is from Rocky Mountain spotted fever.

RUBELLA

Rubella, commonly known as German measles, is characterized by pale pink morbilliform macules, smaller than those of rubeola, and posterior cervical, suboccipital, and postauricular lymphadenitis. After an incubation period of two to three weeks, a faint macular eruption appears upon the face and spreads onto the trunk, disappearing in three days. The mouth may have red macules on the soft palate, but the characteristic Koplik's spots of rubeola are absent.

German measles is caused by the rubella virus, an ether-sensitive RNA pleomorphic paramyxovirus varying in size from 50 to 70 nm.

Congenital Rubella Syndrome

Infants born to mothers who have had rubella during the first trimester of pregnancy may have congenital cataracts, cardiac defects, and deafness. Numerous other manifestations such as glaucoma, microcephaly, and various visceral abnormalities may emerge. Among the cutaneous expressions are thrombocytopenic purpura; hyperpigmentation of the navel, forehead, and cheeks; bluish red infiltrated 2–8 mm lesions ("blueberry muffin" type) which represent dermal erythropoiesis; chronic urticaria; and reticulated erythema of the face and extremities.

Live attenuated rubella virus vaccine is available

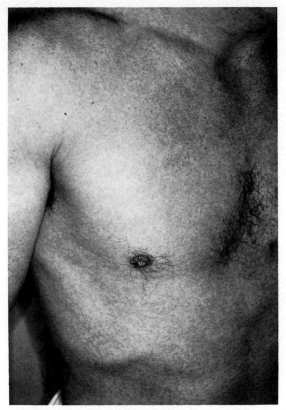

Figure 19–48. Rubella.

for vaccination. In the United States, immunization has been recommended for children between the ages of 15 months and puberty, and adolescent girls and women who are known to be seronegative and in whom pregnancy can be prevented for at least three months thereafter.

Bloch AB, et al: Measles outbreak in a pediatric practice: airborne transmission in an office setting. Pediatrics 1985, 75:676.

Castrow FF II, et al: Congenital rubella syndrome. Arch Dermatol 1968, 98:260.

Current trends in measles—1987. Arch Dermatol 1988, 124:1627.

Davis RM, et al: Transmission of measles in medical settings, 1980 through 1984. JAMA 1986, 255:1295.

Fine J-D, et al: The TORCH syndrome: a clinical review. JAAD 1985, 12:697.

Jones PH: Measles vaccination in infants (letter). JAMA 1982, 247:1273.

Markowitz LE, et al: Patterns of transmission of measles outbreaks in the United States 1985–1986. N Engl J Med 1989, 320:75.

Measles prevention. JAMA 1989, 261:827.

Welliver RC, et al: Typical, modified, and atypical measles. Arch Intern Med 1977, 137:39.

Wilkins J, et al: Additional evidence against measles vaccine administration to infants less than 12 months of age: altered immune response following active-passive immunization. J Pediatr 1979, 94:865.

PAPOVAVIRUS GROUP

Some of the viruses in this group are oncogenic, including several types of human papilloma virus (HPV). They are all ether-resistant DNA-containing viruses characterized as slow-growing, and replicating inside the nucleus. In humans only the wart virus or HPV is manifest, in any of over 50 serologically distinguishable strains. Papilloma viruses of rabbits and cattle, polyoma viruses of mice, and vacuolating viruses of monkeys are some of the other viruses in this group.

WARTS (Verrucae)

CLINICAL FEATURES. The wart, also known as verruca vulgaris, may be separated into a number of varieties depending upon the location on the skin. Certain numbered types of human papilloma virus correspond to clinical subtypes.

Verruca Vulgaris. The common wart, occurring chiefly in children, is usually located on the hands. It is an elevated rounded tumor with a rough, grayish surface so characteristic that it has given us the word "verrucous" to describe it and others like it.

In childhood, warts reach their most profuse growth, being usually multiple and numerous. In adults they are rarely so numerous, two or three lesions being a common number. Warts may occur any place on the skin: even on the lips, in the nostrils or auditory meatus, on the edges of the eyelids, or on the tongue. Generally they are spread to the tongue by the habit of biting the fingernails, about and under which warts frequently grow. On the surfaces of the eyelids, on the scalp, and occasionally about the mouth and chin a special variety called

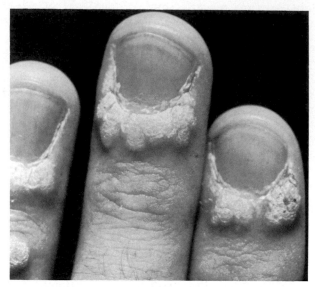

Figure 19–50. Periungual warts. (Courtesy of Dr. Axel W. Hoke.)

verruca filiformis (filiform wart) is encountered, in which the lesions are single, soft, thin, threadlike or shrub-shaped projections. The scalp is also a common site of involvement for the digitate variety of warts, and in this place the affection is difficult to eradicate because new ones develop on other portions, spread by combing or scratching. Meat handlers (butchers) have a high incidence of common warts of the hands.

In the beginning common warts are pinhead-sized, smooth, shiny, translucent, usually discrete hyperkeratoses. They gradually grow in the course of several weeks or months to pea-sized, rough, papillary, dirty brown, gray, or black, horny excrescences. The warts, particularly those about the nails (*periungual warts*) are apt to become fissured, inflamed, and tender. In some instances a single wart (*mother wart*) appears and grows slowly for a long time and then suddenly many new warts erupt. Rarely, extensive or even generalized eruptions of these warts are seen, but such cases must be differentiated from acrokeratosis verruciformis of Hopf and keratosis follicularis (Darier's). HPV types 1, 2, 4, and 7 are most frequently responsible for the common warts.

Myrmecia Warts. Lyell et al in 1951 described these and named them *myrmecia* ("anthill") after Celsus's name for them, or "Type I" (for Inclusion). Myrmecia are deep, dome-shaped, often inflamed and tender, and occur mostly on the palms or soles, beside or beneath the nails, or less often on the pulp of the digits or on the face. They are caused by HPV type 1, and in a transmission experiment Lyell showed that inoculation of material from Type I warts produced a Type I wart in the recipient, and that from Type B (for "banal") produced Type B warts.

They are distinctively dome-shaped, and much

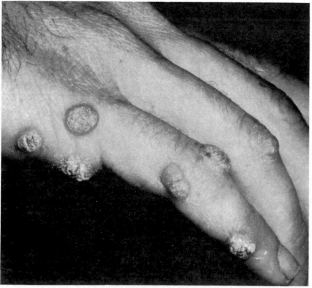

Figure 19–49. Verrucae vulgares. (Courtesy of Dr. Axel W. Hoke.)

A

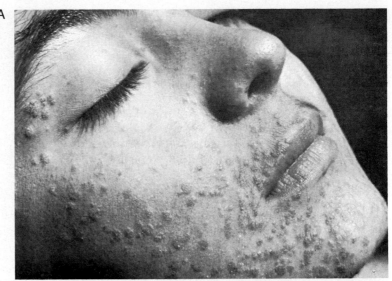

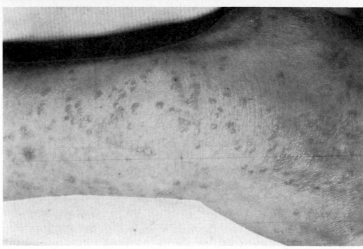

Figure 19–51. A, *Verruca plana juvenilis. Unusually florid example. (Courtesy of Dr. A. Kaminsky.) B, Verruca plana of forearm and hand. Note "Koebner" streak. (Courtesy of Dr. Axel W. Hoke.)*

B

bulkier beneath the surface than they appear to be. Their bulk consists of material which Lyell likened to wet tow (flax fibers). Histologically they are characterized by eosinophilic inclusion bodies, at first intracellular, later extracellular as well, increasing in size as the surface is approached.

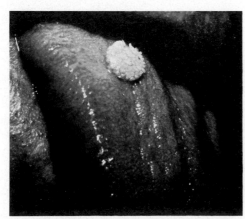

Figure 19–52. Verruca on tongue.

Flat Wart (Verruca Plana Juvenilis). Also known as juvenile warts, these are 1–3-mm, smooth, slightly raised, flat-surfaced lesions.

These warts are generally multiple and numerous, being grouped on the face, neck, dorsa of the hands, wrists, or knees. The forehead, cheeks, and nose, and particularly the area about the mouth and the backs of the hands, are the favorite locations. In men who shave their beards and in women who shave their lower legs numerous flat warts may develop as a result of autoinoculation. In these areas they are often excoriated or conglomerate, making the differential diagnosis from verrucous nevus, lichen planus, and molluscum contagiosum a matter of some difficulty. They tend to spread within scratch marks by autoinoculation and thus form linear, slightly raised, papular lesions. Their color is usually that of normal skin, pink, or light brown. Hyperpigmented lesions occur and when scarcely elevated may be confused with lentigines or ephelides. Although children are the favorite subjects, these warts also occur in adults, usually under 30.

HPV types 3, 10, 28, and 41 have been most often associated with flat warts.

Plantar Wart (Verruca Plantaris). This wart generally forms at points of pressure on the ball of the foot, especially over the midmetatarsal area. It may, however, be anywhere on the sole, irrespective of pressure. Frequently there are several lesions on one foot. Sometimes they are grouped, or several contiguous warts fuse so that they appear as one until the keratotic surface is shaved off and the multiple cores are revealed. Such a patch is known as a *mosaic wart*. The soft, pulpy cores are surrounded by a firm horny ring; they occur in no other form of wart, but resemble somewhat the cores in corns.

Over the surface of the plantar wart, most clearly if the top is shaved off, may be seen multiple small black points. They are dilated capillary loops within hugely elongated dermal papillae.

Plantar warts may be confused with corns or calluses, but plantar warts have a soft central core and black or bleeding points ("seeds"), not present in the latter. Shaving off the top will disclose either the soft core and "seeds" of a wart, or the horny central core of a corn.

The **myrmecia** type of verrucae may occur as deep palmo-plantar warts, or occasionally as smooth-surfaced, often inflammatory papules at the base of a nail. The biopsy of this type of wart is remarkable for the large number of eosinophilic inclusions.

HPV types 1, 2, and 4 are the ones most commonly associated with plantar warts.

Condyloma Acuminatum. These small pointed or cauliflowerlike projections, which multiply to form large vegetating clusters, are sexually transmitted.

They occur in men anywhere on the penis or, usually if acquired by rectal intercourse, about the anus; in women on the mucous surfaces of the vulva, cervix, on the perineum, or about the anus. They are especially numerous during pregnancy and when there is a profuse vaginal discharge. Although usually few, cauliflowerlike masses may develop and, as a result of accumulation of purulent material in the clefts, may be malodorous. Their color is generally gray, pale yellow, or pinkish.

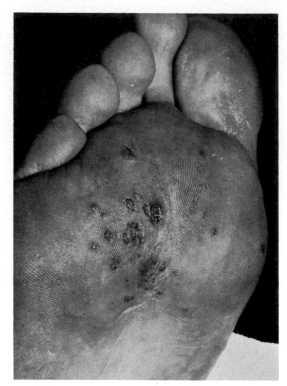

Figure 19–54. Multiple plantar verrucae.

There has been a large increase in the incidence of this lesion over the past 20 years. It is three times as common as herpes simplex and affects chiefly young adults between 18 and 35. There is a 50 per cent chance of transmission of the disease by a single sexual contact.

The occurrence of condyloma acuminatum in the anogenital area in children is strong presumptive evidence of sexual abuse, and warrants a VDRL, gonococcal cultures, and inquiry into the behavior of adults with whom they are associated. A recent

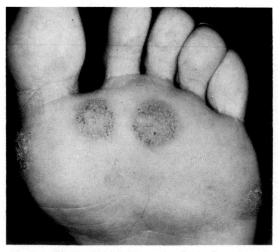

Figure 19–53. Verrucae plantaris.

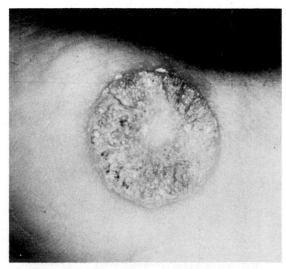

Figure 19–55. Development of a "doughnut" wart after liquid nitrogen treatment.

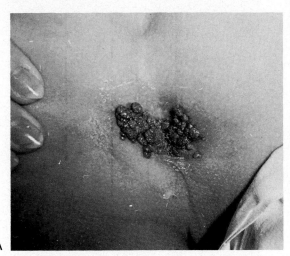 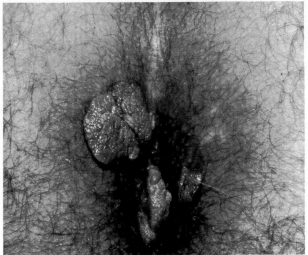

Figure 19–56. A *and* B, *Perianal verrucae (condylomata acuminata).* (B, *Courtesy of Dr. Axel W. Hoke.*)

report by Rock et al strongly suggests that transmission of adult genital tract viruses to children occurs primarily by the sexual route: five cases analyzed by HPV typing proved to be due to types 6, 11, or 16—the same types that cause adult condylomata.

Numerous minute vulvar condylomas associated, at times, with pruritus, pain, or burning may easily be overlooked unless they are soaked with 3 to 5 per cent acetic acid for two or three minutes, which turns them white (acetowhitening) and makes them easily identifiable. This procedure is recommended in men as well as women.

Franceschi et al found that over 8 per cent of women attending a clinic for sexually transmitted diseases because of genital warts had dysplastic changes in cervical smears; less than 2 per cent of women with gonorrhea or trichomoniasis had such changes. Chuango et al found that condylomata acuminata were a highly significant risk factor for cervical dysplasia.

Many studies have provided strong links between condylomata and cervical carcinoma. HPV types found in condylomata are 6, 11, and 16, but also 18, 30, 31, 32, 42, 51 to 54, 13, 43, 44, 55, and 33. HPV types 16 and 18, and less often 30, 31, 34, 35 to 39, and 48, are found in 90 per cent of cases of carcinoma of the cervix and its precursors. Newer associated types include 35 and 39. All women with external condylomata, or with sexual partners who have condylomata, need a Papanicolaou smear of the cervix and endocervix. Frequent follow-ups of negative smears are advisable. HPV has been detected in clinically normal tissue adjacent to both condylomata and genital cancer, as reported by Ferenczy et al and by Macnab et al.

Figure 19–57. Unusually large perianal condyloma acuminatum.

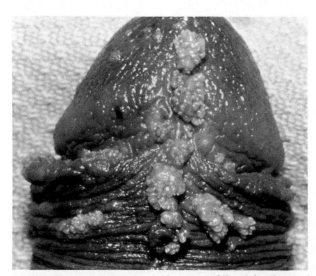

Figure 19–58. Penile warts. (Courtesy of Dr. John Reeves.)

Carcinomas of the penis have now been documented to occur in association with HPV infection, and a direct etiologic association is postulated. Anal cancer in HPV-infected homosexual males has also been reported.

Bowenoid Papulosis. These are dome-shaped, usually rough-surfaced, often pigmented papules a few mm in diameter occurring singly or more often multiply on the penile shaft or on or near the vulva, usually too cornified to respond well to topical podophyllum. Histologically they show as much cellular atypia as Bowen's disease. Though progression or invasive cancer may occur, spontaneous resolution is common, and they rarely recur after conservative excision with fulguration. Gross et al found HPV type 16 in all of 12 lesions; Obalek confirmed this finding and found cervical dysplasia in the female patients, and in the sexual partners of the male patients. HPV 16 and 18 have been found in 80 per cent of Bowenoid papulosis lesions—types associated with malignant transformation. HPV types 34 and 48 are also associated with this condition.

Giant Condyloma Acuminatum (Buschke-Löwenstein Tumor). Giant condyloma acuminatum is a rare, aggressive, wartlike growth, which penetrates into the dermis. It occurs most often on the glans or prepuce of uncircumcised men; less often it may occur on perianal skin or the vulva. Clinically it behaves like a carcinoma, yet histologically it appears remarkably benign. It may be a verrucous carcinoma, but from the evidence we can only classify it as an unusually massive and aggressive wart, produced by HPV types 6 or 11, and containing cytoplasmic inclusions.

The prognosis for the Buschke-Löwenstein giant condyloma is excellent, provided it is completely removed.

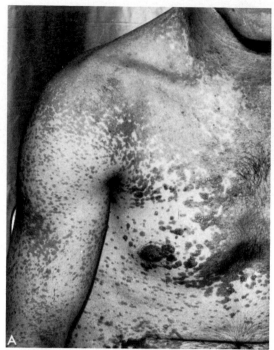
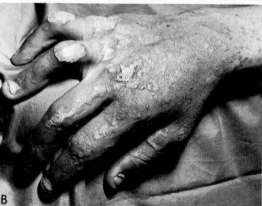

Figure 19–60. A, *Epidermodysplasia verruciformis. Verrucous plaques can be seen, especially on the sternum. B, Lesions consist of flat papules and hyperkeratotic scaly patches, especially over the knuckles. (Courtesy of Drs. M. Ruiter and P. J. Van Mullem.)*

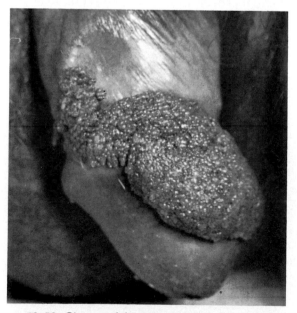

Figure 19–59. Giant condyloma acuminatum. (Courtesy of Dr. V. Beltrani.)

Epidermodysplasia Verruciformis. This rare disorder, described by Lewandowsky and Lutz in 1922, was regarded as an epidermal nevus until papillomavirus was found in the lesions. It is characterized by widespread flat and common warts, which begin in childhood and almost never regress. Squamous cell carcinomas supervene in 30 to 80 per cent of patients, most often on sun-exposed surfaces.

Consanguinity is common in the parents of such patients, and though about 25 per cent of cases appear to be inherited in autosomal dominant fashion, Androphy et al recently reported a kindred with X-linked recessive inheritance. The patients have a selective immunologic defect limited to HPV.

Many virus types have been isolated from patients with this condition. They include types 1, 2, 3, 4, 7, 9, 10, 12, 14, 15, 17 to 25, 36 to 38, 46, 47, 49, and

50. Importantly, two other types, HPV 5 and 8, are found in the skin cancers of these patients, further supporting the oncogenic potential of HPV.

Several immunodeficiency syndromes have increased frequency of HPV infection. These include renal transplant patients, patients on immunosuppressive therapy for other diagnoses such as systemic lupus erythematosus, patients with primary immunodeficiency diseases such as those reported by Barnett et al, and patients with AIDS.

Heck's Disease. Small white to pinkish papules occur diffusely in the oral cavity in this disease, also known as *focal epithelial hyperplasia*. HPV 13 has been linked to this condition by Pfister et al.

Respiratory (Laryngeal) Papillomatosis. HPV-associated papillomas may occur throughout the respiratory tract from the nose to the lungs in both infants and adults. The children are frequently born to mothers with condylomata. The HPV types found in these lesions, 6, 11, 16, and 30, are those types seen in genital condylomata.

Oral Hairy Leukoplakia. This condition appears as a slightly raised, corrugated plaque on the lateral aspect of the tongue of patients with the acquired immunodeficiency syndrome. Although the Epstein-Barr virus is also present in these lesions, Greenspan et al found that 49 of 67 (77 per cent) biopsy specimens were positive for HPV by immunohistochemical staining. Several studies have failed to confirm the reported finding of HPV in this oral lesion, and its contribution to the formation of the white plaque is not well defined.

ETIOLOGY. Verrucae and their mucocutaneous counterpart, condylomata, are caused by the human wart virus, human papillomavirus (HPV), which belongs to the papovavirus group. It contains DNA. Eosinophilic intranuclear and cytoplasmic inclusions are common in plantar warts and much less so in verruca vulgaris; they have been identified as keratohyalin.

Human papovavirus is an ether-resistant virus measuring 52–55 nm in diameter, with 72 capsomeres in its outer shell. Kreider et al have recently cultured HPV Type 11 in the laboratory, by grafting human skin infected with it beneath the renal capsule of athymic mice.

HISTOPATHOLOGY. In common warts the epidermis shows the principal histologic features. There is a prominent circumscribed acanthosis with elongated interpapillary projections and an overlying thickening of the horny layer due to hyperkeratosis and parakeratosis. Mitoses may be present near the basal cell layer. In flat warts the main change is in the rete, while the stratum corneum has a basket-weave appearance. In the acuminate and filiform warts the alteration is principally acanthosis, with slight hyperkeratosis, and a lymphocytic infiltrate in the dermis. Typically HPV papillomas have large keratinocytes with pyknotic eccentric nuclei surrounded by a clear halo—"koilocytes." Large eosinophilic cytoplasmic and smaller basophilic intranuclear inclusions are commonly found. Both appear to be keratohyalin granules. Lesions of Bowenoid papulosis show irregularly arranged dyskeratotic keratinocytes typical of Bowen's disease.

DIFFERENTIAL DIAGNOSIS. Infrequently giant condylomata of Buschke may develop, especially on the glans penis. This may be difficult to distinguish from epidermoid carcinoma. Warts upon the fingers may be confused with tuberculosis verrucosa cutis (anatomic "wart"), but in the latter the lesion is single and larger than the common wart. Molluscum contagiosum may closely resemble the common wart. Spraying with ethyl chloride reveals the central keratin plug in molluscum.

TREATMENT. Some warts respond to simple treatment, or disappear spontaneously and rather suddenly, while others are stubbornly recurrent. Messing found in a two-year study that two thirds of warts in children regressed, apparently spontaneously.

Countless local remedies might be mentioned as potential therapy. At present treatment options consist of modalities which selectively destroy the infected cells, or suggestive-type noninvasive therapy. The choice of the treatment method will be influenced by the location of the warts, their size and number, the presence of secondary infection, the amount of tenderness when pressed, the age and sex of the patient, the history of previous treatment, and the degree to which the physician subscribes to the view that destruction of the wart, if thorough, can be equated to success.

Electrodesiccation. Electrodesiccation and curettage of warts is a widely used method of treatment. It is quick, and impresses the patient as definitive; but even in skilled hands it may leave an unsightly atrophic scar. Warts recur in perhaps 20 to 40 per cent of cases, and the extent and depth of the procedure are no guarantee of success. It gives one pause to realize that Gibson et al treated plantar warts with acyclovir cream, with a placebo cream, and with electrodesiccation, and there was no difference between acyclovir and the placebo cream, but *both* were far superior to electrodesiccation!

Cryotherapy. Refrigeration therapy either with liquid nitrogen or solid carbon dioxide is another very widely used, though painful, way of treating warts. A cotton applicator is dipped into liquid nitrogen and then applied to the wart long enough to turn the wart and a small 1–2 mm halo of surrounding tissue white. The procedure is repeated a few times, depending upon the site, depth, and width of the lesions. A liquid nitrogen spray is also popular.

The object of the treatment is to produce epidermal necrosis. A small blister, which usually becomes hemorrhagic, then dries and peels off together with the wart, is a desired effect.

Both liquid nitrogen and solid carbon dioxide are used for the common warts on the fingers, face, penis, vagina, and anus. It is also excellent for periungual warts, where a finger block type of local anesthesia may be performed. Better cosmetic results are usually achieved with this method than by electrodesiccation.

Acids. Mary Bunney reported a striking reduction in the number of cases of warts requiring specialist referral by instituting primary treatment with applications of salicylic acid and lactic acid in flexible collodion (Duofilm, Duoplant, Occlusal-HP, Viranol, Salactic Film) painted on warts daily. Nearly 70 per cent of common warts and 84 per cent of plantar warts were cured. This liquid is applied, allowed to dry, and occluded with tape. After 24 hours this may be removed with the whitened keratin, and then reapplied. This treatment requires a committed therapeutician in the home environment.

Trichloroacetic acid may be applied to the wart with a wooden stick.

A conservative method for large and multiple plantar warts, where electrodesiccation is contraindicated, is the application of 40 per cent salicylic acid adhesive plaster (Duke). The plaster is cut to the size of the pared wart, the backing of the plaster is removed and the plaster applied. This is removed after 48 hours, the whitened necrotic mass is rubbed off and a new plaster reapplied. Applications are continued for several weeks. This type of therapy is especially effective for treating mosaic warts on the sole.

Podophyllum. Podophyllum USP—often misidentified as "podophyllin" or "resin of podophyllin"—is a resinous mixture, highly effective when applied as a 25 per cent solution in compound tincture of benzoin to the surface of not overly cornified acuminate condylomas, or to warts whose surface keratin has been removed with trichloroacetic acid. Serious poisoning has occurred from treating large areas or applying it inside the vagina. It should be used on lesions not over 3 cm in diameter, and washed off after four to six hours. It is contraindicated for use in pregnancy and should not be applied to vaginal or oral mucous membranes, or used in infants.

Laser. CO_2 laser treatment is quite useful in the therapy of condylomata. Cure rates of up to 90 per cent have been reported. Photocoagulation need be only very superficial; however, several millimeters of grossly uninvolved tissue should be treated to minimize recurrences. Healing occurs in three to four weeks, and cosmesis is excellent. Large areas of treatment require regional or general anesthesia. Warts occurring in the vaginal mucosa, on the cervix, in the anorectal area, in the distal urethra, or on the oral mucosa respond similarly well. Wart virus DNA is present in the "plume" of steam from the operative field; the potential hazard of this is obvious.

5-Fluorouracil. Five per cent 5-FU ointment either alone or in combination with salicylic acid has been reported to be effective in common and plantar warts. Also, it is used as a 5 per cent cream in the treatment of distal urethral lesions, with application four times daily for 14 days.

Retinoids. Topical tretinoin (Retin A), oral isotretinoin (Accutane), and etretinate (Tigosan) have all been anecdotally reported to have resulted in cures of otherwise resistant verrucae.

Interferon. Numerous reports of use of both intralesional and systemic interferon are appearing. While regression of warts is being seen in 60 to 80 per cent of cases, side effects and cost are problems. Research is continuing, to ascertain its potential place in the therapy of warts.

Cantharidin. A 0.7 per cent solution of cantharidin in acetone and flexible collodion (Cantharone) may be effective in the treatment of common and plantar warts. It is applied directly to the wart after preliminary paring. After drying, adhesive tape is applied and removed 24 hours later. In a week the wart is debrided and re-treated if wart tissue is still evident. Tingling, burning, and even extreme pain and tenderness may develop in patients who are sensitive to cantharidin. It is not unusual for common warts to recur in a doughnut-shaped ring surrounding the treated—and often abolished—original wart. We do not recommend the method except for plantar warts, for which Odom finds it very effective.

Formalin. This may be successful in the treatment of recalcitrant plantar warts. After paring, the wart is soaked daily for 30 minutes in 4 per cent formalin solution. An eyecup, a saucer, or a shallow dish may be used as the container for the solution. The skin about the wart is protected with petrolatum. The effect of formalin soaking may be enhanced by weekly applications of cryotherapy. Instead of the formalin solution some prefer the application of 8 ml of formalin solution in 30 gm of Aquaphor. The development of allergic contact dermatitis is a possible complication of this treatment.

Roentgen Rays. Because of recent evidence of the oncogenic potential of certain HPV types, and the epidemiologic and clinical suggestion that radiation and ultraviolet light may enhance these tumor-forming effects, *x-ray therapy should not be given to warts.*

DNCB. An effective if tedious method of treatment is sensitization to dinitrochlorobenzene (or better squaric acid dibutyl ester, to avoid the carcinogenicity associated with DNCB) in the usual manner, followed by painting the wart with it. Erikson reported 80 per cent success in 43 patients; average time to cure was two months, and the recurrence rate after 6–12 months was zero. Complement-binding wart antibodies, present in 15 per cent of the patients before treatment, rose to 43 per cent afterward. It may be worth trying in very large and resistant warts.

Bleomycin. Intralesional injection of bleomycin, introduced as an antibiotic for treatment of cancer, has been repeatedly reported as 60 to 95 per cent successful against warts, and it is worth trying in recalcitrant ones. Still unapproved by the FDA, it is nevertheless in wide use. It is quite painful. One noteworthy side effect, first reported by Bovenmeyer in 1983 and 1984, is the induction of Raynaud's syndrome in the treated digit when bleomycin is injected into paronychial warts. Ernst Epstein also reported this side effect in 1985. It has also been reported rarely to induce onychodystrophy in the adjacent nail. If it is injected too deeply, or into a vessel, digital gangrene may be produced.

Rees uses it by dissolving the contents of a 15-unit vial of Blenoxane in 30 ml of bacteriostatic saline solution; it will keep at least four months. A 1-ml plastic disposable Luer syringe with a ½-inch 30-gauge needle is used to inject 0.1 ml of the solution into warts, at multiple sites if necessary. Mary Bunney advises waiting four weeks before reinjecting.

Other. The placebo effect and the ability of the therapist to positively influence the course of treatment through suggestion should not be underestimated. Any method which does no harm is worthy of trial in certain situations. One of us (HLA) has cured many cases by having patients rub the wart with a piece of raw meat every day for two weeks, and had similar success with some large paronychial and plantar (as well as ordinary) warts by having patients apply the cut end of an *Aloe vera* leaf to the wart every morning. Hypnosis may, in some instances, be successful: one of us (HLA) has had good experience with this modality, and Straatmeyer used hypnosis successfully in six cases of recalcitrant acuminate condylomas.

If "spontaneous disappearance" is invoked (as it often is) to explain these apparent cures, then the responses should occur at random intervals after the treatment. They do not: they occur, in general, in about the epidermal turnover time: two to three weeks.

Abramson, AL, et al: Laryngeal papillomatosis: Clinical, histopathologic and molecular studies. Laryngoscope 1987, 97:678.

Amer M, et al: Therapeutic evaluation for intralesional injection of bleomycin sulfate in 143 resistant warts. JAAD 1988, 18:1313.

American Academy of Dermatology Task Force on Pediatric Dermatology: Genital warts and sexual abuse in children. JAAD 1984, 11:529.

Androphy EJ, et al: X-linked inheritance of epidermodysplasia verruciformis. Arch Dermatol 1985, 121:864.

Idem: Response of warts in epidermodysplasia verruciformis to treatment with systemic and intralesional alpha interferon. JAAD 1984, 11:197.

Baran R: Onychodystrophie induite par injection intralésionnelle de bleomycine pour verrue periungueale. Ann Dermatol Venereol 1985, 112:463.

Barnett N, et al: Extensive verrucosis in primary immunodeficiency diseases. Arch Dermatol 1983, 119:5.

Barrasso R, et al: High prevalence of papillomavirus-associated penile intraepithelial neoplasia in sexual partners of women with cervical intraepithelial neoplasia. N Engl J Med 1987, 317:916.

Beutner KR: Podophyllotoxin in the treatment of genital human papillomavirus infection: A review. Semin Dermatol 1987, 6:10.

Idem: Human papillomavirus infection. JAAD 1989, 20:114.

Black HS, et al: The mutagenicity of dinitrochlorobenzene. Arch Dermatol 1985, 121:348.

Bovenmeyer DA: Can intralesional bleomycin induce Raynaud's phenomenon? The Schoch Letter 1983, 33:107, and Cold-sensitive fingers from bleomycin. The Schoch Letter 1984, 34:31, and "Reply," JAAD 1985, 13:470.

Boyle J, et al: Treatment of extensive virus warts with etretinate in a patient with sarcoidosis. Clin Exp Dermatol 1983, 8:33.

Bunney MH: Viral Warts: Their Biology and Treatment. Oxford, Oxford University Press, 1982.

Idem: Wart treatments. Semin Dermatol 1983, 2:101.

Idem: Treatment of resistant warts with intralesional bleomycin. Br J Dermatol 1984, 110:197.

Idem, et al: The treatment of resistant warts with intralesional bleomycin: A controlled clinical trial. Br J Dermatol 1984, 110:197.

Cassidy DE, et al: Podophyllum toxicity: A report of a fatal case and a review of the literature. J Toxicol Clin Toxicol 1982, 19:35.

Chuang T-Y, et al: Condyloma acuminatum in Rochester, Minn., 1950–1978. I. Epidemiology and clinical features. Arch Dermatol 1984, 120:469. II. Anaplasia and unfavorable outcomes. Arch Dermatol 1984, 120:476.

Idem: Condylomata acuminata. JAAD 1987, 16:376.

Comite SL, et al: Colposcopic evaluation of men with genital warts. JAAD 1988, 18:1274.

Crum CP, et al: Human papillomavirus type 16 and early cervical neoplasia. N Engl J Med 1984, 310:880.

Epstein E: Persisting Raynaud's phenomenon following intralesional bleomycin treatment of finger warts. JAAD 1985, 13:469.

Eriksen K: Treatment of the common wart by induced allergic inflammation. Dermatologica 1980, 160:161.

Eron LJ, et al: Interferon therapy for condylomata acuminata. N Engl J Med 1986, 315:1059.

Ferenczy A: Using the laser to treat vulvar condylomata acuminata and intraepidermal neoplasia. Can Med Assoc J 1983, 128:135.

Ibid, et al: Latent papillomavirus and recurring genital warts. N Engl J Med 1985, 313:784.

Finkel ML, et al: Warts among meat handlers. Arch Dermatol 1983, 120:1314.

Franceschi S, et al: Genital warts and cervical neoplasia: an epidemiological study. Br J Cancer 1983, 48:621.

Friedman-Kien AE, et al: Natural interferon alfa for treatment of condylomata acuminata. JAMA 1988, 259:533.

Gal AA, et al: Papillomavirus antigens in anorectal condyloma and carcinoma in homosexual men. JAMA 1987, 257:337.

Gall SA, et al: Interferon for the therapy of condylomata acuminata. Am J Obstet Gynecol 1985, 153:157.

Gibson JR, et al: A comparison of acyclovir cream vs placebo cream vs liquid nitrogen in the treatment of viral plantar warts. Dermatologica 1984, 168:178.

Greenspan JS, et al: Replication of Epstein-Barr virus within the epithelial cells of oral hairy leukoplakia. N Engl J Med 1985, 313:1564.

Growdon WA, et al: Pruritic vulvar squamous papillomatosis: evidence for human papillomavirus etiology. Obstet Gynecol 1985, 66:564.

Gross G, et al: Bowenoid papulosis. Arch Dermatol 1985, 121:858.

Gruber M: Podophyllum versus podophyllin. JAAD 1984, 10:302.

Guillet GY, et al: Bowenoid papulosis. Arch Dermatol 1984, 120:514.

Happle R: The potential hazards of dinitrochlorobenzene. Arch Dermatol 1985, 121:330.

Healy GB, et al: Treatment of recurrent respiratory papillomatosis with human leukocyte interferon. N Engl J Med 1988, 319:401.

Hursthouse MW: A controlled trial of the use of topical 5-fluorouracil on viral warts. Br J Dermatol 1975, 92:93.

Jensen SL: Comparison of podophyllin application with simple surgical excision in clearance and recurrence of perianal condylomata acuminata. Lancet 1985, 2:1146.

Kreider JW, et al: Morphological transformation *in vivo* of human uterine cervix of papillomavirus from condylomata acuminata. Nature 1985, 317:639.

Idem: *In vivo* transformation of human skin with human papillomavirus type 11 from condylomata acuminata. J Virol 1986, 59:369.

Levine RU, et al: Cervical papillomavirus infection and intraepithelial neoplasia: A study of male sexual partners. Obstet Gynecol 1984, 64:16.

Lind PO, et al: Local immunoreactivity and human papillomavirus (HPV) in oral precancer and cancer lesions. Scand J Dent Res 1986, 94:419.

Lookingbill DP, et al: Human papillomavirus type 16 in bowenoid papulosis, intraoral papillomas, and squamous cell carcinoma of the tongue. Arch Dermatol 1987, 123:363.

Lutzner MA, et al: An unusual wart-like skin lesion found in a renal allograft recipient. Arch Dermatol 1981, 117:43.

Idem: Clinical observations, virologic studies and treatment trials in patients with epidermodysplasia verruciformis, a disease induced by specific human papillomavirus. J Invest Dermatol 1986, 83:185.

Idem: The human papillomaviruses: a review (editorial). Arch Dermatol 1983, 119:631.

Lyell A, et al: The Myrmecia: a study of inclusion bodies in warts. Br Med J 1951, p. 912.

Macnab JCM, et al: Human papillomavirus in clinically and histologically normal tissue of patients with genital cancer. N Engl J Med 1986, 315:1052.

McDonnell JM, et al: Demonstration of papillomavirus capsid antigen in human conjunctival neoplasia. Arch Ophthalmol 1986, 104:1801.

McKay M: Vulvodynia. Arch Dermatol 1989, 125:256.

Mertz B: DNA probes for papillomavirus strains readied for clinical cancer screening. JAMA 1988, 260:2777.

Milburn PB, et al: Disseminated warts and evolving squamous cell carcinoma in a patient with AIDS. JAAD 1988, 19:401.

Miller RAW: Nail dystrophy following intralesional injections of bleomycin for a periungual wart. Arch Dermatol 1984, 120:963.

Idem: Podophyllin. Int J Dermatol 1985, 24:491.

Naghashfar Z, et al: Identification of genital tract papillomavirus HPV-6 and HPV-16 in warts of the oral cavity. J Med Virol 1985, 17:313.

Nash G, et al: Atypical lesions of the anal mucosa in homosexual men. JAMA 1986, 256:873.

Obalek S, et al: Bowenoid papulosis of the male and female genitalia: risk of cervical neoplasia. JAAD 14:433.

Oriel JD: Natural history of genital warts. Br J Venereal Dis 1971, 47:1.

Penneys NS, et al: Papillomavirus common antigens: papillomavirus antigen in verruca, benign papillomatous lesions, trichilemmoma, and Bowenoid papulosis: an immunoperoxidase study. Arch Dermatol 1984, 120:859.

Pfister H, et al: Characterization of HPV 13 from focal epithelial hypoplasia. J Virol 1983, 47:363.

Rees RB: Managing warts: the pros and cons of current therapies. Modern Med 1983, p. 141.

Idem: Treatment of warts. Semin Dermatol 1984, 3:130.

Idem: The treatment of warts. Clin Dermatol 1985, 3:179.

Reichman RC, et al: Treatment of condyloma acuminatum with three different interferons administered intralesionally. Ann Intern Med 1988, 108:675.

Rock B, et al: Genital tract papillomavirus infection in children. Arch Dermatol 1986, 122:1129.

Rosenberg SK, et al: Sexually transmitted papillomaviral infections in the male. I. Anatomical distribution and clinical features. Urology 1987, 29:488.

Rudlinger R, et al: Human papillomavirus infections in a group of renal transplant recipients. Br J Dermatol 1986, 115:681.

Sait MA, et al: Condylomata acuminata in children: report of four cases. Genitourin Med 1985, 61:338.

Sand PK, et al: Evaluation of male consorts of women with genital human papillomavirus infection. Obstet Gynecol 1986, 68:679.

Sanders BB: Dinitrochlorobenzene immunotherapy of human warts. Cutis 1981, 27:389.

Schachner L, et al: Assessing child abuse in childhood condyloma acuminatum. JAAD 1985, 12:157.

Schonfeld A, et al: Intramuscular human interferon-B injections in treatment of condyloma acuminatum. Lancet 1984, 1:1038.

Sehgal VN, et al: Genital warts. Int J Dermatol 1989, 28:75.

Shumer SM, et al: Bleomycin in the treatment of recalcitrant warts. JAAD 1983, 9:96.

Silva PD, et al: Management of condyloma acuminatum. JAAD 1985, 13:457.

Simmons PD: Genital warts. Int J Dermatol 1983, 22:410.

Idem, et al: Cryotherapy versus electrocautery in the treatment of genital warts. Br J Venereal Dis 1983, 57:273.

Stiefler RE, et al: Heck's disease. JAAD 1979, 1:499.

Straatmeyer AJ: Condylomata acuminata: results of treatment using hypnosis. JAAD 1983, 9:434.

Tang CK, et al: Congenital condylomata acuminata. Am J Obstet Gynecol 1978, 131:912.

Vance JC, et al: Intralesional recombinant alpha-2 interferon for the treatment of patients with condyloma acuminatum or verruca plantaris. Arch Dermatol 1986, 122:272.

Van der Leest RJ, et al: Human papillomavirus heterogeneity in 36 renal transplant recipients. Arch Dermatol 1987, 123:354.

VonKrogh G: Condylomata acuminata 1983: an up-dated review. Semin Dermatol 1983, 2:109.

PARVOVIRUS GROUP

ERYTHEMA INFECTIOSUM (Fifth Disease)

Erythema infectiosum is a benign infectious exanthem that occurs in epidemics in the spring and summer. The usually asymptomatic disease begins abruptly with erythema of the cheeks and, hence, is referred to as a *slapped cheek* appearance. The redness varies from a diffuse erythema to closely grouped, tiny papules on erythematous bases. It is most intense beneath the eyes and may extend over the cheeks like butterfly wings. The perioral area, lids, and chin are usually free. In a day or two a nonpruritic macular erythema, often lacelike in appearance, appears on the deltoid areas and trunk. After four or five days the redness fades from the cheeks and body, leaving for a short time a retiform network of faintly bluish blood vessels. A characteristic feature of erythema infectiosum is the evanescent nature of the rash, which fades within a week but may briefly recur a few times. The incubation period is 13 to 18 days. Adults, especially women, who acquire the infection may develop pruritus and migratory arthritis, which may last several months. One woman with

these symptoms also developed a vesicopustular eruption. Anemia, aplastic crisis, and chronic bone marrow failure may result, as the virus attacks the bone marrow progenitor cells.

Erythema infectiosum has long been presumed to be due to a virus, but it was not until June 1983 that Mary Anderson et al reported the finding of parvovirus-specific IgM in sera from 33 cases of erythema infectiosum in a school epidemic, taken three weeks after the onset of an illness characterized by vomiting, diarrhea, and a rash on the face and neck in one case and a sore throat for three days followed by a diffuse, recurring rash in another.

In August 1984, Anderson's final report was published. Red cheeks were present in 85 per cent of 162 children; itching in 46 per cent; rash on the arms and legs in three-quarters, on the trunk in half; the "lacy" pattern was present in two thirds. Sore throat was present in one third, headache or fever in one-fourth; cold or cough, and anorexia, in one fifth each; and diarrhea, vomiting, and arthralgia in 7 per cent each.

After the publication of Anderson et al's prelimi-

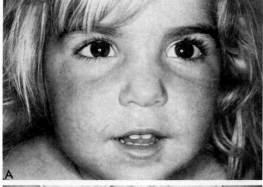

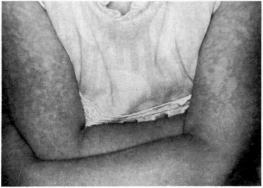

Figure 19–61. A, *"Slapped cheek" appearance, and* B, *retiform erythema of upper extremities, in erythema infectiosum.*

nary report, Plummer et al tested sera taken from 12 patients with erythema infectiosum during a mini-epidemic in 1980, and identified parvovirus B-19 ("the" human parvovirus) in 11. Nunoue in 1985 confirmed this finding in 25 of 34 children with erythema infectiosum.

Anand et al reported in 1987 that two of six pregnant women infected in an outbreak of parvo-virus disease in Scotland had midtrimester abortions; both abortuses were grossly edematous and anemic, and had viral DNA in several tissues.

Anand A: Human parvovirus infection in pregnancy and hydrops fetalis. N Engl J Med 1987, 316:183.
Anderson MJ, et al: Human parvovirus, the cause of erythema infectiosum (fifth disease)? Lancet 1983, 1:1378.
Idem: An outbreak of erythema infectiosum associated with human parvovirus infection. J Hyg Cambridge 1984, 93:85.
Jacks TA: Pruritus in parvovirus infection. JR Coll Gen Pract 1987, 37:210.
Joseph PR: Incubation period of fifth disease. Lancet 1986, 2:1390.
Kurtzman GJ, et al: Chronic bone marrow failure due to persistent B19 parvovirus infection. N Engl J Med 1987, 317:287.
Naides SJ, et al: Human parvovirus B19–induced vesiculopustular skin eruption. Am J Med 1988, 84:968.
Nunoue T, et al: Human parvovirus (B19) and erythema infectiosum. Pediatrics 1985, 107:38.
Plummer FA, et al: An erythema infectiosum-like illness caused by human parvovirus infection. N Engl J Med 1985, 313:74.
Whitley RJ: Parvovirus infection: chance and investigation (editorial). N Engl J Med 1985, 313:111.

ARBOVIRUS GROUP

This group comprises the numerous *a*rthropod-*b*orne viruses (*arbo*viruses). Over 200 different viruses have been isolated and assigned to this group. These viruses multiply in vertebrates as well as the arthropods. The vertebrates usually act as reservoirs and the arthropods as vectors of the various diseases. These are RNA viruses that are lipid-solvent sensitive. They are classified into several groups, the most important of which are Groups A, B, and C.

WEST NILE FEVER

A maculopapular eruption accompanied by lymphadenopathy and fever characterize this disease. The complement fixation test is the test of choice. The disease is seen in the Middle East, especially in Egypt and Israel. The *Culex* mosquito is the vector and, therefore, the disease is most prevalent during the summer months.

SANDFLY FEVER

This is also known as phlebotomus fever and pappataci fever. Small pruritic papules appear on the skin after the sandfly bite and persist for some five days. After an incubation period of another five days

fever, headache, malaise, nausea, conjunctival injection, stiff neck, and abdominal pains suddenly develop. The skin manifestations consist of a scarlatiniform eruption of the face and neck.

Sandfly fever is caused by a virus some 25 nm in diameter belonging to the phlebotomus arbovirus group. The vector, *Phlebotomus papatasii*, is found in the Mediterranean area, Russia, China, and India. The female sandfly transmits the disease to man.

Recovery is slow, with recurring bouts of fever that eventually stop. No specific treatment is available.

DENGUE

Dengue, also known as *break-bone fever*, is characterized by fever, pain, and skin eruptions. The disease begins with a sudden high fever, shaking chills, fatigue, headache, back pain, aching muscles, and a scarlatiniform or morbilliform type of exanthem especially on the face, neck, and chest.

About the fourth day, after a brief remission of fever, a scarlatiniform exanthem appears, most vividly over the trunk, face, and extremities. In some three days the eruption as well as the fever subsides.

Dengue is caused by the dengue virus, belonging to the arbovirus group, and transmitted to man by the *Aedes aegypti* mosquito. The eastern Mediterranean area, Southeast Asia, Africa, India, Hawaii, and some Caribbean islands are a few of the places where dengue may occur. Epidemics occur when the virus is newly introduced into some area by travelers.

The course of the disease is favorable, with complete recovery, although no specific treatment is available at present.

Dengue may exceptionally manifest itself as hemorrhagic fever, with shock, which has a high mortality rate. Sumarmo showed in 97 children, half of whom were treated with a large single dose of hydrocortisone intravenously, that this was ineffective.

Sumarmo, et al: Failure of hydrocortisone to affect outcome in dengue shock syndrome. Pediatrics 1982, 69:45.

RETROVIRUS GROUP

This group of RNA viruses has for many years been known to be the cause of various tumors in animals. Characteristic of these viruses is an RNA-dependent DNA polymerase (reverse transcriptase). Another property associated with the animal tumor viruses is the presence of oncogenes (genes that mediate neoplastic transformation). Human T-cell lymphoma/leukemia virus, type I (HTLV-I) was the first proven link between retroviruses and cancer in humans, being associated with T-cell lymphoproliferative syndromes. HTLV-II, a second virus of this class, is associated with hairy cell leukemia. HTLV-V, the third virus in this group, has been linked to Tac-antigen–negative mycosis fungoides.

Another retroviral disease, the acquired immunodeficiency syndrome (AIDS), is caused by a retrovirus now designated the human immunodeficiency virus (HIV-1). This virus was previously identified as HIV, HTLV-III, lymphadenopathy-associated virus (LAV), or AIDS-related virus (ARV). A second virus has recently been reported to be present in two patients from West Africa with AIDS. It is designated LAV-II in the original article but is now designated by an HIV classification (HIV-2). This is the same virus that had been designated HTLV-IV and is closely related to STLV-III. The syndromes caused by these retroviruses are different from those caused by tumor-forming types of retroviruses in that they do not appear to be oncogenic; rather, they are cytolytic to the target T4 (T helper) cells.

Broder S: Pathogenic human retroviruses. N Engl J Med 1988, 318:243.

Clavel F, et al: Isolation of a new human retrovirus from West African patients with AIDS. Science 1986, 233:342.

Fine RM: HTLV-V. Int J Dermatol 1988, 27:473.

Gibbs WN, et al: Non-Hodgkin lymphoma in Jamaica and its relation to adult T-cell leukemia-lymphoma. Ann Intern Med 1987, 106:361.

Hahlmann R, et al: RNA tumor viruses, in Textbook of Human Virology, Belshe RB (ed), Littleton, Mass., PSG Publishing Company, Inc., 1984, pp. 139–178.

Kalyanaraman VS, et al: A new subtype of human T-cell leukemia virus (HTLV-II) associated with a T-cell variant of cell leukemia. Science 1982, 218:571.

Kanki PF, et al: New human T-lymphotropic retrovirus related to simian T-lymphotropic virus type III. Science 1986, 232:238.

Ligby G, et al: Retroviruses in dermatology. Int J Dermatol 1988, 27:462.

Manzari V, et al: HTLV-V: A new human retrovirus isolated in a Tac-negative T-cell lymphoma/leukemia. Science 1987, 238:1581.

HUMAN T-CELL LEUKEMIA/LYMPHOMA VIRUS I (HTLV-I)

This virus was first isolated in 1978 from humans who were suffering from adult T-cell leukemia or lymphoma. This syndrome is characterized by the presence of pleomorphic mature T lymphocytes with associated cutaneous infiltrates, lymphadenopathy, hepatosplenomegaly, hypercalcemia with or without lytic bone lesions, and interstitial pulmonary infiltrates. Opportunistic infection is common.

Antibody to this virus is present in endemic foci in Japan, the Caribbean, and southeastern United States, where prevalence rates vary between 1 and 15 per cent. In a recent survey of drug abusers in New York City, 9 per cent had antibody to HTLV-I.

The patients identified in the United States have primarily been young (average age of onset 34 years) black men who were born in the southeastern United States. The onset of symptoms is generally acute and related to cutaneous infiltrations or hypercalcemia. Skin lesions—papules, nodules, tumors, erythematous patches or erythroderma—are present in 65 per cent of patients. The onset is acute and the course generally fulminant, as opposed to the insidious onset and chronic course typical of mycosis fungoides. A subset of patients with adult T-cell leukemia/lymphoma who had a chronic, smoldering course has been reported by Yamaguchi et al.

The infected T cells develop moderately condensed nuclear chromatin, inconspicuous nucleoli, and irregular nuclear contour, the nucleus being divided into several lobes. They express large amounts of interleukin-2 cell membrane receptors. On skin biopsy, focal epidermal infiltration or Pautrier-like microabscesses are seen in two thirds of patients. The infiltrating cell is the T helper lymphocyte, but its in vitro function is suppression. Histologically the cutaneous infiltrations mimic mycosis fungoides.

Wantzin et al recently reported that 11 per cent of 315 European patients with cutaneous T-cell lymphoma were positive for HTLV-I antibody. This suggests that HTLV-I may play a role in the pathogenesis of the more classic syndrome seen in cutaneous T-cell lymphoma.

Treatment to date with combination chemotherapy has produced brief remissions, but on relapse the disease is usually nonresponsive.

Blayney DW, et al: The human T-cell leukemia/lymphoma virus in the Southeastern United States. JAMA 1983, 280:1048.

Brew BJ, et al: Another retroviral disease of the nervous system. N Engl J Med 1988, 318:1195.

Broder S, et al: T-cell lymphoproliferative syndrome associated with human T-cell leukemia/lymphoma virus. Ann Intern Med 1984, 100:543.

deShazo RD, et al: Immunologic assessment of a cluster of asymptomatic HTLV-I infected individuals in New Orleans. Am J Med 1989, 86:65.

Dixon AC, et al: Thrombotic thrombocytopenic purpura and HTLV-I. Ann Intern Med 1989, 110:93.

Harper ME, et al: Concomitant infection with HTLV-I and HTLV-III in a patient with T8 lymphoproliferative disease. N Engl J Med 1986, 315:1073.

Robert-Gurott M, et al: Prevalence of antibodies to HTLV-I, -II, and -III in intravenous drug abusers from an AIDS endemic region. JAMA 1986, 255:3133.

Sandler SG: HTLV-I and -II. JAMA 1986, 256:2245.

Takahashi K, et al: Cutaneous type adult T-cell leukemia/lymphoma. Arch Dermatol 1988, 124:399.

Takigawa M, et al: Does adult T-cell leukemia/lymphoma belong to the cutaneous T-cell lymphoma category? JAAD 1988, 18:379.

Wantzin GL, et al: Occurrence of human T-cell lymphotropic virus (type I) antibodies in cutaneous T-cell lymphoma. JAAD 1986, 15:598.

Yamaguchi K, et al: A proposal for smoldering adult T-cell leukemia. Blood 1983, 62:758.

HUMAN IMMUNODEFICIENCY VIRUS (HIV-1)

Infection with this RNA virus is responsible for the acquired immunodeficiency syndrome (AIDS). This disease was first described in 1981 by Gottlieb et al, and 129 cases were diagnosed that year. Since then the epidemic spread has led to the recognition of over 100,000 cases of overt AIDS by the end of July, 1989, with an estimated 2 million people in the United States HIV-1–antibody-positive.

These antibody-positive patients *are infected*, but do not manifest the complete defined syndrome of T helper cell depletion and opportunistic infection; thus statistics that deal only with "AIDS patients" are only reflecting end-stage disease, not the full spectrum of HIV-1 disease. A long-term study in San Francisco has shown that in their population, 50 per cent of HIV-infected patients developed CDC–case-definition AIDS over a 10-year period.

No one who has developed AIDS has recovered, and most AIDS patients die within two years of diagnosis. A subset of HIV-1–infected patients who do not manifest lymphadenopathy, T helper cell depletion, or opportunistic infections (AIDS) develop, and die of, central nervous system disease.

ETIOLOGY. HIV-1 was formerly referred to as HTLV-III, LAV, ARV, or HIV. It infects lymphocytes and monocytes/macrophages: T helper cells are infected and lysed, whereas monocytes/macrophages act as a productive reservoir of virus. Once in the cell, the virions remain there permanently. If the infected lymphocytes are stimulated with antigen, there is enhanced viral replication, and the cells die and release virions.

The virus can be cultured from saliva, tears, breast milk, semen, vaginal secretions, and blood and blood products, but studies on the first three secretions have not defined well the risk of transmission from these sources. In general, the risk is very low, except from blood. To date there are no known reports of transmission via saliva or tears and only five cases of breast milk transmission. HIV is transmitted transplacentally. Infection occurs via intercourse, especially receptive anal intercourse with its inevitable mucosal injury; via contaminated hypodermic needles; and, before serologic tests were available, via blood or blood products in the form of transfusions or clotting factor concentrates.

PATHOGENESIS. The clinical manifestations of HIV infection, with its progressive acquired immunodeficiency, depend upon loss of the functional integrity of the T helper cell. HIV-1 preferentially infects, resides in, and lyses T helper cells. This leads to the inability to adequately fight infection, since depressed T helper cell function impairs T suppressor, T cytotoxic, macrophage, killer-cell, and B-cell function.

Redfield et al presented a classification scheme for adults with HIV-1 infection which recognizes the full spectrum of disease related to this agent. According to this scheme, patients who are seen for clinically suspected HIV-1 disease, or have a positive antibody screen, are given a thorough history and physical examination. The antibody screen, which is usually an ELISA test, is confirmed to be positive. This test is sensitive, but not specific, so Western blot analysis is performed, which is specific for HIV infection. An anergy screen consisting of mumps, tetanus, trichophyton, and monilia antigens is applied. Also a T-helper–lymphocyte count is obtained. Depression of this count below 400 T helper cells per cubic millimeter is considered to be evidence of depletion.

Six stages (Redfield) may be applied to adult patients: WR0 = an antibody negative patient with sexual contact with a patient with HIV infection; WR1 = positive culture for, or 2 positive Western blots to, HIV; WR2 = 2 positive Western blots and chronic lymphadenopathy; WR3 = 2 positive Western blots and persistent T helper cell depletion; WR4 = 2 positive Western blots, persistent T helper cell depletion, and partial defects in delayed hypersensitivity; WR5 = 2 positive Western blots, T helper cell depletion, and either clinical thrush or persistent anergy; WR6 = 2 positive Western blots and an opportunistic infection, as defined normally for a patient with CDC–case-definition AIDS.

Infections included are *Pneumocystis carinii* pneumonia; unusually extensive mucocutaneous herpes simplex of five+ weeks duration; cryptosporidium enterocolitis of four+ weeks duration; esophagitis due to *Candida albicans*, cytomegalovirus, or herpes simplex virus; pneumonia, meningitis, or encephalitis due to one or more of the following: *Aspergillus Sp., C. albicans, Cryptococcus neoformans,* cytomegalovirus, *Nocardia Sp.*, *Strongyloides Sp.*, *Toxoplasma gondii*, zygomycosis, or atypical *Mycobacterium Spp.*; or disseminated histoplasmosis; or isopsoriasis, causing chronic diarrhea (over one month). Other disseminated or chronic nonself-limited infections caused by agents in which deficient cellular immunity is pivotal should be anticipated. Kaposi's sarcoma is accepted as a criterion by the CDC to meet their definition of AIDS, while it is added as a K after the appropriate stage as proposed by Redfield et al.

The Walter Reed (WR) classification (Redfield et al) permits following factors which directly relate to T helper cell function, and therefore the progression of HIV disease. In patients followed at Walter Reed for 18 months or more, those patients entering in stages WR3 to WR6 have had a slow but progressive course to the next stage, or death.

HIV infection may rarely affect only the central nervous system. Progressive multifocal leukoencephalopathy and primary lymphoma of the central nervous system are included in the case definition of AIDS by the CDC, as is the occurrence of non-Hodgkin's lymphoma of high-grade pathologic type and of B cell or unknown immunologic phenotype in a patient with a positive serologic or virologic test for HIV.

INCUBATION PERIOD. In cases where the time of exposure is known, and an acute retroviral syndrome followed, the time period between these events has ranged from two weeks to four months. The time required to develop AIDS after infection with HIV is extremely variable, and at present the precise risk of developing AIDS or neurologic degeneration, or both, is unknown. Most infants who acquire the virus transplacentally manifest AIDS shortly after birth, and virtually all do so by eight months of age. Also, transfusion-associated AIDS in children has a relatively short incubation period (average eight months). In contrast, in adult transfusion cases, the median time between infection and AIDS is 28 months, with a range of one month to seven years. As mentioned above, among the San Francisco gay population, 50 per cent of HIV-positive persons have developed AIDS within 10 years.

RISK FACTORS. Male homosexuals or bisexuals account for 70 to 75 per cent of known cases. The seropositivity among the homosexual population in a high-risk area is 60 to 80 per cent. It is highest among promiscuous practitioners of receptive anal intercourse. Intravenous drug abusers account for another 15 to 17 per cent of cases, with seropositivity in high-risk areas being 40 to 70 per cent. Other groups who were important subsets of patients at relatively high risk early in the epidemic were Haitians, hemophiliacs, and recipients of blood transfusions.

While these groups are at high risk based on past exposure, their relative numbers will diminish as large numbers of others at risk develop the disease. Heterosexual contacts of patients with AIDS or with a person at risk for AIDS are another risk group; the risk of infection for wives of infected men appears to be 10 to 50 per cent. In contrast, older children of patients living in the same household do not appear to be at high risk for infection, as reported by Redfield et al.

CLINICAL COURSE. Two weeks to four months (usually two to four weeks) after infection a brief, self-limited mononucleosis-type syndrome develops. This acute retroviral syndrome is characterized by fever, chills, myalgia, and arthralgia. In several cases it has been accompanied by an erythematous, macular, nonpruritic eruption of the trunk and face which lasts three to seven days. Seroconversion usually occurs within two to three months.

This acute syndrome is then followed by an asymptomatic period lasting a few months to a few years. In those patients who show progressive disease, weight loss, lymphadenopathy, fever, and encephalopathy may appear. During the period of progressive T helper cell depletion it is not uncommon for skin lesions to provide clues to the progressive immunodeficiency, prior to the appearance of opportunistic infection. One factor which may allow the skin to express the T helper cell depletion early in the course of HIV disease is the reduction of the number of Langerhans cells as defined by both Ia and adenosine triphosphatase (ATPase) staining. A functional alteration of these antigen-presenting cells may be yet another factor which depresses the body's ability to fight infection.

CUTANEOUS MANIFESTATIONS. The cutaneous manifestations of HIV infection are numerous. The following lesions may provide an early clue to the dermatologist that HIV disease is present. A history which addresses potential exposure to HIV-infected patients, followed by a physical examination and HIV serology, is appropriate when evaluating these patients.

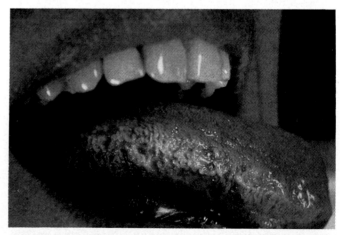

Figure 19–62. Oral hairy leukoplakia. A characteristic whitish verrucous corrugated plaque is commonly seen on the lateral surfaces of the tongue; it may be caused by the Epstein-Barr virus. When scraped with a tongue blade, the lesion does not wipe away. (From Friedman-Kien AE: Color Atlas of AIDS. Philadelphia, WB Saunders International Edition, 1989, p 101.)

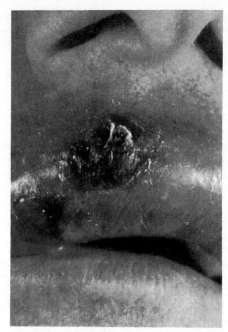

Figure 19–63. Herpes simplex ulcers. (From Friedman-Kien AE: Color Atlas of AIDS. Philadelphia, WB Saunders International Edition, 1989, p 101.)

Oral Hairy Leukoplakia. A distinct corrugated white plaque on one or both sides of the tongue has been well characterized by Greenspan et al. It has been shown to contain candida, human papillomavirus, and Epstein-Barr virus. In one study, 78 of 79 patients with this lesion were HIV-antibody positive.

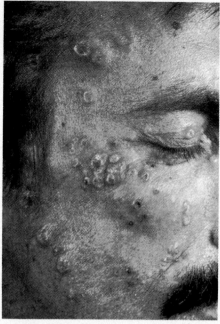

Figure 19–65. Molluscum contagiosum. Numerous large, umbilicated waxy papules have coalesced to form crusted plaques. They may be seen on other body parts as well. (From Friedman-Kien AE: Color Atlas of AIDS. Philadelphia, WB Saunders International Edition, 1989, p 99.)

Herpes Simplex. The ulcerative, chronic form occurs commonly. The perianal location is frequent.

Herpes Zoster. Friedman-Kien et al, in evaluating 48 patients who developed herpes zoster prior to age 50, found 35 serologically positive for HIV. However,

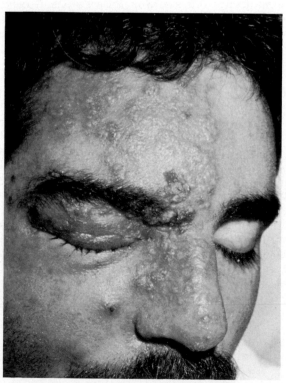

Figure 19–64. Herpes zoster in AIDS.

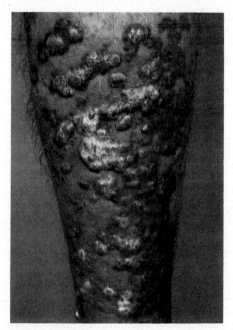

Figure 19–66. Classic Kaposi's sarcoma, nodular stage. Coalescing brown-to-violet plaque-to-nodular lesions with overlying adherent hyperkeratotic scales. (From Friedman-Kien AE: Color Atlas of AIDS. Philadelphia, WB Saunders International Edition, 1989, p 17).

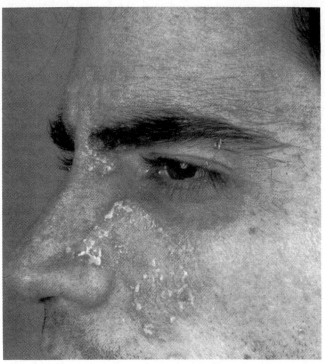

Figure 19–67. Seborrheic dermatitis. Pinkish-red scaly and crusted plaques are seen in the malar areas but also in other locations. (From Friedman-Kien AE: Color Atlas of AIDS. Philadelphia, WB Saunders International Edition, 1989, p 101.)

all but one had known risk factors for infection. Therefore, in a patient at risk for infection, occurrence of zoster may be a signal of progressive T cell depletion. Chronic VZV infection has also been described as nonhealing ecthymatous, papulovesicular, ulcerative, or verruciform lesions.

Molluscum Contagiosum. Several authors have reported the appearance of widespread or severe molluscum contagiosum in HIV disease. In a patient reported by Redfield et al, this was the presenting sign; however, it is usually present only late in the course of the disease.

Condyloma Acuminatum. Perianal lesions, or large, widespread, or numerous lesions, may indicate the need to investigate for HIV infection. Also common warts may grow or disseminate in HIV-infected patients.

Tinea Corporis. Widespread, treatment-resistant lesions may be present in early cases.

Oral Candidiasis (Thrush). One of the criteria listed in the staging of disease, this is present in most cases of progressive HIV disease. Angular cheilitis may be one manifestation.

Psoriasis and Reiter's Syndrome. Winchester et al reported in 1987 13 patients who had Reiter's disease and AIDS or ARC concurrently; in four the two syndromes appeared simultaneously. In two more, administration of methotrexate for Reiter's syndrome was followed by the development of Kaposi's sarcoma and fulminant AIDS, and death. An additional patient with undifferentiated spondyloarthropathy

developed psoriasis in conjunction with the onset of AIDS. Duvic et al reported additional patients with the same experience. They recommend etretinate in treating AIDS-associated psoriasis.

Eosinophilic Pustular Folliculitis. Buchness et al reported six AIDS patients with this disease who responded to UVB phototherapy. There were sterile papules and pustules on the face, trunk, and extremities.

Bacillary Angiomatosis (Cat-Scratch Disease). Disseminated vascular pyogenic-granuloma–like lesions in patients with AIDS have been found by Warthin-Starry stain to be positive for the bacilli of cat-scratch disease (see p. 299). Osseous lesions may occur. Erythromycin, doxycycline, or antimycobacterial antibiotics may be effective.

Kaposi's Sarcoma. In a patient under 60 years of age, this should prompt an investigation into HIV infection. These purple or hyperpigmented patches, papules, nodules, or tumors most often present on the trunk, arms, head, and neck in HIV disease. They are often elongated oval lesions which follow the skin lines. They may be present on mucosal surfaces. They occur more often in white patients and homosexuals, than in black patients or intravenous-drug users.

Kaposi's sarcoma may be the presenting sign of HIV disease. It does not negatively influence survival as much as does the presence of opportunistic infection; however, patients with both Kaposi's sarcoma and opportunistic infection have the worst prognosis.

Seborrheic Dermatitis. Eisenstat et al reported a 46 per cent prevalence in AIDS patients while Mathes et al reported it in 15 of 18 AIDS patients. It may have an abrupt onset and is often severe. It may be an early marker of the disease in the at-risk population. Soeprono et al reports that it is histologically distinctive from seborrheic dermatitis in non-HIV patients.

Papular Eruption. James et al reported the occurrence of 2–5-mm skin-colored, discrete papules of the head, neck, and upper trunk in seven of 35 HIV-infected patients. It was chronic, waxed and waned in severity with time, and was asymptomatic. Histologically a lymphocytic perivascular infiltrate was present in all except one patient, who had perifollicular granulomatous inflammation. This may occur early in the course of HIV infection.

In addition to these early signs of HIV infection, the skin may reflect systemic opportunistic infections. Thus systemic fungal, mycobacterial, parasitic, and viral infections may present with cutaneous macules, papules, nodules, tumors, or ulcerations. These should be biopsied and cultured as appropriate. Organisms isolated with particular frequency are *Cryptococcus neoformans, Histoplasma capsulatum, Candida albicans, Mycobacterium avium-intracellulare, Mycobacterium tuberculosis,* and *Acanthamoeba castellanii.*

Other infections commonly seen in patients at risk for HIV infections may manifest skin lesions such as syphilis (which may be seronegative—Hicks et al), gonorrhea, hepatitis B, and cytomegalic inclusion disease. Staphylococcal folliculitis may be seen in this population with increased frequency. It may progress to septicemia, abscesses, cellulitis, SSSS, or furunculosis. These are reviewed by Ellis et al in their report of neutrophil impairment in AIDS. In syphilis the risk of early progressive CNS involvement is very high, and the regimen for neurosyphilis should be adhered to.

Redfield et al reported the case of a military recruit who had asymptomatic HIV infection and was vaccinated against smallpox. This live-virus vaccine caused progressive, widespread vaccinia.

Non-Hodgkin's lymphoma may manifest itself in the skin. Most lymphomas seen in this population are high-grade B-cell lymphomas. Basal cell carcinomas and squamous cell carcinomas may develop and grow rapidly, as occurs in leukemia patients and organ transplant patients. Dysplastic nevi and melanomas have been reported in HIV-infected patients.

A variety of nonspecific lesions may be seen, such as erythroderma, psoriasiform dermatoses, ichthyotic lesions, and melasma. Reactions to drugs, especially trimethoprim-sulfamethoxazole, are common.

Ultimately death is most often related to opportunistic infection, lymphoma, or encephalopathy.

TREATMENT. Zidovudine (Retrovir) improves survival in advanced cases of AIDS, and treated patients have improved functional ability, weight gain, and fewer opportunistic infections. The drug often causes anemia and leukopenia, and was reported by Gill et al to cause severe bone marrow failure in four patients, with partial recovery after more than six months in only three of them. Close monitoring of the blood count is essential. It also causes a distinctive pigmentation of the nails, especially in black patients.

Ketoconazole for candidiasis; trimethoprim-sulfamethoxazole, pyrimethamine, and sulfadoxine (Fansidar), or inhaled pentamidine for *Pneumocystis* pneumonia; and acyclovir for recurrent herpes have all been used as prophylactic drugs. Other specific antifungal, antibacterial, antiviral, and antiprotozoan agents are used as necessary for concurrent infections.

The preferred treatment for Kaposi's sarcoma is intralesional vinblastine, cryotherapy, or irradiation for accessible individual lesions; but for widespread or inaccessible ones, vinblastine, etoposide, interferon, and "ABV" (Adriamycin, bleomycin, and vinblastine) have been more or less successful. Mintzer et al have reviewed these and reported limited success with vincristine, in 18 cases.

PREVENTION. This disease is most often spread through sexual contact. Therefore, precautions taken to limit spread of venereal disease in general apply to HIV infection. Specifically the use of a latex condom is believed to be important in preventing transmission of this disease, as may spermicides. Counseling of patients and education of the general public

about the ways this virus is and is not transmitted are important in limiting the spread of this infection. Casual contact is clearly not dangerous.

AIDS and HIV update. JAMA 1988, 259:2817.

Alessi E, et al: Mucocutaneous manifestations in patients infected with HIV. JAAD 1988, 19:290.

Amura EF, et al: HIV-associated skin lesions. JAMA 1989, 261:991.

Armstrong D, et al: Treatment of infections in patients with the acquired immunodeficiency syndrome. Ann Intern Med 1985, 103:738.

Azon-Masoliver A, et al: Zidovudine-induced nail pigmentation. Arch Dermatol 1988, 124:1570.

Barre-Sinoussi F, et al: Isolation of a T-lymphotropic retrovirus from a patient at risk for acquired immune deficiency syndrome. Science 1983, 220:868.

Belsito DV, et al: Reduced Langerhans cell Ia antigen and ATPase activity in patients with the acquired immunodeficiency syndrome. N Engl J Med 1984, 310:1279.

Berger RS, et al: Cutaneous manifestations of early human immunodeficiency virus exposure. JAAD 1988, 19:298.

Berk MA, et al: Tubuloreticular structures in a papular eruption associated with HIV disease. JAAD 1988, 18:452.

Berry CD, et al: Neurologic relapse after benzathine penicillin therapy for secondary syphilis in a patient with HIV infection. N Engl J Med 1987, 316:1587.

Blattner WA, et al: Epidemiology of human T-lymphotropic virus type III and the risk of the acquired immunodeficiency syndrome. Ann Intern Med 1985, 103:665.

Bowen DL, et al: Immunopathogenesis of the acquired immunodeficiency syndrome. Ann Intern Med 1985, 103:704.

Bronniman DA, et al: Coccidioidomycosis in the acquired immunodeficiency syndrome. Ann Intern Med 1987, 106:372.

Buchness MR, et al: Eosinophilic pustular folliculitis in AIDS. N Engl J Med 1988, 318:1183.

Burke DS, et al: HIV infections among civilian applicants for United States military service. N Engl J Med 1987, 317:131.

Calabrese LH: Autoimmune manifestations of HIV infection. Clin Lab Med 1988, 8:269.

Centers for Disease Control: Diagnosis and management of mycobacterial infection and disease in persons with HIV infection. Ann Intern Med 1987, 106:254.

Cohen PR, et al: Disseminated herpes zoster in patients with HIV infection. Am J Med 1988, 84:1076.

Idem: Tongue lesions in AIDS. Cutis 1987, 40:406.

Coldiron BM, et al: Prevalence and clinical spectrum of skin disease in patients infected with HIV. Arch Dermatol 1989, 125:357.

Colebunders R, et al: Breastfeeding and transmission of HIV. Lancet 1988, 2:1487.

Conant MA, et al: Prophylactic and suppressive treatment with acyclovir and the management of herpes in patients with AIDS. JAAD 1988, 18:186.

Cooper JS, et al: Initial observations of the effect of radiotherapy on epidemic Kaposi's sarcoma. JAMA 1984, 252:934.

Cordero JF: Issues concerning AIDS embryopathy. AJDC 1988, 142:9.

Coulman CU, et al: Cutaneous pneumocystosis. Ann Intern Med 1987, 106:396.

Creagh-Kirk T, et al: Survival experience among patients with AIDS receiving zidovudine. JAMA 1988, 260:3009.

Curren JW: The epidemiology and prevention of the acquired immunodeficiency syndrome. Ann Intern Med 1985, 103:657.

Idem, et al: Epidemiology of HIV infection and AIDS in the United States. Science 1988, 239:610.

Dassey DE: AIDS and testing for AIDS. JAMA 1986, 255:743.

Denning DW, et al: Oral and cutaneous features of acute human immunodeficiency virus infection. Cutis 1987, 40:171.

DesJarlais DC, et al: HIV-I infection among intravenous drug users in Manhattan, New York City, from 1977 through 1987. JAMA 1989, 261:1008.

Dominey A, et al: Papulonodular demodicidosis associated with acquired immunodeficiency syndrome. JAAD 1989, 20:197.

Dreno B, et al: Prognostic value of Langerhans cells in the epidermis of HIV patients. Br J Dermatol 1988, 118:481.

Duncan WC: Failure of erythromycin to cure secondary syphilis in a patient infected with HIV. Arch Dermatol 1989, 125:82.

Duvic M: Staphylococcal infections and the pruritus of AIDS-related complex. Arch Dermatol 1987, 123:1599.

Idem, et al: AIDS-associated psoriasis and Reiter's syndrome. Arch Dermatol 1987, 123:1622.

Ellis M, et al: Impaired neutrophil function in patients with AIDS and AIDS-related complex. J Infect Dis 1988, 158:1268.

Fauci AS: HIV. Science 1988, 239:617.

FDA Drug Bulletin: Progress on AIDS. JAAD 1986, 14:293.

Ficarra G, et al: Kaposi's sarcoma of the oral cavity. Oral Surg 1988, 66:543.

Idem: Oral hairy leukoplakia among HIV-positive intravenous drug abusers. Oral Surg 1988, 65:421.

Fischl MA, et al: Efficacy of azidothymidine in treatment of AIDS and AIDS-related complex. N Engl J Med 1987, 317:385.

Fischer BK, et al: Cutaneous manifestations of AIDS. Int J Dermatol 1987, 26:615.

Francis DP, et al: The natural history of infection with the lymphadenopathy-associated virus human T-lymphotropic virus type III. Ann Intern Med 1985, 103:719.

Freed JA, et al: Cutaneous mycobacteriosis. Arch Dermatol 1987, 123:1601.

Friedland GH, et al: Transmission of HIV. N Engl J Med 1987, 317:1125.

Friedman-Kien A, et al: Herpes zoster. JAAD 1986, 14:1023.

Fujikawa LS, et al: Isolation of HTL virus type III from tears . . . Lancet 1985, 2:529.

Furth PA, et al: Nail pigmentation changes associated with AZT. Ann Intern Med 1987, 107:350.

Gallo RC, et al: Frequent detection and isolation of cytopathic retroviruses (HTLV-III) from patients with AIDS and at risk for AIDS. Science 1984, 224:500.

Ghadially R, et al: Granuloma annulare in patients with HIV infections. JAAD 1989, 20:232.

Gibson IH, et al: Disseminated ecthymatous herpes varicella-zoster virus infection in patients with AIDS. JAAD 1989, 20:637.

Gill PS, et al: Azidothymidine associated with bone marrow failure in . . . AIDS. Ann Intern Med 1987, 107:502.

Glatt AE, et al: Treatment of infections associated with HIV. N Engl J Med 1988, 318:1439.

Goodman DS, et al: Prevalence of cutaneous disease in patients with AIDS or ARC. JAAD 1987, 17:210.

Gottlieb MS, et al: *Pneumocystis carinii* pneumonia and mucosal candidiasis in previously healthy homosexual man. N Engl J Med 1981, 305:1425.

Greenspan D, et al: Oral "hairy" leukoplakia in male homosexuals: evidence of association with both papillomavirus and a herpes group virus. Lancet 1985, 2:831.

Gretzula J, et al: Complex viral and fungal skin lesions of patients with AIDS. JAAD 1988, 16:1151.

Hicks CB, et al: Seronegative secondary syphilis in a patient . . . [with AIDS]: Ann Intern Med 1987, 107:492.

Hira SK, et al: Cutaneous manifestations of HIV in Luska, Zambia. JAAD 1988, 19:451.

Hirsch MS: The rocky road to effective treatment of HIV infection. Ann Intern Med 1989, 110:1.

Idem: Prospects of therapy for infections with human T-lymphotropic virus type III. Ann Intern Med 1985, 103:750.

HIV infection in the United States. MMWR 1987, 36(Suppl):1.

Ho DD, et al: Primary human T-lymphotropic virus type III infection. Ann Intern Med 1985, 103:880.

Idem: Pathogenesis of infection with HIV. N Engl J Med 1987, 317:278.

Hoff R, et al: Seroprevalence of HIV among childbearing women. N Engl J Med 1988, 318:525.

Hoxie JA: Current concepts in the virology of infection with HIV: a view from the III International Conference on AIDS. Ann Intern Med 1987, 107:406.

Jacobson MA, et al: Serious CMV disease in AIDS. Ann Intern Med 1988, 108:585.

Jaffe HW, et al: Persistent infection with human T-lymphotropic virus type III in apparently healthy homosexual men. Ann Intern Med 1985, 102:628.

James WD, et al: A papular eruption associated with T-cell lymphotropic virus type III disease. JAAD 1985, 13:563.

Janier M, et al: Chronic varicella zoster infection in AIDS. JAAD 1988, 18:584.

Jason JM, et al: HTLV-III/LAV antibody and immune status of household contacts and sexual partners of persons with hemophilia. JAMA 1986, 255:212.

Idem: Risk of developing AIDS in HIV-infected cohorts of hemophilic and homosexual men. JAMA 1989, 261:725.

Johns DR, et al: Alterations in the natural history of neurosyphilis by concurrent infection with the human immunodeficiency virus. N Engl J Med 1987, 316:1569.

Kalish RS, et al: The T4 lymphocyte in AIDS (editorial). N Engl J Med 1985, 313:112.

Kaplan JE, et al: A six-year follow-up of HIV-infected homosexual men with lymphadenopathy. JAMA 1988, 260:2694.

Kaplan LD, et al: Treatment of patients with AIDS and associated manifestations. JAMA 1987, 257:1367.

Idem: AIDS associated non-Hodgkin's lymphoma in San Francisco. JAMA 1989, 261:719.

Idem: Treatment of patients with AIDS and associated manifestations. JAMA 1987, 257:1367.

Kaplan MH, et al: Dermatologic findings and manifestations of AIDS. JAAD 1987, 16:485.

Idem: Antipsoriatic effects of zidovudine in HIV-associated psoriasis. JAAD 1989, 20:76.

Kaslow RA, et al: Infection with HIV: clinical manifestations and their relationship to immune deficiency. Ann Intern Med 1987, 107:474.

Kinchelow T, et al: Changes in the hair in black patients with AIDS. J Infect Dis 1988, 157:394.

Knobler EH, et al: Unique vascular skin lesions associated with HIV. JAMA 1988, 260:524.

Koehler JE, et al: Cutaneous vascular lesions and disseminated cat-scratch disease in patients with AIDS and AIDS-related complex. Ann Intern Med 1988, 109:449.

Koop CE: Physician leadership in preventing AIDS. JAMA 1987, 258:2111.

Kreiss JK, et al: Antibody to HTLV-III in wives of hemophiliacs. Ann Intern Med 1985, 102:623.

Landesman SH, et al: The AIDS epidemic. N Engl J Med 1985, 312:521.

Leaf AN, et al: Thrombotic thrombocytopenic purpura associated with HIV-I infection. Ann Intern Med 1988, 109:194.

LeBoit PE, et al: Epithelioid hemangioma-like vascular proliferation in AIDS. Lancet 1988, 1:960.

Levine AM, et al: Retrovirus and malignant lymphoma in homosexual men. JAMA 1985, 254:1921.

Lupton GP, et al: Oral "hairy" leukoplakia. Arch Dermatol (in press).

Mann JM, et al: AIDS: A global perspective. N Engl J Med 1988, 319:302.

Marcus R, et al: Surveillance of health care workers exposed to blood from patients infected with HIV. N Engl J Med 1988, 319:1118.

Marion RW, et al: Fetal AIDS syndrome score. AJDC 1987, 141:429.

Idem: HTLV-III embryopathy. AJDC 1986, 140:638.

Marx JL: The AIDS virus—well known but a mystery. Science 1987, 236:390.

Matis WL, et al: Dermatologic findings associated with HIV infection. JAAD 1987, 17:746.

Melbye M, et al: Long-term seropositivity for HTLV-III in homosexual men without AIDS. Ann Intern Med 1986, 104:496.

Milbum PB, et al: Disseminated warts and evolving squamous cell carcinomas in a patient with AIDS. JAAD 1988, 19:401.

Mintzer DM, et al: Treatment of Kaposi's sarcoma and thrombocytopenia with vincristine in patients with the acquired immunodeficiency syndrome. Ann Intern Med 1985, 102:200.

Morbidity and Mortality Weekly Report: Revision of the case definition of acquired immunodeficiency syndrome for national reporting. 1985, 34:373.

Murphy PM, et al: Impairment of neutrophil bactericidal capacity in patients with AIDS. J Infect Dis 1988, 158:627.

Needlestick transmission of HTLV-III from a patient infected in Africa (editorial). Lancet 1984, 2:1376.

Norman C: AIDS trends: projections from limited data. Science 1985, 230:1018.

Nzilambi N, et al: Prevalence of infection with HIV over a 10-year period in rural Zaire. N Engl J Med 1988, 318:276.

Pahwa S, et al: Continuous varicella-zoster infection associated with acyclovir resistance in a child with AIDS. JAMA 1988, 260:2879.

Patterson JW, et al: Cutaneous botryomycosis in a patient with AIDS. JAAD 1987, 16:238.

Pearson RD, et al: Pentamidine for the treatment of *Pneumocystis carinii* pneumonia and other protozoal diseases. Ann Intern Med 1985, 103:782.

Penneys NS, et al: Unusual cutaneous lesions associated with acquired immunodeficiency syndrome. JAAD 1985, 13:845.

Peterman TA, et al: Sexual transmission of human immunodeficiency virus. JAMA 1986, 256:2222.

Idem: Risk of HIV transmission from heterosexual adults with transfusion-associated infections. JAMA 1988, 259:55.

Phelan JA, et al: Oral findings in patients with [AIDS]. Oral Surg Oral Med Oral Pathol 1987, 64:50.

Piot P, et al: AIDS: An international perspective. Science 1988, 239:573.

Pyun KH, et al: Perinatal infection with HIV. N Engl J Med 1987, 317:611.

Quinn TC: Perspectives on the future of AIDS (editorial). JAMA 1985, 253:247.

Idem, et al: HIV infection among patients attending clinics for sexually transmitted diseases. N Engl J Med 1988, 318:197.

Quinnan GV, et al: Herpesvirus infection in the acquired immune deficiency syndrome. JAMA 1984, 252:72.

Radolf JD, et al: Unusual manifestations of secondary syphilis and abnormal humoral immune response to *Treponema pallidum* antigens in a homosexual man with asymptomatic HIV infection. JAAD 1988, 18:423.

Rampen FJH: AIDS and the dermatologist. Int J Dermatol 1987, 26:1.

Ratner L, et al: HIV-associated autoimmune thrombocytopenic purpura. Am J Med 1989, 86:194.

Raviglione MC, et al: Fatal toxic epidermal necrolysis during prophylaxis with pyrimethamine and sulfadoxine in an HIV-infected person. Arch Intern Med 1988, 148:2683.

Real FX, et al: Spontaneous remission of Kaposi's sarcoma in patients with AIDS. N Engl J Med 1985, 313:1659.

Redfield RR, et al: Frequent transmission of HTLV-III among spouses of patients with AIDS-related complex and AIDS. JAMA 1985, 253:1571.

Idem: Severe molluscum contagiosum infection in a patient with T-cell lymphotropic (HTLV-III) disease. JAAD 1985, 13:821.

Idem: Disseminated vaccinia in a military recruit with HTLV-III disease. N Engl J Med 1981, 316:673.

Idem: Heterosexually acquired HTLV-III disease. JAMA 1985, 254:2094.

Idem: The Walter Reed staging classification for HTLV-III/LAV infection. N Engl J Med 1986, 314:131.

Resnick L, et al: Regression of oral hairy leukoplakia after orally administered acyclovir. JAMA 1988, 259:384.

Richman DD, et al: Toxicity of azidothymidine . . . N Engl J Med 1987, 317:192.

Idem: The toxicity of AZT in the treatment of patients with AIDS and AIDS-related complex. N Engl J Med 1982, 317:192.

Rico MJ, et al: Interface dermatitis in patients with AIDS. JAAD 1987, 16:1209.

Robert-Guroff M, et al: Prevalence of antibodies to HTLV-I, -II, and -III in intravenous drug abusers from an AIDS endemic region. JAMA 1986, 255:3133.

Rogers MF: AIDS in children. Pediatr Infect Dis 1985, 4:230.

Safai B, et al: The natural history of Kaposi's sarcoma in the acquired immunodeficiency syndrome. Ann Intern Med 1985, 103:744.

Seale J: AIDS virus infection: prognosis and transmission (editorial). J R Soc Med 1985, 78:613.

Simonsen JN, et al: HIV infection among men with sexually transmitted disease. N Engl J Med 1988, 319:274.

Soeprono FF, et al: Seborrheic-like dermatitis of acquired immunodeficiency syndrome. JAAD 1986, 14:242.

Soto-Aguilar MC, et al: Human retroviruses and AIDS. J Allergy Clin Immunol 1988, 81:619.

Stamm WE, et al: The association between genital ulcer disease and acquisition of HIV infection in homosexual men. JAMA 1988, 260:1429.

Steele DR: HTLV-III antibodies in human immune gamma globulin (letter). JAMA 1986, 255:609.

Straka BF, et al: Cutaneous manifestations of AIDS in children. JAAD 1988, 18:1089.

Streicher HZ, et al: HTLV-III/LAV and the monocyte/macrophage. JAMA 1986, 256:2390.

Stricof RL: HTLV-III/LAV seroconversion following a deep intramuscular needlestick injury. N Engl J Med 1986, 314:1115.

Surbone A, et al: Treatment of AIDS and AIDS-related complex with a regimen of AZT and acyclovir. Ann Intern Med 1988, 108:534.

Tindall B, et al: Malignant melanoma associated with HIV infection in three homosexual males. JAAD 1989, 20:587.

Tschachler E, et al: Epidermal Langerhans cells—a target for HTLV/LAV infection. J Invest Dermatol 1987, 88:233.

Ward JW, et al: Transmission of HIV by blood transfusions screened as negative for HIV antibody. N Engl J Med 1988, 318:473.

Warner LC, et al: Cutaneous manifestations of the acquired immunodeficiency syndrome. Int J Dermatol 1986, 25:337.

Weiss SH, et al: HTLV-III infection among health care workers: association with needle-stick injuries. JAMA 1985, 254:2089.

Idem: Screening test for HTLV-III (AIDS agent) antibodies: specificity, sensitivity, and applications. JAMA 1985, 253:221.

Winshester R, et al: The co-occurrence of Reiter's syndrome and acquired immunodeficiency. Ann Intern Med 1987, 106:19.

HUMAN IMMUNODEFICIENCY VIRUS TYPE 2 (HIV-2)

This virus was previously reported as HTLV-IV and STLV-III.

Two West African patients with AIDS were reported in 1986, from whom a related retrovirus, which has been designated HIV-2, was isolated by Clavel et al. In 1987 they reported the isolation of HIV-2 from 30 patients, almost all from West Africa, 17 of whom had AIDS and 7 of whom had died of it at the time of their report. Others had either ARC or no symptoms. HIV-2 was identified in 11 patients by nucleic acid hybridization of retroviral isolates. No HIV-1 was found.

They concluded that some cases of AIDS in West Africa may be caused by HIV-2, but the extent of spread of this virus and its clinical correlates awaits epidemiologic investigations. The nucleotide sequence of HIV-2 was studied by Guyader et al, who found it was distinct from that of HIV-1.

Clavel F, et al: Human immunodeficiency virus Type 2 infection associated with AIDS in West Africa. N Engl J Med 1987, 316:1180.

Guyader M, et al: Genome organization and transactivation of the human immunodeficiency virus type 2. Nature 1987, 326:662.

20

Parasitic Infestations, Stings, and Bites

The major groups or phyla of animal parasites affecting man are the Protozoa, Coelenterata, Nemathelminthes, Platyhelminthes, Annelida, Arthropoda, and Chordata.

Alexander J O'D: Arthropods and Human Skin. Berlin, Springer Verlag, 1984.

Drugs for parasitic infections. The Medical Letter 1986, 28:10.

Fisher AA: Atlas of Aquatic Dermatology. New York, Grune and Stratton, 1978.

Harves AD, et al: Current concepts of therapy and pathophysiology of arthropod bites and stings. Part I Arthropods. Int J Dermatol 1975, 14:543. Part II Insects. Ibid, 1975, 14:621.

Mandell GL, et al (eds): Principles and Practice of Infectious Diseases. New York, John Wiley and Sons, 1985.

Parrish HM: Analysis of 460 fatalities from venomous animals in the United States. Am J Med Sci 1963, 245:129.

Wong RC, et al: Spider bites. Arch Dermatol 1987, 123:98.

1985 STD treatment guidelines. JAAD 1986, 14:707.

PHYLUM PROTOZOA

The protozoa are one-celled organisms, divided into classes according to the nature of their locomotion. Class Sarcodina organisms move by temporary projections of cytoplasm—pseudopods; class Mastigophora by means of one or more flagella; class Ciliata by short hairlike projections of cytoplasm (cilia); and class Sporozoa by no special organs of locomotion.

CLASS SARCODINA

The ameba is the best known in this class. Of medical significance is *Entamoeba histolytica*.

Amebiasis Cutis

CLINICAL FEATURES. Most lesions begin as deep abscesses which rupture and form ulcerations with distinct, raised, cordlike edges and an erythematous halo some 2 cm wide. The base is covered with necrotic tissue and hemopurulent, glairy pus

containing amebae. These lesions are from a few to 20 cm wide. They may occur on the trunk, abdomen, external genitalia, buttocks, or perineum. Those on the abdomen may result from hepatic abscesses. All ages are at risk.

Intestinal amebiasis with bloody diarrhea and hepatic abscesses may be present. Penile lesions are probably sexually acquired. The sole manifestation of early amebiasis may be chronic urticaria.

ETIOLOGY. The causative organism, the trophozoite of *E. histolytica*, may be found in the base of the lesion by direct smear or on shave biopsy.

EPIDEMIOLOGY. Worldwide, an estimated 10 per cent of the population is infected with *E. histolytica*, and an estimated 10 million invasive cases occur annually, most of them in the tropics. In the U.S., the disease occurs chiefly in institutionalized patients, world travellers, recent immigrants, migrant workers, and male homosexuals. As many as 30 per cent of male homosexuals in New York are believed to be infected.

HISTOPATHOLOGY. The histologic findings are those of a necrotic ulceration with many lymphocytes, neutrophils, plasma cells, and eosinophils. *E. histolytica* is found in the tissue, within blood and lymph vessels. The organism measures 50 μ to 60 μ in diameter and has a basophilic cytoplasm in a hematoxylin and eosin stain. It has a single eccentric nucleus with a central karyosome.

LABORATORY FINDINGS. The organism is frequently demonstrable in fresh material from the base of the ulcer. Culture of the protozoa confirms the diagnosis. The indirect hemagglutination test remains elevated for years after the invasive disease, whereas the gel diffusion precipitation test and counter-immunoelectrophoresis become negative at six months and can test for recurrent or active disease in persons coming from endemic areas.

DIFFERENTIAL DIAGNOSIS. When the perianal or perineal areas are involved, granuloma inguinale, lymphogranuloma venereum, deep mycosis, and syphilis must be considered. In chronic urticaria, fresh stool examinations by a trained technician are necessary.

TREATMENT. The treatment of choice is a combination of a specific drug with a luminal amebicide. Metronidazole (Flagyl), 750 mg orally three times a day for five to 10 days, plus iodoquinol (diiodohydroxyquin, Yodoxin), 650 mg orally three times a day for 20 days, is recommended. Abscesses may require surgical drainage, but there is no need for resection of lesions.

El Zawahry M, et al: Amebiasis cutis. Int J Dermatol 1973, 12:305.

Fujita WH, et al: Cutaneous amebiasis. Arch Dermatol 1981, 117:309.

Gullett J, et al: Disseminated granulomatous acanthamoeba infection presenting as an unusual skin lesion. Am J Med 1979, 67:891.

Kean BH, et al: Epidemic of amebiasis and giardiasis in a biased population. Br J Vener Dis 1979, 55:375.

Lin C, et al: Invasive amebiasis in New York City. NY State J Med 1976, 76:574.

Martinez AJ: Acanthamoebiasis and immunosuppression. J Neuropath Exp Neurol 1982, 41:548.

Rimsza ME, et al: Cutaneous amebiasis. Pediatrics 1983, 71:595.

CLASS MASTIGOPHORA

The organisms belonging to this class are known as flagellates. Many have an undulating membrane with flagella along their crest.

Trichomoniasis

Symptoms: Trichomonas vulvovaginitis is a common cause of vaginal pruritus, with burning and a frothy leukorrhea. The vaginal mucosa appears bright red from inflammation and may be mottled with pseudomembranous patches. The male urethra may also harbor the organism; in the male it causes urethritis and prostatitis. Occasionally men may develop balanoposthitis; Michalowski recently reported 16 cases of this, with erosive lesions on the glans and foreskin predominating. Neonates may acquire the infection during passage through the birth canal, but require treatment only if symptomatic or if colonization lasts over four weeks. As this is otherwise nearly exclusively a sexually transmitted disorder, trichomonas vulvovaginitis in a child should make one suspect sexual abuse.

ETIOLOGY. Trichomoniasis is caused by *Trichomonas vaginalis*, a colorless pyriform flagellate 5 to 15 μ long.

DIAGNOSIS. *T. vaginalis* is demonstrated in smears from affected areas. Newer testing by direct immunofluorescence is sensitive and specific.

TREATMENT. Metronidazole 2.0 gm by mouth in a single dose is the treatment of choice. Alternatively 250 mg may be given three times daily for seven days. Male sex partners should be treated also. Metronidazole is contraindicated in pregnancy, and clotrimazole intravaginally may be used in these cases.

Czonka GW: Trichomoniasis and the dermatologist. Br J Dermatol 1974, 90:713.

Krieger JW, et al: Diagnosis of trichomoniasis. JAMA 1988, 259:1223.

Michalowski R: Trichomonal balanoposthitis. Ann Dermatol Venereol (Paris) 1981, 108:73.

Leishmaniasis

Cutaneous leishmaniasis, American mucocutaneous leishmaniasis, and visceral leishmaniasis (kala-

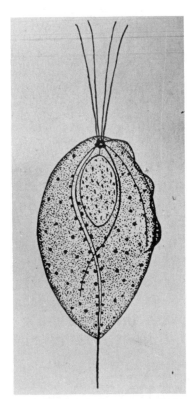

Figure 20–1. Trichomonas vaginalis.

azar), which includes infantile leishmaniasis and post-kala-azar dermal leishmanoid, are all caused by morphologically and culturally indistinguishable protozoa of the family Trypanosomidae, called *Leishmania* (pronounced "Leeshmaynea"). However, the clinical features of these diseases differ and they have, in general, different geographical distributions. These differences are due in large part to the variable cell-mediated immune response of the patient. The development of monoclonal antibodies that discriminate among organisms may lead to a clearer taxonomy, but this is in a state of flux.

CUTANEOUS LEISHMANIASIS

Synonyms: Old World leishmaniasis, Baghdad boil, Oriental sore, leishmaniasis tropica, Biskra button, Delhi boil, Aleppo boil, Kandahar sore, Lahore sore. Other subtypes of New World infection with purely cutaneous involvement are *uta, pian bois,* and bay sore or chiclero ulcer.

CLINICAL FEATURES. There are several types of lesions. One distinct type is the *moist* or *rural* type, a slowly growing, indurated, livid, indolent papule, which enlarges in a few months to form a nodule that may ulcerate in a few weeks to form an ulcer as much as 5 cm in diameter. Spontaneous healing usually takes place within six months, leaving a characteristic scar. This type is contracted from rodent reservoirs such as gerbils.

Another type, the *dry* or *urban* type, develops much more slowly and heals more slowly than the rural type; latent periods may be one to two years before the lesion becomes overt.

New World disease may also induce purely cutaneous lesions, of varied morphology. The primary papule may become nodular, verrucous, furuncular, or ulcerated, with an infiltrated red border. Subcutaneous peripheral nodules (which eventually ulcerate) may signal extension of the disease. Lymphadenopathy may occur, and the nodes may rarely yield organisms, as documented by Berger et al.

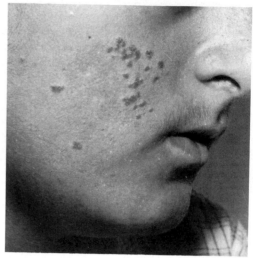

Figure 20–3. Leishmaniasis recidivans. (Courtesy of Dr. S. Ganos, Jerusalem).

Rarely, after the initial or mother lesion is healed, there may appear at the borders of the healed area a few soft red papules covered with whitish scales and having the apple-jelly characteristics of lupus vulgaris. These spread peripherally on a common erythematous base, and are the *lupoid* type. This is also known as leishmaniasis recidivans and occurs with the urban type of disease, caused by *L. tropica minor.*

Chiclero Ulcer. In Yucatán and Guatemala another form exists. The most frequent site of ulceration is the ear. This *chiclero ulcer* occurs most frequently in the workers who harvest chicle for chewing gum in the forests, where there is high humidity. The etiologic agent is *Leishmania mexicana* and the vector, a sandfly, *Lutzomyia flaviscutellata.*

Uta. This is a term used by Peruvians for leishmaniasis occurring in mountainous territory at elevations of 1200 to 1800 meters above sea level. The ulcerating lesions are found upon exposed sites, and mucosal lesions do not occur. The etiologic agent is *L. peruviana.*

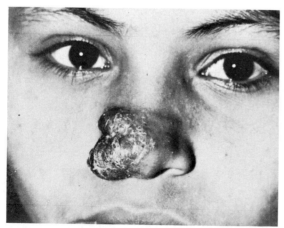

Figure 20–2. Baghdad boil of 5 months' duration. (Courtesy of Dr. G. F. Rahim, Baghdad.)

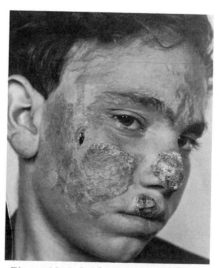

Figure 20–4. Leishmaniasis recidivans.

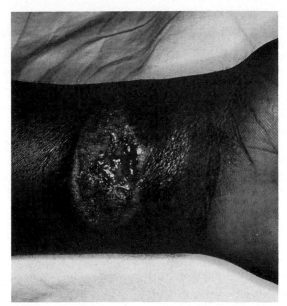

Figure 20–5. Leishmania ulcer of the wrist, acquired in Panama by an American soldier.

Disseminated Cutaneous Leishmaniasis. Convit and his associates described this type in 1957 as disseminated anergic cutaneous leishmaniasis. Multiple nonulcerated papules and plaques, chiefly on exposed surfaces, characterize this type. It is caused by several subspecies of *L. mexicana. L. aethiopica* may cause this type of disease in Ethiopia and Kenya.

The disease begins with a single ulcer, nodule, or plaque from which satellite lesions may develop and disseminate to cover the entire body. The disease is progressive and treatment is usually ineffective.

It is characterized by anergy to the cutaneous test. The Montenegro reaction is negative.

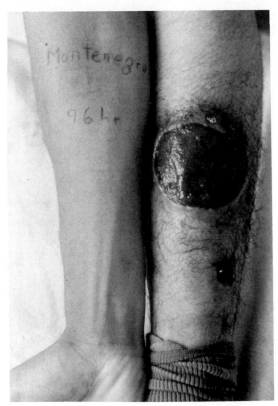

Figure 20–7. Montenegro test in leishmaniasis. (Courtesy of Dr. Axel W. Hoke.)

This type of leishmaniasis must be differentiated from lepromatous leprosy, xanthoma tuberosum, paracoccidioidal granuloma, Lobo's disease, and malignant lymphoma.

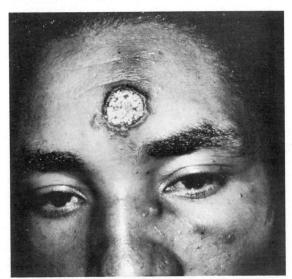

Figure 20–6. Primary inoculation chancre or sporotrichoid form of leishmaniasis. While hunting in the mountains this man was bitten on the forehead. Notice the lymphangitic nodules spreading to the cheek. (Courtesy of Drs. W. F. Schorr and F. Kerdel-Vegas.)

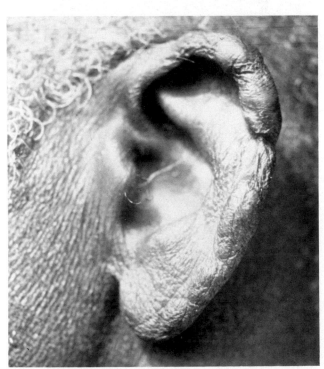

Figure 20–8. Chiclero ulcer in leishmaniasis. (Courtesy of Dr. Axel W. Hoke.)

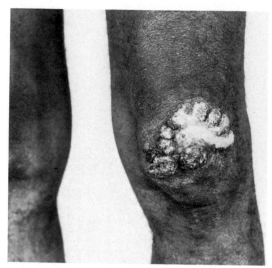

Figure 20–9. Verrucous leishmaniasis on the knee. (Courtesy of Dr. J. Convit.)

EPIDEMIOLOGY. It is endemic in Asia Minor and to a lesser extent in many countries around the Mediterranean Sea. Iran and Saudi Arabia have a high occurrence rate. Purely cutaneous lesions are also found in Central and South America. Nelson et al have documented five cases of cutaneous leishmaniasis who acquired their disease in Texas. Subspecies of *L. brasiliensis* such as *L.b.peruviana* (in Peru) and *L.b.garnhami* (in Venezuela) are associated only with cutaneous disease.

Children are affected most often, since immunity is acquired from the initial infection. Deliberate in-oculation on the thigh is sometimes practiced so that scarring on the face—a frequent site for Oriental sore—may be avoided.

ETIOLOGY. Oriental sore is caused by *Leishmania tropica*, a round or oval parasite 2 to 3 microns wide. It can be demonstrated with Wright's or Giemsa stain in smears from the base of the ulcer, in monocytes, leukocytes, and endothelial cells. Purely cutaneous leishmaniasis is transmitted by several species present in the New World. *L. mexicana* does not induce mucosal disease. *L. brasiliensis guyanensis* and *L. peruviana* cause self-healing lesions called *pian bois* and *uta* respectively, which do not involve the nasopharynx.

PATHOGENESIS. The organism has an alternate life in a vertebrate and an insect host. Man and other mammals, dogs, or rodents, are the natural reservoir hosts. The vector hosts are burrow sandflies, *Phlebotomus caucasicus* and anthropophagous sandflies, *P. papatasii*, and *P. sergenti* in the Old World type, and *Lutzonyia* sandflies for the *L. mexicana* cutaneous leishmaniasis. After the insect has fed on blood, the flagellates (leptomonad, promastigote) develop in the gut over a period of eight to 20 days, after which migration occurs into the mouth parts; from here transmission is made into man by the bite. In man the flagella are lost and a leishmania (amastigote) form is assumed. Rupture of the cells frees the parasites for the invasion of the host's tissues.

HISTOPATHOLOGY. Cutaneous leishmaniasis shows the typical features of an ulcer, with a heavy infiltrate of histiocytes, lymphocytes, and polymorphonuclear leukocytes. Numerous organisms are

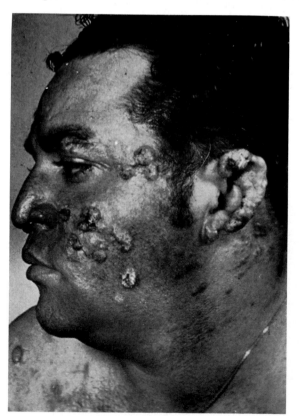

Figure 20–10. Disseminated cutaneous leishmaniasis with nasal lesions, verrucous nodules, and mutilating ulcerations of the ear (chiclero ulcer). (Courtesy of Dr. J. Convit, Venezuela.)

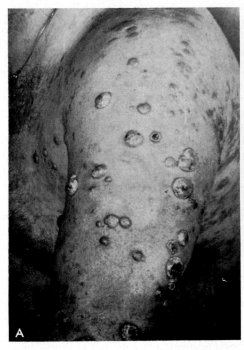
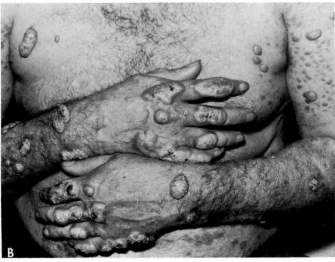

Figure 20–11. A, *Disseminated cutaneous leishmaniasis showing large nodules with one on deltoid area undergoing ulceration. (Courtesy of Dr. J. Convit, Venezuela.)* B, *Disseminated leishmaniasis. (Courtesy of Dr. F. Kerdel-Vegas.)*

present (mostly in histiocytes) which are noncapsulated and contain a nucleus and a paranucleus. The parasitized histiocytes form tuberculoid granulomas in the dermis. Pseudoepitheliomatous hyperplasia may occur in the edges of the ulcer. The leishmania are best seen when Giemsa stain is used.

DIAGNOSIS. In endemic areas the diagnosis is not too difficult. In other localities cutaneous leishmaniasis may be confused with syphilis, yaws, lupus vulgaris, and pyogenic granulomas. The diagnosis is established by the demonstration of the organism in smears.

A hypodermic needle is inserted into the normal skin and to the edge of the ulcer base. The needle is rotated to work loose some material and serum, which is then aspirated. A culture on Nicolle-Novy-MacNeal (NNN) medium at 22 to 35° C is recommended to demonstrate the leptomonads. Hamsters are very susceptible to leishmaniasis, dying three to six months after the intraperitoneal inoculation of infective material.

The leishmanin intradermal test (Leishman-Montenegro-Donovan) is helpful in the diagnosis. It becomes positive some three months after infection.

Newer sophisticated tests now being used to diagnose and classify subspecies are DNA buoyancy, isoenzyme electrophoresis, and radiorespirometry.

TREATMENT. Sodium antimony gluconate (sodium stibogluconate) solution is given intramuscularly or intravenously daily for 10 days. At the Walter Reed Institute of Research a dose of 20 mg/kg/day has been found effective and well tolerated. Ballou et al reviewed this experience. Chulay et al reported success with this high dose of stibogluconate twice daily for 30 days in patients with L. *aethiopica* infection. It is effective in about half the cases. It can be obtained from the CDC Drug Service, Atlanta, GA

30333; telephone (404) 329-3670. Repeated courses may be given. Antimony n-methyl glutamine (Glucantime) is used more often in Central America because of local availability.

El-On et al reviewed treatment of 67 patients in Israel with an ointment containing 15 per cent paranomycin and 12 per cent methyl benzethonium chloride and reported a good response in 67 per cent.

Dapsone, 2 mg/kg/day for 21 days, cured 40 of 50 patients treated by Dogra et al. No controls improved.

Rifampin, 600 mg daily for 21 days, cures about half the cases in which it is used. In combination with antimony, it cured 77 per cent, according to Pareek.

Levamisole, 50 mg t.i.d. on two successive days each week for eight weeks, cured 27 cases treated by Patrick Butler in Saudi Arabia.

Ketoconazole may be very effective, according to Urcuyo and Zaias, who reported on its use in 1982. Bernard Gordon cured three cases in 1986 with 400 mg a day for three months. There were no side effects.

Cryotherapy with solid carbon dioxide or liquid nitrogen is effective, as reported by Leibovici et al. It may cause permanent depigmentation, however. Junaid reported success with infrared heat.

Convit et al reported in 1987 a 94 per cent cure rate in 52 cases of localized leishmaniasis from the administration of two or three intradermal injections over 32 weeks of a vaccine prepared from BCG mixed with cultured promastigotes from a strain of L. *mexicana*. Forty-two controls were treated with intramuscular meglumine antimonate, with a comparable cure rate but many side effects. Cohen reported 100 per cent success with intralesional injections of emetine hydrochloride into 50 lesions.

Spontaneous healing occurs, usually within 12 to 18 months. Chong discusses the rationale of treating an ordinarily self-limited infection. Reasons include avoidance of disfiguring scars in exposed areas, notably the face; avoidance of secondary infection; control of disease in the population; and failure of spontaneous healing: in the diffuse cutaneous and recidivans types the disease may persist for 20 to 40 years if not treated.

Control depends chiefly upon the success of antifly measures taken by health authorities.

MUCOCUTANEOUS LEISHMANIASIS

Synonyms: Leishmaniasis americana, espundia.

CLINICAL FEATURES. The initial lesion, which occurs at the site of the fly bite, may be a destructive ulcer; but in equatorial areas, secondary lesions usually occur at some time during the next five years.

The earliest mucosal lesion is usually hyperemia of the nasal septum with subsequent ulceration, which progresses to invade the septum and later the paranasal fossae. Perforation of the septum eventually takes place. For some time the nose remains unchanged externally in spite of the internal destruction.

At first only a dry crust is observed, or a bright red infiltration or vegetation on the nasal septum, with symptoms of obstruction and small hemorrhages. In spite of the mutilating and destructive character of leishmaniasis, it never involves the nasal bones. When the septum is destroyed, the nasal

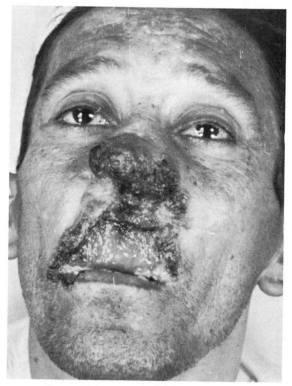

Figure 20–12. Leishmaniasis americana (mucocutaneous). (Courtesy of Dr. J. Convit.)

bridge and tip of the nose collapse, giving an appearance of a *parrot beak* or *camel nose* or *tapir nose*. It is important to recall that the four great chronic infections (syphilis, tuberculosis, leprosy, and leishmaniasis) have a predilection for the nose. The ulcer may extend to the lips and continue to advance to the pharynx, attacking the soft palate, the uvula, the tonsils, the gingiva, and the tongue. The eventual mutilation is called *espundia*.

Escomel described in Peru the so-called *palate cross* of espundia, composed of two perpendicular grooves at the union of the osseous palate and the soft tissues, in the midst of the vegetative infiltration of the entire pharynx.

Only in exceptional cases does American leishmaniasis invade the genital or ocular mucous membranes.

The period between the first attack and the mucous complications varies between three and ten years.

The frequency of mucous membrane involvement is also variable. Whereas in Yucatán and Guatemala it is an exception, in other countries, such as Brazil, it may occur in 80 per cent of the cases.

ETIOLOGY. Mucocutaneous leishmaniasis is caused by *Leishmania brasiliensis*, subspecies *braziliensis* and *panamensis* discovered by Lindenberg in 1909 in Brazil. *L. brasiliensis* has two forms, the nonflagellated form or leishmania, which is found in the tissues of humans and in animals susceptible to the inoculation of the parasite, and the flagellated form or leptomonad, which is found in the digestive tract of the vector insect and in cultures. The typical morphology of leishmania, as found in the vertebrates, is round or oval, usually with one extremity more rounded than the other, measuring 2 to 4 μ by 1.5 to 2.5 μ, with cytoplasm, nucleus, and blepharoplast or kinetoplast.

The association of leishmaniasis in South and Central America with various species of the phlebotomine sandfly, Lutzomyia, is established. *Lutzomyia flaviscutellata, Lu. longipalpis, Lu. verrucarum, Lu. peruensis, Lu. trapidoi, Lu. umbratilis,* and *Lu. intermedia* are a few of the recorded sandfly hosts for leishmanial parasites in South and Central America. Mucocutaneous leishmaniasis is transmitted by *Lu. trapidoi* and *Lu. cruciata* (L.b.panamensis) and *Psychodopygus wellcomei* (L.b.braziliensis).

EPIDEMIOLOGY. Mucocutaneous leishmaniasis is predominantly a rural and jungle disease, endemic in all the tropical American countries. It predominates in damp and forested regions.

The disease can be contracted at any time of the year, but the risk is highest just after the rainy season. All ages and races and both sexes are equally affected.

The majority of cases of leishmaniasis americana have been described in Central and South America, from north latitude 21 degrees (Yucatán peninsula) to south latitude 30 degrees (the north of Argentina). There are many cases in vast regions of Peru, Brazil, and Venezuela.

HISTOPATHOLOGY. In cases of granulomatous infiltration, when intracellular parasites are found in histiocytes, leishmaniasis is one of several diseases to be considered, including rhinoscleroma, histoplasmosis, granuloma inguinale, and toxoplasmosis. The Leishman-Donovan body is noncapsulated and shows a characteristic nucleus and parabasal body. In Wright's-stained smears from the lesions, these L-D bodies can be readily discerned. In sections they are best seen with Giemsa stain.

In the ulcerous type, one can find marked irregular acanthosis and sometimes pseudoepitheliomatous hyperplasia. The dermis shows a dense infiltration of histiocytes, lymphocytes, and plasma cells. In new lesions some neutrophils are observed. Large Langhans giant cells are occasionally seen. Typical tubercles are sometimes observed.

LABORATORY FINDINGS. Leishmania is demonstrated in the cutaneous and mucous lesions and in the glands by direct smears or cultures.

In biopsy material stained with Wright's stain, one sees intracellular and extracellular organisms with typical morphology of two chromatic structures: nucleus and parabasal body. In later mucous lesions the scarcity of parasites makes the identification difficult. The culture is done on Nicolle-Novy-MacNeal medium for leptomonads. They are found in the condensed water of the medium.

The intradermal Montenegro test is performed with a leptomonad suspension of 0.1 to 0.2 ml injected intradermally. The reading is made 48 to 72 hours later. A positive reaction is an area of induration greater than 5 mm in diameter 24 to 48 hours after injection. This test is specific and sensitive, giving 95 per cent positive results, but it can be negative in early cases of the disease, in which, however, it is always easy to find the parasites. Cross reactions occur with certain forms of cutaneous tuberculosis, but they are rare.

Convit performed a number of indirect fluorescent antibody studies, with positive results when the Montenegro test was positive. This immunofluorescent technique is now widely employed and considered to be very reliable.

PROPHYLAXIS. Although it is difficult and impractical to eliminate the insect vector, it is still the only valid measure for the control of this prevalent disease.

TREATMENT. Treatment is the same as described above for cutaneous leishmaniasis except that antimony resistance is common in mucocutaneous disease and amphotericin B is often needed.

VISCERAL LEISHMANIASIS

Synonyms: Kala-azar, dum-dum fever.

CLINICAL FEATURES. The earliest lesion is the cutaneous nodule or leishmanioma, which occurs at the site of the initial sandfly inoculation.

Kala-azar, meaning "black fever," acquired its name because of the patchy macular darkening of the skin due to deposits of melanin that develop in the later course of the disease. These patches are most marked over the forehead and temples, periorally, and on the midabdomen.

Endogenously, the primary target for the parasites is the reticuloendothelial system; the spleen, liver, bone marrow, and lymph nodes are attacked. The incubation period is one to four months. An intermittent fever with temperatures ranging from 39 to 40° C ushers in the disease. There are hepatosplenomegaly, agranulocytosis, anemia, and thrombocytopenia. Chills, fever, emaciation, weight loss, weakness, epistaxis, and purpura develop as the disease progresses.

Susceptibility to secondary infection may produce pulmonary and gastrointestinal infection, ulcerations in the mouth (*cancrum oris*), and noma. Death occurs in about two years from onset in untreated individuals.

American Visceral Leishmaniasis. American visceral leishmaniasis is due to *L. donovani chagasi* and is transmitted by the sandfly *Lutzomyia longipalpis*. This disease is almost always fatal unless treated. American visceral leishmaniasis principally affects domestic dogs, although explosive outbreaks of the human infection occur sporadically, when the number of *Lu. longipalpis* builds up to a high level in the presence of infected dogs. The principal foci of visceral leishmaniasis are in the drier, poorly forested areas of Latin America.

ETIOLOGY. *Leishmania donovani* subspecies *donovani*, *infantum*, and *chagasi* cause visceral leishmaniasis and are parasites of rodents, canines, and man. They are nonflagellate oval organisms some 3 μ in diameter, known as *Leishman-Donovan* bodies. In the sandfly it is a leptomonad form with flagella.

EPIDEMIOLOGY. *L.d. donovani* causes visceral leishmaniasis in India, with the major reservoir being humans and the vector being *Phlebotomus argentipes*. *L.d. infantum* occurs in China, Africa, the Near and Middle East, and the Mediterranean littoral where the major reservoirs are dogs. *L.d. chagasi* occurs in South and Central America, is transmitted by *Lutzomyia longipalpis*, and the major reservoirs are dogs and foxes.

DIAGNOSIS. Leishman-Donovan bodies may be present in the blood in kala-azar of India. Specimens for examination, in descending order of utility, include spleen pulp, sternal marrow, liver tissue, and exudate from lymph nodes. Culture on NNN medium may also reveal the organisms. Complement fixation or immunofluorescence tests may be positive, and the intradermal Montenegro test is also reliable.

TREATMENT. General supportive measures are essential. Pentavalent antimony has long been the drug of choice. However, Hossain reported in 1988 that a combination of monomycine (Paramomycin) and methyluracil (Methacil) promptly cured all of 50 cases of acute cutaneous leishmaniasis. They were all treated for 10 days, and all received 7.5 million units of monomycine intramuscularly and 10 gm of methyluracil. All ulcers healed within one month. Treatment was well tolerated.

Post-Kala-Azar Dermal Leishmanoid. In kala-azar, the leishmanoid (amastigote) forms may be widely distributed throughout the apparently normal skin. During and after recovery from the disease, a special form of dermal leishmaniasis known as post-kala-azar dermal leishmanoid appears. This condition appears during or shortly after treatment in the African form, but it may be delayed up to 10 years after treatment in the Indian form. It is common in India, occurring in up to 20 per cent of patients, whereas in Africa only 2 per cent develop it. There are two constituents of the eruption: a macular, depigmented eruption found mainly on the face, arms, and upper part of the trunk; and a warty, papular eruption in which amastigotes can be found. Since it may persist for up to 20 years, such patients may act as a chronic reservoir of infection. This condition closely resembles leprosy.

Aram H, et al: Recurrent cutaneous leishmaniasis: successful treatment with sodium antimony gluconate. Cutis 1986, 36:177.

Ballou WR, et al: Safety and efficacy of high-dose sodium stibogluconate therapy of American cutaneous leishmaniasis. Lancet 1987, 2:13.

Berger TG, et al: Lymph node involvement in leishmaniasis. JAAD 1985, 12:993.

Idem: Leprosy and leishmaniasis. J Milit Dermatol Assoc 1984, 10:44.

Butler PG: Levamisole and immune response phenomena in cutaneous leishmaniasis. JAAD 1982, 6:1070.

Chong H: Oriental sore. Int J Dermatol 1986, 25:615.

Chulay J, et al: Leishmaniasis. In Spittell JA Jr. (ed.) Clinical Medicine, Philadelphia, Harper & Row, 1986.

Cohen HA, et al: Treatment of leishmaniasis nodosa with intralesionally injected emetine hydrochloride. JAAD 1987, 17:595.

Convit J, et al: Immunotherapy vs. chemotherapy in localized cutaneous leishmaniasis. Lancet 1987, 1:401.

Dogra J, et al: Dapsone in the treatment of cutaneous leishmaniasis. Int J Dermatol 1986, 25:398.

El-On J, et al: Topical treatment of cutaneous leishmaniasis. J Invest Dermatol 1986, 87:284.

Jollife DS: Cutaneous leishmaniasis from Belize—treatment with ketoconazole. Clin Exp Dermatol 1988, 11:62.

Junaid AJN: Treatment of cutaneous leishmaniasis with infrared heat. Int J Dermatol 1986, 25:470.

Kellum RE: Treatment of cutaneous leishmaniasis with an intralesional antimonial drug. JAAD 1986, 15:620.

Kibbi AG, et al: Sporotrichoid leishmaniasis in patients from Saudi Arabia. JAAD 1987, 17:759.

Kubba R, et al: Clinical diagnosis of cutaneous leishmaniasis. (Oriental sore). JAAD 1987, 16:1183.

Idem: Dissemination in cutaneous leishmaniasis. Int J Dermatol 1988, 27:702.

Lainson R, et al: Epidemiology and ecology of leishmaniasis in Latin America. Nature 1978, 273:595.

Leibovici V: Cryotherapy in acute cutaneous leishmaniasis. Int J Dermatol 1986, 25:473.

Lin C-S, et al: Cutaneous leishmaniasis. Int J Dermatol 1986, 25:51.

Livshin R, et al: Efficacy of rifampin and isoniazid in cutaneous leishmaniasis. Int J Dermatol 1987, 26:55.

Nelson DA, et al: Clinical aspects of cutaneous leishmaniasis acquired in Texas. JAAD 1985, 12:985.

Oster CN, et al: American cutaneous leishmaniasis. Am J Trop Med Hyg 1985, 34:856.

Pareek SS: Combination therapy of sodium stibogluconate and rifampin in cutaneous leishmaniasis. Int J Dermatol 1983, 22:70.

Saha SK: Dermal leishmaniasis after kalaazar infection: successful treatment with rifampin. Cutis 1985, 35:81.

Spier S, et al: Sporotrichoid leishmaniasis. Arch Dermatol 1978, 113:1104.

Strick RA, et al: Recurrent cutaneous leishmaniasis. JAAD 1983, 9:437.

Weinrauch L, et al: Cutaneous leishmaniasis: treatment with ketoconazole. Cutis 1983, 32:288.

Human Trypanosomiasis

Three species of trypanosomes are pathogenic to man: *Trypanosoma gambiense* and *T. rhodesiense* in Africa, and *T. cruzi* in America. The skin manifestations are usually observed in the earlier stages of the disease as evanescent erythema, erythema multiforme, and edema, especially angioedema.

In the early stage of African trypanosomiasis a trypanosome chancre may occur at the site of the tsetse fly bite. Then erythema with circumscribed swellings of angioedema, enlargement of lymph glands, fever, malaise, headache, and joint pains ensue. In the West African (Gambian) form, the illness is chronic, lasting several years, with progressive deterioration, whereas the East African (Rhodesian) form is an acute illness, with a stormy fatal course of weeks to months. The Rhodesian form is more often associated with cutaneous signs. Annular lesions and lesions resembling erythema nodosum are frequent manifestations. Lymphadenopathy is generalized, but frequently there is a pronounced enlargement of the posterior cervical group (Winterbottom's sign).

In American trypanosomiasis (Chagas' disease) similar changes take place in the skin. The reduviid bug ("kissing bug," "assassin bug") usually bites at night, frequently at mucocutaneous junctions, where the bug's infected feces are deposited when it feeds. The unsuspecting sleeping person rubs the feces into the bite and becomes infected. If the bite of the infected bug occurs near the eye, *Romaña's sign* de-

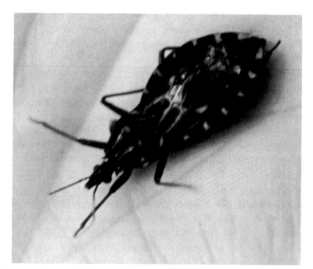

Figure 20–13. Chagas' disease; the reduviid or "assassin" bug. (Courtesy of Dr. Axel W. Hoke.)

velops. This consists of unilateral conjunctivitis and edema of the eyelids, with an ulceration or chagoma in the area. The bite of a "kissing bug" becomes markedly swollen and red whether trypanosomes are involved or not. In chronic Chagas' disease the heart (myocarditis, arrhythmias, thromboembolism, and cardiac failure) and the gastrointestinal system (megaesophagas and megacolon) are the most commonly involved organs.

Rhodesian trypanosomiasis is endemic among the cattle-raising tribes in East Africa, with the savannah habitat of the vectors determining its geographic distribution. Wild game and livestock are reservoir hosts in addition to man. The tsetse fly, *Glossina morsitans*, is the principal vector.

Gambian trypanosomiasis has man as the only vertebrate host and the palpalis group of tsetse flies as the invertebrate host. These flies are found close to the water, and their fastidious biologic requirements restrict their distribution, and thus that of the disease. Incidence is seasonal, with humidity and temperature being determinant factors. The highest incidence is in males 20 to 40 years of age in the tropical areas of West and Central Africa.

Chagas' disease is prevalent in Central and South America from the United States to Argentina and Chile, the highest incidence being in Venezuela, Brazil, Uruguay, Paraguay, and Argentina. Some 29 per cent of all male deaths in the 29 to 44 age group in Brazil are ascribed to Chagas' disease.

Before central nervous system involvement has occurred, suramin, a complex, nonmetal-containing, organic compound, is the treatment of choice for early Rhodesian trypanosomiasis. Pentamidine isethionate is the drug of choice for early Gambian disease. When the central nervous system is involved, melarsoprol is the drug of choice. For American trypanosomiasis no specific therapy is available. Nitrofurans, such as Bayer 2502, pyrimethamine, and primaquine, have been used extensively in acute disease with sporadic elimination of the parasitemia. A second type agent, benzonidazole, a nitroimidazole derivative, appears to have similar efficacy to the nitrofurans. Conservative treatment is most appropriate for the patient with congestive heart failure from Chagas' myocarditis.

Cochran R, et al: African trypanosomiasis in the United States. Arch Dermatol 1983, 119:670.

Lausi L: Investigation regarding Chagas' disease among schoolchildren in Villa Soldati Buenos Aires. Rey Assoc Med Argen 1965, 79:123.

Woody NC, et al: American trypanosomiasis. J Pediatr 1961, 58:568.

Toxoplasmosis

Toxoplasmosis is a zoonosis caused by a parasitic protozoon, *Toxoplasma gondii*, and manifested by mild to severe forms of infection that may terminate in death.

In man the infection may be either congenital or acquired. The congenital infection occurs from placental transmission. Abortion or stillbirth may result. However, a full-term child delivered to an infected mother may be afflicted with a triad of hydrocephalus, chorioretinitis, and cerebral calcification. In addition, there may be hepatosplenomegaly and jaundice. Skin changes in toxoplasmosis are rare and nonspecific clinically. In congenital toxoplasmosis, macular and hemorrhagic eruptions predominate. "Blueberry muffin" lesions, reflecting dermatoerythropoesis, may be seen. Occasionally abnormal hair growth and exfoliative dermatitis have also been observed. In acquired toxoplasmosis skin manifestations consist of cutaneous and subcutaneous nodules and macular, maculopapular, papular, and hemorrhagic eruptions, followed by scarlatiniform desquamation. Pollock reported a case which clinically resembled dermatomyositis. Fine and Arndt reviewed congenital toxoplasmosis and the differential diagnosis of the TORCH syndrome, while Binazzi has reviewed the cutaneous lesions seen in the adult. Roseolalike, erythema multiformelike, and lichen planuslike eruptions are documented. As a rule, the exanthem is accompanied by high fever and general malaise.

Leyva et al reported a man with a widespread pupuric nodular eruption three weeks after a bone marrow transplant for iatrogenic pancytopenia induced by chemotherapy and irradiation for myelogenous leukemia. Biopsy showed many intracytoplasmic organisms within keratinocytes, about 3 μm in diameter. Electron microscopy permitted their identification as *Toxoplasma gondii*. The source of infection was not determined.

As Jones points out, diagnosis of acquired toxoplasmosis is of special importance to three groups of adults: healthy pregnant women concerned about recent exposure; adults with lymphadenopathy, fever, and myalgia, recent or chronic, who might have some other serious disease, such as lymphoma; and immunocompromised persons, such as AIDS patients, in whom toxoplasmosis might be fatal. It is the most common cause of focal encephalitis in AIDS patients. Hirschmann et al also described an AIDS patient with a widespread papular eruption caused by toxoplasmosis.

As to pregnant women, 20 per cent have already had the disease and are thus protected; they are identified by a positive test very early in pregnancy, or before it. A high titer just before the twentieth week of gestation might make abortion advisable, or treatment indicated; or such a test prior to delivery would indicate treatment for the infant. Immunofluorescence or complement fixation tests are both informative.

As to adults with lymphadenopathy, high or rising antibody titers at the time of onset or soon after are diagnostic. Characteristic histologic changes in lymph nodes may provide confirmation.

In congenital cases (and, rarely, acquired ones)

chorioretinitis may occur a decade or more after infection. In congenitally acquired infection, chorioretinitis is usually bilateral, whereas in the acquired type it is usually unilateral.

Toxoplasma gondii is a crescent-shaped, oval or round protozoan that can infect any mammalian or avian cell. The disease is often acquired through contact with animals, particularly cats. The two major routes of transmission of *T. gondii* in man are oral and congenital. Meats used for human consumption may contain tissue cysts, thus serving as a source of infection when eaten raw or undercooked. There is no evidence of direct human-to-human transmission other than from mother to fetus.

The diagnosis cannot be made on clinical grounds alone. The diagnosis of toxoplasmosis may be established by isolation of *T. gondii*, demonstration of the protozoa in tissue sections, smears, or body fluids by Wright's or Giemsa stain; characteristic lymph node histology; and serologic methods. Mouse inoculation with properly prepared tissue such as a lymph node, spinal fluid, or peripheral blood may serve to isolate and identify the parasite if it is stained with Giemsa or Wright's stain. Antibodies are most commonly detected by the Sabin-Feldman dye test, which shows positivity 10 to 14 days after the initial infection. A maximum titer is attained in four to five weeks. The Jacobs-Lunde hemagglutination test, the complement fixation tests, the indirect fluorescent antibody test, and skin tests may also be used to establish the diagnosis.

Toxoplasmosis is worldwide in its distribution, with several areas having over 90 per cent seropositivity. It occurs in the eastern United States more frequently than in the western states. Reservoirs of infection have been reported in dogs, cats, cattle, sheep, pigs, rabbits, rats, pigeons, and chickens.

A combination of pyrimethamine (Daraprim), 25 mg every other day, after a loading dose of 100 mg given in two equal doses for two days, is recommended for adults. In severe cases or in the immunocompromised, 25 mg or even 50 mg may be given daily. Sulfadiazine should be given in combination with the above, with a loading dose of 75 mg/kg, and thereafter 100 mg/kg/day. Total treatment time varies with the type of disease present, but in general it should be continued for at least one month. Daraprim is a folic acid antagonist, so concomitant folinic acid therapy is recommended.

Andreev VC, et al: Skin manifestations in toxoplasmosis. Arch Dermatol 1969, 100:196.

Binazzi M, et al: Profile of cutaneous toxoplasmosis. Int J Dermatol 1986, 25:357.

Cahill KM: Symposium on toxoplasmosis. Bull NY Acad Med 1974, 50:107.

Carey RM, et al: Toxoplasmosis. Am J Med 1973, 54:30.

Fine J-D, et al: The TORCH syndrome. JAAD 1985, 12:697.

Hirschmann JV, et al: Skin lesions with disseminated toxoplasmosis in a patient with AIDS. Arch Dermatol 1988, 124:1446.

Leyva WH, et al: Cutaneous toxoplasmosis. JAAD 1986, 14:600.

Pollack JL: Toxoplasmosis appearing to be dermatomyositis. Arch Dermatol 1979, 115:736.

PHYLUM COELENTERATA

This phylum includes the jellyfish, hydroids, corals, and sea anemones. These are all radial marine animals, living mostly in ocean water. When skin contact is made with these organisms a toxin is released through small spicules.

Portuguese Man-of-War Dermatitis. Stings by the Portuguese man-of-war (*Physalia physalis* in the Atlantic, or the much smaller *Physalia utriculus* or "bluebottle" in the Pacific) are characterized by linear lesions that are erythematous, urticarial, and even hemorrhagic. The forearms, sides of the trunk, thighs, and feet are the usual sites of involvement. The usual local manifestations are sharp stinging and intense pain. Internally there may be severe dyspnea, prostration, nausea, abdominal cramps, lacrimation, and muscular pains. Death may occur if the areas stung are large in relation to the size of the patient.

The fluid of the nematocysts contains toxin, which is carried into the human victim through barbs along the tentacle. The venom is a neurotoxic poison that can produce marked cardiac changes.

Each Portuguese man-of-war is a colony of symbiotic organisms consisting of a blue to red float or pneumatophore with a gas gland, several gastrozooids measuring 1 to 20 mm, reproductive polyps, and the fishing tentacles bearing the nematocysts from which the barbs are ejected. The hydroid is found most frequently along the southeastern Florida coastline and in the Gulf of Mexico, and on windward coasts throughout the mid and South Pacific.

The most effective treatment, said to have been in use for a century or more in Latin America, is to rub the pulp or crushed leaves of the papaya (*Carica papaya*) or pawpaw into the stings. Ordinary unseasoned meat tenderizer sprinkled on the wet skin and rubbed in serves equally well, Arnold has found.

Lacking meat tenderizer, rubbing alcohol may give relief, and lathering the affected area and then shaving it may also help. This beneficial effect is said to be due to the removal of the tentacles in the skin. Antihistaminics given intravenously produce dramatic relief from the vasospasm, visceral cramping, and local flare.

Jellyfish Dermatitis. This produces lesions similar to those of the Portuguese man-of-war, except that the lesions are not so linear. Delayed and persistent lesions were described by Reed et al from stings incurred in the Aegean and Caribbean areas. Burnett

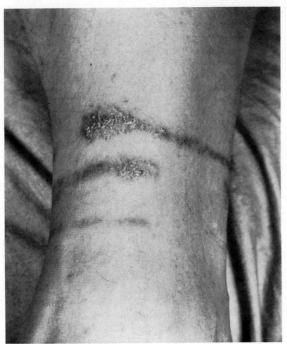

Figure 20–14. Portuguese man-of-war (Physalia physalis) *sting on shin, resembling whip lash.*

et al have reviewed the jellyfish envenomation syndromes, and also have reported prolonged hypersensitivity reactions which were associated with specific antijellyfish immunoglobulins.

The Australian **sea wasp**, *Chironex fleckeri*, which is colorless and transparent, is the most dangerous coelenterate of all, with a sting which is often fatal. Another sea wasp, *Carybdea marsupialis*, much less dangerous, occurs in the Caribbean.

Halecium Dermatitis. This results from contact with the small marine hydroid *Halecium beani*. De Oreo described 52 cases, all of whom had been swimming in the Pacific Ocean near Honolulu and had been in contact with a raft anchored near the beach. The organism grows like a centimeter-thick coat of moss on the submerged portions of vessels or pilings. The rash was noticed in one man as he was being prepared for an appendectomy, so that surgery was unnecessary.

Sponge fisher's dermatitis is caused by a sea anemone, *Sagartia*.

Sea Urchin Injuries. Puncture wounds inflicted by the brittle, fragile spines of sea urchins, mainly of genus *Diadema* or *Echinothrix*, are stained blue-black by the black spines, and may contain fragments of the spines. These are rarely large enough to require removal. Foreign-body or sarcoidlike granulomas may be produced. Burke et al have reported a sea urchin sting which led to a vesicular hypersensitivity reaction 10 days later. Minton says that injuries by spines of the genus *Tripneustes* have been reported

to cause fatal envenomation, but this genus is not found on U.S. coasts.

Coral Cuts. These are injuries caused by the exoskeleton of the corals, *Milleporina*. They have a largely undeserved reputation for becoming inflamed and infected, and for delayed healing. The combination of possible implantation of fragments of coral skeleton, and infection (since they are commonest on the feet), probably accounts almost entirely for these symptoms, and vigorous cleansing as soon as possible after the injury is advisable.

SEAWEED DERMATITIS

Though this is caused by a marine plant (an alga) and not by an animal, it deserves mention with other problems associated with swimming or wading. Grauer and Arnold reported a dermatitis occurring three to eight hours after emerging from the ocean. The distribution is in dependent parts covered by the bathing suit: scrotum, penis, penineum, and perianal area, caused by a marine plant, *Lyngbya majuscula* Gomont. It was observed only in bathers swimming off the windward shore of Oahu, Hawaii.

Seabather's eruption, clamdigger's itch, and swimmer's itch must be differentiated from seaweed dermatitis caused by marine algae.

Prophylaxis is achieved by refraining from swimming in waters which are turbid with such algae. One should shower within five minutes after swimming. Active treatment in severe cases is the same as for acute burns.

Dogger Bank Itch. "Dogger Bank itch" is an eczematous dermatitis caused by the sea chervil, *Alcyondium hirsutum*, a seaweedlike animal colony. These sea mosses or sea mats are found on the Dogger Bank, an immense shelflike elevation under the North Sea between Scotland and Denmark.

Arnold HL Jr: Portuguese man of war ("bluebottle") stings: treatment with papain. Straub Clin Proc 1970, 37:39.

Baden HP, et al: Injuries from sea urchins. South Med J 1977, 79:459.

Burke WA, et al: Delayed hypersensitivity reaction following a sea urchin sting. Int J Dermatol 1986, 25:699.

Burnett JW, et al: Studies on the serologic response to jellyfish envenomation. JAAD 1983, 9:229.

Idem: Recurrent eruptions following unusual solitary coelenterate envenomations. JAAD 1987, 17:86.

Idem: Jellyfish envenomation syndromes. JAAD 1986, 14:100.

Idem: Venomous coelenterates. Cutis 1987, 39:191.

De Oreo GA: Dermatitis resulting from contact with marine animals (hydroids). Arch Dermatol Syph 1946, 54:637.

Grauer FH, Arnold HL Jr: Seaweed dermatitis. Arch Dermatol 1961, 84:720.

Marowitz NR, et al: Cutaneous and systemic reactions of toxins and venoms of common marine organisms. Cutis 1979, 23:450.

Reed KM, et al: Delayed and persistent cutaneous reactions to coelenterates. JAAD 1984, 10:462.

Rosco MD: Cutaneous manifestations of marine animal injuries including diagnosis and treatment. Cutis 1977, 196:507.

PHYLUM PLATYHELMINTHES

This phylum includes the flatworms, of which two classes, trematodes and cestodes, are parasitic to man. The trematodes, or blood flukes, parasitize man in the skin or internally. The cestodes are segmented ribbon-shaped flatworms that inhabit the intestinal tract as adults and involve the subcutaneous tissue, as well as heart, muscle, and eye in the larval form, which is encased in a sac which eventually becomes calcified.

CLASS TREMATODA

Schistosome Cercarial Dermatitis

Schistosome dermatitis is a severely pruritic widespread papular dermatitis caused by cercariae of schistosomes, which are parasitic in waterfowl and rodents such as muskrats. The eggs in the excreta of these animals, when deposited in water, hatch into swimming miracidia. These enter the snail, where further development occurs. From the snail the free-swimming cercariae emerge to invade the human skin on accidental contact. The swimming, colorless, multicellular organisms are a little less than a millimeter long. Exposure to cercariae occurs by swimming or more often wading in water containing them. They attack by burrowing into the skin, where they die. They cannot enter the blood stream.

After coming out of the water, the bather begins to itch and a transient erythematous eruption appears, but after a few hours, the eruption subsides together with the itching. Then after a quiescent period of 10 to 15 hours, the symptoms recur, and erythematous macules and papules develop throughout the parts that were in the water. After several days the dermatitis heals spontaneously. There are two types: one is the freshwater *swimmer's itch*, and the other the saltwater *marine dermatitis* or clam digger's itch. The disease is not communicable.

The disease can be prevented by thorough washing and drying with a towel after exposure. Rubbing the skin with a towel seems to be enough to prevent the disease, although rubbing with alcohol is an additional preventive measure.

Hoeffler has recently summarized the disease, with details of the genera and species of organisms and snails which may be involved.

Seabather's eruption, clinically similar, affects covered areas of the body. This acute dermatitis occurs a few hours after bathing in the ocean. Erythematous macules, papules, and wheals appear, persist for several days and then spontaneously involute. The eruption is largely confined to the area covered by the bathing suit. Often the pruritus and discomfort are intense.

Sams called attention to the influence of pressure on the severity of the eruption. In children and men who wear only bathing trunks, the lesions will be found predominantly on the covered parts, and they will be more pronounced over the buttocks and about the waist, which are pressure areas. In women, in addition to these locations, lesions will occur on the breasts, under the brassiere of a tightly fitting suit, or at other points of pressure.

The disease occurs only in waters off certain Atlantic beaches in the spring months. No definite etiologic agent has been established. Hutton has reported 20 similar cases caused by a needle-shaped pteropod, *Creseis acicula* Rang.

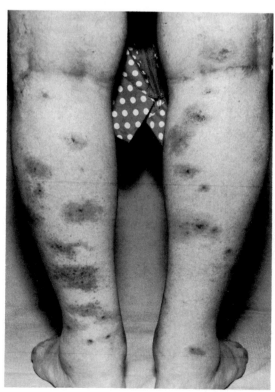

Figure 20–15. Schistosome dermatitis.

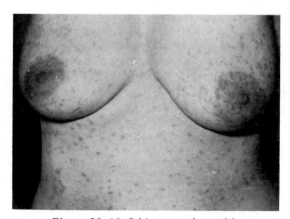

Figure 20–16. Schistosome dermatitis.

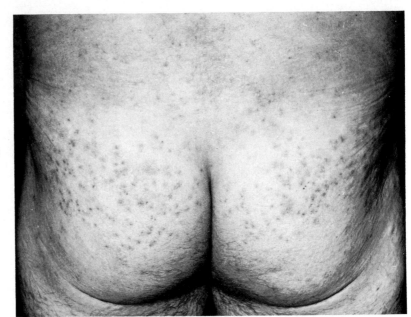

Figure 20–17. Schistosomiasis cutis (swimmer's itch). (Courtesy of Dr. J. Penner.)

VISCERAL SCHISTOSOMIASIS (Bilharziasis)

The cutaneous manifestation of bilharziasis may begin with mild itching and a papular dermatitis of the feet and other parts after swimming in polluted streams containing cercariae. After an asymptomatic incubation period there may be a sudden illness with fever and chills, pneumonitis, and eosinophilia. Petechial hemorrhages may occur.

In Egypt El-Mofty has reported involvement of the perineum and the buttocks. These paragenital granulomas occur frequently in areas endemic for *S. haematobium*. Infections with this organism primarily involve the urinary tract, while those due to *S. mansoni* and *S. japonicum* primarily affect the liver. Here fistulous tracts occur, and extensive hard masses are riddled by sinuses which exude a seropurulent discharge with a characteristic odor. Phagedenic ulcerations and pseudoelephantiasis of the scrotum, penis, or labia are encountered. Histologically, the nodules contain bilharzial ova undergoing degeneration, with calcification and with surrounding cellular reaction of histiocytes, eosinophils, and occasional giant cells.

Schistosomal granulomas (bilharzioma) of the skin have been noted by El-Zawahry in the rural areas of Egypt, especially in girls at the age of puberty. The most frequent site is the external genitalia, especially the labia majora. Vegetating, soft, cauliflowerlike masses occur, which do not usually ulcerate. Eventual malignant changes in these granulomas have been noted.

A severe urticarial eruption known as urticarial fever is frequently present along with *Schistosoma japonicum* infection; it is known as Katayama fever, and occurs with the beginning of oviposition, four to eight weeks after infection. This occurs mainly in China, Japan, and the Philippines. In addition to the urticaria, fever, malaise, abdominal cramps, arthritis, and liver and spleen involvement are seen.

Another type is found mainly on the trunk. This is a papular eruption tending to group in plaques and become darkly pigmented and scaly. It is frequently seen in Egypt with *S. mansoni* infection. Walther et al reported a chronic papular eruption of the scrotum which showed *S. mansoni* on skin biopsy.

Preventive measures, as suggested by Brown, involve reduction of infection sources, prevention of human excreta contamination of snail-bearing

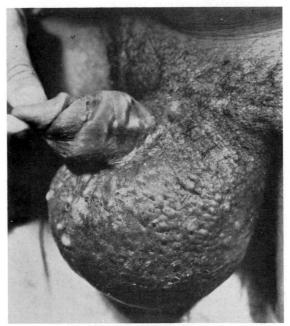

Figure 20–18. Schistosomal granulomas of the scrotum. (Courtesy of Dr. M. El-Zawahry, U.A.R.)

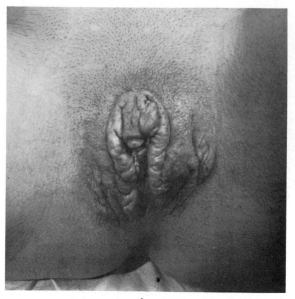 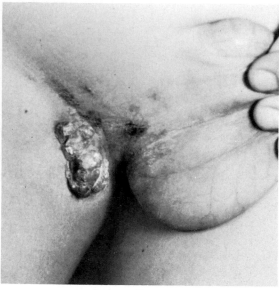

A   B

Figure 20–19. A, *Schistosomal granuloma in a 16-year-old girl. (Courtesy of Dr. M. El-Zawahry, U.A.R.) B, Intercrural granuloma of schistosomiasis. These granulomas are found most frequently in the genital and perineal areas. (Courtesy of Dr. A. M. El-Mofty, U.A.R.)*

waters, control of snail hosts, and avoidance of exposure to cercaria-infested waters.

Prophylactic measures are constantly sought to control one of the world's worst parasitic diseases but as yet none are practical.

TREATMENT. A major advance was the advent of praziquantel (Biltricide) in the early 1980s. Farid et al have demonstrated its effectiveness against both *S. hematobium* and *S. mansoni.* They advise 20 mg/kg

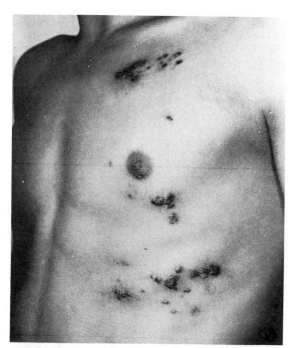

Figure 20–20. Cutaneous schistosomiasis on the trunk, a typical site other than the genital and perineal areas. (Courtesy of Dr. A. M. El-Mofty, U.A.R.)

body weight for each of three treatments in one day, by the oral route. For *S. hematobium* a single oral dose of 30 mg/kg was sufficient.

Schistosomicides exhibit toxicity for the host as well as for the parasite, and the risk of undesirable side effects may be enhanced by concomitant cardiac, renal, or hepatosplenic disease.

Farid Z, et al: Schistosomiasis and praziquantel (letter). Ann Intern Med 1983, 99:883.
Heffler DF: "Swimmer's itch" (cercarial dermatitis). Cutis 1977, 19:461.
King CH, et al: Drugs 5 years later: praziquantel. Ann Intern Med 1989, 110:290.
Sams WM: Seabather's eruption. Arch Dermatol Syph 1949, 60:227.
Torres VM: Dermatologic manifestations of schistosomiasis mansoni. Arch Dermatol 1976, 112:1539.
Walther RR: Chronic papular dermatitis of the scrotum due to *Schistosoma mansoni.* Arch Dermatol 1979, 115:869.

Cysticercosis Cutis

The natural intermediate host of the pork tapeworm, *Taenia solium,* is the pig, but under some circumstances man acts in this role. The larval stage of *T. solium* is *Cysticercus cellulosae.* Infection takes place by the ingestion of food contaminated with the eggs, or by reverse peristalsis of eggs or proglottides from the intestine to the stomach. Here the eggs hatch, freeing the onchospheres. These enter the general circulation and form cysts in various parts of the body such as striated muscles, brain, eye, heart, and lung.

In the subcutaneous tissues the lesions are usually painless nodules, which contain cysticerci. They are more or less stationary, usually numerous, and often calcified, and so demonstrable radiographically. Pain and ulceration may accompany them. The disease is most prevalent in countries where pigs feed on human feces. It may be confused with gumma, lipoma, and epithelioma. A positive diagnosis is established solely by incision and examination of the interior of the calcified tumor, where the parasite will be found.

TREATMENT. Praziquantel in doses as low as 10 mg per kg of body weight is said to cure almost every patient with *Taenia solium*; five times this dose is required if the central nervous system is involved. Levin et al have recently summarized the current status of therapy with this new and valuable drug. King et al have also published a valuable review (v.i.).

Falanga V, et al: Cerebral cysticercosis. JAAD 1985, 12:304.
King CH, et al: Drugs 5 years later: praziquantel. Ann Intern Med 1989, 110:290.
Levin JA, et al: Praziquantel in the treatment of cysticercosis (letter). JAMA 1986, 256:349.
Tschen EH, et al: Cutaneous cysticercosis treated with metrifonate. Arch Dermatol 1981, 117:507

Sparganosis

This disease is caused by the larva of the tapeworm of the species *spirometra*. The adult tapeworm lives in the intestines of dogs and cats. This is a rare tissue infection occurring in two forms described by Strauss and Manwaring.

Application sparganosis occurs when an ulcer or infected eye is poulticed with the flesh of an infected intermediate host. Such poultices are frequently used in the Orient. The larvae become encased in small nodules in the infected tissue.

Ingestion sparganosis occurs when man ingests inadequately cooked meat such as snake or frog, or when he drinks water contaminated with Cyclops infected with plerocercoid larvae. One or two slightly pruritic or painful nodules may form in the subcutaneous tissue or on the trunk and legs.

Man is an accidental intermediate host of the *Sparganum*, which is the alternative name for the plerocercoid larva.

Treatment is surgical removal of the infected nodules. This may be difficult because of the swelling and extensive vascularity.

Sarma DP, et al: Human sparganosis. JAAD 1986, 15:1145.
Strauss WG, et al: Sparganosis. Dermatol Int 1964, 2:73.

Echinococcosis

This is also known as *hydatid disease*. Human infection is produced by the ova reaching the mouth by the hands, in food, or from containers soiled by ova-contaminated feces from an infected dog. This leads to *Echinococcus granulosus* infestation of the liver and the lungs. Soft, fluctuating, semitranslucent, cystic tumors may occur in the skin. These tumors become fibrotic or calcified after the death of the larva. Eosinophilia or intractable urticaria and pruritus may be present. The treatment is excision, with care being taken to avoid rupture of the cyst.

Little JM: Hydatid disease at Royal Prince Alfred Hospital, 1964 to 1974. Med J Aust 1976, 1:903.

PHYLUM ANNELIDA

LEECHES

Ross has reported the dermatologic manifestations of leech attachment. Leeches, of the class Hirudinea, are of marine, freshwater, or terrestrial types. After attaching to the skin they secrete an anticoagulant, hirudin, and then engorge themselves with blood. Local symptoms at the site of the bite may include bullae, hemorrhage, pruritus, whealing, necrosis, or ulceration. Allergic reactions, including anaphylaxis, may result. They may be removed by applying salt, alcohol, or vinegar, or by use of a match flame. Bleeding may be then stopped by direct pressure or by a styptic pencil.

Ross MS: The leech: of dermatologic interest. Arch Dermatol 1983, 119:276.

PHYLUM NEMATHELMINTHES

This phylum includes the roundworms, both the free-living and the parasitic forms. Multiplication is usually outside the host. Both the larval and adult stages may infect man.

CLASS NEMATODA

Enterobiasis

Synonyms: Pinworm infection, seatworm infection, oxyuriasis.

CLINICAL FEATURES. The chief symptom of pinworm infestation, which occurs most frequently in children, is nocturnal pruritus ani. There is intense itching accompanied by excoriations of the anus, perineum, and pubic area. The vagina may become infested with the gravid pinworm. Restlessness, insomnia, enuresis, and irritability are but a few of the many symptoms ascribed to this exceedingly common infestation.

ETIOLOGY. Oxyuriasis is caused by the roundworm *Enterobius vermicularis*, which may infest the small intestines, cecum, and large intestine of the human. The worms, especially the gravid worms, migrate toward the rectum and at night emerge to the perianal and perineal regions to deposit thousands of ova as the worm dries and dies outside the intestine. These ova are then carried back to the mouth of the host on the hands. The larvae hatch in the duodenum and migrate into the jejunum and ileum, where maturity is reached. Fertilization occurs in the cecum, thus completing the life cycle.

EPIDEMIOLOGY. Man is the only known host of the pinworm, which probably has the widest distribution of all helminths. Infection is contracted by hand-to-mouth transmission, from handling of soiled

clothes, bedsheets, and other household articles. Ova under the fingernails are a common source of autoinfection. Ova may also be airborne and collect in dust that may be on furniture and the floor.

Investigation may show that all members of the family of an affected person also harbor the infection. It is common in orphanages and mental institutions and among people living in communal groups.

DIAGNOSIS. The demonstration of the dead pinworm in the stool is only rarely feasible. The diagnosis is made best by the demonstration of ova in smears taken from the anal region early in the morning before bathing. With the patient in the knee-chest position a smear is obtained from the anus with a small eye curette and is placed on a glass slide with a drop of saline solution. It is also possible to use Scotch tape, looping the tape sticky side out over a tongue depressor and then pressing it several times against the perianal region. The tape is then smoothed out on a glass slide. A drop of a solution containing iodine in xylol may be placed on the slide before application of the tape. This will facilitate detection of any ova.

These tests should be repeated on three consecutive days to rule out infection. The examination should be made early in the morning before defecation or bathing. The ova may also be detected under the fingernails of the infected person.

TREATMENT. Pyrvinium pamoate (Povan Film-seals) is probably the best medication available at present. A cure rate of 100 per cent can be expected.

Pyrvinium pamoate (Povan, Parke-Davis) is given in a single dose of 5 mg per kg of body weight. The suspension contains 10 mg per ml. Patients should be warned that the stools will be colored bright red. A second dose may be given one week after the first treatment.

Mebendazole (Vermox, Ortho) in a single dose of 100 mg for all patients (of any age or weight) has been shown to be effective.

PREVENTION. Personal hygiene and cleanliness at home are important. Fingernails should be cut short and scrubbed frequently; they should be cleaned upon arising, before each meal, and after using the toilet. Sheets, underwear, towels, pajamas, and other clothing of the affected person should be laundered thoroughly and separately.

Hookworm Disease

Synonyms: Ground itch, uncinariasis, ancylostomiasis, necatoriasis.

CLINICAL FEATURES. The earliest skin lesions (ground itch) are erythematous macules and papules, which in a few hours become vesicles. These itching lesions usually occur on the soles, toewebs, and ankles, and they may be scattered or in groups. The contents of the vesicles rapidly become purulent.

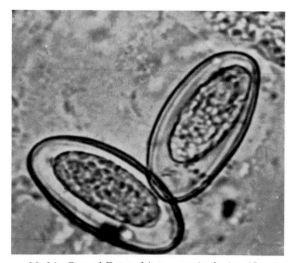

Figure 20–21. Ova of Enterobius vermicularis. *(Courtesy of Dr. H. W. Brown.)*

These lesions are produced by the invasion of the skin by the ancylostoma or necator larvae and precede the generalized symptoms of the disease by two or three months. The cutaneous lesions last less than two weeks before the larvae continue their human life cycle.

The onset of the constitutional disease is insidious and is accompanied by progressive iron deficiency anemia, and debility. During the course of the disease urticaria often occurs. The skin ultimately becomes dry and pale or yellowish.

ETIOLOGY. Hookworm is a specific communicable disease due to *Ancylostoma duodenale* or *Necator americanus*. In the soil, under propitious circumstances, they attain the stage of infective larvae in five to seven days. These tiny larvae (which can scarcely be seen with a small pocket lens), when coming into accidental contact with the bare feet, penetrate the skin and reach the capillaries. They are carried in the circulation to the lungs, where they pass through the capillary walls into the bronchi; they move up the trachea to the pharynx and, being swallowed, eventually reach their habitat in the small intestine. Here they bury their heads in the mucosa and begin their sexual life.

EPIDEMIOLOGY. The disease is prevalent in most tropical and subtropical countries and is often endemic in swampy and sandy localities in the temperate zones. In these latter regions the larvae are killed off each winter, but the soil is again contaminated from human sources the following summer.

Necator americanus prevails in the Western Hemisphere, Central and South Africa, South Asia, Australia, and the Pacific islands.

The defecation habits of infected individuals in the endemic areas are largely responsible for its widespread distribution, as is the use of human feces for fertilization in many parts of the world. In addition, the climate is usually such that people go barefooted because of the heat or because they cannot afford shoes. Infection is thereby facilitated, especially through the toes.

DIAGNOSIS. Finding the eggs in the feces of the suspected individual establishes the diagnosis. The eggs may be found in direct fecal films in heavy infections, but in light infections it may be necessary to resort to zinc sulfate centrifugal flotation or other concentration methods. Mixed infections frequently occur.

There may be as high as 40 per cent eosinophilia around the fifth day of infection, and ova appear in the feces about five weeks after onset of infection.

TREATMENT. Treatment is by expulsion of the parasites from the body and by prevention of reinfection through a proper disposal of human feces. The drug of choice is mebendazole (Vermox chewable), 100 mg b.i.d. for three days. An alternative is pyrantel pamoate (Antiminth, Pfipharmecs) suspension, though the manufacturer recommends it only for ascariasis and enterobiasis. Vermox is effective against roundworm and pinworms as well. The dose is 11 mg/kg body weight in a single dose. No preparation or purging is required with either drug.

Prophylaxis is largely a community problem, which depends upon the prevention of fecal contamination of the soil. This is best attained by proper sanitary disposal of feces, protection of individuals from exposure by education in sanitary procedures, and mass treatment through public health methods.

Creeping Eruption (Larva Migrans)

CLINICAL FEATURES. Creeping eruption is a term applied to twisting, winding linear skin lesions produced by the burrowing of larvae. People who go barefoot at the beaches, children playing in sandboxes, carpenters and plumbers working under homes, and gardeners are often victims. The most common areas involved are the feet, buttocks, genitals, and hands.

The onset is characterized by slight local itching and the appearance of papules at the sites of infection due to the migrations of the larvae. Intermittent stinging pain occurs and thin red tortuous lines are formed in the skin. The migrations begin four days after inoculation and progress at the rate of about 2 cm daily. However, the larvae may remain quiescent for several days or even months before beginning to migrate. The linear lesions are often interrupted by papules that mark the sites of resting larvae. As the eruption advances, the old parts tend to fade, but there are sometimes purulent manifestations due to secondary infection; erosions and excoriations secondary to scratching frequently occur. If the progress of the disease is not interrupted by treatment the larvae usually die in two to eight weeks, with reso-

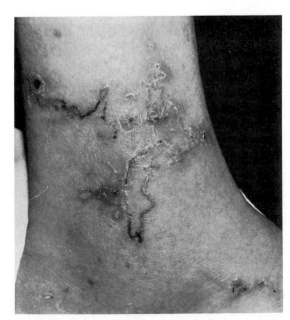

Figure 20–22. Creeping eruption on ankle due to Ancylostoma braziliense.

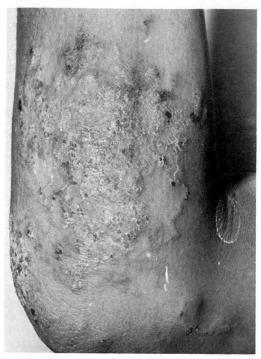

Figure 20–23. Larva migrans on the elbow. Notice extreme eczematization from scratching. (Courtesy of Dr. J. Penner.)

lution of the eruption, although it has rarely been reported to persist for up to one year. At times the larvae are removed from the skin by the fingernails in scratching. Eosinophilia may be present.

Loeffler's syndrome, consisting of a patchy infiltrate of the lungs, with eosinophilia as high as 50 per cent in the blood and 90 per cent in the sputum, may complicate creeping eruption.

ETIOLOGY. The majority of cases in this country are due to penetration by the larvae of a cat and dog hookworm, *Ancylostoma braziliense*, acquired from bodily contact with damp sand or earth contaminated by excreta of dogs and cats. A similar dermatitis is rarely produced by the larvae of *Ancylostoma caninum*, which also infests the dog and the cat. Creeping eruption due to *A. braziliense* is common along the coast of the southeastern United States.

TREATMENT. Thiabendazole (Mintezol) is an effective internal medication. The dose is 50 mg/kg daily by mouth in equal portions every 12 hours for two days with a maximum daily dose of 3 gm. A second course may be given in a few days. Criteria for successful therapy are relief of symptoms and cessation of track extension, which usually occurs within a week.

The oral therapy has largely been replaced by topical treatment due to its convenience and absence of side effects. Davis and Israel reported successful treatment with the topical application four times daily of the suspension alone. Marked relief from pruritus was noted in three days and the tracks were inactive in one week. Ten per cent oral suspension applied four times daily and continued one or two days after the last tracks have resolved is the treatment of choice.

Another condition, not to be confused with this helminthic disease, which also is called creeping eruption (or "sandworm," as it is known in South Africa and particularly in Natal and Zululand), is caused by a small mite about 300 μ in length that tunnels in the superficial layers of the epidermis.

Larva Migrans Profundus

Human gnathostomiasis is characterized by migratory, intermittent, erythematous urticarial plaques. Each episode of painless swelling lasts from seven to 10 days and recurs every two to six weeks. Movement of the underlying parasite may be as much as 1 cm per hour. The total duration of the illness may be 10 years. Histopathologic examination of the skin swelling is that of eosinophilic panniculitis.

The nematode *Gnathostoma spinigerum* is the cause, with most cases occurring in the Orient or South America. Ollague et al reported 15 patients from Ecuador, and Feinstein et al reported another from the same country. Eating raw flesh from the second intermediate host, most commonly freshwater fish in such preparations as sashimi and ceviche, allows man to become a definitive host. As the larval cyst in the flesh is digested, the larva becomes motile and penetrates the gastric mucosa, usually within 24 to 48 hours of ingestion. Symptoms then occur as migration of the parasite continues.

None of the anthelmintics are effective. Surgical removal is the treatment of choice, if the parasite can be located.

Larva Currens

Intestinal infections with *Strongyloides stercoralis* may be associated with a perianal larva migrans syndrome which Arthur and Shelley called "larva currens" because of the rapidity of larval migration (currens means running or racing). This disease is an autoinfection caused by penetration of the perianal skin by infectious larvae as they are excreted in the feces. The features of larva currens include an urticarial band as the prominent primary lesion of cutaneous strongyloidiasis. Strongyloidiasis, and the creeping eruption secondary to it, is often a chronic disease. Pelletier et al reported in 1985 a case acquired in the Vietnam War, and recent studies on prisoners of war from World War II have shown infections may persist for over 40 years. Approximately one third of patients infected are asymptomatic. Symptoms of systemic strongyloidiasis include abdominal pain, diarrhea, constipation, nausea, vomiting, pneumonitis, urticaria, and a peripheral eosinophilia. The skin lesions originate within 30 cm of the anus and characteristically extend as much as 10 cm per day. Von Kuster et al stress widespread petechiae

Therapy is thiabendazole in a dosage of 25 mg/kg/day in two oral doses. Normal patients require only two doses, but immunosuppressed hosts have been treated for five to 15 days.

Amer M, et al: Larva currens and systemic disease. J Invest Dermatol 1981, 20:402.

Edelglass JW, et al: Cutaneous larva migrans in northern climates. JAAD 1982, 7:353.

Eyster WH Jr: Local thiabendazole in the treatment of creeping eruption. Arch Dermatol Syph 1967, 96:620.

Feinstein RJ, et al: Gnathostomiasis, or larva migrans profundus. JAAD 1984, 11:738.

Guill MA, Odom RB: Larva migrans complicated by Loeffler's syndrome. Arch Dermatol 1978, 114:1525.

Kagen CN, et al: Gnathostomiasis. Arch Dermatol 1984, 120:508.

Kalb RE, et al: Periumbilical purpura in disseminated strongyloidiasis. JAMA 1986, 256:1170.

Milder JE, et al: Clinical features of Strongyloides stercoralis infection in an endemic area of the United States. Gastroenterology 1981, 80:1481.

Ollague W, et al: Human gnathostomiasis in Ecuador (nodular migratory eosinophilic panniculitis): first finding of the parasite in South America. Int J Dermatol 1984, 23:647.

Pelletier LL Jr, et al: Chronic strongyloidiasis in Vietnam veterans. Am J Med 1985, 78:139.

Sarubbi FA: Hyperinfection with Stronglyloides during treatment of pemphigus vulgaris. Arch Dermatol 1987, 123:864.

Smith JD, et al: Larva currens. Arch Dermatol 1976, 112:1161.

Von Kuster LC, et al: Cutaneous manifestations of strongyloidiasis. Arch Dermatol 1988, 124:1826.

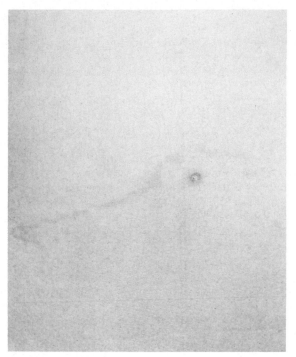

Figure 20–24. *Larva currens of the buttock.* Strongyloides stercoralis *was recovered from the patient's stool specimen.*

and purpura as diagnostic signs of disseminated infection and chronic urticaria as a possible presenting sign.

Amer et al in 1981 reported 26 patients with *S. stercoralis* infection, 10 without systemic symptoms or skin lesions, nine with systemic complaints only, and seven with skin lesions extending as much as several centimeters per hour, with eosinophilia, hunger pain, diarrhea, nausea and vomiting, and pruritus.

Kalb et al and Sarubbi have recently reported fatal cases of hyperinfection in immunocompromised patients. In such patients the parasite load increases dramatically and can produce a fulminant illness.

Dracunculiasis (Guinea Worm Disease)

Synonyms: Dracontiasis, Medina worm.

CLINICAL FEATURES. Guinea worm disease is endemic in India, Southwest Asia, Northeast South America, West Indies, and Africa. It is due to *Dracunculus medinensis,* and is contracted through drinking water contaminated with infected water fleas in which the dracunculus is parasitic. In the stomach the larvae penetrate into the mesentery, where they mature sexually in 10 weeks. Then the female worm

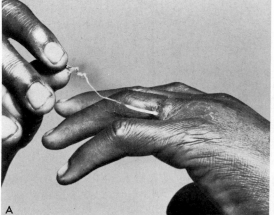
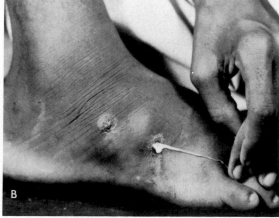

Figure 20–25. A, *Guinea worm disease, dracunculiasis. Guinea worm is protruding from bleb. (Courtesy of Dr. G. H. V. Clarke, Wales.) B, The guinea worm is protruding from one bleb; proximally is another bleb still unbroken. (Courtesy of Dr. M. El-Zawahry, U.A.R.)*

burrows to the cutaneous surface in order to deposit her larvae, and thus causes the specific skin manifestations. As the worm approaches the surface it may be felt as a cordlike thickening and forms an indurated cutaneous papule. The papule may vesiculate, and a painful ulcer develops, usually on the leg. The worm is often visible. When the parasite comes in contact with water, the worm rapidly discharges its larvae, which are ingested by water fleas (*Cyclops*), contaminating the water.

The cutaneous lesion is usually on the lower leg, but it may occur on the genitalia, buttocks, or arms.

In addition to the ulcers on the skin there may be urticaria, gastrointestinal upsets, eosinophilia, and fever.

TREATMENT. The disease may be prevented by boiling the drinking water. Native treatment consists of gradually extracting the worm a little each day, with care not to rupture it, for in the event of such an accident the larvae escape into the tissues and produce fulminating inflammation. Surgical extraction is also practiced. Niridazole, 12.5 mg per kg twice daily for one week, or thiabendazole, 25 mg per kg twice daily, resolves the local inflammation and permits easier removal of the worm. Thiabendazole is probably the best local treatment.

Filariasis

ELEPHANTIASIS TROPICA (Elephantiasis Arabum)

CLINICAL FEATURES. Filariasis is a widespread tropical disorder due to infestation with filarial worms of *Wuchereria bancrofti*, *Brugia malayi*, or *B. timori*. It is characterized by lymphedema, with resulting hypertrophy of the skin and subcutaneous tissues, and by enlargement and deformity of the affected parts, usually the legs, scrotum, or labia majora. The disease occurs more frequently in young men than in women.

The onset of elephantiasis is characterized by recurrent attacks of acute lymphangitis in the affected part, associated with chills and fever (elephantoid fever) which lasts for several days to several weeks. These episodes recur over a period of several months to years. After each attack the swelling subsides only partially, and as recrudescences supervene, thickening and hypertrophy become increasingly pronounced. The overlying epidermis becomes stretched, thin, and shiny, and, in the course of years, leathery, insensitive, and verrucous or papillomatous from secondary pyogenic infection. There may be a dozen or more attacks in a year.

In addition to the involvement of the legs and scrotum, the scalp, vulva, penis, female breasts, and arms are at times affected, either alone or in association with the other regions. The manifestations vary according to the part involved. When the legs are attacked, both are usually affected in a somewhat symmetric manner, the principal changes occurring on the posterior aspects above the ankles and on the

dorsa of the feet. At first the thickening may be slight and associated with edema that pits on pressure. Later the parts become massive and pachydermatous, the thickened integument hanging in apposing folds, between which there is a fetid exudate.

When the scrotum is affected it gradually reaches an enormous size and the penis becomes hidden in it. The skin, which at first is glazed, later is coarse and verrucous or, in the far advanced cases, ulcerated or gangrenous. Resistant urticaria may occur. Filarial orchitis and hydrocele are common. A testicle may enlarge rapidly to the size of an apple and be extremely painful. The swelling may subside within a few days, or the enlargement may be permanent. As a result of obstruction and dilatation of the thoracic duct or some of its lower abdominal tributaries into the urinary tract, chyle appears in the urine, which assumes a milky appearance. Lobulated swellings of the inguinal and axillary glands, called "varicose glands," are due to obstructive varix and dilatation of the lymphatic vessels.

ETIOLOGY. Elephantiasis caused by filariasis is due to *W. bancrofti*, *Brugia malayi*, or *B. timori* and is transmitted by the bites of a variety of mosquitoes, *Culex*, *Aedes*, and *Anopheles* species.

It is important to realize that infestation by the filaria is often asymptomatic and elephantiasis usually occurs only if hundreds of thousands of mosquito bites are suffered over a period of years, with episodes of intercurrent streptococcal lymphangitis. Fi-

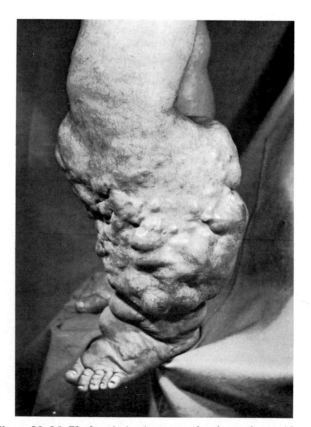

Figure 20–26. *Elephantiasis. An extremely advanced case. (Courtesy of Dr. M. El-Zawahry, U.A.R.)*

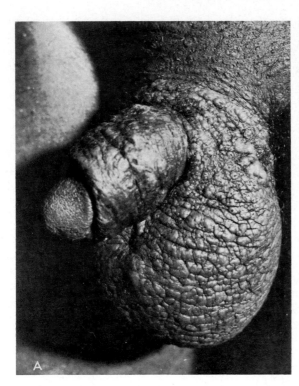
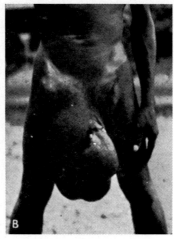

Figure 20–27. A, *Early elephantiasis in onchocerciasis due to* Onchocerca volvulus. *(Courtesy of Dr. G. H. V. Clarke, Wales.)* B, *Elephantiasis of scrotum, with hyperplasia of inguinal glands.*

lariasis has been endemic in the considerable Samoan population of Hawaii for half a century, and only one case of elephantiasis has occurred among this group.

EPIDEMIOLOGY. It is endemic in Africa, India, South China, Japan, Samoa, and Taiwan. It also occurs in the West Indies and Costa Rica. In Malaya, Ceylon, Indonesia, China, and Korea there is Malayan filariasis caused by *Brugia malayi*. *B. timori* is restricted to the eastern Indonesian archipelago.

W. bancrofti or *B. malayi* has been known in India since the sixth century B.C. It is estimated that 250 million people are infected with these parasites. *Culex quinquefasciatus* and *C. fatigans* and 48 other species of mosquitoes transmit these infective larvae.

The adult worms are threadlike, cylindrical, and creamy white. The females are between 4 and 10 cm long. Microfilarial embryos may be seen coiled each in its own membrane near the posterior tip. Fully grown, sheathed microfilariae are 130 to 320 µ long. The adult worms live in the lymphatics, where they produce microfilariae. These either remain in the lymphatics or get into the peripheral blood stream. An intermediate host is necessary for the further development of the parasite.

There is a striking periodicity to the time of the appearance and disappearance of the microfilariae in the skin and superficial vessels. The *Culex fatigans* bites at night and the microfilariae of *W. bancrofti* are found in the peripheral circulation at midnight (nocturnal periodicity) and rarely during the daytime. In the South Pacific it is nonperiodic.

DIAGNOSIS. Search for the microfilariae should be made on fresh coverslip films of blood from the finger or ear and examined with a low power objective. Specimens should be taken at midnight. Demonstration of calcified adult worms may be made by roentgenogram, and sometimes adult filariae are found in abscesses or in pathologic material. The filarial worm can be traced fluorescently, as the microfilariae and adult worms have an affinity for the tetracyclines, which fluoresce in ultraviolet radiation in a dark room. The filarial complement fixation test and skin tests, although only group specific, are useful in seeking the cause of lymphedema.

The prognosis in regard to life is good, but living becomes burdensome unless the condition is alleviated.

TREATMENT. Diethylcarbamazine (Hetrazan, Banocide, Ethodryl), a piperazine, has low toxicity and is effective against *Wuchereria bancrofti*, *Loa loa*, and *Onchocerca volvulus*. It kills the microfilariae and adult *B. malayi*; however, its effect on adult *W. bancrofti* is less certain. On day 1, 50 mg is given; day 2, 50 mg t.i.d.; day 3, 100 mg t.i.d.; days 4 through 21, 2 mg/kg t.i.d. Fever, nausea, vomiting, and rash may occur, as with any drug.

Surgical operations have been devised to remove the edematous subcutaneous tissue from the scrotum and breast.

Prophylactic measures consist of appropriate mosquito control. Diethylcarbamazine has been effective in mass prophylaxis.

Zawahry M: Elephantiasis tropica. Dermatol Int 1966, 5:79.

LOAIASIS

Synonyms: Loa loa, calabar swelling, tropical swelling, fugitive swelling.

CLINICAL FEATURES. Infection with *Loa loa* is often asymptomatic. However, generally more or less painful localized subcutaneous nonpitting edema, or fugitive swellings, called *calabar swellings*, occur. In infected persons the parasite develops slowly and there may even be an interval of as much as three years between infection and the appearance of symptoms, although the usual interval is one year.

Calabar swellings are one or more slightly inflamed, edematous, transient swellings, usually about the size of a hen's egg, on the wrist or forearm or on any area. They usually last a few days and then subside, although recurrent swellings at the same site may eventually lead to a permanent cystlike protuberance. These swellings may result from hypersensitivity to the adult worm or to materials elaborated by it. Eosinophilia may be as high as 90 per cent and often is between 60 and 80 per cent.

The filariae may be noticed subcutaneously in the fingers, breasts, eyelids, or submucosally under the conjunctivae. The worm may be in the anterior chamber of the eye, the myocardium, or other sites. It has a predilection for loose tissues such as the eye region, the frenum of the tongue, and the genitalia. The wanderings of the adult parasite may be noticed by a tingling and creeping sensation. The death of the filaria in the skin may lead to the formation of fluctuant cystic lesions.

ETIOLOGY. Loaiasis is a form of filariasis caused by *Loa loa*, widely distributed in west and central Africa. It is transmitted by the mango fly, *Chrysops dimidia* or *C. silacea*. This fly bites only in the daytime. Humans are the only important gadfly reservoir for the parasite.

DIAGNOSIS. The observation of the worm under the conjunctiva, calabar swellings, and eosinophilia establish the diagnosis. Demonstration of the characteristic microfilariae in the blood during the day is possible in only some 20 per cent of patients. Complement fixation and intradermal tests may be helpful.

TREATMENT. The removal of the adult parasite whenever it comes to the surface of the skin is mandatory. This must be done quickly by seizing the worm with forceps and placing a suture under it before cutting down to it. Worms not securely and rapidly grasped quickly escape into the deeper tissues. Diethylcarbamazine (Hetrazan) kills both adults and microfilariae. For the dose, see under Filariasis.

Nutman conducted a double-blind, placebo-controlled trial of diethylcarbamazine as a chemopreventive, using 300 mg daily, in temporary residents of regions of Africa where *Loa loa* is endemic. It was effective, with only occasional nausea as a side effect.

Marriott WRV: Loaiasis. Int J Dermatol 1985, 25:329.
Nutman TB, et al: Diethylcarbamazine prophylaxis for human loaiasis. N Engl J Med 1988, 319:752.

Onchocerciasis

CLINICAL FEATURES. The first symptoms are constitutional, with an erysipelaslike eruption and marked edema (*erysipelas de la Costa*). These symptoms gradually subside and, after a time, firm subcutaneous nodules, pea size or larger, develop on various sites of the body. These nodules are *onchocercomas* containing myriad microfilariae. These occur in crops and are frequently painful. The site of these onchocercomas varies. In parts of Africa where the native is wholly unclothed the lesions occur on the trunk, axillae, groin, and perineum. In Central and South America the head, especially the scalp, is the usual site of involvement.

The skin lesions are characterized by pruritus, edema, thickening and wrinkling, atrophy, and altered pigmentation of the skin. When the depigmentation is spotted it is known as "leopard skin"; when thickened, as "elephant skin."

Another type of skin involvement may be the generalized vesicopapular eruption, which becomes impetiginized and verrucose. Ichthyotic and hyperkeratotic patches may develop with lichenoid dermatitis.

In about 5 per cent of the affected persons serious eye lesions arise late in the disease, gradually leading to blindness.

ETIOLOGY. Onchocerciasis is caused by *Onchocerca volvulus*, which is transmitted to man by the bite of the black fly of the genus *Simulium*, which breeds in fast-flowing streams of water. When the black fly bites it introduces larvae into the wound. Adulthood is attained in the subdermal connective tissue in about one year. Millions of the progeny migrate back into the dermis and the humor of the eye.

EPIDEMIOLOGY. The disease occurs in Africa on the west coast, in the Sahara, Sudan, and the Victoria

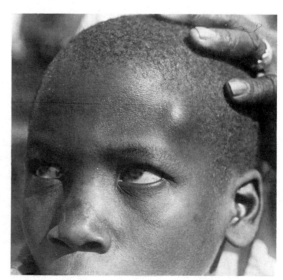

Figure 20–28. Nodule of onchocerciasis on forehead. The skin is of normal appearance. The danger of blinding eye lesions is increased. (Courtesy of Dr. Anthony Bryceson, London.)

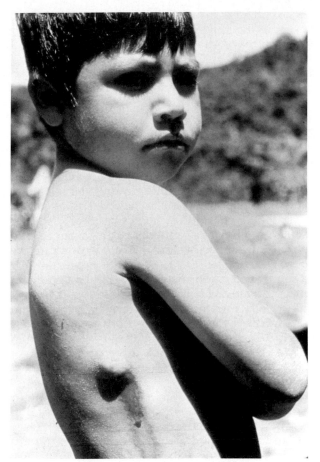

Figure 20–29. Onchocercoma. (Courtesy of Dr. Axel W. Hoke.)

Nile division, where this disease is known as *river blindness*. In Central and South America it is to be found in Guatemala, Brazil, Venezuela, and southern Mexico, where it is endemic in the provinces of Oaxaca and Chiapas. In a recent survey in Chiapas 50 per cent of the population was found to be infected. Onchocerciasis constitutes one of Mexico's major public health problems. Some 20 million people are said to be infected in Mexico.

DIAGNOSIS. The presence of eosinophilia, skin lesions, and onchocercomas with ocular lesions is highly suggestive in endemic areas. Frequently the microfilariae may be found in skin shavings or dermal lymph even when no nodules are detectable. The scapular area is the favorite site for procuring specimens for examination by means of a "skin snip." This is done in the field or office by lifting the skin with an inserted needle and then clipping off a small superficial portion of the skin with a sharp knife or scissors. The specimen is laid in a drop of normal saline on a slide, covered with a coverslip, and examined under the microscope. The filariae wriggle out at the edges of the skin slice.

A patient suspected to have onchocerciasis may be given a single oral dose of 50 mg of diethylcarbamazine. A reaction consisting of edema, itching, fever, arthralgias, and an exacerbation of pruritus is known as a positive Mazzotti test, which supports the diagnosis of onchocerciasis.

TREATMENT. Surgical excision of the nodules may be done whenever feasible. Greene et al treated with ivermectin, a veterinary microfilaricide with low

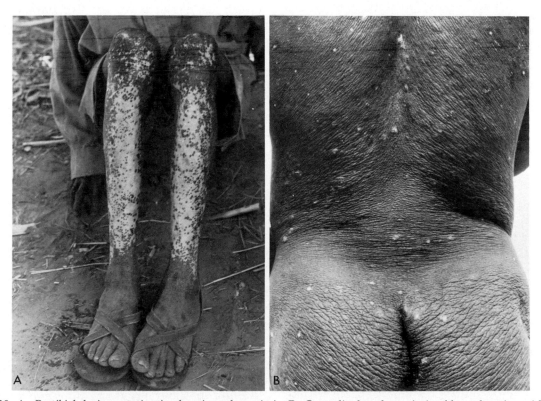

Figure 20–30. A, *Pretibial depigmentation in chronic onchocerciasis.* B, *Generalized onchocerciasis of long duration with thickening, edema, and atrophy of the skin with excoriation. (Courtesy of Dr. Anthony Bryceson, London.)*

toxicity, and saw no adverse reactions to a single oral dose of 200 micrograms per kilo body weight. With ivermectin, skin microfilaria counts remain low at the end of six months' observation. It is the drug of choice. Patients with skin disease only may be treated with the alternative drug, diethylcarbamazine. Neither drug affects adult worms. The doses given are as follows: day 1, 50 mg; day 2, 50 mg three times; day 3, 100 mg three times; and days 4–21, 3 mg/kg three times daily.

Suramin may be used to rid the patient of the adult worms. This drug is quite toxic and should be used only in patients who have recurrent disease after several courses of ivermectin or diethylcarbamazine therapy, or in patients with eye involvement in whom ivermectin fails.

Browne SG: Calcinosis circumscripta of the scrotal wall. Br J Dermatol 1962, 74:136.
Greene BM, et al: Comparison of ivermectin and diethyl carbamazine in the treatment of onchocerciasis. N Engl J Med 1985, 313:133.
Rozenman D, et al: Onchocerciasis in Israel. Arch Dermatol 1984, 120:505.
Somorin AO: Onchocerciasis. Int J Dermatol 1983, 22:182.
Yarzabal L: The immunology of onchocerciasis. Int J Dermatol 1985, 25:349.

Trichinosis

Ingestion of *Trichinella spiralis* larva–containing cysts in inadequately cooked pork, bear, or walrus meat may cause trichinosis. It usually causes a puffy edema of the eyelids, redness of the conjunctivae, and sometimes urticaria associated with hyperpyrexia, headache, erythema, gastrointestinal symptoms, muscle pains, and neurologic signs and symptoms. In 20 per cent of cases a macular or petechial eruption occurs, and splinter hemorrhages are occasionally present. Eosinophilia is not constant but may be as high as 80 per cent. In the average patient eosinophilia begins about a week after infection and attains its height by the fourth week. Rapidly fatal cases of proved trichinosis have been reported without eosinophilia. Gay et al reported a patient, infected from uncooked sausage meat, who died five weeks after onset of brain involvement with right parietal hemorrhage, despite 16 mg of dexamethasone daily. The intradermal skin test gives an immediate (15 minute) response with few false positive reactions, but it usually does not become positive before the third week of infection.

The immunofluorescence antibody test has the greatest value in establishing a diagnosis. The bentonite flocculation test is also reliable. It was negative at the sixth week, however, in Gay et al's fatal case. The serum enzymes—glutamic, oxaloacetic, and pyruvic transaminases—are elevated in the acute stages.

Diagnosis is confirmed by muscle biopsy demonstrating larvae of *Trichinella spiralis* in striated muscle. Unfortunately trichinae cannot usually be demonstrated unless the infection is very heavy, of over a month's duration, and the biopsy is very large. A 2-mm thick slice of the muscle biopsy may be compressed between two glass slides to demonstrate the cysts.

An ELISA test to demonstrate infection in pigs was developed in 1985 by Despommier and the USDA after 35 years of trying. It should be possible soon to have all marketed pork certified as safe from *Trichina* infestation.

Treatment is with thiabendazole (Mintezol), 50 mg/kg body weight daily. The *Medical Letter* recommends 25 mg/kg b.i.d. for five days (maximum 3 gm/day). Corticosteroids are effective as a means of controlling the often severe allergic reactions; 40–80 mg (for an adult) should control these for at least two or three weeks, without side effects.

Gay T, et al: Fatal CNS trichinosis. JAMA 1982, 247:1024.
Labzoffsky NA, et al: Fluorescent test for trichinosis. Can Med Assoc 1964, 90:920.
Testing for trichinosis. Science 1985, 227:621.

PHYLUM ARTHROPODA

The following classes are of dermatologic significance: myriapoda, insecta, and arachnida. This phylum contains more species than all the other phyla put together. Because of its complexity, the class and order of the organisms in this phylum will be given in many instances.

Injury from venoms of the arthropods (envenomization) is a common hazard in temperate and tropical regions. Arthropodal venoms may be mixtures of the following toxin types: vesicating toxin, producing vesicles and bullae; neurotoxins, attacking the nervous system and producing respiratory paralysis and death; hemolytic toxin; and hemorrhagic toxin. Anaphylactic shock is the most serious type of reaction encountered from envenomization; however, this happens but rarely. Scott reported about 25,000 envenomizations per year that caused severe injury, with about 26 deaths.

CLASS MYRIAPODA

Centipede Stings. These are manifested by paired hemorrhagic puncta surrounded by an erythematous swelling that may progress into a brawny edema or lymphangitis and lymphadenopathy. Locally there may be intense itching and pain, sometimes associated with toxic constitutional symptoms.

The western United States species of *Scolopendra*, which will sting, attain a length of 15 to 20 cm; their size is frightening. In the eastern United States the common house centipede, *Scutigera coleopterata*, does not sting man. *Scolopendra subspinipes*, in Hawaii, inflicts a painful sting. Rubbing with raw garlic, using a cut clove, may rapidly relieve the pain, but injection of topical anesthetic into the bite site is more effective.

Millipede Burns. Millipedes' bodies secrete a toxic liquid which, when it comes in contact with human skin, causes a brownish pigmentation which progresses over the next 24 hours to intense erythema and finally vesiculation. Intense stinging and burning pain is present. Washing off the toxin as soon as possible will curb the toxic effects. Topical corticosteroids should be helpful.

CLASS INSECTA

Order Lepidoptera

This order includes the butterflies and moths and their larval forms, the caterpillars.

Caterpillar Dermatitis. Irritation is produced by the nettling hairs coming in contact with the skin, the toxin in the hairs producing local pruritic erythematous macules and wheals at the area of contact. Edwards et al document a case in which both contact urticaria and delayed allergic contact dermatitis resulted from contact with a saddleback caterpillar. If the hairs get into the clothing, widespread dermatitis with conjunctivitis, nausea, and vomiting may result. Not only the caterpillars but their egg covers and cocoons may have the stinging hairs that produce irritation. Stinging caterpillars abound seasonally in the fall and are frequently seen on campers, children playing in trees, and lumberjacks in pine forests.

In the United States the most common caterpillars are the brown-tail moth caterpillar (*Nygmia phoeorrhoea*), puss caterpillar (*Megalopyge opercularis*), saddleback caterpillar (*Sibine stimulae*), crinkled flannel moth (*Megalopyge crispata*), slug caterpillar, and flannel moth (*Norape cretata*). The hairs of the processionary caterpillar (*Thaumetopoea processionea*) of Europe are especially dangerous to the eyes.

Moth Dermatitis. The malady is initiated by the hairs of the brown-tail moth (*Euproctis chrysorrhoea*), the goat moth (*Cossus cossus*), the puss moth (*Dicranura vinula*), the gypsy moth (*Liparis dispar*), and the Douglas fir tussock moth (*Hemenocampa pseudotsugata*).

In Latin America, the moths of the genus *Hylesia* are most frequently the cause of moth dermatitis. Severe conjunctivitis and pruritus are the first signs; shortly afterward erythematous papules and occasional ecthymatous lesions appear over the entire body, including the covered parts. Usually the le-

sions subside in about one week, but a mini-epidemic of *Caripito itch* reported by Dinehart et al lasted for over three weeks in the crew of a ship, which was, however, overwhelmingly infested with dead moths and urticating setae (hairs). Berger detailed an outbreak of Korean yellow moth dermatitis due to *Euproctis flava* Bremer.

Topical applications of various analgesics and antibiotics and oral antihistaminics are of no help. Bathing and changing clothes may help.

Berger TG: Korean yellow moth dermatitis. J Assoc Milit Dermatol 1986, 12:32.

Berman BA, et al: Gypsy moth caterpillar dermatitis. Cutis 1983, 31:251.

Crissey JT: Bedbugs: an old problem with a new dimension. Int Dermatol 1981, 20:411.

DeJong MCJM, et al: Investigative studies of dermatitis caused by larva of the browntail moth. Arch Dermatol 1975, 253:287.

Dinehart SM: Caripito itch: dermatitis from contact with *Hylesia* moths. JAAD 1985, 13:743.

Edwards EK Jr, et al: Contact urticaria and allergic contact dermatitis to the saddleback caterpillar with histologic correlation. Int J Dermatol 1986, 25:467.

Hoover AW, et al: Skin symptoms of tussock moth infestation. Cutis 1974, 13:597.

Rohr AS, et al: Successful immunotherapy for *Triatoma protracta*—induced anaphylaxis. J Allerg Clin Immunol 1984, 73:369.

Order Hemiptera

The bugs represent this order. They have two pairs of wings, usually modified, and a sucking mouth part. Among this order are bedbugs, water bugs, chinch bugs, stink bugs, squash bugs, and conenose bugs (kissing bugs, assassin bugs). The latter are vectors of South American trypanosomiasis.

CIMICOSIS (Bedbug Bites)

The bedbug (*Cimex lectularius*) is a smelly parasite with nonfunctioning wings, found all over the world. It hides in crevices during the daytime and feeds on human blood at night. When the bedbug punctures the skin the bite is painless but saliva is released and resulting hypersensitivity to a protein in the saliva leads to an urticarial or purpuric reaction about the punctum several hours later. One bedbug may produce several bites in the course of the night, chiefly on the exposed surfaces, these often being arranged in a line. The bite is at first painless and some persons react to it scarcely at all. They may not be aware of what has happened until they awake in the morning to find their nightclothing and bed stained with blood. Other persons react violently, with pronounced urticaria and pain. Papular urticaria and even extensive erythemas, urticaria, and even anaphylaxis have been reported, associated with the bites. Itching hives which are worse in the morning than later in the day are suggestive.

The bedbug is an oval, flattened, brown bug, about 5 mm long, with three pairs of legs. The female must

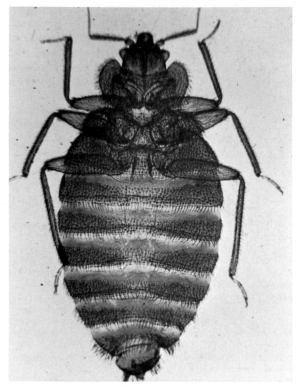

Figure 20–31. Bedbug (Cimex lectularius), *magnified about 15 times. (Courtesy of Dr. H. W. Brown.)*

have a blood meal to lay eggs, which are deposited into the corners of wooden bedsteads and other crevices. The bedbug may survive starvation for many months and is readily transported in baggage and clothing.

The 1-mm operculated eggs are laid at the rate of two daily and hatch in four to 10 days. The bugs mature in about six weeks, after several moltings. The life span is up to a year. Hepatitis B surface antigen has been repeatedly demonstrated in the bugs, and it is thought that hepatitis may be transmitted in this way.

Treatment is by the use of soothing antipruritic lotions containing menthol or phenol. Topical steroid creams are effective, and in extensive reactions systemic antihistaminics are useful. Crevices in the furniture, floor, and walls should be sprayed with 0.1 per cent trichlorfon spray or a pyrethrum spray. Malathion 0.5 per cent spray is also effective. A 0.5 per cent solution of lindane may be used. An infested house may also be treated by methyl bromide fumigation. Crissey urges obtaining the professional services of an exterminator; amateur efforts, he suggests, are likely to be unsuccessful.

KISSING BUG (Reduviid) BITES

The kissing bugs (assassin bugs, or conenoses), do not infest man but descend upon him individually, often when he is asleep, and feed upon an exposed area of skin, often of the face; hence the name "kissing bug." The bite is painless, but somewhat

itchy. The bug immediately defecates, and if the bug is an intestinal carrier of *Trypanosoma cruzi*, the organism is rubbed into the bite—a regular manner of spread of this disease. In nonendemic areas, the bite is often followed by a red swelling suggestive of cellulitis, which soon subsides. Anaphylaxis has also occurred, and Rohr et al have reported successful immunotherapy for immediate hypersensitivity to the bite of *T. protracta*, a variety commonly encountered in Southern California.

Order Anoplura

PEDICULOSIS (Phthiriasis)

Three varieties of these flattened, wingless insects commonly attack man, although others infest the lower animals and may become temporarily deposited upon human hosts. They are *Pediculus humanus* var. *capitis* (head louse), *P. humanus* var. *corporis* (body louse), and *Pthirus pubis* (pubic or crab louse). "*Pthirus*" (which should be *Phthirus*, from Greek, *phtheiros*) is an editorial or typographical error now affirmed as correct by the International Commission on Zoological Nomenclature, for the crab louse.

Each variety of louse has a predilection for certain parts of the body and rarely migrates to other regions. They attach themselves to the skin and live upon the blood that they suck. In piercing the skin the parasites exude an antigenic salivary secretion. This, together with the mechanical puncture, produces a pruritic dermatitis.

In addition, the louse may be a carrier of disease and through its bite or excretions may transmit an infectious disease—epidemic typhus, relapsing fever, or trench fever.

Pediculosis Capitis

This is encountered principally in children, but occurs in adults also. There is usually intense pruritus of the scalp, and the affected hairs become lusterless and dry. Because of the itching, secondary complications with impetigo and furunculosis are common. The pediculi may be seen on the scalp, but more often only the nits are seen. Owing to secondary infection, the cervical lymph glands may become enlarged.

The diagnosis usually presents no difficulties, but occasionally pediculi and nits are so sparse that repeated examination is necessary to discover them. The disease should be suspected in cases of impetigo or furunculosis of the scalp or face in children. It is easy to mistake peripilar keratin ("hair") casts encircling hair shafts, or the breaks of trichorrhexis nodosa, for nits. Scott et al have reviewed peripilar casts in detail.

Treatment of pediculosis capitis aims at destruction of the lice and the ova. Permethrin 1 per cent Creme Rinse contains a synthetic pyrethroid which is a relatively nontoxic and highly efficacious agent. Bowerman et al found it more effective than lindane. It is the drug of choice.

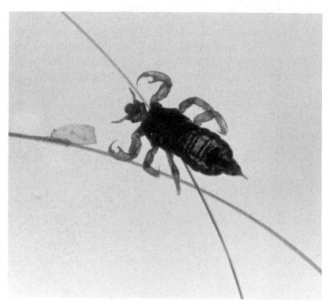

Figure 20–32. Head louse of pediculosis, P. capitis. (Courtesy of Dr. Axel W. Hoke.)

Gamma benzene hexachloride (lindane) shampoo (Kwell) may be thoroughly massaged into the scalp for four or five minutes, well rinsed out, and the hair dried; remaining nits may be removed with a fine-tooth comb, or forceps. Family members and

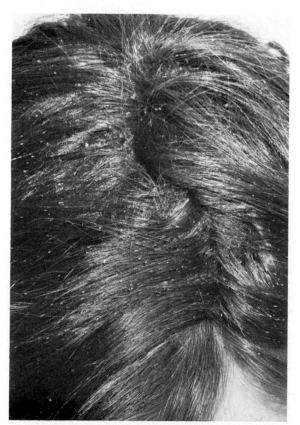

Figure 20–33. Nits on scalp hair infected with Pediculus humanus *var.* capitis.

contacts should be treated. Combs and brushes should be washed. Lindane should not be used on pregnant or nursing women.

Malathion lotion (Prioderm) reliably kills both adult lice and nits, according to Taplin, but it is still not available in the U.S.

Crotamiton (Eurax) in a 10 per cent cream or lotion is effective as a 24-hour application followed by a shampoo, according to Yawalker. Nits should be removed by combing: the effect of crotamiton on them is not known. Crotamiton is far less reliable than lindane.

Pyrethrins combined with piperonyl butoxide (RID, A-200, R+C Shampoo) are sold over the counter and come with a nit comb. They are applied to the scalp for 10 minutes and washed out. Retreatment in 'a week is recommended.

Shashindran et al in 1978 showed that cotrimoxazole by mouth killed all adult lice on the patient taking it, and Burns in 1987 suggested it worked by killing the bacteria in the gut of the lice, on which they are dependent.

Pediculosis Corporis

This is also known as pediculosis vestimenti or vagabond's disease. The lice causing this condition live chiefly in the seams of clothing, especially wherever there is pressure, and therefore warmth, as beneath the belt or the collar, or in bedding. The parasite is rarely discovered on the skin, but obtains its nourishment from it by descending to the skin and piercing it with its teeth. The disease causes generalized itching, which may be accompanied by erythematous macules or urticarial wheals due to the punctures, or by excoriated papules, parallel linear scratch marks, and a pigmented thickening of the skin from continued rubbing. Secondary furunculosis is common.

In the act of feeding the louse bores with its stylets into the skin until a blood space is reached. Instantly the blood of the victim is pumped into the louse with such force that its abdomen is distended and its color changes, so that the young louse appears as a small pink spot. As fresh blood flows in one end, excreta are discharged from the other.

The diagnosis is, as a rule, readily established by the generalized itching, by parallel scratch marks, by hyperpigmentation, and by erythematous macules. It is differentiated from scabies by the freedom of the hands and feet from involvement and by its predilection for the upper back. Pruritus and urticaria may cause some confusion. The diagnosis is positively established by finding the lice or nits in the seams of clothing or in bedding.

Destruction of the lice is accomplished by laundering the clothing and bedding. Dry cleaning destroys lice on wool garments. Pressing woolens, especially the seams, at home is also satisfactory. The patient should bathe thoroughly with soap and water. One per cent malathion powder is dusted onto the inner surface of the underwear, with particular attention being given to the seams.

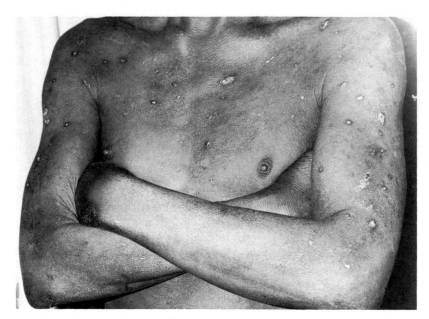

Figure 20–34. Pediculosis corporis. (Courtesy of Dr. J. Stricker.)

Pediculosis Pubis (Crabs)

This disease is contracted chiefly by adults as the result of sexual intercourse, and not infrequently from bedding. *Pthirus* (official spelling) *pubis*, the crab louse, usually limits its incursions to the genital region and hypogastrium or, rarely, the axillae or eyelashes (*pediculosis palpebrarum*). The lice are found on the skin, to which they cling tightly, appearing as yellowish brown or gray specks. Being almost the color of the skin, they are difficult to identify, and for this reason the infestation may exist a long time before its recognition. The nits are attached to the hairs at an acute angle. The symptoms vary from slight discomfort to intolerable itching.

Pediculosis pubis frequently coexists with other sexually transmitted diseases, particularly gonorrhea and trichomoniasis, and to a lesser extent scabies, nongonococcal urethritis, genital warts, candidiasis, and syphilis. The diagnosis of pediculosis pubis should initiate a search for other sexually transmitted diseases. In this setting, HIV infection should be suspected.

Occasionally, peculiar bluish or slate-colored macules that do not itch, or disappear on diascopic pressure, occur in association with pediculosis pubis. These macules, about 0.5 cm in diameter, are located chiefly on the sides of the trunk and on the inner aspects of the thighs. They are most noticeable in blonds. The spots, called *maculae ceruleae*, are probably due to altered blood pigments of the infested human, or to an excretion product from the louse's salivary gland. They may persist for several months.

A recommended treatment is Kwell or Gamene

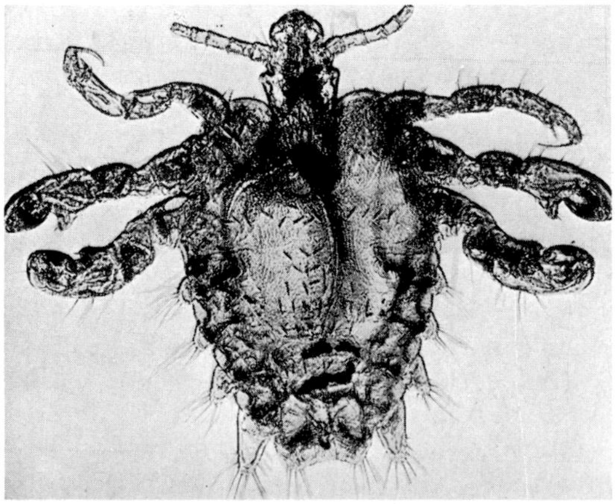

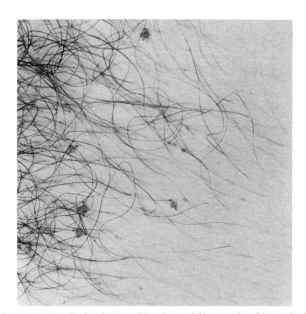

Figure 20–35. Crab louse, female (Pthirus pubis). (×60.) (Courtesy of Army Medical Museum.)

Figure 20–36. Pediculosis pubis. Several lice on the skin and nits on the hair shafts are visible.

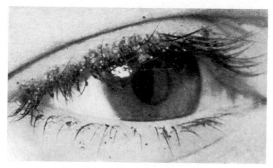

Figure 20–37. Pediculosis palpebrarum in association with pediculosis pubis. (Courtesy of Dr. C. S. Wright.)

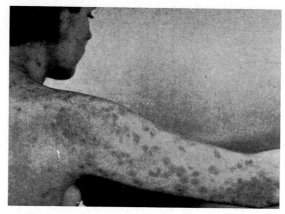

Figure 20–39. Maculae ceruleae. The color is due to saliva of louse, which changes bilirubin to biliverdin.

(lindane) cream, lotion, or shampoo. The lotion or cream is applied to infested areas and washed off eight hours later, or the shampoo is applied for four minutes and washed off. It should not be used in pregnant women or nursing mothers. RID or NIX (permethrin 1 per cent Creme Rinse) is safe and at least as effective as Kwell. They are applied for ten minutes and washed off. A second application is made in ten days. Sexual contacts should be treated simultaneously. Therapy for eyelash involvement is the use of petrolatum applied thickly twice daily for eight days, followed by removing any remaining nits mechanically. Fluorescein drops are also effective. Clothing and fomites should be washed by machine and automatically dried, or laundered and ironed.

Altschuler DZ, et al: Pediculicide performance, profit, and the public health. Arch Dermatol 1986, 122:259.

Baer RL, et al: Current views on the management of pediculosis and scabies. Cutis 1981, Supplement to September issue, pp. 5–31 (7 articles).

Bowerman JC, et al: Comparative study of permethrin 1% creme rinse and lindane shampoo for the treatment of head lice. Pediatr Infec Dis 1987, 6:252.

Burns DA: Action of cotrimoxazole on head lice (letter). Br J Dermatol 1987, 117:399.

Kalter DC, et al: Treatment of pediculosis pubis. Arch Dermatol 1987, 123:1315.

Kucirka SA, et al: The story of lindane resistance and head lice. Int J Dermatol 1983, 22:551.

Mathias RG, et al: Comparative trial of treatment with prioderm lotion and Kwellada shampoo in children with head lice. Can Med Assoc J 1984, 130:407.

Meinking TL, et al: Comparative efficacy of treatments for pediculosis capitis infestations. Arch Dermatol 1986, 122:267.

Robinson DH, et al: Control of head lice in schoolchildren. Curr Ther Res 1980, 27:1.

Rasmussen JE: Pediculosis. In Callen JE, Advances in Dermatology, 1986, 1:109.

Scott MJ Jr, et al: Hair casts. JAAD 1983, 8:27.

Shashindran CH, et al: Oral therapy of pediculosis capitis with cotrimoxazole. Br J Dermatol 1978, 98:699.

Smith DE, et al: Treatment of pubic lice infestation: comparison of two agents. Cutis 1980, 26:618.

Taplin D, et al: Malathion for treatment of pediculus. . .infestation. JAMA 1982, 247:3130.

Urcuyo FG, et al: Malathion lotion as an insecticide and ovicide for head louse infestation. Int J Dermatol 1986, 25:60.

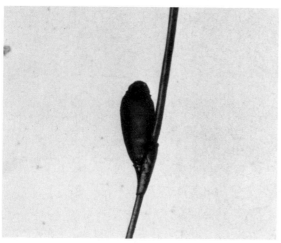

Figure 20–38. Nit attached to hair shaft.

Order Diptera

This order includes the two-winged biting flies. Both the adults and the larvae parasitize man in many ways. Owing to the tremendous number of species, only a few may be mentioned, according to family.

Tabanidae are the horsefly, deerfly, gadfly, and others, which inflict extremely painful bites.

Muscidae include the housefly, stablefly, and the tsetse fly (which transmits trypanosomiasis). Tsetse fly bites usually cause no reaction the first time; however, repeated bites will cause severe reactions so that desensitization may be necessary. Larvae of these flies may infest the skin (myiasis).

Simulidae are represented by the black fly, buffalo gnat, and coffee fly, some being vectors of onchocerciasis. These flies are usually dark-colored and "hunchbacked." They may produce extremely painful bites that may be associated with fever, chills, and lymphadenitis. Black flies are seasonal annoyances in the northern United States and Canada.

Psychodidae are small hairy flies (sandflies). The phlebotomous flies are of importance as vectors of cutaneous leishmaniasis, mucocutaneous leishmaniasis, and verruga peruana.

Culicidae, mosquitoes, are vectors of many important diseases, such as filariasis, malaria, dengue, and yellow fever. Their bites may cause severe urticarial reactions.

Ceratopogonidae, the biting midges or gnats, fly in swarms and produce erythematous edematous lesions at the site of the bite, as described by Steffan.

Three specific problems created by members of the Diptera order will be discussed.

Mosquito Bites. The bloodsucking mosquitoes belong to the subfamily of Culicinae.

The attraction of mosquitoes to hosts has received much study, which A. W. A. Brown has compiled. He finds that numerous factors affect the attraction of mosquitoes to man, notably moisture, warmth, carbon dioxide, and estrogens. Another attracting substance is L-lactic acid in sweat.

The cutaneous reaction to a mosquito bite may be, in its simplest form, a pruritic local wheal which promptly subsides. A more severe reaction is an immediate allergic response, with a subsequent delayed reaction and even with a systemic response. Urticaria is not an unusual reaction, especially in visitors or new residents, and may be intermittent, continuing for approximately one week.

Treatment of mosquito bites usually offers no great problems. For the ordinary bite, application of one of the corticosteriod creams is satisfactory. Meat tenderizer affords rapid relief. The use of mosquito repellents upon the skin and clothing is recommended for those sensitive to mosquito bites. Diethyltoluamide (DEET) has been found to be the most effective. Other good repellents are chlorodiethyl benzamide, ethyl hexanediol, and dimethyl phthalate. DEET is available commercially under the trade name of Off!, Sportsmate II cream, and Cutter Laboratories' Insect Repellent. Ethyl hexanediol, also a good repellent, is available from Union Carbide as 6–12 Plus, liquid, stick, or spray. An excellent repellent is Avon's "Skin-So-Soft" or almost any commercial emollient or moisturizer.

Barnard JH: Cutaneous responses to insects. JAMA 1966, 196:259.
Brown AWA: The attraction of mosquitoes to hosts. JAMA 1966, 196:249.
Gilbert IH: Evaluation and use of mosquito repellents. JAMA 1966, 196:253.
Penneys NS, et al: Mosquito salivary gland antigens identified by circulating human antibodies. Arch Dermatol 1989, 125:219.
Pistone GA: Avon's "Skin-So-Soft" is an effective insect repellent. Schoch Letter 1988, 38:35.

Ked Itch. The sheep ked (*Melophagus ovinus*) crawls into the sheep's wool and feeds by thrusting its sharp mouth parts into the skin and sucking blood. Occasionally it attacks woolsorters and sheepherders, causing pruritic, often hemorrhagic papules, nearly always with a central punctum. The papules are very persistent and may last for up to 12 months. Favorite locations are the hips and the abdomen.

Myiasis. The invasion of mammalian tissues by dipterous (fly) larvae is known as myiasis. The larvae of several varieties of flies produce cutaneous manifestations. The eggs, living larvae, or both are deposited on the skin or mucous membranes, where they hatch and produce larvae, which burrow into the skin and cause mild or severe inflammatory changes. Others migrate to folds of skin and burrow into the subcutaneous tissue, producing an inflammatory reaction which gives the appearance of a furuncle, at whose center maggots may be seen.

Some varieties of flies puncture the skin and extrude the ova beneath the surface (furuncular myiasis), whereas others deposit their eggs on open wounds or ulcers (traumatic or wound myiasis). In

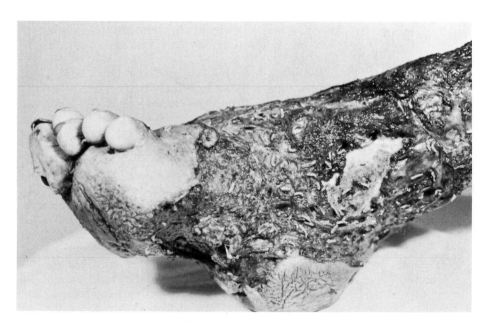

Figure 20–40. Maggots in ulcer on leg. (Courtesy of Dr. F. Kerdel-Vegas.)

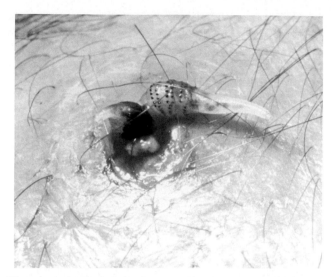

Figure 20–41. Miyiasis; Dermatobia hominis. (Courtesy of Dr. Axel W. Hoke.)

this type of wound myiasis, larvae hatch out on the skin and maggots crawl about in the dirty ulcerated area.

A third type, known as *creeping* eruption, develops when the larvae of the *Gasterophilus* wander intradermally. The most common species are *G. nasalis* and *G. intestinalis*. An itching pink papule develops, followed by a tortuous line extending 1 to 30 cm daily. The larva may be picked out with a needle once localized.

One species of fly that causes furuncular myiasis in North America is the *Wohlfahrtia vigil*. The gravid fly lays its eggs on the skin, then the hatched larvae migrate to folds of skin, into which they burrow. An inflammatory reaction, first as a papule, then as a furuncular lesion, is produced. Maggots may be seen in this lesion, and it seems to pulsate.

They can penetrate infant skin, but not adult. Thus nearly all reported cases have occurred in infants. F. D. Smith et al reported a case in a boy five days old with furuncular skin lesions from the largest of which two larvae were recovered. They were reared on Sabouraud's agar while awaiting identification in the laboratory.

The human botfly *D. hominis* is a common cause of furuncular myiasis in the neotropical region of the New World. It is a serious economic pest when it affects cattle. It has an interesting life cycle. The female glues its eggs to the body of a mosquito, stablefly, or tick. When the unwitting vector punctures the skin by biting, the larvae emerge from the egg and enter the skin through the puncture wound. Over a period of several days a painful furuncle develops in which the larva is present. File et al reported a case seen in a traveller who had been in Brazil.

In tropical Africa the Tumbu fly, or *ver du cayor* (*Cordylobia anthropophaga*), deposits her eggs on the ground, and the active young maggot attacks and

penetrates the skin of its host, especially on the forearm, the scrotum, the upper part of the thigh, and the buttock. Kozminska-Kubarska cured a man with a lesion of the glans penis by extracting a centimeter-long larva from it. The lesion resembles an inflamed tumor, from which the larvae emerge in six or seven days. In the ordinary course of events these tumors do not suppurate. The fly usually attacks mammals other than man.

March reported a case of *ver du cayor* myiasis occurring in New York City in a man who had just returned from Tanzania. A total of 31 maggotlike worms 3 mm in length were found, each in an individual erythematous insect-bitelike lesion. Schorr reported a similar case in Wisconsin in a missionary returned from Tanzania.

According to Scott, other larvae frequently causing furuncular lesions in North America are the screwworm (*Cochliomyia hominivorax*), common cattle grub (*Hypoderma lineatum*), sarcophagid fly (*Wohlfahrtia vigil*), and rabbit botfly (*Cuterebra cuniculi*).

The insect that commonly causes wound myiasis is the screwworm fly (*Chrysomyia macellaria*). This disease occurs in tropical South America, Central America, and Texas, but cases have been reported from as far north as Alaska. *Callitroga americana* is the cause of nearly 90 per cent of cases of human myiasis in the U.S. The black blowfly (*Phormia regina*), which affects principally goats and sheep and occasionally man, is also an important cause in this country. Spigel recently reported such a case. This fly is common around houses, privies, and packing establishments.

Treatment of wound myiasis is by surgical removal of the maggots and douching of the wound for 30 minutes with 15 per cent chloroform dissolved in any light vegetable oil.

Treatment of furuncular myiasis is through the injection of local anesthetic into the skin, which anesthetizes both the skin and the larva. Then the

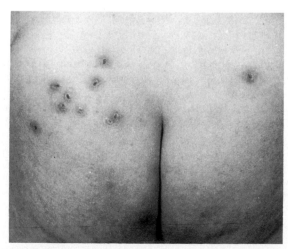

Figure 20–42. Tumbu fly myiasis. Dome-shaped furuncular lesion with central craters through which maggots are evacuated. (Courtesy of Dr. W. E. Schorr and Arch Dermatol 95:61, 1977.)

larva is surgically removed by incising the lesion or by pushing the larva out with pressure from beneath. Sauder et al reported that inhabitants of endemic areas apply pork fat to the skin. This is occlusive, and after 24 hours the larva migrate out of the skin in order to avoid asphyxiation.

Baumhover AH: Eradication of the screwworm fly. JAMA 1966, 196:240.

File TM J Jr, et al: *Dermatobia hominis* dermal myiasis. Arch Dermatol 1985, 121:1195.

Kenney RL, et al: Botfly (*Dermatobia hominis*) myiasis. Int J Dermatol 1984, 23:676.

Kozminska-Kubarska A: *Cordylobia anthropophaga* infestation. Int J Dermatol 1981, 20:495.

Lane RP, et al: Human cutaneous myiasis. Clin Exp Dermatol 1987, 12:40.

Nunzio E, et al: Removal of *Dermatobia hominis* larvae. Arch Dermatol 1986, 122:140.

Sauder DN, et al: Dermal myiasis: the porcine lipid cure (letter). Arch Dermatol 1981, 117:681.

Schorr WF: Tumbu-fly myiasis in Marshfield, Wis. Arch Dermatol 1967, 95:61.

Smith FD, et al: Furuncular myiasis caused by *Wohlfahrtia vigil* (Walker). Arch Dermatol 1981, 117:119.

Spigel GT: Opportunistic cutaneous myiasis. Arch Dermatol 1988, 124:1014.

Steffen C: Clinical and histopathologic correlation of midge bites. Arch Dermatol 1981, 117:785.

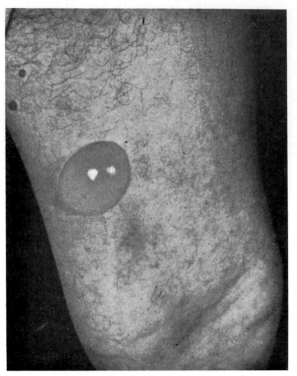

Figure 20–43. Blister beetle bulla above knee. (Courtesy of Dr. C. March.)

Order Coleoptera

Blister Beetle Dermatitis. The Meloidae family contains the blister beetle, which produces injury to the skin by releasing a vesicating agent, *cantharidin*, abundant in its reproductive organs. Cantharidin is sometimes used for the treatment of verruca vulgaris but it often converts a medium-size wart into a much larger annular one. The clematis blister beetle (*Epicauta cinerea*) usually does not excrete cantharidin when it is on the skin except when pressure is placed upon it; then a clear amber hemolymph is excreted from its knee joints, prothorax, and genitalia. Slight burning and tingling of the skin occur in a few minutes, and within a day single or multiple bullae develop, which may be arranged in a linear fashion.

Several species are used medicinally, the best known among these being the "Spanish fly" (*Lytta vesicatoria*), prevalent in southern Europe. Blister beetles are common in all parts of the world. *Epicauta vittata* and *E. pennsylvanica* are found in southern and southwestern United States, according to Burnett et al, who reviewed the subject.

Treatment consists of drainage of the bullae and application of cold wet compresses and topical corticosteroid preparations. Preliminary cleansing with acetone, ether, soap, or alcohol may be helpful.

Paederus Dermatitis. The Staphylinidae family (rove beetles) contain the genus *Paederus*, which is responsible for erythematous vesicular eruptions at the site of contact of the vesicant with the skin. In South America this usually linear or patchy dermatitis is caused by *Paederus brasiliense*, commonly known as "*podo.*" It is frequent during the rainy season and appears predominantly on the neck and exposed parts.

In Venezuela *P. colombinus* causes this same type of blistering dermatitis. "Kissing lesions" are observed when the blister beetle's excretion is deposited in the flexures of the elbows or other folds. Here again a seasonal occurrence is seen, with the greatest incidence just after the rainy season. Paederin is the irritant.

Similar eruptions observed in Indonesia are attributed to *P. peregrinus*, in South India to *P. melampus*. They also occur in Australia, Africa, and France. In 1967, Fan and Chang reported occurrence of this in Taiwan, caused by *Paederus fuscipes*.

Carpet Beetle Dermatitis. Papulovesicular and urticarial dermatitis caused by the common carpet beetle (*Anthrenus scrophulariae*) was reported by Cormia and Lewis. The eruption involved the chest, neck, and forearms. The larvae inhabit warm houses throughout the winter months. They are reddish brown, fusiform, about 6 mm long, and covered by hairs.

A generalized pruritic eruption from larvae of a carpet beetle infesting two wool rugs was reported by Ahmed et al; the beetle was identified as *A. verbasci*. Fumigation of the house with sulfuryl fluoride (Vikane) abolished the larvae and solved the problem.

Ahmed AR, et al: Carpet beetle dermatitis. JAAD 1981, 5:428.

Burnett JW, et al: Blister beetles: "Spanish fly." Cutis 1987, 39:22.

Fan J, et al: Paederus dermatitis. Dermatol Int 1967, 6:203.

Kerdel-Vegas F, et al: Paederus dermatitis. Arch Dermatol 1966, 94:175.

Scott HG: Blister beetle dermatitis produced by *Epicanta cinerea*. J Econ Entomol 1962, 55:145.

Order Hymenoptera

This order includes the bees, wasps, hornets, and ants. Stings by any of these may manifest the characteristic clinical and histologic features of eosinophilic cellulitis (Wells's syndrome) complete with flame figures, as shown by Schorr et al.

Bee Sting. Bees are stinging insects, which produce their sting by the ovipositor of the female abdomen. The venom contains many chemicals. Of importance in producing the clinical effects are histamine, mellitin, mast cell degranulating peptide, and phospholipase A, which cause histamine release from the victim's mast cells. The barbed ovipositor of the honeybee is torn out of the bee and remains in the skin after stinging. The bumble bee, wasp, and hornet are able to withdraw their stinger.

The reaction to these stings ranges from a mild local edema, pain, pruritus, and nausea to severe anaphylactic shock and death. The latter is more likely to occur in the case of multiple stings unless prompt therapy is possible. Hypersensitivity reactions have been shown to be mediated by specific IgE antibodies to individual members of this order. In bees phospholipase A is the principal sensitizing agent. Persons at risk should be warned to keep an emergency treatment kit (Ana-Kit) close at hand at all times.

The imbedded ovipositor containing the poison sac should be scraped away with a sharp knife. Grasping the sac to pull out the sting expresses more poison into the surrounding tissue. Removal is mandatory, since the stinger is not absorbed and will act as an irritant source as long as it remains imbedded. Rubbing with a dilute solution of meat tenderizer (papain) relieves pain very quickly.

Wasps. There are many types of wasps: hunting wasps, social wasps, digger wasps, yellow jackets, and hornets. Many of these can cause severe reactions. Bee and wasp stings may result in secondary infection, generalized allergic reaction, delayed serum-sickness-type reaction, or anaphylactic shock that may lead to death.

Fatal reactions may occur as soon as a few seconds after exposure. Loss of consciousness, cyanosis, involuntary urination, and general collapse leading to death is the usual course of a fatal reaction.

Treatment of local reactions consists of immediate application of ice packs, and antihistaminics to allay pruritus. Analgesics may be necessary for the severe pain, if it is not stopped by rubbing with a dilute solution of meat tenderizer (papain). If meat tenderizer is not available, a pulverized aspirin tablet may be rubbed into the moistened site. Moistening it again will renew the relief. Arnold recommends injecting, into the site of any painful or inflamed sting, 1 or 2 ml of a mixture of equal parts of 1 per cent triamcinolone diacetate (or acetonide) suspension or 0.6 per cent betamethasone solution, and 2 per cent lidocaine or procaine hydrochloride. A 30-gauge needle should be used. Relief is instantaneous and usually permanent.

For severe systemic reactions 0.3 ml epinephrine (1:1000 aqueous solution) is injected subcutaneously. This may need to be repeated for severe reactions. Corticosteroids and epinephrine may be required for several days following the severe reaction.

For persons who are frequently exposed to the hazard, hyposensitization procedures may be indicated. A combination whole-body bee, wasp, hornet, and yellow jacket antigen such as pyridine-extracted alum-precipitated insect antigen (Allpyral, Dome) was shown in the late 70s to be ineffective; venom immunotherapy, which was approved in 1980, is far superior. It is today the only protective treatment recommended. Susceptible persons should also carry a kit (Ana-Kit) containing syringe, epinephrine for injection, and antihistaminics.

Arnold HL Jr: Immediate treatment of insect stings (letter). JAMA 1972, 220:585.

Ewan PW: Allergy to insect stings: a review. J R Soc Med 1985, 78:234

Fikar C: Insect sting treatment. Pediatrics 1981, 68:744.

Frazier CA: The insect sting emergency kit. Drug Ther, June 1976:32.

Golden DBK, et al: Treatment failures with whole-body extract therapy of insect sting allergy. JAMA 1981, 246:2460.

Graft DF, et al: A prospective study of the natural history of large local reactions after hymenoptera stings in children. J Pediatr 1984, 104:664.

Hunt KJ, et al: Diagnosis of allergy to stinging insects by skin testing with Hymenoptera venom. Ann Intern Med 1976, 85:56.

Schorr WF: Eosinophilic cellulitis (Wells' syndrome) in arthropod bite reactions. JAAD 1984, 11:1043.

VonWitt R: Topical aspirin for wasp stings. Lancet 1980, 2:1379.

Ants. The sting of most ants is painful, but that of the fire ants (*Solenopsis saevissima, S. invicta, S. geminata,* or *S. xyloni*) is especially so. *S. saevissima* is especially ferocious and vicious and will produce many burning and painful stings within seconds if its nest is molested. Ginsburg reported on fire ant envenomation in children in the southern United States. The sting causes intense pain, whealing develops, and a hemorrhagic punctum may appear which later develops into a vesicle. Later, umbilicated pustules are seen. Seizures and mononeuropathy have been reported. The sting of *harvester ants* and *soldier ants* may produce similar reactions. Little or nothing can alleviate the severe pain except perhaps intralesional injections of triamcinolone. In the case of multiple stings epinephrine and systemic steroids are of decided benefit.

Triplett reported successful desensitization of 18 sensitive patients using an aqueous whole-body extract of *S. saevissima*. This is not generally accepted therapy, and specific antivenin is not available.

Brown LL: Fire and allergy. South Med J 1972, 65:273.

De Shazo RD, et al: Dermal hypersensitivity reactions to imported fire ants. J Allerg Clin Immunol 1984, 74:841.

Fox RW, et al: Neurologic sequelae following the imported fire ant sting. J Allerg Clin Immunol 1982, 70:120.

Ginsburg CM: Fire ant envenomation in children. Pediatrics 1984, 73:689.

Ross EV, et al: Meat tenderizer in the acute treatment of imported fire ant stings. JAAD 1987, 16:1189.

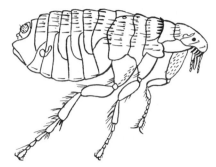

Figure 20–45. Cat flea, female (Ctenocephalides felis). *(Courtesy of C. J. Stojanovich, USPHS.)*

Order Siphonaptera

Fleas are wingless, with highly developed legs for jumping. They are bloodsucking parasites, infesting most warm-blooded animals. The flea's body is armored with chitin, and the mouth is highly specialized for penetration and sucking.

PULICOSIS (FLEA BITES)

Fleas exist universally among animals and human beings. The three species of fleas most commonly attacking man in this country are the human flea (*Pulex irritans*), the cat flea (*Ctenocephalides felis*), and the dog flea (*Ctenocephalides canis*).

Fleas are small, brown, wingless insects about one sixteenth of an inch long, and very flat from side to side, with long hind legs. They slip into the clothing or jump actively when disturbed. They are known to be extraordinary jumpers, which facilitates travel from host to host. They bite especially about the legs and waist and may be troublesome in houses where there are dogs or cats. They extract their blood meal from the superficial capillaries, causing hemorrhagic puncta surrounded by an erythematous and urticarial patch. The lesions are often grouped and may be arranged in zigzag lines. The irritation is produced by the injection into the skin of a fluid secreted by the salivary glands of the parasite. Some persons have hypersensitivity to this secretion and manifest immediate or delayed type reactions at the site of the bite, often assuming the clinical appearance of papular urticaria or, at times, eosinophilic cellulitis (Wells' syndrome).

These lesions may be associated with papular urticaria, extensive excoriations, and furunculosis; they may even resemble purpura.

Vectors of Disease. Fleas are important because the rat flea, *Xenopsylla cheopis*, as well as *X. braziliensis* are vectors of plague and endemic typhus. When the infected rat dies the flea seeks another host, which can be man or other rats. Sylvatic plague is spread by wild rodent fleas. Plague and tularemia are also transmitted by the squirrel flea, *Diamanus montanus*. Several species of fleas are intermediate hosts of the dog tapeworm and rat tapeworm, which may be an incidental parasite of man. The mouse flea, *Leptopsylla segnis*, and the chicken flea, *Ceratophyllus gallinae*, may also attack man.

Flea Control. Liquid and dust sprays are the most effective means of control. Rat nests and sleeping places of cats and dogs should be treated, since the larvae live on excreta of animals, dried blood, and other debris. In extensive rat control measures,

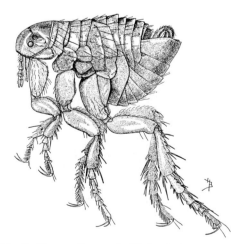

Figure 20–44. Human flea, male (Pulex irritans). *(Courtesy of US Department of Agriculture.)*

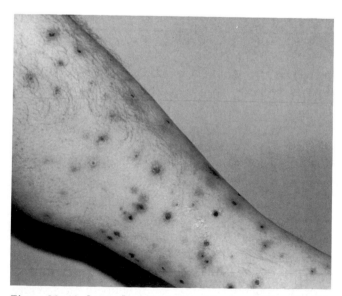

Figure 20–46. Severe flea bites on leg. (Courtesy of Dr. Alex W. Hoke.)

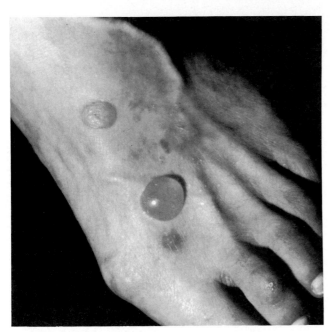

Figure 20–47. Bullae from flea bites.

spraying should be done first so that the fleas do not seek other hosts such as man. Spraying should include carpets, floors, and stuffed furniture. Some of the effective sprays are 5 per cent malathion powder or 1 per cent lindane dust, 0.5 per cent malathion, or chlordane in kerosene.

Insect repellents should be used. Off! and other preparations containing diethyltoluamide (DEET) and pyrethrum are some of the effective repellents.

Soothing lotions, and corticosteroid creams, lotions, or sprays, give prompt relief.

TUNGIASIS

CLINICAL FEATURES. The sand flea or chigoe (*Tunga penetrans*) is a minute parasite, resembling the common flea, which attacks the skin of man, swine, and many other lower animals. The lesions are pruritic swellings the size of a small pea. These usually occur on the ankles, feet, soles, and toes, particularly about the toenails and, less often, about the anogenital areas. The lesions become extremely painful and secondarily infected to produce extensive painful ulcers, which can be crippling.

Although the male and female sand fleas may live on the skin, it is only the impregnated female chigoe that burrows into the skin. The eggs are laid, and they drop to the ground. These eggs develop into larvae, which form cocoons from which the insect emerges in about 10 days. This cocoon when in the skin forms a fibrous sac called *nigua*.

EPIDEMIOLOGY. *Tunga penetrans* is known as nigua in Latin America. In other localities it is also known as chigoe, sand flea, or jigger. It is a reddish brown flea about 1 mm long. It resides in Equatorial Africa and in southern United States but more frequently in Central and South America. In the United States it has been reported in New Orleans. In America the parasite was already known by Columbus. Since that time descriptions by various authors have been numerous, as reported by Reiss. Zalar et al and Wentzell et al have reported cases diagnosed in travellers who acquired the disease elsewhere and presented to clinics in the United States.

TREATMENT. Curettage or excision of the burrows is recommended. Cardoso has described the use of thiabendazole, 25 mg per kg per day, as a successful oral therapy in heavily infested patients. Antibiotics should be used for the secondary infection and tetanus prophylaxis given. These lesions can be prevented by the wearing of shoes. Infested ground and buildings may be disinfested by the use of insecticides.

Cardoso A: Generalized tungiasis treated with thiabendazole. Arch Dermatol 1981, 117:127.
Heng MCY, et al: Pathogenesis of papular urticaria. JAAD 1984, 10:1030.
Milgraum SS, et al: A subungual nodule of recent onset. Arch Dermatol 1988, 124:429.
Reiss F: Tungiasis in New York City. Arch Dermatol 1966, 93:404.
Schorr WF, et al: Eosinophilic cellulitis (Wells' syndrome). JAAD 1984, 11:1043.
Wentzell JW, et al: Tungiasis. JAAD 1986, 15:117.
Zala GL, et al: Infestation by *Tunga penetrans*. Arch Dermatol 1980, 116:80.

CLASS ARACHNIDA

This class includes the ticks, mites, spiders, and scorpions. Adult arachnids have four pairs of legs. Their bodies consist of cephalothorax and abdomen.

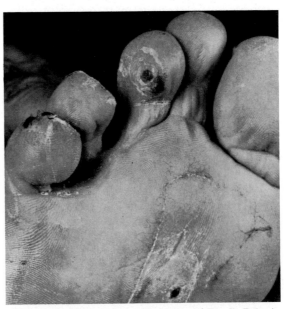

Figure 20–48. Tungiasis. (Courtesy of Dr. F. Reiss.)

Order Acarina

TICK BITE

Several varieties of the family Ixodidae (hard ticks) and Argasidae (soft ticks) occasionally attack human skin. The dog ticks *Dermacentor variabilis* and *Rhipicephalus sanguineus* are two of these. In the United States, the wood tick (*Dermacentor andersoni*) is the chief offender in western United States, having its habitat in wooded districts, being found especially on pine trees and in the underbrush. The ticks are found in the grass or bushes, which they leave to attach themselves to human beings, dogs, and cattle. This and the lone star tick (*Amblyomma americanum*) from Texas are the carriers of Rocky Mountain spotted fever and tick-borne encephalitis. Jones described a case of human "seed tick" infestation with the larva of *Amblyomma americanum*. *Ixodes ricinus* in Europe and *Ixodes dammini* and *I. pacificus* in the United States transmit *Borrelia burgdorferi*, the cause of Lyme disease (see Chapter 14). The kangaroo tick, *Amblyomma trigutatum*, and many other species of the hard ticks transmit Q fever to sheep.

The female tick attaches itself to the skin by sticking its proboscis into it to suck blood from the superficial vessels. The insertion of the hypostome is generally unnoticed by the subject, but in a few hours there appears an urticarial wheal at the place of puncture, which usually itches and is painful for several days. The parasite is engorged after 12 days and then falls off. During this time the patient may suffer from fever, chills, headache, abdominal pain, and vomiting. This is called *tick bite pyrexia*. Removal of the engorged ticks causes a subsidence of the general symptoms in 12 to 36 hours.

If an attempt is made to pull the tick off, the head is likely to be broken off and left in the skin. Hoehn advises tying a slip-knot in a piece of thread, tightening it around the neck of the tick, and pulling gently on it for three or four minutes, till the tick withdraws its head voluntarily. Then it can safely be crushed under foot. It will not (as the late Frances Keddie sagely observed) back into a hot match head or a lighted cigarette! Needham, an acarologist, has confirmed that gentle traction is superior to other methods, in a comparative study. If a portion of the

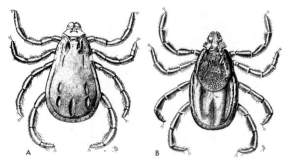

Figure 20–49. American dog tick (Dermacentor variabilis). A, Female; B, male. (Courtesy of the US Department of Agriculture.)

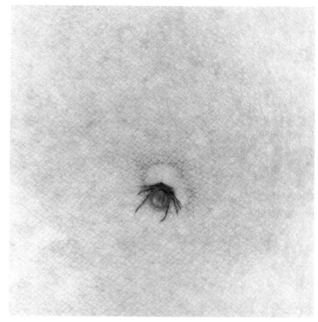

Figure 20–50. Tick bite. (Courtesy of Dr. Axel W. Hoke.)

tick is left in the skin it should be removed by excision.

The bites may be followed by small, severely pruritic, fibrous nodules (tick bite granulomas) that persist for months or even a year or two, or by pruritic circinate and arciform localized erythemas that may continue for months.

Tick Paralysis. This may rarely occur—usually in children—and it may be fatal unless the tick, lodged in the patient's skin, is removed promptly. Paralysis occurs about six days after attachment of the tick, commonly on the neck and back of the head. Usually there is no fever but it may be slight, with rapid pulse and respiration. The paralysis, of the flaccid type, attacks the legs, then the arms, and lastly the neck, resembling Landry-Guillain-Barré syndrome.

Bulbar paralysis, dysarthria, dysphagia, and death from respiratory failure may occur unless the tick is removed. Prompt recovery occurs if the tick is found and removed before the terminal stage.

It is thought that toxins elaborated by the ticks cause a presynaptic neuromuscular blockade with involvement of the peripheral nerves.

Other Tick Bite Disorders. Several species of ticks of the genus *Ixodes* (notably *I. dammini* and *I. ricinus* and *pacificus*) are of importance only as vectors of *Borrelia burgdorferi*, the causative agent of Lyme arthritis or Lyme disease. A skin lesion known as erythema chronicum migrans, annular and concentric with the bite, and spreading centrifugally, occurs at the bite site. It is discussed in Chapter 14.

Ronnen et al reported a case of ornithodoriasis which preceded *Borrelia duttonii* infection, the agent of African endemic relapsing fever. The bite of the tick *Ornithodorus tholozani* produced a typical small inflammatory nodule, surrounded by a zone of normal skin, with a circumferential brownish ring. Other

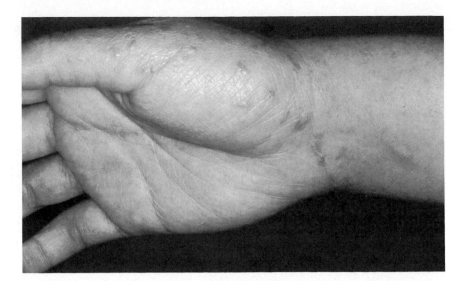

Figure 20–51. *Scabies on the wrist. Note coiled burrow. (Courtesy of Dr. Axel W. Hoke.)*

diseases besides Lyme disease and relapsing fever that are transmitted by ticks include rickettsioses (Rocky Mountain spotted fever, Q fever, boutonneuse fever, tick typhus), tularemia, babesiosis, arbovirus and ungrouped virus encephalitides, and hemorrhagic fevers.

Subcutaneous hemorrhage, chronic ulcerations, malignant lymphomalike tumors, and alopecia are other consequences of tick bites.

Protection from tick bites, according to Gouch, is best accomplished by the use of repellents in clothing, although these are only partially effective. The most effective of these have been found to be diethyltoluamide (DEET), Indalone, dimethyl carbamate, and dimethyl phthalate.

Feder IA: Tick pyrexia. JAMA 1944, 126:293.

Harper A: Tick paralysis. J Med Assoc Ga 1942, 31:422.

Hoehn G: How to remove a wood tick that's embedded. Schoch Letter 1986, 36:15.

Jones BE: Human seed tick infestation. Arch Dermatol 1981, 117:812.

Needham GR: Evaluation of five popular methods for tick removal. Pediatrics 1985, 75:997.

Ronnen M, et al: Ornithodoriasis preceding Borrelia infection. Arch Dermatol 1984, 120:1520.

MITES

Mites may parasitize man in several ways. Both the adult and larval form may invade the skin: some attack the skin only for feeding, others complete their life cycles in the skin.

SCABIES

CLINICAL FEATURES. Scabies is characterized by pruritic papular lesions and also burrows, which house the female mite and her young. Sites of predilection are chiefly the fingerwebs, wrists, antecubital fossae, axillae, areolae and areas around the umbilicus, the lower abdomen, genitals, and buttocks. An imaginary circle intersecting the main sites of election—axillae, elbow flexures, wrists and hands, and crotch—has long been called the *circle of Hebra*. In the adult the scalp and face are spared, but in infants lesions are present over the entire cutaneous surface. In immune-suppressed individuals, too, the face and scalp may be heavily infested.

The burrows form characteristic lesions barely discernible to the naked eye. These are slightly elevated, grayish, straight or tortuous lines in the skin. A vesicle or pustule may be produced at the end of the burrow, especially in infants and children.

The eruption varies considerably, depending on the manner of infection and previous treatment. It may also vary with climate and the host's immunologic status. Elpern raised the question of whether infantile acropustulosis, which may be seen in babies

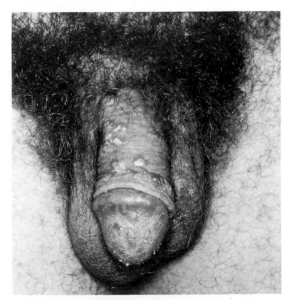

Figure 20–52. *Scabies. Note lesions on glans penis.*

A

B

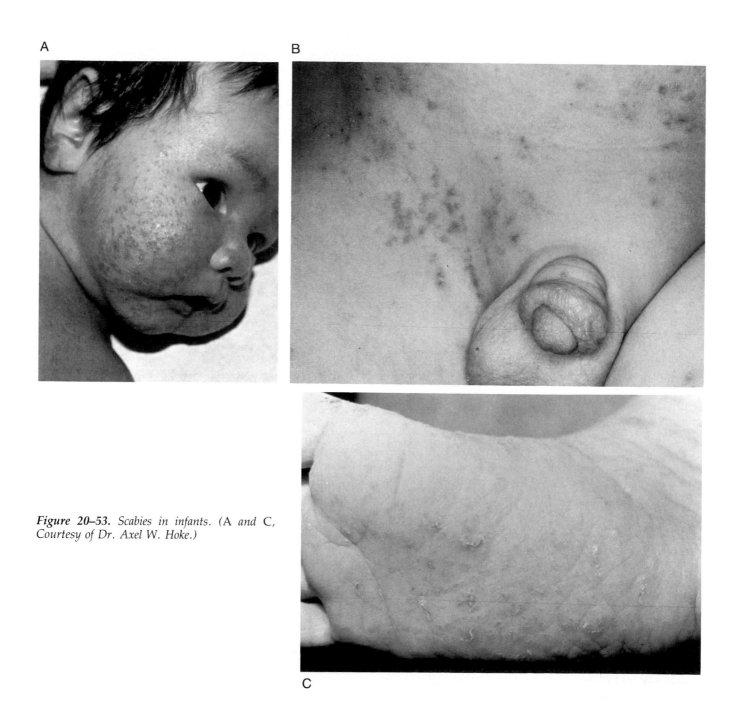

Figure 20–53. Scabies in infants. (A and C, Courtesy of Dr. Axel W. Hoke.)

C

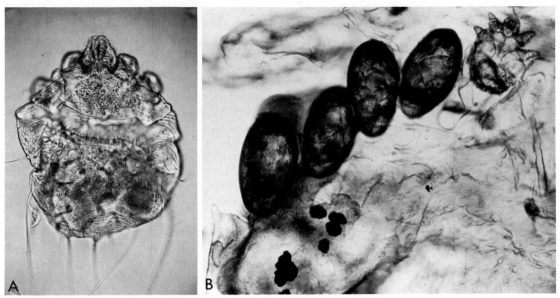

Figure 20–54. A, *Acarus.* B, *Photomicrograph of* Sarcoptes scabiei *burrow. (B, Courtesy of Dr. Axel W. Hoke.)*

who have been treated for scabies, is atypical scabies in nonwhites in the tropics or subtropics. In patients who are clean and bathe frequently the eruption is seldom pronounced, which usually makes the clinical diagnosis much more difficult. Nevertheless, in highly sensitized individuals, it may be profuse and extensive, so much so that scabies may not even be thought of. The diagnosis must often be made, however, from the distribution of the itching and the lesions present. When the disease has been present

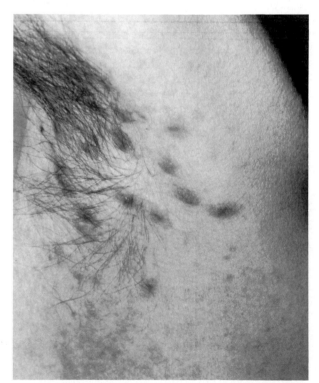

Figure 20–55. Nodular scabies. (Courtesy of Dr. Axel W. Hoke.)

a long time eczematization, lichenification, impetigo, and furunculosis may be present.

Scher called attention to scabies beneath the nails, whence it might emerge and spread. The phenomenon may have been the explanation of a persistent epidemic of two years' duration in two nursing homes.

Shelley has called attention to the fast-developing, transient, small papules formed by the larval stage of the acarus. Scrapings of them, if they are pristine and uninjured, may disclose the larva.

ETIOLOGY. *Sarcoptes scabiei*, the itch mite, is the causative organism. It is an oval, ventrally flattened mite. The female mite is 0.3 to 0.5 mm long. It is the fertilized female which burrows into the stratum corneum and there deposits her eggs. A few hours after the start of the burrow, egg laying begins; two or three eggs are laid daily continuously for nearly four to six weeks. The male dies after copulation; the female dies after laying the eggs. The eggs hatch into larvae in three to four days. The larvae are transformed into nymphs, and these in turn into adults.

EPIDEMIOLOGY. Scabies is usually contracted by close personal contact such as nursing an infested patient, overcrowding, close living quarters as occurs in institutionalized patients, or sleeping together, and only infrequently by the common use of contaminated towels, bed linen, and clothing. The female can survive only two or three days away from warm skin. Arlian et al have reviewed the question of infestivity and survival of *S. scabiei* in detail, and also the question of cross infestation; they concluded that all varieties of the organism prefer certain hosts but do not insist on them. In a related study they found the mites respond to both host odor and thermal stimuli as a means of host-seeking behavior.

PATHOGENESIS. Mellanby points out that sensitization begins about two to four weeks after onset of infection. During this time the parasites may be on the skin and may burrow into it without causing pruritus or discomfort. Severe itching begins with sensitization of the host. In reinfections, itching begins immediately and the reaction may be clinically more intense.

DIAGNOSIS. The diagnosis is usually based upon the presence of fierce itching at night, whereas during the daytime the pruritus is tolerable but persistent. The eruption does not involve the face or scalp in adults. In women, itching of the nipples associated with a generalized pruritic papular eruption is characteristic; in men, itching papules on the scrotum and penis are equally typical. When more than one member of the family has pruritus, a suspicion of scabies should be aroused—and, as scabies cannot be excluded by examination, treatment on presumption of scabies is advisable.

Positive diagnosis is made only by the demonstration of the mite under the microscope with a low-power objective. A burrow is sought and the position of the mite is determined. A surgical blade or sterile needle is used to remove the parasite. A strong light and a magnifying glass are essential to detect the glistening speck with dark margins. The tunnel can be gently slit open by the blade. With the point touching the mite, transfer is made to a glass slide for microscopic examination. Another technique is to place a drop of mineral or immersion oil on a lesion and gently scrape away the epidermis beneath it. Woodley et al prefer the use of black ink applied to the burrow, with subsequent wiping off of the excess. This outlines the burrow in black ink so it may be clearly seen. Scybala, ova, or mites may thus be found. The majority of the mites are found on the hands and wrists, less frequently (in decreasing order) at the elbows, genitalia, buttocks, and finally the axillae.

DIFFERENTIAL DIAGNOSIS. In addition to scabies, other common diseases which usually affect the trunk but not the face are pityriasis rosea, tinea versicolor, pediculosis corporis, and lichen planus, all of which are readily distinguishable from scabies. In pediculosis corporis the interscapular area is the commonest site of lesions.

TREATMENT. Permethrin 5 per cent cream (NIX) appears to be the safest as well as the most effective medication for scabies, although as of this writing it is not yet available in the U.S. Permethrin is a synthetic pyrethroid which is lethal to mites and has extremely low toxicity for humans. Taplin et al have recently reported on its use.

Lindane (gamma benzene hexachloride, Kwell) lotion, which for some years has been the standard drug, is thoroughly rubbed into the skin from the neck to the feet, with particular attention being given to the creases and folds. It is washed off eight hours later. A second application may be made one week later. Clothing and bed linen are changed and laundered thoroughly. Lindane is readily absorbed and its neurotoxicity for infants and even older children

offers a slight hazard. It is not known to be safe in pregnant women or nursing mothers. Davies et al and Friedman have reviewed rare instances of poisoning by lindane.

In babies, and even adults (Rees, 1988), 5 per cent precipitated sulfur in petrolatum is perfectly safe and very effective. Sulfur should be applied nightly for three nights. Crotamiton (Eurax) cream or lotion cures only 50 to 60 per cent of patients. If used it should be applied on two successive nights and washed off 24 hours after the last use.

Persons in close contact with the patient should ideally be closely inspected and treated if affected; however, in practice, since examination cannot exclude the diagnosis, Orkin recommends treatment of all close household and sexual contacts—and we agree. Certainly all contacts who itch should be treated, as well as all family members.

NODULAR SCABIES

Three- to five-mm nodules, dull red, which may or may not itch, may appear during active scabies and persist on the scrotum, penis, or other areas for weeks or months after scabies has been cured, in 5 per cent or so of patients, according to Orkin and Maibach. Intralesional steroids, tar (Estar Gel), or excision are methods of treatment of this troublesome condition.

Histologically the lesions suggest lymphoma.

CRUSTED SCABIES (NORWEGIAN OR HYPERKERATOTIC SCABIES)

This is scabies in the immunocompromised or institutionalized individuals, in whom it assumes a heavily scaling and crusted appearance, with crusts and scales teeming with acari, and involvement of the face and especially the scalp. Look for it in patients immunosuppressed for renal transplantation, with scaling scalps. Itching may be slight. There is in full-blown cases psoriasislike scaling, especially around and under the nails. The tips of the fingers are swollen and crusted; the finger nails are distorted. There are subungual and palmar hyperkeratosis and severe fissuring and scaling of the genitalia and buttocks. Crusted purulent lesions are present on the face and scalp. The pressure-bearing areas are the sites of predilection for the heavy keratotic lesions, in which the mites may abound.

This curious form of infestation is seen most frequently in patients suffering from malnutrition; neurologic disorders, especially mongolism; and in immunosuppressed patients. Several reports of this type of infection have appeared recently in patients with the acquired immunodeficiency syndrome, and Suzumiya et al reported it in a patient with adult T-cell leukemia. Leprosy patients and those living in institutions under unsanitary conditions may manifest this unusual form of scabies. Whereas the patient with ordinary scabies may average a total of some 12 mites, those with keratotic scabies may have thousands of mites in the skin. This type of scabies is believed to be due to a reduced immunologic response.

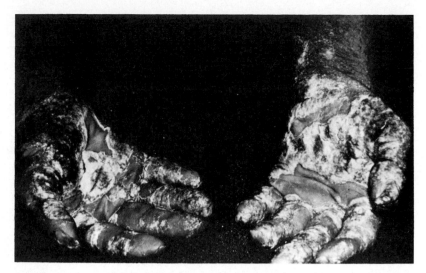

Figure 20–56. Crusted (Norwegian) scabies. (Courtesy of Dr. W. R. Hubler).

Treatment is the same as for ordinary scabies but the hyperkeratotic lesions should be treated also with keratolytics. DePaoli et al have detailed their use of 40 per cent urea to aid in treating nail involvement. Repeated applications of scabicides may be necessary. A short course of oral methotrexate has been reported to be dramatically effective.

ANIMAL SCABIES

Various acari affect animals with which man comes in close contact, and frequently an infection resembling scabies occurs in humans, contracted from dogs, cats, poultry, birds, camels, or horses. The parasites do not find the human skin a favorable habitat, so that human cases contracted from such sources generally run a mild course. They are self-limited, have no burrows, and their mites are not usually found on human cases. Bites are likely to be on surfaces in contact with the owner when the pet is held.

Cheyletiella Dermatitis

Cheyletiella yasguri, *C. blakei*, and *C. parasitovorax* are three species of nonburrowing mites, parasitic on dogs, domestic cats, and rabbits, respectively, which may bite man if there is close contact with the animals, and produce an itchy dermatitis vaguely resembling scabies. The mites are a little smaller than *Sarcoptes scabiei*, and are most easily found by brushing the animal over a dark piece of paper. It may be better to leave its discovery to a veterinarian, to whom the only necessary treatment—treatment of the pet—had best be left anyway.

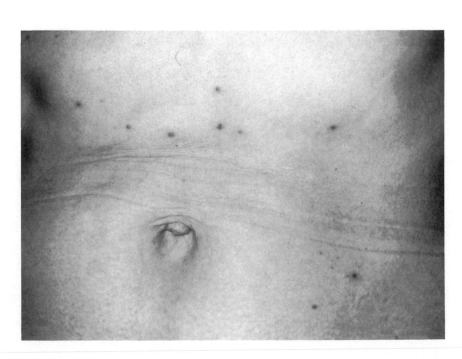

Figure 20–57. Animal scabies. (Courtesy of Dr. Axel W. Hoke.)

Demodicosis

Demodices are usually found in adults over 30 years of age; children but rarely have them. The percentage of the adults in whom at least a few demodex mites are demonstrated varies from investigator to investigator. Marples cites from 27 to 100 per cent. The organisms are not significant unless they are numerous. *Demodicidosis* is an alternative name.

The larval form of *Demodex folliculorum* is a vermiform mite about 0.9 mm long which inhabits the sebaceous glands of the nose, especially the alae nasi, and, to a lesser extent, of the forehead, chin, and scalp. In mammals such as dogs the lesions of demodectic mange contain numerous demodices.

The larva has a flattened head, and on the ventral aspect are four pairs of short peglike legs, behind which is an elongated abdomen. In an extensive and thorough study Spickett described the life cycle as lasting 14 days, of which the egg stage totals 60 hours; larva, 36; several nymph stages, about 132 hours; and the adult, about 120 hours. Fertilization occurs at the pilosebaceous orifice, after which the female burrows down the hair follicle to the sebaceous gland, where the eggs are deposited. After they have hatched there are several stages of moult, in the final of which the deutonymph emerges from the glandular opening and enters another follicle, where fertilization takes place to begin the next generation.

Demodex brevis is a little over half as long, tends to be solitary, and is found in sebaceous glands or ducts. Aylesworth et al have discussed its pathogenicity in detail. It is rare at any age, and especially rare after age 70.

The pathogenicity of the demodex has been conjectural for many years. This is because the demodices may be readily found in adults without any evidence of disease. On the other hand, some rosacea and rosacealike lesions may be caused by the demodex if the number of mites per follicle is large, or if the mite comes in contact with the dermis after rupture of the follicle. A papulonodular eruption caused by *Demodex* in two AIDS patients was re-

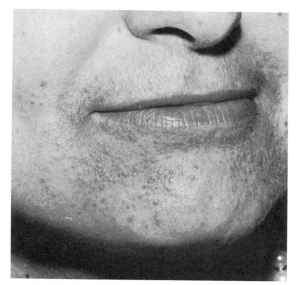

Figure 20–59. Demodicidosis with perioral micropapules from which demodices were demonstrated in groups of four to ten from one lesion.

ported by Dominey et al. Lesions on the head and neck, revealing numerous mites on scraping, were cleared by permethrin creme rinse in one patient and by lindane in the other.

The demodex may be readily demonstrated by expressing the contents of the sebaceous gland duct with a comedo expressor and placing them on a slide with a drop of glycerin. A coverslip flattens out the specimen to make the demodex readily discernible under the microscope with a low-power objective.

Treatment of the eruptions in which demodices have been implicated consists of applying benzyl benzoate emulsion twice daily, or lindane (Kwell). Applying a 5 per cent benzoyl peroxide lotion to which 5 per cent precipitated sulfur has been added is also successful. Usually after three days of therapy, demodex can no longer be demonstrated in the treated area.

Other Mite Diseases

Chigger Bite. The trombiculid mites are known as chiggers, mower's mites, or red bugs.

The chigger mite is a common parasite. The mite is red and 0.3 to 0.5 mm long. In North America *Eutrombicula alfreddugesi* attacks man and animals. In Europe it is the harvest mite, *Neotrombicula autumnalis.*

The attacks occur chiefly during the summer and fall, because of more frequent contact with mite-

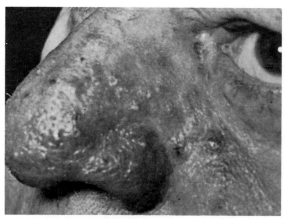

Figure 20–58. Demodicidosis in rosacea.

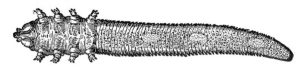

Figure 20–60. Demodex folliculorum, *ventral surface, as seen under the microscope. (× 300.)*

infested grass and bushes. The lesions occur chiefly on the legs and at the belt line, and other sites where clothing causes constriction. They consist of severely pruritic hemorrhagic puncta surrounded by red swellings. At times there are scratch marks, urticarial lesions, and widespread erythema. Tense bullae may be present.

Nuñez of Mexico City has reported cases of trombidiasis due to a new species (*Parascoschoengastia nunezi*) which attacks especially the scalp, neck, back, axillae, and retroaural folds. It causes petechiae, pustules, crusts, scratch marks, scars, and at times high fever, leukocytosis with eosinophilia, and malaise.

Several varieties of trombiculid mites exist and in endemic areas they may be vectors of scrub typhus. In the southwest Pacific the larva of the *Trombicula* transmits *tsutsugamushi fever* ("dangerous bug" fever).

The primary skin lesion is usually on the scrotum, groins, or ankles, where an ulcer a few millimeters in diameter develops. The center becomes black and necrotic and an indurated erythema develops about the ulcer. The draining lymph nodes may become enlarged but do not suppurate. After seven to 14 days' incubation period a high temperature, headache, abdominal pain, vomiting, and diarrhea develop. Conjunctivitis, a dusky flush of the face and neck, and a macular erythematous patchy eruption develop on the face, chest, and abdomen. This usually disappears within seven days, with fever lysing in two to three weeks.

Leptotrombidium deliensis and *Eutrombicula wichmanni* are vectors of scrub typhus in Queensland and New Guinea. According to Belisario, these mites usually attack the legs and ankles, although the buttocks, genitals, and axillae are also favored sites.

A good chigger repellent is dimethylphthalate (DMP) solution. The bite site itself should be washed to get rid of larvae on the skin, and treated with a topical steroid cream to relieve the pruritus.

Gamasoidosis. Those who handle canaries, pigeons, and poultry are especially liable to the disease called *gamasoidosis*. This occurs chiefly on the hands and arms. The bite produces an inflammatory, itchy papule. Any area on the body may be attacked but the more common sites are the groins, areolae, umbilicus, face, and scalp. The diagnosis of urticaria is usually made, but on questioning it may be discovered that other persons similarly exposed are also affected. The mites may wander from birds' nests as soon as the young birds begin to fly, and they may infest terrace cushions and furniture. In large metropolitan areas, especially where pigeons tend to gather, it is not unusual to see pigeons roosting on window ledges. Through the open windows or even through air conditioners the pigeon mites may attack humans and cause urticarial and papular eruptions. The starling mite (*Ornithonyssus bursa*), widely prevalent in wild birds in both continental United States and Hawaii, may do this. Lesions persist and itch for about a week longer than those due to most biting arthropods.

Two genera of mites, *Ornithonyssus* and *Dermanyssus*, commonly infest birds. *O. bursa* and *O. sylvarium* are the two common species of feather mites. They, plus others of the genus, characteristically live throughout their life span in the feathers. *Dermanyssus gallinae*, the red or chicken mite, is also a common parasite of birds. Mites of both genera derive their sustenance from the blood of the host. *Dermanyssus*, however, is found on the bird only at night. It comes out of the cracks and recesses of the poultry house or the bird nest during darkness, feeds on the host, and withdraws again during the daylight hours. It readily attacks man. Apartments may become infested.

Dermanyssus gallinae is killed without direct treatment of the bird. Thorough spraying of the surroundings with malathion is effective. Mites of the *Ornithonyssus* group require, in addition, treatment of the birds themselves.

Grocer's Itch. This is a pruritic dermatitis of the forearms, with occasional inflammatory and urticarial papules on the trunk. It results from the handling of figs, dates, and prunes, when it is due to *Carpoglyphus passularum*, or from the handling of cheese, in which case the infection is due to *Acarus siro* and

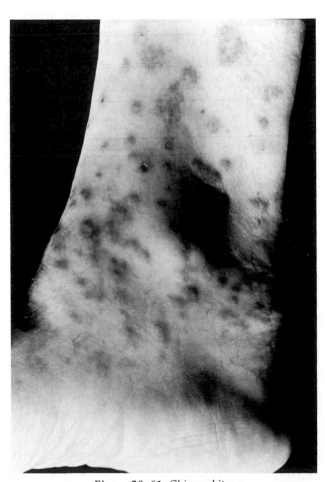

Figure 20–61. Chigger bites.

Tyrophagus longior. This must be distinguished from grocer's eczema due to sensitization to flour, sugar, cinnamon, chocolate, and similar items.

Vanillism. This is a dermatitis caused by *T. siro* and occurs in workers handling vanilla pods.

Copra Itch. Persons handling copra are subject to *Tyrophagus longior* mite bites.

Coolie Itch. This is found in tea plantations in India and is due to *Rhizoglyphus parasiticus.* It causes sore feet.

Rat Mite Itch. *Ornithonyssus bacoti,* the tropical rat mite, may cause an intensely pruritic dermatitis such as reported by Fox. It may transmit endemic typhus and relapsing fever. This papulovesicular urticarial eruption is seen in store, factory, warehouse, and stockyard workers.

Mouse Mite Bite. The house mouse mite, *Liponyssoides sanguineus,* is the vector of *R. akari,* the causative organism of rickettsialpox. Otherwise it does not attack man.

Grain Itch. This is also known as straw itch, barley itch, mattress itch, and prairie itch.

The small causative mite, *Pyemotes tritici,* lives in grain and may temporarily attack the human skin. Those chiefly affected are harvesters of wheat, barley, oats, and other cereals, or farm hands and packers who have contact with straw. Grain itch, as the disease is popularly called, has a typical lesion consisting of an urticarial papule upon which is a small vesicle. There is intense pruritus, with lesions occurring predominantly on the trunk. Frequently there is a central hemorrhagic punctum in the beginning which rapidly turns into an ecchymosis with hemosiderin pigmentation. One report traced a series of straw itch mite dermatoses to a host, the furniture beetle (*Anobium punctatum*), harboring the straw itch mite (*Pyemotes tritici*). This unusual source may help to explain those cases in which there has been no exposure to a straw mattress or grain and in which the mite may not be demonstrable mainly because it resides on the patient only briefly.

They also cite from the literature straw itch mite associated not only with straw mattresses and beetle-infested wood but also with exposure to wheat, straw, hay, bromegrass seed, and termite-infested wood.

In Hawaii, Arnold and Haramoto reported outbreaks of *P. boylei* bites in homes fumigated for termites. Although mites do not appear capable of survival when forced to share an environment with termites, they thrive in locations in which there are termite carcasses. Belisario reported a similar grass itch in Australia from *Odontacarus australiense,* and the bulb itch mite (*Rhizoglyphus hyacinthi*).

House floors should be sprayed with a 2 per cent deodorized malathion emulsion. Beetle infestation of wood should be counterattacked with 10-dichlorobenzene solution spray.

Feather Pillow Dermatitis. Aylesworth et al reported a patient who developed a pruritic papular dermatitis which was traced to the Psoroptid carpet mite, *Dermatophagoides scheremetewskyi,* which had infested a feather pillow.

Anderson CR: Rat mite dermatitis. Arch Dermatol 1944, 50:90.
Arlian LG, et al: Cross infestivity of *Sarcoptes scabiei.* JAAD 1984, 10:979.
Idem: Survival and infestivity of *Sarcoptes scabies* var. *canis* and var. *hominis.* JAAD 1984, 11:210.
Idem: Host-seeking behavior of *Sarcoptes scabiei.* JAAD 1984, 11:594.
Idem: Prevalence of *Sarcoptes scabiei* in the homes and nursing homes of scabietic patients. JAAD 1988, 19:806.
Arnold HL Jr, et al: Grain itch following fumigation for termites. Dermatol Tropica 1962, 1:37.
Aylesworth R, et al: *Demodex folliculorum* and *Demodex brevis* in cutaneous biopsies. JAAD 1982, 7:583.
Idem: Feather pillow dermatitis caused by an unusual mite, *Dermatophagoides scheremetewskyi.* JAAD 1985, 13:680.
Barnes L, et al: Crusted (Norwegian) scabies. Arch Dermatol 1987, 12:95.
Burges I, et al: Aqueous malathion 0.5% as a scabicide. Br Med J 1986, 292:1172.
Chakrabarti A: Human notoedric scabies from contact with cats infested with *Notoedres cati.* Int J Dermatol 1986, 25:646.
Cohen SR: Cheyletiella dermatitis. Arch Dermatol 1980, 116:435.
Davies JE, et al: Lindane poisonings. Arch Dermatol 1983, 119:142.
DePaoli RT, et al: Crusted (Norwegian) scabies. JAAD 1987, 17:136.
Dominey A, et al: Papulonodular demodicidosis associated with AIDS. JAAD 1989, 20:197.
Drabick JJ, et al: Crusted scabies in HIV infection. JAAD 1987, 17:142.
Elpern DJ: Infantile acropustulosis and antecedent scabies (letter). JAAD 1984, 11:895.
Estes SA, et al: Experimental canine scabies in humans. JAAD 1983, 9:397.
Fox JG: Outbreak of tropical rat mite dermatitis in laboratory personnel. Arch Dermatol 1982, 118:676.
Friedman SJ: Lindane neurotoxic reaction in nonbullous congenital ichthyosiform erythroderma. Arch Dermatol 1987, 123:1056.
Frost M, et al: Acral hyperkeratosis with erythroderma. Arch Dermatol 1988, 124:121.
Glover R, et al: Norwegian scabies in AIDS. JAAD 1987, 16:396.
Gupta AK, et al: Chronic pruritus: an uncommon cause (avian mite dermatitis). Arch Dermatol 1988, 124:1101.
Rassmussen JE: Lindane. Arch Dermatol 1987, 123:1008.
Rau RL, et al: Crusted scabies in a patient with AIDS. JAAD 1986, 15:1058.
Rees RB: Five per cent sulfur in vaseline for scabies. Schoch Letter 1988, 38:27.
Rivers JK, et al: Walking dandruff and *Cheyletiella* dermatitis. JAAD 1986, 15:1130.
Scabies in health-care facilities (MMWR). Arch Dermatol 1988, 124:837.
Shelley WB, et al: *Staphylococcus aureus* colonization of burrows in erythrodermic Norwegian scabies. JAAD 1988, 19:673.
Taplin D, et al: Permethrin 5% dermal cream. JAAD 1986, 15:995.
Wolf R, et al: Atypical crusted scabies. JAAD 1987, 17:434.

Order Scorpionidae

Scorpion Sting. Scorpions are different from other arachnids in that they have an elongated abdomen ending in a stinger. There are also the cephalothorax, four pairs of legs, pincers, and mouth pincers. Two poison glands in the back of the abdomen empty into the stinger. Scorpions are found all over the world, especially in the tropics. They are nocturnal and hide during the daytime in closets, shoes, and folded blankets. Ground scorpions may burrow into gravel and children's sandboxes.

Scorpions only sting by accident or in self-defense, but any sting by a large scorpion should be considered dangerous, since they produce both hemolytic and neurotoxic venom. The hemolytic venom causes mostly a painful swelling at the site of the sting, with little or no other effect. The neurotoxic venom may produce numbness at the sting site, laryngeal edema, profuse sweating and salivation, cyanosis, nausea, and paresthesia of the tongue. There is little or no visible change at the site of the sting. Death may occur from cardiac or respiratory failure, especially in children. The sting of the Egyptian scorpion (*Leiurus quinquestriatus*) has a mortality rate of 50 per cent in children. *Centruroides sculpturatus* is the most common cause of scorpion stings in the continental United States. The sting of the now rare small Hawaiian scorpion, *Isometrus maculatus*, is no worse than that of a hornet.

Treatment for systemic reactions involves immediate first aid measures such as the application of a tourniquet if the sting is on an extremity, with refrigeration of the site with ice or ethyl chloride spray. Specific antivenin, if available, should also be given. Phentolamine may be used to block the acute sympathetic and parasympathetic stimulation caused by the Old World species venom, and atropine, to block the cholinergic effect, are useful. Barbiturates best counteract the central nervous system excitability and convulsions most prominent with *Centruroides* stings.

Debris such as loose rocks, mattresses, and boards should be removed from sites of human habitation or sprayed with 2 per cent chlordane and 0.5 per cent dieldrin.

Order Arachnidae

ARACHNIDISM

Spiders are prevalent throughout the world; most of them are beneficial to man in that they trap many insects, including mosquitoes, for food. However, a few among the species may be dangerous to man.

Latrodectism and loxoscelism are the two most important types of clinical manifestions of spider stings. To these one must add the possibility that they will cause eosinophilic cellulitis (Wells' syndrome), flame figures and all, as Schorr et al have pointed out. Campbell et al described the bites of the wolf spider, and Wong et al recently reviewed the cutaneous effects of all types of spider stings, including those due to tarantulas, the orb weaver, the green lynx spider, the broad-faced sack spider, the black jumping spider, the parson spider, and others. This article and an accompanying editorial by King are excellent general references for this subject. Anderson has offered to identify spiders for dermatologists at no cost if they are put into 95 per cent

buffered ethanol and mailed to him at the Division of Dermatology, The University of Missouri Health Sciences Center, Columbia, MO 65212.

Latrodectism

The various species of *Latrodectus* have similar toxins and cause similar reactions in man. Of these the black widow spider, *Latrodectus mactans*, is of chief concern in the continental United States.

It is 13 mm long, coal black, with an orange-red hourglass-shaped marking on its abdomen. The legs are long, with a spread of some 4 cm. The black widow spider inhabits dry dark places under rocks, in cellars, under privy seats, and in wood piles. It avoids strong sunlight and usually bites only when disturbed.

The sting itself is inconspicuous, being located most often on the genitals or buttocks, as a result of being bitten while seated in a privy. Severe pains usually develop within a few minutes and spread throughout the extremities and trunk. Within a few hours there may be chills, vomiting, violent cramps, delirium or partial paralysis, spasms, and abdominal rigidity. The abdominal pains are frequently most severe. These symptoms may be mistaken for appendicitis, colic, or food poisoning. Symptoms begin to subside in about two days; however, such bites may bring death to young children. Toxic morbilliform erythema may occur. The venom of *Latrodectus* is neurotoxic.

Treatment should be immediate. Morphine is usu-

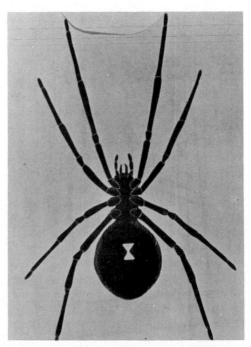

Figure 20–62. Black widow spider (Latrodectus mactans) *with red hourglass shaped patch on abdomen. Magnified 4×. (Courtesy of Drs. H. C. Scott and C. J. Stojanovich.)*

ally necessary for the pain and for sedation. Specific antivenin is efficacious if available. Black Widow Spider Antivenin is highly recommended. It should be given if symptoms are severe, but should always be given to children. Ten per cent solution of calcium gluconate, 10 ml, may be given intravenously. Neostigmine methylsulfate helps to relieve the muscle spasm.

Loxoscelism

Not until 1957 did the toxic effects of the small brown recluse spider (*Loxosceles reclusa*) become known in North America. The house spider (*L. laeta*) has been known for many years in South America for its similar toxic effects.

Two types of reactions occur from the bite of the brown spider. In the localized type, known as *necrotic cutaneous loxoscelism*, a cutaneous lesion with extensive gangrene develops. A painful severe edematous reaction occurs within the first eight hours, with development of a bulla with surrounding zones of erythema and ischemia. In about a week the central portion becomes dark, demarcated, and gangrenous. This may produce a large necrotic ulceration, becoming many centimeters wide and lasting months before healing.

Viscerocutaneous loxoscelism fortunately is rare. There is the same local reaction, but there are fever of 39 to 40°C, chills, vomiting, joint pain, and hematologic pathology. Hematuria almost invariably

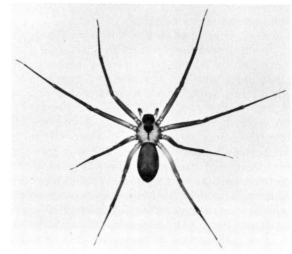

Figure 20–64. Brown recluse spider. Note the inverted violin configuration on the cephalothorax. Magnified 4×. (Courtesy of Dr. G. T. Jansen.)

occurs on the first day, with hemolytic anemia, thrombocytopenia, and other blood dyscrasias. The skin may show a petechial or morbilliform eruption. Shock and death may ensue.

The venom contains a phospholipase enzyme, sphingomyelinase D, which is responsible for both the dermonecrosis and hemolysis. It damages cell membranes.

This shy reclusive spider may be identified by a dark violin-shaped band over the cephalothorax and three pairs of "eyes" on the anterior portion of the cephalothorax. It is light to dark brown, about 1 cm long, and is found in the house in storage closets among clothing. Outdoors it has been found in grass, on rocky bluffs, and in barns. It stings only in self-defense. Most cases of loxoscelism have been found in the southern central United States.

TREATMENT. R. S. Rees et al and King and Rees have had extensive experience with brown recluse spider stings, and they conclude that there is no benefit to be obtained from intralesional injections, or from excision of the bite site. They advise 1) ice bags and elevation, 2) rest, 3) *no* hot packs or surgery, and 4) antibiotics and aspirin. Dapsone seemed to be very effective in a dose of 100 mg b.i.d., starting on the third day, in a proven *L. reclusa* bite. P.H. Ely in a personal communication has suggested that a short course of Accutane might be equally helpful, and without the risk of inducing hemolytic anemia (which may complicate such a spider bite anyway, independently of dapsone), but no studies have been done to date with Accutane. A specific antivenin is available only for *L. laeta*.

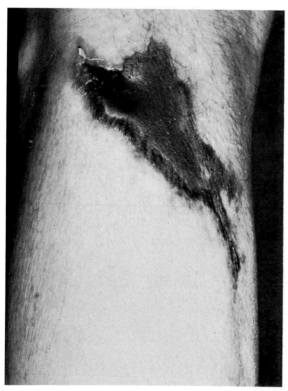

Figure 20–63. Necrotic reaction to bite of the brown recluse spider in the left popliteal space. (Courtesy of Dr. G. T. Jansen.)

Anderson PC: Free identification of spiders for dermatologists. JAAD 1983, 8:562.
Burnett JW, et al: Brown recluse spider. Cutis 1985, 37:197.
Idem: Latrodectism: black widow spider bites. Cutis 1983, 37:121.

Campbell DS, et al: Wolf spider bites. Cutis 1987, 39:113.

Hillis TJ, et al: Presumed arachnidism. Int J Dermatol 1986, 25:44.

King LE Jr, et al: Treatment of brown recluse spider bites (letter). JAAD 1986, 14:691.

Idem: Dapsone treatment of a brown recluse bite. JAMA 1983, 250:648.

Idem: Brown recluse spider bites: stay cool. JAMA 1985, 254:2896.

Idem: Spider bites. Arch Dermatol 1987, 123:41.

Pennell TC, et al: The management of snake and spider bites in the Southeastern United States. Am Surg 1987, 53:193.

Rees RS, et al: Brown recluse spider bites. Ann Surg 1985, 202:659.

Schorr WF, et al: Eosinophilic cellulitis (Wells' syndrome). JAAD 1984, 11:1043.

Wong RC, et al: Spider bites. Arch Dermatol 1987, 123:78.

PHYLUM CHORDATA

Stingray Injury. The two stingray families (*Dasyatidae* and *Myliobatidae*) are among the most venomous fish known to man. Attacks generally occur as a result of an unwary victim stepping on a partially buried stingray. A puncture-type wound, which later ulcerates, occurs about the ankles or feet. Sharp, shooting pain develops immediately, with edema and cyanosis. Symptoms of shock may occur.

Anyone wading in shallow muddy waters where stingray may be found should shuffle his feet through the mud in order to frighten the fish away. Successful treatment is usually attained by immersing the injured part in hot water for 30 to 60 minutes. The water should be as hot as can be tolerated, since the venom is detoxified by heat. Meperidine hydrochloride intravenously or intramuscularly may be necessary. Should the ulcer remain unhealed after eight weeks, excision is indicated.

Snake Bite. Venomous snake bites are a serious problem in some parts of the world. In the United States the rattlesnake, cottonmouth moccasin, and copperhead are the venomous snakes most frequently encountered. There are nearly 30 enzymes found in snake venom, most of which are hydrolases. Snake venom has an anticoagulant action and causes hemolysis and an increase in capillary permeability. These effects may be combated with fresh whole blood transfusions. Neurotoxins are the most toxic of venom constituents. Other toxins include myotoxins and cardiotoxins. Antivenin is of great value.

In all bites on the extremities, if the victim cannot be transported at rest within one hour to a definitive care facility, a tourniquet should be applied so as to obstruct venous and lymph flow but not arterial flow. Incision and suction should be instituted as quickly as possible, since they are effective only during the first 15 to 30 minutes following the bite. The incision is made around the fang marks and the edge of the swelling. Suction should be vigorous; if available, a small piece of thin rubber sheeting may be placed between the mouth and the wound for added protection against ingestion of the venom. It is necessary to use copious amounts of antivenin intramuscularly after a routine skin sensitivity test. In addition, antibiotics should be given and appropriate antitetanus measures begun. Indications for surgical intervention, and a review of snakebite therapy, have been published by Sprenger et al and Burnett et al.

Lizard Bite. Heloderma (Gila monster) is found chiefly in Arizona and New Mexico. Another venomous lizard is the beaded lizard of southwestern Mexico. Bites from these poisonous lizards may cause paralysis, dyspnea, and convulsions. Death rarely ensues. Local treatment is the same as for snake bite.

Burnett JW, et al: Venomous snakebites. Cutis 1986, 38:299.

Russell FE: Stingray injury. JAMA 1966, 195:708.

Sprenger TR, et al: Snakebite treatment in the United States. Int J Dermatol 1986, 25:479.

21

Chronic Blistering or Pustular Dermatoses

There are eight principal chronic blistering (vesicular or bullous) dermatoses: pemphigus, pemphigoid, cicatricial pemphigoid, herpes gestationis (pemphigoid gestationis), linear IgA bullous dermatosis, chronic bullous disease of childhood, dermatitis herpetiformis, and epidermolysis bullosa acquisita. In all of these the cause of blistering is an autoimmune reaction, and the pattern of immunofluorescence, direct or indirect, is generally more authoritative than the clinical findings in establishing the diagnosis. Usually antibodies are bound at the site of the earliest lesions. New categories of blistering disease continue to evolve: for example, Huff has lately described an intraepidermal neutrophilic IgA dermatosis.

For clinical reasons, bullous erythema multiforme is discussed under the far more common nonbullous multiform erythemas; it will be mentioned here only in differential diagnosis. Transient acantholytic dermatosis (Grover's disease) and autoimmune progesterone dermatitis are two vesiculobullous diseases which may be chronic, but show no findings on direct immunofluorescence.

Two chronic pustular eruptions, subcorneal pustular dermatosis and eosinophilic pustular folliculitis (Ofuji's disease), are also presented.

The specific dermatoses of pregnancy are discussed under the differential diagnosis of herpes gestationis.

Beutner EH, et al: Immunofluorescence tests: clinical significance of sera and skin in bullous diseases. Int J Dermatol 1985, 24:405.

Blenkinsop WK, et al: Histology of linear IgA disease, dermatitis herpetiformis, and bullous pemphigoid. Am J Dermatopathol 1983, 5:547.

Callen JP: Internal disorders associated with bullous diseases of the skin. JAAD 1980, 3:107.

Dahl MV: Acquired subepidermal bullous diseases. Austral J Dermatol 1985, 26:93.

Gammon WR, Briggaman RA: Epidermal-dermal junction: Part II. Histologic, immunohistologic, and ultrastructural features of the subepidermal bullous diseases. Prog Dermatol 1981, 15:1.

Katz SI: Blistering skin diseases: new insights (editorial). N Engl J Med 1985, 313:1657.

Katz SI: The epidermal basement membrane zone. JAAD 1984, 11:1025.

Lazaro-Medina A, et al: Limitations in the diagnosis of vesiculobullous diseases. Am J Dermatopathol 1983, 5:7.

Maize JC: Value of immunofluorescent techniques in studies of bullous disease. Am J Dermatopathol 1983, 5:67.

PEMPHIGUS VULGARIS

CLINICAL FEATURES. Pemphigus vulgaris is characterized by thin-walled, relatively flaccid, easily ruptured bullae appearing upon either apparently normal skin and mucous membranes or on erythematous bases. The fluid in the bulla is clear at first, but may become hemorrhagic or even seropurulent. The bullae soon rupture to form erosions, raw surfaces which ooze and bleed easily. The denuded areas soon become partially covered with crusts, with little or no tendency to heal, and enlarge by confluence. The healed lesions often leave hyperpigmented patches; however, there is no scarring.

Pemphigus vulgaris may begin in many ways, but usually the lesions appear first in the mouth and next most commonly in the groin, scalp, face, neck, axillae, or genitals. The nail folds may be involved first, together with mouth lesions. Usually at the beginning the bullae are sparse and seem inconsequential, but extensive generalized lesions may develop in a few weeks or they may be limited to one or more sites for several months.

The *Nikolsky sign* is present; that is, there is an absence of cohesion in the epidermis, so that the upper layers are easily made to slip laterally by slight pressure or rubbing. This sign is variously elicited: The upper layers of the epidermis may easily be removed by a twisting pressure with the fingertip, leaving a moist surface. The lack of cohesion of the skin layers may also be demonstrated with the "bulla-spread phenomenon" by pressure on an intact bulla, gently forcing the fluid to wander under the skin away from the pressure site (the Asboe-Hansen sign).

The mouth lesions appear first in 60 per cent of the cases. The short-lived bullae quickly rupture to involve most of the mucosa in a painful erosion. The lesions extend out onto the lips and form heavy, fissured crusts on the vermilion. Involvement of the throat produces hoarseness and difficulty in swallowing. The mouth odor is offensive and penetratingly unpleasant. The esophagus may be involved, and sloughing of its entire lining in the form of a cast ("esophagitis dissecans superficialis") has been reported. The conjunctiva, nasal mucosa, vagina, penis, and anus may also be involved. Wood et al described a patient in whom hematemesis proved to be due to pemphigus of the esophagus.

EPIDEMIOLOGY. Pemphigus vulgaris occurs with equal frequency in men and women, usually in their fifth and sixth decades, the disease being rare

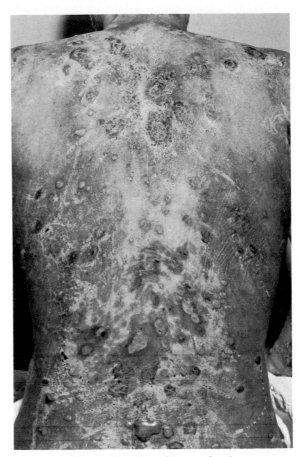

Figure 21–2. Pemphigus vulgaris.

in young persons. In a review published in 1979, Lever reported that nine cases of pemphigus vulgaris in childhood have been published since 1955.

ETIOLOGY. Although the cause of pemphigus vulgaris is unknown, an autoimmune mechanism is clearly the basic fault. Intercellular antibodies (IC)

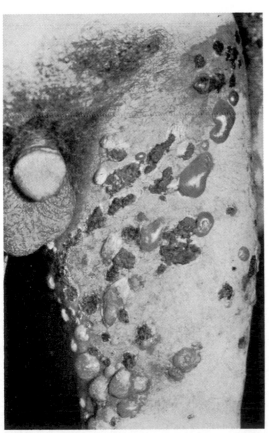

Figure 21–1. Pemphigus vulgaris. Bullous lesions arising from apparently normal skin surface, with crusts.

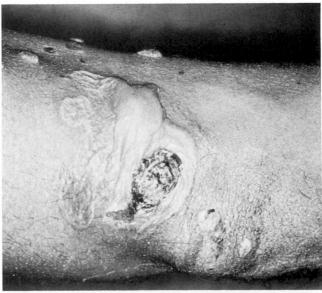

Figure 21–3. Pemphigus vulgaris. Flaccid bullae with crusts.

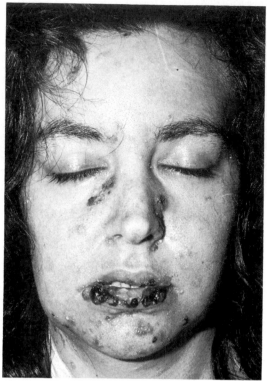

Figure 21-4. Pemphigus vulgaris. (Courtesy of Dr. S. Hochman.)

are demonstrable throughout the epidermis or the oral epithelium, and circulating intercellular antibodies are present in the patient's serum.

Penicillamine treatment of rheumatoid arthritis has induced pemphigus, most often of the foliaceus type. Of the 60 cases of this reported, nearly all had positive direct immunofluorescence and 35 have had positive indirect IF. The doses responsible have ranged from 250 to 1500 mg a day, and were taken for an average of 13 months prior to the onset of pemphigus. Only 13 per cent have had oral lesions. Most such reactions have resolved on discontinuing the medication; some have persisted for many months, however, and a few been fatal. Trotta et al reported drug-induced pemphigus from thiopronine, a sulfhydryl drug similar to penicillamine. Captopril, penicillin, and rifampin have also been reported to induce pemphigus. Ultra-violet light may aggravate the disease.

Other autoimmune diseases have infrequently been reported to occur in association with pemphigus; however, the association of myasthenia gravis and thymoma has been reported by several writers.

Statistical analysis shows a skewed distribution of various HLA antigens among patients with pemphigus. Most patients are of HLA phenotype DRY or DRw6. In addition, a specific HLA-DQ beta restriction fragment has been identified in nearly all patients with pemphigus, which may confer susceptibility to the disease; but in any individual case such findings are meaningless. Sakurai showed that DRw4 was not found in Japanese cases of pemphigus, while

DRw2 was found one third more frequently than in controls.

AUTOANTIBODIES. With the indirect immunofluorescent (IF) technique, circulating intercellular antibodies can be demonstrated in 80 to 90 per cent of patients with pemphigus vulgaris. Indirect IF testing may be negative in patients with early, localized disease at a time when a positive test would be of particular diagnostic value. Using indirect testing as a means of evaluating disease severity has been shown to be unreliable. However, circulating intercellular antibody (IC) titers often parallel disease activity.

Circulating IC antibodies have occasionally been reported in patients with various autoimmune diseases and with burns, bullous drug eruptions, and maculopapular eruptions due to penicillin. These IC antibodies differ from true pemphigus IC antibodies in that they do not fix to the epidermis in vivo, and may be removed from serum samples by absorption with ABO blood-group antigens. On indirect testing it appears coarse, granular, and nonuniform, as was shown by Ahmed et al. In pemphigus there is smooth, uniform staining.

Direct IF is of great value in the early diagnosis of pemphigus vulgaris. The direct IF test shows intercellular IgG throughout the epidermis or the oral epithelium. IgG is found in vivo in nearly all patients with pemphigus. Jordon and coworkers reported finding C3 deposition in the involved skin of 100 per cent of patients with pemphigus. In a study of uninvolved skin in 63 patients with pemphigus vul-

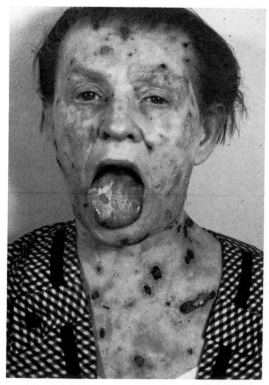

Figure 21-5. Pemphigus vulgaris. *Note membranous sheet on tongue.*

garis or pemphigus foliaceus, Judd and Lever found a positive direct test in 58 patients. IC IgG is found in both involved and clinically normal skin, whereas C3 is usually found only in acantholytic areas. The direct IF test is a very reliable diagnostic test, much more so than the indirect IF test. It becomes positive very early in the disease, often before the indirect IF test has become positive, remains positive for a long time, and may still be positive many years after the disease has subsided and treatment has been discontinued.

These IF tests aid in the differential diagnosis of such bullous dermatoses as bullous pemphigoid, cicatricial pemphigoid, dermatitis herpetiformis, chronic bullous dermatosis of childhood, herpes gestationis, epidermolysis bullosa, erythema multiforme, bullous drug eruptions, toxic epidermal necrolysis, and familial benign pemphigus of Hailey-Hailey.

Stanley et al have immunoprecipitated the pemphigus vulgaris antigen and found all pemphigus vulgaris sera precipitated a complex of polypeptides (PV complex) of 210,000, 130,000, and 85,000 molecular weights after reduction. In addition, 14 of 22 pemphigus vulgaris sera have antibodies to the pemphigus foliaceus complex. The 85 KD peptide is plakoglobin, a plaque protein found in desmosomes and adherens junctions. It is clear from these and other data that the antigen is a specific cell-surface glycoprotein that is synthesized by keratinocytes, but the precise identity of the antigenic substance needs further characterization.

PATHOGENESIS. The pathologic changes in pemphigus vulgaris are acantholysis, cleft and blister formation in the intraepidermal areas just above the basal cell layer, and the formation of acantholytic cells.

Acantholysis is the separation of keratinocytes from one another. The loss of cohesion or contact between the malpighian cells begins with the detachment of tonofilaments from the desmosomes and ends with formation of the intraepidermal cleft or bulla.

Anhalt et al in 1982 induced pemphigus in newborn mice by passive transfer of IgG from patients with pemphigus. Normal IgG caused no pemphigus, but 39 of 55 mice injected with pemphigus antibody reacted with histologically, ultrastructurally, and immunologically typical pemphigus blisters, and the effect was dose-dependent. Buschard et al confirmed the effect in athymic nude mice.

Schlitz et al and Farb et al have shown that pemphigus antibody, when incubated with either normal skin or cultured keratinocytes, binds to the cell surfaces and induces acantholysis. Complement is not required. Hashimoto et al showed that plasminogen activator is released during this process.

Thus it seems that the probable mechanism of blister formation in pemphigus is the binding of circulating antibody to a cell-surface glycoprotein, with resulting activation of plasmin, which causes enzymatic destruction of intercellular cement and desmosomes.

Perry and Brunsting reported a patient who suffered pemphigus erythematosus as a result of emotional stress, and Brenner et al reported two patients who developed pemphigus vulgaris while under severe emotional stress. One was an Ashkenazi Jewish woman of A26, Bw38, and DRw4 type, the other an Iranian Jew of A26, Bw38 type. The woman had an uncle with pemphigus. The concept that pemphigus can be induced by psychogenic immunomodulation continues to be raised.

Storer described a child born with pemphigus vulgaris to a mother who had pemphigus vegetans a year earlier, with remission during pregnancy. Spontaneous remission occurred at two weeks of age, and antibody titers became negative at eight weeks. Wassermann et al documented fetal transmission of pemphigus, with fetal death.

HISTOPATHOLOGY. The characteristic findings consist of acantholysis, intraepidermal cleft and blister formation, and the presence of acantholytic cells lining the bulla as well as lying free in the bulla cavity.

Many of the acantholytic cells are detached or loosely attached to the neighboring cells or lie in clusters within the bulla. These cells are separated and show no intercellular bridges; the large nuclei are surrounded by a lightly staining halo in the cytoplasm and then a darkly staining cytoplasm at the periphery of the cell.

Smears from the base of a bulla stained by the Tzanck method using Giemsa stain will show the typical acantholytic or *Tzanck cells.*

Perry was the first to recognize a collection of eosinophils in the spongiotic epidermis of a patient with pemphigus, a phenomenon which Emmerson and Wilson Jones were later to name "eosinophilic spongiosis." In their cases, and later in many others, it was a harbinger of acantholysis. It far more commonly presages pemphigoid, and exceptionally occurs in a great many other dermatoses. Crotty et al reviewed the Mayo experience in 71 cases of eosinophilic spongiosis.

Biopsy Material. The need for proper specimens for histologic examination has been emphasized by Arundell. Since the bullae of pemphigus become large and flaccid in a short time it is important that a small, early, intact blister be secured. Asboe-Hansen's modification of the Nikolsky test may be used to extend the bulla beyond its original margin to where secondary degenerative changes have not taken place. The site of the biopsy is frozen with an aerosol refrigerant spray so that the punch may include firm tissue. Normal-appearing perilesional skin should be used to obtain tissue for direct immunofluorescence.

TREATMENT. Before the advent of the corticosteroids, treatment was mainly supportive and usually inadequate to combat this severe disease, which was often fatal. Both topical and systemic therapy are essential.

Topical Treatment. The skin lesions are extremely painful in advanced cases. When there are extensive raw surfaces, prolonged daily baths are extremely helpful in removing the thickened crusts and reducing the foul odor. Silver sulfadiazine (Silvadene) 1 per cent, widely used in the local therapy of burns, is an effective topical antimicrobial agent.

Painful ulcerations of the lips and mouth may be benefitted by topical application of a mixture of equal parts of Maalox and elixir of Benadryl or viscous Xylocaine, especially before meals. The various commercial antiseptic mouthwashes are helpful in alleviating discomfort and malodor.

Systemic Therapy. It is agreed that the sooner the diagnosis is established and the sooner treatment is given, the more favorable the prognosis.

Corticosteroids. Arnold has found that corticosteroid therapy is best initiated by giving 80 mg of triamcinolone acetonide (Kenalog IM) intramuscularly, and repeating it on the fourth and seventh days if necessary (as it will probably be). If the clinical response is not good enough, then prednisone is given by mouth in a dose of 120 to 200 mg/day until there is a good clinical response, and then reduced quite rapidly; it can often be halved every two to four days. When the triamcinolone wears off, in about four weeks, it should be repeated, usually just one 80-mg dose; by this time the oral prednisone may have become unnecessary. Thereafter the Kenalog (60 mg) is repeated only as needed. Side effects of steroid therapy are thus almost entirely avoided. Patients may even remain ambulatory.

The addition of an immunosuppressant (azathioprine [Imuran] 100 mg daily is one of the best) is helpful in diminishing the need for corticosteroids. Remember that today the risk of death in pemphigus from the side effects of oral prednisone is greater than the risk of death from the disease itself. The untreated disease, however, is usually fatal, whereas death from sepsis and other complications of therapy occurs in only 5 to 10 per cent of treated cases. Ahmed et al found the primary cause of death is infection, with staphylococcus aureus most commonly isolated; the most common sites of infection are blood, lungs, and skin. Kenalog does not worsen or disseminate staphylococcal or other infections.

Lever recommends 40 mg of prednisone on alternate days in mild cases, and 200–240 mg a day in severe ones. He avoids doses of 40–200 mg a day (except during the transition to lower doses) and he avoids hospitalization when possible. He has not tried Kenalog.

Diaz and Provost recommend institution of oral prednisone, 60 to 100 mg per day, alone or in combination with one or several immunosuppressants (azothioprine, 100 mg/day; cyclophosphamide, 100 mg/day; or methotrexate, 25 mg IM/week) to suppress the blistering disease. They evaluate the therapeutic effects by estimating the number of new vesicles per week and the rate of healing of the new lesions. In addition, pemphigus antibody titers are performed every four weeks, watching for a fall in titer. If after six to eight weeks new blister formation is not suppressed, prednisone is increased to 150 mg per day. They state this is rarely necessary.

Medication is continued until clinical disease is suppressed and pemphigus antibody disappears from the serum. Once the antibody is no longer present, direct immunofluorescence is repeated. After both direct and indirect immunofluorescence become negative, the steroids are gradually, but completely, withdrawn. They then follow with a one to two month gradual withdrawal of immunosuppressives. They find one third of their patients have prolonged clinical and serologic remissions without need of maintenance therapy.

Immunosuppressive Therapy. Immunosuppressants alone have been reported as a successful treatment of early stable pemphigus vulgaris. Lever feels that combined treatment with corticosteroids is superior to treatment with only an immunosuppressant, and we concur.

Gendler reviewed the use of azathioprine in dermatologic disorders. Aberer et al reviewed their own prospective study of 29 patients and found the combination of prednisone and azathioprine to be safe and effective. To it must now be added cyclosporine (Sandimmune), which may be given orally in liquid form, and specifically suppresses T helper cells. The dose is 5–15 mg/kg/day, taken well diluted in fruit juice or chocolate milk. The principal adverse reactions are renal dysfunction, tremor, hirsutism, hypertension, and gum hyperplasia. Thivolet has reviewed its use in pemphigus and pemphigoid. Barthelemy et al found it useful in combination with prednisone.

Methotrexate and cyclophosphamide, in the doses recommended by Diaz and Provost, are other alternatives. Ahmed et al reviewed cases treated with cyclophosphamide and thought it a good alternative to azathioprine failures. They also found dapsone to have helpful additive effects.

Gold. In 1973, Penneys, Frost, and Eaglstein reported that gold sodium thiomalate (Myochrysine) was effective in pemphigus, and this has subsequently been confirmed by them and others, such as Poulin, Perry, and Muller. Aurothioglucose (Solganol) has the advantage of not inducing a nitritoid reaction. They are believed to act through their effect on suppressing both the primary and secondary immune response. They also affect leukocyte function. Pruritic macular and papular eruptions may be produced, though resumption of therapy does not regularly result in reproducing them. Bone marrow suppression may occur. Nephrotoxicity is rare.

Plasmapheresis. In severe cases this modality may be useful if combined with therapy such as high-dose prednisone or immunosuppressants, which will prevent new synthesis of pemphigus antibody.

Pemphigus Vegetans

Pemphigus vegetans is a variant of pemphigus vulgaris and is believed to be connected with the amount of resistance these patients have to their disease. Some authorities formerly recognized two types of pemphigus vegetans. One is the *Neumann type* and the other the *Hallopeau type* (pyodermite végétante).

Despite the benign course of the latter type, and the fact that the lesions are not bullae but pustules, immunofluorescent studies by Nelson et al indicate that both forms are simply mild variants of pemphigus vulgaris, the clinical spectrum of which has to be extended to include them.

Pemphigus vegetans is characterized by flaccid bullae, which become erosions and form fungoid vegetations or papillomatous proliferations, especially in body folds.

Although the onset of the disease may be manifested solely by broken bullae in the mouth or about the genitals or umbilicus, the bullae rupture and their moist bases become exuberant with verrucous vegetations, being capped by crusts and surrounded by a zone of inflammation. At times there is a tendency for the lesions to coalesce to form large patches or to arrange themselves into groups or configurate patterns.

Pemphigus vegetans begins insidiously, usually on the nose or in the mouth, as does pemphigus vulgaris. Other areas frequently affected are the axillae and groin, genitalia and perineum, flexural extremities, and scalp. The subjective symptoms are slight, and there are often long remissions in the course of the disease. At times, however, high fever and other constitutional symptoms develop as a result of sepsis.

The laboratory findings, etiology, epidemiology, pathogenesis, and treatment of pemphigus vegetans are the same as those of pemphigus vulgaris. Storer's report of a child with congenital pemphigus vulgaris born to a mother who had had pemphigus vegetans 16 months earlier is another factor which strongly suggests that pemphigus vegetans is simply modified pemphigus vulgaris.

Histologically, the findings are identical with those of pemphigus vulgaris, but there are an increased papillary proliferation and marked epidermal hyperplasia. Frequently, intraepidermal abscesses filled with eosinophils are present; they are characteristic of this variant of pemphigus.

Pemphigus vegetans must be differentiated from the fungating iodide eruption. The latter occurs without regard to sites of predilection and is not accompanied by the systemic disturbances and other characteristics of pemphigus. Syphilitic condylomata, granuloma inguinale, condyloma acuminatum, and mycotic and amebic granulomas may resemble the disease, especially when it occurs in the anogenital region.

Dermatitis Vegetans

Dermatitis vegetans has also been called *pyodermite végétante* (Hallopeau), pyoderma vegetans, and benign pemphigus vegetans. Having no bullae but rather beginning with pustules, it has long been regarded as a pyoderma. However, Nelson et al showed in 1977 that immunofluorescent findings in cases of this so-called Hallopeau type are typical of pemphigus vulgaris, so it should now be regarded as a variant of pemphigus vulgaris.

Ahmed AR, et al: Death in pemphigus. JAAD 1982, 7:221.

Idem: Pemphigus: current concepts (UCLA Conference). Ann Intern Med 1980, 92:396.

Idem: Anti-intercellular substance antibodies: presence in serum samples of 14 patients without pemphigus. Arch Dermatol 1983, 119:17.

Idem: Use of cyclophosphamide in azathioprine failures in pemphigus. JAAD 1987, 17:437.

Anhalt GJ, et al: Induction of pemphigus in neonatal mice by passive transfer from patients with the disease. N Engl J Med 1982, 306:1189.

Barthelemy H, et al: Treatment of nine cases of pemphigus vulgaris with cyclosporin. JAAD 1988, 18:1262.

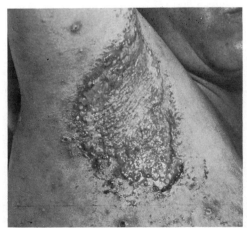

Figure 21–6. Pemphigus vegetans of axilla. (Courtesy of Dr. M. Costello.)

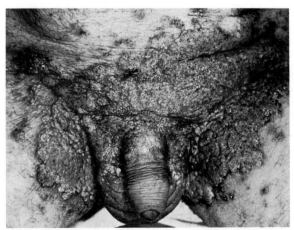

Figure 21–7. Pemphigus vegetans with sharply delineated exudative vegetating lesions.

Bhogal B, et al: The distribution of immunoglobulin and the C$_3$ component in multiple biopsies from the uninvolved and perilesional skin in pemphigus. Clin Exp Dermatol 1986, 11:49.

Brenner S, et al: Pemphigus vulgaris triggered by emotional stress. JAAD 1984, 11:524.

Buschard K, et al: A model for the study of autoimmune diseases applied to pemphigus. J Invest Dermatol 1981, 76:171.

Bystryn JC, et al: Adjuvant therapy of pemphigus. Arch Dermatol 1984, 120:941.

Idem: Plasmapheresis therapy of pemphigus. Arch Dermatol 1988, 124:1702.

Castle WN, et al: Chronic balanitis owing to pemphigus vegetans. J Urol 1987, 137:289.

Enjolras O, et al: Pemphigus induits. Ann Dermatol Venereol 1987, 114:25.

Eyre RW, et al: Identification of pemphigus vulgaris antigen extracted from normal human epidermis and comparison with pimphigus foliaceus antigen. J Clin Invest 1988, 81:807.

Fabbri P, et al: Pathogenesis of pemphigus. Int J Dermatol 1985, 24:422.

Farb RM, et al: Antiepidermal-cell-surface pemphigus antibody detaches viable epidermal cells from plates by activation of proteinase. Proc Natl Acad Sci USA 1978, 75:459.

Fine FD, et al: Pemphigus vulgaris. Arch Dermatol 1988, 124:236.

Fitzpatrick RE, et al: Correlation of disease activity and antibody titers in pemphigus. Arch Dermatol 1980, 116:285.

Gendler E: Azathioprine for use in dermatology. J Dermatol Surg Oncol 1984, 10:462.

Ho VC, et al: Penicillamine-induced pemphigus. J Rheumatol 1985, 12:583.

Korman N: Pemphigus. JAAD 1988, 18:1219.

Krain LS, et al: Pemphigus vulgaris and internal malignancy. Cancer 1974, 33:1091.

Lever W, et al: Treatment of pemphigus vulgaris: results obtained in 84 patients between 1961 and 1982. Arch Dermatol 1984, 120:44.

Parfrey PS, et al: Captopril-induced pemphigus. Br Med J 1980, 281:194.

Poulin Y, et al: Pemphigus vulgaris. JAAD 1984, 11:851.

Provost TT: Pemphigus (editorial). N Engl J Med 1982, 306:1224.

Rodan KP, et al: Malodorous intertriginous pustules and plaques. Arch Dermatol 1987, 123:393.

Roujeau J-C, et al: Plasma exchange in pemphigus. Arch Dermatol 1983, 119:215.

Sakurai M, et al: Absence of HLA-DRW2 in Japanese pemphigus vulgaris. J Invest Dermatol 1981, 76:70.

Sams WM Jr, et al: Mechanisms of lesion production in pemphigus and pemphigoid. JAAD 1982, 6:431.

Schiltz JR, et al: Pemphigus antibody interaction with human epidermal cells in culture. J Clin Invest 1978, 62:778.

Stanley JR, et al: Distinction between epidermal antigens binding pemphigus vulgaris and pemphigus foliaceus autoantibodies. J Clin Invest 1984, 74:313.

Idem: Pemphigus antibodies identify a cell surface glycoprotein synthesized by human and mouse keratinocytes. J Clin Invest 1982, 70:281.

Storer JS, et al: Neonatal pemphigus vulgaris. JAAD 1982, 6:929.

Trotta F, et al: Thiopronine-induced pemphigus vulgaris in rheumatoid arthritis. Scand J Rheumatol 1984, 13:93.

Troy JL, et al: Penicillamine-associated pemphigus. JAAD 1981, 4:547.

Wassermann N, et al: Transplacental transmission of pemphigus. JAMA 1983, 249:1480.

Wood DR: Pemphigus vulgaris of the esophagus. Ann Intern Med 1982, 96:189.

Pemphigus Foliaceus

This relatively mild and chronic variety of pemphigus is characterized by flaccid bullae and localized or generalized exfoliation. Pemphigus foliaceus begins with small flaccid bullae which rupture almost as they evolve to form crusting, below which is a moist surface with a tendency to bleed. After a time the exfoliative characteristics predominate, with few bullae.

The bullae are scattered over the scalp, face, and trunk, or the lesions may spread symmetrically until the entire integument is involved with a moist, red, edematous, exfoliative, and malodorous condition. The Nikolsky sign is present.

Oral lesions are rarely seen and then only as superficial erosive stomatitis.

Generally these patients are not severely ill. They complain of burning and pain and at times of severe pruritus. The lesions may persist for many years without affecting the general health.

Pemphigus foliaceus occurs mostly in adults between the ages of 40 and 50; however, it has been reported occurring in children as young as three. The sexes are affected equally. Ethnic prevalence in people of Jewish heritage is much less in pemphigus foliaceus than in pemphigus vulgaris.

The principal histologic finding consists of acantholysis in the upper epidermis, usually in the granular layer, leading to the formation of a cleft which may develop into a bulla in a superficial, often

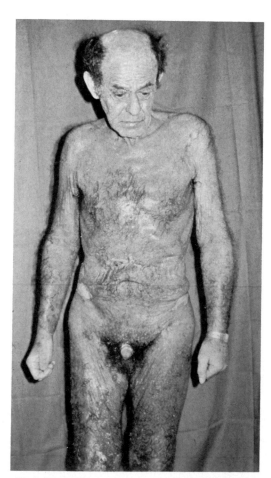

Figure 21–8. Pemphigus foliaceus. Generalized exfoliative erythroderma.

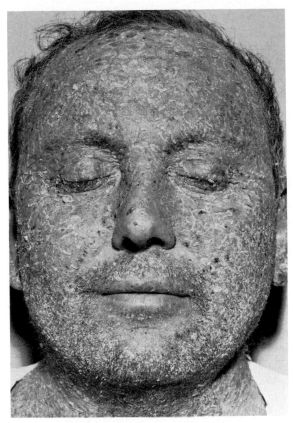

Figure 21-9. Pemphigus foliaceus.

precipitation, consisting of polypeptides of 260, 160, 110, and 85 kD molecular weight. This "PFC" is distinct from that of pemphigus vulgaris in that no PF sera precipitate the PV complex. The pemphigus foliaceus antibody binds to a 160-kD glycoprotein extracted from normal epidermis. This glycoprotein is identical to desmoglein I, a desmosomal glycoprotein.

Treatment is similar to that of pemphigus vulgaris; however, less vigorous treatment is required, which circumvents the side effects common to prolonged oral corticosteroid therapy. Judicious use of topical or intramuscular corticosteroids, or low dose immunosuppressive therapy, or both, may avoid the necessity of oral prednisone in most cases. Additionally, dapsone may be useful, either alone in mild cases or to reduce the steroid dose level.

Brazilian Pemphigus (Fogo Selvagem)

This disease is an endemic form of foliaceous pemphigus found in the tropical regions, mostly in certain interior areas of Brazil. Fifteen per cent of cases are familial. It is also known that fogo selvagem is common in children, adolescents, and young adults, with about one third of cases occurring before 20 years of age and two thirds by age 40. The initial lesions may be flaccid bullae, but later lesions are eczematoid, psoriasiform, impetiginous, or seborrheic in appearance. The midfacial areas may be involved. Azulay says that many cases begin as typical pemphigus erythematosus (Senear-Usher). Melanoderma and verrucous vegetative lesions are not unusual, and exfoliative dermatitis may occur. The mucous membranes are not often involved.

subcorneal, position, with acantholysis present at the floor as well as the roof of the bulla.

Direct immunofluorescence demonstrates intercellular IgG throughout the epidermis, and indirect IF, in most patients, is positive, demonstrating a circulating antibody directed against the cell surface of keratinocytes. Stanley and associates have characterized a "pemphigus foliaceus" complex by immuno-

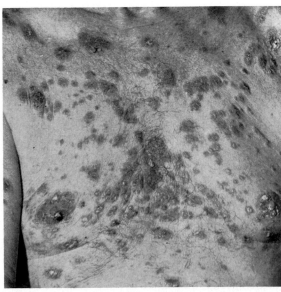

Figure 21-10. Pemphigus foliaceus.

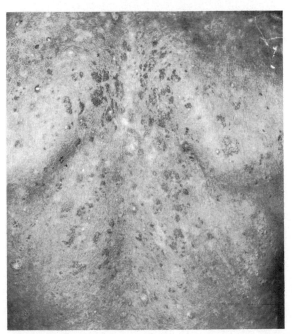

Figure 21-11. Fogo selvagem (Brazilian pemphigus). (Courtesy of Dr. F. Kerdel-Vegas, Venezuela.)

Nikolsky's sign is present. Diaz et al have recently published major clinical and epidemiologic studies of this disease. They feel it is due to an infectious agent, possibly carried by mosquitoes or black flies. Their two major reviews are recommended.

Histologically and immunohistologically fogo selvagem is identical to pemphigus foliaceus. Stanley et al have demonstrated that three of 13 patients with fogo selvagem had serum antibody which specifically bound to desmoglein I, a 160-kD desmosomal glycoprotein. This finding supports the hypothesis that pemphigus foliaceus and fogo selvagem are similar immunopathologically.

The course of this disease is like that of pemphigus foliaceus, of which it is a forme fruste. It may run a chronic course from five to 20 years. Death is usually from some intercurrent disease.

Beneficial effects have been described from administration of quinine and quinacrine, but the corticosteroids are the treatment of choice, as for pemphigus. Movement from their rural environment to the city and potent topical steroids are other adjuvant therapeutic measures.

Pemphigus Erythematosus (Senear-Usher Syndrome)

In the Senear-Usher syndrome, the early lesions are circumscribed patches of erythema and crusting which clinically resemble lupus erythematosus and

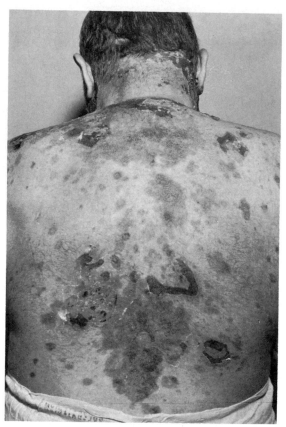

Figure 21–13. Pemphigus erythematosus. Note seborrheic distribution.

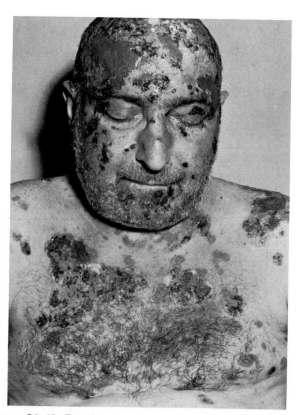

Figure 21–12. Pemphigus erythematosus. Note moon face from oral prednisone. Note also predilection for scalp, and sternal area.

are immunopathologically positive for the lupus band in 60 per cent of patients. The lupus band is present in addition to the universal presence of intercellular IgG on direct immunofluorescence. These are usually localized on the nose, cheeks, and ears—the sites frequently affected by lupus erythematosus. The lesions are erythematous and thickly crusted, bullous, or even hyperkeratotic. In addition to the erythematous crusted lesions on the face, which resemble lupus erythematosus, one sees crusting and impetiginous lesions amid bullae on the scalp, chest, and extremities, and bullae occur on the trunk from time to time. This is a comparatively benign type of chronic pemphigus in which the general health remains unimpaired. Pemphigus erythematosus is a localized, less severe variety of pemphigus, similar to pemphigus foliaceus, combined with discoid LE.

The histopathology is that of pemphigus foliaceus. Immunofluorescent stains show IgG and complement localized in both intercellular and basement membrane sites, adding to the link between this and lupus erythematosus. The biopsy should be taken from sun-exposed skin to maximize the possibility of a positive lupus band test. The antinuclear antibody is present in low titer in 30 per cent of patients.

The dosage of prednisone that has to be administered usually is much smaller than in pemphigus foliaceus. Tye and his associates obtained a favorable response to localized pemphigus erythematosus from the use of topical steroids.

American ML, et al: Pemphigus erythematosus: presentation of four cases and review of the literature. JAAD 1984, 10:215.

Azulay RD: Brazilian pemphigus foliaceus. Int J Dermatol 1982, 21:122.

Basset N, et al: Dapsone in initial treatment of superficial pemphigus. Arch Dermatol 1987, 123:783.

Cruz PD Jr, et al: Concurrent features of cutaneous lupus erythematosus and pemphigus erythematosus following myasthenia gravis and thymoma. JAAD 1987, 16:472.

Diaz LA, et al: Endemic pemphigus foliaceus (fogo selvagem). J Invest Dermatol 1989, 92:4.

Idem: Endemic pemphigus foliaceus (fogo selvagem). JAAD 1989, 20:657.

Eyre RW, et al: Maternal pemphigus foliaceus with cell surface antibody bound to neonatal epidermis. Arch Dermatol 1988, 124:25.

Korman NJ: Pemphigus. JAAD 1988, 18:1219.

Idem, et al: The pemphigus foliaceus and pemphigus vulgaris antigen complexes contain plakoglobulin. J Invest Dermatol 1989, 92:463.

Koulu K, et al: Human autoantibodies against a desmosomal core protein in pemphigus foliaceus. J Exp Med 1984, 160:1509.

Perry HO, et al: Pemphigus foliaceus. Arch Dermatol 1965, 91:10.

Rodan KP, et al: Generalized blistering eruption aggravated by heat. Arch Dermatol 1987, 123:393.

Stanley JR: The enigma of fogo selvagem. JAAD 1989, 20:675.

Stanley JR, et al: Antigenic specificity of fogo selvagem autoantibodies is similar to North American pemphigus foliaceus and distinct from pemphigus vulgaris autoantibodies. J Invest Dermatol 1986, 87:197.

Idem: The monoclonal antibody to the desmosomal glycoprotein desmoglein I binds the same polypeptide as human autoantibodies in pemphigus foliaceus. J Immunol 1986, 136:1227.

PEMPHIGOID

The fundamental criteria in this group of diseases are a subepidermal vesiculobullous eruption, and immunoreactants along the basement membrane zone. Bullae are tense, and the patients are usually elderly.

Bullous Pemphigoid

CLINICAL FEATURES. This entity was identified and named by Lever in 1953. Bullous pemphigoid is characterized by large, tense, subepidermal bullae that may be localized to some part of the body, with a predilection for the groin, the axillae, and the flexor surfaces of the forearms. The reported incidence of oral involvement varies from 8 to 39 per cent, with 20 per cent a frequently quoted incidence. The sex ratio is equal and the age at onset averages 65 to 75 years. After the bullae rupture, large denuded areas are seen, but these do not materially increase in size as they do in pemphigus vulgaris. Instead, the denuded areas show a tendency to heal spontaneously. In addition to the bullae there often are erythematous patches and urticarial plaques with a tendency to central clearing. These patches and plaques may be present without bullae early in the course of the disease.

Bullous pemphigoid may begin at a localized site, frequently on the shins. It may remain localized throughout the course of the disease or eventuate in generalized pemphigoid. Cases of the localized disease in which a vesicular eruption was limited to the soles (*dyshidrosiform pemphigoid*) were reported by Levine et al and Liu et al. Immunofluorescent studies confirmed the diagnosis. Hwang et al reported a patient who had lesions localized to the hands whose circulating antibody immunoprecipitated the bullous pemphigoid antigen. Lever calls this *localized bullous pemphigoid*. Limitation to areas of radiation therapy may also occur.

A vesicular variant of bullous pemphigoid manifested by tense, small, occasionally grouped blisters and termed vesicular pemphigoid was described by Bean et al. Gruber et al also reported a case. Immunofluorescence studies supported bullous pemphigoid, rather than dermatitis herpetiformis.

Many other variants of bullous pemphigoid have been described. Zone et al, Yung et al, and Massa et al have reported patients, mostly women, who have papules and nodules of the scalp and extremities, with sparing of the mucous membranes, sometimes resembling prurigo nodularis. Cases resembling pemphigus vegetans, but with IgG and C3 at the basement membrane zone, were reported by Winkelmann et al and by Kuokkanen et al. Tappeiner et al reported a patient with an erythrodermic form.

Bullous pemphigoid occurs most frequently in the elderly; however, it occurs also in young children. Robison and Odom have reviewed childhood bullous pemphigoid in a study of 14 reported cases.

Bullous pemphigoid has occasionally been reported to be associated with other diseases, such as rheumatoid arthritis (as reviewed by Callen), ulcerative colitis (as mentioned by Barth et al), multiple autoimmune diseases (Lynfield et al), and myasthenia gravis and thymoma in one case reported by James. It has been reported to have been induced by multiple drugs, with furosemide being the most convincingly associated medication. Bullous pemphigoid is seen occasionally with diabetes mellitus, as the case-controlled study by Chuang et al demonstrated. Bullous pemphigoid is not a marker for, or a manifestation of, underlying malignancy.

ETIOLOGY. Circulating basement membrane zone (BMZ) antibodies of the IgG class are present in approximately 70 per cent of patients with bullous pemphigoid. In most instances the antibodies fix complement in vitro, in contrast to pemphigus antibodies, which fail to do so. Complement is activated by both the classical and alternate pathways. No close correlation exists between the titer of antibodies and clinical disease activity. Circulating BMZ antibodies have been reported in pemphigus vulgaris very rarely, in burns quite commonly, and in one patient with Lyell's syndrome.

The direct IF test in bullous pemphigoid is, just as

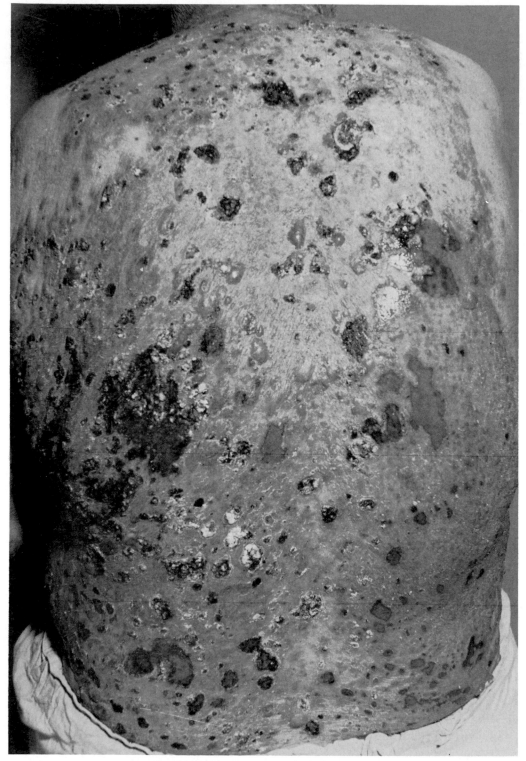

Figure 21–14. Bullous pemphigoid.

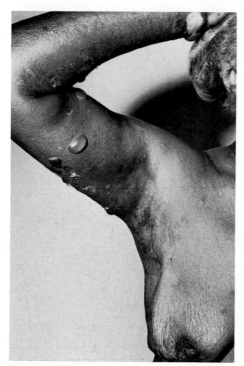

Figure 21–15. Bullous pemphigoid.

in pemphigus, a much more reliable test than the indirect IF test. In a positive test, linear IF is seen along the BMZ. IgG or C3 or both are regularly found in biopsies from involved as well as uninvolved skin. A positive direct IF test is present in nearly 100 per cent of patients, with C3 being most commonly present (approximately 100 per cent of cases), and IgG being present in about 80 per cent of cases. The two immunoglobulins, IgA and IgM, are each occasionally present.

Immunoelectron microscopy has localized the site of IgG binding to the lamina lucida, with some reports of accentuation near hemidesmosomes. Stanley et al have characterized the bullous pemphigoid antigen, which is synthesized by the keratinocyte. By immunoprecipitation of radiolabeled proteins from keratinocytes in culture they identified a protein with disulfide-linked chains of approximately 230 kD molecular weight in 36 of 37 examined.

Such IgG deposition was observed by Fellner and Katz in a case apparently caused by furosemide (Lasix) and therefore classified as a drug eruption until the IF evidence caused the diagnosis to be changed to "bullous pemphigoid induced by a drug."

PATHOGENESIS. The initial event is apparently the binding of the IgG autoantibody to the bullous pemphigoid antigen in the lamina lucida. Complement is activated, which produces factors with anaphylatoxic and chemotactic activity. Mast cells are activated and degranulated, which releases eosinophil chemotactic factors. Eosinophils accumulate in the dermis and eventually adhere to the basement membrane zone, where they release tissue-destructive enzymes and reactive oxygen intermediates.

Resultant injury to this zone causes dermoepidermal separation and blister formation.

HISTOLOGY. The histologic changes are characterized by the subepidermal bulla, by the absence of acantholysis and a superficial dermal infiltrate containing many eosinophils. The amount of inflammatory infiltrate is variable, and, consequently, the subepidermal bullae and the underlying skin may be "infiltrate-poor" or "infiltrate-rich." Often it is pronounced and contains many eosinophils. Eosinophilic spongiosis occurs, with which Crotty et al found bullous pemphigoid to be the most frequently associated disease. In fact Buskell et al reported that peripheral blood eosinophilia is present in 50 per cent of pemphigoid patients. Person and Rogers regard histopathology of minor importance in making a diagnosis.

TREATMENT. Treatment should be the same as for pemphigus, with the expectation that the disease will respond more readily to relatively lower doses of corticosteroids. Immunosuppressives may occasionally be necessary.

In exceptionally severe cases, as Siegel and Eaglstein have reported, an effective measure is pulse therapy with methylprednisolone, giving 15 mg/kg in 16 ml of bacteriostatic water over a period of 30–60 minutes daily for three doses. The sodium succinate salt (Solu-Medrol) is used. It is followed with oral prednisone if necessary, 0.4 mg/kg daily, for at least a week. Blistering stopped completely after the third dose in all eight of the patients in whom they used it.

Person et al reported that 10 per cent of bullous

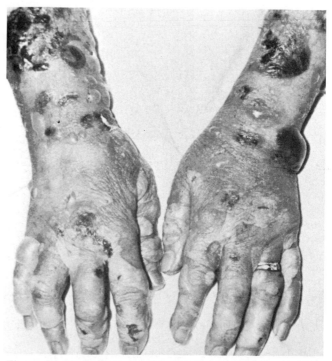

Figure 21–16. Bullous pemphigoid. (Courtesy of Dr. R. Feinstein.)

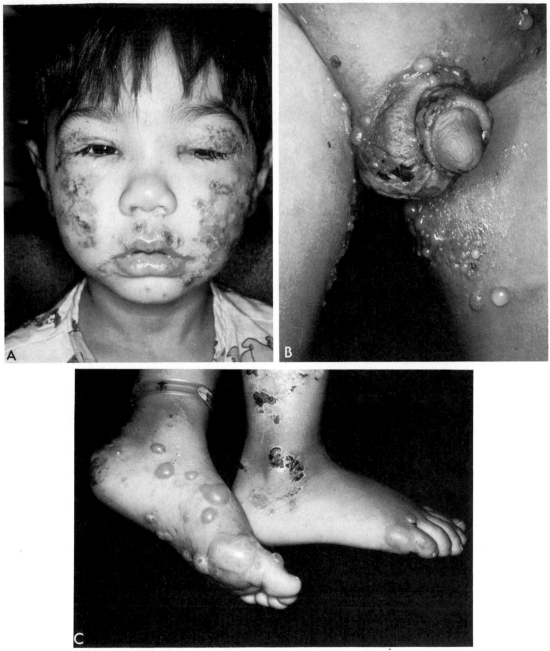

Figure 21–17. Bullous pemphigoid in a 3-year-old child.

pemphigoid patients responded to sulfapyridine or dapsone. The patients who responded tended to be younger (mean age of 54) and tended to have more neutrophils than eosinophils in the infiltrate.

Localized variants may respond to topical steroids alone. Westerhof reported success with topical clobetasol propionate alone in generalized pemphigoid. Fox et al reported two patients treated with erythromycin demonstrated improvement, while Berk et al treated four patients with tetracycline and niacinamide and obtained excellent clinical responses.

COURSE AND PROGNOSIS. Bullous pemphigoid is a relatively benign disease, usually being self-limited over a five to six year period. With adequate therapy response is usually complete: most patients have a lasting remission. Ten to 15 per cent of patients may experience relapses once therapy is stopped.

Cicatricial Pemphigoid (Benign Mucosal Pemphigoid)

In 1953 Lever suggested the designation "benign mucosal pemphigoid" for what had previously been termed ocular pemphigus, cicatricial pemphigoid, or essential shrinkage of the conjunctiva. Because of its

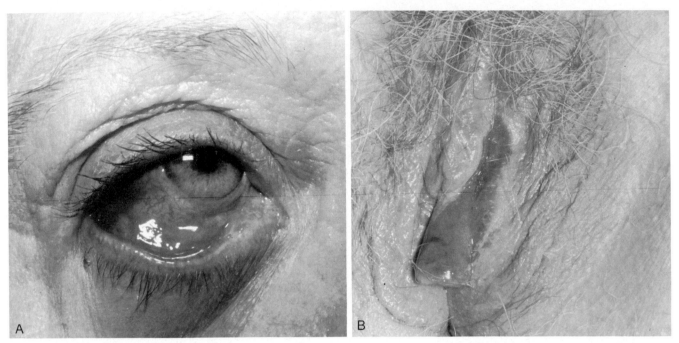

Figure 21–18. A and B, *Cicatricial pemphigoid with ocular and vaginal involvement. (Courtesy of Dr. Axel W. Hoke.)*

scarring nature, the designation cicatricial pemphigoid has gained acceptance.

Cicatricial pemphigoid is characterized by the predilection for evanescent vesicles, which heal by scarring, to occur on the mucous membranes, especially the conjunctiva and oral mucosa. Oral lesions occur in approximately 90 per cent of cases and conjunctival lesions in 66 per cent.

The oral mucosa is almost always involved, and may be the only affected site for years. *Desquamative gingivitis*, a diffuse erythema of the marginal and attached mucosa associated with areas of ulceration, vesiculation, and desquamation, is often the presenting sign, as documented by Rogers et al. The buccal gingivae are almost always involved, the lingual surfaces less regularly. Like cicatricial pemphigoid as a whole, desquamative gingivitis tends to affect middle-aged to elderly women. The female to male ratio is approximately two to one. Of 41 patients with desquamative gingivitis, Rogers et al classified 18 as localized oral pemphigoid (gingival involvement only, without progression over three-year average follow-up), 18 as cicatricial pemphigoid, and only two as pemphigus, one as lichen planus, one as epidermolysis bullosa, and one as contact stomatitis. In contrast, the dental literature and the experience of one of the authors (WDJ) indicate that at least half of all patients presenting with desquamative gingivitis have lichen planus by biopsy and immunofluorescent criteria. Other portions of the oral mucosa which may be involved by cicatricial pemphigold are the palate, tongue, and tonsillar pillars. Oral lesions rarely result in scarring.

The disorder is a chronic benign disease that may lead to a slowly progressive shrinkage of the ocular

mucous membranes and connective tissues, and eventually (untreated) to blindness. It is usually bilateral and associated with redness and flaccid vesicles on the conjunctiva, xerosis, fibrous adhesions (symblepharon), and scarring of the conjunctiva. Entropion, trichiasis, and corneal opacities develop and, ultimately, the adhesions attach both lids to the eyeball and narrow the palpebral fissure. Associated scarring may develop following attacks of

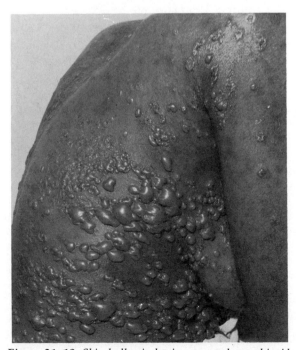

Figure 21–19. Skin bullae in benign mucosal pemphigoid.

inflammation, vesicles and denudation in the pharynx, esophagus, and nose, and on the glans penis and vagina. Stricture of the esophagus may occur. Deafness, suspected of being the result of middle ear involvement, was reported by Thomson et al in one case.

Cutaneous lesions are seen in approximately 25 per cent of patients. These lesions are tense bullae similar to those seen in bullous pemphigoid. The bullae, which heal with or without scarring, occur on the face, scalp, neck, and the inguinal region and extremities. Generalized lesions may also occur. Another type shows only erythema of the face or scalp, where denudation may occur, as reported by Slepyan and his associates. The oral and genital lesions may appear before the ocular signs.

The general health is usually not jeopardized; a chronic course is generally experienced, with deterioration of vision leading to blindness. In contrast to bullous pemphigoid, cicatricial pemphigoid shows little tendency to remission.

Cicatricial pemphigoid may be induced by penicillamine, as reported by Shuttleworth et al, or by clonidine.

In *Brunsting-Perry pemphigoid* there are no mucosal lesions, but one or several circumscribed erythematous patches develop on which recurrent crops of blisters appear. Ultimately atrophic scarring results. Generally, the areas of involvement are confined to the head and neck.

The histologic findings are identical to those of bullous pemphigoid, with the exception that fibrosis and scarring may be present in the upper dermis. The basement membrane separation occurs in the lamina lucida, as is the case in bullous pemphigoid.

Direct IF testing of lesional or perilesional skin or mucosa in cicatricial pemphigoid reveals C3 and IgG at the lamina lucida in 80 to 95 per cent of the patients. The basement membrane zone of mucosal glands stains as well. IgA or IgM or both may be found in about one fourth of cases, and a circulating antibody to the BMZ is found by indirect immunofluorescence in about 20 per cent of cases. Immunoelectron microscopy shows the antibodies to bind to the lamina lucida, and, with suction-blistered or saltsplit skin, binding is seen to occur at a deeper level than with bullous pemphigoid.

In mild cases, topical steroids, either Decadron elixir, 0.5 mg/5 ml, or Temovate ointment mixed with equal parts of Orabase, several times a day, may be effective. More aggressive cases, especially when ocular scarring is threatened, may require dapsone, alone or combined (if 100 mg/day is ineffective) with prednisone or parenteral triamcinolone, plus (if necessary) azathioprine or cyclophosphamide.

Aboobaker J, et al: The localization of the binding site of circulating IgA antibodies in linea IgA disease of adults, chronic bullous disease of childhood and childhood cicatricial pemphigoid. Br J Dermatol 1987, 116:293.

Ahmed AR, et al: Bullous pemphigoid family of autoimmune diseases. Int J Dermatol 1981, 20:541.

Alcalay J, et al: Bullous pemphigoid mimicking bullous erythema multiforme. JAAD 1988, 18:345.

Amato DA, et al: The prodrome of bullous pemphigoid. Int J Dermatol 1988, 27:560.

Anhalt GJ, et al: Mechanisms of immunologic injury: pemphigus and bullous pemphigoid (editorial). Arch Dermatol 1983, 119:711.

Barth JH, et al: Pemphigoid and ulcerative colitis. JAAD 1988, 19:303.

Basset N, et al: Dapsone as initial treatment in superficial pemphigoid. Arch Dermatol 1987, 123:783.

Berk MA, et al: The treatment of bullous pemphigoid with tetracycline and niacinamide. Arch Dermatol 1986, 122:670.

Bernard P, et al: Cicatricial pemphigoid. J Invest Dermatol 1989, 92:402.

Bushkell LL, et al: Bullous pemphigoid: a cause of peripheral blood eosinophilia. JAAD 1983, 8:648.

Chuang T, et al: Increased frequency of diabetes mellitus in patients with bullous pemphigoid. JAAD 1984, 11:1099.

Clayton CA, et al: Systemic lupus erythematosus and coexisting bullous pemphigoid; immunofluorescent investigations. JAAD 1982, 7:236.

Crotty C, et al: Eosinophilic spongiosis: A clinicopathologic review of 71 cases. JAAD 1983, 8:337.

Duschet P, et al: Bullous pemphigoid after radiation therapy. JAAD 1988, 18:441

Fine JD, et al: Immunofluorescence and immunoelectron microscopic studies in cicatricial pemphigoid. J Invest Dermatol 1984, 82:39.

Fine RM: The basement membrane autoantigen in epidermolysis bullosa acquisita. Cutis 1984, 33:646.

Fleming MG, et al: Mucous gland basement membrane immunofluorescence in cicatricial pemphigoid. Arch Dermatol 1988, 124:1407.

Foster CS, et al: Immunosupressive therapy for progressive ocular cicatricial pemphigoid. Ophthalmology 1982, 89:340.

Fox BJ, et al: Erythromycin therapy in bullous pemphigoid. JAAD 1982, 7:504.

Gruber GG, et al: Vesicular pemphigoid. JAAD 1980, 3:619.

Jawitz J, et al: Vesicular pemphigoid vs dermatitis herpetiformis. JAAD 1984, 10:892.

Korman N: Bullous pemphigoid. JAAD 1987, 16:907.

Kuokkanen K, et al: Pemphigoid vegetans: report of a case. Arch Dermatol 1981, 117:56.

Laskaris G, et al: Cicatricial pemphigoid. Oral Surg 1981, 51:48.

Levine N, et al: Localized pemphigoid simulating dyshidrosiform dermatitis. Arch Dermatol 1979, 115:320.

Liu H-N H, et al: Clinical variants of pemphigoid. Int J Dermatol 1986, 25:17.

Lynfield YL, et al: Bullous pemphigoid and multiple autoimmune diseases. JAAD 1983, 9:257.

Massa MC, et al: Bullous pemphigoid with features of prurigo nodularis. Arch Dermatol 1982, 118:937.

Mueller S, et al: A230-KD basic protein is the major bullous pemphigoid antigen. J Invest Dermatol 1989, 92:33.

Murata V, et al: Localized chronic pemphigoid of Brunsting-Perry. Arch Dermatol 1983, 119:921.

Nunzi E, et al: Dyshidrosiform pemphigoid. JAAD 1988, 19:568.

Person JR, et al: Bullous pemphigoid responding to sulfapyridine and the sulfones. Arch Dermatol 1977, 113:610.

Provost TT, et al: Unusual subepidermal bullous diseases with immunologic features of bullous pemphigoid. Arch Dermatol 1979, 115:156.

Rogers RS III, et al: Desquamative gingivitis: clinical, histopathologic, immunopathologic, and therapeutic observations. JAAD 1982, 7:729.

Idem: Treatment of cicatricial pemphigoid with dapsone. JAAD 1982, 6:215.

Shuttleworth D, et al: Cicatricial pemphigoid in D-penicillamine-treated patients with rheumatoid arthritis. Clin Exp Dermatol 1985, 10:392.

Siegel J, et al: High-dose methylprednisolone in treatment of bullous pemphigoid. Arch Dermatol 1984, 120:1157.

Silverman S Jr, et al: Oral mucous membrane pemphigoid: A study of sixty-five patients. Oral Surg 1986, 61:233.

Stanley JR, et al: Characterization of bullous pemphigoid antigen. Cell 1981, 24:897.

Tappeiner G, et al: Erythrodermic bullous pemphigoid. JAAD 1982, 6:489.

Thiers BH: Bullous pemphigoid. JAAD 1982, 6:1103.

Weigand DA: Effect of anatomic region on immunofluorescence diagnosis of bullous pemphigoid. JAAD 1985, 12:274.

Idem: Direct immunofluorescence in bullous pemphigoid. JAAD 1989, 20:437.

Idem, et al: Benign mucous membrane pemphigoid in a wife and husband. Arch Dermatol 1983, 119:59.

Westerhof W: Treatment of bullous pemphigoid with topical clobetasol propionate. JAAD 1989, 20:458.

Yung CW, et al: Pemphigoid nodularis. JAAD 1981, 5:54.

Zone JJ, et al: Bullous diseases. Dermatol Update, 1979:361–379.

Herpes Gestationis (Pemphigoid Gestationis)

CLINICAL FEATURES. Herpes gestationis (HG) has many clinical, histologic, and immunopathologic similarities to bullous pemphigoid, thus the suggested new name of pemphigoid gestationis. It is a rare (approximate incidence 1 in 50,000 pregnancies), pruritic, inflammatory bullous disease with onset either during pregnancy or during the postpartum period.

The onset of the disease is most often during the second trimester (average onset 21 weeks' gestation). Urticarial plaques and papules develop around the umbilicus and extremities, with subsequent spread over the abdomen, back, chest, and extremities, including the palms and soles. The face, scalp, and oral mucosa are usually spared. Within the infiltrated erythematous plaques tense vesicles and bullae erupt, often in an annular or polycyclic configuration. Pruritus is severe and may be paroxysmal (q.v.).

The disease will often flare within a few days after

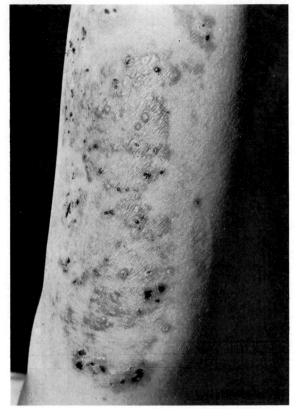

Figure 21–21. Herpes gestationis on left forearm. (Courtesy of Drs. J. A. Tolmach and M. Wolf.)

delivery, and then remit spontaneously, usually within three months. There may be recurrences with the taking of oral contraceptives, with subsequent menstrual periods, and nearly always with subsequent pregnancies. There is no scarring, unless scratching causes scars.

Maternal health is not affected. Lawley et al found a significant adverse effect on fetal survival; however, studies by Holmes et al and Shornick et al failed to confirm this.

Infants may manifest the disease in the form of urticarial lesions or bullae, but this occurs in less than 5 per cent of cases. These cases are of limited extent and severity and clear spontaneously without the need for therapy.

ETIOLOGY. HG is an autoimmune, antibody-mediated disease very like bullous pemphigoid. A complement-fixing IgG antibasement-zone antibody is present in the serum in 75 per cent of cases. This is deposited in the lamina lucida, and fixes complement at the site of dermal-epidermal separation. A 180-kD epidermal protein may be the antigen detected by the HG factor.

Studies have documented an increased frequency of HLA-DR3 and DR 4 in patients with HG. Women may have antibodies directed against their husbands' HLA antigens. Black women rarely manifest HG, and Shornik et al theorize this may be due to the low incidence of HLA-DR4 in American blacks.

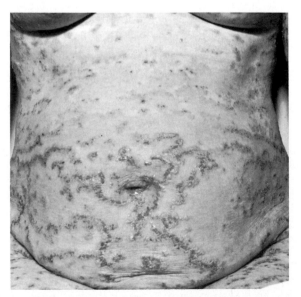

Figure 21–20. Herpes gestationis in fifth month of a seventh pregnancy. During only two pregnancies was patient free of lesions. (Courtesy of Dr. B. M. Kesten.)

Certainly hormonal factors influence the disease manifestation. In addition to being seen with pregnancy, menstruation, and oral contraceptives, the disease may occur in association with hydatidiform mole and choriocarcinoma.

PATHOGENESIS. This is similar to that of bullous pemphigoid (p. 545).

HISTOPATHOLOGY. A subepidermal, teardrop-shaped vesicle with a granulocyte-rich infiltration of the upper dermis with eosinophils and neutrophils is present.

On direct immunofluorescence all patients have C3 deposited in a linear pattern at the dermoepidermal junction. Approximately 25 to 40 per cent have IgG there as well.

By conventional indirect immunofluorescence, approximately 25 per cent of patients have a circulating IgG antibasement zone antibody, but in nearly 75 per cent the "HG factor," a complement-fixing IgG antibody, can be demonstrated by complement-enhanced indirect immunofluorescence.

Immunoelectron microscopy has demonstrated that the blister occurs at the level of the lamina lucida, with deposition of C3 and IgG at this site, exactly as in bullous pemphigoid.

Kelly et al have reported that the IgG autoantibody is directed against an antigen of 180 kD in the placenta. This antigen is also present in the skin. The major antigen they identified differed from the bullous pemphoid antigen, although a few of the sera they examined also identified this molecule, so they felt there was some shared antigenic recognition.

DIFFERENTIAL DIAGNOSIS. The main diagnosis to be considered is pruritic urticarial papules and plaques of pregnancy (PUPPP). There are, however, several diseases which are associated with, or uniquely occur in, pregnancy. Some, like PUPPP, are well-accepted, well-defined clinical entities. Others, such as papular dermatitis of pregnancy, are more controversial in that their very existence as an entity is questioned. All of these pregnancy-related dermatoses will be discussed below so they may be conveniently grouped together.

The differential diagnosis of herpes gestationis also includes diseases which are not specific for pregnancy but which may occur coincidentally. These include erythema multiforme, drug reactions, bullous pemphigoid, and pemphigus. Bronson et al reported a case of acrodermatitis enteropathica which flared in a bullous eruption with each pregnancy.

TREATMENT. Topical steroids may be adequate in some milder cases of herpes gestationis. Oral prednisone in a dose of 40 mg per day will be effective in the remainder, with tapering to the lowest effective dose given on alternate days being ideal; or intramuscular Kenalog, 60 mg initially, may be employed. We do not recommend dapsone, due to possible adverse effects on the fetus. Pyridoxine has been reported to have helped anecdotally; however, systemic steroids are the mainstay of therapy.

PREGNANCY-RELATED DERMATOSES

Pruritic Urticarial Papules and Plaques of Pregnancy (PUPPP). Also reported as *toxemic rash of pregnancy* by Bourne and *prurigo of pregnancy* by Nurse, Lawley et al first reported seven patients under this name in 1979. Holmes and Black prefer the designation *polymorphic eruption of pregnancy*. It is the commonest specific eruption of pregnancy.

This eruption is characterized by erythematous papules and plaques which begin as small 1–2-mm lesions within the abdominal striae. They then spread over the course of a few days to involve the abdomen, buttocks, thighs, and in some cases the arms and legs. The upper chest, face, and mucous membranes are generally spared. The lesions coalesce to form urticarial plaques, sometimes in configurate patterns, and occasionally spongiotic vesicles are present. Intense pruritus is characteristic, but only rarely are there excoriations.

This eruption occurs in primigravidas 75 per cent of the time, and usually does not recur with subsequent pregnancies. It begins late in the third trimester and resolves with delivery. In contrast to herpes gestationis, postpartum onset or exacerbation is rare. Fetal and maternal outcomes are not affected by this eruption, and only one newborn has been reported to be born with transient lesions of PUPPP.

Histologically the findings consist of a perivascular lymphohistiocytic infiltrate in the upper and often mid-dermis with a variable number of eosinophils and dermal edema. The epidermis is usually normal, although focal spongiosis, parakeratosis, or scale/crust may be present. Direct immunofluorescence is invariably negative.

Topical steroids frequently suffice, and if not, systemic steroids may safely be used to bring the eruption under control.

Papular Dermatitis of Pregnancy. This condition is quite controversial, with very few cases reported. It is defined as a pruritic, generalized eruption of 3–5-mm erythematous papules surmounted by a small, firm, central crust. The lesions may erupt at any time during pregnancy and usually resolve with delivery, although a case reported by Michand et al continued to develop papules premenstrually for 11 months postpartum.

A laboratory datum necessary to support the diagnosis of papular dermatitis of pregnancy is a marked elevation of the 24-hour urinary chorionic gonadotropin.

Systemic steroids are reportedly effective in controlling the eruption. The high incidence of fetal deaths reported by Spangler et al is now felt to be overstated. Treatment may prevent whatever adverse effects are seen. There may be recurrence in subsequent pregnancies.

Prurigo Gestationis (Besnier). This eruption consists of pruritic excoriated papules of the proximal limbs and upper trunk, which occur most often between the 20th and 34th week of gestation. It clears post partum and usually does not recur. Therapy with potent topical steroids is recommended. No adverse effects on maternal or fetal health are seen. Holmes and Black believe this eruption is simply an expression of atopic dermatitis in pregnancy.

Pruritic Folliculitis of Pregnancy. Six gravid women with small follicular pustules scattered widely over the trunk, which appeared during the second or third trimester and resolved by two or three weeks postpartum, were reported by Zeberman and Farmer in 1981. Holmes and Black had two identical cases. Acute folliculitis and focal spongiosis with exocytosis of polymorphonuclear leukocytes were seen on biopsy, and direct immunofluorescence was negative. Holmes and Black suspect it of being a type of hormonally induced acne.

Linear IgM Dermatosis of Pregnancy. This may become an additional pregnancy-related dermatosis. It was described by Alcalay et al in 1988 in a woman who developed small, red, follicular papules and pustules that on immunofluorescence showed linear deposits of IgM. More cases will be needed to confirm this as a pregnancy-related dermatosis.

Impetigo Herpetiformis. This is a form of severe pustular psoriasis occurring in pregnancy. It consists of an acute, usually febrile onset of grouped pustules on an erythematous base, which begins in the groin, axillae, and neck. Extension of these lesions occurs until large areas of skin are involved. There is a high peripheral white blood cell count, and hypocalcemia may be present.

The histopathology is that of pustular psoriasis.

There is resolution with delivery, but recurrences with subsequent pregnancies may be expected. Fetal death is not uncommon, due to placental insufficiency.

Treatment is with systemic corticosteroids, 40–60 mg of oral prednisone a day, or 60–80 mg of Kenalog intramuscularly, repeated as needed.

Prurigo Gravidarum. This pregnancy-related disease has no primary lesions, and is usually manifested only by generalized pruritus and jaundice. Secondary excoriations may be present. It is due to cholestasis, occurs late in pregnancy, resolves after delivery, and recurs with subsequent pregnancies. There is an increased incidence of fetal complications.

Ahmed AR, et al: Pruritic urticarial papules and plaques of pregnancy. JAAD 1981, 4:699.

Alcalay J, et al: Linear IgM dermatosis of pregnancy. JAAD 1988, 18:412.

Idem: Pruritic urticarial papules and plaques of pregnancy. J Reprod Med 1987, 32:315

Callen JP, et al: Pruritic urticarial papules and plaques of pregnancy. JAAD 1981, 5:401.

Holmes RC, et al: The fetal prognosis in pemphigoid gestationis (herpes gestationis). Br J Dermatol 1984, 110:67.

Idem: Herpes gestationis persisting for 12 years post partum (letter). Arch Dermatol 1986, 122:375.

Idem: The specific dermatoses of pregnancy. JAAD 1983, 8:405.

Holubar K, et al: Detection by immunoelectronmicroscopy of IgG deposits in skin of immunofluorescence-negative herpes gestationis. Br J Dermatol 1977, 96:569.

Katz SI, et al: Herpes gestationis: immunopathology and characterization of HG factor. J Clin Invest 1976, 57:1434.

Kelly SE, et al: Pemphigoid gestations. J Cutan Pathol 1988, 15:319.

Lawley TJ, et al: Fetal and maternal risk factors in herpes gestationis. Arch Dermatol 1978, 114:552.

Idem: Pruritic urticarial papules and plaques of pregnancy. JAMA 1979, 241:1696.

Lotem M, et al: Impetigo herpetiformis. JAAD 1989, 20:338.

Michaud RM, et al: Papular dermatitis of pregnancy. Arch Dermatol 1982, 118:1103.

Morrison LH, et al: Herpes gestationis autoantibodies recognize a 180-KD human epidermal antigen. J Clin Invest 1988, 81:2023.

Ortonne JP, et al: Localization of herpes gestationis antigen in isolated keratinocytes. J Invest Dermatol 1989, 92:495.

Oumeish OY, et al: Some aspects of impetigo herpetiformis. Arch Dermatol 1982, 118:103.

Rahbari H: Pruritic papules of pregnancy (letter). JAMA 1980, 244:1434.

Reid R, et al: Fetal complications of obstetric jaundice. Br Med J 1976, 1:182.

Shornick JK: Herpes gestationis. JAAD 1987, 17:539.

Idem: Herpes gestationis: Clinical and histologic features of twenty-eight cases. JAAD 1983, 8:214.

Idem: Herpes gestationis in blacks. Arch Dermatol 1984, 12:511.

Winton GB, et al: Dermatoses of pregnancy. JAAD 1982, 6:977.

Epidermolysis Bullosa Acquisita (Dermolytic Pemphigoid)

For many years this nonhereditary bullous dermatosis was considered to be a noninflammatory scarring mechanobullous eruption occurring in the elderly population. Exclusionary criteria for making the diagnosis of epidermolysis bullosa acquisita (EBA) were proposed in 1971 by Roenigk et al to be 1) clinical lesions of dystrophic EB, including increased skin fragility, trauma-induced blistering with erosions, atrophic scarring, milia over extensor surfaces, and nail dystrophy; 2) adult onset; 3) lack of a family history of EB; and 4) exclusion of all other bullous diseases such as porphyria cutanea tarda, pemphigoid, pemphigus, dermatitis herpetiformis, and bullous drug eruption. In 1981 Roenigk et al extended these criteria to include 5) IgG at the basement membrane zone by direct immunofluorescence; 6) the demonstration of blister formation beneath the basal lamina; and 7) deposition of IgG beneath the basal lamina.

Indirect immunofluorescent studies reveal circulating antibasement membrane zone antibodies in approximately half of the cases. Woodley et al by immunoblotting techniques showed that these antibodies are directed against a unique basement membrane zone polypeptide with subunit molecular weights of 290 and 145 kD. It has been shown that the antibodies are directed against type VII procollagen, which is present in anchoring fibrils in the upper dermis in the sublamina densa. Patients with bullous SLE have circulating antibodies with the same specificity.

This noninflammatory clinical presentation of EBA is the most commonly recognized type. It may manifest, in addition to the above mentioned clinical criteria, severe oral and esophageal mucosal scarring. The association of epidermolysis bullosa acquisita with many systemic diseases such as myeloma, granulomatous colitis, diabetes, lymphoma, leukemia, amyloidosis, and carcinoma is well established. In rare instances, cases of this noninflammatory subset may mimic either bullous or cicatricial pemphigoid. Lang et al reported a case in which severe eye involvement so dominated the clinical picture as to lead to an initial diagnosis of cicatricial pemphigoid.

In 1982 Gammon et al described a patient with a generalized, inflammatory bullous disease clinically resembling bullous pemphigoid, but with immunologic and ultrastructural features of EBA. Since that time many cases of this inflammatory subset of disease have been reported. Data collected by Gammon et al suggest that this type of onset of EBA may occur in as many as 50 per cent of all EBA patients. By analyzing 85 sera of patients diagnosed as having bullous pemphigoid they were able to imply that possibly 10 per cent of patients referred to medical centers as having bullous pemphigoid may actually have EBA. Differentiation may be suggested by the fact that histologically EBA patients usually had a predominence of neutrophils over eosinophils, but electronmicroscopic, immunoelectronmicroscopic, or immunoblot techniques, or sodium-chloride-split-skin techniques, are needed to absolutely differentiate this subtype of EBA from bullous pemphigoid.

Since bullous SLE and EBA share anti–basement membrane zone antibodies of identical specificity and there is both clinical and histologic overlap as well, this differential diagnosis may be difficult. The following features help to identify EBA: skin fragility, predilection for traumatized areas, and healing with scars and milia. In SLE sun-exposed skin is involved by preference, and in bullous SLE there is usually a dramatic response to dapsone.

Many of the inflammatory cases have associated diabetes mellitus, are HLA DR2 positive, and progress to the trauma-induced scarring type of EBA on long-term follow-up.

Treatment of EBA is in general unsatisfactory. A few inflammatory patients respond to steroids with or without azathioprine or dapsone, and these are worthy of a trial. Cyclosporin A has been reported effective and deserves further study. The noninflammatory types are best managed by supportive therapy.

Berger T, James WD: Advanced dermatopathology techniques. J Assoc Milit Dermatol 1984, 10:60.

Briggaman RA, et al: Epidermolysis bullosa acquisita of the immunopathological type (dermolytic pemphigoid). J Invest Dermatol 1985, 85 (suppl):79.

Caughman SW: Epidermolysis bullosa acquisita: the search for identity (editorial). Arch Dermatol 1986, 122:159.

Connolly SM, et al: Treatment of EBA with cyclosporin. JAAD 1987, 16:890.

Crow LL, et al: Clearing of EBA with cyclosporine. JAAD 1988, 19:937.

Gammon WR, et al: Epidermolysis bullosa acquisita—a pemphigoid-like disease. JAAD 1984, 11:820.

Idem: Epidermolysis bullosa acquisita presenting as an inflammatory bullous disease. JAAD 1982, 7:382.

Idem: Increased frequency of HLA-DR2 in patients with autoantibodies to epidermolysis bullous acquisita antigen. J Invest Dermatol 1988, 91:228.

Lang PG, et al: Severe ocular involvement in a patient with epidermolysis bullosa acquisita. JAAD 1987, 16:439.

Richter BJ, et al: The spectrum of epidermolysis bullosa acquisita. Arch Dermatol 1979, 115:1325.

Roenigk HH, et al: Epidermolysis bullosa acquisita. Arch Dermatol 1981, 117:383.

Rubenstein R, et al: Childhood epidermolysis bullosa acquisita. Arch Dermatol 1987, 123:722.

Wilson BD, et al: Epidermolysis bullosa acquisita. JAAD 1980, 3:280.

Woodley DT, et al: Identification of the skin basement-membrane autoantigen in epidermolysis bullosa acquisita. N Engl J Med 1984, 310:1007.

Idem: Epidermolysis bullosa acquisita: an autoimmune disease with distinctive immunoultrastructural features. Cutis 1983, 32:521.

Idem: Epidermolysis bullosa acquisita. Prog Dermatol 1988, 22:1.

Zachariae H: Cyclosporine A in EBA. JAAD 1987, 17:1058.

DERMATITIS HERPETIFORMIS
(Duhring's Disease)

CLINICAL FEATURES. Dermatitis herpetiformis is a chronic, relapsing, severely pruritic disease with grouped, symmetrical, polymorphous, erythematous-based lesions. The eruption may be papular, papulovesicular, vesiculobullous, bullous, or urticarial in nature. Upon involution there may rarely be hyperpigmentation and scars. Itching and burning are usually intense, and their paroxysmal quality provokes scratching to the point of bleeding and scars.

Spontaneous remissions lasting as long as a week and terminating abruptly with a new crop of lesions are a highly characteristic feature of the disease.

The eruption is usually strikingly symmetrical, sites of predilection being the scalp, the nuchal area, the posterior axillary folds, the sacral region, the buttocks, the knees, and the forearms, especially the extensor surfaces near the elbows. The lesions are acutely inflammatory and the eruption is characteristically polymorphous.

The manifestations differ widely according to the type of lesions and the distribution. Pruriginous papules are a common feature of most eruptions, and the edema in some of these is sufficient to produce vesicopapules. Mild eruptions may resemble prurigo or urticaria. Vesicular and bullous lesions, if present, are thick-walled and usually tense, and at first have clear contents, but after a time these become somewhat purulent if scratching has not unroofed them. Vesicles are more common than bullae; however, all types of these lesions may be present in one patient, or there may be no vesicles or bullae at all. In late stages of the disease there may be only pigmentation and grouped scars over sites of predilection. Pigmented spots alone over the lumbosacral region should arouse suspicion of dermatitis herpetiformis. The mucous membranes are

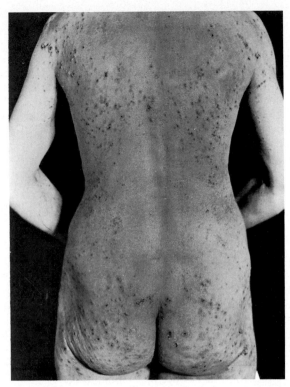

Figure 21–22. Dermatitis herpetiformis. Note large clear areas separating groups of lesions and the symmetry.

involved in rare cases, mostly when bullae are numerous.

The course of the disease is generally lifelong, with prolonged remissions being a rare event. The general health is not directly affected in Duhring's disease. It is remarkable, in view of the frequently associated gluten-sensitive enteropathy (GSE), how very few patients with dermatitis herpetiformis ever have diarrhea. But some do.

Several large series have now been published documenting the occurrence of dermatitis herpetiformis in childhood. The studies by Marsden et al, Reunala et al, and Karapti et al document that children present with disease clinically similar to the adult type, have identical histologic and immunofluoresent findings, and have a high incidence of HLA B8 and DR3 and abnormal jejunal biopsies. Karpati et al reported finding unusual palmar blisters or brown macules in 30 of 47 children with dermatitis herpetiformis, in every one of whom the diagnosis had been confirmed by finding granular IgA deposits in the skin. They were not present in patients who were asymptomatic or who had responded to treatment with a gluten-free diet or dapsone or sulfapyridine. They were seldom found on the feet. These palmar lesions may also be seen in many adult patients. Treatment with sulfones results in prompt response, as in adults; sulfapyridine should be tried first.

Seventy-seven to 87 per cent of patients with dermatitis herpetiformis and IgA deposits in the skin are HLA-B8 positive; the frequency of this specificity

equals that observed in ordinary GSE. Another HLA antigen, DR3, has been shown to occur in ordinary GSE at a higher frequency than the HLA-B8 itself; similarly, HLA-DR3 is as frequent as HLA-B8, or more so, in dermatitis herpetiformis. These HLA markers are associated with other autoimmune diseases and are a marker of patients who appear to have an overactive immune response to common antigens. It is unexpectedly frequent in family members, undoubtedly owing to genetic predisposition.

One common antigen that patients with dermatitis herpetiformis appear to be antigenically stimulated by is gluten, a protein found in cereals, with the exception of rice and corn. In some way as yet to be determined, patients with dermatitis herpetiformis react to gluten in the diet. Villous atrophy of the jejunum and inflammation of the small bowel develop. IgA antibodies are apparently formed. Whether these form IgA immune complexes which are then carried to, and deposited in, the skin, or whether the IgA antibodies bind to antigenically similar skin proteins, is not known.

IgA is bound to the skin, and this apparently activates complement, primarily via the alternate pathway. Once it is activated, the resulting inflammation of the skin with the development of lesions follows.

Patch tests with 50 per cent KI in vaseline produce a bulla in uncontrolled dermatitis herpetiformis, but only exceptionally in patients controlled by a gluten-

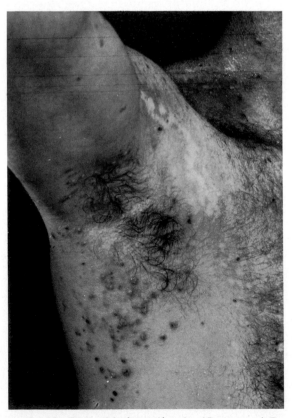

Figure 21–23. Dermatitis herpetiformis. (Courtesy of Dr. H. Shatin.)

free diet or by sulfone therapy. Hafenden et al showed that there was no difference in the presence or amount of IgA or C3 between the induced bullae and the normal skin.

ASSOCIATED DISEASE. Callen reviewed the association of bullous diseases with autoimmune diseases and found thyroid disorders to be increased in dermatitis herpetiformis. Cunningham et al found thyroid disease in 26 of 50 patients examined. Leonard et al found an increased incidence of malignancy in their patients (relative risk 2.38). The incidence of small bowel lymphoma is also increased; Jenkins et al provided a review of 12 cases of this association.

ENTEROPATHY IN DERMATITIS HERPETIFORMIS. It has been found that about 70 per cent of the patients with dermatitis herpetiformis have abnormalities in the jejunal mucosa. If given a high gluten diet, nearly all will develop abnormal findings. Marks and Shuster pointed out that this enteropathy is indistinguishable from celiac disease. The enteropathy seldom reaches the clinical horizon.

The dapsone requirement in dermatitis herpetiformis is not significantly decreased, according to most reports, until a gluten-free diet has been followed for three to six months, and improvement in the skin lesions on the diet alone takes an equally long time to become manifest. Fry et al have shown that nearly all patients who adhere to a strict gluten-free diet, if followed long enough, are able to either stop their medication, or significantly reduce the dosage. The diet is a difficult one, and in successful cases, such expressions as "highly motivated" and "dedicated" occur frequently.

DIAGNOSIS. The distinction between pemphigoid, erythema multiforme, and bullous dermatitis herpetiformis may sometimes be difficult. The distinction from linear IgA bullous dermatosis is often clinically impossible. Other conditions considered in the differential diagnosis at times are scabies, contact dermatitis, nummular eczema, neurotic excoriations, insect bites, and chronic bullous disease of childhood. The finding of IgA in a granular pattern in the dermal papillae in normal skin is specific and pathognomonic for dermatitis herpetiformis.

Autoantibodies. Accetta et al and Beutner et al have found circulating IgA antibodies against the smooth muscle cell endomysium in 70 per cent of dermatitis herpetiformis patients, in nearly all active celiac disease, and almost never in other conditions. Direct IF of noninvolved skin reveals deposits of IgA alone or together with deposits of C3 arranged in a granular pattern in the dermal papillae. IgM and IgG deposits are occasionally observed in association with IgA. Deposits may be focal, so that multiple biopsies may be needed, and the deposits of antibody are more often seen in previously involved skin. By immunoelectron microscopy one observes IgA either alone or in conjunction with C3, IgG, or IgM as clumps in the upper dermis.

INCIDENCE AND PREVALENCE. This disease has equal male to female incidence with the average age of onset between 20 and 40 years. It does occur with some frequency in children. Blacks are rarely affected.

HISTOPATHOLOGY. The initial changes, as described by MacVicar and his associates, are first noted at the tips of the dermal papillae, where edema and an eosinophilic and neutrophilic exudate occur to produce a subepidermal separation. This eventually leads to bulla formation. A degeneration of the papillae tips occurs, the epidermis separates, and the confluence of several dermal tips produces the vesicles. The cellular infiltrate contains many neutrophils and few eosinophils.

The biopsy should always include a good piece of the surrounding erythematous portion of the lesion where there is no apparent vesicle.

The histologic differentiation of linear IgA bullous dermatosis from dermatitis herpetiformis—if indeed they are different—is extremely difficult. Smith et al have devised an elaborate quantitative scheme in which the number of rete tips with neutrophils in basal vacuoles, and the length of the basement membrane zone associated with them (greater in IgA bullous dermatosis), and the number of microabscesses in the dermal papillae (greater in dermatitis herpetiformis) are counted or measured.

TREATMENT. The drugs chiefly used are dapsone and sulfapyridine.

The most effective sulfone is diaminodiphenylsulfone (dapsone). The dose varies between 50 and 300 mg daily, usually starting with 100 mg daily and increasing gradually to an effective level or until side effects occur. Once a favorable response is attained, the dosage is decreased to the minimum that does not permit recurrence of signs and symptoms. Hemolytic anemia, leukopenia, methemoglobinemia, and rarely agranulocytosis or peripheral neuropathy may occur. Acute hemolytic anemia (which may be severe) occurs in patients with glucose-6-phosphate dehydrogenase deficiency, therefore a G6PD level should be done prior to therapy. So rare is this deficiency, however, that many prefer simply to use a low starting dose (50 mg a day) and warn and watch the patient closely for dark urine. The patient should be warned to report by telephone any incident of red or brown urine, or blue nailbeds or lips. A white blood cell count and hematocrit determination should be done weekly for four weeks, bimonthly for the next two months, and every four to six months thereafter. Liver function tests should be monitored bimonthly for the first four months, then checked with the hematologic studies every four to six months.

Sulfapyridine also has long been used for the treatment of Duhring's disease. Sulfapyridine and dapsone response was regarded, prior to the availability of immunofluorescence, as a specific test for the diagnosis; if the patient did not respond to one of them, he did not have Duhring's. After a test dose of 0.5 gm of sulfapyridine, one tablet (0.5 gm) four times daily is given. The dose is then increased if necessary, or reduced if possible. Usually 1 to 4 gm is required for good control.

Griffiths et al found indomethacin worsened the disease in nine of 13 patients challenged prospectively. It may increase sulfone requirements.

Gluten-free diet. If a gluten-free diet is followed strictly, the patient will almost certainly be able to take less medication, or stop it altogether. Also some evidence obtained by Leonard et al suggests this may decrease the incidence of associated malignancy. It is a very difficult diet to follow, and strict adherence is necessary if the desired effects are to be attained.

Accetta P, et al: Anti-endomysial antibodies. Arch Dermatol 1986, 122:459.

Beutner EH, et al: Sensitivity and specificity of IgA-class antiendomysial antibodies for dermatitis herpetiformis and findings relevant to their pathogenic significance. JAAD 1986, 15:464.

Cunningham MJ, et al: Thyroid abnormalities in dermatitis herpetiformis. Ann Intern Med 1985, 102:194.

Emmacora E, et al: Long-term follow-up of dermatitis herpetiformis in children. JAAD 1986, 15:24.

Fry L, et al: Long-term follow-up of dermatitis herpetiformis with and without dietary gluten withdrawal. Br J Dermatol 1982, 107:631.

Griffiths CEM, et al: Dermatitis herpetiformis exacerbated by indomethacin. Br J Dermal 1985, 112:443.

Haffenden GP, et al: The potassium iodide patch test in dermatitis herpetiformis in relation to treatment with gluten-free diet and dapsone. Br J Dermatol 1980, 103:313.

Hall RP, et al: IgA-containing circulating immune complexes in dermatitis herpetiformis. Clin Exp Immunol 1980, 40:431.

Idem: The pathogenesis of dermatitis herpetiformis: recent advances. JAAD 1987, 16:1129.

Idem: Dietary management of dermatitis herpetiformis. Arch Dermatol 1987, 123:1378.

Huff JC: Immunopathogenesis of dermatitis herpetiformis. J Invest Dermatol 1985, 84:237.

Jenkins D, et al: Histiocytic lymphoma occurring in a patient with dermatitis herpetiformis. JAAD 1983, 9:252.

Kalis JB, et al: Dermatitis herpetiformis (commentary). JAMA 1983, 250:217.

Karpati S, et al: Palmar and plantar lesions in children with dermatitis herpetiformis Duhring. Cutis 1986, 37:184.

Katz SI, et al: Dermatitis herpetiformis: the skin and the gut. Ann Intern Med 1980, 93:857.

Idem: The pathogenesis of dermatitis herpetiformis. J Invest Dermatol 1978, 70:63.

Lane AT, et al: Class-specific antibodies to gluten in dermatitis herpetiformis. J Invest Dermatol 1983, 80:402.

Lawley TJ, et al: Small-intestinal biopsies and HLA types in dermatitis herpetiformis patients with granular and linear IgA skin deposits. J Invest Dermatol 1980, 74:9.

Leonard J, et al: Gluten challenge in dermatitis herpetiformis. N Engl J Med 1983, 308:816.

Leonard JN, et al: Increased incidence of malignancy in dermatitis herpetiformis. Br Med J 1983, 286:16.

Marsden RA, et al: A study of benign chronic bullous dermatosis of childhood and a comparison with dermatitis herpetiformis and bullous pemphigoid occurring in childhood. Clin Exp Dermatol 1980, 5:159.

Massone L, et al: Dermatitis herpetiformis. JAAD 1988, 19:577.

Meyer LJ, et al: Familial incidence of dermatitis herpetiformis. JAAD 1987, 17:643.

Pierce DK, et al: Purpuric papules and vesicles of the palms in dermatitis herpetformis. JAAD 1987, 16:1274.

Reunala T, et al: Dermatitis herpetiformis. Arch Dis Child 1984, 59:517.

Idem: Dermatitis herpetiformis, lymphoma, and gluten-free diet (letter). JAAD 1984, 10:526.

Shelley WB: Treatment of dermatitis herpetiformis with cholestyramine. Br J Dermatol 1980, 103:663.

Silvers DN, et al: Treatment of dermatitis herpetiformis with colchicine. Arch Dermatol 1980, 116:1373.

Smith SB, et al: Linear IgA bullous dermatosis vs dermatitis herpetiformis. Arch Dermatol 1984, 120:324.

Zone JJ, et al: Granular IgA is decreased or absent in never-involved skin in dermatitis herpetiformis. J Invest Dermatol 1985, 84:332.

Linear IgA Bullous Dermatosis

Linear IgA deposits, and lack of association with HLA-B8 and with enteropathy, are the chief distinguishing features of this otherwise dermatitis-herpetiformis like blistering disease. Clinically, some patients may have skin lesions resembling pemphigoid more closely than dermatitis herpetiformis. Mucous membrane lesions, very rare in dermatitis herpetiformis, may occur, as in pemphigoid. Several medications have been reported to induce this condition, including vancomycin, lithium carbonate, and diclophenac. By immunoelectron microscopy, IgA is found, either in the lamina lucida or below the basal lamina. When it is present below the lamina densa, according to Rusenko et al, the antibodies are directed against type VII collagen.

Patients are ordinarily treated with dapsone or sulfapyridine, but Aram reported a case in which hemolysis occurred and a switch to colchicine, 500 mg t.i.d., proved completely successful. Systemic corticosteroids are at times necessary—and effective.

Peterson et al have reported a case in a 76-year-old man in which the initial findings were those of bullous pemphigoid, with linear IgG at the basement membrane zone (BMZ) and a low titer circulating IgG anti-BMZ antibody. Three years later this had disappeared and there was linear IgA at the BMZ. Initially he had been treated with prednisone, but at the later time dapsone was effective.

Aboobaker J, et al: The localization of the binding site of circulating IgA antibodies in linea IgA disease of adults, chronic bullous disease of childhood, and childhood cicatricial pemphigoid. Br J Dermatol 1987, 116:293.

Aram H: Linear IgA bullous disease: successful treatment with colchicine. Arch Dermatol 1984, 120:960.

Baden LA, et al: Vancomycin-induced linear IgA bullous dermatosis. Arch Dermatol 1988, 124:1186.

Barnabas MA, et al: Linear IgA bullous dermatosis associated with Hodgkin's disease. JAAD 1988, 19:1122.

Bhogal B, et al: Linear IgA bullous dermatosis of adults and children. Br J Dermatol 1987, 117:289.

Leonard JN, et al: Evidence that the IgA in patients with linear IgA disease is qualitatively different from that of patients with dermatitis herpetiformis. Br J Dermatol 1984, 110:315.

Idem: Linear IgA disease in adults. Br J Dermatol 1982, 107:301.

Long SA, et al: Arciform blistering in an elderly woman. Arch Dermatol 1988, 124:1705.

Peters MS, et al: IgA deposition at the cutaneous basement membrane zone. JAAD 1989, 20:761.

Peterson MJ, et al: A case of linear IgA disease presenting initially with IgG immune deposits. JAAD 1986, 14:1014.

Rusenko KW, et al: Type VII collagen is the antigen recognized by IgA anti–sub lamina densa autoantibodies. J Invest Dermatol 1989, 92:510.

Smith SB, et al: Linear IgA bullous dermatitis vs dermatitis herpetiformis. Arch Dermatol 1984, 120:324.
Wilson BD, et al: Linear IgA bullous dermatosis: an immunologically defined disease. Int J Dermatol 1985, 24:569.

Chronic Bullous Disease of Childhood (CBDC)

This acquired, self-limited bullous disease may begin by age two or three and remits by age 13. The average age at onset is five years. Bullae develop on either erythematous or normal-appearing skin, preferentially involving the lower trunk, buttocks, genitalia, and thighs. Perioral and scalp lesions are common, and oral mucous membrane lesions are not uncommon; indeed, Wojnarowska et al report seeing them in 74 per cent of their 29 patients. Bullae are often arranged in a rosette or annular array, the so-called "cluster of jewels" configuration. Pruritus is often severe.

Histologic findings are the presence of a subepidermal bulla filled with a preponderance of neutrophils. In some cases eosinophils predominate, as in bullous pemphigoid. Direct immunofluorescence reveals a linear deposition of IgA at the basement membrane zone. Indirect immunofluorescence is positive for circulating IgA antibasement-membrane-zone antibodies, usually in low titer, in approximately 50 per cent of cases. Immunoelectron microscopy and immunomapping studies have been conflicting; some cases have had IgA within the lamina lucida, and some have had it below the lamina densa. One revealed the IgA to be deposited both in the lamina lucida and below the lamina densa. Horiguchi et al reported the deposits to be only in the lamina lucida. In two cases subjected by one of us (WDJ) to immunomapping studies, the circulating IGA antibodies were found to bind on the epidermal side of sodium-chloride–split skin, indicating deposition within the lamina lucida.

The untreated disease runs a variably chronic and remitting course, with eventual spontaneous resolution by adolescence. Treatment is most often successful with either sulfapyridine or dapsone, with sulfapyridine being the preferred medication. Occasional cases respond to topical steroids alone. Systemic steroids are necessary in some cases, although a conservative approach is to be followed, since this is a benign, self-remitting disorder.

Aboobaker J, et al: The localization of the binding site of circulating IgA antibodies in linea IgA disease of adults, chronic bullous disease of childhood, and childhood cicatricial pemphigoid. Br J Dermatol 1987, 116:293.
Ayres S Jr: Bullous disease of childhood: possibility of response to vitamin E (letter). Austral J Dermatol 1983, 24:44.
Horiguchi Y, et al: Immunoelectron microscopic observations in a case of linear IgA bullous dermatitis of childhood. JAAD 1986, 14:593.
Marsden RA, et al: A study of benign chronic bullous dermatosis of childhood and comparison with dermatitis herpetiformis and bullous pemphigoid in childhood. Clin Exp Dermatol 1980, 5:159.
Rogers M, et al: Chronic bullous disease of childhood—aspects of management. Austral J Dermatol 1982, 23:62.
Sweren RJ, et al: Benign chronic bullous dermatosis of childhood: a review. Cutis 1982, 29:350.
Wojnarowska F, et al: A comparative study of benign chronic bullous disease of childhood and linear IgA disease of adults. Br J Dermatol 1985, 113 (suppl 29):16.
Idem: Chronic bullous disease of childhood, childhood cicatricial pemphigoid, and linear IgA disease of adults. JAAD 1988, 19:792.

Intraepidermal Neutrophilic IgA Dermatosis

In 1985 Huff et al reported the case of an elderly man with a chronic bullous dermatosis with unique

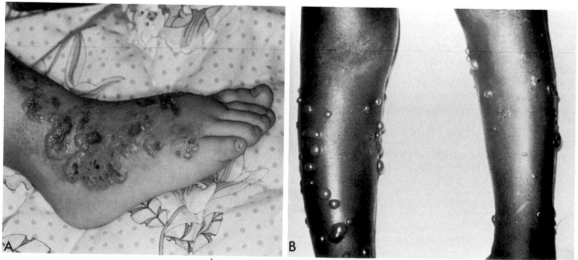

Figure 21–24. Chronic bullous disease of childhood. (A, *Courtesy of Dr. J. Schiffner;* B, *courtesy of Dr. S. Prystowsky.*)

histologic and immunopathologic findings. Clinically there were generalized flaccid bullae which rapidly ruptured and crusted. No scarring was present upon healing. No mucosal lesions were present and the distal extremities, face, and neck were spared. Neither grouping nor symmetry were present. Ten reported cases have been reviewed by Beutner, who feels they belong in the pemphigus category. Some cases manifest acantholysis, and some have circulating autoantibodies. Dapsone, prednisone, and etretinate have all been successful therapeutic agents.

Histologic findings consisted of neutrophilic exocytosis and in some areas neutrophils arranged in a linear fashion at the dermal-epidermal junction. Later, intraepidermal abscesses were formed; no acantholysis was present. Direct immunofluorescence repeatedly showed an intercellular deposition of IgA within the epidermis with minimal staining of the basal layer. No circulating antibodies were found.

Therapy with dapsone was effective at a maintenance dose of 25 mg per day. On discontinuance, however, relapse was the rule. It also responded to high-dose oral corticosteroids prior to the institution of dapsone.

Beutner EH, et al: IgA pemphigus foliaceus. JAAD 1989, 20:89.
Huff JC, et al: Intraepidermal neutrophilic IgA dermatosis. N Engl J Med 1985, 313:1643.

AUTOIMMUNE PROGESTERONE DERMATITIS

A chronic and extensive distinctive vesicobullous eruption resembling dermatitis herpetiformis was reported by Shelley and his associates. The lesions in the 27-year-old woman consisted of flaccid bullae in an arcuate pattern on the back and shins. The bullae were on an erythematous base. Rupture of the bullae resulted in crusting and hypertrophic and depigmented scars.

Although the lesions were almost always present, regular exacerbations occurred a week or 10 days prior to menstruation. In addition, flares could be induced within seven hours after 20 mg of progesterone was given.

There was a satisfactory response to administration of corticosteroids and, later, to oophorectomy.

Hart reported seven patients with autoimmune progesterone dermatitis and emphasized the polymorphous nature of the disease in which urticaria, erythema multiforme, and dyshidrosiform lesions were seen. Intradermal skin testing to progesterone was performed to confirm the diagnosis. Six of the seven patients had a history of use of artificial progesterones prior to the beginning of their eruption. It was postulated that the artificial progesterones may have triggered their autosensitivity. Treatment

with conjugated estrogens resulted in remission of the disease in five of the women.

Hart R: Autoimmune progesterone dermatitis. Arch Dermatol 1977, 113:426.
Shelley WB, et al: Autoimmune progesterone dermatitis. JAMA 1964, 190:35.

TRANSIENT ACANTHOLYTIC DERMATOSIS

Grover in 1970 described a new dermatosis occurring predominantly in persons over 50 years old, consisting of a sparse eruption, often of limited extent and nearly always of limited duration. The lesions were fragile vesicles which rapidly turned to crusted and somewhat dyskeratotic erosions, usually under 1 cm in diameter. The eruption is usually limited to the chest or shoulder girdle area and upper abdomen.

Simon and Bloom in 1976 reported a case persisting for three years and called it "persistent" acantholytic dermatosis. In our experience it is not uncommon for this eruption to follow a prolonged course.

Chalet et al in 1977 proposed division of the entity into four histologic types, resembling, respectively, Darier's disease, pemphigus vulgaris, benign familial pemphigus, and simple spongiosis. Often two or more types can be found in a single biopsy specimen. Direct immunofluorescence studies are negative.

Grover reviewed his 375 patients with the disease in 1984. Many of them were asymptomatic and were discovered in the course of examining the sun-exposed skin of patients with skin cancer. He had only five cases under the age of 40; most were 60–69. Asteatotic eczema was five times as frequent among them as in controls. Skin cancer was almost twice as common, but of course there was a selection bias. The male:female ratio was 3:1.

The treatment of choice is potent topical steroids. In the few cases who do not respond and who are symptomatic, dapsone is an alternative which has been reported to be effective. Paul and Arndt reported a case with extensive skin lesions, only partly controlled with oral prednisone and not at all by 300,000 units/day of vitamin A, in whom 50 mg of methoxsalen and 2 joules/cm^2 of UVA twice a week, increased by 0.5 joule/cm^2 each time, first flared the eruption and then improved it slowly. A shielded control patch 10 cm in diameter did not improve, but it improved when shielding was removed.

Helfman found Accutane effective in three of four cases, with remissions of up to 10 months.

Grover reported in 1989 that in cases with pruritus and a poor response, Grenz radiation—two or three treatments of 300 rads each—is a reliable treatment. One of us (HLA) has confirmed this since being told it by Grover in 1982.

Chalet M, et al: Transient acantholytic dermatosis: a reevaluation. Arch Dermatol 1976, 113:431.

Grover RW: Transient acantholytic dermatosis. Arch Dermatol 1970, 101:426.

Idem: Transient acantholytic dermatosis: electron microscope study. Arch Dermatol 1971, 104:26.

Idem: Transient acantholytic dermatosis. Unit 6–16, vol 2, in Demis DJ: Clinical Dermatology, Philadelphia, Harper & Row, 1985 (revised 1989).

Idem, et al: The association of transient acantholytic dermatosis with other skin diseases. JAAD 1984, 11:253.

Held JL, et al: Grover's disease provoked by ionizing radiation. JAAD 1988, 19:137.

Helfman RJ: Grover's disease treated with isotretinoin. JAAD 1985, 12:981.

Paul BS, et al: The response of transient acantholytic dermatosis to photochemotherapy. Arch Dermatol 1984, 120:121.

Simon RS, et al: Persistent acantholytic dermatosis: a variant of transient acantholytic dermatosis (Grover's disease). Arch Dermatol 1976, 112:1429.

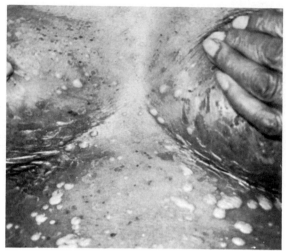

Figure 21–26. Superficial pustules of subcorneal pustular dermatosis.

SUBCORNEAL PUSTULAR DERMATOSIS
(Sneddon-Wilkinson Disease)

Sneddon and Wilkinson in 1956 described this chronic pustular disease, which occurs chiefly in middle-aged women. Johnson and Cripps reported this entity in two three-year-old children. The pustules are as superficial as those of impetigo and are arranged in annular and serpiginous patterns, especially upon the abdomen, axillae, and groins. Sometimes vesicles are present, but these usually change into pustular blebs. Cultures from the pustules are sterile. Oral lesions are rare. Some cases occur in association with an IgA (or infrequently another) monoclonal gammopathy.

Histologically, the pustules form below the stratum corneum, as in impetigo and in pemphigus foliaceus. Acantholysis is absent. The cavity contains many neutrophils. Spongiosis occurs subjacent to the blister, and a perivascular mantle composed of neutrophils and some eosinophils is present in the upper dermis.

Dapsone, 50 to 200 mg daily, appears to be effective in most cases; however, some patients have responded better to sulfapyridine therapy. Etretinate has been helpful in several cases. Without treatment this is a chronic condition with remissions of variable duration.

Chorzelski T, et al: Immunopathologic investigations in subcorneal pustular dermatosis (Sneddon-Wilkinson). Derm Wschr 1967, 153:558.

Hashimoto T, et al: Intercellular IgA dermatosis with clinical features of subcorneal pustular dermatosis. Arch Dermatol 1987, 123:1062.

Ise S: Subcorneal pustular dermatosis. Arch Dermatol 1965, 92:169.

Johnson SAM, et al: Subcorneal pustular dermatosis in children. Arch Dermatol 1974, 109:73.

Kasha EE, et al: Subcorneal pustular dermatosis (Sneddon-Wilkinson disease) in association with a monoclonal gammopathy. JAAD 1988, 19:854.

Sneddon IB: Subcorneal pustular dermatosis. Br J Dermatol 1956, 68:385.

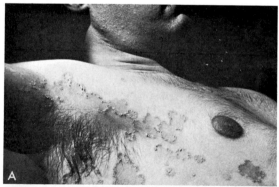

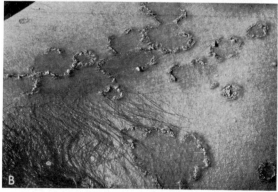

Figure 21–25. A, Subcorneal pustular dermatosis of Sneddon and Wilkinson. Note peripheral pustulation of lesions. B, Close view. (Courtesy of Dr. A. Kaminsky.)

EOSINOPHILIC PUSTULAR FOLLICULITIS

This condition was first described in 1965 by Ofuji. It occurs in males five times more commonly than females and has its peak age of onset in the third decade. It is characterized by pruritic, follicular papulopustules 1 to 2 mm in size. The lesions tend to be grouped: plaques may form. New lesions may form at the edges of the plaques, leading to peripheral extension, while central clearing takes place. Distribution is usually asymmetric, with the face, trunk, and upper extremities most often involved. Twenty per cent have palmo-plantar pustulosis. Many cases have been seen in association with AIDS. Buchness et al reported that UVB was effective in their cases.

Histologically there are spongiosis and vesiculation of the follicular infundibula, with infiltration with eosinophils. There is a peripheral eosinophilia in half the cases.

The typical course is one of spontaneous remissions and exacerbations. Treatment with dapsone or systemic steroids may decrease or clear the lesions.

Buchness MR, et al: Eosinophilic pustular folliculitis in AIDS. N Engl J Med 1988, 318:1183.

Colton AS, et al: Eosinophilic pustular folliculitis. JAAD 1986, 14:469.

Dinehart SM, et al: Eosinophilic pustular folliculitis. JAAD 1986, 14:475.

Jaliman H, et al: Eosinophilic pustular folliculitis. JAAD 1986, 14:479.

Steffen CS: Eosinophilic pustular folliculitis (Ofuji's disease) with response to dapsone therapy. Arch Dermatol 1985, 121:921.

Takematsu H, et al: Eosinophilic pustular folliculitis. Arch Dermatol 1985, 121:917.

22

Nutritional Diseases

A nutritional disease may be defined as a disease caused by lack (or less often, excess) of one or more dietary essentials. Isolated dietary faults are uncommon. In all the deficiency conditions one is impressed with the complex interlinking of one substance with another: more than one substance or vitamin is usually involved in any deficiency condition. In industrialized countries alcoholism is the main cause of these diseases, with some cases seen in patients who have gastrointestinal disease or digestive tract surgery.

There are indications that a group of dermatoses are directly caused by deficiency, and that there is another group of diseases of the skin (and other organs) in which deficiency influences the incidence and course of the disease. Miller presented an excellent review of these. Also, inborn errors of metabolism cause some of the deficiency states. These are discussed in Chapter 25.

Barthelemy H, et al: Skin and mucosal manifestations in vitamin deficiency. JAAD 1986, 15:1263.
Miller SJ: Nutritional deficiency and the skin. JAAD 1989, 21:1.

HYPOVITAMINOSIS A (Phrynoderma)

Numerous specific lesions in the skin due to vitamin A deficiency have been described. In general, the lesions consist of keratotic papules of various sizes, distributed over the extremities and shoulders, surrounding and arising from the pilosebaceous follicles.

The eruption usually begins on the anterolateral aspect of the thighs or the posterolateral aspect of the upper arms. It then spreads to the extensor surfaces of both the upper and lower extremities, shoulders, abdomen, back, and buttocks, and finally reaches the face and posterior aspect of the neck.

The hands and feet are not involved, and only rarely are there lesions on the median portion of the trunk or in the axillary and anogenital areas.

There is hyperkeratosis, especially of the hair follicles, in the form of dry, firm, pigmented papules containing a central intrafollicular keratotic plug. Many of these plugs project from the hair follicles as horny spines or are covered with a loosely adherent scale. When expressed, the plugs leave pits.

On the face the eruption resembles acne because of the presence of many large comedones, but differs from acne in respect to dryness of the skin. The general integumentary surface displays dryness and fine scaling.

In vitamin A deficiency, eye symptoms such as

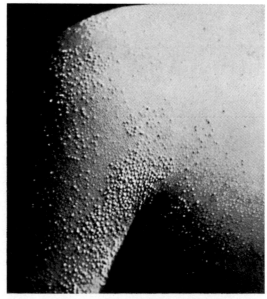

Figure 22–1. Vitamin A deficiency showing a follicular keratotic eruption. (Courtesy of Drs. C. N. Frazier and Ch'uan-K'uei Hu, China.)

night blindness, dimness of sight, xerophthalmia, or keratomalacia predominate and may provide pathognomonic findings. The earliest finding is delayed adaptation to the dark (nyctalopia). Sometimes there are circumscribed areas of xerosis of the conjunctiva lateral to the cornea, occasionally forming a well-defined white spot (**Bitot spot**), or xerosis corneae. These are triangular, with the apex toward the canthus.

Various degrees of severity are encountered, the most authentic and severe cases (phrynoderma, toadskin) having been described in Africa, China, and India. Barr et al reported a woman who developed night blindness and multiple keratotic papules four years after bowel bypass surgery. Biopsy findings were those of perforating folliculitis. The serum vitamin A level was low and treatment with vitamin A led to resolution of her visual and cutaneous disease. A similar case of bowel-bypass phrynoderma was reported by Wechsler in 1979.

The histologic characteristics of avitaminosis A dermatosis are hyperkeratosis, horny plugs in the upper portion of the hair follicle, shrinkage of the sebaceous glands, and, at times, flattening of the secretory cells of the eccrine sweat glands.

The diagnosis may be aided by determination of the vitamin A level in the blood serum. The normal value is over 20 μg per dl. For treatment vitamin A (50,000 IU daily) is recommended until symptoms resolve and the serum vitamin A level is normalized.

Hypervitaminosis A

Hypervitaminosis A symptoms resemble closely those of hypovitaminosis A.

Most of the cases of chronic hypervitaminosis A have been reported in children. There is loss of hair and coarseness of the remaining hair, loss of eyebrows, exfoliative cheilitis, generalized exfoliation and pigmentation of the skin, and clubbing of the fingers. Moderate widespread itching may occur. Hepatomegaly, splenomegaly, hypochromic anemia, depressed serum proteins, and elevated alkaline phosphatase may be present. Bone growth may be retarded by premature closure of the epiphyses in children. Papilledema with pseudotumor cerebri may occur very early, before any other signs appear, apparently by reason of some idiosyncrasy. It is preceded by headache.

In adults the premonitory signs are dryness of the lips and anorexia, which may be followed by joint and bone pains, follicular hyperkeratosis, branny desquamation of the skin, fissuring of the corners of the mouth and nostrils, dryness and loss of scalp hair and eyebrows, dystrophy of the nails, and hyperpigmentation of the face and neck resembling chloasma or Riehl's melanosis. Fatigue, myalgia, anorexia, headache, strabismus, and weight loss commonly occur, if the vitamin is not withdrawn. Schmunes reported that vitamin A intake in patients on dialysis could result in hypervitaminosis A, because dialysis does not remove this vitamin. Silverman et al have emphasized that the major features of hypervitaminosis A are a paradigm of the side effects of the retinoids.

The prognosis is good, with most of the symptoms subsiding in a few days or weeks, as soon as excessive intake is stopped.

Barr DJ, et al: Bypass phrynoderma. Arch Dermatol 1984, 120:919.

Di Benedetto RJ: Chronic hypervitaminosis A in an adult. JAMA 1967, 201:700.

Roels OA, et al: The Vitamins, in Modern Nutrition in Health and Disease, ed. 5, Goodhart RS, and Shils ME, eds. Philadelphia, Lea and Febiger, 1973.

Schmunes E: Hypervitaminosis A in a patient with alopecia receiving hemodialysis. Arch Dermatol 1979, 115:882.

Silverman AK, et al: Hypervitaminosis A syndrome: a paradigm of retinoid side effects. JAAD 1987, 16:1027.

Stimson WH: Vitamin A intoxication in adults. Report of a case with summary of the literature. N Engl J Med 1961, 265:369.

Wechsler HL: Vitamin A deficiency following small-bowel bypass surgery for obesity. Arch Dermatol 1979, 115:73.

VITAMIN B1 DEFICIENCY

Vitamin B1 (thiamine) deficiency results in beriberi. The skin manifestations are limited to edema and a red burning tongue.

VITAMIN B2 DEFICIENCY

Vitamin B2 (riboflavin) deficiency is seen most often in alcoholic patients; however, phototherapy for neonatal icterus has been reported to cause it also.

The classical findings of the oro-ocular-genital syndrome are present. These include angular stomatitis, nasolabial seborrhea, angular blepharitis, cheilosis, atrophic glossitis with a magenta-red tongue, corneal vascularization, hyperpigmentation, and redness and scaling of the scrotum and vulva.

The response to 5 mg of riboflavin daily is dramatic.

Riboflavin under the lights. Lancet 1978, 1:1191.

VITAMIN B6 EXCESS

Friedman et al and Baer et al have reported two patients who ingested large doses of pyridoxine (vitamin B6) and developed a subepidermal vesicular dermatosis and sensory peripheral neuropathy. The bullous dermatosis resembled epidermolysis bullosa acquisita, but direct immunofluorescence was not done in either case. In one patient the neuropathy and vesicular dermatosis resolved after discontinuance of therapy.

Baer RL, et al: Cutaneous skin changes probably due to pyridoxine abuse. JAAD 1984, 10:527.

Friedman MA, et al: Subepidermal vesicular dermatosis and sensory peripheral neuropathy caused by pyridoxine abuse. JAAD 1986, 14:915.

VITAMIN B12 DEFICIENCY

Vitamin B12 (cyanocobalamin) is absorbed through the distal ileum after binding to gastric intrinsic factor in an acid pH. Deficiency is due mainly to digestive malabsorption as in a defect of intrinsic factor, in achlorhydria, in ileal diseases such as malabsorption syndromes due to pancreatic disease or sprue, or in congenital diseases in which intrinsic factor or transcobalamin deficiency is present.

Glossitis, hyperpigmentation, and canities are the main dermatologic manifestations. The tongue is bright red, sore, and atrophic. The hyperpigmentation is generalized, but may be accentuated in exposed areas such as the face and hands. The nails may be pigmented, as in the case reported by Noppakun et al. Premature gray hair may paradoxically occur. Megaloblastic anemia is present.

The mechanism of hyperpigmentation of the skin, nails, and mucous membranes has been postulated to be a decrease in reduced glutathione, which increases tyrosinase activity. Also biopterin, which is increased in vitamin B12 deficiency, may increase hydroxylated phenylalanine and thus lead to hyperpigmentation.

Replacement of vitamin B12 with intramuscular injections leads to a reversal of the pigmentary changes in the skin, nails, mucous membranes, and hair.

Marks VJ, et al: Hyperpigmentation in megalobastic anemia. JAAD 1985, 12:914.

Noppakun N, et al: Reversible hyperpigmentation of skin and nails with white hair due to vitamin B12 deficiency. Arch Dermatol 1986, 122:896.

FOLIC ACID DEFICIENCY

Findings of diffuse hyperpigmentation, glossitis, cheilitis, and megaloblastic anemia, resembling vitamin B12 deficiency, have been described in folic acid deficiency. There may be concomitant B12 and folate deficiency and blood levels of each may be determined. A therapeutic trial of 10 to 30 mg/daily of intramuscular folate may be given to determine if the clinical findings are due solely to folate deficiency.

Downham TF, et al: Hyperpigmentation and folate deficiency. Arch Dermatol 1976, 112:562.

SCURVY

Scurvy, or vitamin C deficiency, is characterized by capillary hemorrhages surrounding hyperkeratotic follicular papules, swollen and bleeding gums, petechiae, ecchymoses, and weakness and tenderness in the lower extremities. Children are most often affected.

The most significant skin manifestation is the keratotic plugging of the hair follicles, chiefly on the anterior forearms, abdomen, and posterior thighs. The hairs are curled in follicles capped by keratotic plugs. This distinctive finding has been named "corkscrew hairs."

Petechiae and ecchymoses, especially on the lower extremities and in perifollicular sites, are common. They appear frequently in pressure areas and hairy portions of the skin.

Hemorrhagic gingivitis is manifested by swelling and bleeding of the gums. The teeth are loosened and the breath is foul.

The subperiosteal, hemorrhage-induced painful and tender nodules on the shins, delayed healing of wounds, nosebleeds, and hematuria are some of the many manifestations of vitamin C deficiency in the human.

An unusual "woody" edema of the legs has been noted by Walker, who found this peculiar hardening of the skin associated with vitamin C deficiency. The edema was associated with pain, ecchymoses, and severe mental depression.

Scurvy may occur in adults, especially in the elderly who live alone on a diet of staple processed foods devoid of fresh vegetables and fruit. Today, in the United States, it is seen quite frequently in malnourished alcoholics. Occasional cases are caused by dietary aberrations, as in the case of a girl (reported by Evans) who lived for a year on tuna fish sandwiches and iced tea. At least one case has occurred in an infant because her mother warmed her orange juice.

Although several tests are available, the diagnosis of scurvy by various laboratory procedures is fraught with inconsistencies. The positive response to a high vitamin C intake is enough to confirm the diagnosis.

Treatment is with ascorbic acid in amounts of at least 200 mg daily. A rapid response of the clinical manifestations is seen in a few days. A diet containing green leafy vegetables and citrus fruits should be taken regularly, together with adequate protein.

Ellis CN, et al: Scurvy. Arch Dermatol 1984, 120:1212.

VITAMIN D-DEPENDENT RICKETS (DDR)

Two types of DDR have been described. Type I is due to an inborn error in the renal metabolism of calcifediol (25-hydroxyvitamin D3) to calcitriol (1,25-

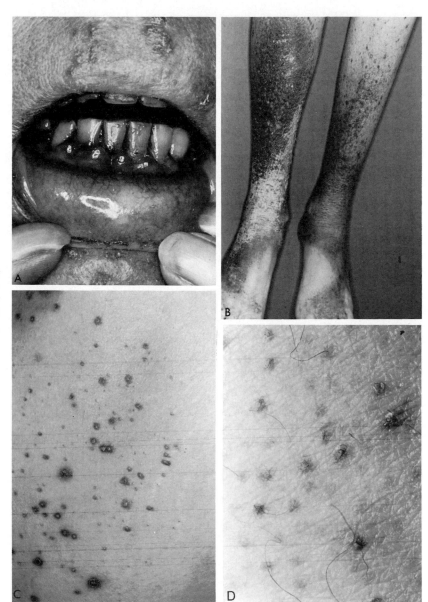

Figure 22–2. Scurvy. A, *Swollen, hemorrhagic gingiva;* B, *extensive ecchymoses of lower extremities;* C, *keratotic plugging and perifollicular hemorrhage of the skin;* D, *corkscrew hairs and perifollicular hemorrhage. (D, Courtesy of Dr. Axel W. Hoke.)*

hydroxyvitamin D3, the biologically active form of this vitamin). This is not associated with skin disease.

Type II DDR is caused by a defect in the target-tissue recognition of calcitriol. It is not a deficiency state, and does not usually respond to vitamin D therapy. It appears to be an autosomal-recessive inherited disease. Hochberg et al reported four children of two kindreds who developed progressive diffuse alopecia in the first year of life. The biochemical and radiologic manifestations developed after the onset of alopecia.

ACQUIRED VITAMIN D DEFICIENCY

The elderly have decreased vitamin D cutaneous photosynthesis by reason of decreased sun exposure (sometimes aggravated by use of sunscreens) and often by poor intake of vitamin D, both of which

predispose to osteomalacia. Others at risk for this include debilitated patients with limited sun exposure, patients taking anticonvulsants, and patients with malabsorption secondary to gastric or intestinal surgery, pancreatic or biliary disease, or celiac disease. Patients in all these risk groups may require an oral vitamin D supplement.

VITAMIN D EXCESS

Therapeutic overdosage of vitamin D is characterized by hypercalcemia and generalized calcinosis. Metastatic calcification may be present in the skin.

Hochberg Z, et al: Calcitriol-resistant rickets with alopecia. Arch Dermatol 1985, 121:646.
Holick MF: Vitamin D resistance and alopecia. Arch Dermatol 1985, 121:601.

Idem: Skin as the site of Vitamin D synthesis and target organ for 1,25-dihydroxyvitamin D₃. Arch Dermatol 1987, 123:1677.
Prystowsky JH: Photoprotection and the Vitamin D status of the elderly. Arch Dermatol 1988, 124:1844.

VITAMIN K DEFICIENCY

Dietary deficiency of vitamin K does not occur; however, in adults, deficiency may occur because of lack of absorption due to biliary disease, malabsorption syndromes, or anorexia nervosa. Liver disease of all causes produces deficiency, with resultant decrease in clotting factors which are dependent upon vitamin K for synthesis or secretion (coagulation factors II, VII, IX, and X). Thus the cutaneous manifestations that result are purpura, hemorrhage, and ecchymosis.

Paradoxically, protein C, a vitamin K-dependent anticoagulant, may be affected, and, as reported by Teepe et al, an acquired deficiency of vitamin K may give rise to coumarin-induced skin necrosis secondary to thrombosis in patients on this medication.

Teepe RGC, et al: Recurrent coumarin-induced skin necrosis in a patient with an acquired functional protein C deficiency. Arch Dermatol 1986, 122:1408.

TRYPTOPHAN AND NIACIN DEFICIENCY

A deficiency of nicotinic acid or its precursor amino acid, tryptophan, produces pellagra, with its characteristic skin lesions.

Pellagra

CLINICAL FEATURES. Pellagra is a chronic, wasting deficiency disease. It affects the alimentary

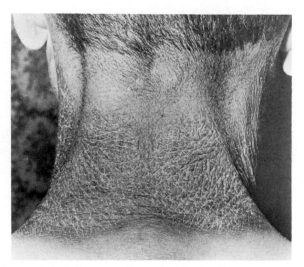

Figure 22–4. Pellagra on the neck. Usually there are two zones of hyperpigmentation at the edge of the involved skin. (Courtesy of Dr. M. El-Zawahry, U.A.R.)

tract, the nervous system, and the skin, where the eruption is influenced by the effect of light. A mnemonic for it is ''DDD'': diarrhea, dermatitis, and dementia.

The dermatitis occurs symmetrically on the face, neck, wrists, and backs of the hands. The affected parts become bright red, with a distinct line of demarcation, which on the wrist is usually higher on the radial than on the ulnar side. The erythema may be accompanied by itching or burning, and thickening of the affected skin. After several weeks or months the epidermis desquamates, leaving the parts deeply pigmented. In protracted cases the skin ultimately becomes atrophic. The eruption has a tendency to be worse in the summer months, after disappearing in the winter and recurring each spring.

The pellagrin's nose is fairly characteristic. There is dull erythema of the bridge of the nose with slight scaling, which resembles seborrheic dermatitis except for its location. The scaling gives a powdery appearance so that the whole suggests a dull red nose partly

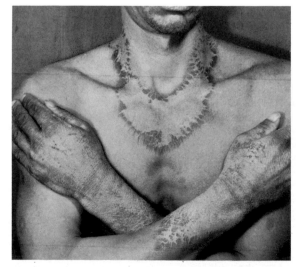

Figure 22–3. Pellagra with typical collarette and lesions on the hands and forearms. (Courtesy of Dr. M. El-Zawahry, Egypt.)

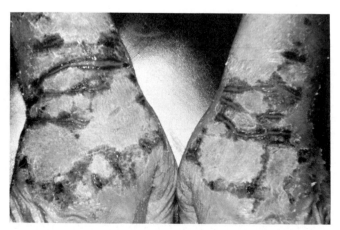

Figure 22–5. Pellagra (US) in an alcoholic patient. (Courtesy of Dr. Axel H. Hoke.)

covered with powder. About the lower neck and extending to the sternal region there is likely to be a collarette of dermatitis *(Casal's necklace)* similar to the eruption on the hands. This is formed because the dermatitis develops in intermittently exposed skin earlier and more severely than in regularly exposed skin, possibly because it has developed less solar-protective alteration. Scrotal erythema is common.

The mucous membranes are affected by painful fissures and ulcerations and by a general tendency to atrophy. The lips and cheeks are thin and pale, the lips and mouth dry, and the tongue red and swollen. There is likely to be fissuring at the commissures. Similar changes occur in the vagina. There may be a swelling of the parotid glands, salivation, toxic psychosis, tabetic symptoms, paralysis, or optic neuritis.

At the onset, there is weakness, loss of appetite, abdominal pain, diarrhea, mental depression, and photosensitivity. Skin lesions may be the earliest sign, with phototoxicity being the presenting symptom in some cases. In the later stages of the disease the nervous symptoms may predominate to such a degree that the identity of the cutaneous lesions is overlooked. The nervous symptoms may be confused with anxiety neurosis, simple depression, melancholia, and manic-depressive insanity. The disease is progressive, the majority of patients dying in four or five years if untreated.

ETIOLOGY. Pellagra is caused by a deficiency of niacin, or its precursor amino acid, tryptophan. Dietary deficiencies of one or both of these occur in patients who eat only maize, who have inadequate animal protein intake (such as vegetarians or alcoholics), or who have inadequate absorption, such as patients with anorexia nervosa. Gopalan reported pellagra in the Decca region of India in populations where jowar (millet) is the principal item of the diet. Jowar has high amounts of niacin and tryptophan, so the reason for the development of pellagra in this population is unclear. It has been speculated that the high leucine content of jowar (or maize) alters tryptophan metabolism.

Hartnup's disease is an autosomal recessive disorder in which there is a defect in the cellular transport of a group of monoamino-monocarboxylic acids. There is a failure of absorption of tryptophan from the gastrointestinal tract, which leads to the appearance of a pellagralike eruption.

The *carcinoid syndrome* may have pellagralike skin lesions associated with it because a high percentage of dietary tryptophan is metabolized by the 5-hydroxyindole pathway, shunting it away from the formation of niacin.

Barthelemy reports that vitamin B6 (pyridoxine) deficiency often produces nicotinic acid deficiency and pellagralike manifestations because it is a coenzyme in tryptophan metabolism. It has also been reported by Katch to have caused a periorificial dermatitis similar to that seen in zinc deficiency.

Several drugs may induce a pellagralike eruption. These include isoniazid, 6-mercaptopurine, 5-fluorouracil, sulfonamides, anticonvulsive drugs and antidepressants.

INCIDENCE. The disease has occurred in many parts of the world. However, in areas where maize is the principal food it has been occurring with greater frequency. Some of the Balkan countries, the southern United States, and Central America are some of the areas where pellagra may be frequently seen. The disease occurs mostly in rural districts, among the poor, who eat an overabundance of corn and an insufficient amount of animal protein, fruits, and vegetables. Alcoholism, with a voluntary reduction of other substances in the diet, produces the same symptoms. It may occur postoperatively, especially if fever and failure to eat occur during this period. Rappaport reported pellagra occurring in a patient with anorexia nervosa.

PATHOLOGY. Histologically, the findings in the skin vary according to the stage of the disease. There is usually hyperkeratosis with patchy parakeratosis; pigmentation is increased. In the upper dermis there is a moderate vascular dilatation accompanied by edema of the collagen and a perivascular infiltration of histiocytes.

DIAGNOSIS. The diagnosis of pellagra is often difficult until the disease is in an advanced stage; however, dermatitis, diarrhea, and dementia, in that order, are fairly diagnostic. The diagnosis is essentially a clinical one, with a therapeutic trial to test it. Rapid clearing of the skin disease upon niacin replacement confirms the clinical impression.

TREATMENT. Dietary treatment to correct the malnutrition is essential. Animal proteins, eggs, milk, and vegetables are beneficial, supplemented with 100 mg nicotinamide four times daily. Fluid and electrolyte loss from diarrhea should be replaced. Within 24 hours after niacin therapy is begun the salivation, nausea, diarrhea, mental symptoms, and fiery redness and swelling of the tongue improve. The erythematous lesions on the skin rapidly blanch, but the scaly, ulcerated, or pigmented lesions respond less promptly.

Horn TD: A photodistributed rash. Arch Dermatol 1987, 123:1225.
Rapaport MJ: Pellagra in a patient with anorexia nervosa. Arch Dermatol 1985, 121:125.

BIOTIN DEFICIENCY

A dermatosis characterized by a patchy reddened periorificial dermatitis of the face, alopecia, glossitis, and sometimes mucocutaneous candidiasis may be caused by total parenteral nutrition without biotin.

Sweetman et al reported a case in a boy, 11, who ingested raw eggs daily. The avidin in the egg white induced biotin deficiency, with a red facial rash, total alopecia, and glossitis. Recovery was complete with treatment.

The dietary deficiency syndrome is identical to that seen with the inherited types of multiple carboxylase deficiencies and has clinical similarities to acrodermatitis enteropathica and essential fatty acid deficiency. Both inherited forms of biotin deficiency are autosomal recessive conditions. The most severe neonatal-onset disease is due to noninheritance of holocarboxylase synthetase formation. In the later-onset, infantile type, biotinidase is lacking. Nyhan has reviewed these uncommon metabolic deficiency syndromes.

Nyhan WL: Inborn errors of biotin metabolism. Arch Dermatol 1987, 123:1696.
Sweetman L, et al: Clinical and metabolic abnormalities in a boy with dietary deficiency of biotin. Pediatrics 1981, 68:553.
Williams ML, et al: Alopecia and periorificial dermatitis in biotin-responsive multiple carboxylase deficiency. JAAD 1983, 9:97.

ZINC DEFICIENCY

Zinc deficiency may be an inherited abnormality, as in *acrodermatitis enteropathica*; more commonly, it may be acquired.

Clinically it is manifested as patchy, red, dry, scaling periorificial dermatitis on the face and anogenital areas, and as an acral papulopustular, psoriasiform, or vesiculobullous eruption. Alopecia is characteristic, and diarrhea is present in most cases. Many abnormalities of the immune response occur in zinc deficiency, and have recently been reviewed in detail by Norris.

Many different clinical situations may lead to acquired zinc deficiency. Premature infants are at risk, because the full complement of neonatal zinc is not received until late in the third trimester. Arlette et al reported ten infants who developed acrodermatitis-type changes when placed on total parenteral nutrition. Several reports of adults on total parenteral nutrition developing zinc deficiency appeared in the mid and late 1970s, before these solutions contained adequate zinc. Acquired zinc deficiency also occurs in alcoholics, as a complication of malabsorption and jejunoileal bypass surgery, in chronic disease, and in adolescents on high phytate-containing diets in the Middle East. Connors et al reported an unusual infant who developed this while being breast fed. The mother's milk had a low level of zinc. It is apparent that oral contraceptives and pregnancy, and possibly cystic fibrosis, predispose to the development of zinc-deficient states.

Arlette JP, et al: Zinc deficiency dermatosis in premature infants receiving prolonged parenteral alimentation. JAAD 1981, 5:37.
Bailly A, et al: Acrodermatitis enteropathica and Crohn's disease. JAAD 1984, 11:525.
Conners TJ, et al: Acquired zinc deficiency in a breast-fed premature infant. Arch Dermatol 1983, 119:319.
Fraker PJ, et al: Zinc deficiency and immune function. Arch Dermatol 1987, 123:1699.
Gaveau D, et al: Cutaneous manifestations of zinc deficiency in alcoholics. Acta Dermatol Venereol 1987, 114:39.
McClain CJ, et al: Severe zinc deficiency presenting with acrodermatitis during hyperalimentation: diagnosis, pathogenesis and treatment. J Clin Gastroenterol 1980, 2:125.
Norris D: Zinc and cutaneous inflammation. Arch Dermatol 1985, 121:985.
West BL, et al: Alcohol and acquired acrodermatitis enteropathica. JAAD 1986, 15:1305.

ESSENTIAL FATTY ACID DEFICIENCY

Prolonged parenteral nutrition may cause, in addition to zinc deficiency, an essential fatty acid deficiency. This may result in periorificial dermatitis, and a generalized xerotic or eczematous dermatitis. There may be a link between biotin deficiency and zinc deficiency, but this is as yet unclear. Classically there is an alteration in the plasma fatty acid profile which occurs in this disease. There is a decrease in linoleic acid levels and an increase in palmitoleic and oleic acids. The serum fatty acid ratio of D_1homo–γ-linolenic acid to arachidonic acid (20:3/20:4) is greater than 4, which is diagnostic. Intravenous lipid therapy (Intralipid 10 per cent) reverses the process, and causes the dry, scaly, easily-bleeding skin lesions to heal.

Hansen RC, et al: Cystic fibrosis manifesting with acrodermatitis enteropathica-like eruption. Arch Dermatol 1983, 119:51.
Riella MC, et al: Essential fatty acid deficiency in human adults during total parenteral nutrition. Ann Intern Med 1975, 83:786.
Skolnik P, et al: Human essential fatty acid deficiency: treatment by topical application of linoleic acid. Arch Dermatol 1977, 113:939.
Ziboh VA, et al: Biologic significance of polyunsaturated fatty acids in the skin. Arch Dermatol 1987, 123:1686a.

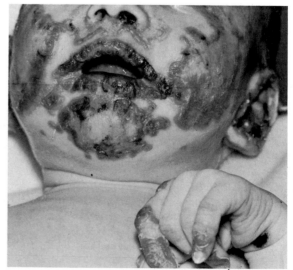

Figure 22–6. Typical perioral and facial lesions of acrodermatitis enteropathica.

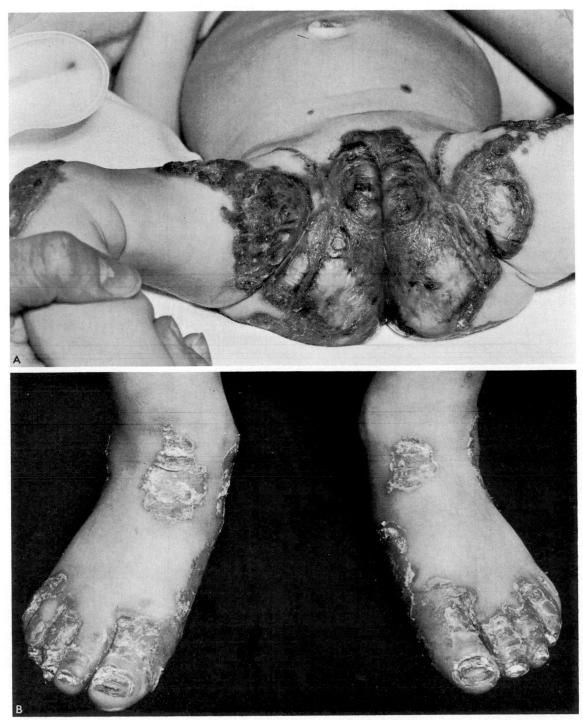

Figure 22–7. Acrodermatitis enteropathica. (A, From Wells BT, Winkelman RK: Arch Dermatol 1961, 84:40–52; B, Courtesy of Dr. D. Bloom.)

PLUMMER-VINSON SYNDROME

Plummer-Vinson syndrome is a combination of microcytic anemia, dysphagia, and glossitis, seen almost entirely in middle-aged women. The lips are thin and the opening of the mouth is small and inelastic, so that there is a rather characteristic appearance. Smooth atrophy of the tongue is pronounced. Koilonychia, "spoon-shaped nails," is present in 40 to 50 per cent of patients. The skin is dry and wrinkled.

There is hypochromic and microcytic anemia and the hair is scanty. Deficiencies resulting from chronic diarrhea associated with achlorhydria and anemia may be present in the Plummer-Vinson syndrome. Difficulty in swallowing is characterized by the feeling of food becoming stuck in the throat. Often a radiologically demonstrable esophageal web or stricture is present in the postcricoid region.

That this syndrome is a precancerosis has been established beyond doubt by Ahlbom, who, in an analysis of 250 cases of carcinoma of the mouth and upper respiratory tract in women, found that 70 per cent occurred in patients with Plummer-Vinson syndrome. About 5 to 10 per cent of patients with an esophageal web develop carcinoma at that site. The

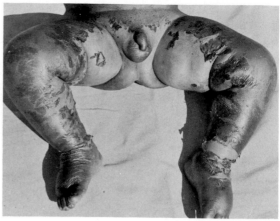

Figure 22–9. Kwashiorkor with distinctive skin changes. (Courtesy of Dr. E. B. Adams, Durban, Natal.)

deficiency is in iron. Treatment is by the use of iron and a high-vitamin diet.

KWASHIORKOR

Kwashiorkor is characterized by a protein malnutrition that produces hair and skin changes, hunger, edema, impaired growth, and characteristic pot belly.

The hair and skin changes are usually striking. The Africans call the victims "red children." The color of the hair may vary from a reddish yellow to gray or even white. The hair is dry and lustreless; curly hair becomes soft and straight; and marked scaling is seen (crackled hair). Especially striking is the flag sign, affecting long, normally dark hair in which the hair grown during periods of poor nutrition is pale, so that alternating bands of pale and dark hair can be seen along a single strand, indicating alternating periods of good and poor nutrition. The nails are soft and thin. The skin changes in severe cases include erythematous scaling and bronzed patches.

Later the patches become hard, scaly, and distinctly elevated ("enamel paint" dermatosis). Angular stomatitis, glossitis, and xerophthalmia often occur.

Children affected by this disease are seriously ill; their height and weight are below normal. They have diarrhea, a swollen abdomen, and edema of the feet and face. The edema may become generalized. Subcutaneous fat disappears and the muscles become wasted.

The treatment of kwashiorkor is centered mostly around a high protein and high vitamin diet. The ever-present infection is treated with proper antibacterials. Electrolytes must be replaced.

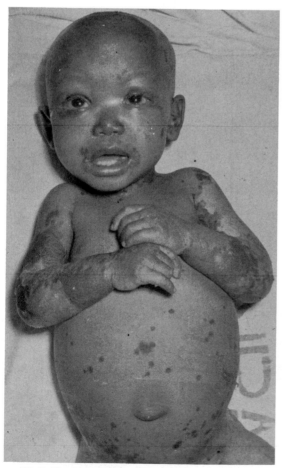

Figure 22–8. Typical potbelly of kwashiorkor. (Courtesy of Dr. E. B. Adams, Durban, Natal.)

Adams EB, et al: Observations on etiology and treatment of anemia in kwashiorkor. Br Med J 1967, 3:451.
El-Hefnawki H: Dermatologic manifestations of kwashiorkor syndrome. Dermatol Int 1966, 5:59.

El-Mofty AM: Dermatological aspects of abnormal protein metabolism. Indian J Dermatol 1964, 10:17.

McLaren DS: Skin changes in protein energy malnutrition. Arch Dermatol 1987, 123:1674.

MARASMUS

Starvation in infancy and early childhood, so common in developing regions of the world, is usually due to weaning problems resulting from ignorance, poor hygiene, and economic and cultural factors. Protein and caloric deprivation soon leads to suppression of growth, negative nitrogen balance due to catabolism of tissue protein for energy, and marasmus (wasting). The skin is dry, wrinkled, and loose, owing to marked loss of subcutaneous fat. The "monkey facies" with loss of the buccal fat pad is characteristic. In contrast to kwashiorkor there is classically no clinical edema or dermatosis.

McLaren DS: Skin changes in protein energy malnutrition. Arch Dermatol 1987, 123:1674.

SPRUE

Sprue is known in two forms, *tropical* and *nontropical*. The latter is also known as *adult celiac disease*. This malabsorption disorder has few distinctive cutaneous manifestations. Its cause is hypersensitivity to gluten, a constituent of wheat, barley, and rye flours. Its chief symptom is fatty, bulky, loose stools. It occurs frequently but usually subclinically in dermatitis herpetiformis (see Chapter 21).

A diffuse brownish pigmentation may appear over the sun-exposed area, purpura may be present, and there may be pallor due to anemia. The tongue reflects the severity of the disease. There may be mild atrophic patches on the tip of the tongue, the papillae may become smooth, and small ulcers may appear. A diffuse alopecia may be present. Clubbing of the fingers is sometimes seen in severe cases. Steatorrhea is a characteristic manifestation, and flattening of the villous pattern of the jejunal mucosa is a constant finding, just as in dermatitis herpetiformis.

CAROTENEMIA AND LYCOPENEMIA

Excessive ingestion of carrots, oranges, squash, spinach, yellow corn and beans, butter, eggs, rutabagas, pumpkins, yellow turnips, sweet potatoes, or papaya may lead to a yellowish discoloration of the skin, which is especially prominent on the palms, soles, and central face. Carotenemia occurs most commonly in vegetarians or food faddists. The sclerae are spared.

In lycopenemia, excess ingestion of red-colored foods such as tomatoes, beets, chili beans, and various fruits and berries leads to a reddish discoloration of the skin.

23

Diseases of Subcutaneous Fat

Deep-seated processes in the skin which produce localized inflammation primarily in the subcutaneous fat are known as *panniculitis*. These may be characterized by inflammation, involving primarily the fibrous septa. The septal panniculitides, such as erythema nodosum, polyarteritis nodosa, and necrobiosis lipoidica, generally have systemic associations, and are discussed elsewhere in this book.

The fat lobules themselves, with inflammation and degeneration of the lipocytes, may also be the site of the primary inflammation. Many types of this lobular inflammation are discussed under the systemic diseases of which they are a part, such as sarcoidosis, lupus erythematosus, and subcutaneous granuloma annulare. Lobular panniculitis associated with vasculitis—nodular vasculitis—is also discussed elsewhere.

There remains a miscellaneous group of diseases in which the primary site of inflammation is the fat lobule in the panniculus. Although many etiologic factors are concerned in this type of panniculitis, the fat reacts in much the same way in all these diseases. There is fat necrosis, the fat staining pink with H&E stain. There are needlelike crystals. Around these there is an infiltrate of polymorphonuclear leukocytes, lymphocytes, plasma cells, and lipophages of foreign-body giant cell type. Mild or severe vascular changes occur. Later, there are fibrosis and calcium deposits.

The lipodystrophies, in which there is either localized or generalized absence of subcutaneous fat, are discussed at the end of this chapter.

WEBER-CHRISTIAN PANNICULITIS

Synonyms: Relapsing febrile nodular nonsuppurative panniculitis, Weber-Christian syndrome.

CLINICAL FEATURES. Weber-Christian panniculitis was first described by Pfeifer in 1892. It is characterized by recurrent attacks of malaise, arthralgia, and fever, associated with localized, inflammatory, tender, 1–4-cm nodules in the panniculus. These nodules appear on the trunk and extremities, chiefly on the thighs. The skin over the nodules may be erythematous, mottled, or somewhat pigmented, and the nodules themselves may be tender. They only very rarely suppurate. Often nodules regress spontaneously and may leave localized atrophy, with round depressions. Each attack is accompanied by fever. In time fewer attacks occur and eventually they stop. The erythrocyte sedimentation rate is

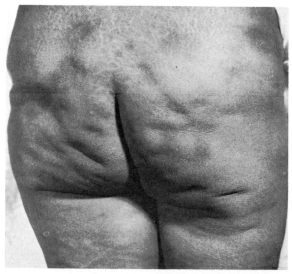

Figure 23–1. Weber-Christian panniculitis in a woman with systemic sclerosis. Outcome was fatal. (Courtesy of Dr. J. Penner.)

570

useful in evaluating the status of the disease: it rises sharply at the onset of each attack and falls to normal at its conclusion.

Systemic Manifestations with Panniculitis. Panniculitis involving simultaneously the omental, mesenteric, and perivisceral fat may occur. Inflammation in these sites may lead to the symptoms of nausea, vomiting, and abdominal pain. Weight loss may occur, and hepatomegaly may be present. If the bone marrow fat is involved, bone pain may be a symptom, and anemia or leukopenia may result.

Liquefying Panniculitis. Liquefying panniculitis is considered to be a form of Weber-Christian panniculitis. Some of the nodules in panniculitis undergo liquefaction and discharge an oily liquid. Aspiration of some fluctuant lesions, not broken down, will show a yellowish fatty fluid, whereas others will show a bloody purulent fluid. Upon involution a saucerlike depression will result from atrophy.

ETIOLOGY. The cause remains elusive. Williams et al reported a case which developed after jejunoileal bypass surgery, suggesting that either a hypersensitivity to bacterial antigens or an immune complex disease was the cause in their patient. Dupont et al reported a case in 1983 which was associated with glomerulonephritis and immune deposits of IgG and IgM on the epithelial side of the glomerular basement membrane, suggesting an immunologic etiology. Several patients with α_1-antitrypsin deficiency have been reported to have Weber-Christian disease, including two reported by Breit et al and one reported by Bleumink et al. The simultaneous occurrence of these two rare conditions suggests an etiologic link. Breit et al postulate this to be a hyperactivity of the immunologic and inflammatory functions found in their patients.

Other cases of panniculitis associated with α_1-antitrypsin deficiency have been reported in which a septal inflammation appeared to be the primary histologic finding. Viraben et al reported a case and reviewed the literature on this subject. They feel that necrotic panniculitis with α_1-antitrypsin deficiency is a distinct entity.

K. C. Smith et al reviewed all 18 cases of panniculitis associated with α_1-antitrypsin deficiency in 1987. Most had a homozygous phenotype z with very low levels of this α_1-proteinase inhibitor. Importantly, dapsone and infusions of α_1-proteinase inhibitor concentrate are effective therapeutic interventions in this genetically determined panniculitis.

INCIDENCE AND PREVALENCE. Weber-Christian panniculitis occurs mostly in women between the ages of 20 and 60 years.

HISTOPATHOLOGY. Lever describes three stages through which lesions evolve. In the first there is degeneration of the fat cells with an infiltrate of neutrophils, lymphocytes, and eosinophils. The second or macrophagic stage shows a histiocytic infiltrate and the formation of lipophages or foam cells. Classic biopsy findings in this stage are diagnostic. In the third stage the foam cells are replaced by fibroblasts, lymphocytes, and plasma cells. Collagen is laid down and fibrosis results. The epidermis and dermis usually show no changes.

TREATMENT. Arnold's case was controlled promptly and specifically on several occasions by sulfapyridine. This drug, or dapsone, would seem well worth trying before resorting to corticosteroids. Moreover, Martin had success with cyclophosphamide, Eravelly with thalidomide (which is relatively innocuous over short periods in men or nonpregnant women), and Leong with tetracycline. Corticosteroids are helpful in high doses; after control is achieved the dosage is decreased as indicated.

Arnold HL Jr: Nodular nonsuppurative panniculitis (Weber-Christian disease). Preliminary report of a case controlled by sulfapyridine. Arch Dermatol Syph 1945, 51:94.

Bleumink E, et al: Protease-inhibitor deficiencies in a patient with Weber-Christian panniculitis. Arch Dermatol 1984, 120:936.

Breit SN, et al: Familial occurrence of α_1-antitrypsin deficiency and Weber-Christian disease. Arch Dermatol 1983, 119:198.

Dupont AG, et al: Weber-Christian panniculitis with membranous glomerulonephritis. Am J Med 1983, 75:527.

Eravelly J, et al: Thalidomide in Weber-Christian disease (letter) Lancet 1977, 1:25.

Leong CH: On treatment of panniculitis with tetracycline (letter). Arch Dermatol 1976, 112:1176.

Lever WF, et al: Histopathology of the Skin, 6th ed. Philadelphia, J. B. Lippincott Co., 1983, pp. 250–251.

Martin RJ, et al: Cyclophosphamide-induced remission in Weber-Christian disease. Milit Med 1977, 142:158.

Panush RS, et al: Weber-Christian disease: analysis of 15 cases and a review of the literature. Medicine (Baltimore) 1985, 64:181.

Patterson JW: Panniculitis. Arch Dermatol 1987, 123:1615.

Smith KC, et al: Panniculitis associated with severe α_1-antitrypsin deficiency. Arch Dermatol 1987, 123:1655.

Viraben R, et al: Necrotic panniculitis with α_1-antitrypsin deficiency. JAAD 1986, 14:684.

Williams HJ, et al: Nodular nonsuppurative panniculitis associated with jejunoileal bypass surgery. Arch Dermatol 1979, 115:1091.

LIPOGRANULOMATOSIS SUBCUTANEA

Lipogranulomatosis subcutanea of Rothmann and Makai is characterized by spherical subcutaneous nodules varying in size from 2 to 30 mm in diameter, most frequently occurring on the legs and sometimes on the trunk and arms. The nodules average about 12 in number and are tender to the touch. There are no systemic symptoms, fever is absent, and the lesions last six to 12 months. New lesions appear singly and only rarely do they break down to form liquefying panniculitis.

Lipogranulomatosis subcutanea is thought by Lever to be a variant of Weber-Christian panniculitis, since their histologic features are the same; however, it differs by the absence of fever, by the appearance of the lesions singly instead of in crops, and by its occurrence mostly in children. It should be differentiated from erythema induratum, erythema nodosum, and nodular vasculitis. The cause is unknown and there is no effective treatment.

Chan HL: Panniculitis (Rothmann-Makai) with good response to tetracycline. Br J Dermatol 1975, 92:351.

CYTOPHAGIC HISTIOCYTIC PANNICULITIS

Winkelmann first described this disorder in 1980. He and others have since described 19 cases of this lobular panniculitis, which is characterized by widespread erythematous, painful subcutaneous nodules, which may occasionally become ecchymotic or break down and form crusted ulcerations. There is a progressive febrile illness, with hepatosplenomegaly, pancytopenia, and liver dysfunction. These result from the proliferation of benign-appearing histiocytes, which have a marked phagocytic capacity.

Histologically there is infiltration of the lobules of subcutaneous fat by histiocytes and inflammatory cells, with fat necrosis and hemorrhage. The typical cell is a "bean bag" cell: a histiocyte stuffed with phagocytized red blood cells, lymphocytes, neutrophils, and platelets.

The patients, 13 of whom were female, usually died of acute hemorrhage after a long illness. Splenectomy and supportive care were of temporary help to the patient reported by Willis et al.

Alegre VA, et al: Histiocytic cytophagic panniculitis. JAAD 1989, 20:177.
Crotty CP, et al: Cytophagic histiocytic panniculitis with fever, cytopenia, liver failure, and terminal hemorrhagic diathesis. JAAD 1981, 4:181.
Peters MS, et al: Cytophagic panniculitis and B cell lymphoma. JAAD 1985, 13:882.
Willis SM, et al: Cytophagic histiocytic panniculitis. Arch Dermatol 1985, 121:910.
Winkelmann RK, et al: Hemorrhagic diathesis associated with benign histiocytic cytophagic panniculitis and systemic histiocytosis. Arch Intern Med 1980, 140:1460.

POSTSTEROID PANNICULITIS

Poststeroid panniculitis is characterized by firm, pruritic, tender, erythematous, subcutaneous nodules occurring on the buttocks, trunk, and extremities of children one to 30 days after cessation of oral prednisone therapy. Approximately 90 per cent of the children had prior acute rheumatic fever and were on prednisone for rheumatic carditis. Fever, joint pain, and heart failure may be present. All reported patients have received a total dosage of at least 2000 mg prednisone or its equivalent. All have been children. The histopathologic changes are confined to the subcutaneous tissue with an inflammatory infiltrate in the interstices of the fat cells. Neutrophils and mononuclear cells are seen in the early lesions. Later, foam cells, histiocytes, lymphocytes, and foreign-body giant cells predominate. The fat cells contain needle-shaped clefts similar to those found in subcutaneous fat necrosis of the newborn.

Poststeroid panniculitis must be differentiated from Weber-Christian panniculitis, rheumatoid nodules, and erythema nodosum.

It is usually transient and disappears spontaneously. If it is severe, steroids may be resumed temporarily; this is seldom necessary

The pathogenesis of this disappearance is unknown.

Roenigk HH Jr., et al: Poststeroid panniculitis. Arch Dermatol 1964, 90:387.
Smith RT, et al: Sequelae of prednisone treatment of acute rheumatic fever. Clin Res Proc 1964, 4:156.

FACTITIAL PANNICULITIS

Self-induced panniculitis is considered rare, and few cases have been reported. Kossard reported focal panniculitis induced by self-injections of procaine povidone. Other chemicals such as organic materials, oils, and silicones may be injected. Medical personnel are at risk because they have ready access to syringes and needles.

Factitial panniculitis can also be produced by trauma. Winkelmann et al reported five cases of this in 1985. Included among them was a case of Secrétan's syndrome, a patient who self-induced edema and hemorrhage in the back of the hand. They point out that when a patient has an obscure panniculitis, drug dependency, and a passive, evasive personality, one should suspect factitial panniculitis. Careful evaluation of the biopsy for foreign material by the polariscope and spectroscope may be helpful.

Nonfactitial, accidental traumatic panniculitis may occur, such as that commonly seen on the breast in 15–60-year-old women, or in children hit during play. Such a firm, indurated breast lesion may mimic carcinoma.

Forstrom L, et al: Factitial panniculitis. Arch Dermatol 1974, 110:747.
Kossard S, et al: Povidone panniculitis. Arch Dermatol 1980, 116:704.
Lever WF, et al: Histopathology of the Skin, 6th ed. Philadelphia, J. B. Lippincott Co. 1983, pp. 253–254.
Winkelmann RK, et al: Factitial traumatic panniculitis. JAAD 1985, 13:988.

SCLEROSING LIPOGRANULOMA

Sclerosing lipogranuloma is a localized fat necrosis that may occur anywhere on the body, but is usually localized to the subcutaneous fat of the genital regions.

Most of the cases occur on the shaft of the penis and scrotum. The lesions appear as painless lumps and persist for years.

Calnan felt that extraneously injected oils might induce this type of lesion. Newcomer et al and Snapper et al confirmed this in their cases.

Histologically there is hyaline necrosis in the septa of the fat cells. An infiltrate of round cells, macrophages, and polymorphonuclear cells is seen. The collagen and the fat are also altered.

In these cases self-induced lesions should always be considered.

Calnan CD, et al: Sclerosing lipogranuloma. Proc R Soc Med 1952, 45:716.
Foucar E, et al: Sclerosing lipogranuloma of the male genitalia containing vitamin E. JAAD 1983, 9:103.
Newcomer VD, et al: Sclerosing lipogranuloma resulting from exogenous lipids. Arch Dermatol 1986, 73:361.
Rees HA: Sclerosing lipogranuloma. Arch Dermatol 1964, 84:277.
Snapper I, et al: Factitious genital sclerogranuloma. Arch Dermatol 1968, 98:30.
Steffen C, et al: Sclerosing lipogranuloma of the male genitalia: a malingerer's malady? Arch Dermatol 1983, 119:791.

NODULAR FAT NECROSIS

Also known as subcutaneous fat necrosis with pancreatitis, or pancreatic panniculitis, in this disorder excessive amounts of circulating pancreatic enzymes (trypsin, amylase, and lipase) and possibly another as yet unidentified factor are responsible for fat necrosis in areas distant from the pancreas.

The skin lesions begin upon the legs as painless, elevated, subcutaneous nodules that resemble erythema nodosum, drug eruption, periarteritis nodosa, or embolic abscesses of staphylococcic bacteremia. The legs are edematous. The nodules may occur on other areas, sometimes being widespread, extremely tender, and fluctuant.

The patients are often extremely ill, with fever, vomiting, and abdominal distension. Sometimes the skin nodules appear before there is any abdominal pain. Joint manifestations are prominent in 60 per cent of patients, especially with pancreatic carcinoma and pancreatitis.

The pancreatic disease may have a number of underlying causes. Goldman states that 50 per cent of cases are caused by pancreatitis. This is most often the result of chronic alcoholism. Thirty per cent are due to pancreatic carcinoma, most often acinous rather than the otherwise more common adenocarcinoma. Pancreatic pseudocysts were present in 15 per cent of one series, and in 5 per cent, traumatic panniculitis was the cause. Detlefs et al reported a case induced by sulindac (Clinoril) in which panniculitis occurred. Haber et al reported a case with pancreas divisum, and Simons-Ling et al reported a case with pancreatitis due to systemic lupus erythematosus. Levine et al reported a patient with acute pancreatitis who developed subcutaneous fat necrosis of the anterior abdominal wall due to leakage of pancreatic enzymes through a rent in the peritoneum following paracentesis.

Laboratory examination shows elevated levels of serum lipase and amylase, and urinary and ascitic fluid amylase. Eosinophilia is present in 25 per cent of cases.

Histology is pathognomonic in the skin, and points to pancreatic disease. In the panniculus, lipocytes

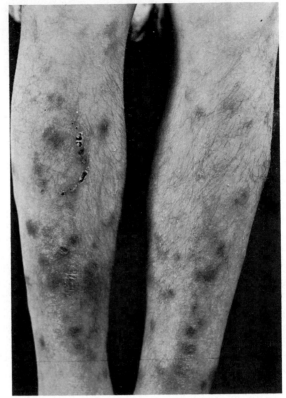

Figure 23–2. Nodular fat necrosis. (Courtesy of Dr. H. Shatin.)

degenerate into "ghostlike" cells with no nuclei, and shadowy walls. There may be granular calcium deposits with surrounding inflammation. Similar changes are found in the pancreas, peritoneum, and omentum. The outcome is dependent on the pancreatic disease.

Berman B, et al: Fatal panniculitis presenting with subcutaneous fat necrosis. JAAD 1987, 17:359.
Detlefs RL: Drug-induced pancreatitis presenting as subcutaneous fat necrosis. JAAD 1965, 13:305.
Goldman MP: Ascites, gastrointestinal bleeding, and leg nodules. Arch Dermatol 1985, 121:673.
Haber RM, et al: Panniculitis associated with a pancreas divisum. JAAD 1986, 14:331.
Hughes PSH, et al: Subcutaneous fat necrosis associated with pancreatic disease. Arch Dermatol 1975, 111:506.
Mullin GT, et al: Arthritis and skin lesions resembling erythema nodosum in pancreatic disease. Ann Intern Med 1968, 68:75.
Simons-Ling N, et al: Childhood systemic lupus erythematosus. Arch Dermatol 1983, 119:491.
Szymanski FJ, et al: Nodular fat necrosis and pancreatic diseases. Arch Dermatol 1961, 83:224.

COLD PANNICULITIS

Exposure to cold may injure the panniculus, causing a lobular inflammatory response within hours to days. Subcutaneous erythematous indurated nodules occur, and resolve spontaneously within a week or two, in the areas exposed to cold. E. H. Epstein et al reported cold panniculitis of the cheeks in children from eating popsicles. Beacham et al reported the disorder on the anterolateral aspects of the thighs in four women who were riding horseback in cold weather. Vickers, and Bleehen, have also reported it.

Fat necrosis of the scrotum is another well-defined entity in the spectrum of cold injury of the panniculus. The typical patient with fat necrosis of the scrotum is a prepubertal (9- to 14-year-old) boy, heavy-set or even obese, with scrotal swelling, usually bilateral, associated with mild to moderate pain. The gait is often guarded and broad-based. There is a lack of systemic complaints and no symptoms related to voiding.

The scrotal masses are bilateral and symmetrical in most cases. However, the lesions may be unilateral and there may be more than two. The masses are firm, tender, and do not transmit light. The overlying scrotal skin will be normal or red. Cryptorchidism is not unusual. The most common location of the necrosis is near the perineum, consistent with the area of greatest concentration of scrotal fat in children. The adult scrotum lacks this fatty tissue.

Pathologically, the lesions are grossly grayish yellow and may be easily dissected free from surrounding tissues. Histology reveals necrosis, early fibrosis, and giant cell formation.

Hypothermia appears to be the most likely cause of the condition. Several reported cases had histories of swimming in very cold water during late winter or early spring within one to five days of the onset of symptoms. Whether the injury from hypothermia is the result of liberation of lipases, a vascular phenomenon, or direct damage from the cold is unknown.

With a firm diagnosis, expectant treatment will allow spontaneous resolution of the lesions during a one- to three-week period. If doubt exists, appropriate surgical intervention is advocated.

Beacham BE, et al: Equestrian cold panniculitis in women. Arch Dermatol 1980, 116:1025.

Bleehen SS: Equestrian cold panniculitis in women. Arch Dermatol 1981, 117:316.

Epstein EH, et al: Popsicle panniculitis. N Engl J Med 1970, 282:966.

Peterson LJ, et al: Bilateral fat necrosis of the scrotum. J Urol 1976, 116:825.

Vickers R: Equestrian cold panniculitis in women. Arch Dermatol 1981, 117:315.

SCLEREMA NEONATORUM

This indurative disease of the subcutaneous tissues begins during the first weeks of life in premature or debilitated infants who usually have an associated severe underlying disease such as sepsis, respiratory distress, diarrhea, congenital heart disease, or dehydration. It is characterized by symmetrical areas of hardening of the subcutaneous fat, particularly on the buttocks, shoulders, calves, and cheeks. The skin on the palms, soles, and genitalia is spared. The skin becomes dry, livid, cold, rigid, and boardlike, so that the mobility of the parts is limited. The skin in the involved areas cannot be picked up. The skin of the entire body may appear half frozen and is yellowish white.

The course of the disease is rapidly downhill, usually with a fatal termination.

ETIOLOGY. Sclerema neonatorum usually arises in marasmic or premature infants who are suffering from a serious underlying illness. Milunsky and Levin believe that the major factor is exposure to cold at birth, which causes sluggish circulation and peripheral vasoconstriction. Although this hypothesis has been repeated often, in most cases the etiology is unclear.

PATHOGENESIS. Kellum and his associates reported a substantial increase in the saturated/unsaturated ratio of the fatty acids of the subcutaneous triglycerides in infants. Also, the ratio of surface area to body fat is high in infants. These factors make the newborn susceptible to cold injury and may be responsible for the dramatic physical changes in the skin in some cases.

The simultaneous occurrence of other disease processes in sclerema neonatorum has suggested possible interference with the enzyme system of the fatty acids to some. Again this remains unproven. Major infection, shock, dehydration, and chilling seem to be influencing agents.

PATHOLOGY. The epidermis and dermis are normal. The subcutaneous tissue is thickened by swollen lipocytes, and wide intersecting fibrous bands are interspersed throughout. There is a notable absence of an inflammatory infiltrate, giant cells, and fat necrosis. Intracellular crystals of triglycerides are present.

DIFFERENTIAL DIAGNOSIS. Subcutaneous fat necrosis of the newborn, scleredema, Milroy's disease, and scleroderma should be differentiated from sclerema neonatorum. Subcutaneous fat necrosis of the newborn usually occurs in healthy infants, is patchy in distribution, and histologically shows inflammation. The other three diseases are rare in newborns, and a biopsy of sclerema neonatorum will reveal characteristic findings.

TREATMENT. No specific treatment is known. Treatment of possible sepsis and meticulous management of fluid and electrolyte problems are of prime importance. Treatment of the underlying disease, if possible, is very important. Because of the grave prognosis, corticosteroids have been advocated as adjunctive therapy.

PROGNOSIS. The disease terminates fatally in at least 70 per cent of cases. If the underlying illness can be successfully treated there may be recovery.

Esterly NB: Sclerema neonatorum and subcutaneous fat necrosis of the newborn. In *Dermatology, 1982*, vol. 2, Demis DJ (ed). Philadelphia, Harper & Row, 1982.

Horsfield GI, et al: Sclerema neonatorum. J Invest Dermatol 1965, 44:326.

Kellum RE, et al: Sclerema neonatorum. Arch Dermatol 1968, 97:372.

Milunsky A, et al: Sclerema neonatorum: clinical study of 79 cases. S Af Med J 1966, 40:638.

SUBCUTANEOUS FAT NECROSIS

Subcutaneous fat necrosis in newborn or young infants is characterized by localized, firm, purple-red, subcutaneous nodules present on the cheeks, back, buttocks, and thighs. These nodules do not pit on firm pressure nor does the induration allow the skin to be pinched up in folds. Softening and absorption of the indurated areas begin about the fifth week and are complete in a few months. The nodules frequently liquefy and may develop calcification.

The cause is unknown but trauma at birth, asphyxia, hypothermia, and diabetes mellitus in the mother have been hypothesized as possible factors, but remain unproven.

Katz et al reported a case with a solitary nodule subsequent to a forceps delivery, which was excised. Silverman et al reported a case which occurred after hypothermic cardiac surgery. Most cases, however, do not have such clear-cut exposure to predisposing factors.

Histologically there is an extensive inflammatory infiltrate in the subcutaneous tissue consisting of lymphocytes, foreign-body giant cells, and histiocytes. Many fat cells are replaced by fibrous tissue. Needle-shaped clefts may be seen within the fat cells.

The prognosis is usually excellent in subcutaneous fat necrosis. It is generally self-limiting and usually heals without scar formation. Thomsen reviewed the literature and found 15 patients, including the young girl he reported, who developed idiopathic hypocalcemia. This may not be present until several months after the onset of the skin disease, and may be a fatal complication. Thomsen recommends serial calcium determinations in following patients with subcutaneous fat necrosis, and observation for signs of hypercalcemia, such as anorexia, constipation, irritability, and failure to thrive. Norwood-Galloway et al in 1987 reported a case with generalized subcutaneous fat necrosis and hypoxic cardiomyopathy at birth, who was found at three weeks of age (with the fat necrosis improving) to be suffering from vomiting, irritability, weight loss, and failure to thrive. Serum calcium was 17 mg/dl, and phosphorus 5.1. Subcutaneous calcitonin, 20 units a day, increased to twice a day, failed to control the hypercalcemia, and oral prednisone was given. Firm nodules continued to appear occasionally until six months of age, but serum calcium had returned to normal and the baby recovered.

Chen TH, et al: Subcutaneous fat necrosis of the newborn. Arch Dermatol 1981, 117:36.

Esterly NB: Sclerema neonatorum and subcutaneous fat necrosis of the newborn. In *Dermatology, 1982,* vol. 2. Demis DJ (ed). Philadelphia, Harper & Row, 1982.

Katz DA, et al: Subcutaneous fat necrosis of the newborn. Arch Dermatol 1984, 120:1517.

Liu DC: Red nodules in an infant. Arch Dermatol 1986, 122:821.

Norwood-Galloway A, et al: Subcutaneous fat necrosis of the newborn with hypercalcemia. JAAD 1987, 16:435.

Silverman AK, et al: Subcutaneous fat necrosis in an infant, occurring after hypothermic cardiac surgery. JAAD 1986, 15:331.

Taieb A, et al: Subcutaneous fat necrosis and brown fat deficiency. JAAD 1987, 16:624.

Thomsen RJ: Subcutaneous fat necrosis of the newborn and idiopathic hypercalcemia. Arch Dermatol 1980, 116:1155.

LIPODYSTROPHY

The lipodystrophies are rare conditions in which there is atrophy of the subcutaneous fat. There is no unanimity on whether the various forms are distinct entities or more closely related conditions. The lipodystrophies include total lipodystrophy, congenital or acquired; partial lipodystrophy; abdominal infantile lipodystrophy; and localized lipodystrophy associated with insulin or other parenteral injections.

Total Lipodystrophy

Total lipodystrophy is also known as *lipoatrophic diabetes, Seip-Lawrence syndrome,* and *congenital lipodystrophic diabetes.*

Lawrence first described a syndrome which he named *acquired lipoatrophic diabetes.* This entity is characterized by loss of adipose issue in late childhood or early adult life, followed by insulin-resistant hyperglycemia, hyperlipemia, and fatty hepatomegaly.

Seip described a congenital syndrome similar to that of Lawrence but without diabetes and with rapid growth, advanced bone age, hepatomegaly, hypermusculature, hyperpigmentation, hypertension, and corneal opacities. Subsequently reported patients with total lipodystrophy have usually had insulin resistance, and many have developed clinically apparent diabetes by the second or third decade. Most reported patients have had the congenital variety of total lipodystrophy.

Reed and his associates reported three patients with the congenital type of lipodystrophy who also had acanthosis nigricans. These patients all attained 90 per cent of their growth in the first 10 years of life; clitoral or penile enlargement was apparent early in life, as were hyperlipemia and hepatomegaly. A fatty liver is present, and may result in cirrhosis and liver failure in some cases of total lipodystrophy. A distinctive facies was apparent in all of Reed's cases, with dolichocephalic skulls, curly scalp hair extending down to the eyebrows, lipodystrophic facies, hirsutism, prominent teeth, and a small chin.

Brunzell and his associates reported a family with

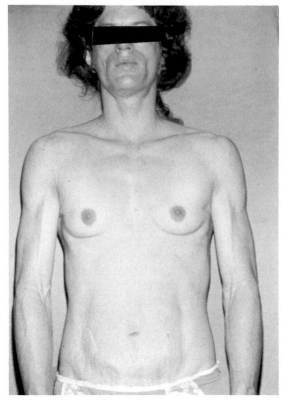

Figure 23–3. *Total lipodystrophy in a patient with insulin-resistant diabetes and hyperlipidemia. (Courtesy of Dr. Axel W. Hoke.)*

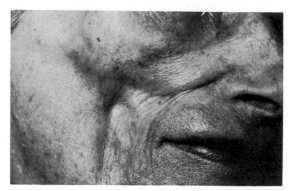

Figure 23–4. *Bilateral lipodystrophy of cheeks. Note preservation of periorbital fat.*

five siblings who had systemic cystic angiomatosis accompanying congenital lipodystrophy.

The characteristic laboratory abnormality is a decreased glucose tolerance. Diabetes may first be detectable only in the second or third decade. The hyperglycemia resists insulin therapy. The insulin resistance appears to be due to a genetic defect in insulin receptor or postreceptor pathways, and is not due to an autoantibody directed against this receptor. The bones are abnormally radiopaque.

Consanguinity is frequently found in these cases. The congenital type is transmitted as an autosomal recessive trait.

Roth et al reviewed the findings in patients born with *leprechaunism*. These patients have decreased or absent subcutaneous fat in a generalized distribution, wrinkled loose skin, acanthosis nigricans, hypertrichosis, rugae at the orifices, hyperkeratosis, dysplastic nails, thick lips, and gingival hypertrophy. They also have insulin resistance, but apparently no organomegaly or liver disease. Also separating them from congenital total lipodystrophy is the presence of muscular wasting, retarded bone age, retarded growth, and early death.

Partial Lipodystrophy

This is also known as progressive lipoatrophy or Barraquer-Simons' syndrome. This progressive fat disorder is characterized by a diffuse and progressive loss of the subcutaneous fat, which usually begins in the face and scalp and progresses downward as far as the iliac crests. It occurs chiefly in children between the ages of five and eight but may begin later in some cases. Girls outnumber boys by 4:1. The upper half of the body seems emaciated. The cheeks sink in, and the skin over the rest of the face is drawn like a death mask. There is an apparent, and possibly a real, adiposity of the buttocks, thighs, and legs.

Most cases are of the cephalothoracic type. A few patients whose condition appears be a separate disease have lipodystrophy of the lower trunk and extremities. Unlike the classic cases, they often have

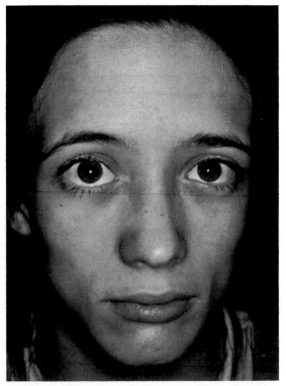

Figure 23–5. *Partial lipodystrophy in a young woman with chronic hypocomplementemic glomerulonephritis.*

a positive family history and may have associated acanthosis nigricans, diabetes, or hepatosplenomegaly. Autografts of normal fat to atrophic sites undergo wasting, while transplants of affected tissue to an uninvolved site accumulate fat.

The onset is insidious, with no discomfort or inflammation in the areas of fat loss. Histologically, the skin is normal except for the absence of fat.

Sissons et al found normal complement profiles, and no renal disease, in three patients with total lipodystrophy, but 17 of 21 with partial lipodystrophy had decreased C3 with normal C1 and C4, and six (all hypocomplementemic) had nephritis. It has since been found that two thirds of patients with classic partial lipodystrophy have in their serum a protein named C3 nephritic factor. This is an autoantibody against the alternate-pathway enzyme, C3 convertase, C3bBb. It increases the half-life of convertase and prevents cleavage of C3b by C3b inactivator. This leads to the development of membranoproliferative glomerulonephritis in many of these patients. How this relates to lipodystrophy has not been determined.

Abdominal Infantile Lipodystrophy

"Lipodystrophia centrifugalis abdominalis infantilis" was the unwieldy name given to this entity by Imamura et al, who first reported it in 1971. It is a disease of childhood: 90 per cent of cases begin by age five. It is characterized by depression of the skin caused by loss of fat, in the abdominal or axillary area, which enlarges slowly centrifugally for three to eight years in most cases. Histologically, most or all of the fat is lost, with minimal inflammatory infiltrate. Regional lymph node swelling occurred in 52 of 86 cases. By the age of 8 to 13 years, the progression stops, and within a year or two, normal contours are restored in almost all cases.

Mysteriously, despite nine publications on the subject, all reported cases have been in Orientals except one, reported by Zachary and Wells in 1984.

Localized Lipodystrophy

Six months to two years after the initiation of insulin injections, localized atrophy of fat may develop at the sites, more frequently in children or women than in men. Valenta et al reported that this dystrophic change resolved in five patients who were switched to human insulin. Much less often, insulin injections may result in lipohypertrophy, as reported by Mier et al.

Lipoatrophia Annularis (Ferreira-Marques)

This is a remarkable atrophy of the subcutaneous fat preceded by a bracelet-shaped swelling, redness,

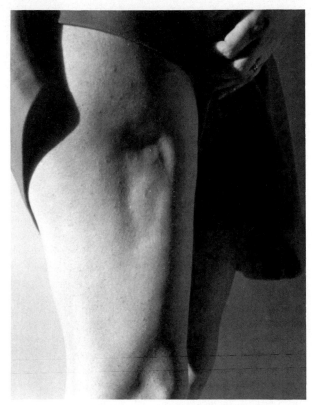

Figure 23–6. Lipoatrophy secondary to insulin injections. (Courtesy of Dr. Axel W. Hoke.)

scaling, and paresthesia about an extremity, followed by loss of subcutaneous fat so that a forearm is divided into two parts by a depressed, atrophic, braceletlike constriction. The cause is unknown. The histology shows massive atrophy of the subcutaneous fat. The collagenous and elastic tissues are also damaged. The vessels show panarteritis and panphlebitis.

Rongioletti et al recently reported a case and distinguished this inflammatory condition from *annular atrophy of the ankles*, in which a wide band of atrophy without clinical evidence of inflammation occurs bilaterally. Another noninflammatory localized lipoatrophy is *semicircular lipoatrophy*, in which semiannular symmetric depressions occur on women's anterior thighs.

Finally, Billings et al reported three cases and reviewed several others of children who developed slowly enlarging erythematous nodules eventuating in lipoatrophy. The disorder is sometimes extensive. They emphasized the frequency of associated autoimmune disease.

Billings JK, et al: Lipoatrophic panniculitis. Arch Dermatol 1987, 123:1662.

Brunzell JD, et al: Congenital generalized lipodystrophy accompanied by cystic angiomatosis. Ann Intern Med 1968, 69:501.

Chartier S, et al: Partial lipodystrophy associated with a type 3 form of membranoproliferative glomerulonephritis. JAAD 1987, 16:201.

Eisinger AJ, et al: Renal disease in partial lipodystrophy. Q J Med 1972, 163:343.

Field LM: Successful treatment of lipohypertrophic insulin lipodystrophy with liposuction surgery. JAAD 1988, 19:520.

Fitch N, et al: Progressive partial lipodystrophy and third-trimester intrauterine fetal death. Am J Obstet Gynecol 1987, 156:1195.

Flier JS: Metabolic importance of acanthosis nigricans. Arch Dermatol 1985, 121:193.

Griebel M, et al: Generalized weight loss in a child. Arch Dermatol 1988, 124:571.

Imamura S, et al: Lipodystrophia centrifugalis abdominalis infantilis. Arch Dermatol 1971, 104:291; JAAD 1984, 11:203.

Ljunghall S, et al: Partial lipodystrophy and chronic hypocomplementemic glomerulonephritis. Acta Med Scand 1974, 195:493.

Mier A, et al: Bilateral abdominal lipohypertrophy after continuous subcutaneous infusion of insulin. Br Med J 1982, 285:1539.

Rongioletti F, et al: Annular and semicircular lipoatrophies. JAAD 1989, 20:433.

Roth SI, et al: Cutaneous manifestations of leprechaunism. Arch Dermatol 1981, 117:531.

Samadaei A, et al: Insulin lipodystrophy, lipohypertrophic type. JAAD 1987, 17:506.

Sissons JGP, et al: The complement abnormalities of lipodystrophy. N Engl J Med 1976, 294:461.

Valenta LJ, et al: Insulin-induced lipodystrophy in diabetic patients resolved by treatment with human insulin. Ann Intern Med 1985, 102:790.

24

Endocrine Diseases

The skin interacts with the endocrine system in many ways. Some of them are discussed in this chapter.

Feingold KR, et al: Endocrine-skin interactions. JAAD 1987, 17:921.
Idem: Endocrine-skin interactions. JAAD 1988, 19:1.

ACROMEGALY

In acromegaly, changes in the soft tissues and in the bones form a characteristic syndrome. In association with the well-known changes in the facial features due to gigantic hypertrophy of the chin, nose, and supraorbital ridges, there is thickening, reddening, and wrinkling of the forehead, and exaggeration of the nasolabial grooves. The lips and tongue are thick. Cutis verticis gyrata is often present. The hands and feet enlarge, and there is gradual growth of the fingertips until they resemble drumsticks. There is diffuse hypertrophy of the skin. Matsuoka et al found this was at least partly due to deposition of colloidal-iron-positive material in the papillary and reticular dermis. Ferguson et al showed that increased skin thickness could be demonstrated radiologically (in lateral radiographs of the heel), with reversal toward normal after treatment. Skin thickness did not correlate well with growth hormone levels at the time of diagnosis. Hypertrichosis, hyperpigmentation, and hyperhidrosis occur in many patients. The clinical changes may suggest the leonine facies of leprosy, as well as Paget's disease, myxedema, and pachydermoperiostosis.

The cause of acromegaly is hypersecretion of growth hormone by the pituitary, usually because of a mixed chromophobe and eosinophilic adenoma of the gland.

The currently preferred treatment is a combination of irradiation and transsphenoidal microsurgical excision of the tumor.

Chalmers RJ, et al: Acne vulgaris and hidradenitis suppurativa as presenting features of acromegaly. Br Med J 1983, 287:1346.
Christy NP: Choosing the best treatment for acromegaly (editorial). JAMA 1982, 247:1320.
Ferguson JK, et al: Skin thickness in acromegaly and Cushing's syndrome and response to treatment. Clin Endocrinol (OXF) 1983, 18:347.
Klein I, et al: Colonic polyps in patients with acromegaly. Ann Intern Med 1982, 97:27.
Matsuoka LY, et al: Histochemical characterization of the cutaneous involvement of acromegaly. Arch Intern Med 1982, 142:1820.

CUSHING'S SYNDROME

In 1932, when Cushing first described pituitary basophilism, relatively little was known about the delicately balanced "HPA" (hypothalamic-pituitary-adrenal) axis. He noted, however, the frequent association of pituitary basophilic tumors with adrenal cortical hyperplasia. Hyperfunction of the adrenocortical tissue is directly responsible for this syndrome when it has not been iatrogenically induced by overdosage with corticosteroid hormones either topically or, more often, systemically.

Among the most prominent features may be mentioned the obesity, affecting the face, neck, the trunk, and markedly the abdomen, but sparing the limbs. There may be deposition of fat over the upper back, or a buffalo hump. The face becomes "moon-shaped," being wide and round. In noniatrogenic cases, women are affected four times more frequently than men, and the peak ages of onset are the twenties and thirties.

The striking and distressing skin changes include hypertrichosis, dryness, and fragility of the skin, with facial acne and susceptibility to superficial dermatophyte and *Pityrosporon* infections; a dusky flushing that may be associated with an actual polycythemia; and the characteristic purplish, atrophic striae on the abdomen and thighs. Ferguson et al have shown that the thinning of the skin can be demonstrated and measured in lateral radiographs of the heels. There is reversal with treatment. Occasionally there may be livedo reticularis, purpura, ecchymosis, or brownish pigmentation. Poikilodermalike changes have been observed. Most women develop facial and body hypertrichosis, with thinning of the scalp hair.

There is usually hypertension and marked generalized arteriosclerosis, with progressive weakness, prostration, and pains in the back, limbs, and abdomen; also kyphosis of the dorsal spine, accentuating the "buffalo" appearance. There is a reduction in the density of the bone, with osteoporosis. There is generally a loss of libido. In 20 per cent of patients a disturbance in carbohydrate metabolism develops with hyperglycemia and glycosuria, and diabetes mellitus.

These varied symptoms indicate a marked and widespread disturbance due to the hyperactive adrenal cortex. When microadenomas of the pituitary produce these clinical findings they are referred to as Cushing's disease. This accounts for only 10 per cent of patients, and contrary to Cushing's original description, most adenomas are chromophobic. Forty to 60 per cent of additional cases are due to an increased ACTH production by the pituitary, but no adenoma is identified. Adrenal adenomas and carcinomas, and ectopic production of ACTH by other tumors, account for the remainder of cases of noniatrogenic Cushing's syndrome.

A rapid screening test for Cushing's syndrome consists of oral administration of 1 mg dexamethasone at 11 PM followed by an 8 AM fluorometric determination of plasma cortisol. A cortisol level below 10 μg per 100 ml essentially rules out Cushing's syndrome, except for the iatrogenic variety, in which there is adrenocortical hypoplasia and the serum cortisol level is very low even without dexamethasone suppression.

Ferguson JK, et al: Skin thickness in acromegaly and Cushing's syndrome and response to treatment. Clin Endocrinol (Oxf) 1983, 18:347.

Sawin CT: Measurement of plasma cortisol in the diagnosis of Cushing's syndrome. Ann Intern Med 1968, 68:624.

Seidensticker JF, et al: Screening test for Cushing's syndrome with plasma 11-hydroxycorticosteroids. JAMA 1967, 202:87.

ADDISON'S DISEASE

Adrenal insufficiency is manifested in the skin primarily by hyperpigmentation. It is diffuse but most prominently observed in sun-exposed areas and sites exposed to recurrent trauma or pressure. The axillae, perineum, and nipples are also affected. Palmar crease darkening in Caucasians; scar hyperpigmentation; and darkening of nevi, mucous membranes, hair, and nails may all be seen. Fibrosis and calcification of the pinnae of the ears are rare complications.

Dunlop D: Eighty-six cases of Addison's disease. Br Med J 1963, 2:887.

PANHYPOPITUITARISM

Pituitary failure results in many changes in the skin, hair, and nails as a result of the absence of the pituitary hormone action on these sites. Pale, thin, dry skin is seen. Diffuse loss of body hair, with axillary, pubic, and head hair being especially thin, is present. The nails are thin, fragile, and opaque and grow slowly.

ANDROGEN-DEPENDENT SYNDROMES

The androgen-dependent syndromes are caused by the excessive production of adrenal androgens by adrenal adenomas, carcinoma, or hyperplasia. The differential diagnosis includes Leydig's cell tumors in men, and arrhenoblastomas and Stein-Leventhal syndrome in women.

The cutaneous signs of excessive androgen include acne, hirsutism, temporal baldness, seborrhea, enlargement of the clitoris, and decreased breast size. Hyperpigmentation of the skin, areolae, genitalia, palmar creases, and buccal mucosa develops in some patients.

In the *congenital adrenogenital syndrome*, excess androgen is produced by an inherited defect in any of the five enzymatic steps required to convert cholesterol to cortisol. The formation of inadequate amounts of cortisol stimulates the pituitary to secrete excessive ACTH, which stimulates excess androgen production. In boys, precocious puberty results. In girls, masculinization occurs, with the prominent cutaneous signs of excess androgen production. Pseudohermaphroditism may occur, with clitoral hypertrophy and (in younger patients) labioscrotal fusion.

Treatment of many of the cutaneous signs of androgen excess, especially acne and hirsutism, with the androgen-blocking agent cyproterone acetate is under investigation in Europe. Holdaway et al confirmed its effectiveness. Schmidt et al evaluated medroxyprogesterone acetate in hirsutism and found it effective when given intramuscularly, subcutaneously, or intralesionally. Topical administration showed only a modest effect. These agents are not now available in the U.S. Spironolactone, which competes for the androgen cytosol receptors, has proved useful as a systemic antiandrogen to hirsutism, acne, adrenal-androgenic female pattern alopecia, and polycystic ovary syndrome. Physiologic doses of hydrocortisone will suffice to control most cases. Studies on topical administration are in progress.

Braithwaite SS, et al: Hirsutism. Arch Dermatol 1983, 119:279.

Holdaway JM: Cyproterone acetate as intitial treatment and maintenance therapy for hirsutism. Acta Endocrinol (Copenh) 1985, 109:522.

Lucky AW: Androgens and the skin. Arch Dermatol 1987, 123:193.

McKenna TJ: Pathogenesis and treatment of polycystic ovary syndrome. N Engl J Med 1988, 318:558.

Price VH: Testosterone metabolism in the skin. Arch Dermatol 1975, 111:1496.

Reingold SB, et al: The relationship of mild hirsutism or acne in women to androgens. Arch Dermatol 1987, 123:209.

Schmidt JB, et al: Medroxyprogesterone acetate therapy in hirsutism. Br J Dermatol 1985, 113:161.

Traupe H, et al: Acne of the fulminans type following testosterone therapy in three excessively tall boys. Arch Dermatol 1988, 124:414.

Wajchenberg BL, et al: Determination of the sources of androgen overproduction in hirsutism associated with polycystic ovary syndrome by simultaneous adrenal and ovarian venous catheterization. J Clin Endocrinol Metab 1986, 63:1204.

Weissmann A, et al: Antiandrogenic effects of topically applied spironolactone on the hamster flank organ. Arch Dermatol 1985, 121:57.

White PC, et al: Congenital adrenal hyperplasia, Parts 1 & 2. N Engl J Med 1987, 316:24, 316:25.

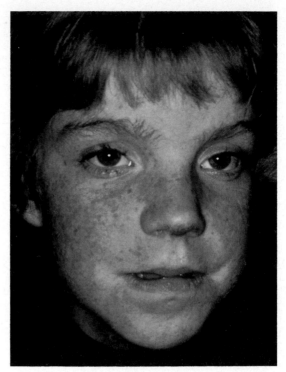

Figure 24–1. Cretinism.

HYPOTHYROIDISM

Hypothyroidism is a deficiency of circulating thyroid hormone, which produces various clinical manifestations, dependent upon the time of life at which it occurs and upon its severity. Middle-aged women are the most commonly affected adults.

Cretinism

Primary thyroid deficiency in fetal life produces the characteristic picture of cretinism at birth and in the next few months of life. Depending upon the degree of thyroid deficiency, a wide variety of signs and symptoms may be evident.

The cretin has a cool, dry, pasty white skin. Disturbances in the amount, texture, and distribution of the hair are common. Pigmentation is less than normal after exposure to sunlight. Sweating is greatly diminished. The lips are pale, thick, and protuberant. The tongue is usually enlarged and there is delayed dentition. The facies is characterized by wide-set eyes, a broad flat nose, periorbital puffiness, and a large protruding tongue. A protuberant abdomen with umbilical hernia is frequently seen.

Myxedema

When lack of secretion of thyroid hormone is severe, a systemic mucinosis called myxedema is produced (see Chapter 9 and Fig. 9–1); the skin becomes rough and dry, and in severe cases of primary myxedema, ichthyosis vulgaris may be simulated. The facial skin is puffy; the expression is often dull and flat; macroglossia is present; and chronic periorbital infiltration secondary to the deposits of mucopolysaccharides frequently develops. Carotenemia may cause a yellow tint in the skin which is especially prominent on the palms and soles. Diffuse hair loss is common and the outer third of the eyebrows is shed. The hair becomes coarse and brittle and the free edges of the nails break easily.

Mild Hypothyroidism

Lesser degrees of deficiency are common and far less easily diagnosed. Coldness of hands and feet in the absence of vascular disease, sensitivity to cool weather (need for a sweater or extra bedcovers when others do not need them), lack of sweating, tendency to put on weight, need for extra sleep, drowsiness in the daytime, or constipation, all suggest possible hypothyroidism and the need for appropriate tests. A T3, T4, and TSH are recommended as the screening tests. Normal or marginal results in the presence of symptoms, however, are untrustworthy, and a brief trial of Synthroid (levothyroxine), 50–100 μg daily, to see whether symptoms are alleviated, is advisable.

Worstman J, et al: Preradial myxedema in thyroid disease. Arch Dermatol 1981, 117:635.

HYPERTHYROIDISM

Excessive quantities of circulating thyroid hormone, produced in a variety of ways, affect various organs. The skin changes are distinctive in hyperthyroidism. Graves's disease has a female-to-male ratio of 7:1, and the peak age at onset is 20 to 30 years.

The cutaneous surface is warm, moist, and smooth textured. Palmar erythema is frequently seen. The hair is thin and has a downy texture. The skin may be diffusely pigmented to produce a bronzed appearance or melanoderma; sometimes even melasma of the cheeks is seen.

Thyroid acropachy is characterized by digital clubbing and diaphyseal proliferation of the periosteum in acral and distal long bones (tibia, fibula, ulna, and radius). It usually occurs in association with past hyperthyroidism, untreated and treated, and frequently accompanies exophthalmos and pretibial myxedema. Thyroid acropachy has been recognized in euthyroid and hypothyroid patients. It can be confused with acromegaly, pachydermoperiostosis, pulmonary osteoarthropathy, or osteoperiosteitis.

Pretibial myxedema (see also Chapter 9 and Figs. 9–2 and 9–3), consisting of localized cutaneous accumulations of glycosaminoglycans, occurs in 5 per cent of patients who have or have had Graves's disease. It may also occur during the course of Hashimoto thyroiditis and primary hypothyroidism. Patients with pretibial myxedema regularly have associated ophthalmopathy and occasionally have thyroid acropachy. Elevated serum levels of long-acting thyroid stimulator (LATS) almost invariably accompany the presence of pretibial myxedema. Worstman et al reported that five of nine consecutively evaluated patients with Graves's disease had mucopolysaccharide deposition in the preradial area of the extensor aspects of the forearms. Improvement in the plaques of pretibial myxedema has resulted from intralesional injections of triamcinolone acetonide.

Vitiligo is associated with hyperthyroidism in 7 per cent of patients with Graves's disease and is seen with an increased frequency in Hashimoto type of thyroiditis.

Goette DK: Thyroid acropachy. Arch Dermatol 1980, 116:205.
Truhan AP, et al: The cutaneous mucinoses. JAAD 1986, 14:1.

HYPOPARATHYROIDISM

Varied changes in the skin and its appendages may be evident. Most pronounced is the faulty dentition when hypoparathyroidism is present during the development of the permanent teeth. The skin is dry and scaly. A diffuse scantiness of the hair and complete absence of axillary and pubic hair may be found. The nails are brittle and malformed. Onycholysis with fungus involvement may be present. Fifteen per cent of patients with idiopathic hypoparathyroidism develop mucocutaneous candidiasis. Hypoparathyroidism with resultant hypocalcemia has been reported to trigger bouts of impetigo herpeti-

formis or pustular psoriasis, as in a case reported by Moynihan et al.

Pseudohypoparathyroidism is an autosomal-dominant inherited disorder characterized by end-organ unresponsiveness to parathyroid hormone. The typical clinical findings include short stature, obesity, round face, short metacarpal and metatarsal bones, delayed dentition, mental deficiency, amenorrhea, and cataracts. Subcutaneous calcification occurs commonly in this disorder; this may occur infrequently in other abnormal parathyroid states such as primary or secondary hypothyroidism.

Kinard RE, et al: Pseudohypoparathyroidism. Arch Intern Med 1979, 139:204.
Lang PG Jr: The clinical spectrum of parathyroid disease. JAAD 1981, 5:733.
Moynihan GD, et al: Impetigo herpetiformis and hyperparathyroidism. Arch Dermatol 1985, 121:1330.
Raimer SS, et al: Metastatic calcinosis cutis. Cutis 1983, 32:543.

ACANTHOSIS NIGRICANS

Acanthosis nigricans is characterized by hyperpigmentation and papillary hypertrophy, which are symmetrically distributed. The regions affected may be the face, neck, axillae, external genitals, groin, inner aspects of the thighs, flexor surface of the elbows and knees, umbilicus, and anus. With extensive involvement, lesions can be found on the areolae, around the umbilicus, and on the lips and buccal mucosa. Rarely the involvement may be almost universal. The color of the patches is grayish, brownish, or black. The palms or soles may show hyperkeratoses. Small papillomatous nonpigmented lesions and pigmented macules may occasionally be found

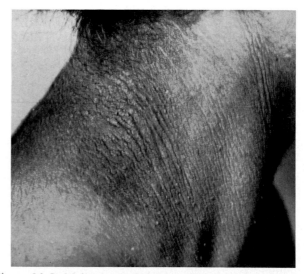

Figure 24–2. Malignant acanthosis nigricans on side of neck in a 26-year-old woman with ovarian carcinoma. (From Fladung G, Heite HJ: Dermatol Wschr 137:1–13, 1958.)

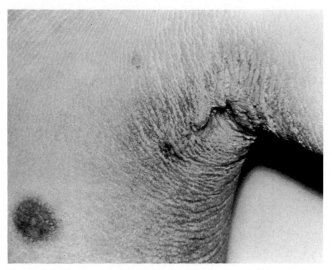

Figure 24–3. Acanthosis nigricans present since childhood. Courtesy of Dr. Axel W. Hoke.)

in the mucous membranes of the mouth, pharynx, and vagina.

Helen Curth has classifed the various forms of acanthosis nigricans into four types. We are amending this classification because of the evidence that most benign types are due to insulin-resistant states.

Type I: Malignant Acanthosis Nigricans

The malignant type of acanthosis nigricans may either precede (18 per cent), or accompany (60 per cent), or follow (22 per cent) the onset of the internal cancer. This rare type generally is the most striking clinically, both from the standpoint of extent of involvement and the pronounced nature of the lesions. Most cases are associated with adenocarci-

noma, especially of the gastrointestinal tract (60 per cent stomach), lung, and breast; less often the gallbladder, pancreas, esophagus, liver, prostate, kidney, colon, rectum, uterus, and ovaries. Other types of cancer, testicular carcinoma, and lymphomas may be seen also. A few cases of this malignant type have been observed in childhood, but most of the cases begin after puberty or in adulthood. This type should be highly suspected if widespread lesions develop in a nonobese male over 40 years of age.

Type II: Familial Acanthosis Nigricans

This exceedingly rare type is present at birth, or may develop during childhood. It is commonly accentuated at puberty. It resembles ichthyosis hystrix clinically, but histologic differences are seen; it is not associated with an internal cancer, and is inherited in an autosomal dominant manner. Tasjian et al recently reported a mother and daughter with this type and presented a good review of the subject.

Type III: Acanthosis Nigricans Associated with Obesity, Insulin-resistant States, and Endocrinopathy

This is the commonest variety of acanthosis nigricans. It presents as a grayish, velvety thickening of the skin of the sides of the neck, axillae, and groins. It occurs in obesity, with or without endocrine disorders, and in acromegaly and gigantism, Stein-Leventhal syndrome, Cushing's syndrome, Addison's disease, hyperandrogenic states, hypogonadal syndromes, and the various well-recognized insulin-resistant states including lipoatrophic diabetes, leprechaunism, pinealoma, the acral hypertrophy syn-

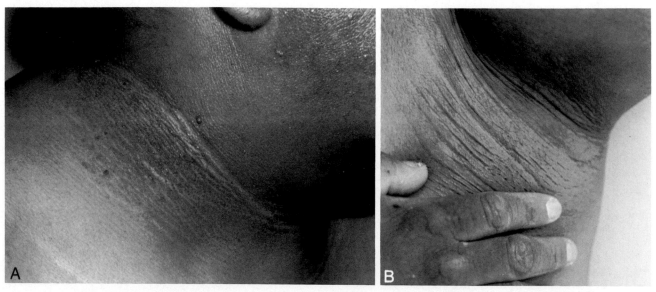

Figure 24–4. A and B, Acanthosis nigricans associated with obesity. (Courtesy of Dr. Axel W. Hoke.)

drome, the Type A syndrome where there is a defect in insulin receptor or postreceptor pathways, and the type B syndrome, where autoantibodies to the insulin receptor are present. This type is reviewed by Ober in a recent article documenting a patient in whom hypothyroidism was also present. Flier, in an accompanying editorial, suggests that most if not all of these cases may have either clinical or subclinical insulin resistance, and recommends investigation of this possibility in these patients. Plourde et al also reviewed this type of acanthosis nigricans.

Acanthosis nigricans may occur in various syndromes such as Bloom's syndrome, Crouzon's syndrome, Rud's syndrome, and Wilson's disease. Drugs known to induce acanthosis nigricans are nicotinic acid, niacinamide, diethylstilbestrol, oral contraceptives, and glucocorticoids. Greenspan et al implicated triazinate, a folic acid antagonist, in their report. Koranda et al found 10 per cent of 200 consecutively examined renal transplant patients had acanthosis nigricans.

The histopathology shows papillomatosis without thickening of the Malpighian layer. The term "acanthosis" was applied here to indicate the clinical, not the histologic, "bristly" thickening of the skin. There is hyperkeratosis, and slight hyperpigmentation of the basal layer is present in most cases; it appears, however, that the clinically observed hyperpigmentation observed is due to hyperkeratosis and clinical acanthosis rather than to melanin.

The differential diagnosis includes ichthyosis hystrix and several disorders of reticulated hyperpigmentation, including confluent and reticulated papillomatosis (Gougerot-Carteaud), Dowling-Degos's disease, Haber's syndrome, and acropigmentatio reticularis of Kitamura. *Dowling-Degos's disease* is a familial nevoid anomaly with delayed onset in adult life. There is progressive, brown-to-black hyperpigmentation of flexures with associated soft fibromas and follicular hyperkeratoses. Pitted acneform scars occur periorally.

Treatment of the malignant type consists essentially of finding the causal malignancy. Early recognition and treatment may be lifesaving. The type occurring with obesity usually improves with weight loss. If there is associated endocrinopathy it must be treated as well. One patient with lipodystrophic diabetes improved markedly during dietary supplementation with fish oil.

Brown WG: Reticulate pigmentation anomaly of the flexures. Arch Dermatol 1982, 118:490.

Curth HO: Classification of acanthosis nigricans. Int J Dermatol 1976, 15:592.

Flier JS: Metabolic importance of acanthosis nigricans. Arch Dermatol 1985, 121:193.

Greenspan AH, et al: Acanthosis nigricans-like hyperpigmentation secondary to triazinate therapy. Arch Dermatol 1985, 121:232.

Holdiness MR: Acanthosis nigricans. Arch Dermatol 1985, 121:588.

Kahn RC, et al: Syndromes of insulin resistance and acanthosis nigricans: insulin receptor disorders in man. N Engl J Med 1976, 294:739.

Kalter DC: Acquired intertriginous pigmentation. Arch Dermatol 1985, 121:399.

Ober KP: Acanthosis nigricans and insulin resistance associated with hypothyroidism. Arch Dermatol 1985, 121:229.

Plourde PV, et al: Acanthosis nigricans and insulin resistance. JAAD 1984, 10:887.

Richards GE, et al: Obesity, acanthosis nigricans, insulin resistance, hyperandrogenemia. J Pediatr 1985, 107:893.

Sherertz EF: Improved acanthosis nigricans with lipodystrophic diabetes during dietary fish oil supplementation. Arch Dermatol 1988, 124:1094.

Tasjian D, et al: Familial acanthosis nigricans. Arch Dermatol 1984, 120:1351.

25

Abnormalities of Dermal Connective Tissue

Several disorders are included in this chapter because they are characterized by abnormalities of the dermal connective tissue fibers. Alterations of mucopolysaccharide ground substance are discussed in Chapter 9 (The Mucinoses) or Chapter 26 (Errors of Metabolism). The collagen and elastin fibers are altered, degenerated, or absent in the diseases that follow. The changes may primarily involve either the elastic fibers or the collagen fibers, and they may be either inherited or acquired. Several miscellaneous conditions characterized by dermal atrophy are included.

The 11 currently recognized types of collagen are shown in Table 25–1, as listed by Uitto et al.

ELASTOSIS PERFORANS SERPIGINOSA (EPS)

In 1953 Lutz described a chronic keratopapular eruption in an arciform shape located on the sides of

Table 25–1. GENETIC HETEROGENEITY OF COLLAGEN

Collagen Type	Tissue Distribution
I	Skin, bone, tendon
I-trimer	Tumors, cell cultures, skin, liver
II	Cartilage, vitreous
III	Fetal skin, blood vessels, intestine
IV	Basement membranes
V	Ubiquitous
VI (intimal)	Aortic intima, placenta
VII (long chain)	Amnion, anchoring fibrils
VIII (endothelial)	Endothelial cell cultures
IX (HMW-LMW)	Cartilage
X (short chain)	Cartilage
1alpha, 2alpha, 3alpha	Cartilage

the nape of the neck. In EPS, the skin-colored keratotic papules, 2 to 5 mm in diameter, are confluently grouped in a serpiginous or horseshoe-shaped arrangement with the area inside of the arc normal or slightly atrophic. Although these lesions typically occur on the neck, other sites may be involved. Such sites are the upper arms, face, lower extremities, and, most rarely, the trunk. Disseminated lesions occur in connection with Down's syndrome.

The etiology is not known. It is postulated that a decrease in the amount of cross-linked elastin and an increase in tropoelastin are the primary pathogenic events. Elastosis perforans serpiginosa (EPS) is commonest in the young adult; however, the ages are known to have varied from five to 84 years. Men outnumber women four to one. It has been reported from all over the world. Woerdeman reported it in three siblings. Several reports have detailed patients with Wilson's disease, under prolonged treatment with penicillamine, who developed EPS.

It may be the local manifestation of a more widespread disease. Approximately one third of cases occur in patients with associated diseases, the most frequent concomitant disorder being Down's syndrome. Rasmussen estimated that 1 per cent of Down's patients have EPS. In this situation the lesions are likely to be more extensive and persistent than when seen without the associated disease. Patterson lists the association of elastosis perforans serpiginosa with the following diseases in addition to Down's syndrome: Ehlers-Danlos syndrome, osteogenesis imperfecta, Marfan's syndrome, Rothmund-Thompson syndrome, and acrogeria. Recent reports have added an association with systemic sclerosis, morphea, and renal disease. Most reports of EPS associated with pseudoxanthoma elasticum are probably examples of perforating pseudoxanthoma elasticum.

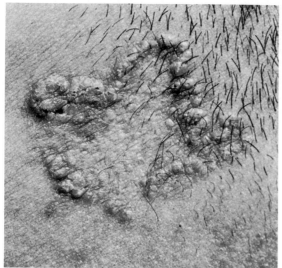

Figure 25–1. Elastosis perforans serpiginosa on neck. (Courtesy of Dr. J. M. Hitch.)

The distinctive histopathologic changes consist of elongated tortuous channels in the epidermis into which abnormal elastic tissue perforates and is extruded from the dermis. There is degeneration and alteration of the elastic tissue, with an inflammatory response.

Elastosis perforans serpiginosa may clinically resemble granuloma annulare, tinea circinata, sarcoidosis, and porokeratosis of Mibelli.

The disease runs a variable course with spontaneous resolution often occurring from six months to five years after onset. Often atrophic scarring remains. Rosenblum reported successful treatment by freezing with liquid nitrogen.

Bergman R, et al: An ultrastructural study of the reactive type of elastosis perforans serpiginosa. Arch Dermatol 1987, 123:1127.

Hashimoto K, et al: Ultrastructure of penicillamine-induced skin lesions. JAAD 1981, 4:300.
Kirsh N, et al: Elastosis perforans serpiginosa induced by penicillamine. Arch Dermatol 1977, 113:630.
Mehregan AH: Perforating dermatoses. Int J Dermatol 1977, 16:19.
Patterson JW: The perforating disorders. JAAD 1984, 10:561.
Rosenblum GA: Liquid nitrogen cryotherapy in a case of elastosis perforans serpiginosa. JAAD 1983, 8:718.
Schamroth JM, et al: Elastosis perforans serpiginosa in a patient with renal disease. Arch Dermatol 1986, 122:82.

REACTIVE PERFORATING COLLAGENOSIS

In 1967 Mehregan et al reported a rare inherited skin disorder characterized by papules on the extremities, face, or buttocks, with onset in infancy or childhood, and involution within six to eight weeks as a rule. There may be recurrent crops for years, however. Damaged collagen fibers are extruded from the keratotic, umbilicated papules. Linear configurations suggestive of a Koebner phenomenon are frequent.

A number of reports attest to an acquired form of this disease occurring with increased frequency in association with diabetes or renal dialysis, or both; Poliak et al, and Cochran et al, have recently published such reports. Cochran et al found UVB effective, while Cullen found lesions improved with 0.1 per cent tretinoin cream nightly.

Cochran RJ, et al: Reactive perforating collagenosis of diabetes mellitus and renal failure. Cutis 1983, 31:55.
Cohen RW, et al: Acquired reactive perforating collagenosis. JAAD 1989, 20:287.
Poliak SC, et al: Reactive perforating collagenosis associated with diabetes mellitus. N Engl J Med 1982, 306:81.

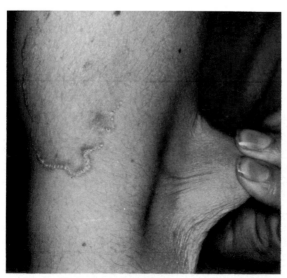

Figure 25–2. Elastosis perforans serpiginosa in a patient with Ehlers-Danlos syndrome.

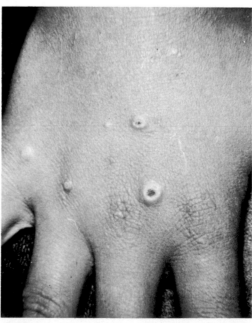

Figure 25–3. Reactive perforating collagenosis. (Courtesy of Dr. A. H. Mehregan.)

PSEUDOXANTHOMA ELASTICUM

The skin, eye, and cardiovascular system are the involved sites in pseudoxanthoma elasticum (PXE). The skin changes are characterized by small, circumscribed, yellowish to cream-colored, crepelike, lax, redundant patches at sites of considerable movement of the skin such as the sides of the neck, axillae, and antecubital spaces. The neck may have redundant folds, causing it to be likened to "chicken neck." The characteristic exaggerated nasolabial folds may remind one of the face of a hound dog. In addition, the inguinal, periumbilical, and periauricular areas may be involved. The mucous membranes of the soft palate, inner lip, rectum, and vagina may also be involved. *Lineae albicantes* similar to those observed after pregnancy may appear on the abdominal skin.

The characteristic retinal change is the *angioid streak*, which is the result of breaks in the elastic membrane of Bruch. The angioid streaks appear earlier than the skin changes, so that most cases are discovered by ophthalmologists. Angioid streaks may be the only sign of the disease for years. In such patients, as shown by Lebwohl et al, biopsies of the midportions of old scars may be diagnostic of PXE. The association of the skin lesions with angioid streaks has been called the Grönblad-Strandberg syndrome. Angioid streaks may also be seen in Ehlers-Danlos syndrome, Paget's disease, sickle cell anemia, trauma, lead poisoning, hyperphosphatemia, pituitary disorders, and intracranial disorders.

On funduscopic examination a reddish brown band is evident around the optic disk, from which glistening streaks extend along the vessels. With fluorescent photography early fluorescence of the angioid streaks and macular lesions are noted. In addition, there may be hemorrhages and exudates. Progressive loss of vision often starts after minor trauma to the eye, such as scratches on the cornea. Ultimately retinal sclerosis and macular degeneration occur, and there is almost total blindness.

Involvement of the cardiovascular system occurs, with a propensity for hemorrhage. Gastrointestinal hemorrhages and hematemesis are common. Epistaxis occurs frequently, hematuria rarely. These vas-

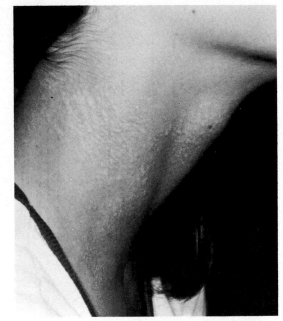

Figure 25–4. Pseudoxanthoma elasticum in a young woman.

cular episodes are caused by the degeneration of the elastic fibers in the media. Angina pectoris is often found in young patients. There is elastic tissue disease in the valves, myocardium, and pericardium. Lebwohl et al found mitral valve prolapse in 71 per cent of 14 patients examined. Hypertension occurs in many patients over 30 years of age as a result of involvement of the peripheral vessels. Any patient with hypertension at a young age should be examined for stigmata of pseudoxanthoma elasticum. Leg cramps and intermittent claudication occur in young persons. The peripheral pulses are diminished or absent. Calcification of peripheral arteries is seen in many patients over 30 years of age, and may be detected by x-ray.

Patients may also suffer from diabetes mellitus, thyrotoxicosis, calcinosis, and osteitis deformans. Cocco and his associates have demonstrated linear yellow nodules in the gastric mucosa through the gastroscope. Repeated gastric hemorrhage is a potential danger in these patients.

Figure 25–5. Pseudoxanthoma elasticum in a 21 year old woman who had a yellowish discoloration with wrinkling of the skin in her axillae (A), sides of the neck (B) and inner thighs for 6 years. No visual abnormalities noted yet. (Courtesy of Dr. V. M. Torres, Puerto Rico.)

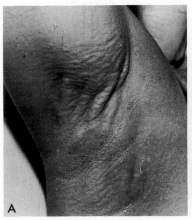

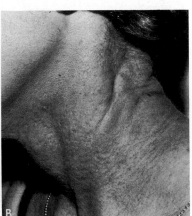

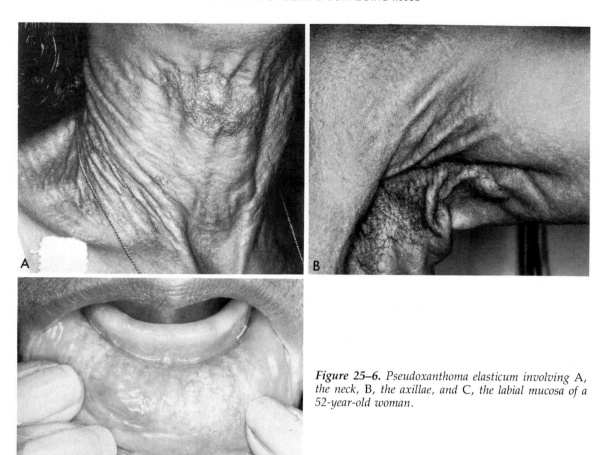

Figure 25–6. Pseudoxanthoma elasticum involving A, the neck, B, the axillae, and C, the labial mucosa of a 52-year-old woman.

A localized acquired type referred to as periumbilical perforating PXE, characterized histologically by transepidermal elimination of altered elastica, was reported in six middle-aged, multiparous black women by Hicks and associates. They suggested that the possible genetic predisposition of these patients to PXE found its expression in the periumbilical skin, a site exposed to the trauma of multiple pregnancies. This acquired perforating form was reported by Nickoloff in a patient with chronic renal failure undergoing renal dialysis.

PXE is an inherited propensity for fragmentation

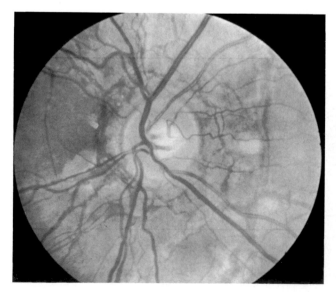

Figure 25–7. Angioid streaks in a patient with pseudoxanthoma elasticum. (Courtesy of Dr. Axel W. Hoke.)

and clumping of the elastic fibers and calcification of their amorphous elastin core. Pope described two forms of autosomal dominant and two forms of autosomal recessive PXE. Both dominant and recessive type I disease show classic skin, eye, and vascular disease, with the former having the most severe vascular disease of all types. Dominant type II has a macular pattern of skin lesions with hyperextensible skin and hypermotile joints, similar to that seen in Ehlers-Danlos syndrome. Funduscopic findings are common, and blue sclerae are present in 40 per cent. Recessive type II, the least common form, has generalized PXE without systemic involvement.

Histologic examination shows an extensive basophilic degeneration of the elastic tissue. Throughout the mid-dermis the elastic fibers are swollen and fragmented or granular. The elastic fibers stain darkly, contain amorphous granules, and are twisted, curled, and broken in individual curls to suggest "raveled wool." Giant cells have been observed around the degenerated tissue. There may be calcification, which is an infiltration of the degenerated elastic tissue with calcium phosphate. Acid mucopolysaccharides are also increased. This is a systemic disease of the elastic tissue, particularly of the vascular elastica, which diffusely involves the aorta and other vessels and is dependent upon genetic factors.

In the differential diagnosis, lichen sclerosus et atrophicus, scleroderma, dermatochalasis, and postzoster scars should be considered. Gordon and associates showed that excised skin from patients with pseudoxanthoma elasticum and their relatives takes up calcium, magnesium, and phosphorus more abundantly than does normal skin. Even subclinical lesions may be identified in this way.

No definitive therapy is available. Usually the skin presents only cosmetic problems; however, there is a progressive loss of vision. Neldner et al advise limiting dietary calcium and phosphorus to minimal daily requirement levels. Plastic surgery is helpful for loose folds.

Fang ML, et al: Cardiac calcifications and yellow papules in a young man. Arch Dermatol 1988, 124:1559.
Gordon SG, et al: In vitro uptake of calcium by dermis of patients with pseudoxanthoma elasticum. J Lab Clin Med 1975, 86:638.
Hicks J, et al: Periumbilical perforating pseudoxanthoma elasticum. Arch Dermatol 1979, 115:300.
Iqbal Q, et al: Pseudoxanthoma elasticum: a review of neurological complications. Ann Neurol 1978, 4:18.
Kazakis AM, et al: Periumbilical perforating pseudoxanthoma elasticum. JAAD 1988, 19:384.
Lebwohl M, et al: Pseudoxanthoma elasticum and mitral valve prolapse. N Engl J Med 1982, 307:228.
Idem: Diagnosis of pseudoxanthoma elasticum by scar biopsy in patients without characteristic skin lesions. N Engl J Med 1987, 317:347.
Nickoloff BJ, et al: Perforating pseudoxanthoma elasticum associated with chronic renal failure and hemodialysis. Arch Dermatol 1985, 121:1321.
Pope FM: Two types of autosomal recessive pseudoxanthoma elasticum. Arch Dermatol 1974, 110:209.
Idem, et al: Patients with Ehlers-Danlos syndrome type IV lack type III collagen. Proc Natl Acad Sci (USA) 1975, 72:1314.
Uitto J, et al: Heritable skin defects with molecular defects in collagen or elastin. Dermatol Clinics 1987, 5:63.

SOLAR ELASTOSIS

This is also known as actinic elastosis and senile atrophy.

Actinic damage to the skin may be apparent in the third decade or may not appear until much later. In the disease xeroderma pigmentosum, it occurs in early childhood. Heredity and exposure to sunlight and wind play a major role in this process. Actinically damaged skin, or prematurely senile skin, inevitable in those who spend much time outdoors, has long been known as *farmer's skin* or *sailor's skin*. Today it might well be called *golfer's skin* instead. It is associated with actinic keratoses in many patients.

Several clinical varieties of solar elastotic change are recognized. As stated above, the diffuse type may lead to coarsely wrinkled, inelastic, yellowish or red skin, and this type is seen in *farmer's neck*. *Elastomas* may be single but more commonly are multiple yellowish papules on the chin, neck, ears, nose, or periorbital areas, where they constitute, together with multiple comedones, the *Favre-Racouchot syndrome*. On the ear they may simulate basal cell carcinomas or nodular chondrodermatitis. On the upper arm a variant similar to Favre-Racouchot syndrome, termed *actinic comedonal plaque*, was described by Eastern et al. Raimer et al noted soft linear lesions of the forearms, which they termed *solar elastotic bands*. Bilateral yellowish, waxy papules may be symmetrically situated at the edges of the thumb, index, and intervening web space. Highet contrasts this type of acquired *acrokeratoelastoidosis* to the inherited type (Costa) discussed in Chapter 10.

Clinically, over-sunned skin is thin, dry, wrinkled, shiny, and slightly scaly. The skin is yellowish, or may be deeply tanned. When pinched it is flaccid, with no recoil. There is a tendency to senile lentigines and senile angiomas.

On the back of the neck, lines cross each other forming diamond-shaped plaques, especially in carpenters, fishermen, construction workers, and farmers. Solar elastosis may cause the skin to become thickened. This is called *cutis rhomboidalis nuchae*.

Microscopic changes show that the papillae and rete pegs become flattened. In the dermis there is basophilic degeneration of connective tissue and fragmentation and swelling of the elastic fibers. The walls of the cutaneous blood vessels become thickened. Chen et al studied the elastotic material by indirect immunofluorescence and found staining positive for elastin, supporting the view that the material is altered elastic fibers.

Chen VL, et al: Immunochemistry of elastotic material in sun-damaged skin. J Invest Dermatol 1986, 87:334.
Eastern JS, et al: Actinic comedonal plaque. JAAD 1980, 3:633.

Highet AS, et al: Acrokeratoelastoidosis. Br J Dermatol 1982, 106:337.

Kligman LH, et al: The contributions of UVA and UVB to connective tissue damage in hairless mice. J Invest Dermatol 1985, 84:272.

Raimer SS, et al: Solar elastotic bands of the forearm. JAAD 1986, 15:650.

Salasche SJ, et al: Cutaneous manifestations of chronic solar exposure. J Assoc Milit Dermatol 1985, 11:3.

EHLERS-DANLOS SYNDROMES

Synonyms: Cutis hyperelastica, India rubber skin, and elastic skin.

Cutis hyperelastica is a group of genetically distinct connective tissue disorders characterized by excessive stretchability and fragility of the skin with a tendency toward easy scar formation, calcification of the skin to produce pseudotumors, and hyperextensibility of the joints, especially the fingers, toes, and knees.

McKusick has classified cases of the Ehlers-Danlos syndromes into 11 types on clinical and genetic grounds, and it has since been found that specific collagen defects underlie many of these.

No specific defect is known for types I ("gravis" type), III (hypermotility only), VIII (bruising, scarring, periodontitis), or XI (familial joint laxity). In type II ("mitis") there is abnormal fibrillogenesis of dermal collagen. In type IV (thin skin, easy bruising), type III collagen is diminished, according to Pope et al; in type V (stretchability and easy bruising), there is lysyl oxidase deficiency; in type VI (severe eye defects and scoliosis) lysyl hydroxylase is deficient; and in type VII (arthrochalasis, short stature, moderate stretchability, periodontosis), there is procollagen peptidase deficiency in the recessive form, and in the dominant form a deficiency in the pro α-2 chain of type I procollagen. In type IX ("X-linked cutis laxa") there are lysyl oxidase deficiency and abnormal copper metabolism; and in type X (easy bruisability and hyperextensible skin and joints), fibronectin is abnormal.

Type IV is further subdivided into the classical (short-lived) type, with pinched face, prominent eyes, thin skin, and proneness to aortic rupture; long-lived, with much milder manifestations; and atypical cases, which are further divided into dominant cases, with normal face and no arterial problems, and recessive cases, with mutant type III collagen, which are like the long-lived ones. Pope et al reported a type III collagen deficiency with normal phenotype.

Type VIII, recognized early by McCusick and confirmed by Stewart et al, is inherited as an autosomal dominant and manifests easy bruising, which is followed on the shins by scarring, and generalized periodontitis. Nelson et al reported such a kindred in 1981.

The skin may be stretched out like a rubber band and snaps back with equal resiliency. This rubbery

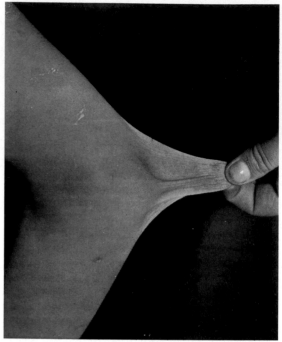

Figure 25–8. *Cutis hyperelastica with stretched skin at elbow. (Courtesy of Dr. F. Ronchese.)*

skin is most pronounced on the elbows, neck, and sides of the abdomen. The skin is velvety in appearance and feels like wet chamois. Minor trauma may produce a gaping "fish-mouth" wound with large hematomas underneath. The subcutaneous calcifications are 2–8-mm oval nodules, mostly on the legs. Trauma over the shins, knees, and elbows produces cigarette-paper-thin scars. Approximately 50 per cent of these patients can touch the tip of the nose with their tongue (Gorlin's sign), compared with 10 per cent of normals.

Other abnormalities may be the following: large frontal bosses, widely spaced eyes, prognathism, flat feet, myopia, and lop ears. Internally the gastrointestinal tract may show diverticula; friability of the intestinal wall can lead to spontaneous rupture. Recurrent gastrointestinal bleeding with hematemesis is common. Aortic aneurysms and diaphragmatic hernias also occur.

Two types of growth may occur in patients with Ehlers-Danlos syndromes. The *molluscum pseudotumor* is a soft, fleshy nodule seen in easily traumatized areas such as the ulnar forearms and shins. *Spheroids* are hard subcutaneous nodules which become calcified and are probably the result of fat necrosis.

It has been demonstrated that types I, II, and III, and one subtype each of types IV, VII, VIII, and XI of Ehlers-Danlos syndrome are transmitted by the autosomal dominant mode; one subtype of types IV, VI, and VII, and type X, by the autosomal recessive mode, and types V and IX by an X-linked recessive inheritance pattern.

Ehlers-Danlos syndromes must be differentiated from Marfan's syndrome, pseudoxanthoma elasticum, osteogenesis imperfecta, and cutis laxa.

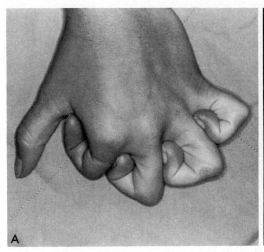
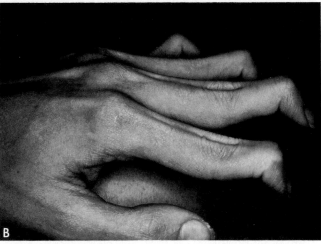

Figure 25–9. Ehlers-Danlos syndrome.

Treatment is supportive, with avoidance of trauma to skin and joints.

Arneson MA, et al: A new form of Ehlers-Danlos syndrome: fibronectin corrects defective platelet function. JAMA 1980, 244:144.

Cullen SI: Localized Ehlers-Danlos syndrome. Arch Dermatol 1979, 115:332.

Holzberg M, et al: The Ehlers-Danlos syndrome. JAAD 1988, 19:656.

Krieg T, et al: Molecular defects of collagen metabolism in the Ehlers-Danlos syndrome. Internat J Dermatol 1981, 20:415.

Maroteaux P, et al: The differential symptomatology of errors of collagen metabolism. Am J Med Genet 1986, 24:219.

McKusick VA: Mendelian Inheritance in Man. 6th ed. Baltimore, Johns Hopkins University Press 1983.

Nelson DL, et al: Ehlers-Danlos syndrome type VIII. JAAD 1981, 5:297.

Pinnell SR: Molecular defects in the Ehlers-Danlos syndrome. J Invest Dermatol 1982, 79:905.

Idem: The skin in Ehlers-Danlos syndrome. JAAD 1987, 16:399.

Pope FM: Type III collagen deficiency with normal phenotype. J Roy Soc Med 1983, 76:518.

Prockop DJ, et al: Hereditable diseases of collagen. N Engl J Med 1984, 311:376.

Rizzo R, et al: Familial Ehlers-Danlos syndrome type II: Abnormal fibrillogenesis of dermal collagen. Pediatr Dermatol 1987, 4:197.

Sasaki T, et al: Ehlers-Danlos syndrome. Arch Dermatol 1987, 123:76.

Uitto J, et al: Heritable skin diseases with molecular defects in collagen or elastin. Dermatol Clin 1987, 5:63.

Idem: Biochemistry of collagen diseases. Ann Intern Med 1986, 105:740.

CUTIS LAXA (Generalized Elastolysis)

Synonyms: Dermatomegaly, dermatolysis, chalazoderma, and pachydermatocele.

Cutis laxa is characterized by loose, redundant skin, hanging in folds. Around the eyelids, cheeks, and neck the drooping skin produces a bloodhound-like facies. Usually the entire integument is involved. The shoulder girdle skin may look like that of a St. Bernard dog. The abdomen is frequently the site of large, pendulous folds.

Generalized elastolysis is a rare systemic disorder of the connective tissue in which the elastic fibers are decreased, disorganized, and fragmented. Besides the skin, the pulmonary, vascular, and gastrointestinal systems may be involved. The pulmonary manifestations may be emphysema, fibrosis of the lungs, and tracheobronchomegaly. The vascular involve-

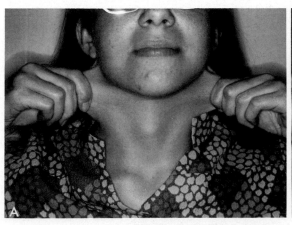
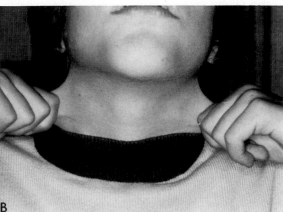

Figure 25–10. Ehlers-Danlos syndrome in a sister and brother.

ment may be in the form of cardiomegaly, congestive heart failure, cor pulmonale, aortic dilatation, or pulmonary artery stenosis. The gastrointestinal system may have esophageal diverticula, esophageal dilation with dysphagia, gastric ulcers, or rectocele. Other changes may be hiatal, femoral, inguinal, or ventral hernias; cystocele; prolapse of the uterus; and ruptured patellar tendons.

Cutis laxa may be genetically determined in a dominant, recessive, or X-linked recessive form. The dominant form is primarily a cutaneous, cosmetic form, with a good prognosis. The recessive cases often have severe internal involvement, and die young. The X-linked recessive form, in which a deficiency in lysyl oxidase has been demonstrated, is classified as type IX Ehlers-Danlos syndrome. Joint laxity is one of its findings. There is also an acquired type, which may appear at any age from early childhood to the late fifties. Randle et al and Tsuji et al have reported such cases and reviewed the literature. No differences have been noted in these two types except the age of onset.

Histologically, there is diminution of the elastic fibers, with those remaining being disorganized and fragmented. The entire dermis is involved. The electron microscope shows granular degeneration of the elastic fibers.

In the differential diagnosis, Ehlers-Danlos syndrome, Marfan's syndrome, and pseudoxanthoma elasticum (type II recessive) must be considered.

Granulomatous slack skin begins with papular and infiltrated plaques, often in the axillae, flanks, or intercrural areas, which become progressively more pendulous. Unlike cutis laxa, there are deep granulomatous infiltrations in the dermis and subcutaneous tissue. Balus et al recently reported such a case, and LeBoit et al have shown it to be an indolent *cutaneous T-cell lymphoma.*

Etiologically, it has been considered that there may be disturbance of the serum elastase inhibitors, chiefly alpha$_1$-antitrypsin. This hypothesis remains unproven and the etiology remains unknown.

Treatment has been generally disappointing. Multiple surgical procedures to remove the sagging tissue have been largely unsuccessful, since new folds develop in time at the sites of removal. ᐟ

Balus L, et al: Granulomatous slack skin. Arch Dermatol 1985, 121:250.
Byers PH, et al: X-linked cutis laxa. N Engl J Med 1980, 303:61.
Gardner LI, et al: Congenital cutis laxa syndrome. Arch Dermatol 1986, 122:1241.
Goltz RW, et al: Cutis laxa congenita: a manifestation of generalized elastolysis. Arch Dermatol 1965, 92:373.
Harris RB, et al: Generalized elastolysis (cutis laxa). Am J Med 1978, 65:815.
Kochs E, et al: Acquired cutis laxa. Pediatr Dermatol 1985, 2:282.
Lally JF, et al: Roentgenographic manifestations of cutis laxa (generalized elastolysis). Radiology 1974, 113:605.
LeBoit PE, et al: Granulomatous slack skin. J Invest Dermatol 1987, 89:183.
Ledoux-Corbuster M, et al: α$_1$-antitrypsin deficiency and skin abnormalities. J Cutan Pathol 1975, 2:25.
Randle HW, et al: Generalized elastolysis with systemic lupus erythematosus. JAAD 1983, 8:869.
Sakati NO: Congenital cutis laxa and osteoporosis. Am J Dis Child 1983, 137:452.
Tsuji T, et al: Acquired cutis laxa concomitant with the nephrotic syndrome. Arch Dermatol 1987, 123:1211.
Verhagen AR, et al: Postinflammatory elastolysis and cutis laxa. Br J Dermatol 1975, 92:183.

BLEPHAROCHALASIS

In blepharochalasis the eyelid skin becomes so lax that it falls in redundant folds over the lid margins. It is an uncommon condition, which occurs in young people at about the time of puberty. Recurrent transitory swellings of the lids, lasting two or three days, are first noted; each is accompanied by a little more stretching, thinning, and wrinkling of the lids, with slowly progressive hyperpigmentation. The condition gives the appearance of fatigue. Most cases are bilateral, but Brazin et al reported a unilateral case. It is generally sporadic, but a dominantly inherited form has been described. Biopsy shows lack of elastic fibers. In elderly patients a similar appearance is induced simply by actinic elastosis.

Ascher's Syndrome is progressive enlargement of the upper lip in association with blepharochalasis. It occurs in at least 10 per cent of cases. The thickening results in superfluous folds of mucosa, giving the appearance of a double lip.

Rarely elastolysis of the earlobes may accompany blepharochalasis, as reported by Cunliffe and recently by Barker et al.

Treatment is by surgical correction.

Barker SM, et al: Elastolysis of the earlobes. JAAD 1986, 14:145.
Brazin SA, et al: Unilateral blepharochalasis. Arch Dermatol 1979, 115:479.

ANETODERMA (Macular Atrophy)

Anetoderma, which means looseness of the skin, is due to the loss of normal elastic fibers without any other apparent changes in the skin.

Anetoderma has been classified as a localized form of elastolysis. Histologically it is characterized by focal loss of normal elastic fibers, as in cutis laxa and blepharochalasis. Patients with anetoderma may also have generalized elastolysis or lid laxity, so some clinical overlap may exist. Clinically the lesions of anetoderma are circumscribed and quite different from cutis laxa.

Based on whether an inflammatory reaction precedes the macular atrophy, two types of primary anetoderma have been generally acknowledged: anetoderma of Jadassohn has a preceding inflammatory reaction, whereas anetoderma of Schweninger-Buzzi has had no preceding discernible inflammatory changes.

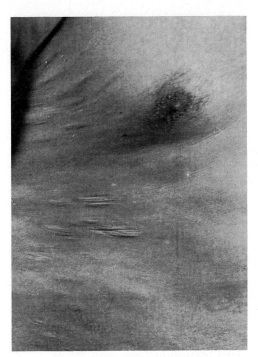

Figure 25–11. Macular atrophy.

Venencie et al reviewed the Mayo Clinic experience in 16 cases, which were of both types, and concluded that there was little reason for separating them. There is no difference between the two types histologically, according to a study of these 16 cases by Venencie and Winkelmann.

Anetoderma of Jadassohn

This form of macular atrophy begins with a well-defined, erythematous, 5–10-mm macule which soon fades at the center and forms a circular lesion within which the epidermis becomes slightly wrinkled. In due course the lesion becomes slightly depressed, and on palpation there seems to be a lessened resistance. Later the surface becomes shiny, white, and crinkly. At this stage, herniation is usually discernible on palpation. The examining finger falls into a distinct hole with definite borders, as in inguinal hernia. This clinical feature, common to all types of macular atrophy, is explained by loss of elastic tissue. The usual locations are on the face and trunk, especially on the shoulders. There are no sensory disturbances and no alterations in the skin between the lesions.

The etiology is unknown.

Histologically, the inflammatory reaction may produce a perivascular infiltrate; however, the main changes take place in the elastic tissue. The elastic fibers become fragmented and eventually completely disappear. Oikarinen et al showed that the concentration of elastin, as determined by radioimmunoassay of desmosine, an elastin-specific cross-linked compound, was markedly reduced in patients with anetoderma.

No treatment seems to be effective.

Anetoderma of Schweninger-Buzzi

This has also been called multiple benign tumorlike new growths of the skin. The disease manifests itself by the appearance of nummular bluish white or slate-tinted, bladderlike lesions beneath the epidermis, some of which have fine telangiectases coursing over them. There are no changes clinically in the overlying epidermis. By pressure with the tip of the finger, lesions can be inverted so that the impinging finger slips into a hollow, much the same as in anetoderma of Jadassohn. These lesions are also situated mostly on the trunk.

The disease is slowly progressive, being maintained by the development of new lesions as the older ones involute spontaneously, leaving depressed soft scars. The cause is unknown. The histologic findings are the same as those of anetoderma of Jadassohn with, as Venencie et al showed, an inflammatory infiltrate present even in the absence of clinical inflammation. Thus these two forms of primary anetoderma appear to be similar, if not identical, pathophysiologically.

No treatment is effective.

SECONDARY MACULAR ATROPHY

Secondary macular atrophy *(atrophoderma maculatum)* is known to occur after macular and papular syphilids, measles, lupus erythematosus, leprosy, sarcoidosis, xanthoma tuberosum involution, acne, varicella, and involution of infiltrative tumors of the reticuloses. In such instances the atrophic spots are often identical with those of primary origin (the Jadassohn or the Schweninger-Buzzi types). Macular atrophy may also be associated with acrodermatitis chronica atrophicans.

Friedman SJ, et al: Familial anetoderma. JAAD 1987, 16:341.
Oikarinen AI, et al: Anetoderma. JAAD 1984, 11:64.
Venencie PY, et al: Anetoderma: clinical findings, associations, and long-term follow-up evaluations. Arch Dermatol 1984, 120:1032.
Idem: Histopathologic findings in anetoderma. Arch Dermatol 1984, 120:1040.

STRIAE DISTENSAE

Also known as *striae atrophicae*, striae (pronounced "strye-ee") distensae are depressed lines or bands of thin, reddened skin, which later become white, smooth, shiny, and depressed. These occur on the abdomen during and after pregnancy *(striae gravidarum)*, on the breasts after lactation, or in those who have suddenly gained weight. Similar striae occur on the buttocks and upper, outer, or inner thighs, in the inguinal areas, and over the knees and elbows, sometimes (especially in children aged nine to 13) without apparent cause. In early striae the color may be pinkish or purplish and an initial urticarial or raised inflammatory component may be present.

Pregnancy, sudden weight gain, rapid growth, and Cushing's disease, endogenous or steroid-induced, are the most frequent causes of striae distensae. Prolonged topical applications of corticosteroid preparations especially under occlusive dressings, or in folds, may also produce striae.

Histologically, there is breakage and retraction of the elastic fibers in the reticular portion of the dermis. The broken elastic fibers curl at the sides of the striae to form a distinctive picture.

There is no effective treatment for atrophic striae. In time they become less noticeable.

Arem AJ, et al: Analysis of striae. Plast Reconstr Surg 1980, 65:22.
Barkey WF: Striae and persistent tinea corporis related to prolonged use of betamethasone dipropionate 0.05% cream clotrimazole 1% cream (lotrisone cream). JAAD 1987, 17:518.
Carr RD, et al: Transverse striae of the back. Arch Dermatol 1969, 99:26.
Chernosky ME, et al: Atrophic striae after occlusive corticosteroid therapy. Arch Dermatol 1964, 90:15.
Peterson JL, et al: Edematous striae distensae. Arch Dermatol 1984, 120:1097.
Pinkus H, et al: Histopathology of striae distensae with special reference to striae and wound healing in Marfan syndrome. J Invest Dermatol 1966, 46:283.
Shelley WB, et al: Striae migrans [sic]. Arch Dermatol 1964, 90:193.
Tsuji T, et al: Elastic fibers in striae distensae. J Cutan Pathol 1988, 15:215.

ACRODERMATITIS CHRONICA ATROPHICANS

This acquired diffuse thinning of the skin begins with an early reddish appearance of the extensor surfaces of the extremities, and progresses to smooth, soft, atrophic skin. This disease is caused by a spirochete, *Borrelia burgdorferi*, and it has been discussed in detail in Chapter 14.

CONCOMITANT ATROPHY

Atrophy of the skin may follow prolonged illness, after which it becomes dry, smooth, and shiny, occasionally with branny desquamation and itching. The hair and nails may be shed.

In chronic acidosis the skin may become dry, scaly, and atrophic with some loss of body hair. Poor wound healing, hemorrhagic diathesis, and bone alterations are other signs of chronic acidosis.

Glossy skin (atrophoderma neuriticum) is a disease secondary to neuritis in which the skin, usually on an extremity, becomes erythematous, but in the course of time develops a grayish, shiny aspect, and eventually looks like ivory. There may be associated alopecia, fissuring, or ulceration. The skin disease tends to improve after the neuritis has subsided. The nails become ridged.

OSTEOGENESIS IMPERFECTA

Osteogenesis imperfecta, also known as *Lobstein's syndrome*, affects the bones, joints, eyes, ears, and skin. There are four recognized forms. Types I and IV are inherited by autosomal dominance, while types II and III are autosomal recessive diseases.

"Brittle bones" is a dramatic feature resulting from a defect in the collagenous matrix of bone. Fractures occur early in life, sometimes in utero. Loose-jointedness may be striking and dislocation of joints can be a problem. Blue sclerae, when present, are a valuable clue to diagnosis. The ocular features are of minimal functional importance. Deafness develops in many by the second decade of life and is audiologically indistinguishable from otosclerosis. Some patients have an element of sensorineural deafness. The skin is thin and rather translucent, and healing wounds result in spreading atrophic scars. Elastosis perforans serpiginosa has been described in patients with osteogenesis imperfecta. Some patients experience unusual bruisability but no consistent defects of the coagulation mechanism have been demonstrated. This is probably due to a structural defect in either the blood vessel wall or the supporting dermal connective tissue.

The basic defect is abnormal collagen synthesis, resulting in type I collagen of abnormal structure. In several patients the precise defect has been identified. In type I (blue scleral dominant) there is diminished type I collagen with an altered pro α_1 (I) gene; in type II (perinatal lethal) there is diminished type I collagen synthesis with a defective pro α_1 (I) gene; in type III (progressive deforming) there is delayed secretion of type I collagen with altered mannosylation; and in type IV (white sclerae dominant) there is simply a defective pro α_1 (I) gene.

Nicholls AC, et al: Biochemical heterogeneity of osteogenesis imperfecta. Lancet 1979, 1:1193.
Sashema K, et al: Osteogenesis imperfecta in twins: case report and review of the literature. Acta Pediatr VPM 1988, Oct 30, 621.
Sykes B, et al: Prenatal diagnosis of osteogenesis imperfecta. Ann NY Acad Sci 1988, 543:136.

HOMOCYSTINURIA

Homocystinuria, an inborn error in the metabolism of methionine, is characterized by the presence of homocystine in the urine and systemic abnormalities of the connective tissue. Activity of the enzyme cystathionine synthetase is deficient and as a result cystine is required in the diet of these patients. Among the signs of homocystinuria are genu valgum, kyphoscoliosis, pigeon breast deformity, and frequent fractures. Generalized osteoporosis, arterial and venous thrombosis, and mental retardation are features of homocystinuria not found in Marfan's syndrome.

The facial skin has a characteristic flush, especially on the malar areas; the color becomes violaceous when the patient is reclining. Elsewhere the skin is blotchy red, suggestive of livedo reticularis. The hair is fine, sparse, and blond. The teeth are irregularly aligned. Downward dislocation of the lens, as opposed to the upward displacement seen in Marfan's syndrome, is a prominent feature.

MARFAN'S SYNDROME

Striae distensae are a prominent feature of Marfan's syndrome. This is an inherited disorder of connective tissue transmitted as an autosomal dominant trait with skeletal, cardiovascular, and ocular involvement. Among the important abnormalities are tallness, loose-jointedness, a dolichocephalic skull, high-arched palate, arachnodactyly, pigeon breast, pes planus, poor muscle tone, and large, deformed ears. The aorta, chordae tendineae, and the aortic as well as the mitral valve are often involved. Ascending aortic aneurysm and mitral valve prolapse are commonly seen. Ectopia lentis, extensive striae over the hips and shoulders, dental anomalies, and, rarely, elastosis perforans serpiginosa may be present. Several case reports document the occasional occurrence of spontaneous pneumothorax and congenital lung abnormalities.

It has long been assumed that an inborn error of protein metabolism, particularly of collagen or elastin, must underlie Marfan's syndrome, but this remains unproven. Gott et al report that prophylactic aortic grafts are useful in the management of patients.

Gott VL, et al: Surgical treatment of aneurysm of the ascending aorta in the Marfan syndrome. N Engl J Med 1986, 314:1070.
Pyeritz RE, et al: The Marfan syndrome: diagnosis and management. N Engl J Med 1979, 300:772.

LICHEN SCLEROSUS ET ATROPHICUS

CLINICAL FEATURES. Also known as lichen albus, Csillag's disease, and white spot disease, lichen sclerosus et atrophicus (LSA) is a chronic atrophic disease of the skin characterized by white angular and flat-topped papules; follicular, black, horny plugs; and an erythematous to violaceous halo about the white papules. The papules are well defined, shiny, and indurated; they appear in close juxtaposition but do not coalesce, so that groups of individual lesions are formed. The papules gradually atrophy and flatten or even become depressed below the surface. Nancy Edwards has described a corymbose configuration of lesions.

Later, the lesions may coalesce into large atrophic patches. Bullae, often hemorrhagic, may occur on the patches. Itching is frequently severe, especially

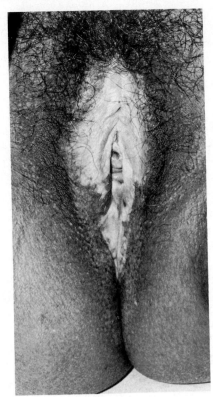

Figure 25–12. Vulvar lichen sclerosus et atrophicus.

in the anogenital area. In the course of time considerable hyperpigmentation develops at the periphery of the patch and the individual papules shrink, leaving the skin smooth, slightly wrinkled, soft, and white.

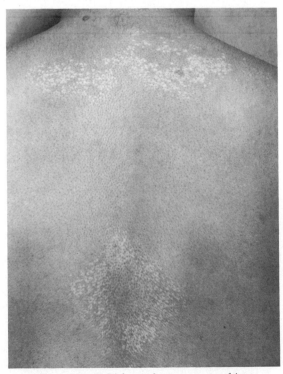

Figure 25–13. Lichen sclerosus et atrophicus.

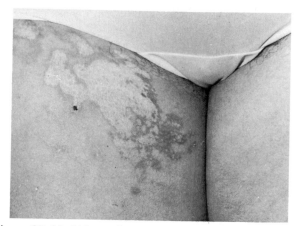

Figure 25–14. Lichen sclerosus et atrophicus in right femoral area. (Courtesy of Dr. H. Curth.)

When the disease appears away from the genital skin, it occurs most frequently in patches on the upper back, chest, and breasts. It almost inevitably involves the anogenital regions, where painful fissures may develop and itching may be a severe and distressing symptom. It occurs predominantly in women. LSA occurs also in children, most frequently in girls two to six years old (Wallace). It has often been overlooked, however, in boys, in whom it is an extremely common cause of scarring phimosis (Chalmers et al). Ledwig et al found that most men with this diagnosis had had circumcision for phimosis, often with meatal stenosis. It involutes, in most girls, before or at menarche.

The tongue may also be involved, either alone or with lesions elsewhere.

The lesions in the anogenital area are similar to those occurring on the trunk. The whitish atrophic area forms a characteristic "hourglass" or "figure-eight" configuration, with the vulva and the anus forming the bulbous parts of the hourglass. The labia minora, the prepuce of the clitoris, and the posterior fourchette may be completely atrophied.

LSA may be present on the anogenital area only. Keratotic and leukoplakic patches may develop in LSA and these may rarely degenerate into cancer.

Kraurosis Vulvae. Previously there were those who thought that LSA and kraurosis vulvae were two separate entities; others thought LSA was kraurosis vulvae. The term kraurosis, like "leukoplakia," has been abandoned in modern gynecologic terminology: diffuse vulvar lesions are now classified as hyperplastic, atrophic, or mixed dystrophic. Tremaine et al have recently reviewed this classification.

Balanitis Xerotica Obliterans. This entity is a manifestation of LSA. It occurs mostly in uncircumcised men who have phimosis and balanitis. Circumcision in infancy appears to protect against its development: Ledwig et al, who recently reviewed the disease, could not find a single case in a man who had been circumcised in infancy. The lesions simulate leukoplakia in appearance, with a whitish plaque on the glans, which may be accompanied by bullae. The

prepuce and the shaft may also be involved. The meatus is affected in over half of the cases. Squamous cell carcinoma, indicated by hyperkeratotic thickening of the lesions, may develop in these plaques. Bart and Kopf's patient had the squamous cell carcinoma removed by Moh's chemosurgery followed by 2.5 per cent testosterone propionate ointment topically.

ETIOLOGY. The etiology of LSA is unknown. It is seen with greatest frequency in menopausal women; however, since it can occur in young girls and also in the male, the hormonal implications are a matter of conjecture. Friedrich reported that women with lichen sclerosus et atrophicus have abnormally low levels of dihydrotestosterone and its precursor, androstenedione. Their testosterone levels do not differ from those of controls. Meyrick et al review its frequent association with autoimmune phenomena, such as alopecia areata, vitiligo, and thyroid disease. In Europe some reports have linked LSA to infection with *Borrelia burgdorferi.*

HISTOPATHOLOGY. The epidermis is thin and rete ridges are effaced. Hyperkeratosis and follicular plugging are prominent. There is hydropic degeneration of the basal layer. The epidermal changes are similar to those of lupus erythematosus, but the dermal changes are diagnostic, consisting of edematous, amorphous collagen in the upper third of the dermis, separated from underlying, normal-appearing collagen by a mid-dermal bandlike lymphocytic infiltrate.

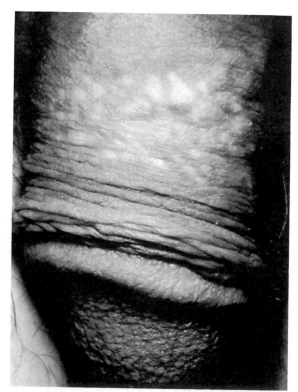

Figure 25–15. Balanitis xerotica obliterans of the penis. (Courtesy of Dr. Axel W. Hoke.)

DIAGNOSIS. The typical locations with the distinctive bone-white patches of atrophy, comedones, and dell formation are characteristic.

DIFFERENTIAL DIAGNOSIS. LSA must be differentiated from guttate morphea, and lichen planus, especially of the atrophic type. When it occurs in the anogenital area both Bowen's disease and extramammary Paget's disease must be kept in mind.

The annular atrophic plaques of the face described by Christianson in 1969 are now thought to be an unusual form of LSA.

TREATMENT. LSA may involute spontaneously, especially in young girls.

For the past ten years it has been generally recognized that 2 or 3 per cent testosterone ointment would give remarkable relief in some cases, and Friedrich has shown that it raises dihydrotestosterone levels. Ely has combined 2 ml of Deladumone, Squibb (containing 360 mg of testosterone enanthate and 16 mg of estradiol valerate in sesame oil) with 30 gm of 0.025 per cent flurandrenolide (Cordran) ointment. An 0.5-gm dab contains roughly 10 mg testosterone and 1.6 mg estradiol. It is used daily till there is a good response, and weekly, indefinitely, for maintenance. In women, if hypertrophy of the clitoris occurs, or hoarseness, treatment should be stopped, and resumed at half strength, weekly, after symptoms subside. Rees still prefers 1 per cent hydrocortisone ointment.

One of us (HLA) had remarkable success in LSA of the trunk with weekly intramuscular injections of 100 mg of bismuth subsalicylate in oil. The medication has no side effects; however, it is no longer marketed and is of chiefly historical interest.

Ratz reported remarkably good results in a case of balanitis xerotica obliterans of great severity unresponsive to topical treatment for over two years, by vaporizing the entire affected area with a CO_2 laser operating at 20 W of power output in the continuous mode; 600W/cm² was delivered to a 2-mm spot. There was burning pain for three weeks, but reepithelization was complete in 12 weeks, and there had been no recurrence 21 months later. Obviously it should not be tried unless Deladumone/Cordran has failed. Circumcision is also effective, if done early.

Romppanen et al reported a good clinical response in 16 women to etretinate 0.6 mg/kg/day for 3 months.

Penneys reported significant clinical improvement in five patients with lichen sclerosus by giving 4 to 12 gm of potassium para-aminobenzoate (Potaba) daily by mouth. Side effects were few and manageable, which is not always the case. Agranulocytosis must be watched for.

Bart RS, et al: Squamous cell carcinoma arising in balanitis xerotica obliterans. J Dermatol Surg Oncol 1978, 4:556.

Chalmers RJG, et al: Lichen sclerosus et atrophicus: a common and distinctive cause of phimosis in boys. Arch Dermatol 1984, 120:1025.

Edwards N, et al: Corymbiform lichen sclerosus et atrophicus (Letter). Arch Dermatol 1979, 116:1035.

Friedrich EG, Jr: Serum levels of sex hormones in vulvar lichen sclerosus, and effect of topical testosterone. N Engl J Med 1984, 310:488.

Garcia-Bravo B, et al: Lichen sclerosus et atrophicus. JAAD 1988, 19:482.

Ledwig PA, et al: Late circumcision and lichen sclerosus et atrophicus of the penis. JAAD 1989, 20:211.

Meyrick RH, et al: Clinical features and therapy of lichen sclerosus et atrophicus affecting males. Clin Exp Dermatol 1987, 12:126.

Idem: Lichen sclerosus et atrophicus and autoimmunity. Br J Dermatol 1988, 118:41.

Pasieczny TAH: Treatment of balanitis xerotica obliterans with testosterone propionate ointment. Acta Dermatol Venereol 1977, 57:275.

Penneys NS: Treatment of lichen sclerosus with potassium para-aminobenzoate. JAAD 1984, 10:1039.

Ratz JL: Carbon dioxide laser treatment of balanitis xerotica obliterans. JAAD 1984, 10:925.

Rees RB: Testosterone ineffective in LS&A, as well as potentially masculinizing? Schoch Letter 1989, 39:21.

Ridley CM: Lichen sclerosus et atrophicus. Arch Dermatol 1987, 123:457.

Romppanen U, et al: Light and electron-microscope findings in lichen sclerosus et atrophicus of the vulva during etretinate treatment. Dermatologica 1987, 175:33.

Shirer JA, et al: Familial occurrence of lichen sclerosus et atrophicus. Arch Dermatol 1987, 123:485.

Tompkins KJ, et al: Persistent bullae on the penis of an elderly man. Arch Dermatol 1987, 123:1391.

Tremaine RDL, et al: Lichen sclerosus et atrophicus. Int J Dermatol 1989, 28:10.

Wallace HJ: Lichen sclerosus et atrophicus. Trans St Johns Hosp Dermatol Soc 1971, 57:9.

PROGRESSIVE IDIOPATHIC ATROPHODERMA OF PASINI AND PIERINI

In 1923 Pasini described a peculiar form of pigmentary atrophoderma that was clinically and histopathologically different from the atrophic stages of localized scleroderma or any other known atrophy.

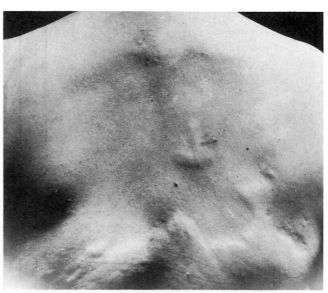

Figure 25–16. Atrophoderma of Pasini and Pierini.

Since then many cases have been reported, mainly from Argentina, and particularly by Pierini. Poché reported two cases in 1980.

The disease consists of brownish, oval, round or irregular, smooth, atrophic macules depressed below the level of the skin. It occurs mainly on the trunk of young individuals, predominantly in females. The lesions are usually asymptomatic. The singly occurring or multiple lesions measure from several to 20 or more centimeters in diameter.

Craps has reported the case of a child with localized patches of congenital anetoderma associated with idiopathic atrophoderma of Pasini and Pierini, and osseous malformations.

The histopathological picture shows slight reduction in the thickness of the epidermis and dermal connective tissue layers and minimal discrete perivascular infiltration in the upper dermis. Because of the minimal changes noted, a biopsy should include an adequate margin of normal-appearing skin so that a comparison may be made.

The course of the disease is benign, terminating spontaneously after several months or a few years although some cases have persisted indefinitely. There is no known effective treatment.

Canizares O, et al: Idiopathic atrophoderma of Pasini and Pierini. Arch Dermatol 1958, 77:42.

Craps L. Anétodermie congenitale. Arch Belg Dermatol Syph 1960, 16:193.

Pierini LE, et al: Atrofodermia idiopathica de Pasini. Rev Argent Dermatol 1944, 28:538.

Poché GW: Progressive idiopathic atrophoderma of Pasini and Pierini. Cutis 1980, 25:503.

26

Errors of Metabolism

LIPID DISTURBANCES

XANTHOMATOSIS

Xanthomatosis is a cutaneous manifestation of lipidosis in which the plasma lipoproteins and free fatty acids are changed quantitatively. It refers to a morphologic change in which there is accumulation of lipids in large foam cells in the tissues. Cholesterol or triglycerides are usually found, but when cholesterol levels are normal, beta-sitosterol, campesterol, or stigmasterol (plant sterols), or cholestanol, may rarely be at fault, as shown by Matsuo et al and others. Parker and Cruz et al have recently reviewed the xanthomas and hyperlipidemias.

CLINICAL FEATURES. The cutaneous manifestations of xanthomatosis are expressed in several distinctive morphologic types.

Xanthoma Tuberosum. Beginning at any age, tuberous xanthomata are variously found as flat or elevated and rounded, grouped, yellowish or orange nodules located over the joints, particularly on the elbows and knees. The lesions are indurated and tend to coalesce. They may also occur over the knuckles, the toe joints, the axillary and inguinal folds, the face, and the buttocks. Solitary lesions may occur. Early lesions are usually bright yellow or erythematous; older lesions tend to become fibrotic and lose their color. Pedunculated, fissured, and suppurative nodules may also be seen.

Xanthoma tuberosum is associated with primary hyperlipoproteinemias with elevated cholesterol levels, such as familial hypercholesterolemia and familial dysbetalipoproteinemia. It also occurs in biliary cirrhosis, myxedema, phytosterolemia, and normocholesterolemic dysbetalipoproteinemia.

Xanthoma Tendinosum. Papules or nodules 5 to 25 mm in diameter are found in the tendons, more especially in extensor tendons on the backs of the hands and dorsa of the feet and in the Achilles tendons. These predominate in conditions with elevated cholesterol, such as the primary hyperlipoproteinemias of familial hypercholesterolemia and familial hyperbetalipoproteinemia. They are seen in association with tuberous xanthomas and xanthelasma. They also occur in obstructive liver disease, diabetes, myxedema, cerebrotendinous xanthomatosis, and phytosterolemia.

Eruptive Xanthoma. *Xanthoma eruptivum* consists of small yellow-orange to reddish brown papules which appear in crops over the entire body. These occur in association with markedly elevated triglycerides. Causes for such elevations are genetic deficiency of lipoprotein lipase, familial deficiency of apoprotein CII, and endogenous familial hypertriglyceridemia. Certain diseases or drugs raise the triglyceride level either by increased production, decreased catabolism, or decreased excretion. These include diabetes mellitus, obesity, pancreatitis, chronic renal failure, hypothyroidism, and treatment with estrogens, corticosteroids, isotretinoin, or etretinate.

The papules may be surrounded by an erythematous halo and may be grouped in various favored locations such as the buttocks, flexor surfaces of the arms and thighs, knees, inguinal and axillary folds, and oral mucosa. Koebnerization may occur. Pruritus is variable.

Xanthoma Planum (Plane Xanthoma). These xanthomas appear as flat macules or slightly elevated plaques with a yellowish tan or orange coloration of the skin diffusely spread over large areas. They are frequently associated with biliary cirrhosis and myeloma but have been described in patients with high-density lipoprotein (HDL) deficiency, monoclonal gammopathy, lymphoma, leukemia, serum lipopro-

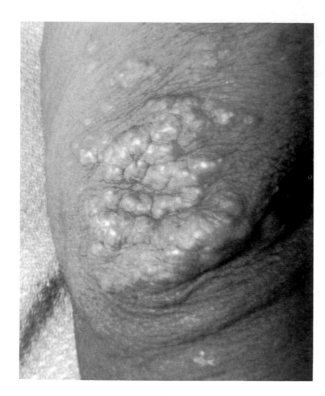

Figure 26–1. Xanthoma tuberosum. (Courtesy of Dr. Axel W. Hoke.)

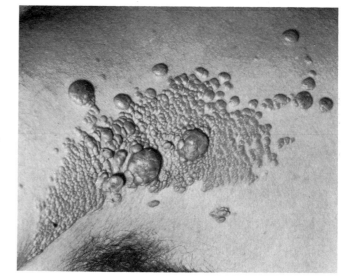

Figure 26–2. Xanthoma tuberosum in axilla.

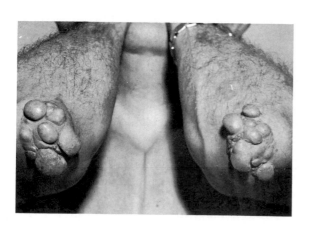

Figure 26–3. Xanthoma tuberosum on elbows.

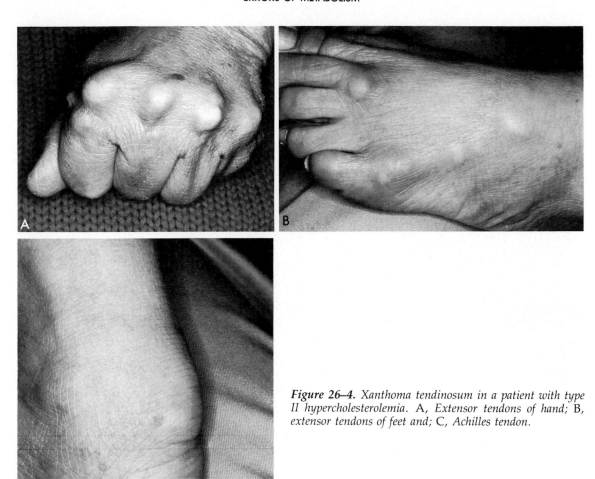

Figure 26–4. Xanthoma tendinosum in a patient with type II hypercholesterolemia. A, Extensor tendons of hand; B, extensor tendons of feet and; C, Achilles tendon.

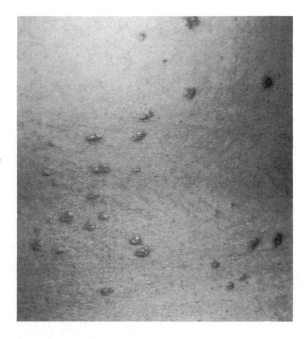

Figure 26–5. Eruptive xanthoma in a patient with adult-onset diabetes mellitus.

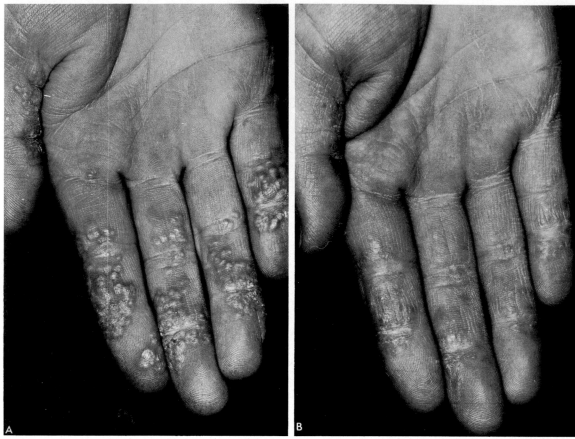

Figure 26–6. A, *Eruptive xanthomata of the palms with hyperprebetalipoproteinemia. B, Same patient after a low calorie and low carbohydrate diet. (Courtesy of Dr. M. K. Polano, The Netherlands.)*

tein deficiency, and in xanthomas following erythroderma. Characteristically, plane xanthomas may occur about the eyelids, neck, trunk, shoulders, or axillae. These well-defined macular patches may be situated on the inner surface of the thighs, and antecubital and popliteal spaces. Xanthelasma palpebrarum may be associated with xanthoma planum elsewhere.

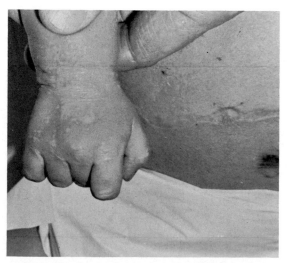

Figure 26–7. *Xanthoma planum on backs of hands and elsewhere in a 9 month old child with biliary atresia.*

Palmar Xanthomas. These consist of nodules and irregular yellowish plaques involving the palms and flexural surfaces of the fingers. *Striated xanthomas* appear as yellowish streaks following the distribution of creases of the palms and soles. These lesions are seen in familial dysbetalipoproteinemia, multiple myeloma, and biliary cirrhosis.

Xanthelasma Palpebrarum (Xanthelasma). This is the most common type of xanthoma. It occurs on the eyelids, being characterized by soft, chamois-colored or yellowish orange oblong plaques, usually near the inner canthi. They vary from 2 to 30 mm in length. Frequent symmetry, with a tendency to be permanent, progressive, multiple, and coalescent, is also characteristic. Frequently xanthelasmata are associated with other types of xanthomas, but they are usually present without any other disease.

The disorder is encountered chiefly during middle age. It is common among women who have hepatic or biliary disorders. Xanthelasma may be seen in the various familial hyperlipoproteinemias, especially in familial hypercholesterolemia; however, half or more of the patients are normolipemic. It is a common finding in generalized xanthoma planum, in obstructive liver disease, myxedema, diabetes, and phytosterolemia.

Douste-Blazy et al measured the apolipoprotein E and apolipoprotein B in the plasma of 10 patients

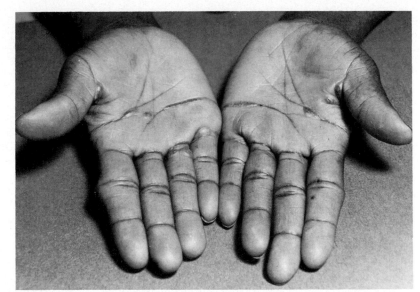

Figure 26–8. Xanthoma striatum palmare.

with normolipidemic xanthelasma of the eyelids and found the levels typical of the heterozygous state for familial dysbetalipoproteinemia, a hyperapobetaproteinemia, or both; some patients had atherosclerosis. Gómez et al, however, found no such associated abnormalities among their group of 50 patients with xanthelasma. Nevertheless, we consider it prudent to evaluate new patients with a full lipoprotein profile as well as a careful history and physical examination.

Treatment of xanthelasma is discussed here because of its uniqueness among the xanthomas in that surgical therapy is often successful. The best method is surgical excision. The anesthetized lesion is grasped with mouse-tooth forceps and clipped off with scissors, and the skin edges undermined and sutured with fine silk. Excellent cosmetic results are obtained, even if the wound is not closed. Fulguration, trichloracetic acid cauterization, and carbon dioxide laser vaporization are other methods. However, complete removal of the lesions does not preclude the possibility of other new lesions' developing.

Tubero-eruptive Xanthomas. These xanthomas are red papules and nodules that appear inflamed and tend to coalesce. They are associated with familial dysbetalipoproteinemia.

Nodular Xanthomas. These are multiple, yellowish, dome-shaped lesions, 4 to 5 mm or larger in diameter, which are discrete or confluent. They may be present on the earlobes, neck, elbows, and knees, and are usually associated with biliary cirrhosis and atresia of the bile ducts.

HISTOPATHOLOGY OF THE XANTHOMAS. The histologic features in all varieties of xanthoma are similar, characterized by fibroblastic proliferation and the presence of numerous large xanthoma or foam cells, which are phagocytes (fat-laden histiocytes). They may be multinucleated. In addition to the foam cells, giant cells of the "Touton" type occur, characterized by a circular arrangement of the nuclei, with deposits of lipids in the cytoplasm outside this ring. Clefts representing cholesterol and fatty acids dissolved by embedding agents may be noted. There is generally a connective tissue reaction about the nests of foam cells, and in old lesions most of the foam cells are replaced with fibrosis.

When the demonstration of lipids in the histologic sections is desired, frozen sections should be stained with lipid stains (scarlet red).

PRIMARY HYPERLIPOPROTEINEMIAS

Cutaneous xanthomas are usually displays of some disorder of lipid metabolism, although they may be attributable to other disorders. The blood lipids, with the exception of free fatty acids, are bound to circulating plasma proteins and are mainly cholesterol, phospholipid, and triglyceride.

The total serum lipids have a range of 400 to 1000 mg per cent. Of this, serum cholesterol values vary according to age. Generally a serum cholesterol below 200 mg/dl is normal, while a level of over 240

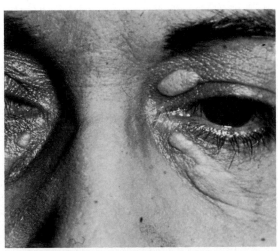

Figure 26–9. Xanthelasma palpebrarum.

mg requires further evaluation. A triglyceride level of over 250 mg/dl is considered abnormal. An approach to the workup and treatment of these disorders is discussed by Hoeg et al.

Lipoprotein fractions may be demonstrated by paper electrophoresis. Four lipoprotein bands may be evident: the alphalipoprotein band (high-density lipoprotein), betalipoprotein (low-density lipoprotein, LDL), prebetalipoprotein (very low-density lipoprotein, VLDL), and the chylomicron band.

When the lipoproteins are subjected to ultracentrifugation it is found that the high-density alphalipoproteins (HDL) are composed mostly of phospholipid and esterified cholesterol. The betalipoproteins (low-density, LDL) are composed mostly of cholesterols. The prebetalipoproteins (VLDL) are fractions of still lower density which are the main carriers of endogenous triglycerides. The lowest density chylomicrons are the exogenous triglycerides.

Frederickson and Lees classified hyperlipoproteinemias into six types on the basis of electrophoretic patterns: type I, excess chylomicrons; type IIa, excess betalipoprotein; type IIb, excess betalipoprotein with slightly elevated VLDL; type III, increased intermediate-density (remnant) lipoprotein; type IV, increased prebetalipoprotein; type V, increased prebetalipoproteins and chylomicrons.

While this phenotypic classification has been useful for many years, advances in the understanding of lipoprotein metabolism and transport, coupled with new knowledge of molecular defects which result in these phenotypes, has led to the use of a genetic classification of lipoproteinemias.

As an introduction to this, lipoprotein metabolism may be viewed as occurring in two cascades: an exogenous and an endogenous category. Exogenous lipids in the diet are absorbed and incorporated into triglyceride-rich chylomicrons. These are hydrolyzed by the action of lipoprotein lipase and certain cofactors, among them apoprotein CII. The resulting remnants are taken up by the liver. Endogenously produced VLDLs are synthesized in the liver and (again through the action of lipoprotein lipase) are connected to cholesterol-rich intermediate-density lipoproteins (IDLs) and eventually into LDLs.

These are then available for uptake by peripheral tissues, as well as by the liver. The uptake of LDL, IDL, and chylomicron remnants is dependent upon specific receptors. Abnormalities of lipoprotein lipase, the apolipoproteins, cofactors, receptors, or stimulators or retarders of endogenous production or catabolism, whether on a genetic or sporadic basis, may accelerate or block the cascade in different areas. If blockade occurs early and results in elevation of triglyceride-rich particles, eruptive xanthoma may result. If a defect occurs later in the cascade, and cholesterol-rich particles accumulate, xanthelasma, tuberous xanthomas, and tendinous xanthomas are to be expected, along with premature atherosclerotic cardiovascular disease.

Parker's tabular presentation provides a clearer understanding of the primary hyperlipoproteinemias (Table 26–1).

A similarly excellent discussion and tables appear in the review by Cruz et al.

Lipoprotein Lipase Deficiency. This causes type I disease (chylomicronemia) early in life. It was described by Bürger and Grutz. As patients grow older they get elevated VLDLs (type V).

Familial Apoprotein CII Deficiency. Patients lack lipoprotein lipase activator, and very high triglyceride levels, up to 10,000 mg/dl, result. It is very rare.

Familial Hypertriglyceridemia. Increased hepatic production of VLDLs occurs first (type IV), but overloaded removal mechanisms result in accumulation of dietary lipids, and chylomicrons accumulate, so a type V pattern results. Eruptive xanthomas are common, and atherosclerotic heart disease may occur. Cholelithiasis is common. Polyarthritis and arthralgia frequently occur.

Familial Dysbetalipoproteinemia (Broad Beta Disease). In this disorder, remnant lipoproteins increase and LDLs and HDLs are reduced, and triglyceride and cholesterol levels are increased. The cholesterol-rich IDLs form a broad band on electrophoresis, extending from prebeta to betalipoproteins: hence "broad beta" disease. Xanthomas (tuberous, eruptive, palmar, or tendinous) are common; xanthelasmas are infrequent. Atherosclerosis is common, as are diabetes, gout, and obesity.

Familial Hypercholesterolemia. This is Frederickson's type II disease: LDLs (betalipoproteins) are found in high levels in the plasma; there may be a moderate increase in VLDLs, and in the triglycerides which they carry. There is overproduction of LDL cholesterol (caused by loss of normal feedback inhibition) and impaired removal of it (because of impaired formation of LDL receptors), so there is elevated plasma betalipoprotein from birth in heterozygotes, and symptoms begin in the third to sixth decade, when tendinous or tuberous xanthomas, xanthelasmas, and atherosclerotic disease appear. Homozygotes generally get coronary atherosclerosis before age 20, and over 40 per cent get xanthelasmas,

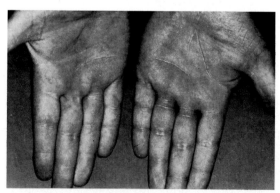

Figure 26–10. Xanthochromia striata palmaris in a patient with hyperprebeta-lipoproteinemia. (Courtesy of Dr. M. K. Polano, The Netherlands.)

Table 26–1. PRIMARY HYPERLIPOPROTEINEMIAS (AFTER PARKER)

Lipoprotein Disorder	Genetic Mechanisms	Lipoprotein Pattern	Estimated Frequency	Expression in Children
Monogenic disorders				
I. Triglyceride removal defects				
1. LPL deficiency	Autosomal recessive	I, V	<1:100,000	Yes
2. Familial apoprotein CII deficiency	Autosomal recessive	I, V	<1:1,000,000	Adolescence
II. Triglyceride excessive production				
1. Endogenous familial hypertriglyceridemia	Autosomal dominant	IV, V	1:500	Rare
III. Lipoprotein removal defects				
1. Broad beta disease; familial dysbetalipo-proteinemia	Autosomal dominant	III	1:100	Rare
2. Familial hyper-cholesterolemia	Autosomal dominant	IIa, IIb	1:500	Yes
Undefined possible monogenic disorders				
Familial combined hyperlipidemia or familial multiple-type hyperlipoproteinemia		IIa, IIb, IV, V	30% of all genetic lipoproteinemias	Seldom

tendinous xanthomas, or tuberous xanthomas in childhood. Cultured amniotic fluid cells permit prenatal diagnosis in homozygotes.

Familial Combined Hyperlipidemia or Multiple-type Hyperlipoproteinemia. This, the commonest of the genetic lipoproteinemias, has a high risk of myocardial infarction and diabetes, and a low incidence of tuberous or tendinous xanthomas.

Parker's therapeutic suggestions are summarized in Table 26–2, taken from his paper.

SECONDARY HYPERLIPOPROTEINEMIA

Obstructive Liver Disease (Xanthomatous Biliary Cirrhosis)

This type of hyperlipoproteinemia shows increase of the serum phospholipid and cholesterol, giving a type II lipoprotein pattern. This is due to the presence of lipoprotein X, which is secreted by the liver in cholestasis. It has the ability to carry large quantities of free cholesterol and phospholipids. The triglycerides are not elevated and the plasma is clear, showing no chylomicrons.

The xanthomatous lesions are plane xanthomas, with lesions on the face, the flexor surfaces of the extremities, and the trunk. Striate palmar and plantar lesions and xanthelasmas are also seen. Tuberous xanthomas may also occur. Pruritus is extremely severe. Hepatomegaly and jaundice are present.

Cholestyramine is of help in allaying pruritus.

Hematopoietic Diseases

Xanthomatoses may occur secondarily in myelomas, Waldenström's macroglobulinemia, cryoglobulinemia and occasionally lymphoma, and hemochromatosis. These xanthomatoses are usually the plane

Table 26–2. THERAPEUTIC SUGGESTIONS

	Diet	Drugs
TG removal defect		
Lipoprotein lipase deficiencies type I	Low fat intake	Medium-chain triglycerides
TG excessive production		
Endogenous familial hypertri-glyceridemia types IV and V	Low calorie; low carbohydrate; low fat; low alcohol	Clofibrate; gemfibrozil (Lopid)
Removal defects		
Broad beta disease type III	Low calorie; low carbohydrate; low alcohol; low cholesterol; unsaturated fats; low saturated fats	Clofibrate
Familial hypercholesterolemia types IIa and IIb		Cholestyramine; colestipol; clofibrate; neomycin; nicotinic acid; D-thyroxine; gemfibrozil; probucol (Lorelco)
Undefined monogenic disease		
Familial multiple or combined hyperlipoproteinemia	Low cholesterol; unsaturated fats; low saturated fats; low calorie	Depending on LP profile found, all the drugs noted above

xanthomas. The lipoproteinemia may be of type I, V, or IIa pattern. In some patients no lipoprotein abnormality is present.

Xanthoma Diabeticorum

Eruptive xanthomas may occur secondarily, especially in young persons unresponsive to insulin. Cardiovascular disease and hepatomegaly are common. Insulin is necessary for the normal plasma triglyceride clearing action of lipoprotein lipase. Therefore in insulin deficiency, an acquired lipoprotein lipase deficiency exists, which leads to impaired clearance of chylomicrons or VLDLs, or both. This results in a type I, IV, or V lipoprotein pattern and hypertriglyceridemia.

When the diabetes is brought under control the triglyceride levels are lowered and prompt involution of the lesions is seen. Weight reduction and carbohydrate intake restriction are also helpful. Identical phenomena may occur in *von Gierke's disease,* a form of glycogen storage disease in which there is a lack of hepatic glucose-6-phosphatase.

Chronic Renal Failure

If plasma protein levels are reduced by urinary loss in the nephrotic syndrome (or by plasmapheresis or repeated bleeding), a compensatory increase of lipoproteins may occur, with hyperlipidemia and various kinds of xanthoma.

Renal failure with or without dialysis may cause hypertriglyceridemia. In long-term dialysis there is increased cardiovascular disease because of increased levels of VLDL as well as lowered HDLs. Type IV and V profiles are most commonly seen.

Myxedema

Lipoprotein lipase needs thyroid hormone to work, and its failure may lead to type I, IV or V disease; or thyroid hormone deficiency may lead to hypercholesterolemia, because thyroid hormone is needed in the oxidation of hepatic cholesterol to bile salts. Xanthelasma and xanthomas are common in myxedema.

Pancreatitis

Hyperlipidemia in the hyperchylomicronemic syndromes (types I and V) may cause pancreatitis; in type V it may be recurrent, and pancreatic necrosis and death may occur. Alternatively, pancreatitis (perhaps initiated by ethanol) may cause type I or V hyperlipoproteinemia by inducing insulin deficiency and a relative lack of lipoprotein lipase activity.

Medication-Induced Hyperlipoproteinemia

Estrogens, by decreasing lipoprotein lipase activity and increasing VLDL synthesis, may cause type I or type IV patterns. Eruptive xanthomas may occur. Oral prednisone may induce insulin deficiency and cause type IV or V patterns to develop. Isotretinoin sometimes increases triglycerides carried in VLDL, and eruptive xanthomas may occur; etretinate has a similar effect.

NONFAMILIAL NORMOLIPOPROTEINEMIC XANTHOMATOSES

The normolipoproteinemic xanthomatoses are various conditions in which serum cholesterol and lipoproteins are normal, yet secondary lipid deposition in the skin occurs. Parker extensively reviewed the many causes of this in 1986.

Cerebrotendinous Xanthomatosis

This autosomal recessive disease is caused by an accumulation of cholestanol in plasma lipoproteins and xanthomatous tissue. It appears that the underlying abnormality is a deficiency of the hepatic enzyme 26-hydrolase, necessary for the complete oxidation of cholesterol to bile acids. Cholestanol, an intermediate, accumulates as a result. It accumulates in tendons, brain, heart, lungs, and the ocular lenses. There may be tendinous xanthomas, especially of the Achilles tendons; progressive neurologic dysfunction; cerebellar ataxia; dementia; spinal cord paresis; cataracts; atherosclerotic coronary disease; and endocrine abnormalities. Bavinck et al reported the value of urinary gas chromatography as a specific test for this disease. Treatment is with chenodeoxycholic acid and cholic acid.

Phytosterolemia

In this rare disorder, plant sterols such as betasitosterol, stigmasterol, and campesterol are absorbed from the gastrointestinal tract in excessive amounts. They accumulate in the body as xanthelasmas, tendinous xanthomas, and cutaneous xanthomas. In most patients there is also type IIa hyperlipoproteinemia. There is a risk of hemolysis, arthritis, and premature atherosclerosis.

Verruciform Xanthoma

This uncommon lesion occurs as a reddish orange or paler hyperkeratotic plaque or papillomatous growth with a pebbly or verrucous surface. The most common site is the oral mucosa, where it was first described by Schafer in 1971. Since then it has been reported on other mucosal surfaces, the genitalia, the lower extremities, and elsewhere. Mountcastle et al have recently reviewed the literature. Histologically there is acanthosis without atypia, parakeratosis, and xanthoma cells in the papillary dermis. The etiology is unknown.

Xanthoma Disseminatum

This rare normolipoproteinemic mucocutaneous xanthomatosis is characterized by small yellowish red to brown papules and nodules, which are discrete and disseminated. They involve chiefly the axillary and inguinal folds, the antecubital and popliteal fossae, face, neck, and flexural surfaces. Diffuse xanthomatous infiltrations may involve the oral mucosa, the oropharynx, the larynx, and the bronchi in 40 per cent of the cases. The conjunctivae may also contain lesions.

Diabetes insipidus may occur from xanthomatous involvement of the pituitary gland. It was present in 39 per cent of the cases reviewed by Altman and Winkelmann.

The serum lipids are normal. It is hypothesized that xanthoma disseminatum is a reactive histiocytic proliferation in which lipids are secondarily deposited into the histiocytes.

Although its occurrence ranges between one and 70 years, xanthoma disseminatum appears mostly in young men. It is a chronic and benign disease, which persists indefinitely, or may involute spontaneously after some years.

Histologic examination shows xanthoma cells, eosinophilic histiocytes, numerous Touton giant cells, and, frequently, an inflammatory cell infiltrate.

Considerable speculation has been made in regard to its relationship to histiocytosis X and its variations.

Xanthoma disseminatum is a non-X histiocytosis and can be differentiated from Hand-Schüller-Christian disease, Letterer-Siwe disease, and eosinophilic granuloma of bone as well as juvenile xanthogranuloma and multiple histiocytomas. This differential diagnosis is fully discussed by Blobstein et al. *Disseminated xanthosiderohistiocytosis* is a variant of xanthoma disseminatum in which there is a keloidal consistency to the lesions; they have annular borders, a cephalad distribution, and extensive iron and lipid deposition in the macrophages and connective tissue. Battaglini et al reported a case in which multiple myeloma supervened.

Generalized Plane Xanthoma (Generalized Xanthelasma)

Xanthoma planum lesions are xanthomatous deposits in the skin characterized by yellow to light brown flat or slightly elevated plaques, which are sharply demarcated from the surrounding skin. The generalized type involves the eyelids, periorbital areas, sides of the neck, shoulders, and upper trunk. Old scars may also contain plane xanthomas.

Plane xanthomas may be associated with familial hyperlipoproteinemia types II and III, and xanthomatous biliary cirrhosis. Generalized plane xanthomas occur primarily, however, with systemic disease associated with the reticuloendothelial system. Xanthoma planum is associated with myeloma, chronic granulocytic leukemia, chronic myeloid leukemia, cryoglobulinemia, Waldenström's macroglobulinemia, lymphoma, and benign monoclonal gammopathy.

Histologically, histiocytic foam cells are diffusely situated in the upper dermis and a few Touton giant cells may also be found.

Familial Alphalipoprotein Deficiency (Tangier Disease)

Waldorf and his associates have reported cutaneous lesions in Tangier disease, which is characterized by markedly hypertrophied tonsils with orange-yellow striations. They reported a generalized papular eruption in one patient. Clinically uninvolved skin showed extracellular deposits of cholesterol esters outside the dermal cells. Generally, however, xanthomas do not occur in this disease, the characteristic finding being yellow enlarged tonsils from accumulation of lipid in this localized area.

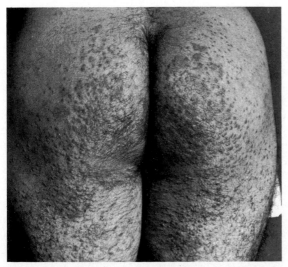

Figure 26–11. Xanthoma disseminatum on the buttocks.

Battaglini J, et al: Disseminated xanthosiderohistiocytosis, a variant of xanthoma disseminatum, in a patient with plasma cell dyscrasia. JAAD 1984, 11:750.

Bickley LK: Yellow papules in a middle-aged woman. Arch Dermatol 1989, 125:287.

Blobstein SH, et al: Bone lesions in xanthoma disseminatum. Arch Dermatol 1985, 121:1313.

Bouwres Bavinc JN, et al: Capillary gas chromatography of urine samples in diagnosing cerebrotendinous xanthomatosis. Arch Dermatol 1986, 122:1269.

Buchner A, et al: Verruciform xanthoma of the oral mucosa. Arch Dermatol 1981, 117:563.

Caputo R, et al: Normolipemic eruptive cutaneous xanthomatosis. Arch Dermatol 1986, 122:1294.

Chyu J, et al: Verruciform xanthoma of the lower extremity. JAAD 1987, 17:695.

Cooper TW, et al: Verruciform xanthoma. JAAD 1983, 8:463.

Cruz PO, et al: Dermal, subcutaneous, and tendon xanthomas. JAAD 1988, 19:95.

Douste-Blazy P, et al: Increased frequency of apo E-ND phenotype and hyperapobetalipoproteinemia in normolipidemic subjects with xanthelasmas. Ann Intern Med 1982, 96:164.

Eckel RH: Lipoprotein lipase. N Engl J Med 1989, 320:1060.

Ellis CN, et al: Etretinate therapy causes increases in lipid levels in patients with psoriasis. Arch Dermatol 1982, 118:559.

Fitzpatrick TB: Xanthelasma of the eyelids in normolipidemic subjects may indicate enhanced atherogenic potential. Dermatol Capsule and Comment 1982 (June-July) p. 8.

Fleischmajer R, et al: Familial hyperlipidemias. Arch Dermatol 1974, 110:43.

Idem: Normolipemic tendon and tuberous xanthomas. JAAD 1981, 5:290.

Friedman SJ, et al: Xanthoma striatum palmare associated with multiple myeloma. JAAD 1987, 16:1272.

Gerber LE, et al: Changes in lipid metabolism during retinoid administration. JAAD 1982, 6:664.

Goldstein GD: The Koebner response with eruptive xanthomas. JAAD 1984, 10:1064.

Gómez JA, et al: Apolipoprotein E phenotypes, lipoprotein composition, and xanthelasma. Arch Dermatol 1988, 124:1230.

Greenberg BH, et al: Primary type V hyperlipoproteinemia: a descriptive study in 32 families. Ann Intern Med 1977, 87:526.

Haggard WR, et al: Broad-beta disease (Type III hyperlipoproteinemia) in a large kindred. Ann Intern Med 1975, 82:141.

Hobbs HH, et al: Deletion in the gene for the low-density lipoprotein receptor in a majority of French Canadians with familial hypercholesterolemia. N Engl J Med 1987, 317:737.

Hoeg JM, et al: An approach to the management of hyperlipoproteinemia. JAMA 1986, 255:512.

Idem: Human lipoprotein metabolism and the liver. Prog Liver Dis 1986, 8:51.

Idem: Cutaneous manifestations of the dyslipoproteinemias. J Assoc Milit Dermatol 1984, 10:55.

Idem: Hyperlipidemia. In Practical Care of the Ambulatory Patient. Stults BM, Dere W (eds). Philadelphia, W. B. Saunders, 1988.

Kimura G, et al: Verruciform xanthoma of the scrotum. Arch Dermatol 1984, 120:1378.

Kraemer BB, et al: Verruciform xanthoma of the penis. Arch Dermatol 1981, 117:516.

Kumakiri M, et al: Xanthoma disseminatum. JAAD 1981, 4:291.

Kushwaha JW, et al: Lipoid proteinosis. Am J Dis Child 1983, 105:81.

Low JR, et al: Xanthomas and lipoproteins. Cutis 1978, 21:801.

Lynch PJ, et al: Generalized plane xanthoma and systemic disease. Arch Dermatol 1966, 93:639.

Matsuo I, et al: Phytosterolemia and Type IIa hyperlipoproteinemia with tuberous xanthoma. JAAD 1981, 4:47.

McCadden ME, et al: Mycosis fungoides associated with dystrophic xanthomatosis. Arch Dermatol 1987, 123:91.

Mishkel MA, et al: Xanthoma disseminatum: clinical, metabolic, pathologic and radiologic aspects. Arch Dermatol 1966, 113:1094.

Mountcastle EA, et al: Verruciform xanthomas of the digits. JAAD 1989, 20:313.

Palestine RF, et al: Verruciform xanthoma in an epithelial nevus. Arch Dermatol 1982, 118:686.

Parker F, et al: Xanthomas and hyperlipidemias. JAAD 1985, 13:1.

Parker F: Normocholesterolemic xanthomatosis. Arch Dermatol 1986, 122:1253.

Rudolph RI: Diffuse "essential" normolipemic xanthomatosis. Int J Dermatol 1977, 14:651.

Sanchez RL, et al: Papular xanthoma. Arch Dermatol 1985, 121:626.

Shulman RS, et al: Beta-sitosterolemia and xanthomatosis. N Engl J Med 1977, 14:651.

Taylor JS, et al: Plane xanthoma and multiple myeloma with lipoprotein-paraprotein complexing. Arch Dermatol 1978, 114:425.

Thomsen RJ, et al: Generalized normolipemic plane xanthoma. Arch Dermatol 1981, 117:521.

Zech LA, et al: Changes in plasma cholesterol and triglyceride levels after treatment with oral isotretinoin. Arch Dermatol 1983, 119:987.

LIPIDOSES

Niemann-Pick Disease

This rare disease most frequently occurs in Jewish infants during the first year of life. It is characterized by hepatosplenomegaly, lymphadenopathy, and the accumulation of foam cells in the bone marrow. Cherry red spots in the maculae retinae, pulmonary infiltration, and mental retardation are also seen. Still rarer are an adult, a juvenile, and a "Nova Scotia" form.

The cutaneous changes consist of distinctive yellowish coloration of the skin and occasionally of lesions resembling eruptive xanthomas. On the mucous membranes black macular patches may occur.

The disease is associated with the accumulation of sphingomyelin and cholesterol in large foam cells throughout the body except in the skin. The enzyme sphingomyelinase is deficient.

The course is progressive, usually ending fatally within the first three years of life. There is no treatment.

Brady RO: The lipid storage diseases: new concepts and control. Ann Intern Med 1975, 82:257.

Crocker AC, et al: Niemann-Pick disease: A review of 18 patients. Medicine (Baltimore) 1958, 37:1.

Gaucher's Disease

In this rare autosomal recessive disorder of the reticuloendothelial system, betaglucocerebrosidase is lacking, with a resulting accumulation of glucocerebrosides in the brain and in the reticuloendothelial cells of the liver, spleen, and marrow. It is characterized by hepatosplenomegaly, rarefaction of the long bones, pingueculae of the scleras, neurologic disturbances, and a distinctive bronze coloration of the skin due to melanin. A deeper pigmentation may extend from the knees to the feet. This is often caused by hemosiderin and may be accompanied by thrombocytopenia and splenomegaly.

The disease occurs at any age, but three forms are recognized: type I, without neurologic involvement; type II disease, with neurologic manifestations; and type III disease, the chronic adult type, with the signs and symptoms described above.

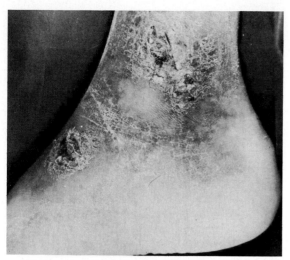

Figure 26–12. Gaucher's disease. (Courtesy of Dr. F. Daniels, Jr.)

The disease occurs most frequently among Ashkenazi Jews. Approximately 1 in 20 carry the defective gene, the lack of which leads to the accumulation of glucocerebroside in histiocytes in the bone marrow and spleen, and Kupffer cells in the liver, forming "Gaucher cells." These are large, 20–100 μ in diameter, with one or a few small nuclei and pale cytoplasm which stains faintly for fat but is PAS-positive. Elevated plasma acid phosphatase occurs, and is a useful clue to the diagnosis. There is thinning of the cortex of the long bones.

Bone marrow transplantation performed before neurologic deficits occur has a high mortality rate (20–50 per cent) but when successful has halted neurologic progression. Otherwise, treatment is symptomatic, with x-ray therapy to the long bones to relieve bone pain, and splenectomy for hypersplenism (anemia and thrombocytopenia, with petechiae and bruising). With the identification of the gene defect, carrier screening and prenatal diagnosis are possible.

Beaudet AL: Gaucher's disease. N Engl J Med 1987, 316:619.
Brady RO: The lipid storage diseases: new concepts and control. Ann Intern Med 1975, 82:257.
Isuji S: A mutation in the human glucocerebrosidase gene in neuropathic Gaucher's disease. N Engl J Med 1987, 316:570.
Kolata G: New understanding of Gaucher's disease. Science 1987, 235:1328.
Rappeport JM, et al: Bone-marrow transplantation in severe Gaucher's disease. N Engl J Med 1984, 311:84.

Lipoid Proteinosis

Also known as *Urbach-Wiethe disease* and *hyalinosis cutis et mucosae*, this rare disturbance is characterized by yellowish white infiltrative deposits on the inner surfaces of the lips, the under surface of the tongue, the fauces, and the uvula. Other parts of the upper respiratory tract are also affected. In the early stage, crops of bullae and pustules occur, which heal, leaving acnelike scars. Changes in the larynx lead to a marked degree of hoarseness, which usually appears within the first few weeks of life. Failure to cry and a hoarse, gravelly voice are suggestive signs.

The tongue is woodlike and movable only with difficulty. The patient is unable to protrude his tongue. Marked changes occur in the epiglottis. The vocal cords are thickened by an infiltration of grayish yellow material, giving rise to the hoarseness so early observed. In some patients similar yellowish and cream-colored deposits are sometimes observed upon the labia majora, the urethral orifice, the scrotum, the gluteal folds, and the axillae. Patchy alopecia is common.

Hyperkeratotic wartlike or nodular lesions are encountered on the dorsal aspects of the hands, fingers, elbows, and knees. The eyelid margins contain small yellowish transparent pearly papules in about two thirds of the patients. Drüsen of Bruch's membrane are seen in the fundi in half of the patients. Sickle-shaped calcifications dorsal and lateral to the sella turcica in skull roentgenograms are pathognomonic, according to Rook. Bauer et al reported a case, with electron microscopic studies and chemical analysis of cultured fibroblasts, in which intracellular hexuronic acid was increased 3–4-fold, strongly suggesting a lysosomal storage disease. The relationship of these findings to the collagen changes discussed below is not known.

The disease is inherited as an autosomal recessive trait.

Distinctive histologic features are extreme dilation of the blood vessels, thickening of their walls, and infiltration of the dermis and subcutaneous tissue with extracellular hyaline deposits, which are also

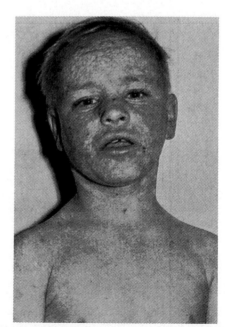

Figure 26–13. Lipoid proteinosis. Yellowish infiltrated plaques over entire face, lips, and buccal mucosa. Notice enlarged tongue. (Courtesy of Dr. J. C. M. Grosfeld and associates, The Netherlands.)

demonstrable in the vessel walls. Normal skin and mucous membranes also show changes of endothelial proliferation of the subpapillary vessels and a homogeneous thickening of the walls of the deeper vessels. Types IV and V collagen are increased around vessels, and types I and III collagen are reduced in quantity and abnormally hydrolyzed in the dermis. Olsen et al found elevated $\alpha 1$ (IV) collagen mRNA levels in lipoid proteins. Thus it is hypothesized that the defect affects endothelial cells, with a resultant increase in the production of basement membrane zone collagen, and it also affects fibroblasts by a decreased synthesis of altered fibrous collagen.

Differentiation from erythropoietic protoporphyria may be difficult, especially histologically; Van der Walt and Heyl found the progressive hyalinization of sweat glands in lipoid proteinosis the most "striking and constant" difference.

Bauer EA, et al: Lipoid proteinosis: in vivo and in vitro evidence for a liposomal storage disease. J Invest Dermatol 1981, 76:119.
Burnett JW, et al: Lipoid proteinosis. Am J Dis Child 1963, 105:81.
Caplan RM: Visceral involvement in lipoid proteinosis. Arch Dermatol 1967, 95:149.
Caro I: Lipoid proteinosis. Int J Dermatol 1978, 17:388.
Harper JI, et al: Lipoid proteinosis: an inherited disorder of collagen metabolism. Br J Dermatol 1985, 113:145.
Moy LS, et al: Lipoid proteinosis: ultrastructural and biochemical studies. JAAD 1987, 16:1.
Olsen DR, et al: Expression of basement membrane zone genes coding for Type IV procollagen and laminin by human skin fibroblasts in vitro. J Invest Dermatol 1988, 90:734.
Rook A: Lipoid proteinosis: Urbach-Wiethe disease. Br J Dermatol 1976, 94:341.
Smith N, et al: Lipoid proteinosis. Brt J Dermatol 1976, 95:48.

ANGIOKERATOMA CORPORIS DIFFUSUM

Also known as *glycolipid lipidosis* and *Fabry's* or *Anderson-Fabry disease*, in this storage disease ceramide trihexoside (galactosyl galactosyl glucosyl ceramide) accumulates in the skin and viscera.

The skin lesions are widespread punctate telangiectatic vascular papules, which on first inspection suggest purpura. Some show hyperkeratotic tops, but this is less prominent than in other forms of angiokeratoma. Myriads of tiny telangiectatic papules are seen, especially on the lower extremities, the scrotum and penis, the lower trunk, the axillae, and the lips, where the small angiokeratomas are most numerous on the midline of the lower lip. Hair growth is scanty.

The deposits of glycolipids (ceramide trihexoside) occur most importantly in the endothelial cells, fibroblasts, and pericytes of the dermis, in the heart, in the kidneys, and in the autonomic nervous system. Cardiac disease (as revealed by abnormal electrocardiogram) and renal insufficiency bring death, usually in the fifth decade. Edema of the ankles, paralyses, paresthesias manifested by a burning sensation of

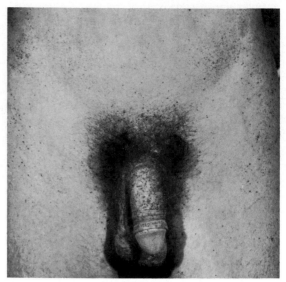

Figure 26–14. Angiokeratoma corporis diffusum. (Courtesy of Dr. H. B. Curry.)

the hands and feet, and hypohidrosis are often present. Abnormal vascular structures are noted in the conjunctiva and eye-grounds. Distinctive whorl-like opacities of the cornea occur in 90 per cent, and 50 per cent develop characteristic spokelike cataracts in the posterior capsular location. The urine in addition to albuminuria may show "Maltese cross" material on polaroscopy, and glycolipids in the form of "mulberry cells" in the sediment.

Brady et al found that the cause of the disease is deficiency of alpha-galactosidase A. Inheritance is by an X-linked recessive route. Female heterozygotes may show evidence of the disease in varying degrees. The diagnosis can be confirmed by finding diminished levels of alpha-galactosidase A in leukocytes, serum, tears, skin fibroblasts, or amniotic fluid cells.

Histologically, there is dilatation of capillaries in the papillary dermis, resulting in endothelial-lined lacunae filled with blood and surrounded by acanthotic and hyperkeratotic epidermis. Electron microscopy reveals characteristic electron-dense bodies in endothelial cells, pericytes, and fibroblasts. These were well illustrated in the case reported by Hwang et al. They have also been found in normal skin in affected adults and in a year-old boy without telangiectases.

There is no treatment, but phenytoin was shown by Lockman et al in a double-blind crossover study to afford significant relief of pain. Infusions of normal plasma, hemodialysis, and renal transplantation have been tried; the latter, however, has not afforded symptomatic relief or overall prognosis, and is not recommended.

Fucosidosis. Angiokeratomas identical with those of Fabry's disease occur in the type III form of this rare disorder. It is distinguished by the presence of granule-filled vacuoles in endothelial and other cells, and lamellar bodies in Schwann cells. The defect, a lack of alpha-L-fucosidase, is transmitted as an autosomal recessive trait. Progressive mental and motor deterioration begins in infancy and progresses, with death by age 18 or 20 as a rule. Among eight cases collected from the literature by Edgar Smith, six had telangiectases of palms and soles, six had coarse thickening of the skin of the face; all had severe mental retardation, weakness, and spasticity. The two oldest had myoclonic seizures.

Sialidosis. Another disease presenting with angiokeratomas is caused by neuraminidase deficiency, which causes intracellular accumulation of sialilated oligosaccharides. Intellectual impairment, psychomotor disturbance, myoclonus, cerebellar ataxia, skeletal abnormalities, and coarse facies have been reported.

Additionally, one patient with beta-galactosidase deficiency, two with betamannosidase deficiency, and several patients without any enzyme deficiency, have been reported to have angiokeratoma corporis diffusum, as reported by Holmes et al and Marsden et al.

Brady RO, et al: Enzymatic defect in Fabry's disease. Ceramide trihexosidase deficiency. N Engl J Med 1967, 276:1163.

Crovato F, et al: Angiokeratoma corporis diffusum and normal enzyme activities. JAAD 1985, 12:885.

Hashimoto K, et al: Angiokeratoma corporis diffusum (Fabry disease). Arch Dermatol 1976, 112:1416.

Holmes RC, et al: Angiokeratoma corporis diffusum in a patient with normal enzyme activities. JAAD 1984, 10:384.

Hwang RY, et al: Fabry's disease. J Assoc Milit Dermatol 1984, 10:26.

Kang WH, et al: Generalized anhidrosis associated with Fabry's disease. JAAD 1987, 17:883.

Marsden J, et al: Widespread angiokeratomas without evidence of metabolic disease. Arch Dermatol 1987, 123:1125.

NECROBIOSIS LIPOIDICA
(Necrobiosis Lipoidica Diabeticorum)

Necrobiosis lipoidica is characterized by well-circumscribed, hard, depressed, waxy, yellow-brown, atrophic patches on the skin of persons (women three times more commonly than men) who may also have diabetes mellitus.

The earliest clinical lesions are sharply bordered, elevated, red papules 2 mm in diameter, which may be capped by a slight scale and which do not disappear under diascopic pressure. Later the lesions develop into irregularly round or oval scleroderma-like lesions with well-defined borders and a smooth glistening (glazed) surface. The center becomes depressed and sulfur-yellow, so that there is formed a firm yellowish plaque surrounded by a broad violet-red or pink border. In the yellow portion numerous telangiectases and small dark macules are evident. Scaling, or more often crusting, may be evident. Ulceration is not unusual.

The commonest location of the lesions is on one or, more often, both shins. About 85 per cent occur

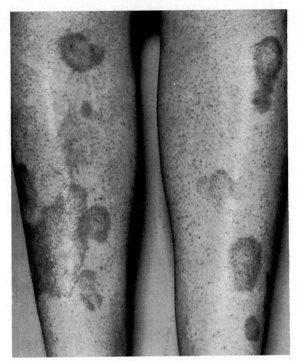

Figure 26–15. Necrobiosis lipoidica.

on the legs. A much less common site is on the forearms; and lesions have been reported on the trunk, face, scalp, and palms and soles.

More than half of the patients have diabetes mellitus, and a portion of the remainder have an abnormal glucose tolerance curve. This may precede the onset of frank diabetes. Control of the diabetes does not influence the course of the disease. Its frequency is three per 1000 diabetic patients, according to Muller and Winkelmann.

The histologic changes arise chiefly in the dermis where there is a replacement of the collagen fiber fasciculi by neutral fat. Present are necrobiotic foci of collagen, elongated and lying horizontally, in which the collagen appears pale, homogenized, and without nuclei. Within these areas the elastic fibers are absent (Weigert), while in the intervening tissue they are fragmented, sparse, and clumped. When stained with Sudan III the thickened fibers in the necrobiotic areas show a diffuse, light brownish red color. Between them are rows of tiny, bright orange-red droplets. A granulomatous infiltrate (palisading granuloma) consisting of Langhans giant cells, histiocytic monocytes, and lymphocytes is greatest near the degenerated collagen. It is predominantly perivascular. The primary injury occurs in the blood vessels where there is a capillary-endothelial proliferation with thickening of the walls. About the vessels and profusely scattered in the upper part of the dermis are fine brown granules of hemosiderin. Sclerosis occurs in the lower reticular dermis.

Miescher's granuloma (granulomatosis disciformis chronica et progressiva) is one or a few yellowish red, sharply marginated, smooth plaques similar in appearance to necrobiosis lipoidica. It occurs usually on the head and neck, hands, or forearms, commonly in middle-aged, nondiabetic women. Histologically there are multinucleate giant cells and granuloma formation without necrobiosis. Because of its clinical findings it is in the differential diagnosis of necrobiosis lipoidica.

Ullmann and Dahl studied necrobiosis lipoidica by direct immunofluorescence microscopy and demonstrated IgM, IgA, C3, and fibrinogen in the blood vessel walls of involved skin and IgM, C3, and fibrinogen at the dermal-epidermal junction in a continuous band. Massive deposits of fibrinogen were seen in necrobiotic areas of all cases studied. They suggested that an immune-complex vasculitis may be involved in the pathogenesis of necrobiosis lipoidica. A more recent study by Quimby et al confirmed these findings.

Treatment, after control of the diabetes is achieved, is not completely satisfactory. The best results have occurred after intralesional injections of triamcinolone suspension into the inflammatory papules. Some cases have benefited by excision and skin grafts, but others have had recurrences in the grafts or at the edges of the grafts.

A combination of dipyridamole (Persantine), 225 mg, and aspirin, 1 gm daily, was reported to be effective by Eldor and his associates in a patient with spontaneous aggregation of platelets. Ely has found that they may have to be continued for three or four months before results are obtained. Trental (pentoxyfylline) may also be helpful in doses of 400 mg t.i.d. as shown by Ely and by Littler et al.

Karkavitsas et al treated seven patients with lesions of six months' to six years' duration, four with diabetes, two ulcerated for four months and two years, with aspirin, about 3 grains (3.5 mg/kg) every 48 hours, or (later) every 72 hours. The ulcerated lesions healed in two months and six months respectively. Improvement occurred in all patients within four months, and in some as early as one month. However, Statham et al were unable to reproduce these optimistic findings in their double-blind controlled study.

Boulton AJM, et al: Necrobiosis lipoidica diabeticorum. JAAD 1988, 18:530.

Christianson HB, et al: Annular atrophic plaques of the face: a clinical and histologic study. Arch Dermatol 1969, 100:703.

Clegg DO, et al: Necrobiosis lipoidica associated with jejunoileal bypass surgery. Arch Dermatol 1982, 118:135.

Clement M, et al: Squamous cell carcinoma arising in long-standing necrobiosis lipoidica. Arch Dermatol 1985, 121:24.

Cohen IK: Necrobiosis lipoidica and granuloma annulare. JAAD 1984, 10:123.

Dahl MV: Immunofluorescence, necrobiosis lipoidica, and blood vessels. Arch Dermatol 1988, 124:1417.

Dubin BJ, et al: The surgical treatment of necrobiosis lipoidica diabeticorum. Plast Reconstr Surg 1977, 60:421.

Eldor A, et al: Treatment of necrobiosis lipoidica with aspirin and dipyridamole. N Engl J Med 1978, 248:1033.

Ely PH: Pentoxifylline in skin ills due to poor vascularity. Skin Allergy News 1986, 17 (No. 5):13.

Karkavitsas K, et al: Aspirin in the management of necrobiosis lipoidica. Acta Dermatover (Stockh) 1982, 62:183.

Littler CM, et al: Pentoxifylline for necrobiosis lipoidica diabeticorum. JAAD 1987, 17:314.

Masotti G, et al: Differential inhibition of prostacyclin production and platelet aggregation by aspirin. Lancet 1979, 2:1213.

Mehregan AH, et al: Miescher's granuloma of the face: a variant of the necrobiosis lipoidica–granuloma annulare spectrum. Arch Dermatol 1973, 107:62.

Quimby SR, et al: Necrobiosis lipoidica diabeticorum. Cutis 1989, 43:213.

Idem: The cutaneous immunopathology of NLD. Arch Dermatol 1988, 124:1364.

Rhodes EL: Fibrinolytic agents in treatment of necrobiosis lipoidica. Br J Dermatol 1976, 95:673.

Stratham B, et al: A randomized double blind comparison of an aspirin dipyridamole combination in the treatment of necrobiosis lipoidica. Acta Dermatol 1981, 61:220.

Ullman S, et al: Necrobiosis lipoidica: an immunofluorescent study. Arch Dermatol 1977, 113:1671.

Wilkin JK: Perilesional heparin injections for necrobiosis lipoidica. JAAD 1983, 8:904.

DIABETIC DERMADROMES

In addition to necrobiosis lipoidica diabeticorum there are many cutaneous signs in this common endocrinopathy. Sibbald and Schachter published an excellent review of these in 1984, as did Huntley in 1982.

Diabetic Dermopathy (Shin Spots). Hyperpigmented and retracted atrophic scars on the shins of young adults are seen more frequently in patients with diabetes mellitus than in normal persons. They are present in 50 per cent of diabetics, most commonly in men.

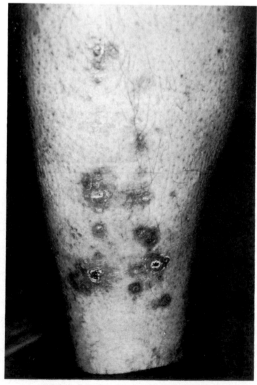

Figure 26–16. Diabetic dermopathy.

Diabetic Bullosis. Noninflammatory blistering, most often in acral locations, characterize these lesions. They heal spontaneously in four to five weeks, usually without scarring.

Collet and Toonstra reported a case of diabetes with spontaneous bullae on the hands alone, and reviewed 44 published cases, in 21 of which biopsy was done. Six were subepidermal and 13 intraepidermal—but might have been subepidermal initially, so quickly does the floor reepithelialize. Electron microscopic studies showed separation at the lamina lucida level in their cases. This process is, then, heterogeneous, and is not well characterized. Immunofluorescence is negative. Ultraviolet light, trauma, neuropathy, and cation imbalance have all been hypothesized to be inciting factors to the blistering.

Bernstein et al reported in 1983 a reduced threshold to suction-induced blistering in insulin-dependent diabetics. Among bullous pemphigoid patients, diabetes is common.

Diabetic Pruritus. Generalized pruritus in diabetics is not unusual; however, some believe that excessively "dry" skin (xerotic eczema) is really the cause rather than some endocrinologic disorder. Pruritus vulvae et ani in the diabetic as well as in the normal person may be due to candidosis.

Carotenosis. This is a yellowish discoloration of the skin, especially of the palms and soles, sometimes seen in diabetics who have carotenemia. Of the 50

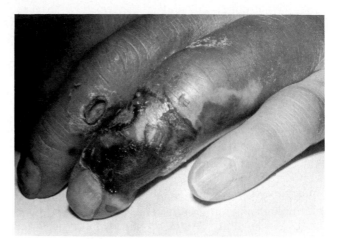

Figure 26–18. Diabetic gangrene. (Courtesy of Dr. Axel W. Hoke.)

per cent of diabetics who have carotenemia, about 10 per cent have carotenosis. The sclerae remain white. There may be night blindness (delayed dark adaptation) as a result of reduced conversion of carotene to vitamin A in the liver.

Diabetic Gangrene. This occurs in diabetics with arteriosclerosis obliterans. The latter condition is seen more frequently in diabetics than in other persons.

Other Associated Conditions. Erysipelaslike erythema of the legs or feet, sweating disturbances, paresthesias of the legs, mal perforans ulcerations, a predisposition to certain infections such as mucormycosis, Group B streptococcal infections, nonclostridial gas gangrene, and malignant external otitis due to *Pseudomonas*, and in addition waxy skin and stiff joints, scleredema, disseminated granuloma annulare, eruptive xanthomas, skin tags, rubeosis of the face, hemochromatosis, lipodystrophies, acanthosis nigricans, cutaneous perforating diseases, Dupuytren's contracture, and finger-pebbling are various abnormalities seen more often in diabetic patients.

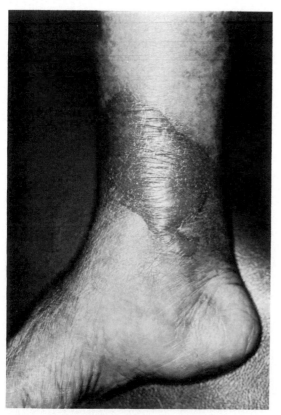

Figure 26–17. Bullous eruption of diabetes mellitus.

Bauer MF, et al: Diabetic dermangiopathy. Br J Dermatol 1970, 83:528.

Idem: Pigmented pretibial patches. Arch Dermatol 1966, 93:282.

Benson PM, et al: Group B streptococcal blistering distal dactylitis in an adult diabetic. JAAD 1987, 17:310.

Bernstein JE, et al: Reduced threshold to suction-induced blister formation in insulin-dependent diabetics. JAAD 1983, 8:790.

Binkley GW: Dermopathy in the diabetic syndrome. Arch Dermatol 1965, 92:265.

Cantwell AR, et al: Idiopathic bullae in diabetes: bullosis diabeticorum. Arch Dermatol 1967, 96:42.

Collet JT, et al: Bullosis diabeticorum: a case with lesions restricted to the hands. Diabetes Care 1985, 8:177.

Flier JS: Metabolic importance of acanthosis nigricans. Arch Dermatol 1985, 121:193.

Hanna W, et al: Pathologic features of diabetic thick skin. JAAD 1987, 16:546.

Huntley AC: The cutaneous manifestations of diabetes mellitus. JAAD 1982, 7:427.

Idem: Eruptive lipofibromata. Arch Dermatol 1983, 119:612.

Idem: Finger pebbles: a common finding in diabetes mellitus. JAAD 1986, 14:612.

Idem: Threshold to suction-induced blister formation in insulin-dependent diabetics. JAAD 1984, 10:305.

James WD, et al: Bullous eruption of diabetes mellitus. Arch Dermatol 1980, 116:1191.

Kahana M, et al: Skin tags: A cutaneous marker for diabetes mellitus. Acta Derm Venereol (Stockh) 1987, 67:175.

Sibbald RG: The skin and diabetes mellitus. Int J Dermatol 1984, 23:567.

Toonstra J: Bullosis diabeticorum: report of a case and review of the literature. JAAD 1985, 13:799.

AMYLOIDOSES

AMYLOIDOSIS

Because of its multifaceted nature, both clinically and etiologically, amyloidosis has been poorly understood. While many recent advances have provided insights as to the types and origins of the deposited material, advances in therapy have not been similarly forthcoming. Amyloidosis has been divided into primary (idiopathic) and secondary amyloidosis, which may be either systemic (visceral) or cutaneous. The following classification is based on material reported from the Armed Forces Institute of Pathology by Brownstein and Helwig.

Classification of Cutaneous Amyloidoses

I. Primary systemic amyloidosis
   Cutaneous—Papules, plaques, nodules, tumefactions, purpura, alopecia, pallor, nail abnormalities, bullae
   Mucous membrane—Macroglossia, dysphonia, dysphagia, glossitis, xerostomia, macrocheilia
II. Secondary systemic amyloidosis
   Absence of cutaneous, mucocutaneous, or subcutaneous lesions
III. Primary localized cutaneous amyloidosis
   A. Macular amyloidosis
   B. Lichen amyloidosis
   C. Nodular amyloidosis
IV. Secondary localized cutaneous amyloidosis
   Microdeposits in association with various cutaneous tumors.

The primary systemic type involves mesenchymal tissue, the tongue, the heart, the gastrointestinal tract, and the skin. Myeloma is also included in this type.

Secondary systemic amyloidosis is the amyloid involvement of the adrenals, liver, spleen, and kidney as a result of some chronic disease such as tuberculosis, lepromatous leprosy, Hodgkin's disease, carcinoma, rheumatoid arthritis, ulcerative colitis, schistosomiasis, or syphilis. The parenchymatous organs are involved but the skin is not. Certain dermatoses such as hidradenitis suppurativa, stasis ulcers, psoriatic arthritis, and dystrophic epidermolysis bullosa may be complicated by systemic amyloidosis.

Primary localized cutaneous amyloidosis refers to clinically significant deposition of amyloid, limited to the skin, unassociated with any underlying dermatologic or systemic disease. Secondary localized cutaneous amyloidosis relates to clinically unrecognizable microdeposits of amyloid sometimes found in association with a variety of skin tumors, without known significance. Hicks et al and Ratz et al have reviewed these types.

Advances in knowledge of the various types of amyloid deposited in each clinical type of disease have provided better insights into their pathogenesis. Despite identical histologic and electron microscopic findings, the protein composition of the amyloid differs in different clinical forms. Amyloid has three distinct components: protein-derived amyloid fibers, a glycoprotein P component, and ground substance.

The amyloid fibril proteins in primary systemic (so-called immunocytic or plasma-cell-dyscrasia-associated) amyloidosis are composed of protein AL. This is derived from the immunoglobulin light chain, usually of the lambda subtype, and is often only a fragment of it, particularly from the aminoterminal end or variable region. This same type of amyloid, AL, is also found in nodular or tumefactive amyloidosis, which may be produced by extramedullary locally present plasma cells.

The amyloid fibrils in secondary systemic amyloidosis, and in the type associated with Muckle-Wells syndrome and with familial Mediterranean fever, are of the type designated AA. This is unrelated to immunoglobulin. Its precursor is serum amyloid A protein, which is an acute phase reactant, increased in various inflammatory states.

In macular amyloidosis and lichenoid amyloidosis, amyloid fibrils are formed by local epidermal damage from tonofilament degeneration and apoptosis (dropping off). Keratinlike material is found in it immunohistochemically, staining positively with EKH4, a monoclonal keratin antibody. It has been named amyloid K, for keratin type. Immunoglobulins, especially IgM, are found in it by direct immunofluorescence, although this is thought to be the result of nonspecific absorption.

Amyloid is weakly PAS-positive and diastase-resistant, Congo-red–positive, purple with crystal violet, negative to slightly reactive with the oil-red-O stain, faintly positive or negative with the aldehyde-fuchsin stain, and positive with the colloidal iron technique. Amyloid stained with thioflavine-T and examined with ultraviolet light exhibits green birefringence under polarized light. By rotation of the polarized light, amyloid fibrils may appear green and then orange (dichroism). Yanagihara and Mehregan reported that amyloid stains an intense, bright orange with Pagoda Red, RIT Scarlet No. 5, or RIT Cardinal Red No. 9; the hyalin of lipoid proteinosis, juvenile hyalin fibromatosis, lichen planus, and discoid LE, and the elastin of elastosis, and the material in three cases of colloid milium did not stain. In hematoxylin and eosin–stained sections, amyloid stains eosinophilic, like collagen. Electron microscopy reveals amyloid to have a characteristic fibrillar structure which consists of straight, nonbranching, nonanastomosing, often irregularly arranged filaments. In general, measurements of the diameters of the fibrillar elements in amyloidosis indicate they are about 100 Å.

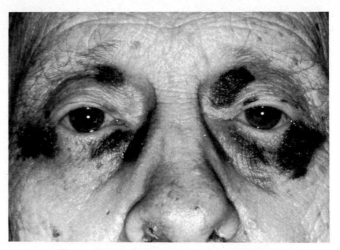

Figure 26–20. Primary systemic amyloidosis.

Systemic Amyloidosis

In *primary systemic amyloidosis*, the cutaneous eruption begins as a shiny, smooth, firm, flat-topped, or spherical papule of waxy color, which because of its tenseness has the appearance of a translucent vesicle. These lesions coalesce to form nodules and plaques of various sizes and, in some cases, bandlike lesions. The regions about the eye, nose, and mouth, as well as the mucocutaneous junctions, are commonly involved. Glossitis, with macroglossia, occurs in at least 20 per cent of cases, and may be an early symptom. The tongue becomes painful and greatly enlarged. Furrows develop, and patches of a necrotic, purulent appearance are seen. The mucous membranes of the lips and cheeks have a similar hypertrophic appearance.

Purpuric lesions and ecchymoses are common,

chiefly on eyelids and limbs and in the mouth. Bullae are a rare but important clinical manifestation of amyloidosis, usually associated with purpura as reported by Westermark et al and Beacham et al. Alopecia (as in Wheeler et al's case), nodular lesions along superficial blood vessels (as in Henry et al's patient), postproctoscopic palpebral purpura from increased intrathoracic pressure (as discussed by Slagel et al), nail dystrophy, pigmentary changes, and sclerodermatous changes, are other types of lesions seen. Winkelmann et al have recently reported *"amyloid elastosis"*—a unique cutaneous and systemic pattern of amyloidosis, with an extensive eruption of yellow-brown, rubbery, discrete papules and nodules, 0.3 to 2 cm in diameter, sparing only the head, hands and feet, and mucosae, in which elastic fibers in both skin and visceral blood vessels were coated with amyloid. Cutaneous manifestations occur in 25 to 50 per cent of cases of systemic amyloidosis. Pains and aches in the back are produced by amyloid changes in skeletal muscles.

Macular Amyloidosis

Typical cases exhibit moderately pruritic, symmetrically distributed, brown, rippled macules characteristically located in the interscapular region of the back, but occasionally the thighs, shins, arms, breasts, and buttocks may be involved. It is a chronic condition of the middle years of life and darker-skinned individuals of Latin, Oriental, or Middle Eastern ancestry seem to be predisposed. Histologically, melanin granules may be found in the stratum corneum and lying free and within melanophages in the papillary dermis. Amyloid masses characteristically are present in several consecutive dermal papillae and these are separated from other affected regions by normal areas of variable length. Involved papillae may present clinically as a unique sort of punctate purpura, black circular macules 0.3 to 0.6 mm in diameter.

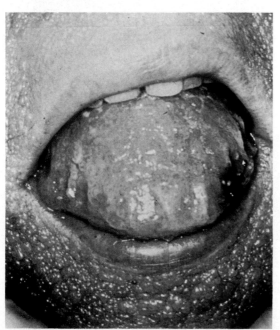

Figure 26–19. Primary systemic amyloidosis: Progressive enlargement of the tongue with translucent papules and purpura of the tongue and skin.

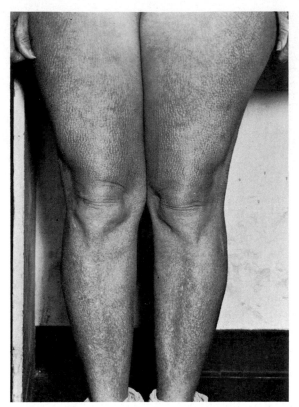

Figure 26–21. Macular amyloidosis cutis of both shins and thighs. Note parallel ripples, defined by rete ridges. (Courtesy of Drs. R. Montgomery and W. B. Hurlbut.)

Lichen Amyloidosis

Lichen amyloidosis is characterized by the appearance of paroxysmally itchy lichenoid papules, typically on the shins, with intense pruritus. The elementary lesions are small, brown, discrete, slightly scaly papules, which group to form infiltrated large moniliform plaques that resemble lichen chronicus simplex. It may occur on the thighs, the forearms, and even on the back, in addition to the shins.

A less frequent form is a large lesion resembling hypertrophic lichen planus. The large papules coalesce to form sharply delineated plaques over the shins. In some cases the eruption is widespread on the trunk and consists of reticulated, pigmented shagreen patches in which the amyloid papules may be discerned.

The histology shows foci of amyloid material situated in the dermal papillae; however, the amyloid is separated from the epidermis by a narrow band of collagen. There may be an inflammatory reaction. The epidermis exhibits nonspecific changes that often include moderate acanthosis, hyperkeratosis, and hyperpigmentation of the basal layer.

In the differential diagnosis, colloid milium, lipoid proteinosis, and the cutaneous manifestations of systemic amyloidosis are to be considered. Clinically, lichen simplex chronicus, hypertrophic lichen planus, and systemic amyloidosis are the diseases to be differentiated.

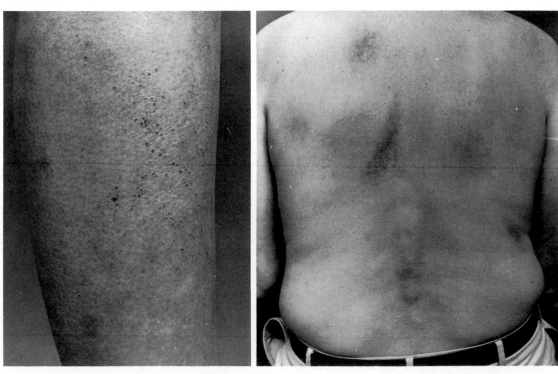

Figure 26–22. Purpuric intrapapillary macular amyloidosis of the shin (left) and back (right).

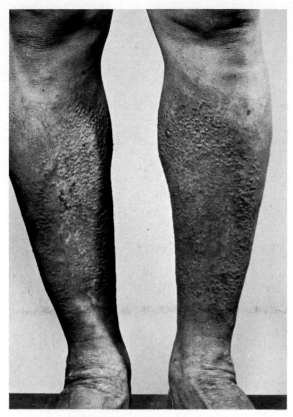

Figure 26–23. Lichen amyloidosis.

Treatment of lichen amyloidosis is frequently unsatisfactory. Marschalko et al reported success with etretinate, and this is worth trying. Wong reported good results with dermabrasion in seven cases, with relief of itching in all and no recurrence in five to seven years. Topical high strength corticosteroids with occlusion are beneficial. Intralesional corticosteroid therapy is effective when small areas are involved. Rubbing undiluted DMSO into the lesions appears to give considerable relief of itching and to do no harm. Baker reported improvement in lesions and relief of pruritus from topical use of DMSO under occlusion, in a man with extensive lichen amyloidosis.

Nodular Amyloidosis

In this rare form of primary localized cutaneous amyloidosis, single or multiple nodules or tumefactions may be found on the extremities, trunk, genitals, or face. The overlying epidermis may appear atrophic or anetodermic and may resemble large bullae. The dermis and subcutis may be seen microscopically to be diffusely infiltrated with amyloid. The lesions may contain numerous plasma cells.

As discussed previously, the amyloid in these patients is immunoglobulin-derived AL, as is seen in primary systemic amyloidosis, and is unrelated to keratinocyte-related amyloid or to AA amyloid. Up to 50 per cent of cases may evolve into systemic amyloidosis, so evaluation at regular intervals for systemic disease is advisable. Northcutt et al and Truhan et al have recently reported patients with this type of disease. Truhan et al's patient was successfully treated with the CO_2 laser.

Familial Syndromes Associated with Amyloidosis

Other familial syndromes have been reported to have types of systemic and localized amyloidosis. They include familial Mediterranean fever, Muckle-Wells syndrome, familial amyloid polyneuropathy, and hereditary cerebral amyloidosis.

Macroscopically, on section, structures infiltrated with amyloid appear to consist of glassy red material. Microscopically, the amyloid appears in the shape of cylinders, flakes, or rods except in the nodular or tumefactive type, in which plasma cells, foreign-body giant cells, and calcification are often present. Some dermal blood vessels are usually dilated and the homogeneous eosinophilic amyloid surrounds and forms a part of the wall of many blood vessels. In generalized amyloidosis the infiltrations are so diffuse that they tend to obliterate the structure of the arterioles. In the skin, amyloid is deposited chiefly in the papillae at the expense of the elastic tissue, which is almost completely destroyed in these areas. The striking change is the homogenization, which may affect the entire dermis. Tissue reaction of a high degree is absent in all lesions of cases seen. Cutaneous involvement in primary systemic amyloidosis occurs in 25 to 50 per cent of cases.

In *secondary systemic amyloidosis* there are no skin lesions attributable to amyloid. Biopsy of normal skin may be positive for perivascular amyloid in slightly over half the cases.

Effective treatment for primary systemic amyloidosis is not yet available. Cardiac insufficiency may result from damage to the musculature of the heart. A progressive and downward course is to be expected in the plasma-cell-dyscrasia–related, or immunocytic, disease. Many patients ultimately develop multiple myeloma or Waldenstrom's macroglobulinemia. In 229 patients studied by Kyle et al, the median survival was 13 months for patients without myeloma, and five months for myeloma cases. In secondary systemic amyloidosis the underlying chronic inflammatory disease state should be treated definitively. Camorian et al reported resolution of factor X deficiency and amyloid adenopathy under treatment with melphalan and prednisone.

Melphalan therapy has had limited success in cases of amyloidosis associated with myeloma. There are several published reports of restoration of lost renal function in cases of secondary systemic amyloidosis by giving 7–15 gm/day of dimethyl sulfoxide (DMSO). The only side effects are mild nausea and an unpleasant breath odor. Ravid et al recently reported success in seven patients. There were no adverse side effects. Secondary infections are treated vigorously with antibiotics, and corticosteroids are of benefit temporarily.

Baher S: Lichen amyloidosus. Int J Dermatol 1981, 20:565.

Beacham BE, et al: Bullous amyloidoses. JAAD 1980, 3:506.

Beber T, et al: Hemorrhagic bullous amyloidosis. Arch Dermatol 1988, 124:1683.

Breathnach SM: The cutaneous amyloidoses. Arch Dermatol 1985, 121:470.

Idem: Amyloid and amyloidosis. JAAD 1988, 18:1.

Brownstein MH, et al: The cutaneous amyloidoses I and II. Arch Dermatol 1970, 102:8.

Idem: Systemic amyloidosis complicating dermatoses. Arch Dermatol 1970, 102:1.

Camoriano JK, et al: Resolution of acquired factor X deficiency and amyloidosis with melphalan and prednisone therapy. N Engl J Med 1987, 316:1133.

De Pietro WP: Primary familial cutaneous amyloidosis. Arch Dermatol 1981, 117:639.

Fritz DA, et al: Unusual longevity in primary systemic amyloidosis. Am J Med 1989, 86:245.

Hashimoto K, et al: Lichen amyloidosus. Arch Dermatol 1971, 104:648.

Idem: Nylon brush macular amyloidosis. Arch Dermatol 1987, 123:633.

Hashimoto K: Progress on cutaneous amyloidoses. J Invest Dermatol 1984, 82:1.

Henry RB, et al: Vascular amyloid in a patient with multiple myeloma. JAAD 1986, 15:379.

Hicks BC, et al: Primary cutaneous amyloidosis of the auricular concha. JAAD 1988, 18:19.

Jambrosic J, et al: Lichen amyloidosus. Am J Dermatopathol 1984, 6:151.

Johnson TM, et al: Bullous amyloidosis. Cutis 1989, 43:346.

Kitajima Y, et al: Nodular primary cutaneous amyloidosis. Arch Dermatol 1986, 122:1425.

Koch SE: Acquired macular pigmentation. Arch Dermatol 1986, 122:463.

Kyle RA, et al: Amyloidosis (AL). Mayo Clin Proc 1983, 58:665.

MacDonald DM, et al: Immunofluorescence studies in primary cutaneous amyloidosis. Br J Dermatol 1977, 96:635.

Marschalko M, et al: Etretinate for the treatment of lichen amyloidosus. Arch Dermatol 1988, 124:657.

Northcutt AD, et al: Nodular cutaneous amyloidosis involving the vulva. Arch Dermatol 1985, 121:518.

Norwood CF: Amyloidosis. J Assoc Milit Dermatol 1985, 11:74.

Piamphongsant T: An immunofluorescent study of cutaneous amyloidosis. Austral J Dermatol 1977, 18:29.

Ravid M, et al: Prolonged dimethylsulphoxide treatment in 13 patients with systemic amyloidosis. Ann Rheum Dis 1982, 41:587.

Ratz JL, et al: Cutaneous amyloidosis. JAAD 1981, 4:21.

Rubinow A: Skin involvement in generalized amyloidosis. Ann Intern Med 1978, 88:781.

Scheinberg MA, et al: DMSO and colchicine therapy in amyloid disease. Ann Rheum Dis 1989, 93:421.

Schwartz BK, et al: Acquired localized pigmentation. Arch Dermatol 1987, 123:633.

Slagel A, et al: Postproctoscopic periorbital purpura. Arch Dermatol 1986, 122:463.

Truhan AP, et al: Nodular primary localized cutaneous amyloidosis: immunohistochemical evaluation and treatment with the carbon dioxide laser. JAAD 1986, 14:1058.

Tuneau A, et al: A waxy plaque on the leg (nodular amyloidosis). Arch Dermatol 1988, 124:769.

Van Rijswijk MH, et al: DMSO in the treatment of AA amyloidosis. Ann NY Acad Sci 1983, 411:67.

Vasily DB, et al: Familial primary cutaneous amyloidosis. Arch Dermatol 1978, 114:1173.

Wang W-J, et al: Response of systemic amyloidosis to dimethyl sulfoxide. JAAD 1986, 15:402.

Westermark P, et al: Bullous amyloidosis. Arch Dermatol 1981, 117:782.

Wheeler GE, et al: Alopecia universalis. Arch Dermatol 1981, 117:815.

Winkelmann RK, et al: Amyloid elastosis. Arch Dermatol 1985, 121:498.

Wong C-K, et al: Dermabrasion for lichen amyloidosus. Arch Dermatol 1982, 118:302.

Yanagihara M, et al: Staining of amyloid with cotton dyes. Arch Dermatol 1984, 120:1184.

PORPHYRIN DISORDERS

Porphyrins are building blocks of all the hemoproteins, including hemoglobin. The photosensitivity of the skin in porphyria is due to the absorption of ultraviolet radiation in the Soret band (400 nm range), with emission of light in the 619–634 nm range: the absorbed energy activates O_2 into "singlet" O, which damages lysosomes and initiates the inflammatory response.

There are three main categories of porphyric disease, based upon the tissue in which the biochemical defect is localized: the erythropoietic, hepatic, and erythrohepatic classes. Congenital erythropoietic porphyria, or Gunther's disease, is the erythropoietic type. Acute intermittent porphyria, hereditary coproporphyria, variegate porphyria, and porphyria cutanea tarda are the hepatic forms. Erythropoietic protoporphyria, erythropoietic coproporphyria, and hepatoerythrocytic porphyria are the erythrohepatic types.

These are all caused by specific defects in the synthesis of heme, which is carried out as follows:

Delta-aminolevulinic acid (dALA) is synthesized in the mitochondrion by action of dALA synthetase. From it are formed, successively, porphobilinogen, uroporphyrin III, coproporphyrin III, and protoporphyrin IX. This reenters the mitochondrion to be acted upon by ferrochelatase to produce heme. Heme, by negative feedback, represses the production, or activity, of dALA synthetase; and if production of heme is blocked, dALA synthetase activity may be multiplied five to seven times over the normal. Heme production may be diminished by a hereditary lack of uroporphyrinogen decarboxylase in porphyria cutanea tarda (PCT) and hepatoerythropoietic porphyria, ferrochelatase in erythropoietic protoporphyria, uroporphyrinogen I synthetase in acute intermittent porphyria, coproporphyrinogen oxidase in hereditary coproporphyria, protoporphyrinogen oxidase in variegate porphyria, or uroporphyrinogen III cosynthetase in erythropoietic porphyria.

Disler et al, of the Porphyria Research Unit of the University of Cape Town, have reviewed the biochemical diagnosis of the porphyrias in detail and tabulated the findings in 11 kinds of porphyria, in red cells, plasma, urine, and feces.

PORPHYRIA CUTANEA TARDA (PCT)

Once known as idiopathic, symptomatic, or hepatic porphyria, PCT is characterized by photosensitivity resulting in bullae, especially on sun-exposed parts or areas subject to friction, trauma, or heat. The bullae rupture easily to form erosions or shallow ulcers. These heal with scarring and dyspigmentation. Lesions on the legs, especially the shins and dorsal feet, occur primarily in young women on birth control pills. There is hyperpigmentation of the skin, especially of the face, neck, and hands, and changes may occur in the hair color, especially from red to black. Hypertrichosis of the face, especially over the cheeks and temples, is seen. The face and neck, especially in the periorbital area, may show a pink to violaceous tint. Sclerodermatous thickenings with calcification may develop on the cheeks, on the back of the neck, in the preauricular areas, the ears, the thorax, the fingers, and the scalp. In the latter instance there is associated alopecia. Friedman et al have reported a direct relationship between the levels of uroporphyrins in the urine and the sclerodermatous change.

Liver cirrhosis or fatty degeneration occurs, with or without icterus. It is estimated that diabetes mellitus is present in 15 to 20 per cent of patients with PCT. PCT has occasionally been reported in association with lupus erythematosus, other autoimmune syndromes, hepatitis, and hepatic tumors. A history of heavy alcoholism is common.

Porphyria cutanea tarda occurs in two forms. A sporadic, nonfamilial form, the most common type, begins in middle age and has normal concentrations of the enzyme uroporphyrinogen decarboxylase; functionally, however, it has diminished activity in the liver. In the second, or familial form, there is an autosomal dominant inherited deficiency of uroporphyrinogen decarboxylase in the liver and red blood cells of patients and also of clinically unaffected family members. In these cases, which may occur at a younger age than the sporadic form, there is an approximate 50 per cent decrease in both the catalytic activity of the enzyme and the quantitative concentration of the protein. Rogers et al recently reported a kindred with reduced levels of erythrocyte uroporphyrinogen decarboxylase (UD) in 10 of 22 paternal relatives of the proband. None of the relatives had clinical PCT. DeSalamanca et al reported 56 cases with 259 relatives, of whom 35 per cent had reduced UD levels and 21 per cent had manifest or subclinical PCT.

PCT may be associated with hemochromatosis, carcinomatosis, Hodgkin's disease, or reticuloendotheliosis. Among the exogenous chemicals known to have caused PCT are the weed-killer 2,4,5-trichlorophenol, the fungicide hexachlorobenzene, ethyl alcohol, and estrogens.

Acquired toxic porphyria cutanea tarda resulting from hexachlorobenzene, a fungicide used on wheat in Turkey, was reported by Cam and Nigogosyan. More than 600 cases were observed during a five-year period, and the total incidence is estimated to have exceeded 4000. The lesions were bullous, became ulcerated, and healed with pigmented scars and epidermal inclusion cysts. Cripps et al have reviewed these cases.

Drug-Induced Porphyria. Drugs known to be ca-

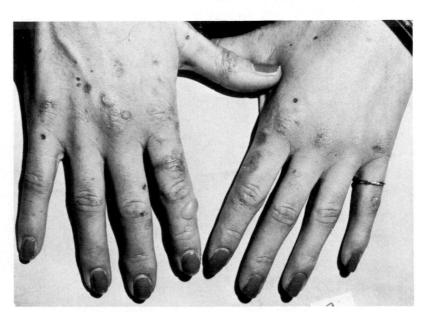

Figure 26–24. Porphyria cutanea tarda. (Courtesy of Dr. Adrian Johnson, Sydney.)

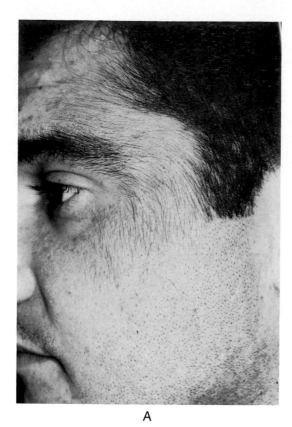

A

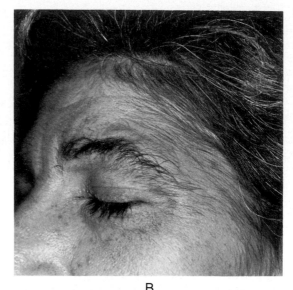

B

Figure 26–25. Hypertrichosis over the forehead, temples, and malar eminences in a man and in a woman, both with porphyria cutanea tarda. (Courtesy of Dr. C. P. De Feo.)

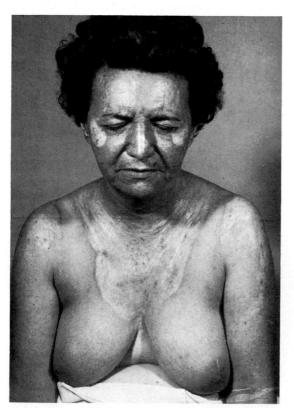

Figure 26–26. Porphyria cutanea tarda with sclerodermoid patches on the sun-exposed areas.

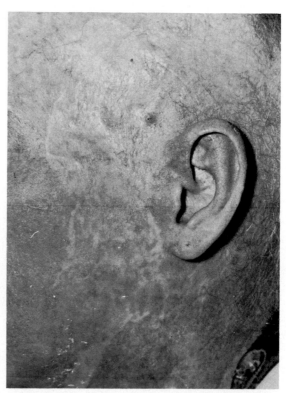

Figure 26–27. Scleroderma, alopecia, and calcium plaques in a 65 year old woman with porphyria cutanea tarda.

pable of inducing PCT are stilbestrol and other estrogens, chloroquine, tetracyclines, furosemide, nalidixic acid, dapsone, pyridoxine, and most recently naproxen (Judd et al). Poh-Fitzpatrick calls attention to the occurrence of marginal elevation of porphyrins in bullous dermatitis of hemodialysis; she points out that it is not really pseudoporphyria (which it has been called) and she hopes it will not be called pseudopseudoporphyria; she suggests the names *drug-induced* or *therapy-induced*. It is noteworthy, as she points out, that patients with these disorders do not develop the associated hypertrichosis, hyperpigmentation, or sclerodermoid features of true PCT.

The laboratory findings of PCT are diagnostic when the urine shows a pinkish or coral red fluorescence under the Wood's light. This denotes the presence in excessive amounts of both uro- and copro-porphyrin. However, it must not be forgotten that lead poisoning can also produce the same type of urine fluorescence. Porphobilinogen (PBG) is not found in abnormal amounts.

The 24-hour urine specimen usually contains less than 100 μg porphyrins in the normal person, whereas in the porphyric it may range from 300 to 70,000 μg. Kalb et al have documented that serum porphyrin levels parallel urinary porphyrin levels both at diagnosis and while on therapy, and this test is a more convenient method of following disease activity than 24-hour urine testing.

Adjarov and Ivanos found serum γ-glutamyl transpeptidase (γGTP) elevated to four times normal in all of 34 new cases of PCT. All patients were men. They reported this in 1973 and confirmed it in 1980. The serum level fell in all cases after repeated phlebotomy.

Histopathology. Biopsy reveals a noninflammatory bulla with an undulating, festooned base. PAS-positive thickening of blood vessel walls occurs. Direct immunofluorescence of sun-exposed skin shows IgG and C3 at the dermoepidermal junction and in the vessel walls in a linear pattern.

Treatment of PCT has advanced considerably in the past few years. Topi et al in 1984 reported 16 cases—14 sporadic and two familial—that recovered completely simply by avoiding hepatic toxins, especially alcohol—a method originally reported by Louis Brunsting in 1954. None appeared to have siderosis. Phlebotomy is effective. J. H. Epstein and Pinski have demonstrated an abnormal iron metabolism in PCT. They suggest that there is increased iron absorption. Chronic alcoholic liver disease is known to produce high serum iron levels through accelerated absorption.

A common procedure is to perform phlebotomy of 500 ml at two-week intervals until the 24-hour uroporphyrin levels are markedly reduced. Usually a total of 3000 to 5000 ml of blood is taken. As the level decreases, the skin lesions also involute. Usually after the second bloodletting a noticeable response is seen, but the response may be much slower

than this, and repeated venesection is a nuisance and may have complications. There is an alternative: low-dose Plaquenil (hydroxychloroquine). Malina et al and Cainelli et al compared the two methods and in general found hydroxychloroquine superior; both groups found it faster.

Chloroquine therapy, rejected initially because the usual dose (250 to 500 mg daily) produces extremely severe systemic reactions, and even death, has enjoyed increasing acceptance since Arnold in 1969 and Hunter in 1970 reported independently a response to very small doses, ranging from 30 mg of hydroxychloroquine daily, slowly increased to 100 mg (Arnold) or 125 mg twice a week (Hunter)—without systemic side effects. Arnold's patient never stopped drinking two 6-packs of beer every day, but despite this he responded well and did not relapse. Malina reported 40 patients thus treated in 1977. Hunter more recently suggests 125 mg twice a week, plus chelation with D-penicillamine if the response is slow. However, Chlumska et al reported clearing in 34 patients on 125 mg of chloroquine twice a week, without significant changes in liver biopsies. This has been confirmed more recently by Ashton et al, who induced 10 remissions in seven patients. One heavy drinker remained in remission. Goetz et al showed that the effect of chloroquine is to reduce the activity of delta-aminolevulinic acid synthetase.

Miyanchi et al have used repeated small-volume plasmapheresis and induced remission after 20 treatments over a 24-week period.

Desferrioxamine subcutaneously is valuable in selected cases, and Rocchi et al showed that it was effective intravenously in doses of 200 mg/kg in 500 ml of saline solution infused over 12 hours, once weekly at first, then every 10 days. Vitamin C, 500 mg three times daily by mouth, is given concurrently.

HEPATOERYTHROPOIETIC PORPHYRIA

Piñol Aguade et al named this rare variant of PCT in 1975; they called it *porphyrie hepato-erythrocytaire*, but it has almost universally been called "hepato-erythropoietic" since.

Thirteen cases were reviewed by S. G. Smith in 1986. Vesicles occur in sun-exposed skin, with onset in infancy, followed by sclerodermoid scarring, hypertrichosis, pigmentation, red fluorescence of the teeth under Wood's light examination, dark urine, and nail damage. There is no hemolysis, a point which helps differentiate it clinically from Gunther's or erythropoietic porphyria. The disease is inherited by autosomal dominance and is due to a homozygous defect of uroporphyrinogen decarboxylase production. DeVerneuil et al found a point mutation in the uroporphyrinogen decarboxylase enzyme that allowed it to be very rapidly degraded. Toback et al reported a three-generation family study in 1987.

ACUTE INTERMITTENT PORPHYRIA

Acute intermittent porphyria (AIP) is also known as *acute porphyria* and Swedish porphyria. It is characterized by periodic attacks of abdominal colic, gastrointestinal disturbances, paralyses, and psychiatric disorders.

Severe abdominal colic is most often the initial symptom of AIP. Usually there is no abdominal wall rigidity, although tenderness and distension are present. Nausea, vomiting, and diarrhea or constipation accompany the abdominal pain. Peripheral neuropathy, mostly motor, is present. Severe pain in the legs occurs. Optic atrophy, diaphragmatic weakness, respiratory paralysis, flaccid quadriplegia, facial palsy, and dysphagia are but a few of the many neurologic signs. Psychiatric disturbances are varied and frequently apparent.

Photosensitivity with skin lesions of vesicles and bullae does not appear in AIP. The only skin sign is a dark pigmentation, which usually appears during an acute episodic attack.

Some of the drugs known to be capable of inducing acute attacks of porphyria are barbiturates, methyprylon, meprobamate, aminopyrine, glutethimide, phenytoin, mephenytoin, sulfonamides, dapsone, griseofulvin, sulfonylureas, estrogens, and ergot preparations.

AIP is inherited as a Mendelian dominant, with onset usually in the third or fourth decade of life.

Uroporphyrinogen synthetase, which converts porphobilinogen to uroporphyrinogen I, is deficient in the liver, red blood cells, cultured skin fibroblasts, whole skin, and cultured lymphocytes of affected individuals and latent carriers of AIP. It appears that the latent carriers of the deficiency must be exposed to precipitating factors, among which are certain drugs, steroid hormones and their metabolites, starvation, and infections, in order to become symptomatic.

Often examination of the urine of apparently healthy parents, or of siblings, will disclose heavy traces of porphobilinogen, suggesting latent porphyria. Fresh specimens of urine may be deep red or of normal color, but on standing in sunlight turn to a burgundy red. This color change can be expedited by acidifying the urine and boiling for 30 minutes.

PBG produces a positive Ehrlich reaction. The Watson-Schwartz modification of the Ehrlich reaction is also frequently used. This test uses 5 ml of Ehrlich's reagent to which 10 ml saturated sodium acetate solution and urine are added. Finally the solution is extracted with chloroform and then with butanol. An intense red color is produced in the water layer. The test is negative in erythropoietic porphyria and PCT.

No specific treatment is available in AIP. Avoidance of precipitating factors such as drugs, sex steroid hormones, and starvation is important. Glucose loading has been used extensively and appears to be beneficial in many cases. Hematin infusions, 200 to 300 mg in saline intravenously once daily, have resulted in clinical improvement and a marked decrease in ALA and PBG excretion. The phenothiazines (chlorpromazine) may be helpful for pain. Tetraethylammonium has been found to give relief from the intense abdominal pain. Opiates and propoxyphene are also useful for analgesia. Rausch-Stroomann and his associates have reported 13 women with AIP who had acute attacks during the premenstrual period. During three years of medication with contraceptive pills containing estrogen and progesterone, none had an acute attack of porphyria. Perlroth and his associates had similar findings in three patients.

HEREDITARY COPROPORPHYRIA

Hereditary lack of coproporphyrinogen oxidase (Elder) causes this rarest of all the porphyrias. Fecal coproporphyrin III is increased; urinary coproporphyrin III, ALA, and PBG are increased only during attacks. Intermittent abdominal pain occurs, with psychiatric symptoms, and both may be precipitated by barbiturates. About one third of patients have photosensitivity.

Harderoporphyria, a variant of hereditary coproporphyrin first described in 1983 by Nordmann et al, is apparently due to a homozygous defect resulting in a lack of coproporphyrinogen oxidase. Harderoporphyrin is the natural intermediate between coproporphyrinogen and protoporphyrinogen.

Treatment is symptomatic.

PORPHYRIA VARIEGATA

This is also known as *mixed porphyria, South African genetic porphyria,* and *mixed hepatic porphyria.* Variegate porphyria is caused by autosomal dominant inheritance—with high penetrance—of protoporphyrinogen oxidase deficiency.

Porphyria variegata is characterized by a combination of cutaneous lesions, abdominal crises, and gastrointestinal and neurologic manifestations either simultaneously or at different times. Relatives may have silent variegate porphyria, in which there is reduced enzyme activity but no clinical lesions. Some cases are easily confused with porphyria cutanea tarda; and as Day et al reported, the two diseases may coexist. They reported 18 such cases. This emphasizes the importance of investigating fecal porphyrins.

The cutaneous lesions are essentially those of PCT mentioned previously. Vesicles and bullae with erosions, especially on the sun-exposed areas, are the chief manifestations. In addition, hypertrichosis is seen in the temporal area, especially in women. Hyperpigmentation of sun-exposed areas is a feature not unlike that of pellagra.

The other signs and symptoms are similar to or

identical with AIP. Poh-Fitzpatrick has described a plasma porphyrin fluorescence marker that can be identified by a simple test on venous blood. The emission wave length specific for variegate porphyria is at 626 nm, as compared to the 619 nm seen in porphyria cutanea tarda, erythropoietic porphyria, acute intermittent porphyria, and hereditary copro-porphyria. Erythropoietic protoporphyria has an emission maximum of 634 nm. Brenner and Bloomer have pinpointed the enzyme defect as a lack of protoporphyrinogen oxidase. Red blood cell ferro-chelatase is decreased approximately 50 per cent in patients with variegate porphyria.

Such persons are also sensitive to the barbiturates and alcohol as well as to the many other substances already mentioned under PCT. The concerned reader should refer to the article by Bickers et al for lists of drugs known to be unsafe, or thought to be safe, in patients with porphyria. Quiroz-Kendall et al reported the onset of this disease in a woman while on the "Scarsdale Gourmet Diet."

Treatment is symptomatic. Various measures have already been outlined.

ERYTHROPOIETIC PROTOPORPHYRIA

This dominantly inherited disorder is characterized by a wide variety of photosensitive cutaneous lesions appearing early in childhood, at from two to five years of age, in boys more often than in girls. Murphy et al have described a man who had his first symptoms of erythropoietic protoporphyria at age 65.

The skin changes may vary from a pruritic or burning sensation to erythema, plaquelike edema, and wheals such as those seen in hydroa aestivale or solar urticaria. These lesions appear solely on sun-exposed areas. They are frequently accompanied by erythema and itching, with vesicles and bullae appearing only rarely. In severe cases purpura is seen in the sun-exposed areas. The skin looks weather-beaten.

Suurmond and his associates also mention shallow scars and waxy thickening of the skin on the nose and cheeks, thickening of the skin over the proximal finger joints, circumoral linear scars, atrophy of the rims of the ears, and a persistent violaceous ery-thema. These are all chronic manifestations. Hepatic cirrhosis, and gallstones containing protoporphyrin, may occur. Several patients with erythropoietic pro-toporphyria (EPP) and hepatic cirrhosis have died in hepatic coma or as a consequence of portal hypertension, with bleeding from esophageal varices. Romslo et al reported such a case.

During the wintertime when there is little or no exposure to sunlight the lesions are completely quiescent.

Ordinary window glass offers these patients no protection from the sun. Photosensitivity is to the longer wavelengths, chiefly in the Soret band (400 to 410 nm). In most cases the action spectrum closely approximates the absorption spectrum of protopor-phyrin, namely, 400 nm.

Histologically, hyperkeratosis is a regular finding, as is PAS-positive material in the upper dermis with perivascular accentuation. This material is type IV collagen. The upper dermal vessels may have a ground-glass appearance, and usually contain a deposit of IgG and often C3 on direct immunofluorescence microscopy.

EPP is characterized biochemically by high levels of protoporphyrin in the red blood cells, plasma, or feces. Erythrocyte protoporphyrin levels in affected persons may range from several hundred to several thousand micrograms per 100 ml of packed RBC (normal values <35 μg/100 ml of packed RBC). Activity of the enzyme ferrochelatase (heme synthetase) has been found deficient in bone marrow, reticulocytes, peripheral erythrocytes, liver, and fibroblast culture preparations from EPP patients. The meta-

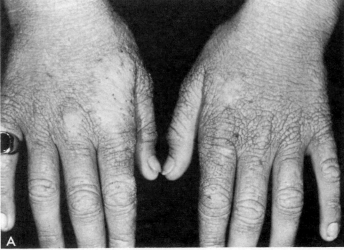
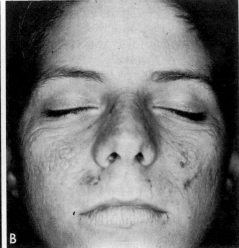

Figure 26–28. Erythropoietic protoporphyria. Note weatherbeaten appearance of hands (A) in this male adolescent, and thickening and shallow scars of face (B).

bolic defect responsible for the overproduction of free protoporphyrin in EPP is lack of ferrochelatase (heme synthetase).

The laboratory findings are distinctive. The urine does not fluoresce under the Wood's light, since porphyrins are present only in normal amounts. In the feces, proto- and coproporphyrins are markedly increased.

Protoporphyrin in the red blood cells is markedly increased. It may also be present in the plasma. These findings strongly point to the diagnosis of erythropoietic protoporphyria. The spectrofluorometric emission maximum is at 634 nm.

A screening test for erythropoietic protoporphyria uses fluorescence microscopy. Several drops of blood diluted one to five with normal saline solution are placed on a microscope slide and examined under the oil immersion objective of a fluorescence microscope. Fluorescing erythrocytes (fluorocytes) suggest erythropoietic protoporphyria.

The diagnosis of erythropoietic protoporphyria is made by the cutaneous lesions of photosensitivity, a raised erythrocyte protoporphyrin content, fluorescent erythrocytes in the peripheral blood, and the absence of porphyrinuria. Several observers have noted that there is no correlation between photosensitivity and serum or erythrocyte protoporphyrin levels.

The treatment consists of prophylactic protection from exposure to sunlight. Betacarotene, 60 to 180 mg daily, to maintain a serum level of from 400 to 600 µg per 100 ml, provides adequate protection for most cases. Bechtel et al successfully treated an eight-year-old boy with transfusions of washed packed red blood cells. Bloomer has emphasized the importance of looking for liver disease, as have Mathews-Roth and Romslo et al. It may be severe and even fatal in these patients.

CONGENITAL ERYTHROPOIETIC PORPHYRIA

This is also known as *Gunther's disease* or *congenital photosensitive porphyria*. It is characterized by the appearance of red urine in early infancy (noticeable on the diapers), photosensitivity, splenomegaly, and hemolytic anemia. Erythrodontia of both deciduous and permanent teeth is also characteristic. This phenomenon is demonstrated by the coral red fluorescence of the teeth when exposed to the Wood's light. The vesicles and subepidermal bullae appear in infancy on the light-exposed skin areas and heal with scarring and hyperpigmentation. Successive bouts of bullae and healing with scarring eventually lead to mutilating scars, especially on the face. This and the always-present hypertrichosis, with hair on the cheeks, profuse eyebrows, and long eyelashes, has prompted the terms "monkey face" or "werewolf" for these unfortunate individuals. Cicatricial alopecia of the scalp may develop. Other chronic findings

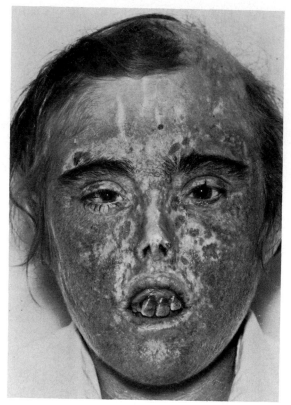

Figure 26–29. *Congenital erythropoietic porphyria (Gunther's disease) in a 17 year old girl with lesions since age 7 months. (Courtesy of Dr. H. R. Vickers, England.)*

include increased fragility of the skin, irregular hyper- and hypopigmentation, photophobia, keratoconjunctivitis, ectropion, and symblepharon.

It is inherited by an autosomal recessive gene. The biochemical deficiency that results is expressed as a deficiency of uroporphyrinogen III cosynthetase.

Less than 100 cases have been reported. Abnormally high amounts of uroporphyrins and coproporphyrin I are found in urine, stool, and red cells. There is stable reddish orange fluorescence of red blood cells. Hemolytic anemia is a constant finding.

On biopsy there are focal inflammation in the upper dermis, and subepidermal bullae.

Treatment is rigid avoidance of sunlight, and sometimes splenectomy for the hemolytic anemia or in the hope of inducing a remission. Primstone et al found activated charcoal efficacious, presumably by retarding the absorption of endogenous porphyrins. Piomelli et al reported in 1986 suppression of all symptoms by repeated transfusions of packed red cells, frequently enough to maintain the hematocrit level at 33 per cent. Chelation with deferoxamine mesylate, 20 to 40 mg/kg/day, may also be helpful. However, if Primstone et al's oral charcoal therapy withstands the test of time, it would clearly seem to be the therapy of choice. Sunscreens, except total blockers, are not much help, but betacarotene orally may be useful.

Arnold HL Jr: Porphyria cutanea tarda: control with small doses of chloroquine. Straub Clin Proc 1969, 35:115.

Ashton RE, et al: Low-dose oral chloroquine in the treatment of porphyria cutanea tarda. Br J Dermatol 1984, 111:609.

Battle AM del C: Tetrapyrrole biosynthesis. Semin Dermatol 1986, 5:70.

Bechtel MA, et al: Transfusion therapy in a patient with erythropoietic protoporphyria. Arch Dermatol 1981, 117:99.

Bickers DR, et al: The treatment of porphyrias. Semin Dermatol 1986, 5:186.

Brenner D, et al: The enzymatic defect in variegate porphyria. N Engl J Med 1980, 302:765.

Cainelli T, et al: Hydroxychloroquine versus phlebotomy in the treatment of porphyria cutanea tarda. Br J Dermatol 1983, 108:593.

Callen JP, et al: Subacute cutaneous lupus erythematosus and porphyria cutanea tarda. JAAD 1981, 5:269.

Chlumska A, et al: Liver changes in PCT patients treated with chloroquine. Br J Dermatol 1980, 102:261.

Clemmensen O, et al: Porphyria cutanea tarda and systemic lupus erythematosus. Arch Dermatol 1982, 118:160.

Collins AG, et al: Porphyria cutanea tarda and agricultural pesticides. Austral J Dermatol 1982, 23:70.

Corey TJ, et al: Variegate porphyria. JAAD 1980, 2:36.

Cram DL, et al: Lupus erythematosus and porphyria. Arch Dermatol 1973, 108:779.

Cripps DJ, et al: Erythropoietic protoporphyria: hepatic cirrhosis. Br J Dermatol 1978, 98:349.

Idem: Porphyria turcica. Arch Dermatol 1980, 115:46.

Day RS, et al: Coexistent variegate porphyria and porphyria cutanea tarda. N Engl J Med 1982, 307:36.

Idem: Severe cutaneous porphyria in a 12-year-old boy. Arch Dermatol 1982, 118:663.

Day RS: Variegate porphyria. Semin Dermatol 1986, 5:138.

Dean G: Porphyria turcica. Arch Dermatol 1981, 117:318.

De Leo VA, et al: Erythropoietic protoporphyria. Am J Med 1976, 60:8.

De Salamanca RE, et al: The genetic basis of porphyria cutanea tarda. Arch Dermatol Res 1985, 8:277.

deVerneuil H, et al: Uroporphyrinogen decarboxylase structural mutant (gly^{281} →glu) in a case of porphyria. Science 1986, 234:732.

Disler PB, et al: The biochemical diagnosis of porphyrias (review). Int J Dermatol 1984, 23:2.

Elder GH: Metabolic abnormalities in the porphyrias. Semin Dermatol 1986, 5:88.

Idem: Decreased activity of hepatic uroporphyrinogen decarboxylase in sporadic porphyria cutanea tarda. N Engl J Med 1978, 299:274.

Ellefson RD: Porphyrinogens, porphyrins, and porphyrias (laboratory report). Mayo Clinic Proc 1982, 57:454.

Epstein JH, et al: Porphyria-like cutaneous changes induced by tetracycline hydrochloride photosensitization. Arch Dermatol 1976, 112:661.

Idem: Porphyria cutanea tarda. N Engl J Med 1968, 279:1301.

Eramo LR, et al: Hydroa vacciniforme. Arch Dermatol 1986, 122:1310.

Eubanks SW, et al: The porphyrias (review). Int J Dermatol 1983, 22:337.

Felsher BF, et al: Decreased hepatic uroporphyrinogen decarboxylase activity in porphyria cutanea tarda. N Engl J Med 1982, 306:766.

Fitzpatrick TB: South Africa porphyria (variegate porphyria) is being discovered in the United States: watch for it–you may save a life. Dermatol Capsule Comment 1980, August, p. 11.

Friedman SJ: Sclerodermoid changes of porphyria cutanea tarda. Possible relationship to urinary uroporphyrin levels. JAAD 1985, 13:70.

Goetz G, et al: Influence of chloroquine on porphyrin metabolism. Arch Dermatol Res 1985, 277:114.

Goldgeier MH, et al: Hydroa vacciniforme. Arch Dermatol 1982, 118:588.

Grossman ME, et al: Porphyria cutanea tarda. Am J Med 1979, 67:277.

Haeger-Aronsen B, et al: Hereditary coproporphyria. Study of a Swedish family. Ann Intern Med 1968, 69:221.

Halasz CL, et al: Hydroa vacciniforme: induction of lesions with ultraviolet A. JAAD 1983, 8:171.

Harber LC, et al: The porphyrias: basic science aspects, clinical diagnosis and management. Yearbook of Dermatology. Malkinson F, Pearson R (eds). Chicago Yearbook Publishers, 1975, p. 9.

Idem: Porphyria and pseudoporphyria. J Invest Dermatol 1984, 82:207.

Judd LE, et al: Naproxen-induced pseudoporphyria. Arch Dermatol 1986, 122:451.

Kalb RE, et al: Correlation of serum and urinary porphyria levels in porphyria cutanea tarda. Arch Dermatol 1985, 121:1289.

Keczkes K, et al: Malignant hepatoma associated with acquired hepatic cutaneous porphyria. Arch Dermatol 1976, 112:78.

Kushner JP: The enzymatic defect in porphyria cutanea tarda. N Engl J Med 1982, 306:799.

Lefer LG, et al: Vesicles in the dorsa of the fingers. Arch Dermatol 1987, 123:105.

Lim HW, et al: Hepatoerythropoietic porphyria: a variant of childhood onset porphyria cutanea tarda. JAAD 1984, 11:1103.

Malina L, et al: A comparative study of the results of phlebotomy therapy and low dose chloroquine treatment in porphyria cutanea tarda. Acta Dermatovenereol 1981, 61:346.

Mascaro JM, et al: Uroporphyrinogen decarboxylase deficiencies: porphyria cutanea tarda and related conditions. Semin Dermatol 1986, 5:115.

Mathews-Roth MM: The consequences of not diagnosing erythropoietic protoporphyria and other photosensitivity diseases. Arch Dermatol 1977, 113:1229.

Miyauchi S, et al: Small-volume plasmapheresis in the management of porphyria cutanea tarda. Arch Dermatol 1983, 119:752.

Muhlbauer L, et al: Variegate porphyria in New England. JAMA 1982, 247:3095.

Murphy GM, et al: Late-onset erythropoietic protoporphyria with unusual cutaneous features. Arch Dermatol 1985, 121:1309.

Mustajoki P: Acute intermittent porphyria. Semin Dermatol 1986, 5:155.

Nordmann Y, et al: Congenital erythropoietic porphyria. Semin Dermatol 1986, 5:106.

Idem: Harderoporphyria: a variant hereditary coproporphyria. J Clin Invest 1983, 72:1139.

Pimstone NR, et al: Therapeutic efficacy or oral charcoal in congenital erythropoietic porphyria. N Engl J Med 1987, 316:390.

Piomelli S, et al: Complete suppression of the symptoms of congenital erythropoietic porphyria by long-term treatment with high level transfusions. N Engl J Med 1986, 314:1029.

Poh-Fitzpatrick MB: Erythropoietic protoporphyria. Semin Dermatol 1986, 5:99.

Idem: The importance of correct diagnosis in variegate porphyria. JAAD 1983, 8:115.

Idem: Porphyria, pseudoporphyria, pseudopseudoporphyria . . . ?. Arch Dermatol 1986, 122:403.

Idem: A plasma porphyrin fluorescence marker for variegate porphyria. Arch Dermatol 1980, 116:543.

Idem, et al: Variegate porphyria. Dermatol Allergy 1982 (Sept).

Idem: The porphyrias. Dermatol Clin 1987, 5:55.

Quiroz-Kendall E, et al: Acute variegate porphyria following a Scarsdale gourmet diet. JAAD 1983, 8:46.

Rocchi E, et al: High weekly doses of desferrioxamine in PCT. Br J Dermatol 1987, 117:393.

Idem: Iron removal therapy in porphyria cutanea tarda: Phlebotomy versus slow subcutaneous desferrioxamine infusion. Br J Dermatol 1986, 114:621.

Rogers M, et al: Familial porphyria cutanea tarda. Austral J Dermatol 1983, 26:58.

Romseo I, et al: Erythropoietic protoporphyria terminating in liver failure. Arch Dermatol 1982, 118:668.

Siepker L, et al: Protoporphyrinogen oxidase in porphyria variegata. S Afr Med J 1986, 70:819.

Sixel-Dietrich F, et al: Hereditary uroporphyrinogen-decarboxylase deficiency predisposing to porphyria cutanea tarda in a female after oral contraceptive medication. Arch Dermatol Res 1985, 278:13.

Smith SG: Hepatoerythropoietic porphyria. Semin Dermatol 1986, 5:125.

Tamayo L, et al: Porphyria cutanea tarda symptomatica in children treated with chloroquine. Dermatol 1985, 12:329.

Toback AG, et al: Hepatoerythropoietic porphyria. N Engl J Med 1987, 316:645.

Topi GC, et al: Recovery from porphyria cutanea tarda with no specific therapy other than avoidance of hepatic toxins. Br J Dermatol 1984, 111:75.

OTHER ERRORS OF METABOLISM

ACRODERMATITIS ENTEROPATHICA

Acrodermatitis enteropathica, an autosomal recessive disorder, is characterized by acral and periorificial dermatitis, alopecia, gastrointestinal disturbances of diarrhea with exacerbations and remissions, and a peculiar apathy during periods of exacerbation. The disease usually begins insidiously in infants between the ages of three weeks and 18 months with a small localized skin eruption near one of the body orifices or on an extremity. At the same time, or shortly afterward, loss of hair and gastrointestinal disturbances, manifested chiefly by diarrhea, occur. Graves et al reported a case lasting 32 years in a woman of 33. Bronson et al reported a 22-year-old woman who had recurrent outbreaks of the acrodermatitis enteropathica eruption with each pregnancy. Pregnancy and birth control pills may exacerbate the underlying genetic disease. During exacerbations there is mental depression with more or less stupidity, listlessness, and loss of appetite. There may be perlèche and blepharitis.

The primary eruption is vesiculobullous, symmetrical, and grouped. It is located about the body orifices and eyes and on the occiput, elbows, knees, hands, and feet. Paronychial infections are common. Crusts form and the patches may become psoriasiform. Cultures from the skin and mouth often reveal

Candida albicans. Cases have incorrectly been diagnosed as moniliasis and epidermolysis bullosa.

The basic defect in acrodermatitis enteropathica appears to be malabsorption of zinc. Plasma zinc levels are at or below approximately 50 µg/100 ml. An absence or deficiency of a specific intestinal transport protein or zinc-binding ligand has been proposed to explain the ultimate genetic defect in acrodermatitis enteropathica. Paneth cells, which are located in the bottom of the crypts of Lieberkuhn and are rich in zinc, may be specifically involved in some phase of zinc transport.

A definite diagnosis of acrodermatitis enteropathica is justified only when all the characteristic symptoms are present, namely, the acral and periorificial eruption and gastrointestinal disturbances with irregular exacerbations and remissions, the mental state during the periods of exacerbation, and the alopecia. Low serum zinc levels are confirmatory, and the patient's response to orally administered zinc also serves as a diagnostic criterion.

All cases respond to treatment with zinc sulfate, 220 mg once or twice a day. Continuous administration of diiodohydroxyquin was used in the past (without realizing it was a source of zinc) to keep patients free from symptoms, but inevitably caused optic atrophy. Acquired dietary deficiencies of zinc occur, and are discussed in Chapter 22.

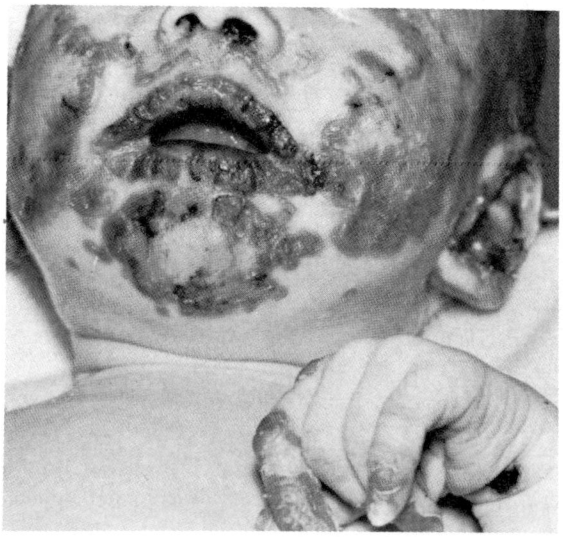

Bronson DM, et al: Acrodermatitis enteropathica. JAAD 1983, 9:140.

Graves K, et al: Hereditary acrodermatitis enteropathica in an adult. Arch Dermatol 1980, 116:562.

McClain CJ, et al: Functional consequences of zinc deficiency. Prog Food Nutr Sci 1985, 9:185.

Neldner KH, et al: Acrodermatitis enteropathica. Int J Dermatol 1978, 17:380.

Prasad AS: Clinical and biochemical manifestations of zinc deficiency in human subjects. J Am Coll Nutr 1985, 4:65.

Robertson AF: Treatment of acrodermatitis enteropathica with zinc sulfate. Pediatrics 1975, 55:738.

Figure 26–30. Typical perioral and facial lesions of acrodermatitis enteropathica.

BIOTINIDASE DEFICIENCY

Multiple carboxylase deficiency has two forms. In the neonatal-onset type, there is an autosomal recessive inherited deficit of holocarboxylase synthetase activity. These patients usually die of lactic acidosis within the first few days of life unless promptly diagnosed.

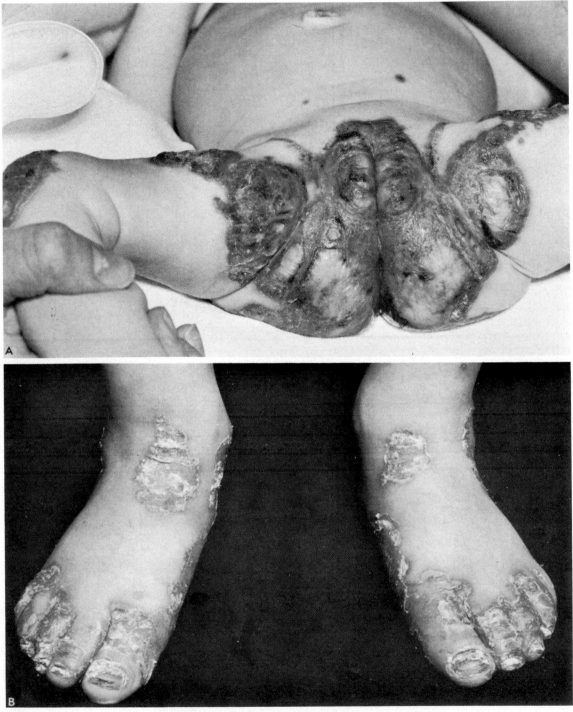

Figure 26–31. *Acrodermatitis enteropathica.* (A, From Wells BT, Winkelmann RK: Arch Dermatol 84:40–52, 1961. B, Courtesy of Dr. D. Bloom.)

The infantile-onset form is caused by an autosomal dominant inherited deficiency of biotinidase, which acts in branched-chain amino acid and carbohydrate metabolism.

Williams et al and Wolf et al have described the clinical manifestations in detail. They include ataxia, seizures, acidosis, recurrent infections, sparseness of hair, and a periorificial dermatitis similar to that seen in acrodermatitis enteropathica.

Biotin supplementation resolves the cutaneous and hair abnormalities and is potentially life-saving.

Nyhan WL: Inborn errors of biotin metabolism. Arch Dermatol 1987, 123:1696.

Williams ML, et al: Alopecia and periorificial dermatitis in biotin-responsive multiple carboxylase deficiency. JAAD 1983, 9:97.

Wolf B, et al: Phenotypic variation in biotinidase deficiency. J Pediatr 1983, 103:233.

Idem: Deficient biotinidase activity in late-onset multiple carboxylase deficiency. N Engl J Med 1983, 308:161.

NEONATAL CITRULLINEMIA

Citrullinemia is an autosomal dominant inherited deficiency of the enzyme argininosuccinic acid synthetase. This enzyme converts citrulline and aspartic acid to argininosuccinic acid, as a part of the urea cycle. Low plasma arginine levels result, and the hypothesis is that since keratin is 16 per cent arginine, dermatitis may occur.

Goldblum et al reported a patient with erosive, erythematous, scaling patches and plaques which were prominent in the perioral, lower abdominal, diaper, and buttock regions. This eruption cleared with arginine supplementation. A similar case was reported by Thoene et al. Two patients with this disease have had short, sparse hair.

In carbamoyl phosphate synthetase deficiency, low plasma arginine levels may also occur, and similar cutaneous findings have been reported in this second metabolic defect of the urea cycle.

Diets high in arginine will heal the skin lesions.

Goldblum OM, et al: Neonatal citrullinemia associated with cutaneous manifestations and arginine deficiency. JAAD 1986, 14:321.

Kline J, et al: Arginine deficiency syndrome. Am J Dis Child 1981, 135:437.

Theone J, et al: Neonatal citrullinemia. J Pediatr 1977, 91:218.

HARTNUP DISEASE

Hartnup disease is an inborn error of tryptophan excretion; it was named after the Hartnup family, in which it was first noted. The outstanding findings are a pellagralike dermatitis following exposure to sunlight, intermittent cerebellar ataxia, psychiatric manifestations, and constant aminoaciduria.

Large amounts of indole-3-acetic acid and indican are secreted in the urine.

The dermatitis occurs upon exposed parts of the skin, chiefly the face, neck, hands, and legs. The erythematous scaly patches flare up into a hot, red, exudative state after exposure to sunlight, followed after subsidence by pigmentation. Stomatitis and vulvitis also occur. The disease becomes milder with increasing age. Hartnup disease is an autosomal recessive trait.

The skin lesions respond to niacinamide, 200 mg a day.

Pahmoush AJ, et al: Hartnup disease. Arch Neurol 1976, 33:797.

Wilcken B, et al: Natural history of Hartnup disease. Arch Dis Child 1977, 52:38.

PROLIDASE DEFICIENCY

This autosomal recessive inherited inborn error of metabolism was described in 1974 by Powell et al. Prolidase cleaves dipeptides containing C-terminal proline or hydroxyproline. When this enzyme is deficient, the normal recycling of proline residues obtained from collagen degradation is impaired. There results a buildup of iminodipeptides, with disturbances in connective tissue metabolism and excretion of large amounts of iminodipeptides in the urine.

Clinically 85 per cent of patients have some dermatologic manifestations. The most important cutaneous signs, which almost always appear before age 12, are skin fragility, ulceration, and scarring of the lower extremities; photosensitivity and telangiectasia; poliosis; scaly, erythematous, maculopapular, and purpuric lesions; and thickening of the skin with lymphedema. Der Kaloustian et al have reviewed these findings in detail. Systemic signs and symptoms include mental deficiency, splenomegaly, and recurrent infections. An unusual facial appearance is noted at times, with low hair line, frontal bossing, and saddle nose.

Prolidase measurement may be determined in erythrocytes, leukocytes, or fibroblasts. Leoni et al have reported structural abnormalities of collagen and elastin after electron microscopic study.

Effective treatment is not available.

Arata J, et al: Prolidase deficiency. Arch Dermatol 1979, 115:62.

Der Kaloustian VM, et al: Prolidase deficiency. Dermatologica 1982, 64:293.

Leoni A, et al: Prolidase deficiency in two siblings with chronic leg ulcers. Arch Dermatol 1987, 123:493.

Rewell GF, et al: A prolidase deficiency in a man with iminopeptiduria. Metabolism 1974, 23:505.

Sheffield LJ, et al: Iminopeptiduria, skin ulcerations and edema in a boy with prolidase deficiency. J Pediatr 1977, 91:578.

PHENYLKETONURIA (PKU)

Also known as phenylpyruvic oligophrenia, PKU, an autosomal recessive disorder of phenylalanine metabolism, is characterized by mental deficiency; epileptic seizures; the presence of phenylpyruvic acid in the urine; pigmentary dilution of skin, hair, and eyes; and dermatitis. Phenylalanine hydroxylase is lacking in the liver and also in peripheral lymphocytes, as shown by Yoshii et al, and phenylalanine is therefore not oxidized to tyrosine.

The affected children are blue-eyed, with blond hair and fair skin. They are usually extremely sensitive to light, and about 50 per cent have an eczematous dermatitis clinically similar to atopic dermatitis, with predilection for the flexures. It is worst in the youngest patients; may improve with dietary treatment; and has been exacerbated by phenylalanine challenge in a carrier of the recessive gene. Skin lesions may be sclerodermatous in nature. Indurations of the thighs and buttocks are present early in infancy and increase with time.

PKU occurs predominantly in Caucasians. The normal pathway for the degradation of phenylalanine and tyrosine in man occurs in a series of separate steps, each of which is catalyzed by an enzyme system. Degradation of phenylalanine to tyrosine is accomplished by phenylalanine hydroxylase. The lack of this enzyme produces the disease PKU.

Blood levels of phenylalanine are high. The presence of phenylpyruvic acid in the urine is demonstrated by a characteristic deep green color when a few drops of ferric chloride solution are added to it. Green diapers occur in histidinemia as well as in phenylketonuria.

Young infants should be treated by a special diet low in phenylalanine; this may bring about normal development if begun shortly after birth. There is now a trend toward stopping the diet at age four to six; however, long-term studies will be needed before we can be sure it does not need to be lifelong.

Fisch RO, et al: Studies of phenylketonurics with dermatitis. JAAD 1981, 4:284.
Yoshii T, et al: Phenylalanine hydroxylase deficiency in peripheral lymphocytes from phenylketonuria. J Dermatol (Tokyo) 1977, 4:49.

ALKAPTONURIA AND OCHRONOSIS

Alkaptonuria, inherited as an autosomal recessive trait, is caused by the lack of renal and hepatic homogentisic acid oxidase, the enzyme necessary for the catabolism of homogentisic acid to acetoacetic and fumaric acids. It is characterized by the excretion of homogentisic acid in the urine to produce a black-staining urine, the deposition of a grossly brown-black pigment in the connective tissue, which is ochre

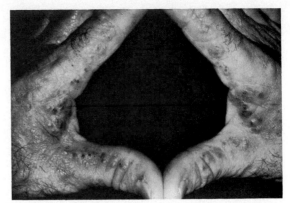

Figure 26–32. *Ochronosis on hands. (Courtesy of Dr. J. M. Hitch.)*

in color microscopically (ochronosis), and ochronotic arthropathy.

In these patients the voided urine is dark and turns black on standing from the homogentisic acid. The dark urine may be the only indication of the presence of alkaptonuria for many years. In the meantime large amounts of homogentisic acid are accumulated in the body tissues.

By the third decade in life the deposition of pigment becomes apparent. Cartilage is a favorite site. The early sign is the pigmentation of the sclera (Osler's sign) and the cartilage of the ears. Later the cartilage of the nose and the tendons, especially those on the hands, become discolored.

Blue or mottled brown macules appear. The bluish macules have a predilection for the fingers, the ears, the nose, the genital regions, the apices of the axillae, and the buccal mucosa. The sweat glands are rich in ochronotic pigment granules, and intradermal injection of epinephrine into the skin of the axillary vault yields brown-black sweat droplets in the follicular orifices. The cerumen is often black. Internally the larynx, the great vessels and valves of the heart, the kidneys, the esophagus, the tonsils, and the dura mater may be involved.

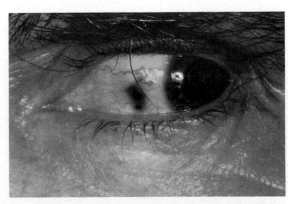

Figure 26–33. *Pigmented macule on sclera—Osler's sign. An early sign of ochronosis. (Courtesy of Dr. J. M. Hitch.)*

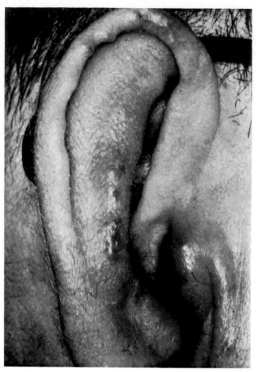

Figure 26–34. Ochronosis on ear. (Courtesy of Dr. J. M. Hitch.)

The ochronotic arthropathy involves the spinal joints first, resembling osteoarthritis, and then is followed by disorders of the knees, shoulders, and hips. Roentgenograms show a characteristic appearance of early calcification of the intervertebral disk and later narrowing of the intervertebral spaces with eventual disk collapse.

There is no effective treatment. However, Murray et al postulate that the inhibition of lysyl hydroxylase activity by homogentisic acid can be counteracted by ascorbic acid, and that long-term ascorbic acid therapy might be helpful.

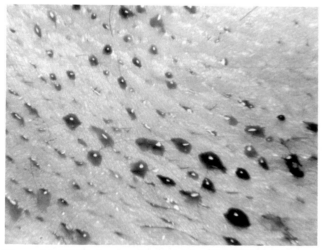

Figure 26–35. Black sweat after intradermal injection of epinephrine in a patient with ochronosis. (Courtesy of Dr. Axel W. Hoke.)

Quinacrine Ochronosis. Antimalarials may induce ochronosislike pigmentation. Although quinacrine was initially implicated, all antimalarials (including quinine, quinacrine, chloroquine, hydroxychloroquine, and amodiaquine) may produce this pigmentation. It is usually first noted on the hard palate and occurs after a mean duration of therapy of 25 months. Topically applied phenolic intermediates such as hydroquinone, carbolic acid (phenol), picric acid, and resorcinol may produce exogenous ochronosis, as reported by Cullison et al, and by Findlay.

Bruce S, et al: Exogenous ochronosis resulting from quinine injections. JAAD 1986, 15:357.

Cullison D, et al: Localized exogenous ochronosis. JAAD 1983, 8:882.

Egorin MJ, et al: Quinacrine ochronosis and rheumatoid arthritis. JAMA 1976, 236:385.

Engasser PG: Ochronosis caused by bleaching creams. JAAD 1984, 10:1072.

Findlay GH: Ochronosis following skin bleaching with hydroquinone. JAAD 1982, 6:1092.

Lawrence N, et al: Exogenous ochronosis in the United States. JAAD 1988, 18:1207.

Murray JC, et al: In vitro inhibition of chick embryo lysyl hydroxylase by homogentisic acid: proposed connective tissue defect in alkaptonuria. J Clin Invest 1977, 59:1071.

O'Donoghue MN, et al: Ochronosis due to hydroquinone. JAAD 1983, 8:123.

WILSON'S DISEASE
(Hepatolenticular Degeneration)

Wilson's disease is an inborn derangement of copper metabolism, an autosomal recessive trait. It comprises hepato- and splenomegaly and neuropsychiatric changes resembling a combination of multiple sclerosis, psychosis, and parkinsonism. Slurred speech, a squeaky voice, salivation, dysphagia, tremors, incoordination, and spasticity may all occur. Physiologically there is progressive, fatal hepatic and central nervous system degeneration. The body retains an excessive amount of copper, leading to damage in the liver, brain, kidney, cornea, and nails. As a result, azure lunulae (sky blue moons) of the nails and the smoky greenish brown Kayser-Fleischer rings develop at the edges of the corneas. Hyperpigmentation may develop on the lower extremities. A vague greenish discoloration of the skin on the face, neck, and genitalia may also be present. The changes of cirrhosis (vascular spiders and palmar erythema) may occur. Low ceruloplasmin level in the serum is diagnostic.

The disease is caused by the inability of the body to synthesize a normal amount of copper protein, ceruloplasmin. D-penicillamine, one of the metabolites of penicillin, effectively removes copper by chelating it. The dose is 1 or 2 gm orally a day. Beware of its many side effects, however! It must be continued for life.

Bearn AG, et al: Azure lunulae. JAMA 1958, 166:904.
Lange J: Long-term treatment of Wilson's disease with D-penicillamine. Deutsch Med Wschr 1967, 92:1657.

TYROSINEMIA II
(Richner-Hanhart Syndrome)

Tyrosinemia is an autosomal recessively transmitted syndrome of mild to severe keratitis, and hyperkeratotic and erosive lesions of palms and soles, often with mental retardation. Serum tyrosine may be from 200 to 300 μmol/100 ml (normal, 10 or less). Tyrosine is elevated because of a deficiency of hepatic tyrosine aminotransferase.

Photophobia and tearing commonly occur as the keratitis begins, and ultimately neovascularization is seen. Palmar and plantar erosions and hyperkeratoses appear at about the same time as the eye lesions. The hyperkeratotic condition appears to be related to regional factors, rather than mechanical. Thigh skin, grafted to the heel by Crovato et al was spared.

No skin lesions occur in tyrosinemia I (tyrosinosis) or neonatal tyrosinemia. A low-tyrosine, low-phenylalanine diet (Mead Johnson 3200 AB) helps the eye and skin lesions and may or may not benefit the problem of mental retardation.

Goldsmith has lately reviewed the subject.

Crovato F, et al: Richner-Hanhart syndrome spares plantar autograft. Arch Dermatol 1985, 121:539.
Goldsmith LA, et al: Tyrosine-induced eye and skin lesions: a treatable genetic disease. JAMA 1976, 236:382.
Idem: Tyrosinemia II. Int J Dermatol 1985, 24:293.

WAARDENBURG'S SYNDROME

Waardenburg's (Waardenburg-Klein's) syndrome, inherited in an autosomal dominant pattern, is thought to be pathogenetically related to a disorder of melanocyte differentiation or migration. The syndrome consists of white forelock, unilateral or bilateral deafness (owing to the absence of the Corti organ), lateral displacement of the inner canthi, a broad nasal root, heterochromia of the iris, and confluent eyebrows. By measuring the intercanthal distance and dividing it by the interpupillary distance, one may document the presence or absence of lateral displacement at the inner canthi. If this ratio is greater than 0.6 it is abnormal, a finding present in 69 per cent of patients. Additional stigmata are partial albinism and pale blue irises. Especially striking is the presence of one blue and one brown eye, or two pale blue eyes in blacks.

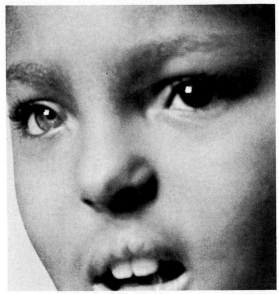

Figure 26-36. Waardenburg's syndrome in an 8 year old girl whose two siblings are similarly affected with deafness, heterochromia of the eyes (right—blue, left—brown), broad nasal root, lateral displacement of inner canthi, and partial albinism. (Courtesy of Dr. Y. Rapp.)

Goldberg F: Waardenburg's syndrome with fundus and other anomalies. Arch Ophthalmol 1966, 76:797.
Soussi-Tsafrir J: Light-eyed Negroes and Klein-Waardenburg syndrome. London, MacMillan, 1974.

HURLER'S SYNDROME
(Mucopolysaccharidosis I)

Hurler's syndrome, or gargoylism, is an inherited disorder of mucopolysaccharide metabolism. It is characterized by mental retardation, hepatosplenomegaly, umbilical and inguinal hernia, genital infantilism, corneal opacities, and skin abnormalities. There are gargoyle features, with broad saddle nose, thick lips, and large tongue.

The skeletal system is deformed, with hydrocephalus and kyphosis and gibbus (cat-back shape). The hands are broad and have claw fingers. The joints are distorted.

The skin is thickened, with ridges and grooves, especially on the upper half of the body. Fine lanugo hair is profuse all over the body. Large coarse hair is prominent, especially on the extremities.

Gargoylism is inherited as an autosomal recessive trait. The two acid mucopolysaccharides, dermatan sulfate and heparan sulfate, are produced excessively so that in many tissues there is an accumulation, which is excreted in the urine in large amounts. A deficiency of α-L-iduronidase was identified by Neufeld and associates as the causative defect in Hurler's syndrome. Dried urine on filter paper will show a purple color when acetic acid followed by toluidine blue reagent is added.

Histologically, the gargoyle cell is found. It is a large histiocyte containing metachromatic granules. These granules are also present in the fibrocytes. The epidermis is normal except for the skin of the hands, which is acanthotic and hyperkeratotic.

Prenatal diagnosis through the study of cultured amniotic fluid cells is possible. However, no treatment is available.

Fratantoni JC, et al: The defect in Hunter's and Hurler's syndromes: faulty degradation of mucopolysaccharide. Proc Natl Acad Sci (USA) 1968, 60:669.
Hambrick GW Jr, et al: Studies of the skin in Hurler's syndrome. Arch Dermatol 1962, 89:455.
McKusick VA, et al: The mucopolysaccharide storage diseases. In The Metabolic Basis of Inherited Disease, 4th ed., Stanbury J. B., et al, (eds). New York, McGraw-Hill, 1978, p. 1282.

Hunter's Syndrome

This syndrome is mucopolysaccharidosis (MPS) II. The clinical features are similar to those of Hurler's syndrome and are characterized by an excessive storage and excretion of mucopolysaccharides. The relative mildness and the mode of inheritance distinguish it from Hurler's syndrome: Hunter's syndrome is transmitted as an X-linked recessive trait. The "pebbly" lesions of MPS II in the skin over the inferior angles of the scapulas represent the only distinctive skin changes of the mucopolysaccharidoses. These are firm, flesh-colored to white papules and nodules, which coalesce. They are most common on the back, but may be seen on the pectoral areas, the nape of the neck, and the lateral aspects of the arms and thighs. They generally occur at about age 10.

The deficient enzyme is iduronate sulfatase. Dermatan sulfate and heparin sulfate are excreted in large amounts.

Prystowsky SD, et al: A cutaneous marker in the Hunter syndrome. Arch Dermatol 1977, 113:602.

Morquio's Disease

This autosomal recessive disorder is characterized by dwarfism, prognathism, corneal opacities, deafness, progressive kyphoscoliosis, flat feet, and knock-knees. The standing position is a crouch. There is increased excretion of keratan sulfate. The enzyme deficiencies are galactosamine-6-sulfate sulfatase in Morquio A and β-galactosidase in Morquio B.

Groebe H, et al: Morquio's syndrome associated with beta-galactosidase deficiency. Am J Hum Genet 1980, 32:258.

UNVERRICHT'S SYNDROME

This syndrome is characterized by convulsive seizures beginning at puberty, myoclonic jerks followed by progressive ataxia, dysphagia, dysarthria, dementia, and death in early adulthood. Medved and his associates described a patient with unusual skin lesions on the ears. Soft, smooth, rubbery, flesh-colored papules and nodules of various shapes were seen, especially on the backs of the ears. Large amounts of acid mucopolysaccharides were demonstrated in the histologic sections of these papules. The syndrome appears to be due to a systemic disturbance of mucopolysaccharide metabolism.

Medved A, et al: Cutaneous findings in Unverricht's syndrome. Arch Dermatol 1967, 95:206.

FARBER'S DISEASE

First described by Sidney Farber in 1952, and also known as *fibrocytic dysmucopolysaccharidosis and lipogranulomatosis*, it is characterized by periarticular swellings, a weak hoarse cry, pulmonary failure, painful joint deformities, and motor and mental retardation. The onset is during the first months of life; death can be expected before the patient reaches the age of two.

The rubbery subcutaneous nodules have a distinct yellowish hue and are 1 to 2 cm in diameter. They are usually located over the joints, lumbar spine, scalp, and weight-bearing areas. Histologically they are granulomas. As Rauch et al reported, the diagnosis can be aided by finding Farber bodies (curvilinear bodies) within the cytoplasm or phagosomes of fibroblasts, histiocytes, or endothelial cells, banana-shaped bodies within Schwann cells, and "zebra" bodies within endothelial cells and neurons.

In Farber's disease an accumulation of ceramide and its degradation products in foam cells and a specific deficiency of acid ceramidase in cultured fibroblasts and white blood cells have been demonstrated.

Rauch HJ, et al: "Banana bodies" in disseminated lipogranulomatosis (Farber's disease). Am J Dermatopathol 1983, 5:263.

ADRENOLEUKODYSTROPHY
(Schilder's Disease)

Adrenoleukodystrophy (ALD) is an X-linked disorder in which cerebral white matter becomes progressively demyelinated and serious adrenocortical insufficiency usually occurs. Skin hyperpigmentation often calls attention to the adrenal disease, and mental deterioration indicates the even graver diagnosis of ALD. Computed tomography may help indicate the site for a diagnostic brain biopsy, but Martin and associates reported that skin biopsies, hitherto thought to show only pigmentation, may show characteristic vacuolation of eccrine secretory coils (duct cells being spared), and both skin and conjunctival biopsies may show diagnostic clefts in Schwann cells surrounding myelinated axons.

There is no known treatment.

Case Records of the Massachusetts General Hospital. N Engl J Med 1979, 300:1037.

Duda EE, et al: Computed tomography in adrenoleukodystrophy. Radiology 1976, 120:349.

Martin JJ, et al: Skin and conjunctival biopsies in adrenoleukodystrophy. Acta Neuropath (Berlin) 1977, 38:247.

Schaumburg HH, et al: Adreno-leukodystrophy: a clinical and pathological study of 17 cases. Arch Neurol 1975, 33:557.

GOUT

In chronic cases of gout (podagra), monosodium urate monohydrate deposits may be formed in the subcutaneous tissues, as a result of which nodules called *tophi* are formed. These vary from a pinhead size to that of a pea or rarely even a baseball and are most commonly found on the rim of the ears. They are of a yellow or cream color. Another common location is over the distal interphalangeal articulations. In the course of time they tend to break down and discharge sodium urate crystals, afterward healing and perhaps breaking down again. The nature of the lesions is verified, on microscopic examination, by finding the characteristic long, needle-shaped crystals of monosodium urate. Since these deposits are dissolved by routine processing, fixation in absolute ethanol or freezing is necessary for their demonstration. Ninety-five per cent of patients are males.

The cause is a metabolic disturbance, not dietary self-indulgence. Both production and clearance of uric acid may be affected. Treatment of the acute attacks is with colchicine. If an overproduction of uric acid is the problem it is treated with allopurinol, a xanthine oxidase inhibitor. If decreased renal excretion is the problem, uricosuric agents such as probenecid (Benemid) are indicated.

Lesch-Nyhan Syndrome

Also known as juvenile gout, this rare X-linked recessively inherited disorder is characterized by childhood hyperuricemia, choreoathetosis, progressive mental retardation, and self-mutilation.

The cutaneous lesions are distinctive. Massive self-mutilation of lips with the teeth occurs. The fingers are also badly chewed. The ears and nose are occasionally mutilated. An early diagnostic clue is orange crystals in the diaper. The blood uric acid is increased and allopurinol, 200 to 400 mg daily, must be given to reduce it to normal and control the disease. There is a marked deficiency in an enzyme of purine metabolism, hypoxanthine-guanine phosphoribosyltransferase (HPRT).

Graham R, et al: Clinical survey of 354 patients with gout. Ann Rheum Dis 1970, 29:461.

Nyhan WL: Clinical features of the Lesch-Nyhan syndrome. Arch Intern Med 1971, 130:186.

Simkin PA: Pathogenesis of podagra. Ann Intern Med 1977, 86:230.

TRIMETHYLAMINURIA (Fish Odor Syndrome)

There have been 18 known cases of this rare metabolic defect, in which trimethylamine, a malodorous gaseous end-product of choline digestion, cannot be converted to the odorless oxide, and im-

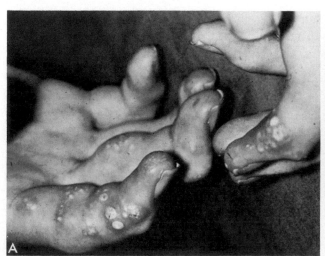 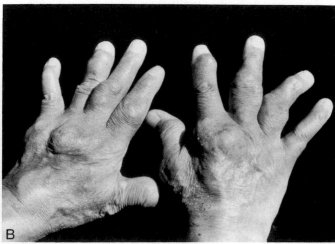

Figure 26–37. Gout.

parts the odor of decomposing fish to the breath, urine, and skin. A reduction of either the choline substrate (by correcting the diet) or of the intestinal bacteria which work on it (by giving neomycin or metronidazole orally) will greatly reduce the odor. The Shelleys reported a case in 1984.

Shelley WB, et al: The fish odor syndrome. JAMA 1984, 251:253.

CALCIUM DISORDERS

CALCINOSIS CUTIS

There are several varieties of calcium deposition in the skin. Calcium may be combined with elements of damaged or altered tissue. Such *dystrophic calcification* may occur in small localized areas (*calcinosis circumscripta*) or in large widespread areas (*calcinosis universalis*). *Traumatic calcinosis* may occur as a result of occupational exposure to calcium-containing materials, as in the cases reported by Wheeland et al and Knox et al in oil field workers. Several idiopathic forms exist, such as solitary congenital subepidermal nodular calcification and tumoral calcinosis. Finally, so-called *metastatic calcification* occurs in association with hypercalcemia or hyperphosphatemia.

Calcinosis Cutis Circumscripta

Deposits of calcium salts (calcium phosphate, apatite) appear in the skin in the form of nodules, plaques, and tumors, and are encountered in sizes varying from 2 to 30 mm. They occur chiefly on the upper extremities, particularly on the fingers or at the wrists, having a tendency to be situated over or along the course of the flexor tendons of the hands and the extensor tendons of the elbows and knees; or, in other words, in locations subject to frequent trauma and motion. Early lesions in the subcutaneous tissues in the immediate vicinity of joints, particularly of the extremities, are covered by skin that is normal in appearance, but as the lesions enlarge the overlying skin becomes adherent and inflamed and later breaks down. Creamy material containing small gritty particles of calcium slowly exudes.

This type of calcinosis is seen in scleroderma and in the *CREST syndrome*, comprising calcinosis cutis, Raynaud's phenomenon, esophageal dysmotility, sclerodactyly, and telangiectasia. Other systemic diseases in which this localized type of dystrophic calcinosis cutis may occur are morphea, dermatomyositis, systemic lupus erythematosus, rheumatoid arthritis, and pseudoxanthoma elasticum.

Circumscribed plaques of calcinosis have already been mentioned as occurring in sclerodermoid porphyria cutanea tarda. Circumscribed calcinosis and "chalk gout" occur frequently in middle-aged women, often beginning at menopause. In calcifying pilomatricoma of Malherbe, in calcified myxoid cysts, and in basal cell nevus syndrome lesions, circumscribed calcinosis may occur. Other cutaneous processes and tumors which may calcify are burn scars, inflamed scrotal epidermal inclusion cysts, trichilemmal cysts, dermoid cysts, hemangiomas, keratoses, neurilemmomas, chondromas, trichoepitheliomas, foreign body granulomas, and miscellaneous inflammatory processes such as acne vulgaris.

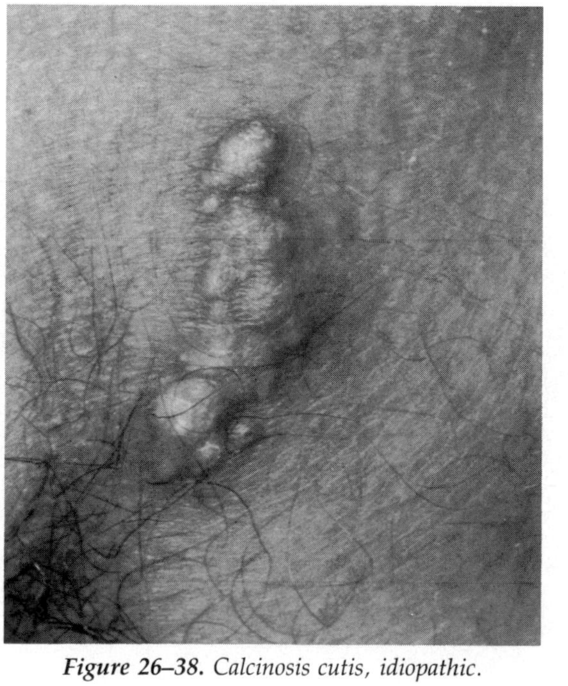

Figure 26-38. Calcinosis cutis, idiopathic.

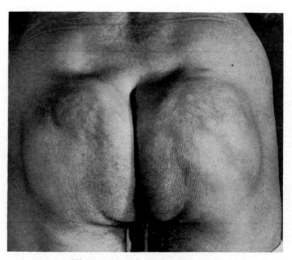

Figure 26-39. Calcinosis cutis.

The intralesional or intramuscular injection of triamcinolone hexacetonide has been known to produce atrophy at the site of injection; however, Baden and Bonar have reported calcinosis cutis occurring after its injection. The calcified lesion allegedly contains a calcified deposit of triamcinolone hexacetonide.

An ingenious method of treatment to relieve the symptoms of localized calcium deposits, especially on the fingers, has been described by MacDowell. A fish-mouthed incision is made over the circumscribed calcium mass, the flap is lifted up and with a dental burr the calcification is broken up and then flushed out with saline. This has proved to be exceptionally useful in treating the nodules of CREST syndrome when ischemic ulcerations have developed over large masses. Wang et al reported a remarkable response to aluminum hydroxide, 15 to 20 mL four times a day for one year, in a patient with dermatomyositis and disfiguring calcinosis cutis.

Calcinosis Universalis

This type of diffuse calcification of the skin usually affects the deeper subcutaneous tissues and the dermis, often in the proximal parts of the extremities and pelvic girdle. It can be associated with the CREST syndrome and dermatomyositis. The muscles and tendons may also be involved, and the joints may become swollen and immobile.

Traumatic Calcinosis Cutis

A rarely reported entity, traumatic calcium deposition in the skin, has been reported as occurring after contact with calcium chloride-containing substances. Prolonged contact with electroencephalogram electrode paste (Clendenning and Auerbach), cloth sacks of calcium chloride, limewater compresses, coal mine exposure to calcium chloride, and exposure to refrigerant calcium chloride have been some of the etiologic agents for this type of calcinosis. Both Wheeland et al and Knox et al have reported that cutaneous exposure to calcium chloride in oil field workers may lead to calcinosis cutis, which appears histologically as transepithelial elimination. Hironaga et al reported a newborn who developed calcinosis cutis after calcium gluconate extravasated into the tissue from the infusion line. Calcifications may occur in neonates following heel sticks.

Solitary Congenital Nodular Calcification

Winer described this entity, in which there is a solitary small raised verrucous nodule, commonly located on the face or extremities. Duperrat and Goetschel reported three patients in whom they found the typical histologic features of calcification

in the upper dermis. Calcium globules were found in nests, and granules were found in the epidermis.

Subepidermal Calcified Nodule

This distinct type of idiopathic calcinosis occurs most frequently as a solitary lesion on the scalp or face of children. Reynaud et al reviewed 41 cases reported since 1952 and found males outnumbered females nearly 2 to 1 and the average age at onset was seven years.

Tumoral Calcinosis

Tumoral calcinosis is a rare familial disease of unknown cause which usually appears early in life, with large subcutaneous masses of calcium overlying pressure areas and joints. The exact mode of inheritance has not been established. Transmission from parent to children has not been observed, but when the disorder occurs in a sibship, about 50 per cent of the members are affected. Skin involvement apart from the tumoral masses is extremely rare but may occur as localized calcinosis cutis. The internal organs are not involved, and serum calcium levels are generally normal. Serum phosphorus levels are often elevated. The masses contain either calcium phosphate or carbonate salts, or both.

Surgical excision has been the mainstay of therapy; however, recurrences are frequent. Various dietary restrictions to lower calcium and phosphorus intake have shown some success.

Metastatic Calcinosis Cutis

This rare entity is characterized by metastatic calcifications to the skin, elevated serum calcium, and hyperphosphatemia. Metastatic calcinosis is usually associated with bone destruction. In calcinosis cutis with hyperparathyroidism, Posey and Ritchie described the skin manifestations as numerous, small, firm, white papules, about 1 to 4 mm in diameter, surrounded by slight edema, occurring symmetrically in the popliteal fossae, over the iliac crests, and in the posterior axillary lines.

This type of calcinosis occurs in those diseases causing chronically elevated serum calcium, hyperphosphatemia, or both. Such are parathyroid neoplasms, primary hyperparathyroidism, hypervitaminosis D, sarcoidosis, excessive intake of milk and alkali, and osteomyelitis with excessive destruction of the bone. Other diseases accompanied by the destruction of bone tissue are leukemia, Paget's disease of the bone, and metastatic carcinoma.

The concomitant association of calcinosis cutis with hyperphosphatemia as seen in chronic renal disease is frequently evident. Other organs involved in addition to the skin are the lungs, kidneys, heart, arteries, eyes, and stomach.

Histologically, the calcium deposits may be found in the subcutaneous fat and in the dermis as black masses when von Kossa's stain is used. A foreign body reaction of an inflammatory infiltrate, giant cells, and fibrosis occurs regularly.

Treatment of metastatic calcinosis cutis associated with chronic renal disease has produced varied results. Eisenberg and Bartholow reported involution of the skin lesions with a diet containing 430 mg phosphorus, 30 gm protein, and 60 ml aluminum hydroxide gel daily.

Osteoma Cutis

Bone formation within the skin may be *primary* in cases where there was no preceding lesion, or *metastatic*, where ossification occurs in a preexisting lesion or inflammatory process. Besides Albright's syndrome, other types of primary osteoma cutis include either widespread or single, plaquelike osteomas present at birth or in early life, single osteomas occurring in later life, or miliary osteomas of the face in women. Some feel the latter are metastatic because they may be occurring in acne scars. Metastatic osteoma cutis occurs most frequently in pilomatricomas; however, other lesions in which bone formation may occur are basal cell epithelioma, intradermal nevi, mixed tumor of the skin, scars, scleroderma, dermatomyositis, and inflammatory diseases of many types.

Anderson HC: Calcific diseases. Arch Pathol Lab Med 1983, 107:341.
Baden HP, et al: Calcinosis cutis following intralesional injections of triamcinolone hexacetonide. Arch Dermatol 1967, 96:689.
Clendenning WE, et al: Traumatic calcium deposition in the skin. Arch Dermatol 1964, 89:360.
Cochran RJ, et al: An unusual case of calcinosis cutis. JAAD 1983, 8:103.
Cornelius CE III, et al: Calcinosis cutis. Arch Dermatol 1968, 98:219.
Coskey RJ, et al: Calcinosis cutis in a burn scar. JAAD 1984, 11:666.
Fisher BK, et al: Idiopathic calcinosis of the scrotum. Arch Dermatol 1976, 114:957.
Goldsminz D, et al: Calcinosis cutis following extravasation of calcium chloride. Arch Dermatol 1988, 124:922.
Hironaga M, et al: Cutaneous calcinosis in a neonate following extravasation of calcium gluconate. JAAD 1982, 6:392.
Knox JM, et al: Acquired perforating disease in oil field workers. JAAD 1986, 14:605.
Leung A: Calcification following heel sticks. J Pediatr 1985, 106:168.
Lim MO, et al: Dysplastic cutaneous osteomatosis. Arch Dermatol 1981, 117:797.
MacDowell F: Digital involvement of extremities in scleroderma. NY State J Med 1969, 69:935.
Mallory SB, et al: Solitary congenital nodule of the ear. Arch Dermatol 1988, 124:769.
Pursley TV, et al: Cutaneous manifestations of tumoral calcinosis. Arch Dermatol 1979, 115:1100.
Quismorio SP, et al: Soft-tissue calcification in systemic lupus erythematosus. Arch Dermatol 1975, 111:352.
Redmond WJ, et al: Keloidal calcification. Arch Dermatol 1983, 119:270.
Reynaud AC, et al: Subepidermal calcified nodule. J Assoc Milit Dermatol 1984, 10:10.
Simons-Ling N, et al: Childhood systemic lupus erythematosus. Arch Dermatol 1983, 119:491.
Song DH, et al: Idiopathic calcinosis of the scrotum. JAAD 1988, 19:1095.
Speer ME, et al: Calcification of superficial scalp veins secondary to intravenous infusion of sodium bicarbonate and calcium chloride. Cutis 1983, 32:65.
Swinehart JM, et al: Scrotal calcinosis. Arch Dermatol 1982, 118:985.
Wang W-J, et al: Calcinosis cutis in juvenile dermatomyositis: Remarkable response to aluminum hydroxide therapy. Arch Dermatol 1988, 124:1721.
Wheeland RG, et al: Calcinosis cutis resulting from percutaneous penetration and deposition of calcium. JAAD 1985, 12:172.

ALBRIGHT'S HEREDITARY OSTEODYSTROPHY

Albright's hereditary osteodystrophy (AHO) includes both pseudohypoparathyroidism and pseudopseudohypoparathyroidism (PHP and PPHP). In PHP there is hypocalcemia and no response to parathyroid hormone. In PPHP serum calcium is normal. Cases may gradually change from PHP to PPHP.

Patients with AHO are short of stature, with short metacarpals and metatarsals; round facies; short, broad nails; and soft tissue calcifications. Cataracts, basal ganglion calcification, mental retardation, defective teeth, tetany, cramps, and various skeletal abnormalities may occur. Actual bone formation commonly occurs in soft tissues.

Barranco VP: Cutaneous ossification in pseudohypoparathyroidism. Arch Dermatol 1971, 104:643.
Eyre WG, et al: Hereditary osteodystropathy with cutaneous bone formation. Arch Dermatol 1971, 104:634.

27

Some Genodermatoses

In many common disorders in dermatology, genetic factors exist that, along with many other influences, may predispose to disease. These are variably expressed, multifactorial diseases such as psoriasis or atopic dermatitis. However, there is another group of diseases, which are comparatively rare and are the result of a single mutant gene. Autosomal (non–sex chromosomal) dominant conditions require only a single gene to produce the phenotype. Usually the patient has one affected parent, and the disease is transmitted from generation to generation. Autosomal recessive traits, on the other hand, require a homozygous state to produce the abnormality. The pedigree here will often reveal parental consanguinity, clinically *unaffected* parents but often affected siblings. X-linked conditions occur when the mutant gene is carried on the X chromosome. If a disease is X-linked recessive it occurs almost exclusively in males, who cannot transmit the disease to their sons, but all of their daughters will be carriers. Carrier females, who are heterozygous (having one normal and one abnormal X chromosome), occasionally may show some subtle evidence of the disease. X-linked dominant disease states, if lethal in male (as incontinentia pigmenti is theorized to be), explain pedigrees where more than one female is affected but no males express the disease. If such conditions are not lethal in males the pedigree may resemble an autosomal dominant pattern of inheritance; however, an affected male will transmit the disorder to all of his daughters but none of his sons. Genetic counseling is a mainstay of the education given to patients and their families in the conditions that follow.

Alper JC (ed): The genodermatoses. Dermatologic Clinics. Philadelphia, W. B. Saunders, 1987.

Alper JC: The genodermatoses and their significance in pediatric dermatology. Dermatol Clin 1986, 4:46.

Emery AEH, et al (eds): Principles and practice of medical genetics. Vol 1 and 2. Edinburgh, Churchill Livingstone, 1983.

Freire-Maia N: Ectodermal dysplasia. New York, Liss, 1984.

Goldsmith LA: Principles of genetics as applied to dermatologic diseases. JAAD 1981, 4:255.

Holbrook KA (ed): Prenatal diagnosis of genetic skin disease. Semin Dermatol 1984, 3:155.

McKusick VA: Mendelian inheritance in man. Baltimore, The Johns Hopkins University Press, 1986.

Wuepper KD, Gedde-Dahl T Jr: Biology of Heritable Skin Diseases. (Curr Probl Dermatol Vol. 17) New York, Karger, 1987.

INCONTINENTIA PIGMENTI

CLINICAL FEATURES. Also known as *Bloch-Sulzberger's disease*, incontinentia pigmenti is characterized by spattered pigmentation on the trunk preceded by urticarial, vesicular, or verrucous inflammatory changes appearing in girls during the first weeks of life. Carney's review of 609 cases showed 96 per cent began by four weeks of age.

The highly distinctive lesions are initially vesicular in 87 per cent of cases. This first stage begins usually before six weeks of age, and while it usually is replaced by verrucous lesions after several months, O'Brien et al reported a patient who developed intermittent vesicles at age six. The second (verrucous) stage follows the blistering in two thirds of patients, occurring in a similar distribution. While these usually resolve by one year of age, lesions may persist for many years.

Following the inflammatory and verrucous stages, the pigmentary phase is seen: pigmented macules, scattered over the trunk, upper arms, and upper legs. The pigmentation is capriciously patterned, dendritic, and bizarre, with irregularly shaped splashes, lines, streaks, whorls, polyangular flecks, and spidery and fountain-spray splatters. The pattern of eruption does not follow the lines of cleavage nor the distribution of the nerves. The inflammatory stages do not necessarily precede the typical pigmentation: there is frequent overlap of the three stages,

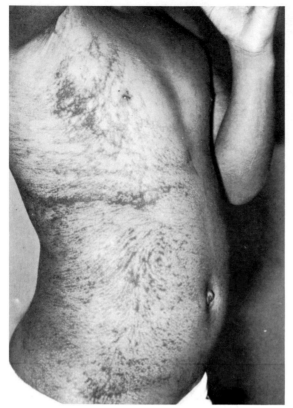

Figure 27–1. *Incontinentia pigmenti with whorls and fountain-spray splatters. (Courtesy of Dr. J. P. Ruppe.)*

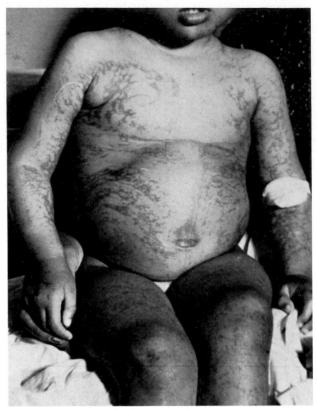

Figure 27–2. *Incontinentia pigmenti. (Courtesy of Dr. H. Curth.)*

and the blistering and verrucous stages may not occur at all in some patients.

The pigmentary stage may last for many years and then fade away, leaving no sequelae except possibly lightly hypopigmented and atrophic lesions, which are the only remains to mark the sites of the previous bizarre lesions.

The general health is good. There is no fever. Other cutaneous changes include patchy alopecia at the vertex of the scalp, atrophic changes simulating acrodermatitis chronica atrophicans on the hands, onychodystrophy, subungual tumors with underlying lytic bone lesions, and palmoplantar hyperhidrosis. Extracutaneous manifestations occur in 70 to 80 per cent of patients. Most commonly involved are the central nervous system, the eyes, the bones, and the teeth. Immune dysfunction with defective neutrophil chemotaxis and elevated IgE has been reported. Eosinophilia is common.

The eye changes, half of them serious, which occur in 35 per cent of cases, according to Carney, include cataract, strabismus (in 18 per cent—Carney), optic atrophy, blue sclerae, and exudative chorioretinitis.

Skeletal abnormalities include syndactyly, skull deformities, dwarfism, spina bifida, clubfoot, supernumerary ribs, hemiatrophy, and shortening of the legs and arms. The teeth may show delayed denti-

tion, pegged or conical crowns, malformation, and missing teeth.

ETIOLOGY. Incontinentia pigmenti is due to an X-linked gene, dominant in females and lethal in males. Some 600 cases have been reported to have occurred in girls as compared to 16 in boys. Boys with one abnormal X chromosome are believed to die in utero with severe disease, and there is an increased incidence of spontaneous abortion in girls with this disease. Affected males are believed to have had a spontaneous mutation during replication in the gamete, resulting in mosaicism after fertilization.

Person has speculated that this disease may be due to an autoimmune attack on antigens limited to the ectoderm.

HISTOLOGY. Histologically, there is an evolutionary process. The vesicles are intraepidermal and associated with marked spongiosis and numerous eosinophils. Small epidermal whorls as well as a dermal inflammatory infiltrate may be evident. Then acanthosis, hyperkeratosis, and papillomatosis occur in the second stage, with epidermal whorls becoming more prominent. The end-stage of pigmentation is manifested by melanin in melanophages in the upper dermis and vacuolar degeneration of the basal cell layer.

Wong and associates at Oxford's Radcliffe Infir-

Carney RG Jr: Incontinentia pigmenti. Arch Dermatol 1976, 112:535.

Jessen RT, et al: Incontinentia pigmenti. Arch Dermatol 1978, 114:1182.

Kegel MF: Dominant disorders with multiple organ involvement. Dermatol Clin 1987, 5:205.

Mascaro JM, et al: Painful subungual keratotic tumors in incontinentia pigmenti. JAAD 1985, 13:913.

O'Brien JE, et al: Incontinentia pigmenti. Am J Dis Child 1985, 139:711.

Peltonen L: Incontinentia pigmenti in four generations. Dermatologica 1986, 172:201.

Person JR: Incontinentia pigmenti. JAAD 1985, 13:120.

Prendiville JS, et al: Incontinentia pigmenti in a male infant with Klinefelter's syndrome. JAAD 1989, 20:937.

Wettke-Schafer R, et al: X-linked dominant inherited diseases with lethality in hemizygous males. Hum Genet 1983, 64:1.

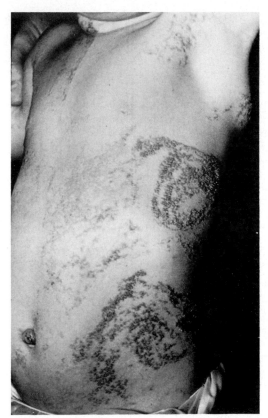

Figure 27–3. Incontinentia pigmenti with whorled verrucous lesions.

mary found giant vacuoles and myelin figures in the melanocytes on electron microscopy, and normal premelanosomes and melanosomes.

DIFFERENTIAL DIAGNOSIS. In the differential diagnosis, epidermolysis bullosa and childhood bullous pemphigoid are easily distinguished. Incontinentia pigmenti differs from the Franceschetti-Jadassohn syndrome in that the latter has a reticular pigmentation rather than sprays or spatters; also no abnormal dentition and no eye lesions are present. Incontinentia pigmenti achromians differs in that it is a negative image, with hypopigmentation; it is autosomal dominant in inheritance; it has no vesicular or verrucous stages; and it has a higher incidence of central nervous system abnormalities.

TREATMENT. There is no treatment. Usually the end-stage of streaks of incontinentia pigmenti start to fade out at age two and by adulthood almost nothing is discernible.

Franceschetti-Jadassohn Syndrome. This, also known as the *chromatophore nevus of Naegeli*, is different from the Bloch-Sulzberger type of incontinentia pigmenti, since the pigmentation is reticular and there are no preceding inflammatory changes or vesiculation or verrucous lesions, except possibly plantar hyperkeratosis. Vasomotor changes and hypohidrosis occur. Both sexes are equally affected. This has been reported only in a Swiss family in which the disease occurred as an autosomal dominant trait.

Incontinentia Pigmenti Achromians (Hypomelanosis of Ito)

This disease is characterized by various patterns of bilateral or unilateral hypopigmentation (instead of hyperpigmentation as seen in the Bloch-Sulzberger incontinentia pigmenti). The lesions suggest the "negative picture" of incontinentia pigmenti. Takematsu et al in 1983 reviewed 32 cases reported from Japan and 41 from the U.S., Europe, the Caribbean, Mexico, and India. The female:male ratio was about 2.5:1 in both groups. Three fourths had associated anomalies of the CNS, eyes, hair, teeth, skin, nails, musculoskeletal system, or internal organs. Takematsu lists 60 defects reported in five organ systems.

No inflammatory changes or vesiculation are found prior to the development of the hypopigmentation, and there is no liquefaction of the basal layer or incontinence of pigment. Peña and Ruiz-Maldonado found Langerhans cells were numerous.

There is no treatment, but eventual repigmentation is the rule, according to Peña and Ruiz-Maldonado.

Cambazard F, et al: Hypomelanosis of Ito. Ann Dermatol Venereol 1986, 113:15.

Jelinek JE, et al: Hypomelanosis of Ito. Arch Dermatol 1973, 107:596.

Pena L, et al: Incontinentia pigmenti achromians. Int J Dermatol 1977, 16:194.

Takemastu H, et al: Incontinentia pigmenti achromians (Ito). Arch Dermatol 1983, 119:391.

KLINEFELTER'S SYNDROME

Klinefelter's syndrome consists of hypogonadism, gynecomastia, eunuchoidism, small or absent testicles, and elevated gonadotropins. The cutaneous changes are minimal, but there may be a low frontal hairline, sparse body hair with only a few hairs in the axillary and pubic areas, scanty or absent facial hair in men, and shortening of the fifth digit of both hands. Dull mentality or misbehavior is frequent.

Many of the patients are tall; some are obese. Psychiatric disorders occur in about one third of the patients.

Klinefelter's syndrome is a problem of male sex differentiation; it is most frequently an XXY sex chromosome pattern, although other variations occur as the number of X chromosomes increases.

Marked improvement in appearance has been achieved by injection of 500 to 1000 mg of testosterone enanthate (Delatestryl) every two weeks, reducing the dose after a few months to once monthly.

XXYY Genotype. Considering it to be a variant of Klinefelter's syndrome, Peterson and his associates described the cutaneous aspects of this genotype. In addition to the changes seen in Klinefelter's syndrome there are vascular changes, such as cutaneous angiomas, acrocyanosis, and peripheral vascular disease leading to stasis dermatitis.

Caldwell PD, et al: XXY syndrome in childhood. J Pediatr 1972, 80:250.
Prendiville JS, et al: Incontinentia pigmenti in a male infant with Klinefelter's syndrome. JAAD 1989, 20:937.

TURNER'S SYNDROME

Turner's syndrome, also known as *gonadal dysgenesis*, is characterized by a webbed neck, low posterior hairline margin, increased carrying angle at the elbow (cubitus valgus), a triangular mouth, alopecia of the frontal area on the scalp, sometimes koilonychia, cutis laxa, cutis hyperelastica, and patchy alopecia on the scalp. Judd and his associates reported hirsutism in a 24-year-old woman with pure gonadal dysgenesis. There may be mental retardation, short stature, infantilism, and retarded sexual development with primary amenorrhea. Sterility does not

always prevent it from becoming a familial problem, as shown by Leichtman and associates.

It has been shown that these patients with gonadal dysgenesis have only 45 instead of a normal 46 chromosomes. An X chromosome is missing to make it 45 XO. Mosaicism, structural abnormalities of the X chromosome, or a partial deficiency of one sex chromosome may account for a number of the variations in gonadal dysgenesis.

No specific treatment is available; however, Tzagournis has reported some growth response to long-term therapy with exogenous human growth hormone.

Leichtman DA, et al: Familial Turner's syndrome. Ann Intern Med 1978, 89:473.
Tzagournis M: Response to long-term administration of human growth hormone in Turner's syndrome. JAMA 1969, 210:2373.

NOONAN'S SYNDROME

Wyre found that the cutaneous findings in this autosomal dominant inherited disease in many respects mimics Turner's syndrome. Males and females are affected, and the chromosome number is normal, in Noonan's syndrome. The major features are a characteristic facies with hypertelorism, prominent ears, webbed neck, short stature, undescended testicles, low posterior neck hairline, cardiovascular abnormalities, and cubitus valgus. The major dermatologic findings are lymphedema, curly short hair, dystrophic nails, tendency to keloid formation, soft elastic skin, and abnormal dermatoglyphics.

Wyre HW Jr: Cutaneous manifestations of Noonan's syndrome. Arch Dermatol 1978, 114:929.

PHAKOMATOSES

The phakomatoses are those various inherited disorders of the central nervous system with congenital retinal tumors and cutaneous involvement. The phakomatoses comprise tuberous sclerosis, von Recklinghausen's disease (neurofibromatosis), von Hippel-Lindau's disease (angiomatosis retinae), ataxia-telangiectasia, basal cell nevus syndrome, nevus sebaceus, and Sturge-Weber syndrome.

Tuberous Sclerosis (Epiloia)

The term "epiloia" (*epi* = epilepsy, *loi* = low intelligence, *a* = adenoma sebaceum) encompasses *adenoma sebaceum*, representing one of the cutaneous changes, and *tuberous sclerosis*, representing the central nervous system involvement.

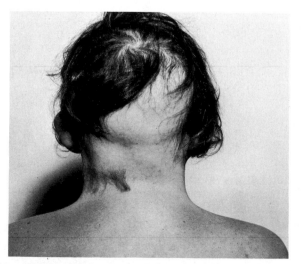

Figure 27–4. Alopecia areata and webbing of the neck in a girl aged 14 with Turner's syndrome.

CLINICAL SIGNS AND SYMPTOMS. This clinical syndrome, also known as *Bourneville's disease*, includes adenoma sebaceum, mental deficiency, and epilepsy. Associated with this triad may be subungual fibromas, shagreen skin, oral papillomatosis, ash-leaf hypomelanotic macules, skin fibromas, and café au lait spots.

Adenoma sebaceum is characterized by pinhead-sized, yellowish red, translucent, discrete, waxy papules situated on the face. These are located principally over the cheeks, nose, and forehead in symmetrical fashion. These pathognomonic lesions of tuberous sclerosis are present in 90 per cent of patients over four years of age, persist indefinitely, and may increase in number. A better name for the facial lesions would be angiofibromas.

Shagreen skin is named for shagreen, meaning leather that is tanned in a particular way to produce greenish knobs on the surface, resembling shark skin. Patches of this type of "knobby" skin varying from 1 to 8 cm are found on the trunk, but most commonly on the lumbosacral area. These are connective tissue nevi. They occur in 40 per cent of patients, and develop in the first decade of life.

Subungual fibromas and *Koenen's periungual tumors* are distinctive when present. These are small, digitate, protruding, asymptomatic tumors. They are angiofibromas histologically, they have their onset at puberty, they affect approximately 50 per cent of adult patients, and similar angiofibromas may occur on the gingiva.

Congenital white leaf-shaped macules, called hypomelanotic macules, have been found to be present in some 85 per cent of patients with epiloia. These may be detected at birth in most patients, although Oppenheimer et al have documented that an occasional patient may not develop them until age six or eight. They may be ash-leaf in shape, but linear and confetti-type white macules may also be present. Wood's light examination should be done when evaluating a patient for tuberous sclerosis. McWilliam and Stephenson document that focal poliosis (localized tufts of white hair) may be present at birth. Although similar lesions are occasionally seen singly in otherwise normal children, they are decidedly unusual. Osburn et al studied 830 consecutive newborns by Wood's light and found none.

Mental deficiency is usually seen early in life, varying over a wide latitude in its manifestations. It is estimated to occur in 40 to 60 per cent of patients.

Epilepsy is also variable in its severity. Myoclonic spells may occur early in life. Eighty to 90 per cent of patients have seizures or nonspecific electroencephalographic abnormalities.

There may be cerebral calcification with *potatolike nodules* or *brain stones* in the cortex. X-ray will visu-

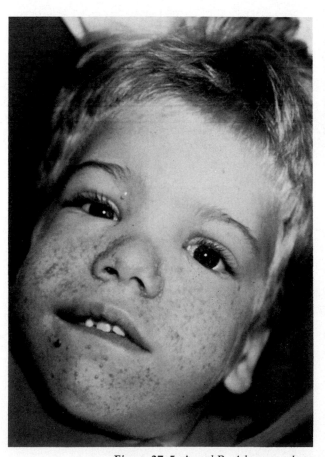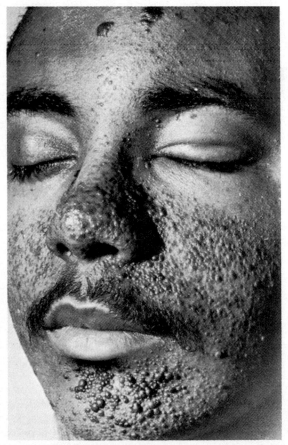

Figure 27–5. A and B, *Adenoma sebaceum.* (B, *Courtesy of Dr. J. McSorley.*)

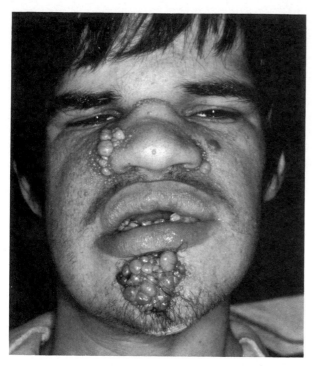

Figure 27–6. Patient with tuberous sclerosis, mental retardation, and a convulsive disorder. (Courtesy of Dr. Axel W. Hoke.)

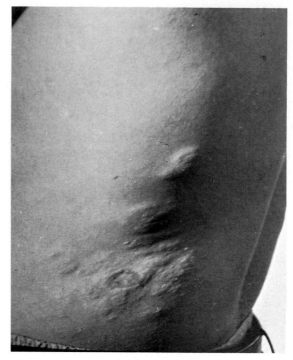

Figure 27–7. Shagreen skin in epiloia on the side of the lower back.

alize these once they are calcified, but computed tomographic (CAT) scans, cranial ultrasound, and magnetic resonance (NMR) imaging may define these lesions as early as six weeks of age and are useful in helping to make an early diagnosis.

Retinal tumors (phakomas) occur, which are optic- or retinal-nerve hamartomas. Various ophthalmologic findings such as pigmentary changes, nystagmus, and angioid streaks occur in 50 per cent of patients.

Renal hamartomas (angiomyolipomas, cystic disease, fibroadenomas, or mixed tumors) and *cardiac tumors* (rhabdomyoma) may also occur.

In the familial variety of tuberous sclerosis, 80 per cent of patients have an angiomyolipoma, which is often bilateral and frequently causes severe problems, including renal failure.

A few patients—all women of childbearing age—have *pulmonary lymphangiomyomas,* and the suggestion has been made by Valensi, Monteforte and others that pulmonary lymphangiomatosis may be a *forme fruste* of tuberous sclerosis.

Almost half of patients have bony abnormalities such as bone cysts and sclerosis, which are seen on x-ray. Pits in the enamel of permanent teeth, when they number five or more, are a marker for this disease.

ETIOLOGY. Tuberous sclerosis is an inherited disease having an autosomal dominant pattern. Its expressivity is varied. One member of the family may have adenoma sebaceum alone, while another may have epilepsy or some other manifestation. Up

to 50 per cent of cases may be a result of spontaneous mutations.

DIAGNOSIS. The "ash-leaf" macules—most easily seen with Wood's light—may be present at birth, and are an indication for skull roentgenograms. If these fail to show calcified intracranial nodules, a CAT scan, which is four times as sensitive, according to Burkhart et al, should be done. Also funduscopic examination, hand and foot x-rays, and renal ultrasound may be considered in the patient, and, as

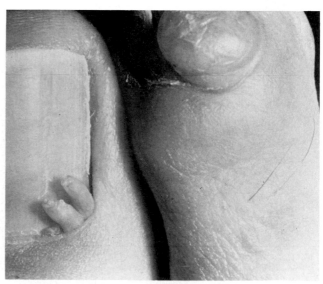

Figure 27–8. Periungual fibromas—Koenen's tumors.

Rogers RS III: Dermatologic manifestations. In Tuberous Sclerosis. Gomez MR (ed). New York, Raven Press, 1979, pp. 95–119.
Valensi QJ: Pulmonary lymphangiomyoma. Am Rev Respir Dis 1973, 108:1411.

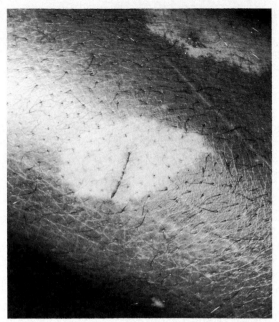

Figure 27–9. "Ash-leaf" macule in a patient with tuberous sclerosis.

Cassidy et al's study would indicate, may even be considered in asymptomatic parents, since they were able to identify 31 per cent of asymptomatic parents as having tuberous sclerosis by using these tests.

PATHOLOGY. The "adenoma sebaceum" is essentially a vascular and connective tissue tumor (angiofibromatous hamartoma). Similar histology is seen with the subungual and gingival tumors.

TREATMENT. The lesions of adenoma sebaceum pose the greatest problem in therapy. The best results have been attained with dermabrasion of the lesions on the face. An excellent cosmetic result is usually attained; however, the lesions tend to recur after a period of months to years.

Bellack GS, et al: Management of facial angiofibromas in tuberous sclerosis. Otolaryngol Head Neck Surg 1986, 94:37.
Burkhart CG, et al: Computed axial tomography in the early diagnosis of tuberous sclerosis. JAAD 1981, 4:81.
Cassidy SB, et al: Family studies in tuberous sclerosis. JAMA 1983, 249:1302.
Fryer AE, et al: Forehead plaque: A presenting skin sign in tuberous sclerosis. Arch Dis Child 1987, 62:292.
Kegel MF: Dominant disorders with multiple organ involvement. Dermatol Clin 1987, 5:205.
Kint A, et al: Histopathologic study of Koenen tumors. JAAD 1988, 18:369.
Lagos JC, et al: Tuberous sclerosis. Mayo Clin Proc 1967, 42:26.
McCarty VS Jr, et al: Pulmonary lymphangiomyomatosis responsive to progesterone. N Engl J Med 1980, 303:1461.
McWilliam RC, et al: Depigmented hair: the earliest sign of tuberous sclerosis. Arch Dis Child 1978, 53:961.
Monteforte WJ Jr, et al: Angiomyolipomas in a case of lymphangiomyomatosis syndrome. Cancer 1974, 34:317.
Oppenheimer EY, et al: The late appearance of hypopigmented macules in tuberous sclerosis. Am J Dis Child 1985, 139:408.
Osburn K, et al: Congenital pigmented and vascular lesions in newborn infants. JAAD 1987, 16:788.
Park Y-K, et al: Cluster growths in adenoma sebaceum. JAAD 1989, 20:918.

Neurofibromatosis (von Recklinghausen's Disease)

SIGNS AND SYMPTOMS. This autosomal dominant inherited syndrome is manifested by developmental changes in the nervous system, bones, and skin. Von Recklinghausen described it in 1882, and Riccardi divided it into seven types almost exactly a century later. Type 1, which comprises over 85 per cent of cases, is "typical" neurofibromatosis, with many neurofibromas from a few millimeters to a few centimeters in diameter and many café au lait spots, widely distributed, and few or no central nervous system lesions. Lisch nodules can be found in the irises in about one fourth of patients under six, and in 94 per cent of older patients.

Type 2, central or acoustic neurofibromatosis, is distinguished by bilateral acoustic neuromas.

Types 3 ("mixed") and 4 ("variant") resemble type 2, but may have more numerous cutaneous neurofibromas, and are at greater risk for developing optic gliomas, neurilemmomas, and meningiomas.

These are all inherited by autosomal dominance, but type 5, segmental (dermatomal) neurofibromatosis, is considered to arise from a postzygotic somatic mutation, and is not generally heritable, though Rubenstein et al reported an instance of apparent genetic transmission. Type 6 has no neurofibromas, only café au lait spots, and must occur in two generations to be diagnosed. Type 7, late-onset neurofibromatosis, begins to manifest neurofibromas no earlier than the twenties. It is not yet known whether it is inherited.

Lisch nodules in only one iris have been reported in a 14-year-old girl with segmental neurofibromatosis by Weleber et al. Roth et al have reviewed segmental neurofibromatosis in detail. And bilateral cases, which are hard to classify, have been reported by Takiguchi et al, Crowe et al, and Roth et al.

The characteristic skin lesions occur in several forms, chiefly neurofibromas, but also café au lait macules, axillary freckles, bronzing, giant pigmented hairy nevi ("neuronevi"), sacral hypertrichosis, cutis verticis gyrata, and macroglossia.

The *cutaneous neurofibromas* are dermal tumors varying in size from pinhead to large, pendulous, flabby masses weighing several kilograms, which may cause great disfigurement. Many of the small soft tumors can be pushed down into the panniculus by light pressure with the finger ("buttonholing"), and spring back when released, which distinguishes them from lipomas. Neurofibromas of the areolae occur in over 90 per cent of women with this disease.

The *subcutaneous neurofibromas* coursing along the nerves occur as discrete, slowly growing nodules along peripheral nerves. These are *plexiform neuromas*.

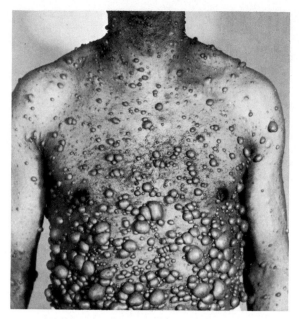

Figure 27–10. Multiple neurofibromas.

Later the single subcutaneous tumor may be associated with other growths, frequently along the same nerve trunk.

The café au lait macule is a hallmark of this disease. Usually it is a uniformly pigmented light brown macule, unevenly round or oval, from 1.5 to 15 cm in diameter, most often present at birth and almost always present by age one. Six or more of these lesions at least 1.5 cm in diameter ("Crowe's sign") is a diagnostic finding, usually indicative of type 1 neurofibromatosis, in light-skinned individuals, though some may be of type 6. Block demonstrated that multiple café au lait spots, and even axillary freckling, may occur without other evidence of neurofibromatosis in the black and "colored" people of South Africa. In children the usual minimum diameter imposed for a significant lesion is 0.5 cm.

Histologically, giant pigment granules may be seen in the malpighian cells and melanocytes.

Axillary freckling may occur, and may extend to the neck and perineal areas. *Bronzing* or hyperpigmentation of the skin may be present. Xanthogranulomas may occur. A plexiform neurofibroma and bony dysplasia may be signalled by a hairy nevus overlying this defect.

CLINICAL FEATURES. Many organ systems may be involved. Endocrine disorders such as acromegaly, cretinism, hyperparathyroidism, myxedema, pheochromocytoma, or precocious puberty may be present, though Riccardi has rarely seen the latter in his patients and feels this is not a major area of overlap with Albright's syndrome. Lisch nodules occur in 94 per cent of postpubertal patients. Bone changes (usually erosive) may produce lordosis, kyphosis, and pseudoarthrosis, as well as spina bifida, dislocations, and atraumatic fractures. Neuromas of spinal nerves may cause various paralyses. The importance of localized and other atypical forms was emphasized in an editorial by Riccardi in 1987.

Mental retardation, dementia, epilepsy, brain tumors, and tumors of cranial nerves may occur. Hypertelorism heralds a severe expression of neurofibromatosis with brain involvement, as Westerhof et al reported.

Finally, diffuse interstitial lung disease was present in 7 per cent of the patients reported by Burkhalter et al.

ETIOLOGY. Neurofibromatosis is of autosomal dominant inheritance, except for type 5, which is believed to be caused by a postzygotic somatic mu-

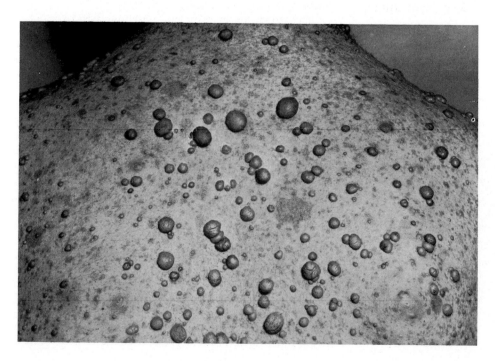

Figure 27–11. Von Recklinghausen's disease. Numerous neurofibromas on the upper back and several café au lait patches are apparent.

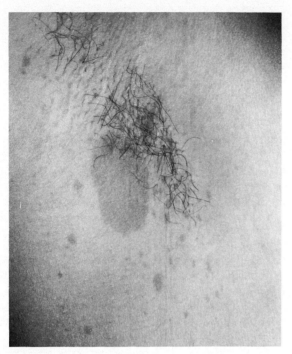

Figure 27–12. Axillary freckles (Crowe's sign) in a patient with neurofibromatosis. (Courtesy of Dr. Axel W. Hoke.)

Barker D, et al: Gene for von Recklinghausen neurofibromatosis is in the periantromeric region of chromosome 17. Science 1987, 236:1100.

Block CH: Cafe au lait spots in colored and Indian children. S Afr Med J 1984, 65:651.

Burkhalter JL, et al: Diffuse interstitial lung disease in neurofibromatosis. South Med J 1986, 79:944.

Case records of the Massachusetts General Hospital. N Engl J Med 1980, 302:736.

Ibid: 1984, 311:520.

Conejo-Mir JS, et al: Segmental neurofibromatosis. JAAD 1989, 20:681.

Fitzpatrick TB, et al: Problems in diagnosing neurofibromatosis. Adv Neurol 1981, 29:245.

Hanke CW, et al: Treatment of multiple facial neurofibromas with dermabrasion. J Dermatol Surg Oncol 1987, 13:6.

Martuza RL, et al: Melanin macroglobules as a cellular marker of neurofibromatosis. J Invest Dermatol 1985, 85:347.

Idem: Neurofibromatosis 2. N Engl J Med 1988, 318:684.

Oranje AP, et al: Segmental neurofibromatosis. Br J Dermatol 1985, 112:107.

Pullara TJ, et al: Cutaneous segmental neurofibromatosis. JAAD 1985, 13:999.

Riccardi VM: Neurofibromatosis and Albright's syndrome. Dermatol Clin 1987, 5:193.

Idem: von Recklinghausen neurofibromatosis. N Engl J Med 1981, 305:1617.

Idem: Pathophysiology of neurofibromatosis IV. JAAD 1980, 3:157.

Idem: Neurofibromatosis. Curr Probl Cancer 1982, 7:1.

Idem: Neurofibromatosis: importance of localized or otherwise atypical forms (editorial). Arch Dermatol 1987, 183:882.

tation. Approximately 50 per cent of cases represent new mutations. The gene for NF-1 has been determined to be in the pericentric region of chromosome 17. The gene for NF-2 has been determined to be on the long arm of chromosome 22.

HISTOPATHOLOGY. The neurofibroma consists of faintly eosinophilic, thin, wavy spindle cells with oval to spindle-shaped nuclei. Most of the cells are Schwann cells.

DIFFERENTIAL DIAGNOSIS. The presence of three or more neurofibromas, six or more café au lait spots 1.5 cm or greater, multiple Lisch nodules, and axillary freckling have been discussed as possible diagnostic criteria by Fitzpatrick et al. The only one which appears to be pathognomonic is the presence of multiple (three or more) neurofibromas.

TREATMENT. There is no treatment for the neurofibromas except excision. Malignant degeneration occurs in only 2 to 5 per cent, though in a cohort of 212 Danish patients reported by Sorensen et al—all severe cases requiring hospitalization—female probands developed malignancy or intracranial tumors four times more often than the others. Incidentally diagnosed relatives may have a better outcome. Deaths have been reported from intracranial meningiomas and gliomas as well as from melanomas and peripheral-nerve sarcomas. The disease tends to worsen during pregnancy, and treatment-resistant hypertension may occur.

The value of dermabrasion for disfiguring facial neurofibromas was emphasized by Hanke et al in 1987.

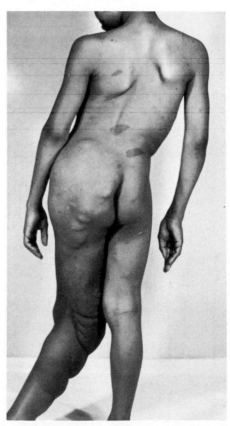

Figure 27–13. Kyphoscoliosis, café au lait macules, and enormous plexiform neuromas (elephantiasis neurofibromatosus).

Idem: Neurofibromatosis. Arch Dermatol 1987, 123:882.

Idem: Mast-cell stabilization to decrease neurofibromatosis growth. Arch Dermatol 1987, 123:1011.

Roth RR, et al: Segmental neurofibromatosis. Arch Dermatol 1987, 123:917.

Idem: Segmental neurofibromatosis. Arch Dermatol 1987, 123:917.

Sorensen SA, et al: Long-term follow-up of von Recklinghausen neurofibromatosis. N Engl J Med 1986, 314:1010.

Takiguchi PS, et al: Bilateral dermatomal neurofibromatosis. JAAD 1984, 10:451.

Toonstra J, et al: Are Lisch nodules an ocular marker of the neurofibromatosis gene in otherwise unaffected family members? Dermatologica 1987, 174:232.

Weleber RG, et al: Iris hamartomas (Lisch nodules) in a case of segmental neurofibromatosis. Am J Ophthalmol 1983, 96:740.

Wertelecki W, et al: Neurofibromatosis 2. N Engl J Med 1988, 319:278.

Westerhof W: Neurofibromatosis and hypertelorism. Arch Dermatol 1984, 120:27.

The Proteus Syndrome

This rare disease, named for the Greek god Proteus (the polymorphous) has protean manifestations which include partial gigantism of the hands and feet, plantar hyperplasia, hemangiomas, lipomas, varicosities, linear verrucous epidermal nevi, macrocephaly, cranial hyperostosis, and hypertrophy of the long bones. Tibbles et al speculate that Joseph Merrick, the Elephant Man, suffered from this disease rather than from neurofibromatosis.

Clark RD, et al: Proteus syndrome. Am J Med Genetics 1987, 27:99.

Costa T, et al: Proteus syndrome. Pediatrics 1985, 76:984.

Samlaska C, et al: Proteus syndrome. Arch Dermatol 1989; 125:1109.

Tibbles JAR, et al: The Proteus syndrome. Br Med J 1986, 293:683.

EPIDERMOLYSIS BULLOSA (EB)

"Epidermolysis bullosa" is a group of rare genetic disorders which have in common the formation of blisters on minor physical injury, and which are manifested in a variety of forms. Jo-David Fine has proposed the following comprehensive classification in a recent article:

Intraepidermal
  EB simplex, generalized (Koebner)
  EB simplex, localized (Weber-Cockayne)
  EB herpetiformis (Dowling-Meara)
  EB simplex (Ogna)
  EB simplex with mottled pigmentation
Junctional (intralamina lucida)
  EB atrophicans generalisata gravis (Herlitz; EB letalis)
  EB atrophicans generalisata mitis
  EB atrophicans localisata
  EB atrophicans inversa
  EB progressiva
  Generalized atrophic benign EB (GABEB)
  Cicatricial junctional EB

Dermolytic or dystrophic (sublamina densa)
  Dominant forms
    Dystrophic EB, hyperplastic variant (Cockayne-Touraine)
    Dystrophic EB, albopapuloid variant (Pasini)
  Recessive forms
    Generalized (gravis or mitis)
    Localized
    Inverse

Three additional less well defined entities will be discussed: Bart's syndrome, Kindler's syndrome, and transient bullous dermolysis of the newborn. Epidermolysis bullosa acquisita is discussed in Chapter 21.

Internal involvement may occur in several of these subtypes of EB. Esophageal involvement and laryngeal involvement are seen primarily in recessive dystrophic EB, but may be present in junctional EB (Herlitz). Pyloric atresia is reported to occur in junctional EB, though one case has been documented with EB simplex. Egan et al reviewed these cases, as has Briggaman. Ocular lesions may be severe in dystrophic EB, and mild lesions have been reported in simplex and junctional disease.

Clinical findings should not be relied upon for diagnosis. Definition of variants with misleading clinical features are becoming quite common: examples are cicatricial junctional EB, Dowling-Meara type EB, and the generalized atrophic benign junctional type. Additionally, routine history is misleading. Definition of disease types must rely on electron microscopic studies. These can identify the level of the epidermal separation, and in addition may define other defects, such as absence of anchoring fibrils or hypoplasia of hemidesmosomes.

Immunofluorescent mapping should be understood, as this technique may define the level of the split without resort to electron microscopy. Katz, and J-D Fine et al, have reviewed this procedure. By staining biopsy specimens for normal components of the basement membrane zone, such as bullous pemphigoid antigen, laminin, type IV collagen, or LDA-1 antigen, as discussed by Fine et al, one may surmise the level of the split by whether the antigen localizes at the roof or base of the blister. In simplex types, all will be at the base; in dystrophic types, all will be at the roof; and in junctional types bullous pemphigoid antigen will be on the roof, while type IV collagen and LDA-1 will be at the base. Finally, another basement membrane zone antigen, KF-1, has been found to be absent or diminished in dystrophic EB.

Epidermolysis Bullosa Simplex (EBS)

CLINICAL FEATURES. The generalized type, dominantly inherited, with complete penetrance, is characterized by the development of vesicles, bullae, and milia over the joints of the hands, elbows, knees, and feet, and other sites subject to repeated trauma. The lesions are sparse and do not lead to severe atrophy. The Nikolsky sign is negative. Usually the mucous membranes and nails are not involved.

The lesions usually appear during the first year of life, but may occur at any age.

HISTOPATHOLOGY. Specimens from rubbed sites show a normal epidermis with the exception of vacuolated basal cells. Separation occurs through the basal layer.

DIFFERENTIAL DIAGNOSIS. EBS differs from the other types of epidermolysis bullosa by its relatively benign course and by the distinctive cleavage of the skin to form bullae at the basal cell level. The basal cells show vacuolation here, but not in the other forms.

TREATMENT. In general with all forms of EB this consists of prevention of trauma, decompression of large blisters, and treatment of infection.

PROGNOSIS. EBS tends to have periods of exacerbation, but with passage of time, skin changes subside markedly.

Localized Epidermolysis Bullosa Simplex

Recurrent bullous eruption of the hands and feet (Weber-Cockayne) is autosomal dominantly determined and appears in a chronic form in infancy or at times later in life. The lesions exacerbate during hot weather and when the patient is subjected to prolonged walking or marching such as is experienced in military service. Hyperhidrosis may be an associated finding. In localized EBS, the bullae are intraepidermal and suprabasal, and healing occurs without scarring.

TREATMENT. Jennings reported using aluminum chloride hexahydrate in anhydrous ethanol (Drysol) on the normal skin of hands and feet twice a day in

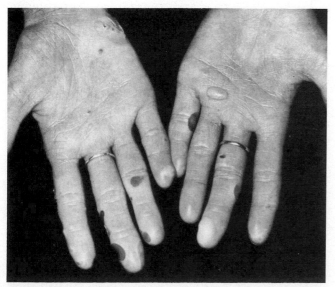

Figure 27–14. Palmar lesions in a patient with epidermolysis bullosa simplex.

a 2½-year-old girl who had had blisters since starting to crawl at age six months. After two weeks no further blisters occurred, and once or twice weekly applications sufficed to prevent blistering after that. Tkach had previously reported this method of treatment. Glutaraldehyde has been reported to be similarly effective.

Junctional Epidermolysis Bullosa (Epidermolysis Bullosa Letalis, Herlitz)

In this rare type of EB, which has autosomal recessive transmission, severe generalized blistering may be present at birth, and extensive denudation may prove fatal within a few months. Separation occurs in the lamina lucida, as shown by electron microscopy. Eventually the lesions heal without scarring or milium formation. Erosions may persist for years, however. Severe oral erosions and dysplastic teeth are common. Laryngeal and bronchial lesions may cause respiratory distress and even death. In patients who survive infancy, there is growth retardation, and moderate to severe refractory anemia is frequent.

TREATMENT. Supportive therapy and intensive systemic corticosteroid therapy are recommended during life-threatening periods.

Carter et al have reported successful treatment of chronic facial erosions by epidermal autografts of cultured keratinocytes taken from clinically uninvolved skin and grown on collagen sponges. Complete reepithelialization was achieved over seven and 10 months in two patients.

Epidermolysis Bullosa Simplex: Other Subtypes

EB Simplex with Mottled Pigmentation. One Swedish family has been reported with EB simplex, whose members were born with scattered hyper- and hypopigmented macules, which faded slowly.

EB Simplex (Ogna). In this single Norwegian kindred, generalized bruising and hemorrhagic blebs occurred.

EB Herpetiformis (Dowling-Meara). Buchbinder et al recently reviewed this disease, in which active blisters with circinate configuration occur in infancy. Milia occur, but there is no scarring. The oral mucosa is involved. Nails are shed, but may regrow, sometimes with dystrophy. Blistering lessens with age. Histologically the split is through the basal layer, and tonofilaments are clumped on electron microscopy.

All of the above types are inherited by autosomal dominance.

Niemi et al have reported two cases of a new histologic group of EB simplex, in which keratinocytes are enlarged and dyskeratotic and have atypical mitoses, and the tonofilaments on EM examination have formed round clumps. Blistering occurred in the lower part of the epidermis.

Generalized Atrophic Benign Epidermolysis Bullosa

Pearson et al in 1974 and Hashimoto in 1976 described adult patients with junctional blistering, and Schnyder et al reported four more in 1979. Hintner and Wolff added eight more, four siblings and four unrelated cases, to establish this entity. The astonishing pedigree was traced through nine generations. Onset at birth, generalized blisters and atrophy, mucosal involvement, and thickened, dystrophic, or absent nails, characterized all cases; all but two had lost most or all teeth, and much hair. Cleavage was within the lamina lucida; hemidesmosomes were reduced or absent; the basal lamina and anchoring fibrils, collagen fibers, and dermal microfibril bundles were unaltered. Inheritance was autosomal recessive in all. Paller et al have reported four American cases.

Cicatricial Junctional Epidermolysis Bullosa

Haber et al described in 1985 another type of junctional EB to which they gave the above name because the blisters heal with scarring, which may produce syndactyly and contractures, and there is stenosis of the anterior nares. Electron microscopy reveals junctional bullae with rudimentary hemidesmosomes. The bases of the bullae are covered by an intact basal lamina with normal anchoring fibrils. They reported three cases.

They present the seven types of JEB in tabular form which outlines the different clinical findings in the types reported. All junctional types are autosomal recessively inherited, and there is no specific therapy available for any of them.

Epidermolysis Bullosa Dystrophic Dominant (EBDD) (Dermolytic Bullous Dermatosis—Dominant)

CLINICAL FEATURES. Upon the extensor surfaces of the extremities appear vesicles and bullae, which are most pronounced over the joints, especially over the toes, fingers, knuckles, ankles, and elbows. Spontaneous, flesh-colored, scarlike (albopapuloid) lesions may appear on the trunk, often in adolescence, in the absence of previous trauma. The nails may be thickened. Usually the Nikolsky sign is present, and frequently the accumulated fluid in a bulla can be moved under the skin several centimeters away from the original site. Healing usually occurs with scarring and atrophy. Epidermal cysts (milia) are often present on the rims of the ears, on the dorsal surfaces of the hands, and on the extensor surfaces of the arms and legs.

The mucous membranes are frequently involved. Bullae, vesicles, and erosions are encountered on the buccal mucosa, tongue, palate, esophagus, and pharynx. The latter involvement is made apparent by the persistent hoarseness in some of these patients. There may be angular contractures at the gingivolabial sulcus, and dysphagia from faucial and pharyngeal scarring. Scarring on the tip of the tongue is typical. The teeth are normal. Usually the conjunctiva is not involved.

Other changes include nail dystrophy, partial alopecia of the scalp, absence of body hair, dwarfism, and the formation of contractures and clawlike hands, with atrophy of the phalangeal bones and pseudosyndactylism. This albopapuloid type (Pasini) is the more severe expression of EBDD. The Cockayne–Touraine type is more limited in extent and severity and no albopapuloid lesions are seen.

HISTOPATHOLOGY. A noninflammatory subepidermal bulla is present. On electron microscopy cleavage occurs beneath the basal lamina and anchoring fibrils are rudimentary and reduced in number. In blistered areas they are not demonstrable.

CARCINOGENESIS. The dystrophic forms of epidermolysis bullosa may predispose to carcinoma of the skin. Both basal and squamous cell types are seen in scarred areas of patients who have had epidermolysis for many years.

TREATMENT. Symptomatic treatment is still the only therapy available.

Epidermolysis Bullosa Dystrophic Recessive (EBDR)

This type of epidermolysis has a recessive form of heredity but its clinical features are similar to those of EBDD. The clinical spectrum ranges from patients with blisters limited primarily to the hands, feet, elbows, and knees to the more severe varieties characteristically beginning at birth with both generalized cutaneous and mucosal blistering. Digital fusion with encasement of the fingers and toes in scar tissues, forming a "mittenlike" deformity, is characteristic of the severe form of EBDR. Esophageal stricture may be present. An inverse distribution may occur. Anemia and growth retardation are frequently seen in the most severe cases. Type VIII collagen is abnormally expressed owing to either inadequate synthesis or excessive breakdown.

On electron microscopy the cleavage occurs beneath the basal lamina and the anchoring fibrils are diminished or absent. KF-1 antigen is absent or markedly diminished.

TREATMENT. Bauer et al reported encouraging results from the use of phenytoin, in 12 of 17 patients, in 1980. In 1984 Cooper and Bauer published a complete report of their experience in 22 patients. Since it is known that in EBDR an increase in colla-

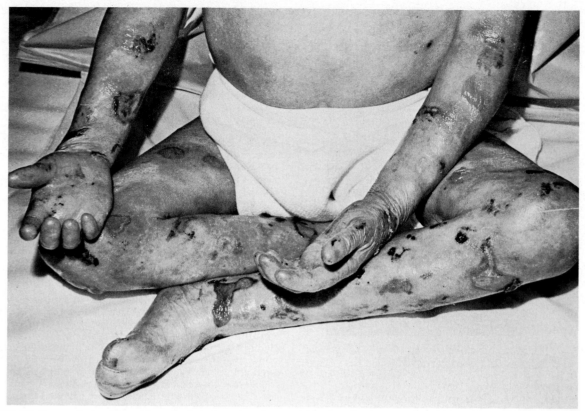

Figure 27–15. *Severe dystrophic epidermolysis bullosa in a 7-year-old boy. Note severe sclerodactylia. (Courtesy of Dr. J. McSorley.)*

genase activity is present, and phenytoin inhibits synthesis and secretion of collagenase by dermal fibroblasts, this therapy is remarkably suited for this disease. Fritsch et al found etretinate ineffective in one case.

Carcinogenesis in Epidermolysis Bullosa. Wechsler and his associates have reported the tendency for

carcinogenesis in polydysplastic epidermolysis bullosa. The pathogenesis is probably similar to that seen with thermal burns and chronic scars with an altered immunologic state.

In a patient of Domonkos, a 46-year-old man who had developed extensive basal and squamous cell carcinomata, Crikelair and his associates performed

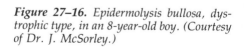

Figure 27–16. *Epidermolysis bullosa, dystrophic type, in an 8-year-old boy. (Courtesy of Dr. J. McSorley.)*

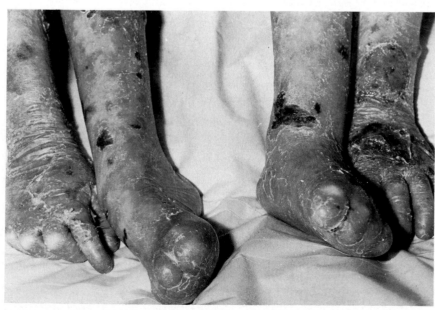

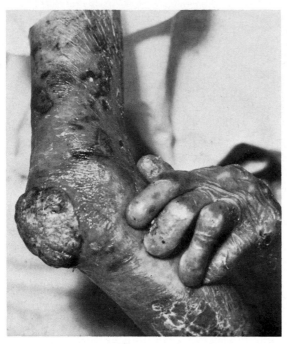

Figure 27–17. Squamous cell carcinoma on elbow of 34-year-old male with epidermolysis bullosa of dystrophic type.

successful skin allografts from his mother's skin. This suggested an attenuation of the immune response to skin allografts in this disease.

Andreano JM, et al: Epidermolysis bullosa simplex responding to isotretinoin. Arch Dermatol 1988, 124:1445.

Bauer EA, et al: Phenytoin therapy of recessive dystrophic epidermolysis bullosa. N Engl J Med 1980, 303:776.

Idem: A perspective on the role of collagenase in recessive epidermolysis bullosa. Arch Dermatol 1988, 124:734.

Idem: Keratinocyte grafting in epidermolysis bullosa (editorial). JAAD 1987, 17:300.

Bergfeld WF, et al: Epidermolysis bullosa letalis and phenytoin. JAAD 1982, 7:275.

Bordas X, et al: Kindler's syndrome. JAAD 1982, 6:263.

Briggaman RA: Hereditary epidermolysis bullosa with special emphasis on newly recognized syndromes and complications. Dermatol Clin 1983, 1:263.

Buchbinder LH, et al: Severe infantile epidermolysis bullosa simplex. Arch Dermatol 1986, 122:190.

Butter DF, et al: Bart's syndrome. Pediatr Dermatol 1986, 3:113.

Callen JP, et al: Bilateral ulcers in a patient with a hereditary bullous dermatosis. Arch Dermatol 1987, 123:811.

Carter DM, et al: Treatment of junctional epidermolysis bullosa with autografts. JAAD 1987, 17:246.

Cooper TW, et al: Therapeutic efficacy of phenytoin in recessive dystrophic epidermolysis. Arch Dermatol 1984, 120:490.

Cowton JAL, et al: Epidermolysis bullosa in association with aplasia cutis congenita and pyloric atresia. Acta Pediatr Scand 1982, 71:155.

Craighead JE: Pathogenesis, clinical features, and management of the nondermatological complications of epidermolysis bullosa. Arch Dermatol 1988, 124:705.

Egan N, et al: Junctional epidermolysis bullosa and pyloric atresia in two siblings. Arch Dermatol 1985, 121:1186.

Fine JD, et al: LDA-1 monoclonal antibody. Arch Dermatol 1986, 122:48.

Idem: Efficacy of systemic phenytoin in the treatment of junctional epidermolysis bullosa. Arch Dermatol 1988, 124:1402.

Idem: Epidermolysis bullosa. Int J Dermatol 1986, 25:143.

Idem: KF-1 monoclonal antibody defines a specific basement membrane zone antigen defect in dystrophic forms of epidermolysis bullosa. J Invest Dermatol 1984, 82:35.

Fine J-D: Antigenic features and structural correlates of basement membranes. Arch Dermatol 1988, 124:713.

Idem: Changing clinical and laboratory concepts in inherited epidermolysis bullosa. Arch Dermatol 1988, 124:523.

Fisher GB, et al: Congenital self-healing mechanobullous dermatosis. Arch Dermatol 1988, 124:240.

Fritsch P, et al: Retinoid therapy of recessive dystrophic epidermolysis bullosa. JAAD 1983, 9:765.

Gryboski JD, et al: Gastrointestinal manifestations of epidermolysis bullosa in children. Arch Dermatol 1988, 124:746.

Guill MF, et al: Junctional epidermolysis bullosa. Am J Dis Child 1983, 137:982.

Haber RM, et al: Hereditary epidermolysis bullosa. JAAD 1985, 13:252.

Idem: Cicatrical junctional epidermolysis bullosa. JAAD 1986, 12:836.

Hashimoto K, et al: Transient bullous dermolysis of the newborn. Arch Dermatol 1985, 121:1429.

Hintner H, et al: Generalized atrophic benign epidermolysis bullosa. Arch Dermatol 1981, 119:375.

Holbrook KA: Extracutaneous epithelial involvement in inherited epidermolysis bullosa. Arch Dermatol 1988, 124:726.

Izumi AK, et al: Familial benign chronic pemphigus. Arch Dermatol 1971, 104:177.

Jennings JL: Aluminum chloride hexahydrate treatment of localized epidermolysis bullosa. Arch Dermatol 1984, 120:1382.

Katz SI: The epidermal basement membrane zone. JAAD 1984, 11:1025.

Kindler T: Congenital poikiloderma with traumatic bulla formation and progressive cutaneous atrophy. Br J Dermatol 1954, 66:104.

Leigh IM, et al: Type VII collagen is a normal component of epidermal basement membrane, which shows altered expression in recessive dystrophic epidermolysis bullosa. J Invest Dermatol 1988, 90:639.

Niemi K-M: Epidermolysis bullosa simplex. Arch Dermatol 1983, 119:138.

Nowak AJ: Oropharyngeal lesions and their management in epidermolysis bullosa. Arch Dermatol 1988, 124:742.

Paller AS, et al: The generalized atrophic benign form of junctional epidermolysis bullosa. Arch Dermatol 1986, 122:704.

Pearson RW, et al: Dermolytic epidermolysis bullosa inversa. Arch Dermatol 1988, 124:544.

Pearson RW: Clinicopathologic types of epidermolysis bullosa and their nondermatological complications. Arch Dermatol 1988, 129:718.

Peltier FA, et al: Epidermolysis bullosa lethalis associated with congenital pyloric atresia. Arch Dermatol 1981, 117:728.

Pfau RG, et al: Blistering eruption in healthy newborns. Arch Dermatol 1986, 122:211.

Schachner L, et al: Epidermolysis bullosa hereditaria letalis. Br J Dermatol 1977, 96:51.

Takamori K, et al: Proteases are responsible for blister formation in recessive dystrophic epidermolysis bullosa and epidermolysis bullosa simplex. Br J Dermatol 1985, 112:533.

Tkach JR: Treatment of recurrent bullous eruption of the hands and feet with topical aluminum chloride. JAAD 1982, 6:1095.

Unamuno P, et al: Harlequin foetus in four siblings. Br J Dermatol 1987, 116:569.

Weary PE, et al: Hereditary acrokeratotic poikiloderma. Arch Dermatol 1971, 103:409.

Wehr RF, et al: Effective treatment of Netherton's syndrome with 12% lactate lotion. JAAD 1988, 19:140.

Williams ML, et al: Ichthyosis induced by cholesterol-lowering drugs. Arch Dermatol 1987, 123:1535.

DERMOLYTIC BLISTERING SYNDROMES

Bart's Syndrome

Bart and his associates reported congenital localized defects of the skin, mechanoblisters, and nail deformities with autosomal-dominant inheritance.

The clinical and histologic picture of this syndrome is one of a mildly scarring mechanobullous dermatosis with a favorable prognosis. Butter et al reported ultrastructural and immunofluorescent mapping studies in a family with Bart's syndrome. They were the same as are seen in EB of dystrophic dominant type, EBDD.

Transient Bullous Dermolysis of the Newborn

Hashimoto et al reported in 1985 a newborn who developed blisters from every minor trauma. Separation was below the basal lamina, with degeneration of collagen and anchoring fibrils. There was rapid healing after four months of age. Nails were not damaged, and there was no scarring.

They consider as criteria for this entity (1) vesiculobullous lesions present at birth or induced by friction; (2) spontaneous recovery at a few months of age; (3) no dystrophic scars; (4) subepidermal blisters beginning in the dermal papillae; (5) ultrastructurally observed collagenolysis and damaged anchoring fibrils; and (6) enormous dilatation of rough endoplasmic reticulum, with stellate bodies of keratinocytes in their vacuoles. They suspect that it is caused by a transient increase in proteases, or decrease in their inhibitors.

Acrokeratotic Poikiloderma (Weary-Kindler)

Kindler reported in 1954 a combination of poikiloderma congenitale and traumatic blistering of the feet from minor trauma, thought to be a form of epidermolysis bullosa dystrophica, and subsequent cases seemed to confirm this as an entity. Weary et al reported a dominantly inherited disorder of very similar nature in 1971. Larrègue et al found 41 published cases with similar features and proposed combining them under the name *acrokératose poikilodermique bulleuse et héréditaire de Weary-Kindler*. Bordas et al reported such a case in 1982 in a 26-year-old man who had had blisters of hands and feet since birth and gradually progressive facial erythema with telangiectasia, wrinkling of the skin, and photosensitivity. The principal histologic change was absence of elastic fibers in the papillary dermis and fragmented ones in the mid-dermis, so it would appear to be dermolytic.

FAMILIAL BENIGN CHRONIC PEMPHIGUS (Hailey-Hailey Disease)

In 1939 Hailey and Hailey described a familial disease characterized by persistently recurrent bullous and vesicular dematitis of the sides of the neck, axillae, flexures, and apposing surfaces. The eruption

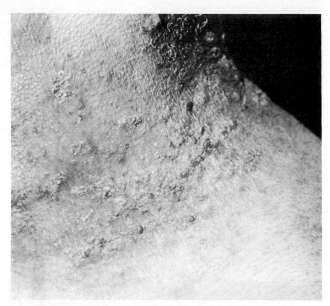

Figure 27–18. Familial benign chronic pemphigus. (Courtesy of Dr. Axel W. Hoke.)

may remain closely localized or may become widespread. The onset is usually in the late teens or early twenties. The primary lesion is a vesicle or bulla arising on seemingly normal skin. After rupture of the bulla, an erosion is seen, and this soon becomes thickly crusted and may resemble impetigo. Sometimes the center becomes dry and crusted and there is an actively inflammatory border that spreads peripherally, producing circinate and configurate patterns. The lesions appear in crops and run their course in several weeks. The original areas are the sites of recurrent lesions. Slight pruritus is the only symptom, although there may be some tenderness and enlargement of the regional lymph glands. The disease is benign. It is more severe in the summer. A papular variant in an affected family was described by Witkowski et al. Esophageal involvement was reported by Kahn and Hutchinson.

Hailey-Hailey disease is frequently hereditary; however, some 30 per cent of patients have been reported with no hereditary background. The disease is transmitted as an autosomal dominant trait.

Morales and his associates have confirmed the general belief that in genetically predisposed persons with Hailey-Hailey, stimulation of the skin by trauma, bacterial or fungal infection, and dermatoses, triggering Koebner's phenomenon, may bring about the overt lesions seen in this disease. Montes and his associates demonstrated carriage of coagulase-positive *Staphylococcus aureus* in most of their patients. Izumi et al were able to induce lesions with a variety of mechanical and chemical stimulants. Cram et al utilized ultraviolet-induced acantholysis to identify clinically normal heterozygotes of FBCP and found the phototest method to be useful in the diagnosis of suspected disease in remission.

The **histopathology** is unique and has some fea-

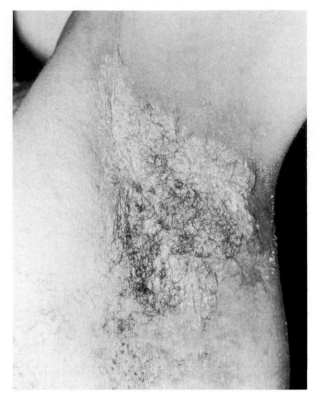

Figure 27–19. Familial benign chronic pemphigus. (Courtesy of Dr. Axel W. Hoke.)

tures that suggest Darier's disease as well as pemphigus. There are prominent intraepidermal vesicles and bullae. There is acantholysis and the formation of clefts above the basal cell layer into which the acantholytic cells "tumble." The basal cell layer remains attached to the dermis. Occasional prematurely keratinized cells may be present. Moderate lymphocytic infiltration is found in the dermis. The defect in this disease may be an abnormality of the intercellular cement substance impairing cellular cohesion. Another theory is that there is an abnormality in the tonofilament-desmosome complex.

In the **differential diagnosis,** infectious eczematoid dermatitis and impetigo should be considered. Usually Darier's disease is easily differentiated.

The **treatment** of Hailey-Hailey poses many problems since the first two or three exacerbations will respond to many different medications. Most cases seem to go into remission with the use of systemic tetracyclines, topical clindamycin, mupirocin, or other antibiotics. Corticosteroids, topically, systemically, or both, have shown the best response. When feasible, the intralesional injection of triamcinolone at weekly intervals brings about a gratifying response. Dapsone was effective in all of three refractory cases treated by Sire and Johnson, and Arnold has had good results with it in two patients, one of whom experienced a remission lasting for three years and a second remission which has now lasted four years.

Shelley et al have reported a case treated by total excision and grafting of the axillae. The groin area was involved and served as a control. Complete absence of lesions in the axillae persisted for four years. Previously, Thorne et al reported excellent results with excision and grafting of the inguinal region in a 29-year-old man. Crotty et al used split-thickness grafts to treat five refractory cases, of whom four showed improvement for follow-up periods of 10 months to nine years.

Cram DL, et al: Ultraviolet-induced acantholysis in familial benign chronic pemphigus. Arch Dermatol 1967, 96:636.
Crotty CP, et al: Surgical treatment of familial benign chronic pemphigus. Arch Dermatol 1981, 117:540.
Don PC, et al: Carbon dioxide laser abrasion. J Dermatol Surg Oncol 1987, 13:1187.
Gottlieb SK, et al: Hailey-Hailey disease. J Invest Dermatol 1970, 54:368.
Hernandez-Perez E: Familial benign chronic pemphigus. Cutis 1987, 39:75.
Izumi AK, et al: Familial benign chronic pemphigus. Arch Dermatol 1971, 104:177.

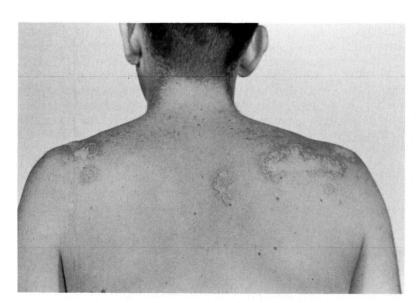

Figure 27–20. Familial benign chronic pemphigus.

Marsch CW, et al: Generalized Hailey-Hailey disease. Br J Dermatol 1978, 99:553.

Michel B: Hailey-Hailey disease. Arch Dermatol 1982, 118:781.

Sire DJ, et al: Benign familial chronic pemphigus treated with dapsone. Arch Dermatol 1971, 103:262.

Witkowski JA, et al: Familial benign chronic pemphigus. Arch Dermatol 1973, 108:842.

CUTIS VERTICIS GYRATA

Cutis verticis gyrata is characterized by folds and furrows on the scalp. Most frequently the vertex is involved, but other areas may have the distinctive furrowing. The folds, according to MacGillivray, may number from two to 20 and be about 1 cm wide. The hair itself is usually of normal growth and black.

Cutis verticis gyrata has been reported occurring mainly in males, with a male-to-female ratio of 6:1. The age at onset is usually in puberty, with over 90 per cent of patients developing it before age 30. The condition may be familial when it occurs as a component of pachydermoperiostosis. Polan and Butterworth found that cutis verticis gyrata may be due to developmental anomalies, inflammation, trauma, tumors and nevi, or proliferative diseases.

In severely involved cases, excision with grafting or scalp reduction, as reported by Garden et al, may be indicated.

Garden JM, et al: Essential cutis verticis gyrata. Arch Dermatol 1984, 120:1480.

MacGillivray RC: Cutis verticis gyrata. Cutis 1968, 4:121.

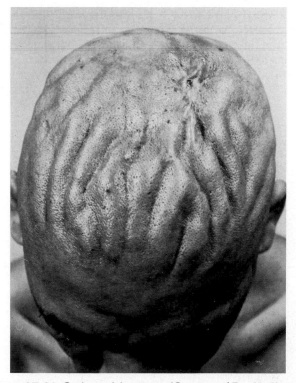

Figure 27–21. Cutis verticis gyrata. (Courtesy of Dr. H. Shatin.)

Polan S, et al: Cutis verticis gyrata. Am J Ment Defic 1953, 57:613.

Tani T, et al: Surgical treatment of cutis verticis gyrata. Br J Plastic Surg 1977, 30:235.

PACHYDERMOPERIOSTOSIS

Pachydermoperiostosis, also known as the Touraine-Solente-Golé syndrome, is characterized by thickening of the skin in folds and accentuation of creases on the face and scalp, clubbing of the fingers, and periostosis of the long bones. The changes are especially prominent on the forehead, where the horizontal lines are deepened and the skin becomes shiny. The eyelids, particularly the upper ones, are thickened. Likewise there is thickening of the ears and of the lips. The tongue is enlarged. The scalp may be thickened and show *cutis verticis gyrata (pachydermie vorticellée)*. The extremities, especially the elbows, knees, and hands, are enlarged and spade-shaped. The fingers become club-shaped. The palms are rough, and the thenar and hypothenar eminences are enlarged. Hyperkeratotic linear lesions of the palms and soles may be present. These lines are rippled "resembling sand of the wind-blown desert" (R. C. Gibbs). Movements of the muscles may be painful.

Clubbing of the fingers and toes and osteoarthropathy have long been known to occur in chronic pulmonary, mediastinal, and cardiac diseases that are associated with chronic low-grade anoxemia in peripheral tissues.

Some cases of pachydermoperiostosis have been associated with bronchogenic carcinoma. When such an association occurs, the enlargement of the forehead, hands, and fingers may antedate the recognition of the tumor, or develop after the tumor is known to be present.

Bronchogenic carcinoma–associated pachydermoperiostosis occurs almost exclusively in men over 40 years of age, whereas the Touraine-Solente-Golé syndrome usually occurs as a familial autosomal dominant disorder, unassociated with malignant disease. Sex influence results in more prominent signs in males, and onset occurs in late adolescence and in the twenties.

The histologic changes of the skin consist of dense collections of fibrocytes and dermal collagen. Acid mucopolysaccharides are found throughout the dermis, according to Hambrick. The epidermal appendages, especially the hair follicles, are hypertrophied.

Treatment is centered mostly around the improvement of the cosmetic appearance of these unfortunate persons. Plastic surgical repair has proved to be quite successful in establishing rehabilitation.

Venencie PY, et al: Pachydermoperiostosis with gastric hypertrophy, anemia, and increased serum bone Gla-protein levels. Arch Dermatol 1988, 124:1831.

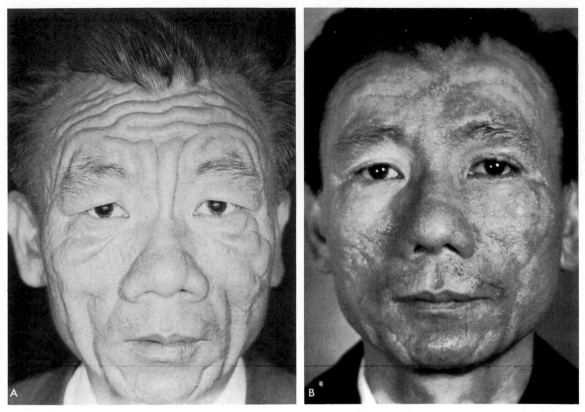

Figure 27–22. A, *Pachydermoperiostosis with marked furrowing on the face and scalp.* B, *Postoperative results. (Courtesy of Drs. F. Reiss and M. M. Shuster.)*

ICHTHYOSES
(Generalized Disorders of Cornification)

Ichthyosis is not one disease but a group of diseases in which the homeostatic mechanism of epidermal cell replacement is accelerated, or that of intercellular detachment is retarded, resulting in the clinical appearance of scale. It has become apparent in recent years that while phenotypic similarities exist, there are multiple genotypically distinct entities.

CLASSIFICATION. Numerous classifications have been proposed. Most include four major ichthyoses (ichthyosis vulgaris, X-linked ichthyosis, lamellar ichthyosis, and epidermolytic hyperkeratosis) followed by several miscellaneous syndromes which have scaling skin as part of the disorder. Williams and Elias have recently split lamellar ichthyosis into

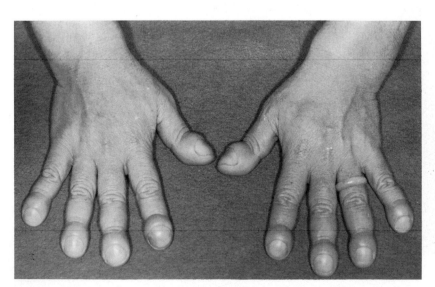

Figure 27–23. Clubbing of the fingertips in patient shown in Figure 27–22. (Courtesy of Dr. F. Reiss.)

two clinically and biochemically distinct entities, and have begun to classify the ichthyoses into a comprehensive scheme of genetically transmitted generalized disorders of cornification. The following is a general discussion of the classic subtypes as well as some of the newly recognized syndromes.

Ichthyosis Vulgaris

Ichthyosis vulgaris has an autosomal dominant mode of inheritance and is characterized by its onset in early childhood, usually between three and 12 months of age, with fine scales that appear "pasted-on" over the entire body. Varying degrees of dryness of the skin may be evident. The scales are coarser on the lower extremities than they are on the trunk. The extensor surfaces of the extremities are most prominently involved. The axillary and the gluteal folds are usually not involved. While the antecubital and popliteal fossae are usually spared by ichthyosis, atopic changes may be present. Accentuated skin markings and hyperkeratosis of the palms are common features. These and keratosis pilaris are markers for ichthyosis vulgaris, not atopy, as has been clearly shown by Mevorah et al. The scalp is involved, with only slight scaling. Follicular keratotic lesions are frequently found on the backs of the hands. Atopy manifested as hay fever, eczema, asthma, or urticaria is frequently present.

The course is mostly favorable, with abatement of signs and symptoms by the time adulthood is reached. Manifestations may be minimal.

Histologically, there is only a moderate degree of hyperkeratosis. The granular layer is reduced or absent, and keratohyalin granules are spongy or fragmented in electron micrographs. The prickle cell layer is of normal thickness. The dermis shows a sparse perivascular lymphohistiocytic infiltrate or no changes at all.

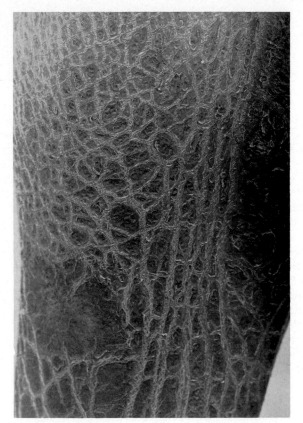

Figure 27–25. *Ichthyosis vulgaris on the thigh of a 23-year-old man. (Courtesy of Dr. H. Shatin.)*

Dole et al have shown there is decreased uptake of histidine, an amino acid characteristic of keratohyaline granules, and its primary protein, filaggrin. Filaggrin is not detectable in severely involved epidermis. This defect, however, is probably not primary, but secondary to abnormal cornification. This is a retention disorder.

Ichthyosis vulgaris is not a steroid-responsive dermatosis. This applies to all forms of ichthyosis. Rather it is best treated with α-hydroxy acids, such as lactic acid. Buxman et al have shown 12 per cent ammonium lactate lotion (Lac-Hydrin) to be helpful symptomatically in ichthyosis vulgaris, as well as lamellar, sex-linked, Netherton's, and epidermolytic hyperkeratotic forms. Other compounds with hydrating and keratolytic properties are also beneficial. Simple lubricating creams, 10 per cent urea cream, and 3 to 6 per cent salicylic acid preparations, may also be useful. Widespread topical salicylic acid use in children may, however, lead to salicylism, and these keratolytic preparations are best reserved for localized thicker areas.

Salt water baths may help by hydrating the horny layer.

A 40–60 per cent solution of propylene glycol in water under an occlusive suit for several nights removes the scales and may give the patient a normal appearance for one to two weeks.

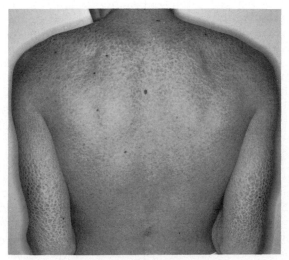

Figure 27–24. *Ichthyosis vulgaris.*

X-Linked Ichthyosis

This type of ichthyosis is transmitted only to males, by heterozygous mothers, as an X-linked recessive trait. In X-linked ichthyosis the scales are large and prominent on the anterior neck, the extensor surfaces of the extremities, and the trunk. The elbow and knee flexures are relatively spared, as are the face and scalp. The palms and soles are nearly always spared. Onset is usually before three months of age. Spontaneous parturition has often failed to occur when these patients were born, owing to a placental sulfatase deficiency. Keratosis pilaris is not present. The incidence of atopy is not abnormally high. Corneal opacities (which do not affect vision) are seen by slit-lamp examination on the posterior capsule or Descemet's membrane in about 50 per cent of affected males and female carriers. Another extracutaneous feature is a 12 to 15 per cent incidence of cryptorchidism, and an independently increased risk of testicular cancer.

Warm weather ameliorates X-linked ichthyosis.

Histologically, the epidermis is hyperplastic and hyperkeratotic. The granular layer is normal or thickened somewhat.

In boys the onset occurs shortly after birth, and if the scalp, ears, neck, and at least one of the flexures are affected, it is highly suggestive of X-linked (rather than autosomal dominant) ichthyosis. The diagnosis is also more likely if the abdomen is more involved than the back and if the ichthyosis extends down the entire dorsum of the leg.

Steroid sulfatase (aryl sulfatase C) is lacking in these patients' fibroblasts, leukocytes, and keratinocytes, and cholesterol sulfate accumulates as a result. This increases corneocyte cohesion, inhibiting the shedding of cells from the horny layer.

The diagnosis can be made (or confirmed) by lipoprotein electrophoresis, because the increase in cholesterol sulfate makes the low-density lipoproteins migrate much more rapidly, and cholesterol sulfate is elevated in serum, erythrocyte membranes, and keratin. The reduced enzyme activity can be assessed in fibroblasts, keratinocytes, leukocytes, and prenatally in amniocytes. The locus of the defective gene is the short arm of the X chromosome.

Unlike ichthyosis vulgaris, X-linked ichthyosis does not improve with age, but gradually worsens in both extent and severity. Ten per cent cholesterol cream has been shown to be effective by Lykkesfeldt. In severe cases etretinate is useful.

Multiple Sulfatase Deficiency

These patients display an overlap of steroid sulfatase deficiency (X-linked ichthyosis), mucopolysaccharidosis, and metachromatic leukodystrophy. This autosomal recessive disorder is caused by a lack of all known sulfatases.

Epidermolytic Hyperkeratosis (Bullous Ichthyosiform Erythroderma)

Epidermolytic hyperkeratosis, once called bullous congenital ichthyosiform erythroderma, is usually manifested by blisters at or shortly after birth. Later, thickened, horny, warty, ridged scales may cover the entire body. Soon after birth the scales are shed to leave a raw surface which forms scales anew. These thick, grayish brown, sometimes verruciform scales prominently involve the flexures and the intertriginous areas. Other parts of the skin may be involved, but to a lesser extent.

Unfortunately, the term epidermolytic hyperkeratosis is still used also as a designation for the histologic process which characterizes the clinical disorder; Ackerman has described it in normal skin and in skin adjacent to benign and malignant epidermal tumors, and Goette et al found it in normal oral mucosa. Still others have reported finding it in a wide variety of situations, which have been summarized by Goette et al.

A wide range of different lesions is inherent to this form of ichthyosis. There may be the intermittent appearance of bullae, flexural lesions alone, or generalized involvement. We view the localized forms of linear verrucous lesions (ichthyosis hystrix, nevus unius lateris) or other configurate lesions as forms of linear epidermal nevi.

While great variability exists, one subtype has been described in enough detail to merit its own name, *ichthyosis bullosa of Siemens*. This is characterized by a lack of erythema, the "mausering phenomenon" (a superficial molting or peeling of the skin), and by confinement of the epidermolytic change to the superficial layers of the epidermis. Traupe et al reported a case in 1986.

The histologic picture is distinctive. Hyperkeratosis is marked. Intracellular edema results in lysis of the epidermal cells to produce an epidermolytic type of pathologic pattern. This process is also described as a reticular pattern of vacuolization. The granular layer is markedly thickened and contains a coarse granular infiltrate. Frequently binucleated epithelial cells are noted in the squamous cell layer. The electron microscope reveals perinuclear halo formation, as described by Wilgram. These findings allow prenatal diagnosis by fetal skin biopsy.

Short intensive therapy with high-dose vitamin A (750,000 units of Aquasol A daily) for two weeks produced modest clinical improvement in a 27-year-old black man treated by Cooke and Winkelmann. Others have tried the retinoids with similar results. Etretinate in effective doses increased bulla formation in three cases treated by El Ramly and Zachariae. The local application of 0.1 per cent retinoic acid (Retin-A cream) has been used successfully. Pyogenic infection is a common problem, and appropriate antibiotics should be administered. Bullous phases may be controlled with systemic steroids.

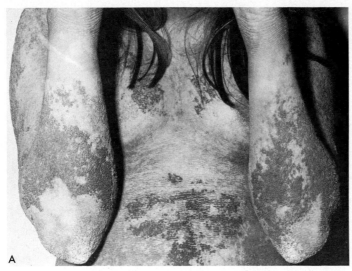

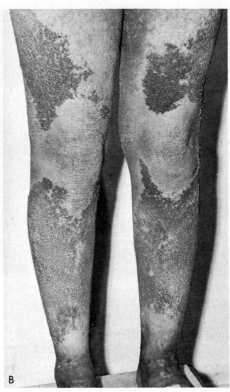

Figure 27–26. A *and* B, *Congenital epidermolytic hyperkeratosis.*

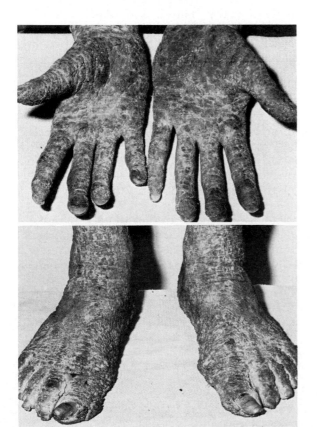

Figure 27–27. Epidermolytic hyperkeratosis on hands and feet. *(Courtesy of Dr. R. Feinstein.)*

A water solution of 10 per cent glycerin and 3 per cent lactic acid has been effective when applied to the wet skin.

The disease tends to become less severe with age.

Recessive Ichthyoses

LAMELLAR ICHTHYOSIS

Lamellar ichthyosis is present at birth or becomes apparent soon thereafter and almost always involves the entire cutaneous surface. Usually a collodionlike membrane encases these babies at birth, but desquamates over the first two to three weeks of life.

It is characterized by large (5 to 15 mm) grayish brown scales, strikingly quadrilateral, free at the edges, and adherent in the center. In severe cases the scales may be so thick that they are likened to armor plate. Moderate hyperkeratosis of the palms and soles is frequently present. The follicles in most instances have a crateriform appearance. Ectropion is almost always present and is a helpful diagnostic sign.

Lamellar ichthyosis is inherited as an autosomal recessive trait.

Distinctive histologic findings are present in this dermatosis: There is marked hyperkeratosis with a prominent granular cell layer. There is acanthosis and papillomatosis of the squamous cell layer and the rete ridges are prominent. Keratin is present in

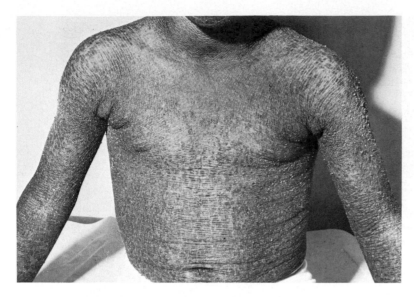

Figure 27–28. Lamellar ichthyosis in a 6-year-old girl.

the follicles and there is a mild perivascular infiltration in the upper dermis.

The underlying metabolic defect is not known; however, *n*-alkanes are normal. Epidermal proliferation rates are normal or only slightly elevated.

Lamellar ichthyosis responds partially to α-hydroxy acids and other creams recommended for ichthyosis vulgaris.

Systemic treatment with orally administered 13-cis retinoic acid (Accutane) is reported by Peck and Yoder and others to have greatly improved patients with lamellar ichthyosis, though the adverse effect of long-term maintenance therapy does not allow for prolonged use. Skeletal hyperostosis is a potential side effect with long-term therapy, and hypertriglyceridemia must be watched for. Pittsley and Yoder in 1983 reported serious symptomatic hyperostosis in four patients taking 3 to 4 mg per kg of tretinoin a day for one to six years. It is irreversible. Etretinate is decidedly more effective, according to El Ramly and Zachariae, who treated five cases with it in 1983. Side effects are numerous, frequently unpleasant, but rarely serious or even severe except for fetal damage. Cheilitis, conjunctivitis, facial dermatitis, xerosis, rhinitis sicca, epistaxis, skin fragility, and dryness of the mouth may all occur.

CONGENITAL ICHTHYOSIFORM ERYTHRODERMA

This disorder was formerly lumped with lamellar ichthyosis. However, Williams and Elias have characterized it as a separate clinical, histologic, and biochemical entity. Hazell and Marks agree. Most infants with it are born enclosed in a constricting parchmentlike or collodionlike membrane, which limits motion, and also ectropion of the eyelids. Within 24 hours, fissuring and peeling begin and large keratinous lamellae are cast off in 10 to 14 days, coincident with rapid improvement. As the membrane is shed, underlying redness and scaling are apparent. Generalized involvement is the rule, including face, palms, soles, and flexures. Cicatricial alopecia, nail dystrophy, and some ectropion are common. Scales may be large and platelike on the legs, but are apt to be fine on the trunk, face, and scalp.

Histologically, there are acanthosis, hyperkeratosis, and parakeratosis. A characteristic staining of the epidermis with PAS is seen. Epidermal turnover rate is increased: this disease is among the hyperproliferative syndromes.

Williams and Elias have documented a constant elevation of the *n*-alkane content of the scales. The source of these hydrocarbons is unknown, and the finding is not specific: however, the level is normal in lamellar ichthyosis.

Bernhardt et al reviewed 42 cases of recessive ichthyoses and they feel that this set of patients is quite heterogeneous. They imply that multiple genetic defects may be found for the many clinical subtypes of recessive disease. As of now, lamellar ichthyosis and congenital ichthyosiform erythroderma (CIE) are the only well-characterized entities.

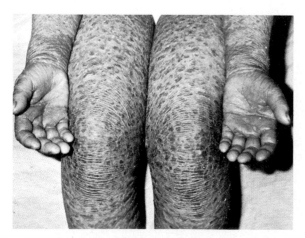

Figure 27–29. Lamellar ichthyosis in a 6-year-old girl. Her sister has a similar skin problem. Note the glazed and thickened palms.

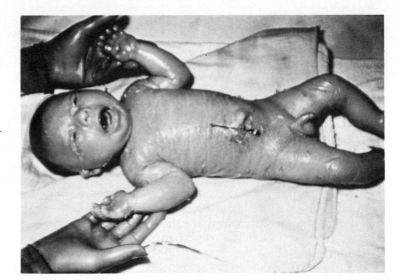

Figure 27–30. Lamellar exfoliation of the neonate (collodion fetus).

"Collodion babies" are most often seen with CIE. The process may also occur, however, with patients who eventually have normal skin (lamellar exfoliation of the newborn) and with lamellar ichthyosis, as well as with isolated cases of other ichthyoses.

TREATMENT. Esterly recommends a humid environment in an isolette, attention to possible infection in fissured areas, and avoidance of keratolytics: simple emollients are safest during the exfoliative stage.

HARLEQUIN FETUS

This severe recessively inherited disorder affects the skin in utero, causing thick, horny, armorlike plates covering the entire surface. The ears are rudimentary or absent and eclabium and ectropion are severe. The child is often stillborn or dies soon after delivery. There is no effective treatment. The longest survival time, 18 months, was reported by Williams et al. Prenatal diagnosis by skin biopsy is possible.

ICHTHYOSIS LINEARIS CIRCUMFLEXA

This is a term applied to a variety of ichthyosis in which bizarre migratory annular and polycyclic patches occur. It is inherited as an autosomal recessive disease. On the trunk and extremities is a widespread polycyclic serpiginous eruption characterized by constantly changing patterns, which from day to day clears in previously involved areas and develops new circinate lesions. In about a week the lesions attain their maximum diameter and involute, leaving no atrophy, scarring, or pigmentation. These patients have bamboo hair (trichorrhexis invaginata). The association of the ichthyosiform dermatitis, hair abnormality, and atopic diathesis is termed *Netherton's syndrome.* Due to atopic involvement, the scalp, face, and eyebrow regions are erythematous and scaly.

The lesions clear almost completely during the summertime, and usually there is little or no discomfort.

Histologic examination shows a remarkable thickening of the horny layer, with parakeratosis and acanthosis. The granular layer is thickened and dyskeratosis is present. In the dermis there are moderate vascular dilatation and round cell infiltration.

Manabe et al reported successful treatment with PUVA, and etretinate may be useful. Otherwise treatment of the ichthyoses is similar among them all, and the useful topical therapies have been described under ichthyosis vulgaris.

NEUTRAL LIPID STORAGE DISEASE

The Chanarin-Dorfman syndrome is an autosomal recessive disorder characterized by an ichthyosiform eruption, myopathy, and vacuolated leukocytes. Lipid vacuoles are present in all circulating granulo-

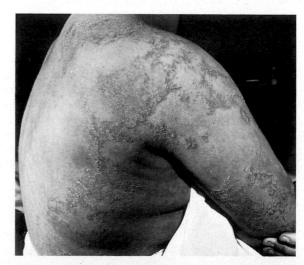

Figure 27–31. Ichthyosis linearis circumflexa. Widespread polycyclic serpiginous circinate lesions in a 12-year-old girl whose brother has same eruption. (Courtesy of Dr. F. J. McCauley.)

cytes and monocytes, as well as dermal cells, keratinocytes, and acrosyringia. The underlying metabolic defect is unknown. Electron microscopic findings of electron-lucent globular inclusions in the lamellar structures of the epidermis suggest a cause for the abnormal keratinocyte cohesion.

ICHTHYOSIS FOLLICULARIS

This syndrome is characterized by striking alopecia, severe photophobia, and generalized cutaneous flesh-colored, spiny, follicular projections. There is xerosis of nonspiny skin. Eramo et al reported two unrelated cases in males in 1985. The main differential diagnostic considerations are the keratitis, ichthyosis, and deafness (KID) syndrome; and keratosis follicularis spinulosa decalvans (KFSD). The disorder may be transmitted by an X-linked recessive pattern. The precise classification of this syndrome is not clear.

PEELING SKIN SYNDROME

Peeling of the stratum corneum above the granular layers associated with pruritus, short stature, and easily removed anagen hairs was reported in two patients by S. B. Levy. Moderate aminoaciduria and low plasma tryptophan were also found. Autosomal recessive inheritance was thought probable, and the authors classified the syndrome with the ichthyoses.

Acquired Ichthyosis

Ichthyosis clinically similar to ichthyosis vulgaris may develop in patients of any age with several systemic diseases. Acquired ichthyosis has been reported to develop in patients with Hodgkin's disease weeks or months after other manifestations of the disease, but it may be a presenting symptom. It has also occurred in association with non-Hodgkin's lymphomas, mycosis fungoides, multiple myeloma, and carcinomatosis. In hypothyroidism, patients may develop fine scaling of the trunk and extremities as well as carotenemia and diffuse alopecia. Characteristic ichthyosiform lesions may develop in patients with sarcoidosis, particularly over the lower extremities, which on biopsy show granulomas. Ichthyosiform changes have also been reported in patients with leprosy, in gross nutritional deficiency, AIDS, lupus erythematosus, and dermatomyositis, and secondary to multiple drugs including nicotinic acid, triparanol, and butyrophenones.

PITYRIASIS ROTUNDA

This remarkable dermatosis is manifested as perfectly circular, hyperkeratotic, hypopigmented macules, characterized by hyperorthokeratosis, on the trunk and extremities. They appear in childhood and extend over most of the skin surface within a few

years, slowly enlarging to as much as 20 cm in diameter. About a third of those over 5 or 6 cm in diameter are slightly oval. Pruritus may occur.

There is a strong ethnic predisposition: cases have been reported only in Japanese, South African and West Indian blacks, an Egyptian woman, and a Korean woman seen by Arnold. The disease persists for many years, except in those few patients with an accompanying malignancy, in whom it has cleared rapidly when the malignancy was treated. Leibowitz et al reported two such cases and implicated malnutrition in its etiology, but DiBisceglie et al found it in association with hepatocellular carcinoma in 10 cases (also in South African blacks) and regard it as a marker for this malignancy. Rubin et al reported two cases in American blacks, one of whom had an abdominal cancer of undetermined nature.

Zina et al reported three siblings with the disease, whose father had ichthyosis vulgaris. Swift and Saxe found 65 cases in 6388 hospital patients, in Cape Town.

Treatment is of no benefit unless there is an accompanying malignancy that can be treated.

Syndromes with Ichthyosis

Ichthyosis is a prominent feature in several genetic disorders. These are mostly of autosomal recessive inheritance and the ichthyosis generally is not of a characteristic type.

SJÖGREN-LARSSON SYNDROME

This syndrome is characterized by ichthyosis, spastic paralysis, oligophrenia, mental retardation, and a degenerative retinitis. The ichthyosis is usually generalized, with little or no involvement of the scalp, hair, or nails. There is a flexural and lower abdominal accentuation. The central face is spared, ectropion is

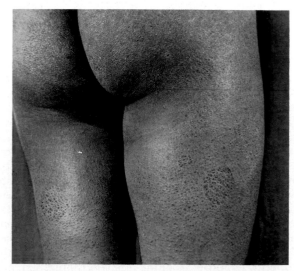

Figure 27–32. Pityriasis rotunda. Three patches are present on the posterior thighs. (Courtesy of Dr. H. El-Hefnawi, U.A.R.)

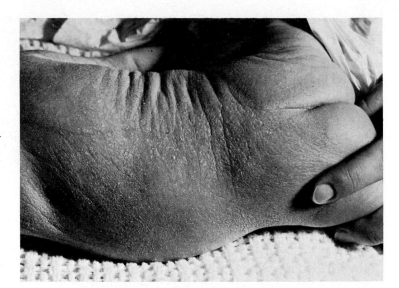

Figure 27–33. Sjögren-Larsson syndrome. Diffuse erythroderma with scaling of the trunk. (Courtesy of Drs. W. B. Reed and A. Heijer.)

unusual, and palms and soles are involved. Beginning by age two or three, there is spastic paralysis consisting of a stiff, awkward movement of the extremities, typical of Little's disease. Electron microscopy by Matsuoka et al revealed prominent Golgi apparatus and increased numbers of mitochondria in keratinocytes, in two siblings. Usually a severe mental deficiency is present; no mentally normal patients have been reported. The epilepsy is of the grand mal type. This is of autosomal recessive inheritance.

RUD'S SYNDROME

This is characterized by ichthyosis, epilepsy, polyneuritis, dwarfism, sexual infantilism, and macrocytic anemia. It is believed to be of autosomal recessive inheritance type, although some patients with this disease have been found to have steroid sulfatase deficiencies of the X-linked variety.

CONGENITAL ICHTHYOSIFORM SYNDROME WITH DEAFNESS AND KERATITIS (KID SYNDROME)

Several reports detail children with a syndrome characterized by an extensive congenital ichthyosiform eruption, neurosensory deafness, hypotrichosis, partial anhidrosis, vascularization of the cornea, nail dystrophy, and tight heel cords. Distinctive leathery, verrucoid plaques involve the central portion of the face and the ears. These changes, with absent eyebrows and eyelashes, and furrows about the mouth and chin, give the children a unique facies. Hazen et al reported that isotretinoin treatment may have exacerbated the corneal vascularization in their patient. This condition is either of autosomal recessive inheritance, or a sporadic disease.

IBIDS SYNDROME (Tay's Syndrome)

Brittle hair, intellectual impairment, decreased fertility, and short stature characterize the BIDS syndrome, and Jorizzo et al have reported a case which also had lamellar ichthyosis. Because there were three previously reported cases, they suggest that this is a subset of the BIDS syndrome—the "IBIDS" syndrome. The brittleness is due to sulfur deficiency, and the alternative designation for the BIDS syndrome is *trichothiodystrophy*.

Rebora et al wish to further split IBIDS syndrome. They classify six patients into this subset, based upon photosensitivity, which is a UV-induced DNA-repair defect related to group D xeroderma pigmentosum. They refer to this autosomal recessive disease as PIBI (D)S.

REFSUM'S SYNDROME

This is ichthyosis with atypical retinitis pigmentosa, hypertrophic peripheral neuropathy, cerebellar ataxia, nerve deafness, and various electrocardiographic changes. The ichthyosis resembles ichthyosis vulgaris. It may be generalized or localized to the palms and soles; it is of delayed onset and shows lipid vacuoles in the basal layer, and the epidermal cell turnover rate is increased. This is an autosomal recessive inheritance disorder. Herndon and his associates found a deficiency of a single enzyme in the α-hydroxylation of phytanate, phytanic oxidase. Reduction of phytanic acid–containing vegetables in the diet affords clinical improvement.

CONRADI'S DISEASE

Also known as *chondrodystrophia congenita punctata* or *chondrodystrophia calcificans congenita*, it is characterized by ichthyosis of the skin similar to that of the collodion baby, followed by hyperkeratotic "whirl and swirl" patterns on an erythematous skin. In addition to the reddening, the waxy, shiny skin has hyperkeratotic scales of a peculiar crushed-eggshell configuration. As the child grows, follicular atrophoderma and pseudopelade develop. Usually the ichthyosis clears within the first year of life but may leave behind temporarily a hyperpigmentation similar to that seen in incontinentia pigmenti. Crovato et al reported a man with such a change, which, while not classifiable as Conradi's disease, appeared to share features of it.

The skeletal defects in Conradi's disease are revealed in x-rays by the appearance of irregular calcified stippling of the cartilaginous epiphyses in the long bones, costal cartilages, and vertebral diaphysis. The stippling occurs in the fetus and persists until age three or four. The humeri and femurs are shortened.

Opacities of the lens, high-arched palate, and a flat-bridged nose constitute other signs of this disease.

Two main types of chondrodysplasia punctata have been described, the rhizomelic dwarf and the Conradi-Huenermann type. Of the three types of Conradi-Huenermann syndrome, type II is the type which manifests the above-described skin changes. This type is seen only in girls.

CONGENITAL HEMIDYSPLASIA WITH ICHTHYOSIFORM ERYTHRODERMA AND LIMB DEFECTS (CHILD Syndrome)

Cullen and his associates have described this entity, present at birth, characterized by unilateral scaling erythroderma and ipsilateral hypoplasia of the bony structures and the brain.

Herbert et al reported the 29th case in 1987. Twenty-eight have been female, which suggests an X-linked dominant gene, lethal in hemizygous males. The ichthyosiform erythroderma is strikingly unilateral and is present at birth or soon after. There are ipsilateral skeletal hypoplastic changes, with cardiovascular and renal defects.

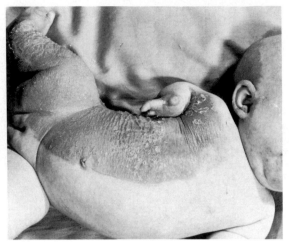

Figure 27–34. Unilateral epidermolytic hyperkeratosis. (Courtesy of Dr. S. I. Cullen.)

Ackerman AB: Histologic concept of epidermolytic hyperkeratosis. Arch Dermatol 1970, 102:253.

Baden HP, et al: Treatment of ichthyosis with isotretinoin. JAAD 1982, 6:716.

Idem: Ichthyosiform dermatosis and deafness. 1988, 124:102.

Banse-Kupin L, et al: Ichthyosiform sarcoidosis. JAAD 1987, 17:616.

Bernhardt, et al: Report of a family with an unusual expression of recessive ichthyosis. Arch Dermatol 1986, 122:428.

Brown BE, et al: Stratum corneum lipid abnormalities in ichthyosis. Arch Dermatol 1984, 120:204.

Bruckner-Tuderman L, et al: Acitretin in the symptomatic therapy for severe recessive X-linked ichthyosis. Arch Dermatol 1988, 124:529.

Burk RD, et al: Early manifestations of multiple sulfatase deficiency. J Pediatr 1984, 104:574.

Buxman MM, et al: Therapeutic efficacy of lactate 12% lotion in the treatment of ichthyosis. JAAD 1986, 15:1253.

Idem: Harlequin ichthyosis with epidermal lipid abnormality. Arch Dermatol 1979, 115:189.

Chung JC, et al: Diazocholesterol-induced ichthyosis in the hairless mouse. Arch Dermatol 1984, 120:342.

Cooke JP, et al: Response of bullous congenital ichthyosiform erythroderma to high-dose vitamin A. Cutis 1982, 29:44.

Dale BA, et al: Ichthyosis vulgaris. J Invest Dermatol 1984, 79:191.

Di Bisceglie AM, et al: Pityriasis rotunda. Arch Dermatol 1986, 122:802.

El Ramly M, et al: Long-term oral treatment of two pronounced ichthyosiform conditions. Acta Derm Venereol 1983, 63:452.

Elias PM, et al: Neutral lipid storage disease with ichthyosis. Arch Dermatol 1985, 121:1000.

Elias S, et al: Prenatal diagnosis of harlequin ichthyosis. Clin Genet 1980, 17:275.

Epstein EH Jr, et al: X-linked ichthyosis. Science 1981, 214:659.

Idem: The epidermal cholesterol cycle. JAAD 1984, 10:864.

Eramo LR, et al: Ichthyosis follicularis with alopecia and photophobia. Arch Dermatol 1985, 121:1167.

Fleckman P, et al: Keratinocytes cultured from subjects with ichthyosis are phenotypically abnormal. J Invest Dermatol 1987, 88:640.

Goette DK, et al: Epidermolytic hyperkeratosis as an incidental finding in normal mucosa. JAAD 1984, 10:246.

Goldsmith LA, et al: Cornification diseases. JAAD 1986, 14:118.

Gorb JJ, et al: Keratosis, ichthyosis and deafness (KID) syndrome. Arch Dermatol 1987, 123:777.

Greene SL, et al: Netherton's syndrome. JAAD 1985, 13:329.

Hazell M, et al: Clinical histologic and cell kinetic discriminants between lamellar ichthyosis and non-bullous ichthyosiform erythroderma. Arch Dermatol 1985, 121:489.

Hazen PG, et al: Corneal effect of isotretinoin. JAAD 1986, 14:141.

Herbert AA, et al: The CHILD syndrome. Arch Dermatol 1987, 123:503.

Holbrook KA, et al: Epidermolytic hyperkeratosis. J Invest Dermatol 1983, 80:222.

Idem: The expression of congenital ichthyosiform erythroderma in second trimester fetuses of the same family. J Invest Dermatol 1988, 91:521.

Hoyer H, et al: Ichthyosis of steroid sulfatase deficiency. Dermatologica 1986, 172:184.

Jobis AC, et al: A new method for determination of steroid sulfatase activity in leukocytes in X-linked recessive ichthyosis. Br J Dermatol 1983, 108:567.

Jorizzo JL, et al: Ichthyosis, brittle hair, impaired intelligence, decreased fertility, and short stature (IBIDS syndrome). Br J Dermatol 1982, 106:705.

Jurecka W, et al: Keratitis, ichthyosis, and deafness syndrome with glycogen storage. Arch Dermatol 1985, 121:799.

Kanerya L, et al: New observations on the finer structure of lamellar ichthyosis and the effect of treatment with etretinate. Am J Dermatopathol 1983, 5:555.

Larreque M, et al: Collodion baby. Ann Dermatol Venereol 1986, 113:773.

Lawlor F: Progress of a harlequin fetus to non-bullous ichthyosiform erythroderma. Pediatrics 1988, 82:870.

Leibowitz MR, et al: Pityriasis rotunda. Arch Dermatol 1983, 119:607.

Levy SB, et al: The peeling skin syndrome. JAAD 1982, 7:606.

Lykksfeldt G, et al: Topical cholesterol treatment of recessive X-linked ichthyosis. Lancet 1983, 2:1337.

Idem: Carrier identification in steroid sulfatase deficiency and recessive X-linked ichthyosis. Acta Derm Venereol (Stockh) 1986, 66:134.

Manabe M, et al: Successful therapy of ichthyosis linearis circumflexa with PUVA. JAAD 1983, 8:904.

Matsuoka LY, et al: Studies of the skin in Sjögren-Larsson syndrome by electron microscopy. Am J Dermatopathol 1982, 4:295.

Mevorah B, et al: The prevalence of accentuated palmoplantar markings and keratosis pilaris in atopic dermatitis, autosomal dominant ichthyosis, and control dermatologic patients. Br J Dermatol 1985, 112:679.

Meyer JCH, et al: Ichthyosis nigricans. Proc XVI Internat Congress Dermatol Tokyo, Tokyo Press, 1983.

Nusbaum BP, et al: Ichthyosiform dermatoses. Semin Dermatol 1983, 2:161.

Paltzik RL, et al: Conradi-Hünermann disease: case report. Cutis 1982, 29:174.

Pittsley RA, et al: Retinoid hyperostosis. N Engl J Med 1983, 308:1012.

Rand RE, et al: The ichthyoses. JAAD 1983, 8:285.

Rebora A, et al: PIBI(D)S syndrome. JAAD 1987, 16:940.

Ross JB, et al: Familial X-linked ichthyosis, steroid sulfatase deficiency, mental retardation, and nullisomy for Xp223-pter. Arch Dermatol 1985, 121:1524.

Rubin MG, et al: Pityriasis rotunda. JAAD 1986, 14:74.

Swift PJ, et al: Pityriasis rotunda in South Africa. Clin Exp Dermatol 1985, 10:407.

Traupe H, et al: X-linked recessive ichthyosis vulgaris rapid identification by lipoprotein electrophoresis. Arch Dermatol Res 1983, 275:63.

Idem: Ichthyosis bullosa of Siemens. JAAD 1986, 14:1000.

Urruta S, et al: Acquired ichthyosis associated with dermatomyositis. JAAD 1987, 16:627.

Van Scott EJ, et al: Ichthyosis and keratinization. Arch Dermatol 1982, 118:860.

Idem: Hyperkeratinization, corneocyte adhesion and alpha hydroxy acids. JAAD 1984, 11:867.

Williams ML, et al: Ichthyosis. Arch Dermatol 1986, 122:531.

Idem: Genetically transmitted generalized disorders of cornification. Dermatol Clin 1987, 5:155.

Idem: The ichthyoses. Pediatr Dermatol 1983, 1:1.

Idem: Elevated n-alkanes in congenital ichthyosiform erythroderma. J Clin Invest 1984, 74:296.

Idem: The dynamics of desquamation. Am J Dermopathol 1984, 6:381.

Idem: Heterogeneity in autosomal recessive ichthyosis. Arch Dermatol 1985, 121:477.

Young L, et al: Acquired ichthyosis in a patient with acquired immunodeficiency syndrome and Kaposi's sarcoma. JAAD 1987, 16:395.

ERYTHROKERATODERMIA VARIABILIS (EKV)

Synonyms: Erythrokeratodermia figurata variabilis; erythrokeratodermia variabilis, Mendes da Costa type.

EKV is a rare genetic disorder characterized by erythematous patches and hyperkeratotic plaques of sparse but generalized distribution. The erythematous patches may assume bizarre geographic configurations that are sharply demarcated and in a short time (hours or days) change their shape or size or involute completely. The keratotic plaques are reddish brown, often polycyclic, and fixed in location. The extensor surfaces of the limbs, buttocks, axillae, groins, and face are most often involved. Keratoderma of the palms and soles sometimes occurs. Hair, nails, and mucous membranes are spared.

The onset is shortly after birth or rarely in early adult life, after which there is usually some improvement with age, particularly after menopause. Exacerbations have been seen during pregnancy. Exacerbations of the configurate erythematous component may result from exposure to heat, cold, or wind; emotional upsets may also be a factor.

The inheritance pattern is a variably expressed autosomal dominant trait. In one family there was linkage to the Rh locus on the short arm of chromosome 1. Vandersteen and Muller found, and Rappaport et al confirmed, that keratinosomes are diminished in number in the hyperkeratotic lesions.

Histologically there is hyperkeratosis and parakeratosis and a diminished granular layer. Acanthosis and elongated dermal papillae may occur. Ultrastructurally, epidermal keratinosomes are diminished.

TREATMENT. Isotretinoin restores the deficient keratinosomes and clears the hyperkeratotic plaques and (partially) the migratory erythematous patches, according to Rappaport, Goldes, and Goltz. But the disease relapses on cessation of therapy.

Cram DL: Erythrokeratodermia variabilis and variable circinate erythrokeratoderma. Arch Dermatol 1970, 101:68.

Luy JT, et al: A child with erythematous and hyperkeratotic patches. Arch Dermatol 1988, 124:1271.

Rappaport IP, et al: Erythrokeratodermia variabilis treated with isotretinoin. Arch Dermatol 1986, 122:441.

Vander Wateren AR, et al: Oral retinoic acid therapy for erythrokeratodermia variabilis. Br J Dermatol 1977, 97:83.

Williams ML, et al: Genetically transmitted generalized disorders of keratinization. Dermatol Clin 1987, 5:155.

Progressive Symmetric Erythrokeratodermia

This rare, autosomal dominantly inherited disorder begins soon after birth, with erythematous, hyperkeratotic plaques symmetrically distributed on the extremities, buttocks, and face, sparing the trunk. Palmoplantar keratoderma may be present. The lesions may regress at puberty. Nazzaro et al reported a good response to etretinate.

Nazzaro V, et al: Progressive symmetric erythrokeratodermia. Arch Dermatol 1986, 122:434.

Rodriguez-Pichardo A, et al: Progressive symmetric erythrokeratodermia. JAAD 1988, 19:129.

Williams ML, et al: Genetically transmitted generalized disorders of keratinization. Dermatol Clin 1987, 5:155.

KERATOSIS PILARIS

Keratosis pilaris is an autosomal dominantly inherited condition which may be limited in mild cases to the posterior upper arms, where the skin appears to be in a state of continual gooseflesh, due to the horny plug in each hair follicle. The thighs are the next most common site. In severe cases the plugs may occur on the face, forearms, and legs, and may become widespread.

The individual lesions are small acuminate follicular papules. These may or may not be erythematous; more often they appear grayish because of the superimposed keratotic cone. The latter is composed of epithelial cells and inspissated sebum collected about a hair shaft, which at times is found coiled within it. Sometimes these corneous plugs are the most prominent feature of the eruption, whereas at other times they are present in only small numbers, and most of the lesions are punctate erythematous papules. Occasionally inflammatory acneiform pustules and papules may appear.

Forcible removal of one of the plugs leaves a minute cup-shaped depression at the apex of the papule, which is soon filled by new keratotic material. The lesions tend to be arranged in poorly defined groups, dotting the otherwise normal skin in a fairly regular pattern.

They are prone, however, to appear in xerotic or atopic subjects. This common dermatosis usually appears between the ages of two and three and then flourishes until age 20, subsiding in adulthood.

Treatment with topical tretinoin, 0.1 per cent cream, is usually beneficial. Twelve per cent lactic acid (Lac-Hydrin Lotion) is the most effective treatment to date, used once or twice daily to the affected area.

Other conditions associated with follicular hyperkeratosis, such as ichthyosis follicularis, atrichia with papular lesions, and the KID syndrome, have been discussed earlier.

Forman L: Keratosis pilaris. Br J Dermatol 1954, 66:279.

FOLLICULAR ATROPHODERMA

Follicular atrophoderma consists of follicular indentations, 1 mm or so broad, without hairs, notably on extensor surfaces of the hands and legs and arms. It has been described repeatedly in association with other genetically determined abnormalities. Curth has summarized these as follows: associated (1) with chondrodystrophia calcificans congenita (Conradi), (2) with Bazex's syndrome, and (3) with keratosis palmoplantaris disseminata.

Bazex et al reported a syndrome of follicular atrophoderma, basal cell carcinoma, and hypotrichosis in which eight members of a family were involved. Viksniks and Berlin reported another, of seven, with follicular atrophoderma, basal cell carcinomas, and localized anhidrosis. Conradi's syndrome has been discussed earlier.

Other diseases associated with follicular atrophoderma include ulerythema ophryogenes, atrophoderma vermiculata, keratosis pilaris rubra faciei, and keratosis follicularis spinulosa atrophicans.

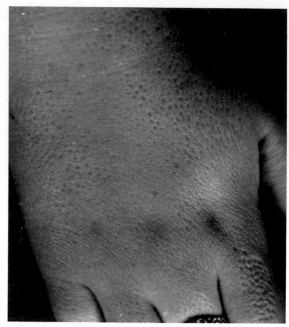

Figure 27–35. Follicular atrophoderma. (Courtesy of Dr. H. Curth.)

Arrieta E, et al: Honeycomb atrophy on the right cheek (atrophoderma vermiculatum). Arch Dermatol 1988, 124:1101.
Burnett JW, et al: Ulerytherma ophryogenes with multiple congenital anomalies. JAAD 1988, 18:437.

Ulerythema Ophryogenes

This disorder is characterized by persistent reticular erythema and small horny follicular papules. Upon involution these leave pitted scars and atrophy with resulting alopecia. Ulerythema ophryogenes occurs most frequently in the eyebrows, from which it may spread to the neighboring skin and even to the scalp. There is often associated widespread keratosis pilaris.

This extremely rare dermatosis is due to a follicular hyperkeratosis of the upper third of the hair follicle. The hyperkeratosis forms a barrier to the outgrowing hair and thereby a chronic inflammatory reaction ensues. A small depressed scar forms when the lesion heals. Mertens has reported this occurring with atopy, and Pierini et al consider it a marker for Noonan's syndrome, which is often associated with it.

Transmission is by an autosomal dominant gene. Ulerythema ophryogenes begins in early childhood, in most cases.

Keratosis Pilaris Rubra Faciei

This is similar to ulerythema ophryogenes except that the lesions begin on the cheeks or temples, rather than the eyebrows.

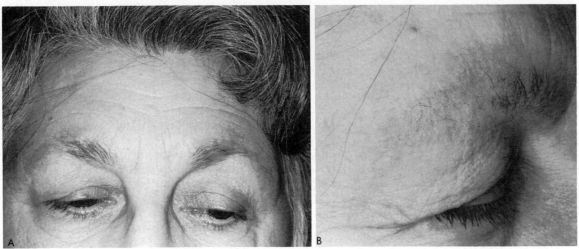

Figure 27–36. A *and* B, *Ulerythema ophryogenes.*

Both disorders begin in early childhood, both are associated with widespread keratosis pilaris, and both are inflammatory and result in scarring.

The lesions appear first on the preauricular regions and spread symmetrically onto the cheeks. The follicles become reddened, then develop papules, later pigmentation, and finally, follicular atrophy.

Histologically there is hyperkeratosis about the follicles, with thinning of the prickle cell layer and flattening of the rete pegs. Horny plugs fill the follicles. In the dermis there is moderate vasodilatation and a cellular infiltrate, usually only sparse. Fibrosis eventually ensues.

Keratolytic ointments or mild tar ointments have been helpful; no doubt Lac-Hydrin Lotion and Retin-A should be tried.

Atrophodermia Vermiculata

This is also known as *atrophodermia ulerythematosa, folliculitis ulerythematosa reticulata*, and *honeycomb atrophy*.

Atrophodermia reticulata is characterized by symmetrical involvement of the face by numerous closely crowded small areas of atrophy separated by narrow ridges, producing a cribriform or honeycomb surface. This almost worm-eaten ("vermiculata") appearance results from atrophy of not only the follicles, but the epidermis and dermis. Each atrophic area is an abrupt, pitlike depression 1–3 mm in diameter. Among the ridges a few milia may be seen.

The skin covering the ridges is even with the normal skin and is contrasted with it by being somewhat waxy, firmer, and apparently stretched. On close inspection through a magnifying glass redness is apparent, which is usually due to a ramification of fine capillaries.

The cause of the disease is undetermined but familial occurrence has been noted, and it may be

associated with other diseases such as congenital heart block and other cardiac anomalies, neurofibromatosis, oligophrenia, or Down's syndrome.

Histologically the epidermis is slightly atrophic with diminution in size of the interpapillary projections. In the dermis the capillaries are dilated and the vessels have a moderate round cell perivascular infiltration. There is slight edema of the collagen with beginning basophilic degeneration in places. Some of the follicles are enlarged, tortuous, dilated, and hyperkeratotic. In addition, there are cystlike cavities lined with epithelium and containing keratin (horn cysts). The sebaceous glands are sparse.

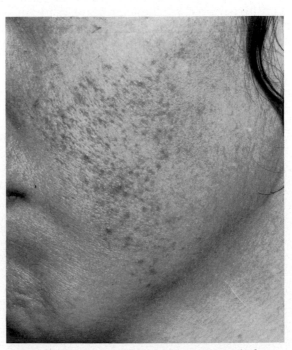

Figure 27–37. Folliculitis ulerythematosa reticulata.

Keratosis Follicularis Spinulosa Decalvans (KFSD)

In this disorder, keratosis pilaris begins on the face and, at any age up to adolescence, progresses to involve the limbs and trunk. Two cases were described by Rand and Baden in 1983.

There is hyperkeratosis of the palms and soles. This is followed by loss of hair and scarring. Cicatricial alopecia of the scalp and eyebrows is a hallmark of the disease. Atopy, photophobia, and corneal abnormalities are commonly associated.

The inheritance is X-linked recessive. Only symptomatic treatment is possible.

Appell ML, et al: A kindred with alopecia, keratosis pilaris, cataracts, and psoriasis. JAAD 1987, 16:89.

Bazex A, et al: Follicular atrophoderma, basal cell carcinoma and hypotrichosis. Ann Dermatol Syph 1966, 94:743.

Corvato F, et al: Acute skin manifestations of Conradi-Huenermann syndrome in an adult male. Arch Dermatol 1985, 121:1064.

Curth HO: The genetics of follicular atrophodermas. Arch Dermatol 1978, 114:1479.

Eramo LR, et al: Ichthyosis follicularis with alopecia and photophobia. Arch Dermatol 1985, 121:1167.

Mertens RLJ: Ulerythema ophryogenes and atopy. Arch Dermatol 1968, 94:743.

Mopper C, et al: Keratosis pilaris rubra faciei. Cutis 1974, 13:257.

Rand R, et al: Keratosis follicularis spinulosa decalvans. Arch Dermatol 1983, 119:22.

POROKERATOSIS (Mibelli)

Porokeratosis is a chronic, progressive disease of hereditary origin. It is characterized by the formation of slightly atrophic patches surrounded by an elevated, warty border. The disorder begins as a small keratotic papule, which spreads peripherally and atrophies in the center, so that eventually there is formed a circinate or serpiginous well-defined plaque surrounded by a keratotic wall or collar, giving rise to a festooned appearance. This wall is grayish or brownish in color and frequently is surmounted by a tiny groove or linear ridge running along its summit. The enclosed central portion of the plaque consists of dry, smooth, atrophic skin, the lanugo hairs generally being absent when the patches occur in hairy areas.

Sometimes minute horny projections are visible, representing follicular orifices. In areas subject to friction and rubbing where the skin is thick, the ridges about the patches are particularly pronounced. In other regions the atrophy is more prominent, chiefly on the hands and ankles, but both the keratosis and the atrophy are less distinct in areas, such as the axillae, where the skin is more delicate. Linear or zosteriform distribution of the lesions may also occur. If the nail matrix is involved, nail dystrophy may develop.

Sites of predilection are the surfaces of the hands and fingers, and the feet and ankles. The disease also occurs on the face and scalp (where it produces bald patches), on the buccal mucosa (where the ridge becomes macerated by moisture and appears as a milky white, raised cord), and on the glans penis (where it causes erosive balanitis).

The onset of the disease is early in life; it persists indefinitely, with a tendency to slow, irregular progress. The disease is twice as common in males as in females, often both father and son being affected.

Histologically, the principal changes are in the epidermis, where there are marked hyperkeratosis, parakeratosis, and acanthosis, and a downgrowth of epidermal plugs, particularly in the raised margin and at the openings of the sweat duct. The stratum corneum and rete may be thinned in the central area. The *cornoid lamella* is a thickened column of keratin

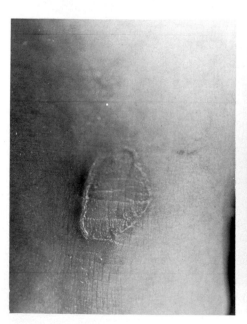
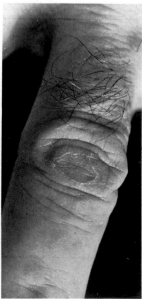

Figure 27–38. Porokeratosis of Mibelli on the antecubital fossa and midfinger. (Courtesy of Dr. H. Shatin.)

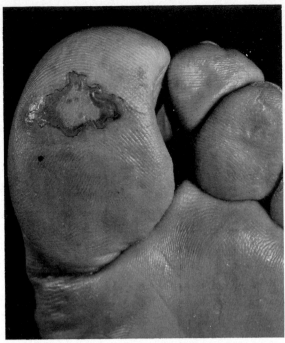

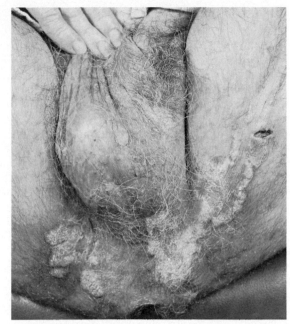

Figure 27–41. *Extensive porokeratosis of Mibelli in the perineal area. Ulceration on posterior thigh is biopsy site. (Courtesy of Dr. H. Shatin.)*

Figure 27–39. *Porokeratosis of Mibelli. (Courtesy of Dr. H. Shatin.)*

containing parakeratotic nuclei extending outward from a notch in the malpighian layer. The granular cell layer is absent beneath the cornoid lamella. Changes in the dermis consist of mild, simple inflammatory infiltration, a complete or relative absence of hair follicles and sebaceous glands, and a tendency to fibrosis.

It has been suggested that porokeratosis develops because of a localized point of faulty keratinization caused by an abnormal clone of keratinocytes with disordered metabolism or increased growth rate. Lederman et al proposed that immunosuppression may be a cause. Appearance or exacerbation of lesions has occurred during chemotherapy for malignancy, after renal transplantation, while on PUVA treatment, or in areas of chronic skin damage. Additionally, Inamoto et al reported that benzylhydrochlorothiazide induced lesions in their case.

Porokeratosis may be simulated by lichen planus, lichen sclerosus et atrophicus, verrucae, actinic keratoses, and epithelial nevi. Histology of a distinctive lesion is diagnostic.

Treatment with topical undiluted 5-FU solution under occlusion, or in the disseminated superficial type by 5 per cent 5-FU cream, has been reported to be effective by McDonald et al, and by Shelley, respectively. Several reports of etretinate and isotretinoin therapy document improvement while on the medication. There is a tendency to recurrence upon discontinuing the retinoid. Carbon dioxide laser ablation and excision are other methods available for localized lesions.

Carcinoma develops in these lesions not infrequently. James et al reviewed the literature in 1986 and found 29 patients in whom squamous cell carcinoma (21 patients), Bowen's disease (8 cases), or basal cell carcinoma (3 occurrences) was found within lesions of porokeratosis. Most occurred in the linear type, and most were on the legs. Lozinski et al reported a patient in whom a squamous cell carcinoma metastasized. Machino et al had previously reported a similar case with a fatal outcome. Lesions of porokeratosis of Mibelli should be either excised or destroyed, or in widespread cases patient education and periodic observation are recommended.

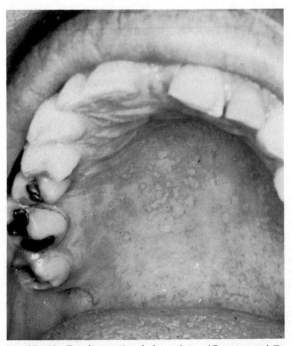

Figure 27–40. *Porokeratosis of the palate. (Courtesy of Dr. G. R. Mikhail.)*

Disseminated Superficial Actinic Porokeratosis (DSAP)

This disease is characterized by numerous superficial, annular, keratotic, brownish red macules found on the sun-exposed areas in persons 20 to 40 years of age. It is transmitted by an autosomal dominant gene, expressed most often in women. The individual lesions enlarge over the years and may be as much as 5 cm in diameter. The centers become depressed and the edge becomes a sharp ridge. Chernosky and Freeman, who called attention to this entity, find the histopathology to coincide with the common form of porokeratosis. The distribution of the lesions on the sun-exposed areas indicates that actinic radiation is an important factor in its pathogenesis, and Chernosky has induced new lesions by exposure to a sun lamp. Exacerbations have occurred in about two thirds of cases during the height of the summer season. However, Schwarz et al point out that lesions rarely occur on the face or ears, and they are skeptical of the importance of actinic radiation in the etiology. Their patient had no improvement on etretinate therapy for three weeks, but cleared after three PUVA treatments at a cumulative dose of 6 joules/cm², and four treatments on the other leg. She had not relapsed after a year. However, Hazen et al reported DSAP beginning during the course of PUVA therapy for psoriasis. Obviously, evidence is contradictory as to this aspect of the disease. Three cases of squamous cell carcinoma occurring in DSAP lesions have been reported.

Porokeratosis Plantaris Discreta

This is discussed under palmoplantar keratoses, in Chapter 6.

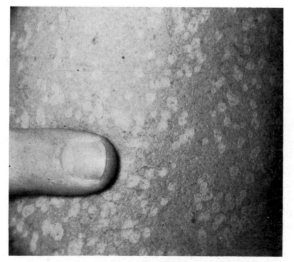

Figure 27–42. Disseminated superficial actinic porokeratosis on upper arm.

Porokeratosis Palmaris, Plantaris, et Disseminata

In this distinctive form of porokeratosis, lesions first appear on the palms or soles, or more often both, of patients in their twenties, and slowly extend over the entire body. Shaw et al reported such a case in 1984, and a fourth kindred was reported by Marschalko in 1986. McCallister et al treated a patient successfully with isotretinoin; however, the condition recurred when medication was stopped.

In *porokeratotic eccrine ostial* and *dermal duct nevus,* the presentation clinically appears as a nevus comedonicus of the palm or sole. However, histologic analysis reveals multiple comedoid lamella-like parakeratotic columns.

In *porokeratosis punctata palmaris et plantaris,* or *punctate porokeratosis,* lesions are limited to the hands and feet. Sakas et al reported such a case in 1985.

Barnett JH: Linear porokeratosis. JAAD 1986, 14:902.
Bencini PL, et al: Porokeratosis. Br J Dermatol 1987, 116:113.
Brodkin RH, et al: Malignant disseminated porokeratosis. Arch Dermatol 1987, 123:1521.
Campbell JP, et al: Etretinate improves localized porokeratosis of Mibelli. Int J Dermatol 1985, 24:261.
Chernosky ME, et al: Disseminated superficial actinic porokeratosis. Arch Dermatol 1969, 99:401.
Idem: Squamous cell carcinoma in lesions of disseminated superficial actinic porokeratosis. Arch Dermatol 1986, 122:853.
Chernosky ME: Porokeratosis. Arch Dermatol 1986, 122:869.
Dover JS, et al: Disseminated superficial actinic porokeratosis. Arch Dermatol 1986, 122:887.
Filho JO, et al: Disseminated superficial actinic porokeratosis in a black patient. Arch Dermatol 1986, 122:852.
Friedman SJ, et al: Punctate porokeratotic keratoderma. Arch Dermatol 1988, 124:1678.
Hacham-Zedeh S, et al: Etretinate in the treatment of disseminated porokeratosis of Mibelli. Internat J Dermatol 1985, 24:258.
Hubler WR, et al: Linear porokeratosis. Cutis 1974, 14:61.
Inamoto N, et al: Porokeratosis of Mibelli. JAAD 1984, 11:357.
James WD, et al: Squamous cell carcinoma arising in porokeratosis of Mibelli. Internat J Dermatol 1986, 25:389.
Lederman JS, et al: Psoralens and ultraviolet A, immunosuppression, and porokeratosis. JAAD 1986, 14:284.
Idem: Immunosuppression: a cause of porokeratosis? JAAD 1985, 13:75.
Lozinski AZ, et al: Metastatic squamous cell carcinoma in linear porokeratosis of Mibelli. JAAD 1987, 16:448.
Marschalko M, et al: Porokeratosis plantaris, palmaris, et disseminata. Arch Dermatol 1986, 122:890.
McCallister RE, et al: Porokeratosis plantaris, palmaris, et disseminata. JAAD 1985, 13:598.
McDonald SG, et al: Porokeratosis (Mibelli). JAAD 1983, 8:107.
Sakas EL, et al: Porokeratosis punctata palmaris et plantaris. JAAD 1985, 13:908.
Schwarz T, et al: Disseminated superficial "actinic" porokeratosis. JAAD 1984, 11:724.
Shelley WB, et al: Disseminated superficial porokeratosis. Cutis 1983, 32:139.
Stoof TJ, et al: Porokeratotic eccrine ostial and dermal duct nevus. JAAD 1989, 20:924.
Witkowski JA: Porokeratosis of Mibelli. Cutis 1982, 29:171.

Porokeratosis Striata (Nekam)

This configurate, linear, lichen planus–like eruption appears to be the same disease as lichen verrucosa et reticularis of Kaposi, and three cases reported by Menter and Morrison all showed histologic changes of lichen planus with leucocytoclastic vasculitis, and serologic evidence of toxoplasmosis. Its nosologic position is not clear, but at least it seems not to be a variety of porokeratosis.

Menter MA, et al: Lichen verrucosus et reticularis of Kaposi (porokeratosis striata of Nekam). Br J Dermatol 1976, 94:645.

DARIER'S DISEASE
(Keratosis Follicularis)

CLINICAL FEATURES. Darier's disease is characterized by dirty, warty, papular excrescences that tend to coalesce into patches on symmetrical areas of the face, trunk, and flexures of the extremities. The early lesions are small, firm papules, almost the color of normal skin. Each of these soon becomes covered with a greasy, gray, brown or black crust that fits into a small concavity in the summit of the papule. As the lesions grow older, their color becomes darker. In the course of years the papules grow and may fuse to form malodorous papillomatous and vegetating growths. These are fissured and eroded and may be covered with an offensive purulent exudate.

The neck and shoulders, the face, the extremities, the front of the chest, and the midline of the back are sites of predilection for the disease, but as the eruption spreads, the entire trunk, buttocks, genitals,

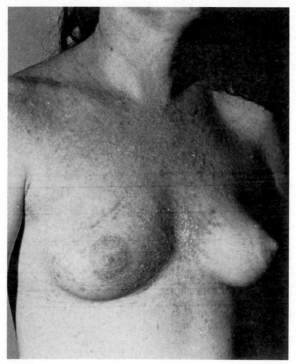

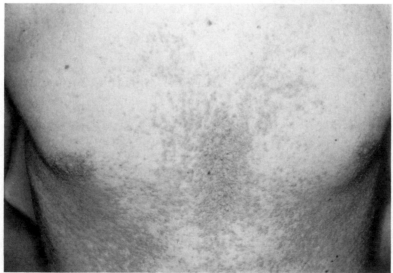

Figure 27–43. Darier's disease.

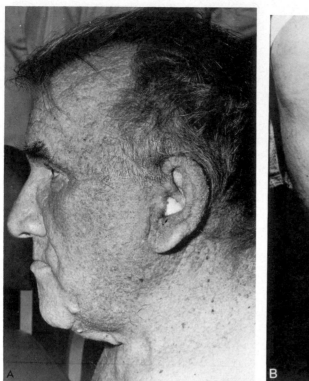
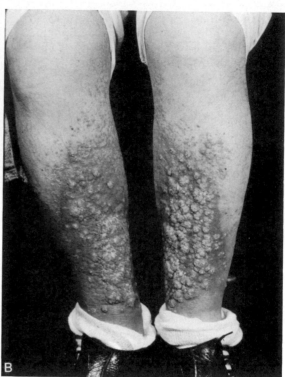

Figure 27–44. A *and* B, *Darier's disease.* (B, *Courtesy of Dr. Axel W. Hoke.*)

and other parts of the skin may be involved. A frequent site for the earliest lesions is behind the ears.

Usually the eruption is symmetrical and widespread, but striking unilateral or zosteriform involvement may also occur. A unilateral case was reported by Moore et al in 1985. These cases of limited or nevoid type distribution may be variants of epidermal nevi, rather than types of familial Darier's disease. Bullae may occur in some cases, as in the patient reported by Hori et al.

Vegetations appear chiefly in the axillae, gluteal

crease, and groins, and behind the ears. The scalp is generally covered with greasy crusts. Lesions on the face are particularly severe about the nose. The lips may be crusted, fissured, swollen, and superficially ulcerated, and there may be a patchy keratosis with superficial erosions on the dorsum of the tongue. Usually small white papules are present on the gingiva and palate, or there may be pebbly areas with verrucous white plaques. Punctate keratoses, either raised or with a central pit, are frequently noted on the palms and soles. A general horny thickening of the palms and soles may be present because of innumerable closely set small papules. On the dorsa of the hands and on the shins the flat verrucous papules may resemble verrucae planae. The nails show subungual hyperkeratosis, fragility, and splintering, with longitudinal alternating white and red streaks, and triangular nicking of the free edges. Involvement with Darier's disease of the oropharynx, esophagus, hypopharynx, larynx, and anorectal mucosa has been reported.

Localized Darier's disease has been found to occur mostly in a linear fashion. The trunk is a favorite site; however, when it occurs elsewhere diagnosis is difficult, so that the biopsy usually establishes the diagnosis. This was true of Wheeland et al's case of localized scalp lesions.

An additional sign was reported in 1981 by Jegasothy et al, who found anergy, and inability to produce leukocyte inhibitory factor, in seven of their eight patients with Darier's disease. Their lymphocytes were totally unresponsive to concanavalin A, but responded normally to phytohemagglutinin and

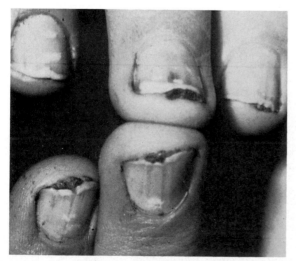

Figure 27–45. Subungual hyperkeratosis in Darier's disease. (*Courtesy of Dr. F. Ronchese.*)

pokeweed mitogen. This report, along with the well-known risk of development of Kaposi's varicelliform eruption, mandates more studies of the immune system in these patients.

Darier's disease is usually worse in the summer months, patients being photosensitive. It may begin after severe sunburn (photo-Koebner). Baba et al were able to reproduce lesions in their patient with suberythema doses of UVB. Most cases tend to improve or clear in winter. The patient usually suffers from severe itching and discomfort, owing to the skin ulcerations, which cause pain, bleed readily, and have an offensive odor.

ETIOLOGY. Darier's disease is a genodermatosis of autosomal dominant inheritance. It has been considered by some to be a disorder of vitamin A metabolism. Reports, however, are conflicting and further investigation is needed to determine the role of vitamin A in the etiology of this disease. Darier's disease represents a familial disorder in the epidermal synthesis and turnover, as shown by the resultant dyskeratosis. Caulfield and Wilgram's electron microscopic studies reveal the defect in the tonofilament-desmosomal complex. The defect may be in either the synthesis, organization, or maturation of this complex.

INCIDENCE. Darier's disease may occur in all races, with males and females affected equally. It usually has its onset during childhood, but it may appear at any time.

HISTOLOGY. Darier's disease shows hyperkeratosis, parakeratosis, acanthosis, formation of suprabasal lacunae, and the upward proliferation of villi into the lacunae. In the lacunae acantholytic dyskeratotic cells, corps ronds, and grains are present. The acantholysis is responsible for the lacunae or cleft formation; the corps ronds are cells with a basophilic nucleus surrounded by a slight halo. Grains are small dark cells with a pyknotic nucleus, seen most frequently in the stratum corneum.

DIFFERENTIAL DIAGNOSIS. Acanthosis nigricans, ichthyosis vulgaris, keratosis pilaris, and seborrheic keratosis are some diseases that may simulate keratosis follicularis.

TREATMENT. Historically, vitamin A has been used for many years to ameliorate the course of the disease, with varying degrees of success. Although the customary dose has been 50 to 100 thousand units daily, 300,000 to 1 million units daily have been more successful. Also the combination of vitamin A and vitamin E has been reported to be effective by Ayres and Mihan. Tretinoin has been used topically for localized lesions. Isotretinoin is very effective; however, prolonged remissions are not seen, thus limiting its use because of the risks of long-term therapy. Orfanos found etretinate rapidly effective in a dose of 50 to 75 mg a day, with 25 to 30 mg a day for maintenance. Mahrle et al, as well as others, support the efficacy of etretinate in this condition.

Local therapy for inflamed lesions includes topical corticosteroid creams or ointments as well as ointments containing salicylic acid, tar, or sulfur. Fulton et al achieved clearing for several months by using 0.1 per cent Retin-A cream under occlusion. Intralesional triamcinolone achieves prompt but transitory relief. For hypertrophic lesions, dermabrasion, laser excision, or excision and grafting should be considered.

Ayres S Jr, et al: Keratosis follicularis. Arch Dermatol 1972, 106:909.

Baba T, et al: UV radiation and keratosis follicularis. Arch Dermatol 1984, 120:1484.

Dicken CH, et al: Isotretinoin treatment of Darier's disease. JAAD 1982, 6:721.

Goldsmith LA, et al: Cornification diseases. JAAD 1986, 14:118.

Hori Y, et al: Bullous Darier's disease. Arch Dermatol 1982, 118:278.

Jegasothy BV, et al: Darier's disease. J Invest Dermatol 1981, 76:129.

Koh HK, et al: Chronic dermatosis in a young man. Arch Dermatol 1987, 123:1071.

Mahrle G, et al: Oral treatment of keratinizing disorders of skin and mucous membranes with etretinate. Arch Dermatol 1982, 118:97.

Moore JA, et al: Unilateral keratosis follicularis. Cutis 1985, 34:459.

Orfanos CE, et al: Oral treatment of keratosis follicularis with a new aromatic retinoid. Arch Dermatol 1978, 114:1211.

Rand R, et al: Commentary: Darier-White disease. Arch Dermatol 1983, 119:81.

Thomas JR, et al: High-dose vitamin A therapy for Darier's disease. Arch Dermatol 1982, 118:891.

Valquist A, et al: Darier's disease and vitamin A. Arch Dermatol 1982, 118:389.

Verner E, et al: Eczema herpeticum in a patient with Darier's disease during treatment with etretinate. JAAD 1985, 13:678.

Wheeland RG, et al: Localized Darier's disease of the scalp complicated by *Trichophyton tonsurans* infection. Arch Dermatol 1985, 121:905.

ACROKERATOSIS VERRUCIFORMIS (Hopf)

This rare genodermatosis is characterized by numerous flat verrucous papules occurring on the backs of the hands, insteps, knees, and elbows. The papules are closely grouped, and resemble warts except that they are flatter and more localized, typically to the backs of the hands. It is inherited as an autosomal dominant trait. Lesions similar to these occur not infrequently in Darier's disease, and in at least one instance, the two diseases were seen in different members of the same family.

Histologically, hyperkeratosis, thickening of the granular layer, and acanthosis characterize the disease. Papillomatosis with a resemblance of the epidermal elevations to church spires is frequently present.

Available treatment methods are liquid nitrogen therapy, shave excision, and carbon dioxide laser ablation. However, recurrence is common.

Panja RK: Acrokeratosis verruciformis (Hopf). Br J Dermatol 1977, 96:643.

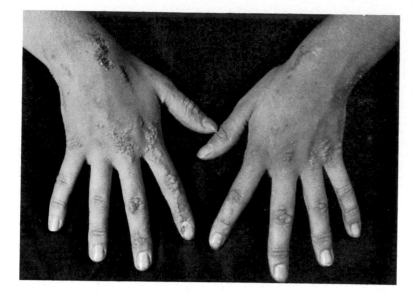

Figure 27–46. Acrokeratosis verruciformis of Hopf.

PACHYONYCHIA CONGENITA

CLINICAL FEATURES. In 1906 Jadassohn and Lewandowsky described a rare, often familial, anomaly of the nails to which they gave the name pachyonychia congenita. It is characterized by distinctively and excessively thickened nails of all fingers and toes; palmar and plantar hyperkeratoses; follicular keratosis of the skin especially on the knees and elbows; blister formation, especially under and around callosities; palmar and plantar hyperhidrosis; and leukokeratosis of the mucous membranes. The nail changes consist of great thickening, which increases toward the free borders. The nail plates are extremely hard and are firmly attached to the nail beds. The nail bed is filled with yellow, horny, keratotic debris, which may cause the nail to project upward at the free edge. Paronychial infection is frequently present.

On the extensor surfaces of the extremities, the buttocks, and the lumbar regions are follicular, keratotic, grayish black papules, having in their centers horny cones that fit into craterlike depressions. The removal of these central cones is fairly easy and leaves a slightly bleeding cavity. The eruption on the outer aspects of the upper and lower extremities is also follicular, resembling keratosis pilaris. This latter condition is not constant and disappears at times.

Painful friction blisters may develop on the plantar aspects of the toes or heels or along the edges of the feet. Cases have been misdiagnosed as epidermolysis bullosa. Leukokeratosis of the tongue and oral mucosa, as well as occasional laryngeal involvement, with hoarseness, may occur.

Schönfeld has divided pachyonychia congenita into three types, the above described type being most common, and designated type I *(Jadassohn-Lewandosky syndrome)*. Type II *(Jackson-Sertoli syndrome)* has the same features as type I, plus natal teeth and steatocystoma multiplex. Type III *(Schafer-Branauer syndrome)* is like type I plus leukokeratosis of the corneas. Tidman et al have described two families with hyperpigmentation around the neck, waist, axillae, thighs, kneebends, buttocks, and ab-

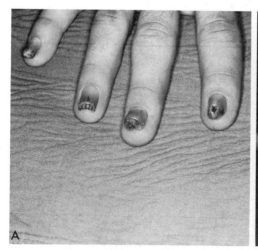
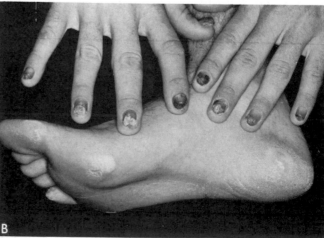

Figure 27–47. A *and* B, *Nail involvement and plantar keratoderma in pachyonychia congenita.*

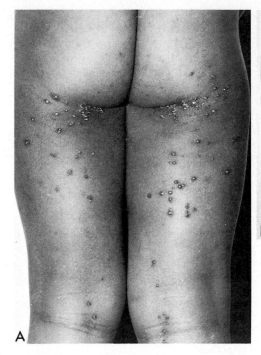

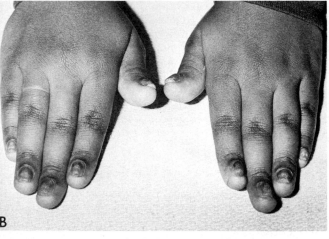

Figure 27–48. A *and* B, *Pachyonychia congenita.*

domen. Pigmentary incontinence and amyloid deposition were seen in biopsy specimens.

ETIOLOGY. Pachyonychia congenita is usually inherited by autosomal dominance. However, Heber et al have described two cases in which it occurred as an autosomal recessive disorder.

PATHOGENESIS. Pinkus and Mehregan aver that the nail plate and the proximal nail matrix are normal; however, the distal matrix and nail bed epidermis produce excessive amounts of keratin and, therefore, produce a condition similar to that of a horse's hoof.

TREATMENT. Numerous measures to relieve the pachyonychia have proved ineffective. Avulsion of the nails brings about only temporary relief. Removal of the nail matrix alone does no good. Thomsen et al reported that vigorous curettage of the matrix and nail bed was the simplest and most effective therapy.

The keratoderma may also produce physical dis-

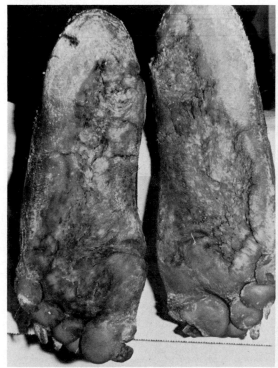

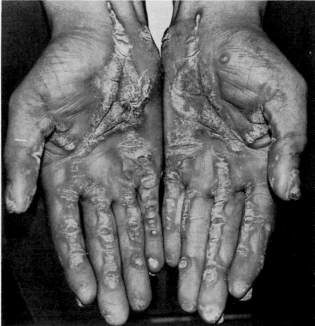

Figure 27–49. Pachyonychia congenita on the palms, soles, and nails of a 21-year-old man.

ability, and topical keratolytics are to date the best treatment for this: lactic acid or Lac-Hydrin (ammonium lactate 12 per cent) lotion, salicylic acid, and urea preparations may all be helpful. Thomas reported that isotretinoin cleared the keratotic papules and the oral leukokeratosis, but did not improve the palms or soles. Burnett reported that the incorporation of 33 per cent lactic acid into Lac-Hydrin (total lactate content 45 per cent) makes it very effective in palmoplantar hyperkeratosis.

Burnett JW: Lac-Hydrin "Forte" for tough hyperkeratosis: 45 per cent! Schoch Letter 1987, 37:22, Item 83.

Feinstein A, et al: Pachyonychia congenita. JAAD 1988, 19:705.

Haber RM, et al: Autosomal recessive pachyonychia congenita. Arch Dermatol 1986, 122:919.

Schonfeld PHIR: The pachyonychia congenita syndrome. Acta Dermatol Venereol 1980, 60:45.

Thomas DR, et al: Pachyonychia congenita. Arch Dermatol 1984, 120:1475.

Thomsen RJ, et al: Pachyonychia congenita. J Dermatol Surg Oncol 1982, 8:24.

Tidman MJ, et al: Pachyonychia congenita with cutaneous amyloidosis and hyperpigmentation. JAAD 1987, 16:935.

DYSKERATOSIS CONGENITA

This rare congenital syndrome is characterized by atrophy and a reticular pigmentation of the skin, dystrophy of the nails, and leukoplakia, together with multisystem ectodermal and some mesodermal changes.

The striking feature of the skin is the tan-gray mottled hyper- or hypo-pigmented macules or reticulated patches that on some areas appear like a fine network. Atrophy and telangiectasia are also present. These lesions are located typically on the upper torso, neck, and face, although the extremities may also be involved.

The nails may be dystrophic, with thinning, tapering, and distortion resulting from atrophy. Ridging and longitudinal fissuring are seen in mild cases. This is the first component of the syndrome to appear, becoming apparent between the ages of five and 15. The other cutaneous lesions follow within three to five years, as a rule.

Leukoplakia may occur, mostly on the buccal mucosa, where extensive involvement with verrucous thickening may be present. The anus, vagina, conjunctiva, and the urethral meatus may also be involved.

Other manifestations of dyskeratosis congenita may be hyperhidrosis of the palms and soles, bullous conjunctivitis, gingival disorders, dysphagia due to esophageal strictures and diverticula, skeletal abnormalities, aplastic anemia, mental deficiency, and hypersplenism. A Fanconi-type pancytopenia may be present, as discussed by Gutman.

Malignant neoplasms of the skin, mouth, nasopharynx, esophagus, rectum, and cervix have been seen in these patients more frequently than in the normal similar age group. These develop within the leukoplakia described above.

The disease usually begins in childhood, with involvement almost completely limited to males. The most likely mode of inheritance is as an X-linked recessive trait: this type is most frequently called the *Zinsser-Cole-Engman syndrome.* Autosomal dominant inheritance has also been reported by Scoggins. Tchou et al reported eight cases in 1982, two of them with only reticulated pigmentation and anemia, from a large French-Canadian family in which it was inherited in autosomal dominant fashion. Ling et al described a girl with dyskeratosis congenita, reviewed the reports of female involvement, and pointed out the clinical and histologic similarities to chronic graft-versus-host disease. Esterly carried this similarity further by pointing out that nail dystrophy similar to dyskeratosis congenita may be present in chronic graft-versus-host disease.

Esterly NB: Nail dystrophy in dyskeratosis congenita and chronic graft-versus-host disease. Arch Dermatol 1986, 122:506.

Gutman A, et al: X-linked dyskeratosis congenita with pancytopenia. Arch Dermatol 1978, 114:1667.

Hitch JM: Dyskeratosis congenita. Cutis 1968, 4:1229.

Ling NS, et al: Dyskeratosis congenita in a girl simulating chronic-graft-versus-host disease. Arch Dermatol 1985, 121:1424.

Tchou PK, et al: Dyskeratosis congenita. JAAD 1982, 6:1034.

Fanconi Syndrome

Also known as *familial pancytopenia* or *familial panmyelophthisis,* the syndrome may be associated with diffuse pigmentation of the skin, absence of the thumbs, aplasia of the radius, severe hypoplastic anemia, thrombocytopenia, retinal hemorrhage, strabismus, generalized hyperreflexia, and testicular hypoplasia. The syndrome is associated with increased risk of myelomonocytic leukemia, squamous cell carcinoma, and hepatic tumors. Chromosome patterns are frequently abnormal.

Johansson et al reported a case surviving to age 27, with chromosomal aberrations, depressed cell-mediated immunity, and numerous recalcitrant viral warts.

In culture, cells from these patients show increased transformation by oncogenic viruses, as well as a marked hypersensitivity to agents that produce DNA interstrand cross-links, such as nitrogen mustard, PUVA, and mitomycin C. Increased cell killing and chromosomal abnormalities occur. The cross-links persist, leading to the hypothesis that there is a defect in the repair of these cross-links in Fanconi patients. No hypersensitivity to UV light, x-rays, or other chemical agents is present.

Johansson E, et al: Fanconi's anemia. Arch Dermatol 1982, 118:249.

Lambert WC: Genetic diseases associated with DNA and chromosomal instability. Dermatol Clin 1987, 5:85.

CONGENITAL ECTODERMAL DEFECT

The ectodermal dysplasia syndromes are characterized by the presence of abnormalities at birth, by being nonprogressive, by diffuse disease, and by involvement of the epidermis plus at least one of the appendages (hair, sebaceous glands, nails, teeth, or mucosal glands). Many families display unique involvement, and many described syndromes exist. An extensive reference source for these is Freire-Maia's book. Solomon et al present the classification table developed by Freire-Maia, which subgroups the syndromes by assigning numbers to the tissues involved. We will discuss only selected syndromes.

Anhidrotic Ectodermal Dysplasia

The classic triad of this disorder consists of hypotrichosis, anodontia, and anhidrosis. This disease is often referred to as the *Christ-Siemens-Touraine syndrome.*

Absent or reduced sweating is a prominent feature. Despite appropriate heat stress, either environmental or fever-induced sweating is absent or slight, and febrile seizures may occur. Biopsy confirms that eccrine glands are absent or rudimentary, and this may be the basis for prenatal diagnosis.

The appearance of these patients is typical and conspicuous, since they have a facies suggestive of congenital syphilis. The cheek bones are high and wide, whereas the lower half of the face is narrow. The supraorbital ridges are prominent; the nasal bridge is depressed, forming a saddle-back nose. The tip of the nose is small and upturned, and the nostrils are large and conspicuous. The eyebrows are scanty. The eyes slant upward, simulating a Mongolian facies. At the buccal commissures there are radiating furrows (pseudorhagades), and on the cheeks there are telangiectases and small yellow papules (sebaceous gland hyperplasia) simulating milium and adenoma sebaceum. The lips are thickened, the upper lip being particularly protrusive.

Hypotrichosis is generalized. This is not a complete alopecia, but rather the hair is scraggly, thin, sparse, and dry. In addition to the scalp, other areas are affected such as the beard area, axillae, pubic area, and trunk. There is partial or total anodontia. Nails may be thinned, brittle, and ridged. The skin is soft and thin, dry, and smooth. Mental retardation is present in some cases, possibly a consequence of hyperthermic episodes in childhood.

The inheritance pattern is almost always expressed through an X-linked recessive gene. Ten per cent of female carriers may have partial overt expression of this affliction. Both autosomal recessive and dominant modes of inheritance have been described.

Hidrotic Ectodermal Dysplasia

The hidrotic type of congenital ectodermal dysplasia is often referred to as *Clouston's syndrome.* Here the eccrine sweat glands are active and the facial features are normal, without the typical saddle nose. An autosomal dominant gene is responsible in these cases. Alopecia, nail dystrophy, palmoplantar hyperkeratosis, and eye changes such as cataracts and

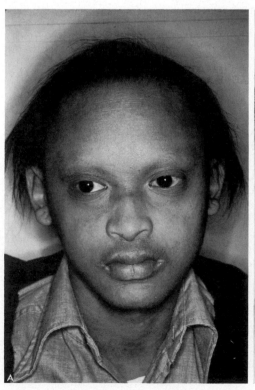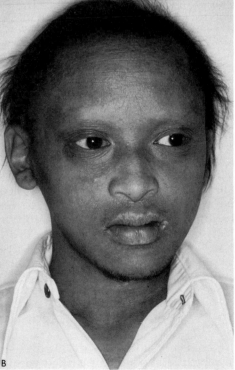

Figure 27–50. A *and* B, *Anhidrotic ectodermal defect and atopic dermatitis in brothers.*

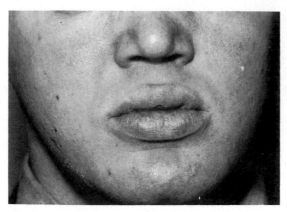

Figure 27–51. Congenital ectodermal defect: saddle nose, up-turned nose tip, thick, protrusive lips. (Courtesy of Dr. D. Bloom.)

strabismus are the features of hidrotic ectodermal dysplasia. Wilkinson et al reported a case with diffuse eccrine poromatosis.

Hazen PG, et al: Premature cataracts in a family with hidrotic ectodermal dysplasia. Arch Dermatol 1980, 116:1385.
Kanzler MH, et al: Atrichia with papular lesions. Arch Dermatol 1986, 122:565.
Katz SI, et al: Sebaceous gland papules in anhidrotic ectodermal dysplasia. Arch Dermatol 1971, 103:507.
McNaughton PZ, et al: Hidrotic ectodermal dysplasia in a black mother and daughter. Arch Dermatol 1976, 112:1448.
Reddy BSN, et al: Anhidrotic ectodermal dysplasia. Int J Dermatol 1978, 17:139.
Sato K, et al: Biology of sweat glands and their disorders. JAAD 1989, 20:713.
Solomon LM, et al: The ectodermal dysplasias. Dermatol Clin 1987, 5:231.
Spiegel J, et al: AEC syndrome. JAAD 1985, 12:810.
Wasserteil V: Fever and hypotrichosis in a newborn. Arch Dermatol 1986, 122:1325.
Wilkinson RD, et al: Hidrotic ectodermal dysplasia with diffuse eccrine poromatosis. Arch Dermatol 1977, 113:472.

AEC Syndrome

*A*nkyloblepharon, *E*ctodermal defects, and *C*left lip and palate constitute the AEC syndrome, of which Spiegel et al reported the eighth and ninth cases in 1985, which she and Colton believed were the first in the United States. It has been called hypohidrotic ectodermal dysplasia with multiple associated anomalies. It has an autosomal dominant pattern of inheritance. There may or may not be fusion or partial fusion of the lids (ankyloblepharon) at birth. Sparse hair, dental defects, cleft palate and lip, dystrophic nails, hypospadias, syndactyly, short stature, absent lacrimal puncta, and stenotic auditory canals and short stature are a few of the possible anomalies.

Atrichia With Papular Lesions

Kanzler et al in 1986 reviewed this rare syndrome in which fetal scalp hair is shed within three months

of birth, and is never replaced. Small keratin-filled cysts are widespread. Teeth and nails are normal.

Aplasia Cutis Congenita

This congenital defect of the skin is a rare anomaly of the newborn, with a predilection for the midline of the vertex of the scalp. A small bleb in fetal life may develop into a coin-sized absence of skin and subcutaneous tissue, very rarely penetrating into the cranium. In a different condition, also rare, multiple symmetrical defects occur on the skin, generally on the lower extremities. There is a tendency for these aplasias to heal spontaneously, making surgical repair unnecessary.

Frieden undertook the all but impossible task of classifying aplasia cutis congenita into nine groups or types according to the number and location of lesions and the presence or absence of associated malformations.

Frieden IJ: Aplasia cutis congenita. JAAD 1986, 14:646.
Guillen PSP, et al: Aplasia cutis congenita. JAAD 1985, 13:429.
Magid ML, et al: Focal facial dermal dysphasia. JAAD 1988, 18:1203.

Focal Dermal Hypoplasia (Goltz's Syndrome)

This is characterized by multiple abnormalities of mesodermal and ectodermal tissues. Reddish tan, atrophic, often linear or cribriform patches in conjunction with herniations of yellowish brown (fat) nodules may be present prominently on the buttocks, axillae, and thighs. The lesions are strikingly linear and often serpiginous. Brown, atrophic, sharply circumscribed patches appear. Telangiectases are commonly present. Papillomas, small and reddish tan, have occurred around the orifices of the mouth, anus, and vagina. They may be misdiagnosed as condylomata acuminata.

The bone changes are concerned mostly with the extremities, where there may be syndactyly, oligodactyly, and adactyly. Scoliosis, spina bifida, and hypoplasia of the clavicle have also been reported. Eighty per cent of patients have skeletal defects. Variable ocular, dental, hair, and nail abnormalities have been described. Forty to 50 per cent of patients have ocular and dental abnormalities. Coloboma is the most common ocular defect. The large majority of reported patients have been female. An X-linked dominant trait is believed to be the hereditary pattern; however, an autosomal dominant trait, but sex limited, is also possible.

Billings JK, et al: Multiple mesodermal defects in an infant. Arch Dermatol 1986, 122:1199.
Goltz RW, et al: Focal dermal hypoplasia syndrome. Arch Dermatol 1970, 101:1.

Cockayne's Syndrome

Cockayne described a syndrome which he named *dwarfism with retinal atrophy and deafness.* The various dermatologic features are photodermatitis due to sensitivity to sunlight resulting in hyperpigmentation and scarring. Other changes are microcephaly, sunken eyes, a facial appearance similar to Mickey Mouse, severe flexion contractures, dorsal kyphosis, cryptorchidism, cataracts, retardation of growth, severe mental retardation, and retinitis pigmentosa with optic atrophy. Dermal fibroblasts and lymphoblastoid cell lines, as well as cultured amniotic fluid cells from an affected fetus, demonstrate impaired colony-forming ability, and decreased DNA and RNA synthesis after ultraviolet light exposure (254 nm). There is progressive neurologic disturbance with shortened lifespan. There is no increased carcinogenesis.

Inheritance is by an autosomal recessive gene with 100 per cent penetrance.

Beauregard S, et al: Syndromes of premature aging. Dermatol Clin 1987, 5:109.

Lambert WC: Genetic diseases associated with DNA and chromosomal instability. Dermatol Clin 1987, 5:85.

WERNER'S SYNDROME
(Adult Progeria)

Werner's syndrome is a premature-aging syndrome characterized by many metabolic and structural abnormalities involving the skin, hair, eyes, muscles, fatty tissues, bones, blood vessels, and carbohydrate metabolism.

The most characteristic findings are premature aging and arrest of growth at puberty, senile cataracts developing in the late twenties and thirties, premature balding and graying, and sclerodermalike lesions of the skin.

An outstanding change is the loss of subcutaneous tissue and wasting of muscles, especially the extremities, so that the legs become spindly and the trunk becomes stocky.

Additional changes may be painful callosities with ulcerations around the malleoli, Achilles tendons, heels, and toes. Hair thins on the eyebrows, axillae, and pubis. The skin over the cheek bones becomes taut to produce proptosis and beaking of the nose. Cataracts develop early. The vocal cords become thickened so that a weak, high-pitched voice ensues. Premature arteriosclerosis and sexual impotence are frequently observed. Diabetes is frequent; and areas of calcinosis circumscripta occur.

Riley and his associates call attention to the high rate of malignancy occurring with Werner's syndrome. Melanotic sarcoma, uterine sarcoma, hepatoma carcinoma of the breast, and thyroid adeno-carcinoma have occurred. Hrabko et al reported a patient with fibrosarcoma and multiple basal cell carcinomas, and reviewed the literature, in 1982.

Histologic changes in the skin may include atrophy of the epidermis and fibrosis of the dermis.

The etiology has not been determined. Consanguinity and familial incidence are encountered, to suggest a mendelian recessive mode of transmission. Endocrinologic involvement, although obvious, is not believed to be connected with the cause of Werner's syndrome.

Werner's syndrome should be differentiated from scleroderma, atopic dermatitis (cataracta dermatogenes), ectodermal dysplasia, dystrophia myotonica, lipoatrophic diabetes, Rothmund's syndrome, progeria with nanism, and Turner's syndrome.

Progeria, or the *Hutchinson-Gilford syndrome,* is characterized by dwarfism, alopecia, generalized atrophy of the skin and muscles, enlarged head with prominent scalp veins, and a high incidence of generalized atherosclerosis, usually fatal by the second decade. There are usually sclerodermatous plaques on the extremities.

Treatment is symptomatic: chiefly, control of diabetes mellitus and treatment of leg ulcerations. Cohn et al achieved normal growth in a boy treated with methyltestosterone from age 14 on.

Aram H, et al: Werner's syndrome. Cutis 1974, 14:215.

Badame AJ: Progeria. Arch Dermatol 1989, 125:540.

Bauer EA, et al: Werner's syndrome. Arch Dermatol 1988, 124:90.

Beauregard S, et al: Syndromes of premature aging. Dermatol Clin 1987, 5:109.

DeBusk FL: The Hutchinson-Guilford progeria syndrome. J Pediatr 1972, 90:697.

Fleishmajer R, et al: Werner's syndrome. Am J Med 1973, 54:111.

Gawkrodger DJ, et al: Werner's syndrome. Arch Dermatol 1985, 121:636.

Hrabko RP, et al: Werner's syndrome with associated malignant neoplasms. Arch Dermatol 1982, 118:106.

Riley TH, et al: Werner's syndrome. Ann Intern Med 1965, 63:285.

Sephel GC, et al: Increased elastin production by progeria skin fibroblasts is controlled by the steady-state levels of elastin m-RNA. J Invest Dermatol 1988, 90:643.

OTHER CONGENITAL ANOMALIES

Congenital Fistulas of the Lower Lip

Variously known as *labial fistulae, lip pits, or congenital pits of the lower lip,* these are characterized as paired circular or slitlike depressions on either side of the center of the lower lip at the edge of the vermilion border. The fistulous tract in the center of the depression may extend 5 to 25 mm into the lip. Frequently these are associated with cleft lip and cleft palate. An autosomal dominant gene is frequently found. Taylor and Lane have also indicated that these pits may be a part of syndromes especially connected with the skeletal system.

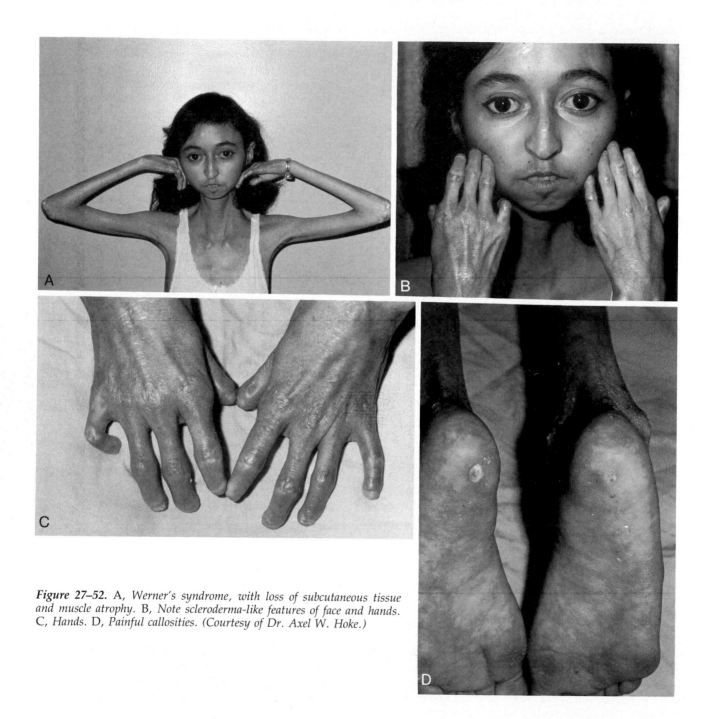

Figure 27–52. A, *Werner's syndrome, with loss of subcutaneous tissue and muscle atrophy.* B, *Note scleroderma-like features of face and hands.* C, *Hands.* D, *Painful callosities. (Courtesy of Dr. Axel W. Hoke.)*

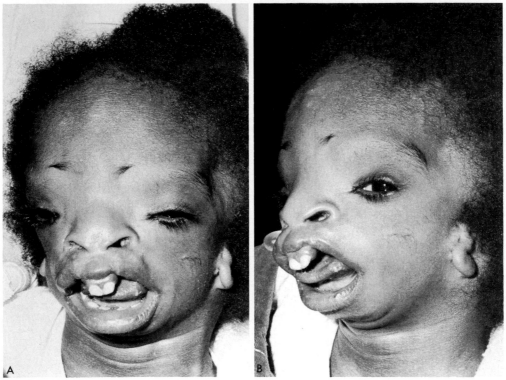

Figure 27–53. A *and* B, *Treacher Collins syndrome (incomplete mandibulofacial dysostosis). Wide-set eyes, deformed nose and ears, enlarged mouth, small lower jaw. (Courtesy of Dr. G. Salinger.)*

Franceschetti Syndrome

The syndrome of Franceschetti and Klein *(dysostosis mandibulo-facialis)* consists, when complete, of palpebral antimongoloid fissures, hypoplasia of the facial bones, macrostomia, vaulted palate, malformations of both the external and internal ear, buccal-auricular fistula, abnormal development of the neck with stretching of the cheeks, accessory facial fissures, and skeletal deformities. The syndrome is inherited as an autosomal dominant trait. Patients who have the complete syndrome usually die in infancy, but in the abortive types they may live to an old age. This abortive type is known as *Treacher Collins syndrome.*

Congenital Auricular Fistula

This anomaly occurs in the preauricular region, often in several members and generations of a family. On each side just anterior to the external ear there is a small dimple, pore, or fistulous opening that may extend even into the middle ear. Occasionally cysts or granulomatous nodules that simulate scrofuloderma or epidermal inclusion cysts may develop at these sites.

Branchial Cleft Cyst

Developmental anomalies of the branchial clefts may occur as cysts, sinus tracts, or cartilage remnants in the skin. These anomalies appear in a line extending from a point anterior to the ears downward on the neck to the insertion of the sternomastoid muscle into the sternum. Most frequently cysts or sinus tracts are seen. They are soft tender lesions from which rancid sebumlike material may exude. Frequently secondary infection calls attention to the disorder.

Wheeler and his associates indicate an autosomal dominant inheritance with incomplete penetrance.

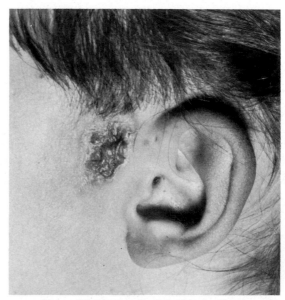

Figure 27–54. *Congenital auricular fistula.*

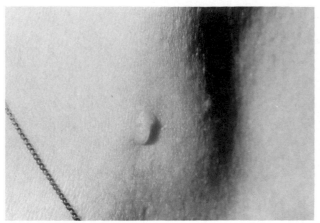

Figure 27–55. Branchial cleft cyst. (Courtesy of Dr. Axel W. Hoke.)

Foote and Anderson have emphasized the importance of differential diagnosis. Tuberculous lymphadenitis, epidermal cyst, and primary as well as metastatic carcinoma must be considered.

Treatment is excision by someone well qualified in head and neck surgery, since the lesions, especially the sinus tracts, may extend deeply into areas encompassing vital structures.

Popliteal Pterygium Syndrome

Pterygia or skin folds may extend from the thigh down to the heel and thus prevent extension or rotation of the legs. In addition, crural pterygia may be present. Cryptorchism, bifid scrotum, agenesis of the labia majora, cleft lip and palate, adhesions between the eyelids, syndactyly, and talipes equinovarus are all commonly seen in this syndrome. An autosomal dominant inheritance trait is presumed.

Apert's Syndrome (Acrocephalosyndactyly)

This autosomal-dominantly inherited disorder is characterized by synostosis of the feet, hands, carpi, tarsi, cervical vertebrae, and skull. The facial features are distorted and the second, third, and fourth fingers are fused into a bony mass with a single nail. Oculocutaneous albinism and severe acne vulgaris have been reported with Apert's syndrome.

Whistling Face Syndrome

Also known as *craniocarpotarsal syndrome*, in this rare disorder the child appears to be whistling all the time. This configuration is due to microstomia, deep set eyes, flattened midface, coloboma, and alterations of the nostrils. Ulnar deviation of the fingers, kyphoscoliosis, and talipes equinovarus may be present. An autosomal dominant trait is responsible for this syndrome.

Familial Autonomic Dysautonomia

Also known as *Riley-Day syndrome*, this is characterized by defective lacrimation (manifested by crying without tears) leading to corneal ulceration, hypertension, excessive hyperhidrosis, drooling, and skin blotching on stress. Erythematous macules 2 to 5 mm in diameter appear over the entire body at times of emotional stress. Shortly afterward the entire skin surface becomes confluently dark red in color. Acrocyanosis with cold, damp hands and feet is usually present.

Dysautonomia is an inherited autosomal recessive trait occurring most frequently in Jewish children.

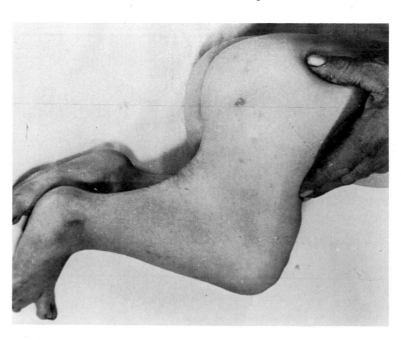

Figure 27–56. Popliteal pterygium syndrome. (Courtesy of Dr. R. J. Gorlin.)

There is evidence that epinephrine and acetylcholine metabolic defects are present in this syndrome.

Fellner MJ: Manifestations of familial autonomic dysautonomia. Arch Dermatol 1964, 84:190.

Guillet G, et al: A linear fibrous cord and ulcer of the lower limb. Arch Dermatol 1988, 124:1443.

McNaughton PZ, et al: Apert's syndrome. Cutis 1980, 25:538.

Steffen C: Acneiform eruption in Apert's syndrome. Arch Dermatol 1982, 118:206.

Taylor WB, et al: Congenital fistulas of the lower lip. Arch Dermatol 1966, 94:421.

Weinstein S, et al: Cranio-carpal-tarsal dysplasia or the whistling face syndrome. Am J Dis Child 1969, 117:427.

Nonne-Milroy-Meige Syndrome (Hereditary Lymphedema)

Milroy's hereditary edema of the lower legs is characterized by a unilateral or bilateral lymphedema present at birth and inherited as an autosomal dominant trait. The edema is painless, pits on pressure, is not associated with any other disorder, and persists throughout life. Most frequently the affection is unilateral and females are predominantly affected.

This type of lymphedema is differentiated from the acquired type, which occurs not only on the

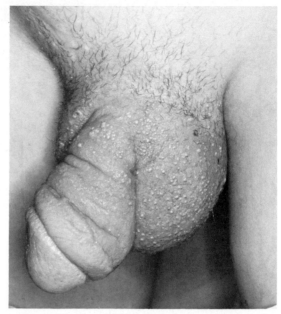

Figure 27–58. *Penile and scrotal lymphedema with lymphangiectases in a patient with Milroy's disease.*

lower extremities but also on the lips, lower eyelids, or other areas where lymph stasis has been produced secondary to other areas of involvement.

Treatment of this particular type of edema is extremely difficult since the disease is an anomaly of the lymph-draining vessels. The Pratt procedure, consisting of the excision of edematous, fibrotic, cutaneous and subcutaneous tissue and fascia, has had varying degrees of success. The Kondoleon operation is similar to the Pratt procedure.

Bastien MR, et al: Treatment of lymphedema with a multicompartmental pneumatic compression device. JAAD 1989, 20:853.

Cook W, et al: Milroy's disease. JAMA 1951, 147:650.

Milroy WF: Hereditary edema of the lower legs. JAMA 1968, 204:166.

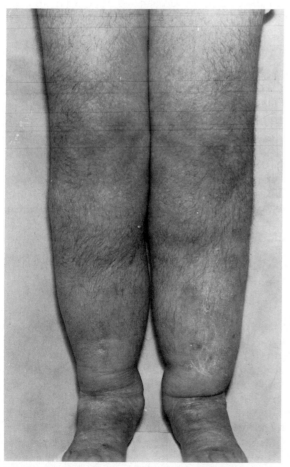

Figure 27–57. *Hereditary lymphedema. (Courtesy of Dr. D. Bloom.)*

RESTRICTIVE DERMOPATHY

Holbrook et al reported two sibs and one unrelated infant in 1987 with this fatal, autosomal recessive inherited disorder, which was named restrictive dermopathy by Witt et al in 1986. The entire integument is thick, hyperkeratotic, and parakeratotic, and so tight and rigid that it causes flexion contractures, and severely restricts respiration, resulting in death at a few hours or weeks after birth. The characteristic facies includes a small, open mouth; small nose; and low-set ears. Probably at least nine cases of the syndrome have been recognized and reported.

Holbrook KA, et al: Arrested epidermal morphogenesis in three newborn infants with a fatal genetic disorder: restrictive dermopathy. J Invest Dermatol 1987, 88:330.

28

Dermal and Subcutaneous Tumors

The dermis and subcutis contain many cellular elements, all capable of both reactive and neoplastic proliferation. In this chapter, such processes—derived from vascular endothelial cells, fibroblasts, myofibroblasts, smooth muscle cells, Schwann cells, and lipocytes—will be reviewed. Also several neoplasms of cells invading or aberrantly present in the dermis, such as metastatic cancer, endometriosis, and meningioma, will be covered.

VASCULAR NEVI

Under this term are included the nevus flammeus, capillary hemangioma, cavernous hemangioma, lymphangioma circumscriptum, and vascular nevi associated with other disorders. "Nevus" araneus (spider "nevus") is not a nevus but an acquired lesion, better called a "vascular spider." An angioma or hemangioma is a benign neoplasm or hamartoma resulting from disturbed development and composed of newly formed vessels. These hemangiomas are so common that a great variety of names have accumulated for each type.

Nevus Flammeus
(Port-wine Stain)

The lesions are usually unilateral and located on the face and neck, although they may be widespread and involve as much as one half of the body. The most common site is a unilateral distribution on the face. They are present at birth and range from small red macules to large red patches, which are partially or completely blanched by diascopic pressure. They vary in color from pink to dark or bluish red. The

mucous membrane of the mouth may be involved. Although the surface of a nevus flammeus is usually smooth, small vascular nodular outgrowths or warty excrescences may be present or develop in the course of life. These lesions often become more bluish or purple with age; however, they sometimes become fainter but rarely disappear.

Nevus flammeus nuchae, or "stork bite," is a common congenital defect of the skin. Osburn et al found it in 29 per cent of 830 patients examined at birth. It may persist in at least 5 per cent of the population. It varies somewhat in appearance but not much in location, being situated on the posterior midline between the occipital protuberance and the tip of the spine of the fifth cervical vertebra. The long axis is usually up and down.

Midline nevus flammeus or "salmon patch" on the glabellar region or on one upper eyelid is common in infants. Osburn et al found them in 13 per cent of newborns. They tend to fade or even disappear during childhood.

Nevus flammeus in the area supplied by the ophthalmic division of the sixth (trigeminal) cranial nerve is a component of the Sturge-Weber syndrome. These larger lesions are uncommon, occurring in less than one-half per cent of patients. In Enjoiras et al's review of port-wine stains they found that 90 of 106 patients had only the cutaneous vascular abnormality, without any leptomeningeal component. Thus the great majority of patients with port-wine stains do not have Sturge-Weber syndrome, this being present only when all or most of the U_1 branch of the trigeminal nerve is involved.

Occasionally nevus flammeus may be associated with nevus anemicus (another vascular anomaly) or with pigmented nevi such as nevus spilus or blue spots. Hasegawa et al have recently reviewed these

682

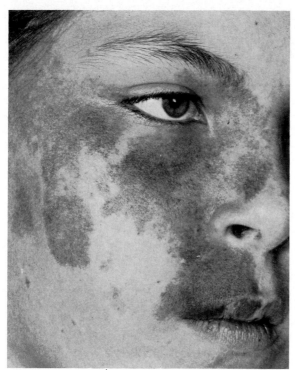

Figure 28–1. Nevus flammeus (port-wine stain).

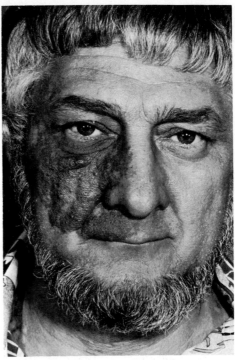

Figure 28–3. Nevus flammeus in an adult. (Courtesy of Dr. J. Cook.)

so-called pigmentovascular phakomatoses. The *Beckwith-Wiedemann syndrome* may comprise facial port-wine stain, macroglossia, omphalocele, visceral hyperplasia, occasionally hemihypertrophy, and hypoglycemia.

The cause of port-wine stain is unknown. It is a developmental defect, which may, as Smoller et al suggest, be due to localized failure of neuromodulation of blood flow.

Histologic changes are not conspicuous: there is only moderate dilatation of capillaries in the subpapillary network.

Treatment has been difficult. Tattooing with skin-colored pigments has been performed for years, but it has been difficult to match the varied, and impossible to match the changing, colors of the normal skin. Grabb and others have fully described the technique of this procedure.

Laser therapy has been used, with increasingly satisfactory results. Many published reports attest to its success. Currently the argon laser is preferred. The best results have been achieved with dark purplish lesions in older patients. Lightening, without scarring, is generally possible. Arndt et al summarized their experience with this method. The CO_2 laser, the neodymium-YAG laser, and the tunable dye laser have also been used.

For most patients, while awaiting a decision as to surgery, tinted creams like Covermark or Dermablend are effective in concealing the lesion.

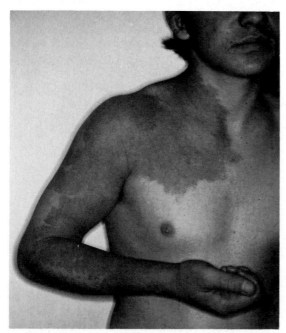

Figure 28–2. Nevus flammeus in a young man.

Arndt KA, et al: Lasers in dermatology. Arch Dermatol 1983, 118:293.

Buecker JW, et al: Histology of port-wine stain treated with carbon dioxide laser. JAAD 1984, 10:1014.

Clodius L, et al: Surgery for the port-wine stain. Ann Plast Surg 1986, 16:457.

Enjoiras O, et al: Facial port-wine stains and Sturge-Weber syndrome. Pediatrics 1985, 76:48.

Finley JL, et al: Argon laser–port-wine interaction. Arch Dermatol 1984, 120:613.

Idem: Port-wine stain. Arch Dermatol 1984, 120:1453.

Garden JM, et al: The pulsed dye laser. J Dermatol Surg Oncol 1987, 13:134.

Grabb WC, et al: Results from tattooing port-wine hemangiomas. Plast Reconstr Surg 1977, 59:667.

Hasegawa T, et al: Phakomatosis pigmentovascularis type IVa. Arch Dermatol 1985, 121:651.

Landthaler M, et al: Neodymium-YAG laser therapy for vascular lesions. JAAD 1986, 14:107.

Osburn K, et al: Congenital pigmented and vascular lesions in newborn infants. JAAD 1987, 16:788.

Polla LL, et al: Tunable pulsed dye laser for the treatment of benign cutaneous vascular ectasia. Dermatologica 1987, 174:11.

Rosen S, et al: Port-wine stain. JAAD 1987, 17:164.

Smoller BR, et al: Port-wine stains. Arch Dermatol 1986, 122:177.

Swerlick RA, et al: Pyogenic granuloma within port-wine stains. JAAD 1983, 8:627.

Tan OT, et al: Treatment of children with port-wine stains using the flashlamp-pulsed tunable dye laser. NEJM 1989, 320:416.

Tian OT, et al: Histologic responses of port-wine stains treated by argon, carbon dioxide, and tunable dye lasers. Arch Dermatol 1986, 122:1016.

Wisnicki JL: Hemangiomas and vascular malformations. Ann Plast Surg 1984, 12:41.

Strawberry Hemangioma (Hemangioma Simplex)

Strawberry ("capillary") hemangiomas may be present at birth (38 per cent in the series reported by Finn et al). Two thirds appear very rapidly, in a hitherto very inconspicuous pale macule, at two weeks to two months of age. The usual size is 1 to 60 mm in diameter, though rarely as much as an entire extremity may be involved. In Finn's series 60 per cent were on the head and neck, but they may occur anywhere.

The dome-shaped lesion is usually a dull red, and when involution begins, streaks or islands of white appear in the lesion as it flattens. The lesions have sharp borders and they are soft and easily compressible. Sites of predilection are the face, shoulders, scalp, and neck, but they also appear frequently in other regions. Generally they tend to grow over the first year or so, remain stable for a while, and then

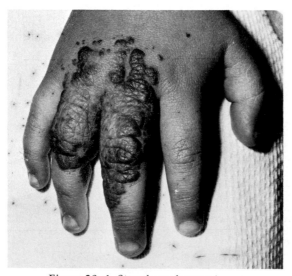

Figure 28–4. Strawberry hemangioma.

in the course of months, or a few years, involute spontaneously. Of 298 lesions followed by Finn et al, all but five had involuted (or were doing so) after five years of observation.

Histologically, strawberry marks are composed of primitive endothelial cells similar to those that are found prior to the embryonic development of true venous channels. Pasyk et al reported that they lack typical Weibel-Palade bodies ultrastructurally, but have crystalloid inclusions typical of embryonic endothelium. They stain positively for vimentin and *Ulex europaeus I* lectin. They proliferate intraluminally. Later, fibrosis becomes pronounced as involution progresses.

TREATMENT. There is general agreement that any intervention at all detracts from the quality of the ultimate cosmetic result. Only when further involution is despaired of, or in special circumstances, should one attempt to treat these lesions. Garcia et al list these indications for intervention: severe hemorrhage, thrombocytopenia, threatened cardiovascular compromise from high-output cardiac failure, or threatened interference with vital functions such as feeding, respiration, passage of urine or stool, limb function, tissue destruction, or vision. Garcia et al and Nelson et al stressed the risk of occlusion amblyopia, astigmatism, and myopia from periorbital hemangiomas. Intralesional steroids or oral prednisone may be employed.

Zarem and Edgerton as well as Fost and Esterly have reported successful treatment of extensive hemangiomas with the use of prednisone. Treatment of rapidly growing capillary hemangiomas requires use of prednisone at the earliest possible age. With daily doses of 20–40 mg of prednisone, one may expect the enlarging hemangioma to stop growing in three to 21 days. Ulcerations will heal within two weeks. Shrinkage of the lesion will usually follow if the treatment is continued for 30 to 90 days. Laryngeal involvement and stridor, if present, are usually dramatically relieved. Repeated courses of treatment may be undertaken if rebound of growth occurs on discontinuation of the steroids. Edgerton reported a better than 90 per cent dramatic response with high-dose, short-course prednisone therapy.

Cavernous Hemangioma

A cavernous hemangioma is usually rounded or flat, bright red or deep purple, and spongy. When it persists into adult life this consistency may be varied by the admixture of fibrous connective tissue. The lesions occur chiefly upon the head and neck, but are found in other regions as well. Frequently two components are noted: the cutaneous part is usually slightly elevated, whereas when the deep structures are involved the subcutaneous portion may be larger than the cutaneous lesion. A mixture of capillary and larger vascular components is often seen. The tumor is readily compressible.

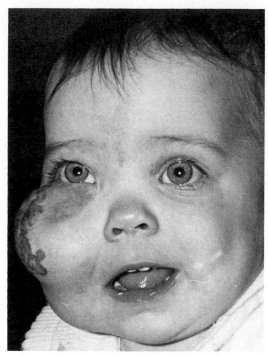

Figure 28–5. Cavernous hemangioma.

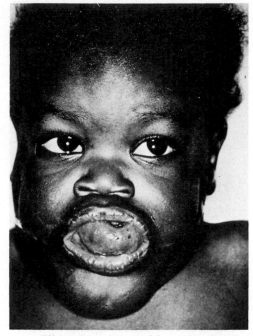

Figure 28–7. Intraoral hemangioma.

Frequently the mass consists of a mixture of imperfectly formed arterial, venous, and lymphatic elements. Occasionally a pigmented or verrucous change may be present in these mixed nevi.

Histologically, large irregular spaces filled with blood may be present in the lower dermis and subcutaneous tissue. These spaces are lined by a single layer of endothelial cells and a fibrous wall of varying thickness. The intermediate filament protein vimentin is expressed by the endothelial cells, as is a marker for endothelial cells, *Ulex europaeus I* lectin.

Cutaneous hemangioma may signal the presence of occult internal hemangiomas; nevertheless, internal hemangiomas need not be accompanied by cutaneous hemangiomas. Segmentally related cutaneous hemangiomas have been found in patients with spinal cord arteriovenous malformations by Doppman and his associates. It is believed that the hemangiomas are the commonest of benign tumors of the liver, as reported by Park and Phillips.

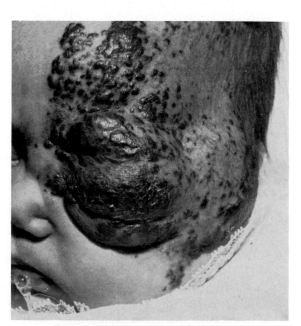

Figure 28–6. Cavernous hemangioma.

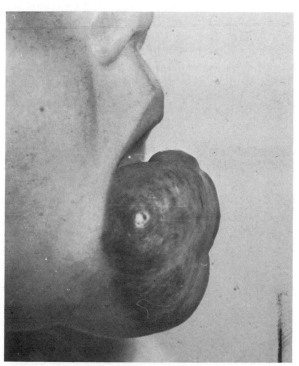

Figure 28–8. Cavernous hemangioma of the lower lip.

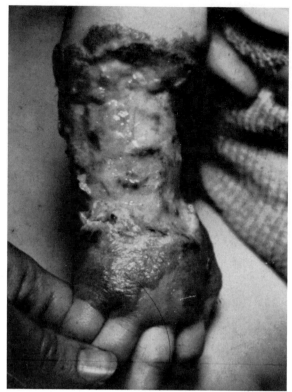

Figure 28–9. Ulcerated and infected cavernous hemangioma of arm.

Several syndromes are associated with capillary and cavernous (or mixed) hemangiomas. Stern et al reviewed *diffuse neonatal hemangiomatosis* in 1981. It is a serious multisystem disorder of multiple cutaneous and visceral hemangiomas with arteriovenous shunts, high-output cardiac failure, thrombocytopenia, and central nervous system involvement. In cases without visceral lesions, the course may be more benign. The *Riley-Smith syndrome* includes multiple cavernous hemangiomas, macrocephaly, and pseudopapilledema. Inheritance is by autosomal dominance. The *Bannayan syndrome* consists of autosomal dominant inherited hemangiomas, lipomas, macrocephaly, growth disturbance, and an increased incidence of intracranial tumors.

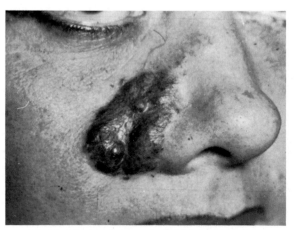

Figure 28–10. Noninvoluting, probably congenital, cavernous hemangioma in 23-year-old woman.

TREATMENT. Often cavernous hemangiomas will spontaneously decrease in size, or even completely involute. This is especially true of mixed (capillary-cavernous) lesions; therefore, procrastination is the safest first course. The same rules for intervention cited above for capillary hemangiomas apply here as well, and the same means of intervention, systemic prednisone, may be employed.

Also, compression therapy may be worth trying. Miller and his associates have described gratifying improvement with this approach in four cases. They recommend customized, snug-fitting garments in preference to elastic bandages.

Surgical excision of isolated hemangiomas of the cavernous type is often feasible, particularly on the scalp, eyelids, and extremities. The relatively large amount of skin and adipose tissue that covers the infant frame permits simple excision of lesions that would offer greater difficulties in adults.

Strawberry and Cavernous Hemangiomas

Barnhill RL, et al: Angiogenesis and the skin. JAAD 1987, 6:1226.

Bowers RE, et al: The natural history of strawberry nevus. Arch Dermatol 1960, 82:667.

Edgerton MT: The treatment of hemangiomas, with special reference to the role of steroid therapy. Ann Surg 1976, 183:517.

Finn MC, et al: Congenital vascular lesions. J Pediatr Surg 1983, 18:894.

Garcia RL, et al: Occlusion amblyopia secondary to a mixed capillary-cavernous hemangioma. JAAD 1984, 10:263.

Glowacki J, et al: Mast cells in hemangiomas and vascular malformations. Pediatrics 1982, 70:48.

Govrin-Yehudain J, et al: Treatment of hemangiomas by sclerosing agents. Ann Plast Surg 1987, 18:465.

Kushner BJ: The treatment of periorbital infantile hemangioma with intralesional corticosteroid. Plast Reconstr Surg 1985, 76:517.

Miettinen M, et al: Antibodies to intermediate filament proteins. Arch Dermatol 1985, 121:736.

Idem: Ulex europaeus I lectin as a marker for tumors derived from endothelial cells. Am J Clin Pathol 1983, 79:32.

Nakayama H: Clinical and histologic studies of the classification and the natural course of the strawberry mark. Int J Dermatol 1981, 8:277.

Nelson LB, et al: Intralesional corticosteroid injections for infantile hemangiomas of the eyelid. Pediatrics 1984, 74:241.

Pasyk KA, et al: Crystalloid inclusions in endothelial cells of cellular and capillary hemangiomas. Arch Dermatol 1983, 119:134.

Sasaki GH, et al: Pathogenesis and treatment of infant-skin strawberry hemangiomas. Plast Reconstr Surg 1984, 73:359.

Spraker MK: The vascular lesions of childhood. Dermatol Clin 1986, 4:79.

Stern JK, et al: Benign neonatal hemangiomatosis. JAAD 1981, 4:442.

Thomson HG, et al: Hemangiomas of the eyelid. Plast Reconstr Surg 1979, 63:641.

Willshaw HE, et al: Vascular hamartomas in childhood. J Pediatr Surg 1987, 22:281.

Wisnicki SL: Hemangiomas and vascular malformations. Ann Plast Surg 1984, 12:41.

Verrucous Hemangioma

This is a vascular malformation with typical features, clinically and histologically, of a hemangioma with a verrucous component. These verrucous hemangiomas are bluish red, well-defined lesions occurring on the lower extremities mostly, but also on the chest or forearm. These lesions are easily mistaken for angiokeratomas. Imperial and Helwig indicate that the verrucous hemangioma is a true congenital hemangioma and develops only later the secondary characteristics of acanthosis and papillomatosis.

Treatment is early excision, since these lesions tend to grow, with no inclination to involute spontaneously.

Sturge-Weber Syndrome (Encephalotrigeminal Angiomatosis)

This is the concurrence of a port-wine stain within the distribution of the ophthalmic division of the trigeminal nerve associated with ipsilateral leptomeningeal vascular anomalies. In a review of 106 cases of facial port-wine stains, Enjoiras et al found that Sturge-Weber syndrome occurred only in the 25 cases with this distribution, and in one with partial involvement of the area.

Symptoms which may occur include glaucoma, contralateral Jacksonian convulsions, paralysis, mental retardation, retinal detachment, and characteristic calcification in the outer layers of the cerebral cortex, consisting of double-contoured "tram lines," following the convolutions of the cerebral cortex.

The port-wine stain is almost always unilateral,

and often involves the buccal mucosa on the same side. It may rarely be bilateral, or in the midline. Kouskoukis et al reviewed the syndrome and reported an almost fully developed example of it in 1982.

Enjoiras O, et al: Facial port-wine stains and Sturge-Weber syndrome. Pediatrics 1985, 76:48.
Kouskoukis CE, et al: The Sturge-Weber syndrome. J Dermatol Surg Oncol 1982, 8:1.
Lasser AE: Sturge-Weber syndrome. Dermatology 1978, 1:27.
Owen LG, et al: Neurocutaneous syndromes. Cutis 1978, 21:848.

Cobb Syndrome (Cutaneous Meningospinal Angiomatosis)

In this nonfamilial disorder, a port-wine hemangioma or angiokeratomas are found in or very close by the dermatome supplied by a segment of the spinal cord also containing a venous or arteriovenous malformation. Angiomas of vertebrae or retinas may be found, and kyphoscoliosis is common. Jessen reviewed this syndrome with the other neurocutaneous syndromes.

Goldberg et al described five cases in 1986 in which vascular nevi of the sacral region were associated, not with an underlying vascular lesion of the spinal cord, but with multiple neurologic, gastrointestinal, urologic, and skeletal abnormalities.

Goldberg NS, et al: Sacral hemangiomas and multiple congenital anomalies. Arch Dermatol 1986, 122:684.
Jessen RT, et al: Cobb syndrome. Arch Dermatol 1977, 113:1586.
Zala L, et al: Cobb syndrome. Dermatologica 1981, 163:417.

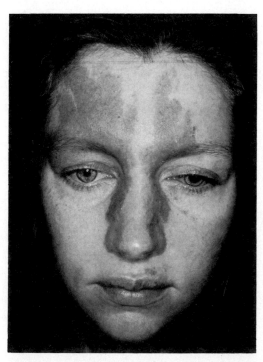

Figure 28–11. Sturge-Weber syndrome, with nevus flammeus, retinal detachment, and cerebral calcification.

Von Hippel-Lindau Syndrome

This disease is an autosomal dominant disorder consisting of retinal angiomas, cerebellar medullary angioblastic tumors, pancreatic cysts, and renal tumors and renal cysts. Usually the skin is not involved in the disorder, although occasionally angiomas may occur in the occipitocervical region.

Ten to 20 per cent of cerebellar hemangioblastomas produce erythropoietin and are accompanied by a secondary polycythemia. Ocular lesions may lead to retinal detachment. Ten per cent of hypernephromas and less than 8 per cent of renal cysts also produce erythropoietin. Pheochromocytoma has been associated in several kindreds with von Hippel-Lindau disease.

Christofferson LA, et al: Von Hippel-Lindau's disease. JAMA 1961, 178:280.

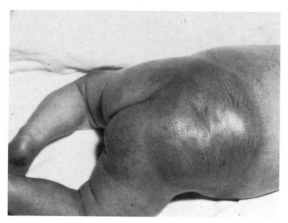

Figure 28–12. Giant hemangioma with thrombocytopenia (Kasabach-Merritt syndrome).

Kasabach-Merritt Syndrome (Hemangioma with Thrombocytopenia)

The hemangiomas in this syndrome are giant hemangiomas, may be single or multiple, may or may not involve the skin, and are most commonly seen in infants. The most striking sign is the bleeding tendency, especially in the hemangioma itself or into the chest or abdominal cavities. The spleen may be enlarged. There is thrombocytopenia, and the bone marrow shows increased megakaryocytes. The majority of patients have petechiae and purpura. Cases of microangiopathic hemolytic anemia have also been described. Repeated episodes of bleeding may occur, and although these may be spontaneous, it is not uncommon for bleeding to be precipitated by surgery, directed either at the hemangioma or elsewhere. The mortality may be as high as 30 per cent, with most deaths being secondary to bleeding complications.

Early investigators thought that the cause of bleeding was secondary to consumption of platelets and other clotting factors by the hemangiomas. Recent evidence suggests that the spontaneous bleeding is due to a disseminated intravascular coagulopathy (DIC) initiated within the hemangioma.

Esterly reported four patients with rapidly growing hemangiomas, thrombocytopenia, microangiopathic hemolytic anemia, and consumption coagulopathy. She stresses that the syndrome is most often seen in infants with hemangiomas of the limbs or trunk, at an average age of five weeks. Hemoglobin, platelets, fibrinogen, and factors II, V, and VIII are all reduced. Prothrombin time and partial thromboplastin time are prolonged, and fibrin split products are elevated. She also emphasizes that it is usually a self-limited disorder: expectant observation is the best approach initially. If steroids, heparin, or antiplatelet drugs are considered, it is well to consult with a hematologist.

Esterly NB: Kasabach-Merritt syndrome. JAAD 1983, 8:504.
Shim WKT: Hemangiomas in infancy complicated by thrombocytopenia. Am J Surg 1968, 116:896.

Hemangiectatic Hypertrophy (Klippel-Trenaunay-Parkes-Weber Syndrome, Angio-osteohypertrophy Syndrome)

Klippel-Trenaunay syndrome is characterized by port-wine hemangiomas, deep venous system abnormalities, superficial varicosities, and bony and soft tissue hypertrophy. When associated with an arteriovenous fistula, it is termed Klippel-Trenaunay-Parkes-Weber syndrome.

The earliest and most common presenting sign is cutaneous hemangiomas, usually of the port-wine variety, confined to the skin of an extremity. They are patchy and may extend over the buttock and trunk and to the thoracic region. They often stop abruptly at the midline with a sharp, linear border. Varicosities become more prominent as the child spends more time in the upright position. In most instances, the lesion is confined to one extremity, although bilateral involvement has been reported. There may be hypoplasia or even atresia of the deep venous system.

Augmented arterial inflow due to hemangiomatosis, and venous stasis and hyperemia, are thought to account for the bony and soft tissue hypertrophy. The involved limb is usually larger and longer than normal.

Other less frequent features include intermittent claudication, varicose ulcers, increased skin temperature, diffuse hair loss, dyskeratosis, lymphedema, and altered sweating, lacrimation, and salivation. Limp and other gait abnormalities have been noted.

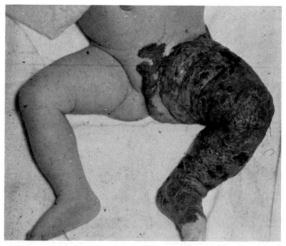

Figure 28–13. Hemangiectatic hypertrophy (Klippel-Trenaunay osteohypertrophic varicose nevus).

Hemihypertrophy of the face, cutaneous lymphangioma, varicose pulmonary veins, and oral complications have also been reported in association with the syndrome.

Treatment has been most unsatisfactory. Clinical evaluation consists of phlebography, arteriography, ortho-roentgenography, and conventional radiography of both extremities. Lindenauer advocates early venography to determine if there are defects that might be amenable to surgical correction. Ligation and stripping of the superficial veins is contraindicated. Surgery should be undertaken only to correct inequality in the length of limbs or to relieve deep venous obstruction.

Mullins found that in 10 per cent of cases the site of involvement was the head or neck. Castro-Magaña et al reported a case with severe involvement of one ear, in which great improvement followed ligation of the ipsilateral external carotid artery.

Castro-Magaña M, et al: Klippel-Trenaunay-Weber syndrome. Cutis 1980, 25:501.
Lindenauer SM: The Klippel-Trenaunay-Weber syndrome. Ann Surg 1965, 162:303.
Mahmoud SF, et al: Klippel-Trenaunay syndrome. JAAD 1988, 18:1169.
Mullins JF, et al: The Klippel-Trenaunay-Weber syndrome. Arch Dermatol 1962, 86:202.
Viljoen D, et al: The cutaneous manifestations of the Klippel-Trenaunay-Weber syndrome. Clin Exp Dermatol 1987, 12:12.

"POEMS" Syndrome
(Crowe-Fukase Syndrome)

Shimpo in 1968 described the first of over 100 subsequently reported cases of "POEMS" syndrome: *Polyneuropathy* (severe sensorimotor), *Organomegaly* (heart, spleen, kidneys), *Endocrinopathy, M* protein, and *Skin* changes (hyperpigmentation, hypertrichosis, thickening, sweating, clubbed nails, leukonychia, and angiomas). Puig et al reported a case in which multiple thinwalled hemangiomas appeared suddenly within a two-month period and persisted; there were associated hyperhidrosis, hypertrichosis, and diffuse thickening of the entire skin. Abnormal production of angiogenic factor was thought to be fundamental in the pathogenesis. Shelley et al reported a case in which taut skin, similar to scleroderma, with hypertrichosis and hyperpigmentation, was the presenting complaint.

Bardwick PA, et al: Plasma cell neoplasia with polyneuropathy, organomegaly, endocrinopathy, M-protein and skin changes. Medicine 1980, 59:311.
Imayamas S, et al: Electron microscope study on the hemangiomas in POEMS syndrome. Int J Dermatol 1984, 11:550.
Kanitakis J, et al: Cutaneous angiomas in POEMS syndrome. Arch Dermatol 1988, 124:695.
Nakanishi T, et al: The Crowe-Fukase syndrome. Neurology 1984, 34:720.

Puig L, et al: Cutaneous angiomas in POEMS syndrome. JAAD 1985, 12:961.
Shelley WB, et al: The skin changes in the Crow-Fukase (POEMS) syndrome. Arch Dermatol 1987, 123:85.
Shimpo S: Solitary myeloma causing polyneuritis and endocrine disturbances. Jpn J Clin Med 1968, 26:2444.

Cherry Angiomas
(Senile Angiomas, De Morgan Spots)

Oval or circular, slightly elevated, 0.5 to 6 mm in diameter, ruby red papules are the commonest of vascular anomalies; it is a rare 30-year-old human who does not have a few, and the number increases with age; probably every 70-year-old has some. Most are on the trunk; they are rarely seen on the hands or feet, or face. Early lesions may mimic petechiae.

They are easily obliterated without scarring by light electrodesiccation or freezing with liquid nitrogen, but most patients accept reassurance and do not request their removal. Aversa and Miller described a method well suited to removal of multiple lesions: freezing with Fluoro Ethyl and removal with a sharp curette. Arndt reported excellent results by laser ablation.

Arndt KA: Argon laser therapy of small cutaneous vascular lesions. Arch Dermatol 1982, 118:220.
Aversa AJ, et al: Cryo-curettage of cherry angiomas. J Dermatol Surg Oncol 1983, 9:11.

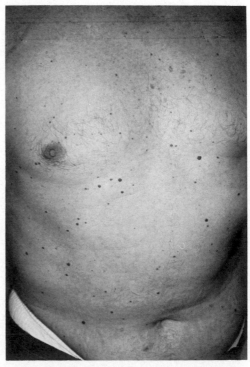

Figure 28–14. Cherry angiomas.

Vascular Spider
(Spider Nevus, Nevus Araneus)

The lesion is suggestive of a red spider; hence, its name. The ascending central arteriole represents the body, and the radiating fine vessels are suggestive of the multiple legs of the spider. These small telangiectases occur singly or severally, most frequently on the face and neck, with decreasing frequency on the upper trunk and upper extremities. In young children the sites of predilection are on the backs of the hands and forearms, and on the face.

Young children and pregnant women show these lesions most frequently. In pregnant women palmar erythema is usually present with the vascular spiders. The presence of vascular spiders in otherwise healthy children is common.

The vascular spiders of childhood usually involute without treatment; however, several years may elapse before that happens. In pregnant women most of the lesions will involute soon after delivery.

Vascular spiders also occur in cirrhosis, malignant disease of the liver, and other hepatic dysfunctions. The common denominator has been shown by Bean to be an elevated blood estrogen level.

When vascular spiders occur with palmar erythema and pallid nails with distal hyperemic bands, cirrhosis of the liver should be considered.

If active therapy is to be done, obliteration by electrodesiccation produces excellent results. It is advisable to anesthetize the area first with an intradermal injection of 0.1–0.2 ml of physiological saline solution, which does not sting on injection as lidocaine or other local anesthetics do, and produces complete anesthesia of the site. Again, Arndt has reported excellent results with the carbon dioxide laser.

Arndt KA: Argon laser therapy of small cutaneous vascular lesions. Arch Dermatol 1982, 112:220.

Bean WB: Spiders and related lesions of the skin. Springfield, Illinois, Charles C Thomas, 1958.

James WD, et al: Hyperpigmentation occurring in vascular spiders. Arch Dermatol 1979, 115:929.

Sudoriparous Angioma

An unusual form of hemangioma, consisting of painful sweating hemangiomas, was first reported by Bier in 1895.

The lesions are dome-shaped, tender, bluish hemangiomas varying from 12 to 20 mm in diameter. The dark red, dusky, moderately soft lesion when stroked or pinched forms characteristic drops or beaded rings of perspiration.

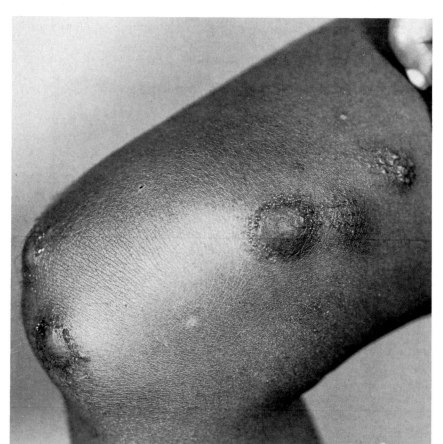

Figure 28–15. Sudoriparous angioma on the thigh of a 3-year-old child. Notice the beads of perspiration on the periphery, induced by stroking. (Courtesy of Dr. Louis Shapiro.)

Histologically, thick-walled blood vessels of varying sizes are present in the mid and deep dermis, surrounded by dilated cystic eccrine sweat gland structures.

Domonkos AN, et al: Sudoriparous angioma. Arch Dermatol 1967, 96:552.
Tharakaram S, et al: Sudoriparous angioma. Int J Dermatol 1983, 32:432.

Angiokeratoma of Mibelli

The lesions consist of 1–5-mm red vascular papules, the surfaces of which in the course of time become hyperkeratotic. The dull red or purplish black, verrucous, rounded papules are usually situated on the dorsum of the fingers and toes, the elbows and knees. Frequently these are called *telangiectatic warts*. The patient often suffers from cold cyanotic hands and feet.

This is a rare genodermatosis with an autosomal dominant trait of vascular lesions located over bony prominences and a family history of chilblains. It is most frequently discovered in prepubertal children.

Histologically, hyperkeratosis, increased thickness of the granular layer, and dilatation of the subpapillary vessels to form lacunae are the chief features. The vascular or lacunar spaces frequently are not lined with endothelium and the epidermis usually forms part of the wall of the vascular space.

Angiokeratoma may be treated with electrocautery, fulguration, carbon dioxide laser ablation, argon laser therapy, or cryotherapy with fairly good results.

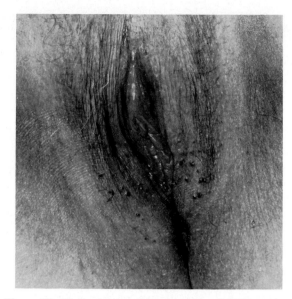

Figure 28–17. Fordyce angiokeratomas on the labia majora.

Angiokeratoma of the Scrotum (Fordyce)

The angiomata are multiple small vascular papules that stud the scrotum and sometimes the vulva in the middle-aged and elderly. Infrequently the keratotic part may be involuntarily scratched off to produce considerable bleeding. They may rarely bleed spontaneously.

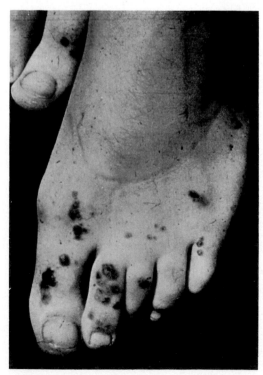

Figure 28–16. Angiokeratoma of Mibelli on feet.

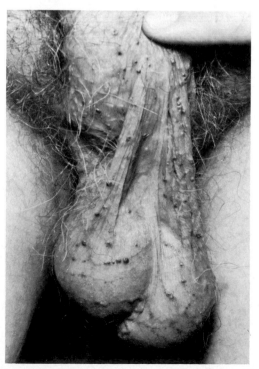

Figure 28–18. Fordyce angiokeratomas of the scrotum. (Courtesy of Dr. E. Kocsard, Australia.)

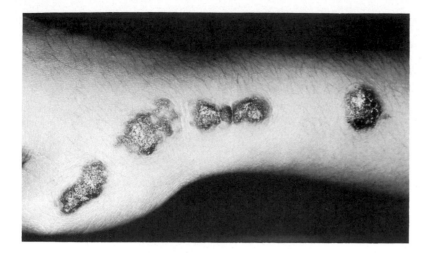

Figure 28–19. Angiokeratoma circumscriptum. (Courtesy of Dr. T. Mathias.)

Histologically, the many communicating lacunae in the subpapillary layer are lined with endothelium and connected underneath by dilated veins.

Treatment is best by cautery, carbon dioxide laser ablation, or fulguration of the more troublesome lesions only, since there may be hundreds of lesions present. The primary therapy is reassurance.

Angiokeratoma Circumscriptum

This rare type of angiokeratoma is characterized by unilateral distribution of discrete papules and nodules, usually localized to a small area on the leg or trunk. The lesions have hyperkeratotic tops so that they resemble red warts. These lesions may also be found in hemangiectatic hypertrophy. Foucar et al reported an acquired lesion which developed overlying a traumatically induced arteriovenous fistula.

Treatment is by fulguration, laser ablation, or simple excision.

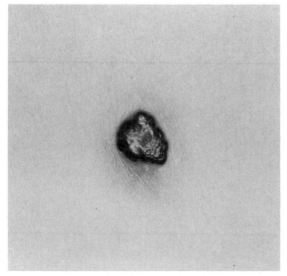

Figure 28–20. Solitary angiokeratoma.

Solitary Angiokeratoma

Described by Imperial and Helwig in 1967, this type of angiokeratoma is a single small, bluish black, warty papule which occurs predominantly on the lower extremities.

It is not a hereditary lesion and probably follows trauma, with subsequent telangiectasia prior to the formation of the angiokeratoma. The mode of acquiring this lesion, the small size, its solitary nature, and its location distinguish it from the other forms of angiokeratoma.

Solitary angiokeratoma is to be considered in the diagnosis of seborrheic keratosis, melanoma, pigmented basal cell carcinoma, and ordinary hemangioma.

Treatment is by electrosurgery, laser ablation, or excision.

Dave VK, et al: Angiokeratoma of Mibelli with necrosis of the fingertips. Arch Dermatol 1972, 106:726.

Foucar E, et al: Angiokeratoma circumscriptum following damage to underlying vasculature. Arch Dermatol 1986, 122:245.

Goldman L, et al: Thrombotic angiokeratoma circumscriptum simulating melanoma. Arch Dermatol 1981, 117:138.

Haye KR, et al: Angiokeratoma of Mibelli. Arch Derm Venereol (Stockh) 1961, 41:56.

Imperial R, et al: Angiokeratoma. Arch Dermatol 1967, 95:166.

Idem: Angiokeratoma of the scrotum. J Urol 1967, 95:379.

Lynch PJ, et al: Angiokeratoma circumscriptum. Arch Dermatol 1967, 96:665.

Newton JA, et al: The treatment of multiple angiokeratomata with the argon laser. Clin Exp Dermatol 1987, 12:23.

Novak NL: Angiokeratoma vulvae. JAAD 1985, 12:561.

Smith RBW, et al: Angiokeratoma of Mibelli. Aust J Dermatol 1968, 9:329.

Granuloma Pyogenicum (Granuloma Telangiectaticum)

Granuloma pyogenicum is a small, almost always solitary, sessile or pedunculated, raspberrylike, neo-

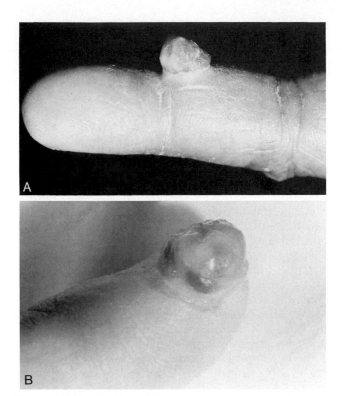

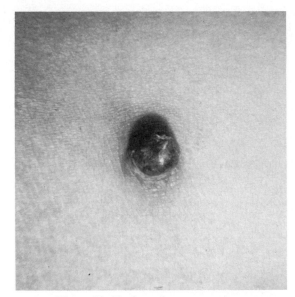

Figure 28–23. *Granuloma pyogenicum.*

Figure 28–21. A, *Granuloma pyogenicum—note collarette at base.* B, *Granuloma pyogenicum occurring in pregnancy. (Courtesy of Dr. Axel W. Hoke.)*

plastic vegetation of exuberant granulation tissue (*"proud flesh"*). It is a dull red color. It occurs most often on an exposed surface: on the hands, forearms, or face. The lesion also occurs in the mouth, especially on the gingiva, oftenest in pregnant women (*granuloma gravidarum*). The sole, or the nail fold of a toe or finger, may also be the site of such a lesion, where it may be mistaken for a melanoma. Such nail

fold lesions may be seen in patients treated with isotretinoin. The lesions bleed easily on the slightest trauma and, if cut off, promptly recur.

Although the lesion occurs mostly in children, other ages are also affected. It usually forms at the site of an injury such as a cut, scratch, or burn.

In rare instances recurring pyogenic granulomas may have one or many satellite lesions. Warner and Wilson Jones reported such a case and found 11 more reported in the literature. These lesions may simulate angioendothelioma with metastatic lesions, or melanoma.

Exceptionally, granuloma pyogenicum may occur subcutaneously; Cooper et al reported five such cases, only one of which was suspected by its bluish color of being a hemangioma, but all of which were identifiable histologically as *lobular capillary hemangiomas*, an alternative name for granuloma pyogenicum.

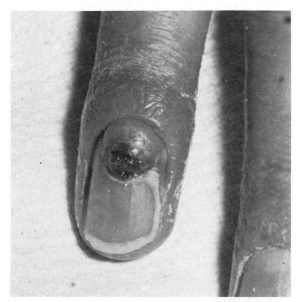

Figure 28–22. Granuloma progenicum resembling malignant melanoma of the nail bed.

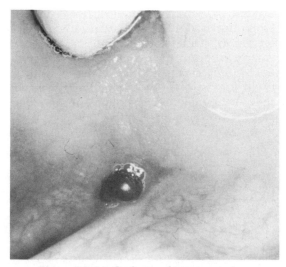

Figure 28–24. Oral granuloma pyogenicum.

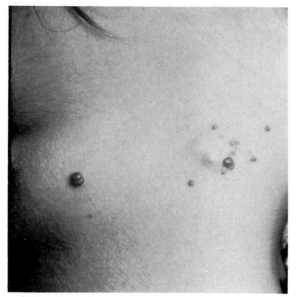

Figure 28–25. Granuloma pyogenicum with multiple satellites.

Histologically, the epidermis is thinned. The growth is composed of numerous newly formed capillaries suggestive of a capillary hemangioma. The capillaries are lined with endothelial cells in a single layer. There is also an edematous fibroblastic proliferation in the stroma that surrounds the vascular tumor. Both Wilson Jones and Fisher have described intraluminal papillary endothelial proliferation in cases with satellite lesions.

Granuloma telangiectaticum is usually easily diagnosed; however, it can be mistaken for Kaposi's sarcoma (especially histologically), melanoma, melanotic whitlow, senile angioma, atypical fibroxanthoma, and metastatic carcinoma. The hemangiomas that occur in disseminated cat scratch disease among AIDS patients may mimic pyogenic granulomas. Usually the histologic findings are distinctive enough to permit a definite diagnosis, although general pathologists (and sometimes dermatologic pathologists) often report them as hemangiomas.

Treatment is the shelling out of the lesion with a dermal curette, followed by destruction of the base by fulguration, under local anesthesia. The smaller lesions may respond to frequent cauterizations with a silver nitrate stick. At other times a recalcitrant lesion will persist after the above therapy has been followed, and excision or laser ablation may become necessary.

Cooper PH, et al: Subcutaneous granuloma pyogenicum. Arch Dermatol 1982, 118:30.

Exner JH, et al: Pyogenic granuloma-like acne lesions during isotretinoin therapy. Arch Dermatol 1983, 119:808.

Kamirsky AR, et al: Multiple disseminated pyogenic granuloma. Br J Dermatol 1978, 98:461.

Leyden JJ, et al: Oral cavity pyogenic granuloma. Arch Dermatol 1973, 108:226.

Miettinen M, et al: Ulex europaeus I lectin as a marker for tumors derived from endothelial cells. Am J Clin Pathol 1983, 79:37.

Okada N: Solitary giant spider angioma with an overlying pyogenic granuloma. JAAD 1987, 16:1053.

Suzuki Y, et al: The value of blood group–specific lectin and endothelial associated antibodies in the diagnosis of vascular proliferations. J Cutan Pathol 1986, 13:408.

Intravascular Papillary Endothelial Hyperplasia

Masson described in 1923, in infected hemorrhoids, intravascular papillary proliferation mimicking angiosarcoma. Hiroshi Hashimoto et al in 1983 reported a study of 91 cases in which they distinguished three categories: a pure form occurring within a dilated vascular space (30 cases); a mixed form occurring as a focal change within a hemangioma (55 cases); and an uncommon third form (six cases). The tumors may occur in the dermis, or subcutis, or intramuscularly. In the skin they appear as red or purplish 5-mm to 5-cm papules or nodules on the head, neck, or upper arms. Reed et al reported a case with multiple leg lesions mimicking classical Kaposi's sarcoma.

Cellular atypia or mitotic figures are rarely present and never prominent.

Excision is curative as a rule.

Barr RJ, et al: Intravascular papillary endothelial hyperplasia. Arch Dermatol 1978, 114:723.

Clearkin KP, et al: Intravascular papillary endothelial hyperplasia. Arch Pathol 1976, 100:441.

Gordon ML, et al: Flesh-colored nodules on the forearm. Arch Dermatol 1988, 124:263.

Hashimoto H, et al: Intravascular papillary endothelial hyperplasia. Am J Dermatopathol 1983, 5:539.

Paslin DA: Localized primary cutaneous intravascular papillary endothelial hyperplasia. JAAD 1981, 4:316.

Wong RC, et al: Intravascular papillary endothelial hyperplasia. JAAD 1984, 10:110.

Tufted Angioma (Angioblastoma)

In 1989, Wilson Jones et al described this lesion, which usually develops in early childhood on the neck and upper trunk. These angiomas are ill-defined, dull, red macules with a mottled appearance, which vary in size from 2 to 5 cm. Some show clusters of smaller angiomatous papules superimposed on the main macular area. Histologic examination reveals small, circumscribed angiomatous tufts and lobules scattered in the dermis. Most lesions slowly extend with time, being progressive but benign in nature.

Wilson Jones E, et al: Tufted angioma (angioblastoma). JAAD 1989, 20:214.

Angioma Serpiginosum

Angioma serpiginosum, first described by Hutchinson in 1889, is characterized by minute, copper-colored to bright red, angiomatous puncta, which have a tendency to become papular. These puncta occur in groups, which enlarge through the constant formulation of new points at the periphery while those at the center fade. In this manner small rings or serpiginous patterns are formed. No purpura is present, but a netlike or diffuse erythema forms the background. In the areas undergoing involution a delicate tracery of rings and lines, a fine desquamation, and, at times, a semblance of atrophy are seen. Slight lichenification and scaling may be evident in the papular lesions. The eruption predominates on the lower extremities but may affect any region of the body except the palms, soles, and mucocutaneous junctions. It is usually slowly progressive and chronic, and although involution may occur it is probably never complete.

The disease affects both sexes at all ages, and the etiology is obscure, but Barabasch and Baur found 90 per cent of cases occurred in girls under 16. It may be regarded as a telangiectasia of existing dermal blood vessels, resulting from a functional abnormality of the capillaries.

Angioma serpiginosum must be differentiated from the progressive pigmentary disease of Schamberg. The latter rarely affects women and the so-called "cayenne pepper spots" are macules which tend to coalesce and form diffusely pigmented patches. Purpura annularis telangiectodes (Majocchi) is bilateral and is characterized by acute outbreaks of telangiectatic points, which spread peripherally and form small rings.

In lichenoid purpuric and pigmentary dermatosis of Gougerot and Blum the primary lesion is a minute, lichenoid, reddish brown papule, which is sometimes hemorrhagic. It has a tendency toward central involution and residual pigmentation.

In angioma serpiginosum the most important histologic finding is the dilated and tortuous capillaries in the dermal papillae and the upper dermis. No inflammatory infiltrate or extravasation of red cells is observed. The dilated capillaries show no alkaline phosphatase activity, in contrast to normal capillaries.

Barker WB, et al: Angioma serpiginosum. Arch Dermatol 1965, 92:613.
Kumakiri M, et al: Angioma serpiginosum. J Cutan Pathol 1980, 7:410.
Marriott PI, et al: Angioma serpiginosum. Br J Dermatol 1975, 93:701.

Elephantiasis Telangiectodes (Virchow)

This is a rare congenital developmental dysplasia characterized by local thickenings of the skin and subcutaneous tissue with great hypertrophy of the blood vessels. The hyperplastic thickenings may cause folds as in neurofibromatosis.

Venous Lakes

Venous lakes (phlebectases) are small, dark blue, slightly elevated blebs, which are easily compressed, located on the face, ears, or lips, or on the forearms and backs of the hands. These venous lakes are markedly dilated blood spaces filled with blood and lined with thin elongated endothelial cells.

Venous lakes may be treated by light electrocautery or fulguration. Sometimes they must be treated because of traumatic bleeding.

Bean WB, et al: Venous lakes. Arch Dermatol 1956, 74:459.

Maffucci's Syndrome

Also known as *dyschondroplasia with hemangiomata*, this is characterized by multiple hemangiomata with dyschondroplasia. During the prepubertal years, 1–2-cm nodules appear on the small bones of the hand

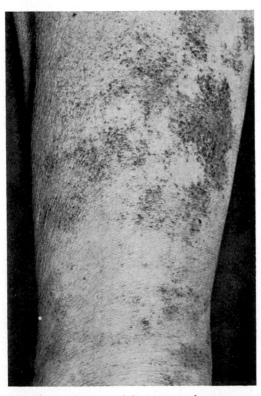

Figure 28–26. Angioma serpiginosum on the upper arm. Note the tiny, individual, slightly elevated vascular tufts. (From Barker LP, Sachs PM: Arch Dermatol 921:613, 1965.)

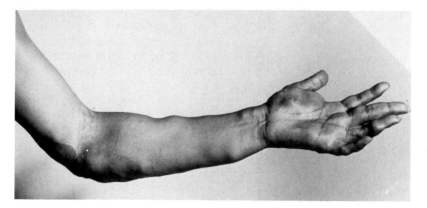

Figure 28–27. Maffucci's syndrome. (Courtesy of Dr. M. Lichtenberg.)

or foot. Later, larger nodules, enchondromas, appear on the long bones. Much later similar lesions appear on the trunk. The distribution of the lesions is mostly unilateral. In addition to the hemangiomata, phlebectases, lymphangiomata, and lymphangiectases may also be present on the skin. Pigmentary changes such as vitiligo and vague skin discoloration have been noted.

The dyschondroplasia is manifested by uneven bone growth due to the defects of ossification, with enchondromatous changes that result in multiple and frequent fractures during the period of bone growth. Sarcomatous degeneration occurs in 50 per cent of patients.

Bean WB: Dyschondroplasia and hemangiomata. Arch Intern Med 1955, 95:767.
Suringa DWR: Cutaneous lymphangiomas with dyschondroplasia (Maffucci's syndrome). Arch Dermatol 1970, 101:472.

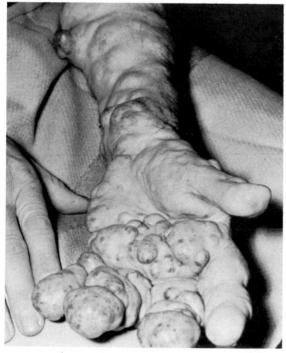

Figure 28–28. Maffucci's syndrome. (Courtesy of Armed Forces Institute of Pathology.)

Blue Rubber Bleb Nevus

This disorder is characterized by bluish hemangiomas, associated with gastrointestinal hemangiomas. The hemangiomas on the skin have a cyanotic bluish appearance with a soft elevated nipplelike center; hence, the name blue rubber bleb. Morris et al pointed out that the lesions can be emptied by firm pressure, leaving them flaccid. Usually the multiple nevi are located predominantly on the trunk and arms.

The gastrointestinal hemangiomas are found throughout the gastrointestinal tract. The most numerous are in the small intestines. Rupture of a lesion may produce melena.

The blue rubber bleb nevus has been traced through five generations of one family. Berlyne concluded that it was an autosomal dominant trait.

Histologically, many dilated vascular spaces are found, with irregular walls producing a papillary appearance.

Treatment is the destruction or excision of the lesions on the skin. These do not involute spontaneously.

McCarthy JC, et al: Orthopedic dysfunction in the blue-rubber-bleb-nevus syndrome. J Bone Joint Surg (Am) 1982, 64A:280.
Morris SJ, et al: Blue rubber-bleb nevus syndrome. JAMA 1978, 239:1887.

Gorham's Disease

Cutaneous hemangiomas occurring with massive osteolysis or "disappearing bones" have been reported by Frost and Caplan. Gorham characterized the disease as osteolysis of multiple areas of the skeletal system, but usually only a single bone is involved. There is complete or partial replacement of the bone with fibrous tissue. Cutaneous hemangioma may be the initial sign of the disease, which appears usually in young children.

Frost JF, et al: Cutaneous hemangiomas and disappearing bones. Arch Dermatol 1965, 92:501.

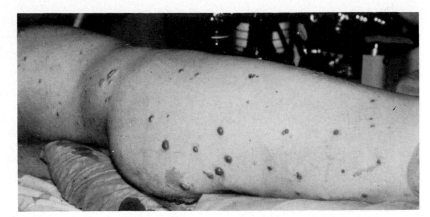

Figure 28–29. Blue rubber bleb nevus. (Courtesy of Dr. L. Goldman.)

Nevus Anemicus

This congenital disorder is characterized by macules of varying size and shape that are paler than the surrounding skin and cannot be made red by trauma, cold, or heat. The nevus resembles vitiligo, but there is a normal amount of melanin. The patches are usually round, and well defined, with irregular edges. Sometimes it occurs as a linear lesion, which may appear in any location. It may rarely occur in neurofibromatosis and epiloia. In nevus anemicus the triple response of Lewis lacks a flare, but outside the nevus a flare does develop after rubbing of the skin.

Histologic, pharmacologic, and exchange transplant studies by Daniel and associates demonstrated donor dominance and suggested that the defect is attributable to increased sensitivity of the blood vessels to catecholamines. Mountcastle et al have recently published a study of three cases by mechanical, histologic, pharmacologic, and electron microscopic technics, which supports this theory.

Daniel RH, et al: Nevus anemicus. Arch Dermatol 1977, 113:53.
Mountcastle EA, et al: Nevus anemicus. JAAD 1986, 14:628.

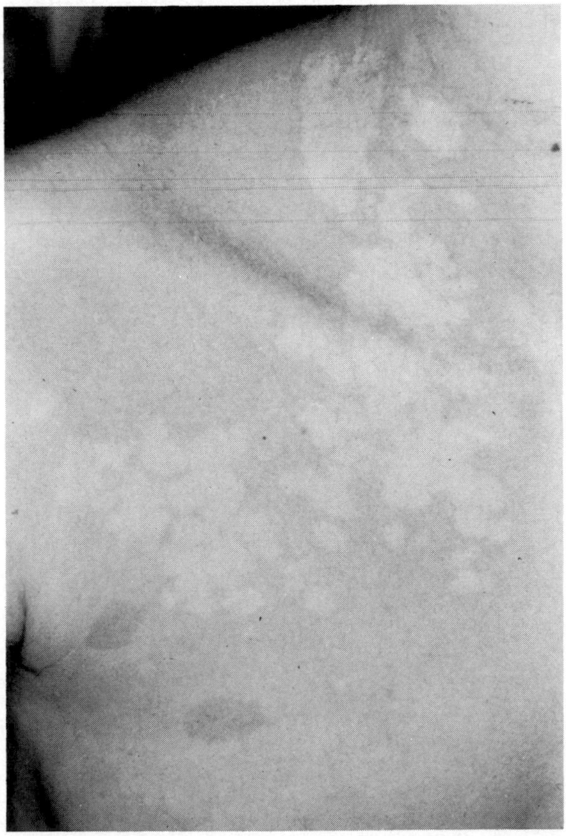

Nevus Oligemicus

Davies et al reported from St. John's Hospital in 1981 a 46-year-old man with a large patch of erythema on the flank, persistent for 14 years, which did not look like an angioma clinically or histologically. It was cooler than normal skin and had decreased blood flow. They believed that this was due to vasoconstriction in deep vessels; the vasodilatation remained unexplained. Surprisingly, they named it *nevus oligemicus*; they considered it a variant of nevus anemicus.

Davies MG, et al: Nevus oligemicus. Arch Dermatol 1981, 117:111.

Lymphangioma Circumscriptum

This nevus is manifest as groups of deep-seated vesiclelike papules resembling frog spawn. The lesions are usually yellowish, but may be pink, red, or dark. When they are punctured, clear, colorless lymph exudes. The papules are arranged irregularly in groups that may be interconnected by sparsely scattered lymph cysts, the entire process, however,

Figure 28–30. Unusually extensive nevus anemicus over the clavicular area. Note the two café au lait patches. (Courtesy of Drs. T. L. Fleisher and I. Zeligman.)

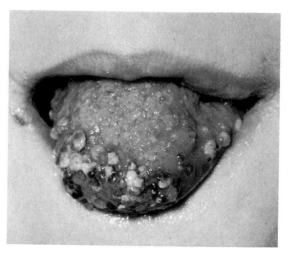

Figure 28–31. Lymphangioma circumscriptum. (Courtesy of Dr. Adrian Johnson.)

being as a rule localized to one region. The sites of predilection are the abdomen, axillae, and the mouth, particularly the tongue. The scrotum is subject to multifocal lymphangiomas presenting as clear, thick-walled, vesiclelike lesions. MacMillan et al and Merka et al discussed this problem. At times the surface is verrucous, in which instance the color may be brownish, and the lesions may be mistaken for warts.

Frequently the lesions consist of a combination of blood and lymph elements so that the term hemolymphangioma is appropriate. Their behavior is that of the lymphangioma circumscriptum. When the lesions are subcutaneous they form small, rounded, compressible, circumscribed tumors, over which the skin may be of normal color, or of a pinkish or yellowish hue, and sometimes telangiectatic. In the course of time, the lymphangiomas show only slight changes; however, the continued proliferation on the tongue poses a space-occupying problem which may not be stopped even by frequent resection.

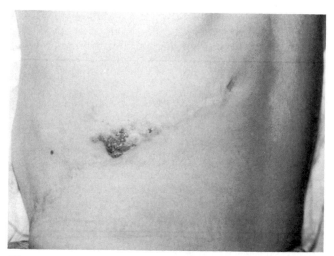

Figure 28–32. Recurrent hemolymphangioma. (Courtesy of Dr. Axel W. Hoke.)

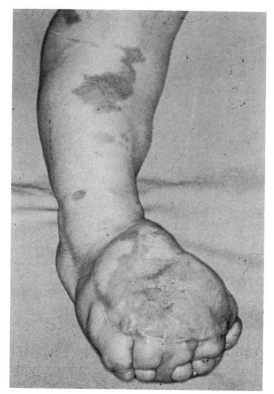

Figure 28–33. Cavernous lymphangioma.

Excision and grafting, fulguration, or coagulation are frequently unsatisfactory because of recurrences. Ian Whimster showed us why: vascular connections between the surface lesions and deeply located lymphatic cisterns are the cause of such failures. If the cisterns are excised in depth, success is the rule.

Bailin reported seven cases treated by vaporization with the carbon dioxide laser, with minimal recurrence after follow-ups ranging from eight months to about two years.

Bailin PL, et al: Carbon dioxide laser ablation of lymphangioma circumscriptum. JAAD 1986, 14:257.
Gupta AK, et al: Chronic zosteriform eruption of the lower extremity. Arch Dermatol 1988, 124:263.
MacMillan RW, et al: Scrotal lymphangioma. Urology 1984, 23:79.
Merka S, et al: Cystic lymphangioma of the scrotum.
Michaud RM: Lymphangioma circumscriptum. Arch Dermatol 1982, 118:692.
Palmer LC, et al: Lymphangioma circumscriptum. Arch Dermatol 1978, 114:394.
Whimster IW: The pathology of lymphangioma circumscriptum. Br J Dermatol 1976, 94:473.

Lymphangiectasis (Acquired Lymphangioma)

Lymphangiectases are acquired dilatations of lymph vessels, whereas lymphangiomas are congenital and appear soon after birth. The lesions are thick-walled vesicles with underlying tubules that appear translucent and slightly pink. Fisher and Orkin believe that the lesions are indistinguishable, clinically and histologically, from lymphangioma. The only difference is that lymphangiectases may be bilateral and develop in adult or late life. These lesions are seen mostly secondary to malignancies that have been irradiated, as reported by Leshin et al following mastectomy and x-ray therapy. DiLeonardo et al reported a case that developed as a sequel of scrofuloderma. Lymphangiectasia is believed to be a consequence of blocked lymphatic drainage.

DiLeonardo M, et al: Acquired cutaneous lymphangiectasias secondary to scarring from scrofuloderma. JAAD 1986, 14:688.
Goldstein JB, et al: Penicillamine dermopathy with lymphangiectases. Arch Dermatol 1989, 125:92.
Leshin B, et al: Lymphangioma circumscriptum following mastectomy and radiation therapy. JAAD 1986, 115:1117.
Ziv R, et al: Lymphangiectasia. Int J Dermatol 1988, 27:123.

Acquired Progressive Lymphangioma (Malignant Lymphangioma)

This term was introduced by Wilson Jones in 1976 to designate a group of lymphangiomas occurring anywhere in young individuals, growing slowly, and presenting (unlike malignant angioendothelioma) as bruiselike lesions or erythematous macules. Watanabe et al, who reported a case in a five-year-old boy, regard it as a slowly developing lymphatic anomaly. They found oral prednisolone caused the lesions to regress.

In 1988, Santa Cruz et al described a lesion in eight patients that was characterized by a small purple papule surrounded by a peripheral ecchymotic ring. On biopsy there was a vascular proliferation that extended into the subcutaneous tissue. They termed it *targetoid hemosiderotic hemangioma*. It shares features with progressive lymphangioma, but its exact place in classification awaits further reports.

Santa Cruz DJ, et al: Targetoid hemosiderotic hemangioma. JAMA 1988, 19:550.
Tudaki T, et al: Acquired progressive lymphangioma as a flat erythematous patch on the abdominal wall of a child. Arch Dermatol 1988, 124:699.
Watanabe M, et al: Acquired progressive lymphangioma. JAAD 1983, 8:663.

Cystic Hygroma

This is a deep-seated, typically multilocular, ill-defined soft-tissue mass in the neck or axilla, consisting of a thick-walled, endothelial-lined, cystic space or spaces filled with lymph. It is to be differentiated from branchiogenic cysts, and from lipomas. Williams et al recently reported such a case.

Williams CM, et al: Cervical bruises—a battered child? Arch Dermatol 1986, 122:1065.

Hemangiopericytoma

Stout and Murray described this rare tumor histologically in 1942. These nontender, bluish red tumors occur on the skin or in the subcutaneous tissues on most any part of the body. The firm, usually solitary nodule may be up to 10 cm in diameter.

Histologically, the tumor is composed of endothelium-lined tubes and sprouts that are filled with blood and surrounded by cells with oval or spindle-shaped nuclei (pericytes).

Wide local excision is the treatment of choice, but x-ray therapy may produce excellent palliation.

A study by McMaster et al showed that nearly half of the malignant hemangiopericytomas of soft tissues metastasize. The rate of metastases from lesions of the skin is closer to 20 per cent. The commonest cause of death is pulmonary metastases.

An exception to the above poor prognosis is found in those tumors arising at birth, or up to seven months of age. These tumors are almost always cutaneous or subcutaneous, and do not metastasize.

Altmeyer P, et al: Das Hämangioperizytom des Säuglings. Hautarzt 1976, 27:272.
Enzinger FM, et al: Hemangiopericytoma. An analysis of 106 cases. Hum Pathol 1976, 7:61.
McMaster MJ, et al: Hemangiopericytoma. Cancer 1975, 36:2232.
Nunnery EW, et al: Hemangiopericytoma. Cancer 1981, 47:906.
O'Brien P, et al: Hemangiopericytoma. Cancer 1965, 18:249.

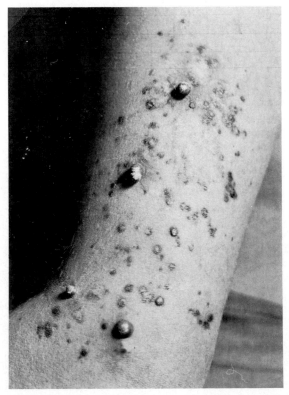

Figure 28–34. Multiple hemangiopericytomata with malignant changes. (Courtesy of Dr. W. Raab, Vienna, and Grosse-Edition, Berlin.)

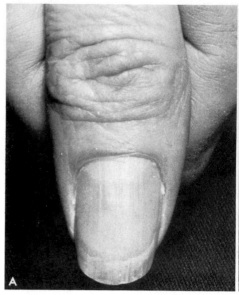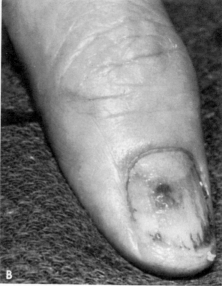

Figure 28–35. Glomus tumor. A, A small area of discoloration under the right side of midline of the nail. B, The lesion showing more prominently after complete avulsion of the nail.

Glomus Tumor (Glomangioma)

The solitary glomus or neuromyoarterial tumor, arising from a normal glomus, is most frequently a skin-colored or slightly dusky blue firm nodule 1 to 20 mm in diameter. The subungual tumor shows a bluish tinge through the translucent nail plate. The tumor is usually extremely tender and painful. The characteristic location is subungual, but it may occur on the fingers and arms, or elsewhere.

Tsuneyoshi et al, in a review of 63 cases, found that 34 of 37 digital lesions were from women, while 19 of 26 lesions in other, widely scattered, sites were from men.

Paroxysmal pain occurs frequently. Sensitivity is likely to be present constantly, and when touched the tumor responds with severe radiating pain. However, nontender glomus tumors are encountered. Progressive growth may lead to ulceration.

Multiple glomangiomas also occur. These usually nontender lesions are generally widely distributed over the body; as many as 90 tumors have been found in one woman. Only two of the tumors were painful. These multiple glomangiomas may be inherited as an autosomal dominant trait. Clinically they may resemble lesions of blue rubber bleb nevus. When grouped in one area they may appear as a confluent mass: Naversen et al reported a case with a single tumor extending from elbow to axilla, which they called a *glomangioma* rather than a glomus tumor.

Histologically, the glomus tumor contains numerous vascular lumina lined by a single layer of flattened endothelial cells. Peripheral to the endothelial cells are a few to many layers of glomus cells, seen in the multiple and solitary types, respectively. Both solitary and multiple glomus tumors are related to the arterial segment of the cutaneous glomus, the Sucquet-Hoyer canal. The glomus cells are smooth-muscle cells, and stain with vimentin.

Treatment of glomus tumors is best carried out by complete excision, which immediately produces relief from pain. The subungual tumors are most difficult to locate and eradicate since they are usually small, seldom more than a few millimeters in diameter.

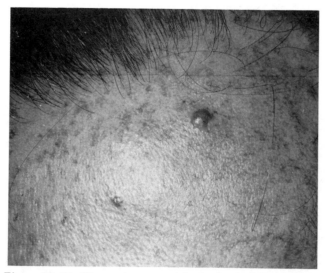

Figure 28–36. Glomus tumors on the forehead of a 64-year-old man.

Goodman TF, et al: Multiple glomus tumors. Arch Dermatol 1971, 103:11.

Heithoff SJ, et al: Glomus tumors of the upper extremity. JAOA 1985, 85:453.

Naversen DN, et al: Giant glomangioma. JAAD 1986, 14:1083.

Rycroft RJG, et al: Hereditary multiple glomus tumors. Trans St Johns Hospital Dermatol Soc 1975, 61:70.

Tsuneyoshi M, et al: Glomus tumor. Cancer 1982, 50:1601.

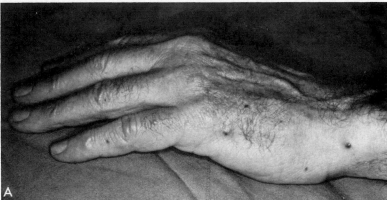

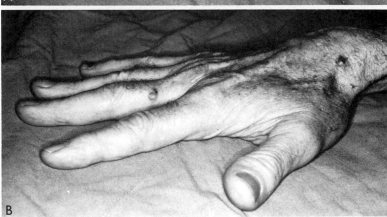

Figure 28–37. A *and* B, *Familial multiple glomangiomas.*

Angiolymphoid Hyperplasia With Eosinophilia (Pseudopyogenic Granuloma, Histiocytoid Hemangioma)

A whole spectrum of eosinophilic-lymphocytic-vascular lesions has gradually grown since Kimura's original report of four cases of nodular lymphoid lesions about the head, with eosinophilia, in 1949. Kawada in 1976 had collected 196 cases, among whom males outnumbered females 7:1; half were under 20; one third had disseminated lesions. The report by Wells and Whimster in 1969 of cases of subcutaneous angiolymphoid hyperplasia with eosinophilia was not immediately taken to be the same disease, but it is now thought that it is.

Wilson Jones and Bleehen described 42 cases of "pseudopyogenic granuloma," of which only five were in males; all occurred about one ear, single lesions in eight cases, multiple in 20; only one was under 20 years of age. Pruritus was present in all, and bleeding was easily induced. Wilson Jones considers now that this is a superficial variant of the deep lesion described by Wells and Whimster.

Olsen and Helwig analyzed the findings in 116 patients with angiolymphoid hyperplasia with eosinophilia. Morphologically all were similar to the above reports: pink to red-brown, dome-shaped, dermal or subcutaneous nodules of the head or neck. Grouped lesions merge to form plaques or grapelike clusters. There was female preponderance, and the average age of onset was 32 years. One third have recurred after excision.

Histologically all showed anomalous vascular hyperplasia with varying degrees of mixed cellular infiltrate, dominated by lymphocytes and eosinophils. Factor VIII staining confirmed the proliferating cells to be endothelial.

Olsen and Helwig found evidence of arteriovenous fistulas in the majority of patients studied, and felt this to be the etiology. They found peripheral eosinophilia in 20 per cent of their series. They believe, unlike most others, that Kimura's disease is part of the spectrum of angiolymphoid hyperplasia with eosinophilia.

Rosai in 1982 coined the term *histiocytoid hemangioma* because the cellular outlines of the endothelioid cells resembled histiocytes, and he desired a broader term to describe some cases with internal-organ lesions, which he felt were part of the spectrum of angiolymphoid hyperplasia. This concept has not been universally accepted; more information is needed. We favor the term angiolymphoid hyperplasia with eosinophilia over its several rivals.

Treatment is surgical excision. Difficult cases have been controlled with vinblastine, and partial responses to intralesional cytotoxic agents were documented by Baum et al. We recommend a surgical approach.

Bamford JT: Coexistence of angiolymphoid hyperplasia with eosinophilia and pulmonary neoplasia. JAAD 1987, 16:142.

Baum EW, et al: Angiolymphoid hyperplasia with eosinophilia. J Dermatol Surg Oncol 1982, 8:966.

Burrall BA, et al: Cutaneous histiocytoid hemangioma. Arch Dermatol 1982, 118:166.

Danno K, et al: Coexistence of Kimura's disease and lichen amyloidosus in three patients. Arch Dermatol 1982, 118:976.

Hobbs ER, et al: Treatment of angiolymphoid hyperplasia of the external ear with carbon dioxide laser. JAAD 1988, 19:345.

Massa MC, et al: Angiolymphoid hyperplasia demonstrating extensive skin and mucosal lesions controlled with vinblastine therapy. JAAD 1984, 11:333.

Olsen TG, et al: Angiolymphoid hyperplasia with eosinophilia. JAAD 1985, 12:781.

Rosai J: Angiolymphoid hyperplasia with eosinophilia . . . in the spectrum of histiocytoid hemangioma. Am J Dermatopathol 1982, 4:175.

Vasquez Botet M, et al: Angiolymphoid hyperplasia with eosinophilia. J Dermatol Surg Oncol 1978, 4:931.

Wells GC, et al: Subcutaneous angiolymphoid hyperplasia with eosinophilia. Br J Dermatol 1969, 81:1.

Wilson Jones E, et al: Inflammatory angiomatous nodules occurring about the ears and scalp. Arch Dermatol 1970, 102:422.

Proliferating Angioendotheliomatosis

This disease may take either a reactive involuting or a malignant, rapidly fatal course. The two types have similar clinical lesions and histologic findings. These diseases appear to be due to different basic mechanisms also, the reactive type being an endothelial proliferation, whereas the malignant type is a manifestation of lymphoma.

The reactive type of angioendotheliomatosis is uncommon. It frequently occurs in patients who have subacute bacterial endocarditis. They present with red to purple patches, plaques, nodules, petechiae, and ecchymoses, usually of the lower extremities. Histologically the capillaries in the dermis and subcutaneous tissue are dilated and are filled with proliferating endothelial cells, usually without atypia. The course in this type is characterized by involution over one to two years. Antibiotic therapy for the endocarditis has been felt to hasten involution.

The malignant type of angioendotheliomatosis is a rapidly progressive disease, usually with death occurring within 10 months of diagnosis. The mean age at onset is 55 years, with reddish purple plaques, nodules, or patches developing in the skin. Multisystem involvement is characteristic, with the central nervous system often involved. There may be progressive dementia or focal signs reflecting ischemic infarcts. Also kidney, heart, lung, and gastrointestinal tract lesions may occur. Cases reported with lymphoma presenting either concomitantly or following the onset of malignant angioendotheliomatosis reflect the truly lymphomatous nature of this disease. The biopsy shows a proliferation of atypical cells which fill the lumen of cutaneous vessels. Immunochemical stains for leukocyte–common-antigen have confirmed the lymphomatous nature of these cells.

Doxorubicin alone, as well as in combination with vincristine, prednisone, and cyclophosphamide, has been reported effective in isolated cases.

Berger TG, et al: Angioendotheliomatosis. JAAD 1988, 18:407.

Bhawan J, et al: Malignant lymphoma and malignant angioendotheliomatosis: one disease. Cancer 1985, 55:570.

Gupta AK, et al: Proliferating angioendotheliomatosis. Arch Dermatol 1986, 122:314.

Kauh VC, et al: Malignant proliferating angioendotheliomatosis. Arch Dermatol 1980, 116:803.

Keahey TM, et al: Malignant angioendotheliomatosis proliferans treated with doxorubicin. Arch Dermatol 1982, 118:512.

Lim HW, et al: Angioendotheliomatosis associated with histiocytic lymphoma. JAAD 1985, 13:903.

Martin S, et al: Reactive angioendotheliomatosis. JAAD 1980, 2:117.

Scott PWB, et al: Proliferating angioendotheliomatosis. Arch Pathol 1975, 99:323.

Sheibani K, et al: Further evidence that malignant angioendotheliomatosis is an angiotropic large cell lymphoma. N Engl J Med 1986, 314:943.

Wick MR: Reassessment of malignant angioendotheliomatosis. Am J Surg Pathol 1986, 10:112.

Wrotnowski U, et al: Malignant angioendotheliomatosis. Am J Clin Pathol 1985, 83:244.

Angiosarcoma

Angiosarcomas of the skin occur in four clinical settings. First, and most common, are those which occur in the head and neck of elderly people. Men outnumber women two to one. The lesion often begins as an ill-defined bluish macule, at which time it may be mistaken for a bruise. Distinguishing features are the frequent occurrence of a peripheral erythematous ring, satellite nodules, the presence of intratumoral hemorrhage, and the tendency for the lesion to bleed spontaneously, or after minimal trauma. The tumor progressively enlarges asymmetrically, often becomes multicentric, and develops indurated bluish nodules and plaques.

Histologically, anaplastic pleomorphic endothelial cells are present, with new vascular channels among them. Immunoperoxidase staining for Factor VIII or with the lectin *Ulex europaeus I* aids in the diagnosis.

Early diagnosis and complete surgical excision offer the best prognosis, as chemotherapy and radiation therapy are only palliative. Because of the multicentricity of lesions, the frequent occurrence on the face or scalp, and the rapid growth with early metastasis, death occurs in most patients within two years.

The second classic clinical situation in which angiosarcoma develops is in chronic lymphedematous areas, such as that which occurs in the upper arm after mastectomy, the so-called *Stewart-Treves syndrome*. This tumor appears approximately 11 to 12 years after surgery in an estimated 0.45 per cent of patients.

The prognosis is poor for these patients, with a mean survival of 19 to 31 months, and a five-year survival rate of 6 to 14 per cent. Metastases to the lungs is the most frequent cause of death. Early amputation offers the best hope.

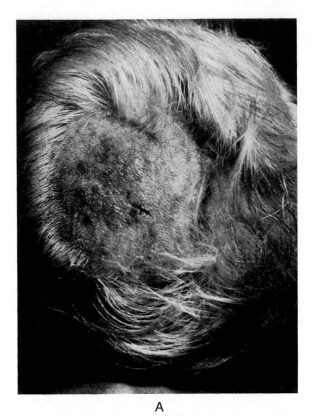

A

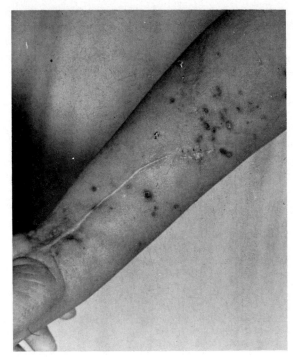

Figure 28–39. *Hemangioendothelioma (angiosarcoma) in a 54-year-old man.*

A third setting includes tumors developing in previously irradiated sites, such as the case reported by Goette et al. If the condition for which radiation was given was a benign one, the average interval between radiation and angiosarcoma development is 23 years; if the preceding diagnosis was a malignant condition, the interval is shortened to 12 years. Again, the prognosis is poor, with survival time generally between six months and two years after diagnosis.

Angiosarcomas develop in settings other than those previously described, and this small miscellaneous subset comprises the fourth category.

Goette DK, et al: Post-irradiation angiosarcoma. JAAD 1985, 12:922.

Hashimoto K, et al: Differentiation of metastatic breast carcinoma from Stewart-Treves angiosarcoma. Arch Dermatol 1985, 121:742.

Holden CA, et al: Angiosarcoma of the face and scalp; Prognosis and treatment. Cancer 1987, 59:1046.

Kettler A, et al: A draining arm lesion in a female adult. Arch Dermatol 1985, 121:1455.

Karuse KI, et al: Anterior abdominal wall angiosarcoma in a morbidly obese woman. JAAD 1986, 15:327.

Kofler H, et al: Hemangiosarcoma in chronic leg ulcer. Arch Dermatol 1988, 124:1080.

Mackenzie IJ: Angiosarcoma of the face. Arch Dermatol 1985, 121:549.

Matsumoto K, et al: Prognosis of angiosarcoma in Japan: A statistical study of 69 cases. Child Plast 1986, 8:158.

Peterman AR: Ulcerating tumor involving the auricular area. Arch Dermatol 1985, 121:927.

Rosai J, et al: Angiosarcoma of the skin. Human Pathol 1976, 7:83.

Scheman AJ, et al: Purple nodules in the lower extremity following above-knee amputation. Arch Dermatol 1988, 124:263.

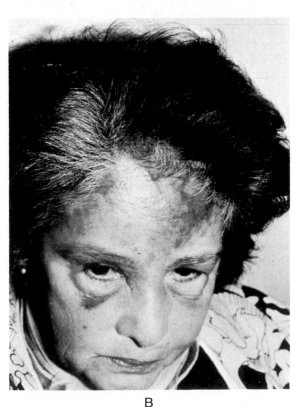

B

Figure 28–38. A, *Angiosarcoma on top of the scalp of a 73-year-old man. The dusky red infiltrated lesion, containing five small nodules, had been present for 3 months.* B, *Angiosarcoma of the forehead and scalp.*

EPITHELIOID HEMANGIOENDOTHELIOMA

In 1982, Weiss and Enzinger described this rare tumor that both clinically and histologically is intermediate between angiosarcoma and hemangioma. It is usually a solitary, slowly growing papule or nodule on the distal extremity. There is a male preponderance and onset is frequently before age 25 years. Histologically, there are two components: dilated vascular channels and spindle cell elements. Some may have cellular pleomorphism and mitotic activity. Wide excision is recommended, and if metastases occur, further surgery may be combined with chemotherapy, radiation, or both. Of the 31 patients from the original series who had follow-up at an average of 18 months, 20 were alive and well.

Lessard M, et al: Spindle cell hemangioendothelioma of the skin. JAAD 1988, 18:393.

Tyring S, et al: Epithelioid hemangioendothelioma of the skin and femur. JAAD 1989, 20:326.

Weiss SW, et al: Epithelioid hemangioendothelioma. Cancer 1982, 50:970.

KAPOSI'S SARCOMA (KS)

Kaposi ("*cop*-o-see") described this vascular neoplasm in 1872 and called it multiple benign pig-

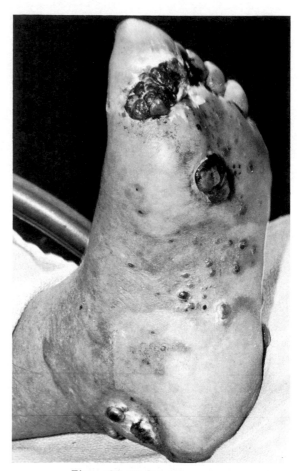

Figure 28–41. Kaposi's sarcoma.

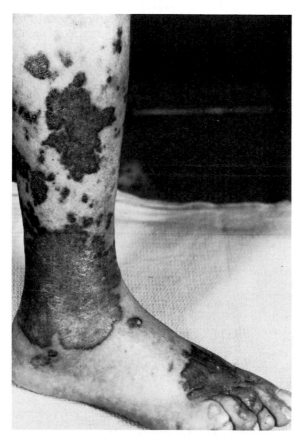

Figure 28–40. Kaposi's sarcoma on the foot where the initial lesions are first seen. Large violaceous plaques, infiltrations, and angiomatous tumors may be present.

mented idiopathic hemorrhagic sarcoma. Since his description, the disease has been reported in five separate clinical settings, with different presentations, epidemiology, and prognoses.

Piette has described the five subtypes: 1) Classical KS, an indolent disease seen chiefly in middle-aged men of Southern and Eastern European origin; 2) African cutaneous KS, a locally aggressive process affecting middle-aged Africans in tropical Africa; 3) African lymphadenopathic KS, an aggressive disease of young patients, chiefly children under 10; 4) KS in the immunosuppressed, by AIDS or 5) lymphoma or chemotherapy.

CLINICAL FEATURES

Classic KS. The early lesions appear most often on the toes or soles as reddish, violaceous, or bluish black macules and patches that spread and coalesce to form nodules or plaques. These have a rubbery consistency and look like dusky, purplish angiomas, which they are. There may be brawny edema of the affected parts. Later, swelling due to lymphedema often develops.

Later the macules or nodules may appear on the arms and hands, and rarely may extend to the face, ears, trunk, or buccal cavity, especially the soft palate. The course is slowly progressive, and may lead to great enlargement of the lower extremities.

There are, however, periods of remission, particularly in the early stages of the disease, when nod-

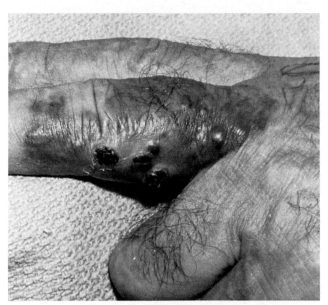

Figure 28–42. Kaposi's sarcoma on the mid-finger. (Courtesy of Dr. M. Simon, Hungary.)

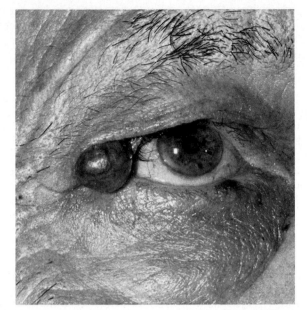

Figure 28–44. Kaposi's sarcoma on eyelid. (Courtesy of Dr. J. Teisch.)

ules may undergo spontaneous involution. After involution there may be an atrophic and hyperpigmented scar.

African Cutaneous KS. Nodular, infiltrating, vascular masses occur on the extremities, mostly of men between 20 and 50. This form of KS is endemic in tropical Africa, and has a locally aggressive but systemically indolent course.

African Lymphadenopathic KS. Lymph node involvement, with or without skin lesions, may occur in children under 10. The course is aggressive, often terminating fatally within two years of the onset.

AIDS-Associated KS. Cutaneous lesions begin as one or several red to purple-red macules, rapidly progressing to papules, nodules, and plaques. There is a predilection for the head, neck, trunk, and mucous membranes. A fulminant, progressive course with nodal and systemic involvement is expected. This may be the presenting manifestation.

Immunosuppression-Associated KS. The lesion's morphology resembles that of classic KS; however, the site of presentation is more variable.

INTERNAL INVOLVEMENT

Classical KS. The gastrointestinal tract is the site of the most frequent internal involvement in classical KS. In addition, the lungs, heart, liver, conjunctiva, adrenal glands, and lymph nodes of the abdomen may be involved.

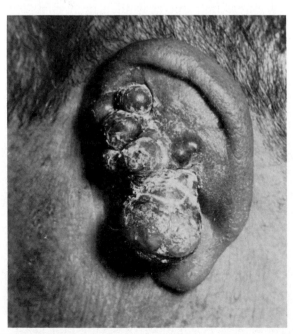

Figure 28–43. Kaposi's sarcoma of the ear, an unusual site.

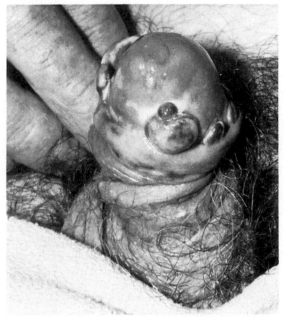

Figure 28–45. Kaposi's sarcoma on glans penis. (Courtesy of Dr. J. Teisch.)

Palmer suggests arteriograms to determine the various locations and extent of the lesions. The lungs rarely show any change except that of congestion. The small intestine is probably the most commonly involved viscus.

Skeletal changes are characteristic and diagnostic. Bone involvement is always an indication of widespread disease. Changes noted are rarefaction, cysts, and cortical erosion.

Radionuclide scanning with ^{99m}Tc (pertechnetate) showed internal lesions in a case reported by Krishnamurthy et al at UCLA; gallium and bleomycin scans were negative.

African Cutaneous KS is frequently accompanied by massive edema of the legs, caused by arborizing infiltrates along cutaneous lymphatics, and frequent bone involvement, often without skin lesions.

African Lymphadenopathic KS. In Bantu children massive involvement of the lymph nodes, especially the cervical nodes, precedes the appearance of skin lesions. Also the children develop lesions on the eyelids and conjunctiva from which masses of hemorrhagic tissue hang down. Eye involvement is often associated with swelling of the lacrimal, parotid, and submandibular glands with a picture of Mikulicz syndrome.

AIDS-associated KS has been studied by several authors, including 24 autopsy studies reported by Lemlich et al. They found that 25 per cent had cutaneous involvement alone, while 29 per cent had visceral lesions only. The most frequent sites of visceral involvement were the lungs (37 per cent), the gastrointestinal tract (50 per cent), and the lymph nodes (50 per cent). Visceral involvement ultimately occurs in over 70 per cent of AIDS-associated KS.

Other immunosuppressed patients with KS may have visceral involvement in a variable percentage of cases.

ETIOLOGY. Kaposi believed this disease to be of multicentric origin and it is still so viewed. Several authors have suggested that it may be the result of two events, one of which may be infection with an as yet undefined oncogenic virus. Friedman-Kien has reported an association with HLA-Dr5 in both classic and AIDS-associated KS, and this has been confirmed by Pollock et al, Rubinstein et al, and Cerimele et al.

EPIDEMIOLOGY. Kaposi's sarcoma is of worldwide distribution. In Europe there appear to be foci of classic KS in Galicia near the Polish-Russian border extending southward to Austria and Italy. In New York City KS has occurred mostly in Galician Jews and southern Italians. Several have occurred in patients who were entirely or partly black. Most have been elderly men.

In Africa, KS occurs largely south of the Sahara. Northeast Congo and Rwanda-Burundi areas have the highest prevalence, and to a less extent West and South Africa. It accounts for 9 per cent of all cancers diagnosed in equatorial Africa.

AIDS-related KS occurs mostly in male homosexuals, with an average age of 35. Very few reports have documented the exceptional occurrence of KS in AIDS patients who acquired their infection from intravenous drug use, or in Haitians or hemophiliacs. Up to 40 per cent of homosexual AIDS patients develop KS, and it accounts for 90 per cent of all cancers diagnosed in this patient population.

Patients at risk for developing KS due to other causes of immunosuppression include those with iatrogenic suppression from oral prednisone or chemotherapy, such as renal transplant patients.

Kaposi's sarcoma is associated with an increased risk of developing second malignancies, such as malignant lymphomas (Hodgkin's disease, T-cell lymphoma, non-Hodgkin's lymphoma), leukemia, and myeloma. Piette has recently reviewed the problem and has found that the risk of lymphoreticular malignancy is about 20 times greater in KS patients than in the normal population.

PATHOGENESIS. Kaposi's sarcoma is formed by proliferation of abnormal vascular endothelial cells. This has been established by histochemical demonstration of Factor-VIII-related antigen in both the cells lining the vascular channels and the spindle-cell component of both classical and AIDS-related KS. This antigen is found only in endothelium and megakaryocytes. Also, Penneys et al measured plasma levels of von Willebrand factor antigen and found consistent elevation of it in otherwise healthy patients with KS. This antigen level is maintained solely by endothelial cell release. The levels correspond to the size of the tumor load. Additionally, the marker *Ulex europaeus* agglutinin I (UEA-I) for endothelial cells is positive in KS.

KS is multicentric in origin; however, it may occasionally invade a vessel and ordinary hematogenous metastasis may then occur.

Recently it has been found that KS-derived cells from AIDS patients express cytokines that have IL-1 and fibroblast growth factor activity, which not only have autocrine but also puracrine growth effects. These factors not only may then be responsible for increasing growth of themselves but also may induce new lesions in a distant site.

HISTOLOGY. There is considerable variation in the histopathology according to the stage of the disease. Early lesions are of a chronic inflammatory or granulomatous nature, with new and dilated blood vessels, edema, hemorrhages, blood pigment, and dense perivascular infiltrations of lymphocytes and plasma and mast cells. The endothelial cells of the capillaries are large and protrude into the lumen, like buds. In the early patch stage, dilated, thin-walled vascular spaces with a jagged outline are present in the upper dermis. Other individual lesions are made up of capillaries and a fibrosarcomalike tissue in greatly varying proportions, and often the capillaries show a marked tendency to anastomose. Extravasation of erythrocytes and deposits of hemosiderin are present. At this stage the lesions look like hemangiomas or angiosarcoma. In the later phases there is a spindle-cell proliferation, which may be difficult to distinguish from sarcoma.

TREATMENT. All types of KS are radiosensitive.

Roentgen therapy has been used with considerable success, either by small fractionated doses, larger single doses, to limited or extended fields, and at times by electron beam radiation. El-Akkad's report may be consulted for details. Local excision or laser ablation has been used for troublesome localized lesions.

Chemotherapy has also been tried, mostly in the aggressive African and AIDS-related forms. Many agents have been found effective, among the best being vincristine, vinblastine, and actinomycin D. Various regimens are under investigation. The response rate initially is high, but recurrent lesions, which are common, are generally less responsive.

Vincristine solution 0.1 mg per ml injected intralesionally, not more than 3 ml at one time at intervals of two weeks, produces involution of tumors, some for as long as eight months. These studies indicate that adequate control of the lesions may be had, at least for periods of six to 12 months. In no instance has complete tumor involution been observed; however, Odom and Goette reported a case of classical KS in which excellent control was achieved in this way over a period of a year. All 31 injected nodules resolved. The development of resistance to medication seems to be inevitable at this time, however.

Krown et al have used recombinant interferon A, and Calvieri et al reported some response to cimetidine. A combined approach using radiation therapy, chemotherapy, and immunotherapy may offer the most hope for the future.

COURSE. *Classic KS* progresses slowly, with rare lymph node or visceral involvement, for long periods. Death usually occurs years later from unrelated causes. *African cutaneous KS* is aggressive, with early nodal involvement, and death from KS is expected within one to two years. *AIDS-related KS,* though widespread, is almost never fatal: nearly all die of intercurrent infection. Patients who develop *immunosuppression-related KS* from other causes than AIDS have a variable course. Removal of the immunosuppression may result in resolution of the KS without therapy.

Ackerman AB: The patch stage of Kaposi's sarcoma. Am J Dermatopathol 1979, 1:165.

Calvieri S, et al: Cimetidine for Kaposi's sarcoma. Clin Exp Dermatol 1985, 10:499.

Cerimele D, et al: Kaposi's sarcoma in Sardinia. Ann NY Acad Sci 1984, 437:216.

Cooper JS, et al: Radiotherapy for epidemic Kaposi's sarcoma. JAMA 1984, 252:934.

Idem: The duration of local control of classic (non-AIDS–associated) Kaposi's sarcoma by radiotherapy. JAAD 1988, 19:59.

El-Akkad S, et al: Kaposi's sarcoma and its management by radiotherapy. Arch Dermatol 1986, 122:1396.

Ensoli B, et al: AIDS-Kaposi's sarcoma–derived cells express cytokines with autocrine and paracrine growth effects. Science 1989, 243:223.

Flotte TJ, et al: Factor VIII–related antigen in Kaposi's sarcoma in young homosexual men. Arch Dermatol 1984, 120:180.

Friedman-Kien AE: Disseminated Kaposi's sarcoma in young homosexual men. JAAD 1981, 5:468.

Idem, et al: Disseminated Kaposi's sarcoma in homosexual men. Ann Intern Med 1982, 96:693.

Harwood AR: Kaposi's sarcoma: update on the results of extended-field radiotherapy. Arch Dermatol 1981, 117:775.

Jaimovich L, et al: Kaposi's sarcoma of the conjunctiva. JAAD 1986, 14:589.

Kriegel RL, et al: Kaposi's sarcoma. Cancer Treat Rep 1983, 67:531.

Krown SE: Preliminary observations on the effect of recombinant leukocyte A interferon in homosexual men with Kaposi's sarcoma. N Engl J Med 1983, 308:1071.

Lee B, et al: Kaposi's sarcoma. South Med J 1986, 79:540.

Lemlich G, et al: Kaposi's sarcoma and acquired immunodeficiency syndrome. JAAD 1987, 16:319.

Lo TMC, et al: Radiotherapy for Kaposi's sarcoma. Cancer 1980, 45:684.

Miettinen M, et al: Ulex europaeus I lectin as a marker for tumors derived from endothelial cells. Am J Clin Pathol 1983, 79:32.

Mintzer DM, et al: Treatment of Kaposi's sarcoma and thrombocytopenia with vincristine in patients with the acquired immunodeficiency syndrome. Ann Intern Med 1985, 102:200.

Modlin RL, et al: Kaposi's sarcoma. Int J Dermatol 1983, 22:443.

Myskowski PL, et al: AIDS-associated Kaposi's sarcoma. JAAD 1988, 18:1299.

Odom RB, et al: Treatment of Kaposi's sarcoma with intralesional vincristine. Arch Dermatol 1978, 114:1693.

Penneys NS, et al: Von Willebrand factor antigen levels in Kaposi's sarcoma. JAAD 1986, 15:1214.

Idem: Confirmation of early Kaposi's sarcoma by polyclonal antibody to type IV collagen. JAAD 1988, 19:447.

Piette WW: The incidence of second malignancies in subsets of Kaposi's sarcoma. JAAD 1987, 16:855.

Pitchenik AE, et al: Opportunistic infections and Kaposi's sarcoma among Haitians. Ann Intern Med 1983, 98:277.

Pollack MS, et al: Frequencies of the HLA and Gm immunogenetic markers in Kaposi's sarcoma. Tissue Antigens 1983, 21:1.

Rieber E, et al: Vincristine and Kaposi's sarcoma. Ann Intern Med 1984, 101:876.

Rubenstein R, et al: Immunologic and immunogenetic findings in patients with epidemic Kaposi's sarcoma. Antibiot Chemother 1984, 32:87.

Volberding P, et al: Chemotherapy in Kaposi's sarcoma. Am J Med 1983, 74:652.

Pseudo-Kaposi Sarcoma (Acroangiodermatitis of Mali, Bluefarb-Stewart Syndrome)

Arteriovenous anomalies in the extremities closely resembling KS both clinically and histologically have been reported by Marshall et al, Goldblum et al, and James et al, among others. These may occur because of congenital malformations, in which case a purplish discoloration of the skin over or distal to the arteriovenous anomaly begins to appear in the second or third decade of life. This type accounts for 80 per cent of cases. The remainder are secondary to traumatically caused fistulas.

Brenner S, et al: Kaposi-like arteriovenous malformation and angiodermatitis. Cutis 1982, 30:240.

DeVillez RL, et al: Acroangiodermatitis of Mali. South Med J 1984, 77:255.

Earhart RN, et al: Pseudo–Kaposi sarcoma. Arch Dermatol 1974, 110:907.

Goldblum OM, et al: Pseudo–Kaposi's sarcoma of the hand associated with an acquired iatrogenic arteriovenous fistula. Arch Dermatol 1985, 121:1038.

James WD, et al: Pseudo–Kaposi's sarcoma. J Assoc Milit Dermatol 1984, 10:14.

Marshall ME, et al: Arteriovenous malformation simulating Kaposi's sarcoma. Arch Dermatol 1985, 121:99.

Angioma Arteriale Racemosum (Cirsoid Aneurysm)

This is a pulsating, tumorlike enlargement composed of newly formed blood vessels that usually develops near the carotid artery and appears on the skin like "a pulsating mass of earthworms." Angioma racemosum is also known as *cirsoid aneurysm.* The growth extends over the neck and scalp and may penetrate into the cranium. This is a manifestation of an arteriovenous shunt.

Biberstein HH, et al: A cirsoid aneurysm in the skin. Dermatologica 1956, 113:129.

KELOID

CLINICAL FEATURES. A keloid is a firm, irregularly shaped, thickened, hypertrophic, fibrous, pink or red excrescence. The growth usually arises as the result of a cut, laceration, or burn—or, less often, an acne pustule on the chest or upper back—and spreads beyond the limits of the original injury, often sending out clawlike ("cheloid") prolongations. The overlying epidermis is smooth, glossy, and thinned from pressure. The early, growing lesion is red and tender and has the consistency of rubber. It is often surrounded by an erythematous halo and the keloid may be telangiectatic. In the course of time the keloid generally becomes brown, sometimes hypesthetic but often extremely tender, painful, pruritic, hard, and stationary.

It is often multiple and varies in size and number. Sometimes keloids are as tiny as pinheads or may be as large as an orange. Those that follow burns and scalds are large. Lesions are often linear, and the surface may be larger than the base so that the edges are overhanging. The most common location is the sternal region, but keloids also occur frequently on the neck, ears, extremities, or trunk, and rarely on the face, palms, or soles. The ear lobes are frequently involved as a result of ear piercing. They are much more common, and grow to larger dimensions, in blacks than in other races.

Onwukwe has described "suppurating keloids," keloids with abscesses. When acute, they are best treated like abscesses; but definitive management requires wide excision, including the abscess in toto. Elston et al and Novick et al have reported additional cases.

ETIOLOGY. Why certain persons develop keloids still remains unsolved. Trauma is usually the immediate causative factor but this induces keloid only in those having a predisposition for its development: blacks, for example. There is also a regional predisposition, as mentioned above. Fibroblasts from keloids have high proline hydroxylase activity, and elevated collagen production. The reason is unknown.

HISTOLOGY. A keloid is a dense and sharply defined new growth of myofibroblasts and collagen in the dermis with a whorllike arrangement of hyalinized bundles of collagenous fibers. The superficial collagen bundles lie parallel to the epidermis but those lower down interlace in all directions. The ribbonlike bundles are more compact and prominent in older lesions. There is a paucity of elastic tissue. By pressure the tumor causes thinning of the normal papillary dermis and atrophy of adjacent appendages, which it pushes aside. Mucopolysaccharides are increased, and often there are numerous mast cells.

DIFFERENTIAL DIAGNOSIS. Keloids are distinctive enough to cause little difficulty in distinguishing them from other dermatoses except perhaps from a hypertrophic scar. The most pronounced distinction is the clawlike projections of the keloid that are absent in the hypertrophic scar. Moreover, the hypertrophic scar does not extend beyond the original wound as the keloid usually does. Frequently there is a spontaneous improvement of the hypertrophic scar during the first six months, whereas in the keloid such does not occur.

TREATMENT. The most gratifying type of treatment has been the intralesional injection of triamcinolone suspension. Using a 30-gauge needle, on a 1-ml tuberculin Luer syringe, 0.02–0.04-ml aliquots of triamcinolone suspension (40 mg/ml) are injected into various parts of the lesion. This treatment is repeated

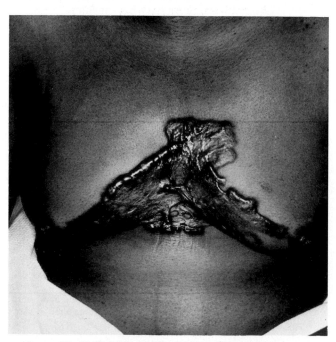

Figure 28–46. Keloids with no history of preceding trauma.

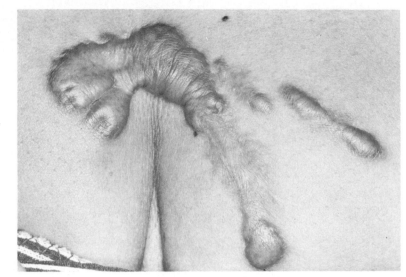

Figure 28–47. Keloids in a Caucasian patient secondary to acne.

at intervals of six to eight weeks as required. Flattening, and cessation of itching, are reliably achieved by this approach. The lesions are never made narrower, however.

If surgical removal by excision is feasible, and if *narrowing* of the keloid is a vitally important goal, the keloid is excised with the use of local anesthesia such as 2 per cent Xylocaine to which an equal part of triamcinolone suspension, 10 mg per ml, may be added. After the excision, the intralesional injection of triamcinolone without the lidocaine may be repeated at weekly or longer intervals. Wilson combined dexamethasone 21-phosphate postoperative treatment with x-ray therapy at two-week intervals. Arnold prefers to shield the normal skin to within 1 mm of the scar, as soon as the sutures are removed, and give 500 rads at 100 to 140 Kv without a filter, every five days, for four doses. There are never any radiation sequelae, and about 85 per cent success can be anticipated, except on the sternal area and shoulder, where it is nearer 20 per cent. Keloids in these areas should almost never be excised. Enhamre et al also reported success with excision and postoperative x-irradiation.

Pierced-ear keloids occur with considerable frequency. When the keloid is young, the intralesional injection of triamcinolone is frequently sufficient to control the problem. In old keloids excision of the lesion using lidocaine with triamcinolone, followed by injections at two-week intervals, produces good results. Laser excision has also been successful in this site, as reported by Kantor et al, though elsewhere it seems almost as unsuccessful as scalpel excision.

Onwukwe, in Nigeria—where, as he says, "keloid is to the African what psoriasis is to the Caucasian"—reports success with surgical excision combined with methotrexate. The methotrexate is given

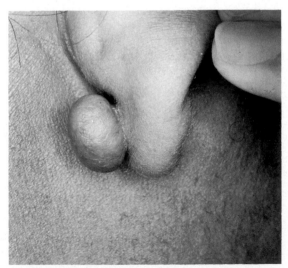

Figure 28–48. Keloid secondary to ear piercing.

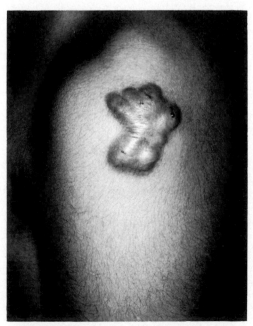

Figure 28–49. Keloid in a vaccination site.

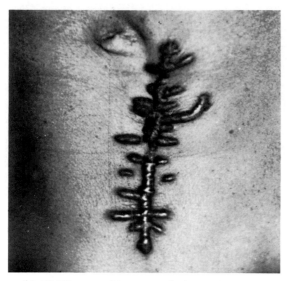

Figure 28–50. Hypertrophic scar on the lower abdomen following laparotomy. Extension into suture marks is conspicuous.

orally or parenterally, 15–20 mg in a single dose, repeated every four days, starting a week before surgery and continuing for about four months.

A future treatment may be retinoids. Abergel et al reported that fibroblasts from keloids, cultured in the presence of tretinoin or isotretinoin, produced less collagen than when cultured without retinoids. Topical tretinoin has been reported to be useful in early studies but these need to be repeated in a larger number of patients. It is ironic that dermabrasion often produces atypical keloids in patients taking isotretinoin.

Abergel RP, et al: Retinoid modulation of connective tissue metabolism in keloid fibroblast cultures. Arch Dermatol 1985, 121:632.
Idem: Skin closure by Nd:YAG laser welding. JAAD 1986, 14:810.
Arnold HL Jr, et al: Keloids: etiology, and management by excision and intensive prophylactic radiation. AMA Arch Dermatol 1959, 80:772.
Bhawan J: The myofibroblast. Am J Dermatopathol 1981, 3:73.
Blackburn WR, et al: Histologic basis of keloid and hypertrophic scar differentiation. Arch Pathol 1966, 82:65.
Elston DM, et al: Suppurative keloids. J Assoc Milit Dermatol 1984, 10:34.
Enhamre A, et al: Treatment of keloids with excision and postoperative x-ray irradiation. Dermatologica 1983, 167:90.
Grabb J, et al: Keloids. Am J Surg 1942, 58:315.
James WD, et al: The ultrastructure of a keloid. JAAD 1980, 3:50.
Janssen de Limpens AMP: The local treatment of hypertrophic scars and keloids with retinoic acid. Br J Dermatol 1980, 103:319.
Idem: A comparison of the treatment of keloids and hypertrophic scars. Eur J Plast Surg 1986, 9:18.
Kantor GR, et al: Treatment of earlobe keloids with carbon dioxide laser excision. J Dermatol Surg Oncol 1985, 11:1063.
Lee CP: Keloids. Int J Dermatol 1982, 21:504.
Maguire HC Jr: Treatment of keloids with triamcinolone acetonide injected intralesionally. JAMA 1965, 192:235.
Murray JC, et al: Keloids. JAAD 1981, 4:461.
Novick NL, et al: Suppurative keloidosis in a black woman. JAAD 1986, 16:1090.
Onwukwe MF: Classification of keloids. J Dermatol Surg Oncol 1978, 4:534.
Rubenstein R, et al: Atypical keloids after dermabrasion of patients taking isotretinoin. JAAD 1988, 15:280.

Salasche SJ, et al: Keloids of the earlobes: a surgical technique. J Dermatol Surg Oncol 1978, 4:534.
Stegman SJ, et al: Cosmetic dermatologic surgery. Arch Dermatol 1982, 118:1013.
Wilson WW: Prophylaxis against post-surgical keloids. South Med J 1965, 58:751.

Dupuytren's Contracture

This is a fibromatosis of the palmar aponeurosis. The lesion arises most commonly in men between the ages of 30 and 50 as multiple firm nodules in the palm. Usually three to five nodules about 1 cm in diameter develop, proximal to the fourth finger. Later the fibromatosis produces contractures, which may be disabling. James et al have reviewed the disease and its associations with alcoholic cirrhosis, diabetes mellitus, and chronic epilepsy, and its familial predisposition. It is also associated with Peyronie's disease, plantar fibromatosis, and knuckle pads. The fibrous nodules are composed of myofibroblasts.

Early intralesional triamcinolone may help, but surgical excision of the involved palmar fascia may be the only way to liberate severely contracted fingers.

Allen PW: The fibromatoses. Am J Surg Pathol 1977, 1:255.
Attali P, et al: Dupuytren's contracture, alcohol consumption, and cirrhotic liver disease. Arch Intern Med 1987, 147:1065.
James WD, et al: The role of the myofibroblast in Dupuytren's contracture. Arch Dermatol 1980, 116:807.

Plantar Fibromatosis

The plantar analogue of Dupuytren's contracture, this occurs as slowly enlarging nodules on the soles, which ultimately cause difficulty in walking or even weightbearing. This is sometimes called *Ledderhose's syndrome*. The usual treatment, as for Dupuytren's, is wide excision of the plantar fascia, but Pentland et al reported in 1985 a case which was symptomatically much improved by the intralesional injection of triamcinolone acetonide, 30 mg/ml, monthly for five months. They diluted the triamcinolone with lidocaine solution, but this is inadvisable, as it has no useful effect and indeed makes the injections briefly extremely painful. Regional block anesthesia is preferable.

Ledderhose G: Ueber Zerreissungen der Plantarfascie. Langenbeck Arch Klin Chir 1894, 48:853.
Pentland AP, et al: Plantar fibromatosis responds to intralesional steroids. JAAD 1985, 12:212.
White S: Plantar fibromatosis. Arch Dermatol 1986, 117:376.

Knuckle Pads

Knuckle pads (heloderma) are well-defined, round, plaquelike, fibrous thickenings that develop on the

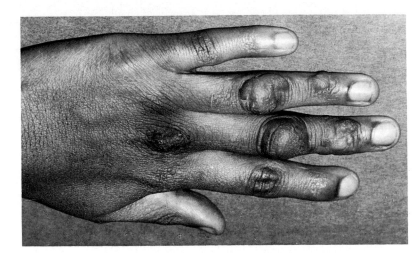

Figure 28–51. Knuckle pads.

extensor aspects of the proximal interphalangeal joints of the toes and fingers, including the thumbs. They develop at any age and grow to be some 10 to 15 mm in diameter in the course of a few weeks or months, then persist permanently. They are of flesh color or somewhat brown, with normal or slightly hyperkeratotic epidermis overlying them and adherent to them. They are a part of the skin and are freely movable over underlying structures.

Knuckle pads are sometimes associated with Dupuytren's contracture and comptodactylia (irreducible flexion contracture of one or more fingers). Some cases are familial.

Histologically, the lesions are fibromas. They are to be differentiated clinically from the nodular type of neurodermatitis and from the small hemispherical pitted papules that may develop over the knuckles after frostbite or in acrocyanosis, and from rheumatic nodules.

Intralesional corticosteroids may be beneficial.

Knuckle Pads, Leukonychia, and Deafness. Bart and Pumphrey reported a family with knuckle pads, mixed hearing loss (sensorineural and conductive), and total leukonychia, inherited as an autosomal dominant trait. This was noted through six generations.

Allison JR Jr, et al: Knuckle pads. Arch Dermatol 1966, 93:311.
Mulvaney MS, et al: Differential diagnosis of multiple dermal acral nodules. J Assoc Milit Dermatol 1985, 11:24.
Ronchese F: Knuckle pads and similar looking disorders. G Ital Dermatol Venereol 1966, 107:1227.

Peyronie's Disease

Plastic induration of the penis is a fibrous infiltration of the intercavernous septum of the penis. This fibrosis results in the formation of nodules or plaques. Owing to these plaques, a *fibrous chordee* is produced: curvature of the penis on erection, sometimes so severe as to make intromission difficult or impossible. Sometimes pain may be severe. The association of this disease with Dupuytren's contracture has been recognized. Intralesional triamcinolone suspension injected into the plaques and nodules may be curative.

Smith BH: Peyronie's disease. Am J Clin Pathol 1966, 45:670.

Desmoid Tumor

A large, deep-seated, well-circumscribed mass arising from the muscular aponeurosis characterizes this lesion. It most commonly occurs on the abdominal wall, especially in women during or soon after pregnancy. They have been divided into five types: abdominal wall, extraabdominal, intraabdominal, multiple, and those occurring in Gardner's syndrome. They recur locally, and can kill if they invade, surround, or compress vital structures. The most dangerous, then, are those at the root of the neck, and the intraabdominal type.

Allen PW: The fibromatoses. Am J Surg Pathol 1977, 1:255, 305.
Enzinger FM, et al: Musculo-aponeurotic fibromatosis of the shoulder girdle (extra-abdominal desmoid). Cancer 1967, 20:1131.

Aponeurotic Fibroma

Aponeurotic fibroma has also been called juvenile aponeurotic fibroma (calcifying fibroma). It is a tumorlike proliferation characterized by the appearance of slow-growing, cystlike masses occurring on the limbs.

Histologically, the distinctive lesions are sharply demarcated and composed of collagenous stroma showing acid mucopolysaccharides infiltrated by plump mesenchymal cells with oval nuclei. Hyalinized areas are also present, suggesting chondroid or osteoid metaplasia.

An aid to the diagnosis is stippled calcification, readily seen on roentgenograms.

Shapiro's 11-year-old female patient with a 1 × 2-cm lesion on the shoulder was treated by excision.

Shapiro L: Digital fibromatosis and aponeurotic fibroma. Arch Dermatol 1969, 99:37.

Congenital Generalized Fibromatosis (Infantile Myofibromatosis)

This uncommon condition, which presents at birth or soon after, is characterized by multiple firm dermal and subcutaneous nodules. Skeletal lesions, primarily of the metaphyseal regions of the long bones, occur in 50 per cent of patients. If only the skin and bones develop fibromas, the prognosis is excellent, with spontaneous resolution of the lesions without complications expected within the first one to two years of life. Some refer to this limited disease as *congenital multiple fibromatosis.*

The fibromas may involve the viscera, including the gastrointestinal tract, breast, lungs, liver, pancreas, tongue, serosal surfaces, lymph nodes, or kidney. Mortality in this more widespread subset is high; 80 per cent die from obstruction or compression of vital organs. Those who survive past four months have spontaneous regression of their disease.

Histologically, fascicles of spindle cells occur in a whorled pattern. The fact that these nodules are composed of myofibroblasts caused Chung et al to suggest the name *infantile myofibromatosis.*

There is a suggestion in the literature of a familial pattern of the disease. Females more commonly get the generalized disease.

Barnes L, et al: Solitary nodule on the arm of an infant. Arch Dermatol 1986, 122:89.
Chung EB, et al: Infantile myofibroblastosis. Cancer 1981, 48:1807.
Rosenberg HS, et al: The fibromatoses of infancy and childhood. Perspect Pediatr Pathol 1978, 4:269.
Spraker MK, et al: Congenital generalized fibromatosis. JAAD 1984, 10:365.

Juvenile Hyaline Fibromatosis

This syndrome begins in early childhood with soft nodular tumors of the scalp, face, and extremities, which may or may not be associated with flexion contractures, hypertrophic gums, osteolytic bone lesions, and stunted growth. Aberrant synthesis of glycosaminoglycans by fibroblasts appears to be present in the nodules, according to Quintal and Jackson, who reported an incomplete case in 1985. The disease has occurred in siblings and in a child from a consanguineous marriage, but it is not established yet as an autosomal recessive disorder.

In two cases reported with long-term follow-up, continued nodule formation, especially in the hands, with disabling contractures, osteolysis of phalanges, and surgical scarring, were the prominent late findings.

Histologically there are fibroblasts with fine intracytoplasmic eosinophilic granules, embedded in a homogeneous eosinophilic dermal ground substance.

Camarasa JG, et al: Juvenile hyaline fibromatosis. JAAD 1987, 16:881.
Finday AY, et al: Juvenile hyaline fibromatosis. Br J Dermatol 1983, 108:609.
Quintal D, et al: Juvenile hyaline fibromatosis. Arch Dermatol 1985, 121:1062.

Infantile Digital Fibromatosis (Infantile Digital Myofibroblastoma)

Infantile digital fibromatosis is a rare neoplasm of infancy and childhood characterized by fibroblastic proliferations. Usually the lesions occur singly or severally on the dorsal or lateral aspects of the distal phalanges of the toes and fingers. The thumb and great toe are usually spared. These asymptomatic, firm, red, smooth nodules, some 1 cm in diameter, occur during the first year of life. Forty-seven per cent occur in the first month of life. Miyamoto et al report the disorder following trauma in an 11-year-old girl. The lesions do not metastasize.

Histologically, the epidermis is normal, but the dermis is infiltrated with proliferating fibroblasts and collagen bundles. In addition, eosinophilic cytoplasmic inclusions in many of the fibroblasts are characteristic. The elongated cells are myofibroblasts ultrastructurally.

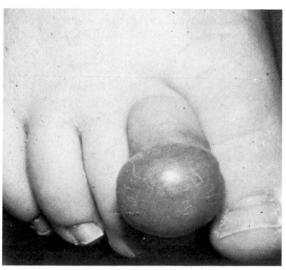

Figure 28–52. Infantile digital fibromatosis. (Courtesy of Dr. L. Shapiro.)

Treatment by surgical excision has a high risk of recurrence. It may be preferable to procrastinate in the hope of spontaneous resolution.

Bhawan J, et al: A myofibroblastic tumor. Infantile digital fibroma. Am J Pathol 1979, 94:19.
Miyamoto T, et al: Posttraumatic occurrence of infantile digital fibromatosis. Arch Dermatol 1986, 122:915.
Ramsdell WM: Recurring digital fibroma of childhood. Arch Dermatol 1983, 119:702.
Ryman W, et al: Recurring digital fibromas of infancy. Aust J Dermatol 1985, 26:113.

Fibrous Hamartoma of Infancy

This is a single dermal or subcutaneous firm nodule of the upper trunk which is present at birth. Biopsy shows a cell-poor fibrous lesion, with immature spindle cells present in a mucoid matrix. There is no recurrence after excision.

Enzinger F: Fibrous hamartoma of infancy. Cancer 1965, 18:241.
King DF, et al: Fibrous hamartoma of infancy. J Dermatol Surg Oncol 1979, 5:482.
Paller AS, et al: Fibrous hamartoma of infancy. Arch Dermatol 1989, 125:88.

Fibromatosis Colli

There is a fibroma tissue proliferation infiltrating the lower third of the sternocleidomastoid muscle at birth, in this entity. Spontaneous remission occurs within a few months. Occasionally some patients are left with a wryneck deformity. This complication, however, is amenable to surgery.

Coventry MB, et al: Congenital muscular torticollis (wryneck). Postgrad Med 1960, 28:383.
MacDonald D: Sternomastoid tumor and muscular torticollis. J Bone Joint Surg 1969, 51-B:432.

Diffuse Infantile Fibromatosis

This process occurs within the first three years of life and is usually confined to the muscles of the arms, neck, and shoulder area. There is a multicentric infiltration of muscle fibers with fibroblasts resembling those seen in aponeurotic fibromas. Calcification does not occur. Recurrence after excision occurs in about a third of cases.

Allen PW: The fibromatoses. Am J Surg Pathol 1977, 1:255, 305.
Fleischmajer R, et al: Juvenile fibromatoses. Arch Dermatol 1973, 107:574.

Aggressive Infantile Fibromatosis

Single or multiple fast-growing masses which are present at birth or within the first year of life is the clinical presentation of this locally recurring, non-metastasizing lesion. It may be seen in any location, although the arms, legs, and trunk are the usual sites. Histologically it mimics fibrosarcoma.

Allen PW: The fibromatoses. Am J Surg Pathol 1977, 1:255, 305.
Balsaver AM, et al: Congenital fibrosarcoma. Cancer 1967, 20:1607.

Giant Cell Tumor of the Tendon Sheath

This tumor most commonly is attached to the tendons of the fingers, hands, and wrists, with predilection for the flexor surfaces. It is firm, measures from 1 to 3 cm in diameter, and does not spontaneously involute. It recurs after excision in approximately 25 per cent of cases. Another tumor of the tendon sheath, the *fibroma of the tendon sheath*, may represent a variant of the giant cell tumor. It also affects the flexural tendons of the fingers and hands and morphologically it and the giant cell tumor are identical. In Chung and Enzinger's series the median age of onset was 31 years, younger than the giant cell tumor patients, and more often male (75 per cent of fibroma patients were male). The recurrence rate after surgery was 24 per cent in their series.

Histologically, the giant cell tumor consists of lobules of densely hyalinized collagen. The characteristic giant cells have deeply eosinophilic cytoplasma and a variable number of nuclei. Lipophages and siderophages may be numerous. The fibroma of the tendon sheath generally lacks the lipophages, siderophages, and giant cells, with the lobules being composed of dense fibrocollagenous tissue.

Carstens PHB: Giant cell tumor of the tendon sheath. Arch Pathol 1978, 102:99.
Chung EB, et al: Fibroma of tendon sheath. Cancer 1979, 44:1945.
Cooper PH, et al: Fibroma of tendon sheath. JAAD 1984, 11:625.
King DJ, et al: Giant cell tumor of the tendon sheath involving the skin. Arch Dermatol 1978, 114:944.

AINHUM

Ainhum is also known as dactylolysis spontanea, bankokerendé, and sukhapakla.

Ainhum is a disease affecting the toes, especially the fifth toe, characterized by a linear constriction around the affected digit, which leads ultimately to the spontaneous amputation of the distal part. It

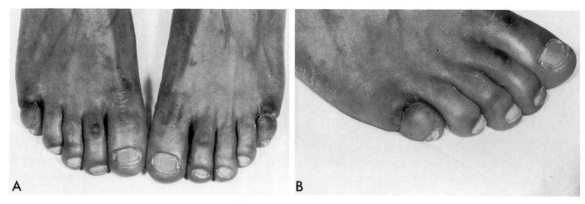

Figure 28–53. Ainhum.

occurs chiefly among black men in Africa. Usually it is unilateral, but it may be bilateral.

The disease begins with a transverse groove in the skin on the flexor surface of the toe, usually beneath the first interphalangeal articulation. The furrow is produced by a ringlike fibrosis and an induration of the corium. It deepens and extends laterally around the toe until the two ends meet, so that the digit becomes constricted as if in a ligature. The constricted part becomes swollen and soft and after a time greatly distended. Ulceration may result in a malodorous discharge, with pain and gangrene. The course of the disease is slow, but in five to 10 years spontaneous amputation occurs, generally at a joint.

The cause is unknown. It may be due to chronic inflammation and fibrosis in fissures. Chronic trauma, fissuring, and walking barefoot in the tropics have been also implicated.

Treatment in the early cases by cutting the constricting band is unsuccessful; in advanced cases amputation of the affected member is advisable. Surgical correction by Z-plasty has produced good results, as reported by Allyn and Leides. Intralesional injection of betamethasone (total, 15 injections) has been successful in one case treated by Merello of Italy.

Grossman J, et al: Ainhum. NY J Med 1968, 68:1741.
McLaurin CI: Psoriasis presenting with pseudoainhum. JAAD 1982, 7:130.

CONNECTIVE TISSUE NEVI

These uncommon lesions, while often very inconspicuous, may present as acquired isolated plaques, as multiple lesions either acquired or congenital, or as one finding in a more generalized inherited disease. The biopsy findings in many cases do not appear very different from normal skin, although in some cases increased amounts of collagen or elastin may be identified.

These lesions characteristically occur on the trunk, most often in the lumbosacral area. They may be solitary, but are often multiple, in which case they may show a zosteriform arrangement. Individual lesions are slightly elevated plaques 1 to 15 cm in diameter, varying in color from light yellow to orange, with a surface texture resembling shagreen leather.

Connective tissue nevi of the acquired type have been classified by Uitto et al as eruptive collagenomas, isolated collagenomas, or isolated elastomas,

PSEUDOAINHUM

Pseudoainhum has been a term used in connection with certain hereditary and nonhereditary diseases in which annular constriction of digits occurs.

Gibbs and Frank have listed conditions capable of causing constriction of the digits. Hereditary disorders are hereditary palmoplantar keratoderma, mal de Meleda, keratosis striata, pityriasis rubra pilaris, pachyonychia congenita, mutilating keratoderma of Vohwinkel, and congenital ectodermal defect.

Nonhereditary disorders associated with constriction of digits are ainhum, leprosy, cholera, ancyclostomiasis, scleroderma, Raynaud's syndrome, syringomyelia, ergot poisoning, and tumors of the spinal cord.

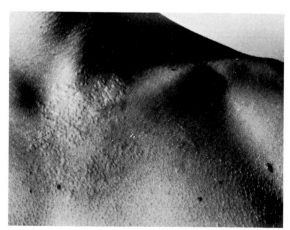

Figure 28–54. Connective tissue nevus over the sternoclavicular junction. (Courtesy of Dr. L. Fragola.)

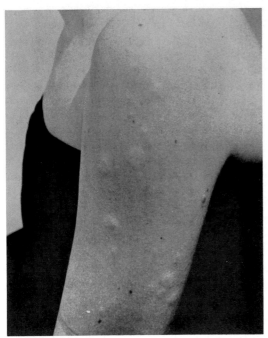

Figure 28–55. Connective tissue nevus on the upper arm of a 12-year-old girl. (Courtesy of Dr. J. Stephens.)

depending on the number of lesions and the predominant dermal fibers present. They cannot be differentiated clinically.

The hereditary types of connective tissue nevi discussed here include dermatofibrosis lenticularis disseminata in the Buschke-Ollendorff syndrome, familial cutaneous collagenoma, and the so-called *shagreen patches* seen in tuberous sclerosis.

The *Buschke-Ollendorff syndrome* is an autosomal dominant inherited disorder in which widespread dermal papules and plaques develop asymmetrically over the trunk and limbs. Various abnormalities of the elastic tissue have been reported in biopsies examined by both light and electron microscopy. Uitto et al found the elastic fibers thickened and of highly variable diameters. Desmosine was increased

3- to 7-fold above normal. The associated feature of osteopoikilosis is asymptomatic, but diagnostic in x-rays. Focal sclerotic densities are seen, primarily in long bones, the pelvis, and the hands.

Familial cutaneous collagenoma is exemplified by numerous asymptomatic cutaneous nodules on the backs of three brothers, described by Henderson et al; one had idiopathic cardiomyopathy, one had atrophy of an iris and severe high-frequency sensorineural hearing loss, and one had recurrent vasculitis. Subsequently Uitto et al reported six patients, from a kindred of 53, with autosomal-dominantly inherited lesions of a similar nature. They all had symmetrically distributed dermal nodules, most commonly on the upper back. The age of onset varied from 15 to 19 years.

Clinically the most important disease associated with connective tissue nevi is *tuberous sclerosis*. The inconspicuous thickened "shagreen plaques" are associated with the classical skin findings of adenoma sebaceum, periungual fibromas, and ash-leaf macules. Since at least half the cases of tuberous sclerosis result from new mutations, all patients with connective tissue nevi should be carefully studied for evidence of tuberous sclerosis, even in the absence of a family history of the disease.

Berberian BB, et al: Asymptomatic nodules on the back and abdomen. Arch Dermatol 1987, 123:811.

Cole GW, et al: An elastic tissue defect in dermatofibrosis lenticularis disseminata. Arch Dermatol 1982, 118:44.

Reinhardt LA, et al: Buschke-Ollendorff syndrome. Cutis 1983, 31:94.

Uitto J, et al: Biochemical and ultrastructural demonstration of elastin accumulation in the skin lesions of the Buschke-Ollendorff syndrome. J Invest Dermatol 1981, 76:284.

Idem: Connective tissue nevi of the skin. JAAD 1980, 3:441.

ELASTOFIBROMA DORSI

Elastofibroma dorsi is a rare benign tumor usually located in the deep soft tissues in the subscapular

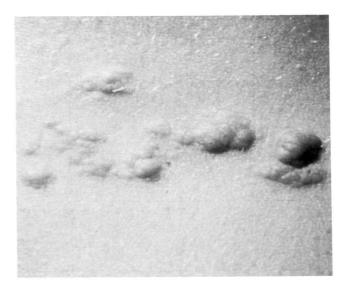

Figure 28–56. Nevus lipomatosus cutaneus superficialis.

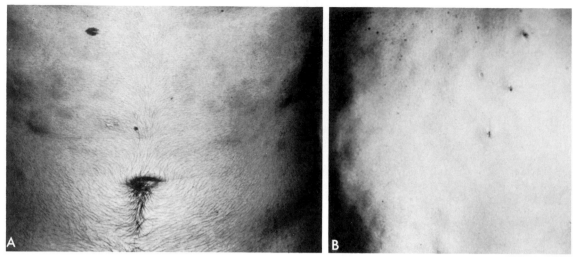

Figure 28–57. Familial cutaneous collagenoma.

region but sometimes at other sites. The tumor is firm, unencapsulated, and measures up to several centimeters in diameter. It is believed to represent an unusual response to repeated trauma. Histologically, the tumor consists of abundant compact sclerotic collagen mixed with large, swollen, irregular elastic fibers, often appearing as globules of elastic tissue. Excision is curative.

FIBROUS PAPULE OF THE NOSE

A dome-shaped, sessile, skin-colored or slightly red papule 3 to 6 mm in diameter, usually solitary, on or near the nose, in an adult, is very likely to be a "fibrous papule of the nose," a harmless lesion first described by Graham and associates in 1965. Graham and others have suggested that it may be a degenerated or involuting nevus, but S-100 protein, which is characteristic of nevus cells and other tissues of nervous system origin, was not found in 20 fibrous papules of the central face studied by Spiegel et al. Two electron microscopic studies involving a total of seven cases failed to find any melanosomes, but rather cells resembling fibroblasts. Most of these lesions, it would appear, are angiofibromas.

Fibrous papule of the nose (or central face) is easily confused with a nevocytic nevus, fibroma, neurofibroma, granuloma pyogenicum, or even a carcinoma. Conservative excision or fulguration is curative; recurrence is rare.

Graham JH, et al: Fibrous papule of the nose. J Invest Dermatol 1965, 45:194.
Meigel WN, et al: Fibrous papule of the face. Am J Dermatopathol 1979, 1:329.
Nemeth AJ, et al: Fibrous papule. JAAD 1988, 19:1102.
Ragaz A, et al: Fibrous papule of the face. Am J Dermatopathol 1979, 1:353.
Saylan T, et al: Fibrous papule of the nose. Br J Dermatol 1971, 85:111.
Spiegel J, et al: Fibrous papule. JAAD 1983, 9:360.

HAMARTOMA MONILIFORMIS

Also known as *linear papular ectodermal-mesodermal hamartoma*, this entity was described by Butterworth and Graham as a flesh-colored papular eruption occurring principally on the forehead. The asymptomatic lesions, which frequently had linear arrangement, were found in young black institutionalized adults. Some 80 cases had forehead involvement; in addition, some also had lesions on the nose and neck.

Histologically, the lesions showed epidermal features of melanocytic nevi; in the dermis were features of subepidermal fibrosis.

Butterworth T, et al: Linear papular ectodermal-mesodermal hamartoma. Arch Dermatol 1970, 101:191.

PEARLY PENILE PAPULES

This term has been given to pearly white, dome-shaped papules occurring on the coronal margin of the glans penis. Another name is *hirsutoid papillomas*. These lesions are not uncommon around the age of 20 to 30 years. Glicksman and Freeman found one case in every five men attending a clinic for sexually transmitted disease.

Histologically, there is a vascular network surrounded by dense connective tissue. As Ackerman and Kornberg point out, these qualify as angiofibromas.

No treatment is necessary, only reassurance.

These lesions should be distinguished from papillomas, hypertrophic sebaceous glands, and condyloma acuminatum.

These lesions do not respond to podophyllin. The absence of symptoms prompts one to refrain from treatment.

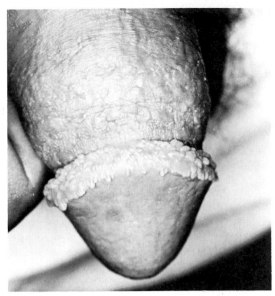

Figure 28–58. Pearly penile papules.

Ackerman AB, et al: Pearly penile papules. Arch Dermatol 1973, 108:673.
Glicksman JM, et al: Pearly penile papules. Arch Dermatol 1966, 93:56.

Perifollicular Fibromas

Zackheim and Pinkus described a rare type of fibroma with a perifollicular pattern. Clinically there are multiple, small, firm papules, either flesh-colored or pink, located on the face and neck. The appearance is not distinctive and may suggest a nevus or trichoepithelioma. They have been reported also as solitary lesions. One report linked it to a colonic villous adenoma, and a second to colonic polyposis.

The pathologic changes are those of a benign fibroma of the connective tissue sheath of the hair follicle. The fibroma stems from the mesodermal portion of the pilary complex. Reports of this entity prior to the elucidation of fibrofolliculoma are difficult to evaluate because many reports of perifollicular fibromas show epithelial proliferation in association with perifollicular fibrosis, a finding characteristic of fibrofolliculomas. This problem is discussed by Ubogy-Rainey et al.

Hornstein OP, et al: Perifollicular fibromatosis cutis with polyps of the colon. Arch Dermatol Res 1975, 253:161.
Ubogy-Rainey Z, et al: Fibrofolliculomas, trichodiscomas, and acrochordons. JAAD 1987, 16:452.
Zackheim H, et al: Perifollicular fibromas. Arch Dermatol 1960, 82:913.

ACRAL FIBROKERATOMA

Acral fibrokeratoma, often called *acquired digital fibrokeratoma*, is characterized by a pinkish, hyperkeratotic, hornlike projection occurring on a finger, toe, or palm; the projection usually emerges from a collarette of elevated skin. Stanton and Wilson reported lesions of the palm in two cases, as did Kint et al. The latter reviewed 50 new cases and found the average age of the patients was 40; 39 lesions were on the fingers, six on the toes; the rest were on the palm, wrist, and calf. Selmanowitz proposed the name acral fibrokeratoma in 1971.

Bart and his associates describe the histologic features as a central core of thick collagen bundles interwoven closely in a vertical position. This is surrounded by capillaries and a fine network of reticulum fibers.

The lesion resembles a rudimentary supernumerary digit, the cutaneous horn, and a neuroma.

Simple surgical excision or ablation at the level of the skin surface, followed by fulguration or cauterization, is effective. However, Shelley reported a case in a 41-year-old woman in which the fingerlike lesion (including a nail, with a lunula!), projecting from a lateral nail fold, had recurred after excision five times in five years. It proved to be a digital (acral) fibrokeratoma. Salasche reviewed the surgical treatment of these lesions in the nailfold.

Berger RS, et al: Dermal papule on a distal digit. Arch Dermatol 1988, 124:1559.
Kint A, et al: Acquired (digital) fibrokeratoma. JAAD 1985, 12:816.
Salasche SJ: Acquired digital fibrokeratoma. J Assoc Milit Dermatol 1985, 11:83.
Shelley WB, et al: Recurring accessory "fingernail": periungual fibrokeratoma. Cutis 1985, 31:451.
Stanton DL, et al: Acquired palmar fibrokeratoma. Cutis 1973, 11:39.

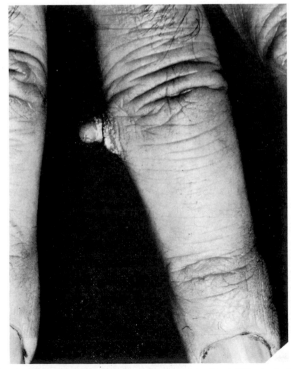

Figure 28–59. Acral fibrokeratoma. (From Bart RS: Arch Dermatol 97:120, 1968.)

FAMILIAL MYXOVASCULAR FIBROMAS

Multiple verrucous papules on the palms and fingers, which on biopsy show focal neovascularization and mucinlike changes in the papillary dermis, have been described by Coskey et al and Peterson et al. These lesions closely resemble warts clinically. They have been reported from several family members, with a probable autosomal dominant inheritance.

Coskey RJ, et al: Multiple vascular fibromas and myxoid fibromas of the fingers. JAAD 1980, 2:425.
Peterson JL, et al: Familial myxovascular fibromas. JAAD 1982, 6:470.

SUBUNGUAL EXOSTOSIS

Subungual exostosis is a solitary fibrous and bony nodule protruding from beneath the distal edge of the nail, most commonly of the great toe. Rarely, the terminal phalanges of other toes, particularly the little toe, or even the fingers may be involved. The exostosis is seen chiefly in women between the ages of 12 and 30. The first appearance is a small pinkish growth projecting slightly beyond the inner free edge of the nail. The overlying nail becomes brittle and either breaks or is removed, after which the tumor, being released, mushrooms upward and distally above the level of the nail. It grows slowly to a maximum diameter of about 8 mm. Pressure of the shoe on the lesion causes great pain.

Subungual exostosis must be differentiated from granuloma pyogenicum, verruca vulgaris, ingrowing nail, glomus tumor, and melanotic whitlow, which should be excluded by biopsy. If subungual exostosis is suspected, the diagnosis can be confirmed by radiographic examination. Complete excision or curettage is the proper method of treatment.

Cohen HJ, et al: Subungual exostoses. Arch Dermatol 1973, 107:431.
James MP: Digital exostosis causing enlargement of the fingertip. JAAD 1988, 19:132.
Lebovitz SS, et al: Subungual exostosis. Cutis 1974, 13:427.

COLLAGENOUS PAPULES OF THE AURAL CONCHAE

Sanchez reported four cases in 1983 of women between 32 and 54 who had multiple 1–4-mm papules in the inner aspects of the aural pinnae which were histologically distinguishable from colloid pseudomilium, fibrous papules, and nodular amyloidosis. They consisted of dense hyalinized sclerotic collagen.

Sanchez JL: Collagenous papules on the aural conchae. Am J Dermatopathol 1983, 5:231.

CHONDRODERMATITIS NODULARIS CHRONICA HELICIS

This is a small, nodular, tender, chronic inflammatory lesion occurring on the outer helix of the ear. Most patients are men. The lesions are not uncommon and sometimes as many as 12 nodules may arrange themselves along the edge of the upper helix. The lesions evolve slowly and are ovoid, well defined, slightly reddish, extremely tender masses, 2 to 4 mm in diameter. They are firmly attached to the underlying cartilage. At times the surface is covered by an adherent scale or a shallow ulcer. After the masses have reached a certain size, growth ceases, but the lesions persist unchanged for years. There is no tendency to malignant change. Barker and his associates have reported similar lesions occurring on the anthelix, predominantly in women.

Often there is a history of frostbite, chronic trauma, or chronic actinic exposure with concomitant actinically induced lesions of the face and dorsal hands.

Histologically, degenerative changes of the collagen are the chief features. In addition, acanthosis and hyperkeratosis with plugging and thinning of the epidermis are noted. On excision one finds a projecting spur of altered cartilage about which the lesion is formed, apparently a chronic inflammatory response. As Goette and others have pointed out, this is a process of transepidermal elimination.

The lesions may be excised, together with the underlying spicule of cartilage. However, Zimmerman has abandoned this approach in favor of intralesional triamcinolone diacetate or acetonide injections, 25 to 40 mg per ml, every month. Wade found it curative in eight cases. Usually two to four injections suffice. Arnold has also found it effective. Kromann

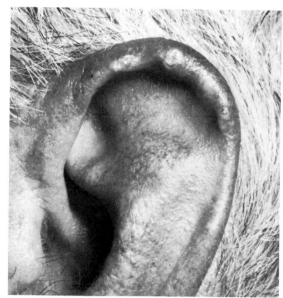

Figure 28–60. Chondrodermatitis nodularis chronica helicis. Painful nodules on the edge of the upper helix. (Courtesy of Dr. I. Abrahams.)

et al reported a 25 per cent in a series of 142 patients subjected to curettage and electrocautery, a figure similar to that reported for excision.

Billon in 1988 reported a lesion, recurrent 2 years after biopsy excision, which cleared promptly during pentoxifylline (Trental) given for vascular insufficiency in the legs. Ely has seen this, and it has been confirmed by two other reports.

Bard JW: Chondrodermatitis nodularis chronica helicis. Dermatologica 1981, 163:376.

Barker LP, et al: Chondrodermatitis of the ears. Arch Dermatol 1960, 81:15.

Billon SF: Trental cleared nodular chondrodermatitis of the helix. Schoch Letter 1988, 38:41.

Goette DK: Chondrodermatitis nodularis chronica helicis. JAAD 1980, 2:148.

Kromann N, et al: Chondrodermatitis nodularis chronica helicis treated with curettage and electrocauterization. Acta Derm Venereol (Stockh) 1983, 63:85.

Wade TR: Chondrodermatitis nodularis helicis. Cutis 1979, 24:406.

DISORDERS OF TRANSEPIDERMAL ELIMINATION

Transepidermal elimination is the name applied by Mehregan to the process whereby various substances are transported from the dermis through the epidermis and thereby excreted. The disorders in which this occurs are often called "perforating," but the process is too complex to be encompassed by this word.

Woo and Rasmussen, who published a valuable review of the process in 1985, suggest that it is the basic pathologic event in elastosis perforans serpiginosa and reactive perforating collagenosis, and a secondary reactive process in many others, such as granuloma annulare, pseudoxanthoma elasticum, and chondrodermatitis nodularis helicis. It occurs also in lichen nitidus, some sarcoidal granulomas, rheumatoid nodules, necrobiosis lipoidica, certain bacterial, fungal, and protozoal disorders, nevocellular nevi and melanomas, calcinosis cutis, porokeratosis of Mibelli, vellus hair cysts, hidradenitis suppurativa, osteoma cutis, and some others. Perforating folliculitis and Kyrle's hyperkeratosis follicularis et parafollicularis in cutem penetrans are not considered examples of this phenomenon by them, but are by others, including Goette.

Barr RJ, et al: Replies in questions to the editorial board. Am J Dermatopathol 1984, 6:89.

Goette DK: Transepithelial elimination disorders. J Assoc Milit Dermatol 1985, 11:28.

Woo TY, et al: Disorders of transepidermal elimination. Int J Dermatol 1985, 24:337.

Submucous Fibrosis of the Palate

A distinctive fibrosis of the palate occurs in India among persons whose diet is heavily seasoned with chili. The irritation produced by this spice causes first a fibrous reaction which acts as a precancerosis. Later, carcinoma results. The lesions are essentially a thickening of the palate, tonsillar pillars, and fauces; later, ulceration and leukoplakic areas develop.

Histologically, an elastotic degeneration of the collagen and epithelial hyperplasia are the main features of this premalignant condition.

Pindborg JJ, et al: Occurrence of epithelial atypia in 51 Indian villagers with oral submucous fibrosis. Br J Cancer 1970, 24:253.

Fascial Hernia

Evanescent herniations in the form of nodules appear in the skin where the deep and superficial veins meet going through the fascia. These herniated nodules, seen most frequently on the lower extremities, become prominent when the underlying muscles contract.

Treatment is not indicated.

ACROCHORDON

Synonyms: cutaneous tag, papilloma colli, fibroma pendulum, cutaneous papilloma, fibroma molluscum, Templeton's skin tags, skin tags.

Small, flesh-colored to dark brown, pinhead-sized and larger, sessile and pedunculated papillomata occur predominantly on the neck. These tags are also seen frequently on the eyelids, less often on the trunk, axillae, and groins, where the soft, pedunculated growths often hang on thin stalks, especially in the axillae. These flesh-colored, tear-drop-shaped tags when palpated feel like small bags. Occasionally, due to twisting of the pedicle, one will become inflamed, tender, and even gangrenous. Lubach et

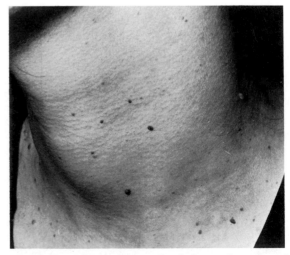

Figure 28–61. "Cutaneous tags" of the neck: pedunculated seborrheic keratoses.

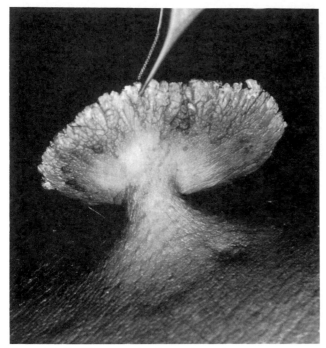

Figure 28–62. Giant acrochordon on buttocks. (Courtesy of Dr. Axel W. Hoke).

al examined 750 patients for skin tags, and found the onset between the ages of 10 and 50. Both sexes had the same incidence, nearly 60 per cent getting them by age 69.

Brown, sessile or pedunculated skin tags on the neck frequently occur with seborrheic keratoses. Waisman indicated a great histologic similarity between the two, and one of us (HLA) has confirmed this on countless occasions during the past 40 years. They increase in number when the patient is gaining weight.

Acrochordons have a documented statistical association with colonic polyps. Leavitt et al reported that the ratio of patients with skin tags to patients without them was about 4:1 in patients with polyps and 1:4 in patients without them. Average age was the same in all four groups. Chobanian et al confirmed this ($p < .001$) in 100 patients undergoing colonoscopy; no mention was made of weight gain. Beitler et al examined 54 patients prior to colonoscopy: of 35 with skin tags, 24 had polyps, whereas of 19 without skin tags, only four had polyps. If skin tags are a marker of polyposis, it is for acquired polyposis, because Luk et al found no such correlation in 187 members of 32 kindreds with familial colonic polyps.

None of these studies address the question of whether the patients with polyps tend to be overweight. Future studies should include this factor. They are certainly common in the corpulent.

Histologically, acrochordons are characterized by a hyperplastic epidermis enclosing a dermal connective tissue stalk composed of loose collagen fibers. The baglike papillomata generally show a flattened epidermis.

Most can be clipped off at the base with either no anesthesia or an intradermal injection of normal saline solution, and 3.8M ferric chloride or light electrodesiccation used for hemostasis. A satisfactory cosmetic result is obtained with this technique.

Arnold HL Jr: Skin tags and colonic polyps (letter). JAAD 1987, 16:402.
Beitler M, et al: Association between acrochordons and colonic polyposis. JAAD 1986, 14:1042.
Chobanian SJ: Skin tags and colonic polyps. JAAD 1987, 16:407.
Idem, et al: Skin tags as a screening marker for colonic neoplasia. Gastrointest Endosc 1986, 32:162.
Idem: Skin tags as a marker for adenomatous polyps of the colon. Ann Intern Med 1985, 103:892.
Huntley AC: Eruptive lipofibromata. Arch Dermatol 1983, 119:612.
Klein I, et al: Colonic polyps in patients with acromegaly. Ann Intern Med 1982, 97:27.
Kune GA, et al: Association between colorectal polyps and skin tags. Lancet 1985, 2:1062.
Leavitt J, et al: Skin tags: a marker for colonic polyps. Ann Intern Med 1983, 98:928.
Lubach D, et al: Skin tags and colonic polyps. JAAD 1987, 16:402.
Luk GD, et al: Colonic polyps and acrochordons do not correlate in familial colonic polyposis kindreds. Ann Intern Med 1986, 104:209.
Margolis J, et al: Skin tags—a frequent sign of diabetes mellitus. N Engl J Med 1976, 294:1184.
Waisman M: Cutaneous papillomas of the neck. South Med J 1957, 50:725.

MASTOCYTOSIS
(Urticaria Pigmentosa)

Mastocytosis is a general term applied to local and systemic accumulations of mast cells. Urticaria pigmentosa is a manifestation of mastocytosis characterized by persistent pigmented, itchy skin lesions of various size that tend to urticate upon mechanical or chemical irritation.

CLINICAL FEATURES. Nettleship first described the disease in 1869. Urticaria pigmentosa may occur from birth to middle age. However, about half the cases have their onset before six months of age and an additional fourth occur before puberty.

The cutaneous lesions may consist of macules, papules, nodules, plaques, vesicles, or bullae. Rarely, telangiectases, petechiae, or ecchymoses may occur. There may be no visible skin lesions at all, even though biopsy will prove the presence of high numbers of mast cells.

At their onset the lesions are similar to urticaria except that they are not evanescent. The lesions of urticaria pigmentosa persist and gradually become chamois- or slate-colored. When they are firmly stroked or vigorously rubbed, urticaria with a surrounding erythematous flare (Darier's sign) usually develops.

Frequently the lesions are slightly elevated; the nodules may be firm and discrete or confluent and are usually of a brownish waxy appearance. Dermographism of clinically uninvolved skin is present in one third to one half of patients. Flushing of a generalized type sometimes accompanied by syn-

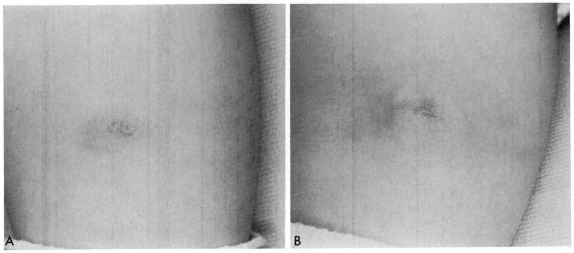

Figure 28–63. Solitary mastocytoma on the leg. A, *Before stroking;* B, *after stroking (Darier's sign).*

cope, may be present at the onset and may gradually decrease during the course of the disease.

Severe symptoms as a result of the massive liberation of histamine from mast cells may occur after ingestion of known mast cell degranulators such as alcohol, morphine, or codeine, or after extended rubbing, or after hymenoptera stings. The latter may induce anaphylaxis, as reported in three patients by Muller et al.

Pruritus, the most frequent symptom, varies from a mild state to an intensity that may interfere with sleep and may be accompanied by fatigue, anorexia, diarrhea, and joint pains. Rarely, diarrhea may be the chief symptom, and Mahood et al reported a case in which it persisted for 40 years. Cromolyn sodium generally controls explosive attacks, though patients may continue to have three or four bowel movements a day.

In the course of time, old lesions tend to disappear without sequelae. Spontaneous involution is especially likely in those patients whose cutaneous disease began in childhood.

The several types of urticaria pigmentosa may be conveniently divided into the juvenile and adult types, with special forms occurring in these two broad categories. These may be the solitary mastocytoma, generalized diffuse mastocytosis, telangiectasia macularis eruptiva perstans, and an erythrodermic form.

CHILDHOOD TYPES. Cutaneous mastocytosis in children begins with a *generalized eruption* or with a solitary tumor or nodule, commonly called *solitary mastocytoma.*

Generalized Eruption. In the generalized form the eruption usually begins during the first weeks of life, presenting with rose-colored, pruritic, urticarial, slightly pigmented macules, papules, or nodules. The lesions are oval or round and vary in diameter between 5 and 15 mm. The color varies from yellowish brown to yellowish red.

Vesicle and bulla formation is a frequent prominent feature early in the disease. Indeed, vesicles and bullae may be the initial presenting signs. They may rarely be unilateral: Arnold followed one such case to spontaneous recovery at about age six. Caplan found the vesicles and bullae to persist no longer than three years. In the older age groups vesiculation rarely occurs.

Usually all pigmentation and evidence of the disease disappear within a few years, generally before puberty. The eruption, however, may persist into adult life. Although systemic involvement is possible, malignant systemic disease is extremely rare.

Pseudoxanthomatous Mastocytosis (Xanthelasmoidea). An uncommon variant of urticaria pigmentosa is xanthelasmoidea, described as such by Tilbury Fox in 1875 and, in a lifelong form, by Griffiths and

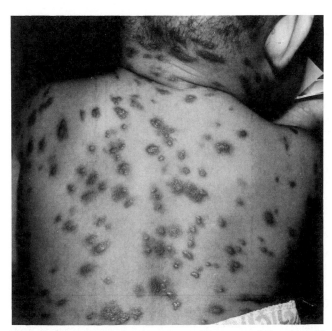

Figure 28–64. Urticaria pigmentosa. (Courtesy of Dr. Axel W. Hoke.)

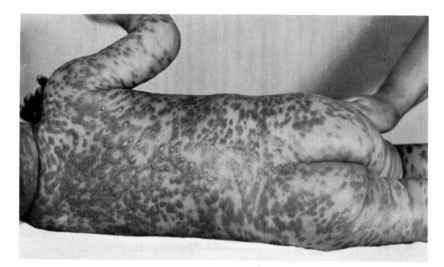

Figure 28–65. Urticaria pigmentosa.

Daneshbod in 1975. Pale yellow nodules 1 mm to 2 cm in diameter had been present in profusion since birth. The spleen was enlarged. Erythema, but no urtication, was elicited by rubbing. A dense mast cell infiltrate was found histologically.

Solitary Mastocytoma. The solitary nodule may be present at birth or may develop during the first weeks of life. The tumor stems from a brown macule which urticates upon stroking. This macule develops into a papule or a raised round or oval plaque up to 20 mm in diameter. It may have a smooth or a slightly warty surface *(peau d'orange)*. Although it may occur anywhere on the body, its favorite location is on the dorsum of the hand near the wrist, according to Lantis and Koblenzer. Edema, urtication, vesiculation, and even bulla formation may be observed in the lesion. Uncommonly, several of these mastocytomas may be present.

Although the disseminated form may begin with a single lesion, dissemination usually occurs within three months of its appearance. Solitary mastocytoma should be of more than three months' duration.

Most solitary mastocytomas involute sponta-

neously by age 10 or earlier. They also respond favorably to excision. Progression to malignant disease does not occur.

Diffuse Cutaneous Mastocytosis. In this form, with diffuse involvement, the entire integument may be thickened and infiltrated with mast cells to produce a peculiar orange color, giving rise to the term *homme orange*. There is infiltrated doughy or boggy consistency to the skin, and lichenification may be present.

ADULT TYPES. Most frequent are the pruritic papular or nodular forms, with typical urtication of the lesion disseminated over most of the body but especially on the upper arms, the legs, and the trunk. Several distinctive forms are seen in the adult types.

Erythrodermic Mastocytosis. This rare form is probably the same as or similar to diffuse cutaneous mastocytosis. There is generalized erythroderma and the skin has a leather-grain appearance. Although this occurs mostly in adults, it also occurs on rare occasions in infants. Brett and his associates described a six-month-old boy who had erythroderma of the entire skin. Urtication could be produced over

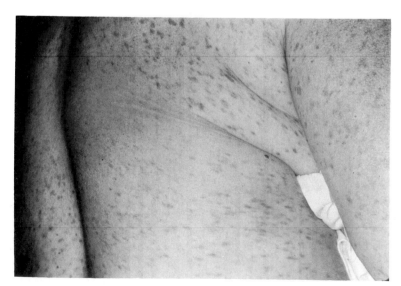

Figure 28–66. Telangiectasia macularis eruptiva perstans.

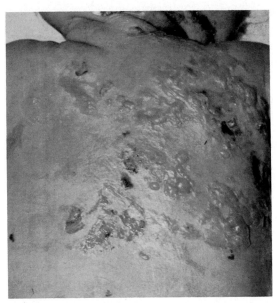

Figure 28–67. Bullous mastocytosis. (Courtesy of Dr. M. Orkin.)

the entire surface. In addition, he had bluish nodules on the trunk.

Telangiectasia Macularis Eruptiva Perstans. This is a persistent, pigmented, asymptomatic macular eruption, with a slightly reddish tinge. Often little or no telangiectasia is evident. It was originally described by Weber and Rust. This form is a benign disorder, of cosmetic import only, in the great majority of cases, although bone lesions and peptic ulcer disease are not uncommon. Darier's sign may not be demonstrable.

Systemic Mastocytosis. Mast cell proliferation not only may occur in the skin but may involve such organs as the lymph nodes, gastrointestinal system, bones, blood, liver, and spleen. In fact, any organ system except the central nervous system may be affected. The process may be progressive or remain stationary. Skin lesions are mostly of the nodular type, and the bone lesions are usually asymptomatic, with x-rays showing areas of radiolucency and radiodensity. A mast cell infiltrate may be present in the bone marrow, and mast cell leukemia may rarely develop. Ridell et al described increased mast cells in the bone marrow, either diffusely or focally, and increased urinary levels of telemethylimidazole acetic acid, as diagnostic of systemic mastocytosis. Cooper et al reviewed malignancies occurring in urticaria pigmentosa, and concluded that nonmast-cell leukemias and lymphomas may complicate this disease.

The gastrointestinal tract may show mucosal changes, which appear to be distinctive. Abdominal pain, nausea, and vomiting are frequently present.

Systemic mastocytosis occurs most frequently in the adult, with about 10 per cent of the juvenile cases going on to systemic involvement.

Excess histamine from the mast cells is believed responsible for reactions, including flushing, headache, and may be manifested by

hematemesis, epistaxis, melena, and ecchymoses. It is believed that elevated plasma heparin levels may be responsible for these signs. Anemia, leukopenia, and thrombocytopenia, with increased prothrombin time, are known to occur.

Malignant mast cell reticulosis occurs when overwhelming infiltration of mast cells in the various organs disturbs their normal functions. Rarely, the cutaneous-visceral type of mast cell reticulosis may be fatal. This is more likely to occur in adults; however, extensive systemic infiltration may produce death in infants also. Death from mast cell leukemia has been reported.

Familial Urticaria Pigmentosa. Mastocytosis of any kind is rarely familial. However, Martin James et al reported cases, in sisters, which were characterized by giant granules, up to 5.8 μm in diameter (mean, 1.58 μm). Such large granules have not been previously described in human skin. Fowler et al reviewed 47 reported cases of familial mastocytosis and concluded that it was usually transmitted by autosomal dominant inheritance with reduced expressivity, although other patterns may occur.

BIOCHEMICAL STUDIES. Human mast cells have been shown to contain histamine. Excess histamine is released from the mast cells into the blood stream. At this time, Demis points out, flushing, tachycardia, hypotension, headache, and gastrointestinal symptoms may occur. The increased amounts of histamine produce histaminuria. Keyzer et al found that while 60 per cent of patients with systemic mastocytosis have an elevated 24-hour urine histamine level, the histamine metabolites methylhistamine and methylimidazole acetic acid are more sensitive and specific indicators.

In 1980 Roberts et al made the important discovery that prostaglandin D_2 was elevated to 120 times normal in one patient and 18 times normal in another. They were able to reduce this about 80 per cent by giving 975 mg of aspirin four times a day. Caution is required: aspirin is probably a histamine releaser, and should not be started in mastocytosis until full doses of H_1 and H_2 blockers have been instituted, and then begun only gradually, and slowly increased. In 1984 Kendall et al were led to the diagnosis of mastocytosis in a case of intractable severe pruritus without characteristic skin lesions by the finding of a PGD_2 metabolite in over 15 times the expected amount in 24-hour urine specimens.

Tissue mast cells also contain heparin, but 5-hydroxytryptamine (serotonin) has not been demonstrated conclusively in human tissue.

Asboe-Hansen and Clausen have demonstrated that mastocytosis is associated with the excretion of acid mucopolysaccharides in the urine. Chondroitin sulfate and hyaluronic acid are probably among the constituents. Heparin was not found in the urine in their studies.

Frieri and associates at the National Institutes of Health reported in 1982 finding an abnormal prebetalipoprotein band in all of six patients with systemic mastocytosis, and in one of four patients with urticaria pigmentosa.

Meggs et al reported the finding of oligoclonal IgG in all four patients with malignant mastocytosis (out of a group of 20) and in only two of 15 patients with benign mastocytosis.

HISTOPATHOLOGY. The typical lesion, histologically, shows a dense dermal aggregate of large mononuclear cells with abundant basophilic cytoplasm. When these large mononuclear cells are stained with Giemsa, azure A, or polychrome toluidine blue, the metachromatic granules are observed. Kasper et al describe a method of counting tissue mast cells using morphometric point counting and a conjugated avidin stain which is useful in establishing the diagnosis.

When blisters are present, the roof of the vesicle or bulla is subepidermal. The mast cells collect in a band below the vesicle and to the sides in the upper dermis.

DIAGNOSIS. The typical case of cutaneous mastocytosis is easily diagnosed. The presence of solitary or multiple pigmented papules or nodules that urticate when irritated by stroking or scratching is suggestive of the diagnosis. This is confirmed by biopsy of the lesion with the demonstration of numerous mast cells. The bullous and vesicular lesions may be difficult to diagnose; however, scrapings from the base of the bulla when stained with Giemsa or Wright stain will show mast cells in profusion.

Keyzer et al reported finding persistently elevated levels of histamine and two of its major metabolites, N-methylhistamine and N-methylimidazole acetic acid, in eight patients with mastocytosis. Elevated levels also occur in chronic myelocytic leukemia and polycythemia vera.

DIFFERENTIAL DIAGNOSIS. Histologically cutaneous mastocytosis is differentiated from Letterer-Siwe disease and eosinophilic granuloma.

Clinically the solitary mastocytoma may most frequently resemble the pigmented nevus or juvenile xanthogranuloma. Urtication establishes the diagnosis.

The disseminated lesions are also distinctive enough to give little or no difficulty in the diagnosis. The nodular form may resemble the xanthomas; however, the presence of urtication is distinctive.

The vesicular and bullous lesions are distinguished from various hereditary and nonhereditary bullous diseases and bullous impetigo.

PROGNOSIS. In all forms of cutaneous mastocytosis without systemic involvement the prognosis is good. In children about one half of the cases clear completely. The others improve or persist indefinitely. The solitary mastocytoma involutes spontaneously, usually within three years of onset.

TREATMENT. Only symptomatic relief may be achieved. Antihistaminics—both H_1 and H_2 blockers—and the antiserotonin drugs such as cyproheptadine (Periactin) may alleviate urtication, pruritus, and flushing.

Christophers reported complete clearing of urticaria pigmentosa—except in small shielded control areas—by oral methoxsalen and UVA (PUVA) therapy, in all of 10 patients so treated. Granerus et al confirmed Christophers' results and also showed that a significant diminution of a major histamine metabolite in the urine occurred at the same time. Zarnetzki et al also found PUVA helpful, but only temporarily.

Dalovich reported control of lifelong diarrhea in systemic mastocytosis by orally administered disodium cromoglycate. Cromolyn sodium (disodium cromoglycate) was also successful in the hands of Evans et al and Welch et al, even though Soter failed to show any diminution of histamine in the urine of treated patients, or in their eosinophilia. Welch gave 20 mg twice a day to a 19-month-old boy, and slowly increased it to 100 mg per day in three divided doses, orally. A bullous case in a 9-month-old girl required 160 to 200 mg daily. In the study by Frieri et al, there was a suggestion that cromolyn is more effective against gastrointestinal manifestations, and the antihistamines better against the cutaneous ones. A single dose of mithramycin resulted in the disappearance of bone pain in one patient, but had little effect on histamine release symptomatology.

Fairley et al have reported a response to nifedipine, an oral calcium-channel blocker, in a dose of 10 mg three times a day. All symptoms ceased within 24 hours. It presumably acts by raising the mast cells' threshold for degranulation.

Burton et al reported that intralesional triamcinolone or potent topical steroids under occlusion cleared cutaneous lesions for long periods. Topical corticosteroids may be valuable in treatment, but clearly one must watch out for systemic effects.

Burklow et al emphasized avoidance of chemical degranulators of mast cells: opiates, large doses of thiamine, polymyxin antibiotics, and D-tubocurarine.

Barton J, et al: Treatment of urticaria pigmentosa with corticosteroids. Arch Dermatol 1985, 121:1516.
Burklow SL, et al: Mastocytosis: one year's experience. South Med J 1987, 80:51.
Idem: Mastocytosis. South Med J 1987, 80:51.
Cainelli T, et al: Monozygotic twins discordant for cutaneous mastocytosis. Arch Dermatol 1983, 119:1021.
Caplan RM: The natural course of urticaria pigmentosa. Arch Dermatol 1963, 87:146.
Christophers E, et al: PUVA therapy for urticaria pigmentosa. Br J Dermatol 1978, 98:701.
Cooper AF, et al: Hematologic malignancies occurring in patients with urticaria pigmentosa. JAAD 1982, 7:215.
Czarnetzki BM, et al: Phototherapy for urticaria pigmentosa. Arch Dermatol Res 1985, 277:105.
Idem: Bone marrow findings in adult patients with urticaria pigmentosa. JAAD 1988, 18:45.
Evans S, et al: Bullous urticaria pigmentosa and sodium cromoglycate. Acta Derm Venereol (Stockh) 1981, 61:572.
Fairley JA, et al: Urticaria pigmentosa responsive to nifedipine. JAAD 1984, 11:740.
Fenske NA, et al: Congenital bullous urticaria pigmentosa. Arch Dermatol 1985, 121:115.
Fowler JF, et al: Familial urticaria pigmentosa. Arch Dermatol 1986, 122:80.
Frieri M, et al: Comparison of the therapeutic efficacy of cromolyn

sodium with that of combined chlorpheniramine and cimetidine in systemic mastocytosis. Am J Med 1985, 78:9.

Idem: An abnormal beta-lipoprotein in patients with systemic mastocytosis. Ann Intern Med 1982, 97:220.

Gordon M, Solitary mastocytosis. Cutis 1971, 7:457.

Granerus G, et al: Decreased urinary histamine metabolite after PUVA treatment of urticaria pigmentosa. J Invest Dermatol 1984, 76:1.

James MP, et al: Familial urticaria with giant mast-cell granules. Arch Dermatol 1981, 117:713.

Kasper CS, et al: Quantification of cutaneous mast cells using morphometric point counting and a conjugated avidin stain. JAAD 1987, 16:326.

Kendall ME, et al: Cutaneous mastocytosis without clinically obvious skin lesions. JAAD 1984, 10:903.

Keyzer JJ, et al: Improved diagnosis of mastocytosis. N Engl J Med 1983, 309:1603.

Lavker RM, et al: Cutaneous mast cell depletion results from topical corticosteroid usage. J Immunol 1985, 135:2368.

Mahood JM, et al: Forty years of diarrhea in a patient with urticaria pigmentosa. Acta Derm Venereol (Stockh) 1982, 62:264; Derm Caps & Com 1983, 1:1.

Meggs WF, et al: Oligoclonal immunoglobulins in mastocytosis. Ann Intern Med 1985, 103:894; Derm Caps & Com 1986, 6:6.

Müller UR, et al: Anaphylaxis after hymenoptera stings in 3 patients with urticaria pigmentosa. J Allergy Clin Immunol 1983, 72:685.

Nickel WR: Clinical spectrum of mastocytosis (urticaria pigmentosa) in man. Arch Dermatol 1967, 96:364.

O'Connell BM, et al: Pigmented papules in the axilla. Arch Dermatol 1988, 124:1421.

Orkin M, et al: Bullous mastocytosis. Arch Dermatol 1970, 101:547.

Parks A, et al: Reddish-brown macules with telangiectasia and pruritus. Arch Dermatol 1988, 124:429.

Prens EP, et al: A rare clinical manifestation of localized cutaneous mastocytosis. JAAD 1986, 15:291.

Ridell B, et al: The bone marrow in urticaria pigmentosa and systemic mastocytosis. Arch Dermatol 1986, 122:422.

Roberts LJ II, et al: Increased production of prostaglandin D_2 in patients with systemic mastocytosis. N Engl J Med 1980, 303:1400; Derm Caps & Com 1981, 4:8.

Schwartz LB, et al: Tryptase levels as an indicator of mast-cell activation in systemic anaphylaxis and mastocytosis. N Engl J Med 1987, 316:1622.

Travis WD, et al: Adult-onset urticaria pigmentosa and systemic mast cell disease. Am J Clin Pathol 1985, 84:710.

Vire G, et al: Urticaria pigmentosa and natural sunlight. JAAD 1986, 14:687.

Webb TA, et al: Systemic mast cell disease. Cancer 1982, 49:927.

Welch EA, et al: Treatment of bullous mastocytosis with disodium cromoglycate. JAAD 1983, 9:349.

DERMATOFIBROMA
(Histiocytoma Cutis)

This common nodular skin lesion has various names because of various interpretations of the histologic findings. Some of these names are fibroma durum, nodulus cutaneus, subepidermal nodular fibrosis, dermatofibroma lenticulare, and sclerosing hemangioma.

CLINICAL FEATURES. The appearance is usually sufficiently characteristic to permit clinical diagnosis. It is generally a single round or ovoid papule or nodule about 1 cm in diameter which is reddish brown, sometimes with a yellowish hue. The surface may be slightly scaly. The sharply circumscribed nodule is more evident upon palpation than is ex-

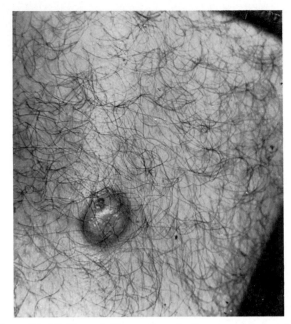

Figure 28–68. Dermatofibroma 2 cm in diameter on inner thigh.

pected from inspection. The larger lesions may present an abrupt elevation at the border to form an exteriorized tumor resting on a sessile base.

The lesions may be elevated or slightly depressed. The hard nodule is adherent to the overlying epidermis, which may be thinner from pressure or even indented, so that there is a dell-like depression over the nodule. In such cases one sees only the depression but on palpation finds the true nature of the lesion. Fitzpatrick proposed the term "dimple sign"

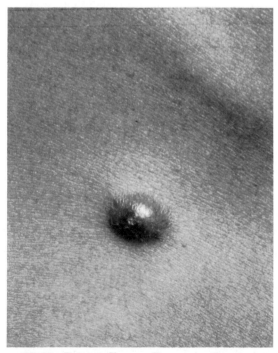

Figure 28–69. Dermatofibroma (8 mm in diameter) on the infraclavicular area of a 12-year-old boy.

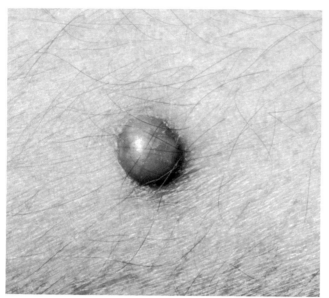

Figure 28–70. Dermatofibroma on the leg. (Courtesy of Dr. Axel W. Hoke.)

for the depression created over a dermatofibroma by grasping it gently between thumb and forefinger.

Dermatofibromas seldom occur in children; they are encountered mostly in middle-aged adults. The size varies from 4 to 15 mm. After reaching this size growth ceases and the harmless lump remains stationary. The principal locations are on the lower extremities, above the elbows, or on the sides of the trunk.

Newman and Walter reported four cases of multiple dermatofibromas in patients with systemic lupus erythematosus receiving prednisone or azathioprine, or both. Lin et al reported three black women with multiple dermatofibromas and SLE; two developed them prior to treatment. Bargman et al reported a patient with myasthenia gravis, under therapy with prednisone and cyclophosphamide, who developed multiple dermatofibromas.

ETIOLOGY. It is suspected that many of these are initiated by various injuries to the skin, such as insect bites.

HISTOPATHOLOGY. The changes in the epidermis are secondary and may be those of pressure atrophy or of acanthosis and hyperkeratosis. In the dermis there is a mass composed of close whorls of fibrous tissue in which are numerous cells with large nuclei rich in chromatin, or elongated spindle cells. The elongated cells are fibroblasts and myofibroblasts. Small or large amounts of pigment, hemosiderin, may be present, or alternatively foam cells and lipid deposits may be seen. There is a great variation in the vascular components. Rarely the vascularization is pronounced and suggests a kind of hemangioma. The tumor is not well circumscribed, and may extend into adjacent structures, especially in the subcutaneous fat.

Goette and Helwig have confirmed Allen's finding of basal cell carcinomas and basal cell carcinomalike changes overlying dermatofibromas; but much more frequently, reactive changes such as acanthosis and pseudoepitheliomatous hyperplasia are seen.

DIFFERENTIAL DIAGNOSIS. The clinical appearance of the lesion and its location, chiefly on the lower extremities and also on the forearms, are distinctive. Clinically granular cell myoblastoma, dermatofibrosis lenticularis disseminata, clear cell acanthoma, and melanoma are some of the lesions to be considered. At times only a biopsy can differentiate these.

Progressive enlargement beyond 2 or 3 cm in diameter suggests a malignant fibrous histiocytoma, and biopsy excision is indicated.

TREATMENT. These lesions do not require treatment, unless they grow, when they may require excision. Involution may occur within a few years if the lesion is left alone. Simple reassurance is suggested.

Bargman HB, et al: Multiple dermatofibromas in a patient with myasthenia gravis treated with prednisone and cyclophosphamide. JAAD 1986, 14:351.

Goette DK, et al: Basal cell carcinomas and basal cell carcinomalike changes overlying dermatofibroma. Arch Dermatol 1975, 111:589.

Hendricks WM: Dermatofibroma occurring in a smallpox scar. JAAD 1987, 16:146.

Lannigan SW, et al: Cryotherapy for dermatofibromas. Clin Exp Dermatol 1987, 12:121.

Lin RY, et al: Multiple dermatofibromas and systemic lupus erythematosus. Cutis 1986, 31:45.

Page EH, et al: Atrophic dermatofibroma and dermatofibrosarcoma protuberans. JAAD 1987, 17:947.

Senear FE, et al: Histiocytoma cutis. Arch Dermatol Syph 1936, 33:209.

DERMATOFIBROSARCOMA PROTUBERANS

Dermatofibrosarcoma protuberans is characterized by bulky, protuberant, neoplastic masses that look like infected keloids. They occur chiefly on the thorax and abdominal wall. Of 30 lesions reported by Gutierrez et al, 20 were on the trunk, four on the proximal limbs, and five on the head or neck.

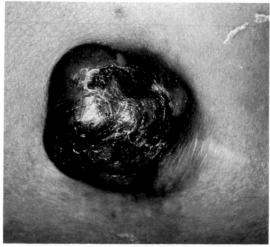

Figure 28–71. Dermatofibrosarcoma protuberans.

The disease begins with one or multiple elevated, erythematous, firm, nodules or plaques associated often with a purulent exudate or with ulceration. Patients, usually middle-aged, complain of a firm painless lump in the skin, which has been slowly increasing in size for several years.

The course is slowly progressive, with pain becoming prominent as the lesion grows, and frequent recurrence after initial surgical intervention. In a series studied by Taylor et al of 115 cases, 49 per cent had local recurrence after surgical resection. There is little tendency for metastasis to develop. The severe pain, contractures, and invalidism gradually deplete the general health. Volpe et al reported the eighth case to metastasize in 1983; the patient died with metastases to lymph nodes, bones, and lungs.

Histologically, the tumor shows a subepidermal fibrotic plaque with uniform spindle cells and variable vascular spaces. In many instances there is a "cartwheel" pattern of spindle cell arrangement surrounding a central area of collagen. Giant cells and histiocytes are also present but only in small numbers. Gutierrez and associates found 30 cases among 2570 sarcomas, in 25 years in Colombia: 11 in males (one was an 8-year-old boy) and 19 in women (one was 13). Both tropocollagen and collagen were abundant. Electron microscopic studies favor a fibroblastic origin, and several lesions have stained positively for vimentin, an intermediate filament protein of mesenchymal cells.

The differential diagnosis, especially in the early stage, is that of keloid and a large dermatofibroma.

Extensive surgical excision is the best form of treatment, since these tumors are radioresistant. Mohs and Robinson have reported successful excision by Mohs's procedure: none of their nine patients had had a recurrence within five years.

Gutierrez G, et al: Dermatofibrosarcoma protuberans. Int J Dermatol 1984, 23:396.

Hashimoto K, et al: Dermatofibrosarcoma protuberans. Arch Dermatol 1974, 110:874.

McLelland J, et al: Dermatofibrosarcoma protuberans arising in a BCG vaccination scar. Arch Dermatol 1988, 124:496.

Miettinen M, et al: Antibodies to intermediate filament proteins. Arch Dermatol 1985, 121:736.

Page EH, et al: Atrophic dermatofibroma and dermatofibromasarcoma protuberans. JAAD 1987, 17:947.

Robinson J: Dermatofibrosarcoma protuberans resected by Mohs surgery. JAAD 1985, 12:1093.

Roses DF, et al: Surgical treatment of dermatofibromasarcoma protuberans. Surg Gynecol Obstet 1986, 162:449.

Taylor HB, et al: Dermatofibrosarcoma protuberans. Cancer 1962, 15:717.

NODULAR FASCIITIS
(Nodular Pseudosarcomatous Fasciitis)

Also known as *subcutaneous pseudosarcomatous fibromatosis*, or *proliferative fasciitis*, this benign mesenchymal neoplasm occurs most often on the arms. Clinically a firm, solitary, sometimes tender nodule develops in the deep fascia, and often extends into the subcutaneous tissue. It measures usually 1 to 4 cm in diameter. The lesion appears suddenly over a period of a few weeks, without apparent cause, in normal, healthy persons. Of 49 cases reviewed by Lubritz and Ichinose, all were adults; all lesions were solitary 1–2-cm nodules on the arm; and less than a third were tender. Chung and Entzinger reported a study of 53 cases, and Shimizu reported 250 cases in 1984. Sex distribution was equal, and the average age at onset was 39.

Microscopic findings consist of myxoid, fibroblastic, and capillary proliferations. Lymphocytic-histiocytic infiltration is present, with many normal-looking mitotic figures. On electron microscopic examination, the component cells in the neoplasm have proved to be myofibroblasts.

The proper treatment is complete excision. Recurrence is rare, and the prognosis is excellent.

Cranial fasciitis of childhood is an uncommon variant of nodular fasciitis manifesting as a rapidly enlarging mass in the subcutaneous tissue of the scalp, which may invade the cranium. It occurs in infants and children, resembles nodular fasciitis histologically, and usually does not recur after surgical excision.

Bernstein KE, et al: Nodular (pseudosarcomatous) fasciitis. Cancer 1982, 49:1668.

Cartwright LE, et al: Rapidly growing asymptomatic subcutaneous nodules. Arch Dermatol 1988, 124:1559.

Chung EB, et al: Proliferative fasciitis. Cancer 1975, 36:1450.

Lauer DH, et al: Cranial fasciitis of childhood. Cancer 1980, 45:401.

Lubritz RR, et al: Nodular fasciitis. Cutis 1975, 15:43.

Patterson JW, et al: Cranial fasciitis. Arch Dermatol 1989, 125:674.

Shimizu S, et al: Nodular fasciitis: an analysis of 250 patients. Pathology 1984, 16:161.

Wirman JA: Nodular fasciitis, a lesion of myofibroblasts. Cancer 1976, 38:2378.

FIBROSARCOMA

Fibrosarcoma usually arises in the subcutaneous fat, where it forms a hard, irregular mass covered by normal epidermis. As the tumor continues to develop, it becomes firm and irregular on palpation and the overlying skin assumes a purplish or brown-red color. Satellite nodules, and ultimately metastases, may appear, but often the growth is slow and the tumor remains localized for years.

These tumors may arise secondary to scarring inflammatory reactions such as chronic radiodermatitis, scars of lupus vulgaris, xeroderma pigmentosum, or burns.

Histologically, the tumor is composed of densely packed, anaplastic spindle-shaped or round cells which vary in staining qualities as well as in the size and shape of their nuclei and cytoplasm. Mitotic figures tend to be bizarre, unlike those seen in pseudosarcomas. The nuclei are mostly spindle-shaped and tend to form bundles or interlacing whorls. In highly malignant tumors collagen is usually sparse.

Wide excisional surgery is the treatment of choice. Recent data place the probability of surviving five years at 60 per cent.

Chung EB, et al: Infantile fibrosarcoma. Cancer 1976, 38:729.
Pritchard DJ, et al: Fibrosarcoma. Cancer 1974, 33:888.
Soule EH, et al: Fibrosarcoma in infants and children. Cancer 1977, 40:1711.

ATYPICAL FIBROXANTHOMA (AFX)

Atypical fibroxanthoma of the skin is a low-grade malignancy related to malignant fibrous histiocytoma, which it resembles histologically. Its smaller size and more superficial location account largely for its more favorable prognosis. The lesion occurs chiefly on the sun-exposed parts of the head or neck in white persons over 50. The tumor is a small, firm nodule often with an eroded or crusted surface without characteristic morphologic features. Fretzin and Helwig's series of 140 patients averaged 67 years of age. A clinical variant, found in 25 per cent of their cases, occurred in a subset with an average age of 39; it occurred as a slowly enlarging tumor on a covered area.

The lesion develops in the dermis and is separated from the epidermis by a thin band of collagen. The tumor consists of bizarre spindle cells mingled with atypical histiocytes. Some spindle cells have a vesicular nucleus. The cytoplasm may be vacuolated to resemble the xanthoma cell. Mitotic figures, prominent eosinophilic nucleoli, and the presence of "biphasic" tumor cell population are characteristic findings. S-100 staining is sparse as compared to melanoma, and prekeratin staining is negative: this helps to distinguish AFX from squamous cell carcinoma.

The treatment of choice is complete surgical excision. While the prognosis is excellent, local recurrence after inadequate excision is usual, and five cases of metastasizing AFX have been reported.

Dahl I: Atypical fibroxanthoma of the skin. Acta Pathol Microbiol Immunol Scand 1976, 84:183.
Fretzin DF, et al: Atypical fibroxanthoma of the skin. Cancer 1973, 31:1541.
Goette DK, et al: Atypical fibroxanthoma masquerading as pyogenic granuloma. Arch Dermatol 1976, 112:1155.
Gonzalesi S, et al: Atypical fibrous histiocytoma. Pathol Res Pract 1982, 174:379.
Kemp JD, et al: Metastasizing atypical fibroxanthoma coexistent with chronic lymphocytic leukemia. Arch Dermatol 1978, 114:1533.
Kuwano H, et al: Atypical fibroxanthoma distinguishable from spindle cell carcinoma in sarcoma-like skin lesions. Cancer 1985, 55:172.

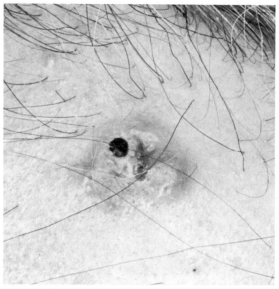

Figure 28–72. Atypical fibroxanthoma.

Pattterson JW, et al: Atypical fibroxanthoma in a patient with xeroderma pigmentosum. Arch Dermatol 1987, 123:1066.
Wesson SK: Solitary nodule on the foot of a 37-year-old man. Arch Dermatol 1986, 122:1325.
Winkelmann RK, et al: Atypical fibroxanthoma. Arch Dermatol 1985, 121:753.

MALIGNANT FIBROUS HISTIOCYTOMA (MFH) (Malignant Histiocytoma)

This lesion resembles dermatofibrosarcoma protuberans: both may present as a protruding rounded tumor from one to several cm in diameter, often reddish or dusky, and progressively enlarging. MFH arises more deeply and is more likely to appear subcutaneous. One third occur on the thigh or buttock. Peak incidence is in the seventh decade. They sometimes (as in the cases of Goette et al and Yamamoto et al) arise in an area of radiodermatitis, or (as in the patient reported by Routh et al) in a chronic ulceration.

Pleomorphic cellular elements and bizarre mitotic figures are characteristic, in contrast to the tightly whorled or "cartwheel" pattern, with uniform cells, seen in dermatofibroma. Atypical fibroxanthomas are smaller and more superficial tumors of the dermis, compared to the deeper or even subcutaneous location of MFH. Epithelioid sarcoma, while it shares with MFH the presence of both polygonal and spindle cell types, lacks the latter's large, bizarre, multinucleated cell types. Several histologic variants of MFH have been described, including myxoid, inflammatory, angiomatoid, and giant cell types. The cells stain positively for vimentin.

The prognosis in MFH is related to the site: deeper and more proximally located tumors have a poorer prognosis. Angiomatoid variants in younger patients have a poorer outlook. The myxoid variant is less prone to metastasize. An especially poor prognosis attends tumors arising in sites of radiodermatitis. Local recurrence after excision is common, and metastasis to the lungs is a frequent cause of death.

Enzinger FM: Angiomatoid malignant fibrous histiocytoma. Cancer 1979, 44:2147.

Farber JN, et al: Malignant fibrous histiocytoma arising from discoid lupus erythematosus. Arch Dermatol 1988, 124:114.

Goette DK, et al: Post-irradiation malignant fibrous histiocytoma. Arch Dermatol 1985, 122:535.

Grabski WJ, et al: Malignant fibrous histiocytoma. J Assoc Milit Dermatol 1985, 11:58.

Kearney MM, et al: Malignant fibrous histiocytoma. Cancer 1980, 45:167.

Routh A, et al: Malignant fibrous histiocytoma arising from chronic ulcer. Arch Dermatol 1985, 122:529.

Weiss SW, et al: Malignant fibrous histiocytoma. Cancer 1978, 41:2250.

Yamamoto Y, et al: Angiomatoid malignant fibrous histiocytoma associated with marked bleeding arising in chronic radiodermatitis. Arch Dermatol 1985, 122:275.

EPITHELIOID SARCOMA

Epithelioid sarcoma occurs chiefly in young adults, the age of onset usually being from 20 to 40 years of age. Two thirds are in men. Nearly all lesions are on the extremities, half of them on the hands or wrists.

The tumor grows slowly among fascial structures and tendons, often with central necrosis of the tumor nodules and ulceration of the overlying skin. Recurrence after attempted excision occurs in two out of three cases, and late metastasis occurs in one out of three cases. Heenan et al reported two cases and reviewed 10 in 1986, with durations ranging from four months to 14 years, emphasizing the wide variation in rate of growth. Initial clinical diagnoses included granuloma annulare, rheumatoid nodule, ganglion, fibroma, and inclusion dermoid cyst. It has also been mistaken for palisading granuloma, chronic inflammation, and squamous cell carcinoma, according to Padilla et al, who reported a carefully studied case and reviewed the literature in 1985.

Histologically, irregular nodular masses of large, deeply acidophilic polygonal cells merge with spindle cells and are frequently associated with large amounts of hyalinized collagen.

Cure may be achieved by wide local excision in the early stage of the disease.

Enzinger FM: Epithelioid sarcoma. Cancer 1970, 26:1029.

Heenan PJ, et al: Epithelioid sarcoma. Am J Dermatopathol 1986, 8:95.

Manivel JC, et al: Epithelioid sarcoma. Am J Clin Pathol 1987, 87:319.

Padilla RS, et al: Epithelioid sarcoma. Arch Dermatol 1985, 121:389.

Puissegur-Lupo ML, et al: Epithelioid sarcoma. Arch Dermatol 1985, 121:394.

Shelley WB: Epithelioid sarcoma, in *Consultations in Dermatology II*. Philadelphia, WB Saunders, 1974, p 70.

Shmookler BM, et al: Superficial epithelioid sarcoma. JAAD 1986, 14:93.

MYXOMAS

These may be considered as two types of lesions, the digital mucous cyst and cutaneous myxomas. The latter may or may not be associated with cardiac myxomas and cutaneous spotty pigmentation.

Digital mucous cysts (mucoceles or "synovial cysts") are taut, shiny, translucent, white-to-pink, dome-shaped lesions characteristically located on the dorsal aspect of the distal interphalangeal articulation. There may be an associated grooving or dystrophy of the nail. Either fingers or toes may be affected. This is an intradermal collection of hyaluronic acid, with no lining present.

Treatment is either by repeated puncturing with a sterile needle and squeezing out the mucin, as recommended by Ernst Epstein; by intralesional steroid injection (after which they recur, as a rule); or as outlined by Arnijo, excision and grafting. They also disappear in about six weeks if the distal interphalangeal joint is splinted (Arnold).

These should be differentiated from *ganglions*, which occur most frequently over the wrists, are herniations of joint linings, are deeper in location, and are often associated with exostoses. These have a lining to the cavity, and require excision and grafting with removal of the cyst, the lining, and the pedicle to the joint. They are also discussed in Chapter 9, Mucinoses.

Cutaneous myxomas may be solitary, and appear as flesh-colored nodules on the face, trunk, or extremities. However, Carney et al have reported 41 patients with a disorder they refer to as myxomas, spotty pigmentation, and endocrine overactivity. This has also been reported under the eponyms NAME (*N*evi, *A*trial myxoma, *M*yxoid neurofibromas, and *E*phelides) and LAMB (*L*entigines, *A*trial myxoma, *M*ucocutaneous myxomas, *B*lue nevi), and simply as *cutaneous lentiginosis with atrial myxoma*.

The complex Carney et al have described consists of patients who have two or more of the following: 1) cardiac myxomas (79 per cent); 2) cutaneous myxomas (not myxoid neurofibromas) (45 per cent); 3) mammary myxoid fibromas (30 per cent); 4) spotty mucocutaneous pigmentation, including lentiginoses and blue nevi (not ephelides) (65 per cent); 5) primary pigmented nodular adrenocortical disease (45 per cent); 6) testicular tumors (56 per cent of male patients); and 7) pituitary-growth-hormone-secreting tumors (10 per cent).

The cutaneous myxomas occur as small (less than 1 cm), multiple, skin-colored papules having a predilection for development by a mean age of 18 years, and a tendency to occur on the ears, eyelids, and nipples. The lentigines are prominent on the face, lips, and genital mucosa. This condition is probably autosomal dominantly inherited. Recognition of this syndrome, with diagnosis and removal of the atrial myxomas, can be lifesaving.

Arnijo M: Mucoid cysts of the finger. J Dermatol Surg Oncol 1981, 7:317.

Atherton DJ, et al: A syndrome of various cutaneous pigmentoid lesions, myxoid neurofibromas, and atrial myxomas: the NAME syndrome. Br J Dermatol 1980, 103:421.

Carney JA, et al: Dominant inheritance of the complex of myxomas, spotty pigmentation, and endocrine overactivity. Mayo Clin Proc 1986, 61:165.

Idem: The complex of myxomas, spotty pigmentation, and endocrine overactivity. Medicine (Baltimore) 1985, 64:270.

Idem: Cutaneous myxomas. Arch Dermatol 1986, 122:790.

Epstein E: A simple technique for managing digital mucous cysts. Arch Dermatol 1979, 115:1315.

Huerter CJ, et al: Treatment of digital mucous cysts with carbon dioxide laser vaporization. J Dermatol Surg Oncol 1987, 13:723.

Johnson WC, et al: Cutaneous focal mucinosis. Arch Dermatol 1966, 93:13.

Idem: Cutaneous myxoid cysts. JAMA 1965, 191:15.

Macpherson M, et al: Ganglia of the ankle. JAAD 1985, 13:873.

Peterson LL, et al: Lentiginosis associated with a left atrial myxoma. JAAD 1984, 10:337.

Reed OM, et al: Cutaneous lentiginosis with atrial myxoma. JAAD 1986, 15:398.

Rhodes AR, et al: Mucocutaneous lentigines, cardiomucocutaneous myxomas, and multiple blue nevi: the "LAMB" syndrome. JAAD 1984, 10:72.

MYXOSARCOMA

This tumor may arise in the subcutaneous fat and the underlying soft tissues.

Pratilas and Arlen described a primary myxosarcoma on the leg of a 70-year-old man. The tumor, some 13 cm in diameter, consisted of multiple, nontender, pale nodules. This tumor was of two years' duration. A wide and deep excision with grafting was performed.

There is a tendency for local recurrence, and the lesion may rarely metastasize.

Pratilas V, et al: Primary myxosarcoma of the leg. NY J Med 1970, 70:309.

Sponsel KH, et al: Myxoma and myxosarcoma of the soft tissues of the extremities. J Bone Joint Surg (Am) 1952, 34:820.

Vidaillet JH Jr, et al: Syndrome myxoma. Br Heart J 1987, 57:247.

SOLITARY NEUROFIBROMA

The ordinary solitary cutaneous neurofibroma may be 2 to 20 mm in diameter. It is soft, flaccid, and pinkish white. Frequently the soft small tumor can be invaginated as if through a ring in the skin by pressure with the finger (this is called "buttonholing").

Neurofibroma is either solitary or multiple. When solitary (one or two lesions) they are spontaneous tumors without any internal manifestations. When three or more are present, the diagnosis of *neurofibromatosis* is made. This genodermatosis is discussed in Chapter 27. Uncommonly, large pendulous masses occur, in which numerous tortuous, thickened nerves can be felt, which have been likened to a "bag of

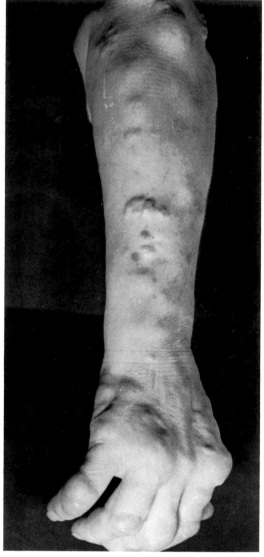

Figure 28–73. Myxosarcoma. (Courtesy of Dr. F. Daniels, Jr.)

worms." These *plexiform neurofibromas*, which often have overlying pigmentation, occur in neurofibromatosis.

The distinctive histopathologic findings are characterized by Winkelmann and Johnson as having three basic features, namely: fibrils, cellular proliferation, and degenerative changes (fatty and myxomatous). The wavy fibrillar tissues with small cells containing ovoid nuclei are arranged in an areolar fashion or are densely packed. Cellular proliferation is in sheets or stellate clumps. Glycosaminoglycans may be greatly increased, and numerous mast cells may be present. Cholinesterase activity is markedly positive in the neurofibromas. Immunochemical staining shows positivity for S-100, vimentin, and myelin basic protein, markers for Schwannian tissue.

Treatment of those lesions that are particularly objectionable is by surgical excision.

Aso M, et al: Immunohistochemical studies of selected skin diseases and tumors using monoclonal antibodies to neurofilament and myelin proteins. Arch Dermatol 1985, 121:736.

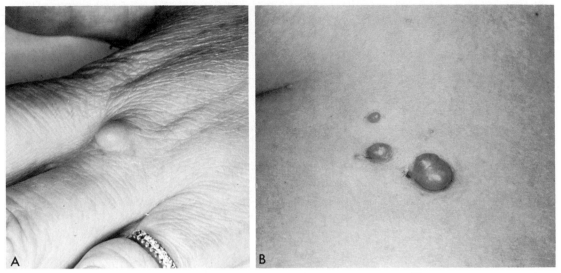

Figure 28–74. A, *Solitary neurofibroma.* B, *Localized neurofibromas.*

Miettinen M, et al: Antibodies to intermediate filament proteins. Arch Dermatol 1985, 121:736.
Oshman RG, et al: A solitary neurofibroma on the finger. Arch Dermatol 1988, 124:1185.
Penneys NS, et al: A survey of cutaneous neural lesions for the presence of myelin basic protein. Arch Dermatol 1984, 120:210.

GRANULAR CELL TUMOR

This was described by Abrikossoff in 1926. It has been called *granular cell myoblastoma* or *schwannoma* for years, but many other synonyms have been used, and Apisarnthanarax, who reported 88 lesions in 16 patients in 1981, prefers "granular cell tumor." About one third of the reported cases have occurred on the tongue, one third involved the skin, and one third occurred in the internal organs. The tumor is usually a well-circumscribed, solitary, firm nodule ranging in size from 5 to 30 mm with a brownish red or flesh tint, depending on the nearness to the surface.

Its surface is usually smooth and glistens, but infrequently it may ulcerate. Although usually soli-tary, it may be multiple in from 7 to 25 per cent of cases. One of Apisarnthanarax's series had 64 lesions in the skin.

The solitary lesion may be located anywhere on the body, but nearly half of all tumors appear on the head or neck. Usually the patients are in the third to fifth decades. About two thirds of patients are black, and two thirds are women. In most cases myoblastoma grows very slowly, and when completely removed does not usually recur. However, local or multicentric recurrence may at times cause confusion in determining if a granular cell tumor is malignant.

The cell of origin has been debated for decades. However, electron microscopic and immunohistochemical studies strongly support a Schwann cell origin. S-100 and myelin protein stains show that the granules are composed of myelin or myelin metabolic products.

The histologic picture is distinctive. The cells are large, pale, and irregularly polygonal, with a poorly defined cellular membrane, and contain coarsely granular cytoplasm. Some of the cells are multinucle-

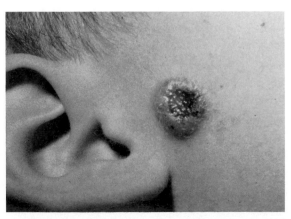

Figure 28–75. Granular tumor cell on cheek of 12-year-old boy.

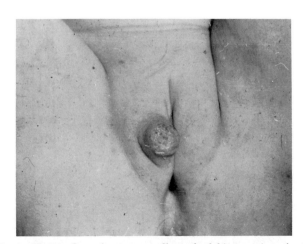

Figure 28–76. Granular tumor cell on the labium majus of a 5-year-old child.

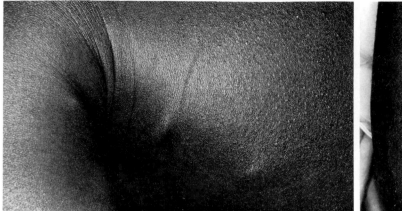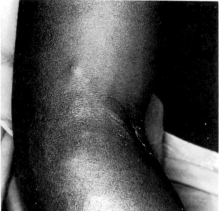

Figures 28–77 and 28–78. Multiple granular cell tumors.

ated or contain vacuoles or small pyknotic or eosinophilic inclusions. At times the arrangement is in cords or sheets, in irregular alveolar masses, or even organoid. The similarity to xanthoma cells has been pointed out. However, with special stains no lipids are demonstrable. Pseudoepitheliomatous hyperplasia is a regular feature, and has often led to a mistaken diagnosis of squamous cell carcinoma associated with xanthoma.

Malignant granular cell tumor is rare. Malignant lesions are much larger, with an average diameter of 9 cm; benign lesions average less than 2 cm. Rapidity of growth and invasion of adjacent tissue are other criteria to be weighed, because the histologic findings are not always reliable.

Aggressive surgery is the treatment of choice, though Baraf and Bender have reported successful treatment with intralesional triamcinolone injections in one of their two patients.

Apisarnthanarax P: Granular cell tumor. JAAD 1981, 5:171.
Berkowitz SF, et al: Granular cell tumor. Cutis 1985, 33:355.
Donhuijsen K, et al: Malignant granular cell tumor. J Cancer Res Clin Oncol 1979, 95:93.
Garancis JC, et al: Granular cell myoblastoma. Cancer 1970, 25:542.
Lack EE, et al: Granular cell tumor. J Surg Oncol 1980, 13:310.
Mukai M: Immunohistochemical localization of S100 protein and peripheral nerve myelin proteins in granular cell tumor. Am J Pathol 1983, 112:139.
Seo IS, et al: Multiple visceral and cutaneous granular cell tumors. Cancer 1984, 53:2104.
Toback AC: Arm tumor resembling a supernumerary nipple. Arch Dermatol 1985, 121:927.
Truhan AP: Firm linear plaque on the lip of a child. Arch Dermatol 1985, 121:1197.

The lesion may be tender or painful, and when scarring has occurred or the distal stump has been removed, a phantom limb syndrome may result. These often occur on the fingers, at sites of amputation of supernumerary digits, or on the sole, usually at the third metatarsal space.

Multiple mucosal neuromas occur as part of Cowden's *multiple mucosal neuroma syndrome* (multiple endocrine neoplasia, type 2b). These patients have a Marfanoid habitus, thickened protruding lips, and multiple neuromas of the oral mucosa (lips, tongue, and gingiva), the conjunctiva, and sometimes the sclera. A few have multiple cutaneous neuromas, usually limited to the face. There is an association with medullary carcinoma of the thyroid and pheochromocytomas.

The *palisaded, encapsulated neuroma* of the skin is a solitary, large, encapsulated tumor, usually of the face. It is a slow-growing, flesh-colored, dome-shaped, firm lesion usually appearing around the mouth or nose. It closely resembles a basal cell carcinoma or an intradermal nevus.

Ayala F, et al: Multiple endocrine neoplasia type IIb. Dermatologica 1981, 162:292.
Dover JS, et al: Palisaded encapsulated neuromas. Arch Dermatol 1989, 125:386.
Gorlin RJ, et al: Multiple mucoid neuromas, pheochromocytomas, and medullary carcinoma of the thyroid. Cancer 1968, 22:293.
Holm TW, et al: Multiple cutaneous neuromas. Arch Dermatol 1973, 107:608.
Reed RJ, et al: Palisaded, encapsulated neuromas of the skin. Arch Dermatol 1972, 106:865.
Rubin Z: Cutaneous neuroma. Arch Dermatol 1982, 118:960.

NEUROMA CUTIS

Cutaneous neuromas are uncommon. Three true neuromas exist in the skin: traumatic neuromas, multiple mucosal neuromas, and solitary palisaded encapsulated neuromas.

Traumatic neuromas result from the overgrowth of nerve fibers in the severed ends of peripheral nerves.

NEUROTHEKEOMA
(Axon Sheath Myxoma)

Gallager and Helwig described a benign cutaneous tumor they called a *neurothekeoma*, meaning a tumor of nerve sheath, composed of cords and nests of large cells packed among collagen bundles in close proximity to small nerves. Mitotic figures and nuclear atypia are sometimes seen, but the tumor is benign.

This is probably the same lesion described by Harkin et al in 1969 as an *axon sheath myxoma*. Also, Burket in 1987 reported a case of localized alopecia overlying a tumor in a young girl; hair growth resumed after the tumor was removed. These benign intradermal or subcutaneous tumors occur in childhood, with a high female preponderance, and a predilection for the head, neck, or shoulders.

Burket JM: Alopecia associated with underlying nerve sheath myxomas. JAAD 1987, 16:209.
Enzinger FM, et al: Soft tissue tumors. St. Louis, C. V. Mosby Co., 1983, pp. 615–617.
Gallager RL, et al: Neurothekeoma. Am J Clin Pathol 1980, 74:759.
Isoda M, et al: Neurothekeoma. Cutis 1988, 41:255.

NEURILEMMOMA (Schwannoma)

The neurilemmoma (neurilemoma or schwannoma) is usually a solitary nerve sheath tumor, most often seen in women. Peripheral neurilemmomas occur almost exclusively along the main nerve trunks of the extremities, especially the flexor surface of the arms, wrists, and knees, but they are also seen on the scalp, sides of the neck, and tongue. Sometimes the tumors are multiple and associated with neurofibromatosis.

Other cases, referred to as *multiple cutaneous neurilemmomas*, occur independently from neurofibromatosis, and belong in an entity reviewed by Shishiba et al in 1984, called *neurilemmomatosis*. Of 33 cases reviewed, 22 were male. Age at onset varied from birth to 41 years. There is no genetic component. Three clinical patterns were described: elevated dome-shaped nodules, pale brown indurated macules, and multiple papules coalescing into plaques from 2 to 100 mm broad, with a predilection for the trunk.

On biopsy, Verocay bodies in tumor nests of Antoni type A tissue are seen.

Neurilemmomas occur in many other organs, and brain tumors such as meningiomas, gliomas, and astrocytomas may occur.

The solitary tumor is a nodule from 3 to 30 mm in diameter. It is soft or firm, pale pink or yellowish; it may or may not be painful.

Neurilemmomas are well encapsulated and composed of two types of tissue, referred to as Antoni types A and B. The diagnosis is affirmed by the finding of Verocay bodies. Bodian stain reveals very few or no nerve fibers. Numerous mast cells may be seen within the tumor. S-100, vimentin, and myelin basic protein stains are positive.

Excision is almost invariably curative.

Berger TG, et al: Agminated neurilemmomas. JAAD 1987, 17:891.
Das Guptas TK, et al: Benign solitary schwannoma (neurilemmoma). Cancer 1969, 24:355.
Izumi AK, et al: Von Recklinghausen's disease associated with multiple neurilemmomas. Arch Dermatol 1971, 104:172.
Prevoo R, et al: Multiple cutaneous neurilemmomas with abnormalities of the eyes and congenital rib deformities. JAAD 1987, 17:1054.
Purcell SM, et al: Schwannomatosis. Arch Dermatol 1989, 125:390.
Shishiba T, et al: Multiple cutaneous neurilemmomas as a skin manifestation of neurilemmomatosis. JAAD 1984, 10:744.

INFANTILE NEUROBLASTOMA

Neuroblastoma is the most common malignant tumor of early childhood. Cutaneous nodules are most often seen in younger patients, being present in 32 per cent of infants with the disease. These occur as multiple 2–20-mm firm, blue nodules that, when rubbed, blanch and form a halo of erythema. The blanching persists for one to two hours and is followed by a refractory period of several hours. Biopsy shows clusters of basophilic cells with large nuclear-to-cytoplasmic ratio, surrounded by eosinophilic fine fibrillar material. Two other findings that may be present are periorbital ecchymoses (the so-called *raccoon eyes*) and heterochromia of the irises.

For patients with skin involvement the prognosis is good, with either spontaneous remission or spontaneous transformation into benign ganglioneuromas expected. Lucky et al reported a classic patient.

Lucky AW, et al: Infantile neuroblastoma presenting with cutaneous blanching nodules. JAAD 1982, 6:389.

GANGLIONEUROMA

This tumor has only rarely been described in the skin as an isolated entity. Geffner et al in 1986 described a solitary cutaneous lesion on the abdomen of a 72-year-old woman.

They are composed of mature ganglion cells commingled with fascicles of spindle cells. They arise most often in von Recklinghausen's neurofibromatosis or with neuroblastomas, being tumors of central nervous system or visceral nervous tissue, which usually occur in childhood. The tissue stains positively for both argyrophilic and argentaffin granules.

Collins JP, et al: Ganglioneuromas of the skin. Arch Dermatol 1972, 105:256.
Geffner RE, et al: Ganglioneuroma of the skin. Arch Dermatol 1986, 122:377.

NASAL GLIOMA

Nasal gliomas are rare, benign, congenital tumors which when they occur extranasally are readily confused with hemangiomas. They are encephaloceles, with the histology of astrocytomas. The tumor is

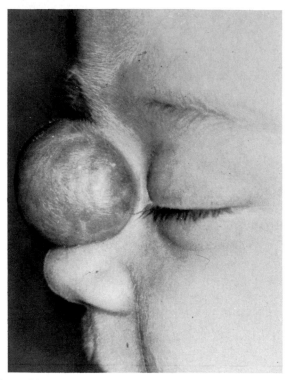

Figure 28–79. Nasal glioma. (Courtesy of Dr. H. C. Christianson.)

usually a firm, incompressible (unlike a hemangioma), reddish blue to purple lesion occurring on the nasal bridge or midline near the root. They may also occur intranasally.

Radiography should be performed to detect possible skull involvement. Neurosurgical consultation is advisable, since some of these lesions are actually encephaloceles. Nasal gliomas differ from encephaloceles in that the latter are connected to the subarachnoid space by a sinus tract, while the former lose this connection prior to birth. Clinically these cannot be differentiated, so biopsy should not be done.

Histologically the nodule consists of glial tissue associated with glial giant cells, fibrous tissue, and numerous blood vessels. It is unencapsulated. Gebhart et al reported a case with electron microscopic studies in 1982.

The lesion does not involute spontaneously.

Christianson HB: Nasal glioma. Arch Dermatol 1966, 93:68.
Gebhart W, et al: Nasal glioma. Int J Dermatol 1982, 21:212.
Kopf AW, et al: Nasal glioma. J Dermatol Surg Oncol 1978, 4:128.

CUTANEOUS MENINGIOMA

This is also known as *psammoma*. Rare cases of primary cutaneous meningiomas have been reported in which small, hard, fibrous, calcified nodules occur along the spine or in the scalp.

Cutaneous meningiomas may develop in the scalp secondary to an intracranial meningioma, either by means of erosion of the skull, or by extension through an operative defect of the skull.

Clinically these lesions have no distinctive appearance. They are firm subcutaneous nodules adherent to the skin.

Diagnosis is made by histologic examination. The tumors consist of strands of cells with large oval vesicular nuclei and granular cytoplasm; these are hyaline bodies *(psammoma bodies)*, which are calcified to some extent. Psammoma bodies have also been found in intradermal nevi, juvenile xanthogranuloma, the pituitary of the fetus and newborn, meninges, choroid plexus, pineal gland, papillary carcinoma of the thyroid, ovarian neoplasms, and mammary intraductal papilloma.

Waterson KW, et al: Meningioma cutis. Int J Dermatol 1970, 9:125.
Weitzner S: Intradermal nevus with psammoma body formation. Arch Dermatol 1968, 98:287.

LIPOMAS

Lipomas are subcutaneous tumors composed of fat tissue, most commonly found on the trunk. They also occur frequently on the neck, forearms, and axillae. They are soft, single or multiple, small or large, lobulated, compressible growths, over which the skin upon traction often becomes dimpled, although otherwise unchanged. They usually stop

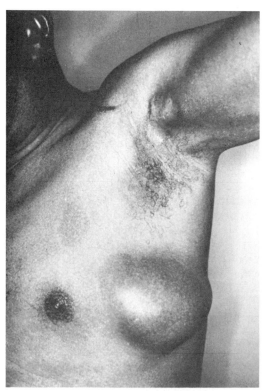

Figure 28–80. Solitary lipoma.

growing after attaining a certain size, to remain stationary indefinitely. Frontalis-associated lipomas of the forehead are relatively large lesions arising either within or deep to the frontalis muscle.

A lipoma located in the midline of the sacral region may be a marker for spinal dysraphism or other embryologic malformation. Other midline lesions, such as tufts of hair ("fawn's tail"), hemangiomas (Cobb's syndrome), skin tags, sinuses, or pigmented lesions should also raise one's suspicion for occult embryologic malformations. At least, x-rays of the lumbosacral region should be obtained. If spinal dysraphism is diagnosed, early treatment may be possible before irreversible damage has occurred. Do not attempt to biopsy a sacrococcygeal lipoma: call a neurosurgeon into consultation. It may be a lipomeningocele, with communicating sinuses to the dura, as in a case reported by Harrist et al.

Histologically, the lipoma is an encapsulated lobulated tumor containing normal fat cells held together by strands of connective tissue.

In the differential diagnosis the epidermoid cyst should always be considered. At times it is difficult to distinguish between the two. Others to be kept in mind are angiolipoma and hibernoma.

Lipomas may be left untreated unless they are large enough to be objectionable. If they are objectionable, trial may be made of intralesional injection of triamcinolone acetonide or hexacetonide in maximum strength into the center of the nodule, in the hope that it will shrink substantially. Far better to have to repeat the injection a time or two than to overdo it and produce an unsightly dimple: inject only a small amount and wait a month or two before repeating it.

Hardin described his method, which consists of introducing a cutting curette through a 3-mm incision over the center of the lipoma and freeing the globular tumor from the surrounding tissue, after which it is compressed laterally and extruded through the incision with gentle traction. Liposuction is another alternative.

Should this fail, simple excision is curative. More advanced surgical technique is necessary to remove the deep lesions on the forehead. Removal of these is discussed in detail by Zitelli and Salasche.

Lipomas should be investigated for malignancy if they become 10 cm in diameter, especially when they occur on the upper thigh.

Multiple Lipomas

Multiple lipomas may occur in groups of two to hundreds of confluent painless tumors of various sizes over any part of the body. These lesions are sometimes painful when growing rapidly.

Three rare conditions are associated with multiple lipomas composed of mature fat cells, with onset in adult life:

Madelung's Disease (Benign Symmetric Lipomatosis, Multiple Symmetric Lipomatosis, Fetthals).

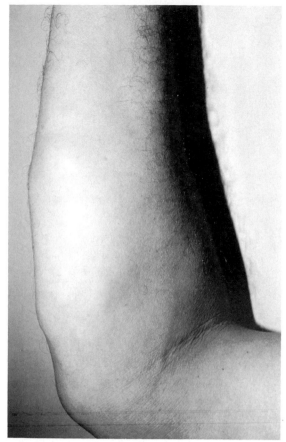

Figure 28–81. Lipomas of arm. (Courtesy of Dr. Axel W. Hoke.)

This occurs most commonly in middle-aged men, who may develop multiple, large, painless, coalescent lipomas around the neck, shoulders, and upper arms.

Dercum's Disease (Adiposis Dolorosa). Obese or corpulent menopausal women may develop symmetric, tender, circumscribed fatty deposits, often accompanied by weakness and psychiatric disturbances. Juhlin obtained relief of pain lasting for weeks in a 60-year-old woman by intravenous infusions of lidocaine, 1.3 gram daily for four days.

Familial Multiple Lipomatosis. In this dominantly inherited syndrome, multiple asymptomatic lipomas of the forearms and thighs appear in the third decade of life. The shoulders and neck are spared, and the lipomas are encapsulated and movable. Leffell et al reviewed the condition in 1986.

Belcher RW, et al: Multiple subcutaneous angiolipomas. Arch Dermatol 1974, 110:583.

Brasfield RD, et al: Liposarcoma. Cancer 1970, 20:2.

Burgdorf WHC, et al: Folded skin with scarring. JAAD 1982, 7:90.

Carlin MC, et al: Multiple symmetric lipomatosis. JAAD 1988, 18:359.

Chung EB, et al: Benign lipoblastomatosis. Cancer 1973, 32:482.

Cocchia D, et al: S100 antigen labels neoplastic cells in liposarcoma and cartilaginous tumors. Virchows Arch (Pathol Anat) 1983, 402:139.

Dardick I: Hibernoma. Human Pathol 1978, 9:321.

Dotz W, et al: Nevus lipomatosus superficialis. Arch Dermatol 1984, 120:376.

Economides NG, et al: Benign symmetric lipomatosis (Madelung's disease). South Med J 1986, 79:1023.

Enzi G, et al: Multiple symmetric lipomatosis. J Clin Invest 1977, 60:1221.

Enzinger FM, et al: Spindle cell lipoma. Cancer 1975, 36:1852.

Field LM: Liposuction surgery for symmetric lipomatosis. JAAD 1988, 18:1370.

Fukamisu H, et al: Large vulvar lipoma. Arch Dermatol 1982, 118:447.

Gardner EW, et al: Folded skin associated with underlying nevus lipomatosus. Arch Dermatol 1979, 115:978.

Gibbs MK, et al: Lipoblastomatosis. Pediatrics 1977, 60:235.

Hall DE, et al: Lumbosacral lesions as markers of occult spinal dysraphism. JAMA 1981, 246:2606.

Hardin FF: A simple technique for removing lipomas. J Dermatol Surg Oncol 1982, 8:316.

Harrist TJ, et al: Unusual sacrococcygeal embryologic malformations with cutaneous manifestations. Arch Dermatol 1982, 118:643.

Hendricks HM, et al: Nevus lipomatosus cutaneus superficialis. Cutis 1982, 29:185.

Herbert AA, et al: Sacral lipomas. Arch Dermatol 1987, 123:711.

Juhlin L: Long-standing pain relief of adiposis dolorosa after intravenous infusion of lidocaine. JAAD 1986, 15:383.

Klein JA, et al: Diffuse lipomatosis and tuberous sclerosis. JAAD 1986, 122:1298.

LaVoo EJ: Noninfiltrating angiolipoma. Arch Dermatol 1982, 118:202.

Leffell DJ, et al: Familial multiple lipomatosis. JAAD 1986, 15:275.

Pursley TV: Nevus lipomatosus cutaneous [sic] superficialis. Int J Dermatol 1983, 32:430.

Ruzicka T, et al: Benign symmetric lipomatosis Launois-Bensaude. JAAD 1987, 17:663.

Salasche SJ, et al: Frontalis-associated lipoma of the forehead. JAAD 1989, 20:462.

Schlappner OLA, et al: Painful and nonpainful piezogenic pedal papules. Arch Dermatol 1972, 106:729.

Shelley WB, et al: Painful feet due to herniations of fat. JAMA 1968, 205:308.

Shmookler BM, et al: Pleomorphic lipoma. Cancer 1981, 47:1126.

Wilson Jones E, et al: Nevus superficialis lipomatosus. Br J Dermatol 1975, 93:121.

Zitelli JA: Subgaleal lipomas. Arch Dermatol 1989, 125:384.

GARDNER'S SYNDROME

This consists of multiple osteomas, fibromas, desmoid tumors, lipomas, fibrosarcomas, epidermal inclusion cysts, and leiomyomas, associated with intestinal polyposis exclusively in the colon and rectum. The coexistence of cutaneous cysts, leiomyomas, and osteomas (mostly on the skull) with intestinal polyposis is frequently not recognized until malignant degeneration of one of the polyps occurs and operative removal brings the syndrome to notice. One half of such patients develop carcinoma of the colon before age 30, and practically all these patients die before 50 unless they have surgical treatment. In general, total colectomy is the safest course to advise.

The bony exostoses occur in 50 per cent of patients, and usually involve the membranous bones of the face and head. Cysts occur in 63 per cent of the patients, which again occur most commonly on the face and in the scalp. Cooper et al found that while histologically these were epidermal inclusion cysts, two thirds had within them foci of pilomatricoma.

Traboulis et al have described pigmented lesions of the ocular fundus in 90 per cent of 41 patients with Gardner's syndrome and 46 per cent of 43 first-degree relatives. They are usually multiple and bilateral, and—having been seen in a three-month-old infant—are probably congenital.

Gardner's syndrome is transmitted as an autosomal dominant disease. In some families polyposis and carcinoma may occur without the skin and bone tumors.

Cooper PH, et al: Pilomatricoma-like changes in the epidermal cysts of Gardner's syndrome. JAAD 1983, 8:639.

Leppard B, et al: Epidermal cysts, polyposis coli, and Gardner's syndrome. Br J Surg 1975, 62:387.

Samitz MH: Clinical significance of skin lesions in the diagnosis of gastrointestinal malignancies. Cutis 1977, 19:649.

Traboulis EI, et al: Prevalence and importance of pigmented ocular fundus lesions in Gardner's syndrome. N Engl J Med 1987, 316:661.

Weary PE, et al: Gardner's syndrome. Arch Dermatol 1964, 90:20.

ANGIOLIPOMA

The angiolipoma is a painful subcutaneous nodule just slightly above the level of the skin, having all the other features of a typical lipoma. It is seen in young adults who have multiple painful lumps in the skin.

Howard and Helwig state that the lesion is an encapsulated fatty tumor with small angiomatous foci; however, no inflammatory features are present. Belcher and associates found numerous mast cells, and large myelinated nerves in the surrounding connective tissue. Multiple subcutaneous angiolipomas, unlike solitary unencapsulated ones, have no invasive or metastatic potential.

PAINFUL PIEZOGENIC PEDAL PAPULES

Shelley and Rawnsley described in 1968 transitory, soft, sometimes painful papules on the sides of the heels, elicited by weight-bearing (hence "piezogenic," produced by pressure) and disappearing when this is stopped. These occur in nearly everyone, but are painful, presumably because of ischemia, in the few persons who complain of the condition. The painful papules are typically large, nearly 1 cm in diameter, and occur mostly in women over 40. They consist of fat lobules forced out of the panniculus by pressure of weight-bearing.

Suitable supportive shoes may alleviate the discomfort. There is no definitive therapy.

NEVUS SUPERFICIALIS LIPOMATOSUS

Soft yellowish papules (see Figure 28–56) or cerebriform plaques, usually of the buttock or thigh, less

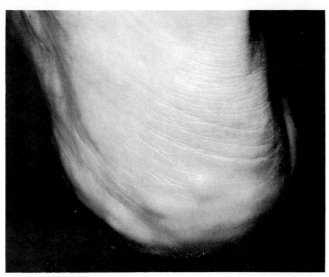

Figure 28–82. Painful piezogenic pedal papules, when bearing weight. (Courtesy of Dr. Axel W. Hoke.)

often of the ear or scalp, with a wrinkled rather than warty surface, characterize this tumor. The distribution may be either zonal (as in the multiple lesions reported by Hoffmann and Zurhelle) or solitary. Solitary ones look rather like a fatty acrochordon. Wilson Jones et al reported a study of 20 cases, plus 44 from the literature.

Onset before age 20 is the rule, but Dotz et al studied a patient whose lesions appeared on the anterior abdominal wall at age 43, and began to enlarge at age 50. He was 68 when seen. Lesions were on the right side and did not cross the midline.

Chanoki M, et al: Nevus lipomatosus cutaneus superficialis of the scalp. Cutis 1989, 43:143.

Wilson-Jones EW, et al: Naevus superficialis lipomatosus. Br J Dermatol 1975, 93:121.

FOLDED SKIN WITH SCARRING
(Michelin Tire Baby Syndrome)

In this rare syndrome, there are numerous deep, conspicuous folds apparently produced by excessive fat, some of which lies high in the dermis. Burgdorf et al reported a case associated with prominent idiopathic pseudoscars, often stellate, in an otherwise normal infant girl. The fat was microscopically and chemically normal. Two published cases were associated with an underlying lipomatous nevus. These two cases, and a third seen by one of us (WDJ), all manifested generalized cutaneous folding, congenital facial and limb abnormalities, and severe neurologic defects.

Collins M, et al: Michelin tire baby syndrome. J Assoc Milit Dermatol 1989, 15:10.

Diffuse Lipomatosis

Diffuse lipomatosis is characterized by an early age of onset, usually before age two; diffuse infiltration of muscle by an unencapsulated mass of histologically mature lipocytes; and progressive enlargement and extension of the tumor mass. It usually involves a large portion of the trunk or an extremity. Some cases are associated with distant lipomas or hemangiomas or with hypertrophy of underlying bone. Klein et al reported a case with associated tuberous sclerosis.

HIBERNOMA

Hibernoma (lipoma of brown fat) is a form of lipoma composed of finely vacuolated fat cells of embryonic type. Hibernomas have a distinctive brownish color and a firm consistency, and usually occur singly. These tumors are benign. They occur chiefly in the mediastinum; but they also occur subcutaneously on the back in the interscapular region, and on the scalp, sternal region, and legs. They are usually about 3 to 12 cm in breadth and the onset is usually in adult life.

PLEOMORPHIC LIPOMA

Shmookler reported a review of 48 cases, 34 followed for a mean period of three years, from the files of the Armed Forces Institute of Pathology. Fat cells of variable size interspersed with characteristic "floret" multinucleated giant cells are seen microscopically. Despite this alarming appearance, the lesions behave in a perfectly benign manner. These lesions, as well as the *spindle cell lipoma*, occur for the most part on the backs or necks of elderly men.

BENIGN LIPOBLASTOMATOSIS

This tumor, frequently confused with a liposarcoma, affects exclusively infants and young children, with approximately 90 per cent occurring before the age of three years. It involves most commonly the soft tissues of the upper and lower extremities. A circumscribed and a diffuse form can be distinguished. The circumscribed form is superficially located and clinically comparable to a lipoma. The diffuse form is more deeply situated and is analogous to diffuse lipomatosis. Microscopically, both forms consist of lobulated immature adipose tissue composed of lipoblasts, a plexiform capillary pattern, and a richly myxoid stroma. Complete local excision is the treatment of choice.

LIPOSARCOMA

Liposarcoma is one of the less common mesenchymal neoplasms of the soft tissue. They usually arise from the intermuscular fascia, and only rarely from the subcutaneous fat. They do not arise from preexisting lipomas. The usual course is an inconspicuous swelling of the soft tissue which undergoes an imperceptibly gradual enlargement.

When a fatty tumor becomes more than 10 cm in diameter Brasfield and Gupta suggest serious consideration of a liposarcoma. The upper thigh is believed to be the most frequent site. Other frequent sites are the buttocks, groin, and upper extremities. Males are affected mostly.

Liposarcomas may be well or poorly differentiated; myxoid or pleomorphic; or dominated by round cells. S-100 stains are positive, and may be helpful in distinguishing pleomorphic liposarcoma from malignant fibrous histiocytoma.

Treatment is adequate radical excision of the lesion. For metastatic liposarcomas, radiation therapy may be effective.

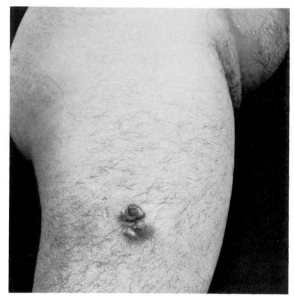

Figure 28–83. Solitary cutaneous leiomyoma on thigh. (Courtesy of Dr. H. Shatin.)

SMOOTH MUSCLE TUMORS

Leiomyoma

Cutaneous leiomyomas are smooth muscle tumors characterized by painful nodules that occur singly or multiply. Leiomyomas have been variously classified. They may be separated conveniently into solitary and multiple cutaneous leiomyomas arising from arrectores pilorum muscles (piloleiomyomas), solitary genital leiomyomas arising from the dartoic, the vulvar, or the mammillary muscle, and solitary angioleiomyomas arising from the muscles of veins.

SOLITARY CUTANEOUS LEIOMYOMA

The typical nodule is a deep, intracutaneous, circumscribed, rounded nodule ranging from 2 to 15 mm in diameter. It is freely movable. The overlying skin may have a reddish or violaceous tint.

Although the lesion is insensitive at first, painful paroxysms may occur. Once pain commences, the tendency is for it to intensify.

MULTIPLE CUTANEOUS LEIOMYOMAS

These brownish, grouped papular lesions vary from 2 to 23 mm in diameter. Two or more sites of the skin surface may be involved. The firm, smooth, superficial, sometimes translucent and freely movable nodules are located most frequently on the trunk and extremities. They often form linear or dermatomal patterns. They may occur on the tongue or, less often, elsewhere in the mouth as well.

These patients often experience pain, especially in cool weather. Engelke et al and Venencie et al re-

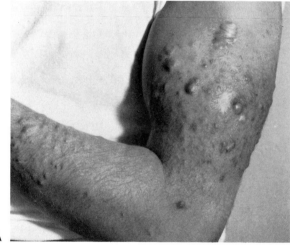

A

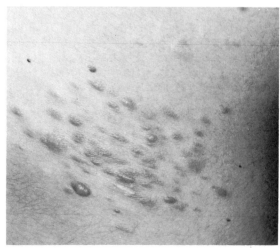

B

Figure 28–84. A and B, Multiple cutaneous leiomyomas.

ported relief of pain by giving phenoxybenzamine (Dibenzyline), an alpha-adrenergic blocker, and Thompson reported one completely relieved by nifedipine (Procardia), 10 mg three times a day, confirming Abraham's report of its effectiveness. These drugs, being calcium channel blockers, act by relaxing smooth muscle. Archer et al reported that an ice cube applied over the lesions would induce pain. They could measure the effectiveness of their therapy by assessing the increasing length of time it took the ice cube to cause pain.

Multiple leiomyomas are sometimes inherited by autosomal dominance, as in Butler's case. Women with this inherited type often have uterine leiomyomas as well.

SOLITARY GENITAL LEIOMYOMA

These lesions are located on the scrotum, on the labia majora, or rarely on the nipples. They may be intracutaneous or subcutaneous in location. Most genital leiomyomas are painless, as were the lesions in the case reported by Livne et al.

ANGIOLEIOMYOMA
(Vascular Leiomyoma)

This variety of leiomyoma arises from the muscle of veins. Pain, either spontaneous or provoked by pressure or cold, occurs in roughly half the cases. It is found mostly on the lower leg in middle-aged women. Inoue reported a case of six years' duration in an 18-year-old man, which resembled a hemangioma clinically. Hachisuga reviewed 562 cases seen in 27 years in his institution. Solid tumors were three times more frequent in women, and cavernous four times more frequent in men. Solid lesions in the extremities were commonly painful; tumors of the head were rarely painful.

Histologically, the leiomyoma is made up of bundles and masses of smooth muscle fibers. Varying amounts of collagen are intermingled. The smooth muscle cells are finely fibrillated and are mostly vacuolated. The nuclei are typically long, thin, and rod-shaped. The muscle bundles are irregularly separated by strands of collagen fibers.

Leiomyomas are benign, and treatment is directed toward the removal of the pain source. Simple excision is the best method of removal of these small lesions.

CONGENITAL SMOOTH-MUSCLE HAMARTOMA

Congenital smooth-muscle hamartoma (CSMH) is typically a skin-colored or lightly pigmented patch or plaque with hypertrichosis. It is often present at birth, usually on the trunk, especially the lumbosacral area, but may also occur on the extremities. Truhan's case showed a particularly widespread distribution. Older patients may have perifollicular papules. They vary in size from 2×3 cm to 10×10 cm.

Clinically a mastocytoma may be mimicked, because transient elevation on rubbing may be seen (pseudo–Darier's sign). A nevocellular nevus is also in the differential diagnosis. Metzker et al report an incidence of one in 2700 newborns at their institution.

Histologically, numerous thick, long, well-defined bundles of smooth muscle are seen in the dermis at various angles of orientation. There may be an increase in hair follicles.

Slifman et al believe this to be part of the spectrum of Becker's nevus. Classically Becker's nevus is a unilateral (rarely bilateral) acquired hyperpigmentation, usually beginning as a tan macule on the shoulder or pectoral area of a teenaged male. Over time hypertrichosis develops within it. It may occasionally be familial, as in the case of Fretzin et al. Biopsy of such lesions classically shows acanthosis, papillomatosis, and increased basal cell pigmentation. Person et al reported a high androgen-receptor level in the tissue of a typical lesion, while normal skin from a contralateral site showed no detectable androgen receptors. Acne has developed within the affected area in rare instances.

Slifman et al point out that occasional congenital lesions of hyperpigmentation and hypertrichosis have shown biopsy findings consistent with those of a Becker's nevus (no smooth muscle proliferation) and lesions with a typical late-onset history compatible with Becker's nevus have occasionally shown smooth-muscle–hamartomalike changes in the dermis.

No treatment is necessary for either lesion. Mechanical epilation may be given to the occasional woman with a Becker's nevus.

Berger TG, et al: Congenital smooth muscle hamartoma. JAAD 1984, 11:709.

Bronson DM, et al: Congenital pilar and smooth muscle nevus. JAAD 1983, 8:111.

Chapel TA, et al: Becker's melanosis. Cutis 1981, 27:405.

Dupre A, et al: Congenital smooth muscle nevus with follicular spotted appearance. JAAD 1985, 13:837.

Fretzin DF, et al: Familial Becker's nevus. JAAD 1985, 12:589.

Metzker A, et al: Congenital smooth muscle hamartoma. JAAD 1986, 14:691.

Idem: Congenital smooth muscle hamartoma of the skin. Pediatr Dermatol 1984, 2:45.

Person JR, et al: Becker's nevus. JAAD 1984, 10:235.

Slifman NR, et al: Congenital arrector pili hamartoma. Arch Dermatol 1985, 121:1034.

Truhan AP, et al: Hypertrichotic skin-colored patches in an infant. JAAD 1985, 121:1197.

LEIOMYOSARCOMA

Leiomyosarcomas of soft-tissue origin are extremely rare; occasionally, however, they may occur as a metastasis from an internal source. A cutaneous leiomyosarcoma appears in the dermis as a solitary nodule. This has a good prognosis, as metastasis to lymph nodes is rare, and rarely fatal. Subcutaneous leiomyosarcomas, on the contrary, have a guarded prognosis, since hematogenous metastases, especially pulmonary, prove fatal in about one third of the cases.

The clinical appearance of these lesions is not distinctive, so that the diagnosis is established by the histopathologic findings. These differ from the leiomyoma only by the nuclear pleomorphism, the numerous mitotic figures, and the disarray of the smooth muscle bundles. Collagen is found only in the septa.

The preferred method of treatment is wide local excision.

Leiomyoma and Leiomyosarcoma

Archer CB, et al: Assessment of treatment for painful cutaneous leiomyomas. JAAD 1987, 17:141.
Brown MD, et al: Genital tumors: Their management by micrographic surgery. JAAD 1988, 18:115.
Burden PA, et al: Piloleiomyoma arising in an organoid nevus. J Dermatol Surg Oncol 1987, 13:1213.
Butler DF: Cutaneous leiomyoma. Arch Dermatol 1984, 120:1618.
Cherrick HM: Leiomyomas of the oral cavity. Oral Surg Med Pathol 1973, 34:54.
Doherty MJ, et al: Immunoenzyme techniques in dermatopathology. JAAD 1989, 20:827.
Fields JP, et al: Leiomyosarcoma of the skin and subcutaneous tissue. Cancer 1981, 47:156.
Hachisuga T, et al: Angioleiomyoma. Cancer 1984, 54:126.
Inoue F, et al: Vascular leiomyoma of the auricle. Arch Dermatol 1983, 119:445.
Livne PM, et al: Leiomyoma of the scrotum. Arch Dermatol 1983, 119:358.
MacDonald DM, et al: Angioleiomyoma of the skin. Br J Dermatol 1974, 91:161.
Miettinen M, et al: Antibodies to intermediate filaments. Arch Dermatol 1985, 121:736.
Moon TD, et al: Leiomyosarcoma of the scrotum. JAAD 1989, 20:290.
Phelan JT, et al: Malignant smooth-muscle tumors of soft tissue origin. N Engl J Med 1962, 266:1027.
Swanson DE, et al: Primary cutaneous leiomyosarcoma. J Cutan Pathol 1988, 15:129.
Thompson JA Jr: Therapy for painful cutaneous leiomyomas. JAAD 1985, 13:865.

CUTANEOUS ENDOMETRIOSIS

Endometriosis of the skin, described by von Recklinghausen in 1885, is characterized by the appearance of brownish papules at the umbilicus or in lower abdominal scars after gynecologic surgery in middle-aged women. In a study of 82 patients, Steck and Helwig noted 28 lesions occurring in the umbilicus, 42 in the lower abdominal wall, and 12 in the inguinal area, labia, and perineum. All but five lesions arose in a scar. Seventy-five per cent occur in women aged 25 to 45.

The tumor, usually solitary, ranges from a few to 60 mm, averaging 5 mm, in diameter. The tender or painful lesion is bluish black from the bleeding that occurs cyclically in many of the patients.

About one third of their cases occurred in postcesarean surgical scars. The major histopathologic findings are glandular structures with two cell types (glands, and decidualized stroma), an infiltrating

margin, and no mitotic figures. It is easily misdiagnosed as a malignant metastasis.

Treatment of mild disease may be by use of hormones such as estrogen, progesterone, or androgen. Extensive disease requires surgical extirpation.

Pellegrini AE: Cutaneous decidualized endometriosis. Am J Dermatopathol 1982, 4:171.
Shwayder TA: Umbilical nodule and abdominal pain. Arch Dermatol 1987, 123:105.
Steck WD, et al: Cutaneous endometriosis. JAMA 1965, 191:101.
Tidman MJ, et al: Cutaneous endometriosis. J Cutan Pathol 1986, 13:89.
Idem: Cutaneous endometriosis. JAAD 1988, 18:373.

TERATOMA

Teratomas may develop in the skin, but are most common in the ovary or testis. They have no characteristic clinical features, but on microscopic examination many types of tissue, representative of all three germ layers, are present. Hair, teeth, and functioning thyroid tissue are examples of fully differentiated tissues that may develop. Occasionally malignancy may occur.

Boughton RS, et al: Malignant melanoma arising in an ovarian cystic teratoma in pregnancy. JAAD 1987, 17:871.

METASTATIC CARCINOMA AND PARANEOPLASTIC SIGNS

Malignant tumors have the ability to grow at sites distant from the primary site of origin; thus, dissemination to the skin may occur with any malignant neoplasm. These infiltrates may result from direct invasion of the skin from underlying tumors, may extend by lymphatic or hematogenous spread, or may be introduced by therapeutic procedures.

The overall incidence of cutaneous metastases probably is in the range of 5 to 10 per cent. The reported incidence figures vary widely according to the type of study undertaken and the site of primary tumor studied. A recent autopsy study from a hematology-oncology referral hospital by Spencer et al found an overall incidence of 9 per cent. The frequency of involvement of the skin is thus low when one considers other sites such as the lung, liver, lymph nodes, and brain. Usually they occur as numerous firm, hard, or rubbery masses, with predilection for the chest, abdomen, or scalp, in an adult over age 40 who has had a previously diagnosed carcinoma. Many variations in morphology, number of lesions, site of growth, age at onset, and timing of metastases exist, however.

Clinically the lesions are most commonly intradermal papules, nodules, or tumors which are firm,

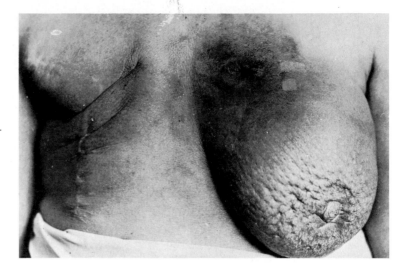

Figure 28–85. Erysipeloid type of metastasis of carcinoma of the breast.

skin-colored to reddish purplish, black or brown; may be fixed to underlying tissues; and rarely ulcerate.

Several unusual morphologic patterns occur. *Carcinoma en cuirasse* is a diffuse infiltration of the skin which imparts an indurated and hidebound leathery quality to it. This sclerodermoid change, also referred to as *scirrhous carcinoma*, is produced by fibrosis and single row lines of tumor cells. This type primarily occurs with breast carcinoma.

Carcinoma telangiectaticum is another unusual type of cutaneous metastases from breast carcinoma which presents as small pink to purplish papules, pseudovesicles, and telangiectases.

Inflammatory carcinoma (carcinoma erysipelatoides) is characterized by erythema, edema, warmth, and tenderness, with a well-defined leading edge, similar to erysipelas in appearance. This is usually due to breast carcinoma, but has been reported with many other types. Most recently Haupt et al described two cases secondary to melanoma, and Schwartz et al reported a patient whose primary tumor originated in the parotid.

Alopecia neoplastica, as reviewed by Baum et al, may present as a cicatricial localized area of hair loss, which on biopsy is usually due to breast metastases in women and lung or kidney carcinoma in men.

The so-called *Sister Mary Joseph nodule* is formed by localization of metastatic tumors to the umbilicus. Powell et al reviewed 85 cases and found the most common primary sites to be stomach, large bowel, ovary, and pancreas.

Zosteriform, linear, or chancroidal ulcerations of the genitalia, and verrucous nodules of the legs, are other rarely reported clinical presentations.

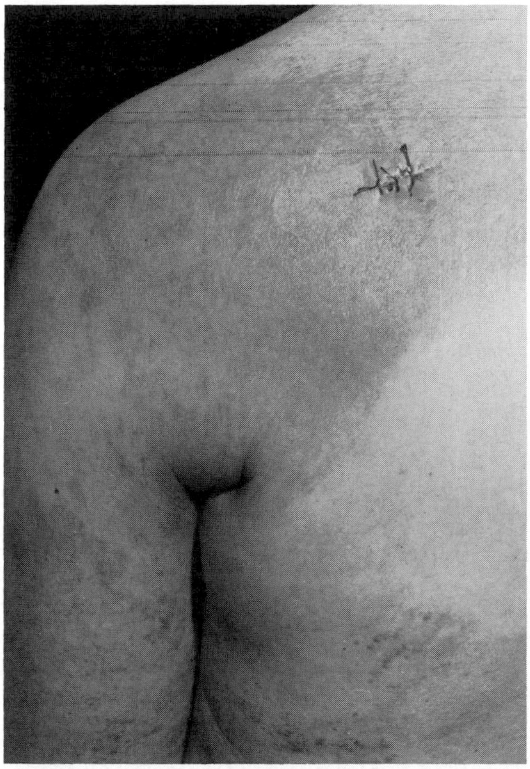

Figure 28–86. Lenticular carcinoma of the chest, back, and arm after removal of carcinoma of the breast. Erysipelas-like, diffuse infiltration of the skin occurred 4 months after breast amputation.

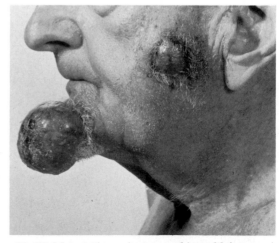

Figure 28–87. Metastatic carcinoma on chin and left preauricular area with primary carcinoma of the lung. (Courtesy of Dr. H. Shatin.)

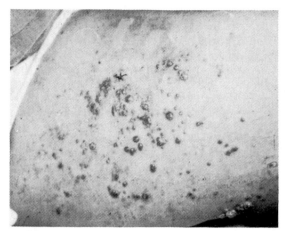

Figure 28–88. Metastatic carcinoma of skin on upper thigh appearing 4 years after removal of carcinomatous uterus.

The primary tumor is usually diagnosed before the appearance of metastases, and dissemination to the skin is often a late finding associated with metastatic disease to other more commonly involved organs such as the lung and the liver. A poor prognosis is thus the rule. Skin infiltrates may, however, be the first harbinger of a malignant visceral neoplasm.

The principal anatomic sites to which metastases localize are the chest, abdomen, and scalp, with the back and extremities being relatively uncommon areas. Involvement of the skin is likely to be near the area of the primary tumor. Thus chest lesions are usually due to breast carcinoma in women and lung carcinoma in men, abdominal or perineal lesions to colonic carcinoma, and the face to squamous cell carcinoma of the oral cavity. Extremity lesions, when they do occur, are most commonly due to melanoma.

Due to its overall high prevalence, breast cancer is the type most commonly metastatic to the skin in women, and lung is the type seen in men. Colon carcinoma is also common due to its high incidence

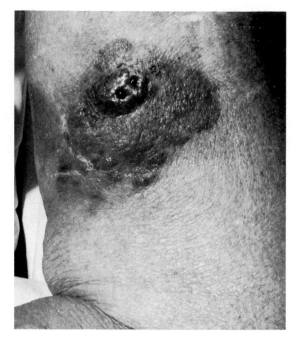

Figure 28–90. Lymphangiosarcoma in Stewart-Treves syndrome on the biceps area of an 84-year-old woman who had had a radical mastectomy followed by ionizing radiation therapy 12 years before.

in both sexes. Hypernephroma, or renal cell carcinoma, while less common, has a predilection for scalp metastases. Lymphangiosarcoma developing in a site of chronic lymphedema is referred to as the *Stewart-Treves syndrome*. Hashimoto et al point to the use of antikeratin and antidesmosomal antibodies to identify metastatic breast carcinoma, while antifactor-VIII antibodies are positive in the Stewart-Treves angiosarcoma.

Some cancers produce reactions in the skin which indicate to the clinician that an underlying internal malignancy may be present. These may range from a specific eruption characteristic of a particular type

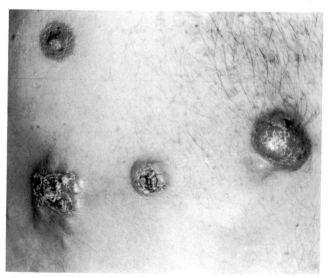

Figure 28–89. Cutaneous metastases from carcinoma of the lung. (Courtesy of Dr. Axel W. Hoke.)

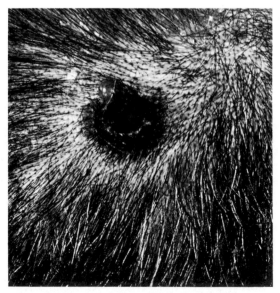

Figure 28–91. Hypernephroma metastatic to the scalp.

of cancer, such as necrolytic migratory erythema, to a nonspecific cutaneous reaction pattern, among the causes of which may be an internal malignancy.

Bazex's syndrome, or *acrokeratosis paraneoplastica*, is characterized by violaceous erythema and scaling of the fingers, toes, nose, and aural helices. Nail dystrophy and palmoplantar keratoderma may be seen. These cases are secondary to primary malignant neoplasms of the upper aerodigestive tract or metastatic cancer to the lymph nodes, as reviewed by Picora et al, Richard et al, and Jacobsen et al.

Necrolytic migratory erythema, or the *glucagonoma syndrome*, is characterized by weight loss, glucose intolerance, anemia, glossitis, erythematous patches with bullae, and light brown papules with scales involving the face, groin, and abdomen. This is seen with glucagon-secreting tumors of the pancreas.

Erythema gyratum repens is a gyrate serpiginous erythema with characteristic wood-grain-pattern scales which is nearly always associated with an underlying malignancy.

Hypertrichosis lanuginosa acquisita, or *malignant down*, is the sudden growth of profuse, soft, nonmedullated, nonpigmented, downy hair in an adult. Jemic's review of 28 cases concluded that the most common sites of associated carcinoma were lung and colon.

The *sign of Leser-Trélat* is the sudden appearance of multiple pruritic seborrheic keratoses, associated with an internal malignancy.

Trousseau's sign, or *migratory thrombophlebitis*, is usually associated with pancreatic carcinoma; it may, however, occur with other tumors, as reviewed by James.

Several cutaneous diseases that are not associated with internal malignancy with the frequency of the above paraneoplastic syndromes, but may be a sign of internal malignancy in some cases, are exfoliative erythroderma (lymphoproliferative disease), acanthosis nigricans (adenocarcinoma), multicentric reticulohistiocytosis, Sweet's syndrome (leukemia), nodular fat necrosis (pancreatic carcinoma), Paget's disease (underlying adnexal or breast carcinoma, or adenocarcinoma of the genitourinary tract or colon), dermatomyositis in patients over 40, and acquired ichthyosis (lymphoproliferative).

A variant of acquired ichthyosis, *pityriasis rotunda*, manifests circular, brown, scaly patches from 1 to 28 cm in diameter and varying in number from one to 20. They may occur on the trunk or extremities. These symptomless patches have been described in the Japanese, and in African and West Indian blacks. Leibowitz et al believe internal malignancy may be seen with increased frequency in these patients.

Ali F, et al: Umbilical metastases of an endometrial carcinoma. JAAD 1985, 12:887.

Archer CB, et al: Metastatic cutaneous carcinoid. JAAD 1985, 13:363.

Baum EM, et al: Alopecia neoplastica. JAAD 1981, 4:688.

Brownstein MH, et al: Patterns of cutaneous metastases. Arch Dermatol 1972, 105:862.

Idem: Patterns of cutaneous metastases. Arch Dermatol 1973, 107:80.

Grimwood RE, et al: Acrokeratosis paraneoplastica with esophageal squamous cell carcinoma. JAAD 1987, 17:685.

Hashimoto K, et al: Differentiation of metastatic breast carcinoma from Stewart-Treves angiosarcoma. Arch Dermatol 1985, 121:742.

Hashizume T, et al: Glucagonoma syndrome. JAAD 1988, 19:377.

Haupt HM, et al: Inflammatory melanoma. JAAD 1984, 10:52.

Hazelrigg DE, et al: Inflammatory metastatic carcinoma. Arch Dermatol 1977, 113:69.

Helfman RJ: Sister Joseph's nodule as the first sign of metastatic adenocarcinoma. J Assoc Milit Dermatol 1985, 111:70.

Holdiness MR: On the classification of the sign of Leser-Trélat. JAAD 1988, 19:754.

Jacobsen FK, et al: Acrokeratosis paraneoplastica. Arch Dermatol 1984, 120:562.

James WD: Trousseau's sign. Int J Dermatol 1984, 23:205.

Jemic GBE: Hypertrichosis lanuginosa acquisita associated with multiple malignancies. JAAD 1985, 12:1106.

Kuols LK, et al: Treatment of malignant carcinoid syndrome. N Engl J Med 1986, 315:663.

Langlois JC, et al: Erythema gyratum repens unassociated with internal malignancy. JAAD 1985, 12:911.

Leibowitz MR, et al: Pityriasis rotunda. Arch Dermatol 1983, 119:607.

McLean DI: Cutaneous paraneoplastic syndromes. Arch Dermatol 1986, 122:765.

Pecora AL, et al: Acrokeratosis paraneoplastica. Arch Dermatol 1983, 119:820.

Poiares-Baptista A, et al: Cutaneous pigmented metastasis from breast carcinoma simulating malignant melanoma. Int J Dermatol 1988, 27:124.

Powell FC, et al: Sister Mary Joseph's nodule. JAAD 1984, 10:610.

Richard M, et al: Acrokeratosis paraneoplastica. JAAD 1987, 16:178.

Scherbenske JM, et al: Prostatic carcinoma with metastases to the nipple. JAAD 1988, 18:391.

Schwartz RA, et al: Inflammatory metastatic carcinoma of the parotid. Arch Dermatol 1984, 120:796.

Spencer PS, et al: Skin metastases in cancer patients. Cutis 1987, 39:119.

Tschen EH, et al: Inflammatory metastatic carcinoma of the breast. Arch Dermatol 1981, 117:120.

Weiss RB: Streptozocin. Cancer Treat Rep 1982, 66:427.

Wilkin JK, et al: Blockade of carcinoid flush with cimetidine and clonidine. Arch Dermatol 1982, 118:109.

Wishner AJ, et al: Psoriasiform dermatitis in a cachectic man. Arch Dermatol 1988, 124:1851.

CARCINOID

Carcinoid is characterized by distinctive involvement of the lungs, heart, gastrointestinal tract, and skin.

The outstanding feature of the skin is the cutaneous flushing, usually of five to ten minutes' duration. The flushing may last as long as 30 minutes.

The flushing involves chiefly the head and neck, producing a diffuse scarlet color, with mottled red patches on the thorax and abdomen. Striking color changes may be present, with salmon red, bluish white, and other colors appearing simultaneously on various portions of the skin. Cyanosis may also be present. As the episodic flushing continues over months to years, telangiectases and plethora appear, as though the patient had polycythemia vera. Gyrate and serpiginous patches of erythema and cyanosis flare up and subside, not only on the face but on all parts of the body and extremities.

The clinical features of the carcinoid syndrome become evident only after hepatic metastases have occurred, or when the primary tumor is a bronchial carcinoid, or if the carcinoid arises in an ovarian teratoma, where the venous drainage bypasses the hepatic circulation.

The release of excessive amounts of serotonin and bradykinin into the circulation produces attacks of flushing of the skin, weakness, abdominal pain, nausea, vomiting, sweating, palpitation, diarrhea, and collapse. These attacks may last a few hours. Such symptoms may be induced in these patients by the injection of epinephrine, at which time kinin peptide is released.

Pellagroid changes due to shunting of dietary tryptophan away from the kynurenin-niacin pathway and into the 5-hydroxyindole pathway. Periorbital swelling, edema of the face, neck, and feet, and ascites may occur.

Rudner and his associates, and more recently, Archer et al, described disseminated deep dermal and subcutaneous nodules that were metastases to the skin from a primary bronchial carcinoid tumor. These occurred without flushing, cyanosis, or pellagroid changes. Bean and Fusaro described another patient with cutaneous nodules; in addition, necrotic ulcers were present. Price and his associates described sclerodermatous changes in carcinoid.

ETIOLOGY. Carcinoid, also called argentaffinoma, is a tumor that arises from the argentaffin Kulchitsky chromaffin cells in the appendix or terminal ileum but also in other parts of the gastrointestinal tract, from the lungs as bronchial adenomas and rarely from ovarian or testicular teratomas. Some of these produce large amounts of serotonin (5-hydroxytryptamine), a derivative of tryptophan, and others do not. The primary lesion is more active in the production of serotonin than are the metastases. The tumor frequently metastasizes to the draining lymph glands or to neighboring organs, especially the liver, rarely to more distal sites.

LABORATORY FINDINGS. The diagnosis may be established by finding a high level of 5-hydroxyindolacetic acid (5-HIAA) in the urine.

The normal urinary excretion of 5-HIAA is 3 to 8 mg daily, but in the presence of carcinoid it may reach 300 mg. Urinary values greater than 25 mg a day are diagnostic of carcinoid. Any value above the normal output is considered suspicious. The ingestion of bananas may cause significant elevations of 5-HIAA in the urine within a few hours, as banana pulp contains serotonin (4 mg per banana) and catecholamines. Tomatoes, red plums, pineapples, avocados, and eggplants also contain serotonin, but in much smaller amounts.

A screening test for 5-HIAA is the addition of nitrosonaphthol to the urine. A purple color is produced when there is 40 mg of 5-HIAA excreted daily. Other serotonin metabolites besides 5-HIAA are found in the urine. The blood also contains serotonin in amounts of 0.2 to 0.4 mg per cent. In the presence of carcinoid the amount may be ten times normal.

TREATMENT. The primary tumor, usually in the small intestine and occasionally in the lung, should be removed. If this is impossible, chemotherapy for metastatic carcinoid is best conducted at the present time with 5-fluorouracil and streptozocin. It induces remission in approximately one third of patients and helps control symptoms in a higher percentage. Serotonin production should be reduced by drugs to inhibit cutaneous flushes, intestinal cramping, hypotension, and bronchospasm. Simultaneous use of H_1 and H_2 antihistamines, cimetidine (Tagamet), and diphenhydramine (Benadryl) has been shown to block the flushes, as have in some instances clonidine, phenothiazines, propranolol, and corticosteroids. A somatostatin analog, SmS 201–995, given subcutaneously three times daily, 150 μg, blocked the flushing and diarrhea in 22 of 25 patients reported by Kvols et al.

Excision of the primary tumor or metastatic lesions in the liver may be curative. Serotonin production may be decreased by restriction of tryptophan-containing foods for short periods of time. Vitamin supplementation with niacin is recommended.

Methysergide maleate (Sansert) has been found to be effective by Mengel. Ionizing radiation and chemotherapy with 5-fluorouracil, methotrexate, or cyclophosphamide have produced varying degrees of improvement. Parachlorphenylalanine controls diarrhea in carcinoid.

Altman AR, et al: Treatment of malignant carcinoid. Arch Dermatol 1989, 125:394.

Camisa C: Somatostatin and a long-acting analogue, octreotide acetate. Arch Dermatol 1989, 125:407.

Kvols LK, et al: Treatment of malignant carcinoid syndrome. N Engl J Med 1986, 315:663.

Maton PN, et al: The carcinoid syndrome. JAMA 1988, 260:1602.

29

Epidermal Nevi, Neoplasms, and Cysts

KERATINIZING EPIDERMAL NEVI

Keratinizing epidermal nevi are described by a great variety of terms; some of these are hard nevus of Unna, soft epidermal nevus, nevus verrucosus (verrucous nevus), nevus unius lateris, linear nevus, systematized nevi, and ichthyosis hystrix. Some of these terms, which denote some distinctive manifestation of the nevus, are described herewith. Hyperkeratosis without cellular atypia characterizes them all: nevus cells do not occur.

Epstein JH: Photocarcinogenesis, skin cancer, and aging. JAAD 1983, 9:487.
Mehregan AH, et al: Benign epithelial tumors of the skin. Cutis 1977, 19:43.

Verrucous Nevus

The individual lesions are verrucous papules of pink, dirty gray, or brown color. Interspersed in the localized patch may be horny excrescences and, rarely, comedones. The age of onset of epidermal nevi is generally at birth or within the first 10 years of life; however, in a study by Submoke et al, lesions appeared between ages 11 and 40 in 27 per cent of 75 patients. In contrast, Rogers et al found that only 5 of 131 patients had an age of onset above 7 years. Their study included not only those with epidermal nevi but also many with nevus sebaceus, nevus comedonicus, and ILVEN.

Nevus Unius Lateris

This is a verrucous nevus ("nevus of one side") arranged in a linear fashion in continuous or broken streaks, bands, or patches. Upon the extremities their course is longitudinal and upon the trunk it is transverse or curved, as if along the distribution of the intercostal nerves, and virtually never extends past

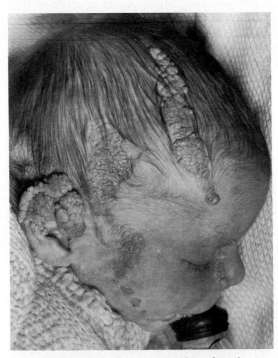

Figure 29–1. Verrucous epidermal nevi.

745

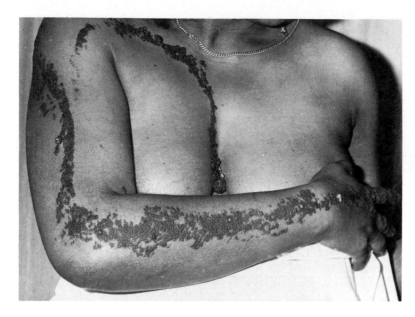

Figure 29–2. Linear epidermal nevus. (Courtesy of Dr. J. Stricks.)

the mid-sagittal line. Blaschko in 1901 published a study of the linear patterns ("Blaschko's lines") followed by these nevi, and by linear lesions of such other diseases as psoriasis and lichen planus, and Jackson has reviewed this study.

More extensive, bilateral systematized lesions are often referred to as ichthyosis hystrix. Since some use this term to suggest a particular histologic appearance or as a subset of ichthyosis, it may impart confusion and is best avoided.

The changes in the epidermis are hyperplastic and affect chiefly the stratum corneum and stratum malpighii. There is variable hyperkeratosis, acanthosis, and papillomatosis. Submoke et al studied the histology of epidermal nevi and found 62 per cent to have this pattern. Another 16 per cent showed epidermolytic hyperkeratosis. Eight other patterns, of lower incidence, were described, including a psoriatic

type, an acrokeratosis verruciformislike type, and a Darier's diseaselike type.

Uncommonly, benign or malignant tumors may develop within epidermal nevi. Some recently reported lesions which have occurred within these lesions have been trichoepithelioma, verruciform xanthoma, keratoacanthoma, basal cell carcinoma, and squamous cell carcinoma. Levin et al's patient with squamous cell carcinoma (SCC) developed metastatic disease.

Therapeutically each lesion presents an individual problem. The age of the patient, the amount of pigment, and the site and extent of the lesions are important. The prime consideration in each case is the therapeutic procedure that will give thorough removal with the least amount of scarring. When the lesions are localized, surgical laser excision is suitable. If more extensive lesions are treated with other modalities it must be considered that partial or complete recurrence is common unless the therapeutic intervention removes at least the papillary dermis. Fulguration or cautery, cryotherapy done repeatedly over a long period of time, or topical tretinoin have been successful in ameliorating the condition. Fox et al compared several modalities and found cryotherapy best for their patient. Five percent 5-fluorouracil ointment has also been found useful by some. It usually produces no scars.

Inflammatory Linear Verrucous Epidermal Nevus (ILVEN)

This epidermal nevus is usually present at birth or appears during the first few years of life, though it may have its onset as late as the forties or fifties. It occurs mainly on an extremity in a girl, is characteristically pruritic, pursues a chronic course, and is generally resistant to topical and intralesional treat-

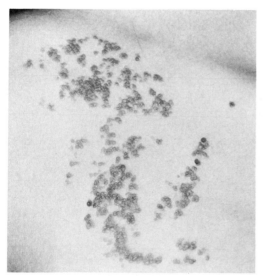

Figure 29–3. Epidermal nevus on thorax.

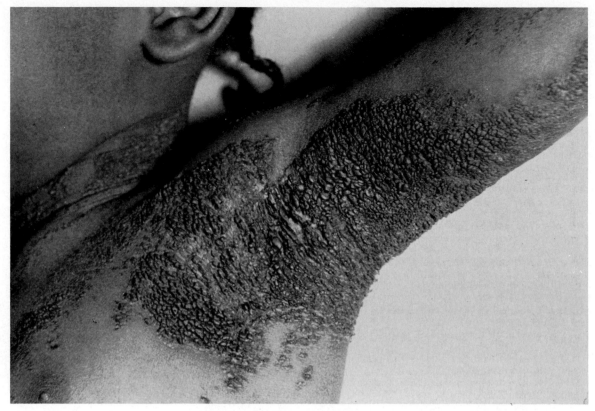

Figure 29–4. Verrucous linear nevus.

ments. It may occur in widely separated areas, usually on only one side of the body. Wong and Wells, however, reported a case in which it was bilateral and generalized.

Because of its psoriasiform histologic appearance, differentiation from linear psoriasis has created some controversy. Baden et al performed polyacrylamide gel electrophoresis in four cases, two of them congenital, and found the epidermal protein pattern different in each case, and always slightly different from the pattern seen in psoriasis. Golitz and Weston reported a female infant with an inflammatory linear verrucous epidermal nevus associated with severe

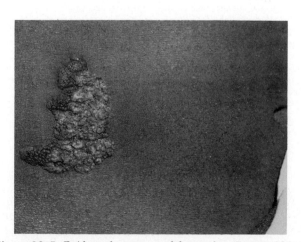

Figure 29–5. Epidermal nevus on abdomen in a 7-year-old boy.

skeletal anomalies of the upper and lower extremities. They concluded that ILVEN (in French, NEVIL) should be considered a component of the epidermal nevus syndrome.

Deep-shave excision or deep dermabrasion may ablate these lesions permanently. Other therapeutic modalities listed for epidermal nevi are applicable to ILVEN.

Epidermal Nevus Syndrome

In 1968 Solomon and associates formulated this syndrome, consisting of extensive epidermal nevi with abnormalities of the central nervous system, skeleton, skin, cardiovascular system, and eyes. Cutaneous lesions other than epidermal nevi which may occur are areas of pigmentary change, multiple nevus cell nevi, café-au-lait spots, and cutaneous hemangiomas. The abnormalities seen are congenitally acquired. Although most cases are sporadic, in some cases an autosomal dominant transmission may occur.

Nevoid Hyperkeratosis of the Nipple

This rare condition, commonest in women, occurs also in men: Kuhlmann et al reported two cases in 1985. It resolved under a keratolytic gel. Vestey reported success with cryotherapy.

Bernhard JD, et al: Inflammatory linear verrucous epidermal nevus. Arch Dermatol 1984, 120:214.

Brownstein MH, et al: Lichenoid epidermal nevus. JAAD 1989, 20:913.

Braunstein BL, et al: Keratoacanthoma arising in a linear epidermal nevus. Arch Dermatol 1982, 118:362.

Fox BJ, et al: A comparison of treatment modalities for epidermal nevus: case report and review. J Dermatol Surg Oncol 1983, 9:879.

Golitz LE, et al: Inflammatory linear verrucose epidermal nevus. Arch Dermatol 1979, 115:1208.

Horn MS, et al: Basal cell epithelioma arising in a linear epidermal nevus. Arch Dermatol 1981, 117:247.

Jackson B: The lines of Blaschko: a review and reconsideration: observations of the cause of certain unusual linear conditions of the skin. Br J Dermatol 1976, 95:349.

Kuhlmann DS, et al: Hyperkeratosis of the nipple and areola. JAAD 1985, 13:596.

Lambert WC, et al: Trichoepithelioma in a systematized epidermal nevus with acantholytic dyskeratosis. Arch Dermatol 1984, 120:227.

Levin A, et al: A squamous cell carcinoma that developed in an epidermal nevus. Am J Dermatopathol 1984, 6:51.

Palastine RF, et al: Verruciform xanthoma in an epithelial nevus. Arch Dermatol 1982, 118:586.

Rogers M, et al: Epidermal nevi and the epidermal nevus syndrome. JAAD 1989, 20:476.

Solomon LM: Epidermal nevus syndrome. Mod Prob Paediatr 1975, 17:27.

Su WPD: Histopathological varieties of epidermal nevus: a study of 160 cases. Am J Dermatopathol 1982, 4:161.

Submoke S, et al: Clinico-histopathologic study of epidermal nevi. Aust J Dermatol 1983, 24:130.

Vestey JP, et al: Unilateral hyperkeratosis of the nipple. Arch Dermatol 1986, 122:1360.

Wong E, et al: Generalized inflammatory epidermal nevus. J R Soc Med 1983, 76:76.

NEVUS COMEDONICUS

This is characterized by closely arranged, grouped, often linear, slightly elevated papules which have at their center keratinous plugs resembling comedones. Cysts, abscesses, fistulas, and scars may develop. It may be localized to a small area, or have an extensive nevoid type of distribution. This lesion occurs mostly on the trunk, in a linear fashion. The lesions may develop any time from birth to middle age, but are usually present by age 10. They are mostly unilateral; however, bilateral cases are also seen. Engber emphasized that the many associated abnormalities of bone, central nervous system, skin, and eyes that may accompany epidermal nevi may also be seen in extensive nevus comedonicus. Nevus comedonicus may be seen with other cutaneous disorders including epidermal nevi.

In nevus comedonicus the pilosebaceous follicles are dilated and filled with keratinous plugs. On the palms, pseudocomedones arise in sweat glands and resemble the changes found in poroma. Histologic examination may also reveal at times well-differentiated cutaneous lesions of follicular origin, as reviewed by Dudley et al, and occasionally epidermolytic hyperkeratosis may be present, as reported by Barsky et al and Lookingbill et al.

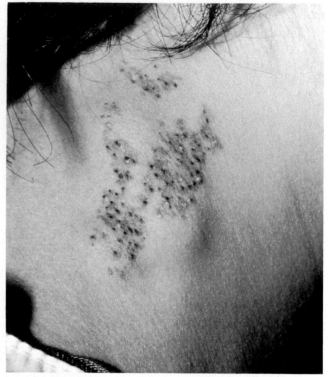

Figure 29–6. Nevus comedonicus with underlying epidermoid cysts. (Courtesy of Dr. Axel W. Hoke.)

Treatment consists of incision and expression of the comedones. Retinoic acid cream, gel, or swabs may be tried. One of the authors (WDJ) treated one patient with isotretinoin, and has knowledge of a second patient so treated. Both patients suffered from recurrent inflammatory cysts prior to therapy. Although the comedolike lesions remained unchanged, the inflammatory lesions improved, becoming less troublesome and less frequent.

Barsky S, et al: Nevus comedonicus with epidermolytic hyperkeratosis. Arch Dermatol 1981, 117:86.

Beck MH, et al: Extensive nevus comedonicus. Arch Dermatol 1980, 116:1048.

Decherd JW, et al: Nevus comedonicus: treatment with retinoic acid. Br J Dermatol 1972, 86:528.

Dudley K, et al: Nevus comedonicus in association with widespread, well-differentiated follicular tumors. JAAD 1986, 15:1123.

Engber PB: The nevus comedonicus syndrome: a case report with emphasis on associated internal manifestations. Int J Dermatol 1978, 17:745.

CLEAR-CELL ACANTHOMA
(Pale Cell Acanthoma)

Also known as Degos acanthoma and *acanthome à cellules claires* of Degos and Civatte, the typical lesion is a circumscribed, reddish, moist nodule with some crusting and peripheral scales; it is usually about 1

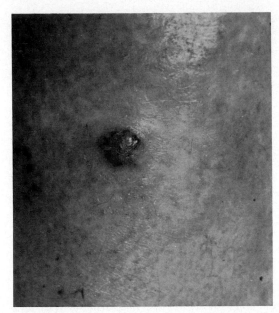

Figure 29–7. Clear cell acanthoma on the shin of a 75-year-old man (actual size).

Boytman M, et al: Giant clear cell acanthoma. JAAD 1987, 17:513.

Desmons F, et al: Multiple clear-cell acanthoma (Degos): histochemical and ultrastructural study of two cases. Int J Dermatol 1977, 16:203.

Goette DK, et al: Multiple clear-cell acanthomas. Arch Dermatol 1983, 119:359.

Lupton GP, et al: Clear cell acanthoma. J Cutan Pathol 1986, 13:85.

Naeyaert JM, et al: Multiple clear cell acanthomas. Arch Dermatol 1987, 123:1670.

Parhizgar B, et al: Pale cell acanthoma of the scrotum. Cutis 1982, 30:231.

Wells GC, et al: Degos' acanthoma (*acanthome à cellules claires*). Br J Dermatol 1967, 79:249.

SEBORRHEIC KERATOSIS

Seborrheic keratoses are multiple, oval, slightly raised, light brown to black, sharply demarcated papules or plaques, rarely over 3 cm in diameter, located mostly on the chest and back but also commonly involving the scalp, face, neck, and extremities. The palms and soles are spared. "Seborrheic keratoses" in these areas are usually eccrine poromas. The individual nummular warty lesions often become crumbly, like a crust that is loosely attached. When this is removed a raw, moist base is revealed.

Seborrheic keratoses are infrequently associated with itching. Some patients have hundreds of these lesions on the trunk. The age of onset is generally in the fourth to fifth decade.

Sanderson describes the pathogenesis of seborrheic keratoses as a development resulting from a local arrest of maturation of keratinocytes which are normal in other respects. They usually originate de novo, but may also evolve from lentigines. In Sanderson's view (Dowling lecture, 1969) they are inherited as an autosomal dominant trait. They may increase in number when the patient is gaining weight and a sudden eruption of many seborrheic keratoses has been associated with inflammatory cutaneous disorders, such as the case of a patient with exfoliative erythroderma described by Berman et al.

cm in diameter. Degos preferred "clear" to "pale" for the English name, and preferred to have Civatte's name joined to his. The favorite site is on the shin, calf, or occasionally the thigh, although in Degos's patient it occurred on the abdomen. Parhizgar and Wood reported a case occurring on the scrotum. The lesion is asymptomatic and slow-growing and can occur in either sex, usually after the age of 40.

Solitary lesions are uncommon, but multiple ones are rare. Goette et al reported a 63-year-old man with six lesions of the lower trunk and legs. The diagnosis by a general pathologist was psoriasis. Intracellular glycogen granules were found. Bonnetblanc et al reported a patient with over 50 lesions.

The acanthotic epidermis consists of pale, edematous cells and is sharply demarcated. The basal cell layer is normal. In the dermis, underneath the acanthoma, dilated blood vessels produce increased vascularity. The clear keratinocytes abound in glycogen, lack phosphorylase, and have reduced amounts of cytoplasmic cytochrome oxidase and succinic dehydrogenase, according to Wells and Wilson Jones. Lupton et al have categorized the histologic appearance into three architectural variants, with most being acanthotic types, followed by exophytic and psoriasiform variants.

The clear-cell acanthoma must be differentiated from eccrine poroma, which appears most frequently on the hair-free part of the foot, and from the clear-cell hidradenoma, which occurs most frequently on the head, especially on the face and the eyelids.

Treatment is the simple removal by fulguration and curettage after a shave biopsy or excision has been performed.

Baden TJ, et al: Multiple clear cell acanthomas. JAAD 1987, 16:1075.

Bonnetblanc JM, et al: Multiple clear cell acanthomas. Arch Dermatol 1981, 117:1.

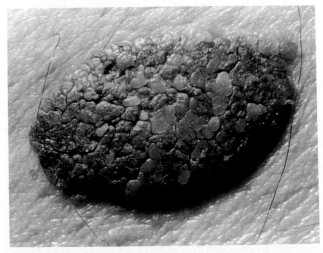

Figure 29–8. Seborrheic keratosis. (Courtesy of Dr. Axel W. Hoke.)

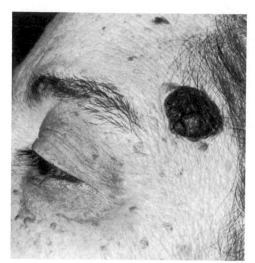

Figure 29–9. *Large and small scattered pigmented seborrheic keratoses.*

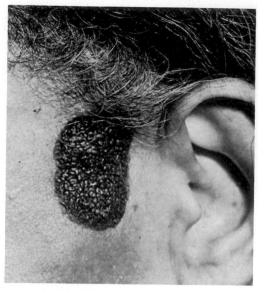

Figure 29–11. *Pigmented seborrheic keratosis resembling pigmented intradermal nevus.*

The seborrheic keratosis is a combined hyperplasia of epidermis and supporting papillary connective tissue. In addition, small horn pseudocysts result from invagination of the stratum corneum. Usually there is some inflammatory reaction in the cutis. Three types, the hyperkeratotic, the acanthotic, and the adenoid keratoses, are distinguished.

The differential diagnosis usually poses no problems. The most difficult, especially for the nondermatologist, is to differentiate the solitary black seborrheic keratosis from melanoma. The regularly shaped verrucous lesion is far different from the smooth-surfaced and slightly infiltrated melanomatous lesion. The actinic keratosis is usually erythematous, more sharply rough, and slightly scaly. The edges are not sharply demarcated and they occur

most often on sun-exposed surfaces, especially the face and backs of the hands, in light-skinned persons. Rarely, intraepidermal nests suggestive of intraepidermal epithelioma of Jadassohn may be seen in the seborrheic keratosis; however, these are regarded as normal parts of the seborrheic keratosis.

Seborrheic keratoses are easily removed with liquid nitrogen or ethyl chloride spray refrigeration and curettage. The spray freezes the lesion to make it brittle enough for easy removal with the curette.

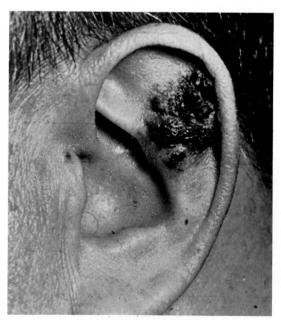

Figure 29–10. *Pigmented seborrheic keratosis resembling melanoma.*

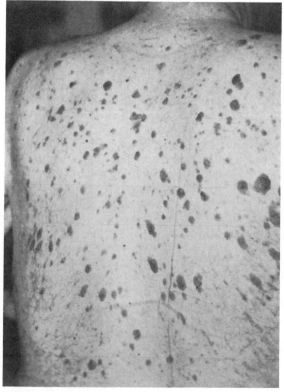

Figure 29–12. *Multiple seborrheic keratoses on the back.*

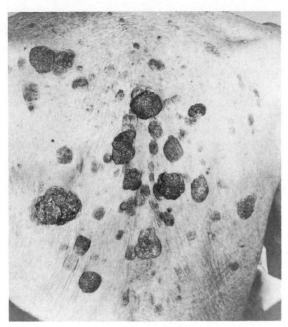

Figure 29–13. Giant seborrheic keratoses.

Scarring is not produced by this method. Light freezing with liquid nitrogen alone is effective. So is simple curettage, either without or with local anesthesia. Ferric subsulfate (Monsel's) solution, or other hemostatic solutions, are suitable for hemostasis. There is no scar. Light fulguration and carbon dioxide laser vaporization are other acceptable methods. Trichloracetic acid is usually not effective, and excision is not necessary. Histopathologic examination of all removed lesions is medically unnecessary but medicolegally indispensable. Baer et al and Kwittken each reported occurrence of a squamous cell carcinoma in a typical seborrheic keratosis, while Mikhail et al reported 14 cases in which a basal cell carcinoma developed within a seborrheic keratosis.

Sign of Leser-Trélat. The sudden appearance of numerous itchy seborrheic keratoses in an adult constitutes this sign of internal malignancy. Sixty per

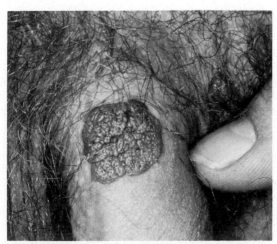

Figure 29–14. Seborrheic keratosis on penis.

cent of the neoplasms have been adenocarcinomas, primarily of the stomach. Holdiness reviewed 51 reported cases and found lymphoma, breast cancer, and squamous cell carcinoma of the lung to be the next most common. In most cases, the dermatosis began at approximately the same time as the development of the cancer, and the processes seemed to run a parallel course in regard to growth and remission. Sperry et al reported an impressive case associated with the recurrence, 10 years after its resection, of a gastric adenocarcinoma. Aylesworth et al reported a patient with Cowden's syndrome who developed endometrial carcinoma and this sign.

DeBersaques reported in 1985 that both Leser and Trélat wrote only of senile angiomas, not of seborrheic keratoses: he states Höllander was the first to associate "seborrheic warts" with internal cancer.

Aylesworth R, et al: Multiple hamartoma syndrome with endometrial carcinoma and the sign of Leser-Trélat. Arch Dermatol 1982, 118:136.

Baer RL, et al: Papillated squamous cell carcinoma in situ arising in a seborrheic keratosis. JAAD 1981, 5:561.

Berman A, et al: Seborrheic keratosis. Arch Dermatol 1982, 118:615.

DeBersaques J: Sign of Leser-Trélat. JAAD 1985, 12:724.

Greer KE, et al: Leser-Trélat associated with acute leukemia. Arch Dermatol 1978, 114:1552.

Holdiness MR: The sign of Leser-Trélat. Int J Dermatol 1986, 25:564.

Idem: On the classification of the sign of Leser-Trétat. JAAD 1988, 19:754.

Kwittken J: Squamous cell carcinoma arising in a seborrheic keratosis. Mt Sinai J Med (NY) 1981, 48:61.

Mikhail GR, et al: Basal cell carcinoma in seborrheic keratosis. JAAD 1982, 6:500.

Sperry K, et al: Adenocarcinoma of the stomach with eruptive seborrheic keratoses: the sign of Leser-Trélat. Cancer 1980, 45:2434.

Venencie PY, et al: Sign of Leser-Trélat: report of two cases and review of the literature. JAAD 1984, 10:83.

Westrom DR, et al: The sign of Leser-Trélat in a young man. Arch Dermatol 1986, 122:1356.

Inverted Follicular Keratosis (Basosquamous-cell Acanthoma)

These benign epithelial tumors occur most frequently on the face or scalp of older persons as firm, skin-colored papules from 2 to 10 mm in diameter. Central scaling with a sharply marginated edge characterizes the lesion. It closely resembles a seborrheic keratosis.

Helwig described this as a benign epithelial tumor related to the infundibulum of the hair follicle. Mehregan described fingerlike projections of squamous cells forming onionlike structures which Helwig calls "squamous eddies." Central funnel-shaped keratinous plugs are present, which correspond to the hair shaft.

This benign lesion responds readily to a shallow shave biopsy with subsequent hemostasis, using any hemostatic solution. Lever considers this lesion to be an *irritated seborrheic keratosis*, a view shared by Wilson Jones and associates and by Malkinson and Pearson, among others—and by us. But others, including Ackerman, believe them to be warts.

Lever WF: Inverted follicular keratosis is an irritated seborrheic keratosis. Am J Dermatopathol 1983, 5:474.
Mehregan AH: Inverted follicular keratosis is a distinct follicular tumor. Am J Dermatopathol 1983, 5:467.
Sim-Davis D, et al: Inverted follicular keratosis: surprising variant of seborrheic wart. Acta Derm Venereol (Stockh) 1976, 56:337.
Spielvogel RL, et al: Inverted follicular keratosis is not a specific keratosis but a verruca vulgaris (or seborrheic keratosis) with squamous eddies. Am J Dermatopathol 5:427, 1983.

DERMATOSIS PAPULOSA NIGRA

This disease occurs in about 35 per cent of blacks and is also relatively common in Orientals. It usually begins in adolescence, showing first as minute, round, skin-colored or hyperpigmented papules that develop singly or in sparse numbers on the malar regions or on the cheeks below the eyes. The lesions increase in number and in size, so that in the course of years the patient may have from 30 to 50 lesions. These closely simulate seborrheic keratoses and verrucae planae in both size and shape. They do not itch or produce other subjective symptoms. Scaling, crusting, and ulceration do not occur, and there is no tendency to disappear.

Microscopically, the chief alterations are in the epidermis and are characterized by an irregular acanthosis and a deposit of uncommonly large amounts of pigment throughout the rete and particularly in the basal layer. There is a resemblance to seborrheic keratoses. The lesions may be a form of epidermal nevus.

Treatment is made difficult by the tendency for the development of dyspigmentation. Light curettage with or without anesthesia; light, superficial liquid nitrogen application; and light electrodesiccation followed by curettage are effective therapeutic modalities in this entity. Aggressive techniques should be avoided in order to prevent pigmentary and scarring complications.

Hairston MA Jr, et al: Dermatitis papulosa nigra. Arch Dermatol 1964, 89:655.

STUCCO KERATOSIS

Keratoelastoidosis verrucosa of the extremities was described by Kocsard and Ofner as "stuck-on" keratoses occurring on the lower legs, especially in the vicinity of the Achilles tendon region. They are also seen on the instep, the dorsa of the feet, the forearms, and backs of the hands. The palms, soles, trunk, and head are never affected. Varying in size from 1 to 5 mm in diameter, they are loosely attached, so that they can easily be scratched off. In numbers there is a variation from two to several score.

The stucco keratoses are common in Australia (the home of Kocsard and Ofner) as well as the United States. They occur mostly in men aged 40 and over.

Histologically, the picture is that of a hyperkeratotic type of seborrheic keratosis.

The treatment, if any is required, consists of emollients which soften the skin and cause the scaly lesions to fall off. Lac-Hydrin (12 per cent ammonium lactate) lotion may be very effective.

Kocsard E, et al: Keratoelastoidosis verrucosa of the extremities (stucco keratosis of the extremities). Dermatologica 1966, 113:225.
Rees RB: For stucco keratoses, Lac-Hydrin. Schoch Letter 1985, 35:45.
Schnitzler L, et al: Stucco keratosis: histologic and ultrastructural study in 3 patients. Ann Dermatol Venereol 1977, 104:489.

MULTIPLE MINUTE DIGITATE HYPERKERATOSIS

This autosomal dominant condition is characterized by multiple minute keratotic papules that are unassociated with follicular orifices. A spiked projection often occurs at the top of the papule. There are no associated abnormalities. Balus et al reported the sixth family with this condition in 1988.

Balus L, et al: Multiple minute digitate hyperkeratoses. JAAD 1988, 18:431.

HYPERKERATOSIS LENTICULARIS PERSTANS (Flegel)

Rough yellow-brown keratotic plaques 2–5 mm in diameter and small psoriasiform discs, on the insteps, tops of the feet, and lower legs, characterize this distinctive dermatosis, described by Flegel in 1958. The palms, soles, and oral mucosa may rarely be involved.

Most of the known cases have begun in men in their thirties and forties. Bean suggests that this is a genodermatosis transmitted as an autosomal dominant trait. In a sibship reported by Beveridge, basal cell carcinomas were an associated finding, but were unrelated to the keratoses.

The histologic findings are distinctive, with hyperkeratosis and parakeratosis overlying a thinned epidermis, and irregular acanthosis at the periphery. A bandlike inflammatory infiltrate occurs in the papillary dermis.

Topical corticosteroid cream may be helpful. Pearson et al found topical 5-fluorouracil effective, and etretinate has been useful. Lac-Hydrin may give relief.

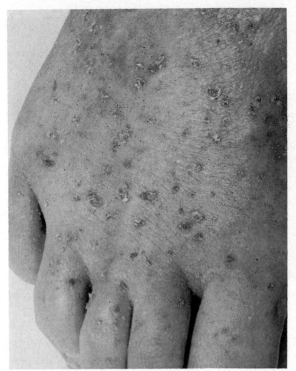

Figure 29–15. Hyperkeratosis lenticularis perstans. (Courtesy of Dr. E. Kocsard.)

The lesions do not recur after shallow shave excision.

Bean SF: Hyperkeratosis lenticularis perstans. Arch Dermatol 1969, 87:91.

Flegel H: Hyperkeratosis lenticularis perstans. Hautarzt 1958, 9:363.

Frenk E, et al: Hyperkeratosis lenticularis perstans (Flegel): biologic model for keratinization occurring in the absence of Odland bodies. Dermatologica 1976, 153:253.

Pearson LH, et al: Hyperkeratosis lenticularis perstans. JAAD 1987, 16:190.

WARTY DYSKERATOMA

Warty dyskeratomas (Szymanski) are found most frequently on the face, neck, scalp, or axilla, and occasionally in the mouth. The lesion is most frequently a brownish red papule with a soft, yellowish, central keratotic plug. Hazelrigg reported three such cases.

Histologically the stratum corneum is hyperkeratotic and crusted. An invagination, filled with a keratotic plug, occurs to produce a cuplike depression. In the intraepidermal lacunae are acantholytic cells and pseudovilli. Corps ronds and grains may be seen in the lining of the crater.

In the differential diagnosis keratoacanthoma, basal cell carcinoma, and syringocystadenoma papilliferum must be considered.

Treatment consists of shave excision of the lesions.

Hazelrigg DE, et al: Warty dyskeratoma. Cutis 1975, 16:63.

Mesa ML, et al: Oral warty dyskeratoma. Cutis 1984, 33:293.

Niren EM, et al: Warty dyskeratoma. Cutis 1982, 29:79.

Rubenstein MH: Warty dyskeratoma. Arch Dermatol 1981, 117:746.

BENIGN LICHENOID KERATOSIS

These usually solitary dusky red to violaceous papular lesions were first described in 1966 by Lumpkin and Helwig and by Shapiro and Ackerman. They occur most often on the distal forearms or hands, or chests, of middle-aged white women. Barranco reported a case of multiple lesions simulating a photodermatitis.

Berman considered this an involuting pigmented lesion, and Berger et al found evidence of preexisting lentigo senilis histologically and by history. The role of sun exposure in the etiology is unsettled.

Histologically there is parakeratosis, a lichenoid infiltrate with occasional plasma cells and eosinophils in addition 'o lymphocytes, and what may be remnants of lentigo senilis at the periphery. Direct immunofluorescence is positive, with clumped deposits of IgM in a lichen-planuslike pattern at the dermoepidermal junction.

Cryotherapy with liquid nitrogen is effective.

Barranco VP: Multiple benign lichenoid keratoses simulating photodermatoses. JAAD 1985, 13:201.

Berger TG, et al: Lichenoid benign keratosis. JAAD 1984, 11:635.

Berman A, et al: The involuting lichenoid plaque. Arch Dermatol 1982, 118:93.

Goette DK: Benign lichenoid keratosis. Arch Dermatol 1980, 116:780.

Lauer WE, et al: Lichen planus–like keratosis. JAAD 1981, 4:329.

Scott MA, et al: Lichenoid benign keratosis. J Cutan Pathol 1976, 3:217.

ARSENICAL KERATOSES

Arsenical keratoses are keratotic, pointed, 2–4-mm wartlike lesions on the palms, soles, and sometimes the ears of persons who have a history of drinking well water or taking "drops" (Fowler's solution) or pills (Asiatic pills), usually for asthma or atopic dermatitis, or psoriasis, often years (average six, in 102 cases reported by Fietz) previously. These lesions resemble verrucae vulgares on the palms and soles. When the lesion is picked off with the fingernails, a small dell-like depression is seen.

Arsenical keratoses may also occur on other areas of the skin, especially the trunk and the extremities. These may or may not be associated with plantar and palmar keratoses and with arsenical hyperpigmentation. The latter is seen in about one half of the patients. In addition to the keratoses and hyperpigmentation, Bowen's disease and invasive arsenical

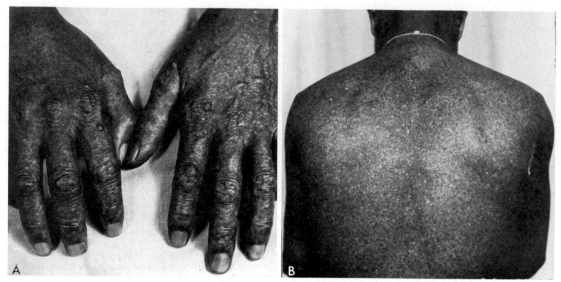

Figure 29–16. A and B, Keratoses ("premalignant") and pigmentary changes following prolonged exposure to insecticide containing arsenic. (From Moschella SI, Hurley HJ: Dermatology. 2nd ed. Philadelphia, WB Saunders, 1985, p 442.)

squamous carcinomata may be present, with the latent period being 10 years and 20 years, respectively. Superficial multicentric basal cell carcinomas may more rarely be seen. Internal carcinoma also occurs with increased frequency, after an average latent period of 30 years, with pulmonary and genitourinary carcinoma being most common.

The etiology of these lesions is inorganic pentavalent arsenic, which was given for many years in the past for medicinal purposes in the form of Fowler's solution or Asiatic pills.

The histopathology shows hyperkeratosis, acanthosis, cellular atypia, and downward proliferation of the rete ridges. The histologic changes are the same as those of actinic keratosis, but without the basophilic degeneration of the dermis frequently associated with actinic damage.

The palmar and plantar keratoses are easily diagnosed if there is hyperpigmentation of the skin, Bowenoid changes, or arsenical cancers. Multiple verrucae and acrokeratosis verruciformis should also be considered.

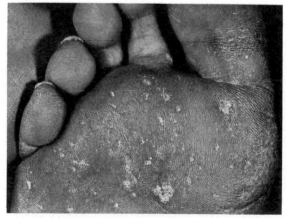

Figure 29–17. Arsenical keratoses on the sole.

Treatment of arsenical keratoses is by cryotherapy, electrodesiccation and curettage, or topical application of 5-fluorouracil.

Fierz U: Katamnestische Untersuchungen über die Therapie mit an organischem Arven bei Haut-Krankheiten. Dermatologica 1965, 131:41.

Jampel RM, et al: Palmar lesions and a nonhealing ulcer of the ear in a former agricultural worker. Arch Dermatol 1987, 123:251.

Miki Y, et al: Cutaneous and pulmonary cancers associated with Bowen's disease. JAAD 1982, 6:26.

Wagner SL, et al: Skin cancer and arsenical intoxication from well water. Arch Dermatol 1979, 115:1205.

Yeh S: Skin cancer and chronic arsenism. Hum Pathol 1973, 4:459.

ACTINIC KERATOSIS
(Solar Keratosis)

Though they are found chiefly on the chronically sun-exposed surfaces of the face, ears, and backs of the hands and forearms, actinic keratoses may occur on any chronically or repeatedly sun-exposed part of the body. They are usually multiple, discrete, flat or elevated, verrucous or keratotic, red, pigmented, or skin-colored. Usually the surface is covered by an adherent scale, but sometimes it is smooth and shiny. The lesions are usually relatively small, measuring 3 mm to 1 cm; however, in the recently described type, the spreading pigmented actinic keratosis, the lesion may be 1 to 2 cm in diameter. Frequently solar keratoses develop into cutaneous horns. This hypertrophic type, which may lead to cutaneous horn formation, is most frequently present on the dorsal forearms and hands, as documented by Billano et al. Squamous cell carcinoma may be present at the base.

Previously known as *senile keratosis* because it is usually seen in elderly persons, now it is known that excessive sun exposure induces the lesions, espe-

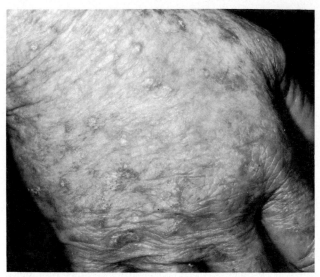

Figure 29–18. Actinic keratoses on back of hand. (Courtesy of Dr. Axel W. Hoke.)

cially in fair-skinned middle-aged and elderly persons. Development of actinic keratoses may occur in the twenties or thirties in patients who live in areas of high solar irradiation, are fair-skinned, and do not use sunscreens for protection. Green et al showed that other clinical signs of solar damage, such as solar lentigines, facial telangiectasia, and actinic elastosis of the neck, were strong risk factors for the development of skin cancer and solar keratoses.

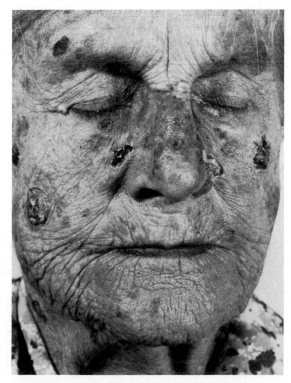

Figure 29–19. Actinic elastosis, basal cell carcinomas on the left ala nasi and cheeks, actinic keratoses on the nose, seborrheic keratosis over each eyebrow, and epidermal cyst on right outer canthus on an 80-year-old woman. (Courtesy of Dr. L. Fragola.)

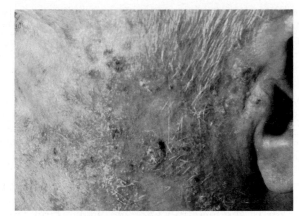

Figure 29–20. Actinic keratoses on left cheek. Patient subsequently died of squamous cell carcinoma metastases.

Histologically, the epidermal changes are characterized by acanthosis and dyskeratosis, and cellular atypia, the keratinocytes differing in size and shape and staining quality. Mitotic figures are common. The histologic picture may resemble *Bowen's disease.* There may be marked hyperkeratosis and areas of parakeratosis, with loss of the granular layer. Six types of actinic keratoses can be recognized histologically: hypertrophic, atrophic, bowenoid acantholytic, pigmented, and lichenoid. There is a dense inflammatory infiltrate: "not-self" is being recognized by T cells.

It is well recognized that squamous cell carcinomas arising from actinic keratoses are nonaggressive and that the prognosis is excellent: metastases are extremely rare. Exceptions to this are those carcinomas developing underlying actinic cheilitis and, as documented by Fukamizu et al, carcinomas occurring in the Japanese appear to be more aggressive and prone to metastasize.

The actinic keratosis is distinguished from discoid lupus erythematosus by the absence of dilated folli-

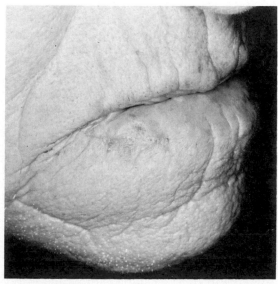

Figure 29–21. Actinic keratosis on vermilion border of lip.

cles and atrophy; from seborrheic keratosis by the absence of the greasy brown crust and sharply demarcated border; from Bowen's disease by the absence of infiltration and sharp outline; and from squamous cell carcinoma by the absence of infiltration and the extremely slow growth.

Vail reported a man with chronic lymphatic leukemia in whom the leukemia was recognized from the fact that he had large, hypertrophic actinic keratoses on all exposed surfaces, by three nondermatologists in his native Bavaria during a visit home.

Treatment should be thorough, as this type of keratosis is precancerous. The treatment methods for actinic keratosis are varied. For the few lesions occurring on the face and back we have found cryotherapy with liquid nitrogen most effective and practical. The individual lesion is frozen for a certain time, depending upon many variables, using a bulky cotton applicator dipped into liquid nitrogen. Lubritz, using a hand-held nitrogen spray, reported a 99 per cent cure rate. Healing usually occurs within the week.

For extensive, broad, or numerous lesions, 5-fluorouracil topically has been found to be extremely effective. Fluoroplex cream or solution, 1 per cent, or Efudex, 2 per cent are recommended for the face; however, for the trunk, scalp, hands, arms, and neck we prefer 5 per cent Efudex cream. It is rubbed in gently twice a day for three to four weeks on the head and neck, four to six weeks for other areas, or until there is a severe inflammatory reaction. The 1 per cent solution is effective on the lips. Breza et al found that application of 0.5 per cent triamcinolone cream immediately after each application of 1 per cent 5-FU solution greatly diminished the painful inflammatory reaction without inhibiting the therapeutic effect at all, but this has not been the experience of Goette, as well as others. The medication should be applied with extreme care near the eyes and mouth. According to the individual's sensitivity, an erythematous burning reaction will occur within several days. Treatment is stopped when a peak response characterized by a change in color from bright to dusky red, by reepithelialization, and by crust formation. Healing usually occurs within another two weeks after treatment has been stopped.

It has been observed that 5-fluorouracil "seeks out" the individual lesions of actinic keratosis even though the lesion is not clinically apparent. Excellent and lasting results are frequently observed. Clinically inapparent basal cell carcinomas may be detected during or upon completion of the treatment. A symposium on the use of 5-fluorouracil was held in 1985. Reprints are available through Howard Maibach at the University of California in San Francisco.

Many other treatments are possible. Winton et al review the arguments for use of dermabrasion for actinic keratoses, and present the results of scalp dermabrasion in five patients. Carbon dioxide laser vaporization is effective. Etretinate was found by Moriarty et al to effect a complete or partial response in 37 of 44 patients, and Edwards et al reported a good response to intralesional α_2-interferon. These latter two modalities are not accepted therapies, but are of interest. Carbon dioxide laser vaporization for actinic cheilitis is an excellent method of treatment.

Daily use of sunscreens is an effective, highly recommended method of preventing further chronic solar damage to the skin of patients with actinic keratoses.

Bennett RG, et al: Current management using 5-fluorouracil. Cutis 1985, 35:218.
Billano RA, et al: Hypertrophic actinic keratosis. JAAD 1982, 7:484.
Dinehart SM, et al: Spreading pigmented actinic keratosis. Arch Dermatol 1988, 124:680.
Dufresne RG, et al: Carbon dioxide laser treatment of chronic actinic cheilitis. JAAD 1988, 19:876.
Edwards L, et al: Effect of intralesional α_2-interferon on actinic keratoses. Arch Dermatol 1986, 122:779.
Epstein E: Treatment of lip keratoses (actinic cheilitis) with topical fluorouracil. Arch Dermatol 1977, 113:906.
Fukamizu H, et al: Metastatic squamous-cell carcinoma derived from solar keratoses. J Dermatol Surg Oncol 1985, 11:518.
Goette DK: Topical chemotherapy with 5-fluorouracil. JAAD 1981, 4:633.
Green A, et al: Skin cancer in a Queensland population. JAAD 1988, 18:1045.
Hughes BR, et al: Clinical response and tissue effects of etretinate treatment of patients with solar keratoses and basal cell carcinoma. JAAD 1988, 18:522.
Johnson TM, et al: Inflammation of actinic keratoses from systemic chemotherapy. JAAD 1987, 17:192.
Marks R, et al: The relationship of basal cell carcinomas and squamous cell carcinomas to solar keratosis. Arch Dermatol 1988, 124:1039.
Idem: Spontaneous remission of solar keratoses. Br J Dermatol 1986, 115:649.
Moriarty M, et al: Etretinate in treatment of actinic keratoses. Lancet 1982, 1:364.
Picascia DD, et al: Actinic cheilitis. JAAD 1987, 17:255.
Subrt P, et al: Spreading pigmented actinic keratoses. JAAD 1983, 8:63.
Tan CY, et al: Lichenoid actinic keratoses. J Invest Dermatol 1982, 79:365.
Vail JT: Hypertrophic solar keratoses: Sign of chronic leukemia? Schoch Letter 1989, 5:17.
Winton GB, et al: Dermabrasion of the scalp as a treatment for actinic damage. JAAD 1986, 14:661.

CUTANEOUS HORN
(Cornu Cutaneum)

Cutaneous horns, sometimes suggesting the horns of animals, are encountered most frequently on the face and the scalp. Lesions may also occur on the hands, the penis, and the eyelids. They are skin-colored, horny excrescences, 2 to 60 mm long, sometimes divided into several antlerlike projections. Their base is usually reddened and slightly thicker than their extremity.

These lesions are most often benign, with the hyperkeratosis being superimposed on an underlying seborrheic keratosis, verruca vulgaris, angioma, or trichilemmoma 50 to 60 per cent of the time. However, 20 to 30 per cent may overlie premalignant

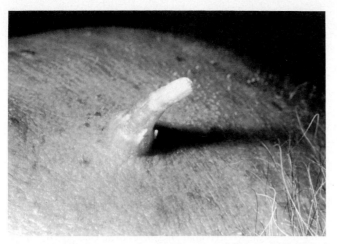

Figure 29–22. Cutaneous horn. (Courtesy of Dr. Axel W. Hoke.)

keratoses and 20 per cent may overlie squamous cell carcinomas or basal cell carcinomas. One third of penile horns are associated with underlying malignancies, as reviewed by Lowe et al. Excisional biopsy of these lesions with histologic examination of the base is necessary to determine the best therapy, which would be dictated by the diagnosis of the underlying lesion and by the apparent adequacy of removal.

Bart RS, et al: Cutaneous horns: clinical and histopathologic study in 35 patients. Acta Dermatovenereol 1968, 48:507.
Lowe FC, et al: Cutaneous horns of the penis. JAAD 1985, 18:369.
Schosser RH, et al: Cutaneous horns: a histopathologic study. South Med J 1979, 72:1129.
Srebrink A, et al: Cutaneous horn arising in cutaneous leishmaniasis. Arch Dermatol 1987, 123:168.

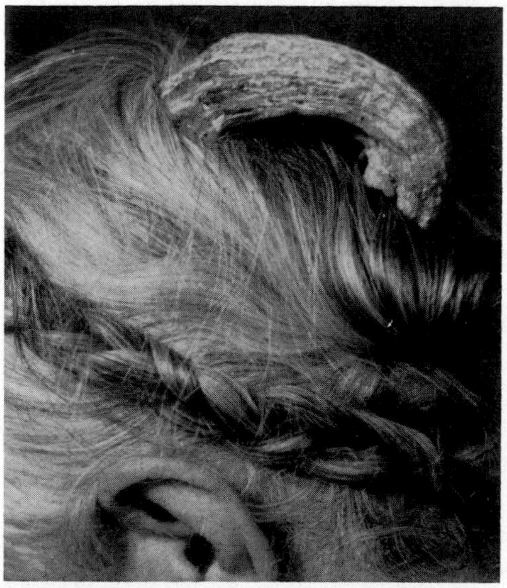

LEUKOPLAKIA

CLINICAL FEATURES. Leukoplakia presents as a whitish thickening of the epithelium of the mucous membranes, occurring as lactescent superficial patches of various shapes and sizes, which may coalesce to form diffuse sheets. The surface is generally glistening and opalescent, often reticulated, and may even be somewhat pigmented. The white pellicle is adherent to the underlying mucosa and attempts to remove it forcibly cause bleeding. At times it is a thick, rough, elevated plaque. The lips, gums, cheeks, and edges of the tongue are the most common sites, but the lesion may arise upon the anus and the genitalia. Leukoplakia is found chiefly in men over 40 years of age.

Biopsy of these white lesions may reveal solely simple orthokeratosis or parakeratosis with minimal inflammation, or there may be evidence of varying degrees of dysplasia. The first type is a benign form which is usually a response to chronic irritation and which has very little chance of conversion into the precancerous dysplastic form. Premalignant leukoplakia, with atypical cells histologically, is present in only about 10 to 20 per cent of leukoplakia. Unfortunately clinically it is not possible to predict the lesions which will histologically be worrisome, except that if ulceration or erosions are scattered throughout, the lesion is most likely precancerous. Therefore biopsy of all leukoplakia is indicated.

The course of the disease is extremely chronic. In time an extensive thick white pellicle may cover the tongue or oral mucosa. In old lesions the epithelium may be desquamated and there may be fissures or ulcerations. Such changes are associated with more

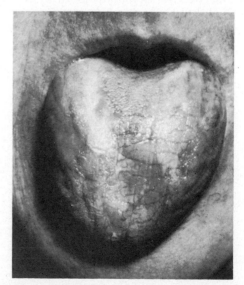

Figure 29–24. Leukoplakia of the tongue. In 10 years this 75-year-old nonsmoking woman developed carcinomas in both tonsillar fossae and on the floor of the mouth. All were successfully treated with ionizing radiation.

Figure 29–23. Cutaneous horn. (Courtesy of Dr. K. G. Higoumenakis, Athens.)

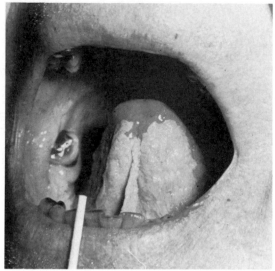

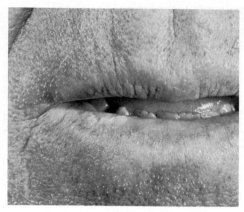

Figure 29–27. Epidermization of right lower lip. Note sharp, irregular proximal edge and undefined distal margin. (Courtesy of Dr. H. Shatin.)

Figure 29–25. Leukoplakia on the tongue. Extensive carcinomas developed in the mouth over the course of 3 years.

or less hyperemia and tenderness, and with a tendency to bleed after slight trauma. If transformation to carcinoma occurs, it generally follows a 1 to 20 year lag time.

When the lesion occurs on the lip, leukoplakia is closely related to chronic actinic cheilitis, which consists of a circumscribed or diffuse keratosis, almost invariably on the lower lip. It is preceded by an abnormal dryness of the lip and may be caused by biting the lips, by smoking (especially pipe smoking), or by chronic sun exposure. This type of leukoplakia is distinguished from squamous cell carcinoma of the lip by the absence of infiltration, from lichen planus and psoriasis of the lips and mouth by the absence of lesions elsewhere, and from lupus erythematosus

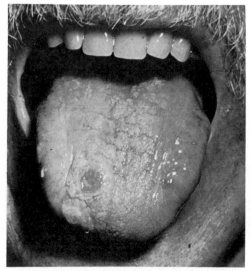

Figure 29–26. Squamous cell carcinoma arising in leukoplakia in late syphilis.

by the absence of telangiectases. Biopsy is necessary, however, to fully differentiate these conditions.

Human papillomavirus has been implicated as a cause of leukoplakia in several studies, such as that of Loning.

Oral hairy leukoplakia is a term used to describe white, corrugated plaques which occur primarily on the sides of the tongue of patients with the acquired immunodeficiency syndrome. This is a virally induced lesion, discussed in Chapter 19, which has a characteristic histology.

One of us (WDJ) has seen a unique case of leukoplakia involving the palate, lips, adjacent gingival mucosa, and labia minora and majora, which, on histologic examination had clusters of large cells with pink cytoplasm and pyknotic nuclei. This was chronic, noninfectious, and unresponsive to therapy.

Leukoplakia of the vulva usually occurs in obese women after menopause as grayish white, thickened, pruritic patches that may become fissured and edematous from constant rubbing and scratching. Secondary infection with edema, tenderness, and pain may occur. It is differentiated from lichen planus by the absence of discrete, rectangular or annular flat papules of violaceous hue in the mucosa outside the thickened patches, or about the anus or on the buccal mucosa. Lichen planus may involve the skin as well as the mucocutaneous areas. Leukoplakia of the vulva is most frequently confused with lichen sclerosus et atrophicus and other vulval atrophies.

On the penis, though leukoplakia may occur, a similar precancerous process called erythroplasia (of Queyrat) is usually seen instead.

ETIOLOGY. Numerous factors are involved in the cause of leukoplakia. It may develop as a result of the excessive use of tobacco, poorly fitting dentures, sharp and chipped teeth, or improper oral hygiene. Extensive involvement of the lips and oral cavity with leukoplakia may exist for years without any indication of carcinoma. On the other hand, small inflamed patches may be the site of a rapidly growing tumor, which, with relatively insignificant local infiltration, may early involve the cervical lymphatics. Carcinoma in leukoplakia usually begins as a localized induration, often about a fissure, or as a warty excrescence or a small ulcer. There is a 6 to 10 per cent transformation rate of intraoral leukoplakia into squamous cell carcinoma. The red lesions of leukoplakia (erythroleukoplakia) have a much higher risk of malignant degeneration than uniform white lesions.

TREATMENT. In the treatment of leukoplakia it must be remembered that cancer develops so frequently upon histologically dysplastic leukoplakia that its complete removal should be the goal in each case: first by conservative measures, then by surgery or destruction, if necessary. The use of tobacco should be stopped, and proper dental care obtained. Fulguration, simple excision, cryotherapy, and carbon dioxide laser ablation are effective methods of treatment. In actinic cheilitis accompanying leukoplakia of the tongue, the mucous membrane of the exposed surface of the lip may be removed and replaced by sliding forward the mucosa from the inner aspect of the lip. Cryotherapy is effected by the use of liquid nitrogen on the lesion. When this is done properly an excellent result will ensue. Odom, Goette, and Epstein have had great success with topically applied 5-fluorouracil. Hong et al reported the beneficial short-term effect of isotretinoin, 1 to 2 mg/kg/day for three months, in 24 patients.

Leukoplakia with Tylosis and Esophageal Carcinoma. Ritter and Petersen reported a case of oral leukoplakia associated with tylosis and esophageal carcinoma, and reviewed previous reports.

Epidermization of the Lip. Relatively smooth leukokeratosis of the lower vermilion, blending evenly into the skin surface distally and having a steep, sharp, irregular proximal margin, may easily be mistaken for precancerous leukoplakia clinically. Histologically, it shows only hyperkeratosis, without parakeratosis or any cellular atypia at all. A shallow shave excision suffices to cure it and to rule out precancerous leukoplakia; no fulguration is required. A histologic examination is, of course, even more important here than in the case of precancerous leukoplakia.

Axéll T: Occurrence of leukoplakia and some other oral white lesions among 20,333 adult Swedish people. Commun Dent Oral Epidemiol 1987, 15:46.

Bouquot JE, et al: Leukoplakia, lichen planus, and other oral keratoses in 23,616 white Americans over the age of 35 years. Oral Surg 1986, 61:373.

Greenspan JS, et al: Oral hairy leukoplakia. Oral Surg 1989, 67:396.

Hong WK, et al: 13-cis-retinoic acid in the treatment of oral leukoplakia. N Engl J Med 1986, 315:1501.

James WD, et al: Acquired dyskeratotic leukoplakia. Arch Dermatol 1988, 124:117.

Loning T, et al: Analysis of oral papillomas, leukoplakias, and invasive carcinomas for human papillomavirus type DNA. J Invest Dermatol 1985, 84:417.

Lupton GP, et al: Oral hairy leukoplakia. Arch Dermatol 1987, 123:624.

Shklar G: Oral leukoplakia. N Engl J Med 1986, 315:1544.

WHITE SPONGE NEVUS (Familial White Folded Mucosal Dysplasia)

Mouth, vagina, or rectum may be the site of this spongy, white overgrowth of the mucous membrane, with acanthosis, vacuolated prickle cells, and acidophilic condensations in the cytoplasm of keratinocytes, which have been shown by electron microscopy to be aggregated tonofilaments. In Jorgenson's review the buccal mucosa was the most common site of involvement. There are no extramucosal lesions.

There is no treatment. Progression of the disorder generally stops at puberty. The disease is inherited as an autosomal dominant disorder.

Jorgenson RJ, et al: White sponge nevus. Arch Dermatol 1981, 117:73.

Reaves CE: White sponge nevus of the tongue. South Med J 1975, 68:1170.

ORAL FLORID PAPILLOMATOSIS

Oral florid papillomatosis was originally described by Rock and Fisher in 1960 as a confluent papillomatosis covering the mucous membranes of the oral cavity.

The distinctive picture is that of a white mass resembling cauliflower, covering the tongue and extending onto the other portions of the mucous mem-

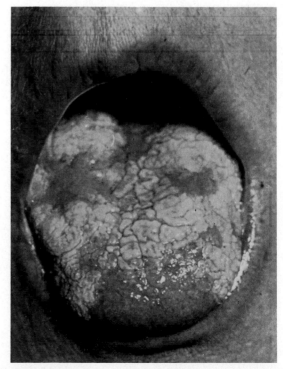

Figure 29–28. *Oral florid papillomatosis of 15 years' duration in a 65-year-old woman.*

branes, including the oropharynx, larynx, and trachea. Usually there is no lymphadenopathy.

The course of the disease is progressive. Some lesions eventuate in squamous cell carcinoma, whereas others continue for many years, the patient dying of some intercurrent disease. Oral florid papillomatosis should be regarded as a verrucous carcinoma, which has been defined as a distinctive, slowly growing fungating tumor representing a well-differentiated squamous cell carcinoma in which metastases occur very late or not at all. The histologic features are those of papillomatosis, acanthosis, and varying degrees of dysplasia of the epithelium, without disruption of the basement membrane.

In the differential diagnosis, leukoplakia, candidiasis, acanthosis nigricans, and condyloma acuminatum should be considered.

Treatment is recommended to be surgical excision; however, it is often followed by recurrence and spread. It is reasonable to expect the eventual development of epidermoid carcinoma in most patients.

Bovenmyer DA: Oral florid papillomatosis. Cutis 1974, 14:701.

Schwartz RA, et al: Florid cutaneous papillomatosis. Arch Dermatol 1978, 114:1803.

ELASTOTIC NODULES OF ANTHELIX

Elastotic nodules of the anthelix of the ear have been described by Carter and his associates. The bilateral, semitranslucent nodules appear exclusively on the upper part of the anthelix. The surface has an "orange peel" appearance.

It is believed that sun damage causes these nodules.

Histologically, a marked hyperkeratosis with a normal granular and malpighian layer characterizes this lesion. Some show basal cell proliferation. In the dermis the collagen is replaced with elastotic fibers and amorphous elastic material is seen.

Elastotic nodules are frequently mistaken for basal cell carcinoma. Other diagnoses frequently considered are rheumatoid nodules, gouty tophi, sarcoid, and calcinosis cutis.

Treatment centers around the removal of the lesions by shave excision and fulgurating the base. The removed specimen serves for biopsy purposes.

Carter VH, et al: Elastotic nodules of anthelix. Arch Dermatol 1969, 100:282.

KERATOACANTHOMA

Synonyms: Self-healing primary squamous carcinoma, molluscum sebaceum, benign keratoacanthoma, and idiopathic cutaneous pseudoepithelio-

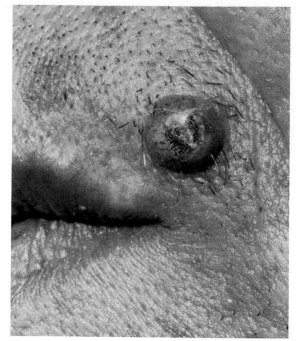

Figure 29–29. Keratoacanthoma.

matous hyperplasia are but a few of the names applied to this tumor.

CLINICAL FEATURES. Baer and Kopf have classified keratoacanthoma into three types: solitary, multiple, and eruptive.

Solitary Keratoacanthoma. This type is a rapidly growing papule, which enlarges from a 1-mm macule or papule to as much as 25 mm in three to eight weeks. When fully developed it is a hemispheric, dome-shaped, skin-colored nodule in which there is a smooth crater filled with a central keratin plug. The smooth shiny lesion is sharply demarcated from its surroundings. Telangiectases may run through the lesion.

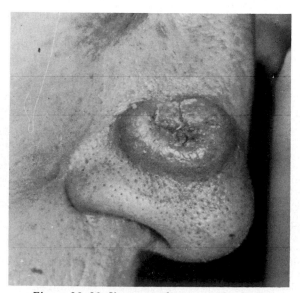

Figure 29–30. Keratoacanthoma on side of nose.

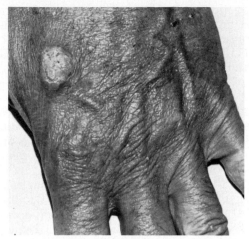

Figure 29–31. Keratoacanthoma resembling epidermoid carcinoma (a typical location). (Courtesy of Dr. L. Shapiro.)

Atypical forms of keratoacanthoma occur frequently. Some resemble seborrheic keratoses or benign acanthomas; others may have a nodulovegetative appearance; some, craterlike depressions. An interesting type is the one in which there is progressive peripheral growth while the center heals at the same time; *keratoacanthoma centrifugum* and *keratoacanthoma centrifugum marginatum* are terms applied to this type. Weedon and Barnett reported such a lesion, 14 × 20 cm, on a woman's calf. *Giant keratoacanthomas* are defined as those larger than 2 cm in diameter. They have been known to attain a diameter of 25 cm, and Piscioli et al reported one 10 cm across which metastasized. This presumably reflects the untrustworthiness of diagnostic criteria rather than the ability of keratoacanthomas to metastasize. An-

other variety is the *coral-reef keratoacanthoma*, in which multiple lesions extend from the original central lesion. Coalescing plaques or nodules occurring on the forehead have been described by Stevanovic and named *keratoacanthoma dyskeratoticum et segregans.*

The solitary keratoacanthoma occurs mostly on sun-exposed skin, with the central portion of the face, the backs of the hands, and the arms being the most commonly involved sites. Less frequently other sites are involved, such as the buttocks, thighs, penis, ears, and scalp. Kingman et al found that women had fewer lesions on the dorsal hands, but keratoacanthomas on the calves and shins were common in women but unusual in men. Rarely, this tumor involves the mucous membranes of the oral cavity or the subungual region. Keratoacanthoma is seen mostly in middle-aged to elderly persons, with men being more frequently involved. Subungual lesions are painful and induce early underlying bony destruction, characterized on x-ray as a crescent-shaped lytic defect without accompanying sclerosis of periosteal reaction.

The most interesting feature of this disease is the rapid growth for some two to six weeks, which is followed by a stationary period for another two to six weeks, and finally a spontaneous involution for another two to six weeks to leave a slightly depressed scar. The stationary period and involuting phase are variable; some lesions may take six months to a year to completely resolve. It has been estimated that some 5 per cent of treated lesions recur.

Invasion along nerve trunks was reported by Lapins and Helwig.

Multiple Keratoacanthomas. This type of keratoacanthoma is frequently referred to as the Ferguson Smith type of multiple self-healing keratoacantho-

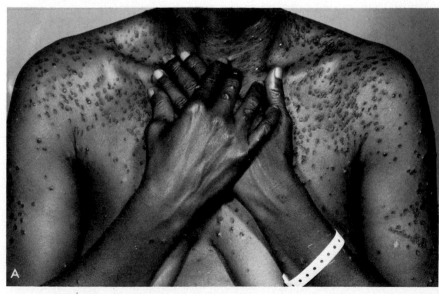
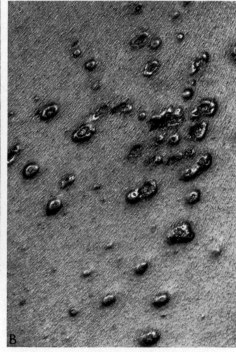

Figure 29–32. A *and* B, *Eruptive keratoacanthoma. (Courtesy of Dr. R. E. Rossman.)*

mas. These lesions are identical clinically and histologically to the solitary type. They may occur in any number, but generally only some three to ten lesions are noted, localized to one site. The commonest sites are the face, trunk, and genitalia. Young men are most frequently affected.

Ereaux and Schopflocher called attention to a familial type of generalized keratoacanthoma, occurring in two siblings, which they called the Ferguson Smith type of self-healing squamous epithelioma. The unusual aspect was the severe pruritus over a number of years, leading to an erroneous diagnosis of prurigo nodularis.

Eruptive Keratoacanthomas. This type of keratoacanthoma is characterized by a generalized eruption of numerous dome-shaped, skin-colored papules from 2 to 7 mm in diameter. The eruption is usually generalized but spares the palms and soles. The oral mucous membranes were involved in four of the seven cases summarized by Winkelmann and Brown and in the case of Snider et al, which was associated with an asymptomatic ovarian carcinoma. Severe pruritus was present in four patients, plus bilateral ectropion and narrowing of the oral aperture. Linear arrangement of some lesions, especially over the shoulders and arms, has also been noted.

ETIOLOGY. Belisario indicated that sunlight plays an important role in the etiology, especially in the solitary types. The high index of sunlight exposure to the incidence of keratoacanthomas is clearly correlated. In addition, light-skinned persons are more apt to develop keratoacanthoma than dark-skinned persons. Human papilloma virus has recently been impugned. Kingman et al found 21 per cent of their 90 patients had associated basal cell or squamous cell carcinomas.

Kopf and Andrade have cited instances of keratoacanthomas seemingly arising from inoculation or as an isomorphic phenomenon. Ghadially et al and Kingman et al found approximately 10 per cent of lesions to have developed in areas of injury or previous skin disease.

The etiology of eruptive keratoacanthomas involves a number of factors. DeMoragas reported an extensive case probably caused by excessive tar therapy (Jamarsan) for pemphigus foliaceus. He also cited other cases caused by tar application. Jolly and Carpenter noted flares in their patient after sun exposure. Claudy and Thivolet found multiple signs of deficient cell-mediated immunity in a 44-year-old man with recurrent episodes of multiple keratoacanthomas. Immunosuppressive treatments were found by Walder et al to predispose patients to more frequent and recurrent keratoacanthomas.

Many reports have suggested an association of keratoacanthoma with internal malignancies. Many appear to be coincidental, and Kingman et al found no increase in internal malignancies in their 90 cases. Two situations may occur when there is an association. In the Muir-Torre syndrome sebaceous tumors and keratoacanthomas occur in association with multiple low-grade malignancies. Inoshita et al reported

one case and reviewed three others in which multiple keratoacanthomas occurred in elderly women who were found to have genital tract cancer.

HISTOPATHOLOGY. The histologic findings of keratoacanthoma and a low-grade squamous cell carcinoma are frequently so similar that it is frequently difficult to make a definite diagnosis on the histologic findings alone. When a properly sectioned specimen is examined under low magnification (10 to 25 times), the center of the lesion shows a crater filled with eosinophilic keratin. Over the sides of the crater, which seems to have been formed by invagination of the epidermis, a "lip" or "marginal buttress" of epithelium extends over the keratin-filled crater. At the base and sides of the crater, acanthosis in the form of pseudoepitheliomatous hyperplasia occurs. The epidermal cells are highly keratinized and have an eosinophilic, glassy cytoplasm. Outside of this keratinocyte proliferation a dense lymphocytic infiltrate is frequently seen.

In the eruptive keratoacanthoma the histologic findings are similar to the solitary type. Many of the lesions will show the typical picture of a keratin-filled crater with an overhanging epidermis which is acanthotic and actively proliferating. Other lesions may show dilated follicles with keratin-plugged orifices. Acanthosis is seen surrounding the follicle.

The keratoacanthoma is distinguished from squamous cell carcinoma by far faster growth (sometimes fully grown in two weeks), and by its typical central core of keratin, which is usually absent in squamous cell carcinoma. Smoller et al have used the immunohistochemical stain for involucrun, a soluble precursor of the envelope of stratified squamous epithelium, as a diagnostic aid in differentiating these tumors. They found keratoacanthomas to show a homogeneous staining pattern, while in squamous cell carcinomas it was highly irregular.

Keratoacanthoma is also to be distinguished from seborrheic keratosis, cutaneous horn, epidermoid cyst, pseudoepitheliomatous hyperplasia, iododerma and bromoderma, prurigo nodularis, verruca vulgaris, and hypertrophic lichen planus. Histologic examination of the lesion is frequently necessary.

The eruptive keratoacanthomas are distinguished from pityriasis rubra pilaris, scleromyxedema, lichen amyloidosus, and Kyrle's disease. It may be necessary to examine several papular lesions before the distinctive features of keratoacanthoma are found.

TREATMENT. Although keratoacanthomas spontaneously involute it is impossible to predict how long it will take. The patient may be faced with an unsightly tumor for as long as a year. More importantly, Grade I squamous carcinoma cannot always be excluded even with a biopsy; therefore, biopsy excision or curettage and fulguration of an ordinary lesion less than 2 cm in diameter can and should be done in most cases. It is the safest course.

The intralesional injection of triamcinolone, especially in the treatment of solitary keratoacanthoma, has been successful in occasional patients, but due to the wide variety of therapies available today this treatment is not recommended.

Odom and Goette have reported excellent results from intralesional injections of 5-fluorouracil solution, straight from the ampoule. For clinically typical lesions this may be tried before resorting to surgical removal, especially if the latter presents any problem. They recommend excision if involution of the lesion is not complete after three consecutive injections one week apart. Parker, Odom, and Goette have all reported its usefulness in lesions in locations difficult to approach surgically.

Cipollaro in 1983 reported cures from the topical use of 25 per cent podophyllum in compound tincture of benzoin in giant keratoacanthomas. Goette, however, had no occasion to try it, since all of his cases treated with 5 per cent 5-fluorouracil (5-FU) cream involuted completely in one to six weeks.

Almost all treatments of eruptive keratoacanthomas have been generally disappointing. Topical vitamin A (retinoic acid) and corticosteroids have been of no avail. Methotrexate internally has shown varied response; Rossman and his associates had a good initial response, whereas Jolly and Carpenter noted no response to methotrexate. Topical 5-FU may be effective.

Goto has reported complete clearing with bleomycin in four cases of keratoacanthoma within 20 days after start of treatment.

Benoldi and Aldovini confirmed earlier reports by Sterry et al and Beretti et al of successful treatment with oral etretinate (Tigason), 1 mg/kg/day for eight weeks, tapered off slowly thereafter. Maintenance doses of 0.5 to 0.75 mg/kg every other day were required to maintain suppression of lesions. Cristofolini et al had excellent results in their patients. Isotretinoin has also been successfully used in a patient reported by Shaw et al.

X-ray therapy may also be used on giant keratoacanthomas when surgical excision or electrosurgical methods are not feasible. We treat these lesions in the same way as squamous cell carcinomas when x-ray therapy is indicated, and Kopf takes the same view. Farina et al reported five cases so treated, using 5000 rads over 15 to 20 days, with satisfactory results in all.

Benoldi D, et al: Multiple persistent keratoacanthomas: treatment with oral etretinate. JAAD 1984, 10:1035.
Cipollaro VA: The use of podophyllin in the treatment of keratoacanthoma. Int J Dermatol 1983, 22:436.
Cooper PH, et al: Perioral keratoacanthomas with extensive perineural invasion and intravenous growth. Arch Dermatol 1988, 124:1397.
Cristofolini M, et al: The role of etretinate in the management of keratoacanthomas. JAAD 1985, 12:635.
Eliezri YD, et al: Multinodular keratoacanthoma. JAAD 1988, 19:826.
Eubanks SW, et al: Treatment of multiple keratoacanthomas with intralesional fluorouracil. JAAD 1982, 7:126.
Fathizadeh A, et al: Aggressive keratoacanthoma and internal malignant neoplasm. Arch Dermatol 1982, 118:112.
Goette DK: Keratoacanthoma and its treatment. J Assoc Military Dermatol 1984, 10:3.
Idem: Treatment of keratoacanthoma with topical fluorouracil. Arch Dermatol 1983, 119:951.
Inoshita T, et al: Keratoacanthomas associated with cervical squamous cell carcinoma. Arch Dermatol 1984, 120:123.
Keeney GL, et al: Subungual keratoacanthoma. Dermatol 1988, 124:1074.
Kingman J, et al: Keratoacanthoma. Arch Dermatol 1984, 120:736.
Lapins NA, et al: Perineural invasion by keratoacanthoma. Arch Dermatol 1980, 116:791.
Macaulay WL: Subungual keratoacanthoma. Arch Dermatol 1976, 112:1004.
Odom RB, et al: Treatment of keratoacanthomas with intralesional 5-fluorouracil. Arch Dermatol 1978, 114:1779.
Parker CM, et al: Large keratoacanthomas . . . treated with intralesional 5-fluorouracil. JAAD 1986, 14:770.
Pelligrini VD, et al: Management of subungual keratoacanthoma. J Hand Surg 1986, 11A:718.
Piscioli F, et al: Gigantic metastasizing keratoacanthoma. Am J Dermatopathol 1984, 6:123.
Shaw JC, et al: Treatment of multiple keratoacanthomas with oral isotretinoin. JAAD 1986, 15:1079.
Smoller BR, et al: Keratoacanthoma and squamous cell carcinoma of the skin. JAAD 1986, 14:226.
Snider BL, et al: Eruptive keratoacanthoma with an internal malignant neoplasm. Arch Dermatol 1981, 117:788.
Wade TR, et al: The many faces of keratoacanthoma. J Dermatol Surg Oncol 1978, 4:483.
Wagner RF Jr, et al: Perineural invasion associated with recurrent sporadic multiple self-healing squamous carcinomas. Arch Dermatol 1987, 123:1275.
Weedon D, et al: Keratoacanthoma centrifugum marginatum. Arch Dermatol 1975, 111:1024.
Yoshikawa K, et al: A case of eruptive keratoacanthoma treated by oral etretinate. Br J Dermatol 1985, 112:579.

BASAL CELL CARCINOMA

Synonyms: Basal cell epithelioma, basalioma, rodent ulcer, Jacobi's ulcer, rodent carcinoma.

CLINICAL FEATURES. Basal cell carcinoma is a tumor composed of one or a few small, waxy, semitranslucent nodules forming around a central depres-

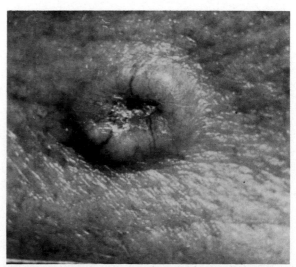

Figure 29–33. Basal cell carcinoma showing rolled waxy edge, telangiectasia, and central ulceration. Approximately 1 cm in diameter.

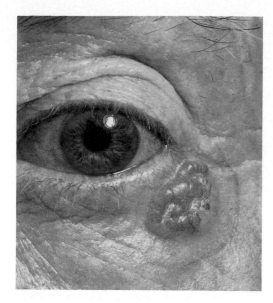

Figure 29–34. Basal cell carcinoma of lower eyelid in a 65-year-old man. (Courtesy of Dr. H. Shatin.)

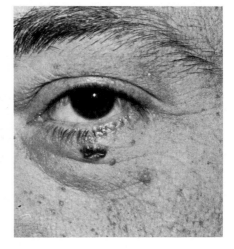

Figure 29–35. Pigmented basal cell carcinoma on lower eyelid. Simple excision yielded excellent results.

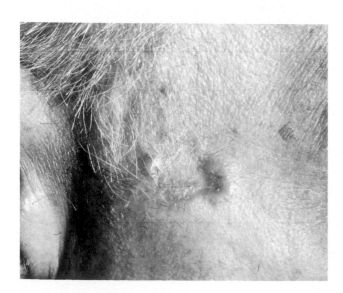

Figure 29–36. Basal cell carcinoma, preauricular area.

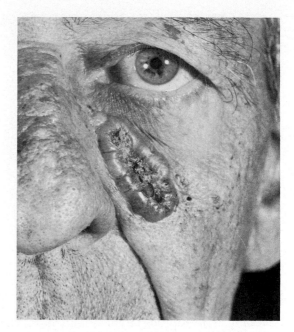

Figure 29–37. Basal cell carcinoma on the cheek. (Courtesy of Dr. H. Shatin.)

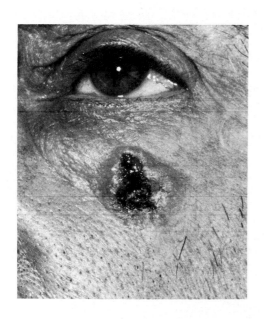

Figure 29–38. Basal cell carcinoma on the cheek with rolled edge and central ulceration.

Figure 29–39. Basal cell carcinomas on the bridge of the nose and left cheek of an 80-year-old woman.

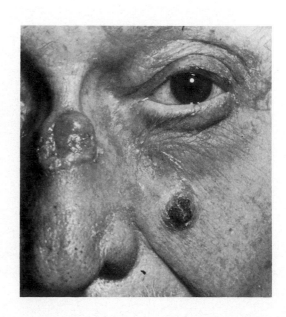
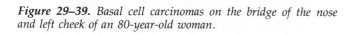

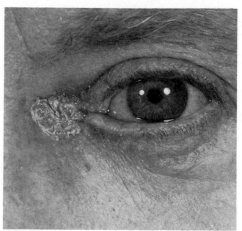

Figure 29–40. Basal cell carcinoma at the inner canthus—a common site when eyelids are involved. (Courtesy of Dr. H. Shatin.)

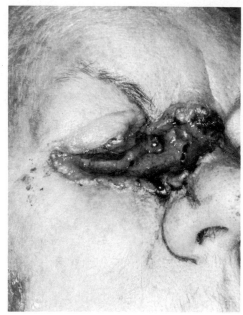

Figure 29–42. Extensive basal cell carcinoma of the orbit and nose.

sion that may or may not be ulcerated, crusted, and bleeding. The edge of larger lesions has a characteristic rolled border. Telangiectases course through the lesion. Bleeding on slight injury is a common sign.

As growth progresses, crusting appears over a central erosion or ulcer, and when the crust is knocked or picked off, bleeding occurs and the ulcer becomes apparent. This ulcer is characterized by chronicity and gradual enlargement as the months and years go by. The lesions are asymptomatic, and bleeding is the only difficulty encountered. They virtually never metastasize, because they are highly dependent on the connective-tissue stroma in which they lie. Metastasizing cases have almost always been subjected to repeated incomplete excisions or are cases which have been so neglected that the lesion reached extremely large size without the benefit of treatment.

The lesions are most frequently found on the face and especially on the nose. The forehead, ears, and cheeks are also often involved as a large review by Roenigk et al has confirmed. Any part of the body may be involved; however, the only other site of major frequency besides the head and neck is the upper trunk, where multiple lesions may occur simultaneously. An interesting observation is that basal cell carcinomas relatively rarely occur on the dorsal hand, where sun exposure and actinic keratoses and squamous cell carcinomas abound. Bean et al, in a review of carcinoma of the hand, showed that squamous cell carcinoma was three times more common than basal cell carcinoma.

In addition to the typical lesion just described, several clinical varieties are recognized. Awareness

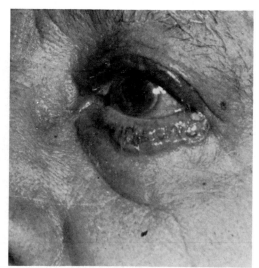

Figure 29–41. Extensive basal cell carcinoma of lower eyelid, which responded well to x-ray therapy.

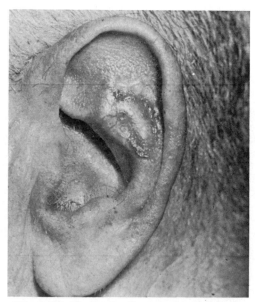

Figure 29–43. Basal cell carcinoma of the ear.

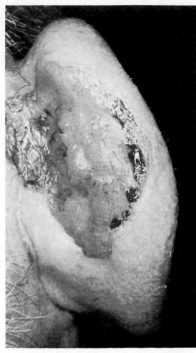

Figure 29–44. Basal cell carcinoma on back of ear.

of these varieties is helpful not only in the diagnosis but also in the management of the tumor.

Pigmented Basal Cell Carcinoma. This variety has all the features of the basal type and, in addition, brown or black pigmentation is present. These are usually extremely slow in evolving. This type is seen more frequently in dark complexioned persons such as Latin Americans or Japanese (not blacks). Carci-

nomas caused by arsenic (Fowler's solution) ingestion are often of the pigmented basal cell variety or the superficial type and occur frequently on the trunk. Domonkos showed that these carcinomas do not contain more arsenic than the surrounding normal skin.

In the management of these lesions it should be known that, if ionizing radiation therapy is chosen as the therapeutic modality, the pigmentation remains at the site of the lesion.

Cystic Basal Cell Epithelioma. Schwartz et al reported two patients with this type of dome-shaped, blue-gray cystic nodules. They point out the clinical similarity to eccrine and apocrine hidrocystomas.

Morphealike Epithelioma. This type of basal cell carcinoma has been described by Howell and Caro as a waxy white sclerotic plaque occurring in the head and neck region, with a conspicuous absence of a rolled edge. Ulceration and crusting are also absent, whereas telangiectasia is prominent.

The unique histologic feature is the strands of basal cells interspersed amidst densely packed connective tissue.

Howell and Caro regard this lesion as being entirely different from that of cicatrizing basal cell carcinoma (see next section). One other feature has been the lack of response to radiotherapy and electrosurgery. The treatment of choice has been scalpel, or Mohs, surgery.

Cicatricial Basal Cell Carcinoma. This type has also been called "field fire" epithelioma by Howell and Caro. It resembles a localized scleroderma which presents a cicatricial surface with nests of active lesions that are usually ulcerated. A fine waxy border or a threadlike raised edge as well as telangiectases

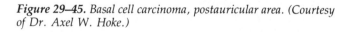

Figure 29–45. Basal cell carcinoma, postauricular area. (Courtesy of Dr. Axel W. Hoke.)

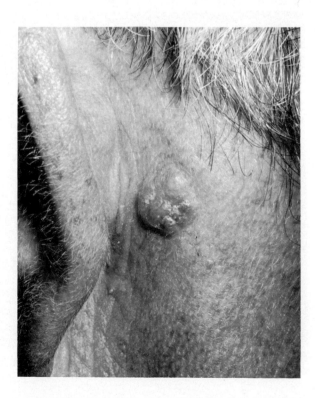

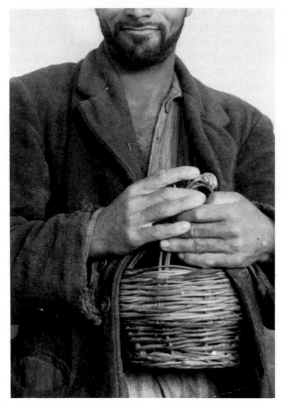

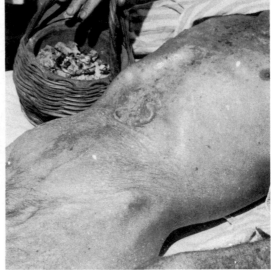

Figure 29–46. A, Kangri (fire basket). B, Kangri cancer (basal cell carcinoma). The "kangri" is a small basket with an earthen pot inside in which glowing coals and Chinan leaves burn. The smoke and the heat on the abdomen are said to induce cancers on the abdomen. (Courtesy of Dr. K. J. Ranadine, Bombay, India.)

are present. In our experience the cicatricial basal cell carcinoma occurs almost exclusively on the cheeks. The only other area noted to be involved has been the forehead. These lesions respond to excision, Mohs surgery, or ionizing radiation therapy.

Rodent Ulcer. Also known as Jacobi's ulcer, this is a penetrating serpiginous ulcer that slowly pro-

gresses for many years to become a large, gnawed-out, mutilating lesion. It is a neglected basal cell carcinoma.

Superficial Basal Cell Carcinoma. This type has been described under various names such as intraepidermal carcinoma, intraepidermal basal cell epithelioma of Borst-Jadassohn, and "multicentric"

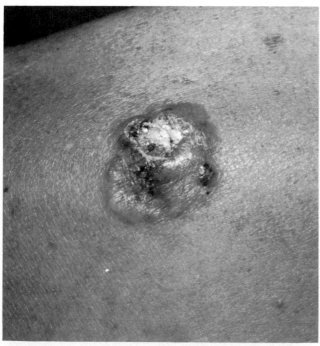

Figure 29–47. Basal cell carcinoma, shoulder. (Courtesy of Dr. Axel W. Hoke.)

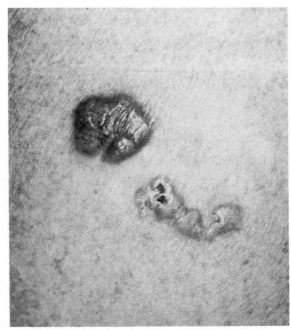

Figure 29–48. Basal cell carcinoma developing in a vaccination site.

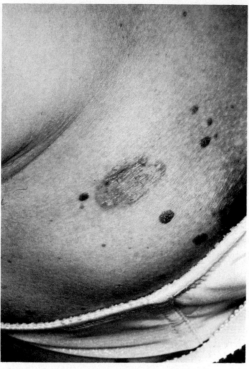

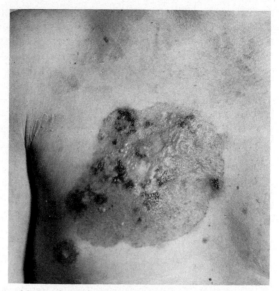

Figure 29–51. Superficial basal cell carcinoma on right pectoral area.

Figure 29–49. Superficial multicentric basal cell carcinoma and smaller seborrheic keratoses on the breast of a black female.

basal cell carcinoma. The multicentricity is merely an illusion created by the passing of the plane of histologic section through the branches of a single, multiply branching lesion. Pinkus has shown that in such lesions the characteristic stroma forms a solid, continuous plate.

This type frequently occurs as several dry, psoriasiform, scaly lesions on the trunk. They are usually superficial flat growths that exhibit little tendency to invade or ulcerate, and enlarge only very slowly. These lesions may grow to be some 10 to 15 cm in diameter without ulceration. Close examination of the edges of the lesion will show a threadlike raised border. These erythematous plaques with telangiectasia may show atrophy or scarring occasionally, and infiltration is conspicuously absent. Sometimes the lesion will heal at one place with a white atrophic scar and then spread actively to the neighboring skin. There may be several dozen lesions, some of which may coalesce to form extensive plaques.

Frequently there is a history of medicinal arsenic ingestion over a long period of time. Domonkos also observed instances of multiple superficial basal cell carcinomas along the spinal column, where fluoroscopic examinations and radiographs had been re-

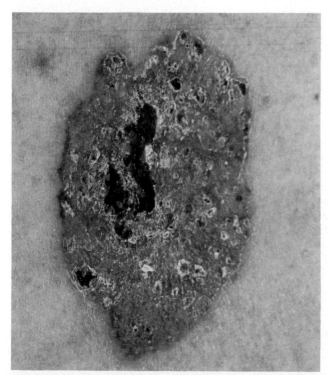

Figure 29–50. Superficial basal cell carcinoma on scapular area.

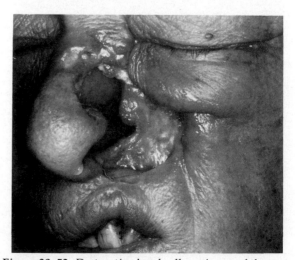

Figure 29–52. Destructive basal cell carcinoma of the nose.

peatedly made. These lesions may occur without concomitant evidence of radiodermatitis. Allison reported four cases in areas of radiation damage and found the lag time between radiation and development of basal cell carcinoma to be 20 years.

These lesions are not only frequently mistaken for plaques of psoriasis but also for Bowen's disease, and extramammary Paget's disease.

Fibroepithelioma of Pinkus. First described by Pinkus as *premalignant fibroepithelial tumor*, the tumor is usually an elevated, skin-colored, sessile lesion on the lower trunk, the lumbosacral area, groin, or thigh. The lesion is superficial and resembles a fibroma or papilloma and may be found occurring together with superficial basal cell carcinomas. Gellin and Bender reported a 7-cm wide lesion on the lower abdomen of a 76-year-old man. The lesion was a thick, sharply outlined, shiny, pinkish gray, eroded tumor.

Occurrence is in middle-aged and older persons. Bryant reported two patients with fibroepitheliomas overlying breast carcinomas.

Histologically, there are interlacing basocellular sheets (not cords, for none are cut into round structures), which extend downward from the surface to form an epithelial meshwork enclosing a hyperplastic mesodermal stroma. A slight inflammatory infiltrate may also be present. Pinkus regarded it as a neoplasm of the stromal element of a basal cell carcinoma.

Simple removal by excision or electrosurgery is the treatment of choice.

Aberrant Basal Cell Carcinoma. Even in the absence of any apparent carcinogenic factor such as arsenic, radiation, or chronic ulceration, basal cell carcinoma may occur in odd sites. McEleney reported one on the scrotum, Lupton one on the nipple, and Simonsen et al reviewed 21 cases on the vulva.

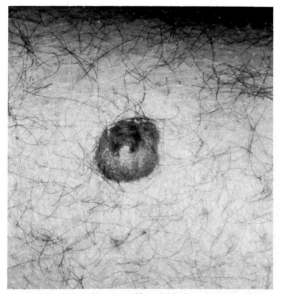

Figure 29–53. Premalignant fibroepithelioma eventuating in a basal cell carcinoma. (Courtesy of Drs. L. Shapiro and J. Penner.)

Solitary Basal Cell Carcinoma in Young Persons. These curious lesions are typically located in the region of embryonal clefts in the face and are often deeply invasive. Deep surgical excision is much safer than curettage for their removal. Rahbari et al reported 40 cases in children and teenagers, unassociated with the basal cell nevus syndrome or nevus sebaceus. Hanke et al studied skin cancer in golfers, all overexposed to sunlight, and found many who developed lesions at an early age.

COURSE. Basal cell carcinomas run a chronic course, during which new nodules develop, crusts form and fall off, and the ulceration enlarges. As a rule, there is a tendency for the lesions to bleed without pain or other symptoms. Some of the lesions tend to heal spontaneously and to form scar tissue as they extend. Peripheral spreading may produce configurate, somewhat serpiginous patches. The ulceration may burrow deep into the subcutaneous tissues, or even into cartilage and bone, causing extensive destruction and mutilation. The floor of the ulcer is covered by viscid necrotic material, crusts, and some serosanguineous discharge. This type is termed rodent ulcer, but in spite of the well-marked tendency to invade locally, it does not usually metastasize.

Metastasis. Although metastasis is extremely rare, more are being reported. Pinkus has shown that supporting stromal tissue is necessary for survival, which explains the infrequency of metastasis. Domarus et al reviewed 170 cases of metastasizing basal cell carcinoma in 1984. The following criteria are now widely accepted for the diagnosis of these rare metastases: 1) the primary tumor must arise in the skin; 2) metastases must be demonstrated at a site distant from the primary and must not be related to simple extension; 3) histologic similarity between the primary tumor and the metastases must exist; and 4) the metastases must not be mixed with squamous cell carcinoma. Males are involved twice as often as females. The head and neck region is the site of the primary tumor in the large majority of cases, with the regional lymph nodes the most frequent site of metastasis, followed by the lung, bone, skin, liver, and pleura. Spread is equally distributed between hematogenous and lymphatic. An average of nine years elapses between the diagnosis of the primary tumor and metastatic disease. The appearance of metastatic deposits indicates a poor prognosis, with a median survival of eight months. Coker et al and Hartman et al have reported response to chemotherapy in patients with metastatic basal cell carcinoma. Hartman et al's case underwent irradiation, surgery, and chemotherapy with cisplatin and was symptom free at 54 months after bony metastases.

ETIOLOGY. Excessive sunlight exposure, chemical cocarcinogens, and genetic determinants are implicated as causes of basal cell carcinoma. For this reason it is seen mostly in middle-aged and elderly persons, since they have had years of cumulative chronic exposure to sunlight. In addition to age, the type of skin and its ability to pigment are important factors. Light-complexioned persons in regions of the world where they are liable to be exposed to large amounts of sunlight (such as in Australia) often demonstrate the effects of that excessive exposure. Dark-skinned persons, other things being equal, are much less susceptible to skin cancers. The carcinogenic rays of the solar spectrum are between 290 and 334 nm. Strickland has confirmed that UVA (315 to 400 nm) alone is carcinogenic, although far less than combined UVB/UVA. It has been shown that the highest incidence of skin cancer occurs among Anglo-Saxons who are fair-skinned and have blue eyes. Sailors, farmers, inveterate sunbathers, and outdoor sportsmen are especially prone to skin cancers.

Excessive chronic exposure to ionizing radiation, especially x-rays, radium, and artificially and naturally occurring radioactive substances, may also cause cancer. Physicians, dentists, technicians, and workers with radioactive substances are at risk, and careful handling, shielding and dosage exposure records should be maintained to minimize danger. X-ray therapy for acne has been responsible for skin cancers 20 or 30 years later.

Ionizing and ultraviolet radiation are carcinogenic; however, some individuals are genetically more at risk than others due to defective DNA repair mechanisms. Xeroderma pigmentosum, an autosomal recessive disorder, is such a disorder, in which cutaneous neoplasms, including basal cell carcinomas, occur with increased frequency, as documented in the review by Kraemer et al.

Certain dermatoses of long standing duration such as linear epidermal nevi, nevus sebaceus, and porokeratosis of Mibelli may degenerate into basal cell carcinoma.

IMMUNOSUPPRESSION. Suppression of defensive immune surveillance by immunosuppressive medications, as in renal transplantation or cancer treatment, increases the risk of skin cancers as well as their aggressiveness. Gupta et al have studied this phenomenon in 523 renal transplant patients. While squamous cell carcinoma is most common, basal cell carcinomas do occur. Local immunosuppression also occurs in areas of the skin exposed to UVB through the damaging action of ultraviolet light on the Langerhans cells. It is theorized that this may lead to a susceptibility to skin cancer formation, because not only are immune responses diminished, but Langerhans cells become tolerant to antigens to which they are exposed after UVB damage. Thus if tumor antigens are present in skin exposed to chronic UVB, they may not respond to these altered antigens, and thus allow the cancer to grow.

INCIDENCE AND PREVALENCE. As already indicated under etiology, the incidence of cancer is highest among middle-aged and elderly people who have been exposed to considerable sunlight.

Basal cell carcinoma is the most common tumor of light-complexioned people. It occurs three to four times as frequently as squamous cell carcinomas, and is more common in men. Approximately 30 to 40 per

cent of patients with a basal cell carcinoma will develop one or more similar lesions within 10 years.

PATHOGENESIS. Pinkus indicated that the basal cell carcinoma belongs to the group of organoid adnexal tumors and that it is the least mature member of this group. It appears that the basal cell carcinomas arise from immature pluripotential cells. These tumors usually originate from the surface epidermis; however, they may also originate from the outer root sheath of the hair follicle.

Some recent observations support the view that the cells of the tumor are arrested in the early stages of epidermal differentiation. Antikeratin stains reveal a lack or decrease of large keratin molecules, which are associated with mature keratinizing epithelium. Also the basement membrane zone is altered; Stanley et al have reported a loss of bullous pemphigoid antigen from this area in basal cell carcinomas.

Grimwood et al have now provided an animal model for studying this tumor, with the transplantation of basal cell carcinoma into athymic mice.

HISTOPATHOLOGY. The early lesion shows small, darkly staining, polyhedral cells resembling those of the stratum germinativum, with swollen nuclei and small nucleoli. These occur within the epidermis as thickenings or immediately beneath the epidermis as downgrowths connected with it. After the growth has progressed, regular compact columns of these cells fill the tissue spaces of the dermis, and a connection with the epidermis may be difficult to demonstrate. At the periphery of the masses of cells, the columnar cells may be characteristically arranged like fence paling (palisading). This may be absent when the tumor cells are in cord arrangement or in small nests. A few mitoses are usually present. Cysts may form. The interlacing strands of tumor cells may present a latticelike pattern.

Subtypes occur histologically in which the immature cells differentiate toward a type of more mature tumor. Pilar, eccrine, apocrine, sebaceous, and squamous types of differentiation may be seen.

Pinkus indicated that the dermal stroma is an integral and important part of the basal cell carcinoma. The tumor does not terminate at the bottom of the epithelial nests but actually extends into its own newly formed connective tissue matrix to constitute a fibroepithelial neoplasm.

Electron microscopic studies show that the cells of the basal cell carcinoma have a greater nuclear/cytoplasmic ratio, fewer filaments, and fewer desmosomes than normal basal cells. No half-desmosomes facing the basement membrane are found in the tumor. On the other hand, the tumor cells are quite similar to the undifferentiated matrix of the human hair follicle.

Differentiation. Occasionally a basal cell carcinoma occurs which has differentiated into structures resembling sweat ducts, hair follicles, or sebaceous gland acini. These are reported under varying names such as the case by Sánchez et al of an eccrine epithelioma, or the tumor reported by Sakamoto et al, entitled apocrine epithelioma.

DIFFERENTIAL DIAGNOSIS. Distinguishing between small basal cell and small squamous cell carcinomas is largely an intellectual exercise, of little practical importance. Both are caused chiefly by sunlight; neither is likely to metastasize; neither is likely to be amenable to ordinary topical therapy with 5-fluorouracil; and both will have to be removed, usually by simple surgical excision or curettage.

Generalizations about location are both helpful and misleading. Both types of lesions may occur anywhere on the skin. However, the basal cell lesions are found chiefly on the face, especially on the nose, forehead, eyelids, temples, and upper lip, whereas the squamous cell growths are found principally on the face, at the mucocutaneous junctions, and on the extremities. Carcinoma primary on the vermilion surface of the lower lip is of the squamous cell type. The lesions on the backs of the hands are usually actinic keratoses, keratoacanthomas, or squamous cell carcinomas. Basal cell carcinomas rarely occur at this site.

The duration of the lesion may serve to differentiate the basal and squamous cell types of carcinoma from keratoacanthoma. If a lesion attains a diameter of 1 cm in less than three months, a diagnosis of squamous cell carcinoma or keratoacanthoma is likely. Cornification is distinctly a property of the squamous cell type and of keratoacanthoma. Horny material is usually clinically undetectable in basal cell lesions.

A waxy nodular rolled edge is fairly characteristic of basal cell growths. The squamous cell carcinoma is a dome-shaped, elevated, hard, and infiltrated lesion.

The early basal cell carcinoma may easily be confused with sebaceous hyperplasia, which has a depressed center with yellowish small nodules surrounding the lesion. These lesions never bleed and do not become crusted.

Bowen's disease, Paget's disease, and actinic and seborrheic keratosis may also simulate basal cell carcinoma. Ulcerated basal cell carcinoma on the shins is frequently considered to be a stasis ulcer, and a biopsy may be the only way to differentiate the two. Pigmented basal cell epithelioma is frequently misdiagnosed as melanoma or as a pigmented nevus. The superficial basal cell carcinoma is easily mistaken for psoriasis. The careful search for the rolled edge of the peripheral nodules is important in differentiating basal cell carcinoma from all other lesions.

TREATMENT. Each lesion of basal cell carcinoma must be thoroughly evaluated individually. Age, sex, and the size, site, and type of lesion are important factors to be considered when choosing the proper method of treatment for an advanced lesion. No single treatment method is ideal for all lesions, be that excision, ionizing radiation, chemosurgery, cryosurgery, curettage, or electrosurgery. The choice of treatment will also be influenced by the experience and ability of the treating physician in the various treatment modalities.

The aim in treatment is for a permanent cure with the best cosmetic results. This is important because the most frequent site of the basal cell carcinoma is the face. Recurrences result from inadequate treatment and are usually seen during the first four to 12 months after treatment. Cure rates are still calculated in five-year periods; however, it is rare to see recurrences later than one year after treatment. Five year follow-up is indicated, however, to continue a search for new lesions, since the development of a second basal cell carcinoma will occur in 35 to 40 per cent of patients, as reported by Epstein, and confirmed by Robinson.

Prophylaxis. All light-skinned individuals, especially those with blue eyes and light hair, should avoid unnecessary exposure to the sun from childhood to old age. Sunscreen lotions and creams that are helpful and effective are available for those regularly exposed. They should be applied every morning and reapplied after swimming or vigorous outdoor activity.

Biopsy. A biopsy should be performed in all these lesions. When the lesion is small enough to be amenable to surgical removal, a biopsy excision is preferable.

Excision. The ideal treatment method for carcinomas over 5 to 7 mm in diameter is simple elliptical excision with suturing, in those areas where this method is feasible. The scalp, ear rim, forehead, cheeks, chin, neck, and the remainder of the body are sites where simple elliptical excision may be indicated. Wedge excision is a method that is ideally performed on the lips, ears, and nostril rims, and even on the eyelids.

When lesions are much too large for simple elliptical excision or where closure is not feasible, excision and skin grafting or the use of skin flaps may be necessary. The skin grafts are either split-thickness or full-thickness grafts. Whether the split-thickness graft is to be thin, intermediate, or thick depends upon the area to be covered. It is reemphasized that the choice of treatment method depends on the probability of achieving a cure with the best possible cosmetic result.

Specimens should be examined histologically to confirm that the margins are clear. If the margins of the excision are involved, reexcision is necessary. The minimal margin generally necessary to totally eradicate the tumor in more than 95 per cent of cases with tumors less than 2 cm in size is 4 mm, as reported by Wolf.

Ionizing Radiation Therapy. The indications for radiation therapy are continually being modified, as chemosurgery evolves and becomes more available. In general, skin cancer should be treated by a modality which insures margin control, such as excision or chemosurgery. For individuals unable to tolerate surgical procedures, such as those with multiple medical problems, or in some cases the extremely elderly, radiation therapy offers an excellent alternative. In cases where surgery would be mutilating this modality may also be considered; however, the ultimate consideration should be the probability of cure, which often then favors surgical intervention.

The amount of x-ray exposure for the treatment of carcinoma is dependent upon the size, depth, and thickness of the lesion and also the type of radiation used. As a rule, ionizing radiation therapy to the ears requires great caution because of possible post-radiation necrosis of the cartilage.

Cancers of the scalp and forehead are near to the skull, and the proximity of the bone to the lesion, as well as the probability of permanent alopecia, modifies the choice of therapy. Heavy radiation exposure is contraindicated because of the danger of bone necrosis. Most carcinomas of the scalp and forehead can be readily treated by surgical measures if these hazards are recognized.

Treatment failures are probably the result of errors in estimating the size and depth of tumors. Recurrence at the periphery of the lesion indicates inadequate field size of irradiation; recurrence in the center of the field results from insufficient tumor depth dose. Radiation should not be used in areas where recurrences might be catastrophic, as in the inner canthus, as discussed by Rosen, or in young patients where radiation sequelae in the treated area will compromise the cosmetic result.

Pseudorecidive. This is a term used to describe the appearance of a pseudoepitheliomatous reaction at the site of a previously irradiated basal cell carcinoma. This reaction occurs some two to four weeks after ionizing radiation therapy has been performed; it may persist for as long as two months before spontaneous disappearance occurs. The lesion may resemble a seborrheic keratosis or, as reported by Poyzer and Delauney, a keratoacanthoma.

Electrosurgery. Many skin cancers are treated satisfactorily with a good cure rate and good cosmetic results by curettage and fulguration. In the hands of an able and experienced operator this form of treatment is probably superior to most other methods. The proper use of various-sized dermal curettes in connection with the fulguration permits the easy seeking out of the cancerous tumor. The large multiple superficial carcinomas found on the trunk are effectively and easily treated by thorough curettage and fulguration. Small lesions, 5 to 20 mm, of the nodular or cystic type, may be treated satisfactorily by this method in most locations.

A pliable, inconspicuous scar is formed with this method and a high cure rate is attained. Knox and his associates and Spiller et al report cure rates of over 96 per cent. Adam and Salasche have both reviewed this method of treatment. Studies by Salasche, d'Aubermont et al, Dubin et al, Lang et al, Roenigk et al, among others, indicate that central facial basal cell carcinomas and those of an infiltrating, micronodular or morpheiform histologic type are prone to recurrence if treated with curettage and desiccation. These lesions are thus better treated by methods which permit examination of the margins such as excision or chemosurgery.

Curettage. McDaniel treated 437 basal cell carcinomas with curettage alone and has followed 328 treatment sites for over five years. Cosmetic results have been excellent. Twenty-eight treatment failures were noted. He avoided utilizing this technique on the eyelids and lips and with morphea type or infiltrating lesions. We recommend this technique in elderly patients with small, well-circumscribed, nodular or superficial lesions. Dermal curettes of varying diameters are necessary.

Mohs Surgery. This method for the removal of accessible forms of cancer under microscope control was introduced by Mohs. His pioneering work began in the late 1930s. For 30 years he microscopically controlled the surgery by fixing the neoplastic tissue in situ with zinc chloride paste, excising a layer of tissue, carefully marking, mapping, and color-coding the margins, cutting horizontal sections, examining them microscopically, and repeating the process until all cancer was removed. This method is time-consuming, but the cure rate is high, determined by Mohs to be 99.3 per cent of 9351 lesions. In 1970 Tromovitch modified the technique by eliminating the fixative paste and doing the procedure on fresh tissue. Tromovitch and Stegman, and others, have done much to popularize this so-called "fresh-tissue" technique. It allows multiple sections to be taken each day, and allows for immediate repair, if desired. This type of surgery has an extremely high cure rate, usually in the range of over 99 per cent for primary basal cell carcinomas, and over 96 per cent for recurrent lesions. The indications for this type of surgery have been expanding, due to its proven cure rate and wider availability. Mohs himself embraced the fresh-tissue modification.

Consideration for Mohs surgery should be allowed for primary tumors occurring in the "H zone" of the face (the nasolabial fold, nasal alae, periorbital region, and periauricular area) and certain scalp tumors, the histologic variants of more aggressive type such as morpheiform or sclerosing types and basal-squamous types, for large lesions (over 2 cm), and for clinical situations such as those lesions occurring in immunosuppressed patients. Recurrent basal cell carcinomas, especially in difficult areas are also candidates for Mohs surgery. Swanson wrote an excellent review of this subject, in 1983.

Topical Cytotoxic Therapy. The topical application of 5-fluorouracil in various concentrations has been reported to be effective in the treatment of basal cell carcinomas, especially the superficial, multicentric type. Some have applied 5-FU after thorough curettage of the lesion. Mohs and associates warn that topical fluorouracil treatment of invasive basal cell carcinoma of the face can result in partial or complete healing of the skin overlying deeper extensions of the neoplasm. This method is not an accepted treatment.

Cryosurgery. Cryotherapy for basal cell carcinomas

as well as other benign and malignant neoplasms has been used since solid carbon dioxide became available. Since liquid nitrogen has become almost universally available, this modality has found increasing application for treatment of basal cell carcinomas. Because nitrogen boils at $-195.8°$ C, a deep penetrating action is attained in a short time when the liquid is applied to the surface of the skin. Zacarian, Torre, and Gloria Graham have all reported on this type of refrigeration therapy. Graham has successfully combined it with curettage. Charles Sheard has recommended the Foster apparatus for administering liquid nitrogen through a shortened 16-gauge needle. He recommends a 90-second freeze, a 60-second thaw, and a 30-second refreeze for a basal cell carcinoma up to 1 cm in diameter. However, cryosurgery is an essentially blind approach, and in general is not indicated except when excision is not feasible and irradiation does not appear to be advisable.

Laser Therapy. Goldman and his associates have pioneered laser beam therapy. Wheeland et al reported their results treating 52 patients with 370 basal cell carcinomas of the superficial type with curettage and carbon dioxide laser vaporization. They had excellent results with the advantages of rapid healing, diminished postoperative pain, and excellent field visualization.

Other Modalities. Greenway et al reported preliminary results in the use of intralesional interferon for treatment. Tse et al have used a hematoporphyrin derivative which localizes the neoplastic tissue and initiates cytotoxic responses after exposure to red light. Guthrie et al reported on the use of cisplatin and doxorubicin for advanced lesions. These methods are all experimental.

PREVENTION. Peck et al have reported preliminary results using isotretinoin as a chemopreventative approach. A large trial is underway to study this question. Sunscreens should be used by all basal cell cancer patients on a daily basis to prevent further solar damage.

Adam JE: The technic of curettage surgery. JAAD 1986, 15:697.

Ahman A, et al: Basal cell epithelioma in black patients. JAAD 1987, 17:741.

Albright SD III: Treatment of skin cancer using multiple modalities. JAAD 1982, 7:143.

Allison JR Jr: Radiation-induced basal cell carcinoma. J Dermatol Surg Oncol 1984, 10:200.

Barr RJ, et al: Multiple premalignant fibroepitheliomas of Pinkus (Case report and review of the literature). Cutis 1978, 21:335.

Bean DJ, et al: Carcinoma of the hand. South Med J 1984, 77:998.

Bryant J: Fibroepithelioma of Pinkus overlying breast cancer. Arch Dermatol 1985, 121:310.

Coker DD, et al: Chemotherapy for metastatic basal cell carcinoma. Arch Dermatol 1983, 119:44.

d'Aubermont PCS, et al: Failure of curettage and electrodesiccation for removal of basal cell carcinoma. Arch Dermatol 1984, 120:1456.

Davis MM, et al: Skin cancer in patients with chronic radiation dermatitis. JAAD 1989. 20:608.

Domarus HV, et al: Metastatic basal cell carcinoma. JAAD 1984, 10:1043.

Dubin N, et al: Multivariate risk score for recurrence of cutaneous basal cell carcinomas. Arch Dermatol 1983, 11:373.

Edens BL, et al: Effectiveness of curettage and electrodesiccation in the removal of basal cell carcinoma. JAAD 1983, 9:393.

Espinoza CG, et al: Immunohistochemical localization of keratin-type proteins in epithelial neoplasms. Am J Clin Pathol 1982, 78:500.

Goette DK, et al: Basal cell carcinomas and basal cell carcinomalike changes overlying dermatofibromas. Arch Dermatol 1975, 111:589.

Goldschmidt H: Radiotherapy of skin cancer: modern indications and techniques. Cutis 1976, 17:253.

Greenway HT, et al: Treatment of basal cell carcinoma with intralesional interferon. JAAD 1986, 15:437.

Grimwood RE, et al: Transplantation of human basal cell carcinoma to athymic mice. Cancer 1985, 56:519.

Gupta AK, et al: Cutaneous malignant neoplasm in patients with renal transplants. Arch Dermatol 1986, 122:1288.

Guthrie TH Jr, et al: Cisplatin and doxorubicin: an effective chemotherapy combination in the treatment of advanced basal cell and squamous cell carcinoma of the skin. Cancer 1985, 55:1629.

Hanke CW, et al: Skin cancer in professional and amateur female golfers. Physician Sportsmed 1985, 13:51.

Hartman R, et al: Long-term survival following bony metastases from basal cell carcinoma. Arch Dermatol 1986, 122:912.

Kaufman D, et al: Basal cell carcinoma. JAAD 1988, 18:306.

Kleinberg C, et al: Metastatic basal cell carcinoma of the skin. JAAD 1982, 7:655.

Kraemer KH, et al: Xeroderma pigmentosum. Arch Dermatol 1987, 123:241.

Kripke ML, et al: Modulation of immune function by UV radiation. J Invest Dermatol 1985, 85:625.

Lang PG, et al: Histologic evolution of recurrent basal cell carcinoma and treatment modalities. JAAD 1986, 14:186.

Lupton GP, et al: Basal cell carcinoma of the nipple. Arch Dermatol 1978, 114:1845.

Matsuoka LY, et al: Basal cell carcinoma in black patients. JAAD 1981, 4:670.

McDaniel WE: Therapy for basal cell epitheliomas by curettage only. Arch Dermatol 1983, 119:901.

Mehregan AH: Aggressive basal cell epithelioma on sunlight-protected skin. Report of 8 cases, one with pulmonary and bone metastases. Am J Dermatopathol 1983, 5:221.

Meyskens FL Jr: Studies of retinoids in the prevention and treatment of cancer. JAAD 1983, 6:824.

Mikhail GR, et al: Metastatic basal cell carcinoma discovered by chemosurgery. Arch Dermatol 1972, 105:103.

Idem: Chemosurgery in the treatment of skin cancer. Int J Dermatol 1975, 14:33.

Mohs FE: Chemosurgery for skin cancer. Arch Dermatol 1976, 113:211.

Idem, et al: Microscopically controlled surgery in the treatment of carcinomas of the scalp. Arch Dermatol 1981, 117:764.

Idem: Micrographic surgery for the microscopically controlled excision of carcinoma of the external ear. JAAD 1988, 19:729.

Nagle RB, et al: The use of anti-keratin antibodies in the diagnosis of human neoplasm. Am J Clin Pathol 1983, 79:458.

O'Dell BL, et al: Diminished immune responses in sundamaged skin. Arch Dermatol 1980, 116:559.

Parnes R, et al: Basal cell carcinomas and lymphoma. JAAD 1988, 19:1017.

Peck GL, et al: Chemoprevention of basal cell carcinoma with isotretinoin. JAAD 1982, 6:815.

Pinkus H: Epithelial and fibroepithelial tumors. Arch Dermatol 1965, 91:24.

Poyzer KG, et al: Pseudorecidivism of irradiated basal cell carcinoma. Austral J Dermatol 1975, 15:77.

Rahbari H, et al: Basal cell epithelioma in children and teenagers. Cancer 1982, 49:350.

Reymann F: Fifteen year's experience with treatment of basal cell carcinoma of the skin with curettage. Acta Derm Venereol (Stokh) 1985, Suppl 120:56.

Richmond JD, et al: The significance of incomplete excision in patients with basal cell carcinomas. Br J Plast Surg 1987, 40:63.

Robins P, et al: Mohs surgery for periorbital basal cell carcinomas. J Dermatol Surg Oncol 1985, 11:1203.

Robinson JK: What are adequate treatment and follow-up care for nonmelanoma cutaneous carcinoma? Arch Dermatol 1987, 123:331.

Roenigk RK, et al: Trends in the presentation and treatment of basal cell carcinomas. J Dermatol Surg Oncol 1986, 12:860.

Sakamoto F, et al: Basal cell tumor with apocrine differentiation. JAAD 1985, 13:355.

Salasche SJ: Status of curettage and desiccation in the treatment of primary basal cell carcinoma. JAAD 1984, 10:285.

Idem: Curettage and desiccation in the treatment of midfacial basal cell epithelioma. JAAD 1983, 8:496.

Sanchez NP, et al: Basal cell tumor with eccrine differentiation. JAAD 1982, 6:519.

Schwartz RA, et al: The blue-gray cystic basal cell epithelioma. JAAD 1980, 2:155.

Shelley WB, et al: Nodular superficial pigmented basal cell epithelioma. Arch Dermatol 1982, 118:928.

Simonsen E, et al: Basal cell carcinoma of the vulva. Acta Obstet Gynecol Scand 1985, 64:231.

Spiller WF, et al: Treatment of basal cell epithelioma by currettage and electrodesiccation. JAAD 1984, 11:808.

Stanley JR, et al: A specific antigenic defect of the basement membrane is found in basal cell carcinomas but not in other epidermal tumors. Cancer 1982, 50:1486.

Strickland PT: Photocarcinogenesis by near-ultraviolet (UVA) radiation in Senar mice. J Invest Dermatol 1986, 87:272.

Swanson NA: Mohs surgery. Arch Dermatol 1983, 118:761.

Torre D: Cryosurgery of basal cell carcinoma. JAAD 1986, 15:917.

Idem: Cryosurgical treatment of basal cell carcinomas. Progr Dermatol 1978, 12:11.

Tromovitch TA, et al: Microscopically controlled excision of skin tumors. Arch Dermatol 1974, 110:231.

Tse DT, et al: Hematoporphyrin-derivative photoradiation therapy in managing nevoid basal cell carcinoma syndrome. Arch Ophthalmol 1984, 102:990.

Wagner RF Jr, et al: Multifocal recurrent basal cell carcinoma following primary tumor treatment by electrodesiccation and curettage. JAAD 1987, 17:1047.

Wheeland RG, et al: Carbon dioxide laser vaporization and curettage in the treatment of large or multiple superficial basal cell carcinomas. J Dermatol Surg Oncol 1987, 13:119.

Wolf DJ, et al: Surgical margins for basal cell carcinoma. Arch Dermatol 1987, 123:340.

Zacarian SA: Cryosurgery of cutaneous carcinomas. JAAD 1983, 9:947.

INTRAEPIDERMAL EPITHELIOMA

This rare neoplasm has also been known as Borst-Jadassohn epithelioma and intraepidermal epithelioma of Jadassohn.

Clinically these single lesions present as a gray to tan-brown, keratotic, scaly, flat, sometimes verrucous, round to irregularly shaped plaque that clinically resembles Bowen's disease, multicentric basal cell carcinoma, epithelial nevus, seborrheic keratosis, nevus cell nevus, and melanotic freckle of Hutchinson. They appear on various parts of the body and may slowly grow to be several centimeters in diameter. Jadassohn's case had several superficial carcinomas at the same time.

Pinkus and Mehregan define intraepidermal epithelioma histologically as a neoplasm in which sharply defined nests of neoplastic cells are surrounded completely by normal keratinocytes. This is in contrast to carcinoma in situ, in which neoplastic cells range from the basement membrane to the epidermal surface. It has been suggested that these lesions may be only seborrheic keratoses, although intraepidermal nests may also occur in intraepidermal poromas and in Bowen's disease. Graham and Helwig believe that intraepidermal epithelioma represents a variety of carcinoma in situ arising from acrosyringium keratinocytes or pluripotential adnexal cells. When the dermoepidermal basement membrane is disrupted, it is considered to represent an adnexal eccrine carcinoma.

Simple local excision, and curettage and desiccation, are acceptable methods of treatment. Lesions showing carcinoma should be treated by wide local excision including subcutaneous fat.

Goltz RW, et al: Borst-Jadassohn epithelioma. Arch Dermatol 1967, 75:117.

Mehregan AH, et al: Intraepidermal epithelioma. Cancer 1964, 17:609.

NEVOID BASAL CELL CARCINOMA SYNDROME

This has frequently been miscalled the basal cell nevus syndrome and nevoid basalioma syndrome.

CLINICAL FEATURES. The nevoid basal cell carcinoma syndrome is a hereditary disorder characterized by basal cell carcinomas; odontogenic cysts of the jaws; pitted depressions on the hands and feet; osseous anomalies of the ribs, spine, and skull; and multiple other disorders. Keratin cysts are frequently

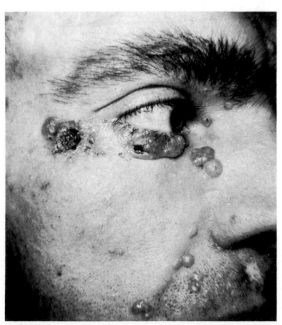

Figure 29–54. Nevoid basal cell carcinoma syndrome in a 39-year-old man with ameloblastoma, multiple cysts of the jaw, calcification of falx cerebri, spina bifida, Marfan's syndrome, and rheumatic heart disease. (Courtesy of Dr. A. M. Lefkovitz.)

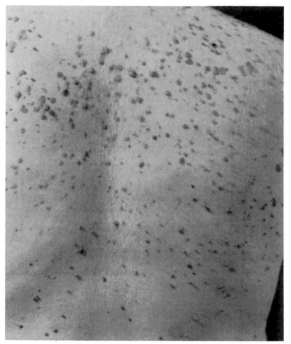

Figure 29–55. Nevoid basal cell carcinoma syndrome in a 10-year-old girl. (Courtesy of Dr. J. B. Howell.)

seen, and calcium deposits in skin, especially in the scalp. A characteristic facies is present, with frontal bossing, a hypoplastic maxilla, a broad nasal root, and true ocular hypertelorism being features.

Skin Tumors. The basal cell carcinomas occur at an early age or any time thereafter as multiple lesions, usually numerous. The usual age of appearance is between the ages of 17 and 35. Although any area of the body may be affected, there is a marked tendency toward involvement of the central facial area, especially the eyelids, periorbital area, nose, upper lip, and cheeks. Any variety of basal cell

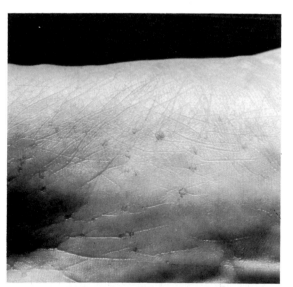

Figure 29–56. Pits on the sole in nevoid basal cell carcinoma syndrome. (From Howell JB: JAMA 190:274–277, 1964.)

carcinoma may be present; among these may be nodular, pigmented, morphealike, or ulcerated types. In children they may be pigmented papules resembling skin tags.

Taylor and his associates have indicated that the basal cell carcinomas in this syndrome may extend into the brain (as in two of their own cases). Metastasis may also occur. It is for this reason that they prefer the designation of "nevoid basal cell carcinoma syndrome" as indicative of the possible mutilating and destructive characteristics of these tumors.

Jaw Cysts. These occur in 70 per cent of patients. Both the mandible and the maxilla may show cystic defects by x-ray, with mandibular involvement occurring twice as often. The patient may complain of jaw pain and tenderness, fever, difficulty in closing the mouth, and swelling of the jaw. The cysts are uni- or multilocular and may occur anytime during life with the first decade being the most common time of appearance. They may have a keratinized lining, and some are ameloblastomas.

Pits of Hands and Feet. An unusual pitting of the hands and feet—not merely the palms and soles—is a distinguishing feature of the disease. They usually become apparent in the second decade of life. Howell and his associates have observed these pits in 70 per cent of their patients with nevoid basal cell carcinoma syndrome. Sulzberger has suggested that they are minimal expressions of a characteristic feature of basal cell carcinomas: inability to keratinize. Howell regards them as intraepidermal basal cell carcinomas which may never become clinically or histologically manifest. If they do, they are remarkably unaggressive.

Skeletal Defects. Numerous skeletal defects are easily detected by roentgenograms; such defects may be spina bifida, deformed ribs, scoliosis, and kyphosis. An interesting finding is shortened fourth metacarpal and metatarsal bones. The shortened fourth metacarpal results clinically in a dimple over the fourth metacarpophalangeal joint (Albright's sign). Radiographic evidence of multiple lesions is highly suggestive of this syndrome, and since most are present congenitally, x-rays may be useful in diagnosing this syndrome in patients too young to manifest other abnormalities. Seventy to 75 per cent of victims manifest skeletal abnormalities.

Disorders of the Central Nervous System. X-rays of the skull may show early lamellar calcification of the falx cerebri, falx cerebelli, and dura or basal ganglia. Varying mental problems may be encountered in patients.

Other Defects. Ophthalmologic abnormalities, mesenteric, ovarian, and mammary cysts, as well as uterine fibromas, lipomas, epithelial cysts, milia, and renal calculi are known to occur at times in these patients. Calcified multinodular ovarian fibromas are characteristic. Gutierrez et al recently reviewed the literature and presented a complete listing of other less common defects.

ETIOLOGY. This is a genetic disorder with an

autosomal dominant pattern. Penetrance may be as high as 95 per cent. The syndrome is seen most frequently in Caucasians. Ringborg et al showed that DNA repair synthesis in peripheral leukocytes is about 25 per cent less than normal.

HISTOPATHOLOGY. The histology of basal cell carcinomas arising in syndrome patients is identical to those arising in nonsyndrome patients, with the solid and superficial types being most common. The cutaneous keratocysts may show histologic finding similar to those seen in jaw keratocysts, and may be another cutaneous marker of this disease, as shown by Barr et al.

DIFFERENTIAL DIAGNOSIS. The skin tumors of the basal cell nevus syndrome have the following unique features which help to differentiate them from other tumors: Usually the lesions are multiple basal cell carcinomas occurring over a span of years from early childhood to late in life. The tumors occur in other than sun-exposed areas, with a history of similar tumors in other family members through several generations.

Two other unique types of presentation of basal cell carcinomas should not be confused with this entity. One is the *linear unilateral basal cell carcinoma* syndrome, in which a linear arrangement of close set papules, sometimes interspersed with comedones, is present at birth. Biopsy reveals basal cell epitheliomas; however, they do not increase in size with age of the patient. The second type, referred to as *Bazex's syndrome*, is a dominantly inherited disease comprising follicular atrophoderma of the extremities, localized or generalized hypohidrosis, hypotrichosis, and multiple basal cell carcinomas of the face, which often arise at an early age.

TREATMENT. The aggressiveness of the carcinomas varies, and owing to this and the multitude of lesions, Mohs surgery provides the best cure rates and cosmetic appearance. Curettage and desiccation of the superficial lesions of the trunk and excision are other effective methods. Genetic counselling is essential.

SQUAMOUS CELL CARCINOMA

Synonyms: Prickle cell carcinoma, epidermoid carcinoma.

CLINICAL FEATURES. This type of carcinoma occurs not only on the skin but also on the mucous membranes. Frequently squamous cell carcinoma begins at the site of actinic keratosis on sun-exposed areas such as the face and backs of the hands. Even though basal cell carcinomas far outnumber squamous cell carcinomas on the facial skin, a large series of carcinomas of the hand reported by Bean et al confirms that squamous cell carcinomas occur three times more commonly than basal cell carcinomas in this location. The lesion may be superficial, discrete, hard, and arises from an indurated rounded elevated base. It is dull red and contains telangiectases. In other instances, the tumors begin as small erythematous, infiltrated, hard, scaly plaques, on skin that has been damaged by x-rays, scars, or chronic ulcers. In the course of a few months the lesion becomes larger, deeply nodular, and ulcerated. The ulcer is at first superficial and is hidden by a crust. When this is removed, a well-defined, papillary base is seen and on palpation a discrete hard disk is felt. In the early phases this tumor is localized, elevated, and freely movable on the underlying structures; later it gradually becomes diffuse, more or less depressed, and fixed. The growth eventually invades the underlying tissues. The tumor above the level of the skin may be dome-shaped, with a corelike center which later ulcerates. The surface in advanced lesions may be cauliflowerlike, composed of densely packed, filamentous projections, between which are clefts filled with a viscid, purulent, malodorous exudate.

Mora et al reviewed 163 cases of squamous cell carcinoma in black patients. They found squamous cell carcinomas to be 20 per cent more common than basal cell carcinomas in blacks of the same patient population. The most common sites were the face and lower extremities, with involvement of non-

Aloi FG, et al: Unilateral linear basal cell nevus associated with diffuse osteoma cutis, unilateral anodontia, and abnormal bone mineralization. JAAD 1989, 20:973.

Barr RJ, et al: Cutaneous keratocysts of nevoid basal cell carcinoma syndrome. JAAD 1986, 14:572.

Gorlin RJ: Nevoid basal cell carcinoma syndrome. Medicine 1987, 66:98.

Gutierrez MM, et al: Nevoid basal cell carcinoma syndrome. JAAD 1986, 15:1023.

Holubar K, et al: Multiple palmar basal cell epitheliomas in basal cell nevus syndrome. Arch Dermatol 1970, 100:679.

Howell JB: Nevoid basal cell carcinoma syndrome. JAAD 1984, 11:98.

Idem, et al: Structure and significance of the pits with their tumors in the nevoid basal cell carcinoma syndrome. JAAD 1980, 2:224.

Johnson AD, et al: Nevoid basal cell carcinoma syndrome. JAAD 1986, 14:371.

Pratt MD, et al: Nevoid basal cell carcinoma syndrome. JAAD 1987, 16:964.

Ringborg U, et al: Decreased UV-induced DNA repair synthesis in peripheral leucocytes from patients with the nevoid basal cell carcinoma syndrome. J Invest Dermatol 1981, 76:268.

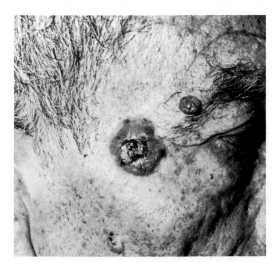

Figure 29–57. Squamous cell carcinoma. (Courtesy of Dr. F. Kerdel-Vegas, Venezuela.)

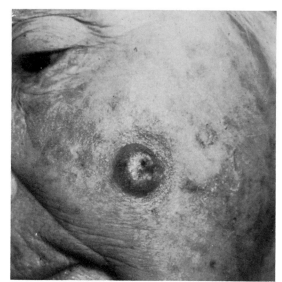

Figure 29–58. Squamous cell carcinoma. Note dome shape of the tumor.

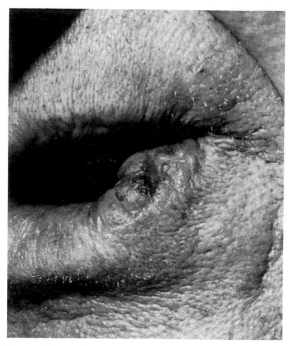

Figure 29–60. Squamous cell carcinoma on the lower lip.

sunexposed areas more common. Thus, as contrasted with white patients, the most common predisposing conditions were scarring processes such as burns, leg ulcers, and hidradenitis suppurativa. As will be discussed later, the incidence of metastases is very low from sites of chronic sun damage, while it is relatively high (20 to 30 per cent) in squamous cell carcinomas occurring in scarring processes. Accordingly, Mora et al found a relatively high mortality rate, 18.4 per cent.

On the *lower lip*, squamous cell carcinoma often develops upon actinic cheilitis. From repeated sunburn the vermilion surface becomes dry, scaly, and fissured, and keratoses develop. Cancer usually arises on such a fissure or keratosis. At the beginning only a local thickening is noticeable. This then becomes a firm nodule. It may grow outward as a

sizable tumor, or grow inward with destructive ulceration. A history of smoking is also frequent and a significant predisposing factor. Fitzpatrick reported a series of 361 lip cancers, 348 of which were squamous cell carcinomas. As in all large series, the lower lip lesions far outnumbered upper lip lesions, men far outnumbered women (ratio 12:1), and the median age was the late sixties. If the carcinoma appears on the upper lip, men outnumber women by a lesser extent. Mora et al reviewed 36 black patients with squamous cell carcinoma of the lip and found 26 were men, and seven lesions occurred on the upper lip. Squamous cell carcinomas occurring on the lower

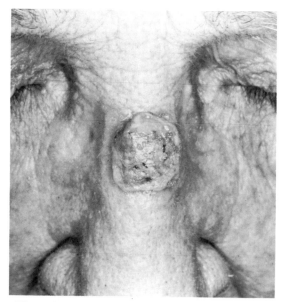

Figure 29–59. Squamous cell carcinoma of the nose.

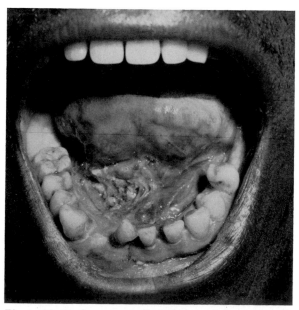

Figure 29–61. Squamous cell carcinoma on floor of mouth.

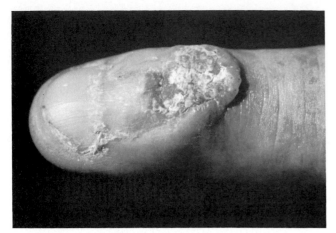

Figure 29–62. Squamous cell carcinoma, subungual, mimicking a wart. (Courtesy of Dr. Axel W. Hoke.)

lip metastasized approximately 10 to 15 per cent of the time, and Mora et al's series confirmed this high frequency in black patients. Martin et al reported the occurrence of squamous cell carcinoma of the lip occurring in areas of discoid lupus in black patients.

Lumpkin et al and Mikhail have reviewed subungual squamous cell carcinoma. They both stress that the early signs are swelling, erythema, and localized pain. It commonly arises in the nail folds of the hands (particularly the thumbs) of patients in the 50 to 69 year old age range. Fifty per cent of those who were x-rayed showed changes in the terminal phalanx. There was a very low rate of metastases, but local excision with Mohs surgery was recommended to save as much normal tissue as possible.

Biopsy of chronic, recalcitrant, indurated lesions in actinically damaged skin of lip, or of similar lesions

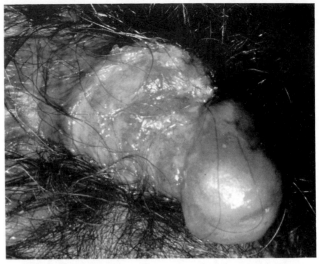

Figure 29–64. Squamous cell carcinoma of the penis. (Courtesy of Dr. Axel W. Hoke.)

of the digits in the subungual area, or of such lesions in chronic scarred sites, should be done to make this diagnosis. Generally incisional or excisional biopsies are recommended. Punch biopsies are of no value if negative.

ETIOLOGY. Many causative factors have been identified in squamous cell carcinoma. Ultraviolet light certainly is a major factor in light-complected individuals. While UVB has long been known to be of prime importance, the role of UVA is just beginning to be realized. It does play some part, as the work of Strickland and Staberg et al shows. UVB may predispose to skin cancer not only through its DNA-damaging action but also via local injury to Langerhans cells. Photochemotherapy, psoralens plus UVA light, as used in this country, is associated with

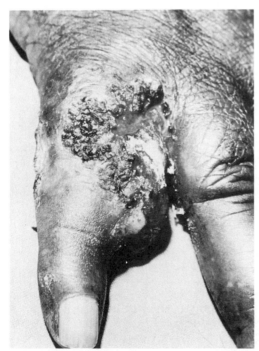

Figure 29–63. Squamous cell carcinoma of the finger.

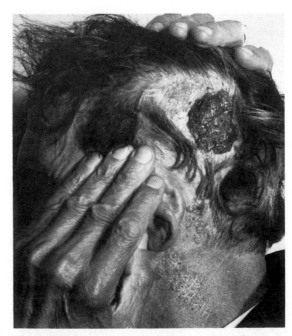

Figure 29–65. Squamous cell carcinoma in nevus sebaceus present since birth. (Courtesy of Dr. J. Penner.)

squamous cell carcinoma formation, following a close relationship curve, as documented by Stern et al. Other situations which reveal the importance of ultraviolet light in squamous cell carcinoma formation include the high incidence of this tumor in African albinos as reported by Launde et al and Okoro et al; in hypopigmented black skin secondary to other dermatoses, as reported by Martin et al; and in patients with genetic inability to repair sun-induced DNA damage, as reviewed by Kraemer et al in their large article on xeroderma pigmentosum.

Thermal injury to the skin may produce thermal keratoses and squamous cell carcinoma. The constant exposure to hot tea as experienced by tea tasters may produce leukoplakia and oral cancer. The *Kangri cancer*, occurring in Kashmir among the natives who use the Kangri jar, a brazier of hot coals carried under the clothing for warmth, develops on the abdomen and upper thighs (see p. 768).

Chemical carcinogenesis is a classic cause of skin cancer. Best known are the effects of polycyclic aromatic hydrocarbons, which include 3,4-benzpyrene. This has been implicated as the cause of scrotal squamous cell carcinoma in mule spinners in the cotton textile industry, as in the case reported by Castiglione et al. Other situations where chemical carcinogenesis can play a role are scrotal cancers in chimney sweeps; patients with mycosis fungoides treated topically with nitrogen mustard, as reported by Lee et al; and potentially psoriatic patients treated with coal tar, as in a patient reported by May et al. Arsenic, paraffin, creosote, anthracene, tobacco smoke tars, and chromates are other important carcinogens.

Chronic radiation dermatitis from x-radiation or radium may produce squamous cell carcinomas, as in several patients who developed carcinoma of the fingers under rings contaminated with radioactive gold. Sarcomas, malignant fibrous histiocytomas, angiosarcomas, and basal cell carcinomas may also appear in these sites.

Human papillomavirus, especially of types 16, 18, 30, and 33, is associated with squamous cell carcinoma. It occurs in sun-exposed areas and with increased frequency in epidermodysplasia verruciformis. This virus is also associated with cervical cancer and may be related to the increase in skin cancer seen in renal transplant patients.

The eponym *Marjolin's ulcer* is used when cancers, most of which are of the squamous cell type, arise in chronic ulcers, sinuses, and scars of various etiologies, although burns are the most common cause. This was reviewed by Applebaum et al. Burns; fistulous tracts such as occur in hidradenitis suppurativa, acne conglobata, or pilonidal sinus; syphilis; lupus vulgaris; stasis ulcers; osteomyelitis sinuses; amputation stumps; smallpox vaccinations; decubitus ulcers; epidermolysis bullosa scars; granuloma inguinale; lymphogranuloma venereum; and discoid lupus scars have been implicated as processes that predispose to the development of squamous cell carcinoma.

Certain dermatoses such as linear epidermal nevi, porokeratosis of Mibelli, and lichen sclerosus et atrophicus have been associated with an increased incidence of squamous cell carcinoma developing in them.

HISTOPATHOLOGY. Squamous cell carcinoma is characterized by irregular nests of epidermal cells invading the dermis in varying degrees. The degree of cell differentiation has been used to grade squamous cell carcinoma. Although interpretations vary, it is believed that the greater the differentiation, the less the invasive tendency, thereby the better the prognosis. The Broders classification has four grades of cell differentiation. In grade I most of the cells are well differentiated, whereas in grade IV most of the cells are undifferentiated or anaplastic. The anaplastic type of tumors may be difficult to differentiate from other tumors such as melanoma, lymphoma, and mesenchymal tumors. This is true also when the tumor is of the spindle-cell type. Kahn et al and Penneys et al report on the value of immunoperoxidase staining for prekeratin or cytokeratin to identify squamous cell carcinoma. Electron microscopy may also be useful when tonofilaments are seen. Immerman et al suggest the use of Clark's anatomic levels to predict the chance of recurrence or metastasis.

DIFFERENTIAL DIAGNOSIS. The squamous cell carcinoma may be difficult to distinguish from keratoacanthoma. The rapid growth and the presence of a rolled border with a keratotic central plug are good indicators that one is dealing with a keratoacanthoma.

The early squamous cell carcinoma may be confused with a hypertrophic actinic keratosis, and, indeed, the two may be indistinguishable clinically. Biopsy to include the base of the lesion is necessary to make the diagnosis.

In the mouth it is to be distinguished from a chancre. The procedure in differentiating the two is to biopsy the lesion. Gummatous lesions of the skin are differentiated in the same manner.

Pseudoepitheliomatous hyperplasia is a histologic diagnosis to be considered. The clinical features are suggestive of a carcinoma occurring in some of the inflammatory diseases, especially in granulomatous reactions and ulcerations. Pseudoepitheliomatous hyperplasia may be seen in granular cell tumor, in bromoderma, blastomycosis, granuloma inguinale, and chronic pyodermas. It is frequently mistaken for squamous cell carcinoma in chronic stasis ulcers, ulcerations occurring in thermal burns, lupus vulgaris, leishmaniasis, and even in sporotrichosis. It may occur in a "dry" socket after dental extraction.

Architecturally the epithelial hyperplasia is suggestive of squamous cell carcinoma; however, the atypical cells are absent and the nuclei show normal staining. Strands of epidermal cells may extend into the reticular dermis. In the dermis a pronounced inflammatory reaction is often present.

METASTASES. Careful attention should be paid to regional lymph nodes draining the site of the squamous cell carcinoma. The propensity of this lesion to metastasize is dependent upon the etiologic factors to some extent. The incidence of metastatic diseases in sun-induced squamous cell carcinoma is low, with the probable overall incidence less than one per cent. In fact Arnold, in 44 years of practice in Hawaii, removing 80 to 100 squamous cell carcinomas a year, did not see one instance. Bickers's and Lund's experiences support this. On the other hand Epstein et al and Moller et al report a 2 to 3 per cent incidence and Fukamizu et al's report supports a higher proportion in Japanese patients.

It is agreed that cancer of the lip, even though it primarily occurs on the sun-exposed lower lip, metastasizes more commonly, with an incidence of 10 to 20 per cent. Mora et al found none of the upper lip lesions in several black patients metastasized, while seven of 25 lower lip lesions metastasized. Squamous cell carcinomas occurring in burn scars, chronic ulcers, and radiodermatitis are more aggressive, with reported incidences of metastases in the 20 to 30 per cent range. Mora et al found an 18 per cent mortality in 163 black patients with squamous cell carcinoma, reflecting the fact that most occurred in areas of chronic scarring. Moller et al and Ames et al, among others, document the poor overall survival of patients with metastatic squamous cell carcinomas. Patients who are immunosuppressed tend to get more aggressive squamous cell carcinomas. On the other hand, patients with porokeratosis of Mibelli who develop squamous cell carcinomas rarely develop metastatic disease.

TREATMENT. Because of the possibility of metastasis from squamous cell carcinoma, treatment should be thorough. Ideally an excisional surgical specimen with margin control should be obtained. Mohs's surgical technique, especially for recurrent disease, large lesions, those in the postauricular sulcus, those in irradiated or scarred skin, or those in areas requiring the salvage of as much normal skin as possible, as on the penis or the finger, is a preferred choice. The results as reported by Dzubow et al are excellent. Radiation therapy is also effective, as attested to by Fitzpatrick's results in lip carcinoma.

For metastatic or advanced disease, Guthrie et al reported their results with cisplatin and doxorubicin. Holnar et al reported on the use of bleomycin alone, or in combination with other agents.

Levine et al found isotretinoin effective within a six-month treatment period, in a patient with multiple carcinomas on sun-exposed skin. There was no recurrence of lesions that were cured by retinoid therapy. Intralesional bleomycin was used by Tanigaki et al in a patient with good results. These therapies should be considered only experimental, however.

PREVENTION. Stern et al estimate that the regular use of a sunscreen with a sun protection factor of 15 for the first 18 years of life would reduce the lifetime incidence of nonmelanoma skin cancers by 78 per cent.

Abel EA, et al: Cutaneous malignancies and metastatic squamous cell carcinoma following topical therapies for mycosis fungoides. JAAD 1986, 14:1029.

Ames FC, et al: Metastasis from squamous cell carcinoma of the extremities. South Med J 1982, 75:920.

Appelbaum J, et al: Acute Marjolin's ulcer. J Assoc Milit Dermatol 1985, 11:57.

Baptiste MS, et al: Health effects associated with exposure to radiatively contaminated gold rings. JAAD 1984, 10:1019.

Bean DJ, et al: Carcinoma of the hand. South Med J 1984, 77:998.

Bickers DR: Reply (letter to editor). JAAD 1981, 4:735.

Castiglione FM, et al: Mule spinner's disease. Arch Dermatol 1985, 121:370.

Cramer SF, et al: Squamous cell carcinoma arising in a linear epidermal nevus. Arch Dermatol 1981, 117:222.

Curry SS, et al: Squamous cell carcinoma arising in dissecting perifolliculitis of the scalp. JAAD 1981, 4:67.

Dzubow LM, et al: Risk factors for local recurrence of primary cutaneous squamous cell carcinoma. Arch Dermatol 1982, 118:900.

Eliezri YD: The toluidine blue test. JAAD 1988, 18:1339.

Epstein E, et al: Metastases from squamous cell carcinoma of the skin. Arch Dermatol 1968, 97:245.

Epstein JH: All-trans-retinoic acid and cutaneous cancer. JAAD 1986, 15:772.

Fitzpatrick PJ: Cancer of the lip. J Otolaryngol 1984, 13:32.

Fukamizu H, et al: Metastatic squamous cell carcinoma derived from solar keratoses. J Dermatol Surg Oncol 1985, 11:518.

Guthrie TH, et al: Cisplatin and doxorubicin. Cancer 1985, 55:1629.

Gupta AK, et al: Cutaneous malignant neoplasms in patients with renal transplants. Arch Dermatol 1986, 122:1288.

Holnar KE, et al: Bleomycin in advanced squamous cell carcinoma. Br Med J 1976, 1:188.

Hubbell CR, et al: Cancer of the skin in blacks. JAAD 1988, 18:292.

Immerman SC, et al: Recurrent squamous cell carcinoma of the skin. Cancer 1983, 51:1537.

Jenson AB, et al: Role of papilloma virus in proliferative squamous lesions. Surv Synth Path Res 1985, 4:8.

Kahn H, et al: Role of immunohistochemistry in the diagnosis of undifferentiated tumors involving the skin. JAAD 1986, 14:1063.

Kraemer KH, et al: Xeroderma pigmentosum. Arch Dermatol 1987, 123:241.

Lee LA, et al: Second cutaneous malignancies in patients with mycosis fungoides treated with nitrogen mustard. JAAD 1986, 14:1029.

Leiter E, et al: Circumcision and penile carcinoma. NY State J Med 1975, 75:1520.

Levine N, et al: Oral isotretinoin therapy: use in a patient with multiple cutaneous squamous cell carcinomas and keratoacanthomas. Arch Dermatol 1984, 120:1215.

Lippman SM, et al: Nonsurgical treatments for skin cancer. J Dermatol Surg Oncol 1988, 14:862.

Luande J, et al: The Tanzania human albino skin. Cancer 1985, 55:1823.

Lumpkin LR, et al: Subungual squamous cell carcinoma. JAAD 1984, 11:735.

Lund HZ: Metastasis from squamous cell carcinoma of the skin: an uncommon event (editorial). J Dermatol Surg Oncol 1984, 10:169.

Lutzner MA: Skin cancer in immunosuppressed organ transplant recipients (editorial). JAAD 1984, 11:891.

Martin S, et al: Metastatic squamous cell carcinoma of the lip. Arch Dermatol 1979, 105:1214.

Mikhail GR: Subungual epidermoid carcinoma. JAAD 1984, 11:291.

Møller R, et al: Metastases in dermatological patients with squamous cell carcinoma. Arch Dermatol 1979, 115:703.

Mora RG, et al: Cancer of the skin in blacks. JAAD 1981, 5:535.

Idem: Cancer of the skin in blacks. JAAD 1982, 6:1005.

Moys LS, et al: Scrotal squamous cell carcinoma in a psoriatic patient treated with coal tar. JAAD 1986, 14:518.

Okoro AN: Albinism in Nigeria. Br J Dermatol 1975, 92:485.

Penneys NS: Immunoperoxidase methods and advances in skin biology. JAAD 1984, 11:284.

Presser SE, et al: Squamous cell carcinoma in blacks with discoid lupus erythematosus. JAAD 1981, 4:667.

Quintal D, et al: Aggressive squamous cell carcinoma arising in familial acne conglobata. JAAD 1986, 14:207.

Staberg B, et al: The carcinogenic effect of UVA irradiation. J Invest Dermatol 1983, 81:517.

Stearns FW: The curious case of the radioactive ring. JAAD 1981, 5:696.

Stern RS, et al: Risk reduction for nonmelanoma skin cancer with childhood sunscreen use. Arch Dermatol 1986, 122:537.

Idem: Cutaneous squamous cell carcinoma in patients treated with PUVA. N Engl J Med 1984, 310:1156.

Strickland PT: Photocarcinogenesis by sun-ultraviolet (UVA) radiation in Senar mice. J Invest Dermatol 1986, 87:272.

Stutzman CD, et al: Squamous cell carcinoma of the skin associated with radioactive gold rings. JAAD 1984, 10:1075.

Swanson NA: Mohs surgery. Arch Dermatol 1983, 119:761.

Tanigaki T, et al: A case of squamous cell carcinoma treated by intralesional injection of bleomycin. Dermatologica 1985, 170:302.

Turner JE, et al: Aggressive behavior of squamous cell carcinoma in a patient with preceding lymphocytic lymphoma. JAAD 1981, 4:446.

ADENOID SQUAMOUS CELL CARCINOMA

Pseudoglandular Squamous Cell Carcinoma

It is characterized by a fast-growing tumor, usually on the sun-exposed areas such as the face, ears, and backs of the hands, although it can occur elsewhere, such as in the instance of a patient of Domonkos's in whom the lesion was on the chest. The lesion has a keratotic verrucous appearance at first, then has ulceration with crusting. The lesion may resemble a keratoacanthoma. Metastases are rare.

Histologically the tumor is basically a squamous cell carcinoma with distinctive adenoid proliferation and acantholytic cells.

In the diagnosis of pseudoglandular carcinoma, keratoacanthoma and rodent ulcer should be considered.

Surgical excision is the preferred treatment. Domonkos found x-ray therapy effective in two cases.

VERRUCOUS CARCINOMA (Carcinoma Cuniculatum)

First described by L. V. Ackerman, verrucous carcinoma is a distinct, well-differentiated variety of squamous cell carcinoma. The term is a collective one, which may include such entities as giant condyloma of Buschke and Lowenstein, epithelioma cuniculatum, and oral florid papillomatosis. Verrucous carcinoma may also be found in the larynx, or on the glans penis, scrotum, vulva, scalp (Baruchin et al), face (Nguyen et al), back (Sanchez-Yas et al), buttocks (Ruppe), and sole. The slow-growing and invading lesion may invade the bony structure around the tumor. Human papillomavirus may be involved in the induction of these tumors.

Histologically, the lesion shows a characteristic picture of bulbous rete ridges, which are topped by an undulating keratinized mass. The squamous epithelium is well differentiated. Pseudoepitheliomatous hyperplasia must always be considered.

Excision is the best treatment. Brownstein and Shapiro reported eight cases with plantar verrucous carcinoma of 14 years' average duration. They agree that only excision is curative. Seehafer et al recently reported on bilateral verrucous carcinoma of the feet, effectively treated with a conservative surgical approach. Mora reported two cases on the sole, effectively managed by Mohs chemosurgery as did Swanson and Taylor, who reported two cases situated on the sole in which Mohs chemosurgery was felt to be the treatment of choice. Radiotherapy has been discouraged in some reports as it was felt to possibly be related to anaplastic transformation of the tumor. Lymph node metastases are extremely rare, so that the prognosis is favorable when complete excision is effected.

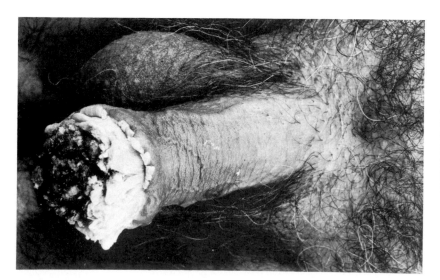

Figure 29–66. Giant condyloma of Buschke-Löwenstein involving the glans penis. [Photograph used by permission of New York University School of Medicine (Skin and Cancer Unit).] (From Andrade R, Gumport SL, Popkin GL, Rees TD [eds]: Cancer of the Skin. Philadelphia, WB Saunders, 1977, p 815.)

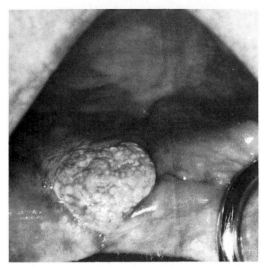

Figure 29–67. Verrucous carcinoma of the postcommissural mucosa in a 52 year old man. There is only slight leukoplakic change of the surrounding mucosal epithelium. (From Andrade R, Gumport SL, Popkin GL, Rees TD [eds]: Cancer of the Skin. Philadelphia, WB Saunders, 1977, p 535.)

Ackerman LV: Verrucous carcinoma of the oral cavity. Surgery 1948, 23:670.

Baruchin AM, et al: Carcinoma cuniculatum capitis: a variant of squamous cell carcinoma of the skin. Int J Dermatol 1984, 23:67.

Grinspan D, et al: Oral florid papillomatosis (verrucous carcinoma). Int J Dermatol 1979, 18:608.

Japaze H, et al: Verrucous carcinoma of the vulva. Obstet Gynecol 1982, 60:462.

Kao GF, et al: Carcinoma cuniculatum (verrucous carcinoma of the skin). Cancer 1982, 49:2395.

Mora RG: Microscopically controlled surgery (Mohs chemosurgery) for treatment of verrucous squamous cell carcinoma of the foot (epithelioma cuniculatum). JAAD 1983, 8:354.

Nguyen KQ, et al: Verrucous carcinoma of the face. Arch Dermatol 1984, 120:383.

Ruppe JD Jr: Verrucous carcinoma. Arch Dermatol 1981, 117:184.

Sanchez-Yas E, et al: Verrucous carcinoma of the back. JAAD 1986, 14:947.

Swanson NA, et al: Plantar verrucous carcinoma: literature review and treatment by the Mohs chemosurgery technique. Arch Dermatol 1980, 116:794.

BOWEN'S DISEASE

Bowen's disease is an intraepidermal squamous cell carcinoma having only lateral, intraepidermal spread. It may ultimately become invasive.

CLINICAL FEATURES. Bowen's disease appears on any part of the body as an erythematous, slightly scaly and crusted, noninfiltrated patch from a few millimeters to many centimeters in diameter. The lesion is sharply defined. The scale is often pronounced, and on its removal the exposed dull red surface may be papillary and moist.

As the lesion slowly enlarges, spontaneous cicatrization may go on in parts of the lesion. When the intraepithelial growth becomes invasive, it does so by forming a nodular infiltration of the lesion, which becomes ulcerated and fungating. Squamous cell carcinoma is the type usually seen and may complicate Bowen's disease in up to 5 per cent of cases. Jacobs reported a sebaceous carcinoma occurring in Bowen's disease of the vulva and an accompanying editorial by Kao stresses the various forms of differentiation these tumors may express.

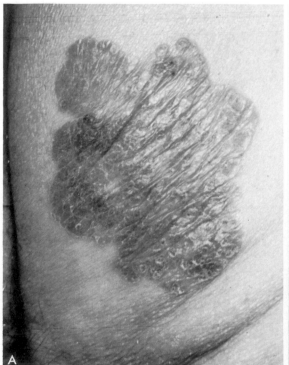

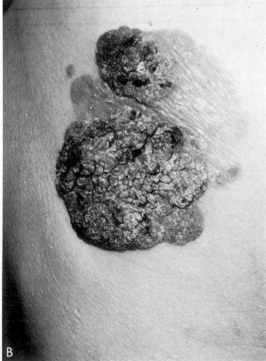

Figure 29–68. A, Bowen's disease. B, Bowen's disease with marked hyperkeratosis. (Courtesy of Dr. D. K. Goette.)

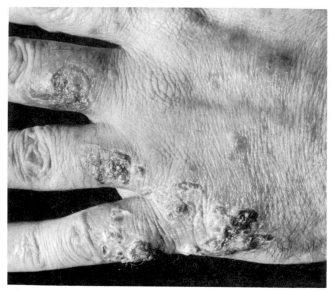

Figure 29–69. Multiple lesions of Bowen's disease. (Courtesy of Dr. Axel W. Hoke.)

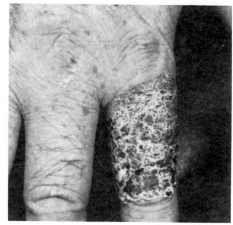

Figure 29–71. Bowen's disease on forefinger.

The mucous membranes may also be involved. The vulva, vagina, nasal mucous membranes, conjunctiva, and larynx are the sites of most frequent involvement on the mucous membranes. When squamous cell carcinoma in situ occurs on the glans penis it is referred to as erythroplasia of Queyrat.

ETIOLOGY. Bowen's disease has its highest incidence in older white men, in whom the lesions occur primarily on sun-exposed surfaces. Thus one etiologic factor is chronic solar damage. Inorganic arsenical exposure predisposes to Bowen's disease in non-sun-exposed areas. A history of ingestion of Fowler's solution or Asiatic pills was found by Peterka and associates in 11 of 33 patients with Bowen's disease on covered surfaces and internal carcinoma, whereas of 20 patients with Bowen's disease on exposed skin,

only one had internal carcinoma and none had a history of arsenic ingestion. Miki et al have documented a group of Japanese patients who developed Bowen's disease and pulmonary cancers years after arsenic ingestion. In many cases of Bowen's disease no etiologic factor is identifiable, as in the 19 black patients reported by Mora et al where neither sun exposure nor arsenic were factors.

A possible relationship of Bowen's disease of the skin to systemic cancer was reported by Graham and Helwig. Many studies have subsequently been published addressing this question and results have been conflicting. While no agreement exists as to the significance of this lesion and malignancy, the following may be concluded. If seen on chronic sun-damaged skin in older white men, other cutaneous carcinomas should be expected to appear, such as squamous cell and basal cell carcinomas. If exposure to arsenic has occurred, internal malignancies may develop with increased frequency, but at a later date, as reported by Miki et al. Finally, if a predisposition

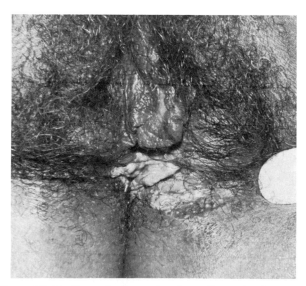

Figure 29–70. Bowen's disease involving the perineal area and extending to the vaginal and perianal areas.

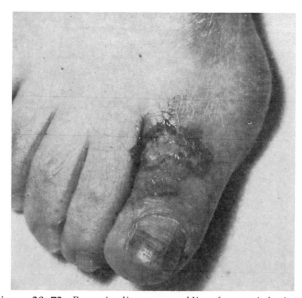

Figure 29–72. Bowen's disease resembling fungus infection of toe.

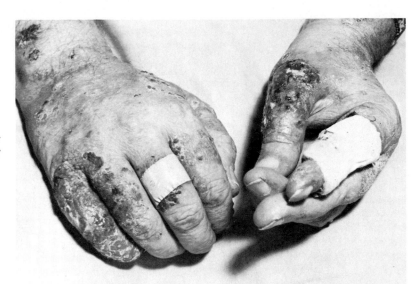

Figure 29–73. Basal cell carcinomas and multiple Bowen's disease in a man with a history of arsenic ingestion for many years.

to develop internal malignancy exists in these patients, it is over their lifetime, and Bowen's disease is not considered to be a marker for concurrently developing malignancy, and thus a full scale cancer search in such patients is not indicated. They should undergo regular physical examinations and testing that would be appropriate for their age or symptoms.

HISTOPATHOLOGY. The epidermis shows hyperkeratosis, parakeratosis, acanthosis, and thickening of the rete ridges. The cellular architecture is disorganized and individually keratinizing cells and atypical cells are seen at all levels of the epidermis. There is, however, a sharp delineation between dermis and epidermis, and the basement membrane is intact. The upper dermis usually shows a chronic inflammatory infiltrate.

DIFFERENTIAL DIAGNOSIS. Bowen's disease is frequently misdiagnosed as psoriasis, superficial multicentric basal cell carcinoma, nummular eczema, and actinic or arsenical keratosis. Paget's disease, especially the extramammary type, not only clinically but also histologically may mimic Bowen's disease. There is no dyskeratosis in Paget's disease, and the intervening nonvacuolated epidermal cells are not atypical in Paget's disease. Stains for mucin are positive in Paget's disease and negative in Bowen's disease, because the material in the vacuolated cells in Bowen's disease is glycogen. Bowen's disease may, at times, be heavily pigmented, especially when occurring in the anogenital region, and may resemble melanoma in these cases. Bowenoid papulosis may histologically mimic Bowen's disease; however, its multicentricity and positive markers for human papillomavirus have revealed it to be a type of viral infection, and this is fully discussed in Chapter 19. When the lesion is in the scalp, seborrheic dermatitis may be simulated. Tinea circinata must also be considered in diagnosing Bowen's disease.

TREATMENT. Simple elliptical excision of small lesions on suitable sites is the best form of treatment.

Fulguration and curettage, electrocautery, cryotherapy, laser ablation, and shave excision may be ineffective even when done thoroughly, owing to extension down the outer root sheaths of hair follicles. When lesions are large and ill defined, or are in sites where preservation of normal tissue is critical, Mohs surgery may be indicated.

Topical treatment with 5-fluorouracil (5-FU) was found to be effective by Jansen, Sturm, and Domonkos. A 5 per cent concentration in propylene glycol or ointment, applied twice daily for one to three months, may be used. Occlusion may be necessary if a marked inflammatory response is not obtained. Post-treatment biopsies and careful follow-up are recommended.

Arbesman H, et al: Is Bowen's disease a predictor for the development of internal malignancy? JAMA 1987, 257:516.

Baran RL, et al: Polydactylous Bowen's disease of the nail. JAAD 1987, 17:201.

Brown MD, et al: Genital tumors. JAAD 1988, 18:115.

Callen JP: Bowen's disease and internal malignant disease. Arch Dermatol 1988, 124:675.

Chuang T-Y, et al: Bowen's disease and internal malignancy. JAAD 1988, 19:47.

Dixon RS, et al: Erythroplasia (Queyrat) of conjunctiva. JAAD 1981, 4:160.

Domonkos AN: Andrews' Diseases of the Skin, ed. 6. Philadelphia, W. B. Saunders Co., 1971, p. 776.

Gross G, et al: Bowenoid papulosis. Arch Dermatol 1985, 121:858.

Jacobs DM, et al: Sebaceous carcinoma arising from Bowen's disease of the vulva. Arch Dermatol 1986, 122:1191.

Kao GF: Carcinoma arising in Bowen's disease. Arch Dermatol 1986, 122:1124.

Kimura S: Bowenoid papulosis of the genitalia. Int J Dermatol 1982, 21:432.

Miki Y, et al: Cutaneous and pulmonary cancers associated with Bowen's disease. JAAD 1982, 6:26.

Mora RG, et al: Cancer in the skin of blacks. III. A review of nineteen black patients with Bowen's disease. JAAD 1984, 11:557.

Obalek S, et al: Bowenoid papulosis of the male and female genitalia. JAAD 1986, 14:433.

Reymann F, et al: Bowen's disease and internal malignant diseases. Arch Dermatol 1988, 124:677.

Sturm HM: Bowen's disease and 5-fluorouracil. JAAD 1979, 1:513.

ERYTHROPLASIA OF QUEYRAT

Queyrat's erythroplasia is histologically Bowen's disease of the glans penis. Clinically it is characterized by single or multiple well-circumscribed, erythematous, moist, velvety or smooth, red-surfaced plaques on the glans penis of uncircumcised men, usually over the age of 40. It resembles Zoon's balanitis, clinically.

Malignant transformation is more common than in Bowen's disease, and the resulting squamous cell carcinomas are more aggressive and tend to metastasize earlier than those which develop in Bowen's disease. There is no evidence of an increase in internal malignancy in patients with erythroplasia. Conservative excision or, preferably, topical 5-fluorouracil, is the recommended treatment. This is effective because of the absence of follicles on the glans.

Goette DK: Erythroplasia of Queyrat. Arch Dermatol 1974, 110:271.
Idem, et al: Erythroplasia of Queyrat: treatment with topically applied 5-fluorouracil. JAMA 1975, 232:934.

BALANITIS PLASMACELLULARIS (Zoon)

This is also known as benign plasma cell erythroplasia and balanoposthitis chronica circumscripta plasmacellularis. Garnier reported vulvar lesions of this disease a year before Zoon's description of a penile lesion, in 1954.

Balanitis plasmacellularis is a benign inflammatory lesion with a plasma cell infiltrate. Clinically it is characterized by a persistent inflammation, which is usually sharply demarcated and usually on the inner surface of the prepuce and the glans penis. The lesion is erythematous, moist, and shiny. It occurs

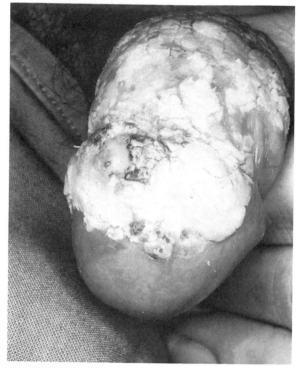

Figure 29–75. Extensive erythroplasia of Queyrat of glans penis and prepuce with eventuation into squamous cell carcinoma.

as a single lesion, but it may consist of several confluent macules. It is asymptomatic and does not produce inguinal adenopathy. Uncircumcised men from 24 to 85 years of age are most often affected.

Plasma cell vulvitis is the counterpart of balanitis in women. The vulva shows a striking lacquerlike lus-

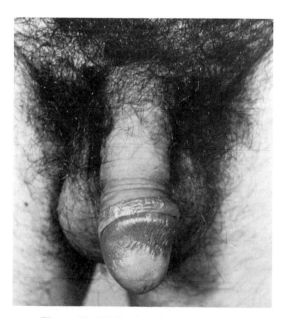

Figure 29–74. Erythroplasia of Queyrat.

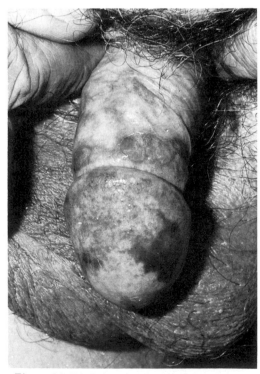

Figure 29–76. Balanitis plasmocellularis (Zoon).

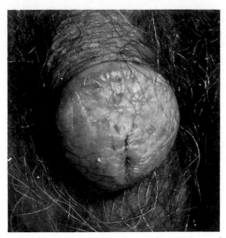

Figure 29–77. Pseudoepitheliomatous keratotic and micaceous balanitis.

ter. Erosions, punctate hemorrhage, synechiae, and a slate-to-ochre pigmentation may supervene.

Plasmacytosis circumorificialis is the same disease on the oral mucosa, lips, cheeks, and tongue, clinically suggestive of squamous cell carcinoma.

Histologically, the epidermis is atrophic with no other changes. In the papillary dermis a band of infiltrate consisting almost exclusively of plasma cells is present. Dilated vessels are also seen. This picture is strikingly different from that of the main clinical differential diagnosis, erythroplasia of Queyrat, in which the epidermis is principally involved, with individual cell keratinization in the thickened prickle cell layer.

Topical steroids are helpful and may even be curative. All 19 patients collected by Souteyrand were uncircumcised, and most were cured by circumcision. Seven cases were reported by Fernandez et al, all uncircumcised; all were cured by circumcision.

Brodin MB: Balanitis circumscripta plasmacellularis. JAAD 1980, 2:33.
Davis J, et al: Vulvitis circumscripta plasmacellularis. JAAD 1983, 8:413.
Souteyrand P, et al: Zoon's balanitis (balanitis circumscripta plasmacellularis). Br J Dermatol 1981, 105:195.
Zoon JJ: Balanoposthitis plasmacellularis. Dermatologica 1952, 105:1.

PSEUDOEPITHELIOMATOUS KERATOTIC AND MICACEOUS BALANITIS

Pseudoepitheliomatous keratotic and micaceous balanitis was described by Lortat-Jacob and Civatte in 1966. The lesions occurring on the glans penis are verrucous excrescences with micaceous scaling. Ulcerations, cracking, and fissuring on the surface of the glans frequently are present. The keratotic scaling is usually micaceous and resembles psoriasis.

The cases have been mostly patients past 50 years of age who have been circumcised for phimosis in adult life. Both of Domonkos's patients had this history.

Histologically, there is marked hyperkeratosis and parakeratosis as well as pseudoepitheliomatous hyperplasia. Acanthotic masses give rise to a craterlike configuration. It may belong to the category of verrucous carcinoma. Treatment may require removal by Mohs surgery, although Mascaro treated four patients with 5-fluorouracil topically with excellent results. If topical chemotherapy is utilized, posttreatment biopsies are recommended.

Bart RS, et al: On a dilemma of penile horns: pseudoepitheliomatous hyperplasia and micaceous balanitis. J Dermatol Surg Oncol 1977, 3:580.
Domonkos AN: Andrews' Diseases of the Skin. 6th ed, Philadelphia, WB Saunders, 1971, p 778.
Jenkins D Jr, et al: Pseudoepitheliomatous, keratotic, micaceous balanitis. JAAD 1988, 18:419.
Lortat-Jacob, E, et al: La balanite pseudoépithéliomateuse keratosique et micacée. Bull Soc Franc Derm Syph 1966, 73:931.

PAGET'S DISEASE OF THE NIPPLE

CLINICAL FEATURES. Paget's disease of the nipple is characterized by a unilateral sharply defined eczema caused by epidermal metastases from underlying ductal adenocarcinoma of the breast. The disease begins as an erythematous crusted or keratotic, circumscribed, pruritic patch. It may simulate unilateral eczematous neurodermatitis. In the course of months or years it may become infiltrated and ulcerated. The nipple may or may not be retracted. The disease is less common, and carries a worse prognosis, in men than in women, according to Satiani and Powell, who collected 22 cases and reported one of their own.

HISTOPATHOLOGY. Paget's disease is characterized by the presence of Paget cells: large, round, clear-staining cells with large nuclei. Intercellular bridges are absent. The cells appear singly or in small nests between the squamous cells. Paget cells undergoing mitosis are frequent. Acanthosis is usu-

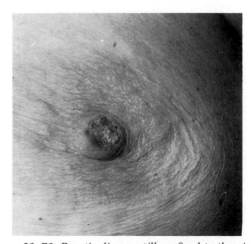

Figure 29–78. Paget's disease still confined to the nipple.

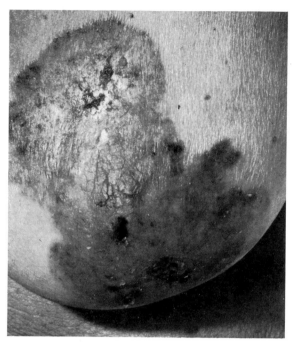

Figure 29–79. Paget's disease of the nipple of 10 years' duration. (Courtesy of Dr. F. Adair.)

with connection to the surface. There is a lining of apocrine type secretory epithelium. Brownstein et al reported 15 cases in 1985. *Hyperkeratosis of the nipple and areola* may occasionally be unilateral, but histologically reveals only hyperkeratosis, acanthosis, and papillomatosis. Kuhlman et al reported prompt response to Keralyt Gel. *Clear cell papulosis* of the skin, newly described by Kuo, occurred as scattered flat, white, flat-topped lesions in two brothers. Histologic examination revealed benign pagetoid clear cells in the basal layer. Immunohistochemical and electron microscopic analysis revealed findings one usually observes in Paget's cells.

TREATMENT. Mastectomy offers the only hope of cure.

PROGNOSIS. Maier and his associates indicate that if the lesions have persisted more than six months without lymph node involvement the prognosis is excellent for a five-year postoperative survival. Lymph node involvement, as always in breast cancer, is the most significant factor affecting the prognosis. In men, who rarely may have this disease, the prognosis is far poorer, as Satiani et al have shown.

ally present, the granular layer is preserved, and usually there is no parakeratosis. Frequently a layer of basal cells separates the Paget cells from the dermis; this is not seen in melanoma. In the dermis an inflammatory reaction is usually present.

The Paget cell may take a periodic acid–Schiff stain even after diastase treatment, unlike the dyskeratotic cells in Bowen's disease. Helwig and Graham, however, prefer the aldehyde fuchsin stain. The cells are DOPA-negative, but may contain some melanin.

Immunoperoxidase stains may also be helpful. Prekeratin stains are negative, whereas carcinoembryonic antigen is positive, as reported by Penneys et al. This latter antigen is found in normal eccrine and apocrine glands and in neoplasms derived from those glands. Also, apocrine epithelial antigen is positive.

DIAGNOSIS. Failures to diagnose Paget's disease are many. The presence of unilateral eczema of the nipple recalcitrant to simple treatment is indicative of Paget's disease, and the lesion should have a thorough biopsy. Bilateral lesions usually mean neurodermatitis, atopic dermatitis, or nummular eczema, and biopsy is seldom required. The biopsy should be through the nipple with the removal of a liberal portion of the nipple. Unless an adequate specimen is obtained, small nests of Paget cells may be overlooked. By keeping in mind that unilateral eczema of the nipple may be the only warning that there is a cancer growing in the breast, one can best understand the nature of Paget's disease.

Papillary adenoma of the nipple clinically closely resembles Paget's disease, but on biopsy shows a papillary and adenomatous growth in the dermis

Extramammary Paget's Disease

The lesions of extramammary Paget's disease are similar to those of the nipple lesions, but may go undiagnosed longer and thus become more extensive. A nonhealing banal eczematous patch may persist in the anogenital or axillary region for several years before it causes concern. Usually a single lesion occurs and is mistaken for a fungus infection, especially in the inguinal region. Intense pruritus is common and sometimes pain is also present. Bleeding is a late sign. Lesions may simulate lichen simplex chronicus or leukoplakia. Murrell and McMullan found that 15 patients had the disease for an average of seven years before a diagnosis was made.

Extramammary Paget's disease is frequently associated with an underlying glandular adnexal carcinoma or a regional internal carcinoma with or without metastasis. Powell et al in 1985 reported eight cases associated with malignancy of the lower urinary tract.

Fligiel and Kaneko reported a case in which a lesion of Paget's disease in the ear of a 63-year-old man was the first evidence of an underlying ceruminous carcinoma.

Chanda published an exhaustive literature review in 1985. He found that 150 of 197 cases reported between 1962 and 1982 were in women. The vulva was most commonly involved, followed by the perianal area, the penis, scrotum, and groin. Twenty-four per cent had an underlying cutaneous adnexal adenocarcinoma, and in these there was a 46 per cent mortality rate. Twelve per cent had an associated concurrent underlying internal malignancy, which was closely related to the location of the extramammary Paget's disease.

Histologically, the findings are similar to those found in the nipple: hyperkeratosis, parakeratosis, acanthosis, and the pale, vacuolated Paget's cells in the epidermis, mostly in the deeper portion of the rete ridges. Sialomucin, diastase-resistant, may be found by PAS stain.

In the anal, perianal, and perineal areas extramammary Paget's disease should be differentiated from other premalignancies and malignancies. These are squamous cell carcinoma, basal cell carcinoma, perianal Bowen's disease, cloacogenic carcinoma, and anorectal melanoma.

In addition to the PAS stain, the Paget cells are positive-staining to mucicarmine and to Alcian blue. Bowen's disease and melanoma do not show this positive staining.

Immunoperoxidase staining is positive with carcinoembryonic antigen, adenokeratin, apocrine epithelial antigen, and gross cystic disease fluid protein-15; all of which signify these cells to be of apocrine gland origin. Keratin staining reveals patterns consistent with the cells being derived from or differentiating to secretory cells.

In the treatment of these patients, surgical removal offers the best prognosis, with Mohs surgery offering the best conservation of normal tissue, and at the same time the best chance of complete surgical removal. The preoperative use of 5-fluorouracil topically may help delineate the tumor margins. Serum carcinoembryonic antigen levels may be useful in prognosticating. Oji et al found that all three patients who had elevated serum levels had widespread metastatic disease.

Brownstein MH, et al: Papillary adenoma of the nipple. JAAD 1985, 12:707.

Chanda JJ: Extramammary Paget's disease. JAAD 1985, 13:1009.

Eliezri YD, et al: Role of preoperative topical 5-fluorouracil in preparation for Mohs micrographic surgery of extramammary Paget's disease. JAAD 1987, 17:497.

Fligiel Z, et al: Extramammary Paget's disease of the ear canal. Cancer 1975, 36:1072.

Hamm H, et al: Extramammary Paget's cells. JAAD 1986, 15:1275.

Kuhlman DS, et al: Hyperkeratosis of the nipple. JAAD 1985, 13:596.

Kuo T-T, et al: Clear cell papulosis of the skin. Am J Surg Pathol 1987, 11:827.

Lancer HA, et al: Paget's disease of the male breast. JAAD 1982, 7:393.

Mazoujian G, et al: Extramammary Paget's disease, evidence for an apocrine origin. Am J Surg Pathol 1984, 8:43.

Oji M, et al: Serum carcinoembryonic antigen level in Paget's disease. Br J Dermatol 1984, 110:211.

Penneys NS, et al: Prekeratin in spindle cell tumors of the skin. Arch Dermatol 1983, 119:476.

Idem: Carcinoembryonic antigen in benign sweat gland tumors. Arch Dermatol 1982, 118:225.

Powell FC, et al: Genital Paget's disease and urinary tract malignancy. JAAD 1985, 13:84.

Rosen L, et al: Bowen's disease, Paget's disease, and malignant melanoma in skin. South Med J 1986, 79:410.

Tazawa T, et al: Immunologic characteristics of keratins in extramammary Paget's disease. Arch Dermatol 1988, 124:1063.

ADNEXAL NEVI AND TUMORS

Brown E: Histologic diagnosis of benign adnexal skin tumors. JAAD 1985, 12:350.

Mehregan AH, et al: Benign epithelial tumors of the skin I. Epidermal tumors. Cutis 1977, 19:43.

Idem: II Benign sebaceous tumors. Cutis 1977, 19:317.

Idem: III Hair follicle tumors. Cutis 1977, 19:595.

Idem: IV Benign apocrine gland tumors. Cutis 1978, 20:53.

SEBACEOUS NEVI AND TUMORS

Nevus Sebaceus
(Organoid Nevus)

Nevus sebaceus of Jadassohn is a sharply circumscribed, yellow-orange, verrucous hamartoma varying from a few millimeters to several centimeters in diameter. The solitary lesion is present at birth, most frequently near the vertex of the scalp but also commonly on the face or neck. The lesions persist throughout life and are usually alopecic. In adulthood the nevus becomes more verrucous.

Basal cell carcinoma may develop in approximately 5 to 10 per cent of the lesion. Wilson Jones and Heyl found nine basal cell carcinomas in 140 lesions of nevus sebaceus, and three were aggressively invasive. A syringocystadenoma papilliferum has been found in approximately 10 per cent of lesions also. Mehregan and Pinkus have reported other tumors occurring in nevus sebaceus, such as solid hidradenoma, sebaceous epithelioma, apocrine cystadenoma, and keratoacanthoma. Domingo and Helwig reported on nine patients who developed aggressive neoplasms, including apocrine carcinomas, adnexal carcinomas with pilar differentiation, and squamous cell carcinoma, associated with nevus sebaceus. Tarkhan et al reported a metastasizing eccrine porocarcinoma which developed in a nevus sebaceus, and reviewed the previous five cases of metastasizing tumors.

Nevus sebaceus lesions, especially when large, may be associated with multiple internal abnormalities, similar to those reported in the linear epidermal nevus syndrome. Associated problems have included intracranial masses, seizures, mental retardation, skeletal abnormalities, pigmentary changes, ocular lesions, and hamartomas of the kidney. Some of these manifestations are reviewed by Marks et al, Moskowitz et al, and Diven et al.

Histologically, papillomatosis is present with hypergranulosis and hyperkeratosis. The hair follicles may range in their development from completely undifferentiated cells of the embryonal type, to just small hair shafts, to normal hair follicles. The sebaceous glands in the early lesion occur as immature lobules with incompletely formed hair follicles. In older lesions, well-developed sebaceous glands may be seen. Apocrine glands are common in the lesions of the adult. The dermis is thickened, with increased vascularity and fibrous connective tissue.

Since malignant changes may occur, the treatment of choice is to remove these nevi early by excision. Wilson Jones and Heyl suggested simple excision at adolescence. We agree.

Diven DG, et al: Nevus sebaceus associated with major ophthalmologic abnormalities. Arch Dermatol 1987, 123:383.
Domingo J, et al: Malignant neoplasms associated with nevus sebaceus of Jadassohn. JAAD 1979, 1:545.
Goldstein GD, et al: Basal cell carcinoma arising in a nevus sebaceus during childhood. JAAD 1988, 18:429.
Marks JG, et al: Linear nevus sebaceus syndrome. JAAD 1980, 2:31.
Moskowitz R, et al: Nevus sebaceus in association with an intracranial mass. JAAD 1982, 6:1078.
Tarkhan II, et al: Metastasizing eccrine porocarcinoma developing in a nevus sebaceus of Jadassohn. Arch Dermatol 1985, 121:413.
Wilson Jones E, et al: Nevus sebaceus: report of 140 patients with special regard to the development of secondary malignant tumors. Br J Dermatol 1970, 82:99.

Sebaceous Hyperplasia

Also known as senile sebaceous hyperplasia and senile sebaceous adenoma, these common lesions are scattered irregularly over the face, having a predilection for the forehead, infraorbital regions, and temples. The lesions are small cream-colored or yellowish umbilicated papules 2 to 6 mm in diameter. The age at onset is usually past age 40, although De Villez et al reported a 29-year-old patient with extensive lesions.

Catalano reported a unique case of a young woman with a confluent yellow thickening of the areolas and nipples bilaterally. On biopsy examination sebaceous hyperplasia was found.

Histologically, the sebaceous glands are hypertrophied, with normal-appearing acini. The glands are multilobulated, each dividing into other lobules to produce a cluster resembling a bunch of grapes.

Recognition of these lesions is imperative since frequently they mimic an early basal cell carcinoma.

Treatment is mostly for cosmetic purposes. Electrodesiccation or an extremely fine fulgurating spark will remove these with good results, though curettage or a shallow shave biopsy may be desirable if there is the least doubt about the diagnosis. Burton et al reported a case with multiple lesions in a man, 37, who responded very well to isotretinoin (Accutane) 40 mg twice a day, but with recurrence three weeks after stopping.

Burton CS, et al: Premature sebaceous gland hyperplasia. JAAD 1985, 12:182.

Catalano PM, et al: Areolar sebaceous hyperplasia. JAAD 1985, 13:867.
DeVillez RL, et al: Premature sebaceous gland hyperplasia. JAAD 1982, 6:933.

Sebaceous Epithelioma

Clinically, sebaceous epitheliomas have the same morphologic characteristics as basal cell carcinomas. In addition the tumor may have a yellowish or orange color. Its location is mostly on the scalp, face, and neck. It may present as a firm intradermal nodule. It may also be associated with the Muir-Torre syndrome, discussed shortly.

Histologically, the tumor consists of neat oval nests of irregularly shaped basaloid cells with differentiation toward sebaceous cells. Also there may be cystic spaces containing vacuolated amorphous hyalinelike material.

Sebaceous Gland Carcinoma

This rare carcinoma may arise on the eyelids from the meibomian or Zeis glands. It usually appears in the tarsal region of the upper eyelids. The scalp, other areas of the face, and the trunk are at times involved. Oppenheim reported a case which occurred in the penis. Fatal metastatic disease occurs in 20 to 30 per cent of eyelid cases, whereas this result is rare when the sebaceous carcinoma originates in other sites. It may also be seen in Muir-Torre syndrome (discussion after next).

Histologically, the lobules contain sebaceous cells and many undifferentiated cells, with numerous mitotic figures with great variations in size and shape of the cells. The cells are eosinophilic and the nuclei are also lighter than those of the sebaceous epithelioma.

Treatment is by wedge resection of the tumor on the eyelid. Mohs surgery is preferable, and has been reported successful by Dixon et al and Ratz et al.

Dixon RS, et al: Sebaceous carcinoma of the eyelid. JAAD 1980, 3:241.
Oppenheim AR: Sebaceous carcinoma of the penis. Arch Dermatol 1981, 117:306.
Page EH, et al: Morpheic plaque of the lower eyelid. Arch Dermatol 1987, 123:653.
Ratz JL, et al: Sebaceous carcinoma of the eyelid treated with Mohs surgery. JAAD 1986, 14:668.

Sebaceous Adenoma

Sebaceous adenoma is usually a solitary, skin-colored or yellowish-papule or nodule of the head or neck, most often occurring in men over 50 or 60 years of age. It may also be seen in Muir-Torre syndrome. Microscopically it is a sharply demarcated tumor in the upper dermis consisting of incompletely differentiated sebaceous lobules. Excision is curative.

Muir-Torre Syndrome

Sebaceous tumors of the skin of any sort at an early age or in large numbers were first reported by Muir in 1967 and Torre in 1968 to be associated with the development of low-grade internal malignancy, a combination which has been called the Muir-Torre syndrome. The internal tumors often occur a decade or two before the cutaneous lesions.

Most often colonic adenocarcinoma, but also neoplasms of the uterus, ovary, and kidney, may occur. The cutaneous lesions may be sebaceous adenomas, sebaceous carcinomas, keratoacanthomas, or basal cell carcinomas with sebaceous differentiation. Burgdorf et al describe these tumors which have varying patterns of sebaceous components. The visceral tumors are usually not aggressive. At times the cutaneous lesions may precede or accompany the internal malignancies. Banse-Kupin et al have reviewed the literature.

Stone et al reported the exacerbation of the syndrome with immunosuppression. Spielvogel et al reported two familial cases whose sebaceous lesions responded well to 40 mg of isotretinoin a day, and on a dose of 10 mg a day developed no new skin or visceral tumors. They believe isotretinoin may be valuable in prophylaxis.

Banse-Kupin L, et al: Torre's syndrome. JAAD 1984, 10:803.
Burgdorf WHC, et al: Muir-Torre syndrome. Am J Dermatopathol 1986, 8:202.
Finan MC, et al: Sebaceous gland tumor and systemic disease. Medicine 1984, 63:232.
Householder MS, et al: Sebaceous neoplasms associated with visceral carcinomas. Arch Dermatol 1980, 116:61.
Jakobiec FA, et al: Unusual eyelid tumors with sebaceous differentiation in the Muir-Torre syndrome. Ophthalmology 1988, 95:1543.
Spielvogel RL, et al: Oral isotretinoin therapy for familial Muir-Torre syndrome. JAAD 1985, 12:475.
Stone MS, et al: Torre's syndrome. JAAD 1986, 15:1101.
Torre D: Multiple sebaceous tumors. Arch Dermatol 1968, 98:549.

Trabecular Carcinoma (Merkel Cell Carcinoma)

This malignant tumor was first described by Toker in 1972. The cell of origin is thought to be a pluripotential cell which may differentiate in a neuroendocrine direction, as evidenced by the typical membrane-bound neurosecretory granules seen within the neoplastic cells by electron microscopy.

Clinically it presents as a rapidly growing nodule on sun-exposed skin, most commonly in elderly patients. In a review of 80 cases by Raaf et al the mean age of onset was 68 years, women outnumbered men 49 to 31, and the primary sites of involvement were the head and neck (44 per cent), leg (28 per cent), arm (16 per cent), and buttock (9 per cent).

No primary tumor appeared on the trunk. The rate of local recurrence was 36 per cent, regional metastases 53 per cent, distant metastases 28 per cent, and death due to tumor 25 per cent.

Histologically the tumor is composed of uniform round cells, with the cells being arranged in sheets. The main differential diagnosis is oat cell carcinoma metastatic to skin. Electron microscopy on properly fixed specimens reveals the granules typical of Merkel cells. These are not seen in formalin fixed tissue; however, characteristic paranuclear whorls of intermediate filaments remain. Immunohistochemically, neuron-specific enolase may be positive, but the most discriminating marker is the antikeratin antibody, which stains the cells in a paranuclear inclusion-bodylike aggregate. The keratin has been shown to be of the simple epithelial type, as is found in Merkel cells.

Complete surgical ablation is the treatment of choice, with Mohs surgery an excellent method, as discussed by Roenigk et al. Both radiation therapy and chemotherapy are effective in palliating unresectable disease, as discussed by Raaf.

Battifora H, et al: The use of antikeratin antibodies in the immunohistochemical distinction between neuroendocrine carcinoma of the skin, lymphoma, and oat cell carcinoma. Cancer 1986, 58:1040.
George TE, et al: Chemotherapy for metastatic Merkel cell carcinoma. Cancer 1985, 56:1034.
Haneke E: Electron microscopy of Merkel cell carcinoma from formalin-fixed tissue. JAAD 1985, 12:487.
Raaf JH, et al: Trabecular carcinoma of the skin. Cancer 1986, 57:178.
Roenigk RK, et al: Merkel cell carcinoma. J Dermatol Surg Oncol 1986, 12:332.
Tazawa T, et al: Immunohistochemical demonstration of simple epithelia–type keratin intermediate filament in a case of Merkel cell carcinoma. Arch Dermatol 1987, 123:489.
Wick MR, et al: Multifocal Merkel's cell tumors associated with a cutaneous dysplasia syndrome. Arch Dermatol 1983, 119:409.

ECCRINE NEVI AND TUMORS

Syringoma

In syringoma small translucent papules develop, yellowish, brownish, or pinkish, globoid, 2 to 3 mm in diameter, discrete and closely set, most frequently—and often exclusively—on the eyelids and upper cheeks. They are disproportionately common, in these sites, in Japanese women. They may also appear in large numbers, however, on the chest, upper arms, and abdomen. They develop slowly and persist indefinitely without symptoms. Occurrence is chiefly in women, after puberty.

Syringomas occur in 18 per cent of adults with Down's syndrome. This is approximately 30 times the frequency seen in other mentally deficient patients.

Microscopically the syringoma is characterized by dilated cystic sweat ducts, some of which have small

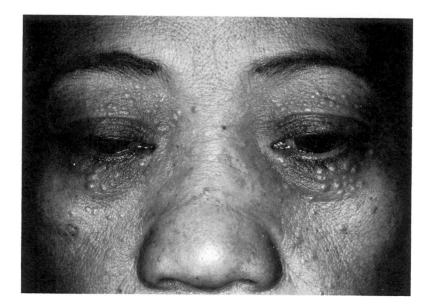

Figure 29–80. Syringomas.

commalike tails to produce a distinctive picture, resembling tadpoles. Strands of epithelial cells may occur independently of the ducts. Usually two rows of epithelial cells line the duct walls. Histochemical studies have shown that syringomas contain phosphorylase and hydrolytic enzymes typical of eccrine origin. Penneys et al have shown strong staining with carcinoembryonic antigen and Hashimoto et al with monoclonal antikeratin antibodies characterizing eccrine ducts. They probably represent adenomas of intradermal eccrine ducts.

Treatment may be desirable because of the unsightly appearance. Electrolysis of each individual lesion, laser ablation, or cryotherapy with liquid nitrogen cautiously applied to each tumor are three methods which usually help without producing unsightly scars.

Clear-cell Syringoma. Twenty-six cases of this variant of syringoma have been reported, nineteen from the U.S., and only one not associated with diabetes mellitus. The last two cases were reported by Furue et al in 1984. Eight were in women. Lesions are clinically identical to syringoma.

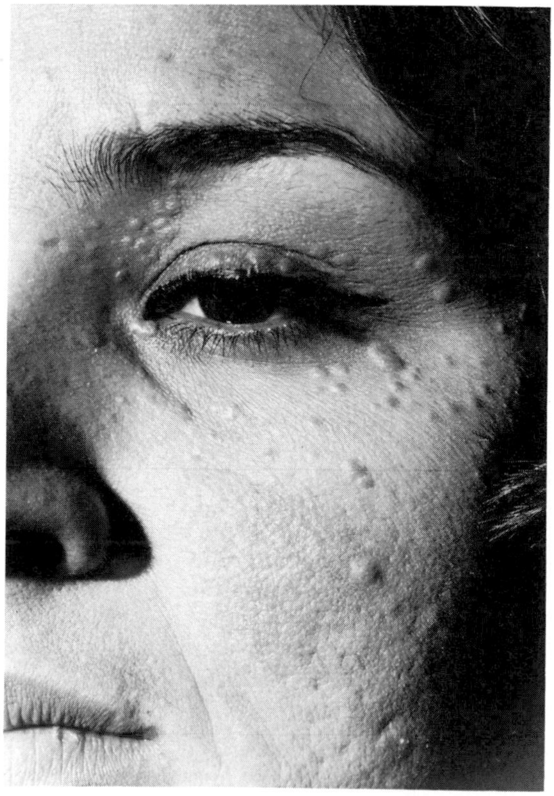

Figure 29–81. Syringomas.

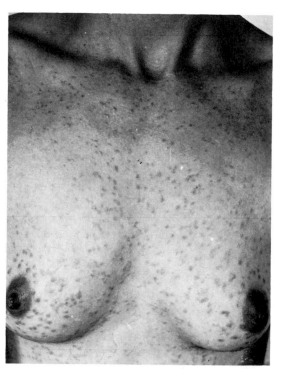

Figure 29–82. Generalized syringomas. (Courtesy of Dr. S. F. Rosen.)

Nests of ordinary syringoma are commingled with nests of cells with clear ground-glasslike material surrounding a small dark oval nucleus. Feibelman and Maize reported electron microscopic studies in two cases, showing numerous glycogen granules in the clear cells in two cases. Nearly all their 18 cases had eyelid lesions; one had lesions of the cheek, one of a labium majus.

Eruptive Syringoma. Hashimoto and his associates called attention to a type of syringoma which was first described by Darier. Eruptive syringoma is histologically identical to syringoma of the eyelid, but occurs in an eruptive form of numerous lesions on the neck, chest, axillae, and upper arms, and periumbilically. The shiny, faintly rose-colored papules closely resemble lichen planus and secondary syphilid. This variant has been reported in Down's syndrome, as a familial trait, and to have occurred in a diabetic woman with the clear-cell histology.

Other Variants. Friedman et al have summarized many individual case reports of unusual clinical variants of syringomas. These include types limited to the scalp, causing alopecia; a unilateral linear or nevoid distribution; those limited to the vulva; those limited to the distal extremities; and the lichenplanuslike and milialike morphologic types.

Diestelmeier MR, et al: Eruptive generalized clear cell syringomas. Arch Dermatol 1983, 119:927.
Dupré A: Syringomas as a causative factor for cicatricial alopecia. Arch Dermatol 1981, 117:315.
Feibelman CE, et al: Clear cell syringoma. Am J Dermapathol 1984, 6:139.
Friedman S, et al: Syringoma presenting as milia. JAAD 1987, 16:310.
Furue M, et al: Clear cell syringoma. Am J Dermatopathol 1984, 6:131.
Hashimoto K, et al: Familial syringoma. Arch Dermatol 1985, 121:756.
Isaacson D, et al: Localized vulvar syringomas. JAAD 1979, 1:352.
Neuman KM, et al: Alopecia associated with syringomas. JAAD 1985, 13:528.
Port M, et al: Syringoma of the ankle. JAAD 1984, 10:291.
Scherbenske JM, et al: Cutaneous and ocular manifestations of Down's syndrome. JAAD (in press).
Idem: Vulvar syringomas occurring in a 9-year-old child. JAAD 1988, 19:575.
Urban CD, et al: Eruptive syringomas in Down's syndrome. Arch Dermatol 1981, 117:374.
Van der Broek H, et al: Syringoma of the upper extremities with onset in the sixth decade. JAAD 1982, 6:534.
Yalisone BL, et al: Multiple penile papules. Arch Dermatol 1987, 123:1391.
Yung CW, et al: Unilateral linear nevoidal syringoma. JAAD 1981, 4:412.

Linear Eccrine Nevus with Comedones

Blanchard et al reported a case appearing to be one of nevus comedonicus but showing on biopsy sharply demarcated islands of cuboidal cells in a glandular pattern. They reviewed other similar cases.

Blanchard LE, et al: Linear eccrine nevus with comedones. Arch Dermatol 1981, 117:357.

Eccrine Hidrocystomas

Eccrine hidrocystomas are 1 to 3 mm translucent papules which occasionally have a bluish tint. They usually are solitary, occur on the face, and are more common in women. In some patients, as in the woman reported by Sperling et al, multiple lesions may be present. They may become more prominent during hot weather. Microscopically a single cystic cavity lined by·two layers of small cuboidal epithelial cells is present. Treatment, if desired, is by excision for solitary lesions. Sperling's case responded to atropine ointment applied topically.

Lesher JL, et al: A tender blue cyst on the leg. Arch Dermatol 1988, 124:935.
Smith JD, et al: Hidrocystomas. Arch Dermatol 1973, 108:676.
Sperling LC, et al: Eccrine hidrocystomas. JAAD 1982, 7:765.

Eccrine Poroma

Eccrine poroma is a benign, slow-growing, slightly protruding, sessile, soft, reddish tumor which may occur anywhere, but most often on the sole or side of the foot. The 2 to 12 mm lesion will bleed upon slight trauma. A striking finding is the frequent cup-shaped shallow depression from which the tumor grows and protrudes. It also may occur on the palms. Although the lesion tends to occur singly, multiple lesions may also occur. A patient of Domonkos's developed a second lesion a year after excision of one located elsewhere on the same foot. Goldner has reported a 65-year-old woman who had more than 100 lesions on her palms and soles. This type, referred to as eccrine poromatosis, may be associated with hidrotic ectodermal dysplasia. Smith and Coburn described intraepidermal poromas under the designation *hidroacanthoma simplex*.

Histologically, solid masses of uniform, very small, basophilic epithelial cells are seen, with intercellular bridging. These cells tend to arrange themselves around cleftlike lumina with formation of a cuticle. Vascular dilatation and hyperplasia of the capillaries may be present. The tumors contain succinic dehydrogenase and amylophosphorylase. Glycogen in the tumor cells may be demonstrable with periodic acid–Schiff stain.

The clinical differential diagnosis is from granuloma pyogenicum, amelanotic melanoma, Kaposi's hemorrhagic sarcoma, basal cell carcinoma, and seborrheic keratosis.

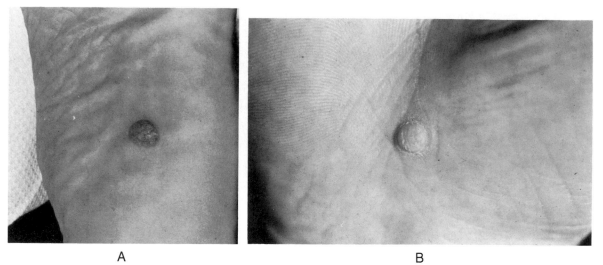

A   B

Figure 29–83. Eccrine poroma on the sole of a 57-year-old man. B, Eccrine poroma on the palm.

The lesions are benign, and the treatment consists of simple excision. This benign tumor has a malignant variant, a case of which was reported in 1983 by Keijiro Kitamura et al. The tumor resembled Bowen's disease or a seborrheic keratosis clinically. Nuclear atypia was marked and there was invasion into the dermis.

Holubar K, et al: Intraepidermal eccrine poroma: a histochemical and enzyme histochemical study. Cancer 1969, 23:262.

Kitamura K, et al: Hidroacanthoma simplex with invasive growth. Cutis 1983, 32:83.

Moeller CA, et al: An enlarging tumor of the foot. Arch Dermatol 1987, 123:653.

Shafrir A, et al: Eccrine poroma. Israel J Med Sci 1974, 10:1133.

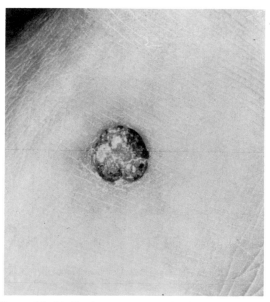

Figure 29–84. Eccrine poroma on the dorsum of the foot.

Chondroid Syringoma

This lesion was formerly called *mixed tumor of the skin*. Clinically, the tumor is usually a firm intradermal or subcutaneous nodule, most commonly located on the nose or cheeks. These tumors are usually asymptomatic and measure 5 to 30 mm in diameter.

Histologically, nests of cuboidal or polygonal epithelial cells in the corium give rise to tuboalveolar and ductal structures and occasionally keratinous cysts. These structures are embedded in a matrix varying from a faint bluish chondroid substance to an acidophilic hyaline material. This tumor is felt to be of eccrine origin. It may be either benign or malignant, with the malignant type often occurring on the extremities rather than the face, and associated with rapid growth and large size.

Devine P, et al: Malignant mixed tumor. Arch Dermatol 1984, 120:576.

Harrist TJ, et al: Cutaneous malignant mixed tumor. Arch Dermatol 1981, 117:719.

Hirsch P, et al: Chondroid syringoma. Arch Dermatol 1961, 84:835.

Milligan MP, et al: Chondroid syringoma: case report. J Assoc Military Dermatol 1984, 10:26.

Clear Cell Hidradenoma (Solid-cystic Hidradenoma)

The wide array of names given to this tumor attest to the confusion surrounding its histogenesis. Some of these names have been hidradenoma, cystic hidradenoma, porosyringoma, dermal duct tumor, sweat gland epithelioma, clear cell myoepithelioma, nodular hidradenoma, and eccrine sweat gland adenoma. On the basis of histochemical studies Winkelmann and Wolff propose the name *solid-cystic hidradenoma*. Johnson and Helwig prefer the name *eccrine acrospiroma*.

The clear-cell hidradenoma occurs as a single nodular, solid or cystic, occasionally protruding cutaneous mass, 5 to 30 mm in diameter. The flesh-colored or reddish lesion may be lobulated, with dome-shaped nodules. Ulceration is frequent. The lesions occur anywhere on the body, such as the axillae, arms, thighs, scalp, and pubic region, but the most common site is the head. Pain on pressure occurs in approximately 20 per cent of patients. Multiple lesions on the eyelids have been reported by Greer. Its incidence is mostly between the ages of 20 and 50 and occurs in women twice as commonly as in men.

Microscopically the tumor is a circumscribed but unencapsulated mass of epithelial cells arranged into irregular or lobular masses extending deeply into the dermis. The distinctive cell is a large cuboidal or polyhedral cell with a clear cytoplasm suggestive of a single transparent vacuole surrounded by a clearly demarcated membrane. The round or oval nucleus is located at the edge of the cytoplasm. A second cell type present is fusiform or polyhedral, with basophilic cytoplasm. No mitoses are seen. This tumor is generally regarded as an eccrine sweat gland neoplasm.

Treatment. The tumor is radioresistant, and extirpation is the treatment of choice.

Headington JT, et al: Malignant clear cell acrospiroma. Cancer 1978, 41:641.
Hernandez-Perez E, et al: Nodular hidradenoma and hidradenocarcinoma. JAAD 1985, 12:15.
Johnson BL, et al: Eccrine acrospiroma. Cancer 1969, 23:641.
Luckasen JR, et al: Clear cell hidradenoma. *In* Demis JR: Clinical Dermatology. Vol 4. Philadelphia, Harper & Row, 1974, pp 22–23.
Winkelmann RK, et al: Solid-cystic hidradenoma of the skin. Arch Dermatol 1968, 97:651.

Eccrine Spiradenoma

Eccrine spiradenoma, first described by Kersting and Helwig, is clinically characterized by a solitary, 1-cm, deep-seated nodule occurring most frequently on the ventral surface of the body, especially over the upper half. Normal-appearing skin covers the nodule, which may be skin-colored, blue or pink. Occasionally multiple lesions may be present and may occur in a linear or zosteriform pattern. A striking symptom is pain appearing in paroxysms.

Eccrine spiradenoma has a generally benign clinical course and occurs most frequently between 15 and 35 years of age. Malignant transformation may occur rarely, as Cooper et al documented in their review of the eight cases reported as of 1985.

Microscopically it is characterized as a multilobu-

lated tumor surrounded by an adherent connective tissue capsule. The lobules are composed of basophilic cells arranged in characteristic small rosettes. Two cell types are those with large pale vesicular and ovoid nuclei and those with small dark nuclei.

When painful, eccrine spiradenoma may be mistaken for leiomyoma, glomus tumor, neuroma, and angiolipoma. It also resembles fibroma, deep hemangioma, and neurofibroma.

Treatment is simple excision.

Castro C, et al: Spiradenoma. Arch Dermatol 1974, 109:40.
Cooper PH, et al: Malignant transformation of eccrine spiradenoma. Arch Dermatol 1985, 121:1445.
Shelley WB, et al: A zosteriform network of spiradenomas. JAAD 1980, 2:59.

Papillary Eccrine Adenoma

This uncommon benign sweat gland neoplasm was originally described in 1977 by Rulon and Helwig. Clinically, dermal nodules located primarily on the extremities of black patients are characteristic. Histologic findings consist of a well-circumscribed, dermal, unencapsulated growth composed of a bilayer of branching tubules. Immunohistochemical analysis of the cells indicates differentiation toward the eccrine secretory coil. Because of its tendency to recur locally, complete surgical excision with clear margins is recommended.

Sexton M, et al: Papillary eccrine adenoma. JAAD 1988, 18:1114.

Syringoacanthoma

Rahbari in 1984 reported 21 cases of this rare seborrheic keratosislike neoplasm, 12 benign and nine malignant. The cells contained fine glycogen particles and small accumulations of glycosaminoglycans.

Rahbari H: Syringoacanthoma. Arch Dermatol 1984, 120:751.

Eccrine Syringofibroadenoma

Mehregan reported the 7th and 8th cases of this rare tumor of eccrine glands in 1985. It is a neoplasm of eccrine acrosyringeal cells, resembling the premalignant fibroepithelial tumor of Pinkus, but with small, uniform, cuboidal cells instead of basaloid cells.

Mehregan AH, et al: Eccrine syringofibroadenoma. JAAD 1985, 13:433.

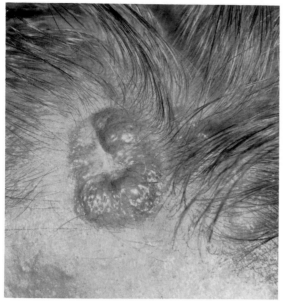

Figure 29–85. Cylindroma on the forehead of a 60-year-old man. (Courtesy of Dr. H. Shatin.)

Cylindroma

Cutaneous cylindroma, also known as turban tumor and tomato tumor, occurs predominantly on the scalp and face as a solitary lesion with a firm but rubberlike nodule, pinkish to blue, and ranging from a few millimeters to several centimeters in size. The solitary cylindroma is considered to be nonhereditary.

The dominantly inherited form manifests itself by the appearance soon after puberty of numerous rounded masses of various sizes on the scalp. The lesions resemble bunches of grapes or small tomatoes. Sometimes they cover the entire scalp like a turban.

Women are affected chiefly, beginning in early adult life. These lesions grow slowly and are benign.

Cylindromas rarely undergo malignant degeneration. Urbanski et al reported a case which was locally aggressive and stress the fact that this aggressive behavior may be predicted by histologic findings such as lack of palisading and diminution or lack of hyalin sheaths. Occasionally multiple lesions of cylindroma are associated with multiple lesions of trichoepithelioma.

It is unclear whether cylindroma is of eccrine or of apocrine origin. Histochemical and electron microscopic analysis has not resolved this.

Histologically, these are cylindrical masses of epithelial cells surrounded and penetrated by a thick band of hyalin substance. Among the groups of epithelial cells are hyalin deposits and cystic cavities.

Cylindroma may be mistaken for epidermoid cyst, but the distinctive appearance and consistency makes diagnosis easy, especially in the multiple type.

Treatment is by excision or electrosurgery. Even if the entire scalp is involved, the disease can be treated successfully by removal of a few tumors at a time.

Baum EW: Cylindroma. Arch Dermatol 1982, 118:692.
Urbanski SJ, et al: Metamorphosis of dermal cylindroma. JAAD 1985, 12:188.
Vernon JH, et al: Autosomal dominant multiple cylindroma associated with solitary lung cylindroma. JAAD 1988, 19:397.

Sweat Gland Carcinoma

Malignant diseases of the sweat gland are rare and those that have been described do not present a characteristic appearance clinically or histologically. They occur predominantly on the head and neck area and in patients aged 50 to 80. Although surgical

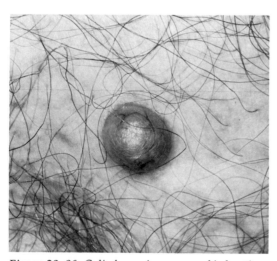

Figure 29–86. Cylindroma in a suprapubic location.

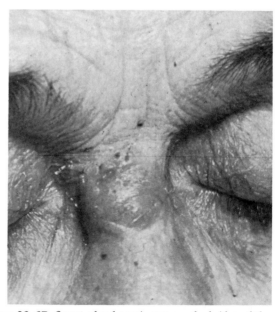

Figure 29–87. Sweat gland carcinoma on the bridge of the nose. It was completely resistant to x-ray therapy.

excision is the treatment of choice, in metastatic disease Whittington et al have suggested the role of chemotherapy and radiation therapy should be re-evaluated as it may show good results in occasional patients. Several varieties have been reported. A listing of some follows.

ECCRINE CARCINOMA

Carcinoma of the eccrine glands does not have a characteristic clinical appearance but does have a high incidence of metastatic spread. It may arise anywhere in the skin. The microscopic pattern is that of an adenocarcinoma, which may create confusion with metastatic adenocarcinoma. In the "classical" type the histologic configuration varies from fairly well-differentiated tubular structures in some areas to anaplastic carcinoma in other areas.

PRIMARY MUCINOUS CARCINOMA OF THE SKIN

This tumor is commonly a round, elevated, reddish, and sometimes ulcerated mass, usually located on the face, head, or trunk. Forty per cent occur on the eyelid. It grows slowly and is usually asymptomatic. Local recurrence is problematic, but the incidence of metastasis is low.

The lesions are often misdiagnosed as sebaceous cysts, hemangiomas, adenocystic basal cell carcinomas, lipomas, melanomas, or neuromas.

Histologically, it is characterized by the presence of large areas of mucin associated with tumor cells in ductlike structures. Histochemically, it has been shown to contain a nonsulfated mucoprotein, sialomucin.

The recommended treatment is local surgical excision.

AGGRESSIVE DIGITAL PAPILLARY ADENOMA AND ADENOCARCINOMA

Kao et al reviewed 57 of these tumors, which usually present as a painless mass on the fingers, toes, or palms and soles. The histologic appearance resembles that of breast carcinoma. There was a marked tendency for recurrence in both types of tumors, and the adenocarcinomas may metastasize and cause death.

Kao GF, et al: Aggressive digital papillary adenoma and adeno-carcinoma. J Cutan Pathol 1987, 14:129.

PRIMARY CUTANEOUS ADENOID CYSTIC CARCINOMA

This rare cutaneous tumor presents usually on the chest or scalp of middle- to older-aged persons. It is identical histologically to adenoid cystic carcinoma of the salivary gland. It may recur locally or, rarely, metastasize.

Seab JA, et al: Primary cutaneous adenoid cystic carcinoma. JAAD 1987, 17:113.

HIDRADENOCARCINOMA

Synonyms: Malignant clear-cell hidradenoma and malignant clear-cell acrospiroma.

Kersting has reported this malignant form of clear-cell hidradenoma occurring in two patients. A man had a dull red 2-cm tumor on the scalp. There was no recurrence for five years following excision. Another man had a recurrent ulcerated dull pink tumor on the nose that resisted ionizing radiation therapy and recurred after excision. Hidradenocarcinoma is a form of eccrine gland adenocarcinoma.

EPIDERMOTROPIC ECCRINE CARCINOMA
(Malignant Eccrine Poroma)

Pinkus and Mehregan reported the case of an 82-year-old woman with an initial lesion on the foot which metastasized two years later. The nodular lesions were rounded, smooth, and reddish or violaceous. Pinkus and Mehregan found these lesions to be malignant eccrine poromas that had metastasized from the original foot lesion of the same character. Subsequent malignant eccrine poromas have metastasized to skin, lymph nodes, and viscera. Mehregan et al reported 18 cases. The tendency for aggressive behavior and lymph node metastases, and the unusual finding of multiple cutaneous metastases were confirmed.

Sweat Gland Cancers

Briscoe KE, et al: Sustained complete remission of metastatic sweat gland carcinoma. JAMA 1978, 240:51.

Cooper PH, et al: Low-grade clear cell eccrine carcinoma. Arch Dermatol 1984, 120:1076.

Holden EA, et al: Loss of membrane B$_2$ microglobulin in eccrine porocarcinoma. Arch Dermatol 1984, 120:732.

Kantor GR, et al: Enlarging ulcerated tumor of the back. Arch Dermatol 1986, 122:585.

Kersting DF: Clear cell hidradenoma and hidradenocarcinoma. Arch Dermatol 1963, 87:323.

Mehregan AH, et al: Eccrine adenocarcinoma. Arch Dermatol 1983, 119:104.

Mezer J, et al: Treatment of sweat gland carcinoma by a four drug combination chemotherapy. Med Oncol Tumor Pharmacother 1986, 3:29.

Mitts DL, et al: Sweat gland carcinoma: a clinicopathological reappraisal. J Surg Oncol 1976, 8:23.

Okada N, et al: Metastasizing eccrine sweat gland carcinoma. Arch Dermatol 1984, 120:768.

Shaw M, et al: Malignant eccrine poroma. Br J Dermatol 1982, 107:675.

Swanson PE, et al: Eccrine sweat gland carcinoma. J Cutan Pathol 1987, 14:65.

Whittington R, et al: Radiation therapy and chemotherapy in malignant sweat gland tumors. JAAD 1986, 15:1093.

MICROCYSTIC ADNEXAL CARCINOMA
(Sclerosing Sweat Duct Carcinoma)

Goldstein et al described in 1982 six cases of "microcystic adnexal carcinoma," closely resembling syringoma, and Nickoloff et al reported immunohistologic studies which suggested both pilar and eccrine differentiation, an observation consonant with the many names that have been given this entity.

The tumor is generally a very slow-growing plaque or nodule. It occurs most commonly on the upper lip in women, but occurs in other facial areas and in men. Histologically it looks rather like a syringoma, with variable development of cords and ducts, embedded in a hyalinized stroma. Perineural infiltration is common and may be extensive. This explains the frequent recurrence after initial excision. Mohs surgery is the treatment of choice. There have been no reports of metastases. Cooper has written a valuable summary of the publications on this lesion.

Cooper PH: Sclerosing carcinomas of sweat ducts. Arch Dermatol 1986, 122:261.
Cooper PH, et al: Microcystic adnexal carcinoma. JAAD 1984, 10:908.
Lupton GP, et al: Microcystic adnexal carcinoma. Arch Dermatol 1986, 122:286.
Nickoloff BJ, et al: Microcystic adnexal carcinoma. Arch Dermatol 1986, 122:290.

APOCRINE GLANDS

Ceruminoma

Ceruminoma is a rare, benign apocrine tumor, which rarely becomes malignant. It is characterized by a firm nodular mass in the external auditory canal. Ulceration and crusting follow, with eventual growth that may obstruct the meatus.

Lynde et al reported seven examples, one benign and six malignant. All were treated by radiation therapy, about half successfully.

Histologically, large masses of tumor cells with pale-staining nuclei are present. Miotic figures may be seen in some cases. There can also be associated adenoid tubular proliferation and cystic spaces.

Treatment is excision; however, recurrences are frequent in the malignant variants, ceruminous adenocarcinoma and adenoid cystic carcinoma, where perineural and neural invasion predispose to recurrence.

Cooper et al reviewed *primary cutaneous adenoid cystic carcinoma*, a tumor closely resembling that type found of salivary gland origin. This subtype of ceruminoma affects older women primarily.

Cooper PH, et al: Primary cutaneous adenoid cystic carcinoma. Arch Dermatol 1984, 120:774.
Lynde CW, et al: Tumors of ceruminous glands. JAAD 1984, 11:841.
Neldner KW: Ceruminoma. Arch Dermatol 1968, 98:344.

Hidradenoma Papilliferum

Hidradenoma papilliferum is a benign solitary tumor that is located almost exclusively in the vulvar and anal areas. The tumor is covered by normal skin. On palpation it is a firm nodule a few millimeters in diameter. Occasionally, bleeding, ulceration, discharge, itching, and pain are noted.

Microscopically this is an adenoma of the apocrine glands. It is encapsulated and lies in the dermis and has no connection with the epidermis. There is a cystlike cavity lined with villi. The walls of the cavity and the villi are lined, occasionally with a single layer but usually a double layer of cells—luminal secretory cells and myoepithelial cells. Tappeiner and Wolff in studies with the electron microscope showed hidradenoma and myoepithelial cells in a hidradenoma papilliferum of the nipple. Their studies confirmed the apocrine origin.

This is a benign lesion, and the diagnosis and treatment are accomplished by biopsy excision.

Goette DK: Hidradenoma papilliferum. JAAD 1988, 19:133.
Santa Cruz DJ, et al: Hidradenoma papilliferum of the eyelid. Arch Dermatol 1981, 117:55.

Syringadenoma Papilliferum (Syringocystadenoma Papilliferum)

This was formerly known as nevus syringocystadenomatosus papilliferus, but Pinkus and Mehregan have discarded this term since they consider that this abnormal apocrine gland growth is not a nevus but a hamartoma.

This lesion most commonly develops in a nevus sebaceus of Jadassohn on the scalp or face, around the time of puberty. About half are present at birth, and approximately 25 per cent arise on the trunk and the genital and inguinal regions during adolescence or adult life, without a preexisting lesion. The lesions

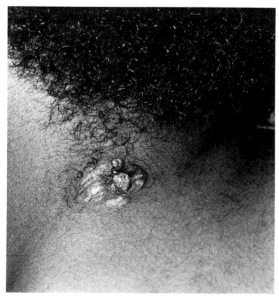

Figure 29–88. Syringoadenoma papilliferum occurring in a nevus sebaceus.

are rose-red papules of firm consistency; they vary in size from 1 to 3 mm and occur in groups. Vesicle-like inclusions are seen, pinpoint to pinhead in size, filled with clear fluid. Some of the papules may be umbilicated and simulate molluscum contagiosum. Extensive verrucous or papillary plaques may also be present.

It is differentiated from syringoma by the grouping of the lesions and by histologic studies, which show dilated and cystic changes in the sweat glands and ducts with numerous papillary projections extending into the lumina. The papillary projections are lined by glandular epithelium, often consisting of two rows of cells. The tumor stains positively for carcinoembryonic antigen by immunohistochemical methods. Lever concurs in Pinkus's opinion that while some lesions are of eccrine origin, most are of apocrine.

Though transition to carcinoma is rare, it has occurred, and excision is advisable. Radiation is ineffective.

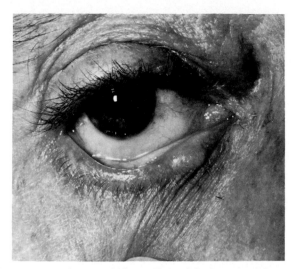

Figure 29–90. Apocrine hidrocystoma of the lower eyelid margin.

Brown FS: Syringocystadenoma papilliferum. Arch Dermatol 1982, 118:202.

Goldberg NS, et al: Linear papules on the neck of a child. Arch Dermatol 1985, 121:1198.

Lever WF, et al: Histopathology of the Skin, ed. 6. Philadelphia, Lippincott, 1983, p. 544.

Pinkus H: Life history of naevus syring adenomatosus papilliferus. Arch Dermatol 1954, 69:305.

Apocrine Hidrocystoma (Apocrine Retention Cyst)

Apocrine hidrocystoma or cystadenoma was described by Mehregan as a single benign tumor occurring chiefly on the face. Those lesions reported on the penile shaft have been reclassified as median raphe cysts. The lesion is a dome-shaped, smooth-surfaced, translucent nodule, frequently bluish or brownish in color. A brownish fluid is noted in some incised lesions.

Microscopically these lesions are an adenomatous cystic proliferation of the apocrine glands. Large cystic spaces lined by apocrine type secretory epithelium are present in the corium. The cysts are surrounded by a fibrous stroma. From the cyst wall papillary projections extend into the cystic cavity.

Apocrine cystadenoma is to be differentiated from pigmented nevus, melanoma, blue nevus, or a cystic basal cell carcinoma.

The lesion is benign, so that when feasible, simple excision is indicated for treatment.

Boddicker ME: Apocrine hidrocystoma. Arch Dermatol 1983, 119:948.

Matsumoto K, et al: Apocrine cystadenoma in a child. Arch Dermatol 1983, 119:182.

Apocrine Gland Carcinoma

Apocrine gland carcinoma, unrelated to Paget's disease, is rare. The axilla is the most common site, but occasionally other areas with apocrine glands, such as the nipples and the vulva, and also the eyelids and the external auditory meatus, where Moll's glands and the ceruminous glands are found, may be involved. Some of these cases from the axillae and nipples may originate from aberrant mammary glands. Widespread metastases may occur.

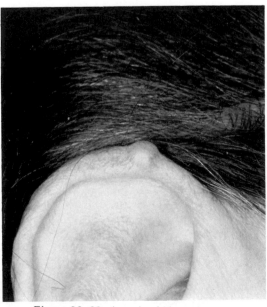

Figure 29–89. Apocrine hidrocystoma.

Burket JM, et al: Tubular apocrine adenoma with perineural invasion. JAAD 1984, 11:639.

Okun MR, et al: Apocrine adenoma versus apocrine carcinoma. JAAD 1980, 2:322.

Warkel RL, et al: Apocrine gland adenoma and adenocarcinoma of the axilla. Arch Dermatol 1971, 103:68.

HAIR FOLLICLE NEVI AND TUMORS

Pilomatricoma
(Calcifying Epithelioma of Malherbe)

Since 1880, when first described, this entity has had various names such as *Malherbe's calcifying epithelioma* and *pilomatrixoma*. Pinkus and Mehregan have corrected this latter term according to the classic rules of etymology to pilomatricoma.

Occurring usually as a single tumor, it is most commonly found on the face, neck, or arms, although it may be located also on the scalp, the trunk, and the lower extremities. Pilomatricoma is an asymptomatic, deeply seated, 0.5–3.0-cm, firm nodule, covered by normal or pink skin, which on stretching may show the "tent sign," with multiple facets and angles.

The lesions may be seen in patients with myotonia atrophica (myotonic muscular dystrophy), together with frontoparietal baldness and Raynaud's phenomenon. A few patients with multiple lesions have been reported. Cooper found pilomatricomalike changes in epidermal cysts in 63 per cent of 57 cysts from patients in one kindred with Gardner's syndrome.

The histopathology shows an encapsulated mass. "Basophilic" and "shadow" cells are seen in solid masses, with a transition from the darkly staining basophilic cells to the shadow cells, which stain eosinophilic. Calcification takes place and in most instances appears as dusting of basophilic substances in the shadow cells or as solid purple amorphous masses. Ossification, melanin deposits, and foreign-body reaction with giant cells may all be present. Pilomatricoma is considered an epithelioma of the hair follicle with cytodifferentiation toward cells of hair matrix, the hair cortex, and cells of the inner sheath.

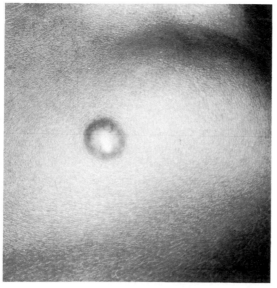

Figure 29–91. Pilomatricoma (calcifying epithelioma of Malherbe) on the chin of a child.

Clinical differential diagnosis is usually impossible. The subcutaneous firm nodule with the normal skin above should suggest the diagnosis, although the epidermoid cyst closely resembles pilomatricoma.

Simple excision of the lesion for biopsy purposes is the best procedure, though curettage of the cyst contents through a small incision or 2-mm punch biopsy hole has been used with success.

Lopanari and Mihm reported a lesion which recurred twice despite wide excision but this seems to be an extremely rare event. It did not occur in series of 100 cases reported in El Salvador by Hernández-Pérez et al, in which female patients outnumbered male by over 2 to 1.

Malignant Pilomatricoma

Margaret Gray Wood and associates reported in 1984 an 86-year-old man with a solitary nodular lesion three months old on the right nape which contained cells with large hyperchromatic nuclei and numerous, frequently atypical, mitoses. Shadow cells were present.

Arnold M, et al: Perforating pilomatricoma. JAAD 1988, 18:255.
Chiaramonti A, et al: Pilomatricoma associated with myotonic dystrophy. Arch Dermatol 1978, 114:1363.
Cooper PH, et al: Pilomatricoma-like changes in the epidermal cysts of Gardner's syndrome. JAAD 1983, 8:639.
Findlay RF: Pilomatricoma. Arch Dermatol 1984, 120:782.
Green DE, et al: Pilomatrix carcinoma. JAAD 1987, 17:264.
Hernandez-Perez E, et al: Pilomatricoma (calcifying epithelioma): a study of 100 cases in El Salvador. Int J Dermatol 1981, 10:491.
Morales A, et al: Pilomatricoma. JAAD 1980, 2:44.
Schwartz BK, et al: Pilomatricomas associated with myotonic dystrophy. JAAD 1987, 16:887.
Wood MG, et al: Malignant pilomatricoma. Arch Dermatol 1984, 120:770.

Trichofolliculoma
(Hair Follicle Nevus)

Originally described by Miescher, trichofolliculoma is a benign, highly structured adenoma of the pilosebaceous unit, characterized by a small dome-shaped nodule some 5 mm in diameter on the face or scalp. From the center of the flesh-colored nodule a small wisp of fine immature hairs protrudes from a central pore. It may occur at any age.

Histologically, the tumor consists of one or more large cystic follicles with smaller radiating follicular structures. The immature hair follicles range from an immature rudimentary matrix to formed hair papillae with fine hairs. Sebaceous glands and even a keratin cyst may be present in the tumor.

The benign nature of the tumor indicates only simple removal such as an excisional biopsy, or fulguration after a suitable shave biopsy has been obtained.

Pinkus H, et al: Trichofolliculoma. Arch Dermatol 1965, 91:46.
Schwartz JL: Trichofolliculoma. Arch Dermatol 1985, 121:262.

Trichoepithelioma
(Epithelioma Adenoides Cysticum)

CLINICAL FEATURES. Described by Brooke in 1892 as epithelioma adenoides cysticum and by Fordyce as multiple benign cystic epithelioma, multiple trichoepitheliomas are hereditary and occur as multiple cystic and solid nodules on the face, especially about the upper lip, the nasolabial folds, and the eyelids. Other sites may be the scalp, the neck, and the trunk.

The lesions are characterized by multiple, small, rounded, smooth, shiny, slightly translucent, firm, circumscribed papules or nodules. The individual lesion is 2 to 4 mm in diameter and flesh-colored or slightly reddish. The center may be slightly depressed. Most frequently the lesions are grouped but discrete. On the face they are often symmetrical. The lesions begin during childhood or at the latest in early adulthood and tend to occur more commonly in the female. Trichoepitheliomas are benign.

The simultaneous presence of multiple trichoepithelioma and cylindroma has been observed repeatedly. Genetic studies have suggested that this occurrence is due to a single autosomal dominant gene capable of phenotypic dimorphism and variable penetrance.

Starink et al reported a patient with generalized trichoepitheliomas, alopecia, and myasthenia gravis. Geffner et al cared for a 10-year-old girl with multiple linear and dermatomal trichoepitheliomas and reviewed the adnexal tumors which may present in this fashion.

Solitary Trichoepithelioma. The singly occurring trichoepithelioma is nonhereditary and occurs mostly

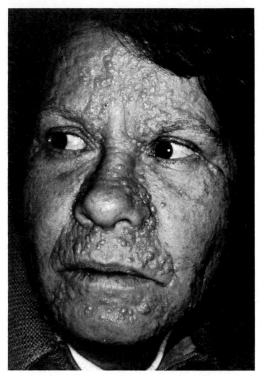

Figure 29–93. Multiple trichoepitheliomas.

on the face; however, it may also be found on the scalp, neck, trunk, upper arms, and thighs.

Desmoplastic Trichoepithelioma. This lesion, which is difficult to differentiate from morpheiform basal cell carcinoma, occurs as a solitary lesion on the faces of young women. Lazorik et al have seen a patient with multiple lesions. They present on the face of young women most commonly, and often have a raised annular border with a central nonulcerated center.

Among the most meaningful histologic criteria are this tumor's differentiation of pilar and sebaceous structures, its lack of any connection with the epidermis, and its noninvasion of cutaneous nerves or muscles. It behaves like an adenoma rather than an invasive malignancy.

HISTOLOGY. Trichoepithelioma shows characteristic keratinous cysts and strands and masses of embryonal cells similar to those of the basal layer or those of the external root sheath of the hair follicle. In proliferating downward these strands form solid epithelial nests showing antlerlike branching. The cell nests contain granular horny or colloid material that forms cysts. The cells are small and mature. Adenoid structures may be present. Calcification of the cystic material and foreign-body giant cell reaction to it may also be seen. Trichoepitheliomas are best classified as an epithelioma of hair germ.

Histologically trichoepithelioma must be differentiated from keratotic basal cell carcinoma.

DIFFERENTIAL DIAGNOSIS. The multiple-lesion type is distinguished from syringoma, which

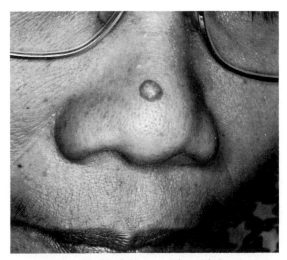

Figure 29–92. Solitary trichoepithelioma.

closely resembles it; in the solitary type it is the basal cell carcinoma with which it may be confused. Undoubtedly, some of the cases of basal cell carcinoma reported in children and adolescents have in fact represented solitary trichoepithelioma.

TREATMENT. Multiple lesions are difficult to treat satisfactorily since only the cosmetic results are of importance. Light fulguration or gentle electrodesiccation seem to be the most acceptable. Cryotherapy with liquid nitrogen is at times satisfactory but an extremely slow process. Dermabrasion is beneficial; however, the lesions tend to slowly recur. Solitary lesions are best removed by excisional surgery or laser.

Fiho GB, et al: Giant solitary trichoepithelioma. Arch Dermatol 1984, 120:797.

Geffner RE, et al: Linear and dermatomal trichoepitheliomas. JAAD 1986, 14:927.

Goldblum OM: Multiple nodules on the face. Arch Dermatol 1985, 121:126.

Lazorik FC, et al: Multiple desmoplastic trichoepitheliomas. Arch Dermatol 1982, 118:361.

Starink TM, et al: Generalized trichoepitheliomas with alopecia and myasthenia gravis. JAAD 1986, 15:1104.

Takei Y, et al: Criteria for histologic differentiation of desmoplastic trichoepithelioma (sclerosing epithelial hamartoma) from morphea-like basal-cell epithelioma. Am J Dermatopathol 1985, 7:207.

in 7 per cent of all cases. Several exhaustive reviews have been published, including those by Elston et al, Salem et al, and Starink et al. The latter author has reported a decreased natural killer cell activity in Cowden's syndrome, as has been reported in a number of other cancer family syndromes. Lazar et al treated a patient with isotretinoin, and while the lesions regressed on medication, they recurred when it was discontinued. Some patients get satisfactory cosmetic results from dermabrasion.

Microscopically, there is typically a verrucous epidermis and lobular acanthosis of glycogen-rich clear cells oriented about a follicle.

Allen BS, et al: Multiple hamartoma syndrome. JAAD 1980, 2:303.

Barax CN, et al: Multiple hamartoma syndrome. JAAD 1987, 17:342.

Brownstein MH, et al: Trichilemmoma. Arch Dermatol 1973, 107:866.

Elston DM, et al: Multiple hamartoma syndrome associated with non-Hodgkin's lymphoma. Arch Dermatol 1986, 122:572.

Lazar AP, et al: Cowden's disease treated with isotretinoin. JAAD 1986, 14:142.

Penneys NS, et al: Papillomavirus common antigen. Arch Dermatol 1984, 120:859.

Salem OS, et al: Cowden's disease. JAAD 1983, 8:686.

Starink TM: Cowden's disease. JAAD 1984, 11:1127.

Velez-Torres R, et al: Facial papules and nodules, thyroid goiter, and acral keratosis. Arch Dermatol 1987, 123:1557.

Trichilemmoma and Cowden's Disease (Multiple Hamartoma Syndrome)

Trichilemmoma is a benign neoplasm of the hair follicle which is derived from or differentiates toward cells of the outer sheath. It may occur as a small solitary papule on the face, particularly the nose and the cheeks. Most lesions are clinically misinterpreted as basal cell carcinoma or verruca. In their report of 40 cases, Brownstein et al found two thirds were men over the age of 40 years. While Ackerman believed these to be verrucae, an immunoperoxidase study by Penneys et al was unable to find papillomavirus common antigen in trichilemmomas.

Trichilemmomas may also occur as multiple lesions. These are a specific cutaneous marker for an autosomal dominant inherited condition associated with multiple benign and malignant tumors: *Cowden's syndrome*. The trichilemmomas are generally limited to the head and neck area; however, Elston et al reported a case with sacral lesions also. Eighty-seven per cent of patients with Cowden's syndrome (the *multiple hamartoma syndrome*) have these facial papules. Other benign features include oral mucosal papules; acral keratotic papules; thyroid goiter, adenomatous or nodular; lipomas; gastrointestinal polyps; and fibrocystic breast disease. Thirty-eight per cent develop malignancies, with breast cancer occurring in 30 per cent of women and thyroid carcinoma

Trichodiscoma, Fibrofolliculoma, and the Birt-Hogg-Dubé Syndrome

Multiple small hamartomas of the mesodermal component of the hair discs (*Haarscheibe*) were identified as trichodiscomas in 1966 by Pinkus. Hundreds of flat or dome-shaped, skin-colored, asymptomatic papules, always in close proximity to a vellus hair, develop at an early age over the face, trunk, and extremities. Histologically there is a richly vascularized stroma, at the periphery of which is a hair follicle.

Starink et al reported *hereditary multiple trichodiscomas*, of early onset and dominant inheritance, in three patients, aged 37, 70, and 73. They analyzed the histologic, histochemical, immunohistochemical, and electron microscopic findings in 27 biopsies. These cases were unassociated with fibrofolliculomas and acrochordons.

Fibrofolliculomas are 2- to 4-mm skin-colored to white papules, which may be solitary, as reported by Scully et al, or more commonly are multiple, scattered over the face, trunk, and extremities. Histologically there is proliferation of the follicular epithelium as epithelial strands extending into well-circumscribed mantle or connective tissue.

The cases in which multiple fibrofolliculomas have occurred have at times been unassociated with other biopsy-proven tumors, but the majority are seen in association with multiple trichodiscomas and acrochordons. This dominantly inherited syndrome, unassociated with any internal disease, is known as the *Birt-Hogg-Dubé syndrome*. This has been reviewed by Ubogy-Rainey et al. Their patient responded well to dermabrasion.

Balus L, et al: Familial multiple trichodiscomas. JAAD 1986, 15:603.
Birt AR, et al: Hereditary multiple fibrofolliculomas with trichodiscomas and acrochordons. Arch Dermatol 1977, 113:1674.
Fujita WH, et al: Multiple fibrofolliculomas with trichodiscomas and acrochordons. Arch Dermatol 1981, 117:32.
Pinkus H, et al: Trichodiscoma: a benign tumor related to Haarscheibe (hair disc). J Invest Dermatol 1974, 63:212.
Scully K, et al: Solitary fibrofolliculoma. JAAD 1984, 11:361.
Starink TM, et al: Familial multiple trichodiscomas. Arch Dermatol 1985, 121:888.
Idem: Fibrofolliculoma. JAAD 1987, 17:493.
Ubogy-Rainey Z, et al: Fibrofolliculomas, trichodiscomas, and acrochordons. JAAD 1987, 16:452.

Proliferating Trichilemmal Tumors (Proliferating Pilar Tumors)

These tumors were first named *proliferating epidermoid cysts* by Wilson Jones. These large (up to 25 cm) and exophytic neoplasms are confined almost exclusively to the scalp and back of the neck. They are approximately five times more common in women, and the mean age of patients is 65 years. They gradually enlarge and may undergo ulceration. These lesions have been misinterpreted both clinically and histologically as squamous cell carcinoma. Rahbari et al reported two cases which developed in nevus sebaceus.

The histologic features include a sharply circumscribed pattern of convoluted lobules with definite margins, frequent continuity with the epidermis, extensive areas of tumor cell necrosis, and trichilemmal type keratinization with abrupt transition to dense keratin but without formation of a granular layer. Patterns of aggressive growth are occasionally present and cytologic atypism may occur.

Carlin MC, et al: Enlarging, painful scalp tumor. Arch Dermatol 1988, 124:935.
Moreland ME, et al: Pathology quiz case 1. Arch Dermatol 1981, 117:440.
Rahbari H, et al: Development of proliferating trichilemmal cyst in organoid nevus. JAAD 1986, 14:123.

Other Hair Follicle Tumors

Other tumors and cysts of the hair follicle have been extensively reviewed and histogenetically classified by Headington and others. These include dilated pore, pilar sheath acanthoma, trichoadenoma, perifollicular fibromas, and generalized hair follicle hamartomas.

Brown AC, et al: Generalized hair follicle hamartoma. Arch Dermatol 1969, 99:478.
Brownstein MH, et al: The pilosebaceous tumors. Int J Dermatol 1977, 16:340.
Headington JT: Tumors of the hair follicle. Am J Pathol 1976, 85:840.
Mehregan AH, et al: Pilar sheath acanthoma. Arch Dermatol 1978, 114:1495.
Winer L: The dilated pore. J Invest Dermatol 1954, 23:181.

EPITHELIAL CYSTS AND SINUSES

Epidermal Cyst (Keratin Cyst, Sebaceous Cyst, Epidermoid Cyst)

The epidermal cyst is a commonly fluctuant, tense swelling varying from one-half to several centimeters in diameter. The surface of the overlying skin is usually smooth and shiny from the upward pressure. These nodules are freely movable over underlying tissue and are attached to the normal skin above them by the remains of the expanded gland duct, the opening of which frequently shows at a central point on the surface as a comedo. The pasty contents of the cysts are formed mostly of macerated keratin and cheesy fatty material. Epidermoid cysts occur commonly on the face, neck, and trunk. Their association with Gardner's syndrome is discussed elsewhere. Those found on the hairy scalp are usually pilar (trichilemmal) cysts (see later).

These cysts may rupture and induce a vigorous foreign body inflammatory response, after which they are most firmly adherent to surrounding structures and are more difficult to enucleate. Rarely lowgrade, nonmetastasizing squamous cell carcinoma may arise in the cyst wall, as reported by Yaffe and others.

Swinehart et al found evidence that *idiopathic scrotal*

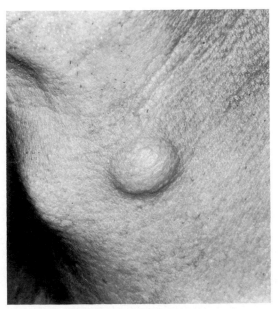

Figure 29–94. Epidermal cyst on the neck.

calcinosis is due to end stage dystrophic calcinosis associated with inflamed scrotal epidermoid cysts. Bhawan et al agreed.

The epidermoid cyst is a keratinizing cyst, the wall of which is stratified squamous epithelium containing keratohyalin granules.

It is differentiated from the pilar cyst by its location. Pilar cysts occur most frequently on the scalp. The lipoma closely resembles the epidermoid cyst, and at times it may be difficult to demonstrate the freely movable property of the cyst. Branchial cleft cysts and nodular fibromas should also be kept in mind.

The fastest and most definitive treatment is enucleation of the cyst through a small incision or even through a hole made with a 4- or even a 2-mm biopsy punch. So trivial is the scar resulting from the use of the 2-mm punch or blade, so easy is the evacuation of the cyst through such a hole by finger pressure, and so often can the sac itself be expressed, or dissected out with iris scissors, that this is one of the best procedures. Inflamed cysts do not lend themselves well to any of these procedures, except simple drainage through a 2-mm punch hole, which is often curative. Injection of intralesional steroids, 3 mg/kg, will resolve an acutely inflamed cyst, and at times may shrink noninflamed lesions.

Bhawan J, et al: The so-called idiopathic scrotal calcinosis. Arch Dermatol 1983, 119:709.
McGavran MH, et al: Keratinous cysts of the skin. Arch Dermatol 1966, 94:499.
Swinehart JM, et al: Scrotal carcinoma arising in an epidermal cyst. Arch Dermatol 1982, 118:961.
Yaffe HS: Squamous cell carcinoma arising in an epidermal cyst. Arch Dermatol 1982, 118:961.

Pilar Cyst
(Trichilemmal Cyst)

The trichilemmal cyst, also known as a *wen*, is similar clinically to the epidermoid cyst except that about 90 per cent of the pilar cysts occur on the scalp, and inheritance by the autosomal dominant mode is common. It has been found rarely on the face, trunk, and extremities. The contents of this type of cyst are more keratinous and not so fatty as those of the epidermoid cyst. They are also odorless.

The trichilemmal cyst has a wall lined by keratinizing epithelium without a granular layer. Pinkus has shown that these trichilemmal cysts originate from the middle portion of the hair follicle epithelium. Brownstein has described lesions which histologically show changes in the cyst wall of both epidermoid and trichilemmal differentiation. He refers to these as hybrid cysts.

Clinically these lesions are indistinguishable from the epidermoid cyst. Differentiation from other lesions is fairly easily established.

Treatment is the same as that for the epidermoid

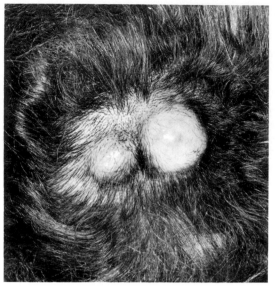

Figure 29–95. *Pilar cysts of the scalp.*

cyst. They are much more easily enucleated, owing to their firm, coherent nature.

Brenner S: Treatment of pilar cysts with solcoderm solution. JAAD 1986, 14:145.
Brownstein MH: Hybrid cyst. JAAD 1983, 9:872.
Kimura S: Trichilemmal cysts. Dermatologica 1978, 157:164.

Dermoid Cyst

Dermoid cysts are congenital in origin and occur chiefly along the lines of cleavage. In the sublingual region the soft, elastic, oval cysts may vary from a few millimeters to several centimeters in diameter. They may also occur about the eyes and at the root of the nose. They are generally not attached to the skin but are freely movable. The contents of the singly occurring tumor usually have a rancid odor.

Histologically, the cyst wall is lined with stratified squamous epithelium containing skin appendages, including lanugo hair. These cysts are the result of sequestration of skin along lines of embryonic closure.

These lesions should be completely excised.

Brownstein MH, et al: Subcutaneous dermoid cysts. Arch Dermatol 1973, 107:237.
Pensler JM, et al: Craniofacial dermoids. Plast Reconstr Surg 1988, 82:953.

Pilonidal Sinus

Pilonidal cyst or sinus is a midline hairy patch or pit in the sacral region with a sinus orifice in the bottom, or a cyst beneath it, in which hair is growing. It usually becomes symptomatic during adolescence, and presents as a foreign body abscess, with hair as the offender. In theory, wide-open cystectomy and thorough debridement should suffice to cure it; but there are many failures. Gustave Hoehn has had great satisfaction for 30 years with a method proposed by Korb in 1951: opening the cyst widely, debriding it, and packing the cavity with silver nitrate crystals. By the third day, the sac has separated and can be lifted out and any remaining sinuses repacked with silver nitrate. The entire procedure is done without hospitalization.

Hoehn GH: A simple solution to the therapeutic dilemma of pilonidal cysts. J Dermatol Surg Oncol 1982, 8:56.

Steatocystoma Simplex

Brownstein reported a solitary steatocystoma in 16 women and 14 men. The site was on the face, limbs, or chest. It appears to be the nonheritable counterpart of the more familiar steatocystoma multiplex. It occurs as a rule between ages 15 and 70 (median age 39). The content of the cyst is an oily yellow fluid. Simple excision is curative.

Brownstein MH: Steatocystoma simplex. Arch Dermatol 1982, 118:409.

Steatocystoma Multiplex

Steatocystoma multiplex consists of multiple, small, yellowish, cystic nodules 2 to 6 mm in diameter, located principally on the upper anterior portion of the trunk, the upper arms, the axillae, and the thighs. In severe cases, the lesions may be generalized, with sparing only of the palms and soles. Nishimura et al reported a patient whose lesions were limited to the face, and Marley et al reported a 70-year-old man with lesions limited to the scalp. These cysts often contain a syruplike, yellowish, odorless, oily material.

Steatocystoma has a high familial tendency and probably has an autosomal dominant mode of transmission. Feinstein et al reported a kindred in which four generations were involved. However, numerous nonhereditary cases have been reported.

Histologically there is a folded cyst wall consisting of several layers of epithelial cells, with flattened sebaceous lobules within or close to the wall. In some instances hair follicle type extensions occur in the wall, and lanugo-sized hairs may be present in the cavity.

In the differential diagnosis steatocystomata are easily differentiated from dermoid and epidermoid cysts by their multiplicity and sites and because of the characteristic oily contents.

The best treatment is excision of the lesions. Elliptical excisions with one or at most two sutures produce excellent results. However, the sheer number of the cysts may preclude this type of treatment. In such instances, incision and thorough expression of the cyst contents is quite effective. The lesions may recur but only after several months.

Marley WM, et al: Steatocystoma multiplex limited to the scalp. Arch Dermatol 1981, 117:673.
Nishimura M, et al: Steatocystoma multiplex. Arch Dermatol 1986, 122:205.

Eruptive Vellus Hair Cysts

Esterly et al described this entity in 1977. Many ensuing publications have characterized it as an au-

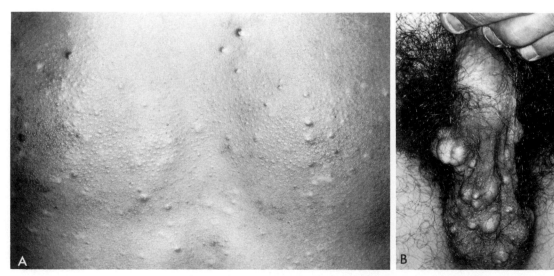

Figure 29–96. Steatocystoma multiplex on the chest (A) and on the scrotum (B).

tosomal dominant inherited disorder which appears as yellowish to reddish brown, small papules of the chest and proximal extremities. They may be congenital, but usually have their onset between 17 and 24 years of age. Disseminated lesions have occurred, as well as lesions limited to the face. Histologically the cystic epithelium is of the stratified squamous type; the cyst contents are composed of laminated keratin and vellus hairs; and folliclelike invaginations may be present in the cyst wall. This is felt to be caused by an abnormality at the infundibular level of the vellus hair. Treatment is usually unsuccessful, but topical retinoic acid, Buf Puf dermabrasion followed by 10 per cent urea cream, or Lac-Hydrin may be tried.

Esterly NB, et al: Eruptive vellus hair cysts. Arch Dermatol 1977, 113:500.
Fisher DA: Retinoic acid in the treatment of eruptive vellus hair cysts. JAAD 1981, 5:221.
Hayashibe K, et al: Eruptive vellus hair cysts. Arch Dermatol 1986, 122:141.
Haynie LS, et al: Blue papules on the chest. Arch Dermatol 1988, 124:1101.
Lee K, et al: Eruptive vellus hair cysts. Arch Dermatol 1984, 120:1191.
Piepkorn MW, et al: A kindred with congenital vellus hair cysts. JAAD 1981, 5:661.
Stiefler RE, et al: Eruptive vellus hair cysts. JAAD 1980, 3:425.

Pigmented Follicular Cysts

Single pigmented lesions occurring in men between 20 and 60, easily mistaken for moles, may be pigmented follicular cysts. These were first described by Mehregan and Medenica in 1982, and a case was reported by Pavlidakey et al in 1986: the seven cases were among 120,000 consecutive biopsy specimens.

The stratified squamous epithelial wall has rete ridges and papillae, and the cyst is full of thick, deeply pigmented hair shafts. Most occurred on the face or neck.

Mehregan AH, et al: Pigmented follicular cysts. J Cutan Pathol 1982, 2:423.
Pavlidakey GP, et al: Pigmented follicular cysts. Int J Dermatol 1986, 25:174.

Milia

Milia are white keratinous cysts, 1 to 4 mm in diameter, appearing chiefly on the face, especially under the eyes. Montgomery described them as "tiny pearly white globoid masses, often appearing like kernels of rice lying beneath a translucent layer of tissue." They may occur in great numbers, especially in middle-aged women.

Milia may originate from the external root sheath of vellus hair follicles. Milialike tiny epidermal cysts can develop in epidermolysis bullosa, pemphigus, porphyria cutanea tarda, and congenital ectodermal defect. They also tend to occur after trauma, such as dermabrasion, or after a bullous or vesicular eruption has healed, or after long-term corticosteroid use, or after 5-FU therapy.

Treatment is incision and expression of the contents with a comedo expresser. No anesthesia is needed, although in sensitive patients an intradermal injection of physiologic saline solution (except in areas of elastosis) will afford anesthesia without the burning pain caused by lidocaine solution.

Brenner S, et al: Mucoid milia. Arch Dermatol 1984, 120:300.
Nunzi E, et al: Milia induced by corticosteroids. Arch Dermatol 1986, 122:139.

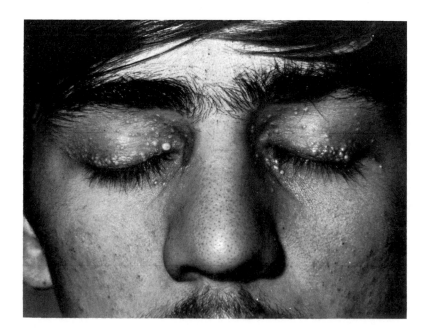

Figure 29–97. Milia on the eyelids.

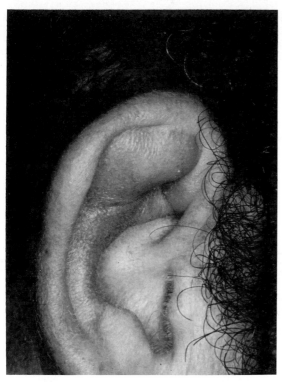

Figure 29–98. Pseudocyst of the auricle.

Pseudocyst of the Auricle

Pseudocyst of the auricle clinically presents as a fluctuant, tense, noninflammatory swelling on the upper half of the ear. Localized degeneration of the cartilage leads to accumulation of fluid. Needle aspiration yields a yellow oily material. Treatment includes drainage of the cavity followed by application of a pressure dressing.

Fukumizu H, et al: Bilateral pseudocysts of the auricles. Arch Dermatol 1984, 120:1238.

Glamb R, et al: Pseudocyst of the auricle. JAAD 1984, 11:58.

Lapins NA, et al: Seroma of the auricle. Arch Dermatol 1982, 118:503.

Cutaneous Columnar Cysts

Four types of cysts which occur in the skin are lined by columnar epithelium. *Branchiogenic cysts* are small, solitary lesions just above the sternal notch. The cells may have cilia, and the wall contains smooth muscle and mucous glands. *Thyroglossal duct cysts* are similar clinically to branchiogenic cysts except they are usually located on the anterior aspect of the neck. Histologically they simulate branchiogenic cysts also, except there is no smooth muscle in the wall, and frequently there are thyroid follicles present. *Cutaneous ciliated cysts* are usually located on the legs in females. The epithelium seen on biopsy resembles that seen in fallopian tubes. *Median raphe cysts of the penis* are developmental defects lying in the ventral midline of the penis, usually on the glans. Asarch et al reviewed the clinical and histologic findings in detail.

Ambiavagar PC, et al: Cutaneous ciliated cyst on the chin. Arch Dermatol 1979, 115:895.

Asarch RG, et al: Median raphe cysts of the penis. Arch Dermatol 1979, 115:1084.

Farmer ER, et al: Cutaneous ciliated cysts. Arch Dermatol 1978, 114:70.

Fraga S, et al: Branchiogenic cysts in the skin and subcutaneous tissue. Am J Clin Pathol 1971, 56:230.

Grabski WJ, et al: Pseudocyst of the auricle associated with trauma. Arch Dermatol 1989, 125:528.

Miller OF, et al: Cutaneous branchiogenic cysts with papilloma and sinus presentation. JAAD 1984, 11:367.

30

Melanocytic Nevi and Neoplasms

The pigmented nevi and neoplasms may be composed of melanocytes or nevus cells. Melanocytes originate in the embryonal neural crest and migrate to the epidermis, the dermis, the leptomeninges, the retina, the mucous membrane epithelium, and the inner ear, cochlea, and vestibular system. Nevus cell precursors enter the epidermis, dermis, and panniculus, where they may aggregate to form clusters of cells, a feature which distinguishes them from melanocytes. They also do not have dendritic processes, whereas melanocytes do.

EPIDERMAL MELANOCYTIC LESIONS

The normal melanocyte occurring at the epidermal-dermal junction is a dendritic secretory cell that supplies all the normal melanin of the skin. These cells contain pigment granules (melanosomes) and stain with dopa reaction and silver stains because they contain melanin. Melanocytes of the epidermis transfer the melanosomes through their thin dendritic processes into surrounding keratinocytes, which migrate outward. The amount of melanin in the keratinocytes determines the pigmentation of the skin and hair. Each melanocyte is associated with approximately 36 keratinocytes to form an *epidermal melanin unit*. The melanocyte has a small dark-staining nucleus and a clear cytoplasm. It rests on the basal lamina between the basal cells of the epidermis.

EPHELIS
(Freckle)

Freckles are tan macules usually less than 5 or 6 mm in diameter, of irregular shape, which form on sun-exposed skin, notably the nose, cheeks, hands, and upper trunk, in genetically predisposed persons who usually have red or sandy hair, white skin, and high susceptibility to sunburn. In freckles, melanocytes are nearly one third less abundant than in adjacent normal skin, but they are larger and contain more, and more mature, melanosomes, whereas those in the pale adjacent skin, though more numerous, contain only small round melanosomes.

TREATMENT. Freckles can be peeled off by cautious painting with trichloracetic acid, a few at a time; but they tend to recur and, like graying hair, are better admired than treated.

Azizi E, et al: Skin type, hair color, and freckles are predictors of decreased minimal erythema ultraviolet radiation dose. JAAD 1988, 19:32.

NEVUS SPILUS

Nevus spilus is a pigmented, light brown or tan macule of varied diameter, speckled with smaller, darker colored macules or papules, and frequently occurs on the trunk and lower extremities, as Kopf et al have reported. They found 14 of 601 patients (2.3 per cent) had such lesions, with no sex predilection.

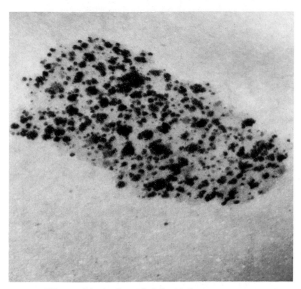

Figure 30–1. Speckled lentiginous nevus.

These lesions may be small, measuring 1 cm in size or may be quite large. When large they may follow a dermatomal or nevoid type distribution, frequently respecting the midline. When this pattern exists the lesion may be referred to as a zosteriform, or sometimes a speckled, lentiginous nevus. There may be multiple sites involved in the same individual, which may be widely separated by normal skin.

Histologically, the tan flat background may show only basilar hyperpigmentation, such as is present in a café-au-lait spot, or may show lentiginous proliferation of the epidermis. The darker speckles usually contain nevus cells.

In the differential diagnosis the café-au-lait patch comes immediately to attention. It is lighter brown and never speckled; other signs of neurofibromatosis may be apparent.

Nevus spilus should be left untreated. Since nevus cells are often present in the dark speckles, it is possible that a melanoma may arise in them; however, this possibility does not necessitate removal.

Cohen HJ, et al: Nevus spilus. Arch Dermatol 1970, 102:433.
Kopf AW, et al: Prevalence of congenital-nevus-like nevi, nevi spili, and café-au-lait spots. Arch Dermatol 1985, 121:766.
Idem: Congenital-nevus-like nevi, nevi spili and café-au-lait spots in patients with malignant melanoma. J Dermatol Surg Oncol 1985, 11:275.
Matsudo H, et al: Zosteriform lentiginous nevus. Arch Dermatol 1973, 107:902.
Stewart DM, et al: Speckled lentiginous nevus. Arch Dermatol 1978, 114:895.
Wagner RF Jr, et al: In situ malignant melanoma arising in a speckled lentiginous nevus. JAAD 1989, 20:125.

LENTIGO

Lentigo Simplex. One, or far oftener many, of these sharply defined, rounded, brown or black macules may appear anywhere on the body surface or the mucosa. The lesions usually arise in childhood, but may appear at any age, and are indistinguishable from junctional nevi. There is no predilection for areas of sun exposure.

Histologically, lentigo simplex shows elongation of the rete ridges, an increase in the number of melanocytes in the basal layer, an increase of melanin in both the melanocytes and basal keratinocytes, and melanophages in the upper dermis.

No therapy is indicated as there is no predisposition to neoplastic change.

Senile Lentigines (Lentigo Senilis, Solar Lentigo). These are commonly known as "liver spots." They are benign, discrete, hyperpigmented macules of irregular shape, occurring upon sun-exposed skin in persons long exposed to the sun. The backs of the hands and the forehead are favorite sites. The knuckles and two distal phalanges are spared.

Histologically, the rete ridges appear club-shaped and show small budlike extensions. There is a marked increase in the number of melanocytes, with increased pigmentation in the basal cell layer and adjacent keratinocytes. The upper dermis often contains melanophages.

Senile lentigines may be accompanied by depigmented macules, senile (actinic) purpura, and other chronic actinic degenerative changes in the skin. Mehregan has documented their evolution into benign lichenoid keratoses and into seborrheic keratoses. The evolution into benign lichenoid keratoses has been since affirmed by many, including Berger et al and Barranco. Light application of liquid nitrogen with a cotton-tip applicator is the most efficient and effective treatment for these lesions of only cosmetic significance. Carbon dioxide laser vaporization or light fulguration are alternative treatment modalities.

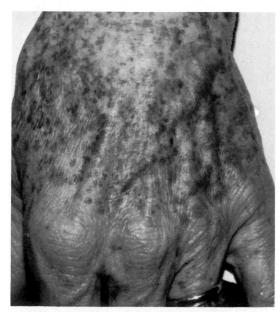

Figure 30–2. Lentigines, "liver spots." Sparing of knuckles is characteristic.

Protective measures, particularly sunscreens, should be taken to prevent excessive exposure to sunlight. Bleaching creams such as 4 or 5 per cent hydroquinone (Eldoquin Forte) may be used over a period of several months. This induces temporary lightening and may be reused as necessary.

Individuals receiving oral methoxsalen photochemotherapy (PUVA) may develop persistent lentigines in which there may be cellular atypia, on sites (such as the penis) which are normally sun-protected, as Abel et al have shown.

Penile and Vulvar Melanosis

These two entities are recently described localized pigmentary alterations that may show lentiginous changes on biopsy, but most often show only basilar hyperpigmentation. Occasionally, atypical melanocytes are also present. Mottling of pigmentation in large patches, which may be quite large, or smaller, well-demarcated lesions may be present on the penis or female genitalia. In the latter location the labia minora is most often affected. Further reports will help better classify these unusual lesions.

Multiple Lentigines Syndrome

Multiple generalized lentigines may occur with a number of associated signs as a dominantly inherited syndrome. The lentigines are dark brown macules from 1 to 5 mm in diameter, with a preponderance on the trunk. However, other areas may also be involved, such as the palms and soles, the buccal mucosa, the genitalia, and the scalp. The lesions appear shortly after birth and form a distinctive speckled appearance which has given rise to the designation of "leopard syndrome" by Gorlin and his associates. "Leopard" is Gorlin's mnemonic acronym for Lentigines, Electrocardiographic abnormalities, Ocular hypertelorism, Pulmonary stenosis, Abnormalities of genitalia, Retardation of growth, and Deafness.

Moynahan's Syndrome

This consists of multiple lentigines, congenital mitral stenosis, dwarfism, genital hypoplasia, and mental deficiency.

Centrofacial Lentiginosis

Centrofacial lentiginosis is characterized by lentigines on the nose and adjacent cheeks, variously associated with status dysraphicus, multiple skeletal anomalies, and central nervous system disorders. Mucous membranes are spared. Onset is in the first

years of life. Dociu et al studied 40 such cases of this autosomal dominant syndrome.

Inherited Patterned Lentiginosis in Blacks

O'Neill and James reported ten light-complexioned black patients who, on an autosomal dominant familial basis, developed numerous lentigines in infancy or early childhood. The lentigines were distributed over the central face, lips, dorsal hands and feet, elbows, and buttocks. The mucous membranes were spared. No internal abnormalities are associated with this newly recognized pigmentary pattern.

LAMB Syndrome

Synonyms are *NAME syndrome* and *Carney's syndrome*. This comprises cardio-cutaneous myxomas, lentigines, blue nevi, and endocrine abnormalities. It is discussed in more detail with myxomas, in Chapter 9.

Peutz-Jeghers Syndrome

This autosomal dominant syndrome consists of pigmented macules on the lips and oral mucosa, and perioral and acral areas. Gastrointestinal polyps, especially prominent in the jejunum, are frequently associated. Further discussion may be found under disorders of pigmentation, in Chapter 36.

Abel EA, et al: PUVA-induced melanocytic atypia. JAAD 1985, 13:761.
Barranco VP: Multiple benign lichenoid keratoses. JAAD 1985, 13:201.
Berger TG, et al: Lichenoid benign keratoses. JAAD 1984, 11:635.
Carney JA, et al: Dominant inheritance of the complex of myxomas, spotty pigmentation, and endocrine overactivity. Mayo Clin Proc 1986, 61:1651.
Idem: The complex of myxomas, spotty pigmentation, and endocrine overactivity. Medicine 1985, 64:270.
Dociu I, et al: Centrofacial lentiginosis. Br J Dermatol 1976, 94:39.
Dormandy TL: Gastrointestinal polyposis with neurocutaneous pigmentation. N Engl J Med 1956, 256:1093, 1141, 1186.
Giardello FM, et al: Increased risk of cancer in the Peutz-Jeghers syndrome. NEJM 1987, 316:1511.
Gorlin RJ, et al: Multiple lentigines syndrome. Am J Dis Child 1969, 117:652.
Jackson R: Melanosis of the vulva. J Dermatol Surg Oncol 1984, 10:119.
Laude TA, et al: Congenital lentiginosis. Cutis 1977, 19:615.
Leicht S, et al: Atypical pigmented penile macules. Arch Dermatol 1988, 124:1267.
Mehregan AH: Lentigo senilis and its evolution. J Invest Dermatol 1975, 65:429.
Moynahan EJ: Multiple symmetrical moles with psychic and somatic infantilism and genital hyperplasia. Proc R Soc Med 1962, 55:959.
O'Neill JF, et al: Inherited patterned lentiginosis in blacks. Arch Dermatol 1989; 125:1231.

Reed OM, et al: Cutaneous lentiginosis with atrial myxomas. JAAD 1986, 15:398.

Revuz J, et al: Penile melanosis. JAAD 1989, 20:567.

Rhodes AR, et al: The PUVA-induced pigmented macule. JAAD 1983, 9:47.

Idem: Mucocutaneous lentigines, cardiomucocutaneous myxomas, and multiple blue nevi. JAAD 1984, 10:72.

Uhle P, et al: Generalized lentiginosis. JAAD 1988, 18:444.

Voron DA, et al: Multiple lentigines syndrome. Am J Med 1976, 60:447.

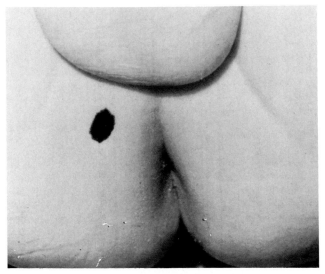

Figure 30–3. Junction nevus near the perineum of an infant.

MELANOACANTHOMA

Cutaneous melanoacanthoma is a rare lesion first described by Bloch and later by Mishima and Pinkus. It is a benign epidermal melanocytic neoplasm, occurring on the head, clinically resembling a pigmented seborrheic keratosis or pigmented basal cell carcinoma. Its onset is slow, and it occurs predominantly in white men over age 60.

Histologically, melanoacanthoma is a benign neoplasm composed of keratinocytes and large dendritic melanocytes, filled with pigment.

Oral melanoacanthoma is also a proliferation of two cell types, melanocytes and epithelial cells; however, it appears to be a reactive lesion. It occurs on the oral tissues, predominantly in young black women, with a rapid onset and spontaneous resolution being typical.

Delacretaz J: Melanoacanthoma. Dermatologica 1975, 151:236.

Goode RK, et al: Oral melanoacanthoma. Oral Surg 1983, 56:622.

CELLULAR NEVI

The common mole, also known as *nevus cell* or *nevocytic nevus* and *cellular nevus*, is not stable; it grows, going through changes of maturation, and even of senescence. They begin to appear in the first years of life and increase in prevalence and number of lesions over the following two to three decades, after which there is a steady decline. Females tend to have more nevi than males, and whites more than blacks. They are seldom seen in doubly covered areas, such as the buttocks, except in the *dysplastic nevus syndrome*, or in other relatively sun-protected sites, such as the inner arms. They typically reach their maximum size within a few years and do not continue to enlarge.

Other types of nevus cell nevi are the giant pigmented nevus (bathing trunk nevus), halo nevus, balloon cell nevus, neuronevus, and spindle and epithelioid cell (Spitz) nevi, formerly called "benign juvenile melanoma."

Walter Lever states: "The typical nevus cell is oval or cuboidal . . . and has a distinctly outlined homogeneous cytoplasm. The nucleus is large, round or oval, pale, and vesicular. Nevus cells, however, show variations in appearance. In the upper dermis they look like epithelial or epithelioid cells, while in the lower dermis, they may resemble histiocytes, fibroblasts, or Schwannian cells." Nevus cells are apparently modified melanocytes without dendrites.

INCIDENCE AND PREVALENCE. The maximum number of nevi are present between the ages of 20 and 25 and the average number is 40. From then on the lesions flatten and fade, until they disappear completely by the age of 90. Nevi begin as small, flat, pigmented macules, junctional nevi. Over time most develop into compound, and finally intradermal, nevi.

Allyn and his associates studied the incidence of pigmented nevi on the palms, soles, nail beds, and conjunctivae. In a study of 1000 patients there was a 9 per cent incidence of plantar nevi, 6 per cent palmar nevi, and 1 per cent conjunctival. None were found in the nail bed. Several prevalence studies by Rampen et al, Stegmaier, Fitzsimons et al, MacKie et al, and Nicholls confirm this. Sun exposure appears to increase the number of moles in the exposed skin,

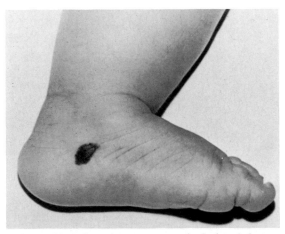

Figure 30–4. Junction nevus near heel of an infant.

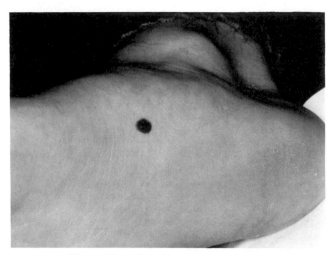

Figure 30–5. Junction nevus on the sole.

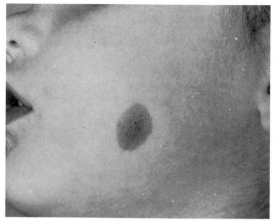

Figure 30–7. Compound nevus. Note fine dark hairs.

as Kopf showed. Australians have more moles than Europeans. Whites have more than blacks, and, as Rampen found, light-complexioned have more than dark-complexioned persons. Also, they found, women tend to have more on the legs, and men more on the trunk, than the opposite sex; sun exposure presumably accounts for this.

Blacks have more nevi than whites on the palms, soles, conjunctivae, and nail beds. Mucous membrane nevi are unusual in either.

PATHOGENESIS. The process by which nevus cell nests apparently descend into the dermis, which was called *Abtropfung* (dropping away or off) by Masson, has been elucidated by Lea et al in an electron microscopic study. They showed that the basement membrane zone continues uninterruptedly to surround the nevus cell nests, and there are no hemidesmosomes along the line of contact of the most superficial nests with the overlying epidermis.

CLINICAL FEATURES. The junction nevus, clinically, is a smooth, hairless, light to dark brown macule, varying in size from 1 to 6 mm in diameter.

It may have the characteristic appearance of a target or a fried egg. It occurs at any site on the body surface. On the palms, soles, or scrotum, pigmented nevi are usually of the junction type. Junction nevi may be present at birth but usually appear between 3 and 18 years of age.

During adolescence and adulthood some of these junction nevi will become compound or intradermal in type. However, junction nevi may persist into, or develop during, adulthood.

The junction nevus usually remains flat until the nevus cells extend into the dermis. The nevus is then said to become "compound": i.e., both junction and intradermal. Later junctional proliferation ceases and the nevus cells become separated from the epidermis by a band of connective tissue to produce the intradermal nevus. In middle-aged people this latter type is the one usually found. The lesions may be dome-shaped, sessile, warty or smooth, flesh-colored or brown, and with or without hairs.

The *junction nevus* is characterized by the presence of single melanocytes, or theques of them, in the lower levels of the epidermis. Pinkus agreed with

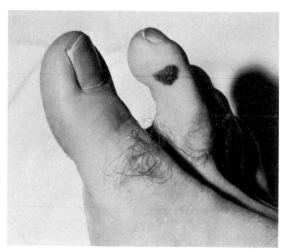

Figure 30–6. Compound nevus. The lesion is slightly elevated.

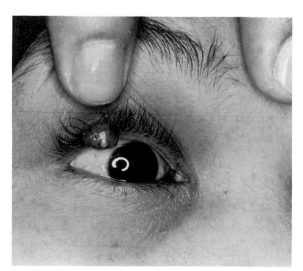

Figure 30–8. Intradermal nevus on the margin of the upper eyelid.

Kopf and Ackerman that neatly circumscribed nests of melanocytes are not reassuring if there is atypia of individual melanocytes: this is simply *melanoma in situ*, and invasive melanoma is not far off.

The *"compound"* nevus is one which is still manifesting so-called "junction activity" (accumulation of melanocytes in theques in the epidermis) but has the formed structure of a cellular nevus in the dermis as well. It is a papule, euchromic to brown to black, with or without a coarse hair or hairs, occurring usually in an older child or an adult.

The pseudovascular spaces found in 10 to 20 per cent of these nevi, and often interpreted as dilated lymphatic spaces, are not vascular, according to Modlin et al, who found that their lining does not stain with an antibody marker for vascular endothelium. They are apparently lined by melanocytes.

The *intradermal nevus* is simply a compound nevus in which "junctional activity" (i.e., theques of melanocytes in the epidermis or at the dermoepidermal junction) has ceased, and all the nevus cells are in the dermis.

MALIGNANT DEGENERATION. The development of a pigmented nevus in a patient over 35 should alert the physician to possible melanoma. The signs of malignant transformation in pigmented nevi are recent enlargement, especially if asymmetric; changes in color (especially red, white, blue, or black); surface changes (scaling, erosion, oozing, crusting, ulceration, or bleeding); development of a palpable thickening; development of pain or tenderness; signs of inflammation; or the appearance of satellite pigmentation.

Features suggesting benignancy are diameter of 3 mm or less; perfectly uniform pigmentation; flaccid epidermis; a smooth, uniform border, unchanging size and color; and on histologic examination, melanocytes all arranged in nests, not singly, and absence of cellular atypia.

Nevocellular nevi may have unusual histologic features during pregnancy, as documented by Foucar et al, or in children, as described by Eng. There may be clinical changes with pregnancy, or with oral contraceptive use. Nevi from normal persons have no estrogen or progesterone receptors; Ellis has shown positive estrogen receptor binding in nevi from pregnant women, as is also found in malignant melanoma.

TREATMENT. The management of nevi is a perplexing problem. Clearly, if all moles were removed, thousands of melanomas would be prevented. Just as obviously, this would be impossibly impractical, and too costly. There are too many. Acquired (as opposed to congenital) nevi should be removed only if they are showing signs of malignant transformation (see above), or if the patient desires removal for cosmetic reasons—and if they are so unsightly that a keloid or hypertrophic scar could look no worse. Neckline and beltline nevi which are actually irritated may be removed to relieve the patient of the irritation, but this is merely an option. Nevi within the hairy scalp should be removed if atypical, because it is impractical to try to watch them.

If removal is solely for cosmetic reasons, a shave removal is the most satisfactory method, as it leaves almost no scar if the shave is skillfully done and the site merely treated with an appropriate styptic such as Monsel's (ferric subsulfate), ferric chloride solution, or 30 per cent aluminum chloride, for hemostasis. This method has served one of us (HLA) well for over 50 years.

Allyn B, et al: Incidence of pigmented nevi. JAMA 1963, 186:890.
Arnold HL Jr: Multiple pigmented nevi. Arch Dermatol Syph 1939, 40:386.
Buchner A, et al: Pigmented nevi of the oral mucosa. Oral Surg 1987, 63:676.
Chaudhuri PK, et al: Incidence of estrogen receptors in benign nevi and human malignant melanoma. JAMA 1980, 244:791.
Christiansen WN, et al: Histologic characteristics of vulvar nevocellular nevi. J Cutan Pathol 1987, 14:87.
Coleman WP, et al: Nevi, lentigines, and melanomas in Blacks. Arch Dermatol 1980, 116:548.
Cullen SI: Incidence of nevi. Arch Dermatol 1962, 86:40.
Eady RAJ, et al: Eruptive nevi. Br J Dermatol 1977, 197:267.
Ellis DL, et al: Increased nevus estrogen and progesterone ligand binding related to oral contraceptives or pregnancy. JAAD 1986, 14:25.
Eng AM: Solitary small active junctional nevi in juvenile patients. Arch Dermatol 1983, 119:35.
Fitzsimons CP, et al: A study of the total number and distribution of melanocytic nevi in a British population. Br J Dermatol 1984, 111(Suppl 26):9.
Foucar E, et al: A histopathologic evaluation of nevocellular nevi in pregnancy. Arch Dermatol 1985, 121:350.
Holly EA, et al: Number of melanocytic nevi as a major risk factor for malignant melanoma. JAAD 1987, 17:459.
Kopf AW, et al: Prevalence of nevocytic nevi on lateral and medial aspects of arms. J Dermatol Surg Oncol 1978, 4:153.
Idem: Eruptive nevocytic nevi after severe bullous disease. Arch Dermatol 1977, 113:1080.
Lea PJ, et al: Human melanocytic nevi. Acta Derm-Venereol, Suppl. 87, 1986.
Lewis MG, et al: The incidence and distribution of pigmented nevi in Ugandan Africans. Br J Dermatol 1968, 80:362.
Mackie RM, et al: The number and distribution of benign pigmented moles in a healthy British population. Br J Dermatol 1985, 113:167.
Modlin RL, et al: Identification of cells lining pseudovascular spaces of benign pigmented nevi. Am J Dermatopathol 1984, 6(Suppl 1):25.
Nicholls EM: Development and elimination of pigmented moles, and the anatomic distribution of primary malignant melanoma. Cancer 1973, 32:191.
Ogawa F, et al: Investigation of skin diseases. J Pediatr Dermatol 1982, 1:111.
Rampen FHJ, et al: Frequency of moles as a key to melanoma incidence? JAAD 1986, 15:1200.
Soltani K, et al: Eruptive nevocytic nevi following erythema multiforme. JAAD 1979, 1:503.
Stegmaier OC: Cosmetic management of nevi. JAMA 1967, 199:917.
Swerdlow AJ, et al: Benign melanocytic nevi as a risk factor for malignant melanoma. Br Med J 1986, 292:1555.

BALLOON CELL NEVUS

The balloon cell nevus is a pigmented nevus, varying in size from 1 to 5 mm, usually occurring on the head, neck, trunk, and occasionally elsewhere, such as the arm and the foot. Clinically the lesions are indistinguishable from the ordinary pigmented or nonpigmented nevus.

Histologically, the lesions are composed of peculiar vesicular cells that appear to be foamy and form large pale polyhedral balloon cells. In addition, nevus cells are also evident. The two types of cells form nests or theques throughout the epidermis and dermis; also, multinucleated giant balloon cells are found in almost all the lesions. Occasionally the lesions are composed entirely of balloon cells.

These nevi are not considered potentially malignant, and treatment is along the conventional lines of other nevi. Balloon cell melanoma does exist, but here the cells are pleomorphic, the nuclei are larger, the cytoplasm is scantier, and mitoses can be observed.

Goette DK, et al: Balloon cell nevus. Arch Dermatol 1978, 114:109.
Lewis BL: Junctional activity recurring over incompletely removed balloon cell nevi. Arch Dermatol 1971, 104:513.

HALO NEVUS

Halo nevus is also known as *Sutton's nevus, perinevoid vitiligo*, and *leukoderma acquisitum centrifugum*.

The halo nevus is characterized by a pigmented nevus, with a surrounding depigmented zone. The nevus is usually a compound or intradermal nevus with a concentric area of depigmentation having a regular, sharply demarcated border. It may be single or multiple and occurs most frequently on the trunk. The lesions develop mostly in teenagers. Chisa has reported them in siblings.

Immunologically induced rejection of melanin or of a melanoma beginning in the nevus has been suggested as the mode of pathogenesis. About one

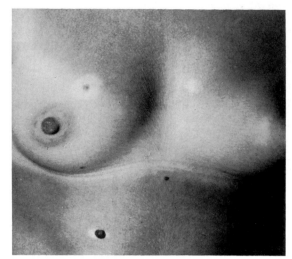

Figure 30–10. Multiple halo nevi.

fourth of cases are associated with vitiligo. Of course, melanoma in a state of regression may have associated leukoderma in the area. This suggests a common etiology, and indeed patients with halo nevi possess antibodies to melanocytes and cell-mediated immunity to melanoma cells.

Although the nevus cell nevus is the tumor most frequently found surrounded by a halo, Kopf and his associates and Smith and Moseley have indicated that many other lesions may also have a surrounding zone of leukoderma. These are the blue nevus, the neurofibroma, the neural nevus, the spindle and epithelioid cell nevus, and melanoma. Garcia, among others, reported a congenital halo nevus.

Histologically, amelanotic dopa-positive melano-

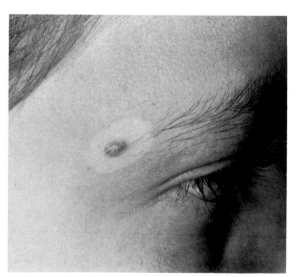

Figure 30–9. Halo nevus on the lateral forehead.

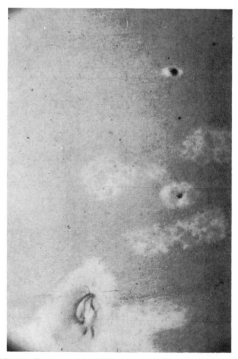

Figure 30–11. Perinevoid vitiligo and vitiligo on upper abdomen.

cytes may be found in the leukodermic halo. In the central lesion the nevus cells form a compound or intradermal nevus with an associated dermal infiltrate.

Treatment of the halo nevus is not indicated. The central nevus will usually disappear in time. The leukodermic area will remain depigmented for an unpredictable time, but eventually repigmentation may take place. Full mucocutaneous examination at the time of diagnosis, to exclude a concurrent melanoma, is indicated.

Berman B, et al: Halo giant congenital melanocytic nevis. JAAD 1988, 19:954.

Brownstein MH, et al: Halo congenital nevus. Arch Dermatol 1977, 113:1572.

Epstein WL, et al: Halo nevi and melanoma. JAMA 1973, 225:373.

Garcia RL, et al: Congenital halo nevus. Cutis 1979, 23:338.

Kikuchi I, et al: Disappearance of a nevocellular nevus with depigmentation. Arch Dermatol 1984, 120:678.

Kopf AW, et al: Broad spectrum of leukoderma acquisitum centrifugum. Arch Dermatol 1965, 92:14.

Larsson P-A, et al: Prevalence of skin disease among adolescents 12–16 years of age. Acta Derm Venereol (Stockh) 1980, 60:415.

Smith WE, et al: Multiple halo neurofibromas. Arch Dermatol 1976, 112:987.

CONGENITAL NEVOCYTIC NEVUS

Giant Pigmented Nevus

Synonyms: Giant hairy nevus and *bathing trunk nevus.*

This distinctive pigmented nevus is characterized by a large darkly pigmented hairy patch in which smaller darker patches are interspersed or present as small satellite lesions. The skin may be thickened and verrucous. A tendency to follow a dermatome distribution results in a typical picture in most instances. The trunk is a favored site, more especially the upper or lower parts of the back.

Giant hairy nevi are present at birth, and grow proportionally to the site of the body on which they are located. They may measure over 20 cm in diameter. The incidence of melanomas developing in giant congenital pigmented nevi is approximately 15 per cent. About 40 per cent of the malignant melanomas seen in children occur in large congenital nevi. Melanoma often occurs in these lesions during early childhood. When a large congenital nevus involves the head and neck, there may be an associated meningeal melanocytosis, sometimes complicated by hydrocephalus or malignant melanoma.

Histologically, giant nevi classically include nevus cells in the lower two thirds of the dermis, occasionally extending into the subcutis, between collagen bundles, and in association with eccrine or pilosebaceous structures in the mid-reticular dermis or below. Immunohistochemical staining or serial sections may at times be necessary to delineate some of these findings. Also estrogen and progesterone binding is present in giant, as well as smaller, congenital nevi. These receptors are present in other precursor

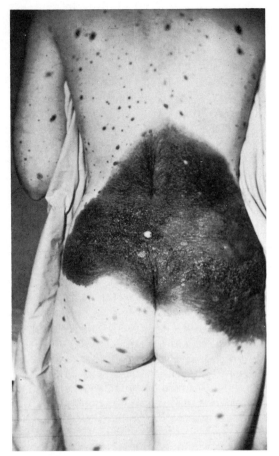

Figure 30–12. Giant pigmented nevus on a 16-year-old girl.

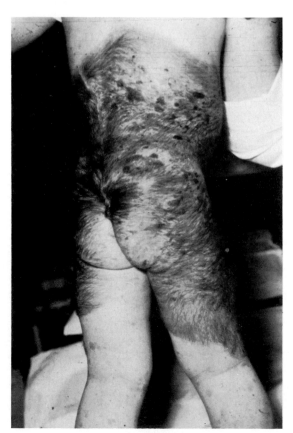

Figure 30–13. Giant hairy nevus.

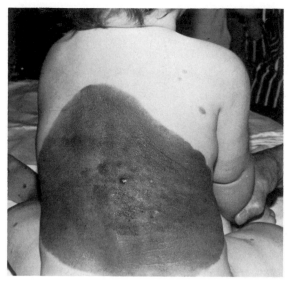

Figure 30–14. Giant pigmented nevus.

lesions of melanoma, such as dysplastic nevi, but are absent from common acquired nevi.

Treatment consists of total removal of the entire giant pigmented nevus and resurfacing with autografts. This should be done whenever possible, in order to prevent malignant degeneration.

Dermabrasion before five months of age was described in 1977 by Johnson; he suggested it only for the removal of pigmentation, for which it appears to be highly effective. Miller et al reported successful dermabrasion of a giant nevus at four weeks of age, and a partially successful one at seven and nine weeks in the same patient; removal with the Reese dermatome followed by dermabrasion removed the pigment permanently but left "a luxuriant growth of hair." Zitelli et al dermabraded four children before three months of age with gratifying cosmetic results, but considered that the leaving of nevus cells in the deep dermis was a serious objection to the procedure. We agree, and regard excision and grafting as the treatment of choice.

Small and Medium-sized Congenital Nevocytic Nevus

These congenital nevocytic nevi are usually more than 1 cm and often more than 1.5 cm in diameter, but less than 20 cm. They are found in about 1 per cent of newborns. About half eventually become hairy. Walton et al found pigmented lesions in 2.5 per cent of newborns, but only about a third were nevocytic nevi.

Histologically they are similar to acquired nevi, but they often have deeper involvement consisting of spindle cells that may extend into the subcutaneous tissue and also may surround the adnexa, vessels, and nerves. This may occur also in acquired nevi.

Since melanoma may be commoner even in these smaller congenital nevi, excision of them—as well as of giant nevi—has been proposed. Illig et al reviewed

52 cases in which melanoma had occurred in congenital nevi less than 10 cm in diameter. All occurred in patients over 18 and originated within the epidermis. Apparently following these lesions until they can be excised under local anesthesia at the end of the first decade is a reasonable course to follow. Since the risk of melanoma, though unknown, is certainly small, indefinitely following lesions which involve unexcisable structures is also reasonable. Kopf points to the public health and economic impact of trying to excise them all, and advises against it.

Alper J, et al: Birthmarks with serious medical significance. J Pediatr 1979, 95:696.

Idem: The incidence and significance of birthmarks in a cohort of 4,641 newborns. Pediatr Dermatol 1983, 1:58.

Alper J: Congenital nevi. Arch Dermatol 1985, 121:734.

Cage GW: Small congenital nevi. JAAD 1982, 7:685.

Clemmensen OJ, et al: The histology of "congenital features" in early acquired melanocytic nevi. JAAD 1988, 19:742.

Coskey RJ, et al: Congenital subungual nevus. JAAD 1983, 9:747.

Elder DE: The blind men and the elephant. Arch Dermatol 1985, 121:1263.

Ellis DL, et al: Estrogen and progesterone receptors in melanocytic lesions. Arch Dermatol 1985, 121:1282.

Idem: Estrogen and progesterone receptors in congenital nevocytic nevi. JAAD 1985, 12:235.

Illig L, et al: Congenital nevi < 10cm as precursors to melanoma. Arch Dermatol 1985, 121:1274.

Jacobs AH: Birthmarks. Pediatr Review 1979, 1:47.

Johnson HA: Permanent removal of pigmentation from giant hairy nevi by dermabrasion in early life. Br J Plast Surg 1977, 30:321.

Keipert JA, et al: Giant pigmented nevi. Aust J Dermatol 1985, 26:81.

Kopf AW, et al: Congenital nevocytic nevi and malignant melanoma. JAAD 1979, 1:123.

Idem: Prevalence of congenital nevus-like nevi, nevi spili, and cafe-au-lait spots. Arch Dermatol 1985, 121:766.

Kroon S, et al: Incidence of congenital melanocytic nevi in newborn babies in Denmark. JAAD 1987, 17:422.

National Institutes of Health Consensus Development Conference. JAAD 1984, 10:683.

Nickoloff BJ, et al: Immunohistologic patterns of congenital nevocellular nevi. Arch Dermatol 1986, 122:1263.

Osburn K, et al: Congenital pigmented and vascular lesions in newborn infants. JAAD 1987, 16:788.

Quaba AA, et al: The incidence of malignant melanoma (0 to 5 years of age) arising in "large" congenital nevocellular nevi. Plast Reconstr Surg 1986, 78:174.

Rhodes AR, et al: A histologic comparison of congenital and acquired nevomelanocytic nevi. Arch Dermatol 1985, 121:1266.

Idem: Prophylactic excision of nevocellular nevi. JAAD 1982, 7:409.

Idem: The malignant potential of small congenital nevocellular nevi. JAAD 1982, 6:230.

Idem: Small congenital nevocellular nevi and the risk of cutaneous melanoma. J Pediatr 1982, 100:219.

Stenn KS, et al: Patterns of congenital nevocellular nevi. JAAD 1983, 9:388.

Sweren RJ: Management of nevocytic nevi. JAAD 1984, 11:629.

Walton RG, et al: Pigmented lesions in newborn infants. Br J Dermatol 1976, 95:389.

Yu H-S, et al: Neurocutaneous melanosis. J Dermatol 1985, 12:267.

Zitelli JA, et al: Histologic patterns of congenital nevocytic nevi and implications for treatment. JAAD 1984, 11:402.

Pseudomelanoma

Kornberg and Ackerman reported six examples of a melanotic lesion resembling a superficial spreading melanoma occurring at the site of a recent removal (usually by shave excision) of a melanocytic nevus. None was actually malignant.

Kornberg R, et al: Pseudomelanoma. Arch Dermatol 1975, 111:1588.

Park HK, et al: Recurrent melanocytic nevi. JAAD 1987, 17:285.

EPITHELIOID AND SPINDLE CELL NEVUS
(Benign Juvenile Melanoma; Spitz Nevus)

CLINICAL FEATURES. Clinically, Spitz nevus is a smooth-surfaced, raised, round, slightly scaly, firm papule with a distinctive pink, brownish red, or purplish red color. Most frequently Spitz nevus occurs during the first two decades of life, although it occurs in adulthood in about a third of the cases. Typical is the firm, rosy papule on the face, especially on the cheek, some 3 to 10 mm in diameter. They are rarely diagnosed in blacks: Bovenmyer reported the second published case of such occurrence.

Infrequently, multiple lesions are present and they may occasionally occur as agminate lesions (clustered papules) in children and adults. When the latter occur, they are termed *multiple agminate spindle and epithelioid nevi.* Prose et al and Lancer et al have reported such cases, which frequently develop on a hyperpigmented base. S. A. Smith et al reported the fourth case of widespread eruptive Spitz nevi.

HISTOPATHOLOGY. Allen emphasizes that Spitz nevus is a variant of the compound nevus. The epidermal changes are mainly those of irregular acanthosis, striking pseudoepitheliomatous hyperplasia, and thinning of the epidermis.

In the upper dermis edema and ectasia of the various vascular elements may be present. The nevus

cells are pleomorphic. They are mostly spindle-shaped (fusiform) cells or, less frequently, polygonal (epithelioid) cells. Giant cells with eosinophilic cytoplasm and a large nucleus may be seen. Multinucleated giant cells are observed less frequently. Many of these giant cells are prominent since they are surrounded by intense edema. In adults, increased fibrosis in the deep dermis may be seen, although no features distinguish the childhood lesion from that of the adult type.

Arbuckle et al in 1982 confirmed the observation of Kamino et al (1979) that eosinophilic globules with fibrillar microstructure are commonly found in Spitz nevi: in 60 per cent (Kamino) to 86 per cent (Arbuckle). Arbuckle found them in melanomas (12 per cent) and compound nevi (8 per cent) as well, but they were fewer and smaller than in Spitz nevi.

DIFFERENTIAL DIAGNOSIS. Most frequently Spitz nevus is misdiagnosed clinically as a pyogenic granuloma, mastocytoma, juvenile xanthogranuloma, or melanoma.

TREATMENT. The Spitz nevus should be completely excised and a specimen examined histologically for completeness of excision. Conservative excision is the procedure recommended by many, including Kopf and Andrade, full excision being recommended to prevent confusion with melanoma if recurrence develops.

Allen AC: Juvenile melanomas. Ann NY Acad Sci 1963, 100:29.

Arbuckle S, et al: Eosinophilic globules in the Spitz nevus. JAAD 1982, 7:324.

Bovenmyer DA: Spitz's nevus in a black child. Cutis 1981, 28:186.

Coskey RJ, et al: Spindle cell nevi in adults and children. Arch Dermatol 1973, 108:535.

Kamino H, et al: Eosinophilic globules in Spitz's nevi. Am J Dermatopathol 1979, 1:319.

Lancer HA, et al: Multiple agminated spindle cell nevi. JAAD 1983, 8:707.

Merot Y: Transepidermal elimination of nevus cells in spindle and epithelioid cell (Spitz) nevus. Arch Dermatol 1988, 124:1441.

Paniago-Perreira C, et al: Nevus of large and spindle or epithelioid cells. Arch Dermatol 1978, 114:1811.

Prose NS, et al: Multiple benign juvenile melanoma. JAAD 1983, 9:236.

Smith SA, et al: Eruptive widespread Spitz nevi. JAMA 1986, 15:1155.

Weedon D, et al: Spindle and epithelioid cell nevi in children and adults. Cancer 1977, 40:217.

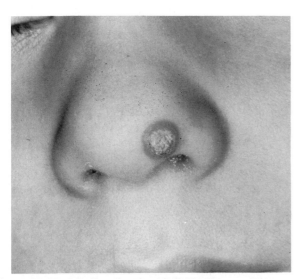

Figure 30–15. Spindle cell and epithelioid cell nevus (Spitz nevus) on the nose of child.

THE FAMILIAL DYSPLASTIC NEVUS SYNDROME (B-K Mole Syndrome)

In 1978 Clark et al described families with unusual nevi and multiple melanomas, a condition they referred to as the B-K mole syndrome (after Family B and Family K). About the same time Lynch et al recognized similar findings in families they were studying and they designated this the familial atypical multiple mole–melanoma syndrome. Since that time our understanding of this autosomal dominant syndrome has grown rapidly. Over the years the most widely accepted term for the precursor lesion is *dysplastic nevus,* with the patients' condition termed the *dysplastic nevus syndrome* (DNS).

Dysplastic nevi differ from common acquired nevi in several respects. The typical dysplastic nevus is clinically characterized by a variegated tan, brown, and pink coloration, with the pink hues seen mainly in the macular portion of the nevus. There is marked lesion-to-lesion variability. The nevi are larger than common nevi, being usually 5 mm to 12 mm in size (common nevi usually measure 6 mm or less in diameter). The shape of dysplastic nevi is very irregular with frequent angulated, indistinct borders. A macular component is always present. The unusual nevi are most commonly seen on the back; however, in diametric contrast to typical nevi, they have a disproportionate predilection for nonsun-exposed areas such as the buttocks, scalp, and breast. Kopf et al have studied the role of sun exposure in the development of these lesions and have shown sun promotes the development of these lesions in individuals afflicted with DNS. The number of lesions per individual varies; however, patients having 75 to over 100 lesions are not unusual. Finally, while the dysplastic nevi may not be evident until puberty in afflicted children, these nevi continue to develop over their lifetime, whereas the common nevocytic nevus usually develops in childhood or early adult years only.

Several categories of DNS occur. Patients with dysplastic nevi who have at least two blood relatives with dysplastic nevi and melanoma have the worst prognosis for development of melanoma, some estimates being a 100 per cent lifetime risk. Crutcher et al have found 5 per cent of unselected patients in a community practice had dysplastic nevi. In some a family history of these lesions or melanoma could not be ascertained. The concept of dysplastic nevi as precursors to melanoma has expanded over time to include a sporadic variety of DNS with a relatively low risk of melanoma development.

Most authorities feel there is a definite histologic correlate to the clinical lesions; however, criteria for its diagnosis vary among dermatopathologists. The NIH consensus conference published the following as typical histologic features: basilar melanocytic hyperplasia with elongation of the rete ridges; spindle-shaped or occasionally epithelioid melanocytes arranged horizontally and aggregating in nests which fuse with adjacent rete ridges; lamellar and concentric superficial dermal infiltrate; and cytologic atypia, usually present but not essential for diagnosis.

When a patient with clinically dysplastic nevi is seen, initial examination should include a total body inspection, including the scalp (especially important in children suspected of having this syndrome, as Tucker et al have shown), and eyes. A family history should be obtained with special attention paid to items such as moles, skin cancer, and melanoma. Evaluation of all first-degree relatives is recommended. Several of the more atypical nevi should be biopsied by deep shave or excision.

If the diagnosis of dysplastic nevus syndrome is made, all lesions which are difficult to follow clinically (especially those of the scalp) should be excised, as well as those with very atypical morphology. There should be prudent sun avoidance and sunscreen use. If familial DNS exists, with a family history of melanoma, the patients should be educated in self-examination techniques and encouraged to examine themselves monthly. Physician examination every three to six months is recommended, with excision of those nevi which change in clinical appearance. Atypical nevi in the hairy scalp are too hard to follow and should be excised early. The use of photographs with measured scale is helpful in following lesions elsewhere. Excision of large numbers of nevi is considered if the patient takes immunosuppressive drugs, if adequate medical care is not available, or if the patient is unable to accept observation in fear of cancer.

Arndt KA: Precursors to malignant melanoma. JAMA 1984, 251:1882.

Barnes LM, et al: The natural history of dysplastic nevi. Arch Dermatol 1987, 123:1059.

Clark WH Jr, et al: Origin of familial malignant melanoma from heritable melanocytic lesions. Arch Dermatol 1978, 114:732.

Clark WH Jr: The dysplastic nevus syndrome. Arch Dermatol 1988, 124:1207.

Crutcher WA, et al: Prevalence of dysplastic naevi in a community practice. Lancet 1984, 1:729.

Elder DE: A phenotypic association of sporadic cutaneous melanoma. Cancer 1980, 46:787.

Fine RM: The dysplastic nevus syndrome—endocrine disease. Int J Dermatol 1985, 25:235.

Greene MH, et al: High risk malignant melanoma in melanoma-prone families with dysplastic nevi. Ann Intern Med 1985, 102:458.

Idem: Acquired precursors of cutaneous malignant melanoma. N Engl J Med 1985, 312:91.

Idem: Managing the dysplastic naevus syndrome. Lancet 1984, 1:166.

Idem: Familial cutaneous malignant melanoma. Proc Natl Acad Sci USA 1983, 80:6071.

Idem: Dysplastic nevus syndrome. Hosp Practi 1984, 19:91.

Haystrom WJ Jr, et al: Dysplastic nevus syndrome. Plast Reconstr Surg 1983, 71:219.

Holly EA, et al: Number of melanocytic nevi as a major risk factor for malignant melanoma. JAAD 1987, 17:459.

Jones RE Jr: Letter to the editor. Am J Dermatopathol 1985, 7(Suppl):213.

Kelly JW, et al: Clinical diagnosis of dysplastic melanocytic nevi. JAAD 1986, 14:1044.

Kopf AW, et al: Relationship of lumbosacral nevocytic nevi to sun exposure in dysplastic nevus syndrome. Arch Dermatol 1986, 122:1003.

Idem: Relationship of nevocytic nevi to sun exposure in dysplastic nevus syndrome. JAAD 1985, 12:650.

Kraemer K: Dysplastic nevi as precursors to hereditary melanoma. J Dermatol Surg Oncol 1983, 9:619.

Kraemer KH, et al: Dysplastic nevi and cutaneous melanoma risk. Lancet 1984, 1:1076.

Lynch HT, et al: Familial atypical multiple mole-melanoma syndrome. J Med Genet 1978, 15:352.

Maize JC: Dysplastic melanocytic nevi in histologic association with primary cutaneous melanomas. JAAD 1984, 10:831.

National Institutes of Health Consensus Development Conference. JAAD 1984, 10:683.

Pehamberger H, et al: Dysplastic nevus syndrome with multiple primary amelanotic melanoma in oculocutaneous albinism. JAAD, 1984, 11:731.

Rahbari H, et al: Sporadic atypical mole syndrome. Arch Dermatol 1981, 117:329.

Rhodes AR, et al: Dysplastic melanocytic nevi in histologic association with 234 primary cutaneous melanomas. JAAD 1983, 9:563.

Rodriguez-Sains RS: Ocular findings in patients with dysplastic nevus syndrome. Ophthalmology 1986, 93:661.

Roush GC, et al: Diagnosis of the dysplastic nevus syndrome in different populations. JAAD 1986, 14:419.

Sagebiel RW, et al: Age distribution and histologic patterns of dysplastic nevi. JAAD 1985, 13:975.

Sterry W, et al: Quadrant distribution of dysplastic nevus syndrome. Arch Dermatol 1988, 124:926.

Tucker MA, et al: Dysplastic nevi on the scalp of prepubertal children from melanoma-prone families. J Pediatr 1983, 103:65.

MELANOMA
("Malignant Melanoma")

There are four recognized clinicohistologic types of melanoma:

1. Lentigo maligna (melanoma in situ, noninvasive melanoma).
2. Superficially spreading melanoma (superficial spreading melanoma).
3. Nodular melanoma.
4. Acral-lentiginous melanoma.

In addition, pedunculated and polypoidal melanomas have been distinguished, and hyperkeratotic and verrucous melanomas may occur.

The subject of melanoma is now enormous and complex enough for a separate textbook, and it will be dealt with only in summary here.

Lentigo Maligna (Melanoma in Situ)

Lentigo maligna was originally described by Hutchinson as *melanotic freckle* or *malignant freckle*. Since then a number of synonyms, all now of historic

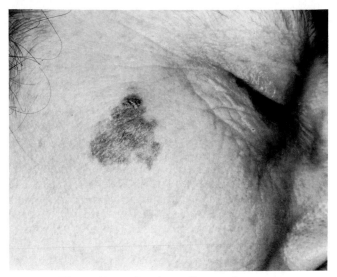

Figure 30–17. *Lentigo maligna melanoma.*

interest only, have been attached to this interesting lesion. These are *precancerous melanosis of Dubreuilh, melanosis circumscripta precancerosa of Dubreuilh,* and *circumscribed precancerous melanosis.*

CLINICAL FEATURES. Lentigo maligna begins as a tan macule that extends peripherally, with gradual uneven darkening, over the course of several years. The spread and darkening are usually so slow that little attention is paid to this insidious lesion. Its edge becomes irregular with time, and its color variegated, due to areas of regression. After a radial growth period of 5 to 20 years, vertically growing melanoma usually develops within it. This is often called *lentigo maligna melanoma,* but it is in reality *nodular melanoma,* and must be treated as such. A palpable nodule within the original macular lesion is

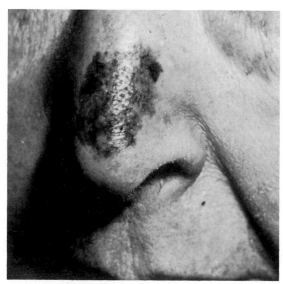

Figure 30–16. *Lentigo maligna.*

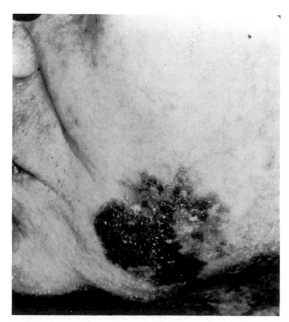

Figure 30–18. *Lentigo maligna melanoma of several years' duration.*

the best evidence that this has occurred, though there may be darkening or bleeding as well.

This occurs equally in men and women, usually in their sixties or seventies, in chronically sun-damaged skin, most often on the face. It accounts for about 5 per cent of all melanomas.

HISTOPATHOLOGY. The findings depend considerably on the age of the lesion. At first atypical melanocytes are found at the dermoepidermal junction. As the melanocytes proliferate, the dermoepidermal border becomes irregular, while the melanocytic cells may form nests at the junction to give it a moth-eaten appearance. There is often extension of these atypical cells down the follicular orifices. As the atypical cells extend into the dermis ("vertical growth"), an invasive melanoma develops and metastasis is a possibility, though unlikely until a palpable nodule is formed, as Hirsch and Helwig have long emphasized.

DIFFERENTIAL DIAGNOSIS. Lentigo maligna may resemble the pigmented seborrheic keratosis, but the latter is usually verrucous and greasy, and seems to rest on the top of the skin. Pigmented basal cell carcinoma is indurated, usually has a rolled edge, and occurs chiefly in deeply pigmented persons. Melanotic freckle is differentiated from the pigmented nevus by its late onset, its steady growth, its slow changes of color, and its mottling.

TREATMENT. Every suspected melanoma should be photographed first and then surgically excised. Removal of the lesion should be thorough so that there will be no doubt regarding the removal of the deeper portions. Extension down the outside of hair follicles is almost invariable. Our recommendation is surgical excision with clear margins. Mohs technique is useful, but not obligatory.

Many other forms of therapy are reported in the literature, and will be briefly discussed here for completeness.

Argon laser treatment has been discussed by Arndt. Close posttreatment clinical and histologic assessment is essential.

Harwood discussed 40 patients treated with radiotherapy. Also Dancuart et al reviewed 23 patients. Results were good. However, Kopf et al abandoned the technique in view of three cases of metastatic melanoma among 16 cases treated. Zacarian reviewed 20 patients treated with cryosurgery. There was a 10 per cent recurrence rate.

Topical 5-fluorouracil has been used successfully in three patients with lentigo maligna by Litwin and associates. It is to be considered experimental.

Although Breathnach states that he has cured some 70 cases in less than 10 years by the inunction of 25 per cent azelaic acid cream, the method is still experimental. Azelaic acid is a 9-carbon dicarboxylic acid which inhibits tyrosinase and is cytotoxic for melanocytes which are actively dividing, but has little if any effect on normal melanocytes. It has no demonstrable toxicity. Approval by the FDA seems unlikely.

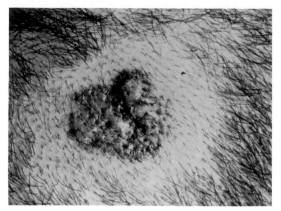

Figure 30–19. Superficially spreading melanoma of the scalp.

Superficially Spreading Melanoma (SSM)

This is commonly called *superficial* spreading melanoma, but Pinkus and Rahbari objected that it merely *spreads superficially*. It is the commonest type of melanoma, constituting 70 per cent of them. It affects adults of all ages, with the median age in the fifth decade. It has no preference—unlike lentigo maligna—for sun-damaged skin. Ackerman says that its location and its more rapid rate of growth are its only distinguishing features. The upper back of both sexes and the shins in women are the commonest sites. It may occur anywhere, however. It tends to be multicolored, not just with different shades of tan, but variegated black, red, brown, blue, and white, as Mihm and Fitzpatrick have emphasized. The border is often notched by focal regression or asymmetric growth.

Trau et al studied 119 melanomas of this type in which regression had occurred and compared them with 297 in which it had not. The former had a slightly better prognosis. The surface is rough and uneven in most older lesions. However, Cooper et al found no correlation between regression and survival, and this is the consensus of studies to date.

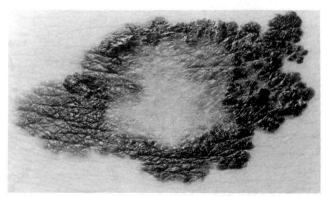

Figure 30–20. Superficially spreading melanoma. (Courtesy of Dr. Axel W. Hoke.)

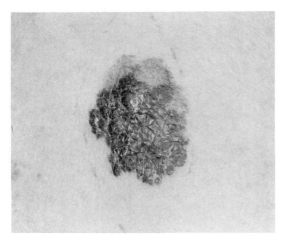

Figure 30–21. Superficially spreading melanoma in a pre-existing nevus of 30 years' duration.

As the vertical growth phase develops, skin markings disappear. If regression occurs, these may reappear. These lesions grow as much in a year as lentigo maligna does in three to five years. Easy bleeding is a sign of malignancy, as is erosion or ulceration. Horizontal or lateral growth into the adjoining epidermis continues for one to five years, before invasion into the dermis takes place.

Acral-Lentiginous Melanoma

This variety, which occurs not merely on acral structures but on *volar*—palmar and plantar—ones, notably the distal phalanges of toes or fingers, lies midway between the lentigo maligna and the superficially spreading melanoma in respect to speed of horizontal growth into adjacent epidermis. Mucosal and subungual lesions are classified with this category. They account for 10 per cent of lesions overall; however, they are the most common type in Japanese, blacks, Hispanics, and American Indians. The median age is 50 years, with equal sex distribution. Reintgen et al found the most common site of melanoma in blacks is the foot with 60 per cent having

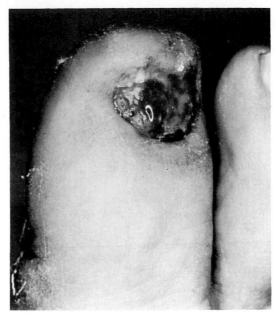

Figure 30–23. Subungual acral-lentiginous melanoma.

subungual or plantar lesions. Several large reviews of this type of melanoma have been published recently, including those by Krementz et al, Gutman et al, Takematsu et al, and Paladusa et al.

It is the same lesion as Hutchinson's "melanotic whitlow" (1886), and was named acrolentiginous melanoma by Reed in 1976. Its interesting history is

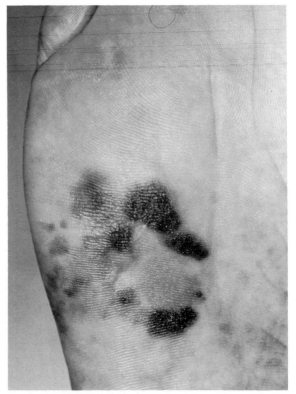

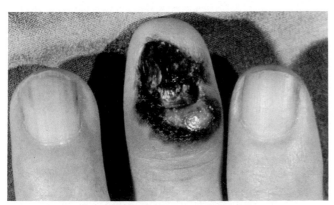

Figure 30–22. Acral-lentiginous melanoma (melanotic whitlow). (Courtesy of Dr. Axel W. Hoke.)

Figure 30–24. Acral-lentiginous melanoma (Courtesy of Dr. Axel W. Hoke.)

reviewed in detail in Kopf's excellent monograph on malignant melanoma. Perhaps its most important feature is that it is so easily overlooked histologically that the first biopsy may give a false impression of a benign lesion. Nevertheless it must be excised in toto or it will, like others, become a nodular melanoma. An irregular, enlarging black macule on palm, sole, digit tip, or nail fold or bed is virtually diagnostic. Hutchinson's sign, a black discoloration of the proximal nail fold at the end of a pigmented streak (melanonychia striata) is ominous, signaling the site of melanoma in the matrix of the nail.

The early changes may be simply a light brown, dark brown, or black discoloration. The thumb and the hallux are more frequently involved than the other digits. In time the lesion becomes nodular and later ulcerates. Metastases to the epitrochlear and axillary nodes develop in the late stage of the disease and are common, as there is often a delay in diagnosis.

Subungual melanoma may be misdiagnosed as onychomycosis, verruca vulgaris, chronic paronychia, subungual hyperkeratosis, pyogenic granuloma, Kaposi's sarcoma, glomus tumor, and subungual hematoma.

Nodular Melanoma

CLINICAL FEATURES. Although a wide variety of clinical lesions of nodular melanoma exist, the typical lesion may be described as a pigmented papule or nodule of varying size, present for a few months. These lesions arise without a clinically apparent radial growth phase, but usually large atypical melanocytes can be found in the epidermis for several rete ridges beyond the region of vertical growth, at all margins of the excised lesion.

Nodular melanoma constitutes about 15 per cent of all melanomas. It is twice as common in men as in women, and occurs primarily on sun-exposed areas of the head, neck, and trunk.

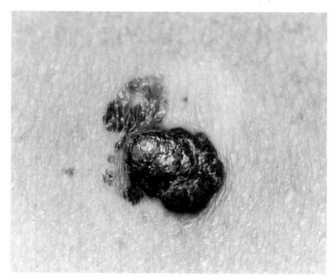

Figure 30–26. Nodular melanoma. (Courtesy of Dr. Axel W. Hoke.)

Although the tumors are at first 1 to 4 mm wide, they may grow much larger and become papillary, fungoid, or ulcerated. Bleeding is usually a late sign. The color is usually not uniform throughout the tumor but is likely to be scattered irregularly, being grayish brown, bluish black, or black. Sepia or coal black spots may appear as if sprayed about the lesion.

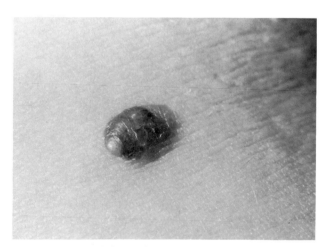

Figure 30–25. Nodular melanoma. (Courtesy of Dr. Axel W. Hoke.)

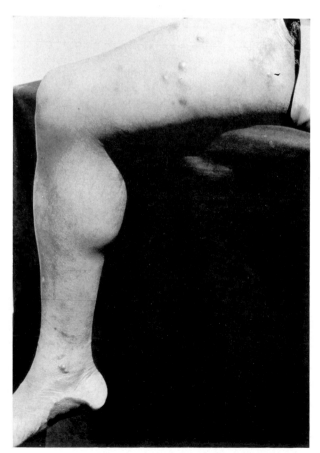

Figure 30–27. Cutaneous metastasis from melanoma of sole. (Courtesy of Dr. Axel W. Hoke.)

Polypoid Melanoma. This variant of nodular melanoma is a pedunculated tumor, which at its base does not appear to descend for any appreciable distance into the dermis. Nevertheless it behaves as a level IV or V tumor; it has only a 42 per cent five-year survival rate, according to Manci et al, as compared to 57 per cent for nodular melanoma.

Verrucous Melanoma. Steiner et al have reviewed this hyperkeratotic, relatively uniformly pigmented, sharply demarcated variant.

Desmoplastic Melanoma. This deeply infiltrating sometimes amelanotic type of melanoma usually has a spindle cell pattern histologically, often necessitating S100 stains for diagnosis. The *neurotropic melanoma* may be a variant of it. Both occur most often on the head or neck, often within a lentigo maligna.

Inflammatory Melanoma. The clinical phenomenon of inflammation in or near the site of a melanoma signifies a poor prognosis. Haupt et al reported two such cases, which metastasized widely in a short time.

Amelanotic Melanoma. The nonpigmented melanoma differs from the other melanomas only in its lack of pigment. The lesion is pink, erythematous, or flesh-colored, but otherwise the appearance of growth and ulceration is the same as that in the pigmented variety. The lesion is easily mistaken for granuloma pyogenicum, even by the experienced. Amelanotic melanoma is the typical variant seen in albinos.

Mucosal Melanoma. Primary melanoma of mucous membranes is rare. It may occur in the nasal mucosa, chiefly as a polypoid tumor, with or without pigment. On the lip it is apt to be an indolent ulcer. In the mouth the lesion is usually pigmented and ulcerated. Rapini et al reviewed 177 cases in 1985 and found that the commonest site was the palate. The

upper jaw was involved more often than the lower. Most patients are elderly and the prognosis is poor. Kato et al reported 13 cases, with a striking preponderance in women. Melanoma of the vulva is manifested by a tumor, often ulcerated, with bleeding and pruritus; however, it is most often detected after metastasis to the groin has occurred. Landthaler et al reviewed 13 cases in 1985.

MELANOMA AND PREGNANCY. During pregnancy pigmented nevi often become darker, and may enlarge. Estrogen and progesterone receptors develop on the melanocytes. Shiu et al and Reintgen et al examined the effect of pregnancy on outcome, and both concluded that there was no adverse effect. However, women who developed melanoma during pregnancy had a shorter disease-free interval following excision.

METASTASIS. In the beginning this is usually manifested by pigmented nodules appearing around the site of the excision. Early remote metastases occur via the lymphatics, and regional lymphadenopathy may be the first sign. The lymph nodes are hard and discrete. Later, metastases occur via the blood stream, and may become widespread. The chief site for metastatic melanoma is the skin, but all other organs are at risk. Central nervous system metastasis is the most common cause of death. In Radaman's series of 18 patients who suffered metastases after 10 years, 16 were premenopausal women. Melanemia, melanuria, and cachexia are likely to occur in terminal disease. In extreme cases the entire integument may become deeply pigmented (*generalized melanosis*). This may be due either to individual melanoma cells, or to melanophages alone. A practical method of assaying the extent of metastases is radiography with tomographic gallium-67 citrate scanning, as Kirkwood et al and Rossleigh et al have shown. Patients seen with metastatic melanoma from an unknown source are estimated to have a 40 per cent chance of five-year survival.

ETIOLOGY. Gellin and his associates are among those who have shown that light complexions, light eyes, and blond or red hair indicate increased risk for melanoma, given comparable sunlight exposure. Their findings have been confirmed by Green, who found that the incidence of melanoma closely paralleled the accumulation of solar exposure throughout life. Schreiber found a close correlation with all forms of sun damage, which disappeared when all diagnoses of lentigo maligna were excluded. Elwood and associates, however, found that even when 70 subjects with lentigo maligna and acral lentiginous melanoma were excluded, light complexion, heavy freckling, and tendency to tan poorly and sunburn easily were significant risk factors for melanoma.

Lew et al found that the occurrence of a blistering sunburn in childhood was correlated with the occurrence of melanoma in adult life. Rampen found blondness and ease of sunburning correlated with number of moles, and that the distribution pattern of these corresponded with the sex and site distribution of melanomas.

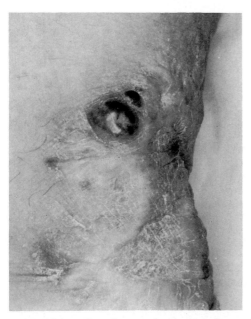

Figure 30–28. Metastatic melanoma developing after excision of a melanoma on the heel of a woman.

Twenty to 50 per cent of melanomas develop in a preexisting nevus, and as Friedman et al showed, this subset of patients has a relatively favorable prognosis. Kopf et al concluded that there is considerable circumstantial evidence that sunlight plays a role in the etiology of melanoma, though a less essential and direct one than in the case of nonmelanoma skin cancer.

Other factors include the presence of precursor lesions such as congenital and dysplastic nevi, as has been discussed; the occasional development of melanoma in large burn scars; and xeroderma pigmentosum, as reviewed by Kraemer et al and by Lynch et al. PUVA treatment remains to be evaluated as a risk factor, though reports of eight atypical lentigines and a melanoma give cause for caution.

An association between administration of levodopa therapy for Parkinson's disease and the onset of melanoma has been implied in some 19 case reports gathered by Rampen, and in a poorly founded warning in the *Physicians' Desk Reference*. Kochar reported another case in 1985. Sober suggests that although the association is unproved, the warning should be respected, for medicolegal reasons.

INCIDENCE AND PREVALENCE. Malignant melanoma is not commonly encountered in the darker races. The lowest incidence is found among the Asians. It occurs most often in light-skinned people. The incidence of melanoma is low until after puberty. Melanomas have increased 1000 per cent in the last 50 years. Currently one in 150 Americans will develop a melanoma.

HISTOPATHOLOGY. Pinkus and Mehregan set forth the following criteria for the diagnosis of malignancy in melanotic tumors: presence of mitoses, inflammatory reaction composed of lymphocytes and perhaps plasma cells, dermoepidermal junctional activity (which is the site of origin for all melanomas except those occurring in the giant pigmented nevus), and the absence of dermal stroma, which is destroyed in malignant melanoma.

Atypical melanocytes are scattered throughout the epidermis, singly and in irregular nests. There is asymmetry, poor circumscription, and failure of melanocytic maturation.

Lever lists the differential points between the junction nevus and malignant melanoma. Melanoma is diagnosed when the melanocytes are widely scattered in the dermis rather than clustered; when melanocytes are pleomorphic, and are present in the upper epidermis; and when melanin granules are present in the papillary dermis. An inflammatory infiltrate, in the absence of trauma or infection, is also highly suggestive of melanoma.

The Clark classification by levels of invasion has been replaced by Breslow's measure of invasion in millimeters of thickness. Thickness correlates with prognosis, in stage I tumors (localized disease without regional node involvement) as follows:

Group I, under 0.85 mm, 99 per cent five-year survival

Group II, 0.85 to 1.69 mm, 94 per cent five-year survival

Group III, 1.70 to 3.64 mm, 78 per cent five-year survival

Group IV, over 3.64 mm, 42 per cent five-year survival.

DIFFERENTIAL DIAGNOSIS. Melanoma may clinically simulate a wide variety of lesions. In our experience melanoma may most frequently resemble the pigmented basal cell carcinoma, darkly pigmented seborrheic keratosis, pyogenic granuloma, and Kaposi's sarcoma.

Other melanoma-simulating lesions are subungual traumatic hematoma, senile angioma, junction and compound nevus.

Biopsy. When the size of the lesion lends itself to simple surgical excision, this is the best method of doing the mandatory biopsy to establish the diagnosis. Should the biopsy show melanoma, then definitive surgery may be performed.

In lesions too large for simple excision, an incisional or punch biopsy, deep enough to permit measurement of thickness, seems to have no effect upon prognosis, and is considered good practice. When melanoma is suspected in the melanotic freckle or in a giant pigmented nevus, biopsy should be done through the thickest and most atypical area, never merely through the border, and multiply sectioned to find the deepest area of involvement.

SPONTANEOUS REGRESSION. Spontaneous regression has been documented in cases of melanoma even with metastases. Nathanson in 1976 reported 33 cases of total regression of a primary melanoma, and 27 cases in which metastatic melanoma spontaneously regressed. Lynch et al reported two instances of this in patients with xeroderma pigmentosum.

TREATMENT. Early diagnosis and excision remain the hope for cure of melanoma. Much debate surrounds the recommendation as to appropriate margins of excision. It appears that the classic 5-cm excision margins are not necessary. With the trend toward smaller margins, survival has remained the same. Presently our recommendations for margins are 0.5 to 1.0 cm margins for melanoma in situ, 1.5 cm margins for lesions of 0.85 mm depth or less, and 3.0 cm margins for all other lesions. A prospective study is currently underway to compare "simple" excision versus "wide" excision.

Regional elective lymph node dissection (ELND) at the time of initial surgery is also controversial. If palpable lymph nodes are present at the time of diagnosis, ELND may be recommended for palliative purposes. Tumors less than 0.8 mm thick so rarely metastasize that ELND is never indicated. For tumors over 4.0 mm thick, survival is uniformly poor and, while ELND may be useful for staging purposes, it is not indicated for therapeutic reasons.

Day et al reviewed the literature in 1985 and recommended the following for other patients, if they could not be entered into a randomized study.

If the tumor ranges from 1.6 to 4.0 mm in depth, ELND is recommended if the patient is in excellent health and there is a clearly defined regional lymph node drainage basin. Likewise for axial lesions of 0.8 mm to 1.5 mm in depth; however, for extremity lesions of this thickness ELND is not recommended owing to good survival rate in these lesions. He also identified a group of melanomas with epithelioid cells in small nests, in which ELND appears to be a lifesaving procedure when the depth of the lesion ranges from 1.70 to 3.64 mm. Other recommendations exist; again, this area is controversial.

Chemotherapy is not very effective in the treatment of melanoma, the most effective agent identified being DTIC (dacarbazine). Combination chemotherapy is undergoing continued trials; however, the response remains poor. Kessinger et al reviewed 105 cases treated with high-dose chemotherapy and autologous bone marrow transplantation and found 48 per cent responded, 34 per cent completely. The patients undergoing this toxic, risky therapy all had widely disseminated melanoma.

Immunotherapy is still under investigation, with local injections of BCG vaccine into cutaneous melanoma being investigated. Rosenberg et al have studied the effects of adoptive immunotherapy with lymphokine-activated killer cells plus interleukin-2, or high-dose interleukin-2 alone. Thirty per cent of 42 patients showed some response to this toxic experimental treatment.

Perfusion chemotherapy has been used for extremity melanoma. This technique establishes a temporary oxygenated and hyperthermic circuit through the vessels supplying the tumor, and limits the distribution of the chemotherapeutic agent via the use of a tourniquet. It is effective for regionally confined advanced disease and has virtually eliminated the need for amputation. Rege et al recently reviewed this technique.

Radiation therapy is not very successful; its use lies largely in symptomatic treatment of metastatic disease to bone or the central nervous system, as discussed by Chan et al.

WORK-UP AND FOLLOW-UP. The initial work-up of a patient with melanoma concentrates on establishing a family history, and examining for evidence of metastatic disease. A thorough physical examination, and a chest x-ray, are indicated in melanoma of less than 0.76 mm. More aggressive work-up is initiated by the oncology referral physician in cases of deeper lesions.

Many schedules are recommended for following patients with melanoma. The principles are increased numbers of visits early in the disease course when spread is most likely, and follow-up for life, since late recurrences and metastases occur in some patients. Chest x-rays are useful in detecting early metastases to the lung. It is worthwhile to detect these since surgical removal of solitary pulmonary metastases may result in cure, as discussed by Heaston et al.

PROGNOSIS. Stage III disease (distant metastasis) uniformly has a grave prognosis. Stage II disease (palpable regional lymph nodes or tumor cells demonstrated in regional lymph nodes) has a 30 per cent five-year survival rate.

In stage I patients several prognostic factors are of interest. Tumor *thickness* is the prime parameter, and the prognostic figures were discussed earlier. The *site* of the melanoma carries significance in that micrometastases in tumors of the head and neck carry a uniformly poor prognosis. The once touted *BANS* (upper *B*ack, posterolateral upper *A*rms, posterior and lateral *N*eck, and posterior *S*calp) area does not appear to affect prognosis, as Cascinelli et al have shown. *Women* with stage I disease have over all better survival. Finally, the development of *leukoderma* is a good prognostic sign. Bystryn et al found that hypopigmentation alone improved five-year survival from 75 per cent to 86 per cent. They concluded that the mechanisms that inhibit or destroy normal melanocytes may also slow the growth of melanoma.

Ackerman AB: Disagreements about the classification of malignant melanomas. Am J Dermatopathol 1982, 4:447.

Idem, et al: Histology of cutaneous melanoma. In Malignant Melanoma. Kopf AW, et al (ed). New York, Masson 1978, p. 25.

Aitken DR, et al: The extent of primary melanoma excisions: how wide is wide? Ann Surg 1983, 198:634.

Albert DM: Vitiligo or halo nevi occurring in two patients with choroidal melanoma. Arch Dermatol 1982, 118:34.

Arndt KA: Argon laser treatment of lentigo maligna. JAAD 1984, 10:953.

Balch CM, et al: Surgical management of regional lymph nodes in cutaneous melanoma. JAAD 1980, 3:511.

Beral V, et al: Cutaneous factors related to the risk of malignant melanoma. Br J Dermatol 1983, 109:165.

Black WC, et al: Melanoma within a Southwestern Hispanic population. Arch Dermatol 1987, 123:1331.

Blake PR, et al: Treatment of malignant melanoma by fast neutrons. Br J Surg 1985, 72:517.

Bondi EE, et al: Skin markings in malignant melanoma. JAMA 1983, 250:503.

Briele HA, et al: Late recurrence of cutaneous melanomas. Arch Dermatol 1983, 118:800.

Briggs JC, et al: Late recurrence of cutaneous melanoma. JAAD 1988, 18:147.

Bukowski RM, et al: Randomized controlled trial of transfer factor in Stage I malignant melanoma. Cancer 1983, 51:269.

Bystryn J-C, et al: Prognostic significance of hypopigmentation in malignant melanoma. Arch Dermatol 1987, 123:1053.

Chanda JJ, et al: Adverse effect of melanoma incision. JAAD 1985, 13:519.

Chang P, et al: Metastatic melanoma of unknown primary. Cancer 1982, 49:1106.

Cooper PH, et al: Regression in thin malignant melanoma. Arch Dermatol 1985, 121:1127.

Cosimi AB, et al: Conservative surgical management of superficially invasive cutaneous melanoma. Cancer 1984, 53:1256.

Dancuart F, et al: Radiotherapy for lentigo and lentigo maligna melanoma of the head and neck. Cancer 1980, 45:2279.

Day CL, et al: Predictors of late death among patients with clinical stage I melanoma who have not had bony or visceral metastases within the first 5 years after diagnosis. JAAD 1983, 8:864.

Idem: Narrower margins for clinical stage I malignant melanoma (editorial). N Engl J Med 1982, 306:479.

Idem: Skin lesions suspected to be melanoma should be photographed: gross morphologic features of primary melanoma associated with metastases. JAMA 1982, 248:1077.

Idem: Prognostic factors for melanoma patients with lesions 0.76–1.69mm thick: an appraisal of "thin" level IV lesions. Ann Surg 1982, 195:30.

Idem: Prognostic factors for patients with clinical stage I melanoma of intermediate thickness (1.51–3.99mm). Ann Surg 1982, 195:37.

Idem: A multivariate analysis of prognostic factors for melanoma patients with lesions over 3.65mm thick. Ann Surg 1982, 195:40.

Idem: Malignant melanoma prognostic factors, 3: surgical margins. Dermatol Surg Oncol 1983, 9:797.

Idem: Malignant melanoma prognostic factors, 5: clinical staging. J Dermatol Surg Oncol 1984, 10:351.

Idem: Malignant melanoma prognostic factors, 6: distant metastases and length of survival. J Dermatol Surg Oncol 1984, 10:686.

Idem: Malignant melanoma prognostic factors, 7: elective lymph node dissection. J Dermatol Surg Oncol 1985, 11:233.

Elder DE, et al: Optimal resection margin for cutaneous malignant melanoma. Plast Reconstr Surg 1983, 71:66.

Idem: Melanoma classifications: testable hypotheses. Am J Dermatopathol 1982, 4:443.

Elwood JM, et al: Pigmentation and skin reaction to sun as risk factors for cutaneous melanoma: Western Canada melanoma study. Br Med J 1984, 288:99.

Epps RL: Malignant melanoma: a review. JCE Dermatol 1979, 18:(5)13, (6), 13(7) 11.

Fox C: Azelaic acid. Cosmetics and Toiletries 1985, 100:19.

Friedman RJ, et al: Favorable prognosis for malignant melanomas associated with acquired melanocytic nevi. Arch Dermatol 1983, 119:455.

Funk W, et al: Prognostic classification of malignant melanoma by clinical criteria. Br J Dermatol 1984, 111:129.

Green A: Sun exposure and the risk of melanoma. Austral J Derm 1984, 25:99.

Gupta AK, et al: Cutaneous melanomas in patients treated with psoralens plus ultraviolet light. JAAD 1988, 19:67.

Gussack GS, et al: Cutaneous melanoma of the head and neck. Arch Otolaryngol 1983, 109:803.

Gutman M, et al: Acral melanoma. Br J Surg 1985, 72:610.

Harwood AR: Conventional radiotherapy in the treatment of lentigo maligna and lentigo maligna melanoma. JAAD 1982, 6:310.

Haupt HM, et al: Inflammatory melanoma. JAAD 1984, 10:52.

Heaston DK, et al: Solitary pulmonary metastases in high-risk melanoma patients. AJR 1983, 141:169.

Heenan PJ: Nodular melanoma: a distinct entity or a common end stage? (letter). Am J Dermatopathol 1982, 4:477.

Hena MA, et al: Effect of surgical treatment on stage IV melanoma. Am J Surg 1987, 153:270.

Hill NO, et al: Interferon and cimetidine for malignant melanoma. N Engl J Med 1983, 307:286.

Holly EA, et al: Cutaneous melanoma in relation to exogenous hormones and reproductive factors. J Nat Canc Inst 1983, 70:827. Dermatol Caps and Comment 1983, 5:1.

Johanson CR, et al: Radiotherapy in nodular melanoma. Cancer 1983, 51:226.

Johnson OK, et al: Comparison of prognostic factors for survival and recurrence in malignant melanoma of the skin, clinical stage I. Cancer 1985, 56:1107.

Kahn HJ, et al: Value of immunohistochemical studies using antibody to S100 protein in dermatopathology. Int J Dermatol 1984, 23:38.

Kahn MS, et al: Management of malignant melanoma. Clin Radiol 1984, 35:151.

Kato T, et al: Malignant melanoma of mucous membranes. Arch Dermatol 1987, 123:216.

Kelly JW, et al: The frequency of local recurrences and microsatellites as a guide to reexcision margins for cutaneous melanoma. Ann Surg 1984, 200:759.

Idem: Frequency and duration of patient follow-up after treatment of primary malignant melanoma. JAAD 1985, 13:756.

Kersey PA, et al: The value of staging and serial follow-up investigations in patients with completely resected primary cutaneous malignant melanoma. Br J Surg 1985, 72:614.

Kessinger A: High-dose chemotherapy with autologous marrow transplantation for malignant melanoma: case report and literature review. JAAD 1985, 12:337.

Kirkwood JM, et al: Tomographic Gallium-67 citrate scanning: useful new surveillance for metastatic melanoma. Ann Intern Med 1982, 97:694.

Kochar AS: Development of malignant melanoma after levodopa therapy for Parkinson's disease. Am J Med 1985, 79:119.

Koh HK, et al: Possible association between malignant melanoma and breast cancer. Arch Dermatol 1987, 123:713.

Kopf AW, et al: Sun and malignant melanoma. JAAD 1984, 11:694.

Idem: Factors related to thickness of melanoma: multifactorial analysis of variables correlated with thickness of superficial spreading malignant melanoma in man. J Dermatol Surg Oncol 1981, 7:8.

Idem: Thickness and malignant melanoma. J Dermatol Surg Oncol 1987, 13:345.

Idem: Cutaneous malignant melanoma. JAAD 1987, 16:610.

Idem: Treatment of melanotic freckle with x-rays. Arch Dermatol 1976, 112:801.

Kopf AW, et al: Prognostic index for malignant melanoma. Cancer 1987, 59:1236.

Kossard S, et al: Neurotropic melanoma. Arch Dermatol 1987, 123:907.

Kraemer KH, et al: Xeroderma pigmentosum. Arch Dermatol 1987, 123:241.

Krementz ET, et al: Acral lentiginous melanoma. Ann Surg 1982, 195:632.

Kuehnl-Petzoldt CH, et al: Verrucous-keratotic variations of malignant melanoma: a clinicopathological study. Am J Dermatopathol 1982, 4:403.

Landthaler M, et al: Malignant melanoma of the vulva. Dtsch Med Wochenschr 1985, 110:789.

Lederman JS, et al: Skin markings in the diagnosis and prognosis of cutaneous melanoma. Arch Dermatol 1984, 120:1449.

Idem: Does biopsy type influence survival in clinical stage I melanoma? JAAD 1985, 13:983.

Lerner AB, et al: Vitiligo and melanoma. JAAD 1984, 11:696.

Lew RA, et al: Sun exposure habits in patients with cutaneous melanoma. J Dermatol Surg Oncol 1983, 9:981.

Lieblich L: Classification of malignant melanoma. Am J Dermatopathol 1982, 4:435.

Lynch HT, et al: Xeroderma pigmentosum. Arch Dermatol 1984, 120:175.

Macy-Roberts E, et al: A critique of techniques for biopsy of clinically suspected malignant melanomas. Am J Dermatopathol 1982, 4:391.

Madejewicz S, et al: Malignant melanoma brain metastases. Cancer 1984, 53:2550.

Maize JC: Primary cutaneous malignant melanoma. JAAD 1983, 8:857.

Idem, et al: Melanomas of palm, sole, and nailbed. Cancer 1980, 46:2493.

Manci EA, et al: Polypoid melanoma, a virulent variant of the nodular growth pattern. Am J Clin Pathol 1981, 75:810.

Marx JL, et al: Malignant melanoma in situ in two patients treated with psoralens and ultraviolet A. JAAD 1983, 9:904.

Michalik EE, et al: Rapid progression of lentigo to deeply invasive lentigo maligna. Report of two cases. Arch Dermatol 1983, 119:831.

Milton FW, et al: Subungual malignant melanoma. Aust J Derm 1985, 26:61.

Miura S, et al: Clinical characteristics of subungual melanoma. J Dermatol 1985, 12:393.

Munz DL, et al: Place of lymphoscintigraphy in treatment of malignant melanoma of the skin. Dtsch Med Wochenschr 1982, 107:86.

Nazzaro-Porro M, et al: Effect of azelaic acid on human malignant melanoma. Lancet 1980, 1:1109.

Nordlund JJ: Hypopigmentation, vitiligo, and melanoma. Arch Dermatol 1987, 123:1005.

Idem, et al: Vitiligo in patients with metastatic melanoma: a good prognostic sign. JAAD 1983, 9:869.

Paladugu RR, et al: Acral lentiginous melanoma. Cancer 1983, 52:161.

Paver K, et al: Amelanotic lentigo maligna. Aust J Dermatol 1981, 22:106.

Penneys NS: Excision of melanoma after initial biopsy. JAAD 1985, 13:995.

Peters MS, et al: Balloon cell malignant melanoma. JAAD 1985, 13:351.

Peterson LL, et al: Plasma 5-S-cysteinyl dopa differentiates patients with primary and metastatic melanoma from patients with dysplastic nevus syndrome and normal subjects. JAAD 1988, 19:508.

Prade M, et al: Malignant melanoma of the skin: prognostic factors derived from a multifactorial analysis of 239 cases. Am J Dermatopathol 1982, 4:411.

Raderman D, et al: Late metastases (beyond ten years) of cutaneous malignant melanoma. JAAD 1986, 15:374.

Rampen FHJ, et al: Frequency of moles as a key to melanoma incidence? JAAD 1986, 15:1200.

Idem: Biopsy and survival of malignant melanoma. JAAD 1985, 12:385.

Rapini RP, et al: Primary malignant melanoma of the oral cavity. Cancer 1985, 55:1543.

Redman JC: Calling malignant melanoma in situ what it is: finding from a recent survey may make this possible. Am J Dermatopathol 1983, 5:297.

Reed KM, et al: Prognosis for polypoidal melanoma is determined by primary tumor thickness. Cancer 1986, 57:1201.

Rege VB, et al: Hyperthermic adjuvant perfusion chemotherapy for stage I malignant melanoma of the extremity, with literature review. Cancer 1983, 52:2033.

Reintgen DS, et al: Metastatic malignant melanoma with an unknown primary. Surg Gynecol Obstet 1983, 156:335.

Idem: Malignant melanoma in Black American and White American populations. JAMA 1982, 248:1856.

Idem: Malignant melanoma and pregnancy. Cancer 1985, 55:1340.

Idem: Sex-related survival differences in instances of melanoma. Surg Gynecol Obstet 1984, 159:367.

Rhodes AR, et al: Risk factors for cutaneous melanomas. JAMA 1987, 258:3146.

Rhodes WL, et al: Dipyridamole for treatment of melanoma. Lancet 1985, 1:693.

Rigel DS, et al: Importance of complete cutaneous examination for the detection of malignant melanoma. JAAD 1986, 14:857.

Rogers GS, et al: Effect of anatomical location on prognosis in patients with stage I melanoma. Arch Dermatol 1983, 119:644.

Idem: Haard-Rate analysis in stage I malignant melanoma. Arch Dermatol 1986, 122:999.

Idem: Influence of anatomic location on prognosis of malignant melanoma. JAAD 1986, 15:231.

Ronan SG, et al: Thin malignant melanoma with regression and metastases. Arch Dermatol 1987, 123:1326.

Rosenberg SA, et al: A progress report in the treatment of 157 patients with advanced cancer using lymphokine-activated killer cells and interleukin-2, or high-dose interleukin-2 alone. N Engl J Med 1987, 316:889.

Idem: Use of tumor-infiltrating lymphocytes and interleukin-2 in immunotherapy of patients with metastatic melanoma. NEJM 1988, 319:1676.

Roses DF: Surgery for primary cutaneous malignant melanoma. The Melanoma Letter 1985, 3:1.

Rossleigh MA, et al: The role of 67 gallium studies in the management of malignant melanoma. Med J Aust 1984, 140:401.

Schreiber MM, et al: Chronic solar ultraviolet damage associated with malignant melanoma of the skin. JAAD 1984, 10:755.

Schwartz BK, et al: Pregnancy and hormonal influences in malignant melanoma. J Dermatol 1987, 13:276.

Shaw HM, et al: Late relapse from cutaneous stage I malignant melanoma. Arch Surg 1985, 120:1155.

Shea TC, et al: Malignant melanoma. Arch Dermatol 1988, 124:878.

Smith T, et al: Regression of melanoma nodules in a patient treated with ranitidine. Arch Intern Med 1987, 147:1815.

Sober AJ: (Comment on Kochar, above). Yearbook of Dermatol 1986, Chicago, Yearbook Publishers, 1986, p. 268.

Stehlin JS Jr, et al: Heat as an adjuvant in the treatment of advanced melanoma. Houston Med J 1988, 4:6.

Steiner A, et al: Verrucous malignant melanoma. Arch Dermatol 1988, 124:1534.

Storm FK, et al: Value of therapeutic hyperthermic limb perfusion in advanced recurrent melanoma of the lower extremity. Am J Surg 1985, 150:32.

Su WPD, et al: Amelanotic lentigo maligna. Arch Dermatol 1980, 116:82.

Swerdlow AJ, et al: Benign melanocytic nevi as a risk factor for malignant melanoma. Br Med J 1986, 292:1555.

Takematsu H, et al: Subungual melanoma. Cancer 1985, 55:2725.

Thiers BH: Immunotherapy of malignant melanoma. JAAD 1982, 6:559.

Idem: Chemotherapy of malignant melanoma. JAAD 1982, 6:411.

Trau H, et al: Regression in malignant melanoma. JAAD 1983, 8:363.

Van der Esch EP, et al: Punch biopsy of melanoma. JAAD 1985, 13:899.

Vaszuez M, et al: Melanoma of volar and subungual skin in Puerto Ricans. JAAD 1984, 10:39.

Veronesi U, et al: Thin stage I primary cutaneous malignant melanoma. NEJM 1988, 318:1159.

Wagner RF Jr, et al: Paraneoplastic syndromes, tumor markers, and other unusual features of malignant melanoma. JAAD 1986, 14:249.

Zacarian SA: Cryosurgical treatment of lentigo maligna. Arch Dermatol 1982, 118:89.

Zappe E: Malignant melanoma: selection of sections of specimens for measurement of maximal thickness. Am J Dermatopathol 1982, 4:399.

DERMAL MELANOCYTIC LESIONS

At birth melanocytes may be present in the dermal portion of the skin of the scalp, the backs of the hands, and the sacrum. These dermal melanocytes are large ameboid cells, which normally disappear shortly after birth.

MONGOLIAN SPOT

The Mongolian spot is a bluish gray macule varying in size from 2 to 8 cm in diameter. It occurs typically in the sacral region of the newborn, in 80 to 90 per cent of Orientals, Southern Europeans, American blacks, and American Indians. The Maya Indians uniquely take great pride in it as an indicator of pure Mayan inheritance. The Mongolian spot may be situated in other locations. It usually disappears during childhood, although rarely it may persist into adulthood. Multiple spots may occur in a widespread distribution.

Histologically, the Mongolian spot shows elongated dermal melanocytes, widely scattered among the collagen bundles.

Widespread lesions referred to as generalized dermal melanocytosis, or dermal melanocytic hamartomas, have been reported by Bashiti et al and Burkhart et al.

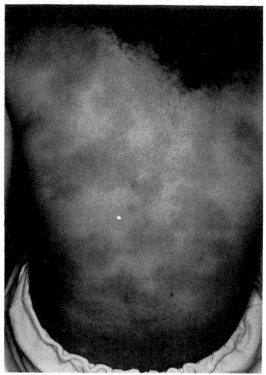

Figure 30–29. Mongolian spots on a young girl.

Bashiti HM, et al: Generalized dermal melanocytosis. Arch Dermatol 1981, 117:791.

Burkhart CG, et al: Dermal melanocytic hamartoma. Arch Dermatol 1981, 117:102.

Fulk CS: Primary disorders of hyperpigmentation. JAAD 1984, 10:1.

Hidano A: Persistent Mongolian spot in the adult. Arch Dermatol 1971, 103:680.

Jacobs AH, et al: The incidence of birthmarks in the neonate. Pediatrics 1976, 58:218.

Kikuchi I: Mongolian spots remaining in schoolchildren. J Dermatol (Tokyo) 1980, 7:213.

Idem, et al: Natural history of the Mongolian spot. J Dermatol 1980, 7:449.

Uribe MGA: The Mongolian spot. Austr J Dermatol 1976, 17:61.

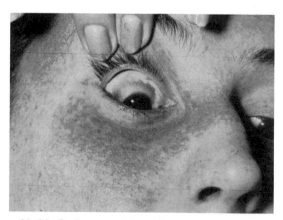

Figure 30–30. Ota's nevus. Nevus fuscoceruleus ophthalmomaxillaris. (Courtesy of Dr. F. Kerdel-Vegas, Venezuela.)

NEVUS OF OTA
(Oculodermal Melanocytosis)

This nevus, described by Ota, is also known as *nevus fuscoceruleus ophthalmomaxillaris.* It is usually present at birth in the two thirds of patients who have ocular involvement. Other lesions may not begin until the teen years. The conjunctiva and the skin about the eye supplied by the first and second branch of the trigeminal nerve, as well as the sclera, ocular muscles, retrobulbar fat, periosteum, and buccal mucosa, may be involved. On the skin, brown, slate gray, or blue-black macules grow slowly larger and deeper in color. It persists throughout life. Eighty per cent occur in females, with 5 per cent being bilateral. Although the lesion is benign, malignant melanoma may rarely occur. Dutton et al reviewed 32 cases of melanoma occurring in nevus of Ota and found it to be proportionally more frequent in white patients, and reported the most common site of malignancy was the choroid. Glaucoma may also occasionally complicate nevus of Ota.

Histologically, elongated dendritic dermal melanocytes are seen scattered in the upper portion of the dermis.

Nevus of Ito

Also known as *nevus fuscoceruleus acromiodeltoideus,* it has the same features as nevus of Ota except that it occurs in the distribution of the posterior supraclavicular and lateral cutaneous brachial nerves, to in-

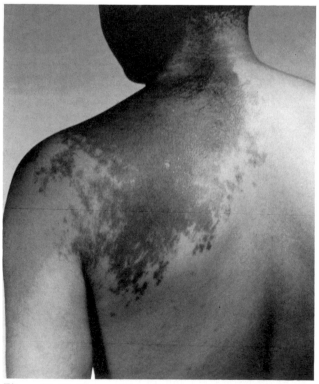

Figure 30–31. Nevus of Ito. (Courtesy of Dr. Axel W. Hoke.)

volve the shoulder, side of the neck, and supraclavicular areas.

Treatment is not possible for either of these lesions except for cosmetic coverup.

Dutton JJ, et al: Orbital malignant melanoma and oculodermal melanocytosis. Ophthalmology (Rochester) 1984, 91:497.

Hidano A: Nevus of Ota with nevus of Ito. Arch Dermatol 1965, 91:357.

Hidano H: Natural history of nevus of Ota. Arch Dermatol 1967, 95:187.

Ito M: Studies on melanoma. Tohoku J Exp Med 1954, 60:10.

Jay B: Malignant melanoma of the orbit in a case of oculodermal melanocytosis. Br J Dermatol 1965, 49:389.

Kopf AW, et al: Nevus of Ota. Arch Dermatol 1962, 85:195.

BLUE NEVUS

The blue nevus consists of two distinct types, the blue nevus of Jadassohn-Tièche (common blue nevus) and the cellular blue nevus.

Blue Nevus of Jadassohn-Tièche

The typical common blue nevus, *nevus ceruleus,* is a steel blue nodule, which begins in early life. The slowly growing lesion is rarely over 2 to 10 mm in diameter. The lesion occurs most frequently on the dorsal hands, feet, forearms, shins, face, and the buttocks. Eruptive lesions were reported by Hendricks in 1981, and one of us (WDJ) has observed a second case. A targetlike appearance was reported by Bondi et al. This type of blue nevus does not become malignant and will persist throughout life.

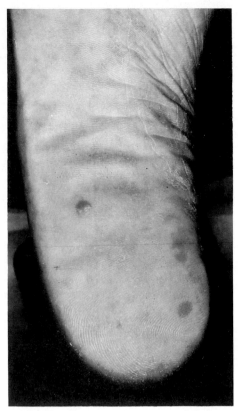

Figure 30–33. Blue nevus resembling a melanoma on the sole of a 36-year-old man.

Histologically, dermal melanocytes, fibrocytes, and melanophages are found to be increased. The nevus cells are situated deep in the dermis. The flattened melanocytes are more abundant than seen in the Mongolian spot.

Because the pigment lies so deep, shave excision is always an unsuccessful and inappropriate method of removal, and in those blue nevi situated near or on the nose, which are not blue but grayish brown, one may be tempted to try it. Excision is necessary for complete removal.

Cellular Blue Nevus

Customarily this is a large, firm, blue or blue-black nodule, most frequently seen on the buttock and sacrococcygeal region, and occasionally present at birth. The nodular tumors are multilobulated and well circumscribed. In a study of 45 cases, Rodriguez and Ackerman found that females had cellular blue nevus 2.5 times as frequently as males; the average age of the patient seen with this lesion was 39 years.

Histologically, in addition to deeply pigmented dendritic melanocytes, one observes cellular islands, composed of large spindle-shaped cells with ovoid nuclei and abundant pale cytoplasm, containing little or no pigment.

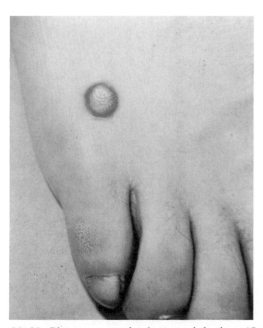

Figure 30–32. Blue nevus on the dorsum of the foot. (Courtesy of Dr. G. Sorensen.)

Malignant Blue Nevus

The cellular blue nevus may rarely undergo malignant transformation into malignant melanoma. Clinically there is a sudden increase in size, and ulceration. Pleomorphism of nuclei, mitotic figures, and invasion of clusters of malignant cells into the deep dermis and fatty tissue are seen; there is no junctional activity in the malignant blue nevus.

Treatment is the same as for a malignant melanoma.

Bondi EE, et al: Target blue nevi. Arch Dermatol 1983, 119:919.

Draelos ZK, et al: Trunk tumor resembling a congenital nevus. Arch Dermatol 1986, 122:1065.

Goldenhersh MA, et al: Malignant blue nevus. JAAD 1988, 19:712.

Hendricks WM: Eruptive blue nevi. JAAD 1981, 4:50.

Hernandez FJ: Malignant blue nevus. Arch Dermatol 1973, 107:741.

Hindano A: Persistent Mongolian spot in the adult. Arch Dermatol 1971, 103:680.

Kwitten J, et al: Malignant blue nevus. Arch Dermatol 1966, 94:64.

Lambert WC, et al: Nodal and subcutaneous cellular blue nevi. Arch Dermatol 1984, 120:367.

Mishima Y: Cellular blue nevus. Arch Dermatol 1970, 101:104.

Reiss RF, et al: Malignant blue nevus. NY State J Med 1975, 75:1749.

Rodriguez HA, et al: Cellular blue nevus. Cancer 1968, 21:393.

Shenfield HT, et al: Multiple agminated blue nevi. J Dermatol Surg Oncol 1980, 6:725.

31

Macrophage/Monocyte and Lymphocytic Infiltrates

Several disorders are characterized by proliferation of cells of macrophage lineage. Headington effectively argues against the use of "histiocyte" in modern-day conceptual thinking, pointing out that through use of electron microscopic and immunohistochemical studies, cell types may be identified more specifically. In the past any cell that was mononuclear and located in the skin or soft tissue, and had a reniform or oval nucleus, a cell diameter of 10 to 25 micrometers, and a nuclear-to-cytoplasmic ratio of about 1, might be called a histiocyte. Thus previous histiocytic syndromes in some classifications included such disease entities as fibrous "histiocytomas," which are derived from fibrocytes ("dermal dendrocytes"—Headington), and "histiocytic" lymphomas, many of which are of B cell origin.

Nonetheless, certain syndromes that are well defined clinically, histologically, and (ever increasingly) immunohistochemically and electron microscopically carry with them the term "histiocyte." We have discussed many of these entities in other chapters, preferring to include dermatofibroma (histiocytoma) and fibrous histiocytoma in the "Dermal Tumors" section, and xanthoma disseminatum and verruciform xanthoma in the differential diagnosis of xanthomas.

The following entities are benign disorders characterized by a proliferation of microscopically "histiocytic"-appearing cells. In the discussion of each entity we will specify the known markers present on or within the prominent cellular infiltrate.

Fowler JF, et al: Cutaneous non-X histiocytosis. JAAD 1985, 13:645.
Gianotti F, et al: Histiocytic syndromes: a review. JAAD 1985, 13:383.
Groopman JE, et al: The histiocytic disorders: a pathophysiological analysis. Ann Intern Med 1981, 94:95.
Headington JT: The histiocyte. Arch Dermatol 1986, 122:533.
Ringel E, et al: Primary histiocytic dermatoses. Arch Dermatol 1985, 121:1531.
Winkelmann RK, et al: Cutaneous syndromes of non-X histiocytosis. Arch Dermatol 1981, 117:667.

BENIGN CEPHALIC HISTIOCYTOSIS

This eruption is characterized by the onset of raised, multiple, reddish yellow papulonodules, limited generally to the face and scalp, in the first year or two of life. Spontaneous involution in two to five years' time is the rule, leaving behind atrophic pigmented lesions. Some view it as a localized variant of generalized eruptive histiocytoma.

Histologically there is a diffuse proliferation of histiocytic-appearing cells. S-100 stains are negative. By electron microscopy about 20 per cent of these cells contain clusters of comma-shaped bodies, which are characteristic but not specific for this disease. Barsky et al and Eisenberg et al reported such cases.

Barsky BL, et al: Benign cephalic histiocytosis. Arch Dermatol 1984, 120:650.

Eisenberg EL, et al: Benign cephalic histiocytosis. JAAD 1985, 12:328.

Gianotti F, et al: Singulière histiocytose infantile à cellules avec particles vermiformes intracytoplasmiques. Bull Soc Franç Dermatol Syphil 1971, 78:232.

SELF-HEALING RETICULOHISTIOCYTOSIS

This has been described in two forms, a solitary and a multinodular variant. In 1973 Hashimoto and Pritzker described a condition characterized by generalized brownish, pink, or dusky red papulonodules, which are present at birth, are asymptomatic, do not involve internal structures, and heal spontaneously.

On histologic examination large mononuclear cells and multinucleated giant cells with ground-glass or foamy cytoplasm are present in the dermis and epidermis. Immunoperoxidase staining is positive for CD1, HLA-DR, and S-100. By electron microscopy 10 to 25 per cent of cells have Langerhans cell granules and the large histiocytic-appearing cells contain dense bodies, regularly laminated bodies, and unique phagolysosomes.

In the solitary variant, of which Berger et al reported four cases, a single congenital, rapidly growing, spontaneously ulcerating tumor is present on the face, trunk, or extremities. Histology and electron microscopy yield the findings described previously, and spontaneous involution occurs.

This is a proliferation of Langerhans cells. Since histiocytosis with systemic involvement may present in identical fashion, systemic evaluation is recommended, including a physical examination, complete blood count, liver function tests, and bone survey. Liver-spleen scan and bone marrow biopsy should be considered.

Berger TG, et al: A solitary variation of congenital self-healing reticulohistiocytosis. Pediatr Dermatol 1986, 3:230.

Bonifazi E, et al: Congenital self-healing histiocytosis. Arch Dermatol 1982, 118:267.

Hashimoto K, et al: Electron microscope study of reticulohistiocytoma. Arch Dermatol 1973, 107:263.

Idem: Congenital self-healing reticulohistiocytosis. Internat J Dermatol 1986, 25:516.

Idem: Congenital self-healing reticulohistiocytosis. JAAD 1984, 11:447.

Taïeb A, et al: Solitary Langerhans cell histiocytoma. Arch Dermatol 1986, 122:1033.

GENERALIZED ERUPTIVE HISTIOCYTOMA

In 1963 Winkelmann and Muller reported and named this syndrome, which occurs in otherwise healthy adults. According to Umbert et al, 23 cases had been reported by 1989. The major characteristics of the syndrome include widespread, essentially symmetrical papules, particularly involving the trunk

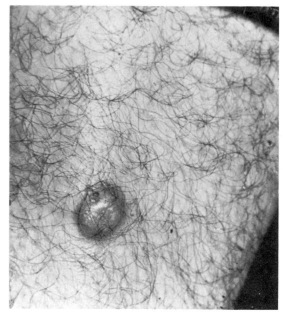

Figure 31–1. Histiocytoma, 2 cm in diameter, on inner thigh.

and proximal extremities, and rarely the mucous membranes; progressive development of new lesions over several years with eventual spontaneous involution toward brown macules; and a benign histologic picture of mononuclear, histiocytic-appearing cells. Caputo et al reported four children with the syndrome and found the major differences from the disease in adults were asymmetry, sparing of mucosae, and progression to xanthomatosis.

Electron microscopy reveals dense multivesicular

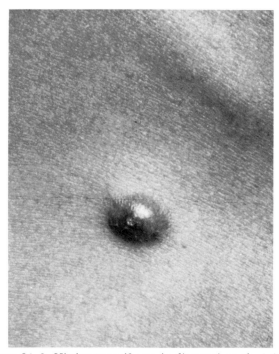

Figure 31–2. Histiocytoma (8 mm in diameter) on the infraclavicular area of a 12-year-old boy.

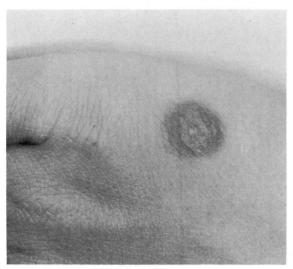

Figure 31–3. Dermatofibroma on the hand.

bodies as well as regularly laminated bodies. S-100 staining is negative.

No treatment is required: it is a self-limited disease.

Caputo R, et al: Generalized eruptive histiocytoma: a clinical, histologic, and ultrastructural study. Arch Dermatol 1981, 117:216.
Idem: Generalized eruptive histiocytoma in children. JAMA 1987, 17:449.
Sohi AS, et al: Generalized eruptive histiocytoma. Dermatologica 1979, 159:471.
Umbert IJ, et al: Eruptive histiocytoma. JAAD 1989, 20:958.
Winkelmann RK, et al: Generalized eruptive histiocytoma. Arch Dermatol 1963, 88:586.
Idem: Eruptive histiocytoma of childhood. Arch Dermatol 1980, 116:565.

PROGRESSIVE NODULAR HISTIOCYTOMA

This condition is clinically characterized by a widespread, papulonodular, essentially symmetrical eruption interspersed with telangiectatic nodules measuring up to 5 cm in diameter. Typically the face is heavily involved by merging lesions, giving a leonine appearance. There is no visceral, mucous membrane, or articular involvement, and the general health is good. New lesions progressively appear, and spontaneous resolution does not occur.

Histologically there is a massive infiltrate of histiocytic-appearing cells admixed with masses of lymphocytes. Giant cells are rare. Ultrastructurally many cells contain pleomorphic cytoplasmic inclusions identical to those found in multicentric reticulohistiocytosis. Some authors consider that this may be a form of multicentric reticulohistiocytosis with limited expression.

Chemotherapy and electron beam may lead to remission of lesions. Burgdorf et al reported success by excision of multiple nodules over the three-year period of observation.

Burgdorf WHC, et al: Progressive nodular histiocytoma. Arch Dermatol 1981, 117:644.
Taunton OD, et al: Progressive nodular histiocytoma. Arch Dermatol 1978, 114:1505.
Winkelmann RK, et al: Response of nodular non-X histiocytosis to vinblastine. Arch Dermatol 1982, 118:913.

HEREDITARY PROGRESSIVE MUCINOUS HISTIOCYTOSIS IN WOMEN

Bork and Hoede described three female patients in a family who began to develop generalized, pea-sized histiocytic tumors in adolescence. These were slowly progressive and remained confined to the skin. The histologic picture was similar to that of progressive nodular histiocytoma, except that with time there was a marked production of mucinous material.

Bork K, et al: Hereditary progressive mucinous histiocytosis in women. Arch Dermatol 1988, 124:1225.

REGRESSING ATYPICAL HISTIOCYTOSIS

Flynn et al in 1982 reported two cases in which multiple fungating, ulcerative papulonodules developed, which on histologic examination showed bizarre, malignant-appearing large mononuclear cells in the dermis. Erythrophagocytosis, mitotic figures, and multinucleated giant cells were present. Both cases resolved spontaneously. McCormick et al reported a third patient in 1984 who had a single lesion.

Caution regarding the diagnosis of this newly described disease is recommended, however, as it awaits further characterization. A patient reported by Flynn et al had inguinal node involvement late in the course. Rogel et al have observed a patient in whom a lymphocytic lymphoma developed, and Headington considers it to be a polymorphic subset of T-cell lymphoma. He reported finding T-cell receptor rearrangement in one case.

Dehner LP: Regressing atypical histiocytosis: The controversy continues. Arch Dermatol 1988, 124:319.
Flynn KJ, et al: Regressing atypical histiocytosis. Am J Dermatopathol 1984, 6:259.
Headington JT: The histiocyte. Arch Dermatol 1986, 122:533.
Idem, et al: T-cell gene rearrangement in regressing atypical histiocytosis. Arch Dermatol 1987, 123:1183.
Moayed MJ, et al: Regressing atypical histiocytosis (of Flynn). Dermatologica 1987, 174:253.
Ringel E, et al: The histiocytic dermatoses. Arch Dermatol 1985, 121:1531.

SINUS HISTIOCYTOSIS WITH MASSIVE LYMPHADENOPATHY

Rosai et al described this disease in 1969. It appears in patients in the first or second decade of life as a febrile illness accompanied by massive cervical (and commonly other) lymphadenopathy, leukocytosis, anemia, and an elevated sedimentation rate. Males, and blacks, are especially susceptible. Ten per cent of patients have isolated or disseminated red-brown or yellow-brown papules or nodules. Most patients with skin lesions are older (40 years) at presentation.

Histologically the dermal infiltrate is composed of histiocytic-appearing cells, often in clusters resembling lymph node sinuses. Comma-shaped bodies and phagosomes are seen on electron microscopy. The histiocytes are S-100 and CD1 negative.

Although it may take several years, spontaneous resolution is expected. Penneys et al reported success with the use of vinblastine-loaded platelets coated with idiopathic thrombocytopenic purpura antibodies to poison the phagocytic cells. Systemic steroids and cyclophosphamide, together or alone, also have been reported to be effective.

Foucar E, et al: Sinus histiocytosis with massive lymphadenopathy. Arch Dermatol 1988, 124:1211.

Olsen EA, et al: Sinus histiocytosis with massive lymphadenopathy. JAAD 1988, 18:1322.

Penneys NS, et al: Sinus histiocytosis with massive lymphadenopathy. Cancer 1982, 49:1994.

Rosai J, et al: Sinus histiocytosis with lymphadenopathy: a pseudolymphomatous disorder. Analysis of 34 cases. Cancer 1972, 30:1174.

Suster S, et al: Histiocytic lymphophagocytic panniculitis. Arch Dermatol 1988, 124:1246.

Thawerani H, et al: The cutaneous manifestations of sinus histiocytosis with massive lymphadenopathy. Arch Dermatol 1978, 114:191.

SEA-BLUE HISTIOCYTOSIS

This disease may occur as a familial inherited syndrome, or as a secondary or systemic infiltration with these peculiar macrophages which, due to their cytoplasmic granules, stain blue-green with Giemsa stain. The disorder is characterized by infiltration of these cells into the marrow, spleen, liver, lymph nodes, and lungs, as well as, in some cases, the skin. The granules appear to be a glycophospholipid, probably a ceroid. Zina et al reported two related patients, one with nodular plaques and one with slight induration of the skin. The condition is probably due to an as yet unidentified metabolic defect.

Zina AM, et al: Familial sea-blue histiocytosis with cutaneous involvement. Br J Dermatol 1983, 108:355.

RETICULOHISTIOCYTOMA

Reticulohistiocytoma is characterized by local and systemic manifestations, with cutaneous and mucous membrane nodules, arthritis, and a distinctive histology of multinucleated histiocytic giant cells. Two distinct forms occur: *multicentric reticulohistiocytosis* and *reticulohistiocytic granuloma*. The two forms are not distinguishable histologically; however, clinically their manifestations are quite distinct.

Multicentric Reticulohistiocytosis

The cutaneous lesions of multicentric reticulohistiocytosis are part of a generalized process that is characterized histologically by aggregates of macrophages and histiocytic giant cells.

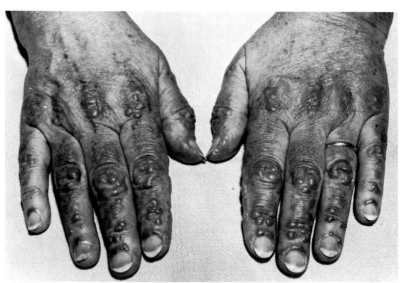

Figure 31–4. Multicentric reticulohistiocytosis on hands of 45-year-old woman. (Courtesy of Dr. T. A. Labow.)

CLINICAL FEATURES. There may be a few or a hundred firm, red, brown, and yellow nodules 2 to 10 mm wide. These occur most frequently on the fingers and hands, with a tendency to cause paronychial lesions. In about half the cases lesions will be arranged about nail folds, giving a so-called "coral bead" appearance. The arms, scalp, face, ears, and neck are also common sites. Characteristic are nodular and papular involvement of the paronychial areas and the ears, and the symmetrical distribution of the lesions, especially over joints. The nodules on the arms, elbows, and knees may resemble rheumatoid nodules or juxta-articular nodes of syphilis.

Mucous membrane involvement is seen in half the cases and is most frequently present on the lips; other sites are the nasal mucosa, the tongue, the palate, and the buccal mucosa. One third of cases have hypercholesterolemia and xanthelasma.

These lesions may involute spontaneously after a few years, leaving no trace, but this is the exception: most cases are progressive.

In about one half to two thirds of patients, polyarthritis and arthralgia are the initial manifestations. In many cases there is rapid progression to arthritis mutilans, with the most severe involvement often being in the distal interphalangeal joints.

In other instances the cutaneous nodules precede mutilating arthritis, with demineralization, absorption, and telescopic shortening of the phalanges and digits—*doigts en lorgnette*, opera-glass fingers. The joint involvement may also resemble rheumatoid arthritis, with a severe inflammatory reaction. Tendon sheath swellings on the wrists occur in the late stages. Weight loss and fever are frequently present. The onset is usually during the third and fourth decades, with three quarters of cases being women.

Other organs and tissues may be involved, such as bone, muscle, lymph nodes, heart, stomach, eye, salivary gland, and thyroid gland. Furey et al proposed gallium scans as a screening method to assess the extent of disease.

The clinical course varies. In some instances there is complete involution; in others the disease remains stationary or progresses to eventual death. One of the authors (RBO) had a patient with multicentric reticulohistiocytosis and acute myelogenous leukemia. This case was reported in 1982 by Goette et al under the title *diffuse cutaneous reticulohistiocytosis,* so called because there were no systemic or skeletal lesions. Cotterall found that 19 (24 per cent) of 74 reported cases of multicentric reticulohistiocytosis developed carcinoma within a few months to four years after the onset: bronchus, stomach, breast, and cervix, three each (and three malignant lymphomas); ovary, colon, and an axillary sarcoma, one each; and one undetected primary. Many other types of cancer have been reported, including a mesothelioma.

ETIOLOGY. No cause has been found.

HISTOPATHOLOGY. Histologically the lesion is a granulomatous proliferation of histiocytic cells and giant cells. The latter may contain many nuclei in a pink-staining cytoplasm resembling ground glass. The smaller cells surrounding the giant cells are histiocytic-appearing cells and lymphocytes, and are separated by intervening fibrous connective tissue strands. When the sections are pretreated with diastase and then stained by the PAS technique, a red positive-staining material may be seen in some of the giant cells. Caputo et al reported in 1981 finding evidence of phagocytosis of collagen fibers (identified by their typical periodic banding) in the lesions. By electron microscopy 40 per cent of the histiocytic cells contain unique highly complex structures called pleomorphic cytoplasmic inclusions. Davies and his associates demonstrated polysaccharides and phospholipids in the giant cells. This material represents glycolipids and glycoproteins.

DIFFERENTIAL DIAGNOSIS. Lesher compiled a valuable tabular summary of the differentiation of the disease from rheumatoid arthritis, lepromatous leprosy, sarcoidosis, xanthoma disseminatum, xanthoma tuberosum, fibroxanthoma, self-healing reticulohistiocytosis, eruptive histiocytoma, histiocytosis X, histiomonocytosis, lipoid proteinosis, disseminated lipogranulomatosis, and familial histiocytic dermatoarthritis.

TREATMENT. About one fourth of the reported cases have been found to involute spontaneously within six to eight years. It appears alkylating agents such as cyclophosphamide or nitrogen mustard may help to prevent disfiguring arthritis and skin lesions. Brandt et al reported a case with bone lesions, in which skin lesions resolved within two weeks on topical nitrogen mustard therapy; the bone lesions responded only to cyclophosphamide, 50 mg per day. Furey et al had only partial remission in a case with salivary gland involvement and pericardial effusion treated with prednisone, vincristine sulfate, and cyclophosphamide. Aldridge et al reported a patient whose cutaneous lesions benefitted from PUVA.

Reticulohistiocytic Granuloma

This variant of reticulohistiocytoma, described by Purvis and Helwig, is characterized by solitary lesions without systemic involvement. In contrast to multicentric reticulohistiocytosis, these lesions have been found mainly in men.

Histologically the lesions are identical to those of multicentric reticulohistiocytosis.

These solitary lesions are to be distinguished from juvenile xanthogranuloma, histiocytoma, sclerosing hemangioma, granuloma annulare, and granular cell tumor.

No specific treatment except destruction or excision of the lesion is feasible.

Aldridge RD, et al: Multicentric reticulohistiocytosis and cancer. JAAD 1984, 10:296.
Berti E, et al: Reticulohistiocytosis of the dorsum. JAAD 1988, 19:259.

Brandt F, et al: Topical nitrogen mustard in multicentric reticulohistiocytosis. JAAD 1982, 6:260.

Caputo R, et al: Collagen phagocytosis in multicentric reticulohistiocytosis. J Invest Dermatol 1981, 76:342.

Idem: Diffuse cutaneous reticulohistiocytosis in a child with tuberous sclerosis. Arch Dermatol 1988, 124:567.

Cotterall MD, et al: Multicentric reticulohistiocytosis and malignant disease. Br J Dermatol 1978, 98:221.

Coupe MO, et al: Multicentric reticulohistiocytosis. Br J Dermatol 1987, 116:245.

Finelli LG, et al: A case of multicentric reticulohistiocytosis with thyroid involvement. JAAD 1986, 15:1097.

Furey N, et al: Multicentric reticulohistiocytosis with salivary gland involvement and pericardial effusion. JAAD 1983, 8:679.

Goette DK, et al: Diffuse cutaneous reticulohistiocytosis. Arch Dermatol 1982, 118:173.

Honeybourne D, et al: A mesothelioma presenting with multicentric reticulohistiocytosis. Postgrad Med J 1955, 61:57.

Kuramoto Y, et al: Multicentric reticulohistiocytosis in a child with a sclerosing lesion of the leg. JAAD 1989, 20:329.

Lesher JL Jr, et al: Multicentric reticulohistiocytosis. JAAD 1984, 11:713.

LYMPHOCYTOMA CUTIS
(Spiegler-Fendt Sarcoid; Pseudolymphoma of Spiegler-Fendt)

Lymphadenosis benigna cutis of Bäfverstedt (LABC) occurs in localized and disseminated forms. It is now generally called *lymphocytoma cutis*.

In the localized form it may appear as a pea-sized or larger discrete, firm, cutaneous nodule or group of nodules, principally on the face, particularly on

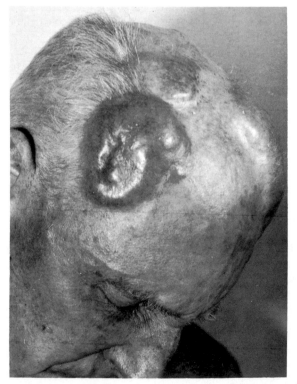

Figure 31–5. Lymphadenosis benigna cutis (lymphocytoma cutis).

the forehead or ear lobes. The epidermis over the nodules is usually smooth and flesh-colored, reddish or yellowish brown, or violaceous. Rarely these lesions may occur on other parts of the body. Most of the cases have occurred on the scalp, especially at the anterior scalp line. Women are most frequently affected.

No internal manifestation or blood changes are noted. The infiltrations are usually superficial; they may involute spontaneously but usually only after months or even a year or two.

The disseminated form, known as *lymphadenosis benigna dispersa*, is found in middle-aged adults in the form of miliary papules or large indurated nodules located mainly on face, trunk, and extremities. These lesions remain for years, but may spontaneously involute. When progression to lymphoma appears to occur, it is considered to have been lymphoma from the outset. In some cases lymphoma may be excluded only after long follow-up ensures that no lymph node or visceral lesions develop.

The cause of this uncommon dermatosis is unknown. Tattoo reactions, insect bites, and trauma have been implicated. At least some cases may be attributed to borreliosis, as is the case with morphea and lichen sclerosis et atrophicus. These reports emanate largely from Europe and may not be applicable to *B. burgdorferi* infection in the United States. Weber et al reported four cases in 1985 in which indirect immunofluorescence tests revealed IgG or IgM antibodies against both *Ixodes dammini* and *Borrelia burgdorferi*. Lasthein Andersen et al reported two cases in 1981 which were histologically diagnosed as malignant but which both responded readily to penicillin. Mach and Wilgram regard lymphocytoma cutis as a localized hyperplasia of lymphoreticular tissue, induced by external factors.

Histologic examination reveals a densely cellular nodular infiltrate composed chiefly of mature lymphocytes of uniform size, with little stroma. They are accompanied by more or less numerous histiocytes. Overlying the infiltrate is a clear Grenz zone separating it from the epidermis. In the deeper portions well-defined germinal centers are usually seen, or the cells may be commingled. Van Hale et al have shown by monoclonal antibody studies that there may be either a polyclonal T cell proliferation, or a nodule composed of B cells with T cells in the periphery.

In the differential diagnosis lymphocytoma cutis must be differentiated from cutaneous lymphoma, leukemia cutis, mycosis fungoides, lymphocytic infiltration of the skin, and polymorphous light eruption. If many nuclei are deeply indented it may be an immunocytoma, which Van der Putte et al (who reported a case) believe to be a low-grade B-cell lymphoma. There is a solid infiltrate in such a lesion, with few or no germinal centers. In the disseminated type, sarcoidosis, lupus vulgaris, lichen nitidus, and leukemia cutis are to be considered. Usually the histologic picture and the strikingly good response to x-ray therapy are sufficient to differentiate it from the possible alternatives already mentioned.

Treatment is x-ray therapy: 100 rads at 100 kv (HVL 1–3 mm Al). Lesions are likely to clear within one to two weeks. In the event of early recurrence it may be necessary to repeat the dose.

Alternative therapies have been reported only infrequently. Stoll reported resolution after treatment with hydroxychloroquine (Plaquenil). Proquazone, a nonsteroidal anti-inflammatory drug, was effective in 8 patients treated by Johansson. Wheeland et al reported using the argon laser with cosmetically satisfactory results in one case. If antibody tests for *Borrelia* or *Ixodes* are positive, as occasionally happens in Europe, the lesion may be due to borreliosis, and penicillin may be rapidly curative.

Andersen BL, et al: Lymphocytoma cutis: a pseudomalignancy treated with penicillin. Acta Dermatovener (Stockh) 1981, 62:83.

Blumental G, et al: Pseudolymphomatous reaction to tattoos. JAAD 1982, 6:485.

Caro WA, et al: Cutaneous lymphoid hyperplasia. Cancer 1969, 24:487.

Evans HL, et al: Differential diagnosis of malignant and benign cutaneous infiltrates. Cancer 1979, 44:699.

Goldberg NS, et al: An extensive papular eruption on the face of a 10-year-old girl. Arch Dermatol 1986, 122:931.

Hormark A, et al: The spirochetal etiology of lymphadenosis benigna cutis solitaria. Acta Derm Venereol (Stockh) 1986, 66:479.

Johansson EA: Proquazone. Dermatologica 1987, 174:117.

Stoll DM: Treatment of cutaneous pseudolymphoma with hydroxychloroquine. JAAD 1983, 8:696.

Van der Putte SCJ, et al: Solitary nonepidermotropic T cell pseudolymphomas of the skin. JAAD 1986, 14:444.

Idem: Immunocytoma of the skin simulating lymphadenosis benigna cutis. Arch Derm Res 1985, 26:277.

Van Hale HM, et al: Nodular lymphoid disease. JAAD 1985, 12:455.

Wantzin GL, et al: Evolution of cutaneous lymphoid hyperplasia to cutaneous T-cell lymphoma. Clin Exp Dermatol 1988, 13:309.

Weber K, et al: Lymphocytoma—a borreliosis? Hautkrankheit 1985, 60:1585.

Wheeland RG, et al: Role of the argon laser in lymphocytoma cutis. JAAD 1986, 14:267.

LYMPHOCYTIC INFILTRATION OF THE SKIN

Jessner and Norman Kanof were the first to describe this entity, characterized by pink to reddish brown, flat discoid papules. These papules enlarge to form elevated plaques, which occur most frequently on the face, neck, and upper back. The eyelids and zygomas are the sites most frequently involved. The asymptomatic lesions are well defined, slightly elevated, firm, erythematous plaques with a smooth surface, with no follicular plugging.

Lymphocytic infiltration is seen more frequently in men. No specific cause has been found for this entity, which in the past has been regarded by some to be a variant of chronic discoid lupus erythematosus and by others to be a form of lymphocytoma cutis. It has

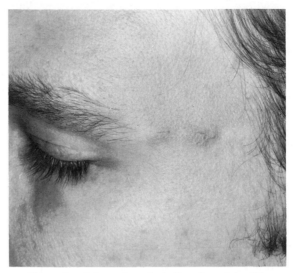

Figure 31–6. Lymphocytic infiltration of the skin.

also been regarded as a dermatophytid, curable by antifungal treatment of the feet, or by griseofulvin. Our view is that this is an entity sui generis, which may be indistinguishable in early stages from—and may therefore eventuate in—discoid LE, polymorphous light eruption, or lymphocytoma cutis.

Histologically, minimal changes are apparent in the epidermis; however, in the dermis an intense perivascular infiltration of lymphocytes is present. Epidermal involvement and follicular plugging are absent. Willemze et al found CD1-positive Langerhans and HLA-DR positive (i.e., activated) T cells in most lesions of discoid LE, and in no patients with Jessner's lymphocytic infiltration, which argues strongly against any relationship with lupus erythematosus.

Blaylock advises chloroquine, but various measures such as ionizing radiation, cryotherapy, antimalarials, and corticosteroids topically, intralesionally, and internally have all produced varied results. With or without treatment, most of these lesions involute after several years.

Calnan CD: Lymphocytic infiltration of the skin (Jessner). Br J Dermatol 1957, 69:169.

Gottlieb B, et al: Lymphocytic infiltration of the skin. Arch Dermatol 1962, 86:626.

Jessner M, et al: Lymphocytic infiltration of the skin. Arch Dermatol Suppl 1953, 68:447.

Patterson JW, et al: Lymphocytic infiltration of the skin (Jessner and Kanof). In Clinical Dermatology, Vol 4, Demis J (ed.). 20:3, 1986.

Willemze R, et al: Immunohistochemical studies in lymphocytic infiltration of the skin and discoid LE. JAAD 1984, 11:832.

GRANULOMA FACIALE

A red-brown or violaceous plaque or plaques on the face, which may be crusted, suggests granuloma faciale. Lesions have also occurred on the trunk or limbs, and two disseminated cases have been reported. Lesions evolve slowly and are usually asymptomatic.

Histologically there is an infiltrate of eosinophils, neutrophils, lymphocytes, histiocytes, and plasma cells, separated from the epidermis by a Grenz zone. Evidence of vasculitis is usually present, and there may be extravasation of red cells. Schroeter reported thick deposits of IgG, IgA, and IgM in the epidermal basement membrane zone in all of three cases.

Nothing that has been tried has worked as well as low-dose dapsone therapy. Milligan et al (1984) duplicated the success of Anderson and Guill et al. As little as 25 mg a day may be effective, though 100 mg a day is usually very well tolerated and is the dose most often employed.

Hudson in 1983 reported success with PUVA after dapsone had failed. Many treatments are successful in selected patients. Intralesional steroids are useful in many cases. Apfelberg et al reported success with the argon laser.

Apfelberg DB, et al: Granuloma faciale. Arch Dermatol 1983, 119:573.

Guill MA, et al: Facial granuloma responsive to dapsone. Arch Dermatol 1982, 118:332.

Horn T: Longstanding erythematous facial plaques. Arch Dermatol 1985, 121:1553.

Hudson LD: Granuloma faciale: treatment with PUVA. JAAD 1983, 8:559.

Milligan MP, et al: Dapsone-responsive granuloma faciale. J Assoc Milit Dermatol 1984, 10:30.

CHEILITIS GRANULOMATOSA

Miescher in 1945 reported six cases of swelling of the lips with progressive changes resulting in permanent macrocheilia. Cheilitis granulomatosa is

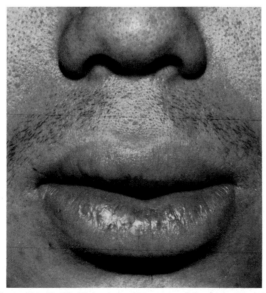

Figure 31–7. Cheilitis granulomatosa of 1 year's duration.

characterized by a sudden onset and progressive course terminating in chronic enlargement of the lips. Usually the upper lip becomes swollen first; several months may elapse before the lower becomes swollen. Usually enlargement only is present, without ulceration, fissuring, or scaling. The swelling remains permanently. It may be a part of the Melkersson-Rosenthal syndrome when associated with facial paralysis and plicated tongue.

The etiology is unknown. Laymon in 1961 showed that it is not sarcoidosis, nor is it a reaction to a foreign body or infectious agent.

Histologically, it is characterized by an inflammatory reaction and a tuberculoid granuloma. The noteworthy finding is the presence of tuberculoid granulomas consisting of epithelioid and Langhans giant cells. The infiltrate consists of lymphocytes, histiocytes, and plasma cells.

In the differential diagnosis solid edema, angioedema, cheilitis glandularis, sarcoidosis, oral Crohn's disease, infectious granulomas, and Ascher's syndrome must be considered.

Treatment with intralesional injections of corticosteroids is sometimes successful. In the firmly established case plastic repair of the involved lip through a mucosal approach should be considered. In some cases concomitant intralesional steroids and surgical repair give best results.

Hines H: Facial swelling in a female adult. Arch Dermatol 1985, 121:127.

Rhodes EL, et al: Granulomatous cheilitis. Arch Dermatol 1965, 92:40.

Venable CE, et al: Persistent swelling of the lower lip. Arch Dermatol 1988, 129:1705.

MELKERSSON-ROSENTHAL SYNDROME

Melkersson in 1928 and Rosenthal in 1930 described a triad consisting of recurring facial paralysis or paresis, soft nonpitting edema of the lips, and scrotal tongue. There may be recurring edema of the upper face, the buccal cavity, the tongue, and even other parts of the body. The facial paralysis, usually unilateral, is a peripheral seventh nerve palsy, which may be transitory or permanent. The macrocheilia may also be transitory. The syndrome may be familial.

Attacks usually start during adolescence, with paralysis of one or the other, or even both, facial nerves, with repeated migraine attacks, and with edema of the upper lip, cheeks, and occasionally the lower lip and circumoral tissues. The first symptoms are the swelling of the skin and mucous membranes of the face and mouth. In order of frequency the swelling occurs first on the upper lip, then the lower lip, and then other regions.

Extrafacial swellings appear on the dorsal aspect of the hands and the feet and in the lumbar region.

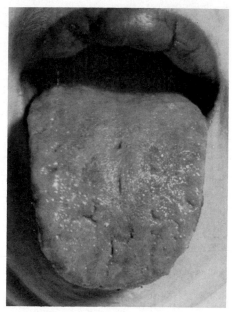

Figure 31–8. Melkersson-Rosenthal syndrome. Note furrowed and swollen tongue.

The pharynx and the respiratory tract may be involved, with thickening of the mucous membrane. The relapsing condition produces an overgrowth of connective tissue, edema, atrophy of the muscle fibers, and round cell infiltration, with permanent deformities of the lips, cheeks, and tongue.

The etiology is unknown. The association at times with megacolon, otosclerosis, and craniopharyngioma supports the theory of neurotrophic origin.

The histopathology shows a tuberculoid type of granuloma with lymphedema and a banal perivascular infiltrate. Yuzuk et al reported a case in which the histology was indistinguishable from sarcoidosis.

In the differential diagnosis a number of diseases characterized by edema of the lips must be considered. *Ascher's syndrome* consists of swelling of the lips with edema of the eyelids (blepharochalasis) and is inherited. It must also be differentiated from the acute swellings produced by angioedema, trauma,

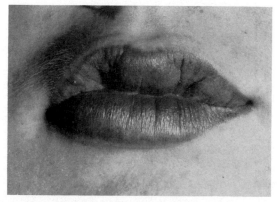

Figure 31–9. Melkersson-Rosenthal syndrome. Note swelling of right side of lower lip.

and infections of all sorts. Lymphangioma, hemangioma, neurofibroma, and sarcoidosis are some of the diseases to be considered on a clinical basis.

There is no satisfactory treatment, although intralesional injections of corticosteroids may be beneficial. Decompression of the facial nerve may be indicated in those with recurrent attacks of facial palsy. In the case of Yuzuk et al the swollen upper lip was made much more presentable by plastic surgery. Combining surgery with intralesional steroid injections may be more successful than either alone. Worsaae et al reported that 11 of 16 patients improved upon treatment of coexistent odontogenic infection.

El-Zawahry M, et al: Melkersson-Rosenthal syndrome: review of the literature and report of a case. Int J Dermatol 1972, 11:86.

Minor MW, et al: Melkersson-Rosenthal syndrome. J Allergy Clin Immunol 1987, 80:64.

Worsaae N, et al: Melkersson-Rosenthal syndrome and cheilitis granulomatosa. Oral Surgery 1982, 54:404.

Yuzuk S, et al: Melkersson-Rosenthal syndrome. Int J Dermatol 1985, 24:456.

MIDLINE GRANULOMA

Midline granuloma, still called by many *lethal midline granuloma*, manifests itself as a progressive, destructive granulomatous ulceration of the face, especially the nose and the upper respiratory tract. The first sign may be a chronic mucoid nasal discharge which later becomes purulent. The necrotic ulceration usually appears first on the nasal septum. Eventually there is necrosis of the facial bones and the base of the skull, and frightful mutilating destruction of the central face. Victims are most often men between 20 and 50.

Fauci et al characterize the condition as a disorder of the central face with acute and chronic inflammation, necrosis, and granuloma formation, which destroys soft tissue, cartilage, and bone. They clearly distinguish it from Wegener's granulomatosis (which used to be included in the entity) by pointing out that in midline granuloma perforation is common, the lungs and kidneys are spared, and disseminated vasculitis rarely occurs.

Many other disorders, such as lymphoma, syphilis, sarcoidosis, and leishmaniasis, may destroy the central face, but when these have been excluded the diagnosis is midline granuloma. Arnold had one case in which "reticulum cell sarcoma" was diagnosed by deep excisional biopsy after two unsuccessful attempts. By then the central face was destroyed.

TREATMENT. DeRamee et al found x-ray therapy effective in 13 of 20 cases, and Fauci et al in 8 of 10. The latter urge a dose of 5000 rads, and define it as the treatment of choice in this rare disease. Lober in 1982 reported a case involving just the distal nose, in which x-ray therapy was effective.

Crissman JD, et al: Midline granuloma syndromes. Am J Surg Pathol 1982, 6:335.

DeRamee RA, et al: Polymorphic reticulosis, lymphomatoid granulomatosis: two diseases or one? Mayo Clin Proc 1978, 53:634.

Fauci AF, et al: Radiation therapy of midline granuloma. Ann Intern Med 1976, 84:140.

Kornblut AD, et al: Idiopathic midline granuloma. Otolaryngol Clin North Am 1982, 15:685.

Lober CW, et al: Midline granuloma, Stewart type. Arch Dermatol 1982, 118:52.

Tsokos M, et al: Idiopathic midline destructive disease. Am J Clin Pathol 1982, 77:162.

SARCOIDOSIS

Sarcoidosis has also been known as *Besnier-Boeck-Schaumann disease*: Boeck's *sarcoid,* Besnier's *lupus pernio,* and Schaumann's *benign lymphogranulomatosis.* Jonathan Hutchinson described this disease in 1869.

Sarcoidosis is a systemic granulomatous disease of undetermined etiology and pathogenesis, which involves the skin and many of the internal organs with a persistent course interrupted by remissions and relapses.

The disease begins at a mean age of 39 in "classic" sarcoidosis, and nearly two thirds of patients are women. In addition to the skin, which is involved in about one fourth of cases, other sites of involvement are lungs, mediastinal and peripheral lymph nodes, eyes, phalangeal bones, myocardium, central nervous system, kidneys, spleen, liver, and parotid glands. In a study of sarcoidosis in Danish Caucasians, 50 of 188 patients fulfilled all of the criteria of D. G. James et al for the diagnosis, but had no demonstrable systemic involvement.

SKIN MANIFESTATIONS. The cutaneous manifestations of sarcoidosis are quite varied, and several morphological lesions have been described—papules, nodules, plaques, subcutaneous nodules, and scar sarcoidosis; erythroderma; ulcerations; and verrucose, ichthyosiform, hypomelanotic, psoriasiform, and alopecic lesions. The lesions are usually multiple and firm and elastic when palpated, and extend deeply to involve the entire thickness of the dermis. The overlying epidermis may be slightly thinned, discolored, telangiectatic, or scaly. The color is faint, showing dull tints of red, purple, brown, or yellow according to the stage of development. Usually the lesions are asymptomatic, but approximately 10 to 15 per cent of patients itch.

Cutaneous involvement may be classified as specific skin lesions, which reveal granulomas on biopsy, or nonspecific lesions, which are mainly reaction patterns, such as erythema nodosum.

Papular Sarcoid. This type of eruption is characteristic in generalized sarcoidosis, in which small papules are predominant. This is also known as *miliary sarcoid.* The papules are especially numerous over the face, eyelids, neck, and shoulders. Lichenification and central pitting are sometimes present. In time the lesions involve to faint macules. The

lesions may resemble syringoma, xanthelasma, lichen planus, or trichoepithelioma.

Hypopigmented Sarcoidosis. Hypopigmentation, which may be the earliest sign of sarcoidosis in blacks, was reported in a West Indian by Thomas et al in 1981. It is more common than is reported.

Lupus Pernio. These are violaceous smooth and shiny plaques on the acral portions of the body: ears, forehead, nose, fingers, and toes. Lupus pernio is frequently associated with granulomas in the bones (punched-out cysts). These cysts are present most commonly in the fingers. Spiteri et al reported 35 patients from a total of 818 sarcoid patients. Those with lupus pernio were commonly women in their fourth or fifth decade of life, and it was associated with other forms of chronic fibrotic sarcoid, especially upper respiratory tract lesions. The skin lesions rarely involute.

Psoriasiform Sarcoidosis. These skin lesions consist of sharply delineated plaques upon which a psoriasiform scaling is present. The trunk and extremities are usually involved.

Verrucose Sarcoidosis. The rare occurrence of exuberant verrucose lesions as the exclusive cutaneous sign of sarcoidosis has been reported only in black patients.

Ulcerative Sarcoidosis. Though Boeck said in 1899 that exudation and ulceration "never take place," a

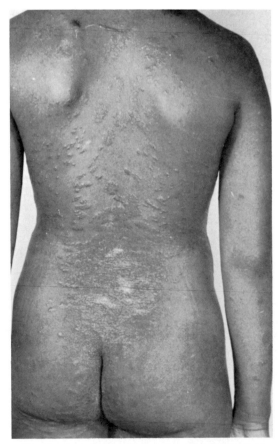

Figure 31–10. Sarcoid, papular type. (Courtesy of Dr. C.T. Nelson.)

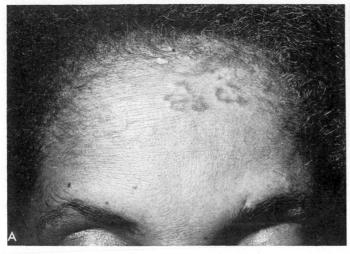

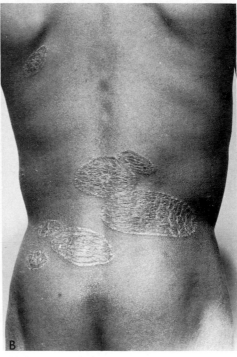

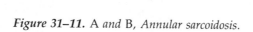

Figure 31–11. A and B, *Annular sarcoidosis.*

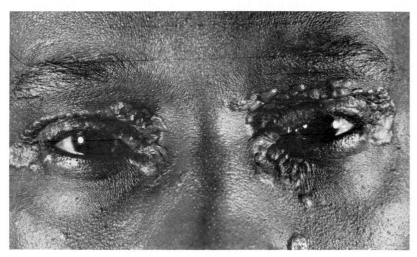

Figure 31–12. Sarcoidosis. *(Courtesy of Dr. H. Shatin.)*

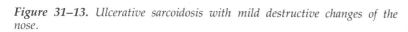

Figure 31–13. Ulcerative sarcoidosis with mild destructive changes of the nose.

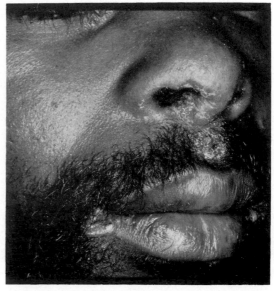

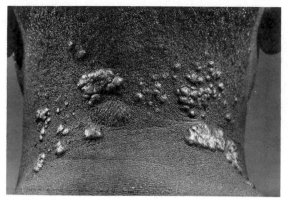

Figure 31–14. Sarcoidosis resembling acne keloidalis nuchae. *(Courtesy of Dr. H. Shatin.)*

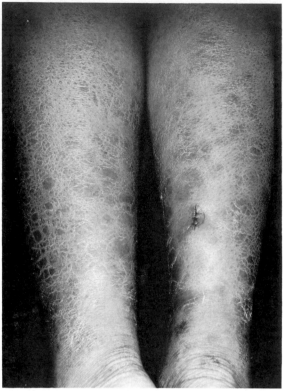

Figure 31–16. Sarcoidosis presenting as acquired ichthyosis.

half-dozen authors, such as Hzura et al, Verdegem et al, Mitchell et al, and Schwartz et al, have described ulcerative lesions in sarcoidosis.

Subcutaneous Sarcoidosis. This is better known as *Darier-Roussy sarcoid* and consists of a few 1–3-cm deep-seated nodules on the trunk and extremities; only rarely do they appear on the face. The lesions are usually attached to the overlying skin. The epidermis may be slightly violaceous. Only biopsy can distinguish these from LE profundus. Five percent or fewer patients with sarcoidosis have subcutaneous nodules; most of these have acute sarcoidosis and have a favorable prognosis for early disease involution. Vainsencher et al reviewed this form of sarcoidosis and reported four cases in 1984, and Kalb et al reported six cases in 1988.

Sarcoidosis in Scars. Sarcoid lesions may develop in old scars from various sources of trauma such as

burns, folliculitis, and herpes zoster. These lesions closely resemble keloids. Ivor Caro reviewed scar sarcoidosis in 1983 and Bisaccia et al reported a case with lesions occurring in zoster scars in the same year.

Hutchinson's Plaques. These distinctive lesions, first reported by Hutchinson, consist of flat-surfaced, slightly elevated, large, lobulated, nodular plaques, which appear with greatest frequency on the cheeks, the nose, and the arms, in a symmetrical fashion.

Erythrodermic Sarcoidosis. Rarely a diffuse infiltrative erythroderma of the skin is seen in sarcoidosis. The eruption usually begins as erythematous, scaling patches on the extremities. While Banse-Kupin et al could document only nine cases in their literature review, it appears to be much more common than reported.

Ichthyosiform Sarcoidosis. Scaling patches, usually of the lower extremities, will often yield granulomatous infiltrates, even when no clinically evident nodularity is present.

Mucosal Sarcoid. The lesions in the mouth are characterized by pinhead-size papules, which may be grouped and fused together to form a flat plaque. A frequent site is the hard palate, where violaceous papules may be present. The uvula and tonsillar pillars may also be involved. The palpebral conjunctiva may be the site of such papules.

Erythema Nodosum in Sarcoidosis. Sarcoidosis may first appear with fever, polyarthralgia, uveitis, bilateral hilar adenopathy, fatigue, and erythema

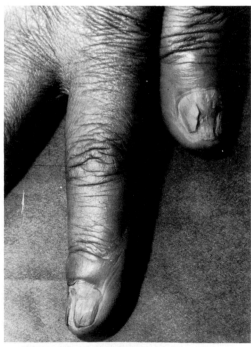

Figure 31–15. Sarcoidosis of the nail beds.

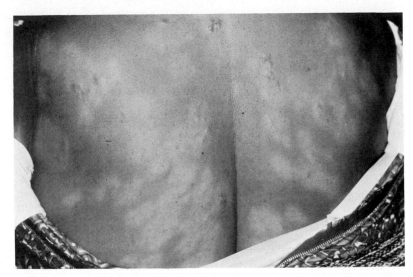

Figure 31–17. Hypopigmented sarcoidosis. (Courtesy of Dr. K. Stein.)

nodosum. This combination, known as *Löfgren's syndrome*, occurs frequently in Scandinavian Caucasian cases, is uncommon in American blacks, and is associated with a good prognosis, involuting within six months of onset in 80 per cent of cases. These typical red, hot, and tender nodes in the skin are distinctive and are most frequently seen on the shins of young women. The face, upper back, and extensor surfaces of the upper extremities may be involved. There is a strikingly elevated erythrocyte sedimentation rate, frequently above 50 mm in the first hour. The histologic features of these skin lesions are those of erythema nodosum.

Other Skin Lesions. Subcutaneous calcium deposits, prurigo, and erythema multiforme have also been noted in association with sarcoidosis. Golitz and associates reported four women with cicatricial alopecia due to sarcoidosis. Greer has reported palmar and follicular lesions, nonscarring alopecia, and widespread plaques in sarcoidosis, all identified only by biopsy. Diestelmeir et al reported a patient whose presenting sign was eyelid swelling. Scott et al reported nodular lesions of the palms and soles. Occasionally nail dystrophy may occur, as described by Patel. Rasmussen reviewed sarcoidosis in children under age six and reported that a characteristic triad of involvement of the skin, joints, and eyes is a common combination in this subset of patients.

Systemic Sarcoidosis. Many instances of sarcoidosis are asymptomatic, and it is only when routine x-rays of the chest reveal some abnormality that sarcoidosis is suspected. Fever may be the only symptom of the disease. In other instances the disease begins insidiously, with fever, weight loss, fatigue, and malaise.

Pulmonary changes are common in sarcoidosis. The changes, usually bilateral, consist of large dense shadows with extensions radiating outward and with reticulation of the lower lobes. The large dense shadows may resemble metastatic tumor. Hilar adenopathy is usually present. Hilar adenopathy alone is often associated with a good prognosis; however,

chronic pulmonary fibrosis, associated with lupus pernio, rarely involutes. *Aspergillus* mycetoma may complicate pulmonary parenchymal cysts.

Lymphadenopathy, especially of the mediastinal and hilar nodes, and generalized adenopathy, or adenopathy confined to the cervical or axillary areas, may be an initial sign of sarcoidosis. Intrathoracic lesions, including lung lesions and hilar adenopathy, are the most common manifestation of the disease.

Osseous involvement is often present. The more characteristic changes are found radiographically in the bones of the hands and feet, particularly in the distal phalanges, and consist of round punched-out spots. These are seen frequently in patients with lupus pernio. These cystlike lesions consist of masses of epithelioid cells similar to those found in the cutaneous lesions.

Ocular involvement is present in some 25 to 30 per cent of patients, with granulomatous uveitis the most frequent lesion. The lacrimal gland may be involved unilaterally or bilaterally by painless nodular swellings. With lacrimal gland changes there may be associated enlargement of the submaxillary, salivary, and cervical lymph glands, or the parotid glands may become involved (*Mikulicz's syndrome*). Lesions of the iris are nodular and painless. Large keratotic precipitates of "mutton fat" type may occur. There may also be lesions of the retina, choroid, sclera, and optic nerve. Ophthalmic disease is highly correlated with systemic involvement.

Parotid gland and lacrimal gland enlargement with uveitis and fever may occur in sarcoidosis; this is known as *uveoparotid fever* or *Heerfordt's syndrome* and usually lasts two to six months if not treated. Facial nerve palsy and central nervous system disease frequently are seen in this syndrome.

Liver involvement occurs in about 20 per cent of patients clinically; however, a blind liver biopsy will reveal granulomas in 60 per cent of cases. Hepatic tubercles, hepatomegaly with marked elevation of serum alkaline phosphatase, biliary cirrhosis with hypercholesterolemia, and portal hypertension with esophageal varices are some of the manifestations. Liver biopsy showing hepatic tubercles is an excellent means of confirming the diagnosis of sarcoidosis.

Kidney involvement produces impaired function as a result of hypercalcemia. Nephrolithiasis may result.

Other sites may be involved. Among these are the heart, with primary myocardial sarcoidosis; the spleen, with hypersplenism; the muscles, with sarcoidal granulomas; the joints, with chronic migratory arthritis and transient effusions; and the nervous system, with peripheral and central nervous system involvement.

LABORATORY FINDINGS. Most patients with sarcoidosis have an increased erythrocyte sedimentation rate, leukopenia, and eosinophilia; rarely, thrombocytopenia, hypercalcemia, and hyperproteinemia may occur.

The serum level of angiotensin-converting enzyme (ACE) was shown by Lieberman in 1975 to be elevated in 15 of 17 patients with untreated sarcoidosis. Shultz et al confirmed this, but showed that false positive tests are common; they found 11 elevations among 47 patients who did not have sarcoidosis. Hara et al found ACE levels to be high in all granulomatous skin disease, but not in other types of inflammatory lesions. Callen and Hannó found a normal ACE level cannot be used to rule out sarcoidosis, and that an elevated level did not necessarily indicate the presence of multisystem involvement. Nosal and associates state that the combination of an assay of antiotensin-converting enzyme and gallium scan increases diagnostic specificity without sacrificing sensitivity.

Elevated serum proteins occur because of increased serum globulin. The elevated alpha-2, beta, and gamma globulins may produce a steplike electrophoretic pattern. With liver or bone lesions, serum alkaline phosphatase is usually elevated.

If hypercalcemia is present, severe anorexia, vomiting, muscle weakness, and polyuria may occur as a result of the severe renal involvement. This occurs most frequently in men, and is felt to be due to increased gastrointestinal absorption of calcium secondary to hypersensitivity to vitamin D.

X-ray studies will frequently show hilar adenopathy and the typical "punched-out" lesions of the distal phalanges.

Pulmonary function tests of vital capacity and oxygen and carbon dioxide diffusing capacity often show early changes in pulmonary sarcoidosis.

An electrocardiogram may provide evidence of an arrhythmia or heart block.

IMMUNOLOGIC ABNORMALITIES. Cell-mediated immune responses in sarcoidosis (Daniele et al) are altered in the following respects: skin-test responses are lost or at least diminished; the proliferative response of lymphocytes to antigens and mitogens is reduced; circulating T helper cells are reduced more than the suppressor cells are increased, with resulting lymphocytopenia; activated T cells are increased.

Humoral (B cell) reactions are increased, with polyclonal elevation of serum immunoglobulin; there is an exaggerated humoral response to certain antigens; serum antibodies to *Mycoplasma* and several viruses are increased; circulating immune complexes occur in the blood in about half the patients with acute disease; autoantibodies to rheumatoid factor, antinuclear antibody, and T cells occur.

D. G. James points out that all this suggests a vigorous host defense against a still unrecognized antigen.

The Kveim-Siltzbach test is performed by the intradermal injection of 0.2 ml Kveim antigen in the forearm. The site is identified for future reference by measuring the distance from the distal crease of the wrist. The antigen is a 10 per cent suspension of proved sarcoid tissue in normal saline solution. After six weeks the site of injection is excised for histologic examination. The presence of typical "naked" epithelioid cell tubercles signifies a positive Kveim reaction.

The Kveim reaction is expected to be positive in about 80 per cent of active cases of sarcoidosis. The test becomes negative when the patient goes into remission. The test is quite specific for sarcoidosis, with only 2 per cent false positives. It is not usually performed in the United States.

ETIOLOGY. That this is a form of tuberculosis has been suspected for many years. It was suggested in 1963 by Mankiewicz that certain mycobacteria may be at least one of the causes of sarcoidosis. She postulated that certain lysogenic mutants of tubercle bacilli may be the cause of sarcoidosis.

A variety of other organisms and substances causing granulomatous reactions has been considered. Some of these have been fungi, *Mycobacterium leprae*, zirconium, beryllium, pine pollen, and microresin-containing hair sprays.

The cause of sarcoidosis remains elusive. It appears to be a reaction to an as yet unidentified antigen or infectious agent. A genetic predisposition may play a part. Sarcoidosis is rare in Hawaii, and cutaneous sarcoidosis almost unknown. Arnold identified only one case in 45 years there.

INCIDENCE AND EPIDEMIOLOGY. Sarcoidosis occurs worldwide. In Europe it is most prevalent in the Scandinavian countries, especially in Sweden, where up to 140 cases per 100,000 occur in certain rural forested areas. In the United States the southeastern states and certain areas in New York City show the largest incidence. The rarity of sarcoidosis in Hawaii is unexplained.

Sarcoidosis has been found to be most prevalent in American blacks; however, Orientals and Caucasians also have the disease. The disease is seen usually between the ages of 20 and 40 years and is predominant in women among blacks; there is no sex predominance in whites. Sarcoidosis shows definite familial aggregation attributable to genetic factors, as it is more common among siblings than spouses. Children may also have sarcoidosis. The average age is 13 years, with a sex ratio of 1:1. In a comparison of the occurrence of sarcoidosis in London and New York, James found women outnumbering men two to one in New York, whereas in London women made up only 56 per cent of the cases.

HISTOLOGY. The characteristic finding is that of the "naked tubercle" composed of islands of large, pale-staining, epithelioid cells intermingled with histiocytes, lymphocytes, and Langhans giant cells. Sometimes the cells are spread diffusely, sometimes they occur in strands or groups; however, the tubercle arrangement is characteristic and is present in at least some parts of the lesion. The predominance of epithelioid cells and the scarcity of lymphocytes, the sparseness or absence of Langhans giant cells, or their poor development, and the lack of caseation necrosis at the centers of the granulomas are important features. There is also an absence of inflammatory reaction in the surrounding tissue.

Occasionally asteroid inclusion bodies, residual bodies, or *Schaumann bodies,* are found in the giant cells. The Schaumann bodies contain calcium and have alkaline phosphatase activity.

At times distinction must be made between sarcoidosis and tuberculoid leprosy. The histologic demonstration of nerve invasion occurs only in tuberculoid leprosy, and lymphocytes are more abundant around the tubercles in leprosy than they are in sarcoidosis. However, absence of anesthesia in the lesions of sarcoid is the most conclusive differential point.

DIAGNOSIS. The diagnosis may be established by the demonstration of systemic involvement consistent with sarcoidosis, a histologic picture of sarcoidosis, and a positive Kveim test. Any two of these factors suffice for a positive diagnosis.

Evaluation of a patient suspected of having sarcoidosis should include a complete history and physical examination, slit-lamp examination, electrocardiogram, serum and 24-hour urine calcium examination, serum protein electrophoresis, serum angiotensin-converting enzyme level, skin tests for anergy and evaluation for tuberculosis, and, of course, biopsy of any skin lesions not incompatible with sarcoid.

Referral for the evaluation of pulmonary function is appropriate in all patients whose chest x-ray shows intrathoracic involvement by the disease. As Bower points out, pulmonary involvement may be asymptomatic. Gallium scan, conjunctival biopsy, scalene node biopsy, or biopsy of minor salivary glands, skeletal muscle, lung, liver, or spleen are potentially supplemental to evaluation by an internist, and may afford a positive diagnosis.

DIFFERENTIAL DIAGNOSIS. Chiefly in Scandinavian countries, an erythrodermic form of Boeck's sarcoid occurs in which many of the lesions are surrounded by a bluish border, suggesting the lilac ring of scleroderma. The lesions of tuberculoid leprosy or syphilis may at times clinically resemble

sarcoid and, histologically, there may be a sarcoid type of reaction in these diseases. Sarcoid must also be differentiated from malignant lymphoma and from lupus vulgaris, lymphadenosis benigna cutis of Bäfverstedt, and leishmaniasis of the lupoid type. Sarcoid reactions in which the lesions are localized, especially to the sites of possible trauma or to foreign bodies, should also be considered. Generalized granuloma annulare may mimic cutaneous sarcoidosis. Frieden et al reported a *granulomatous perioral dermatitis* in children: tiny euchromic papules showing a granulomatous tissue reaction on biopsy. None had systemic involvement, and all lesions resolved spontaneously within months to years.

TREATMENT. The uneven course of the disease makes therapy difficult to evaluate. Lupus pernio, because of its chronic course, is the best measure of success of treatment. Disfiguring skin lesions represent the only indication for systemic steroid treatment for cutaneous disease alone. In acute sarcoidosis, on the other hand, 80 to 90 per cent spontaneous resolution may be expected, so therapy is seldom indicated.

The corticosteroids in both topical and systemic forms are helpful in sarcoidosis by suppressing the inflammatory reaction and producing symptomatic relief. Corticosteroid therapy is indicated when there is acute systemic involvement with fever and weight loss, in active eye disease, in sarcoidal involvement of the myocardium, in active pulmonary disease with functional disability, in hypersplenism, in hypercalcemia, and in symptomatic central nervous system involvement. When the skin involvement is the only manifestation, corticosteroids are generally not used and only careful observation is indicated unless the skin lesions are disfiguring. Hillerdal et al confirmed this conclusion by a 15-year study in Sweden; longterm benefit from corticosteroid therapy, they said, remains to be proved. It is notably effective only in uveitis, arthritis, and hypercalcemia.

The skin lesions respond readily to intralesional corticosteroids. The place of immunosuppressives such as methotrexate and azathioprine is not yet certain, but Fanburg says they have no substantial advantages over oral prednisone. Veien and Brodthagen concluded that methotrexate is a useful alternative to systemically administered glucocorticoids in the treatment of disfiguring cutaneous sarcoidosis and sarcoid uveitis.

Antimalarials, especially chloroquine (Aralen) in doses of 250 mg twice or three times daily, have not produced uniformly favorable results. The hazard of irreversible eye damage with the prolonged use of chloroquine has limited its use. But it is worth trying, as James has emphasized, if steroids are inadvisable, especially in lupus pernio cases.

Waldinger et al reported a patient who responded to isotretinoin. This and other reports of isolated responses (to allopurinol, e.g.) require confirmation before they can be recommended. Certainly vitamin D and ultraviolet light should be avoided for fear of hypercalcemia, and total-block sunscreens might be helpful if sun exposure is inevitable for any reason.

While sarcoidosis is rarely fatal, a heart lesion may cause cardiac arrest, the most common lethal event. Morbidity due to eye, skin, joint, renal, pulmonary, or central nervous system involvement may be severe.

Banse-Kupin L, et al: Ichthyosiform sarcoidosis. JAAD 1987, 17:616.

Bisaccia E, et al: Cutaneous sarcoid granuloma formation in herpes zoster scars. Arch Dermatol 1983, 119:788.

Bower JS: Pulmonary evaluation of patients presenting with cutaneous manifestations of sarcoidosis. Int J Dermatol 1981, 20:385.

Buechner SA, et al: T-cell subsets in cutaneous sarcoidosis. Arch Dermatol 1983, 119:728.

Callen JP, et al: Serum angiotensin I–converting enzyme level in patients with cutaneous sarcoidal granuloma. Arch Dermatol 1982, 118:232.

Idem: Sarcoidosis. In Cutaneous Aspects of Internal Medicine. Callen JP (ed.) Chicago, Year Book Medical Publishers, Inc., pp. 311–22, 1981.

Caro I: Scar sarcoidosis. Cutis 1983, 32:531.

Chapelon C, et al: Sarcoidosis (letter). JAMA 1986, 255:2024.

Daniele RP: Immunologic abnormalities in sarcoidosis. Ann Intern Med 1980, 92:406.

DeRemee RA, et al: Serum angiotensin-converting enzyme activity in evaluating the clinical course of sarcoidosis. Ann Intern Med 1980, 92:361.

Diestelmeier MR, et al: Sarcoidosis manifesting as eyelid swelling. Arch Dermatol 1982, 118:356.

Epstein WL: What begot Boeck? Arch Dermatol 1982, 118:721.

Greer KE, et al: Unusual manifestations of sarcoidosis. South Med J 1977, 70:666.

Hara A, et al: Tissue angiotensin-converting enzyme and lysosomal enzyme levels in skin diseases. Arch Dermatol 1982, 118:468.

Hillerdal G, et al: Sarcoidosis: epidemiology and prognosis. Am Rev Resp Dis 1984, 130:29.

Hruza GJ, et al: Generalized atrophic sarcoidosis with ulcerations. Arch Dermatol 1986, 122:320.

James DG, et al: Immunology of sarcoidosis. Am J Med 1982, 72:5.

Kalb RE, et al: Sarcoidosis with subcutaneous nodules. Am J Med 1988, 85:731.

Kerdel FA, et al: Sarcoidosis: an updated review. JAAD 1984, 11:1.

Lieberman J: Elevation of serum angiotensin-converting enzyme (ACE) level in sarcoidosis. Am J Med 59:365, 1975.

Mitchell IC, et al: Ulcerative and hypopigmented sarcoidosis. JAAD 1986, 15:1062.

Nosal A, et al: Angiotensin-converting enzyme and gallium scan in noninvasive evaluation of sarcoidosis. Ann Intern Med 1979, 90:328.

Olive KE, et al: Cutaneous manifestations of sarcoidosis. Arch Intern Med 1985, 145:1811.

Paller AS, et al: Cutaneous sarcoidosis associated with sarcoidosis of the upper airway. Arch Dermatol 1983, 119:592.

Patel KB, et al: Nails in sarcoidosis. Arch Dermatol 1983, 119:272.

Rasmussen JE: Sarcoidosis in young children. JAAD 1981, 5:566.

Sahn EE: Pruritic white papules in a pregnant woman. Arch Dermatol 1987, 123:1557.

Schwartz RA, et al: Generalized ulcerative sarcoidosis. Arch Dermatol 1982, 118:931.

Scott TH, et al: Sarcoidosis with nodular lesions of the palm and sole. Arch Dermatol 1984, 120:1239.

Spiteri MA, et al: Lupus pernio. Br J Dermatol 1985, 112:315.

Thestrup-Pedersen K, et al: Serum angiotensin-converting enzyme in sarcoidosis and psoriasis. Arch Dermatol Res 1985, 277:16.

Thomas RHM, et al: Hypopigmented sarcoidosis. J R Soc Med 1981, 74:921.

Vainsencher D, et al: Subcutaneous sarcoidosis. Arch Dermatol 1984, 120:1028.

Veien NK: Cutaneous sarcoidosis treated with methotrexate. Br J Dermatol 1977, 97:213.

Idem: Cutaneous sarcoidosis: prognosis and treatment. Clin Dermatol 1986, 4:75.

Idem: Cutaneous sarcoidosis in Caucasians. JAAD 1987, 16:534.

Verdegem TD, et al: Cutaneous ulcers in sarcoidosis. Arch Dermatol 1987, 123:1531.

Waldinger TP, et al: Treatment of cutaneous sarcoidosis with isotretinoin. Arch Dermatol 1983, 119:1003.

Weltfriend S, et al: Subcutaneous sarcoidosis in a patient with malignant carcinoid tumor of the colon. JAAD 1989, 20:507.

RECURRENT GRANULOMATOUS DERMATITIS WITH EOSINOPHILIA (Wells's Syndrome)

Wells described in 1971 four patients with acute eosinophilic cellulitis followed in a few days by the formation of an indolent, infiltrative, granulomatous dermal and subcutaneous mass, persisting for many weeks and finally involuting. In the granulomatous phase, dermal eosinophils and histiocytes are seen around central masses of fibrinoid and collagen, which form what Spigel and Winkelmann call "flame figures." In the final stage the histology is characterized by histiocytic necrobiosis, with persistence of the flame figures.

Wood et al, defining flame figures as discrete foci of extracellular granules of eosinophils adherent to, and altering the staining of, collagen fibers, reported these in five cases unlike Wells's syndrome, and Schorr et al reported them in five cases of arthropod bites (two ticks, one bee, one spider, and one mosquito). Three of their cases had features strongly suggesting erythema chronicum migrans. Steffen, in an editorial, emphasized that flame figures are not peculiar to Wells's syndrome; they occur in many skin lesions. A classic case was reported in 1984 by Mitchell et al, responsive to hydroxyzine and prednisone, but recurrent intermittently on several occasions during the next four or five months.

Fisher et al reviewed the 22 published cases and added two of their own. One of their cases (and one previous case) cleared on dapsone after doing poorly on prednisone.

Aberer W, et al: Wells' syndrome is a distinctive disease entity and not a histologic diagnosis. JAAD 1988, 18:105.

Brehmer-Andersson E, et al: The histogenesis of the flame figure in Wells' syndrome based on five cases. Acta Derm Venereol (Stockh) 1986, 66:213.

Burket JM, et al: Eosinophilic panniculitis. JAAD 1985, 12:161.

Dijkstra JWE, et al: Eosinophilic cellulitis associated with urticaria. JAAD 1986, 14:32.

Fisher GB, et al: Eosinophilic cellulitis (Wells's syndrome). Int J Dermatol 1985, 24:101.

Mitchell AJ, et al: Recurrent granulomatous dermatitis with eosinophilia: Wells's syndrome. Int J Dermatol 1984, 23:198.

Steffen C: Eosinophilic cellulitis (editorial). Am J Dermatopathol 1986, 8:185.

Wells GC: Recurrent granulomatous dermatitis with eosinophilia. Trans St Johns Hosp Dermatol Soc 1971, 57:46.

JUVENILE XANTHOGRANULOMA

McDonagh in 1906 named this benign disorder nevoxanthoendothelioma. Helwig renamed it *juvenile xanthogranuloma*. It is characterized by the appearance at birth (30 per cent of cases) or in the first few months of life of one, or oftener many, yellow, reddish yellow, or brown 4–20-mm papules or nodules on the face, scalp, trunk, and, mostly, the extensor surfaces. Approximately 25 cases have been reported as beginning in adulthood. Rarely the lesions are generalized. Xanthogranulomas may become large tumors 4 or more cm in diameter. In another type the lesions are rough, semiglobular infiltrations.

Internal manifestations may develop in skeletal muscle, salivary gland, stomach, periosteum, pericardium, myocardium, the meninges, testes, and an eye. Eye involvement consists of lesions in the iris or bulb. Flach et al and Ringel et al have reviewed the extracutaneous manifestations. Uncommonly there is an association with neurofibromatosis and, as Cooper et al reported, with chronic juvenile myeloid leukemia.

The skin lesions usually disappear without treatment. The usual course is spontaneous remission in three to six years. Blood lipid values are normal.

The histopathology varies in accordance with the stage of the lesion. In very early lesions there may be only an infiltration of histiocytic cells without any lipid infiltration. Usually the histiocytes have a pale, vacuolated cytoplasm that stains positive with fat stains. S-100 stains are negative. In mature lesions, foam cells are found. Multinucleated foam cells (Touton giant cells) and foreign-body giant cells are also present. Fibrosis occurs in the older lesions. The inflammatory infiltrate is sparse, consisting of a few lymphocytes and eosinophils. The absence of plasma cells and lymphophagocytosis histologically, and of lymphadenopathy clinically, distinguish it from sinus

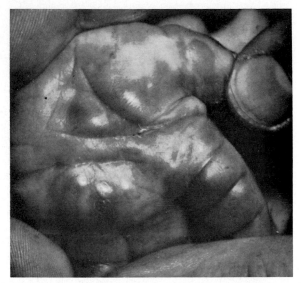

Figure 31–19. Juvenile xanthogranuloma on palm of 6-month-old child.

histiocytosis with massive lymphadenopathy, which it otherwise closely resembles histologically.

Campbell L, et al: Giant juvenile xanthogranuloma. Arch Dermatol 1988, 124:1723.
Cooper PH, et al: Association of juvenile xanthogranuloma with juvenile myeloid leukemia. Arch Dermatol 1984, 120:371.
Flach DB, et al: Juvenile xanthogranuloma with central nervous system lesions. JAAD 1986, 14:405.
Gianotti F, et al: Histiocytic syndromes. JAAD 1955, 13:383.
Helwig EB, et al: Juvenile xanthogranuloma. Am J Pathol 1954, 30:625.
Jensen NE, et al: Naevoxanthoendothelioma and neurofibromatosis. Br J Dermatol 1971, 85:326.
Newell GB, et al: Juvenile xanthogranuloma and neurofibromatosis. Arch Dermatol 1973, 102:262.
Rodriquez J, et al: Xanthogranuloma in adults. Arch Dermatol 1976, 112:43.
Sonoda T, et al: Juvenile xanthogranulomas. Cancer 1985, 56:2280.
Webster SB, et al: Juvenile xanthogranuloma with extracutaneous lesions. Arch Dermatol 1966, 93:71.

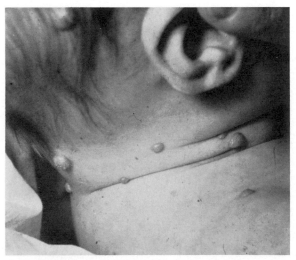

Figure 31–18. Juvenile xanthogranuloma on neck and scalp.

NECROBIOTIC XANTHOGRANULOMA

Kossard and Winkelmann described eight cases of this distinctive entity in 1980. The skin lesions present as sharply demarcated, indurated plaques and nodules, which are usually yellow and have a predilection for the periorbital area, trunk, and proximal extremities. These inflammatory lesions often ulcerate, leading to atrophic scarring. There is always an accompanying monoclonal IgG paraproteinemia, and it thus joins a list of cutaneous diseases that should alert the clinician to the possible presence of a paraprotein. These conditions include amyloidosis, angioimmunoblastic lymphadenopathy, pyoderma gangrenosum, generalized plane xanthoma, scleromyxedema, hyperglobulinemic purpura, and Raynaud's phenomenon.

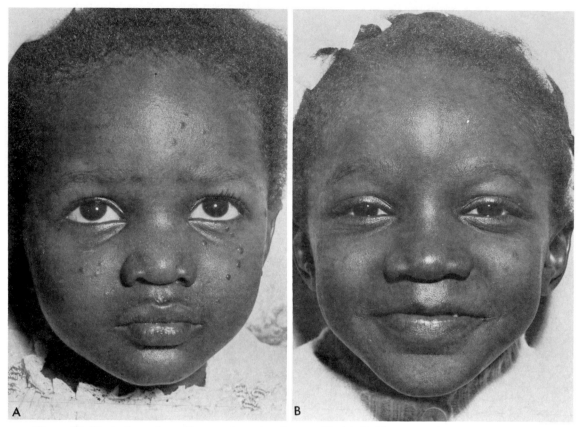

Figure 31–20. A, *Juvenile xanthogranuloma in a 3-year-old girl.* B, *Three years later with no treatment.*

The biopsy reveals intense necrobiosis with a diffuse granulomatous infiltrate of Touton giant cells, foreign body giant cells, foam cells, and lymphocytes. The course is chronic and progressive. Treatment options, which have generally met with limited success, are systemic steroids, cytotoxic drugs, and plasmapheresis.

Finan MC, et al: Necrobiotic xanthogranuloma with paraproteinemia. Medicine (Baltimore) 1986, 65:376.
Finelli LS, et al: Plasmapheresis, a treatment modality for necrobiotic xanthogranuloma. JAAD 1987, 17:351.
Furner BB, et al: Diffuse, ulcerating plaques and nodules. Arch Dermatol 1989, 125:287.
Holden CA, et al: Necrobiotic xanthogranuloma. Br J Dermatol 1986, 114:241.
Kossard S, et al: Necrobiotic xanthogranuloma. Austral J Dermatol 1980, 21:85.
Venencie PY, et al: Necrobiotic xanthogranuloma with myeloma. Cancer 1987, 59:588.

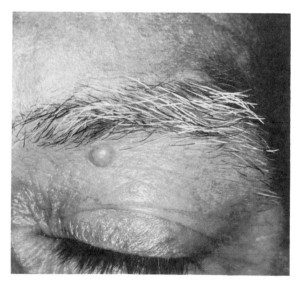

Figure 31–21. Solitary juvenile xanthogranuloma on the upper eyelid of an adult male.

MALIGNANT HISTIOCYTOSIS
(Histiocytic Medullary Reticulosis)

This rare, often fatal, malignant reticulosis is characterized by the acute onset of a widespread papular and nodular skin eruption in about 10 per cent of cases, according to Morgan et al. Marshall et al found that 13 per cent of reported cases had skin lesions. Fever and splenomegaly are usually present. Extensive erythrophagocytosis by histiocytes in marrow, liver, spleen, and lymph nodes is classically seen although it is not often seen in the skin. Skin biopsy early in the course of disease may make the diagnosis when malignant histiocytes are present in the dermis, as in Stone et al's case.

Grönhagen-Riska et al showed that angiotensin I–converting enzyme may be elevated.

Tseng et al reported 22 patients treated with cyclophosphamide, doxorubicin, vincristine, and prednisone ("CHOP"), with complete remission in 68 per cent. The best indicator of prognosis was the platelet count: if it was below 150,000/mm^3, patients did badly. With other treatment, or none, patients usually die in a mean of six months. Grönhagen-Riska et al reported three-year survival in one of three patients (all of whom had elevated serum angiotensin I–converting enzyme levels) as a result of the same combined therapy, substituting methotrexate for doxorubicin. The enzyme levels fell to normal or lower in all three. The other two patients died. Morgan et al's five cases all died within two to seven months. Winkelmann et al's eight cases had an average survival time of 11.8 months.

Grönhagen-Riska, et al: Elevated angiotensin-I converting enzyme in histiocytic medullary reticulosis (letter). N Engl J Med 1983, 308:283.
James WD, et al: Malignant histiocytosis with cutaneous lesions and eosinophilia. J Assoc Milit Dermatol 1984, 10:16.
Marshall ME, et al: Cutaneous involvement in malignant histiocytosis. Arch Dermatol 1981, 117:278.
Morgan NE, et al: Clinical and pathological cutaneous manifestations of malignant histiocytosis. Arch Dermatol 1983, 119:367.
Stone MS, et al: Malignant histiocytosis. Cutis 1985, 34:42.

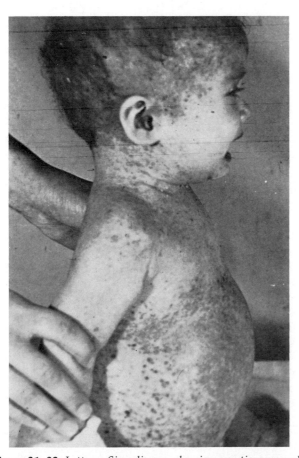

Figure 31–22. Letterer-Siwe disease, showing eruptions on scalp, neck and abdomen similar to seborrheic dermatitis, with protruding abdomen as result of hepatosplenomegaly. (Courtesy of Babies Hospital, New York.)

Tseng A, et al: Treatment of malignant histiocytosis. Blood 1984, 64:48.
Warnke RA, et al: Malignant histiocytosis. Cancer 1975, 35:215.

GRANULOMA GLUTEALE INFANTUM

Tappeiner and Pfleger described six cases of oval, cherry-to-plum–sized bluish red nodules in the diaper area of infants, lying in normal-looking skin. Similar lesions, confined to the buttocks, were described by Kelly and Campbell and by Bazex et al.

Histologically, hyperkeratosis and acanthosis are seen, with a polymorphonuclear infiltrate mixed with plasma cells, histiocytes, and macrophages throughout the dermis.

The etiology remains obscure. Bromidism and starch granules have been suspected. All reported patients have been on rather prolonged application of fluorinated corticosteroids for preexisting diaper eruption, and all slowly cleared on discontinuing the treatment.

Bazex A, et al: Infantile gluteal granuloma. Ann Dermat Syphiligr 1972, 99:121.
Bonifazi E, et al: Granuloma gluteale infantum with atrophic scars. Clin Exp Dermatol 1981, 6:23.
Kelly R, et al: Granuloma gluteale infantum with starch granules in the lesion. Med J Austral 1973, 2:438.
Tappeiner J, et al: Granuloma gluteale infantum. Hautarzt 1971, 22:383.

HISTIOCYTOSIS X
(L-Cell Granulomatosis)

Histiocytosis X is a disease characterized by a granulomatous proliferation of the Langerhans cells, identifiable in electronmicrographs by their unique racquet-shaped organelles, the Birbeck (Langerhans) granules, and by positive staining for S-100 protein, CD1, and CD4.

These disorders can involve the skin, bones, lungs, and nervous system as well as other organs. Several entities have been grouped under the heading of histiocytosis X, which have a great deal of overlap despite being separated into distinct entities in the following classification: Letterer-Siwe disease, Hand-Schüller-Christian disease, and eosinophilic granuloma.

The demonstration of the characteristic racquet-shaped organelles of Langerhans cells in the "histiocytes" in all three syndromes has proved that they are all manifestations of one basic disorder. Hermann Pinkus preferred the term "L-cell granulomatosis" to "histiocytosis X."

Esterly et al in 1985 reviewed 32 patients with histiocytosis X seen in seven years. Twelve had bone lesions only, and in three these were multifocal. The

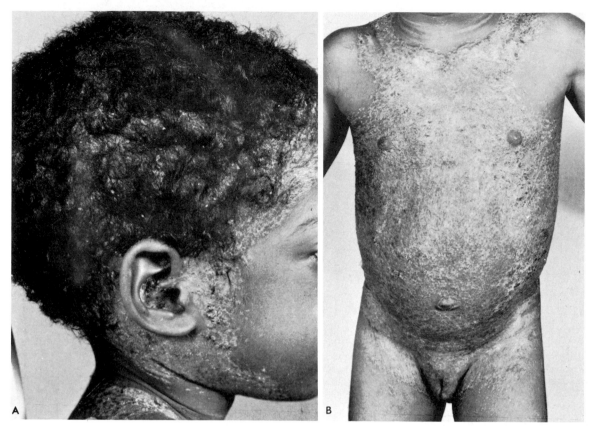

Figure 31–23. A and B, *Letterer-Siwe disease showing typical seborrheic dermatitis-like lesions. (Courtesy of Dr. N.B. Esterly.)*

youngest was eight months, the oldest, 15 years. Nine were treated by curettage, and two were irradiated, following which all were stable or in remission. Three had diabetes insipidus with exophthalmos in addition to bone lesions. These were irradiated and their diabetes insipidus controlled with vasopressin (Pitressin). All were stable or in remission. Seventeen had skin lesions, or visceral and bone lesions, or both. Ten of these received chemotherapy (two were also irradiated); two received prednisone only; one received radiation and

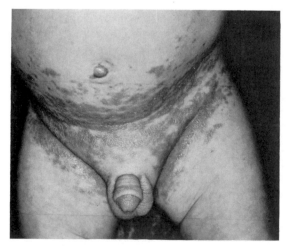

Figure 31–24. Letterer-Siwe disease in the diaper area. (Courtesy of Dr. T. Van Ravenswaay.)

intralesional steroid injections to bone lesions. Three received no therapy. Two died; three were lost to follow-up; the remainder were either improved with treatment, or well. Only one black was involved; 28 were white (nine of them Hispanic), three were Asian.

Purpura, including petechiae, is associated with a poorer prognosis. Lesions on the trunk may be suggestive of Darier's disease. Many patients have reddish, firm papules scattered over the trunk. Hurwitz regards purpuric nodules of the palms and soles as a grave prognostic sign. Timpatunapong et al reported nail lesions: onycholysis, subungual debris, and onychodystrophy. They regarded these as a poor prognostic sign. Holzberg et al found histologic signs of histiocytosis X in a baby who showed only nail dystrophy clinically.

The oral mucosa may show white plaques. Esterly et al state that gingival lesions should be looked for, and dental evaluation done, in all patients. Nodular infiltrates, necrosis, displaced teeth, and loss of alveolar bone are characteristic findings. Ulcerations and weeping eczematoid dermatitis are commonly present in major folds in late stages of the disease. Other lesions include vesicopustules and hemorrhagic lesions.

The etiology and pathogenesis of all forms of histiocytosis X are unknown.

TREATMENT. Corticosteroids, vinblastine, and x-ray therapy have all been helpful. Esterly et al recommend the following guidelines for therapy: Skin involvement only, observation. Extensive or severe skin involvement, oral prednisone only; if the response is poor, vinblastine. Solitary bone lesion, curettage or intralesional steroids. Multiple bone lesions, intralesional steroids with three-drug chemotherapy (vinblastine, prednisone, and methotrexate). For multiple bone or visceral lesions, or both, combination chemotherapy. Radiation therapy is reserved for nonresponders. This aggressive therapy is controversial: some experts, such as Greenberger et al, feel chemotherapy is unlikely to significantly change the course of the disease.

Zachariae reported that two infants with histiocytosis X responded well to topically applied mechlorethamine, 10 to 40 mg in 40 ml of saline. The only side effect was hyperpigmentation. Nethercott et al reported a sustained remission in one case with skin involvement only, and a six weeks' remission in another with systemic lesions, with this therapy.

Prognosis is guarded at the time of onset. The report by Esterly et al suggests that it is fairly good. Thorough clinical and laboratory evaluation, careful management and treatment, and meticulous follow-up are important. Bad prognostic signs, as reviewed by Timpatanapong et al, include onset under six months, extraosseous lesions, multiple organ involvement (especially lungs, liver, and bone marrow) and combined symptoms.

While there is a great deal of overlap among the subgroups of histiocytosis X, short discussions of the three classically described forms follow.

Letterer-Siwe Disease

Generally this subset of patients occurs in infants. It is aggressive, with widespread lesions in various organs such as the lungs, lymph nodes, liver, spleen, and bone marrow. Eighty percent develop cutaneous lesions, which consist of petechiae and papules. Crusted lesions in the scalp, groin, face, and trunk are common. Generally treatment in widespread disease consists of combination chemotherapy with vinblastine, methotrexate, and prednisone. Radiation therapy may be given in cases failing to respond to other measures. The prognosis is generally poor if the disease is extensive.

Hand-Schüller-Christian Type

This usually occurs in children, but may develop in adults. It is characterized by a triad of exophthalmos, diabetes insipidus, and defects in the membranous bones, especially of the skull. Cystic changes in the skull, mandible, or other parts of the entire skeletal system characterize the disease.

Cutaneous lesions are present in about one third of the patients. These may occur with eye and oral lesions. A diffuse icteric tint of yellowish or pale brown color is a typical manifestation. Different types of skin manifestations are attributed to this disorder. They are a bronze pigmentation, a maculopustular rash, a hemorrhagic eruption, seborrheic lesions, lipid infiltration of the eyelids, and ulcerations. There may be crusting of the scalp and a papular and crusted eruption on the trunk resembling seborrheic dermatitis or Darier's disease. Petechiae and larger purpuric spots and even hemorrhagic nodules have also been observed. Rarely, lesions resembling juvenile xanthogranuloma are seen.

Visceral lesions may occur in the liver, spleen, kidneys, brain, and lungs. Hepatosplenomegaly and lymph node enlargement may be present. Stomatitis, gingivitis, and growth abnormalities may also occur.

The disease runs a chronic progressive course that ends fatally in 20 to 50 per cent of cases, although spontaneous involution may also occur. Management of end-organ failure, and vasopressin for diabetes insipidus, are necessary. Due to its chronic course, chemotherapy should be only used judiciously, with prednisone and vinblastine being the most commonly used. Surgical treatment, intralesional steroids, and radiation in selected cases are useful in bone lesions.

Dolezal and Thomson successfully treated a 76-year-old woman with Hand-Schüller-Christian disease with daily applications of 10 mg of nitrogen mustard dissolved in 60 ml of water.

Eosinophilic Type (L-Cell Granuloma)

This disease affects children and young adults and is the most benign type of Langerhans histiocytosis. It is insidious and usually asymptomatic. It is characterized by granulomas of skin or rarely lungs, and osteolytic lesions, without other visceral involvement.

Cutaneous lesions are infrequent. They may consist of crusting of the scalp and one or more brownish red papules on the body, which may become hyperkeratotic, ulcerate, or coalesce to form tumorlike growths resembling the skin lesions of Letterer-Siwe or Hand-Schüller-Christian type. Periorificial involvement is characteristic. There may be ulcerations on the buccal mucosa as in the case reported by Hashimoto et al. Low-grade fever and spontaneous fractures may occur.

Histologic examination shows an inflammatory granuloma with histiocytic-appearing cells, foreign-body giant cells, and varying numbers of eosinophils and neutrophils; it is the presence of the latter in a chronic lesion, according to Pinkus and Mehregan, that is the most prominent and distinctive histologic feature.

The usual course of the disease is benign though often chronic; only rarely does a patient develop signs of fulminating Letterer-Siwe disease.

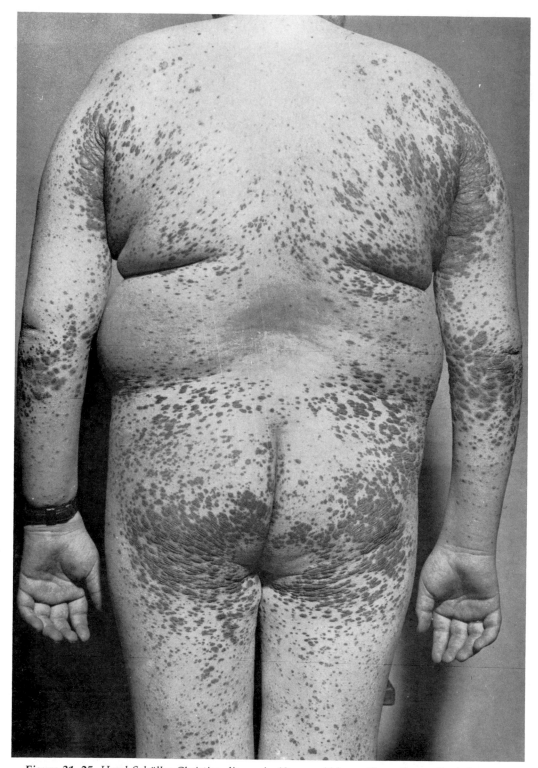

Figure 31–25. Hand-Schüller-Christian disease in 12-year-old boy with xanthoma disseminatum.

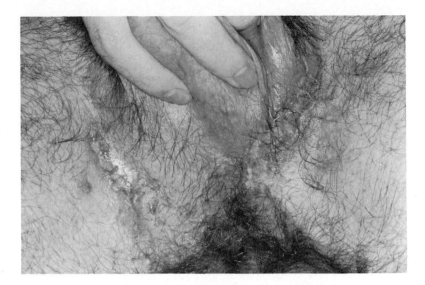

Figure 31–26. *Ulcerative lesions of eosinophilic granuloma in the inguinal folds of a young adult man.*

Treatment consists of curettage of the solitary granulomas, although in many instances the lesions remain unchanged for many years. Some cases, not suitable for curettage, respond well to x-ray treatment. Intralesional steroids may also be helpful.

Dufresne RG Jr, et al: Histiocytosis X mimicking the follicular occlusion syndrome. JAAD 1987, 16:385.

Esterly NB, et al: Histiocytosis X: a seven-year experience at a children's hospital. JAAD 1985, 13:481.

Favara BE, et al: Histiocytosis X. Hum Pathol 1983, 14:663.

Fitzpatrick R, et al: Histiocytosis X. Arch Dermatol 1981, 117:253.

Foucar E, et al: Urticating histiocytosis X. JAAD 1986, 14:867.

Gianotti F, et al: Histiocytic syndromes. JAAD 1985, 13:383.

Goldberg NS, et al: Histiocytosis X. Arch Dermatol 1986, 122:446.

Greenberger J, et al: Results of treatment of 127 patients with systemic histiocytosis (Letterer-Siwe syndrome, Schüller-Christian syndrome and multifocal eosinophilic granuloma). Medicine 1981, 60:311.

Groopman JE, et al: The histiocytic disorders. Ann Intern Med 1981, 94:95.

Harrist TJ, et al: In situ characterization of cutaneous infiltrates with monoclonal antibodies. Am J Clin Pathol 1983, 79:294.

Hashimoto K, et al: Eosinophilic granuloma. Arch Dermatol 1985, 121:770.

Holzberg M, et al: Nail pathology in histiocytosis X. JAAD 1985, 13:523.

Hurwitz S: Clinical Pediatric Dermatology. Philadelphia, W.B. Saunders Co., pp 424–427, 1981.

Ide F, et al: Immunohistochemical and ultrastructural analysis of the proliferating cells in histiocytosis X. Cancer 1984, 15:917.

Kashihara-Sawami M, et al: Letterer-Siwe disease. JAAD 1988, 18:646.

Kilpatrick RJ: Histiocytosis X. J Assoc Milit Dermatol 1980, 6:18.

Kobayashi T, et al: Granules of Langerhans cells in Letterer-Siwe's disease. Acta Dermatol Venereol 1972, 52:257.

Komp DM, et al: A staging system for histiocytosis X. Cancer 1981, 47:798.

Levin MW, et al: Disseminated adult histiocytosis X with unusual manifestations. J Assoc Milit Dermatol 1984, 10:29.

Lichtenstein L: Histiocytosis X. Arch Pathol 1953, 56:84.

Lindelof B: Histiocytosis X in an adult. JAAD 1988, 19:426.

Lipton JM: The pathogenesis, diagnosis and treatment of histiocytosis syndromes. Pediatr Dermatol 1983, 1:112.

Lookingbill DP: Histiocytosis X confined to the skin of the scalp. JAAD 1984, 10:968.

Matus-Ridley M: Histiocytosis X in children. Med Pediatr Oncol 1983, 11:99.

Nethercott JR, et al: Histiocytosis X in two adults: treatment with topical mechlorethamine. Arch Dermatol 1983, 119:157.

Neumann C, et al: Interferon gamma is a marker for histiocytosis X cells in the skin. J Invest Dermatol 1988, 91:280.

Ornvold K, et al: Disseminated histiocytosis X. Acta Path Microbiol Immunol Scand 1985, 93:311.

Risdall RJ, et al: Histiocytosis X. Arch Pathol Lab Med 1983, 107:59.

Rivera MA: Ulcerating papulosquamous eruption and constipation in a 75-year-old man. Arch Dermatol 1985, 121:674.

Roper SS, et al: Cutaneous histiocytosis syndromes. Pediat Dermatol 1985, 3:19.

Rowden G, et al: Cutaneous histiocytosis X. Arch Dermatol 1983, 119:553.

Scarpelli DG: Histiocytosis X. Arch Dermatol 1986, 122:402.

Storer JS, et al: Histiocytosis X and skin scraping cytology. JAAD 1983, 8:913.

Timpatanapong P, et al: Nail involvement in histiocytosis X. Arch Dermatol 1984, 120:1052.

Zachariae H: Histiocytosis X in two infants treated with topical nitrogen mustard. Br J Dermatol 1979, 100:433.

32

Mycosis Fungoides, Other Malignant Lymphomas, and Allied Diseases

The term "malignant lymphoma" has been used widely to designate various malignant neoplastic diseases of the lymph node–forming tissues.

This chapter will deal with mycosis fungoides, other cutaneous malignant lymphomas, the leukemias and allied diseases, and the pseudolymphomas.

Edelson R, et al: Cutaneous lymphoma (periodic synopsis). JAAD 1986, 14:1073.
Mann RB, et al: Malignant lymphomas. Ann J Pathol 1979, 94:105.

CUTANEOUS T-CELL LYMPHOMAS (CTCL)

All the lymphoproliferative disorders characterized by cells with deeply convoluted nuclei on electron microscopy are grouped under one name, "cutaneous T-cell lymphomas." Those diseases are mycosis fungoides, Sézary syndrome, actinic reticuloid, pagetoid reticulosis, and lymphomatoid papulosis.

Mycosis Fungoides

Mycosis fungoides was first described by Bazin in 1851, although Alibert in 1806 had called attention to this skin malady. The name "mycosis" was given it under the misapprehension that it was of fungal origin, and was so widely used that it cannot now be changed. It is a malignant neoplasm of T-lymphocytic origin, specifically, the T helper cell subset. It is an uncommon, chronic, itching, usually fatal disease, running a progressive course. The speed of progression and relative aggressiveness of disease are highly variable.

The course may be divided generally into several stages: premycotic, consisting of severe pruritus and nondescript erythematous, eczematous, or psoriasiform eruptions; patches; infiltrated plaques; tumors; and erythroderma. It may begin with any of these manifestations, and exist without the others. Except in the *d'emblée* type, which begins with tumors, the onset is insidious and does not suggest the gravity of the process, so that the true nature is in many cases not recognized for some time.

CLINICAL FEATURES. In the *premycotic stage*, cutaneous eruptions simulating various forms of dermatitis, such as nondescript eczema, psoriasis, allergic contact dermatitis, nummular eczema, and pityriasis rubra pilaris may occur, being formed by macules, papules, urticarial lesions, or scaly patches. Barnhill et al reported three patients with pigmented purpuric eruptions that eventuated in mycosis fungoides. Ten per cent of patients with large-plaque parapsoriasis and most with poikiloderma vasculare atrophicans eventually develop mycosis fungoides. The eruptions at first may show no distinctive clinical features of mycosis fungoides. They may be transitory or persist for a long time; or they may possess from the beginning, or develop, suggestive charac-

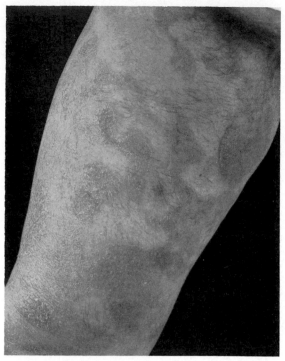

Figure 32–1. Mycosis fungoides in premycotic stage, showing erythematous branny scaling patches with only slight infiltrations into the lesions. (Courtesy of Dr. H. Shatin.)

teristics such as severe pruritus, reticulation, bizarre configuration, polymorphism, or vivid coloration.

The configuration may assume bizarre forms such as doughnut-shaped rings, rounded patches, curled ribbons of varying width, semicircles, large wavy or lobulated crescents, and other unusual patterns. Sometimes a single lesion precedes the outbreak of the premycotic eruption by several weeks. The eruptions may be polymorphous. A bluish or yellowish tinge may be present. The lesions are often of unusual colors, with various vivid shades of red often predominating. Zackheim et al in 1982 reported three cases in which all lesions were hypopigmented macules, which became repigmented following topical therapy with carmustine (BCNU), 50 mg in dilute

alcohol, applied every two days for 16 days, and mechlorethamine. Breathnach et al reported five similar cases, also in 1982.

The *telangiectatic* or *poikilodermic* variety may be localized or generalized. The skin assumes a dusky, reddish brown hue upon which numerous telangiectatic vessels occur. Itching may at first be slight, but later extreme pruritus is predominant.

Plaquelike infiltrations develop only after several years of this premycotic phase as a rule. The earliest clinical lesions that may show histologic features of mycosis fungoides are patches. These are most commonly seen on the buttocks, thighs, abdomen, and breasts. The patches then progress to infiltrated plaques. These are well demarcated, and if present on the scalp may be associated with alopecia. The surface of the plaques may be smooth, scaly, or eczematous, and a few cases with a verrucous or severely hyperkeratotic surface have been reported, like the case of Lupton et al. The plaques may involve an area of less than 10 per cent of the body, or may become widespread.

The infiltration of the plaques, at first recognized by light palpation, may be present in only a few of the lesions. It is a manifestation of diagnostic importance. Different degrees of infiltration may exist even in the same patch, and sometimes it is more pronounced peripherally, the central part of the plaque being depressed to the level of the surrounding skin. The infiltration becomes more marked and leads to discoid patches or extensive plaques, which may be as much as 30 cm in width.

Eventually, through coalescence of the various plaques, the involvement becomes widespread, but there are usually patches of apparently normal skin interspersed. When the involvement is advanced, painful superficial ulcerations may occur. During this phase enlarged lymph nodes usually develop. They are nontender, firm, and freely movable.

The *tumor stage* is characterized by large, various sized and shaped nodules on infiltrated plaques and on apparently healthy skin as well. They have a tendency to break down early and to form deep oval ulcers, with bases covered with a necrotic grayish

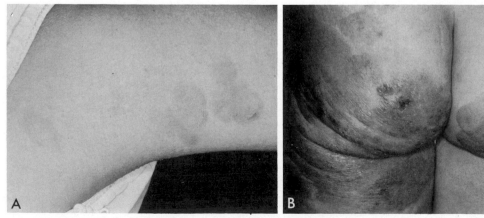

Figure 32–2. Infiltrated plaques of mycosis fungoides in a 28-year-old woman. A, Upper arm; B, buttocks and posterior thigh.

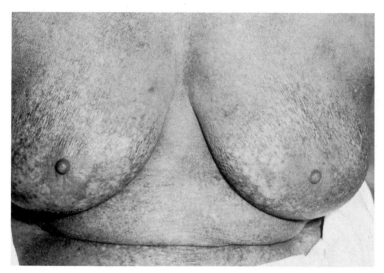

Figure 32–3. *Generalized poikiloderma in mycosis fungoides.*

substance and with rolled edges. The lesions generally have a predilection for the trunk, although they may be seen anywhere on the skin or may involve the mouth and upper respiratory tract. Uncommonly, tumors may be the first sign of mycosis fungoides. These cases are referred to as *tumeur d'emblée.*

The *erythrodermic* variety of mycosis fungoides is a generalized exfoliative process, with universal redness. The hair is scanty, nails dystrophic, palms and soles hyperkeratotic, and at times there may be generalized hyperpigmentation. In these cases the proportion of circulating Sézary cells should be determined, and if it is over 10 per cent of cells the diagnosis becomes *Sézary syndrome.* Erythroderma may be the presenting feature.

The course of the untreated disease during the tumor stage may be grave or mild. Death, as a rule, ensues from exhaustion, septicemia, or intercurrent bronchopneumonia in a few months or years after the beginning of the tumor stage. The development of nodal disease or symptomatic visceral involvement is a poor prognostic sign. In exceptional cases, however, the tumors may remain localized and stationary for many years, even without treatment.

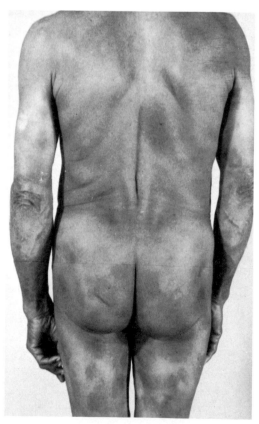

Figure 32–4. *Mycosis fungoides with poikilodermatous changes and minimal infiltrated lesions. (Courtesy of Dr. R. Ames.)*

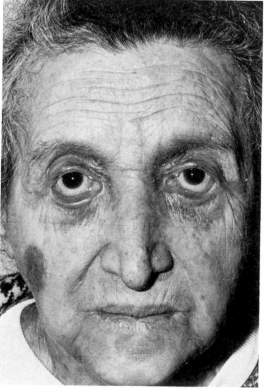

Figure 32–5. *Ectropion of mycosis fungoides.*

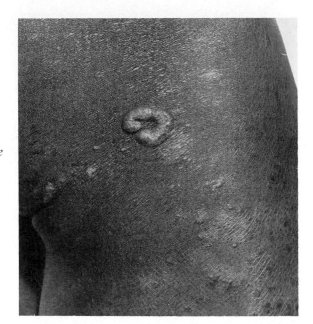

Figure 32–6. Typical kidney-shaped tumor of mycosis fungoides on the lateral upper thigh.

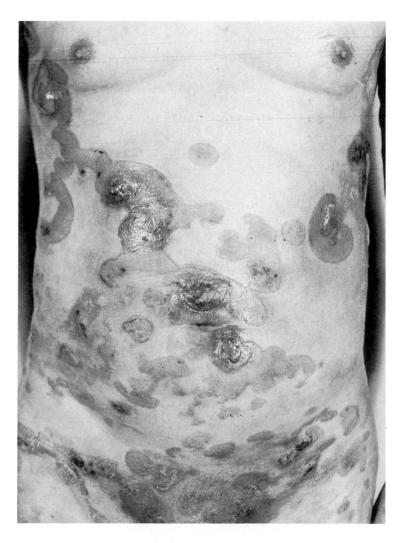

Figure 32–7. Mycosis fungoides showing fungating tumors, bizarrely shaped tumors, and plaques. Note the kidney-shaped lesions on the lateral chest.

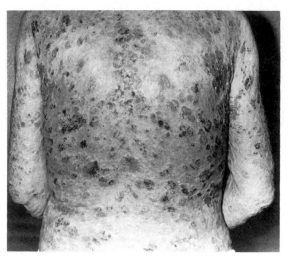

Figure 32–8. Mycosis fungoides.

SYSTEMIC MANIFESTATIONS. Mycosis fungoides is a cutaneous form of malignant lymphoma. Visceral involvement is commonly encountered in cases coming to autopsy. The lymph node is the most frequent site involved with lymphoma, second only to the skin.

The study of 144 patients at the National Institutes of Health by Ervin Epstein Jr et al showed that lymphadenopathy, tumors, or cutaneous ulceration are cardinal prognostic factors: no patient died without having developed one of them, and patients with all three (in any order) survived a median of one year.

Other organs frequently involved with mycosis fungoides at autopsy were, in order of descending frequency: spleen, lungs, liver, bone, kidney, tongue or epiglottis, heart, pancreas, and thyroid. Numerous other organs were infrequently involved.

Zackheim in 1983 reviewed 23 cases of CNS invasion. He points out that cranial (especially facial) nerve paralysis is a sign of this, and in such patients, cytologic examination should be done on the spinal fluid after centrifugation.

CLINICAL AND LABORATORY EVALUATION. In evaluating new patients with possible mycosis fungoides, multiple shave or excisional biopsy specimens from skin lesions should be obtained. A complete history and physical examination should be done. On histologic confirmation of the diagnosis, a complete blood count, serum chemistries, liver function and renal function tests, calcium and phosphorus determinations, a chest x-ray, a peripheral blood smear analysis for atypical circulating lymphocytes (over 20 percent is positive), and a node biopsy of palpable nodes in patients with plaque disease, tumors, or erythroderma, are indicated. Organ evaluation is undertaken if indicated by abnormalities on history or physical examination.

Once the extent of disease is determined, staging may be done according to the summary by Sausville et al. Three prognostic groups have been identified:

plaques (limited or generalized) without adenopathy or peripheral blood involvement, median survival over 12 years; with lymph node effacement or visceral disease, median survival less than 3 years; all others, median survival 5 years.

Parapsoriasis en Plaques and Mycosis Fungoides. Mycosis fungoides may frequently be preceded by parapsoriasis en plaques of the large-plaque type. Approximately 10 per cent of such cases evolve into mycosis fungoides after many years' duration. The color of the lesions may be yellowish brown, yellowish red, or even purple. The trunk and thighs are mostly involved, with patches that are not infiltrated. Its transition into mycosis fungoides may be heralded by infiltration and reticulation of the round or oval plaques. Onset of pruritus is also suggestive.

It is discussed at greater length in Chapter 11.

Alopecia Mucinosa and Mycosis Fungoides. Alopecia mucinosa (follicular mucinosis) may be present in mycosis fungoides. It is an accumulation of acid mucopolysaccharide in the follicular outer root sheath and in sebaceous glands, together with an inflammatory infiltrate.

While alopecia mucinosa associated with mycosis fungoides usually has a lymphomatous infiltrate from the beginning, Pinkus mentioned in one of his last published articles three personal cases of alopecia mucinosa in patients over 40 that terminated in mycosis fungoides. Gibson et al reported 17 patients with follicular mucinosis eventuating in mycosis fungoides.

PATHOGENESIS. Braverman believes that mycosis fungoides is a progressive proliferation of cutaneous lymphoreticular tissue together with a polymorphous mature cell infiltrate that represents a host defense against the neoplasm.

Another theory is that the polymorphous cellular proliferation is a reaction to various stimuli to pro-

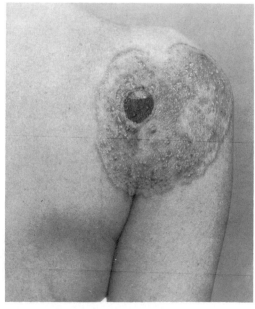

Figure 32–9. Mycosis fungoides, d'emblée type.

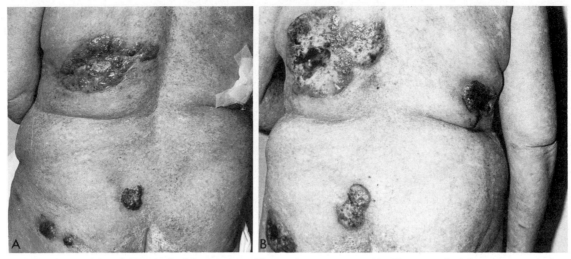

Figure 32–10. A, *Mycosis fungoides, early tumor stage.* B, *Three months later.*

duce a histiocytic response that eventually becomes malignant. Experimentally, evidence has accumulated to support this concept. Tan and associates suggest that mycosis fungoides is a chronic response to persistent unidentified antigens, upon which immune imbalance can develop, resulting in the emergence of a lymphoreticular neoplasm.

Edelson has proposed a theory that takes into account the immunologic microenvironment of the skin and its normal T cell interactions. He proposes that alterations in them may explain cutaneous T-cell lymphoma. T cells normally circulate, differentiate, and proliferate in the skin under the influence of several factors, such as interleukin-1 (IL-1) and a thymopoietin like substance. IL-1 acts to induce production of interleukin-2, which stimulates propagation of antigen-stimulated T cells. Malignant helper

T cells in cutaneous T-cell lymphoma also require IL-2 for clonal expansion. This may account for the epidermotropism seen early in this disease. It is proposed that a clone then develops which makes its own IL-2, thus gaining independence from the skin's microenvironment, and explaining the non-epidermotropic, visceral, and nodal disease seen late in the course of the disease.

As discussed in Chapter 19 (Viral Diseases), HTLV-1 infection may induce adult T-cell lymphoma/leukemia, with skin lesions resembling mycosis fungoides. HTLV-1–infected T cells may produce their own interleukin-2. Other environmental factors have occasionally been implicated as inducers of mycosis fungoides, but a study by Tuyp et al found none to be significantly associated with it.

INCIDENCE AND COURSE. Mycosis fungoides is approximately twice as common in men as in women, and twice as common in blacks as in whites, as shown in a study by Weinstock et al. It is most frequently seen in adults between the ages of 30 and 70. Approximately 400 new cases are diagnosed per year in the United States, and the incidence appears to be steadily increasing.

The onset of mycosis fungoides is insidious and, untreated, it follows a slow, relentless course. In some cases the disease may terminate in two or three years and in others persist for several decades. Levi found the median survival rate to be less than five years. Ervin Epstein Jr, et al found the median survival, if tumors, ulcers, and lymphadenopathy are all present, to be about one year. Redmond and Rahbari found the average overall survival was 7.9 years after onset of lesions. Of 340 patients reported by Lambey et al, one third died during the 54-month follow-up period. On the other hand, Samman's series of 245 (mostly ambulatory) patients in England had a mortality of only 10 per cent in ten years. Infection is the most frequent complication that leads to death. Septicemia and bronchopneumonia are usually present at the time of death.

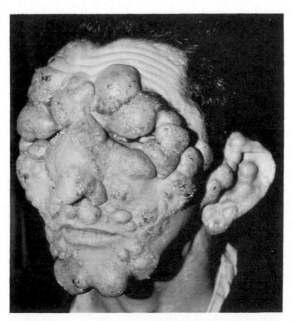

Figure 32–11. Extensive tumors of mycosis fungoides of the face and ears.

HISTOPATHOLOGY. In the *premycotic stage* the histologic appearance is that of subacute or chronic dermatitis. There may be an inflammatory infiltrate consisting of small round cells; however, when histiocytes are present in the infiltrate, Lever suggests that one's suspicion of mycosis fungoides should be aroused.

In the *infiltrative stage* a characteristic pleomorphic cellular infiltrate is found in the dermis. In the epidermis, distinctive focal collections of mononuclear cells containing large amounts of clear cytoplasm and small dense nuclei are found. These are *Pautrier's microabscesses*, whose presence is considered to be pathognomonic for mycosis fungoides. In addition, acanthosis, intracellular edema, and parakeratosis may be present. Spongiosis is absent.

The characteristic mycosis cell is a large cell with a single hyperchromic infolded cerebriform nucleus, an abnormal T helper lymphocyte. Many studies have documented the loss of differentiation antigens with progression of disease. Antibodies that initially seemed specific for cutaneous T-cell lymphoma (BE1 and BE2) have been found in AIDS patients and in B-cell leukemia.

Under the electron microscope the mycosis fungoides cell is seen to have a large nucleus with scanty cytoplasm, with a dense, homogeneous chromatin pattern. The nucleus has from 1 to 12 deep, narrow invaginations. The nuclear contour index, a measure of its irregularity, is high in mycosis fungoides, as compared to benign diseases, as discussed by Shum et al. Payne et al analyzed these nuclei by planigraphy and determined that in benign disorders, no nuclear invaginations are found in at least 19 per cent of lymphocytes, whereas the highest proportion of lymphocytes with zero invaginations in mycosis fungoides was 15 per cent. Computerized planimetry, however, is still a research procedure. DNA cytophotometry and chromosomal analysis, as described by van Vloten, is also not readily available. It can be used to document aneuploidy (abnormal number of chromosomes) or polyploidy (two or more sets of chromosomes).

In the *tumor state* the dermal infiltrate becomes extremely dense and may extend into the subcutaneous layers as well as extend upward into the epidermis to produce ulceration. The polymorphous infiltrate contains mycosis cells in great abundance.

DIFFERENTIAL DIAGNOSIS. In the premycotic stage mycosis fungoides is difficult to diagnose. Pruritus, with or without skin lesions, may be the only symptom. The skin lesions are usually some nondescript form of eczema with some scaling. Interestingly, despite the itching, scratch marks and lichenification are usually absent. This same severe pruritus without skin lesions may be present in Hodgkin's disease for many years.

Clinical differentiation from other forms of malignant lymphoma or pseudolymphomas is usually not possible. Histologically, the same difficulties may also be present. The presence of generalized erythroderma may pose difficulties since it may be present in malignant lymphomas as well as in pityriasis rubra pilaris and psoriatic erythroderma. Mycosis fungoides of the d'emblée type is a rare presentation, and the tumors show on histologic examination a polymorphous infiltrate.

TREATMENT. Effective therapy that reliably prolongs survival has not yet been documented. Many forms of therapy induce remissions of variable length. The choice among them depends on extent of disease, the physician's experience and preference, and the availability of various options. Topical nitrogen mustard, electron beam, and PUVA are generally good choices for early disease. We favor treatment of all advanced cases (lymphadenopathy, tumors, or extensive skin involvement) with electron beam therapy combined with chemotherapy. Extracorporeal photochemotherapy appears to be best for erythrodermic cases.

X-ray Treatment. In erythematous, urticarial, or eczematous types treatment with 50 or 100 rads, unfiltered, to the affected areas will clear most lesions. However, Cotter et al have shown that tumor doses equivalent to 3000 rads (at 200 rads per treatment, five treatments per week) are needed to prevent recurrences, especially in deeper lesions. This local-field approach is good for treating lesions located in difficult areas such as the scalp, palms and soles, or mucous membranes, as well as for deep-seated lesions. Not more than six or eight areas should be treated in one day until the patient's tolerance is known, as nausea and malaise follow more extensive irradiation. After the patient's tolerance has been established, the dosage is regulated by the character of the lesions. Treatment intervals are one to two weeks. Upon isolated patches, 200 rads (unfiltered) at intervals of three weeks may be employed. Indurated plaques should be treated similarly. The tumor stage requires increased dosage, usually 800 to 1200 rads (HVL 1.0 mm Al) in fractionated doses; for extremely thick lesions, 1000 rads at 135 kV filtered through 3 mm Al (HVL 4.0 mm Al). During these exposures the skin about the lesions is shielded by lead.

Teleroentgen Therapy. An effective mode of therapy has been the use of low-voltage x-ray therapy given at a 2-meter target-skin distance to the entire body. Goldschmidt has reviewed this subject.

Electron Beam Therapy. Fromer of the Lahey Clinic reported success with generalized electron beam treatment for mycosis fungoides, especially in patients in whom other forms of therapy have failed. Complete involution of lesions was permanent in some patients. Fromer saw continued suppression of lesions for as long as 14 years before death occurred from other causes. Hoppe et al's Stanford experience was similarly impressive. At 1.5 meV the radiation is almost entirely absorbed in the first 3 to 7 mm of skin. Because of the limited penetration by electrons, damage to underlying structures is avoided. Nisce et al have reviewed this topic. Tadros et al reported their results in 106 patients. Most received 30Gy of 3-meV electrons, divided into 12 sessions in three weeks. Complete remission was induced in 83 per cent. Acute side effects limited treatment schedules in only five patients. Hamminga et al compared electron beam therapy with topical mechlorethamine; they were equally effective in early cases, but in later stages, electron beam was better. However, topical nitrogen mustard was very helpful in reducing the many relapses seen with electron beam alone.

Ultraviolet Therapy. Roenigk's early success with PUVA has withstood the test of time. Current experience indicates 90 per cent of pretumorous patients will respond. Abel et al found long-term maintenance necessary. Patients with erythroderma overreacted, and tumors did not respond well. Kubba et al reported total remission in five plaque-stage cases and 95 per cent clearing in two, and improvement in six, with PUVA therapy. Powell et al found PUVA effective in all cases of parapsoriasis en plaques and beneficial in most of 19 cases of mycosis fungoides. Hönigsmann et al in 1984 obtained long remissions with PUVA in 44 early cases.

Milstein et al in 1982 reported preliminary observations on the use of home ultraviolet therapy in 34 patients, at least 22 of whom had an established diagnosis of mycosis fungoides; they achieved remissions lasting three to 20 months.

Interferon. Recombinant leukocyte A interferon, given intramuscularly in a dose of 50×10^6 units/m^2 three times weekly, was beneficial to most of 20 patients with mycosis fungoides or Sézary syndrome reported by Bunn et al in 1984. Twenty-seven percent of 22 patients reported by Olsen et al responded completely to interferon alpha-2a. Braath et al reported complete remission in three of six patients given a combination of interferon and etretinate.

Topical Nitrogen Mustard (NH$_2$). Sipos and Jaksó and later Haserick and his associates demonstrated beneficial effects from topical applications of NH$_2$ in the premycotic and infiltrative plaque stages. The contents of a 10 mg vial of mechlorethamine hydrochloride (Mustargen-MSD) are dissolved in 60 ml of tap water and applied to the entire skin surface except the genitalia with a 2-inch paint brush. Daily applications are made until complete clearing occurs and for six months thereafter, and every two days for six more months, then weekly for six more months. This is the regimen followed by Ramsey et al. Vonderheid et al follow a similar regimen, with long-term total-body treatments. Both investigators report excellent responses, control, and long-term survival in most patients over a long period of treatment and observation. Topical nitrogen mustard is a proven mainstay of therapy for patch or plaque stage mycosis fungoides without lymphadenopathy. Allergic contact dermatitis is frequently experienced after repeated courses of treatment.

Solutions of mechlorethamine are stable for many months, Taylor et al reported in 1980; they do not need to be "used immediately" as is specified for intravenous use. It is presumably better to keep them refrigerated.

In 1970 Van Scott and Winters reported complete remission of the infiltrative plaque stage in a majority of patients intensively treated with whole body applications over an extended period of several months. Periods of remission varied from two to 12 weeks. Vonderheid et al have reported on a larger group of cases treated for periods of seven or more years.

Price et al, trying to reduce the frequency of hypersensitivity reactions to aqueous solutions of mechlorethamine, used a 10 per cent strength in Aquaphor, incorporating a 10 per cent alcoholic solution in absolute alcohol into 900 gm of Aquaphor. Only one of 31 patients never previously exposed developed hypersensitivity. Ramsey et al reported a long-term follow-up on patients treated with topical nitrogen mustard. They used dilute solutions to treat through episodes of allergic contact dermatitis.

About 80 per cent of patients with patch and plaque disease will get complete remission. It is to be continued as maintenance therapy for one to three years after remission.

Lee et al reported squamous cell carcinomas developing apparently as a result of topical nitrogen mustard therapy as have others.

BCNU. Zackheim and Epstein Jr reported good results with nitrosourea compounds, carmustine (BCNU) and lomustine, in 26 patients, 13 of whom had become allergic to mechlorethamine, and in 1983 Zackheim et al reported their results of 10 years' experience with BCNU. They reported a 65 to 70 per cent complete response rate in pretumorous patients, thus providing an alternative therapy for those unable to tolerate topical nitrogen mustard. Their publication provides physician guidelines for its use. For topical use, the thin film of BCNU powder (it is immaterial if it has liquefied, as it does at room temperature) is dissolved in 50 ml of 95 per cent ethyl alcohol; 5 ml of this in 60 ml of tap water is applied to the entire body surface daily for eight to ten weeks, unless an erythematous reaction occurs earlier.

Topical Corticosteroids. The response to the various corticosteroid topical applications is highly varied. The premycotic and early infiltrative stages often respond temporarily to high-potency topical corticosteroids without occlusion.

Systemic Chemotherapy. The popular cellular poisons of yesteryear, such as arsenic (Fowler's solution, potassium arsenite), antimony, and urethane, have been supplanted by the alkylating agents and the antimetabolites.

These forms of chemotherapy are advisable only in those advanced cases in which internal involvement is clearly indicated. The general response to these drugs is usually favorable in the beginning, but later they are less effective.

Winkler et al summarized experience with systemic chemotherapy, both single agents and combined therapy. Cyclophosphamide, chlorambucil, and methotrexate are the most commonly administered cytotoxic agents. The combination type therapies have higher response rates and longer remission times.

Zakem et al reported some success with a combination of systemic chemotherapy and topical nitrogen mustard for advanced-stage disease, and Braverman et al combined a different chemotherapeutic regimen with electron beam therapy. They showed significant improvement in the duration of complete remission for earlier-stage patients, as compared to the outlook with electron beam alone.

Extracorporeal Photochemotherapy. Edelson et al treated 37 patients with advanced disease, most with erythrodermic CTCL, by giving methoxsalen orally, and two hours after ingestion leukapheresing them. Leukocyte-enriched blood was then exposed to UVA and returned to the patient. Twenty-seven of 37 patients with otherwise resistant disease responded. This exciting new approach requires special equipment and more investigation, but may be useful in the future. Trials are under way with this approach combined with electron beam in less advanced cases.

Hormones. Therapy with corticosteroids may produce antitumor effects on mycosis fungoides; however, the large doses usually required reduce the desirability of this type of therapy. On the other hand, small amounts may contribute greatly to the general comfort of the patient, especially in the erythrodermic and poikilodermic varieties. Triamcinolone acetonide intramuscularly is worth a trial as an adjunct to more effective therapy.

Immunotherapy. Zachariae achieved an apparent cure with x-ray therapy and transfer factor, with no remaining evidence of mycosis fungoides at autopsy, on the patient's death from coronary infarction five years later, and has reported on three years' further experience with this therapy. Vonderheid et al and Wolff et al have reported some effect of intralesional interferon injected into plaques of mycosis fungoides. Systemic administration of interferon induces remission in some patients, as discussed above.

Retinoids. Doses of 13-*cis*-retinoic acid of up to 3 mg/kg/day were very effective in four patients with mycosis fungoides treated by Kessler et al. Kessler et al extended this investigation to 44 patients and found significant clinical benefit. Its use may be as an adjuvant to other approaches. Molin et al reported that isotretinoin and etretinate are equally effective. Arotinoid promises to be even more helpful, according to Mahrle et al. Tousignant et al reported controlling a case with it.

Antibiotics. Though antibiotics are not effective against the disease, patients with mycosis fungoides are susceptible to infection, and septicemia accounts for one fourth to one half of the deaths. Posner et al emphasized the importance of this in 1981, and advised empiric therapy for *S. aureus* septicemia at the first sign of this complication. Gram-negative bacteria should also be investigated.

Acyclovir. Resnick et al reported remission of tumor-stage mycosis fungoides following intravenously administered acyclovir in 1984, but Mahrle et al treated two patients, with no benefit in one and worsening in the other. A multicenter trial of the drug is being conducted.

Abel EA: Clinical features of cutaneous T-cell lymphoma. Dermatol Clinic 1985, 3:647.

Idem, et al: Cutaneous malignancies and metastatic squamous cell carcinoma following topical therapies for mycosis fungoides. JAAD 1986, 14:1029.

Idem, et al: PUVA treatment of erythrodermic and plaque-type mycosis fungoides. Arch Dermatol 1987, 123:897.

Barnhill RL, et al: Progression of pigmented purpura–like eruptions to mycosis fungoides. JAAD 1988, 19:25.

Beyer CL, et al: Diagnosis of cutaneous T-cell lymphoma by use of monoclonal antibodies reactive with tumor associated antigen. J Clin Invest 1982, 70:1205.

Blayney DW, et al: The human T-cell leukemia-lymphoma virus in the Southeastern United States. JAMA 1983, 250:1048.

Braverman IM, et al: Combined total body electron beam irradiation and chemotherapy for mycosis fungoides. JAAD 1987, 16:45.

Idem: Light-activated drugs. Sci Am 1988, 259:68.

Idem: Update on photopheresis. Prog Dermatol 1989, 23:1.

Buechner SA, et al: T-cells and T-cell subsets in mycosis fungoides and parapsoriasis: a study of 18 cases with anti–human–T-cell monoclonal antibodies and histochemical techniques. Arch Dermatol 1984, 120:897.

Idem: Pre-Sézary erythroderma evolving to Sézary syndrome: report of 7 cases. Arch Dermatol 1983, 119:285.

Bunn PA Jr, et al: Recombinant leukocyte A interferon: an active agent in cutaneous T-cell lymphomas. Ann Intern Med 1984, 101:484.

Idem: Clinical course of retrovirus-associated adult T-cell lymphoma in the U.S. N Engl J Med 1983, 309:257.

Idem: Prospective staging evaluation of patients with cutaneous T-cell lymphoma. Ann Intern Med 1980, 93:223.

Caputo R, et al: A verrucoid epidermotropic OKT-8 positive lymphoma. Am J Dermatopathol 1983, 5:159.

Cotter GW, et al: Palliative radiation treatment of cutaneous mycosis fungoides. Int J Radiat Oncol Biol Phys 1983, 9:1477.

Edelson RL: Pathogenesis of T-cell lymphoma of skin. JAAD 1983, 9:857.

Idem, et al: Treatment of cutaneous T-cell lymphoma by extracorporeal photochemotherapy. N Engl J Med 1987, 316:297.

Epstein EH Jr, et al: Mycosis fungoides: survival, prognostic features, response to therapy, and autopsy findings. Medicine 1972, 15:61.

Fitzpatrick JE, et al: Treatment of mycosis fungoides with isotretinoin. J Dermatol Surg Oncol 1986, 12:626.

Gibson LE, et al: Follicular mucinosis. JAAD 1989, 20:441.

Goldschmidt H, et al: Teleroentgen therapy for mycosis fungoides. J Dermatol Surg Oncol 1978, 4:601.

Hamminga B, et al: Treatment of mycosis fungoides: total skin electron beam vs topical mechlorethamine. Arch Dermatol 1982, 118:150.

Haynes BF, et al: Differentiation of human T lymphocytes: II phenotypic difference in skin and blood malignant T cells in cutaneous T-cell lymphoma. J Invest Dermatol 1982, 78:323.

Heald PW, et al: Newer therapies for cutaneous T-cell lymphoma. Arch Dermatol 1987, 123:169.

Holden CA, et al: Differential loss of T lymphocyte marker in advanced cutaneous T-cell lymphoma. JAAD 1982, 6:507.

Hönigsmann H, et al: Photochemotherapy for cutaneous T-cell lymphoma: a follow-up study. JAAD 1984, 10:238.

Jimbow K, et al: Cutaneous T-cell lymphoma and related disorders. Int J Dermatol 1986, 25:485.

Kardashian JL, et al: Lymphomatoid papulosis associated with plaque-stage and granulomatous mycosis fungoides. Arch Dermatol 1985, 121:1175.

Kessler JF, et al: Isotretoin and cutaneous helper T-cell lymphoma (mycosis fungoides). Arch Dermatol 1987, 123:201.

Koch SE, et al: Mycosis fungoides beginning in childhood and adolescence. JAAD 1987, 17:563.

Kubba R, et al: Immunologic evaluation in mycosis fungoides. Arch Dermatol 1980, 116:178.

Lamberg SI, et al: Clinical staging for cutaneous T-cell lymphoma. Ann Intern Med 1984, 100:187.

Lambert WC: Premycotic eruptions. Dermatol Clin 1985, 3:629.

Lee LA, et al: Second cutaneous malignancies in patients with mycosis fungoides treated with topical nitrogen mustard. JAAD 1982, 7:590.

Lindae ML, et al: Poikilodermatous mycosis fungoides and atrophic large-plaque parapsoriasis exhibit similar abnormalities of T-cell antigen expression. Arch Dermatol 1988, 124:366.

Lupton GP, et al: Hyperkeratotic and verrucous mycosis fungoides. J Assoc Milit Dermatol 1984, 10:19.

Lutzner M, et al: Cutaneous T-cell lymphomas. Ann Intern Med 1975, 83:534.

Madison JF, et al: Lymphomatoid papulosis terminating as . . . mycosis fungoides. JAAD 1983, 9:743.

Mahrle G, et al: Mycosis fungoides treated with acyclovir (letter). JAMA 1985, 253:977.

Idem: OKT9 reactivity in mycosis fungoides and . . . parapsoriasis. Cancer 1983, 51:1407.

Idem: Treatment of cutaneous T-cell lymphoma with arotinoid. Dtsch Med Wchnschr 1983, 108:1753.

McFadden NC: Mycosis fungoides: unsolved problems of diagnosis and choice of therapy (review). Int J Dermatol 1984, 23:523.

Idem: Demonstration of OKT6-reactive cells in mycosis fungoides. JAAD 1982, 6:880.

McMillan EM, et al: In situ demonstration of T-cell subsets in atrophic parapsoriasis. JAAD 1982, 6:32.

Milstein HJ, et al: Home ultraviolet phototherapy of early mycosis fungoides: preliminary observations. JAAD 1982, 6:355.

Molin L, et al: Oral retinoids in mycosis fungoides and Sézary syndrome. Acta Derm Venereol (Stockh) 1987, 67:232.

Nasu K, et al: Immunopathology of cutaneous T-cell lymphoma. Am J Pathol 1985, 119:436.

Olsen EA, et al: Interferon alpha-2a in the treatment of cutaneous T-cell lymphoma. JAAD 1989, 20:395.

Payne CM, et al: Quantitative electron microscopy in the diagnosis of mycosis fungoides: a simple analysis of lymphocytic nuclear convolutions. Arch Dermatol 1984, 120:63.

Pineda AA, et al: Leukopheresis in Sézary syndrome. JAAD 1981, 5:544.

Pinkus H: Commentary: alopecia mucinosa: additional data in 1983. Arch Dermatol 1983, 119:698.

Posner LE, et al: Septicemic complications of the cutaneous T-cell lymphomas. Am J Med 1981, 71:210.

Powell FC, et al: Treatment of parapsoriasis and mycosis fungoides: the role of . . . PUVA. Mayo Clin Proc 1984, 59:538.

Price NM, et al: Ointment-based mechlorethamine treatment for mycosis fungoides. Cancer 1983, 52:2214.

Idem: The treatment of mycosis fungoides with ointment based mechlorethamine. Arch Dermatol 1982, 118:234.

Ralfkiaer E, et al: T-cell growth factor receptor (Tac-antigen) expression in cutaneous lymphoid infiltrates. JAAD 1986, 15:628.

Ramsay DL, et al: Topical mechlorethamine therapy for early stage mycosis fungoides. JAAD 1988, 19:684.

Rebora A, et al: Baccaredda-Sézary syndrome (letter). JAAD 1984, 11:907.

Resnick L, et al: Remission of tumor-stage mycosis fungoides following intravenously administered Acyclovir. JAMA 1984, 251:1571.

Ringel E, et al: Localized mycosis fungoides not manifesting as Woringer-Kolopp disease. Arch Dermatol 1983, 119:756.

Rosenbaum MM, et al: Photochemotherapy in cutaneous lymphoma and parapsoriasis en plaques. JAAD 1985, 13:613.

Rotstein H: The management of minimal-extent mycosis fungoides. Int J Dermatol 1983, 22:515.

Sausville EA, et al: Histopathologic staging at initial diagnosis of mycosis fungoides and the Sézary syndrome. Ann Intern Med 1988, 109:372.

Shum DT, et al: The value of nuclear contour index in the diagnosis of mycosis fungoides. Cancer 1986, 57:298.

Slevin NJ, et al: Mycosis fungoides. J Dermatol 1987, 116:47.

Stadler R, et al: Interferons in dermatology. JAAD 1989, 20:650.

Tadros AAM, et al: Total skin electron irradiation for mycosis fungoides: failure analysis and prognostic factors. Int J Radiat Oncol Biol Phys 1983, 9:1279.

Taylor JR, et al: Mechlorethamine hydrochloride solutions and ointment: prolonged stability and biological activity. Arch Dermatol 1980, 116:783.

Thiers BH: Controversies in mycosis fungoides. JAAD 1982, 7:1.

Thomsen K, et al: 13-cis-retinoic acid effective in mycosis fungoides. Acta Derm Venereol (Stockh) 1984, 64:563.

Tomsick RS: Hyperkeratosis in mycosis fungoides. Cutis 1982, 29:621.

Toback AC, et al: Pathogenesis of cutaneous T-cell lymphoma. Dermatol Clinics 1985, 3:605.

Tousignant J, et al: Treatment of cutaneous T-cell lymphoma with the arotinoid Ro 13-6298. JAAD 1987, 16:167.

Tuyp E, et al: Case-controlled study of possible causative factors in mycosis fungoides. Arch Dermatol 1987, 123:196.

Tyring SK, et al: Development of verrucous plaques and gross hematuria in advanced cutaneous T-cell lymphoma. Arch Dermatol 1988, 124:655.

Van Vloten WA, et al: New techniques in the evaluation of cutaneous T-cell lymphoma. Dermatol Clin 1985, 3:665.

Idem: Total skin electron beam irradiation for cutaneous T-cell lymphoma. Br J Dermatol 1985, 112:679.

Vonderheid EC, et al: Treatment of cutaneous T-cell lymphoma. Dermatol Clin 1985, 3:673.

Idem: Diagnostic and prognostic significance of Sézary cells in peripheral blood smears from patients with cutaneous T-cell lymphoma. Blood 1985, 66:358.

Idem: Recombinant interferon alpha-2b in plaque-phase mycosis fungoides. Arch Dermatol 1987, 123:757.

Idem: Clinical implications of immunologic phenotyping in cutaneous T-cell lymphoma. JAAD 1987, 17:40.

Idem: Long-term efficacy, curative potential, and carcinogenicity of topical mechlorethamine chemotherapy in cutaneous T-cell lymphoma. JAAD 1989, 20:416.

Waddell CC, et al: Acute myeloblastic leukemia following chemotherapy for mycosis fungoides. Arch Dermatol 1982, 118:179.

Wantzin GL, et al: Occurrence of human T-cell lymphotropic virus (type I) antibodies in cutaneous T-cell lymphoma. JAAD 1986, 15:598.

Weinstock MA, et al: Mycosis fungoides in the United States. JAMA 1988, 260:42.

Weiss LM, et al: Clonal rearrangement of T-cell receptor genes in mycosis fungoides and dermatopathic lymphadenopathy. N Engl J Med 1985, 313:539.

Winkelmann RK, et al: Pre-Sézary syndrome. JAAD 1984, 10:992.

Wolff JM, et al: Intralesional interferon in the treatment of early mycosis fungoides. JAAD 1985, 13:604.

Yamamura T, et al: The cutaneous lymphomas with convoluted nucleus: analysis of 39 cases. JAAD 1984, 10:796.

Zachariae H, et al: Topical nitrogen mustard in early mycosis fungoides. Acta Derm Venereol (Stockh) 1985, 65:53.

Zackheim HS, et al: Mycosis fungoides of the mastoid, middle ear, and CNS. Arch Dermatol 1983, 119:311.

Idem: Mycosis fungoides presenting as areas of hypopigmentation: report of 3 cases. JAAD 1982, 6:340.

Idem: Topical carmustine (BCNU) for mycosis fungoides and related disorders: a 10-year experience. JAAD 1983, 9:363.

Zackheim HS: Topical mechlorethamine and carmustine for cutaneous T-cell lymphoma. Semin Dermatol 1983, 2:307.

Zakem MH, et al: Treatment of advanced stage mycosis fungoides with bleomycin, doxorubicin and methotrexate with topical nitrogen mustard. Cancer 1986, 58:2611.

SÉZARY SYNDROME

Baccaredda described the syndrome and the cells in detail in 1937 and 1939; Montgomery and Watkins described it as a variant of monocytic leukemia in

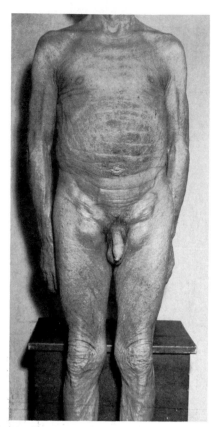

Figure 32–12. Sézary syndrome with lipomelanotic reticulosis (dermatopathic lymphadenopathy).

1937; and Sézary and his associates in 1938 and 1942 described it as *réticulose érythrodermique avec réticulémie*, and it is Sézary's name that has come to be used as its eponymic designation. Essentially, it is the leukemic phase of cutaneous T-cell lymphoma (CTCL).

Also known as malignant reticulemic syndrome, Sézary syndrome is characterized by generalized erythroderma, splenomegaly, superficial lymphadenopathy, and atypical cells in the circulating blood, in the cutaneous infiltrate, and in the lymph nodes. Itching is severe.

The skin shows a generalized erythroderma of a typical fiery red color, with leonine facies, eyelid edema, ectropion, diffuse alopecia, hyperkeratosis of the palms and soles, and dystrophic nails. The symptoms are those of severe pruritus and burning, with episodes of chills and profuse perspiration.

Chronic erythroderma, evolving from previous severe dermatitis, especially in patients with a personal or family history (or both) of atopy, may be a pre-Sézary syndrome; Buechner and Winkelmann reported seven such cases, which evolved to Sézary syndrome. Winkelmann reported 17 such cases in 1984, most of which responded to low-dose chlorambucil and prednisone. They had recurrent cycles of circulating Sézary cells of less than 1000 cells/mm[3]. They lived about twice as long as expected (about 6.6 years from the onset of erythroderma) with this treatment.

Superficial lymphadenopathy is usually found in the cervical, axillary, and inguinal areas. Leukocytosis up to 30,000 is usually present. In the peripheral blood, in the skin infiltrate, and in the lymph nodes, helper T cells with deeply convoluted nuclei are found: the Sézary cells. An absolute number of greater than 1000 atypical cells, or greater than 10 per cent of the circulating cells, is used to delineate the criteria for Sézary syndrome, as these cells may be seen in the skin, blood, and lymph nodes in other diseases.

Buechner et al studied skin biopsies from 39 patients with Sézary syndrome and found two main patterns: a subepidermal band infiltrate of atypical cells, and a lymphocytic band infiltrate which was polymorphous. Fifteen per cent showed epidermal infiltration of atypical cells and 18 per cent showed only chronic dermatitis.

The erythroderma of Sézary syndrome must be distinguished from that seen in mycosis fungoides, chronic lymphocytic leukemia, monocytic leukemia, Hodgkin's disease, and non-Hodgkin's lymphoma. This is done primarily by histopathologic and immunopathologic examination. Other erythrodermas to be kept in mind are exfoliative dermatitis, psoriatic erythroderma, and pityriasis rubra pilaris, especially when there is hyperkeratosis of the palms and soles.

The disease is resistant to most forms of treatment, and death may occur within five years after onset. Extracorporeal photochemotherapy, as discussed above under mycosis fungoides, appears to be a major advance in treatment of this condition. Systemic steroids may relieve itching for short periods, and electron beam therapy may produce remission lasting some months. Cyclophosphamide, 3 to 4 mg/kg a day, orally, may give relief, and a maintenance dose of 50 to 200 mg a day may maintain the remission.

Pineda and Winkelmann used prednisone and low-dose chlorambucil with leukopheresis in five patients and established its safety in patients with normal white blood cell counts and its potential usefulness in Sézary syndrome. Winkelmann et al have since reported on its use in 40 patients. Median survival was 6.2 years. This regimen appears to be an excellent form of treatment.

Aratari et al reported arrest and partial clearing in a case reported as Sézary syndrome, with features of actinic reticuloid, using beta-carotene and canthaxanthine, 90 and 135 mg a day, respectively. Zugerman et al also reported a case which had its onset as actinic reticuloid.

Aratari E, et al: Beta-carotenoids in Sézary syndrome. Ital Gen Rev Derm 1983, 20:4.
Buechner SA, et al: Pre-Sézary erythroderma evolving to Sézary syndrome. Arch Dermatol 1983, 119:285.
Idem: T-cells in cutaneous lesions of Sézary syndrome and T-cell leukemia. Arch Dermatol 1983, 119:895.
Buzzanga J, et al: Lymph node histopathology in Sézary syndrome. JAAD 1984, 11:880.
Kinoshita K, et al: Clinical, hematologic, and pathologic features of leukemic T-cell lymphoma. Cancer 1982, 50:1554.

Oliver GF, et al: Unilesional mycosis fungoides. JAAD 1989, 20:63.

Sentis HJ, et al: Histopathologic studies in Sézary syndrome and erythrodermic mycosis fungoides. JAAD 1986, 15:1217.

Venencie PY, et al: Monoclonal gammopathy in Sézary syndrome. Arch Dermatol 1984, 120:605.

Winkelmann RK, et al: The treatment of Sézary syndrome. JAAD 1984, 10:1000.

Idem: Pre-Sézary syndrome. JAAD 1984, 10:992.

Wood GS, et al: T-cell antigen deficiencies and clonal rearrangements of T-cell receptor genes in pagetoid reticulosis. NEJM 1988, 318:164.

Zugerman C, et al: Photosensitivity and Sézary syndrome. Cutis 1980, 25:495.

ACTINIC RETICULOID

Men between 45 and 70 with severe, recalcitrant photodermatitis, poorly responsive to steroids and not helped by sunscreens, may be suspected of having actinic reticuloid. It was first described and reported by Ive et al in 1969. The skin presents a burning, itching, erythematous, hyperpigmented, eczematized dermatitis, which in later stages may become generalized. The histology suggests lymphoma or mycosis fungoides but mitoses are infrequent and eosinophils often quite numerous. Giannelli et al, testing fibroblast strains from six patients, found they were abnormally sensitive to UVA, to an extent not found in normals, in Bloom's syndrome, or in xeroderma pigmentosum.

There is hypersensitivity, and a pseudolymphomatous response, to UVA, and irradiation of a test site on uninvolved skin, with biopsy, is the best diagnostic test. Frain-Bell showed that repeated attacks of allergic contact dermatitis, especially to plant oleoresins and certain fragrances, frequently precede the appearance of actinic reticuloid.

Systemic steroids may be unavoidable, but even they are far from optimally effective unless the patient remains indoors. Arnold has used 60 mg of Kenalog-IM monthly with fair success and no side effects over a two-year period. Prednisone is effective only in dangerously high doses. Sunscreens are not sufficiently protective. Morison et al found PUVA therapy effective. Fitzpatrick found installation of E-Z Bond Film (Solar Screen Transparent Window Coverings, Corona, NY 11368) in the car extremely helpful in one severely affected man. Kingston et al reported successful therapy with azathioprine in a black patient.

Evolution into any form of lymphoma may occur.

Brody R, et al: Actinic reticuloid. Int J Dermatol 1981, 20:374.

Frain-Bell W: Photosensitivity dermatosis and actinic reticuloid. Semin Dermatol 1982, 1:161.

Giannelli F, et al: Cellular hypersensitivity to UV-A: a clue to the aetiology of actinic reticuloid. Lancet 1983, I:88.

Kingston JP, et al: Actinic reticuloid in a black man. JAAD 1987, 16:1079.

Vandermaesen J, et al: Light on the persistent light reaction–

photosensitivity dermatitis–actinic reticuloid syndrome. JAAD 1986, 115:685.

PAGETOID RETICULOSIS

Woringer and Kolopp reported in 1939 a solitary plaque on a boy's wrist, of six years' duration, in which the epidermis was the seat of a pagetoid infiltration by mononuclear cells. "Localized epidermotropic reticulosis" has been proposed as a name for such cases, with solitary lesions. Since then similar cases have been reported, as well as cases (Ketron-Goodman type) differing only in having a more generalized distribution; and Andreev has suggested that both may simply be variants of mycosis fungoides.

Ioannides et al in 1983 reaffirmed the identity of the cell in Woringer-Kolopp disease as the same one found in mycosis fungoides, reporting a case of 16 years' duration on the foot, which recurred and enlarged after excision. Wood et al found T-cell antigen deficiencies and clonal rearrangements of T-cell-receptor genes, indicating that pagetoid reticulosis is a T-cell lymphoproliferative disorder.

Deneau et al reported four typical cases in which enzyme histochemistry indicated that the infiltrating cells were helper T cells in three cases and suppressor T cells in one. They consider the question of whether Woringer-Kolopp disease is a T-cell lymphoma, or a syndrome with various causes, to be still unsettled.

As Zackheim says, for the present, localized epidermotropic reticulosis should be regarded as a potentially aggressive disease, and treated vigorously from the beginning. Local irradiation is recommended treatment.

Verrucoid Epidermotropic Volar Lymphoma. Caputo et al reported in 1983 a man with verrucoid palmoplantar lesions with pagetoid cells in the epidermis, of which 70 per cent were OKT8 positive lymphocytes. It resolved within a few months.

Deneau DG, et al: Woringer-Kolopp disease. Arch Dermatol 1984, 120:1045.

Edelson RL, et al: Treatment of cutaneous T-cell lymphoma by extracorporeal photochemotherapy. NEJM 1987, 316:297.

Ioannides G, et al: Woringer-Kolopp disease (pagetoid reticulosis). Am J Dermatopathol 1983, 5:153.

Lever WF: Localized mycosis fungoides with prominent epidermotropism: Woringer-Kolopp disease. Arch Dermatol 1977, 113:1254.

Mandojana RM, et al: Localized epidermotropic reticulosis. JAAD 1983, 8:813.

Medenica M: Pagetoid reticulosis (Woringer-Kolopp disease). Arch Dermatol 1978, 114:262.

Tan RS-H, et al: Pagetoid reticulosis, epidermotropic mycosis fungoides, and mycosis fungoides: a disease spectrum. Br J Dermatol 1987, 116:67.

Zackheim HS: Is "localized epidermotropic reticulosis" (Woringer-Kolopp disease) benign? JAAD 1984, 11:276.

Idem: Localized epidermotropic reticulosis (letter). JAAD 1984, 11:904.

LYMPHOMATOID PAPULOSIS

In 1968 Macaulay described a self-healing but chronic, recurrent eruption of hemorrhagic papules, some attaining a diameter of as much as 12 mm, which spontaneously involuted after three to eight weeks. The lesions usually spare the face and scalp and cluster on the trunk and limbs. Clinical similarity to Mucha-Habermann syndrome (pityriasis lichenoides et varioliformis acuta) may be striking. The average age at onset is 38. Male patients slightly outnumber female. No more than some 20 lesions are usually present at any one time, although any particular patient may have only large solitary lesions, or uncommonly, there may be over 100. The disease is in constant activity, with lesions involuting and new ones developing at the same time. Mild pruritus is the only symptom.

Willemze separates these cases histologically into Type A (in which the atypical cell is "histiocytic") and Type B, where the proliferating cell is an activated T helper cell. In both, the histologic appearance is that of a malignancy—despite which, most patients follow a benign clinical course. The infiltrate is generally dense, with either atypical lymphocytes or histiocytic cells; neutrophils are usually present; and in Type B, epidermotropism is seen. Cell phenotyping reveals antigens associated with lymphoma, rather than benign inflammation, and DNA analysis (looking for T-cell receptor rearrangements) also supports the view that this is a T-cell lymphoma.

This view finds support in many reports of its eventual evolution into various types of lymphoma, including mycosis fungoides, Hodgkin's disease, and non-Hodgkin's lymphoma, appearing in the recent literature. Approximately 10 per cent of cases will eventuate, perhaps only after 10 to 20 years, in an aggressive lymphoma.

TREATMENT. Therapy is often unsatisfactory. Wantzin et al found PUVA effective in four cases, though all required maintenance treatment. Zackheim et al treated seven patients with topically applied carmustine (BCNU), 10 mg daily for four to 17 weeks, with satisfactory suppression of lesions (short of complete clearing) in all. Bone marrow depression did not occur.

Topical, intralesional, and systemic corticosteroids are seldom helpful. Zackheim et al reviewed all reported types of therapy, and felt that of all systemic oncologic agents, methotrexate gave the most dependable response. Thomsen et al, in their report of 30 patients, also found methotrexate useful—but maintenance therapy was required.

Espinoza CG, et al: Lymphomatoid papulosis: a premalignant T-cell disorder. JAAD 1985, 13:736.

Everett MA: Lymphomatoid papulosis (editorial). JAAD 1986, 15:507.

Kadin ME: Characteristic immunological profile of large atypical cells in lymphomatoid papulosis. Arch Dermatol 1986, 122:1388.

Idem: Clonal composition of T-cells in lymphomatoid papulosis. Am J Pathol 1987, 126:13.

Kardashian JL, et al: Lymphomatoid papulosis associated with plaque-stage and granulomatous mycosis fungoides. Arch Dermatol 1985, 121:1175.

Lederman JS, et al: Lymphomatoid papulosis following Hodgkin's disease. JAAD 1987, 16:331.

Madison JF, et al: Lymphomatoid papulosis terminating as cutaneous T-cell lymphoma (mycosis fungoides). JAAD 1983, 9:743.

Patterson JW, et al: Lymphomatoid papulosis. South Med J 1986, 79:850.

Sanchez NP, et al: The dimiopathologic spectrum of lymphomatoid papulosis. JAAD 1983, 8:81.

Scheen SR, et al: Lymphoma-associated papulosis. JAAD 1981, 4:451.

Sina B, et al: Lymphomatoid papulosis: case reports and literature review. Arch Dermatol 1983, 119:189.

Thomsen K, et al: Lymphomatoid papulosis. JAAD 1987, 17:632.

Tokura Y, et al: Lymphomatoid papulosis. Arch Dermatol 1986, 122:1400.

Wantzin GL, et al: PUVA treatment in lymphomatoid papulosis. Br J Dermatol 1982, 107:687.

Idem: Lymphomatoid papulosis. Arch Dermatol 1985, 121:792.

Weiss LM, et al: Clonal T-cell populations in lymphomatoid papulosis. N Engl J Med 1986, 315:475.

Willemze R, et al: Clinical and histologic differentiation between lymphomatoid papulosis and pityriasis lichenoides. JAAD 1985, 13:418.

Willemze R: Lymphomatoid papulosis. Dermatol Clin 1985, 3:735.

Wood GS, et al: Lymphomatoid papulosis expresses immunophenotypes associated with T-cell lymphoma, but not inflammation. JAAD 1986, 15:444.

Zackheim HS, et al: Topical carmustine therapy for lymphomatoid papulosis. Arch Dermatol 1985, 121:1410.

NON-HODGKIN'S LYMPHOMA

The classification of non-Hodgkin's lymphoma has been summarized by Krüger and standardized by the National Cancer Institute. Most cutaneous non-Hodgkin's lymphoma is of T cell origin. These types have been discussed above. B cell types involving the skin, and the uncommon true histiocytic and null-cell lymphomas, will be discussed here.

CLINICAL FEATURES. All are so similar that they can hardly be differentiated clinically. Lymphoma of the skin may be primary or, more usually, associated

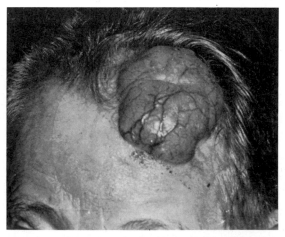

Figure 32–13. Lymphosarcoma of 1 year's duration. Complete involution occurred after 800 rads were given in divided doses.

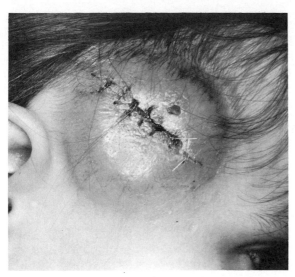

Figure 32–14. Lymphocytic lymphoma in a 6-year-old girl who subsequently developed leukemia.

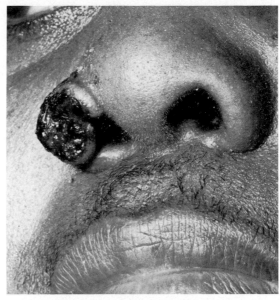

Figure 32–16. Lymphosarcoma. Complete involution occurred after x-ray therapy. (Courtesy of Dr. J. Teisch.)

with lymph node disease. The skin manifestations may be specific or nonspecific.

Specific lesions are solitary, or oftener multiple, plum-colored papules or deep-seated firm nodules from a few millimeters to a few centimeters in diameter. The plum-colored nodule is distinctive. Such nodules may ulcerate, especially if they enlarge progressively. Solitary nodules, especially on the scalp, may be present for several years before they cause symptoms. They are usually firm and rubbery.

Cutaneous lesions of B-cell lymphoma may be contrasted with those of T-cell lymphoma. Generally B-cell lymphoma has a short history—one to two years—compared to the insidious onset and slow evolution seen in T-cell lymphoma. They are often solitary tumors, without scale or ulceration, and

rapidly growing. Nodal disease tends to develop early, but it may be long delayed, as in the report by Marti et al.

Among 1186 patients with non-Hodgkin's lymphoma, 5 to 10 per cent had skin involvement.

Histiocytic Lymphoma. This neoplasm is composed of large atypical transformed B lymphocytes, which are easily mistaken for histiocytes, and have given it its other name: *large-cell lymphoma*. It was formerly called *reticulum-cell sarcoma*. Often it presents as a solitary lesion, but it may be a widespread nodular eruption clinically very much like mycosis

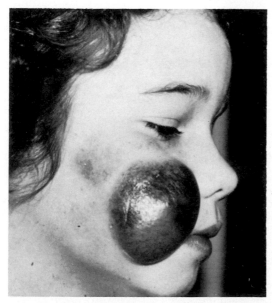

Figure 32–15. Plum-colored tumor of lymphosarcoma in 7-year-old girl.

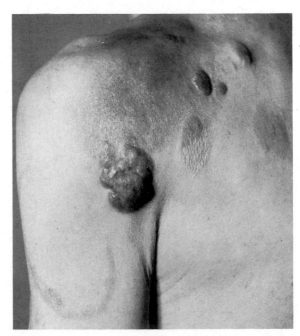

Figure 32–17. Lymphosarcoma with configurate, slightly elevated lesions and large, plum-colored tumors.

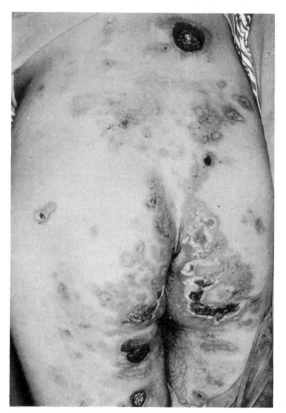

Figure 32–18. Ulcerative lesions of histiocytic lymphoma in a young man.

fungoides. Leukemic transformation may rarely occur. Furukawa reported a case which was apparently cured by a total dose of 4400 rads of superficial x-rays in four weeks. Ultmann says that 80 to 100 per cent of cases of diffuse histiocytic lymphoma can be cured by radiotherapy, chemotherapy, or a combination of the two.

Sheibani was the senior author of a multicenter study of three cases of malignant endotheliomatosis in which the cells filling the vessels had the immunophenotype of T cells in one case and B cells in two cases, and these researchers state that malignant angioendotheliomatosis should be designated as *angiotropic large-cell lymphoma*. This has been confirmed in further publications (see Chapter 28, Dermal Tumors).

The nonspecific lesions are similar to those of Hodgkin's disease; however, pruritus occurs less frequently in non-Hodgkin's lymphoma. Herpes zoster and exfoliative dermatitis are also seen less frequently than in Hodgkin's disease.

PATHOGENESIS. It is likely that multiple factors are concerned in the pathogenesis of lymphoma. Bierman has noted that some of the lymphomas may be induced by oncogenic viruses, chemical carcinogens, and epidemiologic influences. He further notes that immunologic disorders may predispose to, induce, or be associated with the various malignant lymphoproliferative disorders.

There is also an increasing frequency of lympho-proliferative diseases in association with such autoimmune disorders as Hashimoto's thyroiditis, systemic rheumatoid disease, systemic lupus erythematosus, dermatomyositis, and Sjögren's syndrome.

HISTOPATHOLOGY. The non-Hodgkin's lymphomas are classified according to the histologic architecture and the various cell types. The classification of the specific subtype depends on the pattern found in lymph nodes.

The B-cell histologic pattern is a nonepidermal infiltration of lymphocytes, lymphoplasmacytoid cells, and small and large follicular-center cells. Acid phosphatase and acid esterase are absent, but enzyme phenotyping shows a reaction for alkaline phosphatase in some subtypes. The lymphoid cells are predominantly HLA-Dr/Ia+, C3+, and Leu 14+, and stain for surface immunoglobulins and kappa and lambda chains on immunophenotyping. Monoclonality of surface immunoglobulin markers helps differentiate malignant infiltrates from reactive ones, as reported in the case of Hanno et al.

TREATMENT. If involvement of the skin is primary (no disease found in node and bone marrow biopsies, and nodal or organ involvement is excluded) local radiation therapy or excision may be curative. When skin lesions are a part of systemic lymphoma, combination chemotherapy is necessary.

PROGNOSIS. The National Cancer Institute's classification divides the subtypes of lymphoma into low, medium, and high grade malignancy. In general, the higher the grade, the worse the prognosis. Also, skin involvement often occurs in the advanced stages and usually indicates a poor prognosis. Extranodal dissemination to sites other than skin indicates a better prognosis than extranodal disease with skin lesions.

Burg G, et al: Cutaneous non-Hodgkin's lymphoma. Int J Dermatol 1978, 17:496.

Idem: Cutaneous B-cell lymphoma. Dermatol Clin 1985, 3:689.

Descalzi ME, et al: Sebaceous adenomas and keratoacanthomas in a patient with (non-Hodgkin's) malignant lymphoma. Cutis 1981, 28:169.

Fathizadeh A, et al: Morbilliform eruption in non-Hodgkin's lymphoma. Arch Dermatol 1982, 118:353.

Furukawa F, et al: True histiocytic lymphoma. Arch Dermatol 1980, 116:915.

Green PHR, et al: Cure of histiocytic lymphoma. Ann Intern Med 1982, 97:274.

Hanna W, et al: Signet-ring lymphoma of the skin. JAAD 1986, 14:344.

Hanno R, et al: Cutaneous B-cell lymphoma: diagnostic use of monoclonal antibodies. JAAD 1985, 13:373.

Krüger GRF: Concepts in lymphoma classification. J Dermatol Surg Oncol 1984, 10:247.

Long JC: Malignant lymphoma of the skin: clinicopathologic study of lymphoma other than mycosis fungoides diagnosed by skin biopsy. Cancer 1976, 38:1282.

Mann RB, et al: Malignant lymphomas: a conceptual understanding of morphologic diversity. Am J Pathol 1979, 94:105.

Marti RM, et al: Primary cutaneous lymphoplasmacytic lymphoma. JAAD 1987, 16:1106.

Miller RA, et al: Treatment of B-cell lymphoma with monoclonal anti-idiotype antibody. N Engl J Med 1982, 306:517.

National Cancer Institute–sponsored study of classifications of non-Hodgkin's lymphoma. Cancer 1982, 49:2112.

Ralfkiaer E, et al: Immunocytochemical characterization of cutaneous lymphomas other than mycosis fungoides. J Clin Pathol 1986, 39:553.

Ralfkiaer E, et al: Immunocytochemical characterization of cutaneous lymphomas other than mycosis fungoides. J Clin Pathol 1986, 39:553.

Saekow M, et al: Lymphoma *en cuirasse*. JAAD 1986, 14:1096.

Sheibani K, et al: Further evidence that "malignant angioendotheliomatosis" is an angiotropic large-cell lymphoma. N Engl J Med 1986, 314:943.

Sterry W, et al: Skin involvement of malignant B-cell lymphomas. J Dermatol Surg Oncol 1984, 10:276.

Wantzin GL, et al: Cutaneous lymphomas: clinical and histologic aspects. Acta Dermatol Venereol 1984, 62:119.

Wilkel CS, et al: Cutaneous B-cell lymphoma. Arch Dermatol 1987, 123:1362.

Willemze R, et al: Primary cutaneous large-cell lymphomas of follicular center cell origin. JAAD 1987, 17:518.

HODGKIN'S DISEASE

Hodgkin's disease of the skin originates in the lymph nodes, from which extension may take place in contiguity or elsewhere to the skin. These skin lesions may be either specific or nonspecific. Skin lesions are rarely the initial presentation; Silverman et al reported such a case in 1982.

The *specific lesions* may be circumscribed infiltrations, but more commonly are papules. These appear in crops on the extremities or on the trunk, and often enlarge and become ulcerated. The lesions are accompanied (or even long preceded) by itching, and generalized pruritus may be the presenting sign of Hodgkin's disease. J. L. Smith et al reported that only nine (0.5 per cent) of 1810 patients had specific histology, whereas White et al found histologic specificity in 16 (3.4 per cent) patients seen at their institution over a 30-year period. These skin lesions usually arise from retrograde lymphatic spread distal to the involved node; rarely, there may be direct extension from an underlying node, or even hematogenous spread.

Many reports of cutaneous Hodgkin's disease actually represent Type A lymphomatoid papulosis. The relationship between these two diseases is close: many cases of lymphomatoid papulosis eventuate in Hodgkin's disease. Primary cutaneous Hodgkin's disease without nodal involvement is difficult if not impossible to prove, and no acceptable cases have been published to date.

Histologically, the specific skin lesions are similar to affected lymph node changes and show the Reed-Sternberg cell. A Reed-Sternberg cell is a large cell with two or more, often mirror-image, nuclei, each containing a single prominent nucleolus. The cytoplasm is abundant and chromatin is usually condensed at the nuclear membrane. There are also numerous eosinophils and areas of necrosis and fibrosis. Mitotic figures are common. Weiss et al found Epstein-Barr viral genomes in these cells.

The Rye modification of the Lukes-Butler classification divides Hodgkin's disease into four subcategories: *nodular sclerosing, lymphocytic predominance, mixed cellularity*, and *lymphocytic depletion*. White et al found that the histologic classification of cutaneous lesions corresponded with that of the lymph nodes in only eight of 16 cases.

The *nonspecific lesions* are presumably of a toxic nature and may be erythematous, urticarial, vesicular, or bullous, frequently resembling erythema multiforme. Pruritus is outstanding in one fourth of patients, and it may be the initial symptom in 5 to 10 percent, appearing even before any cutaneous lesions are seen. Unexplained persistent generalized pruritus in young adults should suggest roentgenograms of the chest for signs of Hodgkin's disease. Feiner et al found a positive correlation in their patients between severe pruritus and more aggressive disease.

Ichthyosiform atrophy or acquired ichthyosis in an

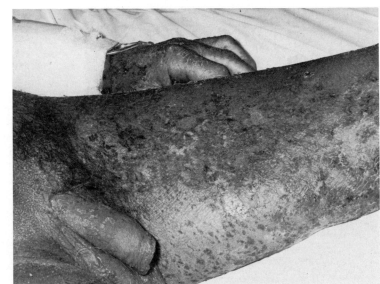

Figure 32–19. Hodgkin's disease. (Courtesy of Dr. F. Rosenberg.)

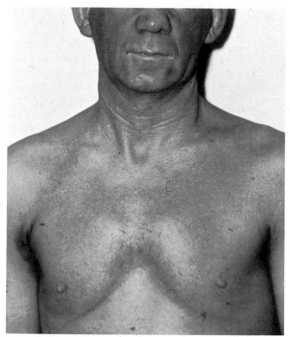

Figure 32–20. Universal erythema (homme rouge) for 3 years before other signs of Hodgkin's disease became overt.

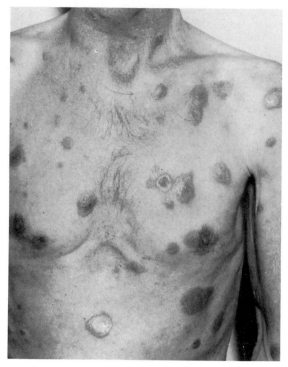

Figure 32–22. Hodgkin's disease granulomas.

adult may indicate Hodgkin's disease. Herpes zoster generalisata and other severe gangrenous and hemorrhagic types of zoster occur frequently in patients who have Hodgkin's disease.

Hodgkin's disease is treated by ionizing radiation therapy and chemotherapy. When specific skin lesions are present, stage IV (advanced) disease is said to be present. It has a poor prognosis, and in this stage chemotherapy is necessary. MOPP therapy (mechlorethamine, vincristine, procarbazine, and

prednisone) and modifications of it are effective in 70 to 80 per cent of patients, and ABVD (doxorubicin, bleomycin, vinblastine, and dacarbazine) is effective in more than half of those with MOPP-resistant disease, according to Santoro et al.

Feiner AS, et al: Prognostic importance of pruritus in Hodgkin's disease. JAMA 1978, 240:2738.

Jaffe ES: The elusive Reed-Sternberg cell. NEJM 1989, 320:529.

Kadin ME: Characteristic immunologic profile of large atypical cells in lymphomatoid papulosis. Arch Dermatol 1986, 122:1388.

Kaufman D, et al: Successfully treated Hodgkin's disease followed by mycosis fungoides. Cutis 1987, 39:291.

Moretti S, et al: In situ immunologic characterization of cutaneous involvement in Hodgkin's disease. Cancer 1989, 63:661.

Mueller W, et al: Hodgkin's disease and Epstein-Barr virus. NEJM 1989, 320:689.

Santoro A, et al: Salvage chemotherapy with ABVD in MOPP-resistant Hodgkin's disease. Ann Intern Med 1982, 96:139.

Idem: Alternating drug combinations in the treatment of advanced Hodgkin's disease. N Engl J Med 1982, 306:770.

Silverman CL, et al: Cutaneous Hodgkin's disease. Arch Dermatol 1982, 118:919.

Smith JL, et al: Skin involvement in Hodgkin's disease. Cancer 1980, 45:354.

Weiss LM, et al: Detection of Epstein-Barr viral genomes in Reed-Sternberg cells of Hodgkin's disease. NEJM 1989, 320:502.

White RM, et al: Cutaneous involvement in Hodgkin's disease. Cancer 1985, 55:1136.

Willemze R: Lymphomatoid papulosis. Dermatol Clin 1985, 3:735.

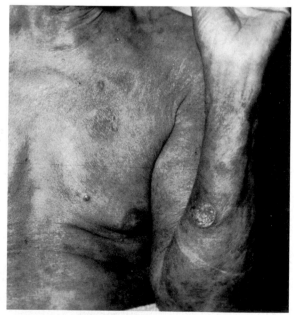

Figure 32–21. Hodgkin's disease with granuloma on forearm. Patient had pruritus and macular skin lesions for 4 years before fungating granuloma appeared.

LEUKEMIA CUTIS

CLINICAL FEATURES. The cutaneous manifestations in lymphocytic, granulocytic, and monocytic leukemia have many similarities. The eruption may

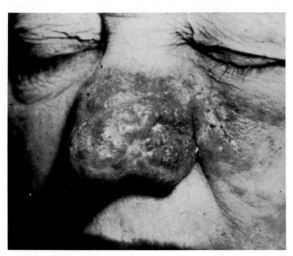

Figure 32–23. Lymphocytic leukemia on nose appearing 25 years after hematologic involvement. Prompt involution of nose lesion was attained with x-ray therapy.

be the first discernible symptom of leukemia, appearing even before the abnormalities in the peripheral blood, bone marrow, or other locations.

The cutaneous eruptions of leukemia may be divided into the specific and nonspecific lesions (leukemids). These may occur separately or in combination.

Specific Eruptions. True leukemic infiltrations of the skin consist of nodular, diffuse, or plaquelike infiltrations with swelling, macules, papules, ecchymoses, palpable purpura, erythroderma, and ulcerations, and as Su et al have shown, these have been seen in all types of leukemia. Both acute monocytic leukemia (AMOL) and acute myelomonocytic leukemia (AMML) have the highest incidence of specific lesions. These are present in 33 per cent of AMOL patients, and 15 per cent of AMML, while 50 per cent of AMOL and 25 per cent of AMML cases have gingival infiltration.

Lymphocytic Leukemia. Leukemic infiltrations ap-

pear in 8 per cent of the chronic type and uncommonly in the acute type. Su et al reported on 16 patients with chronic leukemia (CLL) and three with acute (ALL) who had specific infiltrations of the skin. There are discrete nodules or tumors and, at times, a widespread symmetrical and diffuse swelling and infiltration, with erythroderma. The nodular variety begins as one or more discrete bluish red or plum-colored painless cutaneous nodules of rubbery consistency, or as subcutaneous nodular infiltrations under an apparently normal skin. The most frequent location is on the face (leonine facies), but they may occur on other parts, especially the extensor surfaces of the extremities, the breasts, and the shoulders. The lesions may be rounded tumors or flat-topped raised plaques. The nodules tend to grow to the size of a hen's egg and then to remain stationary or to involute without ulceration or scarring. The infrequently occurring plaques tend to occur on the face. Tumors and plaques may become ulcerated, especially those on the genitalia. Both Rosen et al and Côté et al have reported a vesiculobullous eruption occurring in CLL patients. Su et al noted that in their series of 42 cases, erythrodermic and bullous lesions were observed only in CLL. Frix et al reported an acantholytic bullous disease resembling pemphigus foliaceus in their patient.

Diffuse *infiltrated erythroderma* is manifested by a general and symmetrical swelling and redness of the skin associated with severe pruritus. The skin surface may be simply stretched and smooth, slightly scaly, severely exfoliative, eczematous, or lichenified. There is an enlargement of all palpable lymph glands. There may be shedding of the hair and nails. This is only rarely seen in lymphocytic leukemia. Clinically the differentiation from mycosis fungoides, Hodgkin's disease, and pityriasis rubra pilaris may be a difficult task. A positive diagnosis is made only histologically.

Hairy-cell Leukemia. Skin involvement is a rare exception in this curious form of leukemia, which may be a neoplasm of B cells or monocytes; Li

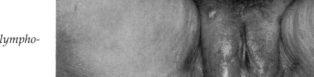

Figure 32–24. Vulvar infiltrates of chronic lymphocytic leukemia.

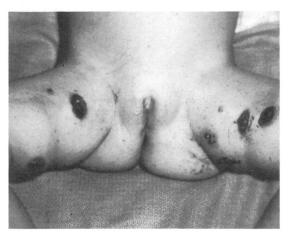

Figure 32–25. Acute monocytic leukemia in a 2-year-old child.

reviewed the evidence. Lawrence et al reported a case diagnosed by biopsy of the skin, and Finan et al reported one case, among 113 cases of hairy-cell leukemia in the Mayo Clinic files, with violaceous skin nodules on the scalp and chest. Acid-phosphatase–positive, tartrate-resistant staining characterizes the neoplastic cells. Connely et al reported a third patient, in whom the lips were infiltrated. Nonspecific lesions, especially of the opportunistic infectious type, are common.

Adult T-Cell Leukemia/Lymphoma. Chan et al reviewed the findings in that condition, and it has been discussed in the retroviral section, as well as under mycosis fungoides.

Monocytic and Myelomonocytic Leukemia. As mentioned previously, infiltrations into the skin and gingiva occur in many patients with AMOL and AMML. Baden et al review possible explanations of this, with retained deformability of the leukemic cells being the most likely explanation. While the chronic varieties rarely involve the skin, Pozo-Román et al report a patient whose skin involvement appeared when he was going into a blastic crisis.

Granulocytic Leukemia (Granulocytic Sarcoma). Although eruptions appear that are similar to those of lymphocytic leukemia, they occur infrequently. The cutaneous nodules have a predilection for the trunk, although they may also occur on the extremities and the face. The nodules may be firm or elastic and may be livid red or mahogany in color.

Sun et al reported a case diagnosed by skin biopsy in the preleukemic phase, in 1980, eight months before her death from granulocytic leukemia. Horan reported a skin lesion originally misdiagnosed as granuloma faciale in which acute granulocytic leukemia supervened three weeks after the appearance of the skin nodule, which was then reexamined and found to be a granulocytic sarcoma.

It is generally agreed that *chloroma (granulocytic sarcoma)* is a form of acute granulocytic leukemia characterized by the presence of tumors on the face, seen primarily in children and adolescents. The lesions result from the infiltration of granulocytic cells into the orbital and cranial periosteum. An enzyme, myeloperoxidase, causes the green pigment, which is visible on the cut surface of the tumors.

Leukemid. The nonspecific eruptions (leukemids) are polymorphous. Urticarial, bullous, and erythema multiforme manifestations; papulonecrotic, eczematous, and zosteriform lesions; diffuse erythroderma, hemorrhagic lesions, xanthomas, pruritus, pallor, acral lividosis, vasculitis, Sweet's syndrome, pyoderma gangrenosum, erythema nodosum, ichthyosis, hyperpigmentation, opportunistic infections, and ulcerations may all be seen.

Pruritus is possibly the most frequent nonspecific manifestation of the leukemias, especially in the lymphocytic type. It may be accompanied by prurigolike papules, which are pale and edematous and show pin-point vesiculation. There may be unbearably severe pruritus with exfoliative erythroderma, and loss of hair and nails.

Hemorrhagic exanthems and *enanthems* are frequent in all types of leukemia. Hemorrhage in lymphocytic

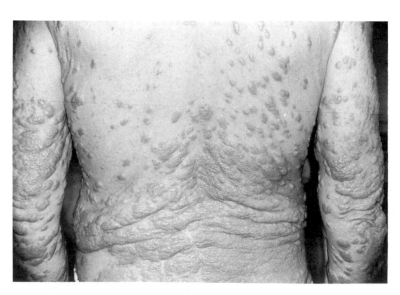

Figure 32–26. Extensive infiltrates in a man with monocytic leukemia.

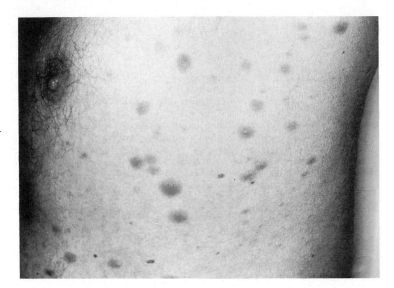

Figure 32–27. Skin infiltrates of acute myelogenous leukemia.

leukemia may be an early sign. There may be purpura, ecchymoses, epistaxis, bleeding gums, and intestinal hemorrhage.

Erythroderma in leukemia may be a specific or nonspecific eruption, but usually is generalized. Pruritus is usually present.

Herpes zoster occurs especially in lymphocytic leukemia, Hodgkin's disease, and myeloma. The zoster may be gangrenous or hemorrhagic, and frequently becomes generalized. Large bullae may be present in the mouth, so that the eruption simulates pemphigus.

Herpes simplex may be ulcerative and often chronic. Many opportunistic infections occur, and some may be fatal.

A subset of chronic granulomatous leukemia, *juvenile CGL,* has been reported to be associated with neurofibromatosis and juvenile xanthogranulomas. Cooper et al and Heskel et al reviewed these reports.

Sweet's syndrome may herald the appearance of leukemia, most often of the AMML type. Bullous pyoderma gangrenosum is another neutrophilic dermatosis that may be associated with a myeloproliferative disorder.

Two reactions to the therapy of leukemia have been described recently. Neutrophilic eccrine hidradenitis may occur as papules or plaques during the second week of therapy for AML. It has a unique histologic appearance. Cytarabine has been implicated as a potential cause. Acral erythema, while it may occur in leukemia without treatment, has been reported to occur most commonly after treatment has been begun.

ETIOLOGY. The cause of leukemia is still a perplexing enigma. Chromosomal aberrations have been carefully studied in the various leukemias. The Philadelphia chromosome is an abnormal chromosome believed to be specifically seen in chronic myelogenous leukemia. The abnormality is the loss of a segment in the twenty-first chromosome. Of course adult T-cell leukemia/lymphoma has a viral cause, the human T-cell lymphoma/leukemia virus (HTLV-1). See Chapter 19, Viral Diseases.

HISTOPATHOLOGY. The circumscribed lesions in leukemia cutis are formed by a single spheroid mass of cells, or of multiple, small, dense, focal accumulations of lymphocytes occurring either diffusely in the upper dermis or as nodules and tumors in the dermis or subcutis. Immature forms may be present. The infiltration is perivascular. In all stages, at the edges of the infiltration, it is possible to demonstrate its tendency to adhere closely to the vessels, about which it frequently forms a cylindrical structure. Mitosis is usually absent. At times plasma cells and fibroblasts are present.

In lymphocytic leukemia the cells are solely lymphocytes, differing only in size, in the shape of the nucleus, and in protoplasmic content. In granulocytic leukemia the cells are large mononuclears with neutrophilic, granular cytoplasm, being eosinophilic myelocytes, myeloblasts, and other immature forms. With them are multinucleated cells, eosinophils, and mast cells, which give a positive oxidase reaction. These cells infiltrate within the connective tissue, which acts as a supportive stroma. In the diffuse variety of infiltration with erythroderma, there is a dense, uniform or nodular, infiltrating band of the characteristic cells in the subpapillary zone and middermis, which is separated almost completely from the basal cell layer by a narrow band of normal connective tissue. The cells of the infiltration follow the vascular channels exactly, but do not encroach upon the papillary bodies.

TREATMENT. Antileukemic therapy consists of ionizing radiation and chemotherapy. For the skin lesions x-ray therapy is probably the most effective. Tumoricidal amounts of x-rays may be given; however, since palliation is mostly desired, small doses may be just as effective. For the nonspecific lesions, therapy is directed to the relief of symptoms.

Chemotherapy has been employed in all the types of leukemia with varying degrees of success. Specific skin lesions are associated with a poor prognosis.

Baden TJ, et al: Leukemia cutis in acute myelomonocytic leukemia. Arch Dermatol 1987, 123:88.

Burgdorf WHC, et al: Peculiar acral erythema secondary to high-dose chemotherapy for acute myelogenous leukemia. Ann Intern Med 1982, 97:61.

Caughman W, et al: Neutrophilic dermatosis of myeloproliferative disorders. JAAD 1983, 9:751.

Chan HL, et al: Cutaneous manifestations of adult T-cell leukemia/lymphoma. JAAD 1985, 13:213.

Cohen PR, et al: Infiltrated blue-gray plaques in a patient with leukemia. Arch Dermatol 1987, 123:251.

Connelly TJ, et al: Leukemic macrocheilitis associated with hairy-cell leukemia and the Melkersson/Rosenthal syndrome. JAAD 1986, 14:353.

Cooper PH, et al: Association of juvenile xanthogranuloma with juvenile myeloid leukemia. Arch Dermatol 1984, 120:371.

Côté J, et al: T-cell chronic lymphocytic leukemia with bullous manifestations. JAAD 1983, 8:874.

Finan MC, et al: Cutaneous findings in hairy-cell leukemia. JAAD 1984, 11:788.

Flynn TC, et al: Neutrophilic eccrine hidradenitis. JAAD 1984, 111:584.

Frankel DH, et al: Acral lividosis—a sign of myeloproliferative diseases. Arch Dermatol 1987, 123:921.

Frix CD III, et al: Pemphigus foliaceus-like, immunologically negative dermatitis in a patient with T-cell chronic lymphocytic leukemia. JAAD 1988, 18:1197.

Hansen RM, et al: Aleukemic leukemia cutis. Arch Dermatol 1986, 122:812.

Heskel NS, et al: Aleukemic leukemia cutis. JAAD 1983, 9:423.

Horan DB: Granulocytic sarcoma preceding granulocytic leukemia. Cutis 1984, 33:285.

Lawrence DM, et al: Cutaneous lesions in hairy-cell leukemia. Arch Dermatol 1983, 119:32.

Levine LL, et al: Distinctive acral erythema occurring during therapy for severe myelogenous leukemia. Arch Dermatol 1985, 121:102.

Leyden JJ: Infection in the immunocompromised host. Arch Dermatol 1985, 121:855.

Margolis RJ, et al: Erythema multiforme in a patient with T-cell chronic lymphocytic leukemia. JAAD 1986, 14:618.

Nielsen M: Painful palmar-plantar erythema in myeloproliferative disease. Arch Dermatol 1985, 121:1240.

O'Donnell JR, et al: Acute myelomonocytic leukemia presenting a xanthomatous skin eruption. J Clin Pathol 1982, 35:1200.

Pozo-Román T, et al: Specific cutaneous involvement in the course of chronic myelomonocytic leukemia simultaneously with blastic crisis. JAAD 1985, 12:943.

Prystowsky JH, et al: Treatment of cutaneous granulocytic sarcoma in a patient with myelodysplasia. Am J Med 1989, 86:477.

Rosen LB, et al: A characteristic vesiculobullous eruption in patients with chronic lymphocytic leukemia. JAAD 1986, 15:943.

Shaikh BS, et al: Histologically proven leukemia cutis carries a poor prognosis in acute nonlymphocytic leukemia. Cutis 1987, 39:57.

Shalen L, et al: Progressive cutaneous herpes simplex infection in acute myeloblastic leukemia. Arch Dermatol 1984, 120:922.

Spann CR, et al: Cutaneous leukocytoclastic vasculitis complicating hairy-cell leukemia. Arch Dermatol 1986, 122:1057.

Stawiski MA: Skin manifestations of leukemias and lymphomas. Cutis 1978, 21:814.

Su WPD, et al: Clinicopathologic correlations in leukemia cutis. JAAD 1984, 11:121.

Sun NCJ, et al: Granulocytic sarcoma of the skin. Arch Dermatol 1980, 116:800.

Vail JT, et al: Cutaneous xanthomas associated with chronic myelomonocytic leukemia. Arch Dermatol 1985, 121:1318.

tutes the hypereosinophilic syndrome. Organ involvement may be in bone marrow, heart, skin, or nervous system. Over 90 per cent of patients reported have been men, mostly of middle age. The usual presenting complex includes fever, weight loss, fatigue, malaise, and a skin eruption. A variety of skin manifestations were described in eight of 15 cases reported by Kazmierowski and associates, ranging from angioedema, through papular lesions on the extremities, sometimes pruritic, to ulcerated nodules; the latter were present in one of the two patients who actually had eosinophilic leukemia. Seven patients had no skin lesions. Cardiomegaly, liver enlargement, diarrhea, neurologic abnormalities, lymphadenopathy, pulmonary infiltrates, and abnormal echocardiograms were found singly or in various combinations. Cardiac disease is the commonest cause of morbidity and mortality. Biopsies show mixed cell populations with numerous eosinophils in a perivascular distribution.

Complement activation products C3a and C5a, and an eosinophilic-chemotactic precursor substance, elaborated by antigen-stimulated lymphocytes, may cause the eosinophilia.

Systemic steroids (alternate-day prednisone) are the drug of choice beginning at 60 mg per day, with downward adjustments as response indicates. Many who do not respond to oral steroids improve on hydroxyurea, 1 to 2 gm per day. In some cases neither is effective. In cases where organ disease is not severe, a trial of less toxic therapy may be undertaken.

Nir et al reported a case in which dapsone was very effective, and this or intramuscular triamcinolone should be tried. PUVA cleared a patient treated by van den Hoogenband et al; he remained clear for two years following 25 treatments totalling 156 joules/cm^2.

The overall five-year survival rate is 80 per cent.

Chusid MJ, et al: The hypereosinophilic syndrome. Medicine 1975, 54:1.

Fauci AS, et al: The idiopathic hypereosinophilic syndrome. Ann Intern Med 1982, 97:78.

Kazmierowski JA, et al: Dermatologic manifestations of the hypereosinophilic sydrome. Arch Dermatol 1978, 114:531.

Nir MA, et al: Hypereosinophilic dermatitis. Dermatologica 1981, 162:444.

Spry CJ: The hypereosinophilic syndrome. Allergy 1982, 37:539.

Van den Hoogenband HM, et al: PUVA therapy in . . . the hypereosinophilic syndrome. Arch Dermatol 1985, 121:450.

Idem: Skin lesions as the first manifestation of the hypereosinophilic syndrome. Clin Exp Dermatol 1982, 267.

Whittaker SJ, et al: Lymphomatoid papulosis and its relationship to "idiopathic" hypereosinophilic syndrome. JAAD 1988, 18:339.

HYPEREOSINOPHILIC SYNDROME

Unexplained eosinophilia of over 1500 eosinophils per cubic millimeter for over six months, with some evidence of parenchymal organ involvement, consti-

ANGIOIMMUNOBLASTIC LYMPHADENOPATHY

This disorder, first clearly described in the late 1970's, is a rare lymphoproliferative disorder, between benign lymphoid proliferation and lymphoma. While it may occur at any age, the usual age at onset is 60, with women and men affected in equal frequency. Most of the 45 percent of patients with cutaneous lesions have them a few weeks before systemic symptoms appear. The lesions are nonspecific, being usually described as widespread erythematous macules and papules. Petechiae, purpura, and nodules may also be seen. Biopsy specimens of these lesions show perivascular collections of histiocytic-appearing cells with variable numbers of lymphocytes.

Lymphadenopathy, fever, malaise, hepatosplenomegaly, and weight loss are present. The lymph node histology is the diagnostic feature. Laboratory findings include anemia, thrombocytopenia, and hypergammaglobulinemia.

Seventy-five percent of patients die within two years or develop a lymphoid malignancy. Treatment with systemic steroids and immunosuppressive agents appears better than no therapy, but response is generally poor.

The etiology of this disease is unknown. Early in the course, activated T-cells stimulate B-cell proliferation, whereas later, increased suppressor function may cause immune suppression. T-cell receptor beta-chain gene or immunoglobulin gene clonal rearrangements are seen in all patients.

Azevedo SJ, et al: Angioimmunoblastic lymphadenopathy. Am J Hematol 1985, 20:301.
Bernstein JE, et al: Cutaneous manifestations of angioimmunoblastic lymphadenopathy. JAAD 1979, 1:227.
Frizzera G, et al: Angioimmunoblastic lymphadenopathy. Am J Med 1975, 59:803.
Goldberg NC, et al: Cutaneous manifestations of angioimmunoblastic lymphadenopathy. Arch Dermatol 1980, 116:41.
Matloff RB, et al: Angioimmunoblastic lymphadenopathy. Arch Dermatol 1978, 114:92.
Nathwani BN, et al: Malignant lymphoma arising in angioimmunoblastic lymphadenopathy. Cancer 1970, 41:578.
Schauer PK, et al: Angioimmunoblastic lymphadenopathy. Cancer 1981, 48:2493.
Seehafer JR, et al: Cutaneous manifestations of angioimmunoblastic lymphadenopathy. Arch Dermatol 1980, 116:41.
Steinberg AD, et al: Angioimmunoblastic lymphadenopathy with dysproteinemia. Ann Intern Med 1988, 108:575.

POLYCYTHEMIA VERA (Erythremia)

This myeloproliferative disorder has also been known as Vasquez's or Osler's disease. It is characterized by an absolute increase of circulating red blood cells ranging between 6.5 and 10 million, a hematocrit of 55 to 80 per cent, and hemoglobin of 18 to 25 gm per cent. The leukocytes and platelets are also increased. Further, there is splenomegaly.

The skin changes are characteristic. There is a tendency for the skin to be red, especially on the face, neck, and acral areas. The mucous membranes are engorged and bluish. The remark "red as a rose in summer and indigo blue in winter" has been

ascribed to Osler in describing polycythemia. Telangiectases, ruby spots, bleeding gums, and epistaxis are frequently encountered. Cyanosis, purpura, petechiae, hemosiderosis, and macroglossia may be present. Severe rosacea is common. Koilonychia may also be present. Grob et al reported a patient with disseminated pustular lesions, which they felt were a reactive pattern that fit into the neutrophilic dermatosis of myeloproliferative disorder.

The onset is insidious. There may be headache, dizziness, ringing of the ears, and dyspnea as well as innumerable other symptoms. Pruritus may be severe. This is typically triggered by contact with water, and the feeling induced may be itching, burning, or stinging. There is a concurrent elevation of blood histamine. The discomfort usually persists for 15 to 60 minutes. Greaves, Steinman, and Kligman regard polycythemia as a primary consideration in pruritus of unknown cause. Forty-three of 325 untreated patients with polycythemia suffered from it. Polycythemia is manifested by an increase of all the bone marrow elements, but there is particularly excessive production of red blood cells.

Treatment is by venesection of approximately 480 ml twice weekly until the packed red blood cell volume becomes normal. Radioactive phosphorus intravenously, and chemotherapeutic drugs such as melphalan, busulfan, and hydroxyurea are used. Antihistamines, such as cyproheptadine hydrochloride, alone or in combination with cimetidine, has been recommended for bath pruritus. Other measures that may help the pruritus are aspirin and PUVA.

Berlin NI: Polycythemia I. Semin Hematol 1975, 12:335.
Easton P: Cimetidine treatment of pruritus in polycythemia vera. N Engl J Med 1978, 299:1134.
Fjellner B, et al: Pruritus in polycythemia vera: treatment with aspirin and the possibility of platelet involvement. Acta Dermatol 1979, 59:505.

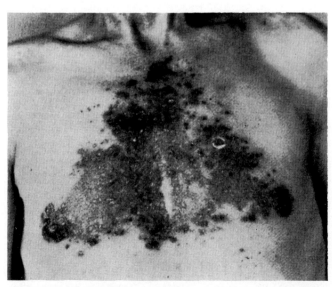

Figure 32–28. Erythematous pustular eruption in polycythemia vera, which healed after treatment by fractional x-ray therapy.

Grob JJ, et al: Disseminated pustular dermatosis in polycythemia vera. JAAD 1988, 18:1212.

Horowitz J, et al: Treatment of polycythemia vera with melphalan. Harefuah 1974, 87:351.

Kligman AM, et al: Water-induced itching without cutaneous signs. Arch Dermatol 1986, 122:183.

Steinman HK, et al: Aquagenic pruritus. JAAD 1985, 13:91.

Swerlick RA: Photochemotherapy treatment of pruritus associated with polycythemia vera. JAAD 1985, 13:675.

PLASMACYTOMA
(Multiple Myeloma)

Multiple myeloma is a plasma cell neoplasm associated with lytic bone lesions and infiltration of plasma cells in the bone marrow. In addition, it is frequently associated with anemia, hyperglobulinemia, hypercalcemia, impaired renal function, and increased susceptibility to infections.

Specific skin lesions (also called plasmacytomas) in patients with myeloma may occur by direct extension into the skin from underlying bone lesions, or as metastatic extramedullary plasmacytomas. The former type is most common, and they are often soft and skin-colored, as in the case reported by W. D. James. The latter are usually hard, violaceous subcutaneous or intradermal masses, which occur late in the course of the disease, although occasionally, as in the case reported by Shah et al, they may be the presenting sign. These extramedullary plasmacytomas may also involve the respiratory, genitourinary, and gastrointestinal tracts.

Plasmacytomas may occasionally occur in the skin without evidence of myeloma. These primary plasmacytomas are rare. Burke et al have reported a patient with multiple lesions, and Canlas et al a solitary one. These patients generally have a better prognosis than those with myeloma.

Nonspecific skin lesions that occur in patients with multiple myeloma include amyloidosis, purpura, toxic erythema, alopecia; ichthyosiform or finely desquamative, pruritic dermatitis; Raynaud's phenomenon, cold urticaria, pyoderma gangrenosum, planar xanthomas, generalized anhidrosis, and scleroder-

malike lesions. Lukitsch et al reported a patient with marked follicular hyperkeratosis. This seems to be a characteristic paraneoplastic sign for myeloma, since its appearance with other malignancies is rare. Schallreuter reported migratory thrombophlebitis as the presenting symptom in a patient who developed myeloma.

In addition, signs and symptoms of hyperuricemia, neurologic manifestations of bilateral and symmetrical paralysis, neuropathies, and root symptoms associated with other evidence of amyloidosis, such as macroglossia, cardiopathy, and carpal tunnel syndrome, may be noted.

The bone involvement is manifested by finding in the roentgenogram "punched out" lesions that may lead to spontaneous pathologic fractures, especially in the rib cage, skull, clavicles, and proximal long bones.

The laboratory findings include hypercalcemia, hyperuricemia, normocytic anemia, erythrocyte rouleau formation, leukopenia, thrombocytopenia, and eosinophilia. The erythrocyte sedimentation rate is usually markedly increased. Blood serum viscosity may be so high as to demand correction, as in four cases reported from Cardiff by Tuddenham and associates. Plasmapheresis was effective.

M component serum globulins with cryoglobulinemia and Bence Jones proteins in the urine are specific changes found frequently in multiple myeloma. Other diseases in which the M component may be found are Waldenström's macroglobulinemia, heavy chain disease, lichen myxedematosus, leukemia, and cancer—and even infrequently in healthy persons. The M component is a narrow band appearing in any part from the very slow gamma globulin region to the faster alpha-1 zone in the electrophoretic pattern.

Histologically, the finding of a massive infiltrate of normal and abnormal plasma cells, which may be multinucleated, is a diagnostic feature.

Treatment of cutaneous plasmacytomas depends on the presence or absence of systemic myeloma. Radiation or chemotherapy is used to treat plasmacytomas occurring with systemic myeloma. Extramedullary lesions generally recur after surgical excision and are relatively unresponsive to radiotherapy and chemotherapy, separately or together.

Cutaneous plasmacytomas metastatic to the skin in patients with myeloma are a poor prognostic sign.

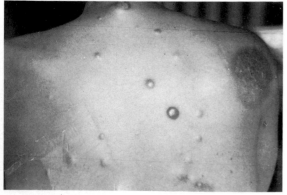

Figure 32–29. Plasmacytomas on back. Note hyperpigmented patch due to x-ray therapy.

Bluefarb SM: Cutaneous manifestations of multiple myeloma. Arch Dermatol 1955, 72:506.

Burke WA, et al: Disseminated extramedullary plasmocytomas. JAAD 1986, 14:335.

Canlas MS, et al: Primary cutaneous plasmacytoma: review of the literature and report of a case. Arch Dermatol 1979, 115:722.

James WD: Plasmacytoma. Arch Dermatol 1982, 118:62.

Kyle RA: Multiple myeloma: review of 869 cases. Mayo Clin Proc 1975, 50:29.

Lukitsch O, et al: Follicular hyperkeratosis and cryocrystalglobulinemia syndrome. Arch Dermatol 1985, 121:795.

Patterson JW, et al: Cutaneous involvement of multiple myeloma and extramedullary plasmacytoma. JAAD 1988, 18:879.

Schallreuter KU: An uncommon onset of myeloma. JAAD 1985, 13:819.

Shah A, et al: Multiple myeloma first observed as multiple cutaneous plasmacytomas. Arch Dermatol 1982, 118:922.

Sirot G: Cutaneous manifestations of multiple myeloma. Cutis 1979, 23:174.

Swanson NA, et al: Extramedullary IgM plasmacytoma presenting in skin. Am J Dermatopathol 1981, 1:79.

Wiltshaw E, et al: The natural history of extramedullary plasmacytoma and its relation to solitary myeloma of bone and myelomatosis. Medicine 1976, 55:217.

PSEUDOLYMPHOMA

Heavy lymphoid infiltrates of the skin may connote cutaneous lymphoma; however, a heterogeneous group of benign lesions occur which are suggestive of malignant lymphoma both clinically and histologically. The subtype of pseudolymphoma most closely resembling true lymphoma is a condition referred to by various names, of which the most frequently used are *lymphocytoma cutis, cutaneous lymphoplasia,* and *Spiegler-Fendt sarcoid.* Clinically, these lesions are most often skin-colored, red-brown, or violaceous nodules or plaques on the face. They may, however, be multiple or even disseminated. Women are affected more often than men.

Histologically there are two variants. One shows a heavy lymphocytic infiltrate in the dermis, with follicular germinal centers. The other subtype lacks follicular germinal centers and contains more or less numerous large, pleomorphic cells with frequent mitoses. At times only long-term follow-up of a patient who fails to develop lymph node involvement will exclude lymphoma.

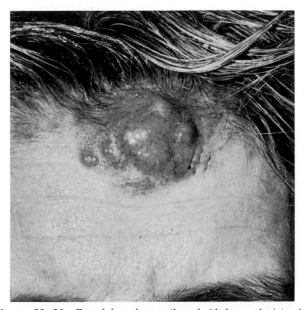

Figure 32–30. Pseudolymphoma (lymphoid hyperplasia) of 3 years' duration in a 45-year-old woman. Complete clearing followed administration of 150 rads (HVL 4 mm Al) at weekly intervals for four treatments.

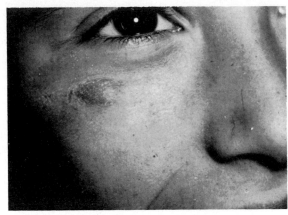

Figure 32–31. Insect bite granuloma resembling malignant lymphoma of the skin both clinically and histologically.

These lesions are probably reactive lymphoid proliferations elicited by external factors such as insect bites, trauma, tattoos, sun exposure, or prolonged contact with an antigen, such as gold earrings.

Treatment consists of topical or intralesional steroids, and at times local x-ray therapy. Stoll reported a good response to hydroxychloroquine.

Drug-Induced Pseudolymphomas

Olmos and Laugier have reported cases of pseudolymphoma induced by analgesics (incriminated by blast transformation tests), gold, and aspirin. Ultrastructural studies showed lymphocytes, many with cerebriform nuclei, and many histiocytes, together with intermediate cell forms. Cellular atypia and mitotic figures were conspicuous by their absence, and vascular changes, usually absent in lymphomas, were always present. The latter often produce epidermal changes. Discontinuing the responsible medication is curative.

Pseudolymphoma Syndrome

Under this term Schreiber and McGregor described a pseudolymphomatous reaction to anticonvulsant drugs such as phenytoin and mephenytoin and related drugs. Such cases consist classically of the triad of fever, lymphadenopathy, and an erythematous eruption: papules, nodules, or a plaque if localized, or in some instances diffuse erythema. Other clinical findings commonly include malaise, arthralgia, hepatosplenomegaly, eosinophilia, and abnormal liver function tests.

Histologically lymphoma may be simulated in biopsies of both lymph nodes and skin. There may be mimicry of either non-Hodgkin's lymphoma or mycosis fungoides.

While most cases resolve after stopping the anticonvulsant, steroid therapy is advisable and may be necessary. Only a few cases have been reported to convert to lymphoma. Whether this is related to suppressor T cell activation and impaired immunologic function, as suggested by the case reported by Lillie et al, or some other mechanism, is not known.

Bhanot P, et al: Primary malignant lymphoma cutis in an infant. Pediatrics 1979, 64:478.

Blumental G, et al: Pseudolymphomatous reactions to tattoos. JAAD 1982, 6:485.

Brodell RT, et al: Cutaneous pseudolymphomas. Dermatologic Clin 1985, 3:719.

Burg G, et al: Differentiation between malignant B-cell lymphomas and pseudolymphoma of skin. J Dermatol Surg Oncol 1984, 10:271.

Evans HL, et al: Differential diagnosis of malignant and benign cutaneous infiltrates. Cancer 1979, 44:699.

Iwatsuki K, et al: Lymphadenoid structure induced by gold hypersensitivity. Arch Dermatol 1982, 118:608.

Idem: Benign lymphoplasia of the earlobes induced by gold earrings. JAAD 1987, 16:83.

Lillie MA, et al: Erythroderma, hypogammaglobulinemia, and T-cell lymphocytosis. Arch Dermatol 1983, 119:415.

Payne CM, et al: An ultrastructural morphometric and immunohistochemical analysis of cutaneous lymphomas and benign lymphocytic infiltrates of the skin. Arch Dermatol 1986, 122:1139.

Silverman AK, et al: Cutaneous and immunologic reactions to phenytoin. JAAD 1988, 18:721.

Stedinger S: Lymphocytic infiltration of the skin. Arch Dermatol 1984, 120:112.

Stoll DM: Treatment of cutaneous pseudolymphoma with hydroxychloroquin. JAAD 1983, 8:696.

Wolf R, et al: Mycosis fungoides-like lesions associated with phenytoin therapy. Arch Dermatol 1985, 121:1181.

33

Diseases of the Skin Appendages

DISEASES OF THE HAIR

Normal human hairs can be classified according to cyclical phases of growth. Anagen hairs are growing hairs, catagen hairs are those undergoing transition from the growing to the resting stage, and telogen hairs are resting hairs, which remain in the follicles for variable lengths of time before they fall out.

Anagen hairs grow for some three years (1000 days—Orentreich), with the limits generally set between two and six years. The follicular cells grow, divide, and become keratinized to form growing hairs. The base of the hair shaft is soft and moist. A darkly pigmented portion is evident just above the hair bulb.

Catagen hairs are in a transitional phase, lasting a week or two, in which all growth activity ceases, with the formation of the "club" hair.

Telogen hairs, also known as club hairs, are resting hairs, which continue in this state some three to four months (100 days—Orentreich) before they are pushed out of the hair follicle by the hairs growing underneath them, or pulled out by a hair brush or other mechanical means.

Among human hairs plucked from the normal scalp, 90 per cent are anagen hairs and 10 per cent catagen or telogen hairs. It has been estimated that the scalp normally contains 100,000 hairs, therefore the average number of hairs shed daily is 100. The hair growth rate of terminal hairs is about 0.37 mm daily. Contrary to popular belief, neither shaving nor menstruation has any effect upon hair growth rate. The average uncut scalp hair length is estimated to be 25 to 100 cm, although exceptional hairs may be as long as 170 cm (70 inches).

Human hair is also designated as lanugo, vellus, or terminal hair. Lanugo hair is the fine hair present on the body of the fetus. This is replaced by the vellus and terminal hairs. Vellus hairs are fine (fuzz), usually light-colored, and characteristically seen on children's faces and arms. Terminal hairs are coarse, thick, and dark, except in blonds. Hair occurs on all skin surfaces except the palms, soles, glans, and prepuce. Terminal hairs are always present on men's face, chest, and abdomen, but vellus hairs usually predominate on these sites in women.

Bergfeld WF: Hair loss: a practical approach to diagnosis. Cutis 1978, 21:497.
Caserio RJ: Diagnostic techniques for hair disorders. Parts I, II, III. Cutis 1987, 40:265, 321, 442.
Idem: Disorders of hair. JAAD 1989, 19:895.
Ebling FJG: The biology of hair. Derm Clin 1987, 5:467.
Hordinsky MK: General evaluation of the patient with alopecia. Derm Clin 1987, 5:483.
Mehregan AH: Histopathology of alopecias. Cutis 1978, 21:249.
Modly CE, et al: Evaluation of alopecia. Cutis 1989, 43:148.
Rook A, Dawber R: Diseases of the Hair and Scalp. Oxford, Blackwell Scientific Publications, 1982.
Stroud JD: Diagnosis and management of the hair loss patient. Cutis 1987, 40:272.

ALOPECIA

Alopecia Areata

CLINICAL FEATURES. Alopecia areata (in French, *pelade*) is characterized by rapid and complete loss of hair in one, or more often several, round or oval patches, usually on the scalp, the bearded area, the eyebrows, the eyelashes, and rarely on other

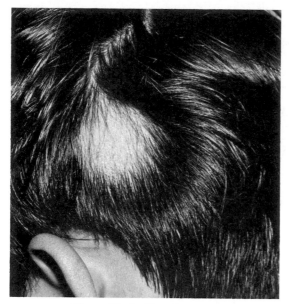

Figure 33–1. Alopecia areata.

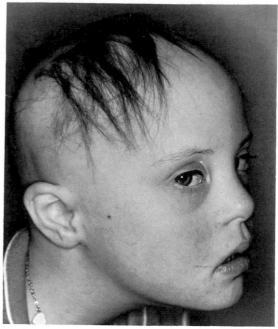

Figure 33–3. Alopecia areata in a child with Down's syndrome.

hairy areas of the body. Commonly the patches are from 1 to 5 cm in diameter. A few resting hairs may be found within the patches, and the surface may be slightly depressed. Early in the course there may be sparing of grey hair. Nearly always the hair loss is patchy in distribution; however, cases may present in a diffuse pattern. At the periphery of the bald patch are loose hairs that may be broken off near the scalp, leaving short stumps. When they are pulled out a tapered, attenuated bulb is seen as a result of

atrophy of that portion: hence the term "exclamation point" hair. These telogen hairs are usually located at the periphery of the bald patch. However, the problem arises in the anagen phase when damage to the hair shaft induces early catagen and telogen phases. The tendency is for spontaneous recovery in patients whose age at onset was after puberty. At first the regrowing hairs are downy and light in color; later they are replaced by stronger and darker hair with full growth. In some patients there is

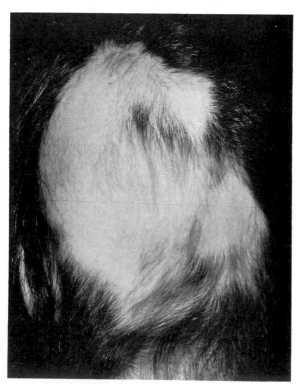

Figure 33–2. Alopecia areata.

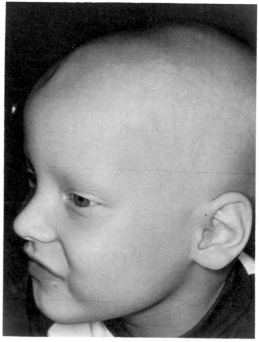

Figure 33–4. Alopecia universalis.

progression of the disease, with the development of new bald patches, until there is a total loss of scalp hair (*alopecia totalis*). When hair has been lost over the entire body, including the scalp, the designation is *alopecia universalis*. Alopecia areata usually occurs without associated disease. However, there is a higher incidence than usual in patients with atopic dermatitis, Down's syndrome, and such autoimmune diseases as thyroiditis and vitiligo.

In about 10 percent of cases of alopecia areata, especially in those of long standing with extensive involvement, the nails develop uniform pits that may form transverse or longitudinal lines. Dotz et al reported a case with leukonychia punctata and pitted nails, and Brown et al reviewed several cases associated with ocular and testicular abnormalities.

ETIOLOGY. Although Celsus described and named alopecia areata some 20 centuries ago, its cause is still unknown. Most evidence points toward its being an autoimmune disease modified by genetic factors and aggravated by emotional stress.

Many studies have documented abnormal cell-mediated immune factors in alopecia areata. There is an increased suppressor T-cell function in patients experiencing regrowth. In the inflammatory perifollicular infiltrate seen in active cases, helper cells predominate. Stress has been regarded for years as a possible initiator, and if it does play a role, it may be as an instigator of an immune mechanism.

Genetic susceptibility appears to be a factor, as suggested by a possible HLA association. Nearly 25 per cent of patients have a positive family history; there are reports of twins with alopecia areata; and certain populations may be at higher risk. Hordinsky et al reported a white American family in which three members from two generations had alopecia, areata in one and universalis in two.

Of 135 cases seen by Arnold in Hawaii from 1942 to 1952, 61 per cent were Japanese, in a practice with 35 per cent Japanese patients. In a morbidity survey by the Hawaii Chapter of the American College of Physicians, the respective proportions were 55 per cent among 69 cases of alopecia areata and 31 per cent overall.

Alopecia areata has been associated with several autoimmune diseases, including chronic lymphocytic thyroiditis (Hashimoto's disease), pernicious anemia, Addison's disease, vitiligo, and several of the connective tissue diseases. The presence of antibodies against thyroglobulin, parietal cells, adrenal cells, and thyroid cells has been demonstrated. Zauli et al and Milgraum et al report two of the more recent series documenting these associations.

HISTOLOGY. Sections of skin at sites of alopecia areata show hairs that are either in early anagen (which often predominate even in long-standing cases) or in dystrophic telogen structures. The hair follicles vary in size but tend to be small and immature. The hair bulbs are higher in the dermis and are surrounded by a chronic lymphocytic inflammatory infiltrate, especially in the early stage of develop-

ment. These infiltrating cells are 90 per cent T helper subtypes. Punch biopsy may be essential for diagnosis in some cases, as Bergfeld has pointed out.

DIFFERENTIAL DIAGNOSIS. The sharply circumscribed patch of alopecia with exclamation point hairs at the periphery and the absence of scarring are indicative of alopecia areata. Tinea capitis, early lupus erythematosus, and trichotillomania should be kept in mind when alopecia areata is considered. Tosti reported 14 cases of congenital triangular alopecia, which may easily be confused with alopecia areata. Schorr and his associates call attention to alopecia neoplastica, occurring in circular areas resembling alopecia areata, caused by metastatic adenocarcinoma of the breast. Indeed, they indicate that alopecia areata–like baldness may be the first sign of metastatic breast cancer.

TREATMENT. It is not known why some patches will regrow in a few weeks without any treatment and others will completely resist all forms of therapy. Intralesional injections of corticosteroid suspensions are the treatment of choice for persistent or rapidly enlarging patches, or conspicuous patches in an eyebrow. In total or universal alopecia, systemic steroids (using intramuscular triamcinolone) should be seriously considered. Both Unger and Winter have shown that side effects in patients treated with oral prednisone (on alternate days) are serious, and very common.

The literature is replete with data from studies using various therapeutic approaches, none of which is clearly superior to another, or to intralesional triamcinolone. Arrazola et al treated 11 patients (six of them totalis) and achieved a cure in seven and improvement in two, using mechlorethamine, 0.2 mg/ml daily, and three times weekly after regrowth began.

Induction of contact sensitivity to dinitrochlorobenzene (DNCB) has also been reported to be effective by Happle and Echternacht, and others, but Cordero says it is difficult and messy, and de Prost et al had only seven successes and 35 failures in 42 chronic cases, 22 of them total or universal. Happle, who was among the first to recommend DNCB, regards it as unacceptably hazardous (as a mutagen) in its present impure form, and Wilkin agrees—and says that squaric acid dibutyl ester and diphenylcyclopropenone have not been adequately studied for this risk. Nelson et al found it ineffective in 11 cases.

Chaudy et al, Mitchell et al, and Brown have reported success with topical or oral methoxsalen and ultraviolet A (PUVA) therapy. Schmoeckel and associates reported good cosmetic results in 18 of 24 patients treated with anthralin in 0.2 per cent to 0.8 per cent concentrations in vehicles such as petrolatum or ointment bases applied daily. Fiedler-Weiss et al agree it is a reasonable option for severe disease.

Topically applied minoxidil (Rogaine) is only feebly effective in alopecia totalis, according to White et al. Many studies have been reported and our conclusion is that it is of minimal, if any, usefulness in this disease. Fiedler-Weiss et al used it orally and found only an 18 per cent cosmetic response in a noncontrolled study.

Inosiplex, a synthetic immunomodulator, was found to be a safe and effective treatment by Galbraith et al.

Arnold found, in his series of 63 consecutive responders to a follow-up questionnaire, that—after reassurance only—hair had regrown in all but four patients after one year, and in all but one after two years. The great majority had recovered in three months after their only office visit. So any treatment may seem to be effective. Spontaneous recovery is extremely common. That is presumably why all treatments, in uncontrolled trials, give high response rates. It is only when patients in a poor prognostic category, such as those with prepubertal onset, or cases of total or universal involvement, or concomitant atopic disease, are considered, that the real lack of efficacy surfaces.

Ophiasis. If alopecia areata becomes confluent along the temporal and occipital scalp ("ophiasis"), the outlook for recovery is poor. Other factors associated with a poor prognosis for regrowth are atopy, and a duration of over five years.

Arnold HL Jr: Alopecia areata: prevalence in Japanese and prognosis after reassurance. Arch Dermatol Syph 1952, 66:191.

Arrazola JM, et al: Treatment of alopecia areata with topical nitrogen mustard. Int J Dermatol 1985, 24:608.

Barth JH, et al: Squaric acid esters in the treatment of alopecia areata (letter). JAAD 1986, 14:845.

Beard HO: Social and psychological implication of alopecia areata. JAAD 1986, 14:697.

Brown AC, et al: Ocular and testicular abnormalities in alopecia areata. Arch Dermatol 1982, 118:546.

Case PC, et al: Topical therapy of alopecia areata with squaric acid dibutylester. JAAD 1984, 10:447.

Caserio RJ: Treatment of alopecia areata with squaric acid dibutylester. Arch Dermatol 1987, 123:1036.

Claudy AL, et al: PUVA therapy of alopecia areata. Arch Dermatol 1983, 119:975.

DeProst Y, et al: Dinitrochlorobenzene treatment of alopecia areata. Arch Dermatol 1982, 118:542.

Dotz WI, et al: Leukonychia punctata and pitted nails in alopecia areata. Arch Dermatol 1985, 121:1452.

Dunagin WG: Potential hazards of dinitrochlorobenzene disputed (letter). Arch Dermatol 1986, 122:11.

Fiedler-Weiss VC, et al: Evaluation of anthralin in the treatment of alopecia areata. Arch Dermatol 1987, 123:1491.

Idem: Evaluation of oral minoxidil in the treatment of alopecia areata. Arch Dermatol 1987, 123:1488.

Idem: Topical minoxidil dose-response effect in alopecia areata. Arch Dermatol 1986, 122:180.

Flowers FP, et al: Topical squaric acid dibutylester therapy for alopecia areata. Cutis 1982, 30:733.

Galbraith GMP, et al: Immunological profiles in alopecia areata. Br J Dermatol 1984, 110:163.

Idem: A randomized double-blind study of inosiplex therapy in patients with alopecia totalis. JAAD 1987, 16:977.

Gilhar A, et al: Hair growth in scalp grafts from patients with alopecia areata and alopecia universalis grafted onto nude mice. Arch Dermatol 1987, 123:44.

Happle R, et al: Potential hazards of dinitrochlorobenzene disputed (reply). Arch Dermatol 1986, 122:11.

Hordinsky MK, et al: Suppressor cell number and function in alopecia areata. Arch Dermatol 1984, 120:188.

Idem: Familial alopecia areata: HLA antigens and autoantibody formation in an American family. Arch Dermatol 1984, 120:464.

Jillson OF: Alopecia. I. Alopecia areata. Cutis 1983, 31:262.

Lowy M, et al: Clinical and immunologic response to isoprinosine in alopecia areata and alopecia universalis: association with autoantibodies. JAAD 1985, 12:78.

Messenger AG, et al: Alopecia areata. Br J Dermatol 1986, 114:337.

Milgraum SS, et al: Alopecia areata, endocrine function, and antoantibodies in patients 16 years of age or younger. JAAD 1987, 17:57.

Mitchell AJ, et al: Topical photochemotherapy for alopecia areata. JAAD 1985, 12:644.

Idem: Alopecia areata: pathogenesis and treatment. JAAD 1984, 11:763.

Idem: Alopecia areata. Derm Clin 1987, 5:553.

Nelson DA, et al: Anthralin therapy for alopecia areata. Int J Dermatol 1985, 24:606.

Price VH: Double-blind placebo-controlled evaluation of topical minoxidil in extensive alopecia areata. JAAD 1987, 16:730.

Tosti A: Congenital triangular alopecia. JAAD 1987, 16:991.

Idem, et al: Therapies versus placebo in the treatment of patchy alopecia areata. JAAD 1986, 15:209.

Idem: Retinal pigment epithelium function in alopecia areata. J Invest Dermatol 1986, 86:553.

Idem: Ocular abnormalities occurring in alopecia areata. Dermatologica 1985, 170:69.

Unger WP, et al: Corticosteroids in the treatment of alopecia areata. Arch Dermatol 1978, 114:1466.

Valsecchi R, et al: Familial alopecia areata. Acta Derm Venereol (Stockh) 1985, 65:175.

Weiss VC, et al: Alopecia areata treated with topical minoxidil. Arch Dermatol 1984, 120:457.

White SI, et al: Topical minoxidil lacks efficacy in alopecia areata (letter). Arch Dermatol 1985, 121:591.

Wilkin JK, et al: Motives and dinitrochlorobenzene (letter). Arch Dermatol 1986, 122:13.

Idem: Squaric acid esters in treatment of alopecia areata (reply). JAAD 1986, 14:846.

Winter RJ, et al: Prednisone therapy for alopecia areata: a follow-up report. Arch Dermatol 1976, 112:1549.

Zauli D, et al: Alopecia areata (letter). Arch Dermatol 1985, 121:169.

Telogen Effluvium

Kligman has defined telogen effluvium as the early and excessive loss of normal club hairs from normal resting follicles in the scalp. This excessive hair loss results from the traumatization of the normal hair by some stimulus (e.g., surgery, parturition, fever, drugs, traction) which precipitates the anagen phase into catagen and telogen phases in short order. Kligman points out that during this process the follicle itself is not diseased, and inflammation is absent.

Whatever the cause, telogen effluvium usually has a latent period of from two to four months; the hair loss is noted by the patient as "lots of hairs coming out by the roots." Loss is diffuse and only infrequently causes noticeable thinning of the hair, since it only rarely involves more than 50 per cent of the hairs. Increased hair loss is noted by the patient before signs of alopecia. The normal telogen count may vary from 5 to 20 per cent; the diagnosis of telogen effluvium is usually justified only if the telogen count is over 25 per cent.

The normal average daily hair loss is influenced by such factors as age, sex, race, and probably other genetic factors. The total number of hairs on the scalp is estimated to be about 100,000; of these, approximately 100 hairs are lost daily. In telogen effluvium estimates of loss vary from 120 to over 400.

Histologic changes are absent, or at most minimal. In telogen effluvium the majority of the follicles continue in the anagen phase. The club hair is shed because the new hair generated in the anagen phase is pushing out the old club hair.

There is no specific therapy for telogen effluvium; it will stop spontaneously within a few weeks and the hair will regrow. If it threatens to become cosmetically significant, it can be arrested promptly in the majority of cases by a single dose of 40 to 60 mg of triamcinolone intramuscularly. Regrowth begins within a week or so. The prognosis is good if a specific event can be pinpointed as a probable cause.

Traction telogen effluvium was emphasized by Steck; it results chiefly from tight braiding, or winding hair too tightly on curlers or otherwise.

Postpartum telogen effluvium has been found to begin between two and five months postpartum. Often the hair loss is first noted over the anterior third of the scalp, although loss is in a diffuse pattern. Lynfield found a telogen count that varied between 24 and 46 per cent. The hair loss continues for some two to six months or longer. A complete regrowth eventually occurs.

Postnatal telogen effluvium of infants may occur between birth and the first four months of age. Usually regrowth occurs by six months of age. Telogen counts by Kligman in six infants varied from 64 to 87 per cent. He also found a tendency for the alopecia to occur in the male-pattern distribution.

Psychogenic telogen effluvium has been found by Kligman to differ from ordinary telogen effluvium: it persists longer, and there may be repeated episodes of lessening loss. The sudden loss of all the scalp hair after shock is believed to be of alopecia areata type.

Postfebrile telogen effluvium is familiar after febrile illnesses such as pneumonia. Here again hair loss begins some two to four months after the febrile episode. Telogen counts may be well over 50 per cent. Regrowth is the course.

Drug-induced telogen effluvium has been noted with heparin, coumarin, triparanol, thioureas, carbamazepine, lithium carbonate, indomethacin, allopurinol, gentamicin, metoprolol, isotretinoin, etretinate, levodopa, and propranolol.

Other causes of telogen effluvium have been noted. The most dramatic has been kwashiorkor, but Kaufman et al reported telogen effluvium secondary to a starvation diet. Goette and Odom have reported telogen effluvium in people on weight reduction programs and crash diets, secondary to protein deprivation.

Anagen Effluvium

Kligman has observed that anagen effluvium is seen frequently following the administration of cancer chemotherapeutic agents such as the antimetabolites, alkylating agents, and mitotic inhibitors. Severe loss is frequently seen with doxorubicin, the nitrosoureas, and cyclophosphamide. When high doses are given, loss of anagen hairs occurs almost immediately or in one or two weeks. It becomes clinically most apparent in one to two months. The hair shafts are abruptly thinned at the time of maximum drug effect, and when the very thin portion reaches the surface, the hair shafts all break at about the same time. Many hairs may also, if the bulb itself is damaged, separate at the bulb itself and come out. It is to be noted that only growing ("anagen") hairs are subject to this type of change. With cessation of drug therapy the follicle resumes its normal activity within a few weeks; the process is entirely reversible. It is apparent that mitotic inhibition only stops the reproduction of matrix cells, but does not permanently destroy the hair. A pressure cuff applied around the scalp during chemotherapy can prevent such anagen arrest. Scalp hypothermia has also been reported by Johansen to prevent this type of alopecia. In addition to the cytotoxic agents, various chemicals such as thallium and boron may induce anagen effluvium.

Bonner AK, et al: Cutaneous complications of chemotherapeutic agents. JAAD 1983, 9:648.
Goette DK, et al: Alopecia in crash dieters. JAMA 1976, 235:262.
Johansen LV: Scalp hypothermia in the prevention of chemotherapy-induced alopecia. Acta Radiol (Oncol) 1985, 24:113.
Kligman AM: Pathologic dynamics of human hair loss. Arch Dermatol 1961, 83:175.
Steck WD: Telogen effluvium. Cutis 1978, 21:543.

Male Pattern Alopecia (Androgenetic Alopecia)

Male pattern alopecia or male pattern baldness (common baldness) was called androgenetic alopecia by Orentreich in 1960. It shows itself during the twenties or early thirties by gradual loss of hair, chiefly from the vertex and frontotemporal regions. At any time after puberty the process may begin subtly, and the presence of "whisker" hair at the temples may be the first sign of impending male pattern alopecia. The anterior hair line recedes on each side, in the "Geheimratswinkeln" ("professor angles"), so that the forehead becomes high. Eventually the entire top of the scalp may become devoid of hair. Several patterns of this type of hair loss occur, but the most frequent is the biparietal recession with loss of hair on the vertex. The rate of hair loss varies among individuals. A sudden hair loss may occur in the twenties and then proceed relentlessly though very slowly for a number of years. The follicles produce finer and lighter terminal hairs until a complete cessation of terminal hair growth results. Vellus hairs on the scalp, however, continue to grow and become more prominent because of the absence of terminal hairs. The parietal and occipital areas are usually spared permanently.

The exact mechanisms responsible for androgenetic alopecia are still unknown; however, there is no doubt that inherited factors and the effect of androgens on the hair follicle are most responsible. Küster and Happle (1984) offer five arguments for regarding this inheritance as polygenic: high prevalence; Gaussian curve of distribution in the population; increase of risk with number of affected relatives; increased risk in relatives of severely affected women as compared to mildly afflicted; and greater import of an affected mother than of an affected father.

In addition to heredity, male-pattern alopecia is dependent upon adequate androgen stimulation at a particular age of the individual. Hamilton has shown that eunuchs do not develop baldness provided they are castrated before or during adolescence; if they are given androgen therapy, baldness may develop.

Vera Price has extensively reviewed testosterone metabolism in the skin. The 5α-reduction of testosterone is increased in the scalp of balding individuals, yielding increased dihydrotestosterone. It has been suggested that high dihydrotestosterone levels in the genetically marked hair follicles initiate baldness by inhibiting adenyl cyclase. Pitts found elevated levels of dehydroepiandrosterone sulfate in young men with male pattern baldness, and suggested that adrenal hyperactivity may initiate alopecia in genetically susceptible men.

The pathogenesis is centered around the lengthening of the telogen phase and the shortening of the anagen phase of hair growth. The shorter the anagen phase, the shorter the hair growth.

Minoxidil, an oral hypotensive drug that causes hypertrichosis when given systemically, is available in a 2 percent topical solution (Rogaine). Many reports of success in early cases (less than 10 years) of limited extent (less than 10 cm diameter bald area) are somewhat encouraging. Still, at best only about one third of cases grow cosmetically useful hair, and they must continue to use minoxidil indefinitely to maintain a response. Hopefully more potent congeners of minoxidil, or other more effective medications, will become available.

Sadly, none of our medical treatments are effective, and as a result, with the cosmetically esthetic emphasis upon the image of hair, numerous solutions for the problem, both medical and paramedical, have been tried. Unger has reviewed many of these. Hair transplantation of small plugs of scalp hair follicles from the occipital area to the anterior scalp line has been successfully developed by Orentreich and Ayres III for restoring hair to the balding area. The Orentreich technique is the most effective one for transplanting hair from the occipital to the frontal area. Ayres III has reported extensively on this method and the problems of multiple punch scalp autografts for male pattern alopecia. Minoxidil topically may prevent the shedding of hairs that ordinarily occurs

two to four weeks after the hair-bearing "plug" is transplanted. Other surgical approaches include scalp reduction by excision of bald areas, and the use of hair-bearing flaps. Stough et al reviewed the various combinations of punch autografts with these two procedures. Excellent cosmetic results are achievable in male-pattern alopecia by surgical intervention.

Implantation of colored synthetic fibers, knotted to keep them in place, was in vogue for a short time in the late seventies. Schwartz et al reported a case in which severe infection and foreign-body reaction was induced. This reaction was quite common, and this procedure should not be used.

Androgenetic Alopecia in Women

The pattern of hair loss is quite different in women. Women generally have diffuse hair loss throughout the mid-scalp, sparing the frontal hair line except for slight recession. Mortimer found the same changes—reduced hair density and diameter, and diminished anagen and increased telogen hair—in women as in men.

The cause is now believed to be a genetic predisposition in combination with an excessive androgen response, even though levels of circulating testosterone are as a rule not elevated. If other evidence of androgen excess is present, such as hirsutism or acne, evaluation as outlined for hirsutism (see below) should be performed. Rook and Ebling classify this form of alopecia with the androgen-dependent syndromes.

Therapy is empirical and will be until an androgen blocker, such as cyproterone acetate, becomes available. Mortimer et al reported the effectiveness of cyclic antiandrogen therapy in three women: the hairs increased in number and thickness. Spironolactone is the usual alternative used in the United States. Progesterone-dominant contraceptives may aggravate the problem. The combination of antiandrogenic

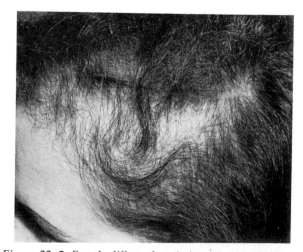

Figure 33–5. Female diffuse alopecia in a 37-year-old woman.

and antiinflammatory effects of intramuscular triamcinolone, 60 mg once every four weeks, may also result in regrowth of hair. Conjugated estrogens-equine (Premarin) in lotion form applied topically in small amounts may decrease the rate of hair loss. The amount of application should be kept minimal to prevent systemic reactions of breakthrough bleeding. Thyroid deficiency and anemias should be corrected and physical condition improved if found to be abnormal.

Adson MH, et al: Scalp expansion in the treatment of male pattern baldness. Plast Reconst Surg 1987, 79:906.
Aram H: Treatment of female androgenetic alopecia with cimetidine. Int J Dermatol 1987, 26:128.
Ayres S III: Conservative surgical management of male pattern baldness. Arch Dermatol 1964, 90:492.
Bazzano GS, et al: Topical tretinoin for hair growth promotion. JAAD 1986, 15:880.
Bergfeld WF: Diffuse hair loss in women. Cutis 1978, 22:190.
Idem: Androgenic alopecia. Derm Clin 1987, 5:491.
Cryer PE: Androgen excess in women. Progr Dermatol 1983, 17:1.
De Villez RL: Topical minoxidil therapy in hereditary androgenetic alopecia. Arch Dermatol 1985, 121:197.
Franz TJ: Percutaneous absorption of minoxidil in man. Arch Dermatol 1985, 121:203.
Jerums G, et al: Androgens in women: source, nature, and investigation. Austral J Dermatol 1985, 26:14.
Kassimir JJ: Use of topical minoxidil as a possible adjunct to hair transplant surgery. JAAD 1987, 16:685.
Katz HI: Topical minoxidil. Cutis 1989, 43:94.
Idem, et al: Long-term efficacy of topical minoxidil in male pattern baldness. JAAD 1987, 16:711.
Knowles WR: Hair transplantation. Derm Clin 1987, 5:515.
Koperski JA, et al: Topical minoxidil therapy for androgenetic alopecia. Arch Dermatol 1987, 123:1483.
Kreindler TG: Topical minoxidil in early androgenetic alopecia. JAAD 1987, 16:718.
Küster W, et al: The inheritance of common baldness. JAAD 1984, 11:921.
Ludwig E: Classification of types of androgenetic alopecia (common baldness) occurring in the female sex. Br J Dermatol 1977, 68:201.
Mortimer CH, et al: Effective medical treatment for common baldness in women. Clin Exp Dermatol 1984, 9:342.
Norwood OT: Micrografts and minigrafts for refining grafted hairlines. Derm Clin 1987, 5:545.
Idem: Scalp reduction in the treatment of androgenic alopecia. Derm Clin 1987, 5:531.
Olsen EA, et al: Topical minoxidil in early male pattern baldness. JAAD 1985, 13:185.
Idem: Dose-response study of minoxidil in male pattern baldness. JAAD 1986, 15:30.
Idem: Long-term follow-up of men with male pattern baldness treated with topical minoxidil. JAAD 1987, 16:688.
Idem: Topical minoxidil in male pattern baldness. JAAD 1987, 17:97.
Pitts RL: Serum elevation of dehydroepiandrosterone sulfate associated with male pattern baldness in young men. JAAD 1987, 16:571.
Price VH: Hormonal control of baldness. Int J Dermatol 1976, 15:742.
Rietschel RL, et al: Safety and efficacy of topical minoxidil in the management of androgenetic alopecia. JAAD 1987, 16:677.
Roberts JL: Androgenetic alopecia. JAAD 1987, 16:705.
Rook AW: Androgen-dependent syndromes (president's address). Int J Dermatol 1980, 19:357.
Savin RC: Use of topical minoxidil in treatment of male pattern baldness. JAAD 1987, 16:696.
Schwartz RS, et al: Dangers of synthetic fiber implantation for male pattern baldness. Cutis 1980, 25:491.
Storer JS: Review: topical minoxidil for male pattern baldness. Am J Med Sci 1986, 291:328.
Stough DB, et al: A contemporary approach to male pattern alopecia. J Dermatol Surg Oncol 1987, 13:756.
Tosti A: Topical minoxidil useful in 18 per cent of patients with androgenetic alopecia. A study of 430 cases. Dermatologica 1986, 173:136.
Weiss VC, et al: Topical minoxidil therapy and hair regrowth (editorial). Arch Dermatol 1985, 121:191.

Other Forms of Alopecia

Complete or partial loss of scalp hair is found in various forms and is caused by many factors. Some forms of alopecia are herewith described briefly.

Trichotillomania is a neurotic practice of plucking or breaking hair from the scalp or eyelashes. This is seen mostly in girls under 10, but boys, and adults of either sex, may do it too. Oranje et al discussed the psychosocial factors in their review of 21 children.

Jillson suggested that one ask the child in a friendly way, when alone with him, how removal of the hair is done. If it fails, close observation for catching the patient in the act may help; or shave a 3x3 cm area in the involved part of the scalp, and watch the hair regrow normally. Finally, a biopsy may confirm the diagnosis.

Hot comb alopecia is seen in black women who straighten their hair with hot combs for cosmetic purposes. Lo Presti and his associates state that the alopecia develops characteristically on the crown and spreads peripherally to form a large oval area of partial hair loss. The hot petrolatum used with the iron causes thermal damage to the hair follicle, leading ultimately to destruction of the entire follicle and a follicular scar. In time significant hair loss occurs if this type of hair straightening is continued.

Traction alopecia is probably of the same mechanism as that of telogen effluvium, but is limited to areas thus traumatized. It occurs from prolonged tension on the hair either from wearing the hair tightly braided or in a ponytail, pulling the hair to straighten it, rolling curlers too tightly, or from the habit of twisting the hairs with the fingers.

Pressure alopecia occurs frequently on the occipital areas in babies lying on their backs. In adults it is seen most often after prolonged pressure on the scalp during general anesthesia, with the head fixed in one position. It may also occur in chronically ill persons after prolonged bed rest in one position, which causes persistent pressure upon one part of the scalp. Wiles et al propose that it arises because of pressure-induced ischemia—a plausible cause.

Loose anagen syndrome, described by Price in 1989, is a disorder in which anagen hairs may be pulled from the scalp with little effort. Price reported that it occurs mostly in blond girls. It improves with age.

Alopecia syphilitica has a typical motheaten appearance on the occipital scalp. Other areas such as

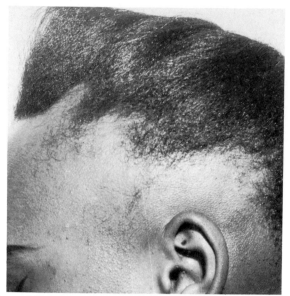

Figure 33–6. Traction/traumatic alopecia in a 14-year-old girl.

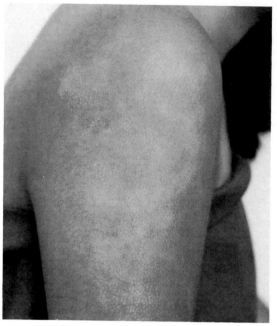

Figure 33–8. Follicular mucinosis (alopecia mucinosa) of arm. Note abundance of vellus hairs outside the clusters of discrete, hypopigmented follicular macules.

the eyebrows and eyelashes and body hair may be involved. The alopecia may be the first sign of a syphilis infection. Its distinct appearance is specific.

Follicular mucinosis (alopecia mucinosa) most commonly occurs on the scalp or beard area and manifests as deposition of mucin in the outer root sheath and sebaceous glands. The inflammatory reaction produces alopecia, and at times hypopigmentation. The sometimes accompanying hypesthesia to cold has on occasion led to a mistaken diagnosis of leprosy.

The primary cases (i.e., unassociated with underlying disease) occur either as localized lesions of the head or neck that usually resolve within a year, or as more generalized lesions with a longer course. Young people are primarily affected.

A secondary type exists, in which there is associated lymphoma, most often mycosis fungoides. Usually, in these cases, lesions are widespread and chronic, and occur in older patients.

When it occurs on the outer aspects of the upper arms, as is not uncommon in adolescent girls in Hawaii, it becomes conspicuous by preventing a tan, and is a cosmetic problem. It is distinguishable from pityriasis alba by the distinctively follicular involvement, the alopecia of vellus hairs, and (occasionally) dysesthesia to cold. A single small dose of triamcinolone acetonide intramuscularly, 20 or 30 mg, usually permits pigmentation to be regained within three weeks, and it may not recur for two or three months, or longer (HLA). Persistent recurrence beyond two to five relapses is seldom seen.

Hempstead and Ackerman would use "follicular mucinosis" only as a histologic diagnosis, but Montgomery, Ebling and Rook, Lever and others regard it as synonymous with alopecia mucinosa. So do we.

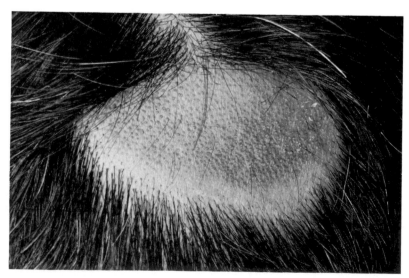

Figure 33–7. Pressure alopecia developing after a prolonged surgical procedure.

Inflammatory alopecia may be seen in lichen simplex chronicus and various eczematous changes on the scalp, including kerion. Discoid lupus erythematosus, lichen planopilaris, sarcoidosis, and folliculitis decalvans are the commonest inflammatory causes of cicatricial alopecia.

Vascular or neurologic alopecia, most often of the lower extremities, may be seen in diabetes mellitus or atherosclerosis. In meralgia paresthetica there may be alopecia of the anesthetic area of the outer thigh.

Tinea capitis is usually manifested by one or several patches of alopecia with scaling, erythema, or pustulation. The hairs are broken off just above the scalp. *Microsporum audouini* and *M. canis* infections fluoresce under the Wood's light, but *Trichophyton tonsurans* does not.

Endocrinologic alopecia may occur in various endocrinologic disorders. In *hypothyroidism* the hair becomes coarse, dry, brittle, and sparse. Freinkel and Freinkel found in six such cases that the proportion of telogen hairs was three to seven times higher than the normal 10 per cent. In *hyperthyroidism* the hair becomes extremely fine and sparse. *Oral contraceptives* have been implicated in some instances of androgenetic alopecia. It develops in predisposed women who are usually taking androgenic progestogens. It is advisable to discontinue the androgen-dominant pill and substitute an estrogen-dominant oral contraceptive. Some women develop telogen effluvium two to four months after discontinuing anovulatory agents, which is analogous to postpartum alopecia.

Tumor alopecia refers to hair loss in the immediate vicinity of either benign or malignant tumors of the scalp. Syringomas, nerve sheath myxomas, and steatocystoma multiplex are benign tumors that may be limited to the scalp and cause alopecia. **Alopecia neoplastica** is the designation given to hair loss from metastatic tumors, most often from breast carcinoma.

Menopausal alopecia is held to be identical with male-pattern (androgenic) baldness by Maguire and Kligman.

Drug alopecia resulting from use of thallium, colchicine, and various antineoplastic cytotoxic agents such as vinblastine, chlorambucil, nitrogen mustard, busulfan, 5-fluorouracil, or actinomycin D is anagen hair loss. There is cessation of mitosis in the hair bulb, with thinning and constriction of the hair shafts (*Pohl-Pinkus constrictions*) and breaking at these points. However, these are reversible hair changes, and hair continues to grow. Other drugs that cause alopecia are prolonged, or single high, doses of vitamin A, heparin, coumarin, triparanol, thiourea, carbamazepine, allopurinol, indomethacin, gentamicin, levodopa, propranolol, isotretinoin, etretinate, lithium, and metoprolol.

Stress alopecia after severe and acute emotional upset has been documented. The severe stress of war conditions or acute illness may induce complete hair loss in a matter of a few weeks. It is believed that this is alopecia areata, which may be diffuse, and is identifiable by easy removal of exclamation-point hairs, in children aged one to four or five who have experienced a serious fright.

Congenital alopecia occurs either as total or partial loss of hair, accompanied usually by other ectodermal defects of the nails, teeth, and bone. The hair is light and sparse, and grows slowly. Congenital triangular alopecia and aplasia cutis congenita are examples of congenital localized absence of hair, while hidrotic ectodermal dysplasia is an example of "diffuse abnormality" of hair associated with dental and nail changes.

Aranoff SM, et al: Alopecia in meralgia paresthetica. JAAD 1985, 12:176.
Arnold HL Jr: Dysesthesia in alopecia mucinosa: a possible diagnostic sign. Arch Dermatol 1962, 85:409.
Birnbaum PS, et al: Intermittent hair follicle dystrophy. JAAD 1986, 15:54.
Brodin MB: Drug-related alopecia. Derm Clin 1987, 5:571.
Burket JM: Alopecia associated with underlying nerve sheath myxoma. JAAD 1987, 16:209.
Freinkel RK, et al: Hair growth and alopecia in hypothyroidism. Arch Dermatol 1972, 106:349.
Frieden IH: Aplasia cutis congenita. JAAD 1986, 14:646.
Gibson LE, et al: Follicular mucinosis. JAAD 1989, 20:441.
Graeber CW, et al: Metoprolol and alopecia. Cutis 1981, 28:633.
Guillén PS, et al: Aplasia cutis congenita. JAAD 1985, 13:429.
Hamm H, et al: Loose anagen hair of childhood. JAAD 1989, 20:242.
Hempstead RW, et al: Follicular mucinosis: a reaction pattern in follicular epithelium. Am J Dermatopathol 1985, 7:245.
Jillson OF: Alopecia. III: diffuse hair loss (nonscarring). Cutis 1983, 31:465.
Idem: Alopecia. II: Trichotillomania (trichotillohabitus). Cutis 1983, 31:383.
Krull EA: Hair replacement techniques. Derm Clin 1987, 5:509.
Lancer HA, et al: Follicular mucinosis. JAAD 1984, 10:760.
LoPresti P: Hot comb alopecia. Arch Dermatol 1968, 98:234.
Mortimer PS, et al: Hair loss and lithium. Int J Dermatol 1984, 23:603.
Muller SA: Trichotillomania. Derm Clin 1987, 5:595.
Neuman KM, et al: Alopecia associated with syringomas. JAAD 1985, 13:528.
Oranje AP, et al: Trichotillomania in childhood. JAAD 1986, 15:614.
Price VH, et al: Loose anagen syndrome. JAAD 1989, 20:249.
Raab B, et al: Follicular mucinosis in childhood. Cutis 1982, 30:87.
Shelley WB, et al: Occult syringomas of scalp associated with progressive hair loss. Arch Dermatol 1980, 116:843.
Snyder RA, et al: Alopecia mucinosa. Arch Dermatol 1984, 120:496.
Spencer LV, et al: Hair loss in systemic disease. Derm Clin 1987, 5:565.
Tosti A: Congenital triangular alopecia. JAAD 1987, 16:991.
Wiles JC, et al: Postoperative (pressure) alopecia. JAAD 1985, 12:195.

Syndromes That Include Abnormalities of the Hair

Polyostotic fibrous dysplasia (Albright's disease) may present—as it did in a case reported by Shelley and Wood—as slowly progressive lifelong unilateral hair loss: scalp, pubic, axillary, and palpebral.

Sickle cell disease is often characterized by scantiness of body and facial hair, according to Prasad et al.

The Cronkhite-Canada syndrome is characterized by alopecia, skin pigmentation, onychodystrophy, malabsorption, and generalized gastrointestinal polyposis.

Marinesco-Sjögren syndrome consists of cerebellar ataxia, mental retardation, congenital cataracts, inability to chew food, thin brittle fingernails, and sparse hair. The dystrophic hairs do not have the normal layers (cortex, cuticle, and medulla), and 30 percent of the hair shafts show narrow bands of abnormal incomplete keratinization. There is an autosomal recessive type of inheritance in this syndrome.

Trichothiodystrophy features brittle hair with a markedly reduced sulfur content. The hair, with sulfur reduced to 50 per cent of the normal value, has distinctive features under polarizing, light, and scanning electron microscopy. With polarizing microscopy, the hair shows alternating bright and dark regions which give a striking striped appearance. With light microscopy, trichoschisis (clean fractures), and trichorrhexis nodosalike fractures may be seen; in addition, the hair is markedly flattened and folds over itself like a thick ribbon, the hair shaft outline is irregular and slightly undulating, and the melanin granules are distributed in a wavy pattern. With scanning electron microscopy, the surface shows marked ridging and fluting, and the cuticle scales may be absent or greatly reduced.

In addition to the hair findings, which are present in all cases, other variable features of the syndrome include short stature, mental deficiency, ichthyosis, nail dystrophy, ocular dysplasia, and infertility. An autosomal recessive inheritance has been suggested in all reports involving more than one family member. The presence of brittle hair with a markedly reduced sulfur content is common to all cases and is an important clinical marker. Thus, Price and Odom proposed the term trichothiodystrophy (Gk. *tricho*, hair + *thio*, sulfur + *dys*, faulty + *trophe*, nourishment) as a useful designation.

Generalized trichoepitheliomas, alopecia, and myasthenia gravis has been reported by Starink et al; it may be a variant of the **generalized hair follicle hamartoma syndrome**.

Crow-Fukase ("POEMS") syndrome is characterized by polyneuropathy, organomegaly, endocrinopathy, M-protein, and skin changes such as diffuse hyperpigmentation, dependent edema, skin thickening, hyperhidrosis, and hypertrichosis.

Cartilage-hair hypoplasia consists of short-limbed dwarfism and abnormally fine and sparse hair in children. They are especially susceptible to viral infections and recurrent respiratory infections. A functional defect of small lymphocytes, with impaired cell-mediated immunity, was reported by Lux. Most patients are anergic to skin-test panels and have increased numbers of natural killer cells.

Acquired Immunodeficiency Syndrome. Many black patients with AIDS have experienced softening, straightening, lightening, and thinning of their hair.

Tricho-rhino-phalangeal syndrome is a genetic disorder consisting of fine and sparse scalp hair, thin nails, pear-shaped broad nose, and cone-shaped epiphyses of the middle phalanges of some fingers and toes. There is an autosomal dominant and also recessive inheritance type.

Lipidematous alopecia associated with skin hyperelasticity and hyperlaxity of the joints has been reviewed by Curtis and Heising. The alopecia consists of shortened hairs, with thickening of the scalp associated with an increase in subcutaneous fat, so that the scalp may be as much as 15 mm thick. Curtis and Heising stated that their patient did not represent a true Ehlers-Danlos syndrome. All cases reported to date have been in blacks.

Hallermann-Streiff syndrome is a rare syndrome of birdlike facies with a pronounced beak-like nose, microphthalmia, micrognathia, congenital cataracts, and hypotrichosis. The hair is diffusely sparse and brittle. Baldness may occur frontally or at the scalp margins, but *sutural alopecia*, hair loss following the lines of the cranial sutures, is characteristic of this syndrome. The small face is in sharp contrast with a disproportionately large-appearing head. The lips are thin; some of the teeth may be absent while others are dystrophic, resulting in malocclusion. Nystagmus, strabismus, and other ocular abnormalities are present.

In Domonkos's patient there was complete hair loss in the frontal areas, whereas the occiput was well covered. This patient had greatest difficulty with her eyesight.

Progeria, also known as Hutchinson-Gilford syndrome, is characterized by premature old age. It is marked by failure to develop normally in growth after the first year of life. The large bald head and

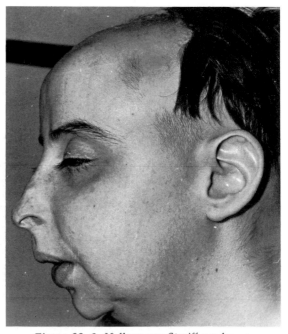

Figure 33–9. Hallermann-Streiff syndrome.

lack of eyebrows and eyelashes are distinctive. The skin is wrinkled, pigmented, and atrophic. The nails are thin and atrophic. Most patients lack subcutaneous fat, which produces the appearance of premature senility. The intelligence remains intact. Arteriosclerosis, anginal attacks, and hemiplegia may occur, followed by death from coronary heart disease at an early age.

Papillon-Lefèvre syndrome is characterized by hyperkeratosis palmaris et plantaris, periodontosis, and sparsity of the hair. Hyperhidrosis and the other signs and symptoms begin early in life. Inheritance of this disease is of an autosomal recessive type.

Klippel-Feil syndrome consists of a low posterior scalp hair line extending onto the shoulders, with a short neck, limiting movement of the neck and suggestive of webbing. The cervical vertebrae are fused. This syndrome is caused by faulty segmentation of the mesodermal somites between the third and seventh weeks in utero. Strabismus, nystagmus, cleft palate, bifid uvula, and high palate are some other features. This syndrome occurs mostly in girls.

McCusick's syndrome includes short-limbed dwarfism and fine, sparse, hypoplastic and dysmorphic hair, as Paul Porter has pointed out.

Turner's syndrome is a distinctive clinical picture comprising short stature, webbing of the neck, low posterior hair line margin, increased carrying angle at the elbow (cubitus valgus), and infantile development of the breasts, vagina, and uterus. Coarctation of the aorta is frequently found. A triangular-shaped mouth, alopecia of the frontal area of the scalp, and cutis laxa are also seen.

Turner's syndrome is caused by ovarian dysgenesis. Only 45 chromosomes are present; the sex chromosomes have an XO pattern.

Noonan's syndrome consists of short stature with typical webbing of the neck, low hair line in the back, prominent and low-set ears, and cubitus valgus.

The syndrome is similar to Turner's syndrome and has been frequently termed "male Turner's syndrome," in which a normal chromosome pattern is

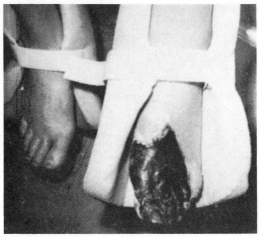

Figure 33–10. Werner's disease. Scleroderma-like plaques and gangrene. (From Moschella SI, Hurley HJ: Dermatology. 2nd ed. Philadelphia, WB Saunders, 1985, p 1157.)

assumed. In addition to its occurrence in the male rather than the female, it is differentiated from Turner's syndrome by the absence of coarctation of the aorta; the typical heart lesion is a valvular pulmonary stenosis.

Werner's syndrome has the essential features of shortness of stature, cataracts, skin changes, premature graying and alopecia, atrophy of muscles and subcutaneous tissues, and bone atrophy of the extremities to produce "spindly extremities." Osteoporosis and aseptic necrosis are frequent in the small bones of the hands.

The skin changes include poikiloderma, scleroderma, atrophy, hyperkeratoses, and leg ulcers. The skin shows a dark gray or blackish diffuse pigmentation. A high-pitched voice and hypogonadism in both sexes are distinctive in this syndrome. Diabetes mellitus is frequently present.

Since most of these signs are not fully manifested before the age of 30 the diagnosis is usually made in middle age. These patients show marked senescence. It has an autosomal recessive mode of inheritance.

Figure 33–11. Werner's syndrome. (Courtesy of Dr. Elaine DeGrande.)

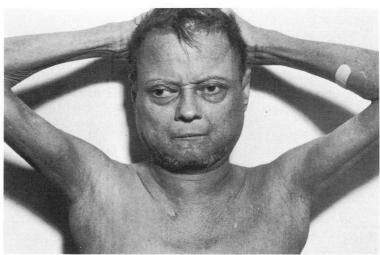

These patients usually die before they are 50 years of age from malignant disease or vascular accidents.

Rothmund-Thomson syndrome is characterized by early-onset poikiloderma, short stature, sun sensitivity, bone defects, and hypogonadism. Cataracts are seen in some families (Rothmund type), and sparseness of eyelashes, eyebrows, or scalp hair has been reported in 60 per cent of cases.

Badame AJ: Progeria. Arch Dermatol 1989, 125:540.

Bey E, et al: Rothmund-Thomson syndrome. JAAD 1987, 17:332.

Brennan TE, et al: Abnormal elastic tissue in cartilage-hair hypoplasia. Arch Dermatol 1988, 124:1411.

Gorlin RJ, Pindborg JJ: Syndromes of the Head and Neck, 2nd ed. New York, Blakiston Division, McGraw-Hill Book Company, 1976.

Kinchelow T: Changes in the hair of black patients with AIDS. J Infect Dis 1988, 157:394.

King MD, et al: Trichothiodystrophy—neurocutaneous syndrome of Pollitt. J Med Genet 1984, 21:286.

Leonidas JR: Hair alterations in black patients with the acquired immunodeficiency syndrome. Cutis 1987, 39:537.

Petrohelos M: Werner's syndrome: a survey of three cases with reviews of the literature. Ann J Ophthalmol 1968, 56:941.

Price VH, et al: Trichothiodystrophy—sulfur-deficient brittle hair. Arch Dermatol 1980, 116:1375.

Rook A, Dawber R: Diseases of the Hair and Scalp. Oxford, Blackwell Scientific Publications, pp 146–178, 1982.

Shelley WB, et al: Alopecia with fibrous dysplasia and osteomas of skin: sign of polyostotic fibrous dysplasia. Arch Dermatol 1976, 112:715.

Idem: The skin changes in the Crowe-Fukase syndrome. Arch Dermatol 1987, 123:85.

Starink TM, et al: Generalized trichoepitheliomas and alopecia and myasthenia gravis. JAAD 1986, 15:1104.

White MC, et al: Trichothiodystrophy. J Assoc Milit Dermatol 1987, 13:4.

Pseudopelade

Pseudopelade (French for pseudo–alopecia areata) of Brocq, also known as **alopecia cicatrisata**, is a rare form of scarring alopecia in which destruction of the hair follicles produces multiple round, oval, or irregularly shaped, hairless, cicatricial patches of varying sizes. They are usually coin-sized and are white or slightly pink in color, with a smooth, shiny, marble-like or ivory, atrophic, "onion skin" surface. Interspersed in the patches may be a few dilated follicles with hairs growing from them. Inflammation is completely absent. No pustules, crusts, or broken-off hairs are present.

The onset is, as a rule, insidious, with one or two lesions appearing on the vertex. It affects females three times more commonly than males, and has a prolonged course. In advanced cases large patches may be formed by coalescence of some of the many small macules. The alopecia is permanent and the disease is slowly progressive. It was reviewed by Braun-Falco et al in 1986. Histologically, there is no inflammation; sebaceous glands are decreased or absent; the epidermis is normal or atrophic; and fibrotic "streams" are seen in the subcutaneous tissue. Direct immunofluorescence is negative.

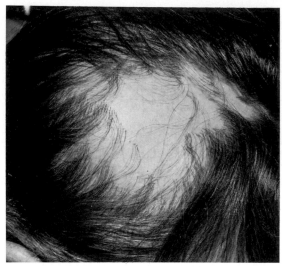

Figure 33–12. Pseudopelade. Note intact follicles and single hairs growing.

The differential diagnosis requires the ruling out of other causes of cicatricial alopecia such as chronic suppurative folliculitis, scleroderma, sarcoidosis, favus, and lupus erythematosus. Folliculitis decalvans is frequently accompanied by inflamed marginal follicles and marginal crusting. Alopecia areata may be simulated; however, the presence of scarring rules this out. Graham-Little syndrome consists of lichen planus, acuminate follicular papules, and scarring alopecia of the scalp and noncicatricial alopecia of other areas. Clinically familial focal alopecia resembles pseudopelade; however, the absence of scarring on biopsy and the pattern of inheritance distinguish it.

Treatment is not available for this scarring alopecia.

Braun-Falco O, et al: Pseudopelade of Brocq. Dermatologica 1986, 172:18.

Gay Prieto J: Pseudopelade of Brocq. J Invest Dermatol 1955, 24:323.

Headington JT, et al: Familial focal alopecia. Arch Dermatol 1987, 123:234.

Graham Little Syndrome (Piccardi-Lassueur-Graham Little Syndrome)

This rare syndrome is characterized by cicatricial patches of alopecia of the scalp with prominent follicular plugging and follicular keratoses on the trunk and limbs, sometimes associated with noncicatricial alopecia of the axillae, pubes, trunk, and limbs. Horn and Odom have demonstrated large subepidermal clumps of IgG and IgM with direct immunofluorescence, supporting the concept that this entity is a variant of lichen planus.

Horn RT, et al: Immunofluorescent findings and clinical overlap in two cases of follicular lichen planus. JAAD 1982, 7:203.

Kubra R, et al: The Graham Little syndrome. Br J Dermatol 1975, 93:53.

HAIR COLOR

On the basis of the ultrastructure of hair pigment, Mottag and Zelickson have reported the variations in the melanocytes and melanosomes as seen in the different colored hairs. Melanin in the hair follicles is produced in the cytoplasm of the melanocytes, in which are involved the endoplasmic reticulum, ribosomes, and the Golgi apparatus. Melanin synthesis begins on the matrix fibers of the premelanosomes, forming in the cytoplasm of the melanocytes. Hair color will depend upon the degree of melanin synthesis, on matrix fibers and in the intervening spaces between the fibers. When all tyrosinase activity halts, the premelanosome becomes a melanosome.

The pigment in black and dark brown hair is composed of eumelanin, whereas in blond and red hair it is pheomelanin. In **black hair** the melanocytes contain the densest melanosomes, with lightened areas that show a "moth-eaten" appearance. **Brown hair** differs only by its smaller melanosomes; light brown hair consists of a mixture of the melanosomes of dark hair and the incomplete melanosomes of **blond hair**. Many of the melanosomes in blond hair develop only on the matrix fibers and not in the spaces between the fibers.

Red hair shows incomplete melanin deposits on the matrix fibers to produce a "splotchy" appearing melanosome. Pheomelanin is distinguished by its relatively high content of sulfur, which results from the addition of cysteine to dopaquinone along the biosynthetic pathway of melanin synthesis.

Changes in hair color occur in various metabolic disorders. The hair becomes blond in *phenylketonuria* because of inadequate amounts of tyrosine; in *homocystinuria* a bleaching effect on the hair is noted; light hair is also seen in *oast-house disease; albinism* is associated with white or yellowish hair; *triparanol* is associated with hypopigmented hair; *minoxidil* (by changing vellus to terminal hairs) causes darkening of hair; another hypotensive agent, *diazoxide*, gives the hair a reddish tint; in *Menkes's kinky hair syndrome* the hair is light; in *kwashiorkor* the hair assumes a red-blond color in infants; with *chloroquine* therapy depigmentation may occur, usually in redheads and blonds, not in brunettes. Segmental heterochromia, with alternating light and dark bands, may occur in iron deficiency anemia. The disorder has been called *canities segmentata sideropenica*. It responds completely to iron supplementation.

In **gray hair** (canities) melanogenic activity is decreased as a result of fewer melanocytes and melanosomes as well as a gradual loss of tyrosinase activity. Graying of the scalp hair is genetically de-termined and may start at any age. Usually it begins at the temples and progresses with time. The beard usually follows, with the body hair coming last.

Early graying (before age 20 in whites or before age 30 in blacks) is usually familial; however, it may occur also in progeria, in the syndromes of Rothmund and Thomson, in Böök's syndrome, and in Werner's syndrome.

In poliosis, gray hair occurs in circumscribed patches. This may occur in Waardenburg's syndrome and piebaldism and is frequent in tuberous sclerosis. Poliosis is also found in association with vitiligo and Vogt-Koyanagi syndrome and may be seen in alopecia areata when the new hairs grow in. Other syndromes which include poliosis are Tietz's syndrome, Alezzandrini's syndrome, and neurofibromatosis.

Green hair was traced by Lampe and Hansen to copper in the water of a swimming pool. As Goette has pointed out, this occurs only in blond or light hair. Melnick et al recommend the following treatments: EDTA topically; penicillamine-containing shampoos; or 1.5 per cent aqueous 1-hydroxyethyl diphosphonic acid. Tars, and chrysarobin, stain light hair brown.

Premature *whitening* of scalp hair is usually due to vitiligo, sometimes without recognized, or actually without, lesions of glabrous skin.

Cline DJ: Changes in hair color. Derm Clin 1988, 6:295.

Dupré A, et al: Chloroquin-induced hypopigmentation of hair and freckles. Arch Dermatol 1985, 121:1164.

Goette DK: Swimmer's green hair. Arch Dermatol 1977, 114:127.

Juhlin L, et al: Red scalp hair turning dark brown at 50 years of age. Acta Dermatol Venerol (Stockh) 1986, 66:71.

Lampe RM, et al: Green hair. JAMA 1977, 237:2092.

Melnick BC, et al: Green hair. JAAD 1986, 15:1065.

Person JR: Green hair. Arch Dermatol 1985, 121:717.

Rees RB, et al: Chloroquine. Arch Dermatol 1963, 88:280.

Rogers MJ, et al: Yellow hair discoloration due to anthralin. JAAD 1988, 19:320.

Sato S, et al: Segmented heterochromia in black scalp hair associated with iron-deficiency anemia. Arch Dermatol 1989, 125:531.

HAIR STRUCTURE DEFECTS

The examination of hairs for structural defects is greatly facilitated by a method devised by Shelley: putting a piece of double-stick tape (Catalogue No. 136, Minnesota Mining and Manufacturing Co., St. Paul, MN 55101) on a microscope slide and aligning 5-cm segments of hair in parallel upon it. KOH examination and even gold-coating and scanning electron microscopy can be done on hairs so mounted.

Hair Casts

This unusual but far from rare disorder, first described by Kligman, mimics nits so closely that it is important to be aware of it. Many scalp hairs bear a white keratinous sleeve about 3 to 5 mm long, which lies within 1 to 3 cm of the scalp surface and can—unlike a nit—be slid along the hair shaft. Their bluish yellow fluorescence under Wood's light may cause confusion with tinea capitis. They have been seen in sisters, and Arnold has seen them in mother and daughter.

They are formed by retention and desquamation of segments of the root sheaths. Taïeb et al reviewed 36 published cases (and reported two of their own, with electron micrographs) and distinguished two groups: (1) girls between two and eight with diffuse involvement and no scalp disease, and (2) children and adults with psoriasis, lichen planus, seborrheic dermatitis, or trichotillomania. Keiper made a similar distinction, separating a large group of cases with some keratinizing disorder of the scalp and dark, oddly shaped masses of keratin adherent to or surrounding the hairs (often three or four together), which he would call *parakeratotic hair casts*; and lighter colored tubular casts, 2 to 4 mm long, which he would call *peripilar hair casts*. We would not call the group with an underlying keratinizing disorder "hair casts," but simply retained scale. Scott and Roenigk propose a more complex nomenclature based upon which of these (or both) are retained; however, we prefer the classifications of Taïeb et al and Keiper et al.

Taïeb et al found 0.025 per cent tretinoin lotion effective.

Pili Torti

Also known as *twisted hairs*, this malformation of hair is characterized by twisting of the hair shaft on its own axis. The hair shaft is segmentally thickened, and light and dark segments are seen. Scalp hair, eyebrows, and eyelashes may be affected. The hairs are brittle and easily broken.

In the classic type, unassociated with other disorders, onset is usually in early childhood; by puberty, it has usually improved. Clinically, it may be associated with patchy alopecia and short, broken hairs. It usually follows a dominant inheritance pattern, though recessive and sporadic cases have been reported.

Pili torti may be seen with associated abnormalities. The **Björnstad syndrome** consists of congenital deafness of the cochlear type, with pili torti. Pili torti also may occur in **Menkes's kinky hair syndrome, Crandall's syndrome** (pili torti, nerve deafness, hypogonadism), and in **trichothiodystrophy**. It was reported by Patel et al in a girl with developmental defects and **citrullinemia** (argininosuccinate synthetase deficiency), and has been described in **Bazex's follicular atrophoderma** syndrome. It was also reported by Hays et al as an explanation of acquired seeming curliness of the hair, an apparent side effect of both isotretinoin and etretinate given for epidermolytic hyperkeratosis.

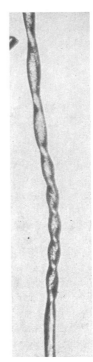

Figure 33–13. Pilus tortus, or twisted hair. (Courtesy of Dr. F. Ronchese.)

Menkes's Kinky Hair Syndrome

Pili torti, and often monilethrix and trichorrhexis nodosa, are all common in the hairs in this sex-linked recessively inherited hair disorder, seen only in boys. It has also been called "steely hair" disease, because the hair resembles steel wool. The characteristic ivory color of the hair appears between one and five months of age. Drowsiness, lethargy, convulsive seizures, and severe neurologic deterioration, with periodic hypothermia, ensue. Hairs become wiry, sparse, fragile, and twisted about their long axes. The skin is pale and the face pudgy, and the upper lip has an exaggerated "Cupid's bow" configuration.

Since no effective treatment is available, the chief importance of diagnosis is for the purposes of prognosis (patients usually die by age four) and genetic counseling.

The cause of the syndrome is still unknown. However, patients have a maldistribution of copper, and an abnormality in the gene regulation of metallothionein, a cysteine-rich metal-binding polypeptide, has been described by Hamer.

Uncombable Hair Syndrome

Shelley and Shelley renewed interest in this syndrome, reported in 1973 by Dupré et al as "*cheveux incoiffable*"—undressable hairs—by their report of three cases in 1985. Stroud and Mehregan had called it "spun-glass" hair in 1974, and *pili triangulati* is another name for this abnormality. Braun-Falco reported 38 cases in 1982.

Clinically the defect is noted in infancy as "dry, blond, shiny hair that stands straight out from the scalp and cannot be combed." On light microscopy it may appear quite normal when viewed lengthwise; but on horizontal sectioning and on scanning electron microscopy it shows longitudinal grooves that make it abnormally rigid. Van Neste et al reported abnormal fibrous proteins in the hair.

One of the Shelleys' cases responded symptomatically (though without apparent change in the hair structure) to biotin orally, 0.3 mg three times daily. Some cases improve spontaneously in late childhood, however.

Monilethrix

This rare hereditary disease is also known as *beaded hairs*. Monilethrix is characterized by dryness, fragility, and sparseness of the scalp hair, with fusiform or spindle-shaped swellings of the hair shaft separated by narrow atrophic segments. The hair tends to break at the delicate internodes. There is an occasional rupture at the node and longitudinal fissuring of the shaft, which also involves the nodes. The disease is often associated with keratosis pilaris of the extensor surfaces, temples, and back of the neck. Hair on regions other than the scalp may be affected. Leukonychia may occur.

Inheritance of monilethrix is an autosomal dominant trait. It has been described in association with Menkes's syndrome.

Solomon and Green have noted that improvement of the hair may occur during pregnancy, but after delivery the hair returns to its original state. They also state improvement may occur with age and that there is seasonal improvement during the summer. A favorable response has been reported with etretinate therapy, but in view of the propensity of etretinate to induce alopecia, we do not recommend treating monilethrix with etretinate. Systemic corticosteroids may be helpful, however, and a trial of four to six monthly 40-mg doses of Kenalog IM is reasonable.

TRICHORRHEXIS NODOSA

The hair shafts may have small white nodes arranged at irregular intervals. These nodes are the sites of fracture of the hair cortex. The splitting into strands produces a microscopic appearance suggestive of a pair of brooms stuck together end to end by their bristles. The hairs soon break at these nodes. The number of these nodes along one hair shaft varies from one to several, depending upon its length. These fractured hairs are found mostly on the scalp, often in just a small area or areas, but other sites such as the pubic area, axillae, and chest may be involved.

Several categories or types of trichorrhexis nodosa have been described. *Proximal trichorrhexis nodosa* involves the proximal shafts of the hairs of blacks who traumatize their hair with styling or chemicals; involved hairs break a few centimeters from the skin surface. It appears to occur in genetically predisposed patients. *Distal trichorrhexis nodosa* occurs primarily in Orientals or white patients, several inches from the

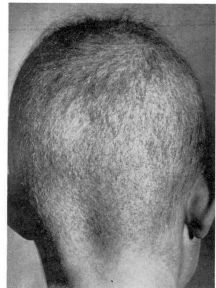

A

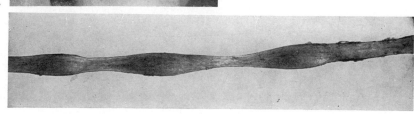

B

Figure 33–14. A, *Monilethrix. Sparse, short, dry hair and follicular keratosis. B, Monilethrix, hair showing alternating constrictions and fusiform enlargements.*

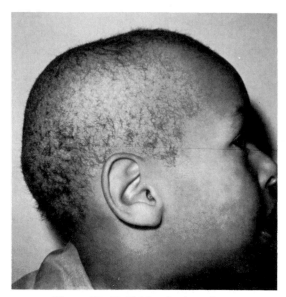

Figure 33–15. Trichorrhexis nodosa.

scalp, and is associated with trichoptilosis, or longitudinal splitting, known as "split ends." *Acquired localized trichorrhexis nodosa* is a common type in which the defect occurs in a localized area, a few centimeters across. Chernosky and Owens found a number of diseases accompanying this type of trichorrhexis nodosa in which pruritus was a prominent symptom; this could be allayed by scratching and rubbing. These were circumscribed neurodermatitis, tinea cruris, contact dermatitis, atopic dermatitis, and lichen sclerosus et atrophicus.

The occurrence of trichorrhexis nodosa in some patients with argininosuccinicaciduria has suggested an etiologic connection. Shelley and Rawnsley have proposed the term **aminogenic alopecia** for a case associated with argininosuccinicaciduria in which a diffuse thinning of the hair occurred, especially over the crown. Brittle nails and trichorrhexis nodosa type of hair changes were present. Other cases with argininosuccinicaciduria association are cited by the same authors. Trichorrhexis nodosa has been de-

scribed in Menkes's kinky hair syndrome and trichorrhexis nodosa–like fractures may be seen in trichothiodystrophy. Trichoschisis, a clean transverse fracture across the hair shaft, is more commonly present in trichothiodystrophy.

Milstein in 1983 reported curly hair as a side effect of Accutane (tretinoin) therapy, and Brauner confirmed it with a report of two cases in 1984, and Ashby with another case. Hughes reported it also, but apparently explained it by the finding of extensive trichorrhexis nodosa in both patients.

Treatment is directed toward the avoidance of traumatization of the hair.

Trichorrhexis Invaginata

Also known as **bamboo hair**, this hair defect is caused by intussusception of the hair shaft at the zone of beginning keratinization. Ito et al concluded from their studies that the invagination was caused by softness of the cortex in the keratogenous zone. The softness may be due to inadequate conversion of -SH to S-S proteins in the cortex. The bamboo hair has nodose ball-and-socket deformities, with the socket forming the proximal and the ball part forming the distal portion of the node along the hair shaft. This type of hair is associated with Netherton's syndrome.

Menne et al reported the bamboo hair defect in very thin, probably vellus, hairs in a seven-year-old boy with short, thin, brittle scalp hairs and no eyebrows. They termed this a "candlestick" deformity.

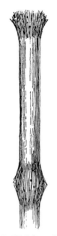

Figure 33–16. Trichorrhexis nodosa.

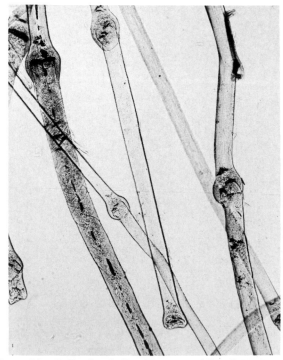

Figure 33–17. Bamboo hairs. (Courtesy of Dr. G.H. Curtis.)

Netherton's Syndrome

Trichorrhexis invaginata (bamboo hairs) associated with congenital ichthyosiform erythroderma or ichthyosis linearis circumflexa, predominantly in females, constitute Netherton's syndrome. Atopic manifestations are commonly present. The bamboo hairs may be present not only on the scalp but also on the eyebrows, eyelashes, and rarely in other hairy areas. Hair sparsity is noted all over the body. The bamboo hairs may become normal within a few years. Other reported findings include pili torti, trichorrhexis nodosa, moniliform hairs, and mental retardation. An autosomal recessive mode of inheritance was suggested by Altman and Stroud.

To this Greene et al added urticaria, angioedema, growth retardation, and recurrent infections. They reviewed 43 published cases. Their own patient had delayed neutrophil phagocytosis and recurrent infections, which were also seen in 12 of the 43 cases. They recommend investigating these patients for immunodeficiency.

Their patients, like some others, were made worse by etretinate; however, Caputo reported improvement with it. PUVA has also been reported to help the circumflex linear ichthyosis.

Pili Annulati (Ringed Hair)

In this peculiar disease the hair seems banded by alternating segments of light and dark color when seen in reflected light. The light bands are due to clusters of abnormal air-filled cavities, which scatter light, as shown by the electron microscope.

The hair growth is normal in these patients and there are no other associated abnormalities of skin or other organ systems. It is inherited by autosomal dominance, begins in infancy, and requires no treatment, since the "spangled" appearance of the hair is not unattractive.

Pili Pseudo-Annulati

Usually miscalled "pseudopili annulati"—as if the hairs, rather than the rings, were false—this anomaly of human hair mimics pili annulati. The two differ in that the light bands in pili annulati are due to internal effects, whereas the bright segments in pili pseudo-annulati are due to reflection and refraction of light by flattened, twisted surfaces of hair. This latter type is a variant of normal hair, according to Price and her associates.

Kinking Hair

Acquired progressive kinking of the hair, first described and named by Wise and Sulzberger in 1932, has a structural abnormality of kinking and twisting of the hair shaft at irregular intervals. The changes typically begin in the late teens or early twenties on the temporal region and then progress to both the parietal and frontal areas. Usually straight, light brown hair becomes woolly, kinky, black hair.

Mortimer et al reported six cases in 1985, and reviewed the scanty literature. Some have regarded this as an androgen-dependent precursor of male-pattern hair loss; however, this outcome is not invariable. "Whisker" hairs, the short dark hairs which grow anterior to the ears in young people who eventually develop androgenic alopecia, is felt to be a variant of acquired kinking of the hair. Cullen reported three women with the disorder in 1989, two of whom experienced reversion to normal hair growth.

Widespread kinking of the hair may be induced by drugs, notably retinoids, and it may also occur, as one of us (WDJ) has noted, in the acquired immunodeficiency syndrome.

Woolly Hair

Woolly hair is present at birth, and is usually severest during childhood, when it is often impossible to brush the hair. In adult life there is a variable amelioration in the condition. There is a clear distinction between the appearance of the affected and nonaffected members of a family. Three subgroups have been identified: *hereditary woolly hair* has evidence of autosomal dominant inheritance; *familial woolly hair* has a distinctive bleached appearance with a reduced diameter and a suspected autosomal recessive mode of inheritance; *woolly hair nevus* has a partial scalp involvement by woolly hair, which has a markedly reduced diameter.

Woolly hairs tend to unite into locks, while hairs of blacks remain individual. The hair may not grow beyond a length of 12 cm, but may attain a normal appearance in adult life. In the familial group the eyebrows and the hairs on the arms, legs, and pubic and axillary regions may be short and pale. There are no associated cutaneous or systemic diseases.

The microscopic findings of the hair include an ovoid shape on cross section, a pili-tortilike twisting about a longitudinal axis, trichorrhexis nodosa, and pili annulati.

Plica Neuropathica

This is a curling, looping, intertwisting, and felting or matting of the hair in localized areas of the scalp. Simpson and Mullins reported a case occurring in a black woman who had tangled and matted hair. Predisposing factors figuring in this condition were kinky hairs and a neurotic mental state. **Plica polonica** is an older name of this condition. Bogaty and Dunlap have induced matting or felting in the laboratory.

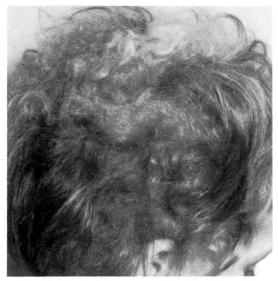

Figure 33–18. Woolly hair nevus, with affected hairs lighter and finer than the normal hair.

Pseudofolliculitis Barbae

These are hairs that, after appearing at the surface, curve back and pierce the skin as ingrowing hairs. The chief cause is close shaving of curly hair, and the cure is to stop this. Solitary hairs may be epilated; however, many hairs are usually involved.

The commonest clinical syndrome resulting is *pseudofolliculitis of the beard*, a serious problem seen chiefly in black men, who must sometimes give up shaving in order to alleviate the disorder. Brauner and Flandermeyer have dealt in depth with this problem, which is common among black soldiers, who are required to shave daily. Shaving of the pubic hair will often result in pseudofolliculitis. Hall et al have described it in three black women and suggest that topical retinoic acid may help. Brown advocates the use of clippers or chemical depilatories, and adjunctive antibiotic therapy. He finds topical tretinoin helpful "in rare instances." Our experience is similar to Brown's. In severe cases keloids may result, in the beard area.

Moore has invented a tiny plastic hook for removing ingrown hairs before shaving, which is very helpful.

Pili Multigemini

This rare malformation of the pilary apparatus is characterized by the presence of bifurcated or multiple divided hair matrices and papillae, giving rise to the formation of multiple hair shafts within the individual follicles. Mehregan and Thompson reported a patient with cleidocranial dysostosis and extensive pili multigemini over the heavily bearded chin and cheek areas. There is no treatment.

Pili Bifurcati

Weary et al described this strange disorder in a three-year old child seen because of hair loss. Bifurcation was found in short segments along the shafts of several hairs. The anomaly was transient.

Trichostasis Spinulosa

This common disorder of the hair follicles clinically gives the impression of follicular keratosis, but the follicles are filled with funnel-shaped, horny plugs within which are bundles of vellus hairs. The hairs are round at their proximal ends and shredded distally. The disease occurs on the nose and forehead of elderly persons and on the shoulders and back and manifests itself by the appearance of little black dots that look like comedones but which on closer examination are seen to be bundles of soft hairs, which project 2 to 3 mm above the skin. Microscopically these tufts are made up of several dozen fine stubby hairs. Even without a magnifying glass the small tufts of vellus hair emerging from the black-dot follicle are apparent.

Goldschmidt et al suggested that trichostasis spinulosa results from retention of telogen hairs which are derived from a single hair matrix. It is primarily due to a hyperkeratosis of the follicular infundibulum. This hyperkeratosis leads to a partial obstruction of the follicular orifice, which does not permit shedding of small telogen hairs.

Sarkany and Gaylarde reported that keratolytics were very effective after using a wax depilatory. Mills et al found 0.05 per cent tretinoin solution, applied daily for two or three months, effective.

Intermittent Hair-Follicle Dystrophy

Birnbaum et al reported in 1986 a new disorder of the hair follicle leading to increased fragility of the shaft, with no identifiable biochemical disturbance.

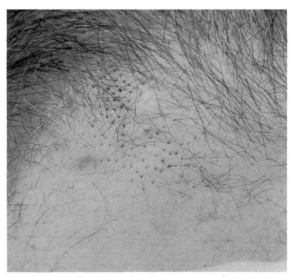

Figure 33–19. Trichostasis spinulosa.

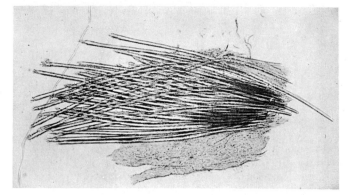

Figure 33–20. Trichostasis spinulosa—the removed plug, full of fine hairs.

Bubble Hair Deformity

Brown et al reported a 16-year-old girl who developed brittle, fragile hairs in localized areas of the scalp. The hairs additionally became straight and stiff. Small bubblelike defects were found within the hair shafts on light and electron microscopy.

Balsa RE, et al: Acquired kinking of the hair. JAAD 1986, 15:1133.

Birnbaum PS, et al: Heritable disorders of the hair. Derm Clin 1987, 5:137.

Brauner GJ: Does accutane make hair curly? Schoch Letter 1983, 33:139.

Idem, et al: Pseudofolliculitis barbae. II: treatment. Int J Dermatol 1977, 16:520.

Brodin MB, et al: Netherton's syndrome. Cutis 1980, 26:185.

Brown LA Jr: Pathogenesis and treatment of pseudofolliculitis barbae. Cutis 1983, 32:373.

Brown VM, et al: An unusual new hair shaft abnormality. JAAD 1986, 15:1113.

Camacho-Martinez F: Localized trichorrhexis nodosa. JAAD 1989, 20:696.

Idem, et al: Hair shaft dysplasias. Int J Dermatol 1988, 27:71.

Caputo R, et al: Netherton's syndrome in two adult patients. Arch Dermatol 1984, 120:220.

Caserio RJ, et al: Diagnostic techniques for hair disorders Part I. Cutis 1987, 40:265.

Idem: Diagnostic techniques for hair disorders Part II. Cutis 1987, 40:321.

Chanwichitrana S, et al: Pili trianguli et canaliculi. Arch Dermatol 1986, 122:977.

Collie WR, et al: Pili torti as a marker for carriers of Menkes' disease. Lancet 1978, 1:607.

Coupe RL, et al: Acquired progressive kinking of the hair. Arch Dermatol 1969, 100:191.

Cullen SI, et al: Acquired progressive kinking of hair. Arch Dermatol 1989, 125:252.

Danks DM: Steely hair, mottled mice, and copper metabolism. N Engl J Med 1975, 293:1147.

Dawber R, et al: Scanning electron microscopy of normal and abnormal hair shafts. Arch Dermatol 1970, 101:316.

Dupré A, et al: A new type of pilar dysplasia. The uncombable hair syndrome with pili trianguli et canaliculi. Arch Dermatol Res 1978, 261:217.

Goldschmidt H, et al: Trichostasis spinulosa. Hautarzt 1975, 26:299.

Goldsmith LA: An approach to the diagnosis of genetic hair disorders. Progr Dermatol 1984, 18:1.

Green SL, et al: Netherton's syndrome. JAAD 1985, 13:329.

Gupta AK, et al: Hair abnormalities and a rash with a double-edged scale. Arch Dermatol 1986, 122:1199.

Hall JC, et al: Pseudofolliculitis: revised concepts of diagnosis and treatment. Report of three cases in women. Cutis 1979, 23:798.

Hamer DH: Metallothionein gene regulation in Menkes' syndrome. Arch Dermatol 1987, 123:1384s.

Hart DB: Menkes' syndrome. JAAD 1983, 9:145.

Hays SB, et al: Acquired pili torti in two patients treated with synthetic retinoids. Cutis 1985, 33:466.

Held JL, et al: Hair casts or pseudonits acquired following psychological trauma. Cutis 1989, 43:380.

Hordinsky MK, et al: Friable hair, urea cycle dysfunction, and trichothiodystrophy. Curr Prob Dermatol 1987, 17:52.

Hughes PSH: Curly hair from Accutane confirmed and explained. Schoch Letter 1984, 34:10.

Hutchinson PE, et al: Woolly hair: clinical and general aspects. Trans St John's Hosp Derm Soc 1974, 60:160.

Ito M, et al: Pathogenesis in trichorrhexis invaginata. J Invest Dermatol 1984, 83:1.

Keipert JA: Hair casts. Arch Dermatol 1986, 122:927.

King MD, et al: Trichothiodystrophy-neurotrichocutaneous syndrome of Pollitt. J Med Genet 1984, 21:286.

Kossard S, et al: Necrobiotic xanthogranuloma with paraproteinemia. JAAD 1980, 3:257.

Laub D, et al: A child with hair loss. Arch Dermatol 1987, 123:1071.

Marshall J, et al: Felted hair untangled. JAAD 1989, 20:688.

Mehregan AH, et al: Pili multigemini. Br J Dermatol 1979, 100:315.

Menne T, et al: Canestick lesions of vellus hair in Netherton's syndrome (letter). Arch Dermatol 1985, 121:451.

Mills OH Jr, et al: Topically applied tretinoin in the treatment of trichostasis spinulosa. Arch Dermatol 1973, 108:378.

Moore MD: Moore tool for lifting ingrown hairs before shaving. Schoch Lett 1989, 39:37, Item 154.

Mortimer PS: Unruly hair. Br J Dermatol 1985, 113:467.

Idem, et al: Acquired progressive kinking of hair. Report of six cases and review of the literature. Arch Dermatol 1985, 121:1031.

Patel HP, et al: Pili torti in association with citrullinemia. JAAD 1985, 12:203.

Price VH: Office diagnosis of structural hair anomalies. Cutis 1975, 15:231.

Idem, et al: Pseudopili annulati. Arch Dermatol 1970, 102:354.

Ravella A, et al: Localized pili canaliculi and trianguli. JAAD 1987, 17:377.

Rebora A, et al: Acquired progressive kinking of the hair. JAAD 1985, 12:933.

Sarkany I, et al: Trichostasis spinulosa and its management. Br J Dermatol 1971, 84:311.

Scott MJ: Hair casts. JAAD 1983, 8:27.

Seay AR, et al: CT scans in Menkes' disease. Neurology 1979, 29:304.

Simpson MH, et al: Plica neuropathica. Arch Dermatol 1969, 100:457.

Shelley WB: Hair examination using double-stick tape. JAAD 1983, 8:430.

Idem, et al: Uncombable hair syndrome: observations on response to biotin and occurrence in siblings with ectodermal dysplasia. JAAD 1985, 13:97.

Steck WD: The clinical evaluation of pathologic hair loss. Cutis 1979, 24:293.

Stroud JD: Hair-shaft anomalies. Derm Clin 1987, 5:581.

Taïeb A, et al: Hair casts: a clinical and morphologic study. Arch Dermatol 1985, 121:1009.

Van Neste D, et al: Abnormal fibrous protein patterns in the uncombable hair syndrome. Arch Dermatol Res 1985, 277:151.

Weary PE, et al: Pili bifurcati. Arch Dermatol 1973, 108:403.

White MC, et al: Trichothiodystrophy. J Assoc Milit Dermatol 1987, 12:4.

Whiting DA: Structural abnormalities of the hair shaft. JAAD 1987, 16:1.

HYPERTRICHOSIS

Hypertrichosis is an overgrowth of hair not localized to the androgen-dependent areas of the skin. Several forms exist.

Localized Acquired Hypertrichosis. Beighton first reported a curious and rare anomaly, *hairy elbows*, in 1970. It is a progressive excessive growth of lanugo hairs initially, in which the hairs may reach (as in Andreev's case) a length of 10 cm. Later they become coarser, but regression has been observed during adolescence. Andreev's case had no endocrine abnormality and was not familial. Rudolph, who reported a case in 1985, emphasized the lack of need for endocrine or other studies, since the condition appears to be of only cosmetic significance.

Lupton and Odom have seen two patients with excessive growth of lanugo hairs on the anterior neck just above the suprasternal notch.

Dermal tumors, such as melanocytic nevi or Becker's nevi, may have excessive terminal hair growth. Repeated irritation, trauma, occlusion under a cast, eczematous states, topical steroid use, linear melorheostotic scleroderma, the Crowe-Fukase (POEMS) syndrome, and pretibial myxedema may be other situations in which there is a localized increase in hair growth. *Porphyrias* generally show a localized hypertrichosis over the malar area such as in porphyria cutanea tarda or variegate porphyria; however, in the Günther variety of erythropoietic porphyria it may be generalized or more diffuse in nature.

Localized Congenital Hypertrichosis. Such cases include congenital nevocytic nevi, simple nevoid hypertrichosis, or as a sign of underlying spinal dysraphism (when occurring over the sacral midline).

Generalized Congenital Hypertrichosis (Congenital Hypertrichosis Lanuginosa). Beighton summarized this rare type of excessive and generalized hairiness, inherited by autosomal dominance. His patient, a boy of five years, was covered over his entire body with fine vellus hairs 2 to 10 cm long. The scalp hair appeared to be normal; otherwise, with the exception of the palms and soles, all areas were covered. *Congenital hypertrichosis lanuginosa* may be associated with dental anomalies and gingival fibromatosis. This type of hairiness has attracted considerable attention over the centuries. These unfortunately afflicted individuals have been billed as "dog-faced boy," "human werewolf," and "human Skye terrier."

Other cases of congenital generalized hypertrichosis may be secondary to drug ingestion by the mother. The *fetal hydantoin syndrome* is characterized by hypertrichosis, depressed nasal bridge, large lips, a wide mouth, and a short, webbed neck. The *fetal alcohol syndrome* includes hypertrichosis, a small face, capillary hemangiomas, and physical and mental retardation. A case of generalized hypertrichosis and multiple congenital defects was reported by Kaler et al in a baby born to a mother who used *minoxidil* throughout pregnancy.

Generalized or Patterned Acquired Hypertrichosis. These cases include those due to acquired hypertrichosis lanuginosa, those associated with various syndromes, and those secondary to drug intake. *Acquired hypertrichosis lanuginosa* has been covered earlier in this book as an ominous sign of internal malignancy. *Syndromes* associated with increased hair growth include lipoatrophic diabetes, Rubenstein-Taylor syndrome (craniofacial dysostosis and patent ductus arteriosus), Cornelia de Lange's syndrome, Hurler's syndrome, Morogu's syndrome, leprechaunism, Winchester's syndrome, and the Schynzel-Giedier syndrome. *Drugs* associated with hypertrichosis include minoxidil, cyclosporine, diphenylhydantoin, diazoxide, streptomycin, penicillamine, corticosteroids, danazol, psoralens, hexachlorobenzene, and topical steroids or topical androgens.

Andreev VC, et al: Hairy elbows. Arch Dermatol 1979, 115:761.

Beighton P: Congenital hypertrichosis lanuginosa. Arch Dermatol 1970, 101:699.

Jemec GBE: Hypertrichosis lanuginosa acquisita: report of a case and review of the literature. Arch Dermatol 1986, 122:805.

Kaler SG, et al: Hypertrichosis and congenital anomalies associated with maternal use of minoxidil. Pediatrics 1987, 79:434.

Miyachi Y, et al: Linear melorheostotic scleroderma with hypertrichosis. Arch Dermatol 1979, 115:1233.

Rampen FHJ: Hypertrichosis in PUVA-treated patients. Br J Dermatol 1983, 109:657.

Roth SI, et al: Cutaneous manifestations of leprechaunism. Arch Dermatol 1981, 117:531.

Rudolph RI: Hairy elbows. Cutis 1985, 33:69.

Shelley WB, et al: The skin changes in the Crowe-Fukase (POEMS) syndrome. Arch Dermatol 1987, 123:85.

Swanson PM: Cornelia de Lange syndrome: an acronymic presentation. Cutis 1972, 10:334.

Wysocki GP, et al: Hypertrichosis in patients receiving cyclosporin therapy. Clin Exp Dermatol 1987, 12:191.

HIRSUTISM

CLINICAL FEATURES. Hirsutism is an excess of terminal hair growth in women in a pattern more typical of men. Androgen-dependent growth areas affected include the upper lip, cheeks, chin, the central chest, the breasts, and the lower abdomen and groins. This altered growth pattern of the hair may or may not be associated with other signs of *virilization*, which include temporal balding, masculine habitus, deepening of the voice, clitoral hypertrophy, and amenorrhea. Acne is an additional associated phenomenon in some cases of hirsutism. When virilization accompanies hirsutism, especially

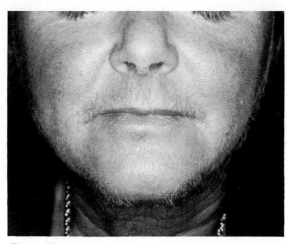

Figure 33–21. Drug-induced (oxymetholone) hirsutism.

when progression is rapid, a neoplastic cause is likely. Neoplastic causes account for only a small minority of hirsute women.

PATHOGENESIS. Racial variation should be considered when evaluating hirsutism. Women of Middle Eastern, Russian, and Southern European countries commonly have facial, abdominal, and thigh hair, whereas Oriental and Indian women generally have little terminal hair growth in these areas.

In women, androgen biosynthesis occurs only in the adrenal and the ovary. The potent androgen testosterone and the androgen precursor androstenedione are secreted by the ovary. The adrenal contributions are preandrogens; dehydroepiandrosterone (DHEA), DHEA sulfate, and androstenedione require peripheral conversion in the skin and liver to testosterone.

Testosterone is converted to dihydrotestosterone, the androgen that promotes androgen-dependent hair growth, in the hair follicle by 5α-reductase. Receptor molecules in the end organ are necessary for binding and hormone action at that level. Since testosterone is normally bound to carrier molecules in the plasma at a 99 per cent level, and it is the unbound testosterone which is active, the levels of free testosterone reflect clinical evidence of androgen excess, rather than total testosterone.

Hirsutism, then, may result either from excessive secretion of androgens from either the ovary or the adrenal gland, or from excessive stimulation by pituitary tumors. The excessive secretion may be from functional excesses or from neoplastic processes. All cases of severe or progressive hirsutism should be investigated for an endocrinopathy.

Ovarian causes include polycystic ovary disease (Stein-Leventhal syndrome), and a variety of ovarian tumors, both benign and malignant. The *Stein-Leventhal syndrome* is characterized by hirsutism (50 per cent), acne (20 per cent), and signs such as amenorrhea, uterine bleeding, anovulation, obesity, and small breasts. The ovaries are frequently palpable on physical examination, as they are polycystic. Pelvic ultrasound is useful also; however, culdoscopy and

colpotomy may be necessary for diagnosis. Serum free testosterone is generally elevated. Luteinizing hormone is also elevated, but follicle-stimulating hormone levels remain normal or may be decreased. *Ovarian tumors* include unilateral benign microadenomas, arrhenoblastomas, Leydig cell tumors, hilar cell tumors, granular–thecal cell tumors, and luteomas. Here the onset is usually rapid, occurs with associated virilization, and begins between the ages of 20 and 40. Again free testosterone is high (generally greater than 2 ng/ml).

Adrenal causes include congenital adrenal hyperplasia and adrenal tumors such as adrenal adenomas and carcinomas. The *adrenogenital syndrome* or congenital adrenal hyperplasia is an autosomal dominant disorder which may result from deficiencies of the following enzymes: 21-hydroxylase (most common form), 11-hydroxylase, and 3b-hydroxy steroid dehydrogenase. Onset is generally in childhood, with ambiguous genitalia, precocious growth, and virilism; however, adult-onset types with partial enzyme deficiencies present generally with hirsutism as a familial trait.

Pituitary causes include Cushing's disease, acromegaly, and prolactin-secreting adenomas. Cushing's disease and acromegaly are dealt with in Chapter 24. Prolactin-secreting microadenomas have a 20 per cent incidence of hirsutism and acne. Other conditions in which prolactin levels may be elevated and which may lead to hirsutism include hypothyroidism, phenothiazine intake, and hepato-renal failure.

Other causes of hirsutism include the exogenous intake of androgens and certain high-progesterone birth control pills (uncommonly). End-organ hypersensitivity may be a mechanism in patients with a normal evaluation. Drugs such as minoxidil, diazoxide, corticosteroids, and phenytoin, which have been reported as causing hirsutism, generally cause hypertrichosis—a generalized increase in hair not limited to the androgen-sensitive areas.

EVALUATION. A careful history and physical examination are essential. The history should focus on onset and progression, virilization, menstrual history, and family/racial background. Physical examination may reveal signs of Cushing's disease or acromegaly. Other signs to be evaluated are the distribution of muscle mass and body fat, clitoral dimensions, voice depth, and galactorrhea.

Laboratory evaluation should include a free testosterone level, a dehydroepiandrosterone sulfate level, a 17-hydroxy progesterone level, and a prolactin level.

DIAGNOSIS. If acromegaly or Cushing's disease is present clinically, referral to an internist or endocrinologist is recommended. The presence of major menstrual irregularities is also an indication for referral to a gynecologist. While 90 per cent of women with hirsutism have an elevated free testosterone level, elevations above 2 ng/ml and rapid onset or progression of virilization suggest serious underlying disease, generally an ovarian neoplasm. Pelvic ultrasound and referral are indicated. A major elevation in the DHEA sulfate level (above 9000 ng/ml) suggests an adrenal neoplasm, and computed tomography of the adrenal gland and referral are recommended. Elevations of the 17-hydroxyprogesterone level (when taken between 0700 and 0900) should suggest congenital adrenal hyperplasia, and ACTH stimulation tests (for levels of 300 to 1000 ng/ml) and referral are recommended. Prolactin levels above 20 ng/ml should be likewise referred for further evaluation.

In all other cases the cause is likely due to a functional disorder and treatment may be instituted. A reevaluation within six to 12 months should be planned.

TREATMENT. Once appropriate testing has led to diagnosis and referral of patients requiring special methods of specific treatment, such as surgical intervention, therapeutic alternatives include cosmetic (mechanical) treatments, nonspecific suppressive therapy, and specific antiandrogens.

Cosmetic or mechanical methods of treatment are the cheapest and easiest methods, and expose the patient to the fewest potential side effects. Shaving is best; however, it is often the most resisted, due to social influences. Wax depilatories, chemical depilatories, bleaching of the hair, and electrolysis are alternatives.

Epilating waxes, usually made of beeswax and rosin, are satisfactory for temporary removal of moderate amounts of cosmetically objectionable hair. It has been proved beyond a doubt that the temporary removal of hairs by waxes, shaving, or plucking does not stimulate their growth or coarsen subsequent growth.

Depilatories containing barium sulfide corrode the projecting hair shaft, but have no destructive action on the intrafollicular growing portion. The barium sulfide may irritate the skin excessively, making this procedure undesirable.

Bleaching with hydrogen peroxide with or without equal parts of strong ammonia makes dark hairs less noticeable and corrodes the finer hairs. Before it is applied, the skin is cleansed with ether to remove any oiliness. It is advisable to begin with one tenth of the usual strength.

Epilation with the use of a high frequency or galvanic current is a safe method for the permanent removal of superfluous hair. A certain number of recurrences (20 to 35 per cent) is inevitable even when it is done by experts. Such hairs must be removed a second time. Referral to an "electrologist" is suggested.

Attempts to cure hypertrichosis by x-rays are about as old as x-rays. Permanent epilation can be effected by x-rays only when sufficient exposure is given to cause subsequent permanent damage to the skin. Numerous sad cases of radiodermatitis, skin keratoses, and cancers have been produced by x-rays used for epilation. It should *never* be done.

These mechanical modalities should be used at least initially, even when medical treatment is planned, in order to achieve some early response, since medical intervention takes many months to give a noticeable response.

Nonspecific suppressive therapies include oral contraceptives and glucocorticoids. Practically, these therapies suppress hirsutism due to adrenal or ovarian causes equally, and hence are utilized based on the individual patient's wants and needs, with particular attention to the specific side effects of each medication. In the case of a young woman who desires contraception and has no contraindications, an oral preparation with low androgenic progestins should be selected. The combination of ethinyl estradiol, 35 mg, and norethindrone, 0.5 mg, is recommended by Rittmaster et al. Birth control pills are helpful in 75 per cent of hirsute women. Glucocorticoids are indicated in the treatment of congenital adrenal hyperplasia, and some recommend the use of dexamethasone at night for other forms of hirsutism; however, in general the use of glucocorticoids is rapidly decreasing and is not recommended by Rittmaster et al except in congenital adrenal hyperplasia.

Antiandrogens include cimetidine, cyproterone acetate, spironolactone, and ketoconazole. Cimetidine is a weak antiandrogen and has not been utilized widely. Ketoconazole is a relatively recent inclusion in the antiandrogens and has not been well evaluated for use in hirsutism.

The efficacy and safety of a combination of the antiandrogen cyproterone acetate combined with ethinyl estradiol has been amply proved in trials in England, Australia, France, and Holland by Ekoe et al, Peereboom-Wynia et al, Thomas et al, and Kuttenn et al. Cyproterone is usually given in a dose of 100 mg a day from days 5 to 14, and ethinyl estradiol 30 mcg a day from day 5 through 25. Acne and hirsutism respond best (80–95 per cent) and alopecia least (50 per cent). Strict contraception is essential. None reported serious side effects. Cyproterone is not approved for use in the United States.

Spironolactone is a stronger antiandrogen than either cimetidine or cyproterone acetate. It is used in doses of 75 mg to 200 mg/day. Cumming et al reported benefit in 10 of 20 women with moderate to severe hirsutism. Board et al studied a combination of spironolactone and oral contraceptives. This useful combination, which is effective in about three of four patients, also limits menstrual irregularities and prevents conception.

Topically applied medications would be an advance, and studies such as that by Weissmann et al, which showed that topically administered spironolactone had only local effects in the hamster, may help lead to further advances in this area. Schmidt et al have used a synthetic progesterone derivative, medroxyprogesterone acetate, topically and intralesionally as well as subcutaneously. It did have a local effect, and further work in this area will be of interest.

Blankstein J, et al: Adult onset familial adrenal 21-hydroxylase deficiency. Am J Med 1980, 68:441.

Board JA, et al: Spironolactone and estrogen-progestin therapy for hirsutism. South Med J 1987, 80:483.

Bouallouche A, et al: Evidence for adrenal and/or ovarian dysfunction as a possible etiology of idiopathic hirsutism. Am J Obstet Gynecol 1983, 147:57.

Braithwaite SS, et al: Hirsutism (editorial). Arch Dermatol 1983, 119:279.

Callan A: Management of hirsutism. Austral J Dermatol 1982, 23:97.

Carvalho D, et al: Treatment of hirsutism with spironolactone. Lancet 1985, 2:560.

Cathelineau G, et al: Adrenocortical 11-B-hydroxylation defect in adult women with postmenarchial onset of symptoms. J Clin Endocrinol Metab 1980, 51:287.

Chang RJ, et al: Steroid secretion in polycystic ovarian disease after ovarian suppression by long acting gonadotropin-releasing hormone agonist. J Clin Endocrinol Metab 1983, 56:897.

Chapman MG, et al: Spironolactone in the treatment of hirsutism. Acta Obstet Gynecol Scand 1986, 65:349.

Cumming DC, et al: Treatment of hirsutism with spironolactone. JAMA 1982, 247:1295.

Ekoe JM, et al: Treatment of hirsutism, acne, and alopecia with cyproterone acetate. Dermatologica 1980, 160:398.

Fine RM: Spironolactone therapy in hirsute women. Int J Dermatol 1989, 28:23.

Frey H, et al: The treatment of essential hirsutism in women with cyproterone acetate and ethinyl estradiol. Acta Obstet Gynecol Scand 1981, 60:295.

Futterweit W, et al: The prevalence of hyperandrogenism in 109 consecutive female patients with diffuse alopecia. JAAD 1988, 19:831.

Holdaway IM, et al: Cyproterone acetate as initial treatment and maintenance therapy for hirsutism. Acta Endocrinol (Copenh) 1985, 109:522.

Kirschner MA, et al: Idiopathic hirsutism—an ovarian abnormality. N Engl J Med 1976, 294:637.

Kuttenn F, et al: Treatment of hirsutism by oral cyproterone acetate and percutaneous estradiol. J Clin Endocrinol Metab 1980, 51:1107.

Idem: Late-onset adrenal hyperplasia in hirsutism. N Engl J Med 1985, 313:224.

Kvedar JC, et al: Hirsutism: evaluation and treatment. JAAD 1985, 12:215.

Lobo RA, et al: The effects of two doses of spironolactone on serum androgens and anagen hair in hirsute women. Fert Steril 1985, 43:200.

Lucky AW, et al: Adrenal androgen hyperresponsiveness to adrenocorticotropin in women with acne and/or hirsutism. J Clin Endocrinol Metab 1986, 62:840.

Lucky AW: Topical antiandrogens. Arch Dermatol 1985, 121:55.

Madanes AE, et al: The vellus index. Fert Steril 1987, 48:1064.

McKenna TJ: Pathogenesis and treatment of polycystic ovary syndrome. NEJM 1988, 318:558.

Pang S, et al: Hirsutism, polycystic ovarian disease, and ovarian 17-ketosteroid reductase deficiency. NEJM 1987, 316:1295.

Pereeboom-Wynia JDR, et al: Effect of cyproterone acetate orally on hair density and diameter and endocrine factors in women with idiopathic hirsutism. Dermatologica 1980, 160:7.

Price VH: Testosterone metabolism in the skin: review of its function in androgenetic alopecia, acne vulgaris and idiopathic hirsutism, including recent studies with antiandrogens. Arch Dermatol 1975, 111:1496.

Reingold SB, et al: The relationship of mild hirsutism or acne in women to androgens. Arch Dermatol 1987, 123:209.

Richards RN, et al: Electroepilation (electrolysis) in hirsutism. JAAD 1986, 15:693.

Rittmaster RS, et al: Hirsutism. Ann Intern Med 1987, 106:95.

Idem: Sensitivity of cortisol and adrenal androgens to dexamethasone suppression in hirsute women. J Clin Endocrinol Metab 1985, 61:462.

Schiavone FE, et al: Elevated free testosterone levels in women with acne. Arch Dermatol 1983, 119:799.

Schmidt JB, et al: Medroxyprogesterone acetate therapy in hirsutism. Br J Dermatol 1985, 113:161.

Seppälä M, et al: Revised serum prolactin levels associated with hirsutism and amenorrhea. J Clin Endocrinol Metab 1980, 51:287.

Sonino N: The use of ketoconazole as an inhibitor of steroid production. NEJM 1987, 317:812.

Thomas AK, et al: The treatment of hirsutism: experience with cyproterone acetate and spironolactone. Austral J Dermatol 1985, 26:19.

Vigersky RA, et al: Treatment of hirsute women with cimetidine. N Engl J Med 1980, 303:1042.

Wagner RF, et al: Electrolysis and thermolysis for permanent hair removal. JAAD 1985, 12:441.

Wajchenberg BL, et al: Determination of the sources of androgen overproduction in hirsutism associated with polycystic ovary syndrome by simultaneous adrenal and ovarian venous catheterization. J Clin Endocrinol Metab 1986, 63:1204.

Weissmann A, et al: Antiandrogenic effects of topically applied spironolactone on the hamster flank organ. Arch Dermatol 1985, 121:57.

TRICHOMYCOSIS AXILLARIS

Trichomycosis axillaris is characterized by 1- to 2-mm nodules of different colors occurring upon the affected hair shafts in the axillary or pubic areas. The color of these discrete nodules attached firmly to the hair shaft may be yellow, red, or black. Hyperhidrosis of the affected regions is usually present. A

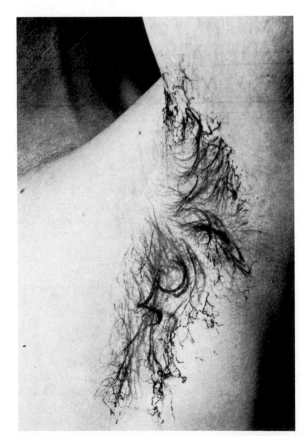

Figure 33–22. Trichomycosis axillaris nigra of the armpit. Note black beaded hairs. (Courtesy of Dr. E. Florian, Budapest.)

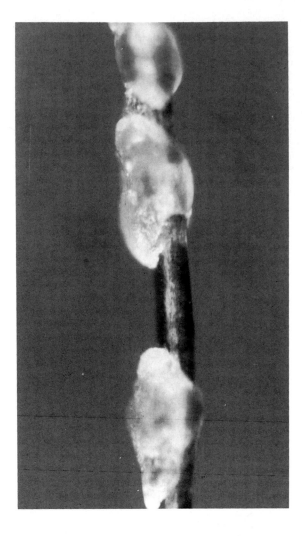

Figure 33–23. Trichomycosis axillaris. Discrete and firmly attached nodules encircle the hair shaft. (From Freeman RG, McBride ME: Arch Dermatol 1969, 100:90.)

yellowish discoloration of the axillae is sometimes noted.

Freeman and his associates have demonstrated three different types of diphtheroids in the nodules or granules and, therefore, believe that the causative organism cannot be identified only as *Corynebacterium tenuis*. Shelley found that although three distinct species were entrapped in adhesive cement substance around the hair, only one species was able to adhere to the hair and colonize it.

Treatment with topical antibiotic preparations such as Cleocin-T lotion or Staticin and with any modality that will decrease the hyperhidrosis is effective, but shaving is faster.

Freeman RG, et al: Pathogenesis of trichomycosis axillaris. Arch Dermatol 1969, 100:90.
Shelley WB, et al: Electronmicroscopy, histochemistry, and microbiology of bacterial adhesion in trichomycosis axillaris. JAAD 1984, 10:1005.

SOME ASSOCIATED HAIR FOLLICLE DISEASES

FOLLICULITIS DECALVANS

Folliculitis decalvans is an inflammatory reaction of the hair follicles that leads to alopecia of the involved area. It is a cicatricial type of alopecia in which small pustules about the follicles, erythema, scaling, and smooth shiny depressed scars are apparent. When the pustules have healed, the condition is identical with pseudopelade. This may occur not only on the scalp but on any other part of the body, such as the axillae and groin.

The cause is unknown. Some have postulated it may be an abnormal host response to an infection of the follicles in a circumscribed patch, usually on the scalp or bearded area.

Histologic findings are intrafollicular abscesses and a perifollicular infiltrate that may contain numerous plasma cells.

Following a Gram stain and bacterial culture of the exudate, therapy is directed toward the elimination

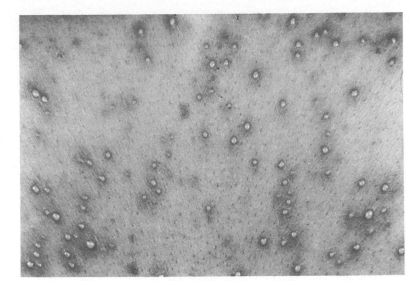

Figure 33–24. Superficial folliculitis.

of infection with antibiotics both internally and externally. Commonly coagulase-positive staphylococci are recovered and should be eliminated, although this seems to not be the primary problem; in many cases no pathogenic organism is cultured. Chronic inflammatory reactions may be helped by topical steroids and by the intralesional injection of triamcinolone.

TINEA AMIANTACEA
(Pityriasis Amiantacea)

Tinea amiantacea is an inaptly named disease manifested by thick, asbestoslike (amiantaceous), shiny

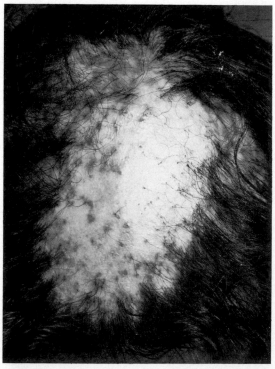

Figure 33–25. Folliculitis decalvans with characteristic infected hair follicles. (Courtesy of Dr. C.P. DeFeo, Jr.)

scales on the scalp. The crusting may be localized or, less often, generalized over the entire scalp, and resembles psoriasis and seborrheic dermatitis. The crusts are silvery white or dull gray. The proximal parts of the hairs are matted together by the laminated crusts. There are no structural changes in the hair, but in some patches where the crusting is thick, there may be some purulent exudate under the crust and temporary alopecia such as occurs after some cases of furunculosis of the scalp.

The cause is probably a secondary infection occurring in seborrheic dermatitis or inverse psoriasis.

The patient should shampoo daily or every other day with selenium sulfide suspension (Selsun or Exsel), or a tar shampoo, for a couple of weeks. Prior application of Baker's P & S liquid a few hours before shampooing facilitates removal of the scales and crusts.

KERATOSIS FOLLICULARIS CONTAGIOSA

Keratosis follicularis contagiosa, also known as epidemic acne and Brooke's disease, is an apparently infectious disease that resembles keratosis follicularis and occurs in children.

The eruption is widespread and symmetrical, affecting chiefly the back of the neck, the shoulders, and the extensor surfaces of the extremities. There is a horny thickening of these areas, especially pronounced about the follicles, where small black corneous plugs may be discerned. The skin is dry and rough. Keratosis follicularis contagiosa is differentiated from Darier's disease by its principal incidence in children, by the histological absence of corps ronds and acantholytic cells, and by the fact that the greasy scaling which is encountered in Darier's disease is never present in this infectious disorder.

Epidemic follicular eruption, reported by Bowers in Cheltenham, England, is a similar disease, known as **epidemic acne**. Approximately 200 cases were recorded. The epidemic lasted about six weeks and seemed to be connected with the use of water from a certain reservoir. The follicular papules occurred chiefly on the face and back without systemic symptoms. They disappeared within ten days without scarring. Lurie and Loewenthal reported an outbreak of epidemic follicular keratosis in South Africa in 1954 and 1955. There were mild constitutional symptoms preceded by small reddish macules on the thighs, trunk, and forearms. Within hours the eruption became generalized. The follicular papules were closely aggregated and resembled keratosis pilaris. The eruption subsided in two weeks and was completely gone in two months. No cause was found in spite of extensive bacteriological and pathological studies.

FOLLICULITIS NARES PERFORANS

Perforating folliculitis of the nose is characterized by small pustules near the tip of the inside of the nose. The lesion becomes crusted, and when the crust is removed it is found that the bulbous end of the affected vibrissa is embedded in the inspissated material. The affected hairs are typical of those occurring inside the nostril. *Staphylococcus aureus* may at times be cultured from the pustules. The hair should be removed, and antibiotic ointment applied.

PERFORATING FOLLICULITIS

Perforating folliculitis is characterized by an asymptomatic eruption of erythematous follicular papules 2 to 8 mm in diameter involving the extensor surfaces of the upper arms, the buttocks, or the upper thighs. When the small whitish keratotic plug is removed from the follicular papule, a small bleeding crater remains behind.

According to Mehregan and Coskey, the histologic examination shows a widely dilated hair follicle in which keratinous debris is encrusted. The follicular epithelium is perforated through with eosinophilic elastic fibers. Degenerated nuclei of inflammatory cells and necrotic connective tissue enter into the hair follicle just above the level of the sebaceous gland. A mild pseudoepitheliomatous hyperplasia surrounds the area of perforation.

This entity may be misdiagnosed as keratosis pilaris, pyogenic folliculitis, or Kyrle's disease. Patterson has suggested that this might be regarded as a phenomenon that may occur in several situations, rather than a specific disease. We agree.

Perforating folliculitis is resistant to treatment. Topical tretinoin (Retin-A) is the only option reported as effective against it.

KYRLE'S DISEASE

This eponymic designation has handily supplanted the original title, **hyperkeratosis follicularis et parafollicularis in cutem penetrans.**

Kyrle's disease is a rare disorder characterized by hyperkeratosis, which forms a horny cone that projects into the dermis, so that when it is removed a pitlike depression remains. Usually the papules are discrete, but they may coalesce to form circinate plaques. There is a predilection for the lower extremities, but the upper extremities, head, and neck may also be involved. Coalescing verrucous plaques are frequently seen, especially on the lower extremities. Koebner's phenomenon may also be observed, in which case plaques or elevated verrucous streaks are formed. The latter are seen only in the antecubital and popliteal spaces. Atrophic scars are seen upon involution of these lesions. Cunningham et al reported 14 cases in 1987.

The disease occurs almost exclusively in adults from the ages of 20 to 63 years with no sex or racial differences noted. Kyrle's disease has been noted to be associated especially with diabetes mellitus. Carter et al and Cunningham et al have found evidence to suggest it is a genodermatosis.

The relationship of Kyrle's disease to chronic renal failure, especially of the type secondary to diabetic vasculopathy, is uncertain. Many cases of perforating lesions in patients with this condition have been reported variably as perforating folliculitis, Kyrle's disease, or reactive perforating collagenosis. There is some difference of opinion as to whether Kyrle's disease, like perforating folliculitis, is a specific entity or a tissue reaction pattern produced by a variety of conditions. Patterson, Ackerman, and Mehregan all favor the latter explanation.

This has led Patterson, after reviewing the reports

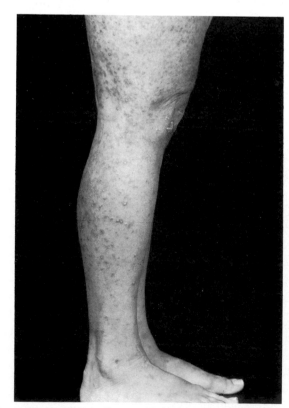

Figure 33–26. Kyrle's disease. (Courtesy of Dr. L.M. Solomon.)

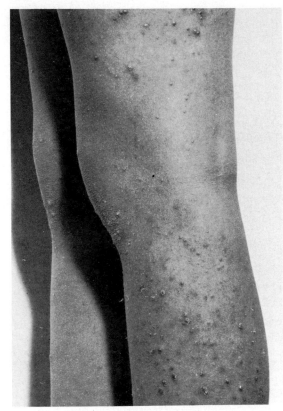

Figure 33–27. Kyrle's disease.

of perforating disease in chronic renal failure, to propose that they not be subclassified further, but simply placed into a category of acquired perforating disease, which would include perforating folliculitis, Kyrle's disease, and most cases of adult acquired reactive perforating collagenosis, with or without renal failure, diabetes mellitus, or both.

The reports of perforating disorders associated with chronic renal failure indicate that between 4 and 10 per cent of dialysis patients develop them. Such lesions are characterized by dome-shaped papules on the legs, or less often on the trunk, neck, arms, or scalp, with variable itchiness. White et al, Hood et al, and Hurwitz et al all reported series of patients with histologic studies. Early lesions may be pustular; late lesions resemble prurigo nodularis both clinically and histologically. One patient (White's) cleared promptly after a renal transplant and stopping dialysis.

Histologically, Kyrle's disease shows large keratotic and parakeratotic plugs penetrating through the epidermis into the dermis. These plugs cause an inflammatory and foreign-body giant cell reaction about the lower end of the plug in the dermis. Mild degenerative changes in the connective tissue with no increase in the elastic tissue also occur.

Kyrle's disease remains stationary for years, with possible clearing of lesions when the associated illness such as diabetes or hepatic disease has been controlled. Ultraviolet treatment, topical corticosteroids, 5-fluorouracil, and keratolytics are usually ineffective. Methotrexate is also ineffective. Aqueous

vitamin A orally in daily amounts of 100,000 units with 400 I.U. of vitamin E (Ayres) may produce improvement after one month of therapy. Topical retinoic acid (0.1 per cent cream) has also been effective in flattening lesions. Cunningham et al had one patient who responded to etretinate, but relapsed promptly when it was stopped.

REACTIVE PERFORATING COLLAGENOSIS

This entity is presented here because of its great similarity to perforating folliculitis and Kyrle's disease.

Reactive perforating collagenosis was described by Mehregan and his associates as pinhead-sized, skin-colored papules that grow to a diameter of 4 to 6 mm and develop a central area of umbilication in which keratinous material is lodged. The discrete papules may be numerous and involve sites of frequent trauma such as the backs of the hands, forearms, elbows, and knees. The lesion reaches a maximum size of about 6 mm in four weeks and then regresses spontaneously in six to eight weeks.

It is believed that this is caused by a peculiar reaction of the skin to superficial trauma. Koebnerization is often observed. Young children are most frequently affected. Most reports support an autosomal recessive mode of inheritance; however, Nair et al reported a family in which it appeared to be inherited by autosomal dominance.

Histologically the epidermis becomes edematous, the granular layer disappears, and parakeratosis develops. Eventually the epidermis becomes atrophic, with disruption of the sites over the papillae. Through these sites necrobiotic connective tissue, degenerating inflammatory cells, and collagen bun-

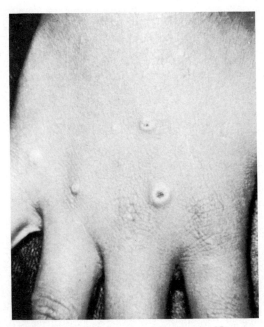

Figure 33–28. Reactive perforating collagenosis. (Courtesy of Dr. A.H. Mehregan.)

dles are extruded into a cup-shaped epidermal depression.

No specific treatment is indicated, since the lesions involute spontaneously. Tretinoin 0.1 per cent cream was effective in a patient reported by Cullen et al.

TRAUMATIC ANSERINE FOLLICULOSIS

Padilha-Gonçalves in 1977 was the first to describe the curious gooseflesh-like follicular hyperkeratosis that may result from persistent pressure and lateral friction of one skin surface upon another. Such friction in his cases was caused by habitual pressure of elbows, chin or jaw, or neck, often while watching television. Two thirds of his cases were atopics.

ERYTHROMELANOSIS FOLLICULARIS FACIEI ET COLLI

Erythromelanosis follicularis faciei et colli is a unique erythematous pigmentary disease involving the follicles. A reddish brown, sharply demarcated, symmetrical discoloration involves the preauricular and maxillary regions. At times the pigmentation may be blotchy. In addition, follicular papules and erythema are present. Under diascopic pressure the reddish brown area, containing telangiectases, becomes pale and the light brown pigmentation becomes more apparent. Pityriasiform scaling and slight itching may occur. Keratosis pilaris on the arms and shoulders is frequently found.

Mishima and Rudner described this occurring in four Caucasians; previously it had been described only in the Japanese. Borkovic et al reported the first

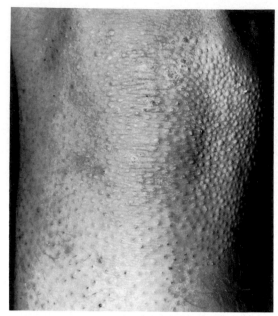

Figure 33–30. Lichen spinulosus in a 14-year-old boy with lesions predominantly on the elbows and knees.

case with unilateral involvement, present for 15 years, in a 30-year-old man of Chinese ancestry.

Histologically, a slight hyperkeratosis occurs, with epidermal hyperpigmentation. The hair follicles are enlarged, especially in the infundibular areas. The sebaceous glands are also hypertrophic. A lymphocytic infiltration surrounds the adnexa.

It is differentiated from ulerythema ophryogenes, erythrose pigmentaire peribuccale, and poikiloderma by its typical location, pigmentation, marked telangiectasia, scaling, and marked atrophy.

DISSEMINATE AND RECURRENT INFUNDIBULOFOLLICULITIS

Hitch and Lund described a disseminate follicular eruption on the torso of a black man that seemed to involve all the pilosebaceous structures. The lesions were irregularly shaped papules pierced by a hair. They likened the eruption to cutis anserina viewed through a magnifying glass.

The eruption is mildly pruritic at times, and is chronic, with recurrent exacerbations. The papules are uniform, 1 or 2 mm in diameter, and involve all the follicles in the affected areas, which are usually the upper trunk and neck, though the entire trunk and proximal extremities may be involved. Rarely, pustules may occur.

Histologically, the infundibular portion of the follicles was chiefly affected, and the lesions were inflammatory rather than hyperkeratotic. Edema, lymphocytic and neutrophilic infiltration, and slight fibroblastic infiltration surround the affected follicles.

Owen and Wood reported vitamin A orally to be effective in five of six cases, even in doses which Kligman has categorized as homeopathic: 50,000

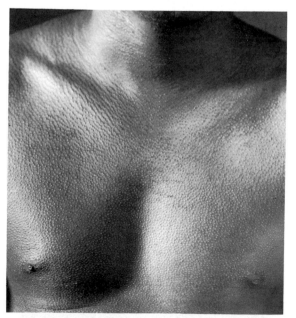

Figure 33–29. Disseminate and recurrent infundibulo-folliculitis. (From Hitch JM, Lund HZ: Arch Dermatol 1968, 97:432.)

units twice a day. We would suggest 150,000 units in a single daily dose, plus vitamin E, 400 I.U. once or twice daily, as recommended by Ayres Jr. Isotretinoin or etretinate might be effective too.

LICHEN SPINULOSUS

Lichen spinulosus (keratosis spinulosa, lichen pilaris seu spinulosus) is a disease chiefly of children and is characterized by minute filiform horny spines, which protrude from follicular openings independent of any papules. The spines are discrete and grouped. The lesions appear in crops and are symmetrically distributed over the trunk, limbs, and buttocks (acne cornée). There is a predilection for the neck, buttocks, abdominal wall, popliteal spaces, and the extensor surfaces of the arms. There is little or no itching.

The histology shows simple inflammatory changes and follicular hyperkeratosis.

The lesions are benefitted by mild keratolytics, such as 3 per cent resorcin or salicylic acid ointment. Tretinoin should be helpful topically as well. Maiocco and Miller reported success with Keralyt (salicylic acid) Gel. Maintenance therapy was needed only twice a week. Tuyp et al achieved complete clearing in a case in a 15-year-old boy with the same therapy. Lac-Hydrin (12 per cent ammonium lactate lotion) may also be worthy of trial.

Some Hair Follicle Diseases

Bogg A: Folliculitis decalvans. Acta Derm Venereol (Stockh) 1963, 43:14.

Borkovic SP, et al: Unilateral erythromelanosis follicularis faciei et colli. Cutis 1984, 33:163.

Cunningham SR, et al: Kyrle's disease. JAAD 1987, 16:117.

Flannigan SA, et al: Recurrent hyperkeratotic papules following superficial trauma. Arch Dermatol 1985, 121:1554.

Goette DK: Transepithelial elimination disorders. J Assoc Milit Dermatol 1985, 11:28.

Hitch JM, et al: Disseminate and recurrent infundibulofolliculitis. Arch Dermatol 1968, 97:432.

Hood AF, et al: Kyrle's disease in patients with chronic renal failure. Arch Dermatol 1982, 118:85.

Hurwitz RM: The evolution of perforating folliculitis in patients with chronic renal failure. Am J Dermatopathol 1985, 7:231.

Knight AG: Pityriasis amiantacea. Clin Exp Dermatol 1977, 2:137.

Mehregan AH: Perforating dermatoses. Int J Dermatol 1977, 16:19.

Idem, et al: Pilar sheath acanthoma. Arch Dermatol 1978, 114:1495.

Owen WR, et al: Disseminate and recurrent infundibulofolliculitis. Arch Dermatol 1979, 115:174.

Padilha-Gonçalves A: Traumatic anserine folliculosis. J Dermatol 1979, 6:365.

Patterson JW: The perforating disorders. JAAD 1984, 10:561.

Idem, et al: Perforating folliculitis and psoriasis. JAAD 1982, 7:369.

Rand R, et al: Keratosis follicularis spinulosa decalvans: report of two cases and literature review. Arch Dermatol 1983, 119:22.

Roenigk R, et al: Tissue expansion in cicatricial alopecia. Arch Dermatol 1987, 123:641.

Salomon RJ, et al: Kyrle's disease and hepatic insufficiency. Arch Dermatol 1986, 122:18.

Shelley WB, et al: Anhydrous formulation of aluminum chloride for chronic folliculitis. JAMA 1980, 244:1956.

Tuyp E, et al: Lichen spinulosus with immunofluorescent studies. Cutis 1984, 33:197.

Watt TL, et al: Erythromelanosis follicularis faciei et colli. JAAD 1981, 5:533.

White CR Jr, et al: Perforating folliculitis of hemodialysis. Am J Dermatopathol 1982, 4:109.

DISEASES OF THE SWEAT GLANDS

The following diseases of the sweat glands are in addition to prickly heat and other diseases discussed elsewhere. The recent extensive review by Sato et al (1989) should be referred to.

HYPERHIDROSIS

CLINICAL FEATURES. Hyperhidrosis, or excessive sweating, may be localized in one area or it may be generalized.

Localized Hyperhidrosis. In the localized type the most frequent sites are the palms and soles and the intertriginous areas; namely, the axillae, the inguinal folds, and the perineal area. The other common sites are the forehead, the tip of the nose, and the sternal area.

The chief cause of such localized hyperhidrosis is emotional. It is also seen with tabes dorsalis and, when unilateral, in hemiplegia or other unilateral nerve disorders.

Emotional Hyperhidrosis. This type is intermittent and is dependent upon the height of emotional excitement that may be triggered by anxiety, anguish, or fear. One of us (W.D.J. et al) found this type of sweating, which is usually limited to the palms, soles, and axilla, to be autosomal-dominantly inherited in some cases.

Generalized Hyperhidrosis. This type of hyperhidrosis may be induced by a hot, humid environment such as a tropical milieu, or by febrile diseases, or vigorous exercise. Hormonal disturbances such as hyperthyroidism, diabetes mellitus, pregnancy, and menopause may also produce generalized hyperhidrosis. Concussion, Parkinson's disease and other disturbances of the sympathetic nervous system, and metastatic tumors producing a complete transection of the spinal cord are additional causes of hyperhidrosis. Acromegaly, pheochromocytoma, hypoglycemia, salicylism, and lymphoma are other causes.

Gustatory Hyperhidrosis. Certain individuals regularly experience excessive sweating of the forehead, upper lip, perioral region, or sternum a few moments after eating spicy foods, tomato sauce, chocolate,

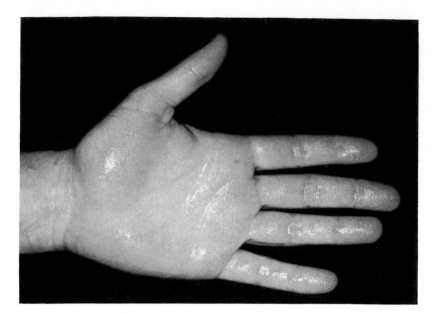

Figure 33–31. Hyperhidrosis.

coffee, tea, or hot soups. Gustatory sweating may also be caused by tumors or other injuries to the parotid gland such as those experienced in the **auriculotemporal syndrome of von Frey**. Chisa and his associates reported a 21-year-old woman in whom this syndrome developed following bilateral subcondylar osteotomy for prognathism. Harper et al reported a man with von Frey's syndrome secondary to trauma which disrupted the postganglionic autonomic innervation in the area.

Olfactory Hyperhidrosis. Eedy et al reported a case of olfactory facial hyperhidrosis in which amitriptyline was effective.

TREATMENT. A number of methods have been used to relieve hyperhidrosis. Most of the following relate to the therapy of localized emotional hyperhidrosis, because the therapy of generalized hyperhidrosis is aimed at underlying systemic disease.

Internal Medication. Most of the currently available internal medications have inherent drawbacks, thus making it difficult to achieve relief from this troublesome malady. The use of anticholinergic agents such as probanthine or glycopyrrolate may be helpful. The dosage of each is regulated by the patient's tolerance and response. Often, sweating is suppressed somewhat just as salivation reaches an intolerably low level, and this approach has to be abandoned. Side effects of acetylcholine blocking agents may also cause or aggravate such conditions as glaucoma, convulsions, and toxic erythema. The effects on sweating generally last four to six hours, and many patients prefer to use the medication to insure dryness for special occasions only, rather than as continuous treatment.

The use of sedatives and tranquilizers has been proved moderately helpful. Some employ Robinul-PH, which is a combination of glycopyrrolate and a sedative, phenobarbital. Indocin, a beta-adrenergic antagonist, is a useful preventive in some patients if taken prior to anticipated stressful circumstances.

Amitriptyline was effective in Eedy's patient with olfactory hyperhidrosis.

W. D. James et al reported success in two patients with diltiazem (Cardizem), a calcium-channel blocker. More research on many patients will be needed, however, to establish its safety and effectiveness. Namer et al found clonidine (0.45 to 0.75 mg/day) effective in 11 of 12 patients with paroxysmal localized hyperhidrosis who tolerated it.

Topical Medication. Many commercial topical applications are available to reduce hyperhidrosis of the axillae. Most of them contain aluminum chloride or aluminum chlorhydroxide. These are highly effective and obviate compounding of prescriptions for topical use. In palmar hyperhidrosis the application of 20 per cent aluminum chloride tincture three times weekly with occlusive plastic gloves has produced good results for some.

Shelley and Hurley reported in 1975 on their use of saturated solution of aluminum chloride hexahydrate in absolute ethanol (DrySol) applied to the carefully dried axillae at bedtime, under snug plastic occlusion. After control is achieved, it is maintained by weekly use.

Cullen found a methenamine gel stick highly effective and safe in control of axillary hyperhidrosis in 26 patients. Only two were not helped.

Other topical treatments include scopolamine, which is rarely effective, and formaldehyde and glutaraldehyde, which sensitize and tan the skin respectively, and are not recommended.

Iontophoresis. Iontophoresis with plain tap water is frequently effective, using a Drionic Device (*Schoch Letter* 1987, 37:Items 117 and 132) or a Fischer unit. Dobson et al found it very effective. The experience of one of us (WDJ) and Hölzle has not been as positive. Levit, Stolman, and Midtgaard have found other devices effective. Treatments generally require 20- to 30-minute sessions daily or twice daily, with current flowing through water-soaked pads. Once response has occurred, treatments may be used intermittently for maintenance.

Surgical Treatment. Upper thoracic sympathectomy has been found to be effective in excessive palmar sweating when all other measures have failed. Sympathetic denervation of the upper extremities is performed by resection of the second thoracic sympathetic ganglion (for the hands) or the fourth (for the axillae). For the axillae, however, this is seldom used, since excision of the affected area is so satisfactory. Sweating of the hands is stopped completely; however, increased (compensatory) sweating elsewhere may be a problem.

Axillary hyperhidrosis has been effectively controlled by the elliptical excision of the most actively sweating portion of the axillary skin, followed by undercutting and subcutaneous resection of the sweat glands for 1 to 2 cm on each side of the elliptical excision. Hurley and Shelley described this procedure, which is virtually always effective. The most significant aspect is the accurate mapping of the most active sweating areas of the axillae.

The axilla is painted with a solution of 2.5 per cent iodine in 95 per cent ethyl alcohol followed by pressure with a blank piece of bond paper (containing starch) for 20 seconds. The areas of hyperhidrosis will show concentrations of bluish black discoloration on the paper.

NEUTROPHILIC ECCRINE HIDRADENITIS

Harrist et al described in 1982 a unique neutrophilic infiltration and degeneration of eccrine glands, especially of the upper trunk, in patients receiving cytarabine for acute myelogenous leukemia. It was clinically manifest as erythematous nodules and plaques. Flynn et al reported two cases, also associated with cytarabine given for acute myelogenous leukemia. Beutner et al reported a case in 1986 occurring in a man receiving his third course of doxorubicin, bleomycin, vinblastine, and dacarbazine for Hodgkin's disease.

ANHIDROSIS

Anhidrosis is absence of sweating. Kay and Maibach have listed the following entities with which generalized anhidrosis may be associated: congenital ectodermal defect, quinacrine anhidrosis, miliaria profunda (thermogenic anhidrosis), Sjögren's syndrome, orthostatic hypotension, diabetic neuropathy, and multiple myeloma. In addition, myxedema, psoriasis, atopic dermatitis, ichthyosis, and pemphigus may be associated with anhidrosis. Mahloudji and Livingstone reported congenital simple anhidrosis in three siblings who had no other signs of congenital ectodermal defect.

Anhidrosis associated with miliaria has been studied by Sulzberger and his associates in military personnel subjected to long periods of heat, humidity, and friction to the skin. Tropical anhidrosis and the sweat retention syndrome are closely related.

A segmental type of anhidrosis has been described by Fisher and Maibach as occurring in lesions affecting the medullary decussation of efferent autonomic fibers and injury to the preganglionic sympathetic nerves. This may occur in poliomyelitis, Horner's syndrome, multiple sclerosis, and diabetic neuropathy. Faden et al reported an extensive case in which segmental anhidrosis was an isolated finding, and in which intradermally injected acetylcholine failed to induce sweating two years after the onset of anhidrosis.

Anhidrosis localized to skin lesions occurs regularly in the hypopigmented macules or frankly granulomatous plaques of tuberculoid leprosy.

BROMIDROSIS

Also known as fetid sweat and malodorous sweating, bromidrosis is chiefly encountered in the axillae. It is considered to be due to bacterial decomposition of apocrine sweat, producing fatty acids with distinctive offensive odors. Various substances such as arsenic and garlic may also affect the odor of perspiration. In many instances, the complaint of bromidrosis is a delusional state which may signal the onset of schizophrenia. True bromidrosis is likely to be unrecognized by the patient.

Antibacterial soaps and many commercial deodorants are quite effective in controlling the malodor. Frequent bathing, changing of underclothes, shaving of the axillae, and aluminum chloride (DrySol) topically are all helpful measures. Surgical removal of the glands, as in axillary hyperhidrosis, is possible, but very rarely indicated.

Plantar bromidrosis is produced by bacterial action on eccrine sweat-macerated stratum corneum. Hyperhidrosis is the chief associated factor. Careful washing with an antibacterial soap and the use of dusting powders on the feet are helpful in eliminating bromidrosis. For malodorous feet, soaking them in 1:5000 potassium permanganate solution for 30 minutes daily for a few days brings about much-needed relief from the fetid odor. Previously described measures to control plantar hyperhidrosis should be instituted.

CHROMHIDROSIS

Chromhidrosis, or colored sweat, is an exceedingly rare functional disorder of the apocrine sweat glands, frequently localized to the face or axilla. It has been less frequently noted on the abdomen, chest, thighs, groin, genitalia, and lower eyelids. The colored sweat may be yellow (most common), blue, green, or black.

The colored secretion appears in response to adrenergic stimuli which cause myoepithelial contraction. Colored apocrine sweat has been shown to fluoresce (**phosphorhidrosis**). Hurley ascribes the abnormal color to alteration in the number or types of lipofuscin granules secreted by normal (or heterotopic) apocrine glands. However, Mali-Gerritis et al report that the fluorescence characteristics of the pigment are incompatible with those of lipofuscin.

Eccrine chromhidrosis is the production of exogenously colored sweat caused by dyes, pigments, or metals on the skin surface. Examples are the blue-green sweat seen in copper workers and the "red sweat" seen in flight attendants in 1980 from the red dye in the labels in life-vests.

Brownish staining of the axillae and undershirt may occur in *ochronosis*, and should be considered in the differential diagnosis.

Periodic manual squeezing out of the colored sweat was Hurley's only therapeutic suggestion.

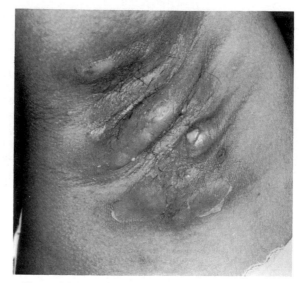

Figure 33–32. Hidradenitis suppurativa in the axilla.

HIDRADENITIS SUPPURATIVA

CLINICAL FEATURES. Hidradenitis suppurativa is a disease of the apocrine gland-bearing areas which occurs in the axillae and groins and on the buttocks. The abscesses may also occur around the areolae of the breasts.

The disease is characterized by the development of tender red nodules, which at first are firm but later become fluctuant and painful. A helpful clinical sign to differentiate early hidradenitis from furunculosis is the presence of comedones in the apocrine areas in the former. Mortimer et al found them in 37 of 42 women evaluated. Rupture of the lesion, suppuration, and the formation of sinus tracts are distinctive for this process. As these heal, recurrent lesions form, so that the course of the disease may be protracted. The disease may eventually lead to

the formation of honey-combed fistulous tracts with chronic infection. The individual lesions contain a thick, viscous, mucoid, suppurative material. When a probe is used to explore the suppurating nodule a burrowing sinus tract is usually detected that may extend for many centimeters, running horizontally just underneath the skin surface.

Hidradenitis suppurativa occurs most frequently in the axillae of young women. Men also are affected, but more frequently the groins and perianal area are the sites of involvement. In its severest form, hidradenitis suppurativa is associated with acne conglobata, pilonidal sinus, and dissecting cellulitis of the scalp. Epidermoid carcinoma and interstitial keratitis have been reported to be associated with hidradenitis suppurativa, but they are extremely rare. Moschella

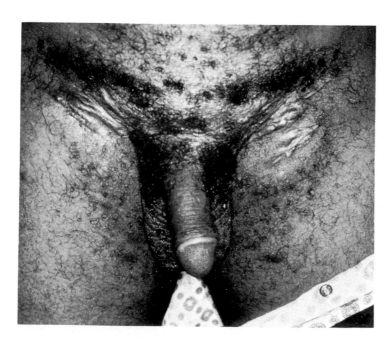

Figure 33–33. Hidradenitis suppurativa in the groins.

reported the development of urethral, vesical, and rectal fistulas, and anemia, hypoproteinemia, amyloidosis, and eventual renal failure and death in an advanced chronic expression of the disease.

ETIOLOGY. Hidradenitis suppurativa represents a poral occlusion disease with secondary bacterial infection of the apocrine glands. The initial event is follicular keratinization with resultant plugging of the apocrine duct, followed by dilatation and a severe inflammatory response in the apocrine gland. The influx of bacteria, usually staphylococci and streptococci as well as opportunistic organisms like *Escherichia coli*, *Proteus*, and *Pseudomonas*, and polymorphonuclear leukocytes, evolves into an abscess which eventually ruptures. Highet et al found *S. milleri* as a factor complicating perianal lesions and recommend erythromycin, 500 mg four times daily, as the antibiotic of choice in these cases.

If the glandular infection persists, the overlying skin may rupture, and considerable fibrosis and sinus tract formation results. As the disease becomes chronic, ulcers evolve, sinus tracts enlarge, fistulas develop, and fibrosis and scarring become more evident. The process smolders and acute episodic eruptions intervene indefinitely. The cause of the initiating events still remains unknown, but hormonal mechanisms are suspected. Rook and Ebling class it with the androgen-dependent syndromes, and Louis Brunsting regarded it as deep-seated axillary cystic acne, not a primarily infectious process. Mortimer et al found higher levels of total testosterone in women with hidradenitis than in controls.

Fitzsimmons et al found that hidradenitis clusters within certain families. One of us (WDJ) observed hidradenitis in identical twins, which lends weight to the supposition that there is a genetic predisposition to the disease.

DIFFERENTIAL DIAGNOSIS. Hidradenitis is to be differentiated from common furuncles, which are typically unilateral and not associated with comedones as hidradenitis is. Hidradenitis must also be differentiated from Bartholin abscess, scrofuloderma, actinomycosis, and granuloma inguinale.

TREATMENT. Despite the numerous forms of treatment available, the possibilities for a permanent cure are elusive. The earliest lesions often heal quickly under intralesional or brief systemic steroid therapy, and this should be tried initially in combination with oral antibiotics. Vigorous treatment with antibiotics is helpful, but does not prevent new lesions unless given on a prophylactic, long-term basis. Antibiotic treatment may have to be carried on for several months. The antibiotics of choice include erythromycin, tetracycline, minocycline, and the cephalosporins. Antibacterial soaps should be used.

Once chronic suppuration and fistulous tracts have become established, incision, drainage, and exteriorization of sinus tracts is helpful, especially when the lining of the sinus tract is cauterized with phenol. This is all performed under local anesthesia.

Ebling has shown complete clearing of a severe, advanced case as a result of therapy with an androgen-blocking agent, cyproterone acetate. Pochi has not found estrogen-dominant contraceptives as effective as in acne. In the light of the results obtained by Mortimer et al, however, it may be worthwhile to investigate antiandrogen treatment further.

Isotretinoin is effective in some cases, but a remission seldom follows its use. Secondary infection with *Staphylococcus aureus* usually occurs, if it has not already.

The chances for permanent cure are best when excision of the affected areas is done. In a series of 45 patients Knaysi and his associates found that the recurrence and complication rates were lowest when, after total excision of the hair-bearing areas of the axillae, the exposed areas were resurfaced with split thickness skin grafts.

Other affected areas are also most amenable to surgical treatment for good results. Paletta has found simple excision in the groin areas to be most feasible.

Fractional x-ray treatment is sometimes helpful in curing the disease. Zeligman has achieved good results with no recurrences for as long as six years by giving 500 rads of superficial x-rays to the axillae in a single dose.

FOX-FORDYCE DISEASE
(Apocrine Miliaria)

Fox-Fordyce disease is a rare disease occurring mostly in women during adolescence or soon afterward. It is characterized by conical, flesh-colored or

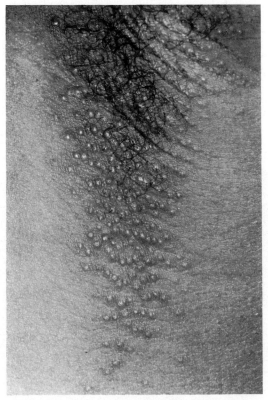

Figure 33–34. Fox-Fordyce disease in the axilla.

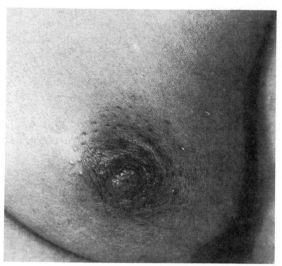

Figure 33–35. Fox-Fordyce disease around the nipple. (Courtesy of Dr. S.F. Rosen.)

grayish, intensely pruritic, discrete follicular papules in areas where apocrine glands occur (the axillae, mammae, umbilicus, pubes, labia majora, and perineum). The hair in these areas is likely to be scanty. From some of the nodules broken hair shafts may protrude, while in the centers of others there are empty follicular openings. In rare cases there is no itching.

Most cases occur in women between the ages of 13 and 35 years. The disease is only one tenth as common in men. It has only rarely been reported before puberty or after menopause. Pregnancy invariably has a beneficial influence.

The disease may be regulated by endocrine factors, but the primary cause of apocrine duct occlusion by a keratinous plug is not known.

Histologically, Fox-Fordyce disease is characterized by obstruction of the apocrine duct at its entrance into the follicular wall. An inflammatory infiltrate surrounds the upper third of the hair follicles. In the dermis the coil glands are dilated.

The treatment of Fox-Fordyce disease includes estrogens, which are helpful in some cases if given cyclically, as for contraception. Kronthal and his associates found contraceptive pills containing norethynodrel and mestranol (Enovid) to be helpful in two cases. A remarkable decrease in pruritus and regression of the papular eruption occurred over several months with this medication. Hermann Pinkus had regular success using weekly erythema doses of UVR from a hot quartz lamp until exfoliation is produced. Intralesional triamcinolone has been reported to induce prolonged remissions. Systemic (oral) prednisone has not been effective.

Giacobetti et al and others have reported success with 0.1 per cent tretinoin (Retin-A) cream applied topically, and it is worth trying as initial therapy. Excision of the affected area is curative, but it should rarely be resorted to.

GRANULOSIS RUBRA NASI

Granulosis rubra nasi is a rare familial disease of children, occurring on the nose, cheeks, and chin. It is characterized by diffuse redness, persistent hyperhidrosis, and small dark red papules which disappear on diascopic pressure. The tip of the nose is red or violet. There may be a few small pustules. The hyperhidrosis precedes the erythema. The tip of the nose is cold and is not infiltrated. The disease disappears spontaneously at puberty without leaving any traces.

Binazzi has reported 20 cases among 94 members of one family in four generations. The cause is unknown.

Histologically, there is a dilatation of the blood vessels and an inflammatory cellular infiltration about the sweat ducts, sometimes accompanied by pressure occlusion of the duct, dilatation, and cyst formation.

Treatment is with local preparations for relief of the inflammation, and reassurance that with puberty there is usually involution of the process.

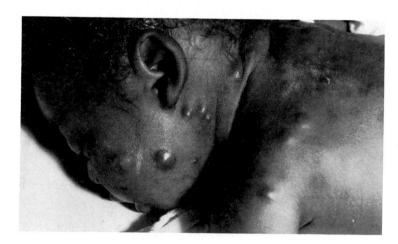

Figure 33–36. Multiple sweat gland abscesses. (From Maibach HI, Kligman AM: JAMA 1960, 174:140.)

MULTIPLE SWEAT GLAND ABSCESSES

Under this title Maibach and Kligman described a disease entity that has previously been called *multiple abscesses of the skin of infants* and *periporitis.*

The disease consists of multiple, dome-shaped, nontender and nonpointing, 2–15-mm abscesses occurring particularly on the occiput, nape, trunk, buttocks, and thighs of infants. Some are superficial and bright red at first, later becoming brownish red. Others are deeper and covered by almost normal skin.

Coagulase-positive staphylococci are regularly recovered from the abscesses. They differ from carbuncles in that they are not centered about the hair follicle, but rather about the eccrine apparatus. This disease may be secondarily infected miliaria profunda.

Diseases of Sweat Glands

Akins DL, et al: Efficacy of the Drionic unit in the treatment of hyperhidrosis. JAAD 1987, 16:828.
Beutner KR, et al: Neutrophilic eccrine hidradenitis associated with Hodgkin's disease and chemotherapy: a case report. Arch Dermatol 1986, 122:809.
Bisbal J, et al: Surgical treatment of axillary hyperhidrosis. Ann Plast Surg 1987, 18:429.
Brown SCW, et al: Surgical treatment of perianal hidradenitis suppurativa, with special reference to recognition of the perianal form. Br J Surg 1986, 73:978.
Cloward RB: Hyperhidrosis. J Neurosurg 1969, 30:545.
Cullen SI: Topical methenamine therapy for hyperhidrosis. Arch Dermatol 1975, 111:1158.
Cunliffe WJ, et al: Gustatory hyperhidrosis. Br J Dermatol 1967, 79:519.
Dicken CH, et al: Evaluation of isotretinoin treatment of hidradenitis suppurativa. JAAD 1984, 11:500.
Dobson RL: Treatment of hyperhidrosis. Arch Dermatol 1987, 123:883.
Duncan WC: Surgical treatment of hidradenitis suppurativa. J Dermatol Surg Oncol 1976, 2:153.
Eedy DJ, et al: Olfactory hyperhidrosis responding to amitriptyline. Clin Exp Dermatol 1987, 12:298.
Faden AI, et al: Progressive isolated segmental anhidrosis. Arch Neurol 1982, 39:172.
Fisher DA, et al: Postural hypotension and hidrosis. Arch Dermatol 1970, 97:327.
Fitzsimmons JS, et al: Evidence for genetic factors in hidradenitis suppurativa. Br J Dermatol 1985, 113:1.
Flynn TC, et al: Neutrophilic eccrine hidradenitis: a distinctive rash associated with cytarabine therapy and acute leukemia. JAAD 1984, 11:584.

Giacobetti R, et al: Fox-Fordyce disease: control with tretinoin cream. Arch Dermatol 1979, 115:1365.
Greenhaig RM, et al: Role of sympathectomy in hyperhidrosis. Br Med J 1971, 1:332.
Harper KE, et al: Delayed onset of Frey's syndrome following trauma. J Assoc Milit Dermatol 1983, 9:32.
Harrison BJ, et al: Recurrence after surgical treatment of hidradenitis suppurativa. Br Med J 1987, 294:487.
Harrist TJ, et al: Neutrophilic eccrine hidradenitis. Arch Dermatol 1982, 118:263.
Highet AS, et al: Bacteriology and antibiotic treatment of perianal suppurative hidradenitis. Arch Dermatol 1988, 124:1047.
Hölzle E, et al: Treatment of hyperhidrosis by a battery-operated iontophoretic device. Dermatologica 1986, 127:41.
Idem: Long-term efficacy and side effects of tap water iontophoresis of palmoplantar hyperhidrosis. Dermatologica 1987, 175:126.
James WD, et al: Emotional eccrine sweating. Arch Dermatol 1987, 123:925.
Jemec GBE: Effect of localized surgical excisions in hidradenitis suppurativa. JAAD 1988, 18:1103.
Maibach HI, et al: Multiple sweat gland abscesses of infants. JAMA 1960, 14:140.
Mali-Gerritis MMG, et al: Axillary apocrine chromhidrosis. Arch Dermatol 1988, 124:494.
McDaniel DH, et al: Furunculosis and hidradenitis suppurativa response. Arch Dermatol 1984, 120:437.
Midtgaard K: A new device for the treatment of hyperhidrosis by iontophoresis. Br J Dermatol 1986, 114:485.
Morgan WP, et al: The role of depilation and deodorants in hidradenitis suppurativa. Arch Dermatol 1982, 118:101.
Mortimer PS, et al: Mediation of hidradenitis suppurativa by androgens. Br Med J 1986, 292:245.
Moschella SL: Hidradenitis suppurativa . . . resulting in death. JAMA 1966, 198:201.
Namer IJ, et al: Idiopathic paroxysmal localized hyperhidrosis. Rev Neurol (Paris) 1986, 142:706.
Pearlstein HH, et al: Chromhidrosis: a rare dermatologic entity. Cutis 1972, 10:41.
Poh-Fitzpatrick MB: "Red sweat." JAAD 1981, 4:481.
Rayner CRW, et al: Axillary hyperhidrosis, 20% aluminium chloride hexahydrate, and surgery (letter). Br Med J 1980, 1:1168.
Sato K, et al: Biology of sweat glands and their disorders. I & II. JAAD 1989, 20:537, 713.
Shelley WB, et al: Studies on antiperspirant control of axillary hyperhidrosis. Acta Dermatol Venereol (Stockh) 1975, 55:241.
Sloan JB, et al: Iontophoresis in dermatology. JAAD 1986, 15:671.
Sparks MK, et al: Hypercalcemia in association with cutaneous squamous cell carcinoma. Arch Dermatol 1985, 121:243.
Spiegel J, et al: AEC syndrome. JAAD 1985, 12:810.
Stolman LP: Treatment of excessive sweating of the palms by iontophoresis. Arch Dermatol 1987, 123:893.
Tsuji T, et al: Acquired generalized anhidrosis. Arch Dermatol 1976, 112:1310.
Wasserteil V, et al: Fever and hypotrichosis in a newborn. Arch Dermatol 1986, 122:1325.
White JW: Treatment of primary hyperhidrosis. Mayo Clin Proc 1986, 61:951.

DISEASES OF THE NAILS

NAIL-ASSOCIATED DERMATOSES

Numerous dermatoses are associated with characteristic, sometimes specific, nail changes. Many are considered elsewhere.

Lichen Planus of Nails

The reported incidence of nail involvement in lichen planus varies from less than 1 per cent to 10 per cent. Lichen planus of the nails may occur without skin changes: Kanwar et al reported such a case in a 10-year-old boy. Zaias enumerated the various types of nail changes in lichen planus. They are irregular longitudinal grooving and ridging of the nail plate, thinning of the nail plate, pterygium formation, shedding of the nail plate with atrophy of the nail bed, subungual keratosis, and subungual hyperpigmentation. Ronchese indicated that, in addition, the nail plate may be markedly thinned, and

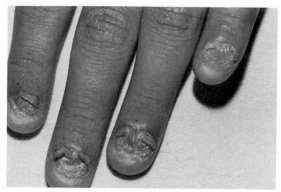

Figure 33–37. *Lichen planus of the nails in a 9-year-old boy with an atrophic patch on his scalp consistent with lichen planus. (Courtesy of Dr. H. Bogaert Diaz, Dominican Republic.)*

at times distinct papules of lichen planus may involve the nail bed. Scher et al have shown that, at times, "20-nail dystrophy" may be the sole manifestation of lichen planus.

The histologic changes of lichen planus may be evident in any individual nail constituent or a combination of them. The one most frequently involved is the matrix. Zaias has correlated the site of pathologic changes with the clinical findings.

Treatment is mostly unsatisfactory. Intralesional injection of corticosteroids has been of little help in our patients. Polyethylene occlusive dressings are also inadequate in our experience. In severe cases, intramuscular injections of 40 to 60 mg of triamcinolone acetonide every four or five weeks may produce enough improvement in two to four months to warrant perseverance in this therapy. Early treatment is mandatory, however.

Psoriatic Nails

Nail involvement in psoriasis is common, with reported incidences varying from 10 per cent to 50 per cent. Zaias has correlated the various manifestations of nail psoriasis and histologic appearances with the disease site. In the nail plate there may be

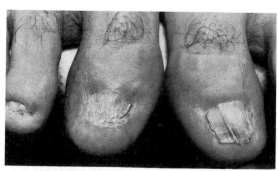

Figure 33–38. *Lichen planus of the toenails. Note almost complete absence of right great toenail, conspicuous longitudinal ridging on left great toenail. (From Ronchese F: Arch Dermatol 1965, 91:347.)*

pits, or much less often, furrows or transverse depressions (Beau's lines), crumbling nail plate, or leukonychia, with a rough or smooth surface. In the nail bed are found splinter hemorrhages, reddish discoloration of a part or all of the nail bed, and horny masses. In the hyponychium yellowish green discoloration may occur in the area of onycholysis. Zaias has also correlated the clinical changes here with the histology.

Pustular psoriasis may produce onycholysis, with lakes of pus in the nail bed or in the perionychial areas. Rarely anonychia may result, as in the case reported by Elston et al.

Other papulosquamous diseases may affect the nails like psoriasis: Reiter's disease, for example. Pityriasis rubra pilaris, Sézary syndrome, and acrokeratosis paraneoplastica produce as a rule hypertrophic nails with subungual hyperkeratosis.

The treatment of psoriatic nails is difficult; all therapies have problems. All too often, avulsion is done under the impression that the condition is onychomycosis. Intralesional injection of triamcinolone acetonide suspension, 3 to 5 mg/ml, with a 30-gauge needle, is frequently helpful; however, it is quite painful, and the condition soon recurs. The intramuscular route is preferable, giving 60 mg monthly for three or four months in order to find whether it is responsive. Side effects are negligible. Topical 1 per cent 5-fluorouracil solution under the nails has been reported to be helpful. Methotrexate, PUVA, or etretinate may be effective.

DARIER'S DISEASE

According to Zaias and Ackerman, and Ronchese, longitudinal, subungual, red or white streaks, associated with distal wedge-shaped subungual keratoses, are the nail signs diagnostic for Darier-White disease. Keratotic papules on the dorsal portion of

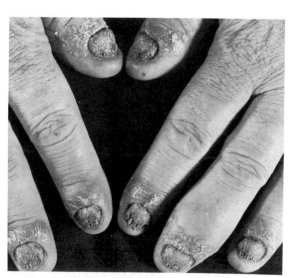

Figure 33–39. *Psoriasis of the nails and proximal nail folds, and paronychia. (Courtesy of Dr. H. Shatin.)*

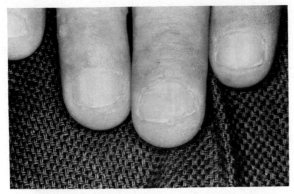

Figure 33–40. Darier's disease of the nails.

the nail fold clinically may resemble acrokeratosis verruciformis but histologically have features of Darier's disease. Other nail findings include splinter hemorrhages and leukonychia. All of these findings are less pronounced on the toenails.

NAIL DISEASES

Clubbing

Zaias divides clubbing into two types: idiopathic, and acquired or secondary.

The changes occur not only in the nails but also in the terminal phalanges. The nails bulge and are convexly curved in both transverse and longitudinal directions like a watch crystal. The eponychium is thickened. The angle formed by the dorsal surface of the distal phalanx and the nail plate (*Lovibond's angle*) is approximately 160°; however, with clubbing this angle is obliterated and becomes 180° or greater. The soft tissues of the terminal phalanx are bulbous, resembling drumsticks. These tissues are mobile upon pressure over the matrix.

Idiopathic clubbing is either of the isolated dominantly inherited type, or of the pachydermoperiostosis type with its associated findings. Secondary (acquired) clubbing is primarily a consequence of pulmonary, cardiac, hepatic, or gastrointestinal disease. Typically there is periostitis, with periosteal new bone formation in the phalanges, metacarpals, and distal ulna and radius: this is called hypertrophic osteoarthropathy, and is responsible for the painful clubbing. It typically occurs in men with bronchogenic carcinoma. Ronchese believed that clubbing is of little diagnostic significance since it has been reported to be associated with at least 50 different diseases, and may occur without any underlying disease at all.

Shell Nail Syndrome

Cornelius and Shelley described this type of nail in association with bronchiectasis. The nail resembles clubbed nail, but the nail bed is atrophic instead of being a bulbous proliferation of the soft tissue.

Koilonychia (Spoon Nails)

Spoon nails are thin and concave, with the edges everted so that if a drop of water were placed on the nail it would not run off.

Koilonychia may result from faulty iron metabolism and is one of the signs of Plummer-Vinson syndrome, as well as hemochromatosis. They have been observed in coronary disease, syphilis, polycythemia, and acanthosis nigricans. Familial forms are

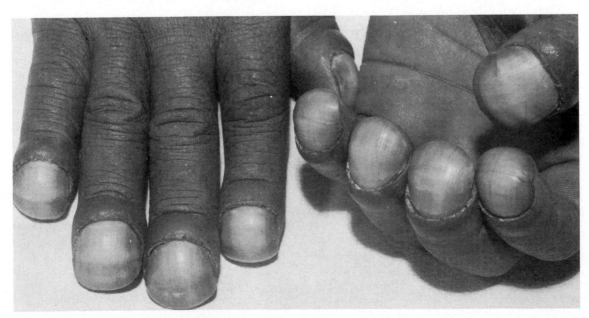

Figure 33–41. Familial clubbed fingers.

also known to occur; one family was reported by Bergeron and Stone.

Other associations include psoriasis, lichen planus, Raynaud's disease, scleroderma, acromegaly, hypo- and hyperthyroidism, monilethrix, palmar hyperkeratoses, and steatocystoma multiplex. A significant number of cases are idiopathic. Leung lists the many causes in his letter.

Congenital Onychodysplasia of Index Fingers

This syndrome (named COIF by Baran in 1980) was first observed by Iso, and categorized and named by Kikuchi in 1974. Baran reviewed 44 cases in 1980 and suggested these criteria for diagnosis: presence at birth, index finger involvement (unilateral or bilateral), variable distortion of nail or lunula, polyonychia, micronychia, anonychia, hemionychogryphosis, or malalignment. Millman et al reviewed published cases in 1982.

Twenty-Nail Dystrophy

All 20 nails may become opalescent, thin, dull, fragile, and finely longitudinally ridged (and as a result, distally notched) at any age from 1½ years to adulthood, although it is most commonly diagnosed in children. Hazelrigg reported six cases in 1977. Horn and Odom believe it can be idiopathic or caused by alopecia areata, psoriasis, lichen planus, or other inflammatory dermatoses.

Arias et al reported a family in which 21 of 37 members in five generations had severe dystrophy of all 20 nails. Inheritance was autosomal dominant. All affected persons had Class 1 malocclusion of teeth.

Donofrio reported a case and reviewed the literature in 1984. Childhood cases may resolve spontaneously by age 20 to 25.

Onychauxis

These nails are much thickened but without deformity (simple hypertrophy). Simple thickening of the nails may be due to trauma, acromegaly, Darier's disease, psoriasis, or pityriasis rubra pilaris. Some cases are hereditary.

Onychogryphosis

Hypertrophy may produce nails resembling claws. This type may be caused by trauma or peripheral vascular disorders. The commonest cause is probably neglect (failure to cut the nails for very long periods), and is most commonly seen in the elderly. Some

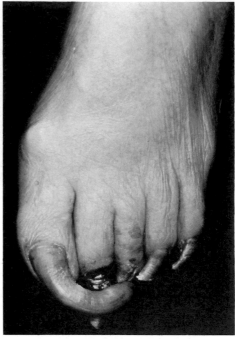

Figure 33–42. Onychogryphosis.

recommend avulsion of the nail plate with surgical destruction of the matrix with phenol or the carbon dioxide laser, if the blood supply is good.

Anonychia

Absence of nails, a rare anomaly, may be due to a congenital ectodermal defect, ichthyosis, severe infection, severe allergic contact dermatitis, Raynaud's phenomenon, lichen planus, or severe exfoliative diseases. Permanent anonychia has been reported as a sequel of Stevens-Johnson syndrome.

Onychoatrophy

Faulty underdevelopment of the nail may be congenital or acquired. The nail is thinned and smaller. Vascular disturbances, epidermolysis bullosa, lichen planus, Darier's disease, multicentric reticulohistiocytosis, and leprosy may cause onychoatrophy. It is also seen in the nail-patella syndrome and as a side effect of etretinate therapy.

Onychomadesis

This is a periodic idiopathic shedding of the nail beginning at its proximal end. The temporary arrest of the function of the nail matrix may cause onychomadesis, as may penicillin allergy. Keratosis punctata palmaris et plantaris may be associated with this type of nail loss.

Beau's Lines

These are transverse furrows that begin in the matrix and progress distally as the nail grows. They are ascribed to the temporary arrest of function of the nail matrix. Various systemic and local traumatic factors may cause this. Some are childbirth, measles, paronychia, acute febrile illnesses, and drug reaction. When the process is intermittent the nail plate may resemble corduroy. They may result from almost any systemic illness or major injury (a broken hip, e.g.). Shelley's "shoreline" nails appear to be a very severe expression of essentially the same transient growth arrest. They have been reported in all 20 nails of a newborn, most recently by Wolf et al.

Half and Half Nails

Half and half nails show the proximal portion of the nail white and the distal half red, pink, or brown, with a sharp line of demarcation between the two halves. Lindsay found this in patients with renal disease associated with azotemia.

Muehrcke's Lines

Narrow white transverse bands occurring in pairs were described by Muehrcke in 1956 as a sign of chronic hypoalbuminemia. In Muehrcke's experience, four patients lost the lines when serum albumin was raised to or near normal. Shearn explains their disappearance: unlike Mees's lines, they are in the nail bed, not in the nail plate. Similar lines have been reported in patients with normal albumin levels, who are receiving chemotherapy.

Mees's Lines

White transverse bands, single or multiple, were described by Mees in 1919 as a sign of inorganic arsenic poisoning. They have also been reported in thallium poisoning, septicemia, dissecting aortic aneurysm, and both acute and chronic renal failure.

Terry's Nails

The distal 1 to 2 mm of the nail shows a normal pink color; the entire nail plate or proximal end has a white appearance due to changes in the nail bed. These changes have been noted in patients with cirrhosis, chronic congestive heart failure, adult-onset diabetes, and the very elderly. Holzberg et al found "Terry's nails" in 25 per cent of 512 consecutive medical patients in a large hospital.

Onychorrhexis (Brittle Nails)

Brittleness with breakage of the nails may result from excessive strong soap and water exposure, from nail polish remover, from hypothyroidism, or after etretinate therapy. *Fragilitas unguium* (nail fragility) is part of this process. Lubach et al found that 12 per cent of 816 men and 27 per cent of 768 women had brittle nails. Beauregard examined 68 patients whose average age was 74 and found 85 per cent had brittle nails. Mulinos, on the basis of a review of the literature and his own findings, believes that daily ingestion of gelatin is effective in correcting brittle nails. This finding is disputed by many. Intralesional injection of triamcinolone suspension into the paronychial tissue is helpful in many cases if done over a period of six months. However, this aggressive approach is generally not recommended—or tolerated.

Onychoschizia

Splitting of the distal nail plate into layers at the free edge is a very common problem among women and represents a dysadhesion of the layers of keratin, possibly due to dehydration. Longitudinal splits may also occur. Nail polish should be discontinued and nail buffing substituted. Frequent application of emollients may be helpful.

Pitted Nails (Stippled Nails)

Small pinpoint depressions in an otherwise normal nail characterizes this type of nail change. They may

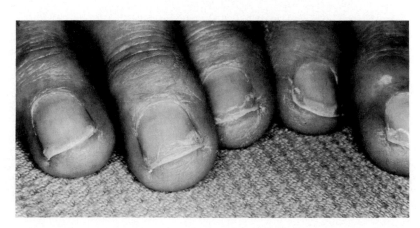

Figure 33–43. Brittle nails.

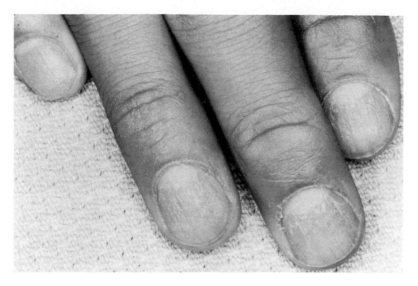

Figure 33–44. Nail dystrophy of alopecia areata.

be the early changes seen in psoriasis. They are also seen with some cases of alopecia areata, in early lichen planus, in psoriatic or rheumatoid arthritis, in chronic eczematous dermatitis, and in some individuals with no apparent disease. The deeper, broader pits are more specific for psoriasis or Reiter's syndrome. The pitting in alopecia areata tends to be shallower and more regular, suggesting a Scotch "plaid" (tartan) pattern.

Racquet Nails (Nail en Raquette)

The end of the thumb is widened and flattened, the nail plate is flattened as well, and the distal phalanx is abnormally short. Racquet nails occur on one or both thumbs and are apparently inherited as an autosomal dominant trait.

Hapalonychia

Softened nails are due to a defect in the matrix which makes the nails thin and soft so that they can be easily bent. This type of nail change is attributed to malnutrition and debility. It may be associated with myxedema, leprosy, Raynaud's phenomenon, etretinate therapy, or radiodermatitis.

Platonychia

The nail is abnormally flat and broad.

Nail-Patella Syndrome (Hereditary Osteo-onychodysplasia, Fong's Syndrome)

This syndrome of numerous anomalies is characterized by the absence or hypoplasia of the patella and congenital nail dystrophy. Triangular lunulae are characteristic. Other bone features are thickened scapulae, hyperextensible joints, radial head abnormalities, and posterior iliac horns. The skin changes may also include webbing of the elbows. Eye changes such as cataracts and heterochromia of the iris may also be present. Hyperpigmentation of the pupillary margin of the iris ("Lester iris") is a characteristic finding which occurs in about half the cases. These patients may exhibit glomerulonephritis with urinary findings of albuminuria, hematuria, and casts of all kinds, especially hyaline casts. Forty per cent of cases have renal dysplasia, and 25 per cent suffer from renal failure. Norton and Mescon have confirmed this syndrome to be a genetically determined autosomal dominant trait. Pechman et al reported a family in which palmar-plantar hyperhidrosis was transmitted, and hypothesized that the locus for the gene controlling this trait was closely linked to the nail-patella syndrome locus.

Median Nail Dystrophy (Dystrophia Unguis Mediana Canaliformis, Solenonychia)

This elaborately named nail disorder consists of longitudinal splitting or canal formation in the midline of the nail. The split, which often resembles a fir tree, occurs at the cuticle and proceeds outward as the nail grows. Trauma has been suspected of being the chief cause; however, many of these cases will persist for years even with scrupulous avoidance of trauma, and this seems to be a specious explanation. Sutton showed that the deformity may result from a papilloma in the nail matrix, forcing the production of a structure like a tube (*solenos*) distal to it. This could hardly account for cases with remissions and recurrences, however.

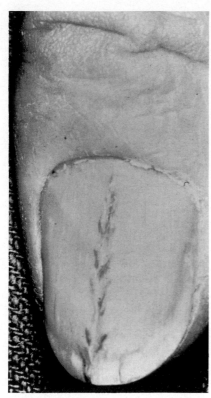

Figure 33–45. Median nail dystrophy.

Pterygium Unguis

This is an abnormal extension of the cuticle over the proximal nail plate. The classic example is lichen planus. Kalb et al reported an unusual case secondary to sarcoidosis. Peripheral circulatory disturbances may also be causative.

Pterygium Inversum Unguis

This entity is characterized by adherence of the distal portion of the nail bed to the ventral surface of the nail plate. The condition may be present at birth or acquired and may cause pain with manipulation of small objects, typing, and close manicuring of the nail. Patterson reported similar findings in four patients with scleroderma. Since the description of this entity in 1973, Odom has had occasion to note this finding in many women without symptoms or evidence of Raynaud's phenomenon, connective tissue diseases, or peripheral vascular disease.

Hangnail

This is an overextension of the eponychium (cuticle), which becomes split and peels away from the proximal or lateral nail fold. These lesions are painful and annoying, so that persistent cuticle biting frequently develops. Trimming these away with scissors is the best solution. The use of emollient creams to keep the cuticle soft is also recommended.

Pincer Nails

Pincer nails, trumpet nails, or omega (from the shape of the Greek letter) nails are alternative terms for a common toenail disorder in which the lateral edges of the nail slowly approach one another, compressing the nail bed and underlying dermis. It may occur (though less often) in the fingernails, and is (surprisingly) usually asymptomatic. No treatment is effective, since the deformity recurs after avulsion unless the matrix is at least partially destroyed.

Onychophagia

Nail biting, a common compulsion neurosis which may markedly shorten the nail bed, and sometimes damages the matrix and leads to pterygium formation, is a difficult habit to cure. If there is strong motivation, application of dimethyl sulfoxide (DMSO) every day or two will provide a reminder and a mild deterrent. Sutton in his textbook advised counselling for the parents.

Onychotillomania

This is a compulsive neurosis in which the patient picks constantly at the nails or tries to tear them off. Hurley et al reported an unusual case: a patient who repeatedly self-avulsed his nails.

NAIL DISCOLORATIONS

The literature on dyschromia of the nails was extensively reviewed by Jeanmougin and Civatte in 1983; their article is a rich source of references. Their article supplements an earlier one by Daniel and Osment published in 1982.

Leukonychia or White Nails

Four forms are recognized: *leukonychia punctata, leukonychia striata, leukonychia partialis*, and *leukonychia totalis*. The punctate variety is common in completely normal persons with otherwise normal nails. Arnold reported three instances of symmetric sympathetic punctate leukonychia, in contralateral or adjacent nails, following a current episode of traumatic leukonychia. Leukonychia striata may be hereditary as well as of traumatic or systemic origin.

Partial leukonychia may occur with tuberculosis, nephritis, Hodgkin's disease, chilblains, metastatic carcinoma, or leprosy, or unassociated with systemic illness.

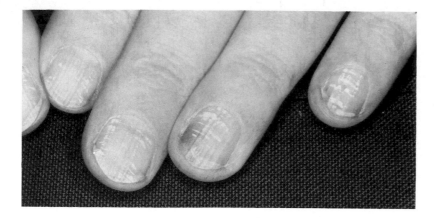

Figure 33–46. Leukonychia striata.

Leukonychia totalis may be hereditary and is of a simple autosomal dominant type. It may also be associated with typhoid fever, leprosy, cirrhosis, ulcerative colitis, nail biting, use of emetine, and trichinosis. Albright and Wheeler, and Zaias believe that leukonychia results from abnormal keratinization, with persistence of keratohyalin granules in the nail plate.

Bushkell and Gorlin reported a syndrome comprising leukonychia totalis, multiple sebaceous cysts, and renal calculi in several generations. Other reports have linked total leukonychia with deafness, or with koilonychia; however, it is most often inherited, or an isolated finding.

Melanonychia

Black or brown pigmentation of the normal nail plate most commonly results from melanin produced by melanocytes in the matrix secondary to inflammatory dermatoses or systemic medications. It may be caused by a benign pigmented nevus in the matrix, malignant melanoma, or use of ionizing radiation therapy. Of greatest importance is to rule out the presence of subungual melanoma. This is fre-

quently confused with subungual hemorrhage. Black nail may be caused by *Proteus mirabilis*, as reported by Zuehlke and Taylor.

Pigmentation of the fingernails occurs with post-inflammatory melanosis such as that due to lichen planus, acanthosis nigricans, Addison's disease, Peutz-Jeghers syndrome, vitamin B_{12} deficiency, phenolphthalein taken internally (fixed drug eruption), PUVA, and as drug-induced pigmentation due most often to antimalarials, minocycline, or gold.

Longitudinal black or brown banding of the nails has been reported to occur in 77 to 96 per cent of blacks and 11 per cent of Orientals.

The combination of longitudinal banding and pigmentation of the nails is referred to as the *Laugier-Hunziker* syndrome. Addison's disease, adrenalectomy for Cushing's syndrome, and Peutz-Jegher syndrome may all lead to pigmented banding of the nails, as may the ingestion of numerous drugs, especially chemotherapeutic agents. Baran reported that friction may cause longitudinal pigmented bands in toenails.

The appearance of a longitudinal band of pigment in one nail in a white patient is unusual, and usually requires biopsy. Retracting the proximal nail fold to expose the origin of the streak at the matrix allows

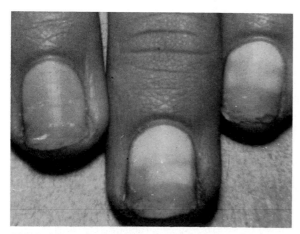

Figure 33–47. Leukonychia. (Courtesy of Dr. H. Curth.)

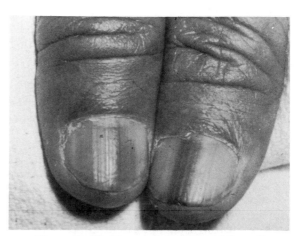

Figure 33–48. Linear pigmentation of the nail.

selection of the best biopsy site. The usual diagnoses are lentigo, nevus, and melanoma.

Green Striped Nails

Shellow and Koplon noted transverse green stripes of the fingernails produced by a paronychial infection with *Pseudomonas aeruginosa*. The stripes were ascribed to intermittent episodes of infection.

Green Nails

When onycholysis is present, a green discoloration may occur in the onycholytic area as a result of an infection with *Ps. aeruginosa*. (See green nail syndrome, Chapter 14.)

Staining of the Nail Plate

Staining of the nail plate may be the result of nicotine, dyes (including hair dyes and nail polish), potassium permanganate, mercury compounds, mepacrine, photographic developer, anthralin, chrysarobin, glutaraldehyde, or resorcin. This is only a partial list, and the article by Jeanmougin et al should be consulted for a complete listing. A helpful diagnostic maneuver to distinguish between nail plate staining from exogenous sources and nail plate pigmentation from melanin or endogenous chemicals is to scrape the surface of the nail plate several times firmly with a glass slide or scalpel blade. Exogenous stains frequently scrape off completely if the agent has not penetrated the entire nail plate. If the stain follows the curvature of the lunulae, it is probably endogenous; if it follows the curvature of the proximal and lateral nail folds, it is exogenous.

Red Lunulae

Dusky erythema confined to the lunulae has been reported in association with alopecia areata, most recently by Misch in 1983. Jorizzo reports seeing the same change in patients with severe rheumatoid arthritis, systemic lupus, and dermatomyositis, all on oral prednisone. Wilkerson et al reviewed this finding in 1989. They feel it is due to vascular congestion from any of several causes.

Spotted Lunulae

Shelley reported this distinctive change in a patient with alopecia areata.

Purpura of the Nail Beds

Purpura beneath the nails usually results from trauma. Chiarello reported a case caused by pressure

on the surfboard by a windsurfer trying to maintain his balance.

Blue Nails

In argyria the lunulae show a distinctive slate-blue discoloration. Lunular blue color, as well as blue discoloration of the whole nail bed, occurs with some chemotherapeutic agents, especially 5-fluorouracil and azidothymidine (Zidovudine), the chemotherapeutic agent used in the acquired immunodeficiency syndrome. Blue discoloration may also result from subungual hematoma and melanotic whitlow. Mepacrine and other antimalarials may stain the nails blue. Blue nails are a normal variant finding in blacks.

A blue discoloration of the lunulae is seen in cases of hepatolenticular degeneration (*Wilson's disease*). The blue color is probably related to the changes in the copper metabolism of the patient.

Yellow Nail Syndrome

The yellow nail syndrome is characterized by marked thickening and yellow to yellowish green discoloration of the nails often associated with systemic disease, most commonly lymphedema and compromised respiration. The nails are typically overcurved both transversely and longitudinally, grow very slowly (less than 0.2 mm per week), are often subject to onycholysis, and lose both lunulae and cuticles. Lymphedema, pleural effusions, chronic pulmonary infections, and chronic sinusitis most commonly precede the nail changes. Pavlioukey et al and Venencie et al have reviewed other states associated with it, to which Chernosky added the acquired immunodeficiency syndrome in 1985.

Following the lead of Ayres and Mihan, who reported success with D-alpha tocopherol in 1973, Norton reported success in two of three cases with 800 IU daily. Two of Venencie's five cases improved greatly, but not while taking vitamin E.

ONYCHOLYSIS

Onycholysis is a spontaneous separation of the nail plate, usually beginning at the free margin and progressing proximally. Rarely the lateral borders may be involved, with spread confined to these. Less often separation may begin proximal to the free edge, in an oval area 2 to 6 mm broad, with a yellowish brown hue ("oil spot"); this is a lesion of *psoriasis*, as is often the case with ordinary onycholysis. The nail itself is smooth and firm with no inflammatory reaction. Underneath the nail a discoloration may occur from the accumulation of bacteria, most commonly *Pseudomonas*, or yeast, most commonly *Candida*. As a result of pyocyanin from *Pseudomonas*, color changes such as green, black, or blue may be seen. One or more nails may be affected.

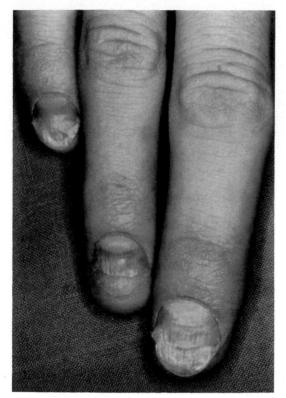

Figure 33–49. Onycholysis due to nail hardener.

matitis from their use. Rarely *photoonycholysis* may occur during or soon after therapy with tetracycline derivatives, psoralens, fluoroquinolones, or chloramphenicol, with subsequent exposure to sunlight.

Trauma should be completely avoided and the nail bed should be kept completely dry. The affected portion of the nail should be kept clipped away. Drying accomplished by exposing the nail bed in this way will rid the area of *Pseudomonas* and assist greatly in eliminating *Candida*. A topical antifungal imidazole should be applied daily. Intralesional or intramuscular triamcinolone acetonide is probably the most effective treatment in cases where every cause except volar (inverse) psoriasis has been excluded.

UNGUIS INCARNATUS
(Ingrown Nail)

Ingrown toenail is one of the most frequent nail complaints. It occurs chiefly on the great toes where there is an excessive lateral nail growth into the nail fold, leading to this painful, inflammatory affliction. The lateral margin of the nail acts as a foreign body and may cause exuberant granulation tissue.

Unguis incarnatus may be caused by wearing improperly fitting shoes and by the improper trimming of the nail at the lateral edges so that the anterior portion cuts into the flesh as it grows distally.

In a series of 88 cases and a review of 80 cases in the literature by Taft, onycholysis was noted almost exclusively in women. The most common cause is probably traumatically induced separation, with rapid secondary infection with the most commonly isolated pathogen, *Candida albicans*, probably being the main reason for lack of the nail to reattach itself. Arnold considers inverse psoriasis to be the commonest cause of onycholysis, and that *Candida* is merely an opportunistic invader, not a pathogen. Intramuscularly injected Kenalog, 40 to 60 mg per month, may be curative of both the onycholysis and the *Candida* infection in such cases, and the psoriasis usually becomes—and remains—latent.

Kechijian reviewed the literature and summarized the causes of onycholysis in 1985. Systemic causes have been enumerated, e.g., hyper- and hypothyroidism, pregnancy, porphyria, pellagra, and syphilis. It has been associated with psoriasis, atopic dermatitis, eczema, lichen planus, and congenital abnormalities of the nails. Other causes may be trauma induced by clawing, pinching, stabbing (manicuring), and foreign-body implantation. It may be due to mycotic, pyogenic, or viral (herpes) infections. Women should be checked for vaginal candidiasis, as that anatomic location may be the source of the infection capable of causing (or opportunistically invading and aggravating) onycholysis. Chemical causes may be use of solvents, nail base coat, nail hardeners containing formalin derivatives, artificial fingernails, and allergic or irritant contact der-

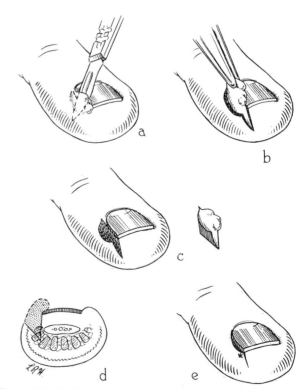

Figure 33–50. Jansey operation. a, Initial linear incision parallel to nail margin. b, Convex portion of incision. c, Involved segment removed. d, Cross section. e, End result approximated with suture or adhesive, encircling the toe. (From Jansey F: Q Bull Northwestern U Med Sch 1955, 29:358.)

Rather than removing the nail to relieve the pressure, Jansey has devised a simple operation of removing the overhanging lateral nail fold so that the nail does not cut into it. When healed, the nail edge resembles that of the thumb and an excellent functional result occurs. The nail is not altered, since it is not touched.

Under local anesthesia and with use of a rubber band tourniquet at the base of the toe a linear incision is made at the edge of the lateral nail fold perpendicular to the nail plate. A convex incision is made in a curvilinear plane parallel to the nail bed to meet the initial incision. The involved wedge of tissue is removed. The lateral flap is then approximated by one or two sutures and a petrolatum gauze dressing is applied. Healing is complete in 10 to 14 days. Another procedure is to apply saturated solution of phenol to the nail matrix after a portion of the ingrown nail has been removed surgically (phenolization). The objective is to permanently ablate the part of the nail matrix producing the nail plate that was ingrowing.

In mild cases, insertion of a cotton pad beneath the distal corner of the offending nail may make surgery unnecessary. Fishman described an elaboration of this technique in detail in 1983. Sonnex and Dawber found liquid nitrogen spray cryotherapy effective.

NEOPLASMS OF THE NAIL BED

Various neoplasms, both benign and malignant, may occur in or overlying the nail matrix and in the nail bed. Signs heralding such neoplasms are paronychia, ingrown nail, onycholysis, pyogenic granuloma, a nail plate dystrophy, bleeding, and discolorations. Symptoms of pain, itching, and throbbing may also occur with various neoplasms.

Benign tumors of the nails include verruca, pyogenic granuloma, fibromas, nevus cell nevi, myxoid cysts, angiofibromas (Koenen's tumors), and epidermoid cysts. Pyogenic-granulomalike lesions may occur during treatment with isotretinoin. Glomangioma is readily recognized by exquisite tenderness in the nail bed. Enchondroma of the distal phalanx has been described by Shelley et al. It often presents as a paronychia. Subungual exostoses may also present as an inflammatory process, but more commonly resemble a verruca or fibroma at the start. Most of these are on the great toe, and an x-ray will aid in the diagnosis of these last two entities.

Squamous cell carcinoma of the nail bed is uncommon, and often mistaken for a pyogenic granuloma initially. X-rays may reveal lytic changes in the distal phalanx. Metastases are rare. Mohs surgery is the treatment of choice. Bowen's disease may occur here, and on more than one digit (eight such cases, seven in men, have been reported), and may be related to papillomavirus infection. When keratoacanthoma occurs, there is often lysis of underlying bone, which fills in after excision of the tumor.

Subungual melanoma is frequently diagnosed late in the course of growth, since it simulates onychomycosis or subungual hematoma, with which it is confused. Eleven occurred on the thumb and five on the great toe in the 16 patients reported by Takematsu et al. Most were deeply invasive, and only 40 per cent survived five years. In five cases a pigmented streak preceded destruction of the nail. Amelanotic melanoma may occur and be mistaken for granuloma pyogenicum.

Diseases of the Nails

Albright SD III, et al: Leuconychia. Arch Dermatol 1964, 90:392.

Arias AM, et al: Familial severe twenty-nail dystrophy. JAAD 1982, 7:349.

Arnold HL Jr: Sympathetic punctate leuconychia: 3 cases. Arch Dermatol 1979, 114:495.

Ayres S Jr, et al: Yellow nail syndrome: response to vitamin E. Arch Dermatol 1973, 108:267.

Azon-Masoliver A, et al: Zidovudine-induced nail pigmentation. Arch Dermatol 1988, 124:1570.

Baran R: Etretinate and the nails (study of 130 cases). Clin Exp Dermatol 1986, 11:148.

Idem: Frictional longitudinal melanonychia. Dermatologica 1987, 174:280.

Baran R, et al: Congenital onychodysplasia of the index fingers. Arch Dermatol 1984, 120:243.

Idem: Melanonychia induced by topical 5-fluorouracil. 1985, 112:621.

Idem: Polydactylous Bowen's disease of the nails. JAAD 1987, 17:201.

Idem: Drug-induced photo-onycholysis. JAAD 1987, 17:1012.

Beauregard S, et al: A survey of skin problems and skin care regimens in the elderly. Arch Dermatol 1987, 123:1638.

Blumenthal G: Paronychia and pyogenic granuloma-like lesions with isotretinoin. JAAD 1984, 10:677.

Bonner AK, et al: Cutaneous complications of chemotherapeutic agents. JAAD 1983, 9:645.

Briggs JC: Subungual malignant melanoma. Br J Plast Surg 1985, 38:174.

Burkhart CG, et al: Nail-patella syndrome. JAAD 1980, 3:251.

Campbell JP, et al: Retinoid therapy is associated with excess granulation tissue responses. JAAD 1983, 9:708.

Chernosky ME, et al: Yellow nail syndrome in patients with acquired immunodeficiency disease. JAAD 1985, 13:731.

Chiarello SE: Toe jam (letter). Arch Dermatol 1985, 121:591.

Clover GB, et al: Is childhood idiopathic atrophy of the nails due to lichen planus? Br J Dermatol 1987, 116:709.

Coskey RJ, et al: Congenital subungual nevus. JAAD 1983, 9:747.

Daniel CR III, et al: Nail pigmentation abnormalities: their importance and proper examination. Cutis 1982, 30:348.

Idem: Nail changes secondary to systemic drugs or ingestants. JAAD 1984, 10:250.

Idem: Nails in systemic disease. Derm Clin 1985, 3:465.

Idem: Pigmentation of nails and systemic disease. Derm Clin 1988, 6:305.

Idem: Dermatologic Clinics, The Nails. Philadelphia, W. B. Saunders Co., Vol. 3, No. 3, July, 1985.

Idem: An approach to initial examination of the nail. Derm Clin 1985, 3:383.

Dawber R, et al: Nail growth. Cutis 1987, 39:99.

Donofrio P, et al: Twenty-nail dystrophy. Acta Dermatovener 1984, 64:180.

Farber EM, et al: Urea ointment in the nonsurgical avulsion of nail dystrophies. Cutis 1978, 22:689.

Feinstein A, et al: Pachyonychia congenita. JAAD 1988, 19:705.

Feldman SR, et al: Unilateral Muehrcke's lines following trauma. Arch Dermatol 1989, 125:133.

Findlay RF, et al: Twenty-nail dystrophy of childhood. J Assoc Mil Dermatol 1984, 10:22.

Fishman HC: Practical therapy for ingrown toenails. Cutis 1983, 32:159.

Furth PA, et al: Nail pigmentation changes associated with azidothymidine (Zidovudine). Ann Intern Med 1987, 107:350.

Greene RA, et al: Nail changes associated with diabetes mellitus. JAAD 1987, 16:1015.

Hanno R, et al: Longitudinal nail biopsy in evaluation of acquired nail dystrophies. JAAD 1986, 14:803.

Hazelrigg DE, et al: Twenty-nail dystrophy of childhood. Arch Dermatol 1977, 113:73.

Held JL, et al: Transverse striate leukonychia associated with acute rejection of renal allograft. JAAD 1989, 20:513.

Holzberg M, et al: Terry's nails. Lancet 1984, 1:896.

Horn RT, et al: Twenty-nail dystrophy of alopecia areata. Arch Dermatol 1980, 116:573.

Hurley PT, et al: Self-inflicted anonychia. Arch Dermatol 1982, 118:956.

Ingram GJ: Reiter's syndrome with nail involvement. Cutis 1985, 36:37.

Jacobsen FK, et al: Acrokeratosis paraneoplastica. Arch Dermatol 1984, 120:502.

James WD, et al: Chemotherapy-induced transverse white lines in the fingernails. Arch Dermatol 1983, 119:334.

Jeanmougin M, et al: Nail dyschromia. J Int Dermatol 1983, 22:279.

Jemec GBE, et al: Ultrasound structure of the human nail plate. Arch Dermatol 1989, 125:643.

Jorizzo JL, et al: Red lunulae in rheumatoid arthritis. JAAD 1983, 8:711.

Kalb RE, et al: Pterygium formation due to sarcoidosis. Arch Dermatol 1985, 121:276.

Kanwar AJ, et al: Lichen planus limited to the nails. Cutis 1983, 32:163.

Kechijian P: Onycholysis of the fingernails: evaluation and management. JAAD 1985, 12:552.

Idem: Brittle fingernails. Derm Clin 1985, 3:421.

Idem: Twenty-nail dystrophy of childhood. Cutis 1985, 35:38.

Kegel MF: Metastasis of pulmonary carcinoma to the nail unit. Cutis 1985, 35:121.

Kitayama Y, et al: Congenital onychodysplasia. Report of 11 cases. Arch Dermatol 1983, 119:8.

Koch SE, et al: Laugier-Hunziker syndrome. JAAD 1987, 16:431.

Kouskoukis CE, et al: The "oil drop" sign of psoriatic nails. Am J Dermatopathol 1983, 5:259.

Leung AN: The many causes of koilonychia. Hosp Pract 1985, 20:29.

Levy DW, et al: Subungual keratoacanthoma. Skeletal Radiol 1985, 13:287.

Lubach D, et al: Incidence of brittle nails. Dermatologica 1986, 172:144.

Lumpkin LR, et al: Subungual squamous cell carcinoma. JAAD 1984, 11:735.

McCormack LS, et al: Benoxaprofen-induced photo-onycholysis. JAAD 1982, 7:678.

Mikhail GR: Subungual epidermoid carcinoma. JAAD 1984, 11:291.

Millman AJ, et al: Congenital onychodysplasia of the index fingers. JAAD 1982, 7:57.

Mostafa WZ: Lichen planus of the nail. JAAD 1989, 20:289.

Mulinos MG: Brittle nail syndrome: treatment with gelatin. Cutis 1968, 4:1089.

Nixon DW: Alterations in nail pigment with cancer chemotherapy. Arch Intern Med 1976, 136:1117.

Norton L: Further observations on the yellow nail syndrome with therapeutic effects of oral alpha-tocopherol. Cutis 1985, 33:457.

Norton LA: Nail disorders. JAAD 1980, 2:451.

Odom RB, et al: Congenital, painful aberrant hyponychium. Arch Dermatol 1974, 110:89.

Peachey RDG, et al: Treatment of psoriatic nail dystrophy with intradermal steroid injections. Br J Dermatol 1976, 95:75.

Pechman KJ, et al: Palmar-plantar hyperhidrosis occurring in a kindred with nail patella syndrome. JAAD 1980, 3:627.

Rabinovitz HS: Response of psoriatic nails to the aromatic retinoid etretinate. Arch Dermatol 1983, 119:627.

Robbins TO, et al: Onycholysis in psoriatic nails. Am J Dermatopathol 1983, 5:39.

Rudolph RI: Subungual basal cell carcinoma presenting as long indexal melanonychia. JAAD 1987, 16:229.

Salasche SJ, et al: Tumors of the nail. Derm Clin 1985, 3:491.

Samman PD, et al: The Nails in Disease. Chicago, Yearbook Medical Publishers Inc., 1986.

Sanusi ID: Subungual myxoma. Arch Dermatol 1982, 118:612.

Scher RK: Cosmetics and ancillary preparations for the care of nails. JAAD 1982, 6:523.

Idem: Lichen planus of the nail. Derm Clin 1985, 3:395.

Idem: Psoriasis of the nail. Derm Clin 1985, 3:387.

Idem, et al: 20-nail dystrophy, a variant of lichen planus. Arch Dermatol 1978, 114:612.

Idem: Disorders of the nails. JAAD 1986, 15:523.

Idem: Subtle clue to the diagnosis of nails by gross pathology: lichen planus. Am J Dermatopathol 1983, 5:373.

Schwartz R, et al: Muehrcke's lines of the fingernails. Arch Intern Med 1979, 139:242.

Shearn MA: Striped nails (letter). Ann Intern Med 1978, 89:577.

Shelley ED, et al: Nail dystrophy and periungual dermatitis due to cyanoacrylate glue sensitivity. JAAD 1988, 19:574.

Shelley WB: The spotted lunula. JAAD 1980, 2:385.

Idem, et al: Onychoschizia. JAAD 1984, 10:623.

Shellow WVR, et al: Green striped nails: chromonychia due to Pseudomonas aeruginosa. Arch Dermatol 1968, 97:149.

Siegle RJ, et al: Phenolalcohol technique for permanent matricectomy. Arch Dermatol 1984, 120:348.

Simmons DA, et al: Subungual tumors in incontinentia pigmenti. Arch Dermatol 1986, 122:1431.

Sonnex TS, et al: Treatment of ingrowing toenails with liquid nitrogen spray cryotherapy. Br Med J 1985, 291:173.

Idem: The nails in adult type 1 pityriasis rubra pilaris. JAAD 1986, 15:956.

Staberg B: Onychonycosis in patients with psoriasis. Arch Dermatol Venereol (Stockh) 1983, 63:436.

Stone OJ: Clubbing and koilonychia. Derm Clin 1985, 3:485.

Sutton RL Jr: Solenonychia (canaliform dystrophy of the nail). South Med J 1964, 58:1143.

Sweren RJ, et al: Multiple Beau's lines. Cutis 1982, 29:41.

Takematsu H: Subungual melanoma. Cancer 1985, 55:2725.

Tom DWK: Melanonychia striata in longitudinum. Am J Dermatopathol 1985, 7(suppl):161.

Vázquez M, et al: Melanomas of volar and subungual skin in Puerto Ricans. JAAD 1984, 10:39.

Venencie PY, et al: Yellow nail syndrome: report of 5 cases. JAAD 1984, 10:187.

Weiss E, et al: PUVA-induced pigmented nails. Int J Dermatol 1989, 28:188.

Weissman K: Beau and his description of transverse depression of the nails. Br J Dermatol 1977, 97:571.

Wilkerson MG, et al: Red lunulae revisited. JAAD 1989, 20:453.

Wolf D, et al: Beau's lines: case report. Cutis 1982, 29:191.

Young MRA, et al: Re-operation rate for ingrowing toe nail treated by phenolization. Br J Surg 1987, 74:202.

Zaias N: The Nail in Health and Disease. New York, SP Medical and Scientific Books, 1980.

34

Disorders of the Mucous Membranes

Lesions on the mucous membranes may be more difficult to diagnose than lesions on the skin, and not merely because they are less easily and less often seen. There is less contrast of color, and greater likelihood of alterations in the original appearance because of secondary factors, such as maceration from moisture, abrasion from food and teeth, and infection. Vesicles and bullae rapidly rupture to form grayish erosions, and the epithelium covering papules becomes a soggy lactescent membrane, easily rubbed off to form an erosion. Grouping and distribution are less distinctive in the mouth than on the skin, and not infrequently it is necessary to establish the diagnosis by the character of associated cutaneous lesions or by the observation of subsequent developments.

Eversole LR: Clinical outline of oral pathology. Philadelphia, Lea and Febiger, 1984.
Rogers RS III (ed): Disorders of Mucous Membranes. *In* Dermatologic Clinics. Philadelphia, WB Saunders, Vol 5, 1987.

CHEILITIS EXFOLIATIVA

This term has been used to designate a primarily desquamative and often only very mildly inflammatory condition of the lips, of unknown etiology, and also a clinically similar reaction secondary to other disease states. The former is a persistently recurrent scaling and sometimes crusting lesion which most often affects the upper lip. The recurrent exfoliation leaves a temporarily erythematous and tender surface.

In the secondary form, the lips are chronically inflamed and covered with crusts that from time to time tend to desquamate, leaving a glazed surface upon which new crusts form. Fissures may be present, and there may be burning, tenderness, and some pain. The lower lip is more often involved, the inflammation being limited to the vermilion part. The cheilitis may be secondary to seborrheic dermatitis, atopic dermatitis, psoriasis, retinoid therapy, pyorrhea, habitual actinic exposure, or the habit of licking the lips. Uncommonly, the initial or only manifestation of atopic dermatitis may be a chronic cheilitis. Irritating substances in lipsticks, dentifrices, and mouthwashes may be causative factors. Dyes in lipsticks may photosensitize. Candidiasis may be present. Cheilitis may be part of the Plummer-Vinson syndrome. Allergic hypersensitivity to nail enamel, after-shave lotion, before-shaving lotion, lipsticks, and a wide variety of other substances may be the cause. Phelan et al reported that nine of 103 AIDS patients had exfoliative cheilitis of undetermined cause.

The only uniformly effective treatment is the elimination of causes when they can be found. Topical corticosteroid creams are usually helpful. When there are fissures, silver nitrate or zinc oxide ointment may be helpful.

ALLERGIC CONTACT CHEILITIS

The vermilion border of the lips is much more likely to develop allergic contact sensitivity reactions than is the oral mucosa. Allergic cheilitis is characterized by dryness, fissuring, edema, crusting, and angular cheilitis. It may result from topical medicaments, dentifrices, other dental preparations, antichap agents, lipsticks, sunscreening lip balms, nail polish, cigarette holders, cosmetics, foods, produce

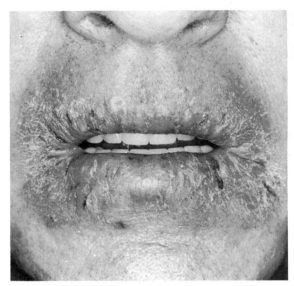

Figure 34–1. Contact cheilitis caused by tooth paste.

such as oranges, lemons, artichokes, and mangoes, rubber, or metals.

Treatment includes discontinuation of exposure to the offending agent, and topical corticosteroid preparations.

ACTINIC CHEILITIS

Actinic cheilitis is an inflammatory reaction of the lips, especially (and often only) the lower, to excessive sunlight exposure over the years. The lips become scaly, fissured, and swollen; leukoplakia and even squamous cell carcinoma may develop. Painful erosions may occur: actual ulceration is very rare unless carcinoma has developed. This type of cheilitis is caused by solar radiation exposure and occurs primarily in outdoor workers and athletes.

While the chronic form is most often seen in the dermatologist's office, the lower lip is singularly vulnerable to acute sunburn. Also, hereditary poly-

morphous light eruption can resemble chronic actinic cheilitis, but it has no malignant potential.

Simple avoidance suffices to prevent most cases, or any of many solar protective lip pomades. Any suspicious thickened areas that persist should be biopsied, preferably by shave excision to avoid scarring, followed by hemostasis with Monsel's solution, ferric chloride, or aluminum chloride. Even a slight scar at the edge of the vermilion may be intolerably conspicuous.

Cryosurgical treatment may be effective, particularly for localized lesions. In severe cases with continued development of leukoplakia, topical 5-fluorouracil may be curative, as Odom and Epstein have shown and Goette has reviewed. Should it fail, vermilionectomy of the lower lip may be necessary. The excision of the exposed vermilion mucous membrane with the advancement of the labial mucosa to the skin edge of the outer lip is a satisfactory procedure. The technique has been described by Burket and Sanchez-Conejo-Mir. In a recent review of actinic cheilitis by Picascia et al, a useful modification of the procedure is described. David described treatment with the carbon dioxide laser, vaporizing the damaged epidermis, with excellent results.

CHEILITIS GLANDULARIS

Cheilitis glandularis is characterized by swelling and eversion of the lower lip, patulous openings of the ducts of the mucous glands, cysts, and general enlargement of the lips. Mucus exudes freely to form a gluey film that dries over the lips and causes them to stick together during the night. When the lip is palpated between the thumb and index finger, the enlarged mucous glands feel like pebbles beneath the surface. The lower lip is the site of predilection.

In general two types are recognized, namely, *cheilitis glandularis simplex* (Puente and Acevedo) and *cheilitis glandularis apostematosa* (Volkman). (Apostematosa means with abscess formation.) The latter

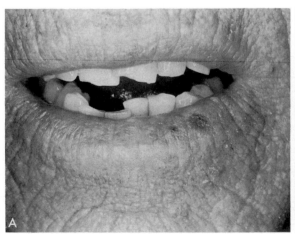
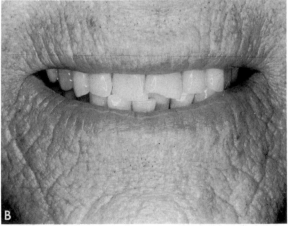

Figure 34–2. Actinic cheilitis. A, Before treatment with topical 5-fluorouracil; B, after treatment.

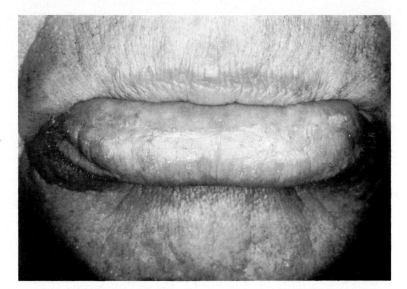

Figure 34–3. Cheilitis glandularis.

form probably stems from the simplex form by the development of infection.

Cheilitis glandularis is a chronic inflammatory reaction that Swerlick et al attribute to an unusual response to chronic irritation, atopic, factitious, or actinic.

On biopsy, there is a moderate histiocytic, lymphocytic, and plasmocytic infiltration in and around the glands, which Swerlick et al found not to be enlarged.

Cheilitis glandularis has been reported to eventuate in squamous cell carcinoma, but these cases may be attributed to chronic sun exposure, which frequently precedes cheilitis glandularis.

Treatment depends upon the nature of the antecedent irritation; in most cases, treatment as described for actinic cheilitis is appropriate. Surgical debulking may be necessary. Schweich achieved excellent results in one patient by intralesional injection of triamcinolone.

ANGULAR CHEILITIS

Angular cheilitis is simply perlèche, often complicated by infection by *Candida albicans*. Moist fissures may radiate downward and outward from the labial commissures.

The disease usually occurs in elderly people who wear dentures, but it may develop simply from overhanging of the upper lip and cheek and recession and atrophy of the alveolar ridges in old age. Measuring the facial dimensions with a ruler and tongue blade will help to objectively assess the importance of decreased vertical facial dimension in the development of perlèche. If the distance from the base of the nose to the lower edge of the mandible is 6 mm or more less than the distance from the center of the pupil to the parting line of the lips, the vertical dimension is decreased.

In these circumstances drooling is usually a factor.

In children, angular cheilitis occurs commonly in thumb suckers and lollypop eaters. Other inciting factors include riboflavin deficiency, or intraoral candidiasis especially in diabetics, patients with AIDS, or patients with chronic mucocutaneous candidiasis.

"Opening the bite" by improving denture fit, capping teeth, replacing lost teeth, or increasing denture height, combined with topical use of nystatin and iodochlorhydroxyquin (Vioform) in hydrocortisone ointment, is usually effective. Chernosky documented the potential effectiveness of injection of collagen to obliterate the angular creases. Symington cured seven of eight patients by excision and a rotating flap graft, but surgery should not be the first treatment tried.

PLASMA CELL CHEILITIS

This type of cheilitis is characterized by a sharply outlined, infiltrated, dark red plaque with a lacquer-like glazing of the surface of the lower lip.

Luger described this lesion on the lip and believes that, histologically, it is the same lesion as Zoon's balanitis plasmacellularis. Histologic alterations include considerable plasma cell infiltration in a band-like pattern. Baughman and associates postulated that plasma cell cheilitis is not a response specific for any stimulus but rather represents a reaction pattern to any one of a variety of stimuli. Jones et al reported success with clobetasol propionate ointment twice daily.

DRUG-INDUCED ULCER OF THE LIP

Mackie reported seven patients with well-defined ulcerations on the lower lip for which no cause could be found, but which healed with the withdrawal of oral medications. The ulceration was tender or painful, without induration, and had been present for several weeks. The ulcers resemble those of discoid lupus erythematosus or squamous cell carcinoma. The causative drugs were phenylbutazone, chlorpromazine, phenobarbital, and methyldopa. Odom has seen several similar cases due to the thiazide diuretics. Solar exposure appears to be a predisposing causative influence; speculatively, this reaction may represent a fixed drug photoeruption.

OTHER FORMS OF CHEILITIS

Cheilitis of Down's Syndrome. A high percentage of these patients have cheilitis of one or both lips. Lip biting may be a contributory factor.

Cheilitis Granulomatosa. This is discussed on page 838.

Leukokeratosis, Leukoplakia. This is seen on the lips, especially on the lower lip. (See p. 757.)

Lichen Planus. Not only the tongue but the buccal mucosa, the gingiva, and the lips may be involved. Typical lesions appear on the buccal mucosa. (See also p. 237.)

Lupus Erythematosus. The mouth and lips may be involved, together with other lesions on the skin. (See also p. 159.)

Psoriasis. The lips may be involved. (See also p. 198.)

Baughman RD, et al: Plasma cell cheilitis. Arch Dermatol 1974, 110:725.

Birt AR, et al: The actinic cheilitis of hereditary polymorphic light eruption. Arch Dermatol 1979, 115:699.

Bouquot JE, et al: Odd lips: The prevalence of common lip lesions in 23,616 white Americans over age 35 years of age. Quintessence Int 1987, 18:277.

Brooke RI: Exfoliative cheilitis. Oral Surg 1978, 45:52.

Burrwell RK: Cheilitis glandularis. J Assoc Milit Dermatol 1982, 8:71.

Butterworth T, et al: Cheilitis of mongolism. J Invest Dermatol 1960, 35:347.

Cataldo E, et al: Solar cheilitis. J Dermatol Surg Oncol 1981, 7:989.

Chernosky ME: Collagen implant in the management of perleche. JAAD 1985, 12:493.

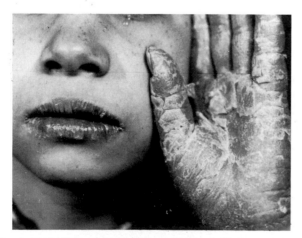

Figure 34–4. "Inverse" psoriasis of the lips and palms. (Courtesy of Dr. M. Zawahry, U.A.R.)

Crotty CP, et al: Factitious lip crusting. Arch Dermatol 1981, 117:338.

David LM: Laser vermilion ablation for actinic cheilitis. J Dermatol Surg Oncol 1984, 11:605.

Dufresne RG Jr, et al: Carbon dioxide laser treatment of chronic actinic cheilitis. JAAD 1988, 19:876.

Epstein E: Treatment of lip keratoses (actinic cheilitis) with topical 5-fluorouracil. Arch Dermatol 1978, 113:906.

Goette DK: Topical chemotherapy with 5-fluorouracil. JAAD 1981, 4:633.

Jansen GT, et al: Candida cheilitis. Arch Dermatol 1963, 88:141.

Jones SK, et al: Response of plasma cell orificial mucositis to topically applied steroids. Arch Dermatol 1988, 124:1871.

LaRiviere W, et al: Clinical criteria in diagnosis of early squamous cell carcinoma of the lower lip. J Am Dent Assoc 1979, 99:972.

Mackie BS: Drug-induced ulcer of the lip. Br J Dermatol 1967, 79:106.

Oliver ID, et al: Cheilitis glandularis. Oral Surg 1980, 49:526.

Phelan JA, et al: Oral findings in patients with acquired immunodeficiency syndrome. Oral Surg 1987, 64:50.

Picascia DD, et al: Actinic cheilitis. JAAD 1987, 17:255.

Sanchez-Conejo-Mir J, et al: Follow-up of vermilionectomies. J Dermatol Surg Oncol 1986, 12:180.

Swerlick RA, et al: Cheilitis glandularis: a re-evaluation. JAAD 1984, 10:466.

Symington JM: A surgical treatment of angular cheilitis. Br J Plastic Surg 1971, 24:315.

Thomas JR III, et al: Factitious cheilitis. JAAD 1983, 8:368.

Venable CE, et al: Persistent swelling of the lower lip. Arch Dermatol 1988, 124:1705.

Wagner G, et al: Mucous membrane involvement in generalized psoriasis. Arch Dermatol 1976, 112:1010.

Weir TW, et al: Cheilitis glandularis. Arch Dermatol 1971, 103:433.

ORAL CROHN'S DISEASE

Crohn's disease is a chronic granulomatous disease of any part or parts of the bowel, to which the names terminal ileitis, regional enteritis, ileocolitis, segmental colitis, and granulomatous colitis have also been given.

Frankel et al reported two patients with diarrhea due to intestinal Crohn's disease and inflammatory hyperplasia of the oral mucosa, with metallic dysgeusia and gingival bleeding. A mouthwash containing triamcinolone acetonide, tetracycline, and lidocaine produced symptomatic and objective improvement. They found 67 reports of oral Crohn's disease, none of them in the American literature.

Reported typical changes included diffuse oral swelling, focal mucosal hypertrophy and fissuring ("cobblestoning"), persistent ulceration, polypoid lesions, indurated fissuring of the lower lip, angular cheilitis, granulomatous cheilitis, or pyostomatitis vegetans. Oral involvement occurs in 10 to 20 per cent of cases of Crohn's disease, and 90 per cent have granulomas on biopsy.

Metastatic Crohn's disease denotes noncaseating granulomatous skin lesions in patients with Crohn's disease. In the absence of bowel involvement, the diagnosis cannot be made; but noncaseating granulomatous inflammatory lesions of the skin in patients with Crohn's disease, of which at least nine cases have been reported, according to Lebwohl et al (who reported two additional cases), are called "metastatic

Crohn's disease." One of their cases had multiple ulcerated granulomas over the abdomen, and the other had a 3 x 5 cm erythematous plaque on the face which responded to 0.01 per cent fluocinonide cream applied twice daily. All reported cases had involvement of the colon or rectum, though over 40 per cent of patients with Crohn's disease have involvement of the small bowel alone.

Curettage and zinc by mouth have resulted in healing in several reported cases. In other cases the course has been prolonged over several years.

Many cases of Crohn's disease with other cutaneous manifestations have been reported, notably pyoderma gangrenosum (more closely associated with ulcerative colitis) and erythema nodosum, polyarteritis nodosa, and necrotizing vasculitis. Direct extension to perianal skin has also been reported.

PYOSTOMATITIS VEGETANS

This inflammatory stomatitis, most often seen in association with ulcerative colitis, was reviewed by van Hale et al. Edema and erythema, with deep folding of the buccal mucosa, characterize it, together with pustules, small vegetating projections, erosions, ulcers, and fibrinopurulent exudate. Of 17 patients reviewed, there was 2:1 male predominance; all were young adults; most had antecedent gastrointestinal involvement; and 10 had concurrent skin lesions. Histologically there were dense aggregates of neutrophils and eosinophils. High-dose systemic steroids were the only effective treatment.

FORDYCE'S DISEASE
(Fordyce's Spots)

Fordyce's spots are ectopically located sebaceous glands, clinically characterized by minute orange or yellowish pinhead-sized macules or papules in the mucosa of the lips, cheeks, and, less often, gums. Similar lesions may occur on the glans penis and the labia minora. Arnold reported a large crateriform hypertrophic sebaceous gland and several comedones among the lesions of this disorder in an otherwise normal young man.

Involvement of the labial mucosa with pseudoxanthoma elasticum may simulate Fordyce's spots.

There are no indications for treatment because the anomaly is asymptomatic and inconsequential, and requires only reassurance.

STOMATITIS NICOTINA

Also known as smoker's keratosis and smoker's patches, and surely caused (despite its name) not by nicotine but by tars and heat in tobacco smoke, stomatitis nicotina is characterized by distinct umbilicated papules on the palate. The ostia of the mucous ducts appear as red pinpoints surrounded by milky white, slightly umbilicated papules, which are completely asymptomatic. The intervening mucosa becomes white and thick and has a tendency to desquamate in places, leaving beefy red raw areas.

This condition is attributed to heavy smoking, especially pipe and cigar smoking, in middle-aged men. Treatment consists of abstinence from the use of tobacco.

Candela pa Den (fire within), a leukokeratosis, appears to be stomatitis nicotina, described by Schoenfeld and Holzberger as occurring among older women in the Netherlands Antilles who smoke cigarettes with the lighted end inside the mouth.

Arnold HL Jr: Fordyce spots (letter). Arch Dermatol 1974, 110:811.
Bernstein ML, et al: Oral lesions in Crohn's disease. Oral Surg 1978, 46:234.
Fisher AA: Allergic contact stomatitis. Cutis 1975, 15:149.
Idem: Contact stomatitis. Derm Clin 1987, 5:709.
Forsey RR, et al: Stomatitis nicotina. Arch Dermatol 1961, 83:945.
Frankel DH, et al: Oral Crohn's disease: report of two cases in brothers with metallic dysgeusia, and review of the literature. JAAD 1985, 12:260.
Hansen LA, et al: The differential diagnosis of pyostomatitis vegetans and its relation to bowel disease. Oral Surg 1983, 55:363.
Lebwohl M, et al: Metastatic Crohn's disease. JAAD 1984, 10:33.
Pindborg JJ, et al: Reverse smoking in Amdhra Pradesh, India: a study of palatal lesions among 10,169 villagers. Br J Cancer 1971, 25:10.
Schwartz DL: Stomatitis nicotina of the palate. Oral Surg 1965, 20:306.
VanHale HM, et al: Pyostomatitis vegetans. Arch Dermatol 1985, 121:94.

TORUS PALATINUS

Torus palatinus is a bony protuberance in the midline of the hard palate, marking the point of junction of the two halves of the palate. It is asymptomatic.

King DR, et al: An analysis of torus palatinus in a transatlantic study. J Oral Med 1976, 31:44.

SCROTAL TONGUE

Also known as furrowed tongue or lingua plicata, scrotal tongue is a congenital and sometimes familial condition in which the tongue is generally larger than normal and there are plicate superficial or deep grooves, usually arranged so that there is a longitudinal furrow along the median raphe. Scrotal tongue is seen in Melkersson-Rosenthal syndrome and in most patients with Down's syndrome.

The condition gives rise to no difficulty, and treatment is not necessary, except that the deep furrows should be kept clean by use of mouthwashes. Fur-

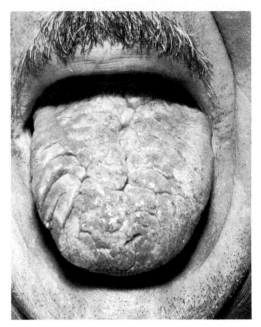

Figure 34–5. Scrotal tongue with candidiasis.

rowed tongue must be differentiated from the "cobblestone" tongue that develops in syphilis.

Chosack A, et al: The prevalence of scrotal tongue and geographic tongue in 70,359 Israeli school children. Community Dent Oral Epidemiol 1974, 2:253.

GEOGRAPHIC TONGUE

This is also known as *lingua geographica, transitory benign plaques* of the tongue, *glossitis areata exfoliativa,* and *benign migratory glossitis*. In some patients, according to Marks et al, it is a manifestation of atopy, and in others, of psoriasis. However, in most it is an isolated finding.

It begins with a small depression on the lateral border or the tip of the tongue, smoother and redder than the rest of the surface. This spreads peripherally, with the formation of sharply circumscribed ringed or gyrate red patches, each with a narrow yellowish white border, making the tongue resemble a map. The dorsal surface of the tongue is usually the affected site. The appearance changes from day to day; patches may disappear in one place and manifest themselves in others. The disease is characterized by periods of exacerbation and quiescence. The lesion may remain unchanged in the same site for long periods. Probably the condition is frequently unrecognized because it occasions no symptoms except for the occasional complaint of glossodynia.

O'Keefe and associates described two clinical variants of geographic tongue. In one type, discrete, annular "bald" patches of glistening, erythematous mucosa with absent or atrophic filiform papillae are noted. Another type shows prominent circinate or annular white raised lines varying in width up to 2 mm. The clinical appearance and histopathologic findings of the tongue lesions in pustular psoriasis, Reiter's syndrome, and geographic tongue are identical, and they suggest the name **annulus migrans** for this entity.

Histologically, the main features are marked transepidermal neutrophil migration with the formation of spongiform pustules in the epidermis and an upper dermal round cell infiltrate.

Although treatment is not usually indicated, Helfman in 1979 suggested tretinoin solution (Retin-A), 0.1 per cent topically: in three cases there was clearing within four to seven days.

Eidelman E, et al: Scrotal tongue and geographic tongue. Oral Surg 1976, 42:591.
Hubler WR Jr: Lingual lesions of pustular psoriasis. JAAD 1984, 11:1069.

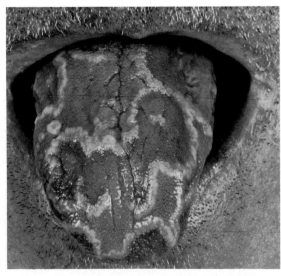
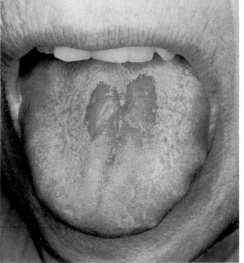

A   B

Figure 34–6. A and B, Geographic tongue. (A, Courtesy of Dr. H. Shatin.)

Kullaa-Mikkonen A, et al: Prevalence of different morphologic forms of the human tongue in young Finns. Oral Surg 1982, 53:152.

Marks R, et al: Geographic tongue: a manifestation of atopy. Br J Dermatol 1979, 101:159.

O'Keefe E, et al: Annulus migrans. Arch Dermatol 1973, 107:240.

Bouquot JE, et al: Odd tongues: The prevalence of common tongue lesions in 23,616 white Americans over 35 years of age. Quintessence Int 1986, 17:719.

Farman AG: Hairy tongue. J Oral Med 1977, 32:85.

Pegum JS: Urea in the treatment of black hairy tongue. Br J Dermatol 1971, 84:602.

Standish SM, et al: Treatment of hair tongue with podophyllum resin. J Am Dent Assoc 1964, 68:335.

Svejda J, et al: Hairlike variations of filiform papillae in the human tongue. Oral Surg 1977, 43:97.

BLACK HAIRY TONGUE

Black or brown hairy tongue occurs on the dorsum of the tongue anterior to the circumvallate papillae, where black, yellowish, or brown patches form, consisting of hairlike intertwining filaments several millimeters long. It represents a benign hyperplasia of the filiform papillae of the anterior two thirds of the tongue, resulting in retention of long conical filaments of ortho- and parakeratotic cells.

Black hairy tongue may be associated with several conditions which may be predisposing factors in its causation. They include excessive smoking, the use of oral antibiotics, and the presence of *Candida* on the surface of the tongue.

This lesion is to be differentiated both clinically and histologically from *oral hairy leukoplakia* seen in HIV-infected patients (see Virus Diseases chapter).

Histologically, there are elongated and stratified filaments originating from abnormal papillae within the epithelial covering of the mucous membrane. Ortho- and parakeratotic cells make up the hairlike processes.

A toothbrush may be used to scrub off the projections either alone or after application of Retin-A gel or 40 per cent aqueous solution of urea. Pegum described the latter method. Predisposing local factors, such as smoking, antibiotics, and oxidizing agents, should be eliminated, if possible, and scrupulous oral hygiene maintained.

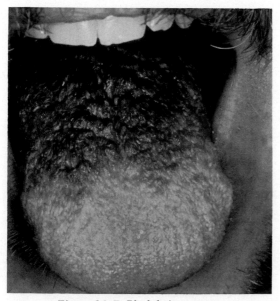

Figure 34–7. Black hairy tongue.

GLOSSITIS

Moeller's Glossitis. Moeller's glossitis (Hunter's glossitis) occurs chiefly on the tip and lateral surfaces of the tongue as intensely red, well-defined irregular patches in which the filiform papillae are absent or thinned and the fungiform papillae are swollen. In these patches the superficial layer of the epidermis exfoliates. The disease is chronic and the patches are painful and sensitive so that eating may be difficult. Moeller's glossitis, painful tongue, and macrocytic anemia are signs of pernicious anemia. The histopathologic changes are those of a nonspecific inflammation.

The treatment is directed against pernicious anemia. With specific therapy an early improvement is to be anticipated in the appearance and sensitivity of the tongue.

Glossitis of Pellagra. Glossitis is a distinctive sign of pellagra, due to a deficiency of niacin or its precursor, tryptophan. The sides and tip of the tongue are erythematous and edematous, with imprints of the teeth. Eventually the entire tongue assumes a beefy-red appearance. Small ulcers appear, and all the mucous membranes of the mouth may be involved. Later the papillae become atrophied to produce a smooth, glazed tongue, as seen in pernicious anemia.

In **malabsorption syndrome**, riboflavin deficiency, and sprue similar changes are noted. Vitamin B complex is curative.

Dreizen S, et al: Oral manifestations of nutritional deficiencies. Dent Clin North Am 1958, July p 429.

Median Rhomboid Glossitis (Glossitis Rhomboidea Mediana). Median rhomboid glossitis is characterized by a shiny oval or diamond-shaped elevation, invariably situated on the dorsum in the midline immediately in front of the circumvallate papillae. The surface is abnormally red and smooth. In some instances a few pale yellow papules surmount the elevation. On palpation the lesion feels slightly firm, but it causes no symptoms. It persists indefinitely with little or no increase in size. There is no relationship whatever to cancer.

Cooke believes the condition is a form of candidiasis. As a result of a literature review and histologic study of 28 cases of median rhomboid glossitis, Wright suggested that this entity is the clinical

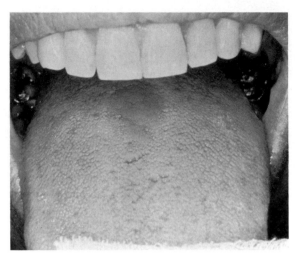

Figure 34–8. Glossitis rhomboidea mediana.

expression of a localized fungal infection with *Candida* species.

Histologically, the changes are those of a simple, chronic inflammation with fibrosis. Cooke and Wright, in separate studies, demonstrated the presence of fungal hyphae in the parakeratin layer in 100 per cent and 85 per cent respectively.

Cooke BD: Median rhomboid glossitis: candidiasis and not a developmental anomaly. Br J Dermatol 1975, 93:399.
Wright BA: Median rhomboid glossitis: not a misnomer. Oral Surg 1978, 46:806.

EOSINOPHILIC ULCER OF THE TONGUE

Eosinophilic ulcer of the tongue may occur anywhere on the tongue, including the ventral surface. It is characterized by an extremely shallow ulcer that is usually covered by a pseudomembrane. A possible traumatic etiology has been postulated for this benign, self-limited disorder. A patient of Domonkos's, a 35-year-old man, had the ulcer in the middle of the tongue. Glossitis rhomboidea mediana had to be considered in the differential diagnosis.

Shapiro and Juhlin described the histopathologic findings in this case as not showing any granulomatous inflammatory changes, but rather a predominantly eosinophilic infiltrate in company with some histiocytes and neutrophils.

Domonkos's patient responded well to liquid nitrogen cryotherapy. Burgess et al emphasize that surgical intervention is unnecessary, in their report of two cases.

Burgess GH, et al: Eosinophilic ulcer of the tongue. Arch Dermatol 1977, 113:644.
Shapiro L: Eosinophilic ulcer of the tongue. Dermatologica 1970, 140:242.

DENTAL SINUS

In dental (or odontogenous) sinus, chronic periapical infection about a tooth produces a burrowing, practically asymptomatic sinus tract, which eventually appears beneath the surface of the gum, palate, or periorificial skin and forms a fistulous opening with a granulomatous nodule at the orifice. It may appear anywhere from the inner ocular canthus to the neck, but is most often seen on the chin or along the jaw line. Hyman and Brownstein reported bilateral odontogenous sinuses, the first recorded case. The differential diagnosis from granuloma pyogenicum is accomplished by dental radiography and often by palpation of a cordlike sinus tract. Actinomycosis must also be considered. Spear et al discuss the differential diagnosis of this frequently misdiagnosed lesion. Conditions to be differentiated are squamous cell carcinoma, osteomyelitis of the mandible, congenital fistulas, the deep mycoses, and foreign-body reactions.

Treatment requires the removal of the offending tooth, or root canal therapy of the periapical abscess.

Fox HH, et al: Cutaneous manifestations of dental sinuses. Cutis 1974, 13:201.
Lewin-Epstein J, et al: Cutaneous sinus tracts of dental origin. Arch Dermatol 1978, 114:1158.
Scott MJ Jr, et al: Cutaneous odontogenic sinus. J Am Acad Dermatol 1980, 2:521.
Spear KL, et al: Sinus tracts to the chin and jaw of dental origin. JAAD 1983, 8:486.

ORAL MYCOSIS

Candidiasis. Also known as *thrush*, this may affect persons of all ages, especially those with wasting

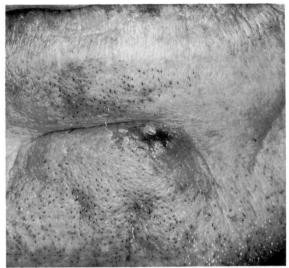

Figure 34–9. Cutaneous sinus tract of dental origin.

illnesses. Usually there is a whitish flaky pseudomembrane on the erythematous mucous membrane. Other distinctive clinical forms of oral candidiasis include denture sore mouth, candidal glossitis, candidal leukoplakia, chronic mucocutaneous candidiasis, and angular cheilitis or perlèche. Cultures may show various types of candida, *C. albicans* appearing most frequently. Nystatin tablet or troches or vaginal suppositories may be allowed to dissolve in the mouth three or four times a day for seven to ten days. Clotrimazole troches may be used in the same way. For infants these may be inserted into a slit pacifier. Topical gentian violet is not effective enough to justify its messiness. Ketoconazole, 200 mg once or twice a day, will always be helpful and may be necessary. Nystatin or clotrimazole ointment may be useful for associated perlèche. Treatment should be continued for at least two days after apparent cure.

Actinomycosis. The mouth is a favored site for actinomycosis. Hard nodules develop, and suppurate, discharging pus containing "sulfur granules."

Blastomycosis. This mycotic infection may resemble actinomycosis or may manifest as firm eroded or ulcerated swellings with a papillated surface.

Cryptococcosis. The tongue is often secondarily involved in systemic cryptococcosis. Mouth lesions may be mistaken for either candidiasis or blastomycosis.

Histoplasmosis. Ulcers are the usual manifestations in the mouth, and occur in 75 per cent of patients with pulmonary histoplasmosis. They are not clinically distinguishable from those of **coccidioidomycosis.**

Goldstein BH, et al: Actinomycosis of the maxilla. J Oral Surg 1972, 30:362.
Holst E, et al: Cervico-facial actinomycosis. Int J Oral Surg 1979, 8:194.
Kirkpatrick GH, et al: Treatment of chronic oral candidiasis with clotrimazole troches. N Engl J Med 1978, 229:1201.
Mackie RM, et al: The relationship between immunological parameters and response to therapy in oral candidiasis. Br J Dermatol 178, 98:343.
Ray TL: Oral candidiasis. Derm Clin 1987, 5:651.
Toth BB, et al: Oral histoplasmosis. Oral Surg 1983, 55:597.
Weir JC, et al: Periapical actinomycosis. Oral Surg 1983, 54:336.
Wright BA, et al: Candidiasis and atrophic tongue lesions. Oral Surg 1981, 51:55.
Young LL, et al: Oral manifestations of histoplasmosis. Oral Surg 1972, 33:191.

NEOPLASMS

Heck's Disease (Focal Epithelial Hyperplasia). These benign, discrete, usually whitish, sessile to papular, soft, nodular elevations of the oral mucosa or lip vary in size from 1 to 5 mm in diameter, are often multiple, may form clusters, and occur most frequently in the lower labial mucosa, followed by the buccal mucosa and the upper labial mucosa. The tongue, upper lip, gingivae, and anterior faucial pillars are infrequently involved. This condition appears to be more common among American Indians and Eskimos. It predominates in children three to 18 years of age. Arnold had a case with a solitary plaque on the upper vermilion.

Histologically, the characteristic features are irregular focal epithelial hyperplasia with blunt and fused rete ridges and enlarged, edematous cells in the stratum spinosum. No viral inclusion bodies are seen. Van Wyk and associates demonstrated intranuclear viral particles by electron microscopy in six of 13 cases studied. Human papillomavirus types 13 and 32 have been identified in these lesions. A family history of focal epithelial hyperplasia is often obtained and recessive inheritance of a predisposition to this infection has been proposed. Lesions may progress or persist; the usual course, however, is spontaneous regression. Solitary lesions seldom recur after shave removal, in Arnold's experience.

Oral Hairy Leukoplakia. This is described under AIDS, in which it occurs, in the chapter on Viral Diseases.

Leukoplakia. Once regarded as precancerous, its name now refers only to whitish plaques or patches in mucous membranes, which may or may not show cellular atypia.

Erythroplakia. This term is applied to leukoplakia which has lost (or not developed) the thick keratin layer which makes leukoplakia white; it is the usual pattern in mucocutaneous junctions. A focal red patch, with no apparent cause, should be suspected of being precancerous when found on the floor of the mouth, soft palate, or buccal mucosa, or under the tongue. Histologically there is cellular atypia, pleomorphism, hyperchromatism, and increased mitotic figures. Carcinoma in situ or invasive carcinoma is found in 90 per cent of lesions.

Squamous Cell Carcinoma. The most frequent sites are the lower lip and the anterior third of the tongue. These lesions frequently develop from leukoplakia or at sites of frequent irritation. Regional lymph node metastasis is a frequent complication. Tobacco smoking is a common cause of carcinoma of the mouth. Snuff dipper's cancer of the mouth may occur in inveterate snuff users.

Sarcoma. Usually this type of tumor arises in the tonsils or tonsillar fossa. These lesions develop quickly and metastasize early. Rapidly fungating masses develop, so that blastomycosis, actinomycosis, or tularemia are frequently considered in the differential diagnosis.

Kaposi's Sarcoma. Dark red to violaceous plaques or solid tumor nodules may be found anywhere; the soft palate is a common site. Similarly hued lesions in an elderly man on the arches of the feet affirm the diagnosis; however, in AIDS-related Kaposi's sarcoma, lesions may occur anywhere, are multifocal, and often quite numerous. They respond readily to x-ray therapy.

Pleomorphic Adenoma. This was formerly referred to as *mixed tumor*. The palate is second only to the parotid and submaxillary glands as a frequent site for pleomorphic adenoma. It may vary in size from a papule to a mass filling the entire oral cavity. The surface is covered with normal mucosa and may be smooth or corrugated.

White Sponge Nevus. This is discussed on page 759.

Molluscum Contagiosum. This umbilicated, papular, poxvirus-induced lesion occasionally occurs in the mouth. In the case of widespread molluscum contagiosum in an AIDS patient, reported by Redfield et al, there were multiple labial lesions.

Verrucae. Human papillomavirus infections may commonly involve the vermilion of the lips and occasionally the tongue, the labial mucosa, and the buccal mucosa. These lesions are frequently filiform and are easily treated by cryotherapy, curettage, shave excision, or scissors excision.

Acquired Dyskeratotic Leukoplakia. This condition, reported by James and Lupton, manifested as distinctive white plaques in the oral mucosa of the palate, gingivae, and lips. There were similar lesions of the genitalia. Histologically there was a unique finding of clusters of dyskeratotic cells in the prickle-cell layer in all sites.

Aggressive laser treatment was followed by recurrence. Etretinate afforded some improvement.

Trumpeter's Wart. This is a firm, fibrous, hyperkeratotic, pseudoepitheliomatous nodule on the upper lip of a trumpet player. A similar "callus" may grow on the lower lip of trombone players.

Melanocytic Oral Lesions. A wide variety of melanocytic lesions appear on the mucous membranes.

Among the melanocytic nevi of the cellular type, the *intramucosal* type is the most frequent, with the *compound nevus* next and the *junction nevus* occurring only rarely. Nevi of the oral mucosa in general are very uncommon. *Ephelis, lentigo, blue nevus,* and *labial melanotic macules* are other types of focal hyperpigmentation. Ephelides darken on sun exposure and are usually limited to the lower lip. The blue nevus has dendritic cells in the submucosa. Lentigenes show acanthosis of rete ridges on biopsy. Spann et al reviewed 41 labial melanotic macules and described them as solitary, sharply demarcated, flat, pigmented lesions, chiefly in young women, which did not change on sun exposure and showed only acanthosis and basal-layer melanin on biopsy.

Oral melanoacanthoma is a simultaneous proliferation of keratinocytes and melanocytes. Goode et al found ten cases, mostly in young (average age, 23) black patients. Most lesions were on the buccal mucosa. It seems to be a reactive process, usually following trauma and resolving spontaneously in 40 per cent of their series.

Melanoma also occurs, rarely, mostly in older patients. It is recognized by being larger than the usual benign pigmented lesion. It is more irregular in shape, with a tendency to ulcerate and to bleed. A peripheral areola of erythema and satellite pigmented spots may be present.

There is a striking predilection for palatal (or less often gingival) involvement. The overall prognosis is poor (less than 5 per cent survival at five years) because the lesions are usually deeply invasive by the time they are discovered.

Oral Melanosis. Pigmentation of the oral cavity tends to occur most frequently in blacks. In other races, the darker the skin the more mucosal pigmentation is to be expected. Oral melanosis may occur with Riehl's melanosis, Albright's syndrome, Peutz-Jeghers syndrome, and Addison's disease. James et al reported a patient with **inflammatory acquired oral hyperpigmentation** which started at age 30 with numerous distinct pigmented macules, similar to those seen in Peutz-Jeghers syndrome. However, she progressed rapidly to a diffuse oral hyperpigmentation. This appeared to be due to some undefined inflammation, and slow partial resolution occurred after several years of observation. Focal, brownish blue macules occur as amalgam tattoo incurred from fragments of silver or amalgam being implanted into the gums. Tar and heavy metal poisoning may also induce such lesions. Bismuth (injected) and lead (ingested or inhaled) may produce a pigmented line along the gums near their margin. Ettinger et al reported the appearance of a gingival platinum line in a patient being treated for osteogenic sarcoma with cis-platinum.

Granular Cell Tumor. This unusual tumor arises in the mucous membranes of the mouth, most typically on the tongue. (See p. 731.)

Epulis. This means any benign tumor situated on the gingiva. Giant cell epulis is a solitary, bluish red, 10–20-mm tumor occurring on the gingiva between or about deciduous bicuspid and incisor teeth. Other varieties may be fibrous, nevoid, and angiomatous epulis, or granuloma telangiectaticum, also known as pyogenic granuloma.

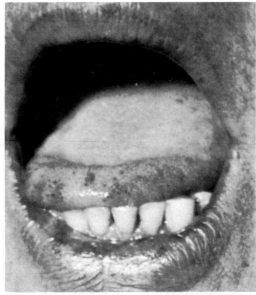

Figure 34–10. Melanosis oris with pigmented macules on the lips and tongue but without intestinal polyposis.

Pyogenic Granuloma (Granuloma Pyogenicum et Telangiectaticum). This lesion is an exuberant overgrowth of granulation tissue, frequently occurring in the oral cavity, most often involving the gingiva but also the buccal mucosa, lips, tongue, or palate. The red to reddish purple, soft, nodular mass bleeds easily and grows rapidly, but is usually not painful. A clinically and histologically identical tumor develops on the gingiva not infrequently during pregnancy. It is referred to as **pregnancy tumor** or **granuloma gravidarum.**

Histologically, vascular proliferation and varying quantities of acute and chronic inflammatory cells are dispersed in an edematous connective tissue stroma.

Treatment is by surgical excision or shave biopsy followed by curettage and electrodesiccation.

Granuloma Fissuratum. This is a circumscribed, firm, whitish, fissured, fibrous granuloma occurring in the labioalveolar fold. The lesion is discoid, smooth, and slightly raised, being about 1 cm in diameter. The growth is folded like a bent coin so that the fissure in the bend is continuous at both sides with the labioalveolar sulcus. Symptoms are slight. It is an inflammatory fibrous hyperplasia that usually results from chronic irritation from poorly fitting dentures. In the dental literature it is *epulis fissuratum*, particularly when there is a deep cleft traversing the lesion. Treatment is by surgical extirpation or electrodesiccation, with biopsy.

Hemangioma. The cavernous type of hemangioma may occur in the mouth as well as other sites. The angles of the mouth and the buccal mucosa are most frequently involved. Fissures and hemorrhage may occur from the trauma to which that site is exposed.

Lymphangioma. The most frequent site in the mouth is the tongue, where numerous Concord-grapelike clusters of lesions may involve the tongue and grow until a space-occupying problem ensues.

Caviar Tongue. William Bean gave this picturesque name to the small, round, purplish capillary telangiectases so commonly found on the undersurface of the tongue after age 50. Kocsard et al studied these in depth and attributed them to elastic tissue deterioration incident to aging.

Osseous Choristoma of the Tongue. Weitzner reported three cases of this rare lesion and found 38 in the literature. It presents as a nodule on the dorsum of the tongue containing mature lamellar bone without osteoblastic or osteoclastic activity. It is called a choristoma and not a hamartoma because bone is not found in the normal tongue. None have recurred after simple excision.

Oral Warty Dyskeratoma. The warty dyskeratoma, an acantholytic dyskeratotic papule histologically resembling Darier's disease, has rarely been reported as an intraoral lesion. It is discussed on page 753. Harrist et al reported a case in 1980, and reviewed eight previously reported cases.

Peripheral Ameloblastoma. Urmacher et al reported a case of this rare invasive neoplasm of the gingivae, oftenest of the lower jaw. Gardner studied 21 cases, including five reported as basal cell carcinoma.

Acevedo A, et al: Focal epithelial hyperplasia. Oral Surg 1981, 51:524.

Angelopoulos AP: Pyogenic granuloma of the oral cavity. J Oral Surg 1971, 29:840.

Bhaskar SN, et al: Pyogenic granuloma. J Oral Surg 1966, 24:391.

Buchner A, et al: Melanotic macule of the oral mucosa. Oral Surg 1979, 48:244.

Idem: Pigmented nevi of the oral mucosa. Oral Surg 1979, 48:131.

Idem: Amalgam pigmentation of the oral mucosa. Oral Surg 1980, 49:139.

Chaudhry AP, et al: Intra-oral minor salivary gland tumors. Oral Surg 1961, 14:1194.

Chuang T-Y: Condylomata acuminata. JAAD 1987, 16:376.

Cutright DE: The histopathologic findings in 583 cases of epulis fissuratum. Oral Surg 1974, 37:401.

Elizeri YD: The toluidine blue test. JAAD 1988, 18:1339.

Ettinger LJ, et al: The gingival platinum line. Cancer 1979, 44:1882.

Eversole LR, et al: Oral Kaposi sarcoma with acquired immunodeficiency syndrome among homosexual males. JAAD 1983, 107:248.

Gardner DG: Peripheral ameloblastoma: a study of 21 cases, including 5 reported as basal cell carcinoma of the gingiva. Cancer 1977, 39:1625.

Goldberg MH, et al: Lymphangioma of the tongue. J Oral Surg 1977, 35:841.

Goode RK, et al: Oral melanoacanthoma. Oral Surg 1983, 56:622.

Harrist TJ, et al: Oral warty dyskeratoma. Arch Dermatol 1980, 116:929.

Horlick HP, et al: Mucosal melanotic macule, reactive type. JAAD 1988, 19:786.

James WD, et al: Inflammatory acquired oral hyperpigmentation. JAAD 1987, 16:220.

Idem: Acquired dyskeratotic leukoplakia. Arch Dermatol (in press).

Kato T, et al: Malignant melanoma of mucous membranes. Arch Dermatol 1987, 123:216.

Khanna JN, et al: Bilateral vascular lesions of the tongue. J Int Dent Assoc 1979, 51:139.

Kocsard E, et al: The histopathology of caviar tongue. Dermatologica 1970, 140:318.

Lupton GP, et al: Oral hairy leukoplakia. Arch Dermatol 1987, 123:624.

Maize JC: Mucosal melanosis. Derm Clin 1988, 6:283.

Mashberg A: Erythroplasia. J Am Dent Assoc 1978, 96:615.

Naeim F, et al: Mixed tumors of the salivary glands. Arch Pathol Lab Med 1976, 100:271.

Nelson JF, et al: Molluscum contagiosum of the lower lip. J Oral Med 1980, 35:62.

Praetorius-Clausen F: Rare oral disorders. Oral Surg 1972, 34:604.

Redfield RR, et al: Severe molluscum contagiosum infection in a patient with human T-cell lymphotropic disease. JAAD 1985, 13:821.

Regezi JA, et al: Granular cell tumors of the head and neck. J Oral Surg 1979, 37:402.

Sexton FM, et al: Melanotic macules and melanoacanthomas of the lip. Am J Dermatopathol 1987, 9:438.

Shafer WG, et al: Erythroplakia of the oral cavity. Cancer 1975, 36:1021.

Shaffer EL Jr, et al: Oral condyloma acuminatum. J Oral Pathol 1980, 9:163.

Shapiro L, et al: The solitary labial lentigo. Oral Surg 1971, 31:87.

Shear M: Erythroplakia of the mouth. Int J Dent 1972, 22:460.

Silverman S Jr: Prevention, early detection and diagnosis of oral cancer. Derm Clin 1987, 5:675.

Sparm CR, et al: The labial melanotic macule. Arch Dermatol 1987, 123:1029.

Stiefler RE, et al: Heck's disease (focal epithelial hyperplasia). JAAD 1979, 1:499.

Trodahl JN, et al: Benign and malignant melanocytic lesions of the oral mucosa. Cancer 1970, 25:812.

Urmacher C, et al: An uncommon neoplasm (ameloblastoma) of the oral mucosa. Am J Dermatopathol 1983, 5:601.

VanWyk CR, et al: Focal epithelial hyperplasia in a group of South Africans: its clinical and microscopic features. Oral Pathol 1977, 6:1.

Weathers DR: Benign nevi of the oral mucosa. Arch Dermatol 1969, 99:688.

Whithen JB: The electron microscopic examination of congenital keratoses of the oral mucous membranes. I: white sponge nevus. Oral Surg 1970, 29:69.

Witkop CJ, et al: Four hereditary mucosal syndromes. Arch Dermatol 1961, 84:762.

Dermoid cyst may occur on the floor of the mouth, especially in the sublingual area.

Catone GA, et al: Sublingual mucous escape phenomenon. J Oral Surg 1969, 27:774.

Gormley MG, et al: Ranulas. J Acad Gen Dent 1973, 21:29.

Harrison JD: Salivary mucoceles. Oral Surg 1975, 39:268.

Lattanand A, et al: Mucous cyst (mucocele). Arch Dermatol 1970, 101:673.

Robinson L, et al: Pathologic changes associated with mucous retention cysts of the minor salivary glands. Oral Surg 1964, 18:191.

MUCOUS CYST
(Mucocele)

A **mucous retention cyst** is most often seen inside the lower lip, but may occur under the tongue or in the buccal mucosa, usually as a soft, rounded projection covered by pale, but otherwise normal, mucosa. The cyst varies from 2 to 10 mm in diameter. It is painless, fluctuant, and tense. Incision of it, or sometimes merely compression, releases sticky, straw-colored fluid, or bluish fluid if hemorrhage has occurred into it.

Mucous cyst is caused by rupture of the mucous duct, with extravasation of sialomucin into the submucosa to produce cystic spaces with inflammation. Granulation tissue formation is followed by fibrosis.

After the cyst is thoroughly evacuated, the point of rupture of the duct is destroyed by the use of phenol, cautery, or fulguration. Carbon dioxide laser ablation or excision are other treatment options. The mucous cyst is frequently encountered in dermatologic practice.

A **ranula** (from *Rana*, the frog genus) is a mucocele of the floor of the mouth.

Parotid duct cyst occurs in musicians who use wind instruments. It develops opposite the upper second molar on the buccal mucosa.

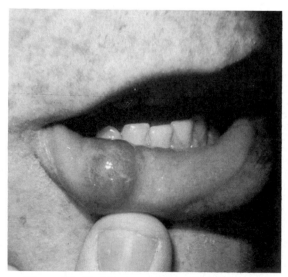

Figure 34–11. Mucous cyst (mucocele) of the lip.

VINCENT'S INFECTION
(Fusospirochetal Gingivitis)

Synonyms: Plaut-Vincent's angina and trench mouth.

Vincent's infection is an acute necrotizing ulcerative gingivitis with a rapid onset of characteristic punched-out ulcerations appearing on the interdental papillae and marginal gingivae. A dirty white pseudomembrane may cover the ulcerations. The lesions may spread rapidly and involve the buccal mucosa, lips, and tongue as well as the tonsils, the pharynx, and the entire respiratory tract. The slightest pressure causes pain and bleeding. The outstanding finding is the characteristic, always-present, foul, fetid odor.

The etiology is thought to be the presence of necrotic tissue, providing an anaerobic environment for the infection by fusospirochetal organisms (*Bacteroides fusiformis*) in association with *Borrelia vincenti* and other organisms. Poor dental hygiene is a predisposing factor; scurvy, pellagra, and poor nutrition are contributory factors. One of us (WDJ) has seen this reaction as an oral finding in AIDS patients.

Acute herpetic gingivostomatitis, occurring as a primary herpes simplex infection, may be confused with Vincent's infection. Young children are susceptible to this severe febrile stomatitis with lymphadenitis.

Noma is a form of fusospirillary gangrenous stomatitis occurring in children with low resistance and poor nutrition. At the onset there is ulceration of the buccal mucosa which rapidly assumes a gangrenous

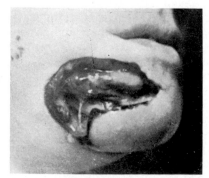

Figure 34–12. Noma of chin. (Courtesy of Dr. L. Goldman.)

character and extends to involve the skin and bones, with resultant necrosis. It may end fatally.

Fusospirillary infection may cause painful, raw, recalcitrant erosions of the penis (*erosive balanitis*) and the vulva (*erosive vulvitis*). These gangrenous ulcerations were once called *cancrum pudendi*.

Treatment consists of thorough dental hygienic measures under the supervision of a dentist. Penicillin, erythromycin, and tetracycline orally are all effective in adequate dosage. Topical application by holding tetracycline oral suspension in the mouth for a few minutes should be done several times daily. Use of 3 per cent hydrogen peroxide as a mouthwash is also helpful.

Coslet RS: The psychological factor in the etiology of acute necrotizing gingivitis. Dent Hyg 1979, 53:257.

PEMPHIGUS VULGARIS

The oral manifestations of pemphigus are described on page 534.

CICATRICIAL PEMPHIGOID

This condition, as well as bullous pemphigoid and desquamative gingivitis are discussed in Chapter 21.

ACATALASEMIA

Acatalasemia (Takahara's disease) is a rare disease in which the enzyme catalase is deficient in the liver, muscles, bone marrow, erythrocytes, and skin. The absence of catalase leads to progressive gangrene of the mouth, with recurrent ulcerations due to increased susceptibility to infection by anaerobic organisms.

Nearly 60 per cent of the affected individuals develop alveolar ulcerations beginning in childhood. A mild type of the disease is characterized by rapidly recurring ulcers. In the moderate type alveolar gangrene develops, with atrophy and recession of the alveolar bone, so that the teeth fall out spontaneously. In the severe type widespread destruction of the jaw occurs. After puberty all lesions heal, even in those individuals who had the severe type.

There is no gross difference in appearance between the blood of an acatalasiac and that of a normal individual. Upon the addition of hydrogen peroxide, however, acatalasic blood immediately turns blackish brown and the peroxide does not foam. Normal blood remains bright and causes the peroxide to foam exuberantly because of the presence of erythrocyte catalase.

Acatalasia is a rare autosomal-recessively inherited trait. Approximately two out of 100,000 Japanese have this disease.

Treatment consists of extraction of the diseased teeth and the use of antibiotics to control the harmful effects of the offending bacteria.

Takahara S, et al: Hypocatalasemia: a new genetic carrier state. J Clin Invest 1960, 39:610.

CR3 DEFICIENCY

CR3 deficiency is the absence or near-absence of the adherence-related glycoproteins which bind C3bi, the opsonic fragment of the third component of complement. The B subunit of this receptor cannot be synthesized because of an autosomal recessive defect which has been mapped to chromosome 21.

Clinically there is delayed separation of the spinal cord and early onset of recurrent bacterial skin infections, mucositis, and otitis. Gingivitis and odontitis occur, with loss of teeth. The common feature is poor chemotaxis, aggregation, and adherence of neutrophil leukocytes.

Anderson DC, et al: Leukocyte adherence deficiency. Annu Rev Med 1987, 38:175.
Buescher ES: Abnormal adherence-related functions of neutrophils, monocytes, and Epstein-Barr virus-transformed B cells in a patient with C3bi receptor deficiency. Blood 1985, 65:1382.
Malech HL, et al: Neutrophils in human disease. N Engl J Med 1987, 317:687.

CYCLIC NEUTROPENIA

Cyclic or periodic neutropenia is characterized by a decrease of circulating neutrophils from the blood, and dermatologic manifestations. At fairly regular intervals (21 days) neutropenia and mouth ulcerations develop, usually accompanied by fever, malaise, and arthralgia. The ulcerations of the lips, tongue, palate, gums, and buccal mucosa may be extensive. The ulcers are irregularly outlined and are covered by a grayish white necrotic slough. The anterior teeth may show a grayish brown discoloration. Premature alveolar bone loss and periodontitis occur. In addition, cutaneous infections such as abscesses, furuncles, and cellulitis may rarely develop. Urticaria and erythema multiforme have been reported.

There is a cyclic depression of neutrophils occurring at intervals of 12 to 30 days (average 21 days) and lasting from five to eight days. The neutrophils in the peripheral blood regularly fall to low levels or disappear at this time. Some cases have been associated with agammaglobulinemia, but in other cases the globulins are normal. Gorlin and Chandhry point out striking similarities between the oral lesions of Sutton's disease and those of cyclic neutropenia.

The cause of cyclic neutropenia is unknown.

Nothing is known that will influence the course of cyclic neutropenia. The use of antibiotics during infections seems to expedite recovery. Careful attention to oral hygiene, including plaque control, helps the mouth lesions and reduces the risk of infections. Death may occur from pneumonia, sepsis, gangrenous pyoderma, or granulocytopenia.

Becker FT, et al: Recurring oral and cutaneous infections associated with cyclic neutropenia. Arch Dermatol 1959, 80:731.
Gorlin RJ, et al: The oral manifestations of cyclic neutropenia. Arch Dermatol 1960, 82:344.
Rylander H, et al: Manifestations and treatment of periodontal disease in a patient suffering from cyclic neutropenia. J Clin Periodontol 1981, 8:77.

RECURRENT INTRAORAL HERPES SIMPLEX INFECTION

Recurrent intraoral herpes simplex infection is characterized by numerous small vesicles occurring in one or a few clusters, almost exclusively on the palate, or infrequently on the gingiva. The grouped vesicles rupture rapidly to form punctate erosions with a red base. Smears from the base prepared with Wright's stain will show giant multinucleated epithelial cells. Immunofluorescent tests and viral cultures are also confirmatory.

The differential diagnosis of this uncommon manifestation of herpes simplex includes oral herpes zoster, herpangina, and oral aphthosis. The latter two involve nonattached mucosa, whereas recurrent herpes simplex involves mucosa fixed to bone. Differentiation from zoster is made on clinical grounds or by culture and immunofluorescent testing.

Griffin JW: Recurrent intraoral herpes simplex virus infections. Oral Surg 1965, 19:209.
Weathers DR, et al: Intraoral ulcerations of recurrent herpes simplex and recurrent aphthae: two distinct entities. J Am Dent Assoc 1970, 81:81.

RECURRENT APHTHOUS STOMATITIS
(Canker Sores; Aphthosis)

CLINICAL FEATURES. Aphthous stomatitis, a painful and recurrent disease of the oral mucous membrane, begins as small discrete or grouped papules or vesicles, which in a few hours become necrotizing ulcerations. They are small, round, shallow, white ulcers (aphthae), generally surrounded by a ring of hyperemia. As a rule, they are tender; they may become so painful that they interfere with speech and mastication. They are mostly about 5 mm in diameter, but may vary in size from 3 to 12 mm. Usually one to three lesions occur per attack; however, they may occur in any number. They are located in decreasing frequency on the buccal and labial mucosa, edges of the tongue, buccal and lingual sulci, and soft palate. Although there is a marked predilection for the nonkeratinized mucosa (any not bound to underlying periosteum) lesions may occasionally be present on the fixed mucosa. Aphthae may also occur on the vagina, vulva, penis, anus, and even the conjunctiva. (See Behçet's syndrome below.)

The lesions tend to involute in two to three weeks, but recurrences are common. These recurrences may be induced by trauma, allergy, emotional stress, or hormonal changes in women such as in menstruation, pregnancy, menarche, and menopause. Lesions may be induced by trauma such as self-biting, toothbrush injury, and dental procedures. Allergy to foods and drugs as well as allergic diseases such as asthma or hay fever may bring about recurrences. It is believed by some that herpes simplex labialis may trigger recurrent aphthae. A familial predisposition tendency has also been noted and described as *familial epidemic aphthosis*.

Rostas et al, in a review, found the prevalence to be about 20 per cent of the population.

Ulcerations such as these may also be the presenting sign in Behçet's syndrome, gluten-sensitive enteropathy, pernicious anemia, cyclic neutropenia,

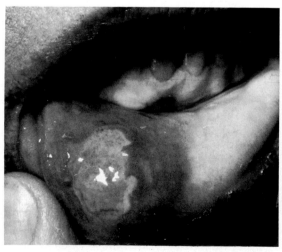
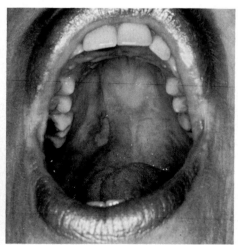

A   B

Figure 34–13. A and B, Aphthous stomatitis.

neutropenia, ulcerative colitis, and Crohn's disease. History, physical examination, complete blood count, and long-term follow-up documenting the recurrent course in the absence of other symptoms will secure the diagnosis. Some patients have aphthosis associated with low folate or iron levels, and these should be included in testing.

ETIOLOGY. Although individual patients often suspect one of the above factors was responsible for precipitating their recurrence, only infectious or immunologic mechanisms are felt to be significant causes.

The highly pleomorphic *Streptococcus sanguis*, with its transitional "L" forms, has been found to have antigenic overlap with human oral mucosa. This might account for the autoantibody and cell-mediated immune factors directed against oral epithelium, which have been demonstrated to be present in a high percentage of patients with recurrent oral aphthae.

R. S. Rogers III and others have presented evidence that aphthosis is a disease of lymphocytotoxic etiology. Lymphocytotoxicity was shown against both autologous and heterologous epithelial target cells. Deposits of immunoglobulin and complement with no consistent pattern are often found on direct immunofluorescence, according to Hale and Rogers.

Histologically, the lesion consists of a lymphocytic inflammatory infiltration with occasional plasma cells and eosinophils, suggestive of delayed hypersensitivity.

DIAGNOSIS. Aphthous stomatitis must be differentiated from mucous patches of early syphilis, candidiasis, Vincent's angina, the avitaminoses (particularly pellagra and scurvy), erythema multiforme, pemphigus, and Behçet's syndrome. Aphthous stomatitis closely resembles primary herpes simplex virus infection of the mouth, recurrent labial herpes, periadenitis mucosa necrotica recurrens (periadenitis aphthae), and recurrent intraoral herpes simplex virus infection (see above). Some believe that Behçet's syndrome and periadenitis mucosa necrotica are the same disease process.

Bell and Rogers have recently emphasized the difficulty of distinguishing aphthous stomatitis from pernicious anemia, pemphigus, cicatricial pemphigoid, and lichen planus. Mechanical injuries and deficiencies of iron and vitamins were emphasized in a National Institutes of Health release.

TREATMENT. At present there is no permanent cure available. Graykowski and his associates found tetracycline suspension the most effective means of treatment. An oral suspension of 5 ml containing 250 mg tetracycline is held in the mouth for two minutes and then swallowed. This is done four times daily for one week. Shelley and Shelley advocate "soft cotton handkerchief packings soaked in freshly made tetracycline suspension (250 mg in 30 ml lukewarm water) for 15 minutes three times a day prior to eating." Colon reported success with topically applied demeclocycline (Declomycin, Lederle) syrup.

Ferguson et al. found a gluten-free diet curative in patients with chronic aphthosis and jejunal mucosal findings of nontropical sprue. Wray found it effective in some patients even in the absence of enteropathy.

Rees B. Rees has had some success with colchicine, 0.6 mg twice a day (personal communication). Gatot et al reported success with it in four patients.

Grinspan reported 15 remissions or marked improvement in 21 severe cases and 19 mild cases—and no failures—using thalidomide, 300 mg daily to start, 200 mg/day after ten days, and 100 mg/day after two months. Relapses were treated with 100 mg/day for 12 days.

Phenelzine (Nardil) being given to alleviate agoraphobia, in a dose of 30 mg/day, wholly relieved severe painful aphthous stomatitis of ten years' duration in a 32-year-old woman treated by Rosenthal. This medication is a monoamine oxidase inhibitor, with many serious side effects which contraindicate its routine use in aphthosis.

A mixture of equal parts of Elixir of Benadryl and Maalox held in the mouth for five minutes prior to meals is soothing.

The lesions may be touched with a silver nitrate stick or cauterized by 95 per cent phenol and neutralized with alcohol.

Lidocaine (Xylocaine Viscous) 2 per cent solution, keeping one teaspoonful in the mouth for several minutes, is helpful in allaying pain. Another useful topical anesthetic is dyclonine hydrochloride (Dyclone) 0.5 per cent applied to the lesions.

A mixture of equal parts of fluocinonide ointment and Orabase applied to the ulcers three or four times a day is effective in aiding the healing of existing ulcers, as shown by Pimlott et al; however, it did not prevent new ulcers. Temovate ointment may be even more effective, according to Contorer and to Odom.

Prednisone incorporated into slowly dissolving lozenges is also helpful. Triamcinolone tablets can be used as lozenges, too, with relief.

Merchant et al found zinc sulfate orally, 220 mg a day, helpful in all of nine aphthosis victims whose serum zinc was initially below 110 µg/dl. None with normal levels was improved.

Wray et al, Tyldesley, and Ferguson et al have reported finding low folate, iron, or B_{12} levels in about 20 per cent of aphthosis patients investigated. Correction of the abnormality cleared or improved the condition in most cases.

Antoon JW, et al: Aphthous ulcers. J Am Dent Assoc 1980, 101:803.

Bell GF, et al: Observations on the diagnosis of recurrent aphthous stomatitis. Mayo Clin Proc 1982, 57:297.

Colon VF: Aphthous stomatitis: treatment with methylchlortetracycline. Cutis 1971, 8:381.

Contorer P: Temovate ointment may help oral aphthae. Schoch Letter 1987, 37:17.

Danby FW: Temovate ointment for oral aphthae confirmed. Schoch Letter 1987, 37:30.

Ferguson MM, et al: Coeliac disease associated with recurrent aphthae. Gut 1980, 21:223.

Gatot A, et al: Colchicine therapy in recurrent oral ulcers (letter). Arch Dermatol 1984, 120:994.

Graykowski EA, et al: Double-blind trial of tetracycline in recurrent aphthous stomatitis. J Oral Pathol 1978, 7:376.

Grinspan D: Significant response of oral aphthosis to thalidomide treatment. JAAD 1985, 12:85.

Idem: Treatment of aphthae with thalidomide. JAAD 1989, 20:1060.

Leiferman KM, et al: Recurrent incapacitating mucosal ulcerations: a prodrome of hypereosinophilic syndrome. JAMA 1982, 247:1018.

Merchant HW, et al: Zinc sulfate supplementation for treatment of recurring oral ulcers. South Med J 1977, 70:559.

National Institutes of Health: Aphthous stomatitis is linked to mechanical injuries and vitamin deficiencies, and certain HLA types. JAMA 1982, 247:774.

Pimlott SJ, et al: A controlled clinical trial of the efficacy of topically applied fluocinonide in the treatment of recurrent aphthous stomatitis. Br Dent J 1983, 154:174.

Rogers RS III: Recurrent aphthous stomatitis: clinical characteristics and evidence for an immunopathogenesis. J Invest Dermatol 1977, 69:499.

Rosenthal SH: Aphthous stomatitis (letter). JAAD 1982, 7:689.

Shore RN, et al: Treatment of aphthous stomatitis by suppression of intralesional streptococci. Arch Dermatol 1974, 109:400.

Tyldesley WR: Stomatitis and recurrent oral ulceration. Br J Oral Surg 1983, 21:27.

VanHale HM, et al: Light and fluorescent microscopic studies of recurrent aphthous ulcers. Cutis 1984, 34:284.

Wray D, et al: Recurrent aphthae. Br Med J 1975, 2:490.

Idem: Role of mucosal injury in initiating recurrent aphthous stomatitis. Br Med J 1981, 283:1569.

MAJOR APHTHOUS ULCER
(Periadenitis Mucosa Necrotica Recurrens)

In *Sutton's disease*, a major aphthous ulcer begins as a small shotlike nodule on the inner lip, buccal mucosa, or tongue, which breaks down into a sharply circumscribed ulcer with a deeply punched out and depressed crater. It is painful. It may at times begin in the faucial pillars or oropharynx. It may persist two to four weeks before healing with a soft, pliable scar. There are seldom more than one to three lesions present at one time. However, remissions tend to be short, and new lesions may appear before old ones have quite healed. The term *major aphthous ulcers* has supplanted the unwieldy Latin name of this disease.

The cause is unknown, but mounting evidence points to an immunologic etiology, as discussed under aphthosis.

Treatment is so difficult that either intralesional or systemic steroids, which may be effective, should be considered. Grinspan's report documents one case which responded to thalidomide, a treatment not available in the United States. Colchicine should be tried, in a dose of 0.6 to 1.2 mg a day.

Grinspan D: Significant response of oral aphthosis to thalidomide treatment. JAAD 1985, 12:85.

Monteleone L: Periadenitis mucosa necrotica recurrens. Oral Surg 1967, 23:586.

BEHÇET'S SYNDROME
(Oculo-Oral-Genital Syndrome)

CLINICAL FEATURES. Behçet's syndrome consists of recurrent oral aphthous ulcerations in the presence of any two of the following: recurrent genital ulcerations, uveitis, cutaneous vasculitis, synovitis, or meningoencephalitis.

The following additional manifestations are observed repeatedly in some but not all cases: erythema nodosum and erythema multiforme–like lesions, acneiform and papulopustular eruptions, furuncle–like pyoderma, subungual abscess, arthritis of knees or toes, thrombophlebitis, cerebral symptoms resembling multiple sclerosis, benign intracranial hypertension, and marked sensitivity to various skin tests, even to sterile saline solution. Tokoro et al have reviewed this in detail.

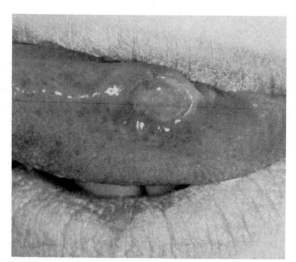

Figure 34–14. Periadenitis mucosa necrotica recurrens on side of tongue. (Courtesy of Dr. L. Cohen.)

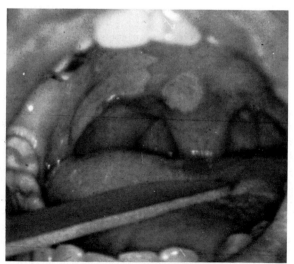

Figure 34–15. Aphthosis in Behçet's syndrome. (Courtesy of Dr. H.O. Curth.)

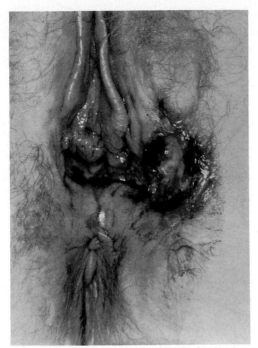

Figure 34–16. Vulvar ulceration of Behçet's syndrome.

The *oral lesions* occur on the lips, tongue, buccal mucosa, soft and hard palate, tonsils, and even in the pharynx and nasal cavity. The lesions are single or multiple, 2 to 10 mm in diameter or larger, and sharply circumscribed, with a dirty grayish base and a surrounding bright red halo. Other patients show deep ulcerations which leave scars resembling those caused by Sutton's major aphthous ulcers.

The lesions are so painful that eating may be difficult. The foul mouth odor is in most instances markedly noticeable.

The *genital lesions* occur in the male on the scrotum and penis, or in the urethra; in the female, on the vulva, cervix, or vagina; they may be found in both sexes on the genitocrural fold, the anus, the perineum, or in the rectum. The ulcerations are similar to those seen in the mouth. In addition, macules, papules, and folliculitis may develop on the scrotum. Lesions in women may lead to deep destruction of the vulva. Swellings of the regional nodes and fever may accompany oral and genital attacks.

The *ocular lesions* start with intense periorbital pain and photophobia. Jorizzo says that retinal vasculitis ("posterior uveitis") is the most classical eye sign and the chief cause of blindness. Conjunctivitis may be an early, and hypopyon a late, accompaniment of uveitis. Iridocyclitis is frequently seen. Both eyes are eventually involved. The disease untreated leads to blindness from optic atrophy or glaucoma or cataracts.

Neurologic manifestations are mostly in the central nervous system and resemble most closely those of multiple sclerosis. Remissions and exacerbations are the rule. O'Duffey and Goldstein reviewed seven such cases in 1976. Systemic steroid therapy was helpful.

Thrombophlebitis occurs with some frequency. Thrombosis of the superior vena cava may also occur.

Arthralgia is present in most cases in the form of polyarthritis.

Cadman has reported on pulmonary manifestations.

Jorizzo believes that in questionable cutaneous lesions (in which he would include only follicular or acneiform lesions), either leukocytoclastic vasculitis or a neutrophilic vascular reaction should be demonstrated, as a minimum diagnostic criterion.

COURSE. Usually the disease starts with one oral ulceration, followed by others. It may take years before additional lesions develop. Therefore, the diagnosis is acceptable in patients with only two classic signs in addition to oral ulcerations. In women anal and genital lesions predominate, often with subsequent involvement of the eyes. Although corticosteroid therapy has been found helpful, death may occur as early as two years after onset of signs and symptoms.

ETIOLOGY. Viral, immunologic, coagulopathic, bacterial, genetic, and ecologic causes have been postulated, but the evidence is still inconclusive for any of these. Haim has reviewed them, and Kaplan has discussed them in detail. Jorizzo et al advanced a theory to explain the cutaneous pustular vasculitis (pathergy). They found five patients who developed this as a reaction to injected histamine, and also found increased neutrophil chemotaxis to Zymosan-activated serum. They postulated that this enhanced chemotaxis would bring numerous neutrophils to the site of any cutaneous or synovial trauma, in response to the release of histamine and other mediators.

Studies of HLA antigens associated with Behçet's syndrome in Turkey revealed a high proportion of HLA-B5 patients. HLA-Bw51 is also associated with susceptibility to this disease, as it is derived from the HLA-B5 antigen. Large British and Japanese studies link disease susceptibility to HLA-B51 and HLA-DRw-52, while there is a decreased incidence of HLA-DR1 and HLA-DOW-1.

INCIDENCE. Both sexes are involved, with male predominance. Young people in the second through fourth decades are affected, with the mean age of onset being 30 years. The disease occurs throughout the world.

HISTOLOGY. The early lesions show a leukocytoclastic vasculitis. There is perivascular infiltration, which is chiefly lymphocytic in older lesions, with endothelial proliferation which obliterates the lumen. Honma in 1981 reported finding atypical lymphocytes indistinguishable from Sézary cells in the oral aphthae of all of four patients with Behçet's syndrome.

DIFFERENTIAL DIAGNOSIS. A *skin puncture* or *pathergy test* is done by injecting 0.1 ml of normal saline solution into the skin, or simply pricking the skin with a sterile needle. A pustule appears at the site within 24 hours. Sharquie used the test to evaluate the effect of dapsone treatment. A negative test should be repeated at two to five points before being accepted. Kaplinsky reported a patient in whom this reaction was misinterpreted as a positive reaction to tuberculin.

Behçet's disease must be differentiated from herpetic or aphthous stomatitis, pemphigus, oral cancer, and Stevens-Johnson syndrome (erythema multiforme).

TREATMENT. Usually the ulcerations heal spontaneously. Mild mouthwashes and restricted use of the toothbrush should be prescribed when there are oral lesions. On the whole, the therapeutic problem of aphthosis is not the healing of the individual lesions but the prevention of new attacks. For that purpose all medications, local and systemic, have generally been unsatisfactory, except for control by systemic corticosteroids, and thalidomide (not available in the U.S.). Saylan et al, using thalidomide 200 mg twice a day for five days and 100 mg twice a day for 15 to 60 days, found that it caused rapid healing of aphthae and reduced recurrences. It had no effect on iridocyclitis.

Fellner and Kantor kept a patient free of lesions for over a year on 15 to 20 mg of prednisone daily. However, this dose will produce osteoporosis within three years, and if it must be continued, efforts should be made to switch to intramuscular triamcinolone, 40 to 60 mg monthly or as often as symptoms require.

Azathioprine (Imuran) has been combined with steroids in many centers in recent years, and Jorizzo says there is a role for chlorambucil in refractory cases. In a dose of 0.1 mg/kg/day, O'Duffy et al found it more effective than steroids; legal blindness occurred in one third of cases during steroid therapy and in only 1 in 12 during chlorambucil treatment. Pezzi et al found it effective against retinal vasculitis.

Cyclosporin (Sandimmune) has had experimental trials, and in Masuda's hands, according to Jorizzo, was more effective for oral lesions than colchicine. Nussenblatt et al found cyclosporin, 10 mg/kg/day, effective over periods of six to 21 months in patients refractory to cytotoxic or steroid therapy, or both.

Levamisole was found effective by Lehner, by de Merieux, and by Hamza et al.

Acyclovir produced prompt and sustained healing of oral ulcerations in a patient treated by Prieto et al.

Hazen and Michel noted improvement in one patient with concomitant vasculitis and Behçet's syndrome treated with 0.6 mg of colchicine three times a day. Both Raynor et al and Harper et al found it effective in a twice-daily dose; Aktulga et al, in a double-blind study, found it ineffective.

Aktulga E, et al: A double bind study of colchicine in Behçet's disease. Haematologica 1980, 65:399.
Arbesfeld SJ, et al: Behçet's disease. JAAD 1988, 19:767.
Cadman EC, et al: Pulmonary manifestations in Behçet's syndrome. Arch Intern Med 1976, 136:944.
Chajek T, et al: Behçet's disease. Medicine 1975, 54:179.
DeMerieux P, et al: Treatment of Behçet's syndrome with levamisole. Arth Rheum 1981, 24:64.
Ffrench-Constant C, et al: Cyclosporine in Behçet's disease. Lancet 1983, 2:454.
Firat T: Results of immunosuppressive treatment in Behçet's disease. Ann Ophthalmol 1978, 10:1421.
Fishel B, et al: Poliomyelitis vaccine in the treatment of Behçet's syndrome (letter). JAMA 1980, 116:1348.
Haim S: Pathogenesis of Behçet's disease. Int J Dermatol 1983, 22:102.
Hamza M, et al: Treatment of Behçet's disease with levamisole. Arth Rheum 1982, 25:714.
Harper RM, et al: Use of colchicine in the treatment of Behçet's disease. Int J Dermatol 1982, 21:551.
Honma T, et al: Intraepithelial atypical lymphocytes in oral lesions of Behçet's syndrome. Arch Dermatol 1981, 117:83.
Jorizzo JL: Behçet's disease: an update based in the 1985 International Conference in London. Arch Dermatol 1986, 122:556.
Idem, et al: Behçet's syndrome: immune regulation, circulating immune complexes, neutrophil migration, and colchicine therapy. JAAD 1984, 10:205.
Idem: Behçet's disease. Arch Dermatol 1986, 122:556.
Idem: Pustular vasculitis. JAAD 1983, 9:160.
Idem, et al: Complex aphthosis. JAAD 1985, 13:80.
Idem: Neutrophilic vascular reactions. JAAD 1988, 19:983.
Kaplan RP, et al: Behçet's disease. In Clinical Dermatology, Vol 2, Demis J (ed.) Hagerstown MD, Harper & Row, 1986.
Kaplinsky N, et al: False-positive tuberculin test in Behçet's syndrome. Cutis 1980, 25:529.
Michelson JB, et al: Behçet's disease. Surv Ophthal 1982, 26:190.
Nussenblatt RB, et al: Effectiveness of cyclosporin therapy for Behçet's disease. Arth Rheum 1985, 28:671.
O'Duffy JD, et al: Chlorambucil in the treatment of uveitis and meningoencephalitis of Behçet's disease. Am J Med 1984, 76:75.
Idem: Neurologic involvement in seven patients with Behçet's disease. Am J Med 1976, 61:170.
Pezzi PP, et al: Prognosis in Behçet's disease. Ann Ophthalmol 1985, 17:20.
Prieto J, et al: Acyclovir and Behçet's disease (letter). Ann Intern Med 1984, 101:566.
Raynor A, et al: Behçet's disease: treatment with colchicine. JAAD 1980, 2:296.
Sander HM, et al: Use of colchicine in Behçet's syndrome. Cutis 1986, 37:344.
Saylan T, et al: Thalidomide in the treatment of Behçet's syndrome. Arch Dermatol 1982, 118:536.
Sharquie KE: Suppression of Behçet's disease with dapsone. Br J Dermatol 1984, 110:493.
Tabbara KF: Chlorambucil in Behçet's disease. Ophthalmology 1983, 90:906.
Tokoro Y, et al: Skin lesions in Behçet's disease. Int J Dermatol 1977, 16:227.
Wilcox CG: Behçet's disease: a review. J Assoc Milit Dermatol 1983, 9:23.
Wong R, et al: Behçet's disease. Int J Dermatol 1984, 23:25.

"ELECTROGALVANIC" NONLESIONS

In 1932, Everett Lain published an account of "electrogalvanic" lesions of the oral mucosa, which he attributed to electric currents generated by dissimilar metals—gold, and mercury or silver—in dental fillings. He used a microammeter between the fillings to demonstrate the existence of the electric current. Currents of 1–40 μA were measured.

Mackert states that a survey of 1000 patients at Northwestern University failed to disclose any lesions in the oral mucosa attributable to or even associated with dissimilar metals in their dental restorations. He also points out that a microammeter gives meaningful readings only when placed in series in a circuit, and that this puts it in parallel, not series. Because of its very low resistance, it gives fictitiously high readings, indicating a current flow large enough (100 μA) to completely destroy a 150-mg amalgam filling in about three weeks.

It seems that Sutton's skeptical reception of this work was sound: he said such currents must be very small, probably inconsequential in intensity, and that it was doubtful if they produced any mucosal lesions. He had never seen any. Nor have we.

Nevertheless, Ayres Jr stated that he had relieved distressing symptoms in the mouths of numerous patients, and caused a variety of lesions to heal, by eliminating dissimilar metallic dental restorations. We feel the evidence is that oral lesions are not caused by such an etiology.

Ayres S Jr: Amalgam and gold dental fillings: reaction from electrogalvanic current. JAAD 1986, 14:277.

Idem: Sore mouth caused by electro-galvanic current. J Soc Med 1984, 77:708.

Idem, et al: Problem of electro-galvanism in the oral cavity caused by dissimilar dental metals. J Am Dent Assoc 1940, 27:1765.

Lain ES: Chemical and electrolytic lesions of the mouth caused by artificial [sic] dentures. Arch Dermatol 1932, 25:21.

Mackert JR Jr: Reply. JAAD 1986, 14:277.

Mills RB, in Reed GJ et al: Galvanism in the oral cavity. J Am Dent Assoc 1940, 27:1471.

Sutton RL Jr: Diseases of the Skin, ed 11, St. Louis, C. V. Mosby Co., p. 1399, 1956.

35

Cutaneous Vascular Diseases

The cutaneous blood vessels are affected in most skin diseases, and circulatory and vascular alterations are the predominant features in many diseases that have been described elsewhere. There remain others for consideration.

VASOMOTOR DISORDERS

RAYNAUD'S PHENOMENON AND RAYNAUD'S DISEASE

"Raynaud's" means either Raynaud's *phenomenon* (in the presence of associated collagen vascular disease) or Raynaud's *disease* (in the absence of such disease). It is a distinction without a difference.

Raynaud's Phenomenon

This is produced by an intermittent constriction of the small digital arteries and arterioles. The digits have varying but symmetrical pallor, cyanosis, and rubor. The involved parts are affected in paroxysms by the attacks of ischemia, which cause them to become pale, cold to the touch, and numb. In time the parts may fail to regain their normal circulation between attacks and become persistently cyanotic and painful.

The phenomenon is more frequently observed in cold weather. When exposed to cold the digits become white (ischemic), then blue (cyanotic), and finally red (hyperemic). Emotional stress can also induce this reaction.

If this phenomenon persists over a long period, punctate superficial necrosis of the fingertips develops; later, even gangrene may occur.

Raynaud's phenomenon occurs most frequently in young to middle-aged women. It occurs with scleroderma, dermatomyositis, lupus erythematosus, mixed connective tissue disease (MCTD), Sjögren's syndrome, rheumatoid arthritis, and paroxysmal hemoglobinuria. Occlusive arterial diseases such as embolism, thromboangiitis obliterans, and arteriosclerosis obliterans may be present. In addition, various diseases of the nervous system, or cervical rib and scalenus anticus syndrome, may be involved. Physical trauma such as pneumatic hammer operation and that incurred by pianists and typists may also induce this phenomenon. Chemicals such as bleomycin or ergot may also be the cause. The clumping of red blood cells is believed to be responsible for the induction of Raynaud's phenomenon in cryoglobulinemia, polycythemia vera, and other disorders with high titers of circulating cold agglutinins. Priollet et al document the frequency of each of these diagnoses in 144 patients with Raynaud's phenomenon. Scleroderma was the underlying diagnosis in over half.

Priollet et al followed 73 patients with Raynaud's phenomenon without apparent underlying cause for nearly five years. They found that simple noninvasive tests could distinguish between those with Raynaud's *disease* (not secondary to an underlying cause) and those with Raynaud's *phenomenon* (secondary to underlying disease, or a forerunner of connective tissue disease). They found that 14 of 24 patients who showed an abnormality on history, physical examination, or serologic tests (sclerodactyly, digital pitted scars, puffy fingers with telangiectases, positive ANA test, acroösteolysis or subcutaneous calcification by x-ray of hands, basilar lung fibrosis on chest x-ray, changes on nailfold capillary microscopy [avascular "skip" areas with irregularly dilated capillary loops]) developed connective tissue disease. This confirmed the experience of Maricq et al that nailfold capillary changes are helpful prognostic indicators. Thompson et al and Scher et al extended this observation by finding PAS-positive globules in the proximal nailfold on biopsy. A search for anticentromere antibodies is part of the workup we recommend.

Raynaud's Disease

Raynaud's disease is a primary disorder of cold sensitivity in young women characterized by intermittent attacks of pallor, cyanosis, hyperemia, and numbness of the fingers, precipitated by emotional stress or by cold. The disease is bilateral, and gangrene occurs in less than 1 per cent of cases.

Diagnosis is made by the absence of any other disease such as those enumerated under Raynaud's phenomenon. The tests outlined above are recommended. In the absence of abnormalities, Priollet found that only one of 49 patients developed a connective tissue disease after being followed for 4.7 years. It may take many years of follow-up to prove this. While the current dictum is that Raynaud's disease should be present for two years before being classified as a primary process, Priollet found that the average time to develop connective tissue disease, in those that did develop it, was 11.5 years. The 97 patients reviewed by Sheiner et al had a very low incidence of associated disease. In the absence of abnormal test results, the prognosis appears to be good.

TREATMENT. The following discussion applies to both Raynaud's phenomenon and Raynaud's disease. Exposure to cold should be avoided as much as possible. This includes avoidance of exposure to cold, not only of the extremities, but also of other parts of the body, since vasospasm may be induced by cooling of the body alone. Warm gloves should be worn whenever possible. Residence in a warm climate is helpful. Trauma to the fingertips should be avoided. Smoking is forbidden.

Nifedipine, 10–20 mg three times a day, benefitted 60 per cent of patients treated by Rodeheffer et al in a randomized, double-blind, crossover trial. This confirmed an earlier similar report by C. D. Smith et al, in which 12 of 17 patients elected to continue the therapy after the trial.

Induction of vasodilatation by immersion of the hands in water at 43°C during exposure of the whole

body to cold (0°C) was shown by Jobe to be effective in relieving the symptoms of Raynaud's syndrome; the effect was attributed to a Pavlovian conditioned response.

Ely has seen symtomatic relief and healing of ulcerations as a result of giving 400 mg of pentoxifylline (Trental) t.i.d. The drug improves the membrane flexibility of red blood cells, reduces blood viscosity, and retards platelet aggregation.

Prazosin (Minipress), an antihypertensive agent, 1 mg t.i.d. increased gradually to 3 mg t.i.d., effected over 50 per cent reduction in frequency of attacks in 20 patients with progressive systemic sclerosis and Raynaud's phenomenon treated by Surwit et al. There were few side effects, none of them serious.

Ketanserin, a selective 5-hydroxytryptamine receptor antagonist, gave good responses in 83 per cent of 18 cases of systemic sclerosis with Raynaud's, according to Seibold et al.

Estrogen therapy has been found to relieve some cases of Raynaud's disease in menopausal women. Tolazoline hydrochloride (Priscoline), 50 mg three times daily, is frequently helpful in mild cases, if the patient does not experience severe side effects.

Charles and Carmick reported benefit in Raynaud's disease in six of seven patients treated with micronized griseofulvin (500 to 1000 mg daily).

Romeo, Whalen, and Tindall achieved excellent results with the intraarterial injection of reserpine. However, Surwit et al were unable to show any response to 1.5 mg of reserpine intra-arterially in 12 subjects with Raynaud's disease, three of them with progressive systemic sclerosis. The systemic vascular effects exceeded the localized effect in both magnitude and duration. This treatment is not recommended.

The local application of 2 per cent nitroglycerin in an ointment base (Nitrobid, Nitrostat) rubbed in well several times will give relief to some patients in two hours or so. Sublingual administration of nitroglycerin was effective in only two of ten patients treated by Peterson et al, while eight of ten were improved by biofeedback training, even eight weeks after the sessions were over. Sublingual nitroglycerin may be more effective if combined with oral sympatholytic agents, as Franks did in his study of topical nitroglycerin. Additionally, sublingual nitroglycerin might be useful in patients with infrequent attacks, as it is convenient and easily administered, and has few side effects.

In severe disabling cases of Raynaud's with trophic changes, sympathectomy has been recommended. Sympathetic ganglionectomy with resection of the sympathetic trunk for both the upper and lower extremities has produced good or excellent results in some 65 per cent of patients in the hands of Allen and his associates. These effects are often only temporary, lasting for some six months to two years.

Adoue D, et al: Raynaud's phenomenon after chemotherapy. Ann Dermatol Venereol (Stockh) 1985, 112:151.

Cohen SR, et al: Vibration syndrome. Arch Dermatol 1985, 121:1544.

Franks AG Jr: Topical glyceryl trinitrate as adjunctive treatment in Raynaud's disease. Lancet 1982, 1:76.

Hoffman GS: Raynaud's disease and phenomenon. Am Family Phys 1980, 21:91.

Jackson R: Raynaud and Molière. Arch Dermatol 1983, 119:263.

Jobe JB: Induced vasodilatation as treatment for Raynaud's disease. Ann Intern Med 1982, 97:706.

Maricq HR, et al: Diagnostic potential of in vivo capillary microscopy in scleroderma and related disorders. Arthritis Rheum 1980, 23:183.

Minkin W, et al: Office nail fold microscopy using the ophthalmoscope. JAAD 1982, 7:190.

Peterson LL, et al: Raynaud's syndrome: treatment with sublingual nitroglycerine, swinging arm maneuver, and biofeedback training. Arch Dermatol 1983, 119:396.

Priollet P, et al: How to classify Raynaud's phenomenon. Am J Med 1987, 83:494.

Rodeheffer RJ, et al: Controlled double-blind trial of nifedipine in treatment of Raynaud's phenomenon. N Engl J Med 1983, 308:880.

Scher RK, et al: The clinical significance of periodic acid–Schiff-positive deposits in cuticle–proximal nail fold biopsy specimens. Arch Dermatol 1985, 121:1406.

Seibold JR, et al: Treatment of Raynaud's phenomenon with ketanserin, a selective antagonist of the serotonin$_2$ (5-HT$_2$) receptor. Arthritis Rheum 1984, 27:139.

Sheiner NM, et al: Isolated Raynaud's phenomenon. Ann Allergy 1987, 58:114.

Smith CD, et al: Controlled trial of nifedipine in the treatment of Raynaud's phenomenon. Lancet 1982, 2:1299.

Strandon E, et al: Treatment of Raynaud's phenomenon with the 5-HT$_2$ receptor antagonist ketanserin. Br Med J 1982, 285:1069.

Statham BN, et al: Quantification of the nail fold capillary abnormalities in systemic sclerosis and Raynaud's syndrome. Acta Dermatol Venereol (Stockh) 1986, 66:139.

Surwit RS, et al: Intra-arterial reserpine for Raynaud's syndrome: systemic reactions without therapeutic benefit. Arch Dermatol 1983, 119:733.

Idem: A double-blind study of prazosin in the treatment of Raynaud's phenomenon in scleroderma. Arch Dermatol 1984, 120:329.

Thompson RP, et al: Nail fold biopsy in scleroderma and related disorders. Arthritis Rheum 1984, 27:97.

Tindall JP, et al: Medical uses of intra-arterial injections of reserpine. Arch Dermatol 1974, 110:233.

ERYTHROMELALGIA

Also called erythermalgia and acromelalgia, this rare form of paroxysmal vasodilation affects the feet with burning, localized pain, redness, and heat, with high skin temperature. Infrequently the upper extremities may be involved.

The burning paroxysms may last from a few minutes to several days; they are usually triggered by an increase in environmental temperature.

The disease may be primary or secondary to a myeloproliferative disease such as polycythemia vera or thrombocythemia. Peripheral neuritis, myelitis, or multiple sclerosis may be present. Secondary erythromelalgia has also been associated with systemic lupus erythematosus, hypertension, and diabetes mellitus. Calcium channel blockers may exacerbate or even induce it. One of us (WDJ) saw it apparently induced by amantadine, given for infectious mononucleosis.

Uno and Parker found that autonomic nerve plexuses in the involved skin of an erythromelalgic patient were sparse and only feebly branching as compared with the plexuses in skin from the patient's own buttock or the skin of a normal foot. They postulated that the local reduction of perivascular adrenergic nerves induced a condition similar to that caused by sympathectomy.

The severe symptoms are relieved by measures (such as immersion in cold water) that cool the skin. Prolonged relief may be obtained by the use of aspirin. However, Cohen et al described two cases in siblings in which 650 mg of aspirin every six hours afforded no relief, and naproxen, dipyridamole, and 2 per cent nitroglycerin ointment all failed.

Michiels et al found aspirin and indomethacin effective in 26 patients, out of 40 with thrombocythemia, presenting with erythromelalgia; busulfan-induced remissions of thrombocythemia also alleviated the erythromelalgia. Good results have been obtained with methysergide, which suggests that this may be a disease of peripheral serotonin activity. Other treatment suggestions have been epinephrine, ephedrine, sublingual isoproterenol hydrochloride, nitroglycerin ointment, prednisone, phlebotomy, sodium nitroprusside, lumbar ganglionectomy, and peripheral nerve block or section.

Cohen IJ, et al: Familial erythromelalgia. Arch Dermatol 1982, 118:953.

Dilmen U, et al: Treatment of erythromelalgia. Arch Dermatol 1983, 119:793.

Michiels JJ, et al: Erythromelalgia caused by platelet-mediated arteriolar inflammation and thrombosis in thrombocytopenia. Ann Intern Med 1985, 102:466.

Ratz JL, et al: Erythermalgia with vasculitis: a review. JAAD 1979, 1:443.

Stern R, et al: Cutaneous adverse reactions associated with calcium channel blockers. Arch Intern Med 1989, 149:829.

Uno H, et al: Autonomic innervation of the skin in primary erythermalgia. Arch Dermatol 1983, 119:65.

LIVEDO RETICULARIS

Livedo reticularis is a mottled or reticulated pink or reddish blue discoloration of the skin, mostly on the extremities, especially the lower legs around the ankles. It also affects the feet, thighs, trunk, and forearms. Exposure to cold usually emphasizes the intensity of discoloration, although the lesions are fixed and remain present on warming. Usually the lesions are asymptomatic; in other instances, coldness, numbness, paresthesia, or a dull ache may be present.

Livedo reticularis may be a manifestation of lupus erythematosus, dermatomyositis, scleroderma, rheumatic fever, or rheumatoid arthritis. It may be seen with cryoglobulinemia, syphilis, meningococcemia, pneumococcal sepsis, tuberculosis, pancreatitis, decompression sickness, various forms of arteritis, polycythemia vera, hypercalcemia, pheochromocy-

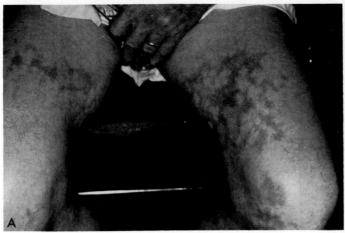
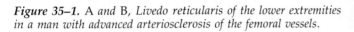
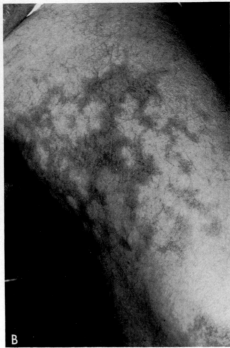

Figure 35–1. A *and* B, *Livedo reticularis of the lower extremities in a man with advanced arteriosclerosis of the femoral vessels.*

toma, mycosis fungoides, and thrombocytopenic purpura. Bruce et al observed it as a photosensitivity phenomenon in a patient who was taking quinidine. Manzi et al reported a similar case in 1989. It has been reported repeatedly as a side effect of amantadine (Symmetrel). Most cases, however, are unassociated with any disease.

Kalter et al reported its occurrence in three patients with advanced arteriosclerotic vascular disease in whom it was caused by *multiple cholesterol emboli.* Falanga et al found that 35 per cent of patients with cholesterol emboli had skin lesions; in half of them, the lesions were livedo reticularis. Some had cyanosis, purpura, nodules, ulceration, or gangrene. Older men with severe atherosclerotic disease are most affected. Patients are often on anticoagulant therapy and many have recently undergone vascular surgery. Differential diagnosis usually includes vasculitis and periarteritis nodosa. There is 72 per cent mortality. Deep biopsy with serial sections usually permits a diagnosis. Livedo reticularis of recent onset in an elderly person warrants consideration of this diagnosis.

Sneddon's syndrome is the association of livedo reticularis, usually in young to middle-aged patients who then develop a cerebrovascular lesion. It may have a genetic component and is likely to be severe and progressive. Deffer et al and Rebollo et al have reviewed this syndrome. Some patients have antiphospholipid antibodies and may have incipient systemic lupus erythematosus (SLE).

Oxalosis may lead to livedo reticularis from deposition of oxalate crystals in and around blood vessel walls. The primary type comprises two rare autosomal recessive disorders, each lacking one specific enzyme. Secondary forms also occur. The character-

istic crystals are seen on biopsy. Gupta et al have recently reviewed this.

Weinstein et al reported that 38 of 78 consecutive patients with *systemic lupus erythematosus* had livedo reticularis, which, when moderately severe, was apt to be associated with more severe disease manifestations such as central nervous system disease, renal disease, vasculitis, and cardiolipin antibodies. The full spectrum of cutaneous changes secondary to cardiolipin antibodies has been reviewed by Sontheimer, and was discussed under lupus erythematosus in Chapter 8.

Livedo reticularis is regarded as endovasculitis in which endothelial proliferation and thrombosis may occur in the more severe cases. It may be a manifestation of a small-vessel angiitis. Rarely, necrosis occurs.

Cutis marmorata is a term applied to skin resembling marble because of its mottled bluish discoloration. It is commonly seen on the lower extremities in young children and women exposed to cold. The mottling disappears when the extremities are warmed. It is a physiological mottling of the skin.

Livedo racemosa implies a mottled branching network which fades into normal skin at the edges. It is due to a patchy arterial disorder.

Bruce S, et al: Quinidine-induced photosensitive livedo reticularis–like eruption. JAAD 1985, 12:332.
Champion RH: Livedo reticularis: a review. Br J Dermatol 1965, 77:167.
Deffer TA, et al: Sneddon's syndrome. JAAD 1987, 16:1084.
Falanga V, et al: The cutaneous manifestations of cholesterol crystal embolization. Arch Dermatol 1986, 122:1194.
Greer KE, et al: Primary oxalosis with livedo reticularis. Arch Dermatol 1980, 116:213.

Gupta AK, et al: Multisystem crystalline deposits. Arch Dermatol 1989, 125:551.

Kalter DC, et al: Livedo reticularis due to multiple cholesterol emboli. JAAD 1985, 13:235.

Kaplan RP, et al: Dermatologic features of fat embolism syndrome. Cutis 1986, 36:52.

Manzi S, et al: An unusual photoactivated skin eruption. Arch Dermatol 1989, 126:417.

Rebollo M, et al: Livedo reticularis and cerebrovascular lesions (Sneddon's syndrome). Brain 1983, 106:965.

Rumpl E, et al: Cerebrovascular lesions and livedo reticularis (Sneddon's syndrome). J Neurol 1985, 231:324.

Rusonis PA, et al: Livedo reticularis and purpura. JAAD 1986, 15:1120.

Sontheimer RD: The anticardiolipin syndrome. Arch Dermatol 1987, 123:590.

Weinstein C, et al: Livedo reticularis associated with increased titers of anticardiolipin antibodies in systemic lupus erythematosus. Arch Dermatol 1987, 123:596.

LIVEDO VASCULITIS

Atrophie Blanche

Livedo vasculitis is a chronic, recurrent, *segmental hyalinizing vasculopathy* of the small blood vessels of the legs. The ulcers that may result from it heal with small stellate white scars called *atrophie blanche*. Other synonyms include *livedo reticularis with summer/winter ulcerations*.

Livedo vasculitis is characterized by initial petechiae, purpuric papules, or hemorrhagic bullae. Some heal without progression, while others pro-

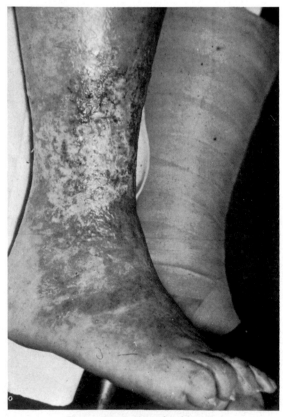

Figure 35–2. Atrophie blanche.

gress to ulcerations covered with an eschar, located around the ankles. Removal of the eschar reveals a deep, punched-out ulcer, which ultimately becomes a glossy white polyangular or stellate scar (atrophie blanche). Fibrin, C3, and IgM are almost always found in vessel walls, according to Schroeter. The surrounding area is discolored, brownish red, or violaceous, and frequently shows telangiectases.

Shornick et al and Milstone et al have both written excellent reviews of this entity. There are cases of idiopathic primary disease (unassociated with other disorders) and a second group with underlying arteriosclerosis, connective tissue disease, diabetes, dysproteinemia, hypertension, or stasis dermatitis. Yasue reported its occurrence in ten of 11 patients with systemic LE who eventually developed CNS involvement, and in three of 26 who had severe nephrotic lupus nephritis; it occurred in no others. He considers it of grave prognostic import.

Schroeter et al found evidence of abdominal aortic atherosclerosis, calcification, or aneurysm in seven of 42 cases (17 per cent). In one, the livedo vasculitis resolved following resection of the aneurysm.

Histologically, the small vessels of the mid and lower levels of the dermis show endothelial proliferations, hyaline degeneration, fibrin plugs, and thrombosis. A perivascular hemorrhage may be present. Because of the absence of polymorphonuclear neutrophils, Shornick et al make the point that this is not a vasculitis, but a vasculopathy, probably secondary to a platelet-aggregating disorder.

The condition has been successfully treated with a combination of phenformin and ethylestrenol, but aspirin and dipyridamole were effective in Kern's hands. He emphasized the importance of low dosage of aspirin, 325 or even 162 mg twice or once daily. To these Yamamoto et al added ticlopidine hydrochloride, a third antiplatelet drug, 200 mg a day. Minidose heparin, as little as 5000 units every three days, was effective in the hands of Jetton et al. Nifedipine, 10 mg three times a day, produced healing in a patient of Purcell et al in whom dipyridamole and aspirin had failed. Gordon Sauer reported six cases in 1986 healed with pentoxyphylline, 400 mg two or three times a day, with 400 mg a day for maintenance. Sams had similar success in his eight patients, as has Ely, who is one of its strongest advocates. Superinfection of ulcers should be treated with systemic antibiotics, and skin grafts to large ulcers, in patients whose disease has responded to therapy, will expedite recovery.

Drucker CR, et al: Antiplatelet therapy in atrophie blanche and livedo vasculitis. JAAD 1982, 7:359.

Ely PH, et al: Therapy of livedo vasculitis with pentoxyfylline. Cutis 1988, 42:448.

Heine KG, et al: Idiopathic atrophie blanche. Arch Dermatol 1986, 122:855.

Jetton RL, et al: Minidose heparin therapy for vasculitis of atrophie blanche. JAAD 1983, 8:23.

Kern AB: Atrophie blanche: report of two patients treated with aspirin and dipyridamole. JAAD 1982, 6:1048.

Milstone LM, et al: Classification and therapy of atrophie blanche. Arch Dermatol 1983, 119:963.

Purcell SM, et al: Nifedipine treatment of idiopathic atrophie blanche (letter). JAAD 1986, 14:851.

Sams WM Jr: Livedo vasculitis. Arch Dermatol 1988, 124:684.

Sauer GC: Pentoxifylline (Trental) therapy for the vasculitis of atrophie blanche. Arch Dermatol 1986, 122:380.

Schroeter AL, et al: The vasculitis of atrophie blanche (livedoid vasculitis) and abdominal aortic pathology. Cutis 1984, 34:298.

Shornick JK, et al: Idiopathic atrophie blanche. JAAD 1983, 8:792.

Yamamoto M, et al: Antithrombotic treatment in livedo vasculitis. JAAD 1988, 18:57.

Yasue T: Livedoid vasculitis and central nervous system involvement in systemic lupus erythematosus. Arch Dermatol 1986, 122:66.

Atrophie Noire

Atrophie noire, as described by Shelley and his associates, is characterized by sharply circumscribed, slate blue-black, pigmented patches on the ankles with small scattered ulcers in the pigmented areas. The pigmented patches result from recurrent episodes of dermatitis with ulceration.

Histologically, fibrosis, hyperkeratosis, and a prominent granular layer are evident. The edematous dermis contains numerous dilated capillaries; extracellular pigment is profuse in the dermis.

Shelley WB, et al: Unique pigment in skin macrophages associated with recurrent painful ankle ulcers: atrophie noire. Arch Dermatol 1969, 99:398.

MARSHALL-WHITE SYNDROME ("Bier's Spots")

The marbled mottling produced in the forearm and hand by occluding the brachial artery with a tight sphygmomanometer cuff is characterized initially, and chiefly, by pale macules 1 or 2 cm in diameter, which were described by Bier in 1898 and are known as "Bier's spots." Wilkin reexamined this phenomenon with laser Doppler velocimetry in 1986 and concluded that the red spots which also appear (chiefly on the hand) are caused by relative vasodilatation, with vasoconstriction in the pale areas.

The Marshall-White syndrome consists of Bier's spots, associated with insomnia and tachycardia. These pale macules are cooler than the surrounding pink skin and become more apparent when the hands are lowered for some time. This syndrome has been noted in white middle-aged men of psychoneurotic disposition.

Marshall W, et al: Dermatologic and psychosomatic aspects of Marshall-White syndrome. Cutis 1965, 1:184.

Wilkin JK, et al: Bier's spots reconsidered: a tale of two spots, with speculation in a humerous vein. JAAD 1986, 14:411.

PURPURA

Purpura is multifocal extravasation of blood into the skin or mucous membrane. It is manifested by distinctive brownish red or purplish macules a few millimeters in diameter resulting from the rupture of the capillary walls at the arteriolar-capillary junction. Several types of purpura are recognized.

Petechiae are superficial, pinhead-sized (less than 3 mm), round, hemorrhagic macules, bright red at first, then brownish or rust colored. They are most commonly seen in the dependent areas, are evanescent, occur in crops, regress over a period of days, and most often imply a disorder of platelets, usually thrombocytopenia. They may also be a sign of a blood vessel disease, such as scurvy or amyloidosis; however, they are not usually indicative of a coagulation factor disorder. These disorders typically give rise to ecchymoses or hematomas.

Ecchymoses are better known as bruises or "black and blue marks." These extravasations signify a deeper and more extensive interstitial hemorrhage, which forms a flat, irregularly shaped, bluish-purplish patch. Such patches gradually turn yellowish and finally fade away.

Vibices (singular, *vibex*) means linear purpuric lesions.

Hematoma designates a pool-like collection of extravasated blood in a dead space in tissue which, if of sufficient size, produces a swelling that fluctuates on palpation. Hematomas are usually walled off by tissue planes and produce massive swellings.

It is useful to classify purpura as thrombocytopenic (caused by decreased platelets) or nonthrombocytopenic (caused by a coagulation defect, vasculitis, or a connective tissue disease).

Lever classifies the purpuras as inflammatory and noninflammatory, depending upon the changes in the walls of the blood vessels. In the noninflammatory group are included stasis purpura, thrombocytopenic purpura, scurvy, senile purpura, coumarin necrosis, autoerythrocyte sensitization purpura, thrombotic thrombocytopenic purpura, and purpura fulminans. In the inflammatory type he places bacterial (meningococcic) purpura, drug allergy purpura, allergic vasculitis, mixed cryoglobulinemia, pityriasis lichenoides et varioliformis acuta, and purpura pigmentosa chronica.

In addition to the above classifications, purpura is also classifiable as flat purpura (noninflammatory) and palpable purpura, as seen in necrotizing angiitis. Sams Jr, Fauci, Braverman, and others have emphasized this valuable clinical clue.

Taylor et al suggest a good working approach to a patient with a bleeding disorder. Evaluation of the presenting complaint may suggest a *platelet defect* (petechiae) or a *clotting defect* (hematoma, or prolonged bleeding). The history should include questions concerning the following: Congenital or acquired? What circumstances lead to bleeding? Is there bleeding from orifices? Prolonged menses? Bleeding after surgery? Previous blood transfusion? Drug history? Family history?

Physical examination should stress the size, type, and distribution of any skin lesions; a search for telangiectases; a joint examination; and an evaluation of skin elasticity, unusual scars, and unusual body habitus. A general screening laboratory examination should include a complete hemogram and platelet count; bleeding, clotting, and partial thromboplastin times; and thrombin clot retraction. After this evaluation, more extensive testing in the suspected area of abnormality (platelets, coagulation disorders, or connective tissue defect) may be indicated.

Rasmussen JE: Puzzling purpuras in children and young adults. JAAD 1982, 6:67.
Taylor RE, et al: Clinical evaluation of the patient with bruising and bleeding. JAAD 1981, 4:348.

THROMBOCYTOPENIC PURPURA

Thrombocytopenic purpura may be classified, as Bithel recommends, into three large categories: states

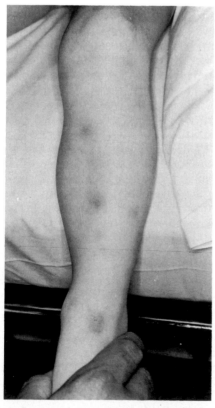

Figure 35–3. Bruises of autoimmune thrombocytopenic purpura in a young child following a viral infection.

due to accelerated platelet destruction, states due to deficient platelet production, and states due to complex, often unknown pathogenesis. The latter two categories will not be discussed here because they are generally in the province of hematologists, being due to such diseases as aplastic anemia and leukemia. Accelerated platelet destruction may be immunologic or nonimmunologic. The former may be due to antibodies (idiopathic or drug-induced thrombocytopenia), isoantibodies (congenital, or posttransfusion), immune complex disease, or other immunologic processes such as erythroblastosis fetalis, neonatal lupus, scleroderma, other connective tissue diseases, or AIDS. The group of thrombocytopenias with accelerated platelet destruction due to nonimmunologic processes includes thrombotic thrombocytopenic purpura and disseminated intravascular coagulation.

Idiopathic Thrombocytopenic Purpura

This is also known as *autoimmune thrombocytopenic purpura,* or Werlhof's disease. It is characterized by either an acute or gradual onset of petechiae or ecchymoses in the skin and mucous membranes, especially in the mouth. Epistaxis, conjunctival hemorrhages, hemorrhagic bullae in the mouth (which was the presenting sign in a case reported by James et al), and gingival bleeding may occur. Melena, hematemesis, and menorrhagia also occur, and the latter may be the first sign of this disease in young women. Chronic leg ulcers occasionally develop.

The presence of splenomegaly usually (but not always) excludes the diagnosis of immune thrombocytopenic purpura. No other noteworthy sign or symptom is present.

Bleeding occurs when the platelet count drops below 50,000. Clear-cut posttraumatic hemorrhage, some spontaneous hemorrhage, and petechiae may appear. The risk of serious hemorrhage is greatly increased at levels below 10,000, and the gravest complication, intracranial hemorrhage, most often occurs with counts below 2,000. Bleeding time is usually prolonged and coagulation time is normal, whereas the clot retraction is abnormal and capillary fragility is increased. Increased numbers of megakaryocytes are found in the bone marrow.

The acute variety most often occurs in children, following a seasonal viral illness in 50 per cent of patients. The average lag between purpura and preceding infection is two weeks. Most of these cases resolve spontaneously or with minimal therapy. A few patients will develop the chronic variety and a few deaths, usually from cerebral hemorrhage, have been reported in patients not treated with steroids.

The chronic form occurs most often in adults; is persistent, lasting years to indefinitely; and has a female:male ratio of between 2:1 and 4:1.

The intermittent variety may occur in childhood or adulthood and is interrupted by intervals free from disease.

Idiopathic thrombocytopenic purpura is the result of platelet injury by antibodies of the IgG class. They coat the platelets, triggering their removal by the spleen after a greatly reduced survival time, which may last from minutes to a few hours.

Hoffman et al reported a patient in whom megakaryocytes were absent from the bone marrow during attacks, apparently as a result of an antibody toxic to megakaryocyte progenitor cells. Immunosuppressive therapy combined with plasmapheresis was effective.

Treatment may be with corticosteroids, immunosuppressive drugs, blood transfusions, and splenectomy. Prednisone in a dose of 60 mg daily is usually effective in bringing about remission. Later the dosage is decreased as indicated.

Four of 14 patients responded to colchicine, 0.6 mg two to four times daily, according to Strother et al. Fourteen days appeared to be an adequate clinical trial.

Danazol was effective in 11 of 22 patients who did not do well on corticosteroids or splenectomy, according to Ahn et al.

Removal of a retroperitoneal accessory spleen identified by radionuclide scanning with Tc99M cured three patients treated by Wallace et al. In one the remission was lasting.

Baumann et al found intravenous high-dose gamma globulin too expensive for long-term use and too slow (at least 72 hours) for urgent use. In children, 90 per cent experience spontaneous remission, and a short course of steroids, or supportive measures alone, may be all that is needed. Adults may require three to four weeks of intensive steroid therapy before tapering is possible. Splenectomy in adults produces a remission in 80 to 85 per cent of cases. In unresponsive cases vincristine- or vinblastine-loaded platelets may be effective.

Platelet transfusions may be lifesaving in acutely ill patients who are actively bleeding. They do not increase the platelet counts and thus are not useful except in emergencies.

Drug-Induced Thrombocytopenia

Thrombocytopenic purpura due to drug-induced platelet antibodies may be caused by drugs such as sulfonamides, digoxin, quinine, quinidine, chlorothiazides, penicillin, phenylbutazone, acetaminophen, allopurinol, methyldopa, furosemide, gold salts, rifampin, and lidocaine.

Weintraub and his collaborators described a rapid diagnostic test to identify a thrombocytopenia-inducing drug by clot retraction studies. They modified the test by admixing the freshly drawn normal blood with small amounts of the patient's serum and the suspected drug.

Treatment consists of the removal of the offending agent. Recovery usually occurs shortly thereafter. Corticosteroids are helpful in moderately high dosage (60 mg prednisone daily) and are usually only necessary as a brief course. Offending drugs are contraindicated for life.

Thrombotic Thrombocytopenic Purpura

Also known as Moschcowitz's syndrome, this is a pentad of thrombocytopenia, hemolytic anemia, renal abnormalities, fever, and disturbance of the central nervous system. Purpura was present in 241 of 251 patients reviewed by Amorosi et al. Multiple ecchymoses, jaundice, pallid mucous membranes, and an enlarged spleen may be found. Other associated findings include arthritis, pleuritis, Raynaud's phenomenon, abdominal pain, and hepatomegaly. Tests may show a decreased hematocrit and decreased platelets. Goodman et al reported that a positive histologic diagnosis of thrombotic thrombocytopenic purpura was possible in seven of 18 gingival biopsies from 16 patients. Diagnostic findings were subendothelial hyaline deposits in capillaries and small arterioles; intraluminal deposits; and lack of inflammation in vessels or stroma. No such subendothelial deposits were seen in 154 control biopsies or in material from 50 unselected autopsies. Bone marrow biopsies probably yield a similar percentage of diagnostic findings. Moake et al reported unusually large Factor VIII:von Willebrand factor multimers in four cases, and suggested a defect in their processing as a reason for the vascular obstruction. Obstruction by platelet aggregates appeared to be the cause of death in a case given platelet transfusion by Harkness et al.

Until exchange plasmapheresis was instituted as the treatment of choice, 80 per cent of these patients died; now, 80 per cent survive. This procedure probably removes the Factor VIII multimers, or "TTP factor." Removal of 3 to 5 liters of plasma for four to ten days is required.

Rose et al reported that 37 per cent of survivors had relapses of their disease, often triggered by pregnancy, infection, or surgery. Most responded to plasma therapy again.

Abrams DI, et al: Antibodies to human T-lymphotropic virus type III and development of AIDS in homosexual men presenting with immune thrombocytopenia. Ann Intern Med 1986, 104:47.

Ahn YS, et al: Danazol for treatment of idiopathic thrombocytic purpura. N Engl J Med 1983, 308:1396.

Amorosi EL, et al: Thrombotic thrombocytopenic purpura. Medicine 1966, 45:139.

Baumann MA, et al: Urgent treatment of idiopathic thrombocytopenic purpura with single-dose gammaglobulin infusion followed by platelet transfusion. Ann Intern Med 1986, 104:808.

Bithel TC: Disorders of Platelets. In Fundamentals of Clinical Hematology, Thorup OAJ (ed.) Philadelphia, Saunders, pp 792–805, 1987.

Braddock SW, et al: Reticular erythematous mucinosis and thrombocytopenic purpura. JAAD 1988, 19:859.

Crain SM, et al: Thrombotic thrombocytopenic purpura. JAMA 1981, 246:1243.

Goodman A, et al: Gingival biopsy in thrombotic thrombocytopenic purpura. Ann Intern Med 1978, 89:501.

Harkness D: Hazard of platelet transfusion in thrombotic thrombocytopenic purpura. JAMA 1981, 246:1931.

Hoffman R, et al: Antibody cytotoxic to megakaryocyte progenitor cells in a patient with immune thrombocytopenic purpura. N Engl J Med 1985, 312:1170.

James WD, et al: Acute idiopathic thrombocytopenic purpura. Oral Surg 1984, 57:149.

Rose M, et al: High incidence of relapse in thrombotic thrombocytopenic purpura. Am J Med 1987, 83:437.

Rosove MH, et al: Ineffectiveness of aspirin and dipyridamole in treatment of thrombotic thrombocytopenic purpura. Ann Intern Med 1982, 96:27.

Stuart MJ, et al: Chronic idiopathic thrombocytopenic purpura: a familial immunodeficiency syndrome? JAMA 1978, 239:939.

Watson R, et al: Thrombocytopenia in the neonatal lupus syndrome. Arch Dermatol 1988, 124:560.

NONTHROMBOCYTOPENIC PURPURA

Dysproteinemic Purpura

PURPURA CRYOGLOBULINEMICA AND CRYOFIBRINOGENEMIA

Abnormal serum proteins behaving as cryoglobulins and cryofibrinogens may be IgG, IgM, or both. Cryoglobulinemic purpura occurs most frequently in multiple myeloma and macroglobulinemia and is of a monoclonal IgM, IgG, or Bence Jones cryoglobulin form. Mixed cryoglobulinemia, in which the cryoglobulins are of various classes, may be seen in systemic lupus erythematosus, rheumatoid arthritis, Sjögren's syndrome, and hepatitis B infection.

Purpura is most apt to occur on exposed surfaces

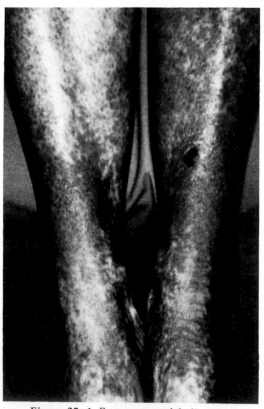

Figure 35–4. Purpura cryoglobulinemica.

after cold exposure in monoclonal disease, and biopsy reveals amorphous eosinophilic material in the vessel lumina. In the mixed type, dependent palpable purpura is present, which on biopsy reveals classic leukocytoclastic vasculitis. In *cryocrystalglobulin syndrome* crystalline deposits are seen in the corneas and joint spaces. Vasculitic skin lesions occur. Lukitsch et al reported a case with follicular hyperkeratosis. Martin described purpura, acral blisters, and ulceration in a patient with cryofibrinogenemia.

Purpura secondary to these abnormal serum proteins tends to be chronic. Plasmapheresis, systemic steroids, immunosuppressors, and colchicine are some options. Boom et al reported a prolonged remission after treatment with high-dose gamma globulin infusion.

Boom BW, et al: Severe leukocytoclastic vasculitis of skin in patients with essential mixed cryoglobulinemia treated with high dose gamma globulin intravenously. Arch Dermatol 1988, 124:1550.

Ellis FA: The cutaneous manifestations of cryoglobulinemia. Arch Dermatol 1964, 89:690.

Fauci AS: The spectrum of vasculitis. Ann Intern Med 1978, 89:660.

Lukitsch O, et al: Follicular hyperkeratosis and cryocrystalglobulinemia syndrome. Arch Dermatol 1985, 121:795.

Martin S: Cryofibrinogenemia, monoclonal gammopathy, and purpura. Arch Dermatol 1979, 115:208.

PURPURA HYPERGLOBULINEMICA

Waldenström's hyperglobulinemic purpura consists of episodic showers of petechiae occurring on all parts of the body, most profusely on the lower extremities. The dorsum of the foot is most intensely involved. The intensity of petechiae diminishes on the ascending parts of the feet. A diffuse "peppery" distribution is noted, resembling Schamberg's disease. The petechiae may be induced or aggravated by prolonged standing or walking, or by wearing constrictive garters or stockings.

The most distinctive laboratory finding is the protein electrophoresis of the serum. The hypergammaglobulinemia is heterogeneous or polyclonal and is demonstrated as a broad-based peak. The bulk of the protein increase is IgG, though occasionally increased amounts of IgA are also found. IgM is usually normal or decreased. Rheumatoid factor in varying amounts is present in almost all patients. Antithyroglobulins, increased rate of erythrocyte sedimentation, leukopenia, antinuclear factors, and proteinuria may be found.

Hyperglobulinemic purpura occurs almost exclusively in women and is frequently seen with Sjögren's syndrome, keratoconjunctivitis sicca, rheumatoid arthritis, and multiple myeloma; or it may be a primary phenomenon when it occurs as a chronic benign illness.

Histologically, the small vessels are the sites of perivascular infiltration of mononuclear cells and deposition of iron pigment. In some cases a necrotiz-

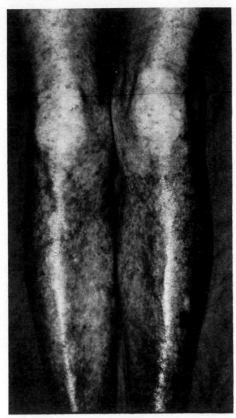

Figure 35–5. Purpura hyperglobulinemica.

ing vasculitis is present. Alexander et al presented evidence that when Waldenström's hyperglobulinemic purpura occurs in Sjögren's syndrome patients, about half show neutrophilic leucocytoclastic vasculitis and half show a mononuclear cell infiltrate. Leucocytoclastic vasculitis was correlated with high titers of Ro and La antibodies and general serohyperreactivity.

The course of the disease is essentially benign, but chronic. Hyperglobulinemic purpura may be a facet or harbinger of connective tissue diseases, and rarely, progression to myeloma has been reported. Steroids are usually not of benefit; however, the case of Hudson et al showed some response to them. Measures to obviate stasis are recommended. Chlorambucil reduces the purpura but does not effect gross changes in the protein abnormality.

Alexander E, et al: Sjögren's syndrome. Arch Dermatol 1987, 123:801.
Hudson CP, et al: Cutaneous leukocytoclastic vasculitis with hyperglobulinemia and splenomegaly. Arch Dermatol 1984, 120:1224.
Kyle RA, et al: Benign hypergammaglobulinemic purpura of Waldenström. Medicine 1971, 50:113.
Olmstead AD, et al: Immune complexes in the pathogenesis of hypergammaglobulinemic purpura. JAAD 1980, 3:174.

WALDENSTRÖM'S MACROGLOBULINEMIA

In 1944 Waldenström described an entity characterized by bleeding from the mucous membranes of the mouth and nose, lymphadenopathy, hepatosplenomegaly, hemorrhage of the retinae, and rarely purpura. Gastrointestinal bleeding, and anemia, may occur. This disease occurs mostly in elderly men who have oronasal bleeding, and represents a plasma cell dyscrasia with lymphocytic infiltration of marrow and lymphoid organs which may be frank malignant lymphoma.

Two types of skin lesion may occur: violaceous to red indurated plaques, infiltrated with atypical lymphoid cells; or alternatively, translucent papules full of amorphous eosinophilic material which has proved on direct immunofluorescence to be IgM. Nonspecific cutaneous findings include Raynaud's, amyloidosis, pruritus, xanthomatosis, and urticaria. Some patients with urticaria and macroglobulinemia *(Schnitzler's syndrome)* satisfy the criteria for Waldenström's macroglobulinemia.

Large amounts of monoclonal IgM are responsible for the variable clinical pattern. Fibrinogenopenia, fibrinolysis, circulating anticoagulants, coagulation factor deficiencies, intravascular or perivascular deposition of paraprotein, or associated cryoglobulinemia or cryofibrinogenemia may result in the bleeding tendencies.

Bouroncle and Doan reported favorable results from treatment with cyclophosphamide and corticosteroids. Plasmapheresis until adequate doses of chlorambucil have been administered is the generally utilized treatment.

Hanke CW, et al: Cutaneous macroglobulinosis. Arch Dermatol 1980, 116:575.
Janier M, et al: Chronic urticaria and macroglobulinemia (Schnitzler's syndrome). JAAD 1988, 20:206.
Mascaro JM, et al: Specific cutaneous manifestations of Waldenström's macroglobulinemia. Br J Dermatol 1982, 106:217.
Pujol RM, et al: Urticarial dermatosis associated with Waldenström's macroglobulinemia. JAAD 1989, 20:855.
Tichenor RE, et al: Macroglobulinemia cutis. Arch Dermatol 1978, 114:280.

PURPURA SECONDARY TO CLOTTING DISORDERS

Hereditary disorders of blood coagulation usually result from a deficiency or qualitative abnormality of a single coagulation factor, as in hemophilia or von Willebrand's disease. Acquired disorders commonly result from multiple coagulation factor deficiencies, as in liver disease, biliary tract obstruction, malabsorption, or drug ingestion, or may also involve platelet and vascular abnormalities, such as disseminated intravascular coagulation. Hemorrhagic manifestations are common and may be severe, especially in hereditary forms. Ecchymoses and subcutaneous hematomas are common, especially on the legs. Severe hemorrhage may follow trauma, and hemarthrosis is frequent. Other hemorrhagic manifestations include respiratory obstruction due to hemorrhage into the tongue, throat, or neck; epistaxis;

gastrointestinal and genitourinary tract bleeding; and rarely central nervous system hemorrhage.

Taylor RE, et al: Clinical evaluation of the patient with bleeding and bruising. JAAD 1981, 4:348.

DRUG PURPURA

A list of drugs has already been given which induce antiplatelet antibodies; however, drug-induced purpura may occur without platelet destruction, as a manifestation of anaphylactoid purpura. Some purpurogenic drugs are the following: aspirin and other nonsteroidal antiinflammatory agents, allopurinol, thiazides, gold, sulfonamides, cephalosporins, hydralazine, phenytoin, quinidine, and penicillin. Cocaine thrombosis with widespread infarctive skin lesions was reported by Heng et al.

Heng MCY, et al: Thrombotic phenomenon associated with intravenous cocaine. JAAD 1987, 16:462.

SOLAR PURPURA
(Senile Purpura, Actinic Purpura)

Solar purpura is characterized by large (1 to 5 cm), sharply outlined, dark purplish red ecchymoses appearing on the dorsa of the forearms and less often the hands. Usually the skin over the forearms is thin and inelastic. The supporting collagen surrounding the small vessels in that area has degenerated, with resulting fragility of vessels. Even slight mechanical trauma may produce a spreading blotch of purpura or actually tear the epidermis open.

Kalivas et al reported under this name a purpuric eruption in a child who developed petechiae after sun exposure. However, this is a different disorder, very likely a variant of polymorphous light eruption.

Corticosteroid purpura has the same clinical appearance and occurs in the same sites as solar purpura: dorsal forearms and shins. Persons on long-term corticosteroid therapy or with Cushing's syndrome are prone to develop this. It is the only steroid side effect (except polymenorrhea) that is seen regularly with triamcinolone acetonide intramuscularly in the elderly, and infrequently with oral prednisone.

Kalivas L, et al: Solar purpura. Arch Dermatol 1988, 124:24.

PURPURA FULMINANS

Also known as *purpura gangrenosa*, this is a severe, rapidly fatal reaction occurring most commonly in children after some infectious illness. The sudden appearance of large ecchymotic areas, especially prominent over the extremities, is characteristic. Fever, shock, and disseminated intravascular coagulation usually accompany the skin lesions, which on biopsy show noninflammatory necrosis, with platelet-fibrin thrombi occluding the blood vessels.

Purpura fulminans usually follows some acute infectious disease such as scarlet fever and, rarely, streptococcal pharyngitis, meningococcal meningitis, or varicella. However, it may occur without any preceding illness, and adults may be affected. Asplenic patients, who are at risk for pneumococcal or meningococcal sepsis, are also predisposed to purpura fulminans. Neonates with homozygous protein C deficiency may suffer purpura fulminans as a result of the lack of this natural anticoagulant. Some infectious or postinfectious patients develop transient deficiencies of proteins C and S, which may be directly related to the pathogenesis of this syndrome. Mitchell et al reported a patient who developed purpura fulminans, whose IgG paraprotein inhibited the functional anticoagulant activity of activated protein C. Other diseases, such as the fibrinolysis syndrome, may have purpura fulminans as part of the symptom complex.

Even with excellent supportive care, treatment of the underlying disease, and the use of heparin, the mortality rate continues to be at least 20 per cent. Waddell and his associates reported encouraging results with the use of hyperbaric oxygenation. Prompt improvement of the involved areas occurred without loss of the gangrenous parts. Dudgeon and associates strongly advocate immediate administra-

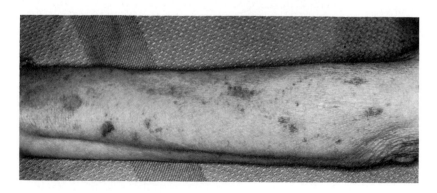

Figure 35–6. Solar purpura.

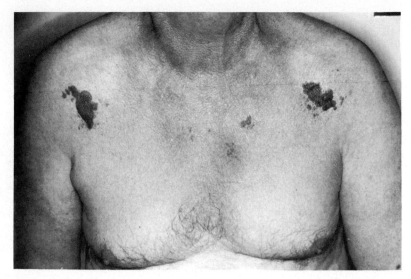

Figure 35–7. *Purpura due to chronic topical application of potent corticosteroids.*

tion of heparin sodium, 100 units/kg every four hours intravenously, with adjustment of the dose to maintain a clotting time of 25 to 30 minutes. Control of the disease may require up to five weeks of heparin therapy.

Auletta MJ, et al: Purpura fulminans: A cutaneous manifestation of severe protein C deficiency. Arch Dermatol 1988, 124:1387.

Benson PM, et al: Purpura and gangrene in a septic patient. Arch Dermatol 1988, 124:1851.

Branson HE, et al: A structured approach to the management of purpura fulminans. J Natl Med Assoc 1983, 75:821.

Dominey A, et al: Purpura fulminans and transient protein C and S deficiency. Arch Dermatol 1988, 124:1442.

Dudgeon DL, et al: Purpura fulminans. Arch Surg 1971, 103:351.

Gladsor CL, et al: Coumarin necrosis, neonatal purpura fulminans, and protein C deficiency. Arch Dermatol 1987, 123:1701a.

Hodge SJ: Purpura fulminans. Cutis 1978, 21:830.

Miller SJ: The dermatologist and protein C. JAAD 1988, 19:904.

Mitchell CA, et al: A fatal thrombotic disorder associated with an acquired inhibitor of protein C. NEJM 1987, 317:1638.

Powars DR, et al: Purpura fulminans in meningococcemia. NEJM 1987, 317:571.

Rusonis PA, et al: Livedo reticularis and purpura. JAAD 1986, 15:1120.

Spicer TE, et al: Purpura fulminans. Am J Med 1976, 61:566.

DISSEMINATED INTRAVASCULAR COAGULATION

Disseminated intravascular coagulation (DIC) may be initiated by a variety of disorders, including septicemic hypotension, hypoxemia, acidosis, cancer chemotherapy, obstetrical crises, or leukemia. Children with giant cavernous hemangioma are at risk for this consumptive coagulopathy (Kasabach-Merritt syndrome).

Minna et al found that two thirds of patients with DIC have skin lesions, which may be the initial manifestation of the syndrome. Minute, widespread petechiae, ecchymoses, ischemic necrosis of the skin, and hemorrhagic bullae may occur. Purpura fulminans may supervene.

Molos et al described symmetrical peripheral gangrene (SPG) as a useful marker for DIC. Many equate SPG with purpura fulminans. DIC is the result of widespread intravascular coagulation in which certain coagulation factors are consumed faster than they can be replaced. Laboratory findings show decreased platelets, decreased fibrinogen, elevated prothrombin time and partial thromboplastin time, and fibrin degradation products. Control of underlying disease is the paramount consideration, together with correction of hemostatic abnormalities through the use of heparin. The dose is adjusted to keep the clotting time two to three times normal.

Feinstein believes that heparin is indicated in purpura fulminans, venous thromboembolism, patients with retained dead fetus and hypofibrinogenemia (prior to induction of labor), bleeding associated with giant hemangioma, and neoplastic disease, particularly promyelocytic leukemia; in other situations he considers its use controversial. It does not seem to diminish morbidity or mortality.

Colman RW, et al: Disseminated intravascular coagulation: a dermatologic disease. Int J Dermatol 1977, 16:47.

Feinstein DI: Diagnosis and management of disseminated intravascular coagulation: the role of heparin therapy. Blood 1982, 60:284.

Molos MA, et al: Symmetrical peripheral gangrene and disseminated intravascular coagulation. Arch Dermatol 1985, 121:1057.

Robboy SJ, et al: The skin in disseminated intravascular coagulation: a prospective analysis of 36 cases. Br J Dermatol 1973, 88:221.

FIBRINOLYSIS SYNDROME (Hypofibrinogenemia, Defibrinating Syndrome)

The fibrinolysis syndrome is characterized by an acute hemorrhagic state brought about by inability of the blood to clot. Massive hemorrhages into the skin produce blackish, purplish swellings, and sloughing. There is an increased tendency to thrombosis as well as to hemorrhage. It occurs as a complication of pregnancy in cases of placenta previa, eclampsia, and fetal death. It may be a complication in certain surgical operations, particularly in lobectomy and during extracorporeal circulation of blood. The syndrome has been repeatedly reported in amyloidosis, thrombotic thrombocytopenic purpura, liver disease, Waterhouse-Friderichsen syndrome, carcinoma of the prostate with metastases to bone marrow, and in other types of malignant disease. It may also follow snake bite. Treatment is by transfusions of whole blood and fibrinogen.

This disease is produced by excessive or inappropriate fibrinolysis.

ANTICOAGULANT-ASSOCIATED PURPURA

This complication of anticoagulant therapy has been increasingly reported in the past several years. Coumarin and heparin may both cause purpura and necrosis of the skin. Coumarin, the orally administered drug, characteristically is associated with a reaction that begins with sudden pain, followed by ecchymoses, and hemorrhagic infarcts appearing between the third and tenth day of anticoagulant therapy. It has been noted mostly in obese, middle-aged women with a predilection for lesions to involve the pendulous breasts, abdomen, buttocks, and thighs, but Stone et al reported a case with acrally located lesions and Gold et al reviewed cases with lesions in other unusual sites. On biopsy most cases show occlusion of dermal and subcutaneous vessels by fibrin thrombi. Following the infarct an eschar forms and sloughing continues down into the deep subcutaneous fat. Healing is difficult and may require grafting or even amputation when the lesions occur on the extremities.

It is likely to be unresponsive to therapy, and responded to neither intravenous heparin nor prednisone (40 mg a day) in a patient reported by Schleicher et al who experienced two attacks, the second after readministration of coumarin in another hospital. Such unresponsiveness is classic; however, several cases have now been reported with recurrent episodes. Several have been associated with either an inherited heterozygous, or an acquired, protein C deficiency. If coumarin anticoagulation is necessary in a patient who has experienced previous necrosis, heparin combined with fresh frozen plasma infusions to maintain normal protein C levels during the critical initial anticoagulation period may be successful, as in the case of Zauber et al.

Heparin has also been associated with cutaneous necrosis, classically associated with sites of injection, such as the abdomen, and beginning six to 13 days afterward. Initial tenderness and erythema progress to necrosis and an eschar. Shelley et al reported such an occurrence in a patient who was felt to have an immunologically induced platelet aggregation. Wide-

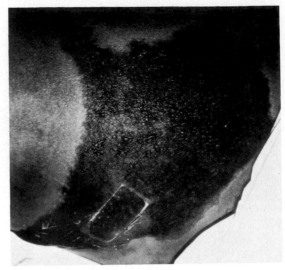

Figure 35–8. Coumarin necrosis.

spread lesions have also been reported, and even intravenously injected heparin may induce skin necrosis, as reported by Levine et al. Biopsy of such reactions usually shows vascular necrosis.

Gold et al and Rosen et al agree that no absolute criteria can distinguish heparin reactions from coumarin reactions when both drugs have been given; however, cutaneous necrosis with fibrin thrombi beginning less than one week after injection favor a coumarin reaction.

Franson TR, et al: Late-onset warfarin-caused necrosis occurring in a patient with infectious mononucleosis. Arch Dermatol 1984, 120:927.

Gladson CL, et al: Coumarin necrosis, neonatal purpura fulminans, and protein C deficiency. Arch Dermatol 1987, 123:1701a.

Gold JA, et al: Coumadin versus heparin necrosis. JAAD 1987, 16:148.

Levine LE, et al: Heparin-induced cutaneous necrosis unrelated to injection sites. Arch Dermatol 1983, 119:400.

Rosen T, et al: Coumadin versus heparin necrosis (reply). JAAD 1987, 16:149.

Schleicher SM, et al: Coumarin necrosis. Arch Dermatol 1980, 116:444.

Shelley WB, et al: Heparin necrosis. JAAD 1982, 7:674.

Stone MS, et al: Acral purpura. JAAD 1986, 14:797.

Teepe RGC, et al: Recurrent coumarin-induced skin necrosis in a patient with an acquired functional protein C deficiency. Arch Dermatol 1986, 122:1408.

Tuneu A, et al: Cutaneous reactions secondary to heparin injections. JAAD 1985, 12:1072.

Zauber NP, et al: Successful warfarin anticoagulation despite protein C deficiency and a history of warfarin necrosis. Ann Intern Med 1986, 104:659.

ITCHING PURPURA

Mosto et al prefer the term *disseminated pruriginous angiodermatitis*. Punctate purpuric macules (petechiae) first appear around the ankles and then ascend to involve the entire body with the exception of the palms and face. These orange-purplish-red petechiae evolve completely and may become confluent in two weeks. Edema of the ankles is present, and severe pruritus is a dominant feature, producing lichenification.

It is seen predominantly in men and has a seasonal predilection for spring and summer. The etiology is unknown. The disease runs its course in three to six months.

Mosto SJ, et al: Disseminated pruriginous angiodermatitis (itching purpura). Arch Dermatol 1965, 91:351.

MISCELLANEOUS PURPURIC MANIFESTATIONS

Postcardiotomy Syndrome. Two to three weeks after pericardiotomy, fever, pleuritis, pericarditis, or arthritis may appear together with petechiae on the skin and palate. This syndrome may be confused with infectious mononucleosis and bacterial endocarditis.

Orthostatic Purpura (Stasis Purpura). Prolonged standing or even sitting with the legs lowered (as in a bus, airplane, or train) may produce edema and a purpuric eruption on the lower extremities. Elevation of the legs and the use of elastic stockings are helpful if prevention is necessary.

Acute Venous Thrombosis. Hirschmann reviewed the ischemic forms of acute venous thrombosis in 1987. Extensive venous thrombosis, almost always affecting at least the femoral vein, can cause reversible ischemia, or frank gangrene. Patients may develop, either abruptly or gradually, severe pain, extensive edema, and cyanosis of an extremity (usually the leg). The left leg is more often affected than the right. Female patients slightly outnumber male, and the mean age is 52 years.

Malignant neoplasms were the commonest underlying condition, with bronchogenic carcinoma by far the most common. In 35 per cent of cancer-associated cases, the thrombosis was the first sign of the cancer.

Immobilization from surgery, extensive trauma, childbirth, or congestive heart failure are other predisposing factors. In addition to the clinical signs, plethysmography, Doppler studies, or radionuclide or contrast phlebography will all demonstrate the lesion reliably.

Treatment involves elevation of the limb, intravenous fluids, and systemic anticoagulation. After these measures are instituted, thrombectomy is often the treatment of choice.

There is a 40 per cent mortality, often from pulmonary emboli or underlying disease. Chronic complications include venous incompetence, with stasis dermatitis or ulcers, as well as venous claudication with leg pain on exercising.

Livedoid Dermatitis. This is an embolic phenomenon (infarction) leading to temporary or prolonged local ischemia as a result of accidental arterial obliteration from the intragluteal injections of various drugs. There is severe local pain and swelling which takes on a waxy, ischemic tint and bluish or reddish mottling. Wheals and plexiform streaks may appear and be followed by purpuric spots resulting from infarcts.

The livedoid changes may arise within a few minutes after the injection but are more pronounced after two or three days. Palpation reveals enormous hard tumefaction, which is very painful, and a local increase of temperature. Fever, tachycardia, dyspnea, and albuminuria may occur. Gangrene may supervene; however, even severe lesions have subsided after a week or two under conservative management.

Perinatal gangrene of the buttock is a similar condition, usually a complication of umbilical artery catheterization, exchange transfusion, or cord injections by means of a syringe. It may also be a spontaneous event.

Bonifazi E, et al: Perinatal gangrene of the buttock. JAAD 1980, 3:596.
Serrano G, et al: Perinatal gangrene of the buttock. Arch Dermatol 1985, 121:23.

Obstructive Purpura. Purpura may also be evoked by mechanical obstruction to the circulation, with resulting stress on the small vessels, as encountered in cardiac decompensation, convulsions, vomiting episodes, the Valsalva maneuver, pertussis, and asthma. Local obstruction of the blood flow may result from compression of the veins by tumors and the gravid uterus; by occlusions from thrombosis; or by a weakening of the elastic coat as in varicose veins; in all these conditions purpura may be observed.

Traumatic Purpura. Rasmussen reviewed some unusual purpuric lesions in children, some of them due to trauma, as in the battered child. "Passion purpura" on the palate may result from fellatio, or on the neck or upper arms (a "hickey") from biting and sucking.

Purpura-associated Diseases. Purpura may be noted at times in erythema multiforme, dermatitis medicamentosa, serum sickness, and herpes zoster. Petechiae or ecchymoses may be associated with measles, scarlet fever, and smallpox and may appear extensively in cerebrospinal meningitis, typhus, and Rocky Mountain spotted fever. Disseminated strongyloidiasis can cause widespread purpura by the passage of the larvae through vessel walls, as in the case reported by von Kuster et al. Purpura may occur also in septicemia, Waterhouse-Friderichsen syndrome, bacterial endocarditis, malaria, miliary tuberculosis, and anthrax.

Calciphylaxis. Acute hypercalcemic crisis can lead to metastatic calcification, and if this occurs in skin vessels it may cause ecchymosis, cordlike nodules, or necrosis. Khafif et al reviewed this syndrome in 1989.

Scorbutic Purpura. In addition to the typical bleeding gums seen in scurvy, cutaneous purpura may be extensive, and severe dissecting subcutaneous hematomas may occur on the legs or abdomen. Deficiency of vitamin C, like solar elastosis, increases the fragility and permeability of the capillaries and accounts for the tendency to purpura and hemorrhage. The petechiae are perifollicular in the skin, which proved a helpful clue to diagnosis in a case reported by Warshauer et al.

Fat Embolism Petechiae. Petechiae associated with systemic fat embolism may be seen after fracture of a long bone. Within 24 to 36 hours after injury, red or brown petechiae may be found on the anterior shoulders, chest, axillae, and conjunctivae. In addition, there may be cerebral, neurologic, or respiratory symptoms, with tachycardia and fever. Progression to livedo reticularis, ecchymosis, or even gangrene may occur. Reports by Kalter et al and Falanga et al stress that cholesterol embolization from dislodged intravascular plaques occurs primarily in elderly men on anticoagulants after a cardiovascular procedure. (See *livedo reticularis*, p. 946.)

Epidemic Dropsy. Bean reported on epidemic dropsy, manifested by eruptive angiomas, purpura, dyspnea, tachycardia, diarrhea, and fever. This occurs in parts of India, Africa, and the Fiji Islands, from mustard oil adulterated with oil of argemone.

Paroxysmal Nocturnal Hemoglobinuria. This acquired intravascular hemolytic anemia usually occurs in young adults. Draelos et al have reviewed the skin findings: the initial erythematous plaques progress to hemorrhagic bullae. Vascular thrombi are found on biopsy. The physiologic drop in pH which occurs with sleep appears to be responsible for the hemolysis and is the basis for the specific Ham (acid hemolysis) test.

Lupus Anticoagulant Syndrome. An antiphospholipid antibody may be responsible for a syndrome which can include thrombosis, spontaneous abortion, neurologic manifestations, pulmonary hypertension, positive Coombs test, and thrombocytopenia. In the skin one may see leg ulcers, distal ischemia, widespread cutaneous necrosis, and livedo reticularis. On biopsy there are microthrombi without vasculitis. Lupus anticoagulant factor is seen in about 40 per cent of lupus patients but is also found in many other diseases, including AIDS, and may also be drug-induced. This is reviewed in more detail in Chapter 8, under lupus erythematosus.

Alcalay J, et al: Mask phenomenon: postemesis facial purpura. Cutis 1986, 38:28.
Bayat-Mokhtari F, et al: Parathyroid storm. Arch Intern Med 1980, 140:1092.
Draelos ZK, et al: Hemorrhagic bullae in an anemic woman. Arch Dermatol 1986, 122:1327.
Ellis CN, et al: Scurvy. Arch Dermatol 1984, 120:1212.
Ely H: White blood cells as mediators of hyperviscosity-induced tissue damage in neutrophilic vascular reactions. Therapy with pentoxifylline. JAAD 1989, 20:677.
Falanga V, et al: The cutaneous manifestations of cholesterol crystal embolization. Arch Dermatol 1986, 122:1194.
Grob J-J, et al: Cutaneous manifestations associated with the presence of lupus anticoagulant. JAAD 1986, 15:211.
Hirschmann JV: Ischemic forms of acute venous thrombosis. Arch Dermatol 1987, 123:933.
Kalter DC, et al: Livedo reticularis due to multiple cholesterol emboli. JAAD 1985, 13:235.
Kaplan RP, et al: Dermatologic features of the fat embolism syndrome. Cutis 1986, 36:52.
Khafif RA, et al: Acute hyperparathyroidism with systemic calcinosis. Arch Intern Med 1989, 149:681.
Rasmussen JE: Puzzling purpuras in children and young adults. JAAD 1982, 6:67.
Sontheimer RD: The anticardiolipin syndrome. Arch Dermatol 1987, 123:590.
Von Kuster LC, et al: Cutaneous manifestations of strongyloidiasis. Arch Dermatol 1988, 124:1826.
Warshauer DM, et al: Scurvy: a clinical mimic of vasculitis. Cutis 1984, 34:539.
Weinstein C, et al: Livedo reticularis associated with increased titers of anticardiolipin antibodies in systemic lupus erythematosus. Arch Dermatol 1987, 123:596.

Easy Bruising Syndrome

Young women who bruise easily despite normal coagulation profiles and normal platelet counts may have antiplatelet antibodies or increased megakaryocytes. Lackner and Karpatkin have divided them into groups I (vasculitis) and II (qualitative platelet function abnormalities).

Lackner H, et al: On the "easy bruising" syndrome with normal platelet count. Ann Intern Med 1975, 83:190.

Painful Bruising Syndrome (Autoerythrocyte Sensitization, Gardner-Diamond Syndrome)

Painful bruising syndrome is a distinctive localized purpuric reaction occurring primarily in young to middle-aged women who usually manifest some emotional or personality disturbance. There may be depression, anxiety, hysterical or masochistic character traits, or inability to deal with hostile feelings. Hällström et al have reviewed this. A recurrent type of eruption, it is characterized by extremely painful and tender ill-defined ecchymoses about the extremities and sometimes on the face or trunk. The lesions evolve in a few hours and resolve within five to eight days. New lesions may appear in crops. Emotional upsets are generally believed to be precipitating factors in the appearance of these painful sheets of purpura. It has been noted that some patients have a premonition as to when they will develop new lesions a few hours ahead of time by the tingling and burning sensation at the site of a future lesion. Both Freedman and Sorenson et al reported cases in children, and the former was able to help the patients with psychotherapy, while Sorenson saw some improvement after discussion of the disorder with the patient and the family. Ratnoff, in his extensive review of 168 patients with whom he was familiar,

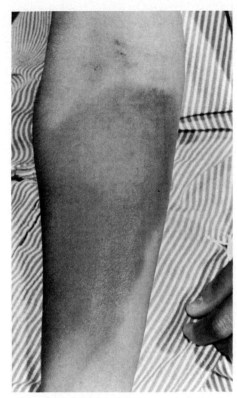

Figure 35–9. Autoerythrocyte sensitization.

Bagot M, et al: Gardner-Diamond syndrome or painful recurrent ecchymotic syndrome. Rev Stomatol Chir Maxillofac 1984, 85:66.

Campbell A, et al: Autoerythrocyte sensitization. J Pediatr 1983, 103:157.

Grace TW, et al: Gardner-Diamond syndrome (letter). JAMA 1981, 245:1909.

Hällström T, et al: Mental symptoms and personality structure in autoerythrocyte sensitization syndrome. Br J Psychiatry 1969, 115:1269.

Hamblin TJ, et al: Plasmapheresis and a placebo procedure in autoerythrocyte sensitization. Br Med J 1981, 283:1575.

Hersle K, et al: Autoerythrocyte sensitization syndrome (painful bruising syndrome): report of 2 cases and review of the literature. Br J Dermatol 1969, 81:574.

Ratnoff OD: The psychogenic purpuras. Semin Hematol 1980, 17:192.

Sorenson RU, et al: Psychogenic purpura in adolescent patients. Clin Pediatr 1985, 24:700.

knew of nine men with this illness. He stresses the extracutaneous somatic symptoms in the diagnosis: headache, paresthesias, transient paresis, syncope, diplopia, abdominal distress, diarrhea, nausea and vomiting, and arthralgia.

The original authors reported that intracutaneous injections of erythrocyte stroma evoked typical lesions. Since then many have reported similar reactions to autologous whole blood, packed or washed red cells, or fractions of erythrocyte stroma. These are hard to assess, because like reactions have been reported to substances as diverse as hemoglobin, phosphatidyl serine, histamine, histidine, trypsin, PPD, autologous serum, and platelets. Blinded, controlled testing, trying to avoid factitial trauma, has given mixed responses. Many believe this syndrome to be artifactual, but Ratnoff feels the lesions are spontaneous, and one of us (HLA), having followed a case for nearly two years, is of the same opinion.

Treatment has been mostly unavailing, though it may be that psychotherapy directed at emotional problems has helped in some cases. The disease follows an irregularly intermittent course, possibly exacerbated by emotional stress or physical injury.

A similar syndrome, reported as DNA autosensitivity, has been described in eight patients who were reactive to intracutaneous injections of purified calf thymus DNA or frozen and thawed buffy coat. Further case studies are needed to fully assess this syndrome. Documentation to date suffers from the same inconsistencies and lack of controlled, blind studies as the Gardner-Diamond syndrome.

Psychogenic Purpura

Psychogenic purpura or factitious purpura presents a similar picture; however, sensitivity to the erythrocytes is absent. Stocker et al have reviewed this type. They proposed that the term psychogenic purpura be broadened to include both purpura resulting from a conversion reaction and purpura resulting from self-inflicted injury.

Ratnoff's classic study also reviewed this as well as religious stigmata, such as the lesions experienced by Louise Lateau, who was said to develop bleeding from the palms, soles, and sides every Friday. Winkelmann et al reported cases of *Sécretan's syndrome*: factitial traumatic edema of the dorsal hand; and *l'oedème bleu*, factitial edema produced by trauma to the upper extremity.

Jørgensen J, et al: Factitious lymphedema, Sécretan's syndrome. Arch Dermatol Venereol 1983, 63:271.

Ratnoff OD: The psychogenic purpuras. Semin Hematol 1980, 17:192.

Stocker WW, et al: Psychogenic purpura. Arch Dermatol 1977, 113:606.

Winkelmann RK, et al: Factitial traumatic purpura. JAAD 1985, 13:988.

Devil's Pinches

Devil's pinches are transitory painful sensations on the upper legs of menopausal women who subsequently develop ecchymoses at the sites of the pain.

Paroxysmal Hand Hematoma (Achenbach's Syndrome)

Spontaneous focal hemorrhage into the palm or the volar surface of a finger has been reported by Achenbach and by Jung. Sharp transitory localized pain, followed quickly by swelling and localized bluish discoloration, constitutes the entire clinical picture. The lesion involuted spontaneously within a few days in both of Arnold's cases. Spontaneous hemorrhage from an arteriole appears to be responsible.

Jung EG: Das paroxysmale Fingerhaematom. Schweiz Med Wchnschr 1964, 94:458.

Winkelmann RK, et al: Factitial traumatic purpura. JAAD 1985, 13:988.

PIGMENTARY PURPURIC ERUPTIONS

The following pigmented purpuric eruptions of the lower extremities are similar. They are all manifestations of capillaritis, but may present in any of several distinctive clinical patterns. Cases with clinical overlap also occur.

Progressive Pigmentary Dermatosis

This is better known as **Schamberg's disease**; the typical lesions are pinhead-sized reddish puncta resembling grains of Cayenne pepper, occurring in irregularly shaped patches on the lower legs. There is a slow proximal extension of the lesions. After a few months the pinhead puncta begin to fade into the surrounding pigmented patches. These lesions seldom itch. The favored sites are around the lower shins and ankles.

Histologically, a lymphocytic infiltrate is present in the upper dermis, especially around the capillaries. Also, small ectatic vessels with swollen endothelium and hyaline degeneration of the vessel walls are seen. Slight red cell extravasation occurs. Hemosiderin is

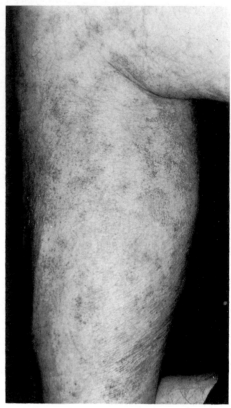

Figure 35–11. Schamberg's disease.

the chief pigment in this dermatosis. The basic process is capillaritis.

Anecdotal reports of benefit from mild topical steroids make a therapeutic trial for four to six weeks not unreasonable. The process can also be stopped by giving 12 mg of betamethasone (Celestone) or 40 mg of triamcinolone intramuscularly—a suggestion of Allan Izumi, confirmed by one of us (HLA). However, it may recur.

Purpura Annularis Telangiectodes

This is better known as **Majocchi's disease**. The early lesions are bluish red annular macules 1 to 3 cm in diameter in which dark red telangiectatic puncta appear. The central part of this annular lesion gradually fades so that the central involution and the peripheral extension form ringed or semicircular lesions. Bean describes these as centrifugally spreading, targetlike, concentric rings such as are seen on the cross-cut section of a tree trunk. The eruption begins symmetrically on the lower extremities and then spreads up the legs and may extend onto the trunk and arms.

Involution usually requires as much as a year, but because of relapses the disease may be prolonged indefinitely. The lesions are asymptomatic.

Histologically, Majocchi's disease is the same as Schamberg's and is believed to have the same pathogenesis: capillaritis.

These lesions tend to clear spontaneously.

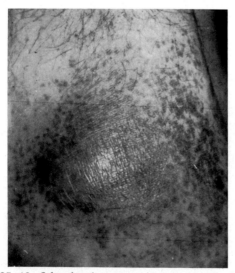

Figure 35–10. Schamberg's progressive pigmentary dermatosis on ankle.

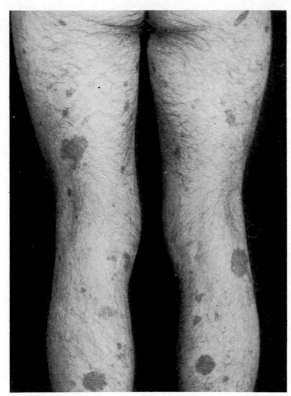

Figure 35–12. Majocchi's disease. (Courtesy of Dr. F. Daniels, Jr.)

Pigmented Purpuric Lichenoid Dermatitis

Better known as **Gougerot-Blum syndrome**, this is characterized by minute, rust-colored, lichenoid papules that tend to fuse into plaques with indistinct borders. The plaques may contain papules of various hues. Favorite locations are upon the legs, thighs, and lower trunk.

Histologically, the upper dermis contains a moderate lymphocyte infiltration and hemosiderin. Ectatic vessels with endothelial proliferations are important findings.

The chief difference between this and Schamberg's disease is in the distribution of the lesions and the presence of lichenoid papular elevations, which are often grouped into plaques, in this disease.

Dermatitis Hemostatica

Stasis dermatitis and erythromelia are synonyms for a blotchy red mottling and a yellowish or light brown pigmentation of the lower third of the lower legs, due to venous insufficiency.

Lichen Aureus

This eruption of the skin is characterized by the sudden appearance of one or several patches of golden-hued or rusty-colored, closely packed lichenoid papules. The patches vary from 2 to 30 cm in width and may occur on any part of the body. They may be solitary or numerous. Ruiz-Esmenjaud et al reported linear segmental lesions on the left arm of a 15-year-old girl. They do not itch, but in the case of Reinhardt et al were associated with severe pain. Adults predominate among reported cases, but children get it too: Kahana et al reported a case in an eight-year-old girl in 1985.

The etiology is unknown. Usually no history of previous injury or drug intake can be elicited.

Shelley et al reported four cases with leg lesions, in three of which an underlying incompetent perforator vein could be demonstrated; but this could hardly account for the many lesions that occurred on the hands or arms.

Price et al regarded it as one of the pigmented purpuric dermatoses. Reinhardt et al demonstrated increased capillary fragility and koebnerization in their case.

Histologically, there are no epidermal changes;

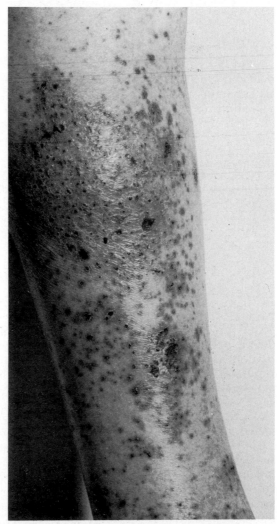

Figure 35–13. Pigmented purpuric lichenoid dermatitis (Gougerot-Blum syndrome).

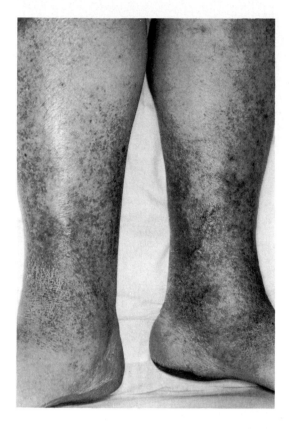

Figure 35–14. Venous ("stasis") dermatitis.

however, in the dermis a broad band of normal dermis separates the epidermis from a zone of lymphocytic infiltration.

There is no effective treatment for lichen aureus.

Aiba S, et al: Immunohistologic studies in Schamberg's disease. Arch Dermatol 1988, 124:1058.
Graham RM, et al: Lichen aureus. Clin Exp Dermatol 1984, 9:393.
Kahana M, et al: Lichen aureus in childhood. Int J Dermatol 1985, 24:666.
Price ML, et al: Lichen aureus: a localized form of pigmented purpuric dermatitis. Br J Dermatol 1985, 112:307.
Reinhardt L, et al: Vascular abnormalities in lichen aureus. JAAD 1983, 8:417.
Rudolph RI: Lichen aureus. JAAD 1983, 8:722.
Ruiz-Esmenjaud J, et al: Segmental lichen aureus. Arch Dermatol 1988, 124:1572.
Shelley WB, et al: Lichen aureus: a hemosiderin tattoo associated with perforator vein incompetence. JAAD 1984, 11:260.
Waisman M: Lichen aureus (Commentary). Int J Dermatol 1985, 24:646.
Wilkin JL: Lichen aureus (letter). JAAD 1985, 12:124.

VASCULITIS

Anthony S. Fauci of the National Institute of Allergy and Infectious Diseases has defined vasculitis as "a clinicopathologic process characterized by inflammation and necrosis of blood vessels," which predominates in some diseases and is only a minor component of others. It may affect any size or type of vessel in any organ system. The basic process involves an immunologically mediated response to antigens that results in vessel-wall damage. The great clinical importance of recognizing the essential unity of this group is that several of the more serious systemic necrotizing vasculitides have been found to be extraordinarily responsive to cyclophosphamide. The small-vessel vasculitis syndromes described under the hypersensitivity group are all relatively refractory to cytotoxic agents, and the risks of oral prednisone are usually not worth the benefits if lesions are limited to the skin. They are best treated less aggressively, with nonsteroidal antiinflammatory agents or antihistamines, if removal of the offending agent or treatment of the underlying disease is not possible or not effective.

The confusion of terminology that has prevailed for the past two decades, and the fact that only a few entities within this group of diseases are sharply defined, as well as the considerable overlap that exists, have prevented and still prevent the emergence of any definitive classification of the group. One of the best classifications is that proposed in 1982 by Fauci:

Systemic necrotizing vasculitis (polyarteritis nodosa group)
    Classic polyarteritis nodosa
    Allergic granulomatosis
    Systemic necrotizing vasculitis ("overlap syndrome")
Hypersensitivity vasculitis
    Serum sickness and serum-sickness–like reactions
    Other drug-related vasculitides
    Henoch-Schönlein purpura
    Vasculitis associated with neoplasms (mostly lymphoid)
    Vasculitis associated with infectious diseases
    Vasculitis associated with connective tissue diseases
    Congenital complement deficiencies
    Erythema elevatum diutinum
Wegener's granulomatosis
Giant-cell arteritis
    Temporal arteritis
    Takayasu's arteritis
Thromboangiitis obliterans (Buerger's disease)
Mucocutaneous lymph node syndrome
Behçet's disease
Miscellaneous vasculitides

Another classification which is clinically helpful is that of Gilliam et al, based on vessel size. Fan et al reviewed this system in detail. Though its usefulness is limited by great overlap, the clinical correlation relating the morphology to the size of the damaged vessel provides a good conceptual approach to the evaluation of the systemic vasculitides. Palpable purpura and urticarial lesions indicate arteriolar or venular involvement, which occurs primarily in dermal leukocytoclastic vasculitis (the *hypersensitivity vasculitis* group). Small muscular (intravisceral) artery involvement usually presents as erythema nodosum in the panniculus. Nearly any group except the giant-cell arteritis group may present in this way; it is most characteristic of the granulomatous group. Involvement of medium-sized muscular arteries, such as the hepatic, coronary, or mesenteric arteries, leads to livedo reticularis, nodule formation, or gangrene; these are characteristic of *classic periarteritis nodosa*. Finally, involvement of large arteries, such as the aorta or the temporal arteries, leads to claudication, congestive heart failure, or stroke: it is characteristic of *giant-cell arteritis*.

PATHOGENESIS. Immunopathogenic mechanisms are either known or strongly suspected to be the cause of the lesions in all the vasculitides. The sequence of events is antigen exposure; formation of circulating soluble antigen-antibody complexes; deposition of these in vessel walls, rendered permeable by vasoactive amines; and activation of complement components. Some of these attract polymorphonuclear leukocytes, which infiltrate the vessel wall and release collagenase and elastase and other lysosomal enzymes, causing necrosis of the wall followed by hemorrhage, thrombosis, occlusion, and surrounding ischemic necrosis of tissue.

Cell-mediated immune reactivity, as Fauci points out, may also be involved in the pathogenesis of vasculitis. This may, by inducing influx and accumulation of macrophages, be one mechanism of inducing granuloma formation.

Christian CL: Vasculitis: genus and species (editorial). Ann Intern Med 1984, 101:862.
Cupps TR, et al: Chronic, recurrent small-vessel cutaneous vasculitis. JAMA 1982, 247:1994.
Idem: The Vasculitides. Philadelphia, WB Saunders Co. 1981.
Fan PT, et al: A clinical approach to systemic vasculitis. Semin Arthritis Rheum 1980, 9:248.
Fauci AS: The spectrum of vasculitis: clinical, pathologic, immunologic, and therapeutic considerations. Ann Intern Med 1978, 89:660.
Idem: Vasculitis. J Allergy Clin Immunol 1983, 72:211.
Idem, et al: Cyclophosphamide therapy of severe systemic necrotizing vasculitis. N Engl J Med 1979, 301:235.
Gilliam JN, et al: Cutaneous necrotizing vasculitis and related disorders. Ann Allergy 1976, 37:328.
Jegasothy BV: Immune complexes in cutaneous disease. Arch Dermatol 1983, 119:795.
Logan W: Periodic synopsis on vasculitis. JAAD 1985, 12:716.
McClusky RT, et al: Vasculitis in primary vasculitides, granulomatous, and connective tissue disease. Human Pathol 1983, 14:305.
Sams WM: Necrotizing vasculitis. JAAD 1980, 3:1.
Sanchez NP, et al: Clinical and histologic spectrum of necrotizing vasculitis. Arch Dermatol 1985, 121:220.
Yancey KB, et al: Circulating immune complexes. JAAD 1984, 10:711.

SYSTEMIC NECROTIZING VASCULITIS (Polyarteritis Nodosa Group)

Classic Polyarteritis Nodosa (Periarteritis Nodosa)

Periarteritis nodosa (PAN) is characterized by necrotizing vasculitis affecting the small and medium-sized muscular arteries of such caliber as the hepatic and coronary vessels and the arteries in the subcutaneous tissue, and sometimes adjacent veins.

CUTANEOUS MANIFESTATIONS. The skin is involved in about 40 per cent of the patients with this grave disease. No single clinical picture is seen. The most striking and diagnostic lesions, which are present in 15 per cent of patients, are 5–10-mm subcutaneous nodules occurring singly or in groups distributed along the course of the blood vessels, above which the skin is normal or slightly erythematous. Such nodules are often painful and may pulsate and, in time, may ulcerate. Common sites are the lower extremities, especially below the knee. Ecchymoses and peripheral gangrene of the fingers and toes may also be present. Livedo reticularis, bullae, papules, scarlatiniform lesions, and urticaria may occur in some patients.

Diaz-Perez and Winkelmann reported 23 patients with biopsy evidence of acute inflammatory periarteritis and no systemic involvement. Nodules, livedo reticularis, and ulcers were the characteristic lesions found. Fever and arthralgia were common findings. No patient died of the disease, but some had inter-

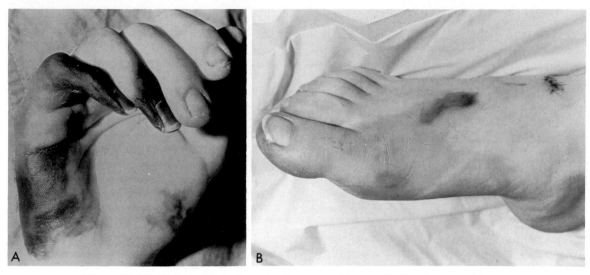

Figure 35–15. Periarteritis nodosa. A, *Gangrene of fingers.* B, *Involvement of foot.*

mittent lesions for 20 or more years. *Cutaneous periarteritis nodosa* represents a characteristic syndrome.

INTERNAL MANIFESTATIONS. Classic systemic periarteritis may involve the vessels throughout the entire body. Hypertension, tachycardia, fever, edema, and loss of weight are cardinal signs of the disease. Hepatomegaly, icterus, lymphadenopathy, hematuria, and leukocytosis are also frequently found. Arthralgia, myocardial and intestinal infarctions, glomerulosclerosis, and peripheral neuritis are also seen. Mononeuritis multiplex, most often manifested as foot drop, is a hallmark of PAN. Involvement of the meningeal, vertebral, and carotid arteries may lead to hemiplegia, convulsions, and various hemorrhages.

The lungs and spleen are rarely involved. In periarteritis nodosa thrombi are frequent, aneurysms are present, and infarcts may occur.

LABORATORY FINDINGS. A leukocytosis of as high as 40,000 may occur. The polymorphonuclears may be 80 per cent; thrombocytosis and progressive normocytic anemia and an elevated sedimentation rate are also present. Hypergammaglobulinemia with macroglobulins and cryoglobulins is usually seen. Urinary abnormalities such as proteinuria, hematuria, and casts are present in 70 per cent of patients.

ETIOLOGY. Periarteritis is four times more common in men than in women and the mean age of presentation is 45 years. Citron et al noted its occurrence among drug abusers, and thought methamphetamine was a possible common denominator.

A second variant was described by Sergent et al in association with serous otitis media. Also, *Cogan's syndrome* (nonsyphilitic interstitial keratitis and vestibulo-auditory symptoms) may be complicated by PAN. Additionally, a small number of hereditary cases have been reported, and several cases have been associated with hepatitis B infection.

PATHOLOGY. The histology is that of an inflammatory necrotizing and obliterative panarteritis that attacks the small and medium-sized arteries. Focal

vasculitis forms nodose swellings which become necrotic, producing aneurysms and ruptures of the vessels. Hemorrhage, hematoma, and ecchymosis may result. Obliteration of the lumen may occur, with ischemic necrosis of surrounding tissue. Characteristically the arteries are affected at their branching points.

The mainstay of diagnosis is the presence of these histologic changes. Obviously, the preferable site for biopsy is an accessible site such as skin, muscle, or testis. If these are not involved, angiography may detect aneurysmal dilatations as small as 1 cm wide in the renal, hepatic, or other visceral vessels, and may be used to direct biopsy to these organs.

TREATMENT. Untreated classic PAN has a five-year survival rate of only 13 per cent, death usually occurring from renal failure or cardiovascular or gastrointestinal-related problems.

Treatment with corticosteroids and cytotoxic agents has increased the survival rate to over 90 per cent. Corticosteroids in the dose range of 1 mg per kg per day are given initially. It is Fauci's practice to begin them in three divided doses, and then once the disease remits or the cytotoxic agents have reached full effect, he tapers the steroid to daily, and then alternate-daily. After an average of three to six months, with the patient in remission, the steroids are slowly tapered to discontinuation.

Cyclophosphamide is given with the steroids, or sometimes as a single agent. Fauci begins with 2 mg per kg as a single daily dose. Twice as much may occasionally be needed, and by the intravenous route, for three or four days in a critically ill patient. It takes ten to 14 days for oral cyclophosphamide to take full effect. The oral dose is then adjusted to maintain the white count between 3000 and 3500 per cubic millimeter, and the neutrophil count above 1500 cells/mm^3. When the disease has been quiescent for at least a year, the cyclophosphamide may be tapered and stopped. On the average, 18 to 24 months of therapy is required.

Citron BP, et al: Necrotizing angiitis associated with drug abuse. N Engl J Med 1970, 283:1003.

Diaz-Perez JL, et al: Cutaneous periarteritis nodosa. Arch Dermatol 1974, 110:407.

Fan PT, et al: A clinical approach to systemic vasculitis. Semin Arthritis Rheum 1980, 9:248.

Fauci AS: Vasculitis. J Allergy Clin Immunol 1983, 72:211.

Goslen JB, et al: Cutaneous polyarteritis nodosa. Arch Dermatol 1983, 119:326.

Jorizzo JL, et al: Neutrophilic vascular reactions. JAAD 1988, 19:983.

Kassis V, et al: Benign cutaneous periarteritis nodosa with nail defects. JAAD 1985, 13:661.

Leib ES, et al: Immunosuppressive and corticosteroid therapy of polyarteritis nodosa. Am J Med 1979, 67:941.

McElgunn PSJ: Dermatologic manifestations of hepatitis B virus infection. JAAD 1983, 8:539.

Sergent JS, et al: Necrotizing vasculitis after serous otitis media. Ann Intern Med 1974, 81:195.

Travers RL, et al: Periarteritis nodosa. Semin Arthritis Rheum 1979, 8:184.

Van de Pette JEW, et al: Cutaneous periarteritis nodosa. Arch Dermatol 1984, 120:109.

Whittaker SJ, et al: Cutaneous polyarteritis nodosa associated with hepatitis B surface antigen. JAAD 1986, 15:1142.

Allergic Granulomatosis

Allergic granulomatosis (Churg-Strauss syndrome) is also known as necrotizing angiitis with granulomata. It is characterized by the distinctive initial manifestation of asthma. A debilitated asthmatic begins after two to 12 years to experience attacks of fever and eosinophilia (20 to 90 per cent) and after a few more months or years, diffuse angiitis involves the lungs, heart, liver, spleen, kidney, intestines, and pancreas. A fatal outcome is likely in most untreated patients, with congestive heart failure due to myocarditis the most frequent cause of death.

Cutaneous lesions are present in two thirds of patients. There may be nodules appearing on the extensor surfaces of the extremities and on the scalp. Firm nontender papules may be present on the fingertips. Purpura is present.

Histologically, Churg and Strauss found necrosis of small arterioles and venules, fibrinoid degeneration, an eosinophilic tissue infiltrate, and granulomas with epithelioid cells, giant cells, and plasma cells, mostly perivascularly, unlike periarteritis nodosa.

The treatment recommended by Fauci for periarteritis nodosa, cyclophosphamide alone or in combination with corticosteroids, is recommended. It has been responsible for a significantly improved prognosis in these patients.

Overlap Syndrome

This is the third disorder in Fauci's polyarteritis nodosa group, and it exists mainly to provide a place for cases of systemic necrotizing vasculitis which fail to fit neatly into either the classic polyarteritis nodosa category, or into that of allergic granulomatosis. It comprises a variety of cases of necrotizing vasculitis, often with hypertension and renal involvement, lung lesions, eosinophilia, granuloma formation, and cryoglobulinemia.

Fauci suggests referring to all these three groups collectively as systemic necrotizing vasculitis of the polyarteritis nodosa group. Therapy for all patients in this group is the same, as discussed under polyarteritis nodosa.

Chumbley LC, et al: Allergic granulomatosis and angiitis (Churg-Strauss syndrome). Mayo Clin Proc 1977, 52:477.

Churg J, et al: Allergic granulomatosis, allergic angiitis, and periarteritis nodosa. Am J Pathol 1951, 27:277.

Crotty CP, et al: Cutaneous clinicopathologic correlation of allergic granulomatosis. JAAD 1981, 5:571.

Fauci AS: Vasculitis. J Clin Allergy Immunol 1983, 72:211.

Gibson LE, et al: Cutaneous granulomatous vasculitis. JAAD 1986, 14:492.

HYPERSENSITIVITY VASCULITIS (Leukocytoclastic Vasculitis)

In this group, Fauci includes the various angiitides of small vessels: anaphylactoid (Henoch-Schönlein)

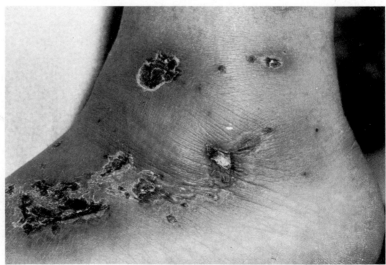

Figure 35–16. Leukocytoclastic angiitis from phenylbutazone.

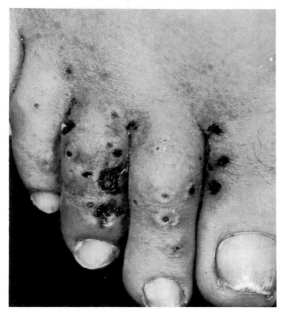

Figure 35–17. Leukocytoclastic angiitis. (Courtesy of Dr. H. Shatin.)

purpura, serum sickness, drug-related vasculitis, erythema elevation diutinum, and vasculitis incidental to cryoglobulinemia, malignancy, infectious diseases, connective tissue diseases, congenital complement deficiencies, or other diseases.

Cutaneous-systemic vasculitis has been variously called allergic cutaneous vasculitis (McCarthy and Kesten); hypersensitivity angiitis (Zeek); allergic angiitis; arteriolitis allergica (Ruiter); dermatitis nodularis necrotica (Werther); nodular dermal allergide (Gougerot); allergic microbid (Miescher and Storck); mono-penta symptom complex (Gougerot); and systemic allergic vasculitis (McCombs).

Braverman indicates that the all-inclusive term of cutaneous-systemic vasculitis is descriptive of leukocytoclastic angiitis, with one end of the spectrum harboring solely the cutaneous forms of vasculitis; the other end, the systemic forms; and the middle, the combination of the two. In the study of 82 patients seen in private practice by Af Ekenstam et al, and in Fauci's experience also, hypersensitivity (leukocytoclastic) vasculitis is usually confined to the skin and does not pose a threat of irreversible dysfunction to vital organs.

The cutaneous manifestations of leukocytoclastic vasculitis are many and varied. Usually the earliest lesions are on the lower legs, which are involved by successive crops. Although there are many different types of lesions, usually only one is present in a given patient. Most often, this is papular, or palpable, purpura. The papules typically flatten, become hyperpigmented, and resolve, over a period of a month or so. They favor the dependent parts: the lower legs in the ambulatory, the buttocks and sacral area in the bedridden. The disease is self-limited, but may recur or become chronic. Hemorrhagic vesicles or bullae may develop. Nodules with ulceration may

occur and persist for months. Rarely, the face, buccal mucosae, and anogenital areas may be involved by petechiae.

Urticarialike lesions are next most common. Lesions are less evanescent than in ordinary hives, and may subside only after a few days, often with residual hyperpigmentation. Other lesions may be pustules on a purpuric base; nodules with purpura, vesicles or bullae; erythematous plaques; livedo reticularis; or necrosis.

Pain and burning and stinging sensations may be present. Edema, especially of the ankles, is usually noted. Fever, malaise, and myalgia are frequently present with the cutaneous manifestations. Arthralgia with hot, tender, and swollen joints occurs. The major kidney manifestation is usually glomerulonephritis. Gastrointestinal involvement may be noted, with the presence of hematemesis, bloody stools, ulcerations in the esophagus and stomach; anorexia, vomiting, nausea, and diarrhea are other features. Infiltrative lung involvement with pneumonitis may also be present. Congestive heart failure and ocular involvement with retinal hemorrhage may supervene. Neural involvement is seen mostly in the severe cases; peripheral neuritis, diplopia, dysphagia, hoarseness, polyneuritis, and peripheral neuritis may be present. The incidence of each of

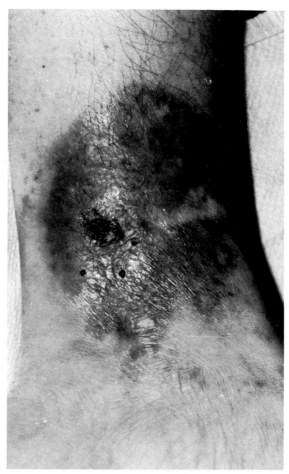

Figure 35–18. Leukocytoclastic angiitis.

these findings varies with the particular subset of presentations of the hypersensitivity vasculitis.

Several identifiable clinical syndromes are recognizable within the general classification of hypersensitivity vasculitis. **Henoch-Schönlein purpura** (HSP), or anaphylactoid purpura, is characterized by intermittent purpura, arthralgia, abdominal pain, and hematuria, in varying combinations. Typically the purpura appears on the extensor aspects of the extremities, including the buttocks. Lesions usually begin as urticarial clusters, which become hemorrhagic within a day and start to fade in about five days. New crops may appear over a period of a few weeks. Urticarial lesions, vesicles, necrotic purpura, and hemangioma-like lesions may also be present at some stage. Piette et al described plaques of palpable purpura with multifocal hemorrhage or superficial necrosis in seven adults with IgA-associated vasculitis and thought it was specific for this, but we have seen it with other types of vasculitis. Green et al documented the occurrence of koebnerization in HSP, and one of us (WDJ) has seen several examples of linear purpura on the legs corresponding to the vertical lines of tight-fitting socks.

Arthralgia is a consistent accompaniment of HSP, and periarticular swelling around knees and ankles may be pronounced.

Abdominal pain and gastrointestinal bleeding may occur at any time during the disease; severe abdominal pain may even suggest—or portend—an acute surgical abdomen. Paralytic ileus may occur. If laparotomy is done (as it was in a case seen by one of us [HLA]) multiple ecchymoses on the visceral peritoneum may be seen. Vomiting, rebound tenderness, and distension are other manifestations. Gastrointestinal x-rays may show "spiking" or a marbled "cobblestone" appearance. Renal involvement manifests as microscopic or even gross hematuria, and may occur in 25 per cent or more of patients. The long-term prognosis in children with gross hematuria is very good; however, progressive glomerular disease and renal failure may develop in a small percentage, so that careful follow-up supervision is necessary for

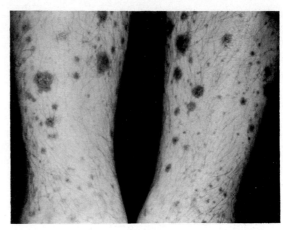

Figure 35–20. Palpable purpuric lesions of the lower extremities of an adolescent male with Henoch-Schoenlein syndrome.

those with hematuria. Guillain-Barré syndrome and mononeuropathies are uncommon but serious associated findings in a few cases of HSP.

Henoch-Schönlein purpura occurs most frequently in the three- to ten-year age group, though it may occur at any age. A viral infection may be the usual triggering event. However, attacks have been attributed to bacterial infections, foods, drugs, chemical toxins, and lymphoma. Phenacetin, penicillin, phenothiazines, sulfonamides, griseofulvin, tetracycline, erythromycin, quinidine, and insect bites have all been incriminated, according to Wenner et al. Aram reported a case precipitated by chlorpromazine.

IgA and C3 depositions have been demonstrated in biopsies of both involved and uninvolved skin by immunofluorescence techniques. VanHale et al suggest that uninvolved skin is a preferable site for biopsy because tissue morphology is better and the hunting is equally good. There may be raised levels of IgA immune complexes irrespective of whether nephritis developed, and even irrespective of whether purpura has made its appearance. One of identical twins, who both had identical renal mesangial deposits of C3 and IgA, had no purpura (**Berger's disease**), while the other had typical Henoch-Schönlein purpura, as reported by Meadow et al. Indeed, Berger's disease (IgA nephropathy) has been shown in several studies to be associated with perivascular deposits of IgA in the skin and is believed by many to be a monosymptomatic form of HSP. The only other condition to be consistently associated with IgA deposition around cutaneous vessels is alcoholic liver disease, as shown by Hené et al.

Treatment is supportive. The usual duration of illness is six to 16 weeks. Between 5 and 10 per cent of patients will have persistent or recurrent disease. Antispasmodics, antibiotics, and anti-inflammatory drugs, including systemic corticosteroids, may be helpful during the course of the disease, which will eventually clear without residua in most cases. Heng found plasmapheresis to be the treatment of choice in the rare severe, progressive cases. Also recom-

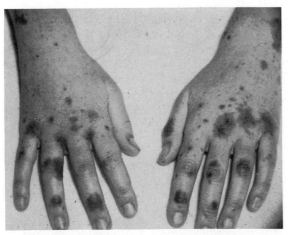

Figure 35–19. Henoch-Schoenlein syndrome.

mended by Heng as helpful in less severe cases are dapsone and corticosteroids. Ephedrine may relieve abdominal pain more effectively than morphine.

Urticarial vasculitis was first described in 1971 and was soon regarded as a distinctive syndrome involving hypocomplementemia, arthritis, arthralgia, angioedema, abdominal or chest pain (or both), and in some cases pulmonary and renal involvement. Sanchez published a series of 40 patients, and divided them into those with hypocomplementemia (severe cases) and those with normal complement. Patients with urticarialike lesions who have leukocytoclastic vasculitis on biopsy may have part or all of the disease manifestations associated with leukocytoclastic vasculitis. Bisaccia et al described a woman in whom urticarial vasculitis was the presenting sign of SLE. Both solar and cold urticaria may manifest leukocytoclastic vasculitis in some cases.

Serum sickness is a clinical syndrome which may occur after primary exposure to heterologous antisera or a nonprotein drug such as penicillin. If the exposure is secondary, an accelerated reaction may occur in two to four days. The patients develop fever, lymphadenopathy, arthralgia, proteinuria, and skin lesions. The latter may be urticarial, or morbilliform; in 12 patients reported by Lawley et al, with bone marrow failure and treatment with IV horse antithymocyte globulin, eight developed a characteristic serpiginous erythematous and purpuric eruption on the edges of the palms and soles.

Pustular vasculitis is a concept lately introduced by Jorizzo to unify certain cases in which there are pustules on purpuric bases. He and McNeely et al have reviewed them and include Behçet's syndrome, disseminated neisserian infections, acute generalized pustular bacterid, *bowel-associated dermatitis-arthritis syndrome*, and their own case of primary idiopathic disease. The dermatitis-arthritis syndrome consists of recurrent pustules occurring episodically on the arms and upper trunk, lasting two or three days and recurring at four to six weeks' intervals. These are associated with fever, arthralgia, and bowel problems, often bowel bypass procedures. Bacterial peptidoglycans are suspected causes, as proposed by Ely. Systemic antibiotics are beneficial.

Erythema elevatum diutinum and **cryoglobulinemia** are discussed elsewhere.

Associated findings and diseases may include drugs, most commonly barbiturates, radiocontrast media, methotrexate, clindamycin, cimetidine, coumadin, propylthiouracil, phenothiazines, sulfonamides, iodides, penicillin, allopurinol, diphenylhydantoin, and acetylsalicylic acid. The reaction generally occurs one to ten days after antigen exposure. Infections are also implicated: upper respiratory infections, pyoderma, and streptococcal infections may trigger leukocytoclastic angiitis. Hepatitis B, mycobacteriosis, and infectious mononucleosis may be associated. Connective tissue diseases associated include lupus erythematosus, scleroderma, dermatomyositis, rheumatoid vasculitis (as reviewed by

Jorizzo et al), and Sjögren's syndrome, as defined by Alexander et al. It is seen in approximately 25 per cent of patients with Sjögren's, usually with high levels of Ro antibody. Malignant neoplasms may also be associated: they accounted for 8 per cent of the cases reviewed by Sanchez et al. The commonest ones are leukemias, lymphomas, and myeloma.

Histologically, the capillaries, arterioles, and (most commonly) the post-capillary venules of the upper dermis are involved. **Leukocytoclasia** (disintegration of polymorphonuclear leukocyte nuclei) and the resultant **nuclear dust** (basophilic particles) are characteristic. Bleeding into the perivascular spaces and fibrinoid necrosis in vessel walls are usually seen. In chronic lesions, massive hyaline changes are likely to occur. On direct immunofluorescence IgM, C3, and fibrin are seen in a speckled perivascular pattern in early lesions.

MANAGEMENT. In view of the many associated conditions and the multiple organ systems which may be affected by hypersensitivity vasculitis, the following evaluation is recommended in patients with skin lesions which show leukocytoclastic vasculitis on biopsy: a thorough history and physical examination with emphasis on drug history; chest x-ray, urinalysis, complete blood count, sedimentation rate, tests for renal and hepatic function, total hemolytic complement, rheumatoid factor, antinuclear antibodies, cryoglobulin, serum protein electrophoresis, hepatitis B antigen and antibody studies, and serum immunoelectrophoresis.

TREATMENT. The treatment of leukocytoclastic angiitis should in general be nonaggressive, since the majority of cases are acute and self-limited, affect only the skin, and do not threaten progressive deterioration of internal organs. Rest and elevation of the legs is likely to be helpful. Analgesics for relief of pain, a good diet, and avoidance of trauma and cold are prudent general measures. An identified antigen or drug should of course be eliminated, and any identified infectious, connective tissue, or neoplastic disease treated.

Among drug therapies one may consider are nonsteroidal antiinflammatory drugs (NSAIDS), antihistamines, dapsone, colchicine, and potassium iodide. Cupps et al and Fauci detail the use of NSAIDS, and Millns et al cleared six of ten patients with urticarial vasculitis with indomethacin. Fredenburg et al treated three cases of leukocytoclastic vasculitis successfully with 100 to 150 mg of dapsone daily. Fortson et al had success with dapsone in urticarial vasculitis, and Bernardet et al report its usefulnes in rheumatoid vasculitis. Callen reviewed his experience with colchicine in 13 patients with leukocytoclastic vasculitis: they were improved, and only three got diarrhea. Wiles et al used it successfully in two cases of urticarial vasculitis. Ely speculates that, because of its effect on white blood cells, pentoxifylline should be investigated in the treatment of neutrophilic vascular reactions.

If progressive systemic disease is present, oral

prednisone or intramuscularly injected triamcinolone acetonide, or pulse methylprednisolone, or long-term immunosuppression, may be tried, although they are often of limited help. Methotrexate in low dosage was helpful in a case of rheumatoid vasculitis reported by Upchurch et al.

Aboobaker J, et al: Urticarial vasculitis. Clin Exp Dermatol 1986, 11:436.

Af Ekenstam E: Cutaneous leukocytoclastic vasculitis: clinical and laboratory features of 82 patients seen in private practice. Arch Dermatol 1984, 120:484.

Alexander E, et al: Sjögren's syndrome. Arch Dermatol 1987, 123:801.

Idem: Cutaneous manifestations of primary Sjögren's syndrome. J Invest Dermatol 1983, 80:386.

Allen DM, et al: Anaphylactoid purpura in children (Schönlein-Henoch syndrome). Am J Dis Child 1960, 99:833.

Aram H: Henoch-Schönlein purpura induced by chlorpromazine. JAAD 1987, 17:139.

Bernard P, et al: Dapsone and rheumatoid vasculitis leg ulceration. JAAD 1988, 18:140.

Bisaccia E, et al: Urticarial vasculitis progressing to systemic lupus erythematosus. Arch Dermatol 1988, 124:1088.

Boom BW, et al: Membrane attack complex of complement in leukocytoclastic vasculitis of the skin. Arch Dermatol 1987, 123:1192.

Callen JP: Colchicine is effective in controlling chronic cutaneous leukocytoclastic vasculitis. JAAD 1985, 13:193.

Idem, et al: Urticarial vasculitis. Br J Dermatol 1982, 107:87.

Idem: Cutaneous leukocytoclastic vasculitis. South Med J 1987, 80:848.

Cupps TR, et al: Chronic recurrent small-vessel cutaneous vasculitis. JAMA 1982, 247:1994.

Curd JG, et al: Potassium iodide sensitivity in four patients with hypocomplementemic vasculitis. Ann Intern Med 1979, 91:853.

Dresnick EJ, et al: Cutaneous lesions after intestinal bypass. Ann Intern Med 1980, 93:557.

Ely PH: The bowel bypass syndrome. JAAD 1980, 2:473.

Idem: White blood cells as mediators of hyperviscosity-induced tissue damage in neutrophilic vascular reactions. Therapy with pentoxifylline. JAAD 1989, 20:677.

Falk DK: Pulmonary disease in idiopathic urticarial vasculitis. JAAD 1984, 11:346.

Fan PT, et al: A clinical approach to systemic vasculitis. Semin Arthritis Rheum 1980, 9:248.

Fauci AS: Vasculitis. J Allergy Clin Immunol 1983, 72:211.

Idem: The spectrum of vasculitis. Ann Intern Med 1978, 89:660.

Feldman D, et al: Cutaneous vasculitis in adult polymyositis/dermatomyositis. J Rheum 1983, 10:85.

Fortson JS, et al: Hypocomplementemic urticarial vasculitis syndrome responsive to dapsone. JAAD 1986, 15:1137.

Fredenberg MF, et al: Sulfone therapy in the treatment of leukocytoclastic vasculitis. JAAD 1987, 16:772.

Gower RG, et al: Small vessel vasculitis caused by hepatitis B virus immune complexes. J Allergy Clin Immunol 1978, 62:222.

Green ST, et al: The Koebner phenomenon in anaphylactoid purpura. Cutis 1986, 38:56.

Hazen PG, et al: Management of necrotizing vasculitis with colchicine. Arch Dermatol 1979, 115:1303.

Hené RJ, et al: The relevance of IgA deposits in vessel walls of clinically normal skin. Arch Intern Med 1986, 146:745.

Heng MCY: Henoch-Schönlein purpura. Br J Dermatol 1985, 112:235.

Jorizzo JL: Pustular vasculitis. JAAD 1983, 9:160.

Idem, et al: Bowel-bypass syndrome without bowel bypass. Arch Intern Med 1983, 143:457.

Idem: Dermatologic conditions reported in patients with rheumatoid arthritis. JAAD 1983, 8:439.

Idem: Neutrophilic vascular reactions. JAAD 1988, 19:983.

Kenny PGW, et al: Leukocytoclastic vasculitis in hairy cell leukemia. Arch Dermatol 1983, 119:1018.

Kerdel FA, et al: Necrotizing vasculitis from [Renografin]. JAAD 1984, 10:25.

Lambert WC, et al: Leukocytoclastic vasculitis induced by clindamycin. Cutis 1982, 30:615.

Lawley TJ, et al: A prospective clinical and immunologic analysis of patients with serum sickness. N Engl J Med 1984, 311:1407.

Ledermann JA, et al: Dapsone in allergic vasculitis. J R Soc Med 1983, 76:613.

Lucas SB, et al: Recurrent vasculitis associated with beta-hemolytic streptococcal infections. Br Med J 1978, 1:1323.

Mackel SE: Treatment of vasculitis. Med Clin North Am 1982, 66:941.

Idem, et al: Leukocytoclastic vasculitis: a cutaneous expression of immune complex disease. Arch Dermatol 1982, 118:296.

Marks CR, et al: Small vessel vasculitis and methotrexate. Ann Intern Med 1984, 100:916.

McNeely MC, et al: Primary idiopathic cutaneous vasculitis. JAAD 1986, 14:939.

Meadow SR, et al: Berger disease: Henoch-Schönlein syndrome without the rash. J Pediatr 1985, 106:27.

Millns JL, et al: The therapeutic response of urticarial vasculitis to indomethacin. JAAD 1980, 3:349.

Mitchell GG, et al: Cimetidine-induced cutaneous vasculitis. Am J Med 1983, 75:875.

Monroe EW, et al: Vasculitis in chronic urticaria: an immunopathologic study. J Invest Dermatol 1981, 76:103.

Newton JA, et al: Leukocytoclastic vasculitis and angioedema associated with inflammatory bowel disease. Clin Exp Dermatol 1984, 9:618.

Piette WW, et al: A cutaneous sign of IgA-associated small dermal vessel leukocytoclastic vasculitis in adults. Arch Dermatol 1989, 125:53.

Popp JW: Cutaneous vasculitis associated with acute and chronic hepatitis. Arch Intern Med 1981, 141:623.

Provost TT, et al: The relationship between anti-Ro (SSA) antibody-positive Sjögren's syndrome and anti-Ro (SSA) antibody–positive lupus erythematosus. Arch Dermatol 1988, 124:63.

Rosenbloom AL, et al: Limited joint mobility in childhood diabetes mellitus indicates increased risk for microvascular disease. N Engl J Med 1981, 305:191.

Sams WM, et al: Leukocytoclastic vasculitis. Arch Dermatol 1976, 112:219.

Sanchez NP, et al: Clinical and histologic spectrum of necrotizing vasculitis. Arch Dermatol 1985, 121:220.

Idem: Clinical and histologic spectrums of urticarial vasculitis: study of 40 cases. JAAD 1982, 7:599.

Schwartz HR, et al: Hypocomplementemic urticarial vasculitis: association with chronic obstructive pulmonary disease. Mayo Clin Proc 1982, 57:231.

Soter NA: Chronic urticaria as a manifestation of necrotizing vasculitis. N Engl J Med 1977, 296:1440.

Idem, et al: Urticaria and arthralgias as manifestations of necrotizing angitis. J Invest Dermatol 1974, 63:485.

Tanay A, et al: Dermal vasculitis due to coumarin hypersensitivity. Dermatologica 1982, 165:178.

Tencati JR, et al: Hypersensitivity angiitis caused by fumes from heat-activated copy paper. Ann Intern Med 1983, 98:320.

Upchurch KS, et al: Low-dose methotrexate therapy for cutaneous vasculitis of rheumatoid arthritis. JAAD 1987, 17:355.

VanArsdel PP: Allergy and adverse drug reactions. JAAD 1982, 6:833.

Van der Horst JC, et al: Urticarial vasculitis in a patient with systemic lupus erythematosus. Clin Exp Dermatol 1981, 6:489.

VanHale HM, et al: Henoch-Schönlein vasculitis. JAAD 1986, 15:665.

Vasily DB, et al: Propylthiouracil-induced cutaneous vasculitis. JAMA 1980, 243:458.

Vollersten RS, et al: Rheumatoid vasculitis. Medicine (Baltimore) 1986, 65:365.

Wanderer AA, et al: Urticarial leukocytoclastic vasculitis with cold urticaria. Arch Dermatol 1983, 119:145.

Wenner NP, et al: Circulating immune complexes in Henoch-Schönlein purpura. Int J Dermatol 1983, 22:383.

Wiles JC, et al: Urticarial vasculitis treated with colchicine. Arch Dermatol 1985, 121:802.

Wintroub BU, et al: Cutaneous drug reactions. JAAD 1985, 13:167.

WEGENER'S GRANULOMATOSIS

Wegener's granulomatosis is a syndrome consisting of necrotizing granulomas of the upper and lower respiratory tract, generalized necrotizing angiitis affecting the medium-sized blood vessels, and focal necrotizing glomerulitis.

By far the commonest initial manifestation is the occurrence of rhinorrhea, severe sinusitis, and nasal mucosal ulcerations, with one or several nodules in the nose, larynx, trachea, or bronchi. There are fever, weight loss, and malaise in these patients, who are usually 40 to 50 years of age and more often male than female (ratio 1.3 to 1). Obstruction in the nose may also block the sinuses. The nodules in the nose frequently ulcerate and bleed. The parenchymal involvement of the lungs produces cough, dyspnea, and chest pain. Granulomas may occur in the ear and in the mouth, where the alveolar ridge becomes necrotic and ulceration of the tongue and perforated ulcers of the palate develop. The "strawberry gums" appearance of hypertrophic gingivitis is characteristic. Israelson et al reported such a case.

Cutaneous findings occur in 45 per cent of patients. Nodules may appear in crops, especially along the extensor surfaces of the extremities. The firm, slightly tender, flesh-colored or violaceous nodules may later ulcerate to form necrotic centers. The necrotizing angiitis of the skin may become evident as purpura in the form of a petechial or hemorrhagic pustular eruption.

Focal necrotizing glomerulitis occurs in 85 per cent of patients. It may be fulminant from the outset or may become more severe as the disease progresses. Renal failure was the most frequent cause of death prior to cyclophosphamide treatment.

Other areas frequently attacked include the joints, with arthralgia in two thirds of cases; eyes (conjunctivitis, episcleritis, and proptosis) in 58 per cent; and central nervous system and cardiac involvement in 22 per cent and 12 per cent of patients, respectively.

The histologic findings show necrotic centers surrounded by granulation tissue with plasma cells, giant cells, and lymphocytes.

Necrotizing granulomas and necrotizing vasculitis are the two types of histologic lesions that may be found, either together or separately. Allergic granulomatosis may also manifest these two types of lesions, but respiratory/renal involvement is most unusual in that condition, whereas asthma commonly precedes it, and eosinophils predominate in the lesions.

In the past, lymphomatoid granulomatosis was included in the granulomatous vasculitides, but Fauci has dropped it from his classification, and one of the authors who originally described the disease (Carrington) now feels it to be a lymphoma. Nichols et al regard it as an angiocentric T-cell lymphoma, and we accept that view.

Untreated Wegener's granulomatosis had a mean survival time of five months, and a 90 per cent mortality over two years. Cyclophosphamide therapy has dramatically changed the prognosis. Fauci et al reported their prospective experience with 85 patients, using 2 mg of cyclophosphamide per kg of body weight, and prednisone, 1 mg/kg/day, followed by tapering of the prednisone to an alternate-day regimen. Complete remission was achieved in 93 per cent, and lasted an average of four years for those patients still living. Twenty-three had been off all therapy for an average of 35 months at the time of the report. Ten of 11 patients who had been on azathioprine failed to achieve satisfactory remission after four to six weeks, and every one achieved complete remission on cyclophosphamide. Nine patients who developed cyclophosphamide-induced cystitis were switched to azathioprine, and all but one went into remission; she responded to a second course of cyclophosphamide.

Generally, in patients with a multisystem disease and a relatively stable clinical course, cyclophosphamide is used alone, at doses discussed above under polyarteritis nodosa. With fulminant vasculitis involving the brain, lungs, peripheral nerves, or kidneys, cyclophosphamide should be used intravenously, 4 mg/kg/day for three days, tapering for the next three days to 1 or 2 mg/kg/day. In fulminant renal or pulmonary disease 60 mg/day of prednisone is added, and tapered over several weeks. Cyclophosphamide is continued for one year after the disappearance of all traces of active disease and the sedimentation rate has returned to normal.

DeRemee reported success in 11 of 12 patients treated with antimicrobial agents, chiefly trimethoprim-sulfamethoxazole. West et al had similar results in their patient.

LYMPHOMATOID GRANULOMATOSIS

This severe systemic disease has as its main component a necrotizing pulmonary angiitis. It is discussed here because it was originally classified as a type of angiitis; however, it is well documented through various studies, including T-cell rearrangement analysis, that this is a clonal T-cell proliferative disease. From its onset, it is a type of T-cell lymphoma.

Cough, shortness of breath, and chest pain are most frequently the presenting complaints. A chest x-ray will characteristically show multiple nodules in the mid and lower lobes bilaterally without accompanying hilar adenopathy. Open lung biopsy will reveal the diagnostic findings of an angiocentric, angiodestructive, atypical lymphohistiocytic infiltrate.

Extrapulmonary manifestations are common, with skin lesions being present in 40 per cent of the cases. Cutaneous involvement may occur at any time during the course of the disease. There is equal frequency of onset before, during, or after pulmonary lesions develop. Types of skin lesions reported are protean; however, subcutaneous or dermal nodules are present in nearly 50 per cent of cases. Macular erythema, papules, ulcers, alopecia, annular lesions, vesicles, and acquired ichthyosis have all been reported. Brodell et al emphasized nodular and annular skin lesions in the diagnosis. Usually the lesions are symmetrical, may involve any area of the body, and may be generalized. They are transient in 80 per cent of the cases, clearing either spontaneously or with minimal therapy within two months after onset. Other frequent sites of involvement are the peripheral and central nervous system and joints.

Systemic complaints of fever, malaise, weight loss, and myalgias are common. Liebow found motor involvement in 22 per cent of cases, and Katzenstein found it was associated with increased mortality (over 80 per cent). Peripheral neuropathy may simulate leprosy. Cranial nerve involvement and central nervous system lesions may be present. Kidney lesions are nodular infiltrations, not the glomerulonephritis type seen in Wegener's. Adenopathy does not occur. Laboratory investigation is generally unremarkable. Occasionally anemia, elevated sedimentation rate, leukocytosis, or mild elevation of liver enzymes may be present.

Histopathologically, skin biopsy nearly always reveals a polymorphous infiltrate centered about blood vessels. Pleomorphism of the infiltrate with angioinvasion and angiodestruction are classic, diagnostic findings seen in some cases. Vessels of any size in the dermis or subcutaneous fat may be involved. The atypical lymphohistiocytic infiltrate is also periappendageal with destruction of eccrine glands, sebaceous glands, and hair follicles seen often.

Prior to the introduction of cyclophosphamide, treatment with systemic steroids alone had a 65 per cent one-year mortality rate with respiratory failure the rule. Seven of 13 cases treated by Fauci et al with cyclophosphamide (2 mg/kg/day) and prednisone (1 mg/kg on alternate days) had complete remissions lasting for an average of five years, though treatment was stopped after an average of one year. Seven of the eight who died had frank lymphoma, which occurs in 12 to 14 per cent of cases.

Early aggressive combination chemotherapy for lymphoma has been advocated by some but we believe this concept is still evolving.

Brodell RT, et al: Cutaneous lesions of lymphomatoid granulomatosis. Arch Dermatol 1986, 122:303.
Camisa C: Lymphomatoid granulomatosis. JAAD 1989, 20:571.
Chyu JYH, et al: Wegener's granulomatosis in childhood. JAAD 1984, 10:341.
Cohen PS, et al: Strawberry gums: a sign of Wegener's granulomatosis. JAMA 1981, 246:2610.
Colby TV, et al: Pulmonary lymphomas. Hum Pathol 1983, 14:884.
Crotty CP, et al: Cutaneous clinicopathologic correlation of allergic granulomatosis. JAAD 1981, 5:571.
DeRemee RA, et al: Wegener's granulomatosis: observations on treatment with antimicrobial agents. Mayo Clin Proc 1985, 60:27.
Fauci AS, et al: Wegener's granulomatosis: prospective clinical and therapeutic experience with 85 patients for 21 years. Ann Intern Med 1983, 98:760.
Idem: Lymphomatoid granulomatosis: prospective clinical and therapeutic experience over 10 years. N Engl J Med 1982, 306:68.
Hu GH, et al: Cutaneous manifestations of Wegener's granulomatosis. Arch Dermatol 1977, 113:175.
Israelson H, et al: The hyperplastic gingivitis of Wegener's granulomatosis. J Periodontol 1981, 52:81.
Jambrosic J, et al: Lymphomatoid granulomatosis. JAAD 1987, 17:621.
James WD, et al: Cutaneous manifestations of lymphomatoid granulomatosis. Arch Dermatol 1981, 117:196.
Katzenstein A, et al: Lymphomatoid granulomatosis. Cancer 1979, 43:360.
Nichols PW, et al: Lymphomatoid granulomatosis: a T-cell disorder? Am J Med 1982, 72:467.
Patton WF, et al: Lymphomatoid granulomatosis: clinicopathologic study of 4 cases and literature review. Medicine 1982, 61:1.
Rongioletti F, et al: Ulcerated plaque and nodules on the thigh of a patient with febrile pulmonary disease. Arch Dermatol 1988, 12:571.
Scully RE, et al: Case records of the Massachusetts General Hospital. N Engl J Med 1987, 317:879.
West BC, et al: Wegener's granulomatosis and trimethoprim-sulfamethoxazole. Ann Intern Med 1987, 106:840.
Whittaker S, et al: Lymphomatoid granulomatosis—evidence of a clonal T-cell origin and an association with lethal midline granuloma. Q J Med 1988, 256:645.

GIANT-CELL ARTERITIS
(Temporal Arteritis)

Giant-cell arteritis is a systemic disease of people over 50. Its best known location is in the temporal artery, where it is known as cranial arteritis and Horton's disease. It is characterized by a necrotizing panarteritis with granulomas and giant cells, which produce unilateral headache and exquisite tenderness in the scalp over the temporal or occipital arteries. Fever, anemia, and a high sedimentation rate are usually present. It is rarely fatal, but Säve Söderbergh et al reported nine fatal cases in 1986. In two a coronary artery was involved; in two the aorta; and in five, the site was a cerebral artery. The disease has also been identified in vessels of the uterus, legs, abdomen, and hand.

The cutaneous manifestations may be only inflammatory, whereby erythema and the affected artery become evident as a hard, pulsating, tender, tortuous bulge under red or cyanotic skin. Another manifestation is gangrene of the scalp. The lesions may first appear as ecchymoses with a zonal distribution over the affected area. Later they may become vesicular or bullous and are followed by gangrene, probably from the thrombosis of the affected vessels. Lingual artery involvement may cause an accompanying red, sore tongue. Blindness may also develop and is the most feared complication of the disease.

Polymyalgia rheumatica has a significant clinical association with giant-cell arteritis, and prompt treatment of it may forestall serious disease. About 10 per cent of central retinal artery occlusions are due to giant-cell arteritis. Biller et al reported a case of this in a man, 48, whose sedimentation rate was normal. It is elevated in over 90 per cent of patients with giant-cell arteritis. Barot et al reported a case of temporal artery involvement with loss of vision, but no pain.

Hitch tabulated the various skin manifestations; in addition to those mentioned previously, ecchymoses, urticaria, purpura, alopecia, tender nodules, lividity, and erythema may be seen. The mouth may show temporomandibular pain and gangrene of the tongue. Temporal artery biopsy is diagnostic.

Treatment is usually begun with prednisone, 60 mg daily, continued for one month or until all reversible clinical and laboratory parameters (such as the sedimentation rate) have become normal. The disease is quite steroid-responsive, and tapering to a dose of 7.5 to 10 mg a day is usually possible. Daily therapy seems important, and is usually necessary for one to two years at least. An effort should probably be made to switch the patient to intramuscular triamcinolone acetonide, while monitoring the sedimentation rate on a daily basis. Most patients achieve complete remission that is often maintained after therapy is withdrawn.

Takayasu's Arteritis

Known also as *aortic arch syndrome* and *pulseless disease*, this is a thromboobliterative process of the great vessels stemming from the aortic arch, occurring generally in young women. Radial and carotid pulses are typically obliterated. Skin changes are due to the disturbed circulation. There may be loss of hair and atrophy of the skin and its appendages, with underlying muscle atrophy. Mousa et al and Perniciaro et al have reviewed the skin findings. Occasional patients with cutaneous necrotizing or granulomatous vasculitis have been reported. Erythema nodosum was seen in four of the 38 patients reviewed by Perniciaro et al.

Treatment with corticosteroids as in temporal arteritis should be given, and followed in the same way. Although it is much less effective here than in that disease, it is the best available treatment at present.

Barot AJ, et al: Temporal arteritis without pain. JAMA 1980, 243:61.

Baum EW, et al: Giant cell arteritis: a systemic disease with rare cutaneous manifestations. JAAD 1982, 6:1081.

Biller J, et al: Temporal arteritis associated with a normal sedimentation rate. JAMA 1982, 247:481.

Fan PT, et al: A clinical approach to systemic vasculitis. Semin Arthritis Rheum 1980, 9:248.

Hitch JM: Dermatologic manifestations of giant-cell (temporal cranial) arteritis. Arch Dermatol 1970, 101:409.

Mousa ARM, et al: Cutaneous necrotizing vasculitis complicating Takayasu's arteritis with a review of the cutaneous manifestations. J Rheumatol 1985, 12:607.

Perniciaro CV, et al: Cutaneous manifestations of Takayasu's arteritis. JAAD 1987, 17:998.

Rosenman HD, et al: Giant cell arteritis with scalp necrosis. Int J Dermatol 1978, 17:643.

Save-Söderbergh J, et al: Giant-cell arteritis as a cause of death: report of 9 cases. JAMA 1986, 255:493.

MALIGNANT ATROPHIC PAPULOSIS

Papulosis atrophicans maligna, also known as Degos's disease, is a fatal cutaneointestinal obliterative arteritis syndrome, described by Degos and his associates in 1942. Clinically it is characterized by the presence of pale rose, rounded, edematous papules occurring mostly on the trunk. Similar lesions may occur on the bulbar conjunctiva and the oral mucosa. Later the lesions become umbilicated, with a central depression, which enlarges. The center becomes distinctively porcelain-white, while the periphery becomes livid red and telangiectatic. Atrophy occurs eventually. The eruption proceeds by crops in which only a few new lesions appear at any one time.

Later, anemic infarcts involve the intestines to

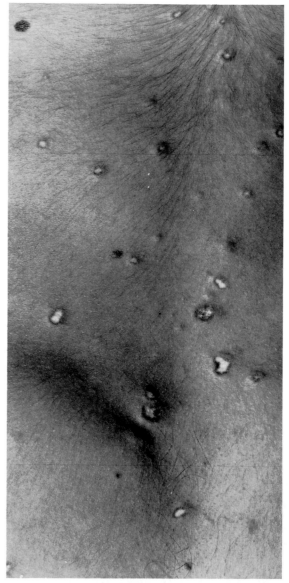

Figure 35–21. Papulosis atrophicans maligna on mid-back. Red papules, some showing umbilication; other papules umbilicated with typical porcelaneous white centers. (From Winkelmann RK, et al: Arch Dermatol 87:54–62, 1963.)

produce acute abdominal symptoms of epigastric pain, fever, and hematemesis. Death is usually due to fulminating peritonitis caused by multiple perforations of the intestine. Less commonly, death occurs from cerebral infarctions. Eye lesions such as episcleritis may also be present. Degos's disease occurs most frequently in men between 20 and 40 years of age. Patients survive untreated an average of two years after the disease has developed.

In a review of the literature in 1971, Wilson Jones and Black stated that 18 of the 45 reported patients were still alive, of which seven with known systemic involvement had survived for periods of one to six years. In 11 cases lesions have been confined to the skin, the longest period of follow-up being 14 years.

Wedge-shaped necroses brought on by the obliteration of arterioles and small arteries account for the clinical lesions. Proliferation of the intima with subsequent thrombosis is the typical histologic picture. Soter et al, using refined techniques of light microscopy, found extensive lymphocytic infiltration and necrotizing vasculitis of the microvasculature, with damage to cutaneous nerves by demyelination. The etiology of this disease is unknown, but seems unlikely to be immunologic or related to immune complexes.

Administration of corticosteroids has not been beneficial, and has even caused gastrointestinal perforation.

Stahl and his associates reported a cure using 0.5 gm acetylsalicylic acid twice a day and 50 mg dipyridamole (Persantine) three times a day, for 20 months. Only one new lesion appeared after treatment was begun. Some have reported success with this combination; however, others have found it ineffective. Anticoagulant therapy has helped on occasion, and heparin, as described by Degos, has been successful.

Pentoxyphylline (Trental), which facilitates blood flow through narrowed capillaries by making the erythrocytes' membranes more flexible, ought to be effective.

Black MM: Malignant atrophic papulosis (Degos's disease). Int J Dermatol 1976, 15:405.
Degos R: Malignant atrophic papulosis. Br J Dermatol 1979, 100:21.
Shwayder TA: Scaly papules with atrophy. Arch Dermatol 1986, 122:89.
Soter NA, et al: Lymphocytes and necrosis of the cutaneous microvasculature in malignant atrophic papulosis: a refined light microscopic study. JAAD 1982, 7:360.
Stahl D, et al: Malignant atrophic papulosis: treatment with aspirin and dipyridamole. Arch Dermatol 1978, 114:1687.
Su WPD, et al: Clinical histologic findings in Degos's syndrome. Cutis 1985, 35:131.
Tribble K, et al: Malignant atrophic papulosis. JAAD 1986, 15:365.

THROMBOANGIITIS OBLITERANS
(Buerger's Disease)

Thromboangiitis obliterans is an obliterative vascular disease affecting the medium- and small-sized arteries, especially those of the feet and hands. It is most often seen in men between 20 and 40 who smoke heavily. The vasomotor changes in early cases may be transitory or persistent; they produce blanching, cyanosis, burning, and tingling. Superficial phlebitis commonly develops in the leg and foot, and attacks tend to come and go every few weeks. The color of the part may change when it is elevated or lowered below the heart level, being red when dependent and white when elevated. Pain is a constant symptom, coming on at first after exercise and subsiding upon resting, instep claudication being the classic complaint. Ultimately pulsation in the dorsalis pedis and posterior tibial arteries, or even others, may cease. In thromboangiitis obliterans, skin supplied by affected arterioles tends to break down, with central necrosis and ulceration and eventual gangrene. Exposure to cold and dampness may have etiologic importance. Histologic examination shows vasculitis of the smaller distal arteries, and foci of necrosis resulting from thrombosis of vessels located at the tip of the necrotic zones. Arteriography should be done to investigate for central atherosclerotic disease, which may be operable, rather than the inoperable distal damage of Buerger's disease.

Treatment is by protection from cold and trauma. Tobacco must be forbidden. Sympathectomy may be tried if vasodilators fail. Ultimately, serial amputations may be necessary.

Giblin WJ, et al: Buerger's disease. Int J Dermatol (in press).
Lie JT: Thromboangiitis obliterans in women. Medicine 1986, 65:65.
McKusick VA, et al: Buerger's disease. JAMA 1962, 181:93.
Mills JL, et al: Buerger's disease in the modern era. Am J Surg 1987, 154:123.

ARTERIOSCLEROSIS OBLITERANS

Arteriosclerosis obliterans is an occlusive arterial disease most prominently affecting the abdominal aorta and the small and medium-sized arteries of the lower extremities. The symptoms are due to ischemia of the tissues. There is intermittent claudication manifested by pain, cramp, numbness, and fatigue in the muscles upon exercise; these are relieved by rest. There may be "rest pain" induced at nighttime when in bed. Also sensitivity to cold, muscular weakness, stiffness of the joints, and paresthesia may be present. Sexual impotence is common.

Impaired pulsation or absence of pulsation in the dorsalis pedis artery is usually evident and is suggestive of the disease. Impaired to absent pulses in the posterior tibial or popliteal areas may be found on physical examination, confirming the diagnosis. The feet, especially the toes, may be red and cold. Striking pallor of the feet on elevation, and redness when dependent, are compatible findings. Decreased to absent hair growth may be observed on the legs. Ulceration and gangrene may supervene. If present, they usually begin in the toes.

Arteriography may be indicated as a preliminary to corrective surgery (arterial grafts).

Kerdel et al called attention to the fact that occasionally subclavian atherosclerosis may give rise to these signs in the distal upper extremity. Their case presented with a painful nail and loss of digital skin.

Claudication and diminished blood pressure in the affected extremity are findings that may lead to earlier diagnosis and thus to curative surgical intervention. Usually bypass of the affected artery, or sympathectomy, or both, are the preferred treatment.

Kerdel FA, et al: Subclavian occlusive disease presenting as a painful nail. JAAD 1984, 10:523.

MUCOCUTANEOUS LYMPH NODE SYNDROME
(Kawasaki's Disease)

Irritable, febrile infants or children (or rarely, adults) with erythema-multiformelike, scarlatiniform, or morbilliform skin lesions accompanied by stomatitis, cheilitis, edema of the hands and feet, conjunctival congestion, and cervical lymphadenitis, probably have mucocutaneous lymph node syndrome (MLNS). An early finding, described in detail by Fritter et al, is the appearance of an erythematous, desquamating perianal eruption. Of their 58 patients, 67 per cent developed it, usually within the first week of symptoms. After a week or two the fingers and toes desquamate, starting around the nails. The disease lasts 10 to 20 days and then subsides, but 1 to 2 per cent of patients may die of myocardial infarction soon after their apparent recovery.

Kawasaki first reported this acute febrile illness in children in 1967, in Japan. Since then it has been diagnosed in increasing numbers worldwide, and by 1980 a review of 580 cases seen in the United States was published by Bell et al. They made several epidemiologic observations: as in Japan, most patients were children under five; there was male predominance (1.5:1); and there was a higher incidence in children of Asian ancestry. They also noted a higher incidence in blacks, a peak incidence between February and May, and no evidence of person-to-person transmission.

DIAGNOSIS. Six criteria have been defined: fever, conjunctival congestion, oropharyngeal lesions, hand and foot lesions, an exanthem, and lymphadenopathy. *Fever* is above 38.3°C, lasting over five days and unresponsive to antibiotics. This is the only essential criterion; four of the other five must be present. Nonpurulent bilateral *conjunctival congestion* occurs early in the course. *Oropharyngeal changes*: (1) Erythema, fissuring, and crusting of the lips; (2) diffuse oropharyngeal erythema; (3) strawberry tongue. *Hand and foot lesions*: indurative erythema of hands and feet; erythema of palms and soles; desquamation

from the tips of the digits about two weeks after onset. Polymorphous *erythematous exanthem* occurs, without vesicles or crusts. The *perianal eruption* occurs in about two thirds of patients. Nonpurulent cervical *lymph node enlargement* reaches at least 1.5 cm in diameter.

Bell et al found the following complications: joint involvement (27 per cent), cardiac abnormalities (22 per cent), and a 1.2 per cent mortality.

PATHOLOGY. Arteritis of the main coronary arteries is the characteristic histopathologic finding in all the fatal cases, though vasculitis may occur in other vessels as well. Some consider the syndrome indistinguishable from infantile polyarteritis nodosa.

ETIOLOGY. The etiology is unknown; an infectious agent is suspected, with a hypersensitivity reaction to it, perhaps genetically determined, leading to the arteritis.

TREATMENT. The best treatment appears to be 100 mg/kg/day of aspirin given from the start for the antipyretic and antiinflammatory effect. Koren et al gave as much as 180 mg/kg during the febrile phase, when absorption is poor. Absorption rises rapidly when temperature becomes normal and the sedimentation rate begins to decline. Steroids are not effective, and may increase the risk of myocardial infarction.

Newburger et al, in a multicenter randomized trial of high-dose intravenous gamma globulin, 400 mg/kg/day daily for four days, found the incidence of coronary-artery abnormalities reduced from 23 per cent to 8 per cent after two weeks, and from 18 per cent to 4 per cent after seven weeks. Both groups received aspirin, 100 mg/kg/day through the 14th day of illness, and then from 3 to 5 mg/kg/day for the antiplatelet effect. There were no ill effects. Rowley et al and Nagashima et al had similar results.

Calabro emphasized the importance of reducing the dose of aspirin once the patient is well, and before the sedimentation rate returns to normal (which often takes a few weeks), lest serum salicylate rise rapidly to toxic levels, probably as a result of increased absorption.

Bell DM, et al: Kawasaki syndrome in the United States. Am J Dis Child 1983, 137:211.

Calabrio JJ, et al: Preventing coronary involvement in Kawasaki disease (letter). JAMA 1986, 255:200.

Everett ED, et al: Acute febrile mucocutaneous lymph node syndrome-Kawasaki syndrome. Int J Dermatol 1982, 21:506.

Fritter BS, et al: The perianal eruption of Kawasaki disease. Arch Dermatol 1988, 124:1805.

Kawasaki T, et al: A new infantile acute febrile mucocutaneous lymph node syndrome (MLNS) prevailing in Japan. Pediatrics 1974, 54:271.

Koren G, et al: Probable efficacy of high-dose salicylates in reducing coronary involvement in Kawasaki disease. JAMA 1985, 254:767.

Landing BH, et al: Are infantile periarteritis nodosa with coronary artery disease and fatal mucocutaneous lymph node syndrome the same? Pediatrics 1977, 59:651.

Melish ME, et al: Mucocutaneous lymph node syndrome in the United States. Am J Dis Child 1976, 130:599.

Nagashima M, et al: High dose gamma globulin therapy for Kawasaki disease. J Pediatr 1987, 110:710.

Nahmias AJ: Kawasaki disease: from children to adults (editorial note). Ann Intern Med 1980, 92:564.

Newburger JW, et al: Treatment of Kawasaki syndrome with intravenous gamma globulin. N Engl J Med 1986, 315:341.

Odom RB, et al: Mucocutaneous lymph node syndrome. Arch Dermatol 1977, 113:339.

Rowley AH, et al: Prevention of giant coronary artery aneurysms in Kawasaki disease by intravenous gamma globulin therapy. J Pediatr 1988, 113:290.

Urbach AH, et al: Kawasaki disease and perianal rash. Am J Dis Child 1988, 142:1174.

Velez-Torres R, et al: Acute febrile mucocutaneous lymph node (Kawasaki) syndrome. Int J Dermatol 1987, 26:96.

MONDOR'S DISEASE

Mondor's disease occurs three times as frequently in women as in men, and most patients have been in the age range of 30 to 60 years. The sudden appearance of a cordlike thrombosed vein, which is at first red and tender and subsequently changes into a painless, tough fibrous band, is characteristic. There are no systemic symptoms. Both sides of the chest have the same incidence of involvement. The cause is unknown. The condition represents a localized thrombophlebitis of the veins of the thoraco-epigastric area. The veins involved are the lateral thoracic, thoracoepigastric, and superior epigastric. In the end stage a thick-walled vein remains which has a hard ropelike appearance and on occasion may result in a furrowing of the breast. Exceptionally, a vein coursing up the inside of the upper arm may be involved and Tanii reported four cases of involvement of the penis, two in the sulcus and two on the dorsum.

Malignancy is associated with hypercoagulability of the blood, and when *superficial migratory thrombophlebitis* exists (which is in the differential diagnosis of Mondor's disease), an underlying cancer should be suspected, especially of the pancreas. This entity is known as *Trousseau's sign*. A case report, discussing the signs and symptoms, as well as the spectrum of associated malignancies, was published by one of us (WDJ). Superficial migratory thrombophlebitis may also occur in hereditary protein S deficiency, anti-thrombin III deficiency, and factor XII deficiency.

Treatment is symptomatic, with hot, moist dressings and analgesics or nonsteroidal antiinflammatory agents. The disease process runs its course in from three weeks to six months.

Bell WR, et al: Trousseau's syndrome. Am J Med 1985, 79:423.

Engesser L, et al: Hereditary protein S deficiency. Ann Intern Med 1987, 106:677.

James WD: Trousseau's syndrome. Int J Dermatol 1984, 23:205.

Miller DR, et al: Mondor's disease associated with metastatic axillary nodes. Cancer 1985, 56:903.

Samlaska CP, et al: Superficial migratory thrombophlebitis and factor XII deficiency. JAAD (in press).

Tanii T, et al: Mondor's phlebitis of the penis. Acta Dermatovener 1984, 64:405.

Weinstein EC: Mondor's disease. West J Med 1975, 123:56.

TELANGIECTASIA

A telangiectasis is a dilated cutaneous blood vessel: venule, capillary, or arteriole. Telangiectases are fine linear vessels coursing on the surface of the skin; the name given to them collectively is telangiectasia.

Telangiectasia may occur in normal skin at any age, in both sexes and anywhere on the skin and mucous membranes. Fine telangiectases may be seen on the alae nasi of most adults.

They are prominent in areas of chronic actinic damage seen in fair-skinned persons long exposed to sunlight. In addition, persons long exposed to wind, cold, or heat are subject to telangiectasia.

Telangiectases can be found in such conditions as radiodermatitis, xeroderma pigmentosum, lupus erythematosus, scleroderma and the CREST syndrome, rosacea, cirrhosis of the liver, AIDS, poikiloderma, basal cell carcinoma, necrobiosis lipoidica diabeticorum, sarcoid, lupus vulgaris, adenoma sebaceum, keloid, angioma serpiginosum, angiokeratoma corporis diffusum, ataxia-telangiectasia, pregnancy, and Bloom's syndrome. A complete review of telangiectasia and the diseases characterized by telangiectases was published in 1987 by Goldman et al, in an excellent article.

Altered capillary patterns on the finger nail folds (cuticular telangiectases) are indicative of collagen vascular disease such as lupus erythematosus, scleroderma, or dermatomyositis. They may infrequently be present in rheumatoid arthritis. Minikin et al and Maricq et al, among others, have reviewed the significance of this helpful sign, and we have discussed it previously in the sections on Raynaud's syndrome and in Chapter 8.

Telangiectases about the nose and cheeks from rosacea or actinic damage are best treated by touching the overlying skin at several points with the tip of the epilating needle, using either monopolar or bipolar current, or with a fine pointed galvanocautery tip. The current should be minimal to avoid scarring. Touch-up treatment of old or newly developing lesions may be necessary on an annual basis. Sclerosing solutions are also effective in the hands of those skilled in their use.

Goldman et al reviewed all types of telangiectasia, treatment of the telangiectases according to type, and the indications for treatment. The principal available modalities include electrosurgery, laser beam, dermabrasion, sclerotherapy, and medical measures (tetracycline, estrogen) for specific types.

Braverman IM: Telangiectasia as a sign of systemic disease. Connecticut Med 1969, 33:42.

Fallon T Jr, et al: Telangiectasias of the anterior chest in homosexual men. Ann Intern Med 1986, 105:679.

Goldman MP, et al: Treatment of telangiectasia: a review. JAAD 1987, 17:167.

Idem: Sclerosing agents in the treatment of telangiectasia. Arch Dermatol 1987, 123:1196.

Jimenez-Acosta F, et al: Response to tetracycline of telangiectasias in a male hemophiliac with HIV infection. JAAD 1988, 19:369.

Maricq HR, et al: Diagnostic potential of in vivo capillary microscopy in scleroderma and related disorders. Arthritis Rheum 1980, 23:183.

Minkin W, et al: Office nail fold capillary microscopy using ophthalmoscope. JAAD 1982, 7:190.

Norris MJ, et al: Treatment of essential telangiectasia. JAAD 1989, 20:643.

Stegman SJ, et al: Cosmetic dermatologic surgery. Arch Dermatol 1982, 118:1013.

GENERALIZED ESSENTIAL TELANGIECTASIA

Generalized essential telangiectasia is characterized by the dilatation of veins and capillaries over a large segment of the body without preceding or coexisting skin lesions. The telangiectases may be distributed over the entire body or be localized to some large area such as the legs, arms, and trunk. They may be discrete or confluent. Distribution along the course of the cutaneous nerves may occur. This type of telangiectasia is not associated with systemic disease.

Generalized telangiectasia develops most frequently in women in their forties and fifties. The initial onset is on the lower legs and then spreads to the upper legs, abdomen, and arms. The dilatations persist indefinitely. Wells et al reported three families with this disorder, and in each it was inherited as an autosomal dominant trait.

McGrae and Winkelmann indicated that generalized essential telangiectasia may be differentiated from telangiectasia associated with systemic disease by the presence of alkaline phosphatase activity. Telangiectatic vessels in generalized essential telangiectasia do not have alkaline phosphatase activity in the endothelium of the terminal arteriole and the arterial portion of the capillary loops.

The etiology of essential telangiectasia is unknown. It is believed that estrogens, serotonin, and adrenocorticosteroids are not causative, such as would be seen in telangiectases of pregnancy, hepatic disease, metastatic carcinoid syndrome, and Cushing's syndrome. Shelley reported a case that cleared on therapy with tetracycline orally. Ayres Jr reported a case that cleared after eradication of a chronic sinus infection and suggested that Shelley's case might have cleared for the same reason. Shelley et al more recently reported a case whose lesions partially responded to oral ketoconazole, only to flare with a bout of acute sinusitis.

McGrae JE Jr, et al: Generalized essential telangiectasia. JAMA 1963, 185:909.

Person JR, et al: Estrogen and progesterone receptors are not increased in generalized essential telangiectasia. Arch Dermatol 1985, 121:836.

Shelley WB: Essential progressive telangiectasia. JAMA 1971, 216:1343.

Idem, et al: Focal intravascular coagulation in focal ascending telangiectasia. JAAD 1984, 10:876.

Wells RS, et al: Hereditary benign telangiectasia. Br J Dermatol 1981, 84:93.

UNILATERAL NEVOID TELANGIECTASIA

In 1983 Wilkin et al reviewed 46 published cases of this disorder and nine cases of their own. In this lesion, fine, threadlike telangiectases develop in a unilateral, sometimes dermatomal, distribution. The areas most often involved are the trigeminal and C3 and C4, or adjacent areas, with the right side slightly more often involved than the left. Onset was congenital in 11 cases, and acquired in 34. Increased estrogen appeared to play a role in the onset of acquired cases: for instance, pregnancy, puberty in women, adrenarche in a man, and hepatitis/alcohol related cases were all reported.

Uhlin et al reported a case in 1983 which began when the patient started to take oral contraceptives and worsened during pregnancy, and in which substantially elevated estrogen and progesterone receptors were found only in involved skin. However, another case studied by Su et al failed to confirm these results.

Su WPD, et al: Unilateral dermatomal superficial telangiectasia. Dermatol Sinica 1984, 2:27.

Uhlin SR, et al: Unilateral nevoid telangiectatic syndrome. Arch Dermatol 1983, 119:226.

Wilkin JK, et al: Unilateral dermatomal superficial telangiectasia. JAAD 1983, 8:468.

HEREDITARY HEMORRHAGIC TELANGIECTASIA (Osler's Disease)

Also known as Osler-Weber-Rendu disease, this hereditary vascular anomaly (HHT) is characterized by small tufts of dilated capillaries scattered over the mucous membranes and the skin. These slightly elevated lesions develop mostly on the lips, tongue, palate, nasal mucosa, ears, palms, fingertips, nail beds, and soles. They may closely simulate the telangiectases of the CREST variant of scleroderma, and Fritzler et al showed that they may be distinguished by one test, for anticentromere antibodies, which can be elevated from the earliest stages in CREST and are not found in HHT.

Frequent nosebleeds and melena are experienced

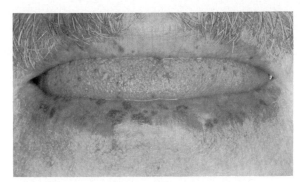

Figure 35–22. Hereditary hemorrhagic telangiectasia.

because of the telangiectasia in the nose and gastrointestinal tract. The spleen may be enlarged. Pulmonary and central nervous system arteriovenous fistulas may appear later in life. Retinal arteriovenous aneurysms occur only rarely. Other sites of bleeding may be the gastrointestinal tract, kidney, spleen, bladder, liver, meninges, and brain.

The telangiectases tend to increase in number in middle age; however, the first appearance on the undersurface of the tongue and floor of the mouth is at puberty. Epistaxis is the most frequent and persistent sign.

Pulmonary or intracranial arteriovenous fistulas and bleeding in these areas may be the cause of death. Waller et al reported three cases with brain vessel anomalies. Conlon et al reported two kindreds in whom hereditary hemorrhagic telangiectasia was associated with von Willebrand's disease, and proved to be a complicating reason for their gastrointestinal bleeding. Solomon and Kleiman reported two cases with associated polycystic kidney disease.

Osler's disease is inherited as an autosomal dominant trait.

The manifestations of this disease are probably due to a systemic weakness in the vascular walls, and endothelial discontinuity and degeneration have been described on electron microscopic study.

Several treatment methods have been recommended. The tendency to epistaxis has been reduced by estrogen therapy. Harrison treated 118 patients over 25 years, 67 with large-dose estrogen therapy using ethinyl estradiol. He stated that it was successful in every patient. Dermoplasty of the bleeding nasal septum may be performed by replacing the mucous membrane with skin from the thigh or buttock. No specific therapy for gastrointestinal bleeding is yet available, and blood transfusions may be necessary.

Conlon CL, et al: Telangiectasia and von Willebrand's disease in two families. Ann Intern Med 1978, 89:921.
Fritzler MJ: Hereditary hemorrhagic telangiectasia versus CREST syndrome: can serology aid diagnosis? JAAD 1984, 10:192.
Gorlin RJ, et al: Hereditary hemorrhagic telangiectasia. Dermatol Surg Oncol 1978, 4:865.
Harrison DFN: Use of estrogen in treatment of familial hemorrhagic telangiectasia. Laryngoscope 1982, 92:314.

BLOOM'S SYNDROME
(Bloom–Torre–Machacek Syndrome)

Originally named *congenital telangiectatic erythema resembling lupus erythematosus in Lorain-Levi dwarfs,* Bloom's syndrome is transmitted as an autosomal recessive trait, chiefly among Jews of eastern European origin. It is characterized by telangiectatic erythema in the butterfly area of the face, sunlight sensitivity, and dwarfism.

Telangiectatic erythematous patches resembling lupus erythematosus develop in the first two years of life. Bullous, crusted lesions may be present on the lips. Exacerbation of skin lesions occurs during the summer months. Other changes that may be noted are café-au-lait spots, ichthyosis, acanthosis nigricans, syndactyly, irregular dentition, prominent ears, hypospadias, and cryptorchidism.

The stunted growth is characterized by normal body proportions, no endocrine abnormalities, and low birth weight at full term. Dolichocephaly and narrow, delicate facies are present. There are abnormal immune functions and frequent gastrointestinal and respiratory infections. Gretzula et al reviewed this syndrome in detail in 1987.

There is a high frequency of chromosomal breakage and rearrangement and sister chromatid exchanges in Bloom's syndrome. Quadrilateral configuration during metaphase is frequently seen, and the rate of sister chromatid exchange in general is increased more than in ataxia-telangiectasia or Fanconi's anemia, which are also chromosome-breakage disorders.

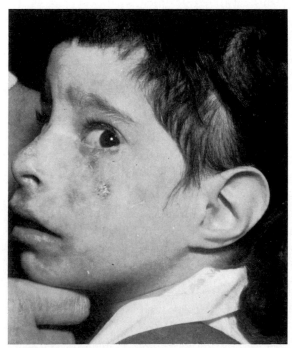

Figure 35–23. Bloom's syndrome with telangiectatic patches resembling discoid lupus erythematosus in a girl dwarf. (Courtesy of Dr. D. Bloom.)

Leukemia, lymphoma, adenocarcinoma of the sigmoid colon, and oral and esophageal squamous cell carcinoma, as well as other malignancies, have been associated with Bloom's syndrome. About one fourth of patients under age 20 have developed a neoplasm, and bone-marrow storage is an excellent precaution because of the high frequency of leukemia. Regular use of a sunscreen is recommended.

Gretzula JC, et al: Bloom's syndrome. JAAD 1987, 17:479.
Oono T, et al: Bloom's syndrome with dimorphism of sister chromatid exchanges in phytohemagglutinin-stimulated lymphocytes. Arch Dermatol 1987, 123:988.

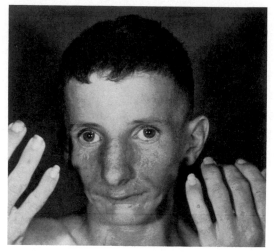

Figure 35–24. Cockayne's syndrome. (Courtesy of Dr. V.J. Derbes.)

COCKAYNE'S SYNDROME

Cockayne's syndrome is characterized by photosensitivity, which leads to telangiectasia, atrophy, scarring, and hyperpigmentation, and dwarfism with microcephaly and mental retardation. The ears are large and protruding, suggestive of a "Mickey Mouse" appearance. The hands, legs, and feet are cyanotic and cold, and disproportionately large. Cataracts, retinitis pigmentosa, partial deafness, and unsteady gait are other components of this autosomal recessively inherited syndrome, which has so far been reported in approximately 40 boys and 10 girls.

It is frequently confused with progeria, but *Cockayne's syndrome* includes ocular defects, and patients' fibroblasts show prolonged decrease in DNA and RNA synthesis rates after UV irradiation, which is the basis for prenatal diagnosis.

Beauregard S, et al: Syndromes of premature aging. Dermatol Clin 1987, 5:109.
Kahn G: Photosensitivity and photodermatitis in childhood. Dermatol Clin 1986, 4:107.
Schmickel RD, et al: Cockayne syndrome: a cellular sensitivity to ultraviolet light. Pediatrics 1977, 60:135.

ATAXIA-TELANGIECTASIA

Also known as the Louis-Bar syndrome, ataxia-telangiectasia consists of cerebellar ataxia, oculocutaneous telangiectasia, and sinopulmonary infection. It is familial and is usually first noted when the child begins to walk. There is awkwardness and a swaying gait, which by about ten years of age results in the child's being confined to a wheelchair. Choreic and athetoid movements and pseudopalsy of the eyes are other features. Fine telangiectases of venous origin appear upon the exposed surfaces of the conjunctivae at about three years of age. Nystagmus is present. Telangiectases also appear later on the butterfly area of the face, inside the helix and over the backs of the

ears, in the roof of the mouth, the necklace area, the bends of the elbows and knees, and over the dorsa of the hands and feet. Other stigmata are café-au-lait patches, hypopigmented macules, seborrheic dermatitis, premature graying and sparsity of the hair, and progeroid features. The skin tends to be dry and coarse, and in time becomes tight and inelastic, as in scleroderma. Early death from bronchiectasis occurs in over half the patients, most of whom suffer from recurrent sinus and lung infections which begin between the ages of three and eight. Many of the remainder (10 per cent of the total) succumb to lymphoma by age 20.

Ataxia-telangiectasia is transmitted as an autosomal recessive trait, and heterozygotes, though they lack clinical findings, are clearly cancer-prone, as Swift et al showed.

Patients have a marked IgA deficiency, with decreased lymphocytes and a small to absent thymus. Eleven of 16 patients studied by Amman et al lacked IgE. Cellular and humoral immune systems are both impaired. Other abnormalities seen include increased chromosome breakage, often involving chromosome 13. Cells are abnormally sensitive to killing by ionizing radiation, but DNA synthesis is radioresistant.

Two specific test findings are cerebellar alterations in computerized tomography scans, and elevated serum alpha-fetoprotein levels. Serum carcinoembryonic antigen levels are also high. These findings support the hypothesis that the primary disorder in Louis-Bar syndrome is one of poor tissue differentiation due to abnormal interaction between the ectodermal and mesodermal germ lines. L.L. Smith et al published a thorough review of this disease in 1985.

Cohen LE, et al: Common and uncommon cutaneous findings in patients with ataxia-telangiectasia. JAAD 1984, 10:431.
Smith LL, et al: Ataxia-telangiectasia or Louis-Bar syndrome. JAAD 1985, 12:681.

Swift M, et al: Malignant neoplasms in the families of patients with ataxia-telangiectasia. Cancer Res 1976, 36:209.

POIKILODERMA VASCULARE ATROPHICANS

Poikiloderma vasculare atrophicans (PVA) is characterized by variegated skin presenting hyper- and hypopigmentation, telangiectasia, and atrophy. The skin changes resemble radiodermatitis; later, ulcerations may occur. The skin is dry and furfuraceous and has cigarette-paperlike wrinkling. Severe pruritus may be present.

PVA is not a disease entity, but rather a manifestation seen in several different diseases. The first well-described case of PVA, which Jacobi reported in 1906, is now considered to have been dermatomyositis. In 1921 Lane described the first American case, which ultimately terminated as Hodgkin's disease. PVA is frequently seen as a form of mycosis fungoides. Other diseases of which PVA may be a characteristic manifestation are large-plaque parapsoriasis (which may eventuate in mycosis fungoides), lupus erythematosus, acrodermatitis chronica atrophicans, xeroderma pigmentosum, poikiloderma congenitale, dyskeratosis congenita, Werner's syndrome, Fanconi's syndrome, Kindler's syndrome (considered by some to be a combination of poikiloderma congenitale and epidermolysis bullosa), and arsenism.

The histologic findings vary according to the stage of the process. Early changes are a dilatation of the superficial vessels, perivascular round cell infiltration, and increase in or loss of pigment, or both. Atrophy ensues, the papillae are flattened, and in

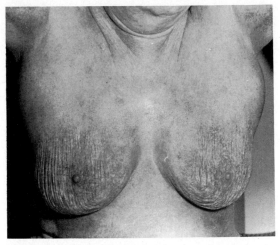

Figure 35–25. Generalized poikiloderma; changes in the skin compatible with mycosis fungoides have been present for 5 years.

the dermis there are degenerative changes in the collagen bundles, as well as in the elastic tissue.

Treatment is that of the disease in which it occurs.

HEREDITARY SCLEROSING POIKILODERMA

Weary and his associates have described a heritable widespread poikilodermatous and sclerotic disorder. It was found in seven members of two unrelated black families.

The skin changes consist of generalized poikiloderma with hyperkeratotic and sclerotic cutaneous bands extending across the antecubital spaces, axillary vaults, and popliteal fossae.

In addition, the palms and soles may show scle-

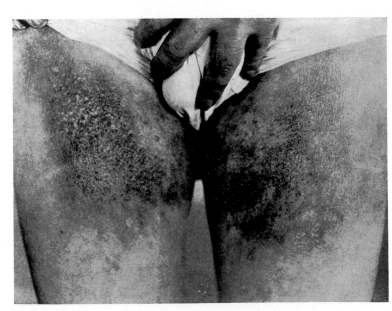

Figure 35–26. Poikiloderma vasculare atrophicans. Note resemblance to chronic radiodermatitis.

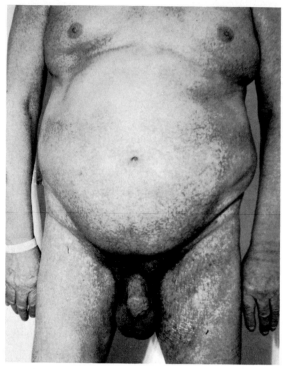

Figure 35–27. *Poikiloderma vasculare atrophicans. (Courtesy of Dr. D. Wolf.)*

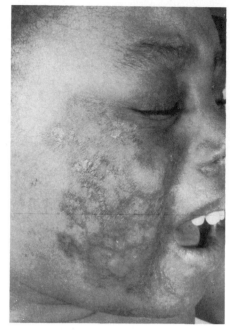

Figure 35–28. *Poikiloderma congenitale. (Courtesy of Dr. J.L. Burton, Bristol, England.)*

rosis resembling shiny scotch-grain leather. Clubbing of the fingers and localized calcinosis of the skin have also been noted.

The dermatosis is transmitted as an autosomal dominant trait. There is no treatment.

Weary PE, et al: Hereditary sclerosing poikiloderma. Arch Dermatol 1969, 100:413.

POIKILODERMA CONGENITALE

This is also known as Thomson's disease (after the dermatologist who described his cases in 1923) and Rothmund-Thomson syndrome (recognizing the ophthalmologist who described his cases in 1868). It is a rare familial syndrome transmitted as an autosomal recessive trait. It occurs predominantly in girls. Poikiloderma begins at three to six months of age with tense, pink, edematous patches on the cheeks, hands, feet, and buttocks; there follows fine reticulated or punctate atrophy associated with telangiectasia and reticulated pigmentation.

Short stature, small hands, absence or sparseness of eyebrows and eyelashes, alopecia of the scalp, and congenital bone defects are frequently observed. Hypogonadism, dystrophic nails, and defective dentition are seen in less than 30 per cent of cases. Sensitivity to sunlight may be manifested by the development of bullae or intense erythema after short

sun-exposure. Berg et al reported normal response to UVB in their case, but striking immediate erythema to small doses of UVA. Squamous and basal cell carcinoma of the skin, bowenoid keratoses, and Bowen's intraepidermal carcinoma occasionally occur, and osteosarcoma of bone has been reported. Juvenile cataracts occur between the ages of three and six in 50 per cent of patients.

Most of the affected children are the offspring of consanguineous marriages. Berg et al reviewed the literature in 1987.

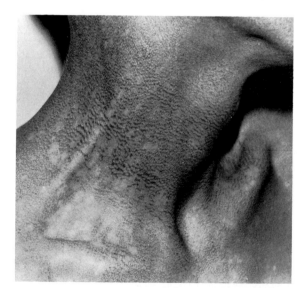

Figure 35–29. *Poikilodermatous lesions in dyskeratosis congenita in one of three siblings. Lesions were generalized. (Courtesy of Dr. V.M. Torres-Rodriguez.)*

Berg E, et al: Rothmund-Thomson syndrome. JAAD 1987, 17:332.
Bordas X, et al: Kindler's syndrome. JAAD 1982, 6:263.

UNIVERSAL ANGIOMATOSIS

Universal angiomatosis, called *generalized telangiectasia* by Bean, is a bleeding disease that affects the blood vessels of the skin and mucous membranes as well as other parts of the body. Bean and Rathe reported a 13-year-old boy who had frequent nosebleeds and ear and upper respiratory infections. He had a mottled skin, with redness that blanched on pressure. Finely dilated blood vessels were universal, suggesting the term "pink man." Some irregular white patches were also present.

This form of total angiomatosis was believed to be due to the lack of self-sealing vascular substance to produce hemostasis. Continual bleeding into the skin was evident despite normal coagulation of the blood. This type of angiomatosis differs from generalized telangiectasia because of its hemorrhagic tendency, especially epistaxis.

VASCULAR ANOMALIES

CAPILLARY ANEURYSMS OF THE SKIN

These usually flesh-colored solitary lesions, resembling an intradermal nevus, may suddenly grow larger and darker and become blue-black or black. They are surrounded by a zone of erythema. The lesions may be clinically indistinguishable from malignant melanoma. Shave excision in stages will expose the clot and eliminate the uncertainty.

Histologically, these are thrombotic, dilated capillaries lying just below the epidermis.

PROMINENT INFERIOR LABIAL ARTERY

Howell and Freeman reported seven cases of a potentially troublesome arterial anomaly of the lower lip characterized by the appearance of a pulsating papule in the lower vermilion, a centimeter or two from the oral commissure, formed by a tortuous segment of the inferior labial artery. In one study, three examples were found among 90 new dermatologic patients, of both sexes, between the ages of 40 and 70 years.

Howell JB, et al: Prominent inferior labial artery. Arch Dermatol 1973, 107:386.
Paslin DA, et al: Acral arteriolar ectasia. Arch Dermatol 1972, 106:906.

CUTIS MARMORATA TELANGIECTATICA CONGENITA
(Congenital Phlebectasia, Van Lohuizen's Syndrome)

Cutis marmorata telangiectatica congenita is characterized by the presence of exaggerated cutis marmorata with a generalized or segmental distribution, phlebectasia, telangiectasia, and at times ulcerations, usually involving the extremities. The mottling is pronounced and is not made more distinct by cold.

Powell et al, who reported nine cases, estimated that they brought the total to 77. There is female preponderance.

Other common anomalies associated with this disorder include varicosities, hemangiomas, and hypoplasia and hypertrophy of soft tissue and bone. These and other more unusual associated anomalies, such as generalized congenital fibromatosis in the case of Spraker et al, and rectal and genital anomalies in the case reported by Del Giudice et al, occur in about 50 per cent of cases.

Andreev VC, et al: Cutis marmorata telangiectatica congenita in two sisters. Br J Dermatol 1979, 101:345.
Del Giudice SM, et al: Cutis marmorata telangiectatica with multiple congenital anomalies. Arch Dermatol 1986, 122:1060.

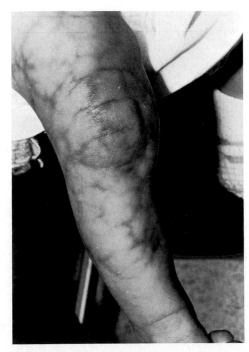

Figure 35–30. Congenital phlebectasia in a 14-month-old child. (Courtesy of Dr. V.M. Torres-Rodriguez.)

Kurczynski TW: Hereditary cutis marmorata telangiectatica congenita. Pediatrics 1982, 70:52.

Powell ST, et al: Cutis marmorata telangiectatica congenita: report of 9 cases and review of the literature. Cutis 1984, 34:305.

Rogers M, et al: Cutis marmorata telangiectatica congenita. Arch Dermatol 1982, 118:895.

Spraker MK, et al: Congenital generalized fibromatosis. JAAD 1984, 10:365.

CONGENITAL ARTERIOVENOUS FISTULA

Arteriovenous (AV) fistulas have acquired a great number of names, too numerous to list here. The AV fistula is a route from artery to vein, bypassing the capillary bed. AV fistulas may be congenital or acquired; the latter are usually the result of wounds, as reviewed by James et al in the discussion of his case, which resulted from a wound received in the Vietnam war. Such iatrogenic AV fistulas as those produced to facilitate hemodialysis may also bring about skin changes, as demonstrated in the case of pseudo–Kaposi's sarcoma reported by Goldblum et al. The condition may be a part of the Osler-Rendu-Weber syndrome (hereditary hemorrhagic telangiectasia).

Congenital AV fistulas occur mostly on the extremities and may be recognized, or at least suspected, in the presence of varicose veins, ulcerations, hemangiomas, and nevus flammeus. The skin over these fistulas is warmer, the hair may grow faster, the affected limb may be larger than the other; thrills and bruits may be discerned in some cases. There may be changes due to stasis, edema, a vascular mass, increased sweating, or paresthesia. At times reddish purple nodules or a plaque may be present, clinically resembling Kaposi's sarcoma (see Pseudo–Kaposi's Sarcoma in Chapter 28, Dermal and Subcutaneous Tumors). Another name for these lesions is *acroangiodermatitis*.

Diagnosis is established by plethysmography, thermography, determination of oxygen saturation of venous blood, or arteriography.

Traumatic AV fistulas are often managed by a surgical approach because they are usually more localized than the more diffuse, congenital, extremity type, which requires conservative management.

Finley JL, et al: Port-wine stains. Arch Dermatol 1984, 120:1453.

Goldblum OM, et al: Pseudo–Kaposi's sarcoma of the hand associated with an acquired iatrogenic arteriovenous fistula. Arch Dermatol 1985, 121:1038.

James WD, et al: Pseudo–Kaposi's sarcoma. J Assoc Milit Dermatol 1984, 10:14.

Lee EB, et al: Ulcers associated with congenital arteriovenous fistulas. Arch Dermatol 1983, 119:949.

Marshall ME, et al: Arteriovenous malformations simulating Kaposi's sarcoma. Arch Dermatol 1985, 121:99.

ACRAL ARTERIOLAR ECTASIA

Paslin and Heaton reported a man with purple serpiginous ectactic arterioles on the backs of his fingers, which appeared in the fifth decade of life.

Paslin DA, et al: Acral arteriolar ectasia. Arch Dermatol 1972, 106:906.

LEG ULCERS

The following discussion of the classification, diagnosis, and treatment of chronic leg ulcers is cursory and attempts to indicate only the highlights of this frequently occurring dermatosis. For more detailed discussion there are excellent recent reviews such as that by Falanga et al (1986); articles by Young and by Lofgren, and the book chapters by Husni and Villavicencio et al may also be consulted.

VENOUS ULCER
("Varicose" Ulcer, "Stasis" Ulcer)

Chronic venous insufficiency in the deep veins of the legs leads to shunting the venous return into the superficial veins, in which pressure and flow rate are increased; its oxygen content is also increased. We call the dermatitis that results *stasis dermatitis*; the British call it *eczema secondary to venous hypertension*, as Burton explained recently in a letter to the editor. "Venous dermatitis" and "venous ulcer," as suggested by Falanga and Eaglstein, would be preferable to either.

Edema and fibrosis develop in the skin over the mesial aspect of the lower third of the shin, and eventually, often as a result of minor trauma, an ulcer forms, and may grow to 8 or 10 cm in diameter. The dermatitis may be weepy or dry, scaling or lichenified; it is almost invariably hyperpigmented by melanin and hemosiderin. Varicose veins are usually present, though they need not be numerous or conspicuous.

Leakage of fibrinogen is believed by Browse and Burnand to eventually coat the skin capillaries with a layer of fibrin which inhibits the passage of oxygen and thus causes anoxia and sets the stage for dermatitis and ulceration. Falanga et al studied skin biopsies, and their findings support this concept.

The cause of varicose veins is not clear; however, there is no doubt about an inherited tendency. Standing in one position for long periods promotes the development of varicosities. Any condition causing

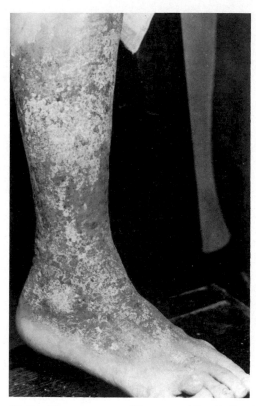

Figure 35–31. Venous eczema. (Courtesy of Dr. F. Daniels, Jr.)

are necessary in the long-term management of venous disease.

Many changes in recommendations for wound care have occurred because of the occlusive permeable biosynthetic wound dressings (such as DuoDERM) now available. They have speeded healing, reduced pain, made dressing changes infrequent, helped debridement, excluded microorganisms, and improved cosmetic results. Advance preparation consists of reduction of edema by leg elevation and use of dextranomer, to reduce the rate of exudation. If a hard eschar is present over the ulcer when first seen, a DuoDERM dressing will assist in its removal. Dressings of this type are highly recommended. Reviews by Eaglstein, Falanga et al, Friedman et al, and Alper et al should be consulted.

Many other techniques of wound care are acceptable. The double-layer bandage described by Eriksson is excellent. Zinc oxide, benzoyl peroxide, antibiotic ointments, and Unna boots are all recommended alternatives for wound care in uncomplicated venous leg ulcers.

All leg ulcers are contaminated with many microorganisms and there is usually nothing gained by cultures unless signs of cellulitis are present. Oral antibiotics are safer than topical as well as more effective, if infection of surrounding tissue requires such therapy.

prolonged intraabdominal pressure against the iliac veins may also cause them: the commonest cause of this is pregnancy. Thrombophlebitis may also cause incompetence of the veins.

Venous ulcers usually occur on the lower medial aspect of the leg. Usually there is preceding venous ("stasis") dermatitis with lipodermatosclerosis. Ninety per cent of all leg ulcers result from chronic venous insufficiency, and perhaps 5 per cent from arteriosclerosis obliterans, with the majority of remaining cases occurring as a complication of diabetes.

When one suspects venous ulceration and it is in an atypical location, is not accompanied by the expected edema/stasis, or does not respond to treatment in six to eight weeks, a biopsy from the edge of the ulcer and the following workup may be considered: complete blood count, serologic test (VDRL) for syphilis, fasting blood glucose, bacterial culture, patch test, rheumatoid factor, sedimentation rate, serum protein electrophoresis, and chest x-ray.

Treatment is primarily to improve circulation by improving venous return. This involves elevation of the leg above the heart as much of the time as possible. Elastic support to the legs, and exercise to improve calf muscle strength, is recommended. The avoidance of long, cramped sitting (in airplanes or cars) or standing is advisable. Avoidance of trauma is important. In some cases venous reconstruction is helpful. A cooperative patient and a patient doctor

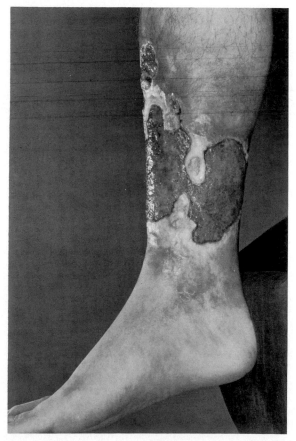

Figure 35–32. Venous ulcer. (Courtesy of Dr. H. Shatin.)

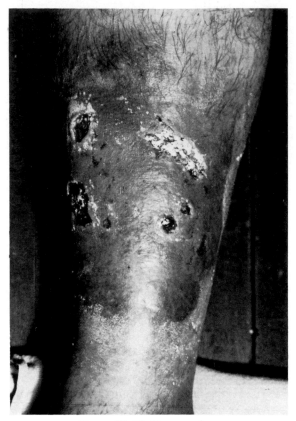

Figure 35–33. Venous ulcers.

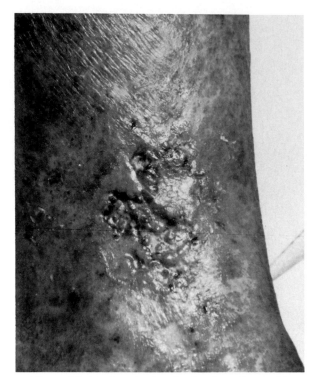

Figure 35–34. Arteriosclerotic ulcer just above ankle.

Oral zinc sulfate, 220 mg t.i.d., has been shown by Hallböök to be useful adjunctive therapy. Falanga et al recommend a trial of Stanazol, 2 to 4 mg a day for three to six months, in patients with recurrent ulcerations. Their article should be consulted for an understanding of the several contraindications before using this.

Grafting may ultimately be necessary in some cases. Pinch grafts or use of a meshed graft are good choices. Hefton et al described the use of cultured autologous epidermal cells. A comprehensive review of the status of cultured skin grafts was published by Phillips in 1988.

HYPERTENSIVE ISCHEMIC ULCER

These ulcers are mostly located on the lateral surface of the ankle and the calf. The initial red painful plaque breaks down into a painful superficial ulcer with a surrounding zone of purpuric erythema. Granulation tissue is minimal, little or no infection is present, and a membranous inactive eschar forms over the ulcer. Patients at risk are those with long-standing hypertension or other signs and risk factors of arteriosclerotic disease.

Such signs and symptoms of arterial disease as the cause of the ulceration include thinning of the skin, absence of hair, decreased or absent pulses, pallor on elevation, coolness of the extremity, dependent rubor, claudication on exercise, and pain on elevation (especially at night) relieved on dependency.

Treatment with topical antibiotic ointments and protection of the affected area from injury, plus avoidance of cold, smoking, and tight socks, are practical measures of importance. Enhancement of the blood supply by raising the head of the bed on 6-inch blocks is advisable.

A vascular surgeon should be asked to consult and advise with regard to arteriography, Doppler arterial flow studies, and ankle and arm blood pressure evaluation. Lumbar sympathectomy may be considered.

If the blood supply can be improved, local wound care (perhaps with a DuoDERM dressing) will heal the ulcer. If the blood supply cannot be improved, little can be done except to prevent infection by the measures described above under venous ulcers. Heng et al reviewed the one alternative, hyperbaric oxygen use by a simplified technique, and was able to heal 18 of 27 ulcers in six to 21 days with it.

LEG ULCERS OF OTHER CAUSES

As mentioned earlier, about 90 per cent of leg ulcers are the result of venous insufficiency, 5 per cent result from arterial disease, and 5 per cent are due to miscellaneous causes. One of the commonest is diabetic microangiopathy. Young has reviewed this long differential diagnostic list. The evaluation suggested above under venous ulcers will aid in identifying many of these other causes.

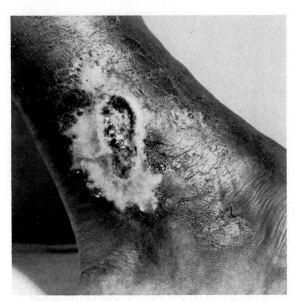

Figure 35–35. Ulcer on ankle in sickle cell anemia.

Hematopoietic ulcers are those occurring with sickle cell anemia, Cooley's anemia (thalassemia), congenital hemolytic anemia, polycythemia vera, thrombocytopenic purpura, macroglobulinemia, and cryoglobulinemia. In addition, cryofibrinogenemia may also be manifested by ulcerations on the lower extremities. Stevens et al have emphasized the importance of thalassemia in the production of leg ulcers and discussed their management.

The ulcers may antedate the overt disease for years. Although the ulcers may appear on any part of the leg, they are most common on the ankle. The single or multiple ulcers are usually discrete, sharply marginated and punched-out, with suppurating bases.

The diagnosis is usually established by the accompanying signs and symptoms of the original disease.

Treatment of the underlying disease should be maximal, and then general measures used for leg ulcers should be followed: avoidance of trauma and hydrocolloid occlusive patch dressings, such as DuoDERM, to provide a moist, infection-free local environment.

Leg ulcers due to collagen vascular disease may be seen with systemic lupus erythematosus, Felty's syndrome, rheumatoid arthritis, scleroderma, porphyria cutanea tarda with scleroderma, and dermatomyositis. The ulcers are deep, indolent, and dry.

Basal cell and squamous cell carcinoma, malignant melanoma, sarcoma, Kaposi's sarcoma, and malignant lymphomas may be the cause of ulcers on the legs. Diagnosis of neoplastic causes of leg ulcers requires biopsy of the ulcer margin.

Burns, radiodermatitis, decubitus ulcers, neurotic excoriations, factitial ulcers, and chrome ulcers are in this category. Versluysen et al discuss the risk factors for production of pressure sores.

Necrobiosis lipoidica, gout, diabetes, pellagra, Gaucher's disease, ulcerative colitis, and primary amyloidosis form another group in which leg ulcers also may be found.

The ulcers of lupus vulgaris, mycobacterial ulcers (Buruli ulcers), sporotrichosis, blastomycosis, coccidioidomycosis, cryptococcosis, histoplasmosis, and schistosomiasis are some of the more important infectious leg ulcers.

The gummatous ulcers of late syphilis should not be forgotten!

Alinovi A, et al: Systemic administration of antibodies in the management of venous ulcers. JAAD 1986, 15:186.

Alper JC, et al: Use of vapor permeable membrane for cutaneous ulcers. JAAD 1984, 11:858.

Alper JC: Recent advances in moist wound healing. South Med J 1986, 79:1398.

Browse NL, et al: The cause of venous ulceration. Lancet 1982, 2:243.

Browse NL: The etiology of venous ulceration. World J Surg 1986, 10:938.

Figure 35–36. Pyoderma gangrenosum. (Courtesy of Dr. Adrian Johnson, Australia.)

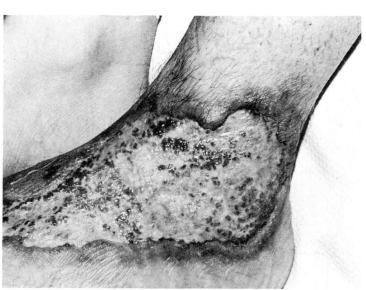

Burton JL: "Quirks" of British nomenclature (letter). JAAD 1985, 13:841.

Clancey JMP, et al: Treatment of leg ulcers with cultured epithelial grafts. JAAD 1988, 18:1356.

Colman GJ, et al: Topical therapy of leg ulcers with 20 per cent benzoyl peroxide lotion. Cutis 1978, 21:491.

Eaglstein WH: Experiences with biosynthetic dressings. JAAD 1985, 12:434.

Eriksson G: Comparison of two occlusive bandages in the treatment of venous leg ulcers. Br J Dermatol 1986, 114:227.

Idem, et al: The clinical significance of bacterial growth in venous leg ulcers. Scand J Infect Dis 1984, 16:175.

Falanga V, et al: A therapeutic approach to venous ulcers. JAAD 1986, 14:777.

Idem: Dermal pericapillary fibrin in venous disease and venous ulceration. Arch Dermatol 1987, 123:620.

Falanga V: Occlusive wound dressing. Arch Dermatol 1988, 124:870.

Friedman SJ, et al: Management of leg ulcers with hydrocolloid occlusive dressing. Arch Dermatol 1984, 120:1329.

Hallböök T, et al: Serum-zinc and healing of venous leg ulcers. Lancet 1982, 2:780.

Hefton JM, et al: Grafting of skin ulcers with cultured autologous epidermal cells. JAAD 1986, 14:399.

Heng MCY, et al: A simplified hyperbaric oxygen technique for leg ulcers. Arch Dermatol 1984, 120:640.

Heng MCY: Venous leg ulcers. Int J Dermatol 1987, 26:14.

Husni EA: Skin ulcer secondary to arterial and venous disease. In Chronic Ulcers of the Skin. Lee BY (ed) New York, McGraw-Hill, pp 93–99, 1985.

Jacobson S: Plastic surgery in management of the peripheral vascular ulcer. Angiology 1978, 29:661.

Kitahama A, et al: Leg ulcer: conservative management or surgical treatment. JAMA 1982, 247:197.

Krull EA: Chronic cutaneous ulcerations and impaired healing in human skin. JAAD 1985, 12:394.

Lim T, et al: Therapy of peripheral vascular ulcers: surgical management. Angiology 1978, 29:654.

Lofgren EP: Chronic venous insufficiency. Cardiovasc Clin 1983, 13:133.

Millard LG, et al: Chronic leg ulcers treated by the pinch graft method. Br J Dermatol 1977, 97:289.

Phillips TJ: Cultured skin grafts: Past, present and future. Arch Dermatol 1988, 129:1035.

Roenigk HH Jr: Leg ulcers; stasis syndrome. Dermatologica 1978, 1:8.

Romasz RS, et al: Application of dextranomer beads (Debrisan) in the treatment of exudating skin lesions: results of a cooperative study. Angiology 1978, 29:175.

Strömberg H-E, et al: Topical zinc oxide treatment improves arterial and venous leg ulcers. Br J Dermatol 1984, 111:461.

Versluysen M: How elderly patients with femoral fractures develop pressure sores in hospital. Br Med J 1986, 292:1311.

Villavicencio JL, et al: Nonsurgical management of lower extremity venous problems. In Surgery of the Veins. Bergan JJ, Yao JST (eds). Orlando, FL, Grune & Stratton, pp 323–345, 1985.

Winton GB, et al: Wound dressings in dermatologic surgery. JAAD 1985, 13:1026.

Witkowski JA, et al: Cutaneous ulcer therapy. Int J Dermatol 1986, 25:420.

Young JR: Differential diagnosis of leg ulcers. Cardiovasc Clin 1983, 13:171.

PYODERMA GANGRENOSUM

Brunsting and his associates described pyoderma gangrenosum in 1930. It is characterized by the rapid appearance of one or more violaceous, boggy, undermined ulcers, most frequently on the legs of persons with ulcerative colitis.

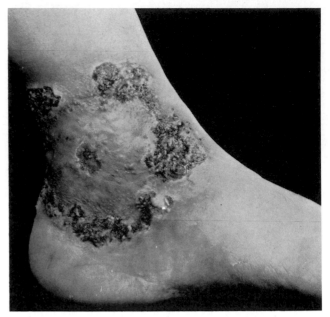

Figure 35–37. Pyoderma gangrenosum. (Courtesy of Dr. H. Shatin.)

First a papulovesicle or pustule appears which rapidly becomes necrotic to produce an ulceration. This is surrounded by an erythematous halo. Many of these ulcers have been described as having distinct rolled edges. These painful gangrenous ulcers may show satellite violaceous papules just peripheral to the border of the ulcer, which break down to fuse with the central ulcer. The lesions may extend laterally to form large peripherally extending phage-

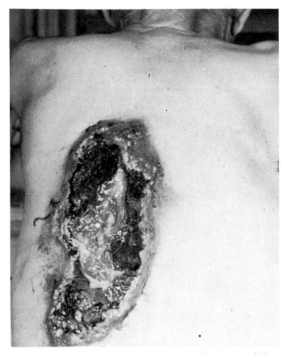

Figure 35–38. Pyoderma gangrenosum. (Courtesy of Dr. S.F. Rosen.)

denic ulcerations. These gangrenous ulcerations heal centrally, forming an atrophic, thin, flexible scar. A primary lesion may not always be seen, as 40 per cent of cases develop a lesion at the site of previous trauma.

Pyoderma gangrenosum is a disease chiefly affecting persons 40 to 60 years old. Powell et al reviewed eight cases occurring in children five to 14 years of age, but the extremely elderly may also develop this condition. In more than 50 per cent of the patients it has been associated with an underlying disease, most commonly ulcerative colitis; but at times only minimal bowel symptoms may be present. In addition to ulcerative colitis, other gastrointestinal manifestations have been polyposis, regional ileitis, and gastric ulcers.

Many other associated conditions may be present. Arthritis (rheumatoid or other), leukemia (chiefly acute or chronic myelogenous), myeloma, monoclonal gammopathy (chiefly IgA), polycythemia vera, myeloid metaplasia, chronic active hepatitis, HIV infection, systemic lupus erythematosus, and Takayasu's arteritis are among the many diseases seen in conjunction with pyoderma gangrenosum.

A bullous variant, which remains more superficial and maintains an expanding bullous margin, is described, primarily in association with hematologic disorders. Powell et al described eight patients with an associated monoclonal gammopathy, seven of whom had an IgA paraproteinemia. All but one developed pyoderma gangrenosum before the onset of the gammopathy.

Finally, almost half the cases of pyoderma gangrenosum occur without any associated causes being discovered. The etiology remains unknown.

The **diagnostic evaluation** should take into account the associated disease states as well as the differential diagnosis, because treatment of an underlying disease may aid in healing the ulceration. A complete blood count, blood chemistries, antinuclear antibody titer, rheumatoid factor, serologic test for syphilis (VDRL), serum bromide and iodide levels, hepatic profile, urinalysis, serum protein electrophoresis, chest x-ray, and gastrointestinal evaluation (even in the absence of symptoms) are advisable. Biopsy of an early lesion or the active edge of a mature one should be obtained, and complete viral, bacterial, fungal, and mycobacterial cultures taken, as well as a smear for amebae, if this is a consideration.

Evidence of impaired immunity has been demonstrated in patients with pyoderma gangrenosum. Abnormalities of humoral immunity, cell-mediated immunity, complement, and neutrophil and monocyte function have been described, but as yet no consistent common defect has been defined. Shands et al reported five cases occurring in one kindred.

Histologic examination reveals marked infiltration with neutrophils, which leads to necrosis.

In the differential diagnosis pyogenic abscesses, hemolytic streptococcal gangrene, blastomycosis, tuberculosis, and late syphilis must be considered.

Treatment of any underlying disease process may be beneficial. Local therapy with Burow's or other compresses or whirlpool baths followed by silver sulfadiazine (Silvadene) ointment is useful. Hyperbaric oxygen therapy has reportedly been successful in several patients. Davis et al used it, and followed it with successful skin grafting in four patients.

Treatment with sulfapyridine or salicylazosulfapyridine has been found helpful in clearing these painful lesions of pyoderma gangrenosum. Perry and Brunsting administered 0.5 gm salicylazosulfapyridine (Azulfidine) every three hours for ten days followed by a ten-day rest period. Dapsone is also often effective, and it or other sulfones are often the preferential treatment in the chronic, slowly progressive form of the disease. Newell et al reviewed their use. Byrne et al reported favorable responses to azathioprine. Michaëlsson et al found clofazimine (Lamprene) effective in eight patients, using 300 or 400 mg daily. Brandt and associates at Lund also reported success with clofazimine, in a young woman with regional enteritis and pyoderma gangrenosum, as did Berbis et al, in a case with hyperglobulinemia E.

Corticosteroids are often effective and have been extensively used. Intralesional steroids were reported by Moschella to be useful, and Odom and Jennings have found them effective in a few cases. High-dose oral steroids are usually required for the rapidly progressing, acute form of the disease. Johnson et al found pulse methylprednisolone effective in three patients, and Prystowsky et al reported that six of eight patients responded to it. Prolonged maintenance therapy is discouraged, unless it can be achieved with 60 mg or less of triamcinolone acetonide intramuscularly, once a month or less often.

Many other medications have been found useful in isolated cases. Kark et al also saw a dramatic response to clofazimine in three patients, but Rasmussen found that it failed in six of seven cases, in a dose of 200–300 mg daily. Newell et al found cyclophosphamide effective in a case which had become recalcitrant to prednisone and dapsone. Saffomi et al found 2 per cent disodium cromoglycate effective topically. Chlorambucil may heal some resistant lesions. Cyclosporine was effective in a patient of Curley et al and one of Magid, and one of the Shelleys, who had failed to respond to several other forms of treatment. Thalidomide has been reported to be effective in a few isolated cases. Lynch and Bergfeld reported four cases responding to minocycline, 300 mg daily.

Malignant pyoderma, which is characterized by ulcers of the head and neck, was originally thought to be a separate disease but is now believed to be simply a variant of pyoderma gangrenosum. Snyder's report of six patients with pyoderma gangrenosum confined to the head and neck, and the excellent review by Wernikoff et al with an accompanying editorial by Malkinson, all support this concept.

Perry et al reported the original three cases, in

which lesions were also present on the trunk. Only corticosteroid therapy was helpful. Arnold, in 1944, had such a patient, a teenage Japanese boy in whom every acne pustule, and every needle puncture, became a circular, spreading, suppurating ulcer. Hydrocortisone by mouth in moderate dosage was rapidly curative. Scarring was severe. Dicken et al in 1985 reported a case, also beginning in lesions of acne, in which they thought isotretinoin was effective, though sulfapyridine was also given. They also reviewed the literature.

Anderson JAR: Malignant pyoderma. Br J Dermatol 1978, 99:211.

Barnes L, et al: Pustular pyoderma gangrenosum associated with ulcerative colitis in childhood. JAAD 1986, 15:608.

Berbis P, et al: Hyperimmunoglobulin E and impaired neutrophil functions in a case of pyoderma gangrenosum. JAAD 1988, 18:574.

Byrne JPH, et al: Pyoderma gangrenosum associated with chronic active hepatitis. Arch Dermatol 1976, 112:1297.

Callen JP, et al: Recurrent pyoderma gangrenosum and agnogenic myeloid metaplasia. Arch Dermatol 1977, 113:1585.

Curley RK, et al: Pyoderma gangrenosum treated with cyclosporin A. Br J Dermatol 1985, 113:601.

Davies MG, et al: Pyoderma gangrenosum. Clin Exp Dermatol 1981, 6:219.

Davis JC, et al: Pyoderma gangrenosum. Plast Reconst Surg 1987, 79:200.

Dicken CH: Malignant pyoderma. JAAD 1985, 13:1021.

Greenberg SJ, et al: Pyoderma gangrenosum. Arch Dermatol 1982, 118:498.

Heng MCY: Hyperbaric oxygen therapy for pyoderma gangrenosum. Aust NZ J Med 1984, 14:618.

Holt PJA, et al: Pyoderma gangrenosum. Medicine 1980, 59:114.

Idem: Pyoderma gangrenosum: clinical and investigative findings in 15 patients. Br J Dermatol 1978, 99(Suppl 16):10.

Jennings JL: Pyoderma gangrenosum: successful treatment with intralesional steroids. JAAD 1983, 9:575.

Johnson R, et al: Pulse therapy . . . in the treatment of pyoderma gangrenosum. Arch Dermatol 1982, 118:76.

Lewis SJ, et al: Atypical pyoderma gangrenosum with leukemia. JAMA 1978, 239:935.

Lynch WS, et al: Pyoderma gangrenosum responsive to minocycline hydrochloride. Cutis 1978, 21:535.

Magid ML, et al: Treatment of recalcitrant pyoderma gangrenosum with cyclosporine. JAAD 1989, 20:293.

Malkinson FD: Pyoderma gangrenosum vs malignant pyoderma. Arch Dermatol 1987, 123:333.

Michaëlsson G, et al: Clofazimine: a new agent for treatment of pyoderma gangrenosum. Arch Dermatol 1976, 112:344.

Newell LM, et al: Pyoderma gangrenosum: response to cyclophosphamide. Arch Dermatol 1983, 119:495.

Idem: Commentary: pyoderma gangrenosum. Arch Dermatol 1982, 118:769.

Perry HO, et al: Pyoderma gangrenosum. Arch Dermatol 1957, 75:380.

Idem: Bullous pyoderma gangrenosum and leukemia. Arch Dermatol 1972, 106:901.

Powell FC, et al: Pyoderma gangrenosum and monoclonal gammopathy. Arch Dermatol 1983, 119:468.

Idem: Pyoderma gangrenosum in childhood. Arch Dermatol 1984, 120:757.

Prystowsky JH, et al: Present status of pyoderma gangrenosum. Arch Dermatol 1989, 125:57.

Rasmussen I: Pyoderma gangrenosum treated with clofazimine: clinical evaluation in 7 cases. Acta Derm Venereol (Stockh) 1983, 63:552.

Rustin MHA, et al: Hairy cell leukemia and pyoderma gangrenosum. JAAD 1985, 13:300.

Saffoni B, et al: Treatment of pyoderma gangrenosum with disodium cromoglycate. Dig Dis 1984, 29:183.

Schwaegerie SM, et al: Pyoderma gangrenosum: A review. JAAD 1988, 18:559.

Shands JW, et al: Pyoderma gangrenosum in a kindred. JAAD 1987, 16:931.

Shelley ED, et al: Cyclosporine therapy for pyoderma gangrenosum associated with sclerosing cholangitis and ulcerative colitis. JAAD 1988, 18:1084.

Snyder RA: Pyoderma gangrenosum involving the head and neck. Arch Dermatol 1986, 122:295.

Thomsen K, et al: Clofazimine in the treatment of pyoderma gangrenosum. Arch Dermatol 1979, 115:851.

Wernikoff S, et al: Malignant pyoderma or pyoderma gangrenosum of the head and neck? Arch Dermatol 1987, 123:371.

Wyrick WJ, et al: Hyperbaric oxygen treatment of pyoderma gangrenosum. Arch Dermatol 1978, 114:1232.

LYMPHEDEMA

Lymphedema is the swelling of soft tissues where an excess amount of lymph has accumulated. Chronic lymphedema is characterized by long-standing nonpitting edema.

Taylor and Young have proposed the following classification of lymphedema:

Primary lymphedema
  Congenital lymphedema (Milroy's)
  Lymphedema praecox
  Lymphedema tarda
  Syndromes associated with primary lymphedema
    Yellow nail syndrome
    Turner's syndrome
    Noonan's syndrome
    Pes cavus
  Cutaneous disorders sometimes associated with primary lymphedema
    Yellow nails
    Capillary hemangiomas
    Xanthomatosis and chylous lymphedema
    Congenital absence of nails

Secondary lymphedema
  Postmastectomy lymphedema
  Malignant occlusion with obstruction
  Extrinsic pressure
  Postradiation therapy
  Following recurrent lymphangitis/cellulitis
  Lymphedema of upper limb in recurrent eczema
  Granulomatous disease
Complications of lymphedema
  Cellulitis of lymphedema
  Elephantiasis nostras verrucosa
  Ulceration
  Lymphangiosarcoma

To these complications Tompkins et al added lymphangioma circumscriptum, localized neurodermatitis, and pseudoacanthosis nigricans. They reported the fifth case of lymphangioma circumscriptum following mastectomy. Also discussed was cutaneous chylous reflux, a viscous liquid discharged from the skin surface. Johnson reviewed this and the problem of lymphedema in an excellent article.

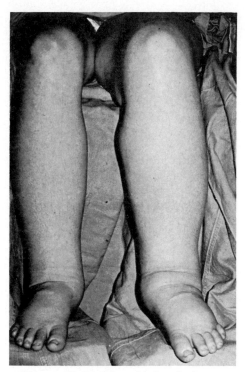

Figure 35–39. Idiopathic lymphedema.

Taylor and Young have reviewed the problem of "the swollen limb" in an admirable article detailing the diagnostic cutaneous clues and appropriate treatment.

TYPES. The primary noninflammatory types in-clude lymphedema praecox and congenital lymph-edema (Milroy's disease and "simple" type). The secondary noninflammatory type consists of lymph-edema caused by malignant occlusion, surgical re-moval of lymph nodes, pressure, or ionizing radia-tion therapy.

The inflammatory types may be caused by recur-rent lymphangitis or cellulitis, dermatophytosis, sys-temic granulomatous disease, or filariasis. Kin-month's book is the most complete source of information regarding the lymphatic system.

Lymphedema Praecox. This type develops in fe-males between the ages of nine and 25 years. A puffiness appears around the ankle and then extends upward to involve the entire leg. With the passage of time the leg becomes painful, with a dull heavy sensation. Once this has evolved the swollen limb remains swollen. Primary lymphedema is caused by a defect in the lymphatic system. Lymphangiography demonstrates hypoplastic lymphatics in 87 per cent, aplasia in approximately 5 per cent, and hyperplasia with varicose dilation of the lymphatic vessels in 8 per cent.

Congenital Lymphedema. Milroy's disease has been described on page 681.

Primary Lymphedema Associated with Yellow Nails and Pleural Effusion (Yellow Nail Syndrome). The primary lymphedema is confined mostly to the ankles, although other areas may be involved. The nails show a distinct yellowish discoloration and transverse ridging. Recurrent pleural effusion requir-ing thoracocentesis may be a feature.

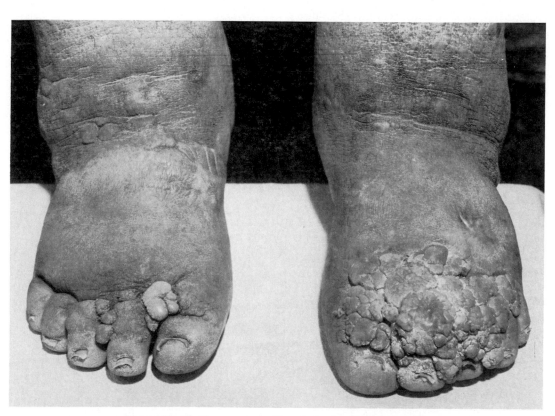

Figure 35–40. Verrucous papillomata in chronic lymphedema.

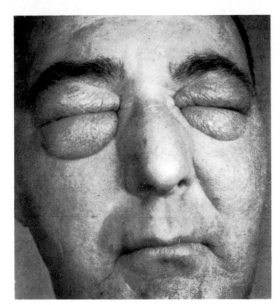

Figure 35–41. Chronic lymphedema, solid.

Secondary Lymphedema. In some malignant diseases the metastases to the lymph nodes will produce blockage and lymphedema. Malignant disease of the breast, uterus, prostate, skin, bones, or other tissues may cause such changes. Hodgkin's disease and, especially, Kaposi's sarcoma may be accompanied by chronic lymphedema. Chronic lymphedema is frequently seen after mastectomy and the removal of the axillary nodes; it may occur after varying lengths of time.

Postmastectomy Lymphangiosarcoma (Stewart-Treves Syndrome). This may arise in chronic postmastectomy lymphedema. Stewart and Treves were the first to describe this complication of simple or radical mastectomy. The lesions are bluish or reddish nodules arising on the arms. Numerous localized lesions may occur, and pulmonary metastasis is frequent. The prognosis is extremely poor.

Inflammatory Lymphedema. The inflammatory reaction is caused by recurrent bouts of acute cellulitis and lymphangitis. Chills, high fever, and swelling and redness of the involved extremity are severe and may last for as long as three or four days. Recurrent attacks of this streptococcic infection increase the likelihood of lymphedema. It is these recurrent attacks, when they complicate filariasis, that eventuate

in elephantiasis arabicum. Baddour et al reported three patients with non–group A beta-hemolytic streptococcus cellulitis following venectomy in patients who had undergone coronary bypass surgery.

TREATMENT. The excellent review article by Schirger should be consulted. The management of chronic lymphedema is centered around the removal of causes, especially in the early stages. Internal cancer should be looked for. Diuretics are highly recommended even in cases of long duration. Elevation of an edematous leg when the patient is in bed, and the wearing of made-to-measure elastic support stockings, applied after maximal treatment to avoid reaccumulation of fluid, is recommended. In those with infections, vigorous antifungal agents and antibiotics, as appropriate, is important. Low-dose, long-term, or intermittent prophylactic use of antibiotics or antifungals is sometimes advisable. Uniform or intermittent pressure by fitted pumps such as the Jobst pump or the Wright linear pump may be of great benefit. Even manual lymphatic massage as described by Zanolla et al is beneficial.

Surgical procedures—the Homans operation, the modified Charles operation, the Pratt procedure, or the Kondoleon operation—produce excellent results in selected cases. The surgical management has been reviewed by Schirger and more recently by Savage. Hettler described lipectomy for congenital lymphedema.

Alexander MA, et al: Lymphedema treated with a linear pump. Arch Phys Med Rehabil 1983, 64:132.

Baddour LM, et al: Non-group A beta-hemolytic streptococcal cellulitis. Am J Med 1985, 79:155.

Haagensen CD, et al: The Lymphatics in Cancer. Philadelphia, W. B. Saunders, 1972.

Hetter GP (ed): Lipoplasty. Boston, Little, Brown, 1984.

Johnson WK: Cutaneous chylous reflux. Arch Dermatol 1979, 115:464.

Kinmonth JB: The Lymphatics, 2nd ed, London, Edward Arnold, 1982.

Savage RC: The surgical management of lymphedema. Surg Gynecol Obstet 1985, 160:283.

Schirger A: Lymphedema. Cardiovasc Clin 1983, 13:293.

Taylor JS, et al: The swollen limb. Cutaneous clues to diagnosis and treatment. Cutis 1978, 21:553.

Tompkins KJ, et al: Lymphangioma circumscriptum following radical mastectomy. J Assoc Milit Dermatol 1987, 13:2.

Vieras F, et al: Lymphedema tarda (letter). JAMA 1978, 236:1116.

Zanolla R, et al: Evaluation of the results of three different methods of postmastectomy lymphedema treatment. J Surg Oncol 1984, 26:210.

36

Disturbances of Pigmentation

This chapter will be concerned with those diseases of abnormal pigmentation which have not been dealt with elsewhere.

Brownness of the skin depends upon transfer of melanosomes from melanocytes into keratinocytes. Melanosomes are cytoplasmic particles formed in melanocytes and then distributed among the basal cells of the epidermis. Each melanocyte in the epidermis secretes melanosomes into the surrounding keratinocytes to form the epidermal melanin unit. The melanosomes are the sites of melanin synthesis by the action of tyrosinase upon tyrosine.

The variations in skin color between persons and between races are due to the degree of melanization of melanosomes, their number, and their distribution in the epidermal melanin unit.

Biossy RE: The melanocyte. Derm Clin 1988, 6:161.
Bolognia JL, et al: Biology of hypopigmentation. JAAD 1988, 19:217.
Fulk CS: Primary disorders of hyperpigmentation (CME article). JAAD 1984, 10:1.
Jimbow K, et al: Some aspects of melanin biology, 1950–1975. J Invest Dermatol 1976, 67:72.
Lucky AW: Pigmentary abnormalities in genetic disorders. Derm Clin 1988, 6:185.
Mosher DB, et al: Disorders of pigmentation. In Dermatology in General Medicine. Fitzpatrick TB, et al (eds.) New York, Mc-Graw-Hill, p. 794, 1987.
Nordlund JJ, et al: Genetic basis of pigmentation and its disorders. Int J Dermatol 1981, 20:621.
Idem: Periodic synopsis on pigmentation. JAAD 1985, 12:359.
Pawelek JM, et al: The biosynthesis of mammalian melanin. Am Scientist 1982, 70:136.
Quevedo WC, et al: Biology of melanocytes. In Dermatology in General Medicine. Fitzpatrick TB, et al (eds.) New York, Mc-Graw-Hill, p. 224, 1987.
Spoor HJ, et al: Hyperpigmentation problems: effectiveness and rationale of therapy. Cutis 1976, 18:799.

PIGMENTARY DEMARCATION LINES

Miura classified the natural pigmentary demarcation boundaries of the skin into five groups, as follows:

Group A: lines along the outer upper arms with variable extension across the chest

Group B: lines along the posteromedial aspect of the lower limb

Group C: paired median or para-median lines on the chest, with midline abdominal extension

Group D: medial, over the spine

Group E: bilaterally symmetrical, obliquely oriented, hypopigmented macules on the chest

James et al reported the occurrence of these lines in a survey of 380 white and black patients. Over 70 per cent of black patients had one or more lines; they were much less common in whites. Type B lines often appear for the first time during pregnancy.

James WD, et al: Pigmentary demarcation lines. JAAD 1987, 16:584.
Idem: Pigmentary demarcation lines associated with pregnancy. JAAD 1984, 11:438.
Selmanowitz VJ, et al: Pigmentary demarcation lines. Br J Dermatol 1975, 93:37.

Abnormal Pigmentation

Normal pigmentation of the skin is influenced by the amount and depth of melanin, by the degree of vascularity, by the presence of carotene, and by the thickness of the horny layer. The amount of melanin

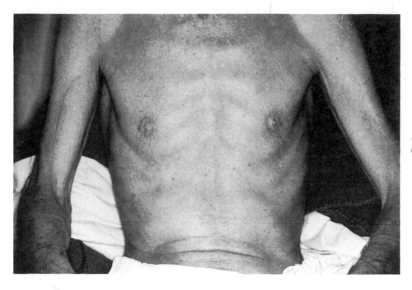

Figure 36–1. Generalized hyperpigmentation due to chronic arsenic ingestion.

produced is influenced by genetic factors, the amount and wavelengths of ultraviolet light received, the amount of melanocyte-stimulating hormone (MSH) secreted, and the effect of melanocyte-stimulating chemicals such as furocoumarins (psoralens). Abnormal pigmentation of the skin is produced by a variety of causes.

Hemosiderin Hyperpigmentation. Pigmentation due to deposits of hemosiderin occurs in purpura, hemochromatosis, hemorrhagic diseases, and stasis ulcers.

Pigmented Lesions. The pigmented nevi exemplify the group caused by the increased production of melanin. Accumulations of melanin occur in malignant melanoma. When metastases are extensive, melanuria also may be present; this can be demonstrated by the ferric chloride test and by the presence of 2,5-hydroxyindoleacetic acid in the urine. Pigmented nevi at the base of the nail may cause longitudinal pigmented bands. Nevus of Ota and

nevus of Ito are isolated blue-gray hyperpigmented lesions. Café-au-lait macules are seen in von Recklinghausen's disease, among many others.

The hyperpigmentation of suntan, freckles, radiodermatitis, and xeroderma pigmentosum results from the deposition of melanin. Macular pigmentation of the face and the backs of the hands and forearms appears in middle and old age (lentigo senilis).

Melanoderma (hyperpigmentation of the skin) may result from long-continued exposure to heat—so-called erythema (really pigmentatio) ab igne—or from prolonged friction, rubbing, scratching, or pressure upon the skin.

Dermatoses with Hyperpigmentation. Hyperpigmentation may be present in lichen planus, dermatitis herpetiformis, incontinentia pigmenti, dyskeratosis congenita, poikiloderma, Riehl's melanosis, photosensitization dermatitis, porphyria cutanea tarda, and xeroderma pigmentosum. Uneven brown pigmentation on the exposed parts of the skin is

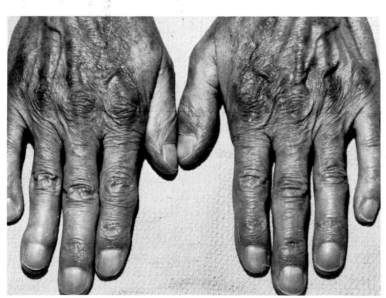

Figure 36–2. Hyperpigmentation of malignancy in a 63-year-old man with hypernephroma. (Courtesy of Dr. J. Shapiro.)

often seen in Gaucher's disease. In Niemann-Pick disease the skin color is grayish brown or yellow. In alkaptonuria, homogentisic acid produces a bluish black pigmentation, especially in the ear cartilage.

Internally Administered Chemicals. The antimalarial drugs may produce pigmentary changes of the skin mucous membranes and nails. Chloroquine binds to melanin. Chloroquine may also produce hypopigmentation of the hair, and freckles, as reported by Dupré. Clofazimine (Lamprene) induces a brown-black discoloration from deposition of the drug in the subcutaneous fat. Amiodarone therapy may produce a slate-gray pigmentation of the sun-exposed skin as well as a yellow-brown stippling of the cornea. Another cardiac drug structurally related to the antimalarials, quinidine, induced a localized blue-gray pigmentation, as reported by Mahler et al. Chemotherapeutic agents such as bleomycin, cyclophosphamide, melphalan, busulphan, daunorubicin, 5-fluorouracil, mechlorethamine, and BCNU may produce hyperpigmentation. Zidovudine (AZT) commonly causes pigmentation of the nails but may also cause oral melanosis and diffuse pigmentation of the skin, as reported by Merenich et al. Chlorpromazine and hydantoin may cause severe hyperpigmentation. Fixed drug eruptions become more deeply pigmented with each recurrent attack. Minocycline has been shown to cause a brown-black pigmentation of the skin, nails, and teeth, in rare instances. Granstein and Sober reviewed drug- and heavy-metal–induced pigmentation in detail in 1981. Topically administered medications also may induce pigmentation. The ochronosislike changes sometimes induced by topical hydroquinone are an example.

Industrial Hyperpigmentation. In industrial dermatoses, melanosis is an important feature. It occurs in coal miners, anthracene workers, pitch workers, and those in similar occupations. Pigmentation of the face may occur from the incorporation in cosmetics of derivatives of coal tar, petroleum, or picric acid, as well as mercury, lead, bismuth, or furocoumarins (psoralens).

Systemic Diseases. Among the causes may be mentioned syphilis, malaria, pellagra, and diabetes, in which there may be a diffuse bronzing of the skin, as well as Addison's disease, in which there is a diffuse melanosis that is pronounced in the axillae, in the palmar creases, about the nipples and the genitals, and on the buccal mucosa. In patients with adrenocortical insufficiency, pituitary activity is increased because the inhibitory action of the adrenal steroids is removed. In cases of virilizing adrenal tumors, hyperpigmentation and hypertrichosis usually develop. In Cushing's syndrome treated by bilateral adrenalectomy, some patients, after a good initial response, later develop extreme hyperpigmentation despite corticosteroid therapy. A pituitary MSH-producing tumor should be suspected. This condition is called *Nelson's syndrome.* Abe and his associates found that plasma MSH was elevated in patients with pituitary-adrenal abnormalities and normal in hyperpigmentation from other causes. Pheochromocytoma, hemochromatosis, amyloidosis, scurvy, pregnancy, menopause, porphyria cutanea tarda, vitamin B_{12} deficiency, kwashiorkor, and vitamin A deficiency are some other conditions in which hyperpigmentation is seen.

Primary biliary cirrhosis produces a diffuse and heavy hyperpigmentation. The triad of diffuse hyperpigmentation, pruritus, and xanthomas is quite specific for this disease. The pigmentation is similar to that seen in Whipple's intestinal lipodystrophy. In abdominal carcinoma, tuberculosis, severe anemias, hepatic and pancreatic disease, hyperthyroidism, chronic encephalitis, and Gaucher's disease various degrees of melanoderma may be present. David et al reported diffuse, progressive hyperpigmentation to be a presenting sign of mycosis fungoides.

Abdel-Malek ZA: Endocrine factors as effectors of integumental pigmentation. Derm Clin 1988, 6:175.

Alinovi A, et al: Cutaneous hyperpigmentation induced by amiodarone therapy. JAAD 1985, 12:563.

Basler RSW: Monocycline-related hyperpigmentation. Arch Dermatol 1985, 121:606.

Benning TL, et al: Microprobe analysis of chlorpromazine pigmentation. Arch Dermatol 1988, 124:1541.

David M, et al: Diffuse progressive pigmentation. JAAD 1987, 16:257.

Dupré A, et al: Chloroquin-induced hypopigmentation of hair and freckles. Arch Dermatol 1985, 121:1164.

Fernandez-Obregon AC, et al: Flagellate pigmentation from intrapleural bleomycin. JAAD 1985, 13:464.

Gordon G, et al: Hyperpigmentation of the skin associated with minocycline therapy. Arch Dermatol 1985, 121:618.

Granstein RD, et al: Drug- and heavy metal-induced hyperpigmentation. JAAD 1981, 5:1.

Held JL, et al: Hyperpigmentation of the lower extremities associated with porphyria cutanea tarda. Arch Dermatol 1989, 125:297.

Hoshaw RA, et al: Ochronosis-like pigmentation from hydroquinone bleaching creams in American Blacks. Arch Dermatol 1985, 121:105.

Kelly TM, et al: Hyperpigmentation with daunorubicin therapy. Arch Dermatol 1984, 120:263.

Klein AD, et al: Blue-gray discoloration of the face. Arch Dermatol 1989, 125:417.

Lerner EA, et al: Chemical and pharmacologic agents that cause hyper- or hypopigmentation. Derm Clin 1988, 6:337.

Mahler R, et al: Pigmentation induced by quinidine therapy. Arch Dermatol 1986, 122:1062.

Masu S, et al: Pigmentary incontinence in fixed drug eruptions. JAAD 1983, 8:525.

Merenich JA, et al: Azidothymidine-induced hyperpigmentation mimicking primary adrenal insufficiency. Am J Med 1989, 86:469.

Miller RAN, et al: Dermal lipofuscinosis associated with amiodarone therapy. Arch Dermatol 1984, 120:646.

Moore TG, et al: Nelson's syndrome. Ann Intern Med 1976, 85:73.

Nordlund JJ: Postinflammatory hyperpigmentation. Derm Clin 1988, 6:185.

Sexton M, et al: Generalized melanosis in occult primary melanoma. JAAD 1989, 20:281.

Trimble JW, et al: Cutaneous pigmentation secondary to amiodarone therapy. Arch Dermatol 1983, 119:914.

Waitzers, et al: Cutaneous ultrastructural change and photosensitivity associated with amiodarone therapy. JAAD 1987, 16:779.

HEMOCHROMATOSIS
(Bronze Diabetes)

Hemochromatosis is characterized by gray to brown skin and mucosal hyperpigmentation, diabetes mellitus, and hepatomegaly. In addition, heart disease, cirrhosis of the liver, and hypogonadism are usually present. The cause is either an inborn error of metabolism of iron, or excessive blood transfusions.

The skin pigmentation is usually generalized, although more pronounced upon the face, the extensor surfaces of the forearms, the backs of the hands, and the genitocrural area. Iron is deposited in the skin, being present as granules around blood vessels and sweat glands and within macrophages. The pigmentation, however, is due to increased basal-layer melanin. The mucous membranes were pigmented in only 20 per cent of the 100 cases studied by Chevrant-Breton and Bourel et al. Koilonychia occurred in 50 per cent, and localized ichthyosis in 40 per cent. Alopecia was common.

The plasma iron level and the serum iron-binding protein are elevated.

Hemochromatosis occurs mostly in men in their sixties. It is extremely rare in the young. However, Escobar reported a family in which a 7-year-old child and a 29-month-old child developed the disease.

Treatment is by phlebotomy of 500 ml at weekly intervals until satisfactory iron levels are attained. Removal of serum iron is the goal of this procedure. The diabetes must also be treated, of course, and the cirrhosis appropriately managed. Hepatomas occur not infrequently as a long-term complication of cirrhosis.

Chevrant-Breton J, et al: Cutaneous manifestations of idiopathic hemochromatosis. Arch Dermatol 1977, 113:16.

Dymock JW, et al: Arthropathy of hemochromatosis. Ann Rheum Dis 1970, 29:469.

Edwards CQ, et al: Prevalence of hemochromatosis among 11,065 presumably healthy blood donors. NEJM 1988, 318:1355.

Escobar GJ, et al: Hemochromatosis in childhood. Pediatrics 1987, 80:549.

Pedrup A, et al: Hemochromatosis and vitiligo. Arch Dermatol 1964, 90:34.

Simon M, et al: Idiopathic hemochromatosis. N Engl J Med 1977, 279:1017.

Williams R, et al: Venesection therapy in idiopathic hemochromatosis. Am J Med 1969, 28:1.

MELASMA
(Chloasma Faciei)

Melasma is characterized by brown patches, typically on the malar prominences and forehead. The upper lip is also frequently involved. The pigmented patches are usually quite sharply demarcated. Increased pigmentation may also occur at the same time on the nipples and about the external genitals.

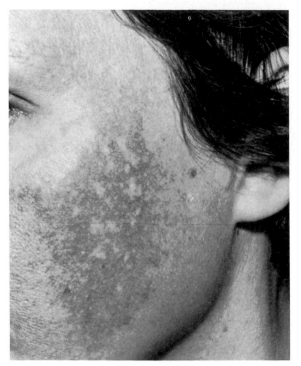

Figure 36–3. Melasma.

Melasma occurs frequently during pregnancy and at menopause. It may also be seen in ovarian disorders and probably occurs in other endocrinologic disorders. It is seen most frequently in young women taking oral contraceptives. Nevertheless, it may occur in the absence of any of these factors, and it is sometimes seen in men. Dilantin may induce melasma, and patients with AIDS may also have an increased incidence of similar hyperpigmentation. Discontinuing contraceptives rarely clears the pigmentation, and it may last as long as five years after stopping them.

The exact pathogenesis is not known. Genetic predisposition and sunlight exposure are undoubtedly important factors, as stated by Pathak et al and Sanchez et al.

Melasma of pregnancy usually clears within a few months of delivery.

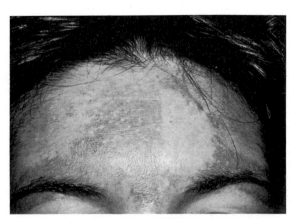

Figure 36–4. Melasma.

Bleaching creams containing hydroquinone may be tried. Pathak et al studied several combinations of hydroquinone and tretinoin for effectiveness and irritancy. They found that a cream containing 2 to 3 per cent hydroquinone and 0.05 to 0.1 per cent tretinoin was most effective. Kenney preferred 5 per cent hydroquinone, 2 or 3 per cent salicylic acid, and 0.025 per cent fluocinonide, which he has used for several years. Kligman et al reported success with 0.1 per cent tretinoin, 5 per cent hydroquinone, and 0.1 per cent dexamethasone, in either hydrophilic base, or equal parts of 95 per cent ethanol and propylene glycol, daily for four to six weeks. Exposure to sunlight should be avoided in any case: a complete sun block should be used daily. Eldopaque Forte and Solaquin both combine a bleaching agent with a sunscreen. Melanex is 3 per cent hydroquinone.

Temporary bleaching may be induced by the careful application of 95 per cent phenol to the pigmented patch. As soon as whitening occurs at the site of application the phenol is neutralized by isopropyl alcohol. The treated area turns first red and then black. The black eschar peels off, usually within a week.

Kligman AM, et al: A new formula for depigmentating human skin. Arch Dermatol 1975, 111:40.
Pathak MA, et al: Usefulness of retinoic acid in the treatment of melasma. JAAD 1986, 15:894.
Sanchez N, et al: Melasma. JAAD 1981, 4:698.

ALBRIGHT'S SYNDROME

Albright's syndrome consists of large pigmented macules of the skin (café-au-lait spots), fibrous dysplasia of the long bones, and precocious puberty in girls. Various associated endocrinopathies have been reported. The café-au-lait spots of Albright's syndrome are present soon after birth, are usually unilateral, stop abruptly at the midline, and involve the forehead, nuchal area, and buttocks most commonly. Albright described them as darker and more jagged in outline than those seen in neurofibromatosis, but this is not always the case. Spotty pigmentation may also occur periorally. The cause of this disorder may be autonomously functioning ovarian cysts. Estrogen receptors in bone may account for the bony lesions.

DiGeorge AM: Albright's syndrome. J Pediatr 1975, 87:1018.
Geffner ME, et al: Treatment of acromegaly with a somatostatin analog in a patient with McCune-Albright syndrome. J Pediatr 1987, 111:740.
Giovannelli G, et al: Mc-Cune-Albright syndrome in a male child. J Pediatr 1978, 92:220.
Kaplan FS, et al: Estrogen receptors in bone in a patient with polycystic fibrous dysplasia. NEJM 1988, 319:421.
MacMahon HE: Albright's syndrome. Pathol Annu 1971, 6:81.
Shelley WB, et al: Alopecia with fibrotic dysplasia and osteomas of skin. Arch Dermatol 1976, 112:715.

ACROMELANOSIS PROGRESSIVA

Acromelanosis progressiva, also known as acropigmentation, is a progressive pigmentary disorder that was first seen in early infancy in a Japanese child by Furuya and Mishima. A diffuse black pigmentation occurring on the dorsum of all the fingers and toes became progressively enlarged and more intensely pigmented. By age four to five the perineum, extremities, and areas of the head and neck were involved. Epileptiform seizures were also present. The history revealed consanguinity.

Furuya T, et al: Progressive pigmentary disorder in a Japanese child. Arch Dermatol 1962, 86:410.
Gonzalez JR, et al: Acromelanosis. JAAD 1980, 2:128.

RETICULAR PIGMENTED ANOMALY OF THE FLEXURES

This rare pigmentary adult-onset disorder, sometimes termed Dowling-Degos disease or "dark dot" disease, should be thought of whenever the diagnosis of acanthosis nigricans is considered in a patient who is not obese and is not known to have internal cancer. Clinically, it does not look velvety: it looks smooth. The pigmentation is reticular; at the periphery, discrete, brownish black macules surround the partly confluent central pigmented area. Typically, axillae, inframammary folds, and intercrural folds are involved. It begins as a rule at 20 to 30 years of age and progresses very gradually. There are frequently pits, sometimes pigmented, about the mouth.

Though the etiology is unknown, Brown reported six cases in one family, and other authors have observed a tendency to familial occurrence. He regards it as an autosomal dominant genodermatosis with variable penetrance and expressivity, and delayed onset.

Crovato et al believe this and Kitamura's *reticulate acropigmentation* are different manifestations of the same disease. Kikuchi considers that *Haber's syndrome* (familial rosacealike dermatitis with warty keratotic plaques on the trunk and limbs) is another manifestation of this disorder.

Histologically, the appearance is distinctive: there is elongation, tufting, and deep hyperpigmentation of the rete ridges, with protrusion of similar tufts even from the sides of the follicles. In Dowling's original case (which was initially thought to be atypical acanthosis nigricans) there was even a trichoepithelioma in one of the areas subjected to biopsy. In the case reported by Howell and Freeman the eruption was most striking on the scrotum, and electron microscopy showed aggregation of normal melanin granules in the keratinocytes.

There is no treatment.

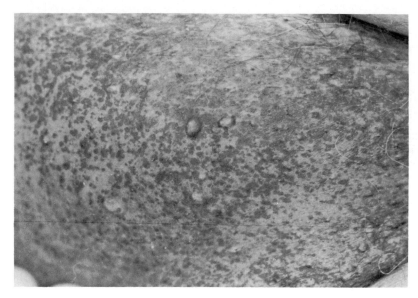

Figure 36–5. Reticulated pigmented anomaly of the flexures. (Courtesy of Dr. James B. Howell, Dallas.)

Brown WG: Reticulate pigmented anomaly of the flexures. Arch Dermatol 1982, 118:490.

Crovato F, et al: Reticulate pigmented anomaly of the flexures associating [sic] reticulate acropigmentation: one single entity. JAAD 1986, 14:359.

Degos R, et al: Dermatose pigmentaire reticulée des plis. Ann Dermatol Syphiligr 1954, 81:147.

Dowling JB, et al: Acanthosis nigricans. Br J Dermatol 1938, 50:467.

Howell JB, et al: Reticular pigmented anomaly of the flexures. Arch Dermatol 1978, 114:400.

Katter DC: Acquired intertriginous pigmentation. Arch Dermatol 1985, 121:401.

Kikuchi I: Haber's syndrome or Dowling-Degos disease? Arch Dermatol 1983, 119:365.

RETICULATE ACROPIGMENTATION OF KITAMURA

Woodley and his associates reported a 17-year-old girl with depressed, pitted, pigmented macules 1 to 4 mm in diameter, of 13 years' duration, on the volar and dorsal aspects of her hands and feet. It is an autosomal dominant disorder. The pitting and the absence of hypopigmented lesions distinguished it from acropigmentation of Dohi. They summarized the differential features of five of these rare acral pigmentary disorders. Fulk, in his review, discusses seven different subtypes of punctate and reticulate hyperpigmentation.

Mizoguchi M, et al: Behavior of melanocytes in reticulate acropigmentation of Kitamura. Arch Dermatol 1985, 121:659.

Woodley DT, et al: Reticulate acropigmentation of Kitamura. Arch Dermatol 1979, 115:760.

TRANSIENT NEONATAL PUSTULAR MELANOSIS

Ramamurthy et al reported infants showing 2- to 3-mm macules, pustules, and ruptured pustules at birth, with central pigmentation persisting for weeks or months after the pustules had healed. They observed it in 4.4 per cent of black and 0.6 per cent of white newborns.

Ramamurthy RS, et al: Transient neonatal pustular melanosis. J Pediatr 1976, 88:831.

Wyre HN, et al: Transient neonatal pustular melanosis. Arch Dermatol 1979, 115:458.

PEUTZ-JEGHERS SYNDROME

Peutz-Jeghers syndrome is characterized by melanin-pigmented macules on the lips and oral mucosa, and polyposis of the small intestine.

The dark brown or black macules appear typically on the lips, especially the lower lip, in infancy or early childhood. Similar lesions may appear on the buccal mucosa, tongue, gingiva, and genital mucosa; macules may also occur around the mouth, on the central face, and on the backs of the hands, especially the fingers, and on the toes and tops of the feet. Banse-Kupin et al reported a patient who developed pigmented macules within preexisting psoriatic plaques.

The associated polyposis involves the small intestine by preference, but hamartomatous polyps may also occur in the stomach and colon. The small-intestinal polyposis may cause repeated bouts of abdominal pain and vomiting. Bleeding is common. Intussusception is a frequent cause for operation.

The incidence of malignancy within the polyps is about 2 to 3 per cent. Ryo and associates reported a case with extensive metastases. Giardiello et al reviewed 31 cases of Peutz-Jeghers syndrome and found that 15 developed cancer—gastrointestinal in only four—an incidence 18 times higher than in the general population.

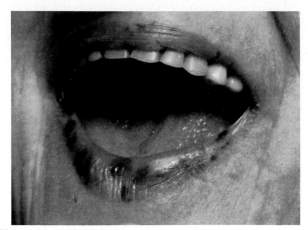

Figure 36–6. *Peutz-Jeghers syndrome. Note melanin-pigmented macules on lips. (Courtesy of Dr. A. Kaminsky.)*

In a case reported by Keeling et al, the pigmented lesions regressed immediately following resection of four large polyps from the ileum. This suggested that these hamartomatous lesions secrete a hormone which provokes the pigmentation.

The syndrome is inherited and is transmitted as a simple mendelian dominant trait. However, sporadic noninherited cases may also occur.

In the differential diagnosis **Cronkhite's syndrome** should be considered. It consists of melanotic macules on the fingers and gastrointestinal polyposis with its attendant symptoms. Also there is generalized, uniform darkening of the skin, extensive alopecia, and onychodystrophy. The polyps that occur are benign adenomas, usually, and may involve the entire gastrointestinal tract. Onset is typically after age 30 in this generally benign, sporadically occurring condition.

Banse-Kupin LA, et al: Localization of Peutz-Jeghers macules to psoriatic plaques. Arch Dermatol 1986, 122:679.

Cronkhite LW, et al: Generalized gastrointestinal polyposis. N Engl J Med 1955, 252:1011.

Dubois RS, et al: Feminizing sex cord tumor . . . in Peutz-Jeghers syndrome. J Pediatr 1982, 101:568.

Giardiello FM, et al: Increased risk of cancer in Peutz-Jeghers syndrome. N Engl J Med 1987, 316:1511.

Johnson GK, et al: Cronkhite-Canada syndrome. Gastroenterology 1972, 63:140.

Keeling PW, et al: Involution of mucocutaneous pigmentation of Peutz-Jeghers syndrome. Br Med J 1977, 1:949.

Kindblom LG, et al: Cronkhite-Canada syndrome. Cancer 1977, 39:2667.

Long JA Jr, et al: The Peutz-Jeghers syndrome: a 39-year clinical and radiological follow-up report. N Engl J Med 1977, 297:1070.

Ryo UY, et al: Extensive metastasis in Peutz-Jeghers syndrome. JAMA 1978, 239:2268.

POIKILODERMA OF CIVATTE

Poikiloderma of Civatte is a reticular pigmentation limited to the face, neck, and upper parts of the chest. The eruption is symmetrical and consists of reddish brown or bronze-colored 1–3-mm macules or papules intermingled with superficial atrophic white spots and telangiectasia.

Sun-exposed areas are involved exclusively, with shaded areas conspicuously free of disease. This is one of the benign, cosmetically disturbing reactions to chronic sun exposure.

There is no treatment. Patients should be advised to routinely apply sunscreens and avoid sun exposure as much as possible.

Salasche SJ, et al: Cutaneous manifestations of chronic solar exposure. J Assoc Milit Dermatol 1985, 11:3.

RIEHL'S MELANOSIS

This pigmentary disease, first described by Riehl, is a photosensitivity, probably a phototoxic dermatitis. It begins with pruritus, erythema, and pigmentation, gradually spreads and, after reaching a certain extent, becomes stationary. The melanosis occurs mostly in women and develops slowly over the course of several months. It is frequently diagnosed in Japan.

The characteristic feature is spotty light to dark brown pigmentation. This is most intense on the forehead, on the malar regions, behind the ears, on the sides of the neck, and on other sun-exposed areas. Pigmentation on covered parts of the body is only on areas exposed to friction, such as the anterior axillary folds and the umbilicus.

In addition to the melanosis, there may be circumscribed telangiectasia and temporary hyperemia. Diffuse hyperkeratosis occurs, making the skin appear as if "dusted with flour."

The cause of Riehl's melanosis is sunlight, generally following the use of some perfume or cream on the skin. Sudan I dye, occurring as an impurity in the cosmetic coloring agent Brilliant Lake Red R, was incriminated by Sugai et al and by Kozuka et al.

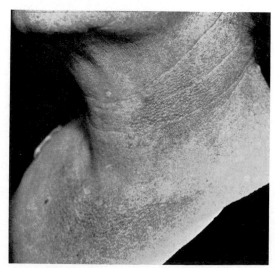

Figure 36–7. Poikiloderma of Civatte.

Tadokor reported a series of 85 cases occurring between 1958 and 1961 and found the female:male ratio to be 77:8. Photosensitivity was demonstrated in 60 per cent.

All treatment methods are of no avail unless the cause of photosensitivity is determined. Eventually the hyperkeratosis and pigmentation disappear spontaneously.

Kozuka T, et al: Brilliant Lake Red R: a cause of pigmented dermatitis. Contact Dermat 1979, 5:297.
Rorsman H: Riehl's melanosis. Int J Dermatol 1982, 21:75.
Sugai T, et al: Pigmented cosmetic dermatitis and coal tar dyes. Contact Dermat 1977, 3:249.

TAR MELANOSIS
(Melanodermatitis Toxica Lichenoides)

This occupational dermatosis occurs among tar handlers after several years' exposure. Severe widespread itching develops and is soon followed by the appearance of reticular pigmentation, telangiectases, and a shiny appearance of the skin. In addition, there is a tendency to hyperhidrosis. Small, dark, lichenoid, follicular papules become profuse on the extremities, particularly the forearms. Bullae are sometimes observed.

This represents a photosensitivity or phototoxicity induced by tar.

FAMILIAL PROGRESSIVE HYPERPIGMENTATION

Familial progressive hyperpigmentation (FPH) is characterized by patches of hyperpigmentation, present at birth, which increase in size and number with age. Later, hyperpigmentation appears in the conjunctivae and the buccal mucosa. Eventually a large portion of the skin and mucous membranes becomes involved.

FPH was described by Chernosky and his associates in four persons in two generations of a black family. Inheritance was believed to be of a dominant mode.

Histologically, the most distinctive finding was the increase of melanin in the basal cell layers, especially at the tips of the rete ridges. In addition, pigmented granules were scattered diffusely throughout the epidermal layers, including the stratum corneum.

FPH is differentiated from other hyperpigmentations mainly by the presence of bizarre, sharply marginated patterns of hyperpigmented skin.

Chernosky ME, et al: Familial progressive hyperpigmentation. Arch Dermatol 1971, 103:58.

UNIVERSAL ACQUIRED MELANOSIS
(Carbon Baby)

Ruiz-Maldonado and associates reported the case of a Mexican child, born white, who progressively became black, with pigmentation of palms, soles, and the mucous membranes. Electron microscopy showed a negroid pattern in the melanosomes of the epidermal melanocytes and keratinocytes. Melanocytes were not increased in number.

Ruiz-Maldonado R, et al: Universal acquired melanosis. Arch Dermatol 1978, 114:775.

ZEBRALIKE HYPERPIGMENTATION

Alimurung and associates reported an unusual pattern of hyperpigmentation in a black male infant with congenital defects that included an atrial septal defect, dextrocardia, auricular atresia, deafness, and growth retardation. The hyperpigmentation was strikingly linear and symmetrical and followed a dermatome distribution, with involvement of the trunk and extremities. An increased number of melanocytes in the bands of hyperpigmentation was demonstrated. The pigmentary anomaly was fading spontaneously. Fulk classified it as a variant of incontinentia pigmenti. The differential diagnosis included incontinentia pigmenti, the Franceschetti-Jadassohn syndrome or Naegeli's reticular pigmented dermatosis, and several other unusual pigmentary disorders.

Alimurung FM, et al: Zebra-like hyperpigmentation in an infant with multiple congenital defects. Arch Dermatol 1979, 115:878.

PERIORBITAL HYPERPIGMENTATION

Maruri and Diaz discuss the nomenclature, pathology, and genetics of the dark circles found around the eyes of some persons. The hyperpigmentation of familial periorbital melanosis, an autosomal dominant disorder, usually involves all four eyelids and may extend to involve the eyebrows and the cheekbones. The pigmentation is due to melanin. Fulk's case had increased basal melanocytes and upper- and mid-dermal melanophages. Goodman et al and Aquilera et al reported their observations of this disease.

Aquilera MA, et al: Periorbital melanosis. Cutis 1969, 5:579.
Fulk CS: Primary disorders of hyperpigmentation. JAAD 1984, 10:1.
Goodman RM, et al: Periorbital melanosis. Arch Dermatol 1969, 100:169.

METALLIC DISCOLORATIONS

Pigmentation may develop from the deposit of fine metallic particles in the skin. The metal may be carried to the skin by the blood stream or may permeate into it from surface applications. Electron microprobe x-ray analysis is a useful, accurate technique of identifying such compounds in the skin.

Argyria. Argyria is a localized or wide-spread slate-colored pigmentation due to the presence of silver albuminate in the skin. The pigmentation is most noticeable in parts exposed to sunlight (the face and hands) and spares the skin folds; however, it also occurs in the conjunctivae, sclerae, mucous membranes, and nails. At first the discoloration is hardly perceptible, being a faint bluish gray tone, but as it becomes more pronounced a slate color develops. The oral mucous membranes and the sclerae are usually pigmented in a distinctive diffuse manner. At one time when silver nitrate was used internally more frequently, argyria was encountered more often than at present. Other causes of argyria include prolonged use of Argyrol, Protargol, and Neo-silvol. These may cause argyria localized to the region of use: for example, the conjunctivae, from eye drops, or a wound, from silver sulfadiazine cream.

Examination of an unstained biopsy section by darkfield illumination provides a brilliant diagnostic picture by demonstrating silver proteinate or sulfide granules outlining the basement membrane of the epidermis and the eccrine sweat glands, as shown by Mitchell and by Arnold.

Staining from the topical application of silver nitrate may be removed by moistening the area with water, then rubbing potassium iodide crystals over it and allowing this to remain on the skin for an hour or two.

Bismuth. When bismuth compounds were used intramuscularly or orally for a long time, it caused (but very infrequently, and only in dirty mouths) the deposition of metallic particles into the gums. This, known as the bismuth line, was usually accompanied by stomatitis. Generalized cutaneous discoloration, as well as oral mucous membrane and conjunctival pigmentation resembling argyria, has rarely occurred from the use of this drug.

Arsenic. Ingestion of inorganic trivalent arsenic (Fowler's solution, Asiatic pills) for some years may produce diffuse bronze pigmentation or, more characteristically, a "raindrop" appearance, with depigmented and hyperpigmented macules interspersed, combined with small hyperkeratotic papules on the palms, soles, and ears. This takes from one to 20 years to develop.

Lead. Chronic lead poisoning can produce a "lead hue," with lividity and pallor, and a deposit of lead in the gums may occur, the "lead line."

Iron. In the past, soluble iron compounds were used in the treatment of allergic contact and other dermatitides. In eroded areas iron was sometimes deposited in the skin, like a tattoo.

Titanium. A titanium-containing ointment caused yellowish papules on the penis in a patient treated by Dupre et al. Titanium was identified by electron-probe microanalysis.

Gold. *Chrysiasis* may be induced by the excessive administration of gold. A gray or lilac-colored pigmentation may develop on the eyelids, face, hands, and other areas (chrysoderma) following the prolonged parenteral use of gold salts. The intensity of the pigmentation is accentuated by exposure to light. In many respects it resembles argyria. The color is produced by the metal itself.

Mercury. Prolonged application of facial creams containing mercurous chloride, ammoniated mercury, or mercurous oxide produced brown-gray or slate-colored pigmentation of the face and neck, especially prominent in folds, such as the periorbital and nasolabial regions and the folds of the neck. Mercury particles were deposited in the skin and shone (see under argyria) brilliantly on darkfield microscopy. The pigmentation results from both mercury and melanin. Topical mercury, however, is no longer available.

Systemic mercury has been reported to cause gingival hypertrophy, comparable to reactions to lead or bismuth.

Arnold HL Jr: Correspondence (on darkfield demonstration of silver in unstained histologic sections of skin, in argyria). Br J Dermatol 1954, 66:334.

Blechen SS, et al: Occupational argyria. Br J Dermatol 1981, 104:19.

Burge JM, et al: Mercury pigmentation. Arch Dermatol 1979, 102:51.

Conners RS, et al: Generalized argyria. Cutis 1973, 11:797.

Dupré A, et al: Titanium pigmentation. Arch Dermatol 1985, 121:656.

Dupuis LL, et al: Hyperpigmentation due to topical application of silver sulfadiazine cream. JAAD 1985, 12:1112.

Granstein RD, et al: Drug- and heavy-metal induced hyperpigmentation. JAAD 1981, 5:1.

Pariseo RJ: Generalized argyria. Cutis 1973, 11:797.

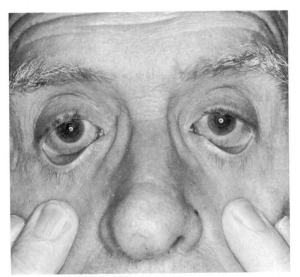

Figure 36–8. Diffuse pigmentation of the sclerae in a man with argyria.

Shelley WB, et al: Argyria. JAAD 1987, 16:211.
Sladin KR, et al: Blue lady: a case of argyria. Cutis 1978, 22:321.
Tanita Y, et al: Blue macules of localized argyria caused by implanted acupuncture needles. Arch Dermatol 1985, 121:1550.

CAROTENOSIS
(Carotenemia)

This is a yellow discoloration of the skin caused by carotene derived from the ingestion of excessive quantities of carrots, oranges, squash, spinach, yellow corn and beans, butter, eggs, rutabagas, pumpkin, yellow turnips, sweet potatoes, or papaya. Beta-carotene ingestion for erythropoietic protoporphyria, or for other reasons, also results in this condition. The color is most noticeable on the palms and soles, in the nasolabial grooves, at the rims of the nostrils, on the forehead and chin, behind the ears and over the knuckles. The sclerae are spared, which easily rules out jaundice.

Carotenemia occurs in diabetes as a result of either dietary intake or of failure of the liver to convert carotene to vitamin A. In the latter case it is accompanied by nyctalopia (night blindness) of varying degrees. It is also seen in myxedema. The disease is commonest in children and in food faddists, especially vegetarians. Excessive amounts of carotene are demonstrable in the bloodstream and in the urine. The detection of carotene depends on two properties, namely, its solubility in alcohol and petroleum-ether, and its failure to be adsorbed by calcium carbonate.

Histologically, the epidermis and papillary layer are yellow. The disease is common in children.

Treatment is the restriction of carotene-containing foods. Porter et al list the foods significantly high in carotenoid pigments.

LYCOPENEMIA

Lycopene is a red carotenoid pigment found in tomatoes, beets, chili beans, and various fruits and berries. High intake of these foods may lead to a reddish discoloration of the skin and abnormal liver function with bizarre vacuoles and crystals in the liver cells.

Orange People. Hughes and Wooten described two interesting patients, a man and a woman, who showed an orange-bronze color of the skin over the entire body, especially the palms. Both had a history of high intake of carrots, tomatoes, and tomato juice. Discontinuation of the ingestion of yellow and red-pigmented food-stuffs brought about resumption of normal color in six months.

Canthaxanthin. This orange-red pigment is present in many plants (notably algae and mushrooms) and in bacteria, crustaceans, sea trout, and feathers. When ingested for the purpose of simulating a tan, its deposition in the panniculus imparts a golden-orange hue to the skin. Stools become brick red and the plasma orange, and golden deposits appear in the retina.

Bilimoria S, et al: Hypercarotenaemia in weight watchers. Clin Exp Dermatol 1979, 4:331.
Everett MA: Carotenemia and carotenoderma. In Clinical Dermatology, vol 2. Philadelphia, Harper & Row, pp. 11–13, 1985.
Lober CW: Canthaxanthin—the "tanning" pill. JAAD 1985, 13:660.
Porter JW, et al: The biosynthesis of carotenes. Arch Biochem 1962, 520—528.
Reich P, et al: Lycopenemia. N Engl J Med 1960, 262:263.

DYE DISCOLORATION

"Blue hands" due to accidental dyeing were reported by Albert in 1976 and by Berton Roueché, in which a man's hands were dyed as a result of warming them in his armpits while wearing a new blue flannel shirt. The dye, insoluble in water, was soluble in sweat.

Albert BL: Blue dye, blue hands, and sweat. Ann Intern Med 1976, 85:541.
Roueché B: Two blue hands. New Yorker, December 22, 1975, p 72.

RUBEOSIS

Rubeosis is a rosy coloration of the face occurring in young people with uncontrolled diabetes mellitus. It may be associated with xanthochromia to produce a "peaches and cream" complexion.

VITILIGO

CLINICAL FEATURES. Vitiligo is an acquired, often disfiguring, pigmentary anomaly of the skin manifested by depigmented white patches surrounded by a normal or a hyperpigmented border; the depigmented skin lacks melanocytes, and has markedly diminished capacity to react to topically applied sensitizing substances as reported by Uehara et al and Nordlund et al, but is normal in all other respects. The hairs in the vitiliginous areas usually become white also. Very rarely the patches may have a red, inflammatory border. The patches are of various sizes and may have various configurations. They are often symmetrically situated in the generalized variety. The most commonly affected sites are the face, upper part of the chest, dorsal aspects of the hands, axillae, groins, eyes, nose, mouth, ears, nipples, umbilicus, penis, vulva, anus, elbows, and knees. The depigmentation may be generalized or universal.

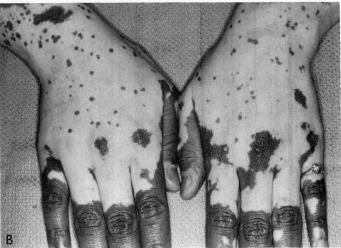

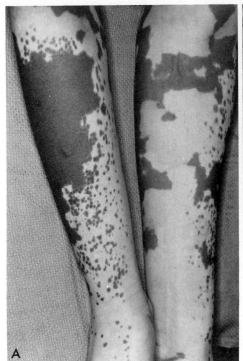

Figure 36–9. A and B, Vitiligo. The symmetry is characteristic.

Four types have been described according to the extent and distribution of the involved areas: localized, including a linear or segmented pattern; generalized; universal; and perinevic (halo nevus). Vitiligolike leukoderma may occur in melanoma patients.

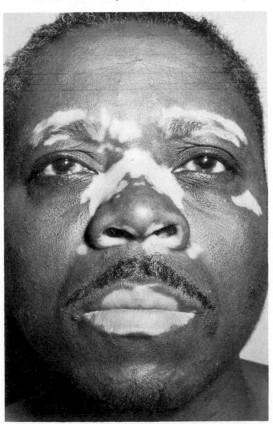

Figure 36–10. Vitiligo.

In those with previously diagnosed melanoma it portends metastatic disease. Paradoxically, however—as the reaction indicates an autoimmune response against melanocytes—patients who develop it have a better survival rate than patients without leukoderma.

The white patches are hypersensitive to ultraviolet light and burn readily when exposed to the sun. It is not unusual to note the onset of vitiligo after a severe sunburn. Lesions tend to develop in trauma-prone areas. A Koebner reaction may occur.

Vitiligo affects all races, and both sexes seem equally vulnerable to the disease. Approximately 50 per cent of patients develop some form of the disease before age ten, but vitiligo may have its onset any time from infancy to senescence.

Halder et al reviewed their experience with childhood vitiligo. They found it to be a distinct subset, showing increased segmental presentation; strong autoimmune or endocrine background, or both; high incidence of premature graying in the families; and a poor response to PUVA therapy.

Nordlund et al and Cowan et al have shown a high percentage of ocular abnormalities, such as abnormal pigmentation in the fundus. Eight per cent of patients with idiopathic uveitis have vitiligo or poliosis. Tosti et al found sensorineural hypoacusis in 16 per cent of vitiligo cases, in Sicily.

Vitiligo has been reported in association with numerous disorders, including insulin-dependent diabetes mellitus, pernicious anemia, hypo- and hyperthyroidism, Down's syndrome, dysgammaglobulinemia, biliary cirrhosis, acromegaly, and carcinoma of the stomach. In some of these conditions, such as the autoimmune diseases, the incidence of vitiligo is significantly higher than in the population at large; in others, such as psoriasis, it is not.

In many cases vitiligo occurs as an inherited disease transmitted as an autosomal dominant characteristic with variable expressivity. About 35 per cent of persons with a family history of vitiligo develop the disorder.

PATHOGENESIS. Four possible mechanisms (which are not mutually exclusive!) are autoimmunity, neurohumoral factors, autocytotoxicity, and exogenous chemical exposure. Except (possibly!) in the neurosegmental type, autoimmunity seems most likely to be the chief cause.

Autoimmunity. The incidence of vitiligo in patients with autoimmune disease is 10 to 15 per cent as compared with 1 per cent in the general population. Patients with vitiligo have increased organ-specific autoantibodies including antibodies against adrenal cytoplasm, thyroid cytoplasm, thyroglobulin, gastric parietal cells, and pancreatic islet cells. Antibodies to intracellular antigens of melanocytes have been demonstrated, and Naughton et al have found (by immunoprecipitation) antibodies to surface antigens of normal melanocytes. They found a correlation between the incidence and level of the antibodies, and the extent of depigmentation. Also, Grimes et al showed a statistically significant decrease in helper T cells and T-cell helper/suppressor ratios in 20 randomly chosen patients with vitiligo as compared with 16 healthy controls.

Neurohumoral. Hypopigmentation or depigmentation may be caused by an excess of some neurotoxic agent released near melanocytes—possibly norepinephrine or some other catecholamine. Disturbances of the autonomic nervous system have been suggested by many investigators. This hypothesis best explains the segmental cases of vitiligo.

Exogenous Chemical Exposure. Thiols, phenolic compounds, catechol, derivatives of catechol, mercaptoamines, and several quinones produce depigmentation through inhibition of tyrosinase and a direct cytotoxic action on the melanocyte. All of the intermediates in the biosynthesis of melanin are phenolic compounds, and it has been suggested that accumulation of these within the melanocyte may damage or kill the cell.

INCIDENCE AND PREVALENCE. Vitiligo occurs in 1 to 2 per cent of the population. Its comparative prevalence in the tropics and in dark-skinned persons may be largely due to its conspicuousness in suntanned or naturally dark skin.

HISTOPATHOLOGY. Few changes in the skin are evident, save for complete absence of dopa-positive melanocytes. Langerhans cells are not increased in number.

DIAGNOSIS. Vitiligo must be differentiated from morphea, in which the skin is ivory-colored, shiny, and adherent to the underlying tissue. Pityriasis alba, tinea versicolor, and pinta might easily lead to diagnostic confusion. Leukoderma following herpes zoster or syphilis may be difficult to distinguish from vitiligo.

TREATMENT. Spontaneous repigmentation occurs in no more than 15 to 25 per cent of cases. Repigmentation by PUVA therapy has been reported to occur in 50 to 70 per cent. It requires a long-term commitment to therapy. But when repigmentation is once begun, it tends to persist and spread. Trisoralen (trimethylpsoralen) is less effective, but for the same reason it is less likely to cause accidental sunburn, and some prefer it for outpatient use.

Mosher et al outline their protocol for oral psoralen plus UVA, and the package insert (or PDR) gives a recommended regimen for starting dosages of both the drug, and joules of UVA, as well as stepwise increases according to response and toxicity.

Repigmentation may begin after 15 to 25 treatments; significant improvement, however, may take as many as 100 to 300. If follicular pigmentation has not appeared after three months of therapy, treatment may as well be stopped.

Khellin, a furanochromone, is being investigated as a photosensitizer, in combination with ultraviolet light. Its chief advantage is that it does not produce phototoxic erythema.

Contraindications. Known photosensitivity, porphyria, liver disease, and systemic lupus erythematosus are contraindications to psoralen therapy. Children under 12 years of age should probably not take it. Overdosage of either psoralen or sunlight may produce painful blistering burns. The distal extremities, lip lesions, and segmental lesions are least responsive to this treatment.

Topical therapy, for isolated small lesions (or occasionally for larger lesions covering less than 20 per cent of the body) is safer and may be more convenient, but it is best to begin with a .01 per cent solution (a 1:100 dilution of the 1 per cent Oxsoralen Lotion) especially in persons of light complexion or (in exposed lesions) in localities with intense sunshine. Grimes et al have described a suitable regimen. Topical psoralens are the only treatment for children.

Systemic Steroids. Indian dermatologists, Desai and others, have long believed that systemic prednisone is a helpful adjunct to therapy. Gokhale reported success in 25 cases, 16 of whom had resisted oxsoralen therapy, using ACTH alone, 40 mg twice weekly for five weeks on and 15 weeks off.

Surgical Therapy. Caver had success, in Hawaii, by dermabrasion of lesions in dark, hairy areas. Falabella et al reported success with autologous minigrafts, and Behl with split-thickness grafts. Tsuji's abrasion method, described below, may work. Suvanprakorn and Koga described a method of inducing blisters and transplanting their roofs onto previously blistered involved skin. Melanocyte cultures from cells of the patient's normal skin injected into blister cavities as described for piebaldism, is being investigated. These surgical methods are likely to be especially useful in segmental vitiligo.

Kumari reported repigmentation of 90 to 100 per cent in facial lesions in Asians and blacks treated with 0.05 per cent clobetasol propionate in paraffin base; it was even used successfully on the eyelids, without inducing glaucoma.

Tsuji et al had equal success with 5 per cent topical 5-fluorouracil cream after dermabrasion of the lesions, and Monk tried 2.5 per cent 5-fluorouracil in 8 per cent dimethyl sulfoxide (DMSO) but without success. Cormane tried phenylalanine, 50 mg/kg/day, plus UVA, 2-12J/cm^2 for four months, progressively increasing the dose. He achieved good repigmentation, without sunburn.

Urbanek reported Zetar bath oil treatments were effective in some cases.

In nearly universal cases, bleaching of residual pigment with monobenzone (monobenzyl ether of hydroquinone) 20 per cent, twice daily for three to six months, was used successfully by Mosher et al. It is the only indication for use of this otherwise dangerous drug, as Becker Jr has emphasized. Nordlund et al have lately reported that six women (out of about 40 patients treated in this way) experienced acute dermatitis confined to the still-pigmented areas; it never occurred in depigmented skin, nor were patch tests positive in depigmented areas.

Tattooing of the achromic patches with gold salts (such as 20 per cent aurothioglucose) has been successfully used by Grinspan and associates in Argentina, and infrequently by Domonkos. The treatments are repeated at weekly intervals. Usually four to 12 treatments suffice. The best results are seen on the face and neck. Tattooing should produce an erythema without bleeding.

Localized vitiligo has been treated successfully with intradermal injections of triamcinolone acetonide by Kandil. The rate of cure is inversely proportional to the duration of the disease. Thirty of the 52 patients treated were cured or almost completely cured.

Vitadye (Paul B. Elder Co.) may be used to color and conceal conspicuous lesions. Covermark (Lydia O'Leary) and Blenderm are excellent and elegant cosmetics which are produced in many shades and afford superior concealment of leukoderma, as well as port-wine stains and scars.

Lerner et al have treated several patients by growing in vitro melanocytes from the patients' normal skin and injecting them into artificially induced blister cavities in the depigmented areas. Gokhale has reported success with fetal and autologous skin grafts.

Barnes L: Vitiligo and the Vogt-Koyanagi-Harada syndrome. Derm Clin 1988, 6:229.

Beck HI, et al: Graft exchange in vitiligo. Acta Derm Venereol (Stockh) 1986, 66:311.

Becker SW Jr: Uses of Benoquin. Schoch Letter 1980, 30:15.

Behl PN: Repigmentation of segmental vitiligo by autologous minigrafting. JAAD 1985, 12:19.

Berterle C, et al: Incidence and significance of organ-specific autoimmune disorders (clinical, latent or only autoantibodies) in patients with vitiligo. Dermatologica 1985, 171:419.

Buckley WR, et al: Vitiligo with raised inflammatory border. Arch Dermatol Syph 1953, 67:316.

Cormane RH, et al: Phenylalanine and UV light in vitiligo. Arch Dermatol Res 1985, 277:176.

Cowan CI, et al: Ocular disturbances in vitiligo. JAAD 1986, 15:17.

Falabella R: Repigmentation of segmental vitiligo by autologous minigrafting. JAAD 1983, 9:514.

Idem: Treatment of localized vitiligo by autologous minigrafting. Arch Dermatol 1988, 124:1649.

Idem: Repigmentation of stable leukoderma by autologous minigrafting. J Dermatol Oncol 1986, 12:172.

Gokhale BB: ACTH for vitiligo. The Schoch Letter 1975, 25:3.

Idem: Fetal and autologous skin grafts equally good for restoring pigmentation. The Schoch Letter 1989, 39:24.

Gould IM: Vitiligo in diabetes mellitus. Br J Dermatol 1985, 113:153.

Grimes PE, et al: T cell profiles in vitiligo. JAAD 1986, 14:196.

Idem: Determination of optimal topical photochemotherapy for vitiligo. JAAD 1982, 7:771.

Halder RM, et al: Childhood vitiligo. JAAD 1987, 16:948.

Hatchome N, et al: Possible functional impairment of Langerhans cells in vitiliginous skin. Arch Dermatol 1987, 123:51.

Howanitz N, et al: Antibodies to melanocytes . . . in vitiligo. Arch Dermatol 1981, 117:705.

Koga M: Epidermal grafting using the tops of suction blisters in the treatment of vitiligo. Arch Dermatol 1988, 124:1656.

Koh HK, et al: Malignant melanoma and vitiligo-like leukoderma. JAAD 1983, 9:696.

Korkij W, et al: Tissue-specific autoantibodies and autoimmune disorders in vitiligo and alopecia areata. J Cutan Pathol 1984, 11:522.

Kumari J: Vitiligo treated with topical clobetasol propionate. Arch Dermatol 1984, 120:6.

Idem: Vitiligo: in reply (letter). Arch Dermatol 1985, 121:22.

Lerner AB, et al: Transplantation of human melanocytes. J Invest Dermatol 1987, 89:219.

Idem: Repopulation of pigment cells in patients with vitiligo. Arch Dermatol 1988, 124:1701.

McBurney ET: Vitiligo. Arch Intern Med 1979, 139:1295.

Monk B: Topical fluorouracil in vitiligo. Arch Dermatol 1985, 121:25.

Mosher DB, et al: Monobenzyl ether of hydroquinone: a retrospective study of treatment of 18 vitiligo patients and a review of literature. Br J Dermatol 1977, 97:669.

Idem: Disorders of pigmentation. In Dermatology in General Medicine. Fitzpatrick TB, et al (eds.) New York, McGraw-Hill, pp. 818–821, 1987.

Naughton GK, et al: Detection of autoantibodies to melanocytes in vitiligo by specific immunoprecipitation. J Invest Dermatol 1983, 81:540.

Idem: Correlation between vitiligo autoantibodies and extent of depigmentation in vitiligo. JAAD 1986, 15:978.

Nordlund JJ, et al: Vitiligo: it is important (editorial). Arch Dermatol 1982, 118:5.

Idem: Dermatitis produced by applications of monobenzone in patients with active vitiligo. Arch Dermatol 1985, 121:1141.

Idem: Vitiligo in patients with metastatic melanoma. JAAD 1983, 9:689.

Idem: Prevalence of vitiligo and poliosis in patients with uveitis. JAAD 1981, 4:528.

Ortel B, et al: Treatment of vitiligo with khellin and ultraviolet A. JAAD 1988, 18:693.

Parrish JA, et al: Photochemotherapy of vitiligo. Arch Dermatol 1976, 112:1531.

Scholtz JR: Vitiligo (letter). Arch Dermatol 1985, 121:22.

Soubiran P, et al: Vitiligo and peripheral T cell subset imbalance as defined by monoclonal antibodies. Br J Dermatol 1985, 113(suppl 28):124.

Suvanprakorn P, et al: Melanocyte autologous grafting for treatment of leukoderma. JAAD 1985, 13:968.

Todes-Taylor N, et al: The occurrence of vitiligo after psoralens and ultraviolet A therapy. JAAD 1983, 9:526.

Tosti A, et al: Audiologic abnormalities in cases of vitiligo. JAAD 1987, 17:230.

Tsuji T, et al: Topical . . . fluorouracil in vitiligo. Arch Dermatol 1983, 119:722.

Uehara M: Diminished contact sensitivity response in vitiliginous skin. Arch Dermatol 1984, 120:195.

Urbauck RW: Tar vitiligo therapy. JAAD 1983, 8:755.

VOGT-KOYANAGI-HARADA SYNDROME

Vogt-Koyanagi syndrome is characterized by a marked bilateral uveitis associated with symmetric vitiligo, alopecia, white eyelashes and brows (poliosis), and dysacousia (diminished hearing). In Harada's syndrome the uveitis is posterior, and there is pleocytosis in the spinal fluid, with fever and encephalitic or meningeal symptoms which precede the uveitis. As this appears to be a different aspect of the same disease, the entire complex is usually referred to as the Vogt-Koyanagi-Harada syndrome.

The disease usually occurs in adults in their third decade. Initially a meningoencephalitis occurs with prodromata of fever, malaise, headache, nausea, and vomiting. The ophthalmic stage is characterized by uveitis, which may appear rapidly and last for several years. The changes in the skin appear three weeks to three months after onset of the uveitis. The scalp, eyebrows, eyelashes, and the hairs of the axillae are the main sites of alopecia and poliosis. There may be deafness and tinnitus. In all patients there is a bilateral uveitis, which tends to be self-limiting in its course. Alopecia invariably occurs; poliosis occurs in about 90 per cent of the patients, vitiligo and temporary deafness in about half. Treatment of the ocular inflammatory disease with systemic steroids may prevent blindness.

The syndrome is believed to be of viral origin or an autoimmune disorder.

Howsden HM, et al: Vogt-Koyanagi-Harada syndrome and psoriasis. Arch Dermatol 1973, 108:395.

ALEZZANDRINI'S SYNDROME

Alezzandrini's syndrome is characterized by a unilateral degenerative retinitis followed after several months by ipsilateral vitiligo on the face and ipsilateral poliosis. Deafness may also be present.

Alezzandrini AA: Manifestation unilatérale de degénérescence tapéto-retinienne, de vitiligo, de poliose, de chève aux blancs et d'hypoacousie. Ophthalmologica 1964, 147:407.

LEUKODERMA

Leukoderma may be defined as a type of acquired skin depigmentation produced by some specific substance or dermatosis. Several types of leukoderma may be seen.

Occupational leukoderma may occur in those who work in rubber garments or wear gloves that contain an antioxidant, monobenzyl ether of hydroquinone. (The antioxidant has been used to retard aging of the rubber.) Many phenolic compounds can produce leukoderma, with or without antecedent dermatitis. It may spread to areas with which they have not come in contact. Examples are paratertiary butylphenol, amylphenol, and butylcatechol; alkyl phenols; and monobenzyl ether of hydroquinone. One source of these is phenolic antiseptic detergents used in hospitals. Adhesives and glues containing them may be in shoes, wristbands, and adhesive tape, and rubber products used in brassieres, girdles, panties, or condoms may also be at fault. Self-sticking bindis (the cosmetic used by many Indian women on the forehead) has been reported to induce leukoderma due to the adhesive material. Also, electrocardiograph electrodes may cause similar round hypopigmented spots at the site of contact.

Occupational leukoderma in 54 of 198 employees exposed to contact with p-tert-butylphenol was reported by O. James et al. Involvement of protected sites suggested a systemic effect. Liver damage occurred in six severe cases. The chemical was used in manufacture of adhesives.

Postinflammatory leukoderma may result from many inflammatory dermatoses; such are pityriasis rosea, psoriasis, herpes zoster, secondary syphilis, and morphea. Sarcoidosis, tinea versicolor, mycosis fungoides, scleroderma, and pityriasis lichenoides chronica may all present with hypopigmented (only rarely actually depigmented) lesions, as may leprosy. In the latter, one or a few lesions over 3 or 4 cm in diameter suggest tuberculoid disease, while numerous lesions under 2 cm across are usually lepromatous. Mathias et al reported an unusual case of perioral leukoderma from a toothpaste containing cinnamic aldehyde.

Burns, scars, postdermabrasion, and intralesional steroid injections with depigmentation are other examples of leukoderma.

Bajaj AK, et al: Bindi depigmentation. Arch Dermatol 1983, 119:629.
Calnan CD: Occupational leukoderma from alkylophenols. Proc R Soc Med 1973, 66:258.
Fisher AA: Vitiligo due to contactants. Cutis 1976, 117:431.
Friedman SJ, et al: Perilesional linear atrophy and hypopigmentation after intralesional corticosteroid therapy. JAAD 1988, 19:537.
James O, et al: Occupational vitiligo induced by p-tert butylphenol: a systemic disease? Lancet 1977, 2:1217.
Kahn G: Depigmentation caused by phenolic detergent germicides. Arch Dermatol 1970, 102:177.
Mathias CGT, et al: Perioral leukoderma simulating vitiligo from use of a toothpaste containing cinnamic aldehyde. Arch Dermatol 1980, 116:1172.
Weigand DA: Contact hypopigmentation from electrocardiograph electrodes. JAAD 1986, 15:1048.

ALBINISM

Albinism is a partial or complete congenital absence of pigment in the skin, hair, and eyes (oculocutaneous albinism), or the eyes alone (ocular albinism).

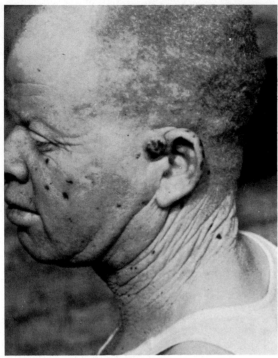

Figure 36–11. Albinism with numerous basal cell carcinomas and epidermoid carcinomas on the ear. (Courtesy of Dr. S.F. Rosen.)

The skin is dry and a milky, pinkish white. There is an excess of lanugo hair, while the regular hair is of a fine silky texture and pale yellow. The eyes are striking because of the red pupils; the irides are pink or bluish; there are photophobia, nystagmus, and astigmatism, with rapid blinking and lacrimation. Some albinos are impaired physically and mentally.

With the absence of pigment protection these individuals suffer from constant threat of sunburn and are prone to actinic cheilitis, actinic dermatitis, actinic keratoses, cutaneous horns, and basal cell and squamous cell carcinomas.

The disease is transmitted as a simple recessive trait with consanguinity playing a prominent role, except in autosomal dominant cases.

Oculocutaneous albinism is classified into 11 types: tyrosinase-negative OCA, tyrosinase-positive OCA, yellow mutant OCA, minimal-pigment OCA, autosomal dominant OCA, brown OCA, rufous OCA, black-locks–albinism-deafness syndrome, Hermansky-Pudlak syndrome, Chédiak-Higashi syndrome, and Cross-McKusick-Breen syndrome. There are five types of *ocular albinism*, in which only the eye pigmentation is abnormal. These include three X-linked types, an autosomal recessive type, and an autosomal dominant type. In the different types of albinism, various defects in the production and distribution of melanin are involved, including enzymes (tyrosinase and permease), melanosome development, and the type of melanin produced (eumelanin versus pheomelanin).

Chédiak-Higashi Syndrome. This is a progressively degenerative, fatal, autosomal recessive familial disease in young children characterized by partial oculocutaneous albinism, azurophilic leukocytic inclusions, susceptibility to infections, hematologic and neurologic abnormalities, photophobia, and early death.

The albinism is due to defective melanocytes containing few and very large melanosomes. Giant lysosomal granules are found in all circulating granulocytes and many other cells. Neutropenia and defective granulocyte migration are common. There is a high incidence of consanguineous marriages. Malignant lymphoma may be the cause of death.

Boxer and associates found that 200 mg ascorbic acid daily restored the defective leukocyte activity in an 11-month-old girl with Chédiak-Higashi syndrome. Leal et al reported a black Venezuelan child with this syndrome, only the third reported case in a black child. Spontaneous repigmentation was complete within a few months.

Hermansky-Pudlak Syndrome. This rare disorder features tyrosinase-positive oculocutaneous albinism, a hemorrhagic diathesis secondary to a platelet defect, and accumulation of a ceroidlike material in the reticuloendothelial system, oral mucosa, and urine. These patients have a history of easy bruisability, epistaxis, gingival bleeding, hemoptysis, and bleeding after various surgical procedures and childbirth. Frenk et al reported two patients who were part of a large Swiss kindred with 13 affected members. Giant melanin granules were visible in each section in skin biopsies.

Cross-McKusick-Breen Syndrome. Also known as Cross syndrome, oculocerebral-hypopigmentation syndrome, or hypopigmentation and microphthalmia, this extremely rare disorder is characterized by white skin, blond hair with a yellow-gray metallic sheen, small eyes with cloudy corneas, jerky nystagmus, gingival fibromatosis, and severe mental and physical retardation.

Cuna Moon Children. The Cuna Indians live on the San Blas islands and on the nearby Atlantic coast in Colombia. The Cuna are a pure race among whom there is frequent inbreeding. The frequency of albinism among these Indians is about one in 100. Cuna Indian albinos are called "moon children" because they have photophobia and prefer to go outdoors only at night. About the age of ten the skin of the "moon children" becomes wrinkled, freckled, and easily blistered by sunshine. The scalp hair is silky and white to straw-colored, sometimes with a reddish tinge. The irides are yellow, gray, or light blue. Nystagmus and other visual anomalies are common. Benign and malignant tumors are common so that their life expectancy is shorter than that of their fellow tribesmen.

Oculocutaneous Albinoidism. This autosomal dominant disorder is characterized by hypomelanosis of skin and hair and blue irides; there is no photophobia, nystagmus, or significant reduction of visual acuity.

Tietz's Syndrome. Tietz's syndrome is characterized by generalized cutaneous hypomelanosis, blond hair, complete deaf-mutism, hypoplasia of the eyebrows, and normal eyes.

Selenium Deficiency. Vinton reviewed four cases with macrocytosis and pseudoalbinism occurring in children during total parenteral nutrition without selenium supplementation. Once selenium was added, pigment returned to the skin and hair and the blood cell volume decreased.

Bedoya A: Pigmentary changes in Chédiak-Higashi syndrome. Br J Dermatol 1971, 85:336.

Bjornberg O: Total albinos in Cuna Indians. J Hist Med 1960, 15:265.

Bolognia JL, et al: Biology of hypopigmentation. JAAD 1988, 19:217.

Boxer LA, et al: Correction of leucocyte function in Chédiak-Higashi syndrome by ascorbate. N Engl J Med 1976, 295:1041.

Depinho RA, et al: The Hermansky-Pudlak syndrome. Medicine (Baltimore) 1985, 64:192.

King RA, et al: Brown oculocutaneous albinism. Ophthalmology 1985, 92:1496.

Idem: Albinism. Derm Clin 1988, 6:217.

Leal I, et al: Chédiak-Higashi syndrome in a Venezuelan black child. JAAD 1985, 13:337.

Nimmo JE, et al: Plasma 5-S-cysteinyldopa concentrations in oculocutaneous albinism. Acta Derm Venereol (Stockh) 1985, 65:169.

Shanahan F, et al: Hermansky-Pudlak syndrome. Am J Med 1988, 85:823.

Stegmaier OC, et al: Chédiak-Higashi syndrome. Arch Dermatol 1965, 91:1.

Tietz W: A syndrome of deaf-mutism associated with albinism showing dominant autosomal inheritance. Am J Hum Genet 1963, 15:259.

Vinton NE, et al: Macrocytosis and pseudoalbinism. J Pediatr 1987, 111:711.

Witkop CJ Jr, et al: Ophthalmologic, biochemical, platelet, and ultrastructural defects in various types of cutaneous albinism. J Invest Dermatol 1973, 60:443.

Wolff SM, et al: The Chédiak-Higashi syndrome: studies of host defenses. Ann Intern Med 1972, 76:293.

Yoshiike T, et al: Macromelanosomes in x-linked ocular albinism. Acta Derm Venereol (Stockh) 1985, 65:66.

Idiopathic Guttate Hypomelanosis (Leucopathia Symmetrica Progressiva)

This curious and very common disorder was first described in 1923 by Matsumoto in natives of Truk. The lesions, which occur chiefly on the shins and forearms, are very much like those of vitiligo except that they never enlarge beyond 6 or 8 mm, rarely become very numerous—a dozen or two at most—and never occur on the trunk or face. Costa in Brazil reported a typical case in 1951; Cummings and Cottell, and Whitehead, unaware of the previous obscure references, reported the disorder in 1966 under the name idiopathic guttate hypomelanosis. Falabella reported in a study of 400 patients that the overall incidence was 46 per cent, with more women affected than men; that it was more common after 40 than before; that there was family clustering; and that while minigrafts did not restore the lost pigment,

intralesional triamcinolone tended to produce repigmentation.

The lesions are irregular in shape and very sharply defined, like depigmented ephelides, and are of only minor cosmetic significance.

Costa OG: Leucopathie symmetrique des extremités. Ann Derm Syphiligr 1951, 78:452.

Cummings K, et al: Idiopathic guttate hypomelanosis. Arch Dermatol 1966, 93:184.

Falabella R, et al: On the pathogenesis of idiopathic guttate hypomelanosis. JAAD 1987, 16:35.

Matsumoto S: On the peculiar, symmetrical hereditary pigment anomaly of the extremities (leukopathia punctata reticularis symmetrica). Acta Dermatologica (Kyoto) 1923, 2:191.

Whitehead J: Idiopathic guttate hypomelanosis. Arch Dermatol 1966, 94:279.

Piebaldism

Piebaldism is a rare, patchy, congenital absence of melanocytes and melanin, associated with white fore-

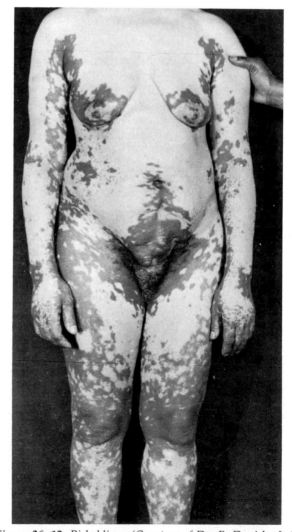

Figure 36–12. Piebaldism. (Courtesy of Dr. F. Daniels, Jr.)

lock. Hyperpigmented macules occur within vitiligolike unpigmented ones.

The striking and characteristic white forelock arises from a triangular or diamond-shaped midline white macule on the frontal scalp or forehead. The medial portions of the eyebrows, and eyelashes, may be white. The depigmented patches typically occur on the abdomen, back, mid-upper arm to wrist, mid-thigh to mid-calf, and shins. A characteristic feature of piebaldism is the presence of hyperpigmented macules within the areas of lack of pigmentation and also on normally pigmented skin. Occasional associated findings include heterochromic irides, deafness, and mental retardation. This combination of findings constitutes the autosomal recessive disease called *Woolf's syndrome*.

Selmanowitz and associates found that 2–4-mm punch grafts of normal skin, transplanted to piebald areas, retained their pigment, and within a year pigment had spread to about three times their diameter, but no farther. Epidermal grafts up to 12 mm in diameter merely retained their pigment. Lerner et al have successfully cultured melanocytes from the patient's normal skin and injected them into blister cavities produced in the depigmented areas.

Breathnach AS, et al: Electronmicroscopy of melanocytes in human piebaldism. J Invest Dermatol 1965, 45:28.

Hayashibe K, et al: Tyrosinase-positive melanocyte distribution and induction of pigmentation in human piebald skin. Arch Dermatol 1988, 124:381.

Jimbow K, et al: Congenital circumscribed hypomelanosis: a characterization based on an electron microscopic study of tuberous sclerosis, nevus depigmentosus, and piebaldism. J Invest Dermatol 1975, 64:50.

Lerner AB, et al: Transplantation of human melanocytes. J Invest Dermatol 1987, 89:219.

Mosher DB, et al: Piebaldism. Arch Dermatol 1988, 124:364.

Ortonne J-P: Piebaldism, Waardenburg's syndrome, and related disorders. Derm Clin 1988, 6:205.

Selmanowitz VJ, et al: Pigmentary correction of piebaldism by autografts. I. Procedures and clinical findings. J Dermatol Surg Oncol 1977, 3:615.

Woolf CM, et al: Congenital deafness associated with piebaldness. Arch Otolaryngol 1965, 82:244.

37

Physical Modalities of Dermatologic Therapy

Roy C. Grekin, M.D.

The practice of dermatology has always involved the performance of surgical procedures. The busy dermatologist will see many skin lesions daily that require biopsy, destruction, or excision. There is a trend now within the specialty toward doing increasingly complex surgical procedures as practiced by both plastic surgeons and competent dermatologic surgeons. Several excellent texts on dermatologic surgery describe these more complicated procedures. However, there are many simpler procedures indicated for small cutaneous lesions, which the dermatologist knows best and is best qualified to treat. In this chapter we will focus on the simpler modalities, with wide clinical application, that all dermatologists should be either competent to do, or at least acquainted with.

CURETTAGE

The dermal curette has long been a standard tool in the dermatologist's surgical armamentarium. This round, semisharp knife is available in sizes from 1 mm to 6 mm, allowing for the removal of a variety of lesions. The proper selection of lesion, its location, and the size of the curette, combined with the surgeon's technique, all play a role in both the therapeutic and the cosmetic outcome.

Because it is not as sharp as a scalpel, the curette does not easily cut through normal epidermis, and will not enter the dermis. Therefore it is best suited for use on soft or friable lesions such as warts, seborrheic and actinic keratoses, the papules of molluscum contagiosum, or selected basal and squamous cell carcinomas.

On the head and neck, lesions in concave areas such as the medial canthi, naso-malar junction, and parts of the ear will heal with a better cosmetic result (since no normal dermis is removed) following curettage than those on more convex surfaces. Below the neck, healing is generally cosmetically acceptable, with some pigmentary change. Anatomic structures with little tissue turgor or without solid bony or cartilaginous undersurfaces (such as eyelids, lips, and genitals) may not afford enough resistance to allow sufficient tissue removal by the semisharp curette.

Appropriate choice of curette size is important. Too small a diameter may cause severe fragmentation of a biopsy specimen and is inefficient. A curette which is too large may cause unnecessary damage to normal tissue as well as miss small extensions of tumor growth into the deeper dermis.

While the use of the curette is a simple technique, quickly learned by first-year residents, there is definitely a necessary degree of expertise to be gained in its use. In 1977 Kopf et al showed that recurrence rates of basal cell carcinomas were far higher when curettage and electrodesiccation were done by residents than when done by attending physicians.

Except for treatment of extremely small or superficial lesions, anesthesia must be used to insure patient comfort when using the curette. This is usually accomplished with infiltration of lidocaine or, if

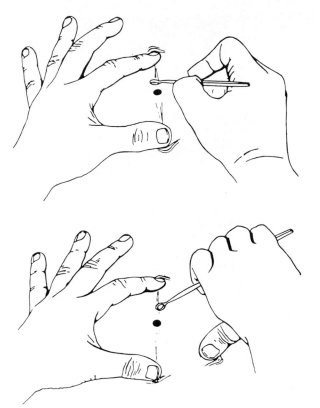

Figure 37–1. Two techniques for holding the curette: the "pencil" technique and the "potato-peeler" method.

preferred, Benadryl solution. However, for some superficial lesions the use of a topical refrigerant such as ethyl chloride can give adequate anesthesia as well as adding tissue turgor to the area to be treated.

In a recent review, Adam discusses two different techniques of holding the curette (Fig. 37–1). The more common procedure, the "pencil" technique, involves holding the curette between the thumb and index and middle fingers as one would hold a pencil. In the "potato-peeler" method, the curette is held between the bent interphalangeal joints of the second through fifth fingers without the thumb, and the surgery performed by flexion of the metacarpalphalangeal joints. Both methods are effective and offer individual advantages relating to strength, flexibility, and fine control.

In general the lesion is removed all at once with a scooping action while the opposite hand stabilizes the skin. Because the most power is delivered toward the operator, initial debulking is done in this direction. However, for completeness of excision the area should be repeatedly curetted in all directions. This also aids in producing symmetric wound margins. Particularly with malignant lesions, initial debulking should be followed by curettage with a smaller curette, 1–3 mm, to track out fine fingerlike tumor extensions.

The consistency of the normal dermis is felt as a "gritty" sensation by the curette and defines the necessary depth of excision. A slight amount of punctate dermal bleeding is easily controlled by 35 per cent aluminum chloride solution, Monsel's solution, or light electrodesiccation.

When treating basal and squamous cell carcinomas, curettage must be followed by vigorous electrodesiccation. There is little agreement as to the requisite number of cycles of curettage and electrodesiccation. It is this author's opinion that the comparatively slight added cosmetic insult, the effort, and the extra time required in performing three cycles are amply justified by the admittedly small percentage increase in cure rate as compared with fewer cycles. Arnold, on the other hand, adheres to Wile's technique and never curettes again after he has done it thoroughly once and electrodesiccated once. His results have compared well with those reported by many using two or three cycles.

SHAVE EXCISION

Shave biopsy or shave excision is a simple and quick technique with high applicability to dermatology. With proper selection of lesion and location, cosmetically acceptable cure or the rapid procurement of adequate biopsy material can be achieved. The lack of sutures and the speed of the procedure may be of great importance to children or anxious adults.

This technique is best suited to pedunculated, papular, or otherwise exophytic lesions. However, using a deep or rolled shave, one can also use this procedure to biopsy macular or indurated lesions, provided the necessary histologic changes reside in the epidermis or papillary dermis. Examples of lesions which are amenable to shave excision include seborrheic and actinic keratoses, intradermal nevi,

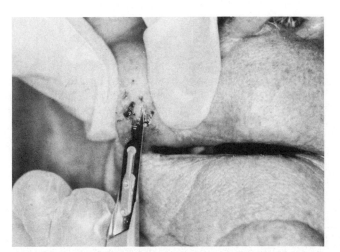

Figure 37–2. Technique for shave excision, using smooth, sweeping strokes.

pyogenic granulomas, warts, and superficial basal and squamous cell carcinomas. Such lesions, if under 2 cm in diameter, should rarely be subjected to mere biopsy, but to "excisional biopsy."

A local anesthetic injection is required prior to a shave excision, for pain control and to aid the procedure. The intradermal instillation of anesthetic will distend and elevate the lesion. This affords greater resistance to the blade, giving better control to the operator, and also facilitates undercutting the lesion.

The shave excision is generally performed with a No. 15 blade on a handle. Bigger lesions may require a No. 10 blade. After injection of the anesthetic, the skin surrounding the lesion is pinched up with the thumb and third finger. This stabilizes the lesion and aids hemostasis. With the blade edge parallel to the skin surface, the excision is then performed with one or more smooth sweeping strokes (Fig. 37–2). A rapid sawing motion may damage the specimen and impair the cosmetic result. Just before the blade exits the skin, the lesion should be stabilized with the index finger to avoid tearing the last bit of tissue. Hemostasis is easily attained with 35 per cent aluminum chloride solution or Monsel's solution, or pressure. Electrofulguration may make the scar less cosmetically acceptable.

A variation of this procedure may be performed with a Gillette Blue Blade razor. Cut in half longitudinally by twisting between two hemostats or with a heavy scissors, this tool is extremely sharp and also bends enough to follow the skin's or the lesion's contour. It is particularly useful for shave removal of lesions on convex surfaces such as the nasal tip or alae, jaw line, or helix of the ear (Fig. 37–3).

Sharp scissors excisions are a variant of shave excisions. In this procedure, essentially, two scissors blades are used simultaneously in opposing directions to remove a lesion parallel to the skin surface. As with the scalpel, an open wound is left which (depending on its depth) may have an excellent cosmetic outcome. The scissors excision is very quickly performed. It is best suited for pedunculated lesions such as skin tags, filiform warts, and baggy nevi. However, it is also an excellent technique for debulking lesions of softer consistency such as basal cell carcinomas and large warts, providing good quality biopsy specimens before performing curettage and electrodesiccation. It has its greatest value in very flaccid, elastotic skin; Arnold has not used a curette in this situation for many years.

For smaller or pedunculated lesions, sharp scissors excision may not require anesthesia, as the sting of the scissors is fleeting and less painful than the injection. The distal lesion is grasped with a fine-toothed forceps and gently elevated. Using the tips of a sharp curved iris scissors or small tenotomy scissors, the base is quickly cut at the skin surface. Hemostasis may not be necessary, but is easily obtained with pressure or a styptic solution.

For larger lesions, and biopsies of more infiltrative lesions, anesthesia is required. In these cases the

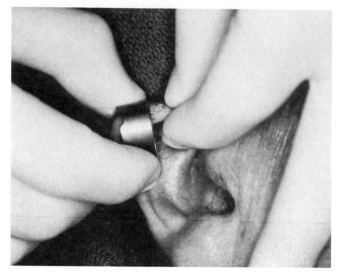

Figure 37–3. Shave excision using a blue blade razor.

lesion is surrounded by the blades and the curvature employed to excise a deep bite of the tumor. The scissor blades will tend (like the curette) to follow the gross cleavage plane between the softer tumor, e.g., wart or basal cell carcinoma, and the underlying normal dermis. This will provide a biopsy specimen with a more normal architecture than that seen in a curettage specimen.

CRYOSURGERY

Over the last 50 years, especially since the ready availability of liquid nitrogen, cryosurgery has become deeply ingrained in the practice of dermatology. This technique offers several advantages to both doctor and patient. It is technically easy to perform, and the reactions heal quickly. Postoperative wound care is simple, and complications are infrequent. Cryosurgery is useful in patients afraid of more directly invasive surgery and electrosurgery, and in those allergic to lidocaine, on anticoagulant therapy, or with contagious diseases such as hepatitis or AIDS.

The first true cryosurgery was performed in the late nineteenth century by dermatologist A. Campbell White, using solid carbon dioxide. Its use did not become widespread within dermatology, however, until modern apparatus was developed by a neurosurgeon, Irving Cooper, in 1962. While there are a number of cryogens available (including ethyl chloride, Freon, carbon dioxide, and nitrous oxide), liquid nitrogen, with a boiling point of $-195.6°C$, is most widely used.

The mechanism of cell death following cryosurgery is not completely understood. Several factors are thought to be important, including mechanical damage to cells due to rapid crystal formation, exposure to high electrolyte concentrations in surrounding nonfrozen or thawing fluids, recrystallization patterns during thaw, and ischemia due to vascular stasis and damage. Experience has shown that rapid freezing followed by a slow thaw results in increased damage, as do repeated freeze-thaw cycles.

It is known that there are differential sensitivities, among different cells and tissues, to freezing. Melanocytes are more sensitive than keratinocytes, which is advantageous in treating lentigo, but may produce permanent hypopigmentation in blacks, or long-lasting reactive hyperpigmentation in Asian patients. Nerves can be damaged, and care must be taken if sensory or functional deficits are to be avoided. Hair follicles are also sensitive; cryosurgery is an excellent therapy for trichiasis. Vascular endothelial cells are also sensitive to freezing. Fibroblasts and stromal structures are less sensitive to the effects of cryosurgery, and this may be an important factor in the lack of scarring seen following superficial procedures.

It is important to grasp the concept of the expanding "ice ball" forming in the tissue during cryosurgery. This must reach an appropriate size in both horizontal and vertical dimensions to effect adequate treatment.

A reasonable estimate of depth of freeze can be made by an experienced operator, based on the surface area of ice formation. However, when treating malignant lesions such as basal and squamous cell carcinomas, it is advisable to employ thermocouples to directly measure the depth and duration of the desired isotherm (temperature level) and insure adequate treatment. In treating benign superficial lesions, some authors believe it is better to undertreat initially. It is better to have to retreat a lesion than to overfreeze the first time and increase the risk of scarring.

There are a number of ways to deliver liquid nitrogen to the skin. The simplest is to use a cotton-tipped applicator. The size may be altered to fit the lesion by removing or adding cotton. The depth of freeze may also be controlled by varying the amount of pressure applied by applicator to the skin; depth of the ice ball increases with increasing pressure. Longer contact will also increase the depth of freeze.

Several models of hand-held liquid nitrogen spray units are made. These come with a changeable nozzle to vary the size of the stream so that very fine control can be achieved.

Cryoprobes are sophisticated instruments that allow for a very precise delivery of liquid nitrogen to the lesion and fine control of tissue temperature over a wide range. The equipment one selects should reflect the experience and training of the cryosurgeon and the complexity of the cryosurgical procedure.

Numerous lesions, benign or malignant, can be effectively treated by cryosurgery (see Table 37–1), either alone or in combination therapy. The bias toward selecting cryosurgery for a particular lesion will certainly be influenced by a physician's training and past experience. It is important to reiterate that cryosurgical treatment of malignant lesions should

Table 37–1. LESIONS TREATED BY CRYOSURGERY

Acne (pustules, small cysts)	Keratoacanthoma
Actinic cheilitis	Leiomyoma
Actinic keratosis	Leishmaniasis
Angiomas	Lentigo
Basal cell carcinoma (especially superficial)	Molluscum contagiosum
	Porokeratosis
Bowen's disease	Prurigo nodularis
Chloasma	Sebaceous hyperplasia
Chondrodermatitis nodularis helicis	Seborrheic keratosis
	Skin tags
Condyloma acuminatum	Steatocystoma
Dermatofibroma	Syringoma
Elastosis perforans serpiginosa	Trichoepithelioma
Epidermal nevi	Warts
Granuloma annulare	Xanthelasma
Keloid	

Modified from Torre D. Reprinted with permission from J Dermatol Surg Oncol 1985, 11:292.

be carefully monitored with thermocouples, and the patient closely followed postoperatively to insure complete tumor extirpation.

Side effects of cryosurgery are generally not severe, but cause some patient discomfort. There is pain associated with the application of liquid nitrogen. Occasionally patients will suffer a vaso-vagal response, so it is advisable to have them lie down, even for small procedures. Postoperatively there will be a throbbing sensation, the duration (a few minutes to several hours) and intensity of which will be dependent on the depth of the freeze. Postoperative inflammation and edema are a function of the intensity of the freeze and also the area. Areas with low tissue turgor such as the eyelids and genitalia will swell more. Bulla formation is common, and the fluid may be quite bloody. If the patient is warned, it should pose no problems. If it is painful, evacuation may help. Infection is uncommon, especially with good wound care.

From two to four weeks after freezing, a hyperplastic or pseudoepitheliomatous healing response may occur. This is self-limited. Hypertrophic scarring can occur, particularly with very deep freezes. However, mildly atrophic scarring is more common. As melanocytes are quite sensitive to freezing, temporary or permanent hypopigmentation or depigmentation can occur. Patients, particularly those with darker natural pigmentation, must be warned of this.

Nerve damage is probably the most worrisome adverse reaction. In areas at risk (e.g., fingers), care should be taken to avoid this. Tenting the skin up and away from the nerve, ballooning the skin with lidocaine, or sliding the skin back and forth over the underlying fascia can help prevent nerve damage, which may rarely be permanent.

THE DERMATOLOGIC PUNCH

The dermatologic punch is a round knife with great versatility. In the experienced hand it can perform many different tasks with speed and cosmetic acceptability. Punches are available in sizes ranging from 2 to 10 mm. Most punches now used are disposable.

The most common use of punches is for skin biopsy. These tools generally provide adequate epidermal and dermal specimens when 3- or 4-mm punches are employed. For biopsies of the scalp, a 6-mm punch is preferred, to insure that an appropriate number of follicles can be examined. Punches are not suitable for biopsy of conditions involving the subcutaneous tissue. A superior cosmetic result can be obtained when compared with any but very shallow shave biopsies, and a far better histologic specimen. The procedure is more quickly performed than fusiform excision, and requires less expertise.

Punches may also be used to completely excise lesions, to treat acne scars, and for hair transplantation. The dermatologic punch is an easy tool to use, but there is some finesse necessary in obtaining optimal specimens and cosmetic results. It is important to choose the right size punch depending on the lesion's size, type, and location. After properly cleansing the skin, an intradermal wheal is raised by injection of local anesthetic. Anesthesia will be achieved immediately, and this will improve the quality of the biopsy specimen by firming up the skin. Care must be taken when using the punch not to apply too much downward pressure. Too much pressure may result in a tapering or conical shape of the specimen removed. This will limit the tissue for histologic examination and may cause artifact.

Before performing a punch excision or biopsy the normal skin tension lines should be determined. Using the thumb and forefinger, stretch the skin perpendicular to these lines. After the punch incision is performed, release of the stretch will result in the formation of an elliptical wound which can be closed within normal skin tension lines without "dogears" (Fig. 37–4).

Grasped between the thumb and the first two fingers, the punch is placed on the skin perpendicular to the surface. While applying gentle pressure, it is rotated back and forth and advanced to the hub. The specimen is then gently grasped with a toothed forceps or a needle tip and elevated. Be careful not to crush the specimen. With an iris scissors, it is cut free in the fat plane. Hemostasis can be obtained by a styptic solution, light electrofulguration, or pressure. Closure should be effected with one or two sutures to avoid a depressed scar.

ELECTROSURGERY

Electrosurgery comprises a variety of surgical techniques, applications, and apparatus. In general the tissue effect is created by heat delivered to or generated in the tissue as a result of an electrical current. Because of this heat, local anesthesia is required for all but the simplest procedures. Some type of electrosurgery is routinely used by dermatologists for

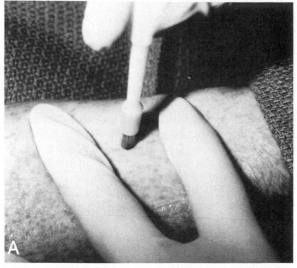

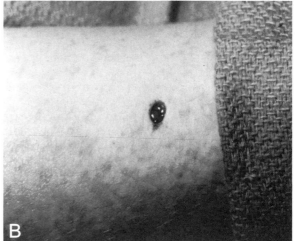

Figure 37–4. A and B, Technique for performing a punch excision.

destruction, hemostasis, or simple or complex excisions. An understanding of the different modalities and their applications can improve the surgical outcome.

Electrocautery. With this technique a step-down transformer is used to pass current through thin platinum tips of various configurations. Resistance to the flow of current through the tip causes heat to be generated. The amount of heat can be controlled by the intensity of the current. No electrical current passes through the patient. The heated electrode can be used to destroy lesions such as verrucae by carbonization, to coagulate small vascular lesions, or to shave-excise small papular or pedunculated lesions such as nevi, seborrheic keratoses, and skin tags. Hemostasis is generally excellent. The current should be controlled to produce a heated surgical tip that cuts easily without accumulating charred tissue, but that at the same time limits destruction of surrounding tissue. Anesthesia is required only if the lesions are large.

Electro-Epilation. One of the first applications of electrical current in surgery was the use of direct (galvanic) current to destroy hair follicles (electrolysis). In this technique heat is actually not a factor. A chemical reaction at the electrode tip, as a result of direct current passing through, causes the evolution of sodium hydroxide (lye) at the hair root. The lye is responsible for follicular destruction. While this is a safe technique with minimal pain or risk of scarring, it is very slow, requiring one minute or more for hair root destruction.

Thermolysis is a form of diathermy in which a high frequency current causes heat in the follicle resulting in tissue destruction. Thermolysis is more painful, may have a higher regrowth rate, and is more likely to cause scarring if not properly used. However, it is very fast in its effect and 100–200 hairs may be treated in a half hour session. For this reason it has generally replaced electrolysis.

Electrodesiccation, Electrofulguration. These techniques represent the most commonly employed uses of electrosurgery in dermatology. While often used to denote the same procedure, there is a subtle technical difference between the two. With electrodesiccation the electrode tip is in contact with the tissue; with electrofulguration there is a 1- to 2-mm separation.

The current is produced by a spark-gap generator. With this device current is supplied to a capacitor, which builds sufficient charge to overcome air resistance, allowing current to cross the spark gap and flow to the patient. A highly damped (decreasing amplitude) wave form is produced, of high voltage and low amperage. This limits the depth of tissue destruction. As this is a monoterminal current, a grounding electrode on the patient is not required. This type of electrosurgery has numerous applications in the daily practice of dermatology.

Using a low power setting and a fine needle, electro-epilation may be performed. While this is slightly painful, it is useful to treat a small number of coarse dark hairs which may trouble the patient, particularly in nevi. Fine telangiectases may also be blanched with this technique. It is important not to overtreat telangiectases, to avoid creating pitted scars. Superficial small dermal tumors such as syringomas may be treated with electrodesiccation. Insertion of the fine epilating needle into the tumor is followed by the application of low current until a surface bubbling occurs. The small amount of char is then removed with a curette, resulting in a smooth surface appearance.

Higher power electrofulguration may be used to destroy seborrheic keratoses, skin tags, or warts. These lesions are then curetted to appropriate depths to insure their removal.

Electrodesiccation or fulguration is commonly employed in treatment of many basal cell and squamous cell carcinomas under 2 cm in diameter. Following thorough, vigorous curettage of the lesion, the base and margins of the defect created should be electro-desiccated for both hemostasis and extension of treatment margins. It is this author's bias that the cycle be carried out three times.

Electrodesiccation/fulguration is very useful in excisional surgery to provide hemostasis. It is important that the field be dry for this to be effective, as the destruction by this current is rather superficial and will not be transmitted through blood (Fig. 37–5).

Electrosection (Cutting Current). The biterminal current used for electrosection is produced by a vacuum tube, resulting in waves with a frequency similar to that of radiowaves. For cutting purposes a sinusoidal undamped (equal amplitude) waveform is generated. The active electrode is cool. Cellular disruption (cutting) occurs as a result of heat produced in response to the wave at the point of contact with the electrode.

When properly used, fine surgical excisions can be produced with minimal trauma to surrounding tissue and excellent hemostasis. Various attachments to the handpiece, including scalpels, needles, wire loops, and balls, can further adapt the instrument to the specific procedure. Most of these devices have the ability to alter their waveform to produce a current which also electrocoagulates and electrofulgurates like spark-gap machines. This makes these instruments quite versatile.

LASERS

The first laser (light amplification by stimulated emission of radiation) was operated in 1960 by Mai-

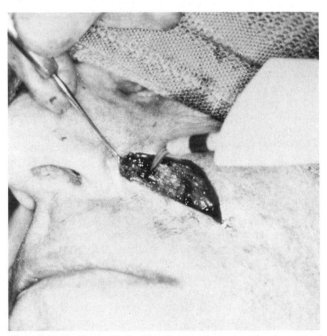

Figure 37–5. Electrodesiccation/fulguration provides hemostasis in excisional surgery.

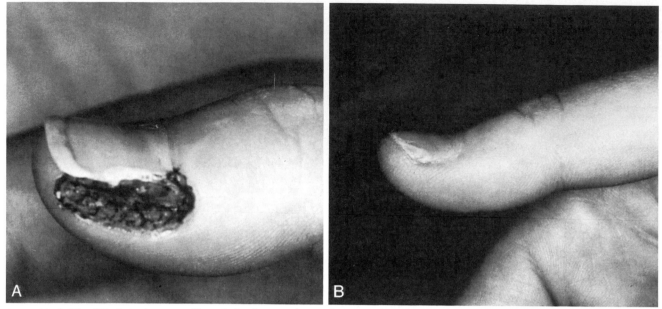

Figure 37–6. The CO_2 laser is an excellent choice for very large plantar and periungual warts that have failed to respond to routine office modalities.

man. Medical application was quickly recognized; Leon Goldman pioneered their dermatologic use.

Lasers are characterized and named by the medium within the laser tube which produces the laser beam. Many different lasers exist but the three with the most applicability to dermatology currently are the argon, carbon dioxide (CO_2), and pulsed or tunable dye lasers. Others are being developed, including the gold and copper vapor lasers.

Lasers produce a light beam which is described as "coherent." This means a beam of one (or a very few) wavelengths (temporal coherence) which travels in a highly collimated fashion (spatial coherence). The beam produces its effect as a result of heat generated following the beam's absorption by specific tissue elements. The CO_2 laser has a wavelength of 10,600 nm and is colorless. Its beam is absorbed by water, which constitutes more than 70 per cent of the skin. The argon laser has its major wavelengths at 488 and 514 nm (blue and green) and is absorbed by both hemoglobin and melanin. While the tunable dye laser can theoretically be set to any wavelength over a wide spectrum, most clinical applications currently involve the use of a 585-nm beam, which coincides with a hemoglobin absorption peak.

The laser is a technologically advanced instrument. However, as with any surgery, side effects can occur. Hypertrophic scarring and pigmentary changes are the most common. Also infection, pain, postoperative bleeding, and recurrent lesions are possible. Laser surgery tends to be more expensive than are more routine modalities applied to similar lesions. It is essential that appropriate instruction and supervision in the use of lasers be obtained by prospective surgeons to insure that optimum safety is provided and the best surgical results are achieved.

The CO_2 *laser* is the most versatile one for dermatologic use. It is an excellent therapeutic choice for very large plantar and periungual warts which have failed to respond to routine office modalities (Fig. 37–6). The CO_2 laser can also remove tattoos in one stage when excision is not feasible. Other lesions amenable to the CO_2 laser include actinic cheilitis, small vascular lesions and some port-wine stains, xanthelasma, adnexal tumors, rhinophyma, and superficial basal cell carcinomas.

The instrument can be used in a highly focused mode to excise lesions in a relatively bloodless fashion with good healing. However, the success obtained in treating keloids is variable and may be related to body region. Earlobe keloids respond well but those on the chest and upper back frequently regrow.

The *argon laser* is best suited to treatment of vascular and pigmented lesions. Because its wavelengths do not correspond to absorption peaks of either hemoglobin or melanin, and also because of its continuous-wave nature, thermal damage to surrounding tissue may be significant. By carefully tracing (under magnification) the individual vessels in a port-wine stain with an 0.1-mm beam diameter, the risk of scarring can be minimized. However, hypopigmentation may still occur. The argon laser is not advised for use before puberty, as the risk of scarring is greater in children.

The *pulsed dye laser* seems to be the most successful instrument to date for treating port-wine stains, telangiectases, and other small, flat, or minimally elevated vascular lesions. The flashlamp pumped rhodamine dye laser emits a beam of yellow light at a wavelength of 585 nm. This is an absorption peak for hemoglobin and is also less well absorbed by melanin. The extremely short pulse-width (time the laser is on) of 500 microseconds permits the delivery of energy and generation of heat to be closely confined to the blood and vessel walls. Damage to surrounding tissues is very slight, and there is virtually no surface damage. Pain is so slight that as a rule no anesthesia is needed. The risk of scarring and pigment change is very slight, and infants as young as 1 month old can be treated.

Adams JE: The technic of curettage surgery. JAAD 1986, 15:697.

Arndt KA, et al (eds): Cutaneous Laser Therapy. New York, John Wiley and Sons, 1983.

Blankenship ML: Physical modalities: electrosurgery, electrocautery, and electrolysis. Int J Dermatol 1979, 18:443.

Epstein E, et al (eds): Skin Surgery. Philadelphia, W. B. Saunders, 1987.

Garden JM, et al: The pulsed dye laser: its use at 577 nm wavelength. J Dermatol Oncol Surg 1987, 13:134.

Jackson R: Basic principles of electrosurgery. Can J Surg 1970, 13:354.

Kopf AW, et al: Curettage-electrodesiccation treatment of basal-cell carcinomas. Arch Dermatol 1977, 113:439.

Kuflik EG, et al: Cryosurgery. Dermatol Clin 1984, 2:319.

Robinson JK: Fundamentals of Skin Biopsy. Chicago, Year Book Medical Publishers, 1986.

Salasche SJ: Status of curettage and desiccation in the treatment of primary basal cell carcinoma. JAAD 1984, 10:285.

Swanson NA: Atlas of Cutaneous Surgery. Boston, Little, Brown, 1987.

Wagner RF, et al: Electrolysis and thermolysis for permanent hair removal. JAAD 1985, 12:441.

Wheeland RG, et al: Dermatologic applications of the argon and carbon dioxide (CO_2) laser. Curr Concepts Skin Disorders 1984, 5:5.

Zacarian SA (ed): Cryosurgery for Skin Cancer and Cutaneous Disorders. St. Louis, C. V. Mosby, 1985.

38

X-Ray Therapy

Herbert Goldschmidt, M.D.

The use of ionizing radiation in dermatologic therapy has decreased markedly owing to the development of more efficient medications and to the increased awareness of potential genetic and somatic hazards of radiation (Goldschmidt, 1975). Because of the public concern about nuclear weapons and nuclear energy, the effects and side effects of x-ray therapy have been investigated more intensively than any other therapeutic modality. The knowledge gained from these studies has made it possible to avoid all major risks formerly associated with dermatologic radiotherapy. Radiotherapy is an integral part of dermatologic therapy, and every skin specialist should be familiar with modern radiotherapeutic indications and radiation techniques.

Today, dermatologic x-ray therapy should be considered only when results from radiation therapy can be expected to be superior to those of other methods. Ionizing radiation should not be administered in children or in pregnant women. Careful selection of patients and rigorous application of radiation protection measures are essential to reduce radiation hazards to a minimum.

RADIATION METHODS

A wide variety of radiation methods is available for various types of neoplasms involving different organs (Goldschmidt and Sherwin, 1980). Table 38–1 summarizes the physical and technical factors of the commonly used radiation techniques, arranged according to their penetration. Most of these methods are not indicated for dermatologic disorders because the radiation beams penetrate deeper than necessary and are likely to cause side effects on underlying organs. Traditionally, the most commonly used x-ray units in dermatology were low-voltage superficial x-ray machines with Pyrex windows (60 to 100 kV). More recently, beryllium-windowed x-ray units have become available for soft x-ray therapy (20 to 100 kV), which is ideally suited for all dermatologic problems. Ultrasoft grenz rays (5 to 20 kV) are not penetrating enough to reach the base of deeper skin tumors but are very useful for superficial skin diseases. Domonkos (1965) was a pioneer in the use of the ultrashort distance, low voltage, contact therapy technique (Chaoul), which offered several advantages in the treatment of skin cancer. However, contact therapy units (50 to 60 kV) have not been commercially available for several years and are now superseded by soft x-ray machines.

Table 38–1. RADIATION METHODS

Therapy	Sources and Synonyms	kV	TSD (cm)	Wavelength (Å) (average)	HVT	D½ (mm tissue) (or average penetration)
Megavoltage	Betatron, particle accelerators	> 1000	80	0.001	> 10 mm Pb	200
Supervoltage	Gamma ray Telecurie sources	400–800	50–80	0.03	5–10 mm Pb	80–110
Orthovoltage	Deep x-ray Conventional x-ray	200–400	50–80	0.14	2–4 mm Cu	50–80
Half-deep	Intermediate	110–130	30	0.1	4 mm Al	30
Contact	Ultrashort distance Chaoul	50–60	1.5–3.0	0.8	2–4 mm Al	4–30
Superficial x-ray	Low voltage Standard x-ray Pyrex-window unit	60–100	15–30	0.5	0.7–2.0 mm Al	7–10
Soft x-ray	Beryllium-window unit	20–100	10–30	0.15	0.1–2.0 mm Al	1–20
Grenz ray	Ultrasoft Supersoft	5–20	10–15	2	0.03 mm Al	0.2–0.8

(From Goldschmidt H, et al: Dermatologic radiation therapy. *In* Dermatology, 2nd ed. Moschella SL, et al. (eds). Philadelphia, WB Saunders, 1985, pp 2048–2081.)

RADIATION FACTORS

Therapeutic x-radiation can be defined by its intensity, its penetrating quality, and its total dose.

INTENSITY (DOSE RATE)

The intensity of a radiation beam is measured by the rate at which it ionizes a confined volume of air in the thimble chamber of a radiation dosimeter ("R-meter"). Such an instrument, placed in the beam at a defined distance from the anode of the tube, reads out the roentgens (R) per minute at that distance, which is usually the distance at which the treatment will be delivered (target skin distance, or TSD). This figure is the intensity (dose rate) of the beam. It is roughly proportional to the peak kilovoltage (kVp).

RADIATION QUALITY

The penetration ("hardness") of an x-ray beam can be described by the half-value thickness (HVT) or the half-value depth (HVD, D½) of the radiation beam.

HALF-VALUE THICKNESS (HVT). The penetration of x-rays is largely determined by two factors: voltage and filtration. Formerly, the combined effect of these factors was expressed by the physical term "half-value layer" (HVL). This was replaced by the new designation "half-value thickness" (HVT). The half-value thickness is defined as that thickness of a given filter material (in dermatology, usually aluminum) that reduces the intensity of the x-ray beam to 50 per cent of the original incident radiation. Figure 38–1 illustrates the range of penetration obtained with various radiation qualities used in dermatology.

HALF-VALUE DEPTH (HVD, D½). The biologic term "half-value depth" is now preferred by many

dermatologists as a more useful definition of the penetration and absorption of x-rays because it relates better to the actual depth of various anatomic structures of the skin (Fig. 38–1). The D½ describes the depth in tissue at which 50 per cent of the surface dose has been absorbed (50 per cent depth dose). "Half-dose depth" (HDD) has been proposed by Kopf and associates (1976) as an alternative term.

The basic rule is to select radiation qualities with a D½ corresponding to the depth of the tumor (Fig. 38–1). Most of the radiation will then be absorbed in the pathologic tissue and therefore be of greater therapeutic benefit. At the same time, the possibility of undesirable radiation effects to underlying uninvolved tissue will be reduced markedly. The depth of the tumor can be reasonably estimated by close inspection and palpation of the tumor. The biopsy specimen can then be used to measure the depth of the tumor. Atkinson (1962) correlated histologic findings and radiation quality by comparing depth of lesion and dose homogeneity in cutaneous carcinomas. He summarized data on depth of lesions from biopsies of cutaneous cancers and found that 50 per cent of all basal cell carcinomas in his large series infiltrated to a depth of only 2 mm or less, and 75 per cent of all tumors infiltrated to 5 mm or less. His findings confirm that deeply penetrating radiation qualities with an HVT over 1 mm of aluminum (Al) are rarely needed in dermatology. The vast majority of "typical" superficially located basal cell carcinomas require a D½ of only 5 mm (HVT 0.2 to 0.4 mm Al); only 25 per cent of all basal cell carcinomas are deeper and need radiation with a D½ of up to 10 mm of tissue (HVT 0.8 to 1.0 mm Al). Because of their limited penetration, beryllium-windowed machines are particularly useful in the treatment of skin cancers.

Even before modern soft x-ray machines were

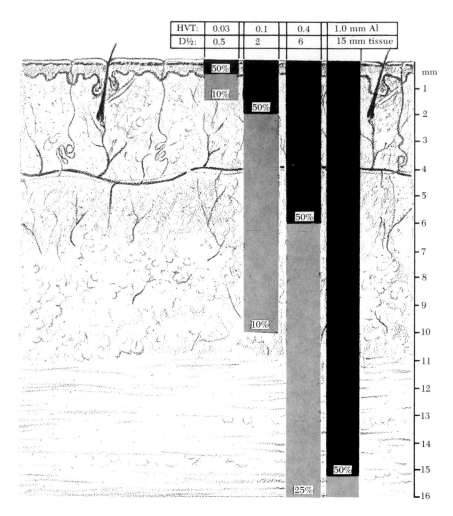

HVT:	0.03	0.1	0.4	1.0 mm Al
D½:	0.5	2	6	15 mm tissue

Figure 38–1. Penetration of x-rays of different half-value thickness (HVT) and half-value depth (D½). (From Goldschmidt H, Sherwin WK: Dermatologic radiation therapy. In Moschella SL, Hurley HJ (eds): Dermatology. 2nd ed. Philadelphia, WB Saunders, 1985, pp 2048–2081.)

available, many dermatologists used radiation qualities similar to the currently recommended radiation qualities. For example, the "unfiltered superficial x-ray technique" with Pyrex-windowed x-ray units utilized half-value layers of 0.6 to 1 mm Al with excellent results. In the past, superficial x-ray machines were sometimes used with a "filtered technique" (100 to 140 kV, 1 to 2 mm Al added filtration) with an HVL of 2 to 3 mm Al and a D½ of 12 to 20 mm skin. This radiation quality would now be considered too penetrating for ordinary and uncomplicated cutaneous cancers.

The application of the D½ rule also eliminates cumbersome calculations from depth-dose charts. The dose reaching the base of the tumor is one half of the surface dose; when 5000 cGy are delivered to the surface of a tumor, the base of the lesion is exposed to 2500 cGy. The known HVT of any radiation can easily be converted to the corresponding D½ value from available charts and curves (Fig. 38–2). Recent measurements by Harley (1982) permit accurate determination of D½ values. Table 38–2 presents calibration data of a beryllium-window machine with five different radiation qualities that have proved adequate for the treatment of the vast majority of cutaneous carcinomas and benign dermatoses. Kilovoltage and filtration have been arranged to produce the same dose rate (100 R/min) for the first four calibration steps. This feature helps to reduce potential errors, particularly when beryllium-window

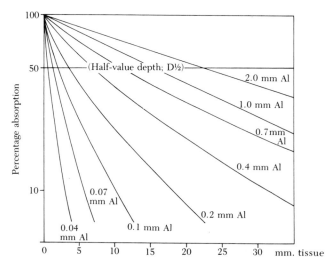

Figure 38–2. Comparative depth-dose curves for radiations of different half-value thickness. (From Goldschmidt H, Sherwin WK: Dermatologic radiation therapy. In Moschella SL, Hurley HJ (eds): Dermatology. 2nd ed. Philadelphia, WB Saunders, 1985, pp 2048–2081.)

Table 38–2. CALIBRATION DATA (50 kV BERYLLIUM-WINDOW UNIT)

D½* (mm Tissue)	HVT* (mm Al)	kV	Filter (mm Al)	mA	TSD* (cm)	Dose Rate (R/min)
0.2	0.02	10	—	25	30	100
3.0	0.15	29	0.3	25	30	100
7.5	0.40	43	0.6	25	30	100
13.0	0.75	50	1.0	25	30	100
18.0	1.40	50	2.0	25	30	45

*D½, half-value depth; HVT, half-value thickness; TSD, target skin distance. (From Goldschmidt et al: Dermatologic radiation therapy. *In* Dermatology, 2nd ed. Moschella SL, et al (eds). Philadelphia, WB Saunders, 1985, pp 2048–2081.)

machines with fixed kilovolt-filter combinations are used.

RADIATION DOSE

The air dose (now called exposure) used to be measured in roentgens and stated in terms of the quantity of radiation measured in air; the original symbol for roentgen was "r," later changed to "R." Since 1975, radiation doses have been expressed not as air doses but as the amount of radiation absorbed in tissue. The term for absorbed dose (the rad), is now called the gray (Gy). One gray means 1 joule of energy absorbed in 1 kg of tissue. One centigray (cGy), or 0.01 Gy, equals 1 rad; and since a rad is almost equivalent to one R, anyone accustomed to expressing radiation doses in roentgen (R) or rad can substitute cGy and use roughly the same numbers. This substitution is possible only in dermatologic radiation therapy, not for more penetrating radiation techniques.

RADIOTHERAPY OF CUTANEOUS NEOPLASMS

The need for ionizing radiation in the treatment of cutaneous neoplasms has decreased because advanced surgical methods, Mohs surgery, and cryosurgery have become available. Although radiotherapy has not been replaced completely, the recent emphasis on surgical treatments has reduced indications for radiotherapy to a well-defined group of skin cancers in specific anatomic locations. Dermatologic radiotherapy still has a place in the treatment of large or complicated cancers of the eyelid, nose, ear, and lip, where properly administered radiotherapy often yields satisfactory therapeutic and cosmetic results. As a general rule, dermatologists should select radiation therapy only for those skin cancers that are not easily amenable to surgical methods.

INDICATIONS FOR RADIOTHERAPY

Theoretically, nearly all skin cancers in all anatomic locations could be effectively treated with x-rays. Experience has shown, however, that functional and cosmetic results of radiotherapy depend on many factors, especially the location and size of the tumor and the age of the patient.

LOCATION. There is general agreement that ionizing radiation is an effective alternative therapy for skin cancers of the eyelids, the medial and lateral canthi of the eyes, the nose, the ears, and the lips. In carcinomas of the nasolabial fold and in preauricular and retroauricular areas (which often have a tendency to deep invasion), radiation therapy may also be considered when surgical methods seem impractical. The skin of the trunk and extremities has a greater tendency to develop unsightly radiation sequelae, particularly telangiectases and pigment changes. Hence, radiation therapy is rarely advisable in these locations, where surgical methods usually are not associated with any special problems. In exceptional cases (e.g., large multiple superficial basal cell tumors of the trunk, or complicated or inoperable tumors in any other skin area, or in patients who refuse surgery), radiotherapy offers an effective therapeutic choice when other methods cannot be used.

SIZE. Radiotherapy is particularly valuable in medium-sized tumors 2 to 6 cm in diameter. Lesions smaller than 1 to 2 cm in diameter can often be treated equally well or better with surgical methods. Tumors larger than 6 to 8 cm in diameter are rarely seen in dermatologic private practice and are best referred to radiation oncologists.

AGE. The age of the patient is also an important consideration in the decision whether or not to use x-ray therapy. In order to minimize the potentiating or additive hazards of solar radiation in later years, sun-exposed areas in patients under 40 years of age should be irradiated only in exceptional cases. In elderly patients irradiation is a more favored option because there is comparatively less danger of late radiation sequelae. In addition, x-ray therapy is psychologically a less traumatic procedure for elderly patients who often fear surgery of any type.

CONTRAINDICATIONS. In general, office x-ray therapy is not recommended for skin cancers that are located in regions other than the head and neck, are over 8 cm in diameter, occur intraorally, invade bone, extend from the upper lip into a nostril, are secondary to radiodermatitis, or are carcinomas secondary to osteomyelitis, chronic ulcers, or burn scars.

ADVANTAGES OF X-RAY THERAPY

PRESERVATION OF TISSUE. The main indications for radiotherapy in the dermatologist's office are medium-sized basal cell carcinomas, squamous cell carcinomas, and keratoacanthomas. Biopsies should be performed in all cases to confirm the clinical diagnosis.

By far the most important advantage of radiotherapy over surgical methods is the preservation of uninvolved tissue. All surgical methods of cancer therapy require that a relatively large margin of normal-appearing skin be included. Inclusion of a sufficiently wide uninvolved border poses no problem to the radiotherapist, since the radiation field can easily be adjusted to the required area of treatment. Tumor margins may be made as generous as necessary, usually extending at least 0.5 to 1 cm on each side of the tumor. Because complicated reconstructive methods are not necessary, the contour of the involved tissue and of the surrounding normal skin will not be changed markedly by radiotherapy. This is especially important in carcinomas of the nose, eyelids, ears, and lips and in other areas in which tissue cannot readily be sacrificed without undesirable cosmetic consequences.

IRREGULAR OR ILL-DEFINED CARCINOMAS. Since the radiation port can be easily adjusted to the shape of the tumor with lead cutouts, radiotherapy is sometimes preferable to surgical methods for lesions with very irregular or ill-defined borders. Multiple biopsies are advisable to determine the true extent of the tumor.

INCOMPLETELY EXCISED CARCINOMAS. Postoperative radiation therapy is a simple and useful alternative following histologically demonstrated inadequate surgical excision of skin cancers. A sufficiently wide border can be included to destroy residual carcinomatous tissue. In most of these cases full tumor doses are indicated.

RECURRENT SKIN CANCERS. Recurrences of surgically treated cancers (residual carcinomas) can be successfully irradiated in patients for whom Mohs surgery is not the choice of treatment.

Menn and associates (1971) have emphasized the high incidence of recurrences following treatment of recurrent skin cancers; the overall recurrence rate after radiotherapy of recurrent skin cancers was 27 per cent. The recurrence rates after excision, and especially after curettage and electrodesiccation, were higher still (40 and 59 per cent, respectively). Only Mohs surgery had a higher cure rate than radiotherapy for recurrent basal cell cancer (90 per cent).

HOSPITALIZATION VERSUS OFFICE THERAPY. In most cases, even large or complicated carcinomas can be irradiated in the office. Since hospitalization is not required, costs can be considerably reduced, and the patient does not have to interrupt daily activities for longer periods of time.

OTHER HEALTH PROBLEMS. Patients in poor health can often be treated with ionizing radiation with fewer complications and less stress than encountered with surgical methods. This applies especially to patients on anticoagulant therapy or with allergies to anesthetics.

DISADVANTAGES OF RADIOTHERAPY

MULTIPLE OFFICE VISITS. Fractionated radiotherapy requires multiple office visits, varying from 5 to 25 treatments. This relative disadvantage is important for working patients but less so for retired patients, who represent the majority of those treated with ionizing radiation.

RADIATION SEQUELAE. Whereas surgical scars often improve over the years, in some patients cosmetic results after radiotherapy tend to worsen, especially when irradiated areas have been exposed to excessive solar radiation without effective sun protection. Undesirable late changes in the treated area may include atrophy and depigmentation, sometimes also hyperpigmentation, often associated with the appearance of telangiectases. The cosmetic changes used to be common but are seen less often after treatment with modern radiation techniques. Pigment changes can be camouflaged with cosmetics, and telangiectases can be electrodesiccated. In hairy skin areas a tumoricidal dose of ionizing radiation will always result in permanent alopecia. It is best to avoid treatment of such areas even though hair transplants can be used effectively in areas of chronic radiodermatitis.

SELECTION OF RADIATION FACTORS

RADIATION QUALITY. In modern dermatologic radiotherapy the basic rule for skin cancers is to select a D½ that closely approximates the actual depth of the tumor (Goldschmidt and Sherwin, 1983). As mentioned previously, microscopic measurements have shown that 50 per cent of all basal cell and squamous cell carcinomas are not deeper than 2 mm, and only 25 per cent extend deeper than 5 mm. Consequently, a HVT ranging from 0.3 to 1.0 mm is sufficient for most skin cancers. Either soft x-ray units or superficial x-ray machines can be used effectively.

DOSE SCHEDULES. Intensive or massive treatment applies the total dose (2000 to 2500 cGy, depending on the size of the tumor) in one sitting, so that the maximum effect is obtained at once, and no repetition of the dose is necessary. This form of treatment is used rarely now for cutaneous neoplasms because fractionated doses yield better cosmetic results.

Fractionated doses are usually given daily, every other day, or twice a week until the total planned therapeutic dose (e.g., 5000 cGy) has been delivered. By dividing the dose into 5 to 10 treatments, it is possible to give a larger total dose than could be given safely in one exposure. The fractionation of x-ray dosage makes it theoretically possible to maintain for one to several weeks a saturation dose lethal to cancer cells in the tissues. Since cells are especially susceptible to x-rays during mitosis, this method of irradiation is highly destructive to cancer. Pathologic cells are, in general, more radiosensitive than normal cells, which usually recover in a short period of time.

The total dose to be applied to a particular carcinoma of the skin is influenced by various factors, especially the size of the lesion. The larger the field, the higher the backscatter produced in the irradiated tissue. The total dose required to kill cancer cells in large tumors is smaller than that required when the field is small.

Time-Dose–Fractionation Factor. Different dose schedules for fractionated therapy have been successfully used in various dermatologic centers (Table 38–3). Schedule A is used widely in Europe and in the United States; schedule B is preferred by dermatologists trained at New York University Skin and Cancer Hospital; and schedule C is traditional in Zurich, Switzerland.

The introduction of the time-dose–fractionation (TDF) factor by Orton and Ellis (1973) allows for the first time a comparison of different factors. According to these authors, the malignancy may be undertreated (and more likely to recur) when the factor is smaller than 90. When it is larger than 110, it may be overtreated (and more likely to develop unsightly radiation sequelae). A comparison of the TDF factor of several commonly used dose schedules listed in Table 38–3 confirms the clinical experience that good therapeutic results can be obtained with markedly different radiation schedules.

Dosage Recommendations for Different Skin Cancers. There is no major difference in radiation methods for treatment of basal cell carcinomas, squamous cell carcinomas, and keratoacanthomas. The recommended dose schedules are applicable to all clinical and histologic variations of basal cell carcinoma. The same dose schedules can also be used for squamous cell carcinomas; however, some authors prefer to add 500 to 1000 cGy to the total dose for squamous cell cancers. Since it is difficult to differentiate keratoacanthomas from squamous cell cancers clinically and histologically, we treat them with the same techniques recommended for squamous cell carcinomas. Shimm and associates recommend lower total doses for typical keratoacanthomas (2500 cGy in five fractions on consecutive days).

Recurrences of cutaneous cancers after surgical excision are also treated with the same techniques. We do not recommend routine treatment by curettage followed by low doses of x-ray therapy because we believe that cutaneous cancers should be treated adequately either by surgical means or by radiotherapy but not by a combination of both modalities. In combining methods there is always the danger of going halfway with either, or of overtreatment.

SHIELDING. Overlay lead shielding around the visible tumor will reduce unnecessary stray and scatter radiation (Gladstein, 1978). A 0.5 to 1 cm–wide healthy margin should always to be included in the irradiated site. Failures are due mainly to improper technique and fall mostly into two categories: insufficient field about the visible part of the tumor and incorrect appraisal of the depth of the lesion.

Treatment cones should always be used. The diameter of the cone depends upon the size of the lesion. When any part of the head is being treated, the eyes should be shielded with lead goggles. The thyroid gland area should also be protected with lead shields. When the eyelids are irradiated, brass eye shields should be placed between the eyelid and the properly anesthetized eyeball.

SKIN REACTION. Beginning 5 to 10 days after the initial dose of radiation, the skin reacts with erythema. By the end of the treatment series, the irradiated site is reddened and continues to become more so until about 2 weeks after the last treatment, at which time the peak of reaction is attained. At this stage there may be desquamation, erosion, and hemorrhagic crusting. The reaction then begins to subside; healing is usually achieved in 4 to 5 weeks after the completion of radiation treatment.

RESULTS OF RADIOTHERAPY. Most reports in the literature indicate cure rates of about 95 per cent (90 to 100 per cent) following radiotherapy of uncomplicated cutaneous cancers (Goldschmidt and Sherwin, 1983) and less favorable results for larger or complicated tumors. The 5-year cure rate published by Bart and associates (1968) of the New York Skin and Cancer Group for 500 histologically proven basal cell carcinomas was 93 per cent. These cure rates are similar to the results obtained with other therapeutic methods in large comparative studies. Only Mohs

Table 38–3. RADIATION SCEDULES USED AT VARIOUS DERMATOLOGIC CENTERS

	Treatment Schedule	Frequency	Total Dose	Duration	TDF Value
Schedule A					
< 4 cm	12 × 4 Gy (400 rad)	3×/week	48 Gy (4800 rad)	3 weeks	100
	10 × 5 Gy (500 rad)	5×/week	50 Gy (5000 rad)	2 weeks	107
> 4 cm	14 × 3.5 Gy (350 rad)	3×/week	49 Gy (4900 rad)	5 weeks	95
Schedule B					
Basal cell carcinoma	5 × 6.8 Gy (680 rad)	3×/week	34 Gy (3400 rad)	2 weeks	95
Squamous cell carcinoma	8 × 6.8 Gy (680 rad)	3×/week	54.4 Gy (5440 rad)	4 weeks	151
Schedule C					
< 2 cm	5 × 8 Gy (800 rad)	1×/week	40 Gy (4000 rad)	5 weeks	145
2–8 cm	12 × 4 Gy (400 rad)	2×/week	48 Gy (4800 rad)	6 weeks	107
> 8 cm	26 × 2 Gy (200 rad)	2×/week	52 Gy (5200 rad)	6 weeks	80

(From Goldschmidt et al: Dermatologic radiation therapy. *In* Dermatology, 2nd ed. Moschella SL, et al (eds). Philadelphia, WB Saunders, 1985, pp 2048–2081.)

surgery yields higher cure rates. Treatment failures are usually the result of errors in estimating the size and depth of tumors. A recurrence at the periphery of the lesion indicates inadequate field size; a recurrence in the center of the field results from insufficient tumor depth dose.

RADIOTHERAPY OF OTHER TUMORS

KAPOSI'S SARCOMA

Ionizing radiation therapy is often effective in the classic type of Kaposi's multiple idiopathic hemorrhagic sarcoma. Since the tumors are relatively radiosensitive, small doses of x-rays can be used from time to time to keep recurrent tumors under control. In many cases, doses of 200 to 300 cGy, given once or twice a week, will cause involution of the lesions after two to eight sessions. Because of their depth, most lesions required more penetrating radiation (D½ 5 to 10 mm) by filtered superficial x-rays, orthovoltage radiation, cobalt treatment, or electron beam therapy. Large tumors may respond to an extended field technique (at least half a limb, with a 15-cm margin) with only a single dose of 800 cGy of cobalt radiation (Harwood, 1981).

The recurrence rate depends on many factors, yet there is evidence that higher total doses are more likely to control individual lesions. A recent study by Cooper and associates (1988) of 82 cases suggests that high total doses result in long-term local control of the disease. These authors advocate a dose of 3000 cGy in 10 fractions over 2 weeks; more than half of all lesions were free of disease for 10 years and longer. Tumors responding rapidly and completely several weeks after therapy were less likely to recur than slowly resolving lesions without complete resolution. Much higher doses are not advisable in acral areas of the lower leg; cumulative doses exceeding 2000 to 3000 cGy may cause considerable radiation sequelae, in rare instances even chronic radiation ulcers.

EPIDEMIC KAPOSI'S SARCOMA IN AIDS

Local irradiation of lesions of AIDS-related Kaposi's sarcoma is an effective palliative treatment in patients with substantial cosmetic disfigurement and for painful, edematous, or ulcerated lesions (Cooper et al, 1984). Compared with other forms of treatment, local radiotherapy has few side effects; in contrast to many systemic therapies, it does not cause immunosuppression and so does not have any potential negative effects on the course of the disease.

Effective control of the lesions can often be achieved with relatively small doses. Most experts agree that there is no major difference between the response of epidemic Kaposi's sarcoma and classic Kaposi's sarcoma to radiotherapy. This also applies to the management of Kaposi's sarcoma related to immunosuppressive drugs (El Akkad et al, 1986). Dose recommendations vary considerably; on average, a dose of 300 cGy given twice a week for three to six times seems to be effective in the majority of patients; doses exceeding 3000 cGy are rarely needed. The D½ depends on the depth of the tumor (D½ 5 to 10 mm); radiation oncologists prefer 100 kV, orthovoltage, or megavoltage radiation.

BOWEN'S DISEASE

When surgical excision is problematic owing to the large size or location of the tumor, radiotherapy with soft x-rays is a useful therapeutic alternative for Bowen's disease (and erythroplasia of Queyrat). Hauss and associates (1978) describe good therapeutic results in 30 patients treated with 5000 to 6000 cGy of a very soft type of radiation (HVT 0.15 mm Al). Blank and Schnyder report treatment of 77 lesions with a primary healing rate of 100 per cent after a cumulative dosage of 3200 to 5000 cGy with a D½ of 5 to 12 mm. Only two recurrences were observed several months later.

LENTIGO MALIGNA

Filtered grenz rays or soft x-rays can be used effectively in the treatment of lentigo maligna when surgical treatment is impractical because of the size or location of the lesion. Reports from European dermatologic centers describing hundreds of cases (Braun-Falco et al, 1975) indicate that the Miescher technique with filtered grenz rays (HVT 0.1 mm Al; D½ 2 mm) will induce slow resolution over a period of several months following doses of 2000 cGy given at 2- to 3-day intervals, with a total dose of 10,000 cGy. Care must be taken to rule out the presence of an early invasive melanoma.

In cases with deeper involvement, soft x-rays or superficial x-rays (D½ 4 to 8 mm; HVT 0.3 to 0.8 mm Al) can be used. The dose schedule is similar to doses used in the treatment of skin cancers (e.g., 500 cGy daily for a total of 5000 cGy). Ionizing radiation is only rarely used in U.S. centers because of a report of three cases of metastatic malignant melanoma observed in a series of 16 patients after radiation therapy (Kopf et al, 1976).

MALIGNANT MELANOMA

Surgical excision is the treatment of choice for various types of malignant melanomas of the skin. In recent years an increasing number of experimental and clinical investigations were published contradicting the formerly accepted claim that melanomas are radioresistant. Instead, it was suggested that cutaneous melanomas have "reduced radiosensitivity" that can be overcome by changes in treatment techniques, especially by the use of higher doses per fraction or multiple fractions per day. There are obvious differences in therapeutic responses depending on the type of melanoma treated. Lentigo maligna melanoma seems to be the most responsive melanoma and nodular melanoma the least responsive subtype (Johanson et al, 1983). Many radiation oncologists feel that all possibilities for the use of ionizing radiation therapy alone have not yet been exhausted (Harwood and Cummings, 1981).

Further research is needed to confirm whether ionizing radiation alone or in combination with chemotherapeutic, immunologic, or radiosensitizing agents can be used as curative therapy for certain types of melanomas (Cooper, 1985). At this time, radiotherapeutic methods are recommended only as palliative treatment for metastatic tumors (Rounsaville et al, 1988). Harwood and Cummings (1981) reported satisfactory results in the primary treatment of lentigo maligna melanoma.

RADIOTHERAPY OF CUTANEOUS T-CELL LYMPHOMAS

X-RAY THERAPY

Localized forms of mycosis fungoides respond well to relatively low doses of ionizing radiation. Infiltrated plaques can be successfully treated with superficial x-rays (80 to 100 kV, HVT 0.7 to 1 mm Al), with a total dose of 1000 to 1200 cGy given in three to four fractions over 3 to 4 days. Markedly infiltrated plaques or isolated tumors require more penetrating therapy (200 to 280 kV orthovoltage radiation) with similar doses.

Cotter (1983) compared various dose schedules for individual tumors and reported complete responses in all tumors treated with total doses of at least 2000 cGy. As expected, lower doses resulted in more frequent recurrences. Eighty-three per cent of these recurrences occurred within the first year of treatment, and none occurred later than 2 years after radiotherapy.

ELECTRON BEAM THERAPY

TREATMENT OF INDIVIDUAL TUMORS. Linear accelerators are available in many radiation oncology centers where electron beams are used to produce penetrating photon radiation for the treatment of internal neoplasms. In some centers, the electron beam itself is utilized not only for localized lymphomatous tumors but also in the treatment of cutaneous malignancies, with dose schedules similar to those used in superficial x-ray or orthovoltage therapy. Theoretically, electron beam therapy is ideally suited for cutaneous carcinomas, since the depth of penetration can be adjusted with some precision, owing to a rapid falloff of energy below the treated area (Tapley and Fletcher, 1973), thereby eliminating unnecessary radiation in deeper underlying tissues. The depth of penetration (7 to 15 mm skin) depends on the energy of the linear accelerator, varying from 2.5 to 15 MeV. Since electron beam therapy is more complicated, more time consuming, and more costly, it is currently not used routinely for cutaneous malignancies.

TOTAL BODY ELECTRON BEAM THERAPY. Electron beam therapy has been used as palliative treatment of widespread cutaneous lymphomas, especially in all stages of mycosis fungoides, for over 30 years. Fromer and associates (1961) initially used a Van de Graaff accelerator at 2.5 MeV with an average penetration of electrons to 7 mm of tissue. Daily doses of 100 to 200 cGy were given to the entire body surface through multiple ports in courses of 600 to 800 cGy, resulting in remissions lasting 6 months or longer. Because of the excellent curative results achieved with high-dose schedules in the treatment of Hodgkin's disease, Hoppe and others (1979) at Stanford University applied electron beams powered by a linear accelerator at 2.5 to 4 MeV (12-mm depth) in an attempt to cure widespread cutaneous T-cell lymphomas with a more aggressive dose schedule. In most patients 400 cGy were administered per week in 32.8 cGy fractions to six fields over a period of 8 to 10 weeks, with the total doses varying between 3000 and 4000 cGy. Long-term remissions were observed, especially in early forms of mycosis fungoides. There is still some controversy whether these lymphomas were cured and whether a life-prolonging effect was achieved. Hoppe (1985) reported complete remissions in 84 per cent of 140 patients. Forty-two per cent of patients in early stages of cutaneous T-cell lymphomas remained disease free for long periods. Depending on the stage of disease, 5-year survival rates ranged from 96 per cent for patients with limited plaques to 28 per cent for patients in the tumor stage. As expected, side effects of higher dose therapy (atrophy, telangiectasia, poikiloderma, and skin fragility) were more severe than those following lower dose therapy.

RADIOTHERAPY OF BENIGN SKIN DISORDERS

Indications for radiotherapy of benign skin diseases have been narrowed to a small list of dermatoses that do not respond well to other forms of treatment (Goldschmidt, 1975). With few exceptions, radiotherapy should be considered only after other therapeutic methods have failed and when active treatment seems essential for the well-being of the patient. This philosophy is in agreement with the recommendations of the National Academy of Sciences, which were endorsed by the Food and Drug Administration (1977). Limitation of the total fractionated dose to 1000 cGy for x-rays (5000 cGy for grenz rays) and the application of meticulous radiation protection measures are essential.

INDICATIONS FOR SUPERFICIAL AND SOFT X-RAY THERAPY (20 to 100 kV)

LYMPHADENOSIS BENIGNA CUTIS. Clinically typical histologically confirmed localized lymphocytomas of short duration, especially of the face, forehead, and scalp, respond remarkably well to small doses of x-rays; older lesions are more radioresistant. In some cases, just one low dose (100 to 250 cGy) of x-rays with an HVT of 0.5 to 1 mm Al will induce prompt resolution of pseudolymphomatous lesions. Olson and associates (1985) confirmed that doses of 150 to 300 cGy given once or twice a week for 2 to 3 weeks are highly effective. Special cytochemical and immunologic studies are often necessary to differentiate pseudolymphomas from malignant lymphomas (which may also respond to radiotherapy).

KELOIDS. Radiotherapy of keloids is indicated only in cases that have not responded to intralesional steroid injections or other forms of treatment. X-ray therapy yields best results if therapy is initiated during the first 6 months; in older cases the therapeutic response is less satisfactory. The narrowly shielded lesion is exposed to doses of 300 cGy at 1- to 3-week intervals for a total of three to five sessions. More penetrating radiation qualities (HVT 1 to 2 mm Al) are often indicated for deeper tumors. In patients with recurrent keloids, surgical excision followed by radiotherapy 3 to 6 days after surgery with a similar dose schedule can often prevent recurrences, with a minimum of side effects.

OTHER BENIGN SKIN DISORDERS. Most benign skin diseases known to respond well to x-rays involve only very superficial layers of the skin and can be effectively treated with grenz rays, which have a large margin of safety. In exceptional cases, however, superficial or soft x-rays with an HVT of 0.3 mm Al yield better results in thicker infiltrated psoriatic or eczematous plaques, especially of the hands and feet. Single doses of 50 to 100 cGy are applied once a week for 3 to 4 weeks. Courses of treatment may be repeated after several months. The total cumulative dose for soft x-ray therapy should not exceed 1000 cGy; doses in excess of 1500 cGy may cause permanent sequelae.

INDICATIONS FOR GRENZ RAY THERAPY

Because of its extremely limited penetration, this type of ionizing radiation is not associated with any conceivable risk when proper radiation safety measures are used. The report of the National Academy of Sciences (FDA, 1977) on the use of ionizing radiation for the treatment of benign diseases in all medical specialties specifically mentions grenz ray therapy as a radiation method with minimal risks.

With few exceptions, grenz ray therapy should not be used as the first form of treatment. Only when other therapeutic attempts have failed and when there is a clear need for further treatment may grenz rays be used, usually in combination with other topical therapies.

Grenz rays are ultrasoft x-rays with an HVT of 0.018 to 0.036 mm Al and a D½ of 0.5 mm skin. Most grenz ray units have a beryllium window and operate at a kV range of 8 to 20 kV. Because of their limited penetration, grenz rays are useful for superficial dermatoses, for example, psoriasis, various pruritic eczematous conditions, and pruritus ani and pruritus vulvae (Hollander, 1968). Recent investigations by Lindelöf and associates (1984, 1986) have demonstrated various effects of ultrasoft x-rays on Langerhans cells and other aspects of the cutaneous immune system. These results clarify the possible mechanism of action of ionizing radiation on the course of benign dermatoses.

Grenz ray therapy is usually administered in weekly or biweekly doses of 100 to 300 cGy, in a course of three to four sessions. Courses can be repeated twice or three times a year up to 1000 cGy per year and a maximum total dose of 5000 cGy per lifetime and area. Recent data from large groups of patients treated in Sweden suggest that even a total dose of 10,000 cGy is not associated with significant major side effects (Lindelöf and Eklund, 1986).

RADIATION RISKS

Most therapeutic modalities are associated with risks. Although more data are available on the theoretical and clinical aspects of radiation side effects than on the risks of any other mode of therapy, there is a large gap between the opinions of experts and the views of the public (Goldschmidt and Sherwin, 1980).

NONSTOCHASTIC EFFECTS

These are effects that vary with the dose of radiation and require a relatively high threshold dose.

CATARACTS. The lens is the most radiosensitive part of the eye. When given in fractionated doses, more than 350 cGy are needed to produce cataracts. In dermatologic therapy, the maximum exposure to the lens is smaller than 50 cGy, even when tumoricidal doses are used for treatment of eyelid cancers, provided that proper radiation protection is used.

FERTILITY. The sperm count may be depressed temporarily by an absorbed dose of 25 cGy. The absorbed dose required to cause permanent sterility is larger by at least an order of magnitude. In contrast to the nonstochastic effects on the sperm count, the potential genetic effects on the descendants of the irradiated individual are considered stochastic and not dependent on a threshold.

CHRONIC RADIODERMATITIS. The cumulative threshold dose for fractionated therapy resulting in chronic radiodermatitis is greater than 1000 cGy for superficial x-ray therapy. This dose was established in the landmark study by Sulzberger and associates at New York University (1952) confirmed by Rowell in England (1973), who found no clinical sequelae following cumulative doses of 1200 cGy. The threshold dose for chronic radiodermatitis for grenz ray qualities is a cumulative dose of over 5000 cGy.

RADIOGENIC SKIN CANCER. The latest recommendations of the International Commission on Radiological Protection (1977) mention an absorbed dose of 2000 cGy for occurrence of skin cancers (basal cell carcinomas and squamous cell carcinomas) when superficial roentgen-ray qualities are used in fractionated doses. Rowell found five cases of skin cancer in 100 patients treated with 1500 to 3000 cGy. Radiogenic skin cancers following grenz ray therapy are very rare. Only a few anecdotal cases were reported in the world literature for patients who received grenz ray doses exceeding 10,000 cGy. A recent retrospective study of over 14,000 Swedish patients by Lindelöf and Eklund (1986) confirms the absence of major side effects following cumulative maximum grenz ray doses between 5000 and 10,000 cGy.

In comparison with the occurrence of cutaneous malignancies following fractionated radiotherapy of benign dermatoses, the incidence of cutaneous neoplasms secondary to superficial radiotherapy of skin cancers with high tumor doses (up to 6000 cGy) is extremely low; this may be related to the relatively small field sizes used for cancer therapy and the cell-killing effect of high individual and total doses administered over a short period of time.

STOCHASTIC EFFECTS

The frequency of stochastic effects is related to the dose without evidence of a threshold. Even very small doses may cause late effects in some individuals when large populations are considered. Most somatic risks of radiation (i.e., leukemogenesis and carcinogenesis of internal organs) are stochastic. Since there is no unequivocal evidence of injury related to low-dose medical treatments (under 50 cGy organ dose), risk estimates are usually based on the linear hypothesis (National Academy of Sciences, 1980). Because dermatologic radiation is relatively nonpenetrating, only two types of noncutaneous carcinomas are of practical importance.

THYROID CANCER. This potential risk has been stressed in numerous articles during the past decade. While there is no doubt that ionizing radiation can cause thyroid cancer (for example, following thymus irradiation in childhood), this risk can be reduced to a minimum by proper radiation protection measures. Our own extensive dose measurements (Goldschmidt et al, 1983) have shown that with lead shields over the thyroid region, the thyroid dose is below 1 cGy when the total facial region is exposed to 1000 cGy at an HVT of 0.75 mm Al. The risk of death associated with this dose can be calculated as 1:1 million; this equals a reduction of life expectancy by 8 minutes. Similar 1:1 million everyday risks of death are associated with smoking 1.4 cigarettes, eating 100 charcoal-broiled steaks, spending 3 hours in a coal mine, or traveling 300 miles by car or 1000 miles by jet.

BREAST CANCER. Excessive exposure of the breast may induce carcinomas (as in patients radiated for mastitis or following numerous fluoroscopies for tuberculosis). In dermatology, the risks are minimal when proper radiation protection standards are used (Goldschmidt et al, 1982). The calculated breast exposure associated with a 1000 cGy skin dose to the facial area (0.05 cGy) is lower than exposures during mammography (xeromammography: 0.1 to 0.2 cGy).

GENETIC EFFECTS. Heritable effects are considered stochastic, and no safe threshold dose is assumed. The gonadal dose is symbolically important to society, not to the patient; it is just one more increment in the total radiation burden of the population. Obviously, it should be kept at a minimum by proper shielding in any patient who might subsequently have a child. In dermatologic therapy, the use of simple gonad shields can effectively reduce doses to the gonad. Measurements by various investigators confirm the protective effect of lead shields; during treatment of facial cancers, the dose to the gonad averages 0.05 cGy. In comparison, the annual background radiation in the United States is higher (0.1 cGy).

General References

Atkinson HR: Skin carcinoma depth and dose homogeneity in dermatological x-ray therapy. Aust J Dermatol 6:208, 1962.

Bart RS, et al: X-ray therapy of skin cancer: Evaluation of a "standardized" method for treating basal cell epitheliomas. Proceedings of the Sixth National Cancer Conference. Philadelphia, JB Lippincott, 1968.

Blank AP, et al: Soft x-ray therapy in Bowen's disease and erythroplasia of Queyrat. Dermatologica 171:89–94, 1985.

Braun-Falco O, et al: Zur behandlung der melanosis circumscripta praecancerosa Dubreuilh. Hautarzt 26:207–210, 1975.

Cooper JS: Radiotherapy of malignant melanoma. Dermatol Clin 3:341–350, 1985.

Cooper JS, et al: Initial observations of the effect of radiotherapy on epidemic Kaposi's sarcoma. JAMA 252:934–935, 1984.

Idem: The duration of local control of classic (non-AIDS-associated) Kaposi's sarcoma by radiotherapy. J Am Acad Dermatol 19:59–66, 1988.

Cotter GW: Palliative radiation treatment of cutaneous mycosis fungoides—a dose response. Int J Radiat Oncol Biol Phys 9:1477–1480, 1983.

Domonkos AN: Treatment of eyelid carcinoma. Arch Dermatol 91:364, 1965.

El Akkad S, et al: Kaposi's sarcoma and its management. Arch Dermatol 122:1396–1399, 1986.

FDA: A review of the use of ionizing radiation for the treatment of benign diseases. Washington, DC, US Dept HEW, Publication 78-8043, 1977.

Fromer JL, et al: Management of lymphoma cutis with low megavolt electron beam therapy. South Med J 54:769–774, 1961.

Gladstein AH: Radiation protection. In Physical Modalities in Dermatologic Therapy. Goldschmidt H (ed). New York, Springer-Verlag, 1978.

Idem, et al: Radiotherapy of cutaneous malignancies. In Physical Modalities in Dermatologic Therapy. Goldschmidt H (ed). New York, Springer-Verlag, 1978, pp 95–121.

Goldschmidt H: Dermatologic radiation therapy. Current use of ionizing radiation in the United States and Canada. Arch Dermatol 111:1511, 1975.

Idem, et al: Dermatologic radiotherapy and breast cancer. Dose measurements and risk quantification. Arch Dermatol Res 272:293, 1982.

Idem: Dermatologic radiotherapy and thyroid cancer. Dose measurements and risk quantification. Arch Dermatol 119:383, 1983.

Goldschmidt H, Sherwin WK: Reactions to ionizing radiation. J Am Acad Dermatol 3:551–579, 1980.

Idem: Office radiotherapy of cutaneous carcinomas. J Dermatol Surg Oncol 9:31–47, 1983.

Idem: Dermatologic radiation therapy. In Dermatology, 2nd ed. Moschella SL, Hurley HJ (eds). Philadelphia, WB Saunders, 1985, pp 2048–2081.

Harley, NH: Determination of half-dose depth in skin for soft x-rays. J Am Acad Dermatol 7:328–332, 1982.

Idem: Kaposi's sarcoma: An update on the results of extended field therapy. Arch Derm 117:775–778, 1981.

Harwood AR, et al: Radiotherapy for malignant melanoma: A reappraisal. Cancer Treat Rev 8:271–282, 1981.

Hauss H, et al: Radiotherapy of lentigo maligna and Bowen's disease. In Physical Modalities in Dermatologic Therapy. Goldschmidt H (ed). New York, Springer-Verlag, 1978.

Holecek MJ, et al: Radiotherapy of Kaposi's sarcoma. Cancer 41:1733–1738, 1978.

Hollander MB: Ultrasoft x-rays. Baltimore, Williams & Wilkins, 1968.

Idem: The role of radiation therapy in the management of the non–Hodgkin's lymphomas. Cancer 55:2176–2183, 1985.

Hoppe RT, et al: Radiation therapy in the management of cutaneous T-cell lymphomas. Cancer Treat Rep 63:625–632, 1979.

ICRP (International Commission on Radiological Protection): Recommendations of the International Commission on Radiological Protection. ICRP Publication 26. Oxford, Pergamon Press, Ltd, 1977.

Johanson CR, et al: Radiotherapy in nodular melanoma. Cancer 51:226–232, 1983.

Kopf AW, et al: Treatment of melanotic freckle with x-rays. Arch Dermatol 112:801, 1976.

Lindelöf B, et al: Incidence of malignant skin tumors in 14,140 patients after grenz-ray treatment for benign skin disorders. Arch Dermatol 122:1391–1395, 1986.

Idem: Effect of grenz rays on Langerhans' cells in human epidermis. Acta Derm Venereol 64:436–438, 1984.

Idem: The effect of grenz rays on the expression of allergic contact dermatitis in man. Scand J Immunol 21:463–469, 1985.

Menn H, et al: The recurrent basal cell epithelioma. Arch Dermatol 103:628–631, 1971.

National Academy of Sciences—National Research Council: The Effect on Populations of Exposure to Low Levels of Ionizing Radiation. Washington, DC, US Government Printing Office, 1980.

Olson LE, et al: Cutaneous lymphoid hyperplasia: Results of radiation therapy. Radiology 155:507–509, 1985.

Orton CG, et al: A simplification in the use of the NSD concept in practical radiotherapy. Br J Radiol 46:529, 1973.

Rounsaville MC, et al: Radiotherapy in the management of cutaneous melanoma: Effect of time, dose, and fractionation. Front Radiat Ther Oncol 22:62–78, 1988.

Rowell NR: A follow-up study of superficial radiotherapy for benign dermatoses. Br J Dermatol 88:583–590, 1973.

Storck H: Radiotherapy of cutaneous cancers and some other malignancies. J Dermatol Surg Oncol 4:573–584, 1978.

Sulzberger MB, et al: Do roentgen ray treatments as given by skin specialists produce cancers or other sequelae? Arch Dermatol Syph 65:639, 1952.

Tapley N, et al: Applications of the electron beam in the treatment of cancer of the skin and lips. Radiology 109:424–428, 1973.

Index

Note: Page numbers in *italics* refer to illustrations; page numbers followed by t refer to tables.